Seminars in General Adult Psychiatry

Second edition

Edited by George Stein and Greg Wilkinson

Gaskell

College Seminars Series

Series Editors

Professor Anne Farmer
Professor of Psychiatric Nosology, Institute of Psychiatry and Honorary Consultant Psychiatrist, South London and Maudsley NHS Trust, London

Dr Louise Howard
Research Fellow, Institute of Psychiatry, London

Dr Elizabeth Walsh
Clinical Senior Lecturer, Institute of Psychiatry, London

Professor Greg Wilkinson
Professor of Liaison Psychiatry, University of Liverpool and Honorary Consultant Psychiatrist, Royal Liverpool University Hospital

Praise for books in the series

'... the series will undoubtedly be a valuable and essential part of the library of trainee, trainer and practitioner alike.'

Journal of Mental Health

'Excellent grounding for the newcomer... "pearls" abound that make it a refreshing read for those of us who are more experienced.'

JAMA

'This very reasonably priced textbook should improve knowledge and stimulate interest in a common and challenging topic.'

BMJ

'Every chapter informs, but also pleases. This is expert teaching by skilled and committed teachers.'

Journal of the Royal Society of Medicine

'The editors state that this book is not intended to be a substitute for supervised clinical practice. It is, however, the next best thing.'

Psychological Medicine

'... this book joins others in the series in being both readily understandable and accessible... should be on every psychiatrist's bookshelf...'

Journal of Psychopharmacology

'... an excellent, up-to-date introductory text. It can be strongly recommended for residents, clinicians, and researchers.'

American Journal of Psychiatry

'Congratulations are due to the editors for the breadth of their vision and to the authors for the thoroughness and liveliness of their contributions.'

Psychological Medicine

Gaskell is an imprint of the Royal College of Psychiatrists
17 Belgrave Square, London SW1X 8PG
http://www.rcpsych.ac.uk

British Library Cataloguing-in-Publication Data.
A catalogue record for this book is available from the British Library.
ISBN13 978-1-904671-44-2

Distributed in North America by Balogh International Inc.

The Royal College of Psychiatrists is a registered charity (no. 228636).
Printed by The Cromwell Press, Trowbridge, Wiltshire, UK.

Contents

Tables, boxes and figures

Tables

Boxes

Figures

Contributors

Muna Adwa, Locum Lecturer, Institute of Psychiatry, De Crespigny Park, Camberwell, London SE5 8AF

Katherine J. Aitchison, Senior Lecturer in General Adult Psychiatry, and Honorary Consultant General Adult Psychiatrist, PO 80 MRC SGDP Centre, Institute of Psychiatry, De Crespigny Park, London SE5 8AF

Hiroko Akagi, Consultant in Liaison Psychiatry, Leeds and West Yorkshire CFS/ME Service, Newsam Centre, Seacroft Hospital, York Road, Leeds LS14 6UH

Spilios Argyropoulos, Consultant Psychiatrist and Honorary Senior Lecturer, South London and Maudsley NHS Trust and Section of Neurobiology of Psychosis, Division of Psychological Medicine, Institute of Psychiatry, De Crespigny Park, London SE5 8AF

Amlan Basu, Specialist Registrar in Forensic Psychiatry, and Honorary Researcher, PO 80 MRC SGDP Centre, Institute of Psychiatry, De Crespigny Park, London SE5 8AF

Morris Bernadt, Visiting Senior Lecturer, Department of Psychiatry, Institute of Psychiatry, De Crespigny Park, London SE5 8AF

Jonathan Bird, Consultant Neuropsychiatrist, Burden Centre for Neuropsychiatry, Frenchay Hospital, Bristol BS16 1JB; Honorary Senior Lecturer, Department of Psychiatry, University of Bristol

Tom Brown, Consultant Liaison Psychiatrist, Department of Liaison Psychiatry, Western Infirmary, Dumbarton Road, Glasgow G11 6NT

Adam Campbell, Senior Clinical Research Fellow and Honorary Consultant Clinical Psychologist, Psychotherapy Evaluation Research Unit, Tavistock and Portman NHS Trust, 120 Belsize Lane, London NW3 5BA

Patricia Casey, MD, FRCPI, FRCPsych, Professor of Psychiatry, University College Dublin, Dublin, Ireland; Consultant Psychiatrist, Mater Misericordiae University Hospital, Eccles Street, Dublin, Ireland

John Cookson, Consultant Psychiatrist, The Royal London Hospital, St Clement's, 2a Bow Road, London E3 4LL

Lynne M. Drummond, Consultant Psychiatrist and Senior Lecturer in Psychotherapy, St George's Hospital Medical School, Cranmer Terrace, London SW17 0RE

Irshaad Ebrahim, Consultant Neuropsychiatrist, The London Sleep Centre, 137 Harley Street, London W1G 6BF

Anne Farmer, Professor of Psychiatric Nosology, SGDP Centre, Institute of Psychiatry, De Crespigny Park, Camberwell, London SE5 8AF, and South London and Maudsley NHS Trust, Denmark Hill, London

Naomi A. Fineberg, Consultant Psychiatrist, Queen Elizabeth II Hospital, Welwyn Garden City, Hertfordshire AL7 4HQ; Visiting Professor, University of Hertfordshire

Frank Holloway, Consultant Psychiatrist, South London and Maudsley NHS Trust, Bethlem Royal Hospital, Monks Orchard Road, Beckenham, Kent BR3 3BX

Matthew Hotopf, Professor of General Hospital Psychiatry, Department of Psychological Medicine, Institute of Psychiatry, Weston Education Centre, Cutcombe Road, London SE5 9RJ

Allan House, Professor of Liaison Psychiatry, Academic Unit of Psychiatry and Behavioural Sciences, University of Leeds, 15 Hyde Terrace, Leeds LS2 9LT

Roger Howells, Consultant Psychiatrist, The Sloane Court Clinic, 11 Sloane Court West, Chelsea, London SW3 4TD

Michael Hunter, Senior Lecturer in Psychiatry, Honorary Consultant Psychiatrist, School of Medicine and Biomedical Sciences, University of Sheffield, Beech Hill Road, Sheffield S10 2RX

Robin Jacobson, Consultant Neuropsychiatrist, Keats House, 24–26 St Thomas Street, London SE1 9RS

Arun Jha, Consultant Psychiatrist, Hertfordshire Partnership NHS Trust, Logandene Care Unit, Ashley Close, Hemel Hempstead, Hertfordshire HP3 8BL

Gill Kirk, Consultant in General Adult Psychiatry, Barnsley District General Hospital, Gawber Road, Barnsley S75 2EP

Michael Kopelman, Professor of Neuropsychiatry, King's College London, Institute of Psychiatry, Adamson Centre, Block 8, South Wing, St Thomas' Hospital, London SE1 7EH

Kezia Lange, Consultant Psychiatrist, Oxleas NHS Foundation Trust, and Institute of Psychiatry, De Crespigny Park, Camberwell, London SE5 8AF

Alan Lee, Consultant Psychiatrist and Special Senior Lecturer, Department of Psychiatry, University Hospital, Queen's Medical Centre, Nottingham NG7 2UH

Julian Leff, Emeritus Professor of Social and Cultural Psychiatry, Institute of Psychiatry and Royal Free and University College Medical School, London; 1 South Hill Park Gardens, London NW3 2TD

Peter F. Liddle, Professor of Psychiatry, University of Nottingham, A Floor, South Block, Queen's Medical Centre, Nottingham NG7 2UH

Clive Mellor, Professor and Chairman of Psychiatry, Memorial University of Newfoundland (retired), PO Box 437, Agassiz, British Columbia, V0M 1A0, Canada

Harold Merskey, Emeritus Professor of Psychiatry, University of Western Ontario, 1001 Adelaide Street North, London, Ontario, Canada

Stirling Moorey, Consultant Psychiatrist in Cognitive Behaviour Therapy, South London and Maudsley Foundation Trust, Denmark Hill, London SE5 8AZ

Gethin Morgan, Emeritus Professor of Mental Health, University of Bristol, Division of Psychiatry, Cotham House, Cotham Hill, Bristol B6 6JL

John Owen, Consultant Psychiatrist, Cossham Hospital, Lodge Hill, Bristol, Avon BS15 1LF

Vikram Patel, Wellcome Trust Senior Clinical Research Fellow in Tropical Medicine, London School of Hygiene and Tropical Medicine, Keppel Street, London WC1E 7HT

Jerson Pereira, Consultant Psychiatrist, South London and Maudsley NHS Trust, Ladywell Unit, Lewisham Hospital, London SE13 6LH

Rosalind Ramsay, Consultant Psychiatrist, South London and Maudsley NHS Trust, Maudsley Hospital, Denmark Hill, London SE5 8AZ

Danny Rogers, Consultant Neuropsychiatrist, Burden Centre for Neuropsychiatry, Frenchay Hospital, Bristol BS16 1JB

Pak Sham, Chair Professor of Psychiatric Genomics, Department of Psychiatry and Genome Research Centre, Faculty of Medicine, University of Hong Kong, 21 Sassoon Road, Pokfulam, Hong Kong

George Stein, Consultant Psychiatrist, Green Parks House, Princess Royal University Hospital, Orpington, Kent; Hayes Grove Priory, Preston Road, Hayes, Kent BR2 7AS

Michael Stone, Professor of Clinical Psychiatry, Department of Psychiatry, Columbia College of Physicians and Surgeons, and Attending Psychiatrist, Mid-Hudson Forensic Psychiatric Hospital, New Hampton, New York 10958, USA

Gregory Stores, Emeritus Professor of Developmental Neuropsychiatry, University of Oxford; North Gate House, 55 High Street, Dorchester on Thames, Oxon OX10 7HN

George Tadros, Consultant Psychiatrist, Queen Elizabeth Psychiatric Hospital, Mindelsohn Way, Birmingham B15 2QZ

Janet Treasure, Professor of Psychiatry, Eating Disorders Unit, Department of Academic Psychiatry, 5th Floor, Thomas Guy House, Guy's Hospital, London SE1 9RT

Peter Trigwell, Consultant in Liaison Psychiatry and Psychosexual Medicine, Department of Liaison Psychiatry, Leeds General Infirmary, Great George Street, Leeds LS1 3EX

Christopher A. Vassilas, Consultant Psychiatrist, Queen Elizabeth Psychiatric Hospital, Mindelsohn Way, Birmingham B15 2QZ

Greg Wilkinson, Professor of Psychiatry, Royal Liverpool University Hospital, Liverpool L69 3GA; Consultant Psychiatrist, 31 Rodney Street, Liverpool L1 9GH

Peter Woodruff, Professor of Academic Clinical Psychiatry, Head of Academic Clinical Psychiatry, Director of the Sheffield Cognition and Neuroimaging Laboratory (SCANLab), University of Sheffield School of Medicine and Biomedical Sciences, University of Sheffield, Beech Hill Road, Sheffield S10 2RX

Preface to the second edition

More than 9 years have passed since the first edition of *Seminars in General Adult Psychiatry* was published and much has changed in that time, although not surprisingly even more has stayed the same. Psychiatric disorder itself has a certain immutable quality and so many of the excellent clinical descriptions of the first edition have been retained here. By contrast, the science of psychiatry has expanded massively on all fronts. At the time of the first edition evidence-based medicine applied largely to the drug-related topics: now it is the rule and, with the advent of the National Institute for Health and Clinical Excellence (NICE), systematic reviews and meta-analyses permeate almost every area of psychiatry as the specialty gradually develops from being a skill reliant on clinical experience to a scientific discipline based on a well-validated body of factual knowledge. As in the first edition we have done our best to be selective and to highlight the more recent and important studies without overwhelming the reader with too much information. The first edition was produced as two volumes, but for the convenience of the reader this second edition is published as a single volume, although it actually contains considerably more text.

The scope of this edition is essentially similar to that of the first, although there are three additional chapters. Two of these, those on liaison psychiatry and sexual medicine, comprised separate books in the first College Seminar Series. The third, on cross-cultural and international psychiatry, might easily have merited a volume in its own right. The text is primarily aimed at doctors training for their Membership of the Royal College of Psychiatrists (MRCPsych) examination but we hope it will also serve as a useful reference volume for those already in practice. It covers the whole of general adult psychiatry with the exception of forensic psychiatry, which is covered in another volume of the College Seminars Series.

For the novice, attempting to read a book of this size will seem a daunting prospect and at least initially it might be better to dip in and out of it. For those starting their training a brief guide is presented below on how best to use this book. The chapters have been arranged in a carefully considered order. The first 19 cover all the conditions commonly encountered in clinical practice and it is best to start with these, so as to acquire a basic knowledge of these disorders. The remaining chapters cover the main sub-specialties of general psychiatry, and the way the psychiatric services are organised.

The early asylum doctors spent the bulk of their professional lives working with people suffering from the major functional psychoses, namely schizophrenia and affective disorder, and so knowledge of these disorders became the core of psychiatry. Gradually, over the 20th century the subject expanded to include a wide range of rather less severe disorders, even to the point where psychiatrists were asked to pontificate on almost any type of human distress. In more recent years this trend towards overinclusion has swung sharply into reverse in the context of publicly funded health services. General psychiatry is returning once more to its older roots and, at least within NHS hospital units and community mental health teams, there is now a much greater focus on people with 'severe and enduring mental illness'.

Most trainee psychiatrists will start their training on an in-patient unit or community mental health team, where the bulk of the clinical work is with people who have schizophrenia or affective disorder. These conditions are described in detail in the first 12 chapters of the book. However, within this core only a small nucleus of topics will be needed from early on. These chapters include: the clinical features of depression, mania and schizophrenia (Chapters 1, 2 and 8) and their drug management (Chapters 4 and 11). Even within these chapters many of the more theoretical topics such as classification or drug receptor action can initially be omitted and studied at a later reading. The most common emergency that a trainee will need to attend is emergency sedation, which may provoke a great deal of anxiety on the part of professionals. An account of the procedure of rapid tranquillisation and its underlying logic is given in Chapter 11. Overall, this nub of information, representing a tiny fraction of the whole, may provide some initial direction for the bewildering first few weeks in acute in-patient psychiatry.

As experience in out-patient work grows, Chapters 12–20 will become more important. People with anxiety disorders, phobias and obsessive–compulsive disorders (Chapters 13–15) commonly present to out-patient clinics, where in fact much of the treatment is now carried out by psychologists or other paramedical staff. It may be helpful for readers to have some clinical contact with people who have the more problematic conditions of conversion, somatisation and the personality disorders (Chapters 16, 18 and 19) before reading about these topics in any depth, because academic knowledge taken in isolation will fail to convey the subtleties and special difficulties posed by these individuals, especially those with personality disorders.

The main sub-specialties follow and these are: liaison psychiatry (Chapter 17), neuropsychiatry (Chapters 20–23), eating disorders, perinatal psychiatry and psychosexual medicine (Chapters 24–26). Few trainees will be fortunate enough to work in all of these sub-specialties, which usually offer a stimulating and varied experience, but the account given here ensures that all these topics are covered to a reasonable depth.

Towards the end of the book are two rather more theoretical chapters, on clinical epidemiology and psychiatric diagnosis (Chapters 27 and 28). The final three chapters are devoted to the psychiatric services in primary and secondary care and cross-cultural perspectives (Chapters 29–31). These five chapters are best appreciated after the reader has worked in the services for some time and is reasonably familiar with the way the system works.

Some issues are intrinsically more difficult to understand than others. In this respect the four most densely presented chapters are those on drug treatments, the first of the neuropsychiatry chapters, and the description of clinical epidemiology (Chapters 4, 11, 20 and 27). These need to be taken slowly and carefully; the reader will need a fresh mind with good powers of concentration and it would be frustrating to try to tackle these topics after a busy day in the clinic.

Four other chapters are also of a theoretical type but are not so difficult to comprehend. The two chapters on the causes of depression and schizophrenia (Chapters 3 and 10) are essentially reviews of the current state of research into the aetiology of these conditions. They address the fundamental issue of 'Why do these disorders occur?' and will arouse a natural curiosity, and as they include the cream of modern psychiatric research they make fascinating reading. However, these fields are constantly changing and so it may not be necessary to commit to memory the multiplicity of genetic or brain scan studies they contain in the same way that it is essential to know the side-effects of a commonly used drug. The psychiatry of neurological and medical disorders (Chapters 21 and 22) also appears to be difficult, but for doctors coming from recent postings in neurology and general medicine much of their content will already be familiar. These four chapters (3, 10, 21 and 22) also need to be taken slowly, but they are not as compactly written as the previously mentioned group of four chapters and perhaps represent an intermediate level of difficulty.

The remaining rather more clinical chapters make absorbing reading and may be rather easier to read than the chapters highlighted above. Also these topics are unlikely to change as much in the future and so becoming thoroughly acquainted with these more clinical aspects is not only an examination requirement but also a wise long-term investment. Examinations such as the MRCPsych require a wide general knowledge of psychiatry, and to acquire the necessary comprehensive coverage, at some point, perhaps neither too early on in the career, nor too late (such as on the eve of the examination!), a reading of the whole book from beginning to end may serve to bring the whole subject together as well as fill in any missing gaps.

Producing a major textbook today is usually the result of a team effort, but a book of this magnitude has required nothing less than a whole orchestra of talent. The reader will soon realise that many of our contributors have given virtuoso performances and have fine-tuned their chapters to a high degree of perfection. We are truly grateful for their scholarship and commitment, which in today's academic climate, dominated by research assessment exercises, otherwise seems largely unrewarded. Much of the editing of this book was done in the Institute of Psychiatry library, a unique national treasure, containing perhaps the largest collection of psychiatric journals and books in the world, and for this we thank the chief librarian Mr Martin Guha and his team for helping us utilise this wonderful resource. Thanks also go to Mrs Penny Nicholson of the Princess Royal University Hospital, Farnborough, Kent, who coordinated much of the work and passed many hours typing and retyping the numerous manuscripts. Especial thanks also go to Mr Ralph Footring the production editor, for the design and superb layout of the chapters and who, through a spell of magic, was able to produce this work as an exquisite single volume.

Our publisher Gaskell, at the Royal College of Psychiatrists, has been a constant source of support as well as of valuable advice, and for this we expressly thank Andrew Morris and David Jago, who have been with us throughout all the trials and tribulations of both editions of these books. Finally, we thank our wives Suzanna and Chris and our families for their support and forbearance, especially for tolerating the sackfuls of typescripts left lying around the house, often for months on end. It is our intention for you to enjoy this book and for your patients to benefit from your reading.

George Stein
Greg Wilkinson

Preface to the first edition

Psychiatry, according to Johann Christian Reil (1759–1813) the German anatomist who first coined the term, consists of the meeting of two minds, the mind of the patient with the mind of the doctor. As patients tell their story, it is the task of the doctor to recognise the tale, and to do so with compassion. Pattern recognition lies at the heart of the diagnostic process; common trends in the rich tapestry of the patient's experiences are summarised in the many clinical syndromes and disorders of psychiatry. This book, intended for doctors in training beginning their career in psychiatry, places its greatest emphasis on detailed descriptions of the common psychiatric disorders. We hope such a clinical descriptive approach will help doctors recognise patterns and so make sound psychiatric diagnoses. Our intention is that this book will be a useful basis for trainees preparing for their Membership examinations, but in addition it should engage those who have passed that hurdle.

Diagnostic acumen separated from therapeutic skill is of little use to patients or their families. When Reil first introduced the word psychiatry, he meant it in a therapeutic sense, in that the psyche of the doctor would act as a healing agent on the mind of the patient. While the initial meetings between doctor and patient usually have a diagnostic purpose, later contacts involve treatment. Throughout the book we have tried to provide guidelines on the management of common disorders. Our approach to treatment has been eclectic, but at the same time we have tried to describe each of the many treatments now available in some depth. The more specialised psychotherapies, once shrouded in a mystique requiring years of specialised training, are now gradually being replaced by briefer, less intensive treatment more readily grasped by trainees. We have described these newer treatments in some detail (for example, with behaviour therapy for the treatment of phobias, or cognitive therapy for depression). Physical treatments are accorded equal weight and separate chapters describe the physical treatments of both depression and schizophrenia.

Our hopes for better understanding and new treatments lie in scientific research. Sometimes, the scientific advances of the previous decades have been spectacular, for example the new drugs to treat depression and schizophrenia; in other cases developments have been less dramatic but as important, such as the gradual realisation that much of the depression found in the community is socially determined. At one time, a medical advance was deemed to have occurred if a charismatic professor at an ancient university announced a new classification; if another professor, perhaps from a different school of psychiatry, disagreed, it was hailed as a medical controversy. Today, this is no longer possible and rigorous scientific evidence is required before any new information can be incorporated into the fabric of existing knowledge. This applies to both the biological and psychosocial dimensions of the spectrum of knowledge.

We have tried to balance the essential clinical descriptive information and its supporting scientific evidence, with some of the more interesting but still speculative recent findings, hopefully without overwhelming the reader with too many studies. In this lies a dilemma, because the needs of the beginner and those with experience can be at variance. The novice must assimilate the body of existing knowledge while the established clinician is more interested in the advancing front of knowledge, even if many of the new findings eventually prove ephemeral.

Our guiding principle in editing the book has been to remain close to clinical issues and to answer the two questions "What disorder is it?" and "How can we help?" The third and often the most tantalising question "Why is it" remains unanswered, at least for most conditions, and so we have tended to focus less on aetiological considerations.

An era is now passing when doctors bear sole responsibility for the treatment of patients under their care. Modern psychiatric treatment is a team effort and this change is to be welcomed, not least because it helps to ease the burden on the doctor. Medical authority no longer rests on a position in the hierarchy, but rather on greater knowledge and wider clinical experience. Increasingly patients, relatives, carers, managers and other members of the psychiatric team question the doctor's decisions and treatment, and as a consequence of these wider changes this book is rooted in an evidence base and comprehensively and extensively referenced.

The College Seminars Series has separate volumes for each of the sub-specialties of psychiatry, and this structure has given the editors and contributors considerable freedom, permitting us to concentrate solely on general psychiatry. General psychiatry is now too vast a subject for a single person to be an expert in all its aspects and this inevitably means a comprehensive text must be multi-authored. We believe that many of the chapters are works of great scholarship by leading experts in their fields, and their length and detail bear witness to long hours of toil. For this the editors express their deepest gratitude. In other chapters the clinical acumen, diagnostic nuances and imaginative therapeutic strategies have an immediacy which brings the whole book to life, while offering the clinician new ways to help patients and their families. We hope our readers will derive both pleasure and wisdom from this book.

We would like to thank the American Psychiatric Association and the World Health Organization for permission to publish tables from DSM–IV and ICD–10. The editors are particularly grateful for the assistance of Dr Rosalind Ramsay throughout the preparation of this book, first for keeping the editors in touch with the needs of the readership, and second for critically scrutinising the text. Much of this book was edited in the library of the Maudsley Hospital, which houses a unique collection of psychiatric journals and books; we would like to thank the librarian, Mr Martin Guha, and his staff for their unfailing support. Numerous junior doctors from Farnborough Hospital, the London Hospital and the University of Liverpool have read earlier drafts of the chapters in this book and their comments have helped us greatly to sharpen the focus of the text. Special thanks are due to Penny Nicholson at Farnborough Hospital who typed and retyped many of the manuscripts as well as coordinating the whole project, ably assisted in this task by Christine Scotcher. The technical and publishing expertise of the staff at the Royal College of Psychiatrists is also acknowledged with much gratitude.

George Stein
Greg Wilkinson

CHAPTER 1

Clinical features of depressive disorders

Alan Lee

Classic phenomenology

Robert Burton published *The Anatomy of Melancholy* in 1621 and it enjoyed great popularity. Samuel Johnson found it to be the only book that ever raised him from his bed 2 hours sooner than he wished to rise. The writings of Milton, Byron and Lamb were all strongly influenced by it. In his account of melancholy, Burton described a state of mind that had been familiar to many before him, and his description must have resonated with the experiences of a large number of his readers. Here was a systematic account of the mental phenomena that had much earlier led the psalmist David to declare:

> 'I am a worm, and no man; a reproach of men, and despised of the people.... I am poured out like water, and all my bones are out of joint: my heart is like wax; it is melted in the midst of my bowels. My strength is dried up ... and thou has brought me into the dust of death.' (Psalm 22: 6–15)

Similarly, Job had described:

> 'wearisome nights are appointed to me ... I am full of tossings to and fro unto the dawning of the day.... When I say, My bed shall comfort me, my couch shall ease my complaint; Then thou scarest me with dreams, and terrifiest me through visions ... I have sinned ... I am a burden to myself ... thou shalt seek me in the morning, but I shall not be.' (Job 7: 3–21)

Melancholy, literally the 'black humour', had been one of Hippocrates' four categories of madness, and it had been established as such throughout medieval teaching. In the 13th century Bartholomeus Angelicus wrote:

> 'The patients are faint and fearful in heart without cause, and oft sorry ... feeling like earthen vessels they dread to be touched lest they should break ... they feel they have the world upon their heads and shoulders for it is about to fall.' (Quoted by Hunter & Macalpine, 1963, p. 2)

For many of Burton's predecessors, melancholy had been regarded with ambivalence. While few welcomed its ravages, many believed it to be a sign of great sensibility, and some even believed that people with melancholy 'are accounted as most fit to attempt matters of weightie charge and high attempt' (Du Laurens, 1599; quoted by Hunter & Macalpine, 1963, p. 52).

In keeping with this, Burton gave to melancholy a bitter-sweet character. In his rhyming prologue, alternate verses had the refrain 'Naught so sweet as melancholy', but he left his readers in no doubt as to the terrifying quality of its most severe forms. He wrote: 'If there is a hell on earth, it is to be found in a melancholy man's heart'.

After Burton, 300 years elapsed before there was an account of the phenomenology of melancholy which matched his in both scope and quality. Emil Kraepelin's *Manic Depressive Insanity and Paranoia*, published in English in 1921, is filled with vivid descriptions which confirm for the reader the appropriateness of Burton's use of the words 'hell on earth'. His text is still widely quoted. A decade after Kraepelin, the *Journal of Mental Science* published Aubrey Lewis's 'Melancholia: a clinical survey of depressive states'. In about 100 pages, this paper combines meticulous phenomenological analysis with an empirical study of 61 carefully documented patients seen in his practice at the Maudsley Hospital. Taken together, these works of Burton, Kraepelin and Lewis render an account of the clinical features of the depressive disorders that is unlikely ever to be equalled.

Psychiatry in the 19th and early 20th centuries saw a shift in terminology from Burton's 'melancholy' to the current usage of the word 'depression'. The nature and context of this change have been well described by Berrios (1992). The term 'depression' was favoured by physicians who heard in it echoes of a more physiological disorder. Kraepelin legitimised its use by giving it adjectival status in 'depressive insanity' and Adolf Meyer was an enthusiast for the more modern usage. The word 'depression', however, still has its passionate opponents. In *Darkness Visible*, a personal account of the illness, William Styron wrote:

> 'Melancholia would still appear to be a far more apt and evocative word for the blacker forms of the disorder, but it was usurped by a noun with a bland tonality and lacking any magisterial presence, used indifferently to describe an economic decline or a rut in the ground, a true wimp of a word for such a major illness ... for over 75 years the word [depression] has slithered innocuously through the language like a slug, leaving little trace of its intrinsic malevolence and preventing by its very insipidity, a general awareness of the horrible intensity of the disease when out of control.' (Styron, 1991, p. 37)

Clinical features of depressive disorders

> 'The Tower of Babel never yielded such confusion of tongues, as the chaos of melancholy doth variety of symptoms.' (Burton, 1621, p. 240)

Many phenomena can be identified as features of depressive disorders. These vary both in the patterns in which they occur and in their intensity. In severe forms symptoms tend to be pervasive and unchanging. In milder forms they may shift constantly, in ways which reflect the dynamic relationships between them.

Some phenomena are exaggerations of normal experience, for example feelings of sadness or guilt. These become significant as symptoms because of their intensity, or their frequency, or their inappropriateness. Other phenomena involve impairments of normal capacities, for example loss of the ability to feel pleasure. A third group emerge as developments from other symptoms, as is seen when marked feelings of guilt evolve into delusions.

There have been many attempts to classify symptoms but none has been widely accepted. This account follows the traditional order of presentation within the mental state, although appearance and behavioural features (including linguistic ones) are considered separately at the end, after an account of histrionic features and depressive stupor. Impaired concentration and memory are discussed alongside other impairments of feeling, energy and thinking; these, together with vegetative (bodily) changes, are often referred to as the 'associated features' of depression.

Painful affects

Depressed mood

> 'Sorrow sticks by them still continuously gnawing as the vulture did....' (Burton, 1621, p. 236)

Depressed mood is the commonest symptom found in depressive disorders. It has an obvious claim to be the central feature, but it is not essential for diagnosis and it is not easy to delineate. Most definitions refer to sadness, misery or dejection. The mood is painful and oppressive, and frequently without apparent cause. It can be distinguished from normal feelings of sadness or unhappiness which accompany loss or failure by its greater intensity, duration and pervasiveness. A special quality is often described, as if a black cloud were descending. Sufferers feel heavy-hearted and weighed down with their miseries. Tears come unexpectedly and at times for no reason. Those who are severely depressed may be beyond tears, in a state of frozen misery.

This extremely unpleasant state is usually coloured by depressive thinking, and is experienced as gloom, hopelessness, despair, insufficiency, loneliness or unwantedness. One sufferer wrote:

> 'The gray drizzle of horror induced by depression takes on the quality of physical pain.... I feel the horror like some poisonous fogbank roll in on my mind, forcing me into bed.' (Styron, 1991, pp. 50, 58)

Some patients successfully conceal their mood change and very few offer their mood as a presenting complaint. It is extremely rare for someone depressed for the first time to use the words 'I feel depressed'. Sometimes depressed mood is absent, or it may be masked by irritability, problems with introspection or a cultural tendency to show depression in forms other than mood disturbance.

Anxiety

> 'A kind of panic and anxiety overtook me ... accompanied by a visceral queasiness.... The flight of birds caused me to stop, riveted with fear ... I have felt the wind of the wing of madness.' (Styron, 1991, pp. 42, 46)

Anxiety is also one of the commonest symptoms in depressive disorders, although sufferers rarely complain of it by name. Often it is experienced as an apprehensive foreboding, as if something terrible is going to happen. Sufferers usually do complain of autonomic accompaniments, which include a dry mouth, palpitations, tremulousness, sweating, blushing, 'butterflies' or a knot in the stomach, choking, difficulty getting breath, dizziness and giddiness. These may be misinterpreted as evidence of a physical illness, which may lead to escalating anxiety. Panic attacks and phobic avoidance may develop. Many sufferers wake early with anxious ruminations and autonomic symptoms, feeling unable to face the day. This is a very useful diagnostic pointer to the presence of a depressive illness.

The feeling of anxiety can be coloured by cognitive features, in particular pessimistic thinking, low self-esteem and a preoccupation with death. Danger is felt to be imminent, as are loss and disgrace. Everyone encountered is a potential thief or is out to pick a quarrel. Friends or relatives will die. The world is upon the sufferer's shoulders and it is about to fall. There is a fear of collapse, of madness, of death or eternal damnation.

Agitation

Agitation is marked anxiety combined with excessive motor activity. Sufferers feel anxious and restless and complain that they cannot keep still. They may continually wring their hands or fidget with a convenient object. They may constantly shift positions. In severe forms they cannot remain seated, and pace up and down, or pick feverishly at their clothes. They often appear scared or startled, with wide eyes and a half open mouth.

Agitation is often accompanied by worrying. The sufferer cannot escape from a round of painful thoughts ridden with anxiety. Agitated patients report feeling frantic, always wanting to be somewhere else but not knowing where to go to. One man described feeling dreadful, badgered and worried. A woman felt she was getting into a terrible state of feverish nervous excitement: 'I know that something has to be done. I don't know what to do.'

Agitation can be distinguished from akathisia (motor restlessness occurring as an extrapyramidal side-effect of neuroleptic medication), from states of gross excitement and from stereotypies. In akathisia, anxiety is usually less prominent than it is in depression and indeed often absent. Gross excitement in depression usually has an aggressive or explosive quality. Motor stereotypies involve the exact repetition of patterns of movement and tend to be comforting, leading to a reduction of anxiety.

Irritability

Alongside sadness and anxiety, those who are depressed may complain of increased irritability, experienced as a lowered threshold for annoyance and anger in the face of frustration. Sufferers may keep it to themselves, or may exhibit increased argumentativeness, uncharacteristic shouting and quarrelling, outbursts of temper, throwing or breaking things or, in extreme cases, violence to others.

Changes in mood

Fluctuations in mood are common, and may be both abrupt and extreme. About 50% of sufferers show a regular pattern. Most feel worse in the mornings but there can be regular mid-afternoon or evening exacerbation. Diurnal variation, with mood lowest in the morning, is often considered typical of the somatic syndrome of depression (see Box 1.1, below), as is loss of reactivity to the environment.

Reactivity is often harder to assess in hospital, but improvements often follow immediately after admission, with further marked changes following visits from relatives, visits home, changes in other patients and attempts at therapy. Reactivity does not imply a less serious depression, for it is not unknown for patients to be cheerful to the point of misleading those around them as to the need for vigilance, and then unexpectedly to hang themselves.

Impairments of feeling, energy and thinking

Anhedonia: loss of capacity for enjoyment

> 'They are utterly unable to rejoice in anything. They cannot apprehend, believe or think of anything that is comfortable to them.' (Richard Baxter, a 17th-century clergyman, quoted by Hunter & Macalpine, 1963, p. 241)

Anhedonia is the second most common symptom in depressive disorders. Whereas painful sadness is the psychological opposite of pleasure, anhedonia refers to its negation – the absence of pleasure. Anhedonia is part of a wider phenomenon; as Jaspers (1963, p. 111) describes: 'the feeling of having lost feelings' is associated with a 'terrible emptiness – a subjectively felt void'. It is closely linked to feelings of dulled perception and depersonalisation, and also to feelings of insufficiency and lack of vitality.

Those with anhedonia do not experience pleasure even if something good happens. They are not cheered by fine weather, receiving a compliment, winning a game or by a surprise windfall, for example. They cannot enjoy the company of friends and are not happy spending time at their previous hobbies and interests (see also 'Loss of interest', below). Kraepelin (1921, pp. 75–76) captures the phenomenon well:

> '[the sufferer is] indifferent to his relatives and to whatever he formerly liked best ... a dull submission ... shuts out every comfort and every gleam of light.... Everything has become disagreeable to him; everything wearies him, company, music, travel, his professional work.... Life appears to be aimless ... and meaningless.... All the joy [of nature] cannot pump a drop of bliss from [his] heart up to [his] brain.'

Lewis (1934) comments on the 'especial distress' experienced by his patients from rural districts when they were unable to enjoy the sight of the fields, the sky, the trees and the flowers.

Anergia: loss of energy

Kraepelin's description of 'total lack of energy' in a depressed man has never been bettered:

> 'He drags himself with difficulty from one day to another ... [he] lacks spirit and willpower.... He cannot rouse himself ... cannot work any longer ... has to force himself to everything.... The smallest bit of work costs him an unheard-of effort; even the most everyday arrangements, household work, getting up in the morning, dressing, washing, are accomplished with the greatest difficulty and in the end indeed are left undone. Work, visits, important letters, business affairs are like a mountain in front of the patient and are just left, because he does not find the power to overcome the opposing inhibitions. Finally [he] gives up all activities, sits all day with his hands in his lap, brooding to himself in utter dullness. Sometimes a veritable passion for lying in bed is developed.' (Kraepelin, 1921, pp. 76–78)

Kraepelin did not view loss of energy as tiredness or fatigue but rather as one manifestation of 'psychic inhibition', the sufferer being unable to overcome inhibitions to action, which themselves may have resulted from excessive fear and pessimism. The French psychiatrist and philosopher Pierre Janet (quoted by Lewis, 1934, p. 298) held a similar view: 'The feeling of inadequacy is essentially a fear of action, a flight from action, a checking regulation which stops one action, seeks to replace it with its opposite, and in doing so causes a failure of the action.'

Today these concepts are often regarded as closer to the phenomenon of obsessional slowness. Loss of energy is now usually framed in terms of unpleasant inappropriate tiredness, listlessness and exhaustion. There may also be an important overlap with hypochondriasis.

Although these observations suggest that anergia is not a unitary phenomenon, the description 'decreased energy or increased fatiguability' is a central element of the ICD–10 criteria for depression (World Health Organization, 1992). A useful probe is: 'Have you been getting exhausted or tired-out during the day or evening, even when you have not been working very hard?'. It is important to distinguish the psychological symptom from anergia due to a physical disorder.

Sufferers complain of sluggishness, of feeling sapped and drained, or of lacking strength. Their limbs feel like lead, they have lost their vitality or they feel insufficient in some way. They may describe themselves as worn out, exhausted or even too weak to move. They may feel slowed down almost to the point of paralysis. Styron (1991) wrote that it was as if psychic energy was throttled back to zero. Informants report neglect of children, meals, housework, personal cleanliness and tidiness. Depressed people are often sent home from work because of inefficiency. The combination of exhaustion with inability to sleep may be particularly hard to bear.

Retardation

About half of depressed patients feel that their movements are slowed down. This phenomenon is termed 'retardation'. Those affected may walk very slowly or may sit perfectly still throughout an interview. Speech may also be slowed, hesitant and laboured, with few sentences longer than ten words, and seldom more than one sentence. There may be long pauses before replying ('response latency') and also between each word.

Inefficient thinking and retardation have often been viewed as being unified by the concept of psychic inhibition. Many textbooks follow this line and refer to an observed slowing of thought and action as psychomotor retardation. This practice has been criticised as leading to an overemphasis on objective signs, as against the core phenomenon of the subjective experience of slowness. Lewis (1934) argued that observed slowness in speech and task performance is usually not due to slowness in thought but rather to inattention, preoccupation or difficulty in thinking. None of his patients said that their thoughts were slower or fewer. Many of those whose talk appeared to be slowed described their thoughts as racing. Conversely, many complaints of slowed movement were not borne out by objective testing. These considerations suggest that the term 'retardation' be reserved for a subjective feeling of slowed movement, but nevertheless observable slowness also remains an element of diagnostic criteria.

Inefficient thinking/impaired concentration

> 'They are inconstant ... persuaded to and fro on every small occasion.... Wavering, irresolute, unable to deliberate through fear.... As a man that's bitten with fleas, their restless minds are tossed and vary.' (Burton, 1621, p. 237)

There are several components to the difficulty in thinking found in depression. These include indecisiveness, a tendency to ruminate and an inability to sustain attention. There is often a difficulty in ordering and calling up thoughts and memories, and occasionally slowness. Most of Lewis's patients described a constant press of thoughts, their thoughts running on, their brain never stopping. Kraepelin similarly described his patients as feeling that too much was in their heads: fresh thoughts were always coming, leading to confusion. As a result their thinking was unclear, muddled and lacking in focus. In many patients apparently laborious and slow thinking is due to disorganisation of thoughts rather than any slowness of the thoughts themselves.

Other patients describe their lack of concentration by saying that their thoughts just drift off. Those who are severely affected cannot read more than a few lines, follow a television programme for more than a few minutes, or follow a conversation. They may feel that they cannot take things in, cannot collect or pull together their thoughts. Their head feels heavy, their mind stupid and confused. They often feel they have no memory and that they have lost their command of previous knowledge. They may have problems remembering where they put things. This difficulty may interact with an increased sensitivity to losses; Styron (1991, p. 57) wrote that 'each momentary displacement filled me with a frenzied dismay'. Indecision may show itself as inconstancy or appear as paralysis, with sufferers considering at length the simplest matters.

Loss of interest

> 'the enthusiast gradually gives up his hobby, the gardener leaves the weeds alone, the golfer lets his clubs rust.' (Hamilton, 1982)

In both major diagnostic systems – ICD–10 (World Health Organization, 1992) and DSM–IV (American Psychiatric Association, 1994) – this symptom is combined in a single criterion with loss of pleasure. Most definitions also refer to a marked reduction in the range and intensity of interests and hobbies, as well as in work and domestic activities, leisure pursuits, keeping well informed and maintaining an interest in clothes, food and personal appearance.

By these definitions the symptom is a composite phenomenon, related to both feeling and activity. It has three components:

1 inability to enjoy interests (anhedonia – see above)

2 loss of anticipatory pleasure and concern (apathy)

3 reduction of activities.

The distinction between the first two of these, anhedonia and apathy, may reflect disorder of different neurophysiological mechanisms. Apathy also has an element of helpless futility. The third component, reduction of activities, follows from anhedonia and apathy, but also may result from inefficient thinking, inability to sustain concentration, phobic avoidance, fatigue and loss of energy, and motor retardation. Despite the fact that it is not a unitary phenomenon, it is loss of interest as defined by behavioural change that is most easily identified and rated, and therefore this is likely to remain in clinical use.

Bodily symptoms

Disturbances of appetite and weight

As a rule there is little appetite for food or drink, and food lacks any flavour. Occasionally, there may be increased appetite or episodes of ravenous hunger and bingeing. Attitudes to eating and drinking may change quickly, and will usually range from a mild disinclination (due to lack of appetite) to outright refusal. Carers may need to use persuasion and cajolery. Reluctance to eat or drink may result directly from a delusional belief that food is poisoned. Refusal to accept fluids can quickly become life-threatening.

Kraepelin described marked fluctuations in body weight, and these are suggestive of changes in fluid balance. Today the most common clinical picture before treatment is of weight loss due to poor appetite rather than dieting or physical illness. Symptom criteria usually specify losses of more than 5% of body weight in a month, or around 1 kg (2 lb) a month for several months. Typically, a depressed person's weight stabilises after a loss of about 6–7 kg (1 stone), unlike the continuing decline seen in anorexia nervosa and occult malignancy. Sometimes weight is lost without any apparent reduction in food intake. In about 10% of depressive episodes there is a similar degree of weight gain, and this is often associated with hypersomnia.

Constipation is a common complaint, which may be due to reduced intestinal motility, to reduced food intake, or to the side-effects of antidepressant drugs. The complaint may also reflect hypochondriacal cognitive distortions in the mental state.

Disturbance of sleep

Hippocrates described his melancholic patients as having little or no sleep (he claimed several had not slept for over 2 years). Kraepelin's patients typically lay sleepless for hours in bed, tormented by painful ideas; if they did sleep, they had confused and anxious dreams, then woke dazed, worn out and weary. They would get up late and might lie in bed for days or even weeks.

Three patterns of sleep in depression are traditionally described. Initial insomnia or delayed sleep is present when there is more than a 1 hour delay in sleeping after settling down. A delay of 2 hours or more marks a severe disturbance. Middle insomnia is also common, with either frequent wakening or a prolonged period of being unable to return to sleep. People with depression frequently fall asleep shortly before they are due to arise. The third pattern, which is traditionally associated with the somatic syndrome, is early-morning wakening. This is defined as waking at least one hour earlier than normal. Waking two or more hours earlier than usual marks a severe disturbance, and this is required to satisfy the 'somatic symptom' criterion in ICD–10. Mood is often lowest after waking early and this is a time when the risk of suicidal behaviour can be high.

Occasionally there is an increased duration of sleep (hypersomnia) or an inverted sleep pattern, with long periods of sleep during the day. There may be discrepancies between observed and reported sleep, which may reflect confusion, histrionic exaggeration, or hypochondriacal and nihilistic features of the mental state. The clinical picture is often distorted by hypnotic medication. A fuller account of the disorders of sleep in depression will be found on page 595.

Loss of libido

This symptom is rarely volunteered but is often present. A tactful approach will help to elicit it, and combining enquiries with routine questions about sleep and appetite is often useful. There is usually a lack of interest in sexual activity compared with normal, and this is often reflected in a diminished frequency of sexual intercourse. Men may suffer from erectile impotence and women may report loss of sexual pleasure. Very occasionally libido is increased.

Disorders of thought content: depressive cognition

Alongside feelings of sadness and anxiety, and together with impaired enjoyment, energy and thinking, and bodily symptoms, there are usually changes in thought content. These include morbid preoccupation and disturbed judgement. In severe depression distorted thinking leads to overvalued ideas and delusions, which may have a melodramatic or even fantastic quality.

Cognitive distortions can relate to the past, present or future, and to the self or to the outside world. Thinking about the past is often dominated by self-reproach and guilt. In the present the self is often viewed as worthless and helpless. Hypochondriacal ideas may be prominent. The outside world is seen as useless, meaningless and, occasionally, persecutory. The future is viewed with apprehension, pessimism, hopelessness and even nihilism. Thoughts of death are common. Suicidal ideas may follow, particularly in the setting of acute hopelessness and despair, but sometimes they arise independently and unexpectedly.

Thoughts and feelings of guilt

> 'Their phantasy most erreth in aggravating their sin.... They are continual Self-Accusers ... apprehending themselves forsaken of God.' (Richard Baxter, 1716, quoted by Hunter & Macalpine, 1963, p. 241)

Guilt is one of the most striking features of depressive disorders. Seventy-five per cent of sufferers feel it to some degree. Three phenomena can be distinguished.

1. *Pathological guilt*. Those affected blame themselves for some action which others would not take very seriously. They often recognise that this is out of proportion but they cannot help feeling self-blame and dwelling upon it. They may blame themselves for neglecting their children, bills having not been paid, duties having been ignored. Sufferers may feel their friends have been let down; their unwise decisions are regretted intensely. They may feel guilty about having stolen sweets as a child or for having been ungrateful to their parents. Characteristically, sufferers also feel blame for bringing an illness upon themselves. Ideas of worthlessness and self-deprecation are closely associated.
2. *Guilty ideas of reference*. Those affected feel that others are blaming them; in more severe forms they feel accused. Insight is preserved and so sufferers recognise the feeling as their own. Intense forms shade into persecutory delusions.
3. *Delusions of guilt*. As depressive states deepen, ideas of guilt become less realistic, and insight into their pathological nature is lost. Patients magnify their own role in events and may give an entirely false account of a serious misdemeanour (delusional memory). Delusional guilt sometimes has the quality of glorifying self-aggrandisement. One patient claimed 'I am the chief sinner; there never was anyone in the world as wicked as me.' Patients may believe that they have committed adultery or incest, that they have killed their families, that they have caused a train crash or air disaster, or that they have become possessed by the Devil. Patients may give themselves up repeatedly to the police. Delusional guilt may also involve feelings of responsibility for others. One patient was convinced that she was making other patients ill. Another believed that whenever he ate someone was executed. Great care should be taken to distinguish between delusional memories and accurate recall of painful events for which feelings of guilt are appropriate. Guilt over past incest may be delusional or it may be a highly significant disclosure.

Thoughts of worthlessness and self-deprecation

> 'But I am a worm, and no man.' (Psalm 22: 6)

In depressive states any premorbid tendency to feelings of inferiority and low self-worth is amplified. Raised standards are applied to the self without a corresponding change with regard to others. Compensatory merits are discounted. People with severe depression often regard themselves as worthless and as total failures. There are occasionally delusions of poverty, such as the false belief that one is bankrupt.

Sufferers describe themselves as unwanted, unloved and not worthy of having friends. They feel discontented with themselves. They lack confidence. They have failed at everything, they will lose their jobs, they face ruin. Requests for lists of personal strengths and weaknesses often result in catalogues of faults with no redeeming features. In severe states, feelings border on self-loathing and self-hatred.

It can be hard to distinguish depressive self-deprecation from insight and from long-standing attitudes to the self. For example, there may have been genuine failure at work as a result of impaired concentration, indecisiveness and lack of energy. There may always have been a lack of confidence and low self-esteem. Depression is identified by a fluctuation in self-deprecation with mood, by its intensity and by the fact that it is a change from the normal.

Hypochondriasis

> 'Some are afraid that they shall have every fearful disease they see others have, hear of or read.' (Burton, 1621, p. 235)

People who are depressed have many good reasons to feel that they are physically ill. They may have experienced low mood, loss of appetite and fatigue during a previous physical illness. Depressed mood or muscular tension may be felt as a physical pain in the chest or head. The autonomic symptoms of anxiety all suggest physical disorder.

These experiences may lead a person to suspect a physical illness, but this does not amount to hypochondriasis. When there is also anxious foreboding and a worried, pessimistic mood, hypochondriacal phenomena are likely to emerge. There may be a heightened awareness of bodily sensations, and an abnormally intense and painful preoccupation with the possibility of a fearful disease, or a growing conviction of an unhealthy, rotten or diseased body. In extreme forms there may be beliefs that the sufferer has one or more physical illnesses in the face of evidence to the contrary. Such hypochondriacal delusions can take on a fantastic and even nihilistic quality. The illness may be viewed as a deserved punishment.

Kraepelin described patients who believed that they were incurably ill and expecting a slow and painful death. Some claimed they had lung disease or cancer; others had tapeworms; others could not swallow. Lewis's patients were particularly concerned with their bowels; one said, for example, 'they have all gone wrong ... the food just wedges in'. One patient had a sudden blank feeling across his forehead and was sure it was a stroke. More fantastic ideas have involved: organs being withered, burnt or rotten; brains melting, leaving skulls full of filth; and bones out of joint and insects breeding inside the cavity. Patients have reported excruciating pains, disfiguring eruptions on the face, testicles being crushed, food falling down between intestines into the scrotum. Nihilistic hypochondriacal delusions have included beliefs that the body is hollow, that stomach and bowels are no longer there, that no urine is passed, and that genitals have disappeared.

Hopelessness, *tedium vitae* and suicidal thoughts, plans and acts

> 'My days are swifter than a weaver's shuttle, and are spent without hope ... so that my soul chooseth strangling, and death rather than my life.' (Job 7: 6, 15)

The future may appear bleak and without comfort. Life can seem pointless and not worth living (*tedium vitae*), there being little or no hope of recovery, so that more pain and anguish will follow. Fleeting thoughts of suicide are common and often plans are made. When hope is lost, suicide may begin to appear as a logical solution, as a relief from intolerable pain or even as an atonement for real or delusional guilt. Thoughts of joining loved ones who have already died are particularly ominous, as is the writing of a suicide note, settling one's affairs and taking precautions against being found. Threats to take the lives of children or a partner to save them from the effects of the suicide should also be taken very seriously. While suicidal acts usually arise out of a sense of extreme despair, they may emerge suddenly and without warning in states of milder depression, often in association with impaired impulse control, and with the sufferer unable to account for the motives.

Many risk factors for suicide have been identified, but these can be difficult to apply in practice. Three useful clinical predictors are hopelessness, suicidal plans and previous attempts. Kraepelin regarded psychic inhibition (see 'Anergia', above) as protective against suicide, and warned against the increasing risk when retarded patients recovered their volition while remaining hopeless. Many clinicians have encountered the unexpected suicide of a patient who appeared to be recovering. The decision to take one's life is often accompanied by a sense of calmness, and suicidal plans may be concealed behind apparently cheerful behaviour. A detailed account of suicide is given in Chapter 7.

Suicidal thoughts and acts are not the only results of depressive thinking about the future. If recovery is felt to be unlikely, or impossible, then concordance with treatment may be poor. Pessimism can interact with perceptions of the world as cruel and desolate, and with an extremely apprehensive mood. The resulting thought content can range from regret that society's values are decaying to a conviction of imminent global catastrophe.

The self may be perceived as potentially dangerous. One patient reported by Du Laurens (1597, quoted by Hunter & Macalpine, 1963), believed that if he were to pass water then his whole town would be drowned by the volume of his urine. He was reportedly treated by his attendants convincing him that the town was engulfed in a raging fire which needed his intervention. Today patients are more likely to be convinced of impending nuclear holocaust or financial ruin, and it may be that altruism can no longer be relied upon for a cure. Delusions of catastrophe have a nihilistic quality: everything will be destroyed, nothing can be done. In extreme forms, as Jaspers (1963) describes, the future vanishes.

Delusions

As already indicated, these will sometimes occur as an end-point of severe cognitive distortion. Five main types can be identified:

1 delusions of guilt
2 delusions of poverty
3 hypochondriacal delusions
4 delusions of catastrophe
5 nihilistic delusions.

All of these are regarded as mood congruent. Persecutory delusions, delusional jealousy and delusions of bodily change are also sometimes found in depressive illnesses. Examples of delusions of guilt, poverty, hypochondriasis and catastrophe have already been given.

Cotard (1882) described a syndrome of nihilistic delusions often associated with hypochondriasis. The central feature is the delusion of negation: for example, a patient goes beyond the belief that his bowels are not working to the point where his bowels cease to exist. Such nihilistic delusions can refer to parts of the body, the self, the world or even the future.

Persecutory delusions commonly take the form of beliefs that the patient is under surveillance, that there is a plot, an organisation such as the CIA is pursuing the patient, other patients are detectives or secret agents, food is poisoned, and so on. The persecution is usually felt to be justified, as a development from guilty ideas of reference, but some patients show resentment at its unjust nature and may even loudly proclaim their innocence.

Disorders of experience

Depersonalisation

Depersonalisation is not a common symptom of depression, but when present it is striking. Sufferers feel unreal, as if they were acting a part, or as if they were a robot. Insight into the abnormality of this phenomenon is retained. The feeling is highly unpleasant but difficult to describe, and hence metaphor is often used. One patient said, 'I've got this dreadful feeling as if I'm unreal, a sort of dead feeling, wooden inside. I've changed; I do things mechanically.' Jaspers analysed depersonalisation as resulting from a loss of sense of awareness: of the self as an active agent; of temporal continuity of the self; and of the distinction between the self and the outside world. Depersonalisation is also closely linked to the phenomenon of anhedonia. It should be distinguished from:

1 a perception of parts of the body as unfamiliar
2 dysmorphophobia (the perception of one's appearance as changed)
3 delusions of bodily change
4 nihilistic delusions of non-existence.

Exploring the reasons behind a person's feelings of depersonalisation sometimes uncovers hidden delusions.

Only about a half of those presenting with depersonalisation are depressed and so it is not a diagnostic sign. It sometimes occurs in healthy persons under stress, in association with intense anxiety, or following sensory deprivation. It may occur in many other psychiatric conditions, including organic disorders (especially temporal lobe seizures), schizophrenia, generalised and phobic anxiety disorders, post-traumatic stress disorder and after the use of hallucinogens. Very occasionally it occurs as a primary phenomena alongside derealisation (see below). It is categorised as such in ICD–10 as depersonalisation disorder, a sub-class of the dissociative disorders.

Theories of the mechanisms underlying depersonalisation have been reviewed by Sierra & Berrios (1998). Functional imaging studies have identified reduced neural responses in emotion-sensitive areas of the brain, accompanied by increased responses in regions associated with emotional regulation. Depersonalisation may have a protective effect in acute anxiety but in depressive disorders it is often associated with a chronic course and it can be difficult to treat. Glutamate hyperactivity has been postulated, but early results from a small randomised controlled trial of lamotrigine, which inhibits glutamate release, were disappointing.

Derealisation

Derealisation is another uncommon but often striking feature of depression. In mild forms, the person's surroundings lack colour and life, and other people may seem to be making a pretence of their emotions. In more severe forms everything seems artificial or unreal, like a stage set populated with actors. One patient described it as follows: 'People seem changed, like machines; things look mysterious. It's as if I were in a dream, watching a film.' Lewis analysed the phenomenon as a combination of various changes, including:

1 altered perceptions of the environment, for example appearances of unreality, mystery, acting and soulessness
2 changes in consciousness, for example bewilderment, muddle, impressions of mystery and confusion
3 loss of the ability to recall images with vividness
4 changes in the experience of time.

Derealisation should be distinguished from nihilistic delusion. Derealisation is an experience, not a belief, and insight into its abnormal nature is retained.

Obsessive–compulsive phenomena

Obsessive–compulsive symptoms occur in 20–35% of depressive episodes, often as an exaggeration of premorbid traits. The core phenomenon is the experience of intrusive thoughts or impulses which are recognised as one's own and which are entertained or carried out against conscious resistance. The sufferer recognises them as senseless and tries to stop but cannot. In time the experience of conscious resistance may fade.

Obsessional thoughts in depressive disorders usually have aggressive or obscene themes. For example, knives may be avoided for fear of harming the self or others, or there may be a strong impulse to shout obscenities while in a church service. There may be recurrent and apparently senseless thoughts of killing one's family. The obsessional nature of such thoughts is usually protective against harmful actions, but any switch from an obsessional to a delusional quality in thoughts with suicidal or homicidal themes is extremely ominous.

Repeated checking is a frequent problem. For instance many people with depression cannot remember whether they have locked doors and may return to check. This is not a true obsessional symptom unless they can remember locking the door but still need to check again to satisfy an inner compulsion.

A few of those who gain obsessional symptoms during a depressive episode fail to lose them on recovery. One interesting hypothesis is that such symptoms may have a dual role in depression, acting both as markers of a propensity for psychosis and also as defences against disintegration of the psyche (Stengel, 1945).

A full account of obsessive–compulsive phenomena is given in Chapter 15.

Hallucinations

In states of normal grief, seeing and hearing the deceased is not uncommon, but in depressive illnesses hallucinations are rare. When they occur they are usually auditory, in the second person and consistent with depressive themes of guilt, death, personal inadequacy, disease, nihilism or deserved punishment. They are often isolated phenomena and are seldom in the foreground of the clinical picture. Often there is little more than an indistinct muttering. Kraepelin reported his patients as hallucinating the crackling of hell or the hammering of a gallows being erected. When a voice is recognised it is often that of a relative or partner. Typically only a few words are distinct. A parent may be heard to say in a condemnatory tone: 'You have let everybody down' or 'You deserve to die'. On closer examination, many of these phenomena are not true hallucinations but rather illusions, auditory misinterpretations, or pseudo-hallucinations (i.e. they are heard within the mind and not located in physical space by the patient). Kraepelin describes vividly how the vascular murmur of the ear becomes a reproach: 'Whore, whore, whore…', which is then attributed to the Devil. When true hallucinations do occur they are often more frequent at night and are often described as emanating from the sufferer's body, for example as a voice speaking from inside the stomach.

Command hallucinations also occur, most often instructing the patient to harm him- or herself, or others. These should be examined carefully for evidence of passivity phenomena, in which the patient feels impelled to act under the controlling influence of an outside force. The association of command hallucinations with passivity phenomena is an extremely dangerous development.

Visual distortions are sometimes seen. Faces can take on an ominous or spectral quality. A shadow may be seen at the window. Worms may swarm in the patient's food. True visual hallucinations are rare, but they can appear as an invitation or enticement to suicide. One patient saw a clear vision of a noose and believed this was a signal that she should hang herself.

Hallucinations in other modalities are even rarer, but can include the perception of a strong smell of putrefaction emanating from a house or from the person's own body. Very occasionally hallucinations occur simultaneously in more than one sensory modality.

Schizophrenia-like and mood-incongruent psychotic features

There are patients whose illnesses appear to be typically depressive but who experience somatic hallucinations, or passivity phenomena, or describe thought insertion, or express bizarre nonsensical or absurd delusions, or delusions of external influence, or persecutory delusions unrelated to deserved punishment. Both Kraepelin and Lewis reported such features in their classic descriptions of melancholy, and they were especially prominent in Kraepelin's categories of 'paranoid' and 'fantastic' melancholy. Many of these phenomena constitute first-rank symptoms of schizophrenia, and if they are prominent they point to an ICD–10 diagnosis of schizoaffective disorder (see Chapter 9).

Delusions or second-person hallucinations that are affectively neutral or not in keeping with a depressed mood occur in up to a third of all patients with psychotic depression and do not in themselves point to schizoaffective disorder. These can be specified in ICD–10 as mood-incongruent psychotic features, although there is little agreement about the value of making such a distinction.

Histrionic features

Kraepelin wrote that hysterical disorders were observed 'extraordinarily often' in melancholia. Aubrey Lewis devoted many paragraphs to 'neurotic features', which comprised a mixture of psychosomatic and conversion symptoms and histrionic behaviours. Although such features are familiar to most clinicians, they now receive scant recognition in many textbooks.

Kraepelin's account included noises in the ears, shivering in the back and special sensitivity to the influence of the weather. He also described fainting fits, giddiness, hysterical convulsions, choreiform clonic convulsions and psychogenic tremor. Lewis portrayed many conversion-type symptoms, such as vomiting or headaches under stress or in unwelcome situations. His account of histrionic behaviour included exaggerated and melodramatic talk, attitudes of extreme dependence, threatening a hunger strike, clutching arms with a very appealing manner, seeking endless sympathy and pedantic formality. He described over-intimacy, letters like novelettes and strong affective relationships which quickly changed from strong attachment to active dislike. Some of his patients were 'always seeking attention, calling out, asking for interviews, self-pitying, and copying symptoms from others'. Others were 'laughing and crying alternately with neither giving the impression of much depth'. One patient was always stealing another patient's pillows; another's eyes kept revolving. Many were worried about their eyes or ears, and multiple pains, which resolved quickly.

Such features can be regarded as pathoplastic effects of a histrionic premorbid personality, or as a re-emergence of childhood and infantile behavioural patterns, with acute fears of abandonment, fierce attachments and possessiveness. One should be cautious about assuming the former, for it is striking how apparently histrionic 'personality' features often disappear completely when a patient recovers fully from a depressive illness.

Depressive stupor

Kraepelin described stupor as a syndrome rather than a symptom. His patients usually lay mute and motionless in bed, at most withdrawing timidly from approaches, sometimes demonstrating catalepsy, sometimes merely aimless resistance. They sat helpless before food but often allowed themselves to be spoon-fed. They held fast what was pressed into their hand, turning it slowly about, without knowing how to get rid of it. Unable to care for their bodily needs they frequently became dirty. Now and then periods of excitement were interpolated. Kraepelin described how, after the return of consciousness, memory was 'very much clouded and often quite extinguished'.

Depressive stupor is usually conceptualised either as an end-point of severe retardation or as an extreme form of psychic inhibition. Severe forms, with a complete failure to respond to the surroundings, are now rarely seen. More commonly patients present in a pre-stuporous phase, having stopped eating and drinking, still speaking a few words, but spending most of their time staring into space. When patients recover they usually give a clear account of their experiences, describing the state as an extremely painful one. The fact that Kraepelin's stuporous patients had only patchy recall on recovery has led to suggestions that some were showing clouding of consciousness, perhaps due to dehydration or nutritional factors. Stupor is included in ICD–10 alongside hallucinations and delusions as a psychotic feature of severe depression. Stupor is also discussed in Chapter 20 (see page 490).

Appearance, behaviour and talk

The appearance of depression is usually easier to recognise than it is to describe. It is often identified directly rather than inferred from any combination of elements. The following features are common, but few may be present, and there may even be smiles and apparent jocularity.

Most sufferers appear sad, dejected, downcast, miserable or guilty, much of the time. They may look stony faced, frightened or apprehensive. Worry may be evidenced by a furrowed brow, and the corners of the mouth may be turned down. Posture is often stooped or drooping and sufferers may sit head in hands, looking at the floor. Tears may be close, or there may be actual crying, weeping or sobbing. Their general manner may signal an attitude of dependency, hostility or even indifference.

Evidence of self-neglect is common. Those affected may be untidy and unkempt, dirty and smelling, with unwashed hair. Clothes may be unusually drab, or dirty and stained. Night-clothes may be worn in the middle of the day. There may be signs of weight loss or dehydration, or evidence of self-harm (e.g. scars or bruises). Agitation or retardation may be apparent, as described above. There may be a poverty of movement, gesture and speech. Talk is likely to be soft or monotonous, and may die away, often with sentences left incomplete. There may be hesitancy, monosyllabic replies or even muteness.

Changes in social behaviour

Depressive illnesses can provoke many changes in social behaviour and these are often the most prominent features of the clinical presentation.

Inefficiency at work may lead to threats of redundancy or to unemployment. Unpaid bills and failure in budgeting may cause financial crises. Irritability, loss of feeling and social withdrawal can lead to a breakdown of relationships with friends or family. Marital discord is a common presenting problem. It may be hard to distinguish between cause and effect in a person with chronic depression who complains of an unhappy marriage.

Alcohol and other drugs are often used to provide relief from depressive symptoms, especially low mood, anxiety and insomnia. A presentation with alcohol or drug misuse may mask an underlying depressive illness. Equally, a hidden alcohol problem commonly underlies treatment-resistant depression. Antisocial behaviours are sometimes released by depressive illnesses. Shoplifting, promiscuity, sexual aberrations, violence and physical and sexual abuse are all ways in which a depressive illness can present itself.

Hypochondriacal features may lead to repeated medical consultations, especially when somatic symptoms closely mimic a physical illness. This is a fairly common mode of presentation of depressive disorders, particularly in those who have difficulty in describing their feelings.

Most importantly of all, depressive illnesses can result in increased risk-taking, self-harm, suicide and even homicide. An episode of deliberate self-harm is one of the commonest ways in which a depressive illness is revealed.

Of course, phenomena such as unemployment, marital discord, antisocial behaviour and deliberate self-harm can have many other causes. They are sometimes associated with depressive illnesses, and when they occur one possibility among many is that the individual is suffering from a primary depressive illness.

Diagnostic criteria and classification

No clinical feature described here is either necessary or sufficient for the diagnosis of a depressive episode. For each, there are episodes where the phenomenon is absent and yet the diagnosis remains one of depression. Conversely, each can occur as a symptom of another disorder. Depressive disorders therefore show a pattern of family resemblance, and diagnoses are best made using polythetic criteria, with multiple elements. Both ICD–10 (World Health Organization, 1992) and DSM–IV (American Psychiatric Association, 1994) employ this approach.

Core features

There have been many attempts to isolate core features. The most obvious candidate is depressed mood, which appears in most accounts, ranging from *The Anatomy of Melancholy* to current textbooks. Burton, however, was very aware that depressed mood was not essential. He wrote: 'Some indeed are sad and not fearful, some fearful and not sad; some neither fearful nor sad' (Burton, 1621, p. 234). Kraepelin did not even view depressed mood as a central feature. He believed the underlying process to be a depression of function: 'simple psychic inhibition'. Bleuler and Janet held similar views, Janet stressing the importance of a feeling of inadequacy (see Lewis, 1934, p. 301). Jaspers (1963) argued for two independent central features: 'an unmotivated profound sadness' and 'a retardation of psychic events'.

Two other features, low self-esteem and anhedonia, have found support as candidates for core features of the disorder. ICD–10 and DSM–IV criteria include both depressed mood and anhedonia as core features. DSM–IV requires that at least one of these must be present for a diagnosis of a depressive syndrome. ICD–10 is closer to the Jasperian tradition, in that it includes increased fatiguability as a third core feature and requires two out of three features for the diagnosis of depression to be made. Thus in both current systems there can be patients diagnosed as depressed who are 'neither fearful nor sad'. Robert Burton would have approved.

Classification

The bewildering range of depressive disorders has led to a search for organising principles. Variation can be accounted for by differences in severity and by the shaping ('pathoplastic') effects of personality and circumstances. However, many psychiatrists believe that there must also be a heterogeneous group of disorders behind the variability, and there have been many attempts to find a useful and valid division into subtypes. Few areas in psychiatry have generated more heated debate and yet remained for so long in a state of confusion. There have been two main themes running through the literature: an endogenous/somatic distinction of subtypes, and a unipolar/bipolar distinction.

From endogenous depression to the somatic syndrome and beyond

First, can depressive illnesses be divided into two main types on the basis of aetiology, clinical features and response to treatment? Timothy Bright (1586, quoted by Hunter & Macalpine, 1963, p. 37) noted 'how diverslie the word melancholy is taken'. He identified cases where melancholy was 'not moved by any adversity present or imminent', in which 'the melancholy humour ... abuseth the mind' and for which physical treatment was needed. He described a second type of melancholy where 'the perill is not of body' but 'proceedeth from the mind's apprehension'; this required 'cure of the minde', that is, psychotherapy. For the four centuries and more since, Bright's distinction between endogenous and exogenous forms has reappeared in various guises, in particular as the division between endogenous and reactive depressions, and that between psychotic and neurotic depression, which had been embodied in the *International Classification of Diseases* until ICD–10, which introduced the somatic syndrome (see below).

With hindsight we can see how this simple and apparently sensible distinction led to confusion. Three main elements characterise Bright's 'melancholy humour' or what we would now term the endogenous category:

1 the absence of an external cause

2 a biological clinical picture

3 response to physical treatment.

Problems arise whenever cases meet one of these criteria but not the others. For example, Paykel *et al* (1984) have shown that the clinical picture of depressive illnesses is mostly independent of the presence or absence of an external cause. It follows that the aetiological division between endogenous and reactive depression may bear little relation to the biological clinical picture or to response to particular forms of treatment.

Further problems have arisen from the use of the terms 'psychotic' and 'neurotic' to attempt to identify the distinction that Bright made. Kendell (1968) has discussed how the patients encountered in asylum practice by Kraepelin, and identified as suffering from manic–depressive psychosis, differed from those seen in the consulting rooms of early psychoanalysts, who described their patients as suffering from depressive neuroses. This selective experience by different groups of clinicians with very different aetiological models may have led to an artificial polarisation between two forms of what may nevertheless have been the same illness.

In addition, both 'psychotic' and 'neurotic' have had several meanings. A diagnosis of 'manic–depressive psychosis' or 'psychotic depression' according to Kraepelin and the tradition of the *International Classification of Diseases* (again, before ICD–10) did not require the presence of hallucinations or delusions. For most psychiatrists now the word 'psychotic' is used to convey precisely the fact that hallucinations or delusions are present. The term 'neurotic' has been used to refer to milder depressive episodes, to episodes showing 'neurotic' clinical features, to 'reactive' episodes, to chronic fluctuating depressive disorders, to depressive disorders that respond to psychotherapeutic interventions or to depressive episodes arising on the background of a neurotic personality. It has been no surprise to find that the diagnosis of 'neurotic' depression lacks both reliability and validity.

One escape route from this confusion would be to adopt the position argued by Lewis (1938), namely that all the variability in depressive illness is due to the effects of severity and pathoplastic factors, together with a variation between episodic and chronic forms. This unitarian approach has been central to the development of DSM criteria and also underpinned the tenth revision of ICD, in which the neurotic–psychotic distinction was finally abandoned.

It was the advent of the Research Diagnostic Criteria (RDC) in the United States that marked the first step in this direction (Spitzer *et al*, 1978). Neurotic depression was rejected on the grounds that it was an amorphous category, and depressions were divided into major and minor on the basis of severity. 'Psychotic' major depression was restricted to cases showing delusions or hallucinations. Subtypes were proposed, including endogenous depression (RDC) or melancholia (in the subsequent DSM criteria), and operational criteria for these included pervasive anhedonia, loss of reactivity, early-morning wakening and weight loss. DSM–III–R (American Psychiatric Association, 1987) further introduced a classification of depressions into three levels

Box 1.1 ICD–10 criteria for the somatic syndrome

At least four of the following:
- marked loss of interest or pleasure
- loss of emotional reactions
- waking in the morning 2 hours or more before usual time
- depression worse in the morning
- objective evidence of marked psychomotor retardation or agitation
- marked loss of appetite
- weight loss (5% or more of body weight in the past month)
- loss of libido

of severity – mild, moderate and severe – and this has remained in DSM–IV.

A similar approach was taken in ICD–10, with four main levels of severity (see Box 1.2, below), with 'psychotic' being restricted to hallucinations, delusions or depressive stupor. 'Melancholic' features were designated as 'somatic' (an optional 'syndrome'). 'Biological features' had been considered as an alternative term to 'somatic symptoms' and this would reflect the usage of many psychiatrists, but 'somatic symptoms' remained in the final version.

It is the somatic syndrome (ICD–10) (see Box 1.1) or melancholic subtype (DSM–IV) that has the strongest echoes of Bright's endogenous form of depression. The clinical features identifying this symptom cluster have emerged consistently from discriminant function and factor analytic studies, and have been repeatedly shown to predict both response to physical treatments (including electroconvulsive therapy and antidepressants) and an increased risk of recurrence. Most proponents claim that pervasive anhedonia and loss of reactivity are central defining characteristics and that these probably reflect a distinct pathophysiology. Others have suggested that retardation is the central phenomenon.

Critics of the approach taken by ICD–10 and DSM–IV continue to argue against the relegation of what they feel to be a crucial diagnostic distinction to merely an optional subtyping into melancholic or somatic features, while perhaps less meaningful distinctions based on severity are promoted. It is probably true that most psychiatrists can cite criteria to separate major and minor depression, whereas only a minority will reliably identify the somatic syndrome. Contrary to the hopes expressed in ICD–10 and DSM–IV, most depressive episodes previously described as 'neurotic' or 'reactive' cannot be classified as minor depressions or dysthymia (see below), but fall squarely into the major depressive category, so that samples of patients with major depression ascertained for research purposes may be unduly heterogeneous.

While the unitarian approach has found support from the longitudinal studies of Angst and colleagues, who present evidence for a spectrum of depressive disorders (Angst & Merikangas, 1997), others still remain strongly wedded to the notion of two distinct illnesses, and have accused DSM and ICD–10 of leading depression research into a blind alley. To be fair, the authors of ICD–10 have acknowledged that while the status and future of the biomedical pole of Timothy Bright's distinction is still uncertain, there remains widespread clinical and research interest in its survival.

Unipolar and bipolar disorders

The second major theme running through the history of the classification of the affective disorders involves the relationship between mania and depression. Kraepelin believed that mania and depression were definitely 'manifestations of a single morbid process' and he argued strongly for their unification in a single disorder, manic–depressive insanity. This term was to be used even where no manic attacks ever occurred. Many believe that this synthesis was as significant as his separation of manic–depressive insanity from dementia praecox, but it has always had its critics. Diagnoses in ICD–9 (World Health Organization, 1978) followed Kraepelin, so that a single episode of severe depression was described as 'manic–depressive psychosis: depressed type'. This often misled the lay public, who wrongly interpreted the diagnosis as implying that manic attacks were to be expected.

Leonhard (published in English in 1979) has been credited with rediscovering the distinction between unipolar and bipolar affective disorders. Two further independent empirical studies embodying this distinction appeared almost simultaneously (Angst, 1966; Perris, 1966) (see also Chapter 3, page 51) and their remarkably consistent findings have had a major effect on the subsequent psychiatric literature, which has emphasised the differences between those patients who show unipolar depressive histories and those who show bipolar histories (i.e. of both depression and mania).

Despite these findings, as yet there has been no clear difference shown in clinical features or pathophysiology between unipolar and bipolar depressive episodes. Most of the evidence remains consistent with the hypothesis that bipolar illness represents no more than an increased genetic loading for a unitary affective disorder. There is also increasing support for the concept of a bipolar spectrum (Akiskal *et al*, 2000). Kraepelin may yet be proved to have had an equally penetrating insight, but the unipolar/bipolar distinction is now widely regarded as the most robust sub-classification of the affective disorders. It was no surprise to find that ICD–10 followed the DSM approach in distinguishing between unipolar and bipolar disorders.

The two main classificatory systems

ICD–10

As indicated above, the ICD–10 classification is a radical departure from its predecessors in finally abandoning the distinction between manic–depressive psychosis and depressive neurosis. An operational definition is given for a depressive episode (outlined in Box 1.2), which is based on a 2-week duration of symptoms. Four levels of severity are defined, mainly on the basis of symptom numbers, but also taking into account functional impairments.

A useful distinction can be made between symptoms, syndromes, episodes and disorders. Symptoms comprise the clinical features described earlier in this chapter,

Box 1.2 An outline of ICD–10 criteria for a depressive episode

A

- Depressed mood most of the day, nearly every day
- Loss of interest or pleasure
- Decreased energy or increased fatiguability

B

- Loss of confidence or self-esteem
- Unreasonable self-reproach or guilt
- Recurrent thoughts of death, or suicide, or any suicidal behaviour
- Impairments of thinking (subjective or objective)
- Agitation or retardation (subjective or objective)
- Sleep disturbance of any type
- Decreased or increased appetite with corresponding weight change

The symptoms should not be attributable to psychoactive substance use or to any organic disorder.

For a mild episode: At least four symptoms are present during the same 2-week period. At least two of these should be from group A. The patient is usually distressed by the symptoms but will probably be able to continue with most activities.

For a moderate episode: At least six symptoms are present during the same 2-week period. At least two of these will be from group A. The patient is likely to have great difficulty in continuing with ordinary activities.

For a severe episode: At least eight symptoms are present during the same 2-week period, including all three from group A. Suicidal thoughts and acts are common.

For a severe episode with psychotic symptoms: As for a severe episode, but with the additional presence of either hallucinations or delusions or stupor so severe that social activities are impossible. There may be danger to life from suicide, dehydration or starvation.

Adapted with permission from ICD–10.

differing from the normal by virtue of their intensity, pervasiveness and inappropriateness. These can be combined, as in ICD–10, as elements of operational criteria to define mood syndromes. Mood syndromes can occur as part of any disorder, but when they occur on the basis of a mood disorder the result is a mood episode. Episodes occurring singly or in combination define a mood disorder.

In ICD–10, the move from depressive episodes to bipolar and unipolar disorders appears complicated but follows simple rules. If a manic or hypomanic episode has already occurred, then the present episode is classified as 'bipolar disorder, current episode mild/moderate/severe/severe with psychotic symptoms', as defined in Box 1.2. If only episodes of depression have occurred previously, then the present episode is classified as 'recurrent depressive disorder, current episode mild/moderate/severe/severe with psychotic symptoms', defined similarly. If no previous affective episode has occurred, then a current episode of depression remains classified at the episode level, again with definitions as in Box 1.2. ICD–10 also allows for the specification of the presence within mild and moderate episodes of the somatic syndrome (Box 1.1), but assumes that in severe episodes this syndrome will almost invariably be present. Severe episodes with psychotic symptoms can be further divided on the basis of mood congruence. ICD–10 also provides provisional criteria for seasonal pattern (see Box 1.3, below).

DSM–IV

The DSM–IV classification of the affective disorders is similar to that in ICD–10. This reflects both a conscious effort by the authors of each to bring the two systems together, and also the fact that the two approaches share a common ancestry in DSM–III–R. In general, the DSM–IV system is simpler and avoids making a distinction between single and recurrent episodes. It also includes a wider range of useful specifiers, including seasonal pattern, atypical features, catatonic features, rapid cycling and postpartum onset (within 4 weeks of childbirth). Longitudinal characteristics can also be identified, including the degree of any remission and chronicity.

DSM–IV criteria for a mild depressive episode are more stringent than those in ICD–10, in that they require five symptoms rather than four. In DSM–IV diagnosis requires one out of two essential features (sadness, anhedonia) compared with two out of three (sadness, anhedonia, anergia) in ICD–10. There is an additional requirement of clinically significant distress or impairment of functioning. Depressive episodes induced by a drug of misuse or medication, or by an organic factor or as part of normal bereavement are excluded. The somatic syndrome is called melancholia, and the criteria for this differ from those in ICD–10. Psychotic features do not include stupor but are restricted to delusions and hallucinations.

Seasonality: seasonal affective disorder

For over 2000 years there has been speculation about seasonal influences on the incidence of mania and melancholia, and in particular about the possible connection between the winter months and depression. Most clinicians can identify patients with bipolar illnesses or recurrent depressive illnesses that show a remarkably consistent seasonal pattern, and it is possible that these constitute a significant subtype of the mood disorders. During the decade 1980–90 this idea received a major impetus from the finding that winter depression may respond to a specific treatment, phototherapy (see below). As a result, criteria for seasonal pattern were incorporated into DSM–III–R and these have been modified in DSM–IV and ICD–10 (Box 1.3). Community and clinic surveys show that about 10% of all patients with major mood disorders meet these criteria.

Summer and winter depressions have been recognised, but it is winter depression that has been most studied; it has been popularised as 'seasonal affective disorder' (SAD) (Wehr & Rosenthal, 1989). Patients with

Box 1.3 An outline of the ICD–10 criteria for seasonal affective disorder

- Three or more episodes of mood disorder must occur with onset within the same 90-day period of the year for 3 or more consecutive years.
- Remissions also occur within a particular 90-day period of the year.
- Seasonal episodes substantially outnumber any non-seasonal episodes that may occur.

SAD typically describe lowered levels of energy and activity, anxiety, dysphoria and irritability, impaired concentration, social withdrawal and decreased libido. Most also report a distinctive constellation of symptoms, which include hypersomnia, increased appetite and overeating and carbohydrate craving. Most are mild to moderate in severity but a significant number (11% in one series) require in-patient treatment. In Washington, DC, at latitude 38.9, the illness has been reported as beginning in November, when the hours of daylight fall below 10. Patients in the United States typically report their worst months as January and February, compared with November and December for those in Europe. Untreated episodes usually resolve by springtime and some sufferers report mild euphoria and increased levels of energy, activity and libido, with decreased need to sleep, in the summer months. Most meet the criteria only for unipolar disorders, although some meet bipolar II criteria and very occasionally bipolar I disorders are found (see Chapter 2 on bipolar I and II disorders). Familial risks of affective disorders in SAD are similar to those found in non-seasonal depressive illnesses. It is not clear whether SAD is inherited as a distinct entity or whether seasonality and depression are separate heritable traits that happen to coincide in certain individuals.

The underlying pathophysiology of SAD remains a fascinating intellectual and scientific puzzle. Early hopes that the seasonal pattern and response to phototherapy could be explained in terms of changes in melatonin secretion have not been fulfilled. These have been replaced by theories of disordered brain serotonin regulation, or phase-advanced circadian rhythms. There is likely to be biological and genetic heterogeneity. One intriguing hypothesis is that patients with SAD generate a biological signal of change of season that is absent in healthy volunteers but is similar to that which mammals use to regulate seasonal changes in their behaviour.

Prevalence estimates for SAD vary between 0% and 10%. Studies within the United States have shown consistently higher rates at northern latitudes, but wider comparisons suggest that the influence of latitude on prevalence is relatively small, with other factors such as climate, genetic vulnerability and sociocultural context playing a more important role. Estimates within Europe cluster around a mean of about 3%. Follow-up studies show diagnostic instability, with only about a third of cases remaining seasonal after 5–8 years. In Switzerland two-thirds of those where the picture had changed reported improvement, which suggests that SAD is not necessarily the prodrome of a more serious disorder.

Phototherapy

About a half of patients studied have shown a clinically significant response to a week of treatment with bright light. Early studies found response to be dependent on both the intensity of light and its duration. While 2500 lux for 2 hours daily was initially recommended, 10000 lux for 30 minutes has proved a more practical and equally effective option. There may be a differential response, with the typical depressive symptoms in SAD responding to bright light whereas the atypical symptoms respond to light treatment at all intensities. Exposure of the eye to the light is important; skin absorption does not modify circadian rhythms and is ineffective in SAD. Early-morning treatment is superior but leads to an increase in reported side-effects, including jumpiness, headaches and nausea, which occur in up to 15% of those treated. Dawn simulators (which produce a gradually increasing signal over 1.5 hours, peaking at 250 lux) may be an effective alternative approach.

Patients who respond to light treatment are usually advised to continue this until springtime and prophylactic treatment beginning in the autumn has been advocated.

Conventional antidepressant treatments have also been reported to be effective in SAD.

Recurrent brief depressive disorder

Not all episodes of depression last for 2 weeks or more, and some remit after just a few days. Thus, while some brief episodes can meet criteria for mild, moderate or even severe depressive syndromes, they may fail to be classified as depressive episodes because of their short duration. When such brief depressions recur frequently, the cumulative morbidity can be very significant.

Criteria for recurrent brief depressive disorder are included in ICD–10: brief depressive episodes must have occurred at least once a month over the previous year, and not solely in relation to the menstrual cycle. A prevalence rate of 10% has been estimated, with only half of those affected seeking treatment.

In contrast to dysthymia (see below), patients with recurrent brief depressive disorder are not depressed most of the time. The occurrence of this disorder in those who also have histories of more prolonged depressive episodes has been shown to carry a particularly high risk of suicidal behaviour.

Although recurrent brief depressive disorder may yet prove to be an important clinical diagnosis, it has not been widely used and its significance has perhaps been overshadowed by the development of the depressive spectrum concept and a focus on the importance of all forms of sub-threshold depressive syndromes.

Persistent disorders: dysthymia/cyclothymia

In Chapter 7 of his *Manic Depressive Insanity*, Kraepelin (1921) identified four fundamental states which he viewed as 'permanently slighter' forms of the disorder. These were described as depressive, manic, irritable and cyclothymic 'temperaments'. He maintained that these occurred in about one-third of his manic–depressive patients, and that they provided evidence of the illness even during the 'free' intervals between attacks. He also believed that such states occur in others who have never experienced an episode of illness.

Box 1.4 An outline of the ICD–10 criteria for dysthymia

A period of at least 2 years with constant or constantly recurring depressed mood. Intervening periods of normal mood rarely lasting longer than a few weeks. No episodes of hypomania.

Very few of the individual episodes of depression within the 2-year period are sufficiently severe or long lasting to meet the criteria for recurrent mild depressive disorder.

During at least some of the periods of depression at least three of the following are present:
- reduced energy or activity
- insomnia
- loss of self-confidence or feelings of inadequacy
- difficulty concentrating
- frequent tearfulness
- loss of interest in enjoyment of sex and other pleasurable activities
- feelings of hopelessness
- perceived inability to cope with routine responsibilities
- pessimism about the future or brooding over the past
- social withdrawal
- reduced talkativeness.

Early onset: late teens or 20s.
Late onset: 30–50 years of age, often after an affective episode.

Box 1.5 An outline of the ICD–10 criteria for cyclothymia

A period of at least 2 years of instability of mood involving several periods of both depression and hypomania.

None of these periods meets the criteria for a manic episode, or moderate or severe depressive episodes, although such episodes may precede or follow the period of mood instability

During at least some of the periods of depression at least three of the following have been present:
- reduced energy or activity
- insomnia
- loss of self-confidence or feelings of inadequacy
- difficulty in concentrating
- social withdrawal
- loss of interest in or enjoyment of sex and other pleasurable activities
- reduced talkativeness
- pessimism about the future or brooding over the past

During at least some of the periods of mood elevation at least three of the following have been present:
- increased energy or activity
- decreased need for sleep
- inflated self-esteem
- sharpened or unusually creative thinking
- increased gregariousness
- increased talkativeness or wittiness
- increased interest and involvement in sexual and other pleasurable activities
- over-optimism or exaggeration of past achievements

Early onset: late teens or 20s.
Late onset: 30–50 years of age, often after an affective episode.

Two of Kraepelin's fundamental states can be found in modern classifications: 'depressive temperament' emerges as 'dysthymia' and 'cyclothymic temperament' as 'cyclothymia'. The ICD–10 criteria are summarised in Boxes 1.4 and 1.5. There is no consensus on how these disorders should be regarded; they probably include a mixture of subclinical mood disorders, chronic reactions to adverse circumstances, partial remissions of mood episodes and disorders of personality structure (Akiskal, 1983). The term 'double depression' has been coined to describe a depressive episode occurring against the background of dysthymia (Keller & Shapiro, 1983). Follow-up studies (Angst & Merikangas, 1997) suggest that there is little diagnostic stability over the long term for many subtypes of depression, including dysthymia and brief recurrent depressive disorder. There is increasing support for the concept of a spectrum of manifestations within depressive disorders. In this way an individual might experience a depressive episode as either an antecedent to or as a sequel to sub-threshold disorders, such as dysthymia.

Dysthymia has a 1-year prevalence of 1–3% in general population surveys, and is more common in women, the unmarried and those with low income. Comorbid psychiatric disorder is found in over two-thirds of those affected and there is familial aggregation with other depressive disorders. Early-onset cases begin typically in adolescence or early adult life; it has been hypothesised that these are the consequence of either traumatic developments in childhood or an inherited liability to mood disorder. Cases of later onset often arise following an episode of major depression or are associated with enduring health problems and chronic life difficulties. Both forms can give rise to considerable subjective distress and disability, and cumulative levels of morbidity have been estimated as equivalent to those resulting from major depressive disorders.

There is an increasing consensus that treatment of dysthymia is warranted. All classes of antidepressants have been found to achieve symptom response rates of the order of 65%, with residual impairments of social adjustment improving further with cognitive, group and interpersonal psychotherapies. Particular claims have been made for low doses of sulpiride and amisulpride; indeed, in Italy the first marketing authorisation for amisulpride was with the sole indication of dysthymia. There is emerging evidence supporting the use of other atypical antipsychotics, such as olanzapine and risperidone.

Cyclothymia typically begins early and shows a chronic course. Its lifetime prevalence has been estimated at 0.4–3.5%, with men and women equally affected. Cyclothymia may be over-represented in psychiatric out-patient clinics. There is a familial aggregation with both unipolar and bipolar disorders, and some of those with cyclothymia go on to develop frank bipolar illnesses. Mood swings are typically unrelated to life events and cyclothymia may be difficult to diagnose without prolonged assessment or an exceptionally good account of previous behaviour. Misuse of psychoactive substances is a frequent concomitant. Low doses of mood stabilisers have been suggested as a rational treatment for cyclothymia but evidence for their efficacy is limited.

It has long been recognised that cyclothymia is likely to be a heterogeneous condition, with at least some cases being a mild or subclinical form of bipolar disorder. Akiskal and Angst, among others, have advanced the concept of the bipolar spectrum (see, e.g., Akiskal *et al*, 2000). About half the spectrum is occupied by bipolar illness or closely related disorders, while the remainder (including most of those diagnosed with cyclothymia) fall into the 'soft' bipolar spectrum, intermediate between bipolarity and normality. The combination of cyclothymia with a depressive disorder, characterised by increased risk taking and irritability, has been identified as a likely bipolar subtype that can be easily mistaken for an emotionally unstable personality disorder.

Classification on the basis of family history

The best way to resolve the problem of classifying depressive disorders would be to demonstrate genetic heterogeneity. There have been tantalising glimpses of this possibility. Winokur *et al* (1971) distinguished two groups on the basis of age at onset. The group with age at onset before 40 years was predominantly female. This group showed a higher incidence of alcoholism and sociopathy in male relatives, and a high incidence of depression in female relatives. The other group showed a predominance of males with a family history of depressive disorders alone. On this basis, the authors proposed a division into those with a family history of depression alone (pure depressive disease), those with a history of alcoholism or sociopathy in first-degree relatives (depressive spectrum disease) and 'non-genetic' cases (sporadic depressive disease). This classification has received some support from clinicians. Neuroendocrine treatment and outcome correlates have been found, but attempts to replicate these validating studies have been inconsistent. Research with twins shows that the familial patterns observed are mainly due to environmental rather than genetic factors, which undermines the 'genetic' basis of the hypothesis. Recent developments in molecular genetics have opened up promising horizons for new hypotheses along similar lines to Winokur's proposal, but no practical classification has yet emerged.

Other classifications

'Agitated' and 'retarded' depressions have often been identified but criteria to separate these show little validity and they have been dropped from classificatory systems. The adjectives 'agitated' and 'retarded' are still used as clinical descriptors and both phenomena may occur at the same time. 'Involutional melancholia' was a term used by Kraepelin to describe depression occurring in late middle age with agitated and hypochondriacal features, often on the background of an obsessional personality. This diagnosis has been shown repeatedly not to meet validating criteria and is now obsolete. Researchers in the United States favoured a distinction between 'primary' depression (occurring *de novo*) and 'secondary' depression (following on from other disorders). While this approach enabled the definition of more homogeneous groups of depressive disorders for research purposes, it was received with little enthusiasm in the UK. The distinction is difficult to apply rigorously in clinical practice, and the validating evidence to support it is weak.

Measurement

The severity of a depressive syndrome depends on the number of symptoms, their intensity, their frequency, their duration and their pervasiveness. Subjective distress and impairments in functioning are also relevant. Not all of these factors covary and some may be negatively correlated. Despite this, experienced clinicians and their patients are able to make global assessments of severity which correlate surprisingly well. An example of guidelines for global assessment is given in the ICD–10 criteria for distinguishing mild, moderate and severe depressive episodes (see Box 1.2).

Most scientific approaches to the measurement of depression involve rating instruments. These are of two types. Observer ratings involve an examination of the subject, and ratings are completed by the interviewer. Self-ratings are made directly by the subject. While self-rating scales are more economical and are therefore useful for large-scale surveys, they have disadvantages. Those with milder depression tend to overrate their symptoms, while those with psychotic depression underrate them.

Good scales show test–retest and inter-rater reliability and have face validity, predictive validity and internal consistency (see Chapter 27, page 698). Data should be available for normative populations and to enable comparison with other instruments. Effective scales are short, clear and easy to administer, but if they are too short then reliability is sacrificed. A few of the better scales are discussed below.

Hamilton Rating Scale for Depression

After over 40 years of use, the Hamilton Rating Scale for Depression (HRSD; Hamilton, 1960) remains the most popular observer rating scale for measuring the severity of depression. It meets most of the above criteria, although it has been criticised for being too long. Seventeen items are rated on scales of either 0–4 or 0–2, using a clinical interview and all available information. The assessment refers to the previous 1–2 weeks, and this limits its usefulness as a repeated measure of progress. Some argue that it is biased towards biological features of depression: over half the 17 items relate to anxiety, somatic features or insomnia. Nevertheless, it remains for many the instrument of choice for rating severity in those diagnosed as suffering from a depressive episode. The accuracy of other scales is often tested by the strength of their correlation with the HRSD. Concerns have been raised that the scale is not always used according to its instructions, and that it is often used inappropriately as a diagnostic tool to screen for the presence of a depressive episode.

Montgomery–Asberg Depression Rating Scale

The Montgomery–Asberg Depression Rating Scale (MADRS; Montgomery & Asberg, 1979) is a shorter observer rating scale than the HRSD. It was derived from the Scandinavian Comprehensive Psychiatric Rating Scale. Ten items were selected as the most sensitive to response to treatment. It satisfies most of the above criteria and although it also requires a clinical interview, it is in theory easier to administer than the HRSD, and can be completed in under 20 minutes. It is widely used to measure change in depressed patients.

Beck Depression Inventory

The Beck Depression Inventory (BDI; Beck *et al*, 1961) is probably the best-known self-rating scale for depression, and it too has retained its popularity for over 40 years. It was designed to be read to the subject, who chose from set responses. In this way it overcame the main objection to self-rating scales, namely the uncertainty that the subject is following the instructions correctly. Now it is usually given in a self-report form. It satisfies most criteria mentioned above, but lacks discriminatory power among those with very severe depression. In contrast to the HRSD, all but 6 of the 21 items relate to psychological phenomena. It can be repeated after short intervals and can be seen as complementary to the HRSD and the MADRS.

Hospital Anxiety and Depression Scale

The Hospital Anxiety and Depression Scale (Zigmond & Snaith, 1983) is a brief self-assessment scale that was designed to detect states of depression and anxiety in hospital medical out-patient clinics. Questions are carefully worded to avoid response bias, and refer to the previous week. Five of the seven items in the depression sub-scale relate to loss of the pleasure response, in order to avoid confounding with symptoms of physical illness, and on the basis that anhedonia may be the central feature of a biogenic depressive illness. The scale is easy to administer and it can be used both as a screening instrument and as a measure of severity.

Visual Analogue Scale

The Visual Analogue Scale (Zealley & Aitken, 1969) is one of the easiest ways of estimating global severity or the severity of individual symptoms. The rating can be made by either a clinician or the subject. A line 10 cm long is drawn and the end-points are identified as the extremes of the phenomenon to be measured. When rating sadness the end-points might be 'Not sad at all' and 'As sad as I can imagine'. The rater makes a mark at the point on the line that best represents the present state. Despite its simplicity, this technique can produce useful information that correlates well with results from more sophisticated instruments. It is very useful for making repeated measures of a rapidly changing phenomenon such as diurnal variation in mood. One drawback is that ratings suffer from contrast effects, rapid changes being rated higher than slower ones.

Course and outcome

In *The Anatomy of Melancholy*, Burton devoted most of his chapter on 'prognostics' to suicide. Suicide does remain 'the greatest, most grievous calamity', which is 'a frequent thing and familiar' among depressed people, and is 'the doom of all physicians' (Burton, 1621, p. 260). It is considered in Chapter 7 in the present book.

Regarding the course and outcome of depression, Burton (p. 260) quoted Montanus:

> 'This malady doth commonly accompany them to the grave: Physicians may ease it, and it may lay hid for a while, but they cannot quite cure it, but it will return again more violent and sharp than at first.'

Three hundred years later, a more optimistic perspective was provided by Kraepelin, who separated manic–depressive insanity from dementia praecox on the grounds that it was a 'remitting' disorder.

Throughout most of the 20th century an optimistic view held sway, despite follow-up studies in the first three decades which catalogued an impressive array of long-term morbidity and mortality (e.g. Poort, 1945). The advent of modern 'effective' treatments and the promising results of short-term therapeutic trials reinforced that optimism and it was widely assumed that the prognosis of depressive illnesses had improved. However, few of the therapeutic trials lasted longer than 2 years, so that if later recurrence and long-term chronicity were a feature of the natural history of depressive disorders, they would rarely have been recorded. More recent long-term follow-up studies of depressed in-patients from Sydney (Kiloh *et al*, 1988) and London (Lee & Murray, 1988) revealed a picture similar to that found in the earlier era (before the advent of pharmacotherapy). These studies, taken together with prospective studies from the US National Institute of Mental Health (NIMH) that showed cumulatively high rates of relapse and failure to recover (Keller *et al*, 1986) led to a less sanguine but perhaps more realistic appraisal of the serious long-term import of a severe depressive illness. This has been followed by a reframing of severe depressive illnesses as lifelong disorders more akin to hypertension or diabetes.

Clinical prognosis studies

Knowledge of the course and outcome of psychiatric disorders is gained by combining clinical experience with the findings of clinical prognosis studies. Ideally, the follow-up of a typical cohort of sufferers will allow useful estimation of the rates at which patients recover, of the likelihood of recurrence, of the chances of chronicity and other complications, and of the risks of increased mortality from suicide and other causes.

While shorter-term follow-up studies (1–5 years) give a fairly accurate picture of recovery and early relapse, they underestimate recovery among those with apparently chronic illnesses. More importantly, they also underplay the long-term risks of recurrence. Longer follow-up studies give a clearer picture of the lifetime impact of a disorder, by showing the risks of poor outcome due to repeated recurrences, cumulative chronicity, accumulating secondary handicaps and the evolution of secondary disorders. While longer-term studies will almost always be naturalistic, with no attempt to control for treatments, this has the advantage of giving a clearer picture of the likely ranges of outcomes under normal clinical conditions.

A well-designed follow-up study will identify prospectively a representative cohort, will make diagnoses according to well-established criteria, and will follow this series closely and comprehensively. Outcomes will be established according to clearly defined criteria, and analyses will use actuarial techniques in order to allow for deaths and patients lost to follow-up. There should be sufficient numbers to allow for generalisable findings, but not so many that intensive follow-up becomes impossible. Where predictors of outcome are sought, then the follow-up examinations should be conducted blind to initial assessments.

Since the NIMH, London and Sydney studies were published in the 1980s, several other long-term outcome studies of depression have met most of these criteria. There has been a growing understanding of the importance of comprehensive follow-up, as investigators have found up to half of severely ill survivors had lost contact with mental health services and so were difficult to trace. Studies using comparable methods have enabled us to explore whether there were improvements in outcome between 1960 and 2000. There is surprisingly little evidence that modern treatment approaches and prophylactic strategies are affecting either recovery or recurrence rates, although there are some grounds for hoping that they may be modifying episodes and ameliorating some of their more disabling and enduring consequences.

Recovery

Kraepelin (1921) described depressive episodes which ranged in length from days to more than a decade. Durations of several years were commonplace. Since 1945 the median length of depressive episodes has fallen to 6 months. Recovery rates are often thought to depend on severity of illness but there has been no convincing demonstration that out-patients or even those seen in primary care recover at different rates to in-patients.

In the early months of episodes of depression the cumulative likelihood of recovery rises quickly, so that by 6 months about half will have remitted. By 2 years about three-quarters will have remitted, and the remainder are defined as chronic. Chronic depressive episodes continue to remit slowly, so that by 5 years a further 15% of the initial cohort will have recovered, making 90% in all. The remaining 10% of episodes may be very prolonged, but the chances of eventual remission never disappear entirely.

Recovery has been shown to be faster for bipolar patients and from episodes with somatic features. Secondary depressive episodes are slow to remit, although successful treatment of underlying disorders or substance misuse can lead to rapid recovery. The presence of hallucinations or delusions predicts a slower recovery, as do neurotic personality traits. Mood-incongruent and hypochondriacal features have also been shown to predict longer episodes. While the pattern of previous episodes is a useful guide to future course, this can be misleading, as a recurrent disorder with short episodes can unexpectedly become chronic.

The bodily symptoms of depression often remit more rapidly than cognitive features such as pessimism and low self-esteem. Cognitive distortion can be persistent and troublesome, as may continuing phobic avoidance, obsessional features and impairments of concentration. Symptoms often remit in a gradual and fluctuating way, which can be disheartening. Social impairments can also persist, with loss of confidence, social withdrawal, and difficulties both at work and in personal relationships. These social changes are sometimes found even where there is complete symptomatic remission. About a quarter of all those who have apparently recovered from depressive episodes show significant and enduring residual problems of one kind or another.

Relapse and recurrence

Many of those who recover from a depressive episode experience a return of symptoms, and the risks of this occurring are best described using survival analysis, a technique borrowed from the life-table approach used by insurance companies. There are two phases to the cumulative risk of symptom return. The first phase, within a few months, can be seen as signifying a re-emergence of the original episode. It has been proposed that the term 'relapse' be kept for this pattern, while 'recurrence' be used for those cases where a new episode of illness occurs after a longer period of full remission.

As many as one-third of depressive episodes may show the phenomenon of relapse. Predictors of relapse differ from those of recurrence and include severity, chronicity and premorbid personality difficulties, together with older age, poor social support, continuing adversity and further life events.

Estimates of recurrence rates vary with the samples studied and the length of follow-up. Most community studies show lifetime risks of around 50%. Angst (1988) argued that if followed long enough and closely enough virtually all moderate and severe depressive episodes would lead to recurrence. Recent studies suggest that, provided only genuinely first-episode cases are followed, as many as 50% of patients will suffer only a single episode, even in hospital series. This is an important message for clinicians and patients alike.

Two powerful predictors of recurrence emerge consistently from follow-up research. The first is the presence of residual symptoms after apparent recovery, which increases the recurrence risk threefold to about 75% in 2 years. The second factor is previous episodes of depression. This doubles the recurrence risk, with each new episode increasing the risk again by a further 16%. Other factors identified as likely to increase recurrence risks include the presence of somatic or psychotic features, an early age of onset, occurrence as part of a bipolar disorder and having a first-degree relative admitted with depression. Many of these factors have been shown to have independent effects. In both the London and Sydney series discussed above, in-patients with somatic features and previous admissions had a 50% risk of being readmitted again within 2 years. Findings such as these suggest that for some depressed people little may have changed since Burton's quotation from Montanus.

Very poor global outcome

One of the most alarming findings from recent follow-up research is the extent of the cumulative risk of poor long-term outcome. It appears that each new episode of depression brings with it a renewed and considerable risk of chronicity. The cumulative risk of experiencing an episode lasting over 2 years may be as high as one in three. Factors predicting chronicity (i.e. slow recovery) are outlined above under 'Recovery'. A positive family history, previous episodes and thyroid disorder in women have also been implicated.

Very poor long-term outcome can result from failure to recover or from an interaction between residual symptoms and secondary handicaps such as unemployment, divorce and social isolation. Alcoholism may be a complicating factor. A very small number of sufferers also develop chronic schizophrenic illnesses, or chronic paranoid states, and very occasionally a chronic defect state occurs without other schizophrenic symptoms. In the London series up to a quarter of the survivors showed one or other of these various forms of very poor outcome after 18 years. Those with very poor outcome fell into two groups: the divorced and single, who had multiple hospital admissions; and those with very unhappy marriages, few admissions and a relative isolation from mental health services.

Mortality

The mortality risk for depressed in-patients is doubled (Tsuang & Woolson, 1977), through both suicide and an increased risk of physical disorders, especially arterio-sclerotic and other vascular disorders (Angst, 1988). It was long held that 15% of in-patients with depression eventually ended their lives by suicide, but this figure was probably inflated as a result of bias from recurrent cases admitted to specialist centres. The estimated lifetime risk has been lowered to 6% (Inskip *et al*, 1998) and this may still be an overestimate when considering all cases in secondary care. Most suicides occur outside hospital. The risk for in-patients is at its highest in the 2 years following discharge.

Switches from unipolar to bipolar disorder

One in ten of those who begin with a depressive episode go on to develop an episode of mania. The likelihood of such a switch drops markedly after the third episode of depression, by which time more than two-thirds of those who will show a bipolar disorder have already done so. The two main predictors of a switch are an early age at onset and a family history of bipolar disorder. Other predictive factors include retardation, hypersomnia, hypomania precipitated by antidepressants, melancholia, delusions and hallucinations, and occurrence in the year after childbirth.

Differences in course and outcome between unipolar and bipolar disorders

There are surprisingly few differences, but those that exist are clear cut. Bipolar disorders tend to begin at an earlier age and have shorter episodes (with a median duration of 4 months) but more frequent recurrences. There appear to be no differences in rates of recovery, chronicity, suicide or overall mortality. After onset, the average proportion of lifetime spent ill has been estimated as 20% for both bipolar and unipolar patients (Angst, 1988). Outcomes among bipolar patients tend to be either very good or very poor. Mixed episodes and rapid-cycling disorders (four or more episodes in a year) are more likely to have very poor outcomes, but otherwise there are no reliable predictors among bipolar patients.

Prognosis for the individual patient

The best predictions of future course are often based on knowledge of a person's previous history, together with baseline risks for the disorder. Clinicians will also weigh the predictive factors outlined above, and consider personal strengths and vulnerability alongside the continuing supports and stresses in the environment. Maintaining factors and further life events will contribute to delays in recovery. Vulnerability factors such as unemployment and a lack of a confiding relationship will increase the risk of recurrence. Therapeutic factors are also important. Delay in adequate treatment is strongly associated with a chronic course. Outcome will very much depend on concordance with treatment and on whether adequate biomedical and psychosocial measures are available, both for immediate treatment and for prophylaxis in recurrent disorders. The task of translating therapeutic approaches with demonstrated efficacy into effective treatment programmes in clinical settings remains a major public health challenge.

Bereavement

> 'The chambers of the mansion of my heart, in every one whereof thine image dwells, are black with grief eternal for thy sake.' (James Thomson, 1932)

Human grief is universal and many of the experiences of bereaved people overlap with clinical features of depression. In 'Mourning and melancholia' Freud (1917) based an aetiological theory of depression on these similarities. This was the first of many models of the process of mourning, which have drawn on diverse perspectives, including psychoanalysis, behaviourism, ethology, social anthropology and developmental psychology. Of these, attachment theory (Bowlby, 1982) has been particularly influential in shaping understanding of the painful process of adjusting to the death of a loved person.

A helpful distinction can be made between the *situation* of bereavement, the *process* of mourning and the *experiences* of grief. Thus, bereavement describes the situation of having lost someone significant through his or her death. Mourning is the process of adjusting to bereavement. Grief refers to the personal experience of mourning. Among the bereaved there are very wide cultural variations in the practices and rituals of mourning. These are both derived from and serve to reinforce existing religious and social conventions. By contrast, many of the phenomena of grief are ubiquitous; for example, weeping and feelings of painful sadness occur throughout the world.

Uncomplicated mourning

Many authors have attempted to describe stages in the mourning process. In a very influential account, Lindemann (1944) studied the phenomenology of normal grief in 101 bereaved subjects. Robertson & Bowlby (1952) observed 2–3-year-old children temporarily separated from their mothers and identified a progression from preoccupation and protest, through despair, towards detachment, and this has proved to be a valuable analogy. One of the best syntheses of different models has been that of Brown & Stoudemire (1983), who combined the work of Lindemann and Bowlby, as well as others. They distinguished three phases:

1 shock

2 preoccupation with the deceased

3 resolution.

In the first phase, shock, intense mental and somatic distress is defended against by mechanisms of numbing, denial and disbelief, with associated feelings of depersonalisation and derealisation. Bereaved people at this time may appear dazed or immobile. They will often describe intermittent feelings of intensely distressing mental pain, tension and anxiety, which may be experienced as tightness in the throat, choking with shortness of breath, a need for sighing, empty feelings in the abdomen or a lack of muscular power.

Usually within about 2 weeks the first phase evolves into a second, of intense preoccupation with the deceased. More structured phenomena of separation occur, such as pining and yearning, searching behaviours in the hope of reunion, and anger directed at third parties, the self and the deceased. The bereaved person will spend long periods thinking about the deceased and will dream frequently of that person. One in ten will report brief hallucinatory experiences. Past conflicts will be reviewed and intense guilt will be experienced by at least one person in three. Mechanisms of identification may be evidenced by the appearance of traits and activities of the deceased. This second phase is also characterised by social withdrawal and a range of fluctuating depressive symptoms, including sadness, anhedonia, fatigue, insomnia and anorexia. The tasks of this second phase of the mourning process have been described as reliving memories, working through feelings, reparation and gradually restructuring the representation of the lost person from one of reality to one of memory. This process of internalisation involves a freeing of the self from the bondage of the deceased, and the formation of a new adjustment to the environment.

Over a period of months to years, this process gradually merges into a third and final phase, characterised by a subjective feeling of acceptance, the capacity to remember the deceased without excessive pain, and a reorganisation of life towards the possibility of new attachment. Phenomena from the second phase may sometimes re-emerge, and these are often more sharply focused at times of significant anniversaries.

Relationship with depressive disorders

Although clinical depression and mourning share many phenomena, and the boundary between them is not always clear, this does not imply that they are the same syndrome. Clayton & Darvish (1979) found that 42% of bereaved spouses examined at 1 month showed sufficient depressive symptoms to meet criteria for a depressive episode. By 1 year this figure had fallen to 15%. When depressive episodes do occur after bereavement, they have been shown to be no different in form from those precipitated by other major life events, but there is still controversy as to whether they warrant a different treatment approach using models of the mourning process. Parkes (1985) and others have described features that may distinguish normal mourning from depressive disorders: pangs of grief, angry pining, anxiety when confronted by reminders of loss, brief hallucinations, somatic symptoms and identification-related behaviours all point to normal mourning; the presence of retardation, generalised guilt and suicidal thoughts after the first month all suggest the development of a depressive episode.

Complicated mourning

The development of a depressive episode is only one of the ways in which mourning can be complicated. Compared with normal cultural patterns, mourning can be absent, delayed or abnormally prolonged; there may also be unusual behaviours, such as extreme preoccupation with the deceased. There may be excessive identification with, or idealisation of the lost person. Patterns of extreme denial, avoidance and compulsive self-reliance can emerge. Health-related behaviours such as smoking and drinking alcohol may increase to pathological levels. Mourning may be further complicated by secondary physical and other psychological disorders, which in turn may modify and colour the experience of grief. Several studies have shown widowers to have increased risks of death, particularly from cardiovascular disorders, in the year following bereavement.

Criteria that describe complicated mourning, or traumatic grief, have been proposed, and two factors have been identified: 'separation distress', which features searching, yearning and loneliness; and 'traumatic distress', which includes numbness, distrust, anger and a sense of futility about the future. These two factors can be separated from the depressive syndrome and are independently associated with enduring functional impairments. It has been proposed that the presence of complicated mourning at 6 months or longer after bereavement suggests a need for professional intervention.

In non-clinical samples about 10% of bereaved people show complicated mourning, usually in the form of chronic grief. Delayed or absent mourning is relatively rare. In a large survey of consecutive referrals to a general psychiatric clinic, about one-third of all patients met criteria for either moderate or severe traumatic grief, with an average duration of almost 10 years. Conversely, in one traumatic grief clinic, 52% of attendees met criteria for major affective disorders and 30% met criteria for post-traumatic stress disorder.

Risk factors for complicated mourning

Freud (1917) predicted that mourning would be complicated by depression in those whose relationships were marked by intense ambivalence, but Bowlby (1982) observed that the loss of ambivalently loved persons was often consistent with healthy mourning. He stressed the role of anxious attachments to parents as precursors of insecure adult relationships and subsequent difficulties in negotiating mourning. In this way overdependence might lead to chronic grief, while patterns of compulsive self-reliance would result in the denial of loss and the delayed onset of grief. Indeed, empirical research has shown that, contrary to Freud's hypothesis, high levels of ambivalence are associated with lower intensities of grief, whereas the predictions of Bowlby appear to be confirmed.

Parkes (1985) identified clinging behaviours and inordinate pining as early signs of prolonged grief. Other factors that have been suggested as increasing the risks of complicated grief include a sudden, unexpected or unlikely bereavement, potentially stigmatised losses such as abortions, suicides and deaths from AIDS, and deaths where the bereaved may be held to be to blame. Violent or severely traumatic deaths may induce symptoms in the bereaved that resemble those of post-traumatic stress disorder. Multiple losses and deaths resulting from negligence appear to be very hard to cope with. Mourning may also be complicated if previous losses remain unresolved, and in the presence of pre-existing physical and mental health problems, including substance misuse. Low socio-economic status, perceived lack of social support, poor coping skills, absence of contact with organised religion and the need to care for dependent children are also risk factors.

The loss of a child has been shown to result in more intense grief, greater somatisation and an increased risk of secondary depressive disorders. Feelings of guilt and powerlessness are common. The outcome may be increasing marital stresses, overprotection of other children, idealisation of the lost child or unreal expectations of a 'replacement' child.

The loss of a spouse may bring with it many practical problems. These include increased responsibilities for dependent children, financial hardship and social isolation. Persisting sexual feelings can cause frustration, conflict and guilt. Elderly people who lose their partners may be particularly vulnerable to social isolation and the loss of support and care. Those bereaved after a lifetime together commonly experience extremely prolonged feelings of grief.

The death of an elderly parent seems to be the least likely form of bereavement to result in complicated mourning. Painful but healthy grief is often followed by a period of increased creativity and fruitful reparation.

Appendix. A practical scheme for diagnosing and describing depression

- Do the clinical phenomena amount to depressive symptoms?
- If they do, then are they sufficient to constitute a depressive syndrome?
- Can one then exclude other disorders and bereavement, so that one can say that a depressive episode is present?
- Is the episode mild, moderate or severe?
- Are there psychotic features?
- If so, are they mood congruent or mood incongruent?
- Does the episode show the somatic syndrome?
- Are there any other very prominent features (agitation, retardation, panic attacks, obsessional or histrionic features)?
- Does the episode show chronicity, having lasted for more than 2 years?
- Is this the only episode, or is the episode part of a recurrent depressive disorder or a bipolar disorder?
- Is there evidence of a seasonal pattern, rapid cycling or a post-partum onset?
- If the depressive symptoms do not amount to a depressive syndrome or episode, is the patient suffering from dysthymia or cyclothymia, or recurrent brief depressive disorder? Or is this a depressive episode in partial remission?

References

Akiskal, H.S. (1983) Dysthymic disorder: psychopathology of proposed chronic depressive subtypes. *American Journal of Psychiatry*, **140**, 11–20.

Akiskal, H. S., Bourgeois, M. L., Angst, J., *et al* (2000) Re-evaluating the prevalence of and diagnostic composition within the broad clinical spectrum of bipolar disorders. *Journal of Affective Disorders*, **59**, suppl. 1, S5–S30.

American Psychiatric Association (1987) *Diagnostic and Statistical Manual of Mental Disorders* (3rd edn, revised) (DSM–III–R). Washington, DC: APA.

American Psychiatric Association (1994) *Diagnostic and Statistical Manual of Mental Disorders* (4th edn) (DSM–IV). Washington, DC: APA.

Angst, J. (1966) *Zur Atiologie und Nosolgie Endogener Depressiver Psychosen. Monographien aus dem Gesamtgebiete der Neurologie und Psychiatrie*. Berlin: Springer.

Angst, J. (1988) Clinical course of affective disorders. In *Depressive Illness: Prediction of Course and Outcome* (eds T. Hegalson & R. J. Daly). Berlin: Springer-Verlag.

Angst, J. & Merikangas (1997) The depressive spectrum: diagnostic classification and course. *Journal of Affective Disorders*, **45** (1–2), 31–40.

Beck, A. T., Ward, C. H., Mendelson, M., *et al* (1961) An inventory for measuring depression. *Archives of General Psychiatry*, **4**, 561–571.

Berrios, G. E. (1992) History of the affective disorders. In *Handbook of Affective Disorders* (2nd edn) (ed. E. S. Paykel). Edinburgh: Churchill Livingstone.

Bowlby, J. (1982) Attachment and loss: retrospect and prospect. *American Journal of Orthopsychiatry*, **52**, 664–678.

Bright, T. (1586) *A Treatise of Melancholie*. London: Vautrollier.

Brown, J. T. & Stoudemire, G. A. (1983) Normal and pathological grief. *Journal of the American Medical Association*, **250**, 378–382.

Burton, R. (1621) *The Anatomy of Melancholy*. Oxford: Cripps. (Page numbers quoted in the text are from the fifth edition published in Philadelphia by J. W. Moore in 1853.)

Clayton, P. J. & Darvish, H. S. (1979) Course of depressive symptoms following the stress of bereavement. In *Stress and Mental Disorder* (eds J. Barret, R. M. Rose & G. L. Klerman). New York: Raven Press.

Cotard, M. (1882) Du delire de negations. *Archives de Neurologie, Paris*, **4**, 152–170. Translated into English by M. Rohde in *Themes and Variations in European Psychiatry* (eds S. R. Hirsch & M. Shepherd), pp. 353–373. Bristol: Wright.

Freud, S. (1917) Mourning and melancholia. *The Standard Edition of the Complete Psychological Works*, Vol. XIV, pp. 243–258. London: Hogarth Press.

Hamilton, M. (1960) A rating scale for depression. *Journal of Neurology, Neurosurgery and Psychiatry*, **23**, 56–62.

Hamilton, M. (1982) Symptoms and assessment of depression. In *Handbook of Affective Disorders* (1st edn) (ed. E. S. Paykel). Edinburgh: Churchill Livingstone.

Holy Bible. Authorised King James Version (1967). London: Oxford University Press.

Hunter, R. & Macalpine, I. (1963) *Three Hundred Years of Psychiatry (1535–1860)*. London: Oxford University Press.

Inskip, H. M., Harris, E. C. & Barraclough, B. (1998) Lifetime risk of suicide for affective disorder, alcoholism and schizophrenia. *British Journal of Psychiatry*, **172**, 35–37.

Jaspers, K. (1963) *General Psychopathology*. Translated into English by J. Hoenig & M. W. Hamilton from *Allgemeine Psychopathology* (7th edn). Manchester: Manchester University Press. (Page numbers quoted in the text are from the edition published by Johns Hopkins University Press in 1997.)

Keller, M. B. & Shapiro, R. W. (1983) Double depression: superimposition of acute depressive episodes on chronic depressive disorders. *American Journal of Psychiatry*, **139**, 438–442.

Keller, M. B., Lavorie, W., Rice, J., *et al* (1986) The persistent risk of chronicity in recurrent episodes of nonbipolar major depressive disorder: a prospective follow-up. *American Journal of Psychiatry*, **143**, 24–28.

Kendell, R. E. (1968) *The Classification of Depressive Illnesses*. Maudsley Monograph, No. 18. London: Oxford University Press.

Kiloh, L. G., Andrews, G. & Neilson, M. (1988) The long-term outcome of depressive illness. *British Journal of Psychiatry*, **153**, 752–757.

Kraepelin, E. (1921) *Manic Depressive Insanity and Paranoia*. Translated into English by R. M. Barclay from the 8th edn of *Lehrbuch der Psychiatrie*, Vols III and IV. Edinburgh: E. & S. Livingstone. (Page numbers quoted in the text are from the Classics in Psychiatry edition published by Ayer Company Publishers.)

Lee, A. S. & Murray, R. M. (1988) The long-term outcome of Maudsley depressives. *British Journal of Psychiatry*, **153**, 741–751.

Leonhard, K. (1979) *The Classification of Endogenous Psychoses*. Translated into English by R. Berman from the 8th edn of *Aufteiling der Endogenen Psychosen*. New York: Irvington.

Lewis, A. J. (1934) Melancholia: a clinical survey of depressive states. *Journal of Mental Science*, **80**, 277–378.

Lewis, A. J. (1938) States of depression: their clinical and aetiological differentiation. *BMJ*, *ii*, 875–878.

Lindemann, E. (1944) Symptomatology and management of acute grief. *American Journal of Psychiatry*, **101**, 141–148.

Montgomery, S. A. & Asberg, M. (1979) A new depression scale designed to be sensitive to change. *British Journal of Psychiatry*, **134**, 382–389.

Parkes, C. M. (1985) Bereavement. *British Journal of Psychiatry*, **146**, 11–17.

Paykel, E. S., Rao, B. M. & Taylor, C. N. (1984) Life stress and symptom pattern in out-patient depression. *Psychological Medicine*, **14**, 559–568.

Perris, C. (1966) A study of bipolar (manic depressive) and unipolar recurrent depressive psychoses. *Acta Psychiatrica Scandinavica*, **42**, suppl. 194.

Poort, R. (1945) Catamnestic investigations on manic–depressive psychoses with special reference to the prognosis. *Acta Psychiatrica et Neurologica*, **20**, 59–74.

Robertson, J. & Bowlby, J. (1952) Responses of young children to separation from their mothers. *Courrier de la Centre Internationale de l'Enfance*, **2**, 131–142.

Sierra, M. & Berrios, G. E. (1998) Depersonalisation: neurobiological perspectives. *Biological Psychiatry*, **44**, 898–908.

Spitzer, R. L., Endicott, J. & Robins, E. (1978) Research Diagnostic Criteria: rationale and reliability. *Archives of General Psychiatry*, **35**, 773–782.

Stengel, E. (1945) A study of some clinical aspects of the relationship between obsessional neurosis and psychotic reaction types. *Journal of Mental Science*, **91**, 166–187.

Styron, W. (1991) *Darkness Visible*. London: Jonathan Cape.

Thomson, J. (1932) *The City of the Dreadful Night*. London: Methuen.

Tsuang, M. T. & Woolson, R. F. (1977) Mortality in patients with schizophrenia, mania, depression and surgical conditions: a comparison with general population mortality. *British Journal of Psychiatry*, **130**, 162–166.

Wehr, T. A. & Rosenthal, N. E. (1989) Seasonality and affective illness. *American Journal of Psychiatry*, **146**, 829–839.

Winokur, G., Cardoret, R., Dorzab, J., *et al* (1971) Depressive disease: a genetic study. *Archives of General Psychiatry*, **24**, 135–144.

World Health Organization (1978) *Mental Disorders: Glossary and Guide to Their Classification in Accordance with the Ninth Revision of the International Classification of Diseases* (ICD–9). Geneva: WHO.

World Health Organization (1992) *International Classification of Diseases and Related Health Problems* (10th revision) (ICD–10). Geneva: WHO.

Zealley, A. K. & Aitken, R. C. P. (1969) Measurement of mood. *Proceedings of the Royal Society of Medicine*, **62**, 993–996.

Zigmond, A. S. & Snaith, R. P. (1983) The Hospital Anxiety and Depression Scale. *Acta Psychiatrica Scandinavica*, **67**, 361–370.

CHAPTER 2

Mania, bipolar disorder and their treatment

John Cookson

History

The writers of ancient Greece used the terms 'mania' and 'melancholia'. Their descriptions included what we would now regard as mania, but encompassed a broader grouping of mental disorders. Hippocrates (5th to 4th century BC) argued that such disorders were due to physical (humoral) imbalance and not to supernatural forces. Aretaeus of Cappadocia (2nd century AD) was probably the first to see mania and depression as manifestations of the same disorder. With the dominance of the monasteries in Europe in the Middle Ages, mental illness was attributed to sin or supernatural forces, until clinical science began to re-emerge in the 17th century. In that century, 'madness' began to rank as one of the problems of the cities. Places of confinement were developed which grouped the poor and the unemployed with criminals and the insane. Within such places, when the insane became dangerous, their rages were dealt with by mechanical restraint, iron chains, cuffs and bars – leading Foucault to conclude that they were treated as animals, or wild beasts.

The history of 'psychiatry' began with the custodial asylum – an institution to confine raging individuals who were dangerous or a nuisance (see Shorter, 1997). The discovery that the institution itself could have a therapeutic function led to the birth of psychiatry as a medical specialism. Pinel in Paris in the 1790s, at the Salpêtrière for women and the Bicêtre for men, in particular, anticipated several trends, abolishing the use of restraining chains and recognising a group of 'curable lunatics' (mainly with melancholia or mania without delusions), for whom a more humanitarian approach might be therapeutic.

Falret, who described *folie circulaire*, and Baillarger, who described *folie à double forme* in 1854, recognised that mania and depression could occur in the same episode of illness – the modern concept of a 'cycle'. Kahlbaum (1874) described cyclothymia, as well as the association between states of excitement, some resembling mania, and catatonia. Kraepelin, basing his views upon both the pattern of symptoms and the longitudinal course, developed, in successive editions of his textbook, the concept of *manisch–depressives Irresein* (manic–depressive insanity) from 1893. He unified various forms of depression and mania under this name in 1899, and later distinguished these from dementia praecox. Bleuler in 1920 used the term 'affective illness' to describe the condition.

Kraepelin's concept of manic–depressive illness was too broad and, in 1957, Leonard proposed the distinction between bipolar depressed patients (those with a history of mania or hypomania) and unipolar depressed patients. Later, those patients with recurrent depression who have hypomanic episodes (not requiring hospitalisation), especially on recovery from depression, were described as BP-II (bipolar) and those with a history of mania as BP-I (Dunner *et al*, 1976*b*).

The history of the concept of bipolar disorder from classical to modern times is reviewed in depth by Marneros (2000).

Diagnostic criteria

The manic syndrome is one of the most clearly defined in psychiatry, but the diagnosis is frequently missed, or mistaken for schizophrenia or personality disorder. Box 2.1 shows the inclusion criteria for the diagnosis according to DSM–IV (American Psychiatric Association, 1994). The majority of patients exhibit all the listed symptoms, although hypersexuality, flight of ideas and distractibility are less frequent, and a minority of patients have delusions or hallucinations.

Box 2.1 DSM–IV diagnostic criteria for mania

A Distinct period of elated or irritable or expansive mood, lasting at least 1 week (or any duration if hospitalisation is necessary)

B Three of the following:
  1 inflated self-esteem or grandiosity (which may be delusional)
  2 decreased need for sleep
  3 increased talkativeness or pressure of speech
  4 flight of ideas or racing thoughts
  5 distractibility
  6 increase in goal-directed activity (e.g. social or at work) or psychomotor agitation
  7 indiscreet behaviour with poor judgement (sexual, financial, etc.)

C Symptoms do not meet criteria for mixed episode

D Marked impairment in occupational or social function

E Not due to a drug (of misuse or other medication) or a physical illness such as hyperthyroidism

Table 2.1 Glossary of terms used to describe states of excitement

Term	Definition
Mania	A severe illness, characterised by excitement, disinhibition and increased motor activity, usually resulting in hospitalisation
Hypomania	Similar to mania, but less severe, usually not resulting in hospitalisation
Cyclothymia	Cycles of depression which usually terminate with a brief (a few days only) elated period, with some hypomanic symptoms but the 'high' is much less than hypomania, and the depression is less severe and briefer than a major depressive episode
Bipolar I disorder	A severe recurrent illness with at least one episode of mania, and episodes of depression
Bipolar II disorder	Recurrent depression with hypomanic phases
Bipolar III disorder	States of excitement following a course of antidepressants or other drugs, or electroconvulsive therapy. Not an official category and a little-used diagnosis
Mixed affective state	Presence of depression and mania in the same episode with symptoms of depression and mania occurring together
Unipolar depression	Recurrent episodes of depression
Unipolar mania	Recurrent episodes of only mania, i.e. with no depression. A subtype of bipolar I disorder, but rare
Schizoaffective disorder (manic type)	Manic symptoms combined with schizophrenic symptoms. Psychotic symptoms may be mood incongruent
Mania with psychotic symptoms	An episode of mania with psychotic symptoms where the psychotic symptoms are usually mood congruent, e.g. grandiose delusions
Manic depression	An older historical term incorporating mainly bipolar I and bipolar II disorder, but which some medical authors use to describe any or all of the above disorders and in the lay press is sometimes used to describe almost any type of mental disorder

The criteria for mania in ICD–10 are similar (World Health Organization, 1992). They differ by the inclusion of loss of social inhibitions as an explicit symptom. Also, ICD–10 places mania with Schneider's first-rank symptoms or bizarre delusions as schizoaffective, whereas DSM–IV retains its classification as mania, and ICD–10 has a broader definition of mixed states.

Both DSM–IV and ICD–10 exclude the presence of delusions for hypomania; thus, if delusions are present the diagnosis is mania.

Many different terms have been used to describe recurrent excited states, some recent and some historical, and this may be a source of confusion. Table 2.1 therefore provides a glossary with a brief explanation of these terms, while more detailed descriptions of each item are given in the text.

Clinical features

Mood

The essential criterion for the diagnosis of mania is elevation of mood, in the form of elation or irritability. The elation is described by the patient in terms such as 'never felt better', 'on top of the world', 'full of energy', 'marvellous'. It may be accompanied by a sense of limitless optimism, exaltation or religious revelation. Often there is an infectious quality to the good humour – it cheers other people and leads to laughter.

However, the sustained elation is wearing on those around the patient. Any frustration of the patient's ambitious plans provokes anger and a sense of persecution, which may lead to abusiveness and aggression. Often the mood is labile and capricious. Tearful swings of mood occur, especially when the patient is confronted with personal problems. These swings of depression or hostility tend to be fleeting, but in some cases the irritability or depression can mask the elation. Some patients report that their excitement is unpleasant (dysphoric).

Appearance

The patient often appears overdressed or garish. Those with more severe illnesses may look untidy and neglected (they may appear in bare feet). Many patients have signs of infection, especially of the chest. Fluid retention and peripheral oedema may develop. Excessive consumption of alcohol may also complicate the picture (see below).

Overactivity

This is apparent in an excessive use of gestures, and the patient's tendency to leave the chair during the interview. Sometimes this excessive energy is used in purposeful activities, but in more severe phases actions are hurried and clumsy, and ultimately can be repetitive and stereotyped. General overactivity tends to diminish if the environment is calm and not too stimulating but offers distractions. Extreme overactivity may continue for days, with the patient taking little sleep or food, which can lead to exhaustion and physical debility.

Behaviour

Indiscreet behaviour may result from a loss of normal social inhibitions. Patients may become overfamiliar, outspoken, abusive or assaultative. They may have overspent either on excessive quantities of everyday items or on luxuries. One patient whose first episode followed the death of his father, a greengrocer, purchased hundreds of crates of apples with the aim of relieving starvation in India. The effects on patients and their families may be ruinous, with all savings spent and debts accumulated within the space of a few days or weeks. Those in sensitive jobs may have behaved with such poor judgement in planning or finance or in relation to their superiors as to jeopardise their careers. A junior manager in a well-known theatre used the ward telephone to invite international figures to a conference which he planned to hold at his theatre, without the knowledge of his director.

Vegetative signs

There is a decreased need for sleep; patients often awaken from a short sleep feeling energetic. The patient in mild mania takes longer to go to sleep and wakes earlier than usual. Increased appetite occurs but is not necessarily accompanied by increased food intake or weight gain because the patient may be too distracted to finish a meal. Likewise, there may be an increased interest in and enjoyment of sexual activity, leading to flirtatiousness, and new or promiscuous relationships. In more severe states the patient is too distractible to consummate the relationship.

Speech

Many patients appear to feel a great need to seek out other people and to talk to them at length. They talk at an increased rate and excessively, and it is difficult to interrupt them ('pressure of speech'). Their voice is often raised, which can lead to hoarseness. Others demonstrate such pressure by voluminous writings.

In 'flight of ideas' the association of thoughts proceeds in a fast and lively but usually understandable way, and puns and other sorts of word play are common. It differs from schizophrenic thought disorder in that connections can be seen as the patient jumps from one topic to another. The links may be in the content, although it sometimes appears as if a connecting thread has been left out, probably because the patient is thinking faster than he or she can speak. Alternatively, the links may be through sounds, as in rhymes, puns or clang associations. Patients may describe their own thoughts as being fast or racing. The term 'prolixity' is used to describe milder abnormalities of speech in mania. In severe mania, flight of ideas may degenerate into incoherent speech.

Case example

A West Indian woman, named Mrs Samuel, who was transferred to a psychiatric intensive therapy unit, introduced herself to the doctor as follows: 'I'm Samuel. I'm not a mule. I'm a new parent. I pay rent. I can just whisk myself off to Dominica. I'm a woman of leisure. When I came up here, I didn't want to come to England at the age of three. I didn't want to go to school, the intense therapy of developing from 11 to 13. At the age of 16 I burst out of school uniform into chiffon and lace, 'cos I'm a teenager, young lady, and I went to work.'

Increased self-esteem, grandiosity

The thought content reflects the mood and displays increased self-esteem and ambitiousness. Patients have an increased estimation of their abilities, wealth or status.

Delusions

The grandiosity may become delusional, with some patients becoming convinced that they have great wealth, have some special mission to fulfil, or are of royal descent or have some special relationship or identity with a great leader, politician, religious figure or even a deity. Patients may falsely believe that they are pregnant, and perhaps bearing a prophet or messiah.

In keeping with the mood state, the content of delusions in mania is, typically, grandiose or persecutory. Such delusions are 'congruent' with altered mood. Persecutory ideas may develop when patients' grandiose plans are frustrated, although in other cases the clinical picture is dominated by paranoia. Sometimes the ideas are overvalued rather than delusional and seem metaphorical or exaggerated expressions of the patient's wishes or frustrations.

Hallucinations

Auditory hallucinations may occur in the form of voices addressing the patient with a content that is either reassuring or exciting, for instance the comforting voices of dead relatives or God's voice encouraging the patient to perform religious acts.

Mood-incongruent psychotic features and catatonia

Some patients who meet the criteria for the diagnosis of mania have in addition one or more of the 'first-rank symptoms' of schizophrenia described by Schneider (see Chapter 8, page 168). Disagreement can arise about the diagnosis. According to the Research Diagnostic Criteria (Spitzer *et al*, 1978), the diagnosis is 'schizoaffective disorder' (schizomania). Likewise, ICD–10 calls mania with Schneider's first-rank symptoms or bizarre delusions 'schizoaffective disorder'. According to DSM–IV, if the content of the delusions or hallucinations is congruent with raised mood the diagnosis is 'mania with psychotic features'; otherwise the diagnosis is 'mania with mood-incongruent psychotic features'. Delusions of control and other first-rank symptoms occur in 10–20% of patients with mania.

Catatonic symptoms (e.g. stereotypies, mannerisms, posturing, negativism, mutism) were originally described by Kahlbaum (1874) in association with mania. According to DSM–IV such patients have 'mania with mood-incongruent psychotic features'. Recent studies have confirmed the frequency of catatonic symptoms in bipolar disorder.

Mania should not be diagnosed if psychotic features were present before the manic syndrome developed or after it remitted; according to DSM–IV, such patients have schizoaffective disorder.

Cognition

Patients are distractible – their thoughts and behaviour are easily distracted by changes in the environment, such as extraneous noises. Distractibility may lead to forgetfulness, as well as suspiciousness, for example that others are taking their belongings. Patients are correctly oriented for time and place except at the height of a severe manic episode.

Insight

Mania is the most insightless form of mental illness and patients not only believe but also behave in accordance with their increased self-esteem. For example, a woman with mania introduced herself to the doctor as the Queen of England. She responded to his friendly but informal return of greetings by slapping his face. It was no way to speak to the Queen.

Only a small proportion of patients admitted with mania recognise that they are ill, but others will sometimes acknowledge that there has been a change in their behaviour or that they might benefit from a 'rest'. As their condition improves in hospital, patients are usually amenable to explanations about their condition and the need for treatment, but this insight can soon be lost if the manic state re-emerges.

Self-reports of mania

The subjective experience of depression is relatively easy to grasp, partly because most people will have had some personal experience of depression and also because patients with the condition will readily explain how they feel. Gaining access to the subjective experience of an episode of mania is far more difficult, but several writers have described their experiences after a manic episode and some of these seem generally applicable. The main features of the subjective experience are an intense sense of well-being, a heightened sense of reality, a sense of communion and of mystical revelation, inhibition of the sense of repulsion, loss of normal sexual and social inhibitions, and grandiose ideas. These are illustrated in the following extracts reported by Lerner (1980):

> 'The intense sense of well-being which is physical as well as mental is not wholly illusory. My digestive system works particularly well, without the slightest hint of constipation or diarrhoea and I have an inordinate appetite.'
>
> 'The sense of communion extends to all fellow creatures with whom I come into contact.'
>
> 'When in a manic state I have no objection to being more or less herded together – as is inevitable in public Mental Hospitals – with men of all classes and conditions.'
>
> 'The question of selecting an attractive girl, which normally plays a large part in sexual adventures, did not trouble me in the least. I was quite content to leave it to chance.'
>
> 'I have no repulsion to excreta, urine and so on. I have no distaste of dirt. I do not care in the least whether I am washed or not.'
>
> 'My thoughts ran with lightening-like rapidity from one subject to another. I had an exaggerated feeling of self-importance. All the problems of the universe came crowding into my mind, demanding instant discussion and solution.'
>
> 'Your eyes are unblinded more and more and your ears are undeafened more and more.'

An American psychoanalyst said that a person who has not experienced mania 'has not lived', whereas a British psychiatrist recalled, 'You learn who your friends are in mania; they arrange a compulsory treatment order if necessary'.

A visitor to the poet Robert Lowell (1917–77) wrote (see Jamison, 1993):

> 'Meanwhile he writes and revises translations furiously and with a kind of crooked brilliance, and talks about himself in connection with Achilles, Alexander, Hitler and Christ, and breaks your heart.'

Lowell himself wrote afterwards (see Hamilton, 1982):

> 'it is fierce facing the pain I have caused, and humiliating to think that it has all happened before and that control and self-knowledge come so slowly, if at all.'

The following extracts from the letters of the poet Sylvia Plath (1932–63) to her mother reveal changes in her mood following separation from her husband and preceding her suicide (see Plath & Schober Plath, 1992):

> 12 October 1962: 'Every morning when my sleeping pill wears off, I am up at about five, in my study writing like mad – have managed a poem a day before breakfast.... I am a genius of a writer; I have it in me.'
>
> 7 November 1962: 'I am so happy and full of fun and ideas and love.... Living apart from Ted [her husband Ted Hughes] is wonderful.'
>
> 21 December 1962: 'I have never been so happy in my life. I have found the most fantastic store – Dickens and Jones – which knocks Harrods out of the window. I spent the rest of Mrs. Prouty's clothes money and feel like a million. I haven't had a new wardrobe for seven years. You should see me nipping around London in the car!'
>
> 4 February 1963: 'I just haven't written to anybody because I have been feeling a bit grim – the upheaval over, I am seeing the finality of it all. I'm going to start seeing a woman doctor free on the National Health to whom I've been referred by my very good local doctor.'

Sylvia Plath died on 11 February 1963.

Types of mania

Kraepelin divided manic states into hypomania, acute mania, delirious mania and chronic mania. The term 'hypomania' has been used inconsistently; if it is to be used at all it should probably be reserved for conditions that would be recognised as pathological only by those who are familiar with the patient or with psychiatry (Goodwin, 2002).

Carlson & Goodwin (1973) described three stages of mania through which an episode may develop, corresponding to mild, moderate and severe levels of symptoms. At moderate severity the euphoric mood is increasingly interrupted by periods of irritability and depression, and thinking becomes delusional. In the severe stage, there is frenzied overactivity; mood is experienced by the patient as unpleasant (dysphoric) or even terrifying, delusional thinking becomes bizarre and hallucinations appear, and in some cases there is disorientation.

Beigel & Murphy (1971) found that patients with repeated manic attacks tend to exhibit similar behaviour and mood patterns during subsequent episodes.

Delirious mania

Occasionally patients with mania become disoriented or have other symptoms suggestive of a confusional state, including visual hallucinations. These are more likely to occur in severe mania or where self-neglect and physical exhaustion develop. Evidence of chest infection and cardiac failure should be sought. If left untreated such patients become increasingly ill and may die.

The term 'delirious mania' or 'Bell's mania' is used for cases with confusional symptoms without evidence of underlying physical illness; such cases usually have a rapid onset.

Chronic mania

In rare cases mania runs an unremitting course. This seems to have occurred more commonly in the 19th century. Kraepelin described the chronic form as featuring some intellectual and emotional blunting compared with acute mania. Hare (1981) attributed the decline of this condition to improvements in general health and public hygiene. Some cases of chronic mania seen today may be secondary to organic brain disease. Magliano *et al* (1997) described chronic mania (continuing for more than 2 years) in 13% of a series of 155 in-patients in Italy with mania. They differed from the other patients with mania in their higher ratings of psychosis, and less severe excitement, insomnia and hypersexuality.

Dysphoric mania

This term has been used to describe patients in whom classical manic symptoms are accompanied by marked anxiety, depression or anger (Post *et al*, 1989). Although these symptoms tend to emerge in more severe stages of the illness, some patients present throughout with a 'destructive–paranoid' pattern rather than the classic 'elated–grandiose' type.

Mixed affective states

Transient depressed mood is very common in mania and so the term 'mixed state' is best reserved for cases in which symptoms of both mania and depression are consistently present. Depression occurs as an integral part of bipolar disorder, and often either precedes or succeeds an episode of mania. The switch between mania and depression may occur suddenly, but it is usually more gradual, with an intervening mixed state or period of normality.

Kraepelin (1921) distinguished 'autonomous' mixed episodes from those occurring during transitions from one mood phase to another and thought 'autonomous' mixed states had a poor prognosis: 'the most unfavourable form of manic–depressive insanity'. Kraepelin thought that three areas of functioning (mood, activity and thinking) could be altered independently to produce 'mixed states'. He recognised six mixed states, the most common being depressive or anxious mania, excited depression, and depression with flight of ideas. Others were manic stupor, mania with poverty of thought, and inhibited mania (without flight of ideas).

The description 'mixed state' has been used in more than a dozen ways, each of which carries different implications for treatment (Cookson & Ghalib, 2005).

Bipolar affective disorder and subtypes in DSM–IV and ICD–10

The criteria of ICD–10 for mania are very similar to those of DSM–IV. They differ by including loss of social inhibitions as an explicit symptom. ICD–10 has a broader definition of mixed states.

In DSM–IV the minimum criteria for bipolar affective disorder is a single episode of mania (or mixed disorder). ICD–10 specifies at least two separate episodes, one of which must have been hypomanic, manic or mixed, but the other episode may be depression. Both schemes require that the current episode be classified. ICD–10 has different subtypes but DSM–IV has a slightly different terminology and uses the word 'specifier' instead.

Hypomania is a less severe condition than mania. The criteria are similar to those for mania but DSM–IV specifies a minimum duration of 4 days, as compared to 1 week for mania. Hypomania impairs social function to a lesser degree than mania, but more than cyclothymia.

DSM–IV defines BP-I disorder as episodes of mania (with or without depression) and BP-II disorder as recurrent episodes of major depression with hypomanic episodes. ICD–10 merely classifies BP-II disorders under the heading of 'other bipolar affective disorders'. Unipolar mania accounts for 5–10% of bipolar disorder but has not been established as being different in any way from BP-I disorder.

ICD–10 describes bipolar affective disorder with the current episode being:

- hypomanic
- manic without psychotic symptoms
- manic with psychotic symptoms
- mild or moderate depression
- severe depression without psychotic symptoms
- severe depression with psychotic symptoms
- mixed episode
- in remission.

DSM–IV also describes 'mixed episodes' where the patient fulfils criteria both for mania as described above and criteria for major depression, and the condition lasts for at least 1 week. ICD–10 'mixed' includes patients showing a mixture *or alternation* of manic and depressive symptoms for 2 weeks; this would include people who might also be classified as having rapid-cycling bipolar disorder.

DSM–IV has three groups of 'specifiers', the first group describing severity, the second group the clinical type, and the third longitudinal course. Thus, bipolar affective disorder may be: mild; moderate; severe without psychotic features; severe with psychotic features, in partial remission, in full remission; with catatonic features; with a post-partum onset. If the most recent episode is depressive it may be chronic; melancholic; or with atypical features. Longitudinal course specifiers are: with or without full inter-episode recovery; with a seasonal pattern; or with rapid cycling. All of the above specifiers may be associated with either bipolar I or bipolar II disorder.

Other classificatory schemes

Before the official DSM–IV and ICD–10 schemes, there were many other classificatory schemes. These each emphasised a different aspect of the phenomenology of bipolar disorder. They included schemes based on the severity of the episodes (Angst, 1978); the order of the episodes (Koukopoulos, 2002); the diversity of the presentations as a spectrum disorder (Akiskal, 2002), a concept similar to the spectrum disorder as described for schizophrenia, as well as schemes based on the factor analysis of the symptoms of mania. A brief overview of these classifications is given below, but it should be emphasised that these classifications were never official and are rarely applied in clinical practice today.

Because of the different combinations of severity of manic and depressive episodes, Angst (1978) proposed three categories of patients:

- MD (in which both manic and depressive episodes are severe enough to require hospitalisation)
- Md (recurrent mania with only mild depression)
- Dm (BP-II) (hypomania with severe depression)

To these might be added:

- md (cyclothymia)
- M (unipolar mania)

People with unipolar depression with a family history of mania are sometimes said to have BP-III or pseudo-unipolar disorder. Others use BP-III to describe hypomania occurring during treatment (see below).

Koukopoulos (2002) has used the *sequence* of mood changes to distinguish:

- patients in whom mania is followed by depression, followed by a well interval (MDI)
- patients with depression followed by mania (DMI)
- patients with a continuously circular pattern (CC)
- patients with completely separate affective swings.

This follows the tradition of Falret concerning 'cycles' of mood. There is extensive overlap between patients with the DMI pattern and those with BP-II, and slightly less overlap between those with the MDI pattern and BP-I.

Within an individual, the episode duration tends to be stable through the course of the illness but the onset may become more rapid in later episodes. Post *et al* (1988) distinguished patients who switched rapidly (within 24 hours) into mania from those in whom the change was more gradual. The former had been ill longer and had experienced more affective episodes.

The inclusion of sub-syndromal forms of depression or mania into diagnostic categories led Akiskal to postulate eight or more different forms of bipolar disorder, some of which are manifest only when patients with unipolar depression receive antidepressant drugs (see Akiskal, 2002). The conditions in the bipolar spectrum are: schizoaffective disorder (schizomania), BP-I, depression with protracted hypomania, BP-II, depression superimposed on cyclothymia, anti-depressant-associated hypomania (BP-III), prominent mood swings in association with stimulant and alcohol use, and depression superimposed on hyperthymia.

Between major episodes, patients with recurrent affective disorder are frequently seen with fewer symptoms or symptoms that are less severe than necessary to meet the standard criteria for the definitions of an episode of major depression or hypomania. These 'sub-syndromal' forms may herald the development of a full-blown form. Keller *et al* (1992) found that symptoms of mood elevation led to mania twice as often as sub-syndromal depressive symptoms led to full depression.

Factor analysis of manic states

Factor analysis reveals yet another way of classifying mania. Thus, in a factor analysis of results drawn from rating scales administered in the first 3 days of admission, Double (1990) found factors reflecting overall severity, and other factors that separated elation from aggression, but no evidence of a bimodality that would support the existence of two distinct types of mania. Irritability was more closely associated with overall severity than was elation.

A larger study using a broader range of items identified five factors, corresponding to mood (from elation to dysphoria), psychomotor acceleration, psychosis, hedonism (including euphoria and grandiosity) and irritable aggression (including paranoia) (Cassidy *et al*, 1998). In this analysis psychosis, aggression and dysphoria were separately identifiable. Only the first factor (mood) showed bimodality, giving support to the idea that mixed mania is a separate state.

Sernetti *et al* (1999), analysing the results of interviews for lifetime symptoms excluding depression, identified three factors: excitement, psychosis and irritability.

Dilsaver *et al* (1999) identified four factors: manic activation, depression, insomnia and irritability/paranoia. Cluster analysis then suggested a separation into classical mania and mixed mania, but the classical group could be further divided according to their levels of 'dysphoria' (anger, worry and irritability).

Mania in childhood and adolescence

Mania is rare before puberty. This suggests a hormonal interaction with the brain that occurs around puberty among those with a predisposition to mania. The onset of the first symptoms of bipolar disorder is frequently in adolescence, with the emergence of sub-syndromal mood swings or cyclothymia. The diagnosis of bipolar disorder is commonly delayed by as much as 10 years. Recognition of these prodromal features is particularly important in young people with a family history of major affective disorder. Recently there appears to have been an increase in the frequency of mania in children (Geller *et al*, 2001); it has been suggested that this is linked to substance misuse and to the therapeutic use of stimulant and antidepressant drugs in young people thought to have attention-deficit hyperactivity disorder or depression, respectively (Reichart *et al*, 2000).

Adolescents show similar symptom profiles in mania to adults, except that psychotic symptoms may be more common in patients with an earlier age of onset. An onset before the age of 20 has not been found consistently to affect the prognosis by comparison with an older onset. Their education and training are liable to be interrupted.

Risk studies

Studies of children at high risk of developing bipolar disorder by virtue of their family history have found associations with increased aggressiveness and greater affective expression; the children also demonstrated some strengths, such as more involvement in activities. Cyclothymia was much more common in the high-risk group, developing at the age of 12–14 years, and a large proportion of these presented within 3 years with bipolar disorder. Examination of children who subsequently became manic revealed a superior level of motor development and intelligence than in controls and no greater risk of obstetric complications (Cannon *et al*, 2002).

Mania among those with learning difficulties

Mania occurs with the usual frequency in persons with learning difficulties. In those with severe learning difficulties, verbal expressions are less but the diagnosis can be based upon the cyclical nature of the disorder, changes in mood and irritability, activity, sleep and the family history. Among those with mild and moderate degrees of learning difficulty, the manifestations of mania are similar to those among people without such difficulties.

Measurement

The measurement of mania must be by observer ratings, as self-ratings are unreliable. The first validated rating scale for mania was that of Beigel *et al* (1971). Specially trained nurses scored 26 items for intensity and frequency. Blackburn *et al* (1977) modified that scale for use by doctors, rating 28 items for severity on 6-point scales, but without defined anchor points. This scale is comprehensive but time-consuming and depends for reliability upon a structured interview. Young *et al* (1978) provided a scale consisting of 11 items, each with 5-point sub-scales and defined anchor points. Completion of the scale requires a 15- to 30-minute interview. This instrument is convenient for following the progress of mania in an individual patient during treatment.

Natural history

Prevalence

The lifetime prevalence of BP-I disorder is about 0.8% and BP-II disorder about 1%. If other conditions in the bipolar spectrum are included the total is 3–6% or more.

Age of onset

The peak age of first hospitalisation for mania is in the late teens, the median in the mid-20s and the mean age of first hospitalisation about 26. There have often been earlier affective episodes sufficient to cause some impairment or for the patient to receive treatment outside hospital. There is a greater prevalence of affective illness among the first-degree relatives of those whose first episode of mania occurs by the age of 20 than among the relatives of patients whose mania begins later. There is a slight secondary peak of onset in women aged 45–50 years, and first episodes of mania continue to be seen in late life. An onset over the age of 60 is more likely to be associated with organic brain disease.

Number of episodes

The great majority of patients have more than one episode of mania, confirming the view that bipolar disorder is a recurrent illness. It follows a relapsing, often chronic course, with, in some studies, an average of approximately eight episodes over the 10 years following diagnosis.

Duration of episodes

The duration of manic episodes in the pre-treatment era was usually 3–12 months, with a mean of 6 months. Treatment shortens this duration. Remission from mania occurred in 50% of manic episodes by 12 weeks in one modern series (Kupfer *et al*, 2000). After the first episode of mania, 93% had recovered within two years in terms of the syndrome of mania, but only 35% had recovered in terms of personal and occupational functioning (Tohen *et al*, 2000).

Frequency of episodes

The interval from one episode to the next tends to decrease during the first five episodes (see Kessing *et al*, 1998). For instance, in Kraepelin's series the average time between the first and second episode was 5 years, but this had fallen to 2 years between the fifth and sixth episode. A series of patients with first-episode mania with 2-year follow-up found that major depression had occurred previously in 24%, and further depression followed immediately after mania ('post-manic depression') in 16%. There was a recurrence of mania or depression within 2 years in 36%, but 40% had no recurrence within 5 years (Tohen *et al*, 2003).

In an individual there is great variability in the length between episodes, and a tendency for episodes to be clustered at particular times in the patient's life, for instance when he or she has difficulties coping with children, or when relationships are ending. Antidepressant treatments may increase the tendency to switch from depression to mania, and may have altered the natural course of the illness towards more frequent episodes. The work of Angst (1985) is cited in support of this; he found an increase in the incidence of manic switches in the era after the introduction of electroconvulsive therapy (ECT) and antidepressant drugs compared with the earlier period. However, in Angst's view such upswings of mood represent the natural course of recovery, speeded by effective treatment.

Rapid cycling

Rapid cycling is included as a course specifier of bipolar disorders in DSM–IV and defined as 'At least four episodes of a mood disturbance in the previous 12 months that meet criteria for manic episode, a hypomanic episode, or a major depressive episode'. Episodes are demarcated by either partial or full remission for at least 2 months, or a switch to a mood state of opposite polarity. Rapid cycling can occur at the onset of illness but more commonly later in its course, perhaps in up to 15% of patients at some stage. It is also commoner in females. It may come and go rather than being an end-stage of bipolar disorder (Maj *et al*, 1994). About 70% cease to show rapid cycling within a year of diagnosis (Coryell *et al*, 2003).

Antidepressant medication can increase the frequency of cycling, and withdrawal of antidepressants can restore normal cycling (Wehr & Goodwin, 1979). Some cases of rapid cycling are associated with clinical or sub-clinical hypothyroidism, although a causal relationship has not been proved; lithium treatment can contribute to this. Rapid cycling has been described in secondary mania associated with organic brain disease and among those with learning difficulties.

'Ultra-rapid cycling' describes four or more episodes a month. Rare cases exist – about 20 in the world literature – of patients who oscillate from mania to depression and back again every 48 hours.

Ultradian cycling

Ultradian cycling has been described in otherwise typical bipolar patients (Kramlinger & Post, 1996). Mood changes in such patients occur in a matter of minutes or hours and resemble the mood swings in people with borderline personality disorder (see Chapter 18, page 448) but the latter present additionally with extensive difficulties in maintaining relationships.

Seasonal pattern

There is a slight excess of manic episodes in summer months in temperate climates. There is rarely evidence of a regular seasonal pattern in individual patients with BP-I illness (Hunt *et al*, 1992*b*). Patients with seasonal affective disorder and winter depression are more commonly of the BP-II type (Rosenthal *et al*, 1984).

Outcome

Before effective treatment was available, about 20% of patients hospitalised with mania died, many from exhaustion. With modern treatment, increased mortality from natural causes occurs only in those with a pre-existing physical illness. However, later death by suicide occurs in about 15–20% of cases.

Some patients become socially and economically disadvantaged. In a US study of patients referred to a tertiary centre, less than half returned to their previous jobs (Carlson, 1980). In a Canadian study patients lost 11% of their productive time in the 15–20 years after their index admission (Bland & Orn, 1982). However, in a study from Belgium comparing bipolar with unipolar patients and normal controls, bipolar patients in remission showed only mild social maladjustment (Bauwens *et al*, 1991).

There can be a considerable social and economic burden on the family.

Cognitve impairment, particularly in attention and concentration, may persist in some patients even when their mood has apparently recovered (Clark *et al*, 2002).

Psychosocial factors

Life events and expressed emotion

Episodes of mania may develop following major life events such as bereavement, personal separation, work-related problems and loss of role (Ambelas, 1987). An interesting example of an 'independent' event precipitating mania was described after a hurricane; the only patients in a lithium clinic who relapsed were those who had been less stable ('meta-stable') before the event (Aronson & Shukla, 1987). A prospective study showed an increased rate of life events in the month before mania, but the proportion of patients so affected was small (Hunt *et al*, 1992*a*). The first episode is more likely to be triggered by life events than later episodes (Sclare & Creed, 1987). This view is in keeping with the suggestion that a process of 'kindling' occurs: a facilitation of the development of subsequent episodes (see below). Post (1992) has reviewed the possible biochemical substrates for the progressive effects of stress in recurrent affective disorders.

Psychological stress may also arise from 'high expressed emotion' in the environment in which the patient lives. Patients with bipolar disorder who return to such environments show an increased rate of relapse. This may, however, be a secondary phenomenon rather than a causative one.

Insomnia or sleep deprivation is an important factor that may trigger a manic episode (Wehr *et al*, 1987). This is relevant to the observation that flying overnight from west to east is more likely to lead to mania than travel in the opposite direction (Jauhar & Weller, 1982), and to cases of mania in fathers following childbirth. A short course of an antipsychotic or a sedative may reduce the risk of mania for patients with bipolar disorder and transient sleep disturbance.

Marriage and parenting

Manic symptoms tend to be destructive to existing relationships. Although spouses may at first be attracted by mildly manic behaviour, such as increased sociability and sexual activity, a full-blown manic episode is embarrassing and frightening. Assortative mating occurs in bipolar disorder, the choice of marital partner being an individual with a matching or complementary temperament. During depression patients may seem excessively dependent on their spouses but in mania they may assert their independence and humiliate the spouse. Although marriages often survive individual episodes of mania, the divorce rate where one partner has bipolar disorder is very high – in one series, 57% compared with 8% where a partner had a unipolar disorder (Brodie & Leff, 1971). Very few of the spouses of patients with bipolar disorder have seen the patient during a manic episode before marriage. Fortunately, treatment often improves the quality of the marriage.

Bipolar disorder in the mother may adversely affect attachment patterns with younger children. However, the development of abnormal patterns is less if there is a father in the household.

Alcohol and drug misuse in bipolar disorder

Some patients increase and some decrease alcohol or drug misuse when manic compared with euthymic. Alcohol and stimulants, such as amphetamine and cocaine, are used by patients to restore hypomania during a dysphoric phase, or to heighten existing states of elation. These drugs can alter the course of bipolar disorder by triggering mania; they diminish impulse control and impair judgement and are serious risk factors for suicide. Therefore the recognition and treatment of alcohol or drug misuse is a matter of urgency.

Cannabis has been associated with an increase in psychotic symptoms in mania, and with the induction of mania.

Secondary mania

A manic state may develop following a physical disturbance by drugs or disease. When this occurs in clear consciousness, in patients without any past history of affective disorder, it is called secondary mania (Krauthammer & Klerman, 1978). Box 2.2 shows the commonest causes of secondary mania.

Drugs

Low doses of amphetamines in normal people produce a state resembling mild mania but with reduced hunger and appetite and anomalous endocrine effects (Jacobs & Silverstone, 1986).

Dopamine agonists, such as bromocriptine, used in the treatment of pituitary tumours and Parkinson's disease or to suppress lactation can lead to psychotic states, including mania (Turner *et al*, 1984).

Box 2.2 Common causes of secondary mania

Drugs

Psychostimulants
- Amphetamines
- Cocaine

Recreational drugs
- Cannabis
- Alcohol

Medication
- Dopamine agonists (bromocriptine, etc.)
- L-dopa
- Corticosteroids
- Anabolic steroids
- Thyroid hormone
- Anticholinergics (benzhexol, procyclidine)

Drug withdrawal
- Fenfluramine
- Baclofen
- Clonidine

Endocrine/metabolic conditions
- Thyrotoxicosis
- Cushing's disease
- Childbirth: puerperal psychosis

Organic brain disease
- HIV/AIDS
- Cerebrovascular disease
- Head inury
- Cerebral tumour
- Epilepsy
- Multiple sclerosis
- Dementia

The dopamine precursor L-dopa can trigger mania, but this is far more likely to occur in individuals with a bipolar predisposition. Likewise, a manic episode may be triggered by amphetamine in predisposed individuals (Gerner *et al*, 1976).

Benzhexol and procyclidine are liable to be misused for their psychostimulant effects and can produce a state resembling mania (Coid & Strang, 1982) or a confusional state. In addition to their anticholinergic properties, these drugs also block dopamine reuptake (Horn *et al*, 1971) and this may be relevant to their stimulant properties.

Endocrine causes

Corticosteroids in high doses can produce elated psychotic states resembling mania, although Cushing's disease is associated with depression in some 40% of cases and with mania in only 2%.

Anabolic steroids can produce character changes resembling mania.

Thyrotoxicosis is often accompanied by hyperactivity and irritability. The main diagnostic similarity is with anxiety states rather than mania, although mania can be precipitated in predisposed individuals. The commencement of treatment of myxoedema with thyroid hormone leads in some cases to a worsening of pre-existing psychotic symptoms and to the emergence of mania (Josephson & Mackenzie, 1979). There are also neuroendocrine changes during mania (Cookson, 1985).

Stroke

In contrast to secondary depression, mania is associated with right-sided cerebral vascular lesions and is more likely to occur if there is a family or personal history of affective disorder. The frontal and temporal regions are most often involved.

Head injury

Patients in whom mania follows head injury tend to have damage to the right hemisphere rather than the left. In contrast to post-stroke mania, a family history is not more likely; the mania tends to be characterised by irritability rather than euphoria.

The non-pharmacological treatment of mania

The need for admission

Patients with milder degrees of mania may be treated in the out-patient department or at home. Patients should be admitted if their mania is associated with aggressive behaviour, and also when other aspects of their behaviour – particularly sexual indiscretion or substance misuse – threaten health or safety.

The loss of insight, grandiosity and hyperactivity often preclude voluntary admission. Compulsory admission should be considered before the situation deteriorates.

Whatever the means of admission, patients should always be reassured that admission will enable them to rest and have relief, for instance from their excessive activities and personal conflicts, and from their 'over-excitement'.

Milieu management

There should be stable external control, and administrative issues should be handled in a firm and non-negotiable manner. Firm and consistent limits should be set in order to prevent behaviour that is dangerous or disruptive to the patient or others. All the staff should be consistent in this. Patients will often require either individual attention or nursing in a (locked) psychiatric intensive-care setting to prevent them leaving the ward. The emphasis should be on calming the patient. Restrictions on visiting and time spent alone help to reduce stimulation. When speaking with the patient the voice should be lowered, with slightly slower cadence than usual. Argument about the content of delusions should be avoided.

A structured timetable may be helpful, and writing or colouring materials should be available if the patient can concentrate sufficiently to use them. Other reality-based diversionary activities should be provided. The patient should be addressed tactfully and care should be taken to avoid provocation or pressure.

Specific issues to be addressed are the alienation of family members, the progressive testing of limits by the patient, overinvolvement with other patients and the tendency to dominate the ward. Janowsky *et al* (1974) described these tendencies as 'the manic game' and implied that the manic patients demand care without having to admit their need for it. Staff need to understand these manoeuvres in order to avoid becoming too personally involved, for instance in angry exchanges. Community meetings are helpful as they allow the responses of other patients to the person's manic behaviour to be recognised and guided.

As the patient's condition improves, individual work should be aimed at identifying factors that may have contributed to the present episode, and at helping the patient to tolerate feelings of depression or distress that may emerge. Patients may need help to re-establish personal and occupational relationships. Empathic meetings between a member of the ward team and relatives can help them to understand explanations that the patient's condition is a treatable illness which, in the longer term, needs their support and may benefit from prophylactic medication.

Before being left to supervise their own medication, patients should begin 'psycho-education' about their condition and the drugs they may need.

ECT in mania

Early reports of the use of ECT in mania showed that about two-thirds of patients responded. More recently, in a retrospective study, 78% of patients treated with ECT showed marked improvement, compared with 62% on lithium (Black *et al*, 1987). In a double-blind trial, ECT was superior to lithium during the first 8 weeks, especially for severe mania and for mixed states (Small *et al*, 1988).

In some countries, clinicians reserve ECT for patients with the most severe and drug-resistant mania, whereas elsewhere it is regarded as generally helpful in mania and used often. The use of lithium during ECT is discussed below (under contraindications to lithium); neurotoxic complications have been reported.

Drug treatment of mania

A physical examination and tests of the blood and urine should, wherever possible, precede drug treatment or take place soon after the patient is sedated, in order to elucidate any intercurrent physical illness, especially infection, and any causes of secondary mania (e.g. drugs), and to determine baseline renal, hepatic and thyroid function. An electrocardiogram (ECG) should be done if high doses of medication are to be used.

Acute tranquillisation

Treatment begins with control of the severe and agitated patient by 'acute' or 'rapid' tranquillisation. This requires an antipsychotic such as haloperidol (5–10 mg)

Table 2.2 Guidelines for treatment of mania

Source	Recommendations
APA (1994)	Mood stabiliser: lithium, valproate or carbamazepine Antipsychotic or benzodiazepine 'adjunct' for psychosis, agitation, violence
APA (2002) (Hirschfeld *et al*, 2002)	Severe mania: lithium or valproate plus antipsychotic in combination Mild mania: lithium or valproate or atypical antipsychotic
BAP (2003) (Goodwin & BAP, 2003)	Less ill: lithium, valproate, or carbamazepine Severe: antipsychotic (preferably atypical) or valproate Psychotic: antipsychotic (preferably atypical)
WFSBP (2003) (Grunze *et al*, 2003)	Lithium or valproate or atypical antipsychotic with or without benzodiazepine or low-potency classical antipsychotic

APA: American Psychiatric Association.
BAP: British Association for Psychopharmacology.
WFSBP: World Federation of Societies of Biological Psychiatry.

or olanzapine (5–10 mg), either of which may be given intramuscularly. Often a benzodiazepine such as lorazepam (1–2 mg) is also required. The more disturbed patient may be given haloperidol (5–10 mg) intramuscularly at hourly intervals until he or she is calm. Larger intramuscular doses are discouraged because they are excessive in some patients and because their effect may last for several days and may therefore obscure the diagnosis and make further management difficult; the patient may no longer appear very disturbed but is likely to deteriorate unless treatment is continued. Large doses of antipsychotic drugs have been associated with sudden deaths in disturbed young patients, probably through cardiac dysrhythmias. A Royal College of Psychiatrists consensus statement applies to the use of doses above those in the *British National Formulary* (see Chapter 11, Box 11.8, page 279).

Once calmed, the patient then requires treatment over 2–4 weeks to achieve more gradual further improvement.

A third consideration is to avoid the phase of post-manic depression.

Treatment guidelines for mania

Numerous guidelines exist for the management of bipolar disorder, including mania (see Table 2.2), perhaps reflecting the uncertainty that has prevailed about the efficacy and side-effects of treatments. Although differences remain in approaches to the treatment of bipolar depression and to prophylaxis, there has been a convergence of views about the treatment of mania between North American and European guidelines (Hirschfeld *et al*, 2002; Goodwin & BAP, 2003). These now recommend that severe mania is treated with an antipsychotic, with or without lithium or valproate. Some include starting with high doses of valproate alone (20–30 mg/kg). Less severe mania should usually be treated initially with monotherapy with either an antipsychotic, preferably an atypical, or valproate or lithium; carbamazepine is an alternative.

The notable difference is that American guidelines (2002) favour starting with a combination of an antipsychotic with valproate or lithium, whereas other guidelines include options for monotherapy at the start.

Antipsychotic drugs

Moderate or severe mania is usually most rapidly controlled by antipsychotic drugs (Cookson, 2006*a*,*b*). Phenothiazines (e.g. chlorpromazine) and thioxanthines (e.g. zuclopenthixol) are effective but the butyrophenone haloperidol is often particularly useful in a dose of 5–10 mg three times a day. Atypical antipsychotics with proven efficacy in mania include olanzapine (15–20 mg/day), risperidone (up to 6 mg/day), quetiapine (at least 600 mg/day), aripiprazole and ziprasidone. Sulpiride and amisulpride are also used.

Mild mania may be treated with atypical antipsychotic drugs or an older drug such as haloperidol 5–10 mg daily; valproate is an alternative. Lithium treatment may also be useful, but improvement takes up to 2 weeks.

Haloperidol tends to produce initial sedation, which wears off after a day or so during continued treatment (Cookson *et al*, 1983). If the patient remains very behaviourally disturbed, chlorpromazine may be more useful because, having anti-histaminic properties, it is more sedative than haloperidol. However, many patients with mania resent being made to feel drowsy and this limits the dose of chlorpromazine that they will accept. Chlorpromazine is hypotensive and should be used cautiously with elderly patients.

Extrapyramidal side-effects seem less of a problem with larger doses of haloperidol but may emerge as the dose is reduced or a few days after it is discontinued. Antiparkinsonian medication should therefore be continued for up to 7 days after haloperidol is stopped.

Rapid improvement in mania occurs 1–3 days after antipsychotic medication is begun; the manic state tends then to improve more gradually over the next 2 weeks. There is no clear evidence that increasing the dose of haloperidol above 30 mg per day achieves greater improvement.

For patients with mania whose failure to improve is due to poor compliance, depot antipsychotic medication including haloperidol or zuclopenthixol decanoate can be used. Zuclopenthixol acetate is a depot formulation which has a duration of action of up to 3 days, and a more rapid onset of action than the decanoates; it is useful in disturbed patients who persistently refuse oral medication, during the first few days of treatment.

Mechanism of action

The mechanism of the antimanic effect of these drugs is thought to be largely through blockade of dopamine (DA) receptors (Cookson *et al*, 1981). It is possible that the DA pathways and receptor subtypes relevant to the antimanic effect are different from those involved in the antischizophrenic effect of these drugs. Blockade of histamine H_1 and noradrenaline α_1 receptors may contribute to the initial effects, including sedation (Cookson *et al*, 1985).

Table 2.3 Drug and placebo response rates[a] in Bowden *et al*'s (1994) 3-week placebo-controlled clinical trial of lithium and valproate for the treatment of mania

Treatment	Number of patients	Drop-outs due to inefficacy (%)	Drop-outs due to adverse events, etc. (%)	Response (%)	Difference from placebo (%)	Number needed to treat (95% CI)
Valproate	68	30	6	48	23	5 (3–14)
Placebo	73	51	3	25		
Lithium	35	33	11	49	24	5 (3–22)

[a]The criterion for clinical improvement was a 50% reduction in score on the mania component of the Schizophrenia and Affective Disorders Scale.

Other sedative drugs

For patients with mania who are not adequately sedated by antipsychotic drugs, or to avoid prescribing such drugs, sedation may be achieved by diazepam (10–20 mg intravenously or 30 mg orally). For intramuscular use the benzodiazepines lorazepam and midazolam are absorbed faster, cause less local pain and are useful in the control of acutely agitated patients. The anticonvulsant benzodiazepine clonazepam (4–16 mg a day) is sedative and may improve mania. However, in a double-blind comparison, patients with mania on clonazepam alone showed little improvement, whereas those on lorazepam alone (6–24 mg/day) showed marked improvement. Lorazepam has also been used as an adjunct to other antimanic drugs. Depersonalisation and dissociation are potential problems during treatment with benzodiazepines, and dependence and symptoms of withdrawal occur during longer-term treatment.

Antipsychotic-resistant mania

A proportion of patients with mania show only partial improvement or initial improvement followed by partial relapse with antipsychotic drugs. There is little evidence that increasing the dose will produce further improvement. Clozapine may exert effects through an action on a different subtype of DA receptors, and this drug may prove to be useful in resistant mania as in resistant schizophrenia (Suppes *et al*, 1999). However, at present the main alternatives or adjuncts to the antipsychotic drugs are lithium and the anticonvulsants valproate and carbamazepine.

Lithium

History

Amdisen has described two eras of lithium's medicinal use. The earlier included the use of lithium salts in the 19th century for 'gouty diseases', among which Garrod in 1876 included mania; Hammond in 1871 recommended the use of lithium salts in mania. However, by 1920 this notion was rejected and with it the use of lithium. The toxicity of lithium salts received prominence in 1949 when, following several deaths, they were banned in the USA for use as salt substitutes for people with heart disease.

The modern era of lithium began in 1949 with the reinvestigation by Cade (1949) in Australia of the use of lithium in severe psychosis. Working first with guinea pigs and later with patients with a psychosis, he found that in 10 patients with mania there was a positive response. Problems with toxicity remained, until by the late 1960s the importance of serum monitoring below specific levels became established. Cade's findings were confirmed and extended, particularly by Schou in Denmark.

Open studies

In open studies, 81% of 443 patients showed some improvement on lithium, usually beginning within a week of starting treatment.

Placebo-controlled studies

Among the first placebo-controlled studies to use a cross-over design were those by Schou and his colleagues in Denmark (Schou *et al*, 1954), by Maggs in England (Maggs, 1963) and by Stokes and colleagues in the USA (Stokes *et al*, 1976). In a total of 116 patients on lithium there was an overall response rate of 78%, much greater than on placebo; but recent experience suggests the figure is lower. Lithium requires 2 weeks or more to approach a full effect on mania.

Parallel-group randomised controlled trials

One published (Bowden *et al*, 1994: see Table 2.3) and at least three unpublished randomised controlled trials (RCTs) have confirmed the efficacy of lithium in mania. However, in these studies it was seldom sufficient in monotherapy to achieve remission.

Prediction of antimanic response to lithium

Used alone, lithium is more useful in mild than in severe cases. Patients who respond tend to have classical mania rather than mixed or schizoaffective disorders. There are no data to confirm whether a family history of bipolar disorder predicts an antimanic response as it does for prophylaxis. Patients in a rapid-cycling phase tend not to respond to lithium (Dunner & Fieve, 1974; Dunner *et al*, 1976*a*). Dysphoric mania is less likely to improve (Post *et al*, 1989). Patients who have benefited previously from lithium are more likely to do so again.

Doses in mania

The narrow gap or overlap between therapeutic and toxic blood levels of lithium necessitates careful monitoring of lithium levels, usually based on samples taken 12 hours after the last dose. The pharmacokinetics of lithium involve rapid absorption, with a peak at 4 hours, followed by distribution in body fluids and slow penetration of the intracellular space and brain. Elimination is largely by the kidney, and the plasma half-life varies from 7 to 20 hours in physically healthy individuals but is longer in the elderly and physically unwell. Thus, on a regular dose, steady-state blood levels would be reached after a period of between 2 and 9 days. Many of the features of toxicity may reflect high intracellular rather than extracellular levels; hence, in assessing toxicity and efficacy, clinical judgement rather than blood levels should be paramount.

In mania salt metabolism is altered, and lithium is distributed in bone and other sites; hence higher doses are needed for a given blood level.

Plasma levels of lithium of up to 1.4 mmol/l are associated with higher rates of response in mania, but levels above 1.2 mmol/l require special care in monitoring to avoid toxicity (Stokes *et al*, 1976).

Mode of action of lithium

Lithium has numerous effects on biological systems, especially at high concentrations. It is unclear which of these are relevant to its therapeutic effects.

Ionic mechanisms

As the smallest alkaline cation, lithium can substitute for sodium, potassium, calcium and magnesium in several ways. It penetrates cells via sodium and other channels, but is extruded less efficiently than sodium by the sodium–potassium active transport system and other transporters. Thus, the cell:plasma ratio for lithium (about 0.5 in red blood cells) is much higher than that for sodium. Within the cell, lithium can interact with systems that normally involve other cations, including transmitter release and second-messenger systems.

Second-messenger systems: adenylate cyclase

Many neurotransmitters and hormones – luteinising hormone (LH), thyroid stimulating hormone (TSH), antidiuretic hormone (ADH) at V_2 receptors, dopamine at D_1 receptors, noradrenaline at β-receptors, etc.) interact with receptors that use cyclic adenosine monophosphate (cAMP) as the second (intracellular) messenger. Lithium is known to inhibit cAMP production in these systems. In humans, therapeutic levels of lithium have been shown to inhibit the adrenaline-induced rise in plasma cAMP. The inhibition by lithium of ADH-linked adenylate cyclase is thought to contribute to the polyuria and polydipsia (nephrogenic diabetes insipidus) which are side-effects of lithium. Goitre and hypothyroidism are due in part to interference with the action of TSH at its receptors in the thyroid. Noradrenaline beta-receptors and dopamine D_1 receptors are also linked to adenylate cyclase and lithium inhibits these, although it is not certain that this occurs at therapeutic concentrations.

Phosphoinositide turnover

This second-messenger system involves the release and uptake of inositol phosphates, which control intracellular calcium levels. The phosphoinositide cycle is the second messenger for several neurotransmitters, including thyrotrophin-releasing hormone (TRH) in the pituitary, acetylcholine at muscarinic M_1 receptors, noradrenaline at α_1, and 5-HT at S_2 receptors. Lithium inhibits inositol monophosphatase and has an inhibitory or stabilising effect on responses for instance to acetylcholine.

Lithium also lowers levels of the intracellular messenger protein kinase C.

Effects on monoamines and monoamine receptors

Lithium reduces presynaptic release of dopamine transmission, as well as blocking D_1 receptors.

Lithium potentiates the uptake of L-tryptophan, the precursor of 5-HT, can potentiate release of 5-HT and can potentiate 5-HT_1 responses; for instance, in humans the rise in prolactin levels induced by L-tryptophan but not that induced by d-fenfluramine is potentiated by lithium.

Lithium can block the development of dopamine receptor super-sensitivity, which normally occurs during prolonged treatment with dopamine-blocking (antipsychotic) drugs. It has been suggested that lithium may reduce the development of tardive dyskinesia in patients with bipolar disorder on antipsychotic drugs. Although in two studies tardive dyskinesia was more common in patients who had a briefer exposure to lithium, in a third study the opposite was found (Dinan & Kohen, 1989).

Side-effects of lithium

At therapeutic doses lithium has actions on many bodily systems. These are important, as some require intervention and they contribute to non-compliance. The majority of patients on lithium will experience at least one side-effect. All should be informed about side-effects and signs of toxicity, and about the risks of abrupt discontinuation.

Gastrointestinal

About one-third of patients experience mild abdominal discomfort, sometimes with loose motions during the first few weeks of treatment, especially with higher doses. By using divided doses, these side-effects can usually be avoided. Sometimes a slow-release preparation is tolerated better, but occasionally these themselves irritate the lower bowel. Severe or persistent diarrhoea suggests toxicity.

Kidney

Polyuria and excessive thirst with polydipsia are noted by about one-third of patients on lithium. The condition is usually reversible but after long-term treatment it is not always so (Bucht *et al*, 1980). Giving lithium once daily as opposed to in divided doses was associated with lower daily urine volumes in some studies, although others found no difference (Bowen *et al*, 1991). For patients in whom a reduction in dose is not appropriate in order to avoid polyuria, the loop diuretic frusemide or amiloride may be helpful.

In 1977, histological changes were reported in patients on lithium, including glomerular damage, interstitial fibrosis and tubular atrophy (focal interstitial nephropathy). However, similar findings were later made in patients who had received no lithium treatment. Much further work has shown that, during long-term treatment with lithium, monitored at therapeutic doses, no deterioration occurs in glomerular filtration rate in the vast majority of patients. Episodes of lithium toxicity may produce renal damage with reduced glomerular filtration rates. However, occasional cases of chronic renal failure have been reported and attributed by nephrologists to lithium, even in patients whose lithium levels have been monitored carefully; this is thought to be a rare idiosyncratic reaction to lithium. In such cases, lithium levels should be kept as low as possible using alternative medications, and regular monitoring of glomerular function with a nephrologist is advised before determining to stop lithium altogether.

Thyroid

Lithium tends to reduce thyroid function. The most sensitive laboratory index, increased TSH, occurs in 23% of patients. Thyroid enlargement (goitre) develops in about 5%, and clinical hypothyroidism in 5–10% of patients, depending upon the dose and duration of treatment. Patients with pre-existing thyroid antibodies or a family history of thyroid disease are at greater risk of developing hypothyroidism, and lithium treatment can increase antibody levels.

The development of hypothyroidism is often signalled by weight gain and lethargy and should be distinguished from depression. Treatment with L-thyroxine is usually straightforward. Thyrotoxicosis during lithium treatment has also been described, and there may be a rebound exacerbation when lithium is discontinued.

Central nervous system

A fine tremor of the hands occurs in about 25% of patients, and is similar to that in anxiety. Tricyclic antidepressants and selective serotonin reuptake inhibitors (SSRIs) can worsen the tremor. Beta-blockers such as propranolol (starting at 10 mg twice daily) reduce this and are probably best taken intermittently.

Lithium can increase extrapyramidal (Parkinsonian) side-effects in patients on antipsychotic drugs (Tyrer *et al*, 1980) and can itself produce cogwheel rigidity in a small minority of patients (Asnis *et al*, 1979). In contrast to antipsychotic-induced parkinsonism, this does not improve with anticholinergic drugs. Cerebellar tremor and incoordination are signs of toxicity, as are more severe forms of fine tremor and parkinsonism.

Mental and cognitive effects

There is some objective evidence of an effect of therapeutic levels of lithium upon memory, but not all studies show this. Patients interviewed about possible side-effects frequently affirm memory problems.

The possible effect of lithium upon creativity was explored by Schou (1979), who interviewed 24 successful artists and professionals taking lithium. Some did not want to continue lithium because of this effect, but the majority, although missing some hypomanic swings, considered that their long-term productivity and creativity were higher under lithium treatment. Only six thought they were diminished.

The use of ECT for patients on lithium has been associated with acute organic brain syndrome or prolonged confusional states, but a small retrospective case–control study did not find a higher frequency of adverse effects of ECT in patients on lithium (Jha *et al*, 1996).

In therapeutic doses lithium does not impair psychomotor coordination and is not a bar to driving private motor vehicles, although a diagnosis of manic-depressive illness excludes patients from driving certain public service vehicles in the UK and the USA. After an admission for mania, the patient may not drive for 6–12 months according to the UK Driver and Vehicle Licensing Agency.

Skin

Lithium can produce or exacerbate acne and psoriasis. Tetracyclines should be used with caution because of their interaction with lithium, but retinoids can be used. Hair loss and altered texture may also occur in about 6% of patients. Hair loss is sometimes associated with thyroid impairment but can occur in the presence of normal thyroid function. There may also be a golden discolouration of the distal nail plates.

Metabolic effects and weight gain

About 25% of patients gain more than 4.5 kg in weight. The mechanism is unknown. Although increased consumption of sweet drinks is cited, an increase in food intake and altered metabolism are also possible. Lithium produces subtle alterations in glucose and insulin metabolism. It may occasionally worsen control of diabetes. In a study over 1 year, more patients reported weight gain as a side-effect on valproate (21%) and on lithium (13%) than on placebo (7%) (Bowden *et al*, 2000).

Fluid retention and oedema may occur, especially with higher doses. Lithium may antagonise aldosterone and increase angiotensin levels.

Cardiovascular effects

Lithium can produce benign reversible T-wave flattening or inversion, a pattern similar to that with hypokalaemia. Cardiac dysrhythmias are rare at therapeutic doses, especially in younger patients, but sinus node arrhythmias have been described (sick sinus syndrome) (Mitchell & MacKenzie, 1982). Caution should be exercised in using lithium in patients with cardiac failure and the elderly. Higher rates of arrhythmia should be expected when lithium is used in combination with carbamazepine than with either drug alone. Lithium treatment ameliorates the excessive cardiovascular mortality found in untreated patients with bipolar disorder.

Blood and bone marrow

Lithium produces a benign reversible leucocytosis, probably by an effect on marrow growth factors. This effect can be useful in some patients on clozapine, particularly Africans, who have a benign lowering of the white cell count.

Parathyroid, bones and teeth

Lithium produces mild increases in parathyroid hormone level and serum calcium. Clinical hyperparathyroidism in patients on lithium has been reported but this may have been coincidental.

No long-term effects on bone have been found in animals or humans. It is unknown whether this applies to the growing bones of children. There is no evidence of a direct effect of lithium upon the teeth, but increased consumption of sweet drinks will lead to caries.

Sexual function

Impairment of sexual drive, arousal and ejaculation have been attributed to lithium, but are thought to be rare. The LH response to luteinising hormone releasing hormone (LHRH) is potentiated by lithium treatment, as is the potentiation of the TSH response to TRH.

Neuromuscular junction
Lithium reduces acetylcholine release and impairs neuromuscular transmission. Normally the safety factor in neuromuscular transmission is sufficient to overcome these effects. Lithium potentiates neuromuscular blocking agents, including succinyl choline, and exacerbates myasthenia gravis.

Respiratory effects
Lithium can produce respiratory depression in patients with chronic obstructive airways disease, especially at toxic blood levels. Lower therapeutic levels reduce the reactivity of bronchial smooth muscle and may benefit some patients with asthma.

Contraindications

There are no absolute contraindications to lithium treatment but caution is required in people with renal failure, heart failure, recent myocardial infarction, electrolyte imbalance, the elderly and in patients who are unreliable in taking medication.

In the USA lithium is generally withheld before ECT to reduce the risk of arrhythmia. Kellner *et al* (1997) advise stopping lithium 36–48 hours before ECT and withholding it until after the final ECT treatment, to avoid delirium or prolonged seizures. Many clinicians withhold solely the dose of lithium immediately proceeding an ECT session, and some simply continue routine lithium dosing.

Pregnancy

Initial concern about the risk of teratogenicity was based largely on the frequency of abnormalities reported to the Lithium Information Center in Wisconsin. These voluntary reports included particularly high rates of Ebstein's cardiac anomaly and suggested that foetal exposure to lithium, especially in the first trimester, carried substantially greater risk of other malformations as well. Recent cohort studies suggest the risk of major congenital abnormalities may be 4–12%, compared with 2–4% in women taking other drugs not known to be teratogenic (Kallen & Tandberg, 1983; Jacobson *et al*, 1992; Cohen *et al*, 1994). As Cohen & Rosenbaum's (1998) review notes, first-trimester exposure to lithium is associated with a risk of Ebstein's anomaly 10–20 times that of the general population. However, the absolute risk, at 0.05–0.1%, is low.

Screening tests, including high-resolution ultrasound and echocardiography examination of the foetus at 16–18 weeks' gestation, are advisable in women exposed in early pregnancy to lithium.

Perinatal toxicity is reported in neonates delivered to mothers taking lithium. Hypotonicity and cyanosis characterise this 'floppy baby syndrome'. A naturalistic study (Cohen *et al*, 1995), however, found no evidence of neonatal toxicity in the newborns of bipolar women treated with lithium at the time of labour and delivery. Before delivery, lithium should be restarted to reduce the risk of puerperal psychosis (Cohen *et al*, 1995). A 5-year follow-up of children with second- and third-trimester exposure to lithium born without congenital malformations found no significant behavioural toxicity.

Lithium is secreted in breast milk and serum lithium levels in nursing infants are reported to be 10–50% of the mother's serum level. It remains unclear what effect this low lithium intake might have on well-hydrated, breast-feeding infants. Women accepting this risk and wishing to breast-feed should be counselled to provide supplemental fluids and discontinue breast-feeding under circumstances of increased fluid loss or decreased intake.

A switch from lithium to an anticonvulsant medication for prophylaxis during pregnancy is not recommended. The risks of teratogenicity associated with valproate and carbamazepine are higher than with lithium, and a lithium-responsive patient may not be protected by these anticonvulsants.

Even the remote possibility of teratogenicity or developmental effects upon the child causes understandable concern among those planning to conceive. Pregnancy in a woman with bipolar disorder may be managed acceptably without psychotropic drugs. However, the risk of lithium discontinuation mania applies even during pregnancy (Viguera *et al*, 2000). This risk is likely to be lowest in women with only one previous episode (Cohen & Rosenbaum, 1998). Women choosing to discontinue lithium should be encouraged to taper medication gradually (over several weeks or months) and only after a euthymic period of 1 year or more. If alternative medication is needed when pregnancy is planned, antipsychotics or antidepressants are probably the safest. There is a risk of transient extrapyramidal side-effects in the neonate if antipsychotics are continued up to delivery.

Lithium toxicity

Clinical features
Lithium toxicity is indicated by the development of three groups of symptoms: gastrointestinal, motor (especially cerebellar) and mental (Table 2.4). Nausea and diarrhoea progress to vomiting and incontinence. Marked fine tremor progresses to a coarse (cerebellar or Parkinsonian) tremor, giddiness, cerebellar ataxia, and slurred speech, and to gross incoordination with choreiform movements and muscular twitching (myoclonus), upper motor neuron signs (spasticity and extensor plantar reflexes), abnormalities on electroencephalography (EEG) and seizures. In mild toxicity there is impairment of concentration but this deteriorates into drowsiness and disorientation, and in more severe toxicity there is marked apathy and impaired consciousness leading to coma. A Creutzfeldt–Jakob-like syndrome with characteristic EEG changes, myoclonus and cognitive deterioration has been described, but was in these cases reversible (Smith & Kocen, 1988).

Diagnosis of toxicity
Lithium toxicity should be assumed in patients on lithium with vomiting or severe nausea, cerebellar signs or disorientation. Lithium treatment should be stopped immediately, and serum lithium, urea and electrolyte levels measured. However, the severity of toxicity bears little relationship to serum lithium levels

Table 2.4 Symptoms of lithium toxicity

Severity	Gastrointestinal	Motor/cerebellar	Mental
Mild	Nausea Diarrhoea	Severe fine tremor	Poor concentration
Moderate	Vomiting	Coarse tremor Cerebellar ataxia Slurred speech	Drowsiness Disorientation
Severe	Vomiting Incontinence	Choreiform/Parkinsonian movement General muscle twitching (myoclonus) Spasticity and cerebellar dysfunction EEG abnormalities and seizures	Apathy Coma

(Hansen & Amdisen, 1978) and neurotoxicity can occur with serum levels in the usual therapeutic range (West & Meltzer, 1979). Diagnosis should be based upon clinical judgement and not upon the blood level. Lithium should be restarted (at an adjusted dose) only after the patient's condition has improved, or an alternative cause of the symptoms has been found.

Treatment of lithium toxicity

Often, cessation of lithium and provision of adequate salt and fluids, including saline infusions, will suffice. In patients with high serum levels (greater than 3 mmol/l) or coma, haemodialysis can speed the removal of lithium and reduce the risk of permanent neurological damage.

Outcome

Patients who survive episodes of lithium toxicity will often make a full recovery. However, some will have persistent renal or neurological damage with cerebellar symptoms, spasticity and cognitive impairment. This outcome is more likely if patients are continued on lithium while showing signs of toxicity, or during intercurrent physical illnesses (Schou, 1984). Those patients who develop persistent neurological damage have more severe signs of toxicity in their episode of toxicity (Hansen & Amdisen, 1978). Signs of toxicity develop gradually, over several days, during continued lithium treatment and, in some cases, continue to develop for days after treatment is stopped. Serum lithium levels may also continue to rise after treatment is stopped, probably because of the release of lithium from intracellular stores (Sellers *et al*, 1982).

Factors predisposing to lithium toxicity

Conditions of salt depletion (diarrhoea, vomiting, excessive sweating during fever or in hot weather) can lead to lithium retention. Drugs that reduce the renal excretion of lithium include thiazide diuretics (but not frusemide or amiloride), certain non-steroidal anti-inflammatory drugs (ibuprofen, indomethacin, piroxicam, naproxen and phenylbutazone, but not aspirin, paracetamol or sulindac) and some antibiotics (erythromycin, metronidazole and probably tetracyclines) and calcium antagonists. These drugs should be avoided if possible; if they are used, the dose of lithium should be reduced and blood levels monitored.

In patients with serious intercurrent illnesses, especially infections, lithium should be stopped or reduced in dose, and carefully monitored until the patient's condition is stable. Gastroenteritis is particularly liable to lead to toxicity. In the elderly, renal function is decreased, lower doses are required and toxicity can develop more readily.

Lithium–antipsychotic combination

Combinations of high levels of lithium with high doses of antipsychotics, including haloperidol, have been associated with severe neurological symptoms, hyperthermia, impaired consciousness and irreversible brain damage (Cohen & Cohen, 1974; Loudon & Waring, 1976). The conditions reported resemble both lithium toxicity and neuroleptic malignant syndrome. Antipsychotic drugs can increase intracellular lithium levels, suggesting a possible mechanism for this interaction (Von Knorring, 1990). Subsequent series have demonstrated the safety of combining haloperidol (up to 30 mg per day) with lithium at levels of up to 1 mmol/l (see Johnson *et al*, 1990).

In practice, when combining lithium with antipsychotics, the blood levels should generally be maintained below 1 mmol/l, staff should be advised to observe and report the development of neurological symptoms, and lithium should be temporarily discontinued if symptoms do develop. The combination of antipsychotics and lithium in patients with bipolar disorder can also lead to troublesome somnambulism, requiring dosage reduction (Charney *et al*, 1979).

Valproate in mania

Valproate is a branched-chain fatty acid. It is also available as a non-covalent dimer (two identical molecules held together by hydrogen bonding) called divalproex in the USA (Depakote, known in the UK as semi-sodium valproate). This formulation was used in several clinical trials after the company was granted a patent separate from that for valproate.

Valproate in acute mania

Valproate is effective in a proportion of patients with acute mania, including non-responders to antipsychotic drugs and lithium. Patients who respond to valproate do not necessarily respond to carbamazepine and vice versa. In the first large parallel-group placebo-controlled study (which included only patients who were unresponsive to or intolerant of lithium), 59% of patients on valproate improved, compared with only 16% of those on placebo (Pope *et al*, 1991). Most of the improvement occurred within 1–4 days of the patient achieving therapeutic levels.

The results of a second and larger study comparing divalproex with lithium or placebo in a 3-week parallel-group double-blind study are summarised in Table 2.3 (see above). Half the patients had been unresponsive to lithium previously. Valproate was as effective in patients with rapid-cycling mania as in patients with other types of mania, and equally effective in the patients previously judged responders or non-responders to lithium. However, few patients in the study returned to normal functioning within 3 weeks.

In a direct comparison of valproate and the atypical antipsychotic olanzapine (Tohen *et al*, 2002), the latter produced faster and slightly greater improvement in mania. This advantage was seen in patients with pure (non-psychotic) mania, although in psychotic mania the drugs were equally effective.

Dosage

The starting dose is 200 mg two to three times daily, rising by 200 mg at 3-day intervals, towards 2000 mg daily according to clinical response. For more rapid control a starting dose of 20 mg/kg is used. The modified-release form is started at 500 mg daily and increased.

Side-effects

Valproate is generally well tolerated but side-effects include vomiting, tremor, ataxia, weight gain, rash, hair loss – usually transient – and, potentially, acute liver damage in children. A confusional state with asterixis (flapping tremor) occurs rarely, and high blood ammonia levels confirm the cause; liver damage is not involved. Pancreatitis has occasionally been reported, as has spontaneous bruising or bleeding.

A foetal valproate syndrome has also been described with cardiac and other congenital abnormalities and with jitteriness and seizures in the neonate.

The modified-release form is associated with fewer side-effects.

Mechanism of action

Valproate is thought to reduce dopamine turnover, perhaps by increasing the function of the inhibitory transmitter gamma-aminobutyric acid (GABA); there is little direct evidence for increased GABA levels but GABA-B receptors may be upregulated by valproate. The drug may also enhance central serotonin activity, and may reduce levels of adrenocorticotrophic hormone (ACTH) and cortisol.

Pharmacokinetics

Valproate is metabolised in the liver and has a plasma half-life of 8–20 hours, which may be prolonged by cimetidine.

It inhibits cytochrome enzymes and thereby tends to raise the blood levels of lamotrigine.

Selection of patients for valproate and combinations

Patients with mania who do not respond to antipsychotics alone should be tried on a combination with valproate or lithium. Those with mixed affective disorders may be given valproate in preference to lithium. Although side-effects, including weight gain, tremor and drowsiness, may be greater, the combination is generally safe.

The drug should be avoided during pregnancy.

Monitoring and testing

The recommended plasma concentration is in the range 50–150 mg/l. In children and patients with a history of liver disease, liver function tests should be done before treatment and occasionally during the first 6 months.

Carbamazepine in mania

The mood-stabilising effect of carbamazepine was initially recognised in epilepsy. Japanese psychiatrists were the first to report that carbamazepine improved mania, even in patients who were resistant to other drugs (Okuma *et al*, 1973). Ballenger & Post (1980) independently studied carbamazepine in bipolar disorder; they had developed the theory that affective illness might involve a 'kindling' process in limbic brain areas, such as they had found with cocaine-induced behavioural changes in animals. Small placebo cross-over studies confirmed the antimanic efficacy of carbamazepine, and studies comparing carbamazepine with antipsychotic drugs or lithium show it to be approximately as effective as lithium, with about 60% of patients doing well. There is some delay in its action, but less so than with lithium. Only recently have parallel-group placebo-controlled studies been reported (Weisler *et al*, 2004, 2005).

Predicting response to carbamazepine

Patients who respond to carbamazepine differ somewhat from those who respond to lithium, and a history of non-response to lithium does not reduce the chances of a response. More severe, including dysphoric, mania can benefit from carbamazepine, as can mixed mania. Patients with no family history of mania or with mania secondary to brain damage can also benefit.

Doses of carbamazepine

The dose of carbamazepine for mania is similar to that for epilepsy, except that the drug's introduction has to be less gradual if considerable delay is to be avoided. (Gradual introduction reduces the incidence of side-effects, discussed below.) The recommended starting dose is 100 mg twice daily, increasing by 200 mg every 2 or 3 days, up to 400 mg twice daily or more, depending on response in mania. For prophylaxis the increase should be at weekly intervals. For most people with mania, 800–1200 mg is sufficient, but a few may require up to 1600 mg a day. For prophylaxis the range is usually 400–600 mg per day. Modified-release tablets (200 mg and 400 mg) are associated with reduced peak plasma levels, can help to reduce side-effects and are taken once or twice daily at the same total daily dose as above.

Side-effects of carbamazepine

The commonest side-effects are nausea, dizziness, ataxia and double vision. Others include headache, drowsiness and nystagmus. At higher doses confusion may occur.

A maculopapular itchy rash develops within 2 weeks in about 10% of patients and requires great caution and usually cessation of the drug, and a full blood count should be performed. Carbamazepine must be discontinued if the rash worsens, the blood count is abnormal or other symptoms develop. Serious toxic side-effects are agranulocytosis, aplastic anaemia, Stevens–Johnson syndrome and water intoxication. A moderate leucopenia occurs in 1–2% of patients, and often transiently at the start of treatment. Agranulocytosis and aplastic anaemia can develop suddenly, and occur in about eight patients per million treated.

Carbamazepine regularly lowers the white-cell count via a pharmacological effect on the marrow. Hyponatraemia and water intoxication may occur and are due to potentiation of ADH, and may lead to malaise, confusion and fits. Fluid retention may occur.

Patients should be warned of side-effects, and advised particularly to report any rashes, fevers or severe sore throats, which may herald agranulocytosis and require immediate discontinuation of the drug.

Because of the possibility of foetal neural tube defects, carbamazepine should be avoided in pregnancy; folate supplements are essential if it is continued.

Oxcarbazepine
A related drug, oxcarbazepine, carries a lower risk of bone marrow toxicity. Its efficacy in mania is disputed.

Pharmacokinetics and drug interactions

Carbamazepine induces liver enzymes. This results in the lowering not only of its own blood levels after 3 weeks of treatment, but also increasing the metabolism of other drugs such as haloperidol, risperidone, valproate, lamotrigine, oral contraceptives, clonazepam and tricyclic antidepressants. Its own plasma half-life may shorten from 48 hours to 7 hours during long-term treatment. The dose of oral contraceptives needs to be raised, or an alternative method of birth control should be used. The dose of warfarin may also need increasing. Thyroid hormone metabolism is increased and blood levels lowered; carbamazepine may precipitate hypothyroidism, particularly in combination with lithium.

Carbamazepine is itself metabolised by CYP IIIA4. A metabolite (carbamazepine 10,11-epoxide) has similar pharmacological activity. Barbiturates and phenytoin induce enzymes and lower plasma levels of carbamazepine. On the other hand, the blood level of carbamazepine is increased by some drugs, including erythromycin, verapamil, dextropropoxyphene (in Co-Proxamol), cimetidine, valproate and some SSRIs (e.g. fluoxetine).

Being of tricyclic structure, carbamazepine should not be given in combination with a monoamine oxidase inhibitor, as serotonin syndrome is a risk.

Mechanism of action

An anti-kindling effect may underlie some of the actions of carbamazepine, but the pharmacological mechanism of action in mania is unknown. Carbamazepine reduces L-type calcium channel activation by depolarisation, and may block the excitatory transmitter glutamate at NMDA-type receptors. Carbamazepine potentiates central 5-HT transmission in normal subjects, as judged by the prolactin response to L-tryptophan.

Blood tests

No clear relationship has been found between blood level and antimanic effect. A range of 15–30 μmol/l (5–10 mg/l) is generally cited in epilepsy. A target of above 7 mg/l provides some guidance in affective disorders but the dose should be determined mainly by clinical response and tolerance of side-effects, as in epilepsy.

The differential blood count and electrolyte levels should be monitored in the first few weeks. Hyponatraemia requires a reduction of dose or discontinuation. Carbamazepine should be stopped immediately if the total white-cell count is less than 3000 per mm^3 or the neutrophil count is less than 1500.

Combination treatment

Many patients who fail to improve when taking carbamazepine alone do improve when lithium is added. This combination may – as with antipsychotics – increase the risk of lithium neurotoxicity (see above).

Other drugs in mania

While it is of theoretical interest that the cholinesterase inhibitor physostigmine has antimanic properties, its side-effects preclude clinical use (Janowsky *et al*, 1973). Likewise, the addition of lecithin (a precursor of acetylcholine) may potentiate other antimanic medication but its value in clinical practice is doubtful. The antiepileptic drugs lamotrigine, topiramate and gabapentin do not improve mania.

Prophylaxis of bipolar disorder

Selection of patients

Maintenance treatment should be considered after a second major episode of bipolar disorder, especially if the interval between episodes is less than 5 years. Because the intervals between the first and second episode tends to be longer than between subsequent episodes, maintenance treatment should be used after a first episode only if the dangers of a subsequent episode are thought to justify it, for instance if the episode was severe and disruptive, had a relatively sudden onset and was not precipitated by external factors, or if the person's job is in jeopardy, or if there is a high suicide risk.

Sequence within cycles

In those patients in whom a prolonged episode of mania is generally followed by a phase of depression and then a well interval ('MDI' – see page 27), prompt treatment of the manic phase may reduce the severity of subsequent depression. Koukopoulos (2002) suggested this might be a mechanism by which lithium reduces depression in BP-I disorder. The same could be suggested for the use of antipsychotic drugs in this condition. However, some patients exhibit cycles of hypomania followed by major depression.

Lithium prophylaxis

Predicting response to lithium

Patients with typical bipolar disorder and complete recovery between episodes are more likely to benefit (Grof *et al*, 1993). A family history of bipolar disorder is strongly predictive of prophylactic efficacy, but in contrast it is questionable whether 'secondary' bipolar disorder ever responds to lithium; indeed, neurological signs predict a poor response to lithium. Patients whose first episode was manic rather than depressive also do better on lithium, and the MDI pattern predicts a better response than the DMI pattern (Faedda *et al*, 1991). A good response to lithium in mania or depression may predict prophylactic efficacy. Patients with a rapid-cycling phase of illness are less responsive to lithium (Dunner & Fieve, 1974). Other factors militating strongly against prophylactic efficacy are poor adherence to treatment and drug misuse.

In the prophylaxis of unipolar depressive disorder, a good response to lithium is predicted by a family history of bipolar disorder, premorbid personality with low neuroticism and good inter-episode functioning.

Blood levels and monitoring

Blood levels lower than those formerly used are sufficient in prophylaxis. Thus, efficacy is preserved until levels are below 0.6 mmol/l. For some patients lower levels than this would suffice, although Gelenberg *et al* (1989) found that a group with levels of 0.8–1.0 mmol/l had a better outcome than a group with levels of 0.4–0.6 mmol/l. For elderly patients, a level of 0.5 mmol/l is recommended. Recommendations vary about monitoring lithium, renal and thyroid function tests, but even in the most stable patient these tests should be performed at least once a year, and during less stable phases lithium levels should be determined more frequently.

Lithium prophylaxis: open studies

The first major report indicating the prophylactic efficacy of lithium in recurrent affective disorders (Baastrup & Schou, 1967) was a retrospective analysis involving 88 patients. While they were taking lithium, the patients' total annual duration of affective episodes was reduced from an average of 13 weeks to 2 weeks. These observations were widely confirmed, but the study design was criticised by Blackwell & Shepherd (1968); the natural history of the illness might have been for improvement after a period of frequent episodes, and a double-blind design would be needed to eliminate the effect of bias in the observer and the patient. The methodological considerations are outlined in Box 2.3.

Box 2.3 Trial design in studies of prophylaxis

The methodology for demonstrating the efficacy of a drug such as lithium in long-term prophylaxis is the double-blind placebo-controlled trial with random allocation. The trial should select patients with known bipolar disorder, who may be stratified according to the number and pattern of previous episodes – so that, for instance, rapid-cyclers or older patients would be assigned equally to the two treatments. The patients should be in remission and receiving no other medication, or steps should be taken to avoid the possibility of withdrawal problems complicating the commencement of the trial – either by weaning off before or tapering the medication after the start of the trial. The patients should be sufficient in number to avoid the possibility of a type 2 statistical error (false negative result). Each patient should give informed consent and the trial should have the approval of the regional and local ethics committees and be conducted according to national and European Community (1991) requirements, with the possibility of external audit. If an effective treatment already exists, patients can be admitted ethically to the trial only if they are non-responding, or have unacceptable side-effects with that treatment, or if they recognise the risk of relapse on placebo and agree to this.

The patients should be assigned randomly to receive either placebo or the study medication (e.g. lithium). The dosage may be variable according to blood levels, perhaps within preset limits. Dose changes should be made without revealing the nature of the medication to the rating doctor; this can be achieved by making adjustments to the dose in patients in each treatment group. The use of more than one dose range of the active treatment allows dose–response relations to be explored, and compared with side-effect incidence. Blood tests also confirm adherence to treatment. The trial should be of sufficient duration to show the benefit of the active treatment compared with placebo, for instance 1 year.

Patients should be assessed regularly using validated clinical rating skills for depression and mania. The criteria for relapse should be defined before the study starts. Patients who relapse during the study should be withdrawn and given appropriate treatment. During the study other medication should be avoided, although special arrangements may be made for the treatment of intercurrent illnesses not related to the side-effects of the medication under study. In a study of a new treatment, enquiries should be made throughout the study about possible side-effects, but in the case of a medication with a well-established side-effect profile this procedure may undermine the trial by revealing (to the blinded rater) the nature of the patient's medication.

All the data should be collected before the trial code (showing which patient received which medication) is broken. Patients who drop out of the study because of side-effects rather than relapse should be included in the analysis only up to the time of withdrawal. The results should be analysed using appropriate statistical methods (e.g. survival analysis), preferably by a statistician independent of the investigators. A sequential method of analysis should be considered, to minimise the number of patients exposed to placebo.

Lithium prophylaxis: placebo-controlled studies

There have been 14 major double-blind comparative trials of lithium versus placebo in bipolar patients. Three types of design have been used. Two studies used double-blind discontinuation, patients already on lithium being assigned randomly either to continue on lithium or to switch to placebo. However, this design is weakened by the occurrence of lithium withdrawal mania (see below). One study used a cross-over design, which also involved a lithium withdrawal phase. A prospective design was used by Coppen *et al* (1971) in the UK and by Prien *et al* (1973) in the USA and in five other studies. However, some studies included patients with unipolar depression and some (including Prien *et al*, 1973) did not report whether the recurrences were manic or depressive.

A meta-analysis of prophylactic studies that included lithium and placebo confirmed that lithium is effective in preventing relapses in total and in preventing mania, but the effect in preventing depression appeared slightly smaller and failed to reach statistical significance (Geddes *et al*, 2004). Overall, in 369 patients on lithium, 40% relapsed in the study period (which varied from 4 months to 2 years) compared with 60% of 401 patients on placebo.

Lithium reduces both the severity and frequency of episodes. Usually it also stabilises the mood between major episodes.

It is noteworthy that the marked efficacy of lithium in the study by Prien *et al* (1973) was accompanied by a very low rate of drop-outs through side-effects, a finding that cannot be generalised to modern psychiatric clinics (Maj *et al*, 1998).

Antidepressants and lithium

Depression occurring during lithium treatment can be treated with monoamine reuptake inhibitors. Other drugs that have antidepressant effects in bipolar depression are quetiapine and lamotrigine. The former is licensed for this indication in the USA.

In people experiencing a current episode of depression and who have a history of mania (BP-I) it is advisable to combine the antidepressant with an antimanic drug. For those who do not have a current episode of depression, or whose episode is satisfactorily resolving, the antidepressant should be discontinued gradually, in order to reduce the risk of triggering a manic episode, as well as to avoid the induction of rapid cycling.

For patients with a predominantly depressive pattern of bipolar disorder (BP-II) the combination of lithium and a monoamine reuptake inhibitor may be more effective in preventing depression than either drug alone.

The SSRI class of antidepressants carries a lower risk of triggering mania than broader-acting drugs, such as the older tricyclics amitriptyline and imipramine or the newer drug venlafaxine.

The drug treatment of bipolar depression is further discussed in Chapter 4 (see page 102).

Discontinuation of lithium

Symptoms of anxiety, irritability and emotional lability can occur following sudden discontinuation of lithium. In a double-blind placebo-controlled cross-over study, sudden cessation of lithium in patients with bipolar disorder led to the development of mania 2–3 weeks later in 7 out of 14 patients (Mander & Loudon, 1988). Discontinuation of lithium should therefore be gradual and certainly over more than 2 weeks, for example at the rate of one-quarter to one-eighth of the original dose every 2 months. Patients whose mood has been stable are less likely to relapse on stopping lithium than those who have continued to show mild mood swings.

Natural outcome on lithium

Dickson & Kendell (1986) reported a threefold increase in admissions for mania in Edinburgh during the period 1970–81, when the use of lithium increased. This highlights the difficulty of delivering an effective treatment to a community. A large proportion of patients at risk do not seek treatment, and many who do adhere poorly to lithium. In addition, there is the risk of withdrawal mania in those who stop treatment too abruptly, for instance during a mild upswing of mood when patients generally feel they do not need any medication. Some naturalistic follow-up studies found no difference in outcome between patients with bipolar disorder discharged on or off lithium. However, under circumstances where special steps are taken to encourage and check adherence, relapse rates and affective morbidity on lithium as low as those in controlled trials can be achieved (McCreadie & Morrison, 1985; Coppen & Abou-Saleh, 1988). This is part of the rationale for specialist lithium or affective disorder clinics.

During careful follow-up in a well-staffed lithium clinic in Naples, only 23% of patients with bipolar disorder remained free of recurrence on lithium for 5 years, but only 61% were still on lithium by that time and only 39% were receiving lithium alone (Maj *et al*, 1998).

A case record study of patients with manic–depression treated with lithium showed that mortality was reduced to the same level as in the general population (Coppen *et al*, 1991). Lithium appears to confer protection against suicide that may be separate from its effects on mania or depression.

Adherence to treatment

In the UK the use of lithium is only about 0.8 per 1000 population, even in centres with active lithium clinics (McCreadie & Morrison, 1985); about half the patients who start taking lithium discontinue it within 1 year, but a quarter remain on it for over 10 years.

The patients who are less likely to adhere tend to be younger, male and to have had fewer previous episodes of illness. The reasons they give for stopping are side-effects, missing periods of elation, feeling well and in no need of treatment, feeling depressed or less productive, or not wanting to depend on medication. The side-effects most often given as reasons for non-adherence are excessive thirst and polyuria, tremor, memory impairment and weight gain. Hair loss may be significant for women.

In order to increase adherence, the doctor should take side-effects seriously, keep lithium levels as low as possible, educate patients and their families about their illness and the use of lithium, and discuss adherence. For non-adherent patients, the regular contact provided by counselling or psychotherapy can be useful and has been shown to improve compliance and affective morbidity. It may be helpful to plot a 'life chart' with the patient.

Alternatives to lithium in prophylaxis

As indicated above, for many patients lithium will either lack efficacy or have intolerable side-effects, and so alternative treatments to lithium are clearly needed (Cookson & Elliot, 2006).

Valproate

Sodium valproate has been studied less but may be useful for prophylaxis in those who are resistant to lithium and antipsychotics (on which see below). Some patients may benefit from the combination of lithium and valproate if they have not responded to either drug alone.

Continuation treatment with valproate after remission of mania or hypomania was investigated in a comparative trial with lithium or placebo (Bowden *et al*, 2000). This failed to show a benefit from either drug in preventing relapses of mania or depression. However, some 40% of the patients considered for the study were previously known to be non-responders to lithium. There was a possible small benefit of valproate in preventing milder depressive symptoms. The combination of lithium and valproate produces fewer neurological problems than the combination of lithium with carbamazepine.

The benefit in preventing suicide is less with valproate than with lithium (Goodwin *et al*, 2003).

Guidelines from the National Institute for Health and Clinical Excellence (2006) on the management of bipolar disorder advise that valproate prophylaxis should not be used routinely for women of child-bearing potential, because of the risk of foetal malformation and of impaired intellectual development in the child, and in young women because of the risk of polycystic ovary syndrome.

Carbamazepine

The first controlled studies of the use of carbamazepine in prophylaxis were those of Okuma *et al* (1981) and Post *et al* (1983). Several small studies suggested it was of similar efficacy to lithium (Davis *et al*, 1999) but larger, more naturalistic studies have suggested that lithium is in fact superior (Greil & Kleindienst, 1999; Hartong *et al*, 2003). Rapid-cycling patients and others resistant to lithium may benefit from carbamazepine (Greil *et al*, 1998). In longer-term use there may be partial loss of efficacy by the third year of treatment, although it is not clear to what extent poor adherence to medication is responsible.

Side-effects

These can be minimised by starting treatment with low doses (100–200 mg at night) and increasing every few days to the maximum dose that is well tolerated (usually 400–600 mg, maximum 1600 mg daily). Patients should be informed of the risk of side-effects, including blood disorders (see above), and told to report to the doctor symptoms such as sore throat, rash or fever.

Lithium and carbamazepine in combination

Some patients appear to benefit more from the combination than from either drug alone. There have been reports of reversible neurological side-effects, characterised mainly by confusional states and cerebellar signs (Shukla *et al*, 1985).

Lamotrigine

Treatment of BP-I patients with lamotrigine after recovery from mania or hypomania has been investigated in a large comparative study with lithium and placebo (Bowden *et al*, 2003). The greatest effect of lamotrigine was in preventing subsequent depression. It was also effective in rapid-cycling patients with BP-II but not BP-I disorder (Calabrese *et al*, 2000).

Antipsychotic drugs

Because of their sedative effects and long-term neurological side-effects, classical antipsychotic drugs should be used cautiously in the long-term management of patients with bipolar disorder. However, there is growing evidence that their continued use after an episode of mania helps to prevent recurrences of mania and, to a lesser extent, depression. Also, for those who have frequently recurring episodes, and either do not benefit from or do not adhere to oral medication, depot formulations of antipsychotic drugs can provide a period of stability (Lowe & Batchelor, 1990; Littlejohn *et al*, 1994).

It has been suggested that patients with bipolar disorder are particularly susceptible to developing tardive dyskinesia. Other authors have found a prevalence (about 20%) similar to that among patients with chronic schizophrenia (Hunt & Silverstone, 1991). However, tardive dyskinesia may be more preventable in patients with bipolar disorder since they have less need for continuous long-term antipsychotic drug treatment.

Studies indicate that continuation of treatment with an antipsychotic (olanzapine) after remission of mania helps to reduce the risk of relapses or recurrences, especially of mania, in the following year, even in patients who are also continued on lithium or valproate (Tohen *et al*, 2004, 2006). One of the trials, in which more than 40% of patients had a history of rapid cycling, found that treatment with olanzapine alone reduced recurrences of both mania and depression. In comparison with lithium, continued treatment with olanzapine was associated with higher compliance, fewer recurrences of mania, similar recurrences of depression and lower rates of rehospitalisation in the year after an episode of mania.

Adjunctive thyroid hormone

There is evidence from placebo-controlled studies that L-thyroxine or tri-iodothyronine in replacement doses can potentiate the antidepressant effect of monoamine reuptake inhibitors in patients with resistant depression. However, in long-term prophylaxis this treatment eventually loses efficacy (Wehr *et al*, 1988). High-dose thyroid hormone treatment has also been advocated for patients with resistant bipolar disorder, especially rapid-cyclers, but prospective placebo-controlled studies are required (Bauer & Whybrow, 1990).

Leucotomy in bipolar disorder

Stereotactic subcaudate tractotomy for patients with intractible bipolar disorders appears to offer a good result (Poynton *et al*, 1988).

The psychology of mania

Psychoanalytical views

Freud (1917) saw the psychological precipitant of mania (and depression) as the loss of an ambivalently regarded 'object'. Instead of depressive anxiety and guilt, mania is the 'festival of the ego', released from its domination by the super-ego with which it now becomes fused.

Astute clinical observations led Karl Abraham (1924) to regard the basis of all manic symptoms as increased oral drives with accompanying fantasies of cannibalistic incorporation. Patients who were manic seemed to identify with what is incorporated, including both parents. This led symbolically to phallic identification, which could be viewed as a central feature of the psychology of mania.

Winnicott and Klein (see Segal, 1975), who had herself been analysed by Abraham, introduced the idea of the 'manic defence' against depressive anxiety. The manic defences (omnipotent control, triumph and contempt) protect the ego against despair, but interrupt the process of reparation and produce a vicious circle by further attacks upon the 'object'. However, a manic form of reparation can occur and some of the identifications made in mania can be seen as potential advances in individual development.

Lewin (1951) wrote of the 'oral triad' of the wishes to eat, be 'eaten' (or taken in) and to sleep. In mania the second component is resisted because of a dread of phallic rivalry; oral devouring is prolonged and sleep postponed.

These ideas are sometimes helpful in understanding the content of manic ideas. However, their aetiological significance is less clear, a fact recognised by Freud, who referred to the 'economic problem' of the libido in mania and depression.

Dependence

Fromm-Reichmann emphasised the contrast between the dependence of the depressive and the assertiveness, rivalry and independence of the manic state. These changes in feelings of dependence are relevant to the marital difficulties and the tendency to substance misuse in patients with bipolar disorder.

Beliefs

Religious and other beliefs can be altered by pathological mood states and can become important parts of the individual's identity. Martin Luther, the leader of the Reformation in Germany, experienced marked depressive and hypomanic swings. He composed hymns of joy and strength and revived the doctrine of justification by the faith of the individual. The mechanisms behind his ambivalent rejection of the Pope's authority are open to psychoanalytical interpretation and his life was the subject of a book by Erikson (1958).

Leadership and creativity

There has been a view held at periods in history that madness and genius are related. Much of the evidence is based on individual biographical accounts, but recent work has investigated the association critically (see Goodwin & Jamison, 1990).

Leadership

Among military leaders Achilles in legend, Alexander the Great and Napoleon have all shown features of cyclothymia. Oliver Cromwell's biographer, Christopher Hill (1970), describes the evidence for hypomanic phases as well as depression. Among wartime political leaders, Churchill, Roosevelt and Mussolini exhibited features of hypomania, and Churchill was prone also to periods of depression, which he called 'black dog'. Driving energy, sense of purpose and right, confidence and the ability to convey this to others are relevant traits, together with varying degrees of grandiosity. In peacetime leaders, these traits tend to be less important or even disadvantageous. Even in war it is likely that they lead to rash or catastrophic decisions.

Artistic creativity

Among visual artists, Michelangelo, Van Gogh and many others showed severe mood swings and some died by suicide. The composers Schumann, Bruckner, Tchaikovsky and Mahler were cyclothymic or manic–depressive. Schumann's creative output was greatly increased during two hypomanic periods and diminished during depression, and he died of self-starvation in an asylum. In these individuals the intense feelings associated with mood swings may have increased a desire to express themselves in art. Freedom from normal restraints and heightened sensory perceptions may have contributed to their originality.

The poets Shelley, Byron and Chatterton were manic–depressive, Robert Lowell had BP-I disorder, and Sylvia Plath had BP-II disorder and possibly borderline personality disorder, and committed suicide. The novelists and playwrights Balzac, Ruskin, Hemingway, Fitzgerald and Woolf were cyclothymic or manic–depressive. In the case of Virginia Woolf the writing of her most original ('stream of consciousness') novels led usually into a psychotic breakdown. In the interval between these novels she wrote less original 'novels of fact' or 'holiday books'. Her husband, Leonard Woolf, had a steadying influence on her. Her nephew and biographer Quentin Bell described her imagination as being 'furnished with an accelerator but no brakes', an admirable description of a manic trait (Lehmann, 1987).

In Churchill's case, Storr (1969) emphasised the creative use of words and ideas; his writing, painting and oratory were 'manic defences' against the depressive tendencies which could be traced in the family to the first Duke of Marlborough. His daughter, however, has stated that her mother 'very largely kennelled the black dog', except in Churchill's old age (Soames, 1993).

Among performing artists, comedians seem particularly likely to have bipolar conditions, and this association has been described in detail in one case (Milligan & Clare, 1993). In some cases the long intervals between major works suggest a link with affective swings. Joseph Conrad considered writing 'a sort of mental revulsion' and described his completion of *Nostromo* as a 'recovery from a dangerous illness'.

Critical studies

Andreasen (1987) found a lifetime prevalence of bipolar disorder of 43% among a group of American writers, compared with 10% among matched controls. Alcoholism was also more prevalent in the writers. In their first-degree relatives, affective disorder had occurred in 18% of writers and 2% of controls, usually in the form of major depression.

Jamison (1989) investigated the link between creativity and affective swings in 47 outstanding British artists and writers. Of this sample, 38% had been treated for an affective illness, 6% for BP-I disorder. Poets were the most commonly treated with medication, and were the only group to have BP-I disorder (17%). Playwrights were the most commonly treated with psychotherapy. Biographers and visual artists had somewhat lower rates than the other writers, although these were still greater than in the general population. Of all the participants, 90% reported intense creative episodes; these usually lasted about 2 weeks but a quarter lasted more than 1 month and were characterised by many of the features of hypomania, although not usually by increased talkativeness or sociability.

Conclusion

Mania can affect people of all social and occupational groups and is usually a phase in a recurring bipolar illness. Hypomanic traits and episodes can be associated with successful leadership, productivity and creativity but can also be disruptive. Manic episodes are very disruptive and there is a high rate of divorce and successful suicide in patients with bipolar disorder. Treatment will often minimise or allow such disruptions to be avoided, and reduce the suicide risk.

During an episode of mania, the treating team should strive to establish and maintain a therapeutic alliance. When insight returns, efforts should be made to educate the patient and carers about bipolar illness and the treatments that are available. The patient should be helped to formulate an action plan, designed to help with recognition of the early signs of recurrence of mania or depression and how to respond.

Options for drug treatment of mania include antipsychotics, lithium, valproate and carbamazepine. Drugs recommended by the National Institute for Health and Clinical Excellence (2006) for maintenance treatment, in combination with psycho-education, are lithium, the atypical antipsychotic olanzapine, valproate and lamotrigine. Maintenance with an antidepressant may also be needed in people with predominantly depressive forms of the illness, but is best combined with an antimanic drug to reduce the risk of mania. Quetiapine and lamotrigine also have antidepressant properties.

References

Abraham, K. (1924) A short study of the development of the libido, viewed in the light of mental disorders: mania. In *Selected Papers of Karl Abraham* (trans. D. Bryan & A. Strachey), pp. 470–475. London: Hogarth (1949).

Akiskal, H. (2002) Classification, diagnosis and boundaries of bipolar disorders: a review. In *Bipolar Disorder* (eds M. Maj, H. S. Akiskal, J. J. Lopez-Ibor, *et al*), pp. 1–52. Chichester: Wiley.

Ambelas, A. (1987) Life events and mania: a special relationship? *British Journal of Psychiatry*, **150**, 235–240.

American Psychiatric Association (1994) *Diagnostic and Statistical Manual of Mental Disorders* (4th edn) (DSM–IV). Washington, DC: APA.

American Psychiatric Association (2000) *Diagnostic and Statistical Manual of Mental Disorders* (4th edn, text revision) (DSM–IV–TR). Washington, DC: APA.

Andreasen, N. C. (1987) Creativity and mental illness: prevalence rates in writers and their first-degree relatives. *American Journal of Psychiatry*, **144**, 1288–1292.

Angst, J. (1978) The course of affective disorders II: Typology of bipolar manic–depressive illness. *Archiv für Psychiatrie und Nervenkrankheiten*, **226**, 65–73.

Angst, J. (1985) Switch from depression to mania: a record study over decades between 1920 and 1982. *Psychopathology*, **18**, 140–155.

Aronson, T. A. & Shukla, S. (1987) Life events and relapse in bipolar disorder: the impact of a catastrophic event. *Acta Psychiatrica Scandinavica*, **75**, 571–576.

Asnis, G. M., Asnis, D., Dunner, D. L., *et al* (1979) Cogwheel rigidity during chronic lithium therapy. *American Journal of Psychiatry*, **136**, 1225–1226.

Baastrup, P. C. & Schou M. (1967) Lithium as a prophylactic agents. Its effect against recurrent depressions and manic-depressive psychosis. *Archives of General Psychiatry*, **16**, 162–172.

Ballenger, J. C. & Post, R. M. (1980) Carbamazepine in manic depressive illness: a new treatment. *American Journal of Psychiatry*, **137**, 782–790.

Bauer, M. S. & Whybrow, P. C. (1990) Rapid-cycling bipolar affective disorder. II. Treatment of refractory rapid-cycling with high dose levothyroxine: a preliminary study. *Archives of General Psychiatry*, **47**, 435–440.

Bauwens, F., Tracy, A., Pardoen, D., *et al* (1991) Social adjustment of remitted bipolar and unipolar out-patients. A comparison with age- and sex-matched controls. *British Journal of Psychiatry*, **159**, 239–244.

Beigel, A. & Murphy, D. L. (1971) Assessing clinical characteristics of the manic state. *American Journal of Psychiatry*, **128**, 688–694.

Beigel, A., Murphy, D. L. & Bunney, W. E. (1971) The Manic-State Rating Scale: scale construction, reliability, and validity. *Archives of General Psychiatry*, **25**, 256–262.

Black, D. W., Winokur, G. & Nasrallah, A. (1987) Treatment of mania: a naturalistic study of electroconvulsive therapy versus lithium in 438 patients. *Journal of Clinical Psychiatry*, **48**, 132–139.

Blackburn, I. M., Loudon, J. B. & Ashworth, C M. (1977) A new scale for measuring mania. *Psychological Medicine*, **7**, 453–458.

Blackwell, B. & Shepherd, M. (1968) Prophylactic lithium. Another therapeutic myth? *Lancet*, *i*, 968–971.

Bland, R. C. & Orn, H. (1982) Course and outcome of affective disorders. *Canadian Journal of Psychiatry*, **27**, 573–578.

Bowden, C., Brugger, A. M., Swann, A. C., *et al* (1994) Efficacy of divalproex vs lithium and placebo in the treatment of mania. *JAMA*, **271**, 918–924.

Bowden, C. L., Calabrese, J. R., McElroy, S. L., *et al* (2000) A randomized, placebo-controlled 12-month trial of divalproex and lithium in treatment of outpatients with bipolar I disorder. Divalproex Maintenance Study Group. *Archives of General Psychiatry*, **57**, 481–489.

Bowden, C. L., Calabrese, J. R., Sachs, G., *et al* (2003) A placebo-controlled 18-month trial of lamotrigine and lithium maintenance treatment in recently manic or hypomanic patients with bipolar I disorder. *Archives of General Psychiatry*, **60**, 392–400.

Bowen, R. C., Grof, P. & Grof, E. (1991) Less frequent lithium administration and lower urine volume. *American Journal of Psychiatry*, **148**, 189–192.

Brodie, H. K. H. & Leff, M. J. (1971) Bipolar depression: a comparative study of patient characteristics. *American Journal of Psychiatry*, **127**, 1086–1090.

Bucht, G., Wahlin, A., Wentzel, T., *et al* (1980) Renal function and morphology in long-term lithium and combined lithium–neuroleptic treatment. *Acta Medica Scandinavica*, **208**, 381–385.

Cade, J. F. J. (1949) Lithium salts in the treatment of psychotic excitement. *Medical Journal of Australia*, **36**, 349–352.

Calabrese, J. R., Suppes, T., Bowden, C. L., *et al* (2000) A double blind placebo controlled, prophylaxis study of lamotrigine in rapid cycling bipolar disorder. *Journal of Clinical Psychiatry*, **61**, 841–850.

Cannon, M., Caspi, A., Moffitt, T. E., *et al* (2002) Evidence for early-childhood pan-developmental impairment specific to schizophreniform disorder. *Archives of General Psychiatry*, **59**, 449–456.

Carlson, G. A. (1980) Manic depressive illness and cognition immaturity. In *Mania: An Evolving Concept* (eds R. H. Belmaker & H. M. Van Praeg), pp. 281–289. New York: Spectrum Books.

Carlson, G. A. & Goodwin, F. K. (1973) The stages of mania: a longitudinal analysis of the manic episode. *Archives of General Psychiatry*, **28**, 221–228.

Cassidy, F., Forest, K., Murry, E., *et al* (1998) A factor analysis of the signs and symptoms of mania. *Archives of General Psychiatry*, **55**, 27–32.

Charney, D. S., Kales, A., Soldatos, C., *et al* (1979) Somnambulistic-like episode, secondary to combined lithium–neuroleptic treatment. *British Journal of Psychiatry*, **135**, 418–424.

Clark, L., Iverson, S. D. & Goodwin, G. M. (2002) Sustained attention deficit in bipolar disorder. *British Journal of Psychiatry*, **180**, 313–319.

Cohen, L. S. & Rosenbaum, J. F. (1998) Psychotropic drug use during pregnancy: weighing the risks. *Journal of Clinical Psychiatry*, **59**, suppl. 2, 18–28.

Cohen, L. S., Friedman, J. M., Jefferson, J. W., *et al* (1994) A reevaluation of risk of in utero exposure to lithium. *JAMA*, **271**, 146–150.

Cohen, L. S., Sichel, D. A., Robertson, L. M., *et al* (1995) Postpartum prophylaxis for women with bipolar disorder. *American Journal of Psychiatry*, **152**, 1641–1645.

Cohen, W. J. & Cohen, N. H. (1974) Lithium carbonate, haloperidol, and irreversible brain damage. *JAMA*, **230**, 1283–1287.

Coid, J. & Strang, J. (1982) Mania secondary to procyclidine (Kemadrin) abuse. *British Journal of Psychiatry*, **141**, 81–84.

Cookson, J. C. (1985) The neuroendocrinology of mania. *Journal of Affective Disorder*, **8**, 233–241.

Cookson, J. C. (2006*a*) Haloperidol and risperidone in mania. In *Bipolar Pharmacotherapy: Clinical Management* (eds H. Akiskal & M. Tohen). Chichester: Wiley.

Cookson, J. C. (2006*b*) Management of mania. In *Handbook of Bipolar Disorder* (eds R. Hirshfeld & S. Kasper). Boca Raton, FL: Taylor & Francis.

Cookson, J. C. & Elliot, B. (2006) The use of anticonvulsants in the aftermath of mania. In Managing the aftermath of mania. *Journal of Psychopharmacology*, **20**, suppl. 2.

Cookson, J. C. & Ghalib, S. (2005) The treatment of bipolar mixed states. In *Bipolar Disorders: Mixed States Rapid Cycling and Atypical Forms* (eds A. Marneros & F. K. Goodwin), pp. 324–352. Cambridge: Cambridge University Press.

Cookson, J. C., Silverstone, T. & Wells, B. (1981) A double-blind comparative clinical trial of pimozide and chlorpromazine in mania: a test of the dopamine hypothesis. *Acta Psychiatrica Scandinavica*, **64**, 381–397.

Cookson, J. C., Moult, P. J. A., Wiles, D., *et al* (1983) The relationship between prolactin levels and clinical ratings in manic patients treated with oral and intravenous test doses of haloperidol. *Psychological Medicine*, **13**, 279–285.

Cookson, J. C., Silverstone, T., Williams, S., *et al* (1985) Plasma corticol levels in mania: associated clinical ratings and change during treatment with haloperidol. *British Journal of Psychiatry*, **146**, 498–502.

Coppen, A. & Abou-Saleh, M. T. (1988) Lithium therapy: from clinical trials to practical management. *Acta Psychiatrica Scandinavica*, **78**, 754–762.

Coppen, A., Noguera, R., Bailey, J., *et al* (1971) Prophylactic lithium in affective disorders: controlled trial. *Lancet*, *ii*, 275–279.

Coppen, A., Standish-Barry, H., Bailey, J., *et al* (1991) Does lithium reduce the mortality of recurrent mood disorders? *Journal of Affective Disorders*, **23**, 1–7.

Coryell, W., Solomon, D., Turvey, C., *et al* (2003) The long-term course of rapid-cycling bipolar disorder. *Archives of General Psychiatry*, **60**, 914–920.

Davis, J. M., Janicak, P. G., Hogan, D. M. (1999) Mood stabilizers in the prevention of recurrent affective disorders: a meta-analysis. *Acta Psychiatrica Scandinavica*, **100**, 406–417.

Dickson, W. E. & Kendell, R. E. (1986) Does maintenance lithium therapy prevent recurrences of mania under ordinary clinical conditions? *Psychological Medicine*, **16**, 521–530.

Dilsaver, S. C., Chen, R., Shoaib, A. M., *et al* (1999) Phenomenology of mania: evidence for distinct depressed, dysphoric, and euphoric presentations. *American Journal of Psychiatry*, **156**, 426–430.

Dinan, T. G. & Kohen, D. (1989) Tardive dyskinesia and bipolar affective disorder: relationship to lithium therapy. *British Journal of Psychiatry*, **155**, 55–57.

Double, D. B. (1990) The factor structure of manic rating scales. *Journal of Affective Disorders*, **18**, 113–119.

Dunner, D. L. & Fieve, R. R. (1974) Clinical factors in lithium prophylaxis failure. *Archives of General Psychiatry*, **30**, 229–233.

Dunner, D. L., Fleiss, J. L. & Fieve, R. R. (1976*a*) Lithium carbonate prophylaxis failure. *British Journal of Psychiatry*, **129**, 40–44.

Dunner, D. L., Gershon, E. S. & Goodwin, F. K. (1976*b*) Heritable factors in the severity of affective illness. *Biological Psychiatry*, **11**, 31–42.

Erikson, E. H. (1958) *Young Man Luther.* New York: W. W. Norton.

Faedda, G. L., Baldessarini, R. J., Tohen, M., *et al* (1991) Episode sequence in bipolar disorder and response to lithium treatment. *American Journal of Psychiatry*, **148**, 1237–1239.

Freud, S. (1917) Mourning and melancholia. Reprinted (1953–1974) in *Standard Edition of the Complete Psychological Works of Sigmund Freud* (trans. and ed. J. Strachey), vol. 14, p. 239. London: Hogarth Press.

Geddes, J. R., Burgess, S., Hawton, K., *et al* (2004) Long-term lithium therapy for bipolar disorder: systematic review and meta-analysis of randomized controlled trials. *American Journal of Psychiatry*, **161**, 217–222.

Gelenberg, A. J., Kane, J. M., Keller, M. B., *et al* (1989) Comparison of standard and low serum levels of lithium for maintenance treatment of bipolar disorder. *New England Journal of Medicine*, **321**, 1489–1493.

Geller, B., Craney, J. L., Bolhofner, K., *et al* (2001) One-year recovery and relapse rates of children with a prepubertal and early adolescent bipolar disorder phenotype. *American Journal of Psychiatry*, **158**, 303–305.

Gerner, R. H., Post, R. M. & Bunney, W. E. (1976) A dopaminergic mechanism in mania. *American Journal of Psychiatry*, **133**, 1177–1180.

Goodwin, F. K. & Jamison, K. R. (1990) *Manic–Depressive Illness*. Oxford University Press.

Goodwin, F. K., Fireman, B., Simon, G. E., *et al* (2003) Suicide risk in bipolar disorder during treatment with lithium and divalproex. *JAMA*, **290**, 1467–1473.

Goodwin, G. M. (2002) Hypomania: what's in a name? *British Journal of Psychiatry*, **181**, 94–95.

Goodwin, G. M. & BAP (2003) Evidence-based guidelines for treating bipolar disorder: recommendations from the British Association for Psychopharmacology. *Journal of Psychopharmacology*, **17**, 149–173.

Greil, W. & Kleindienst, N. (1999) Lithium versus carbamazepine in the maintenance treatment of bipolar II disorder and bipolar disorder not otherwise specified. *International Clinical Psychopharmacology*, **14**, 283–285.

Greil, W., Kleindienst, N., Erazo, N., *et al* (1998) Differential response to lithium and carbamazepine in the prophylaxis of bipolar disorder. *Journal of Clinical Psychopharmacology*, **18**, 455–460.

Grof, P., Alda, M., Grof, E., *et al* (1993) The challenge of predicting response to stabilising lithium treatment. The importance of patient selection. *British Journal of Psychiatry*, **163**, suppl. 21, 16–19.

Grunze, H., Kasper, S., Goodwin, G., *et al* (2003) World Federation of Societies of Biological Psychiatry (WFSBP) guidelines for the biological treatment of bipolar disorders, part II: treatment of mania. *World Journal of Biological Psychiatry*, **4**, 5–13.

Hamilton, I. (1982) *Robert Lowell: A Biography*. New York: Random House.

Hansen, H. E. & Amdisen, A. (1978) Lithium intoxication (report of 23 cases and a review of 100 cases from the literature). *Quarterly Journal of Medicine*, **47**, 123–144.

Hare, E. (1981) The two manias: a study of the evolution of the modern concept of mania. *British Journal of Psychiatry*, **138**, 89–99.

Hartong, E. G., Moleman, P., Hoogduin, C. A. L., *et al* (2003) Prophylactic efficacy of lithium versus carbamazepine in treatment-naïve bipolar patients. *Journal of Clinical Psychiatry*, **64**, 144–151.

Hill, C. (1970) *God's Englishman*. London: Weidenfeld and Nicholson.

Hirschfeld, R. M. A., Bowden, C. L., Gitlin, M. J., *et al* (2002) American Psychiatric Association Practice Guideline for the Treatment of Patients with Bipolar Disorder (revision) (2nd edn). *American Journal of Psychiatry*, **159**, 1–50.

Horn, A. S., Coyle, J. T. & Snyder, S. H. (1971) Catecholamine uptake by synaptosomes from rat brain. Structure–activity relationships of drugs with differential effects on dopamine and norepinephrine neurones. *Molecular Pharmacology*, **7**, 66–80.

Hunt, N. & Silverstone, T. (1991) Tardive dyskinesia in bipolar affective disorder: a catchment area study. *International Clinical Psychopharmacology*, **6**, 45–50.

Hunt, N., Bruce-Jones, W. & Silverstone, T. (1992*a*) Life events in bipolar affective disorder. *Journal of Affective Disorders*, **25**, 13–20.

Hunt, N., Sayer, H. & Silverstone, T. (1992*b*) Season and manic relapse. *Acta Psychiatrica Scandinavica*, **85**, 123–126.

Jacobs, D. & Silverstone, T. (1986) Dextroamphetamine-induced arousal in human subjects as a model for mania. *Psychological Medicine*, **16**, 323–329.

Jacobson, S. J., Jones, K., Johnson, K., *et al* (1992) Prospective multi-centre study of pregnancy outcome after lithium exposure during first trimester. *Lancet*, **339**, 530–533.

Jamison, K. R. (1989) Mood disorders and seasonal patterns in British writers and artists. *Psychiatry*, **52**, 125–134.

Jamison, K. R. (1993) *Touched with Fire: Manic–Depressive Illness and the Artistic Temperament*. New York: Simon and Shuster.

Janowsky, D. S., El-Yousef, M. K., Davis, J. M., *et al* (1973) Parasympathetic suppression of manic symptoms by physostigmine. *Archives of General Psychiatry*, **28**, 542–547.

Janowsky, D. S., El-Yousef, M. K. & Davis, J. M. (1974) Interpersonal manoeuvers of manic patients. *American Journal of Psychiatry*, **131**, 250–255.

Jauhar, P. & Weller, M. P. I. (1982) Psychiatric morbidity and time zone changes: a study of patients from Heathrow Airport. *British Journal of Psychiatry*, **140**, 231–235.

Jha, A. K., Stein, G. S. & Fenwick, P. (1996) Negative interaction between lithium and electroconvulsion therapy. A case-controlled study. *British Journal of Psychiatry*, **168**, 241–243.

Johnson, D. A. W., Lowe, M. R. & Batchelor, D. H. (1990) Combined lithium–neuroleptic therapy for manic–depressive illness. *Human Psychopharmacology*, **5** (suppl.), 262–297.

Josephson, A. M. & Mackenzie, T. B. (1979) Appearance of manic psychosis following rapid normalization of thyroid status. *American Journal of Psychiatry*, **136**, 846–847.

Kahlbaum, K. L. (1874) *Catatonia*. Baltimore, MA: Johns Hopkins University Press (1974).

Kallen, B. & Tandberg, A. (1983) Lithium and pregnancy: a cohort study on manic–depressive women. *Acta Psychiatrica Scandinavica*, **68**, 134–139.

Keller, M. B., Lavery, T. W., Kane, J. M., *et al* (1992) Sub syndromal symptoms in bipolar disorder. A comparison of standard and low-serum levels of lithium. *Archives of General Psychiatry*, **49**, 371–376.

Kellner, C. H., Pritchett, J. T., Beale, M. D., *et al* (1997) *Handbook of ECT*. Washington, DC: APA.

Kessing, L. V., Anderson, K. A., Mortensen, P. B., *et al* (1998) Recurrence in affective disorder. I. Case register study. *British Journal of Psychiatry*, **172**, 23–28.

Koukopoulos, A. (2002) Prognosis and manic–depressive cycle. In *Bipolar Disorder* (ed. M. Maj, H. S. Akiskal, J. J. Lopez-Ibor & N. Sartorius), pp. 168–171. WPA Series: Evidence and Experience in Psychiatry. Chichester: Wiley.

Kraepelin, E. (1921) *Manic Depression Insanity and Paranoia* (trans. R. M. Barclay, ed. G. M. Robertson). Edinburgh: E. & S. Livingstone. (Reprinted New York: Arno Press, 1976).

Kramlinger, K. G. & Post, R. M. (1996) Ultra-rapid and ultradian cycling in bipolar affective illness. *British Journal of Psychiatry*, **168**, 314–323.

Krauthammer, C. & Klerman, G. L. (1978) Secondary mania: manic syndromes associated with antecedent physical illness or drugs. *Archives of General Psychiatry*, **35**, 1333–1339.

Kupfer, D. J., Frank, E., Grochocinski, V. J., *et al* (2000) Stabilization in the treatment of mania, depression and mixed states. *Acta Neuropsychiatrica*, **12**, 112–116.

Lehmann, J. (1987) *Virginia Woolf*. London: Thames and Hudson.

Lerner, Y. (1980) The subjective experience of mania. In *Mania: An Evolving Concept* (eds R. H. Belmaker & H. M. Van Praag), pp. 77–88. Jamaica, NY: Spectrum Publications.

Lewin, B. (1951) *The Psychoanalysis of Elation*. London: Hogarth Press.

Littlejohn, R., Leslie, F. & Cookson, J. (1994) Depot antipsychotics in the prophylaxis of bipolar affective disorder. *British Journal of Psychiatry*, **165**, 827–829.

Loudon, J. B. & Waring, H. (1976) Toxic reactions to lithium and haloperidol. *Lancet*, *ii*, 1088.

Lowe, M. R. & Batchelor, D. H. (1990) Lithium and neuroleptics in the management of manic–depressive psychosis. *Human Psychopharmacology*, **5**, 267–274.

Magliano, L., Pirozzi, R., Marasco, C., *et al* (1997) Chronic mania: family history, prior course, clinical picture and social consequences. *British Journal of Psychiatry*, **173**, 514–518.

Maggs, R. (1963) Treatment of manic illness with lithium carbonate. *British Journal of Psychiatry*, **109**, 56–65.

Maj, M., Magliano, L., Pirozzi, R., *et al* (1994) Validity of rapid cycling as a course specifier for bipolar disorder. *American Journal of Psychiatry*, **151**, 1015–1019.

Maj, M., Pirozzi, R., Magliano, L., *et al* (1998) Long-term outcome of lithium prophylaxis in bipolar disorder: a 5-year prospective study of 402 patients at a lithium clinic. *American Jouranl of Psychiatry*, **155**, 30–35.

Mander, A. J. & Loudon, J. B. (1988) Rapid recurrence of mania following abrupt discontinuation of lithium. *Lancet*, *ii*, 15–17.

Marneros, A. (2000) Bipolar disorder: roots and evolution. In *Bipolar Disorders. 100 Years After Manic Depressive Insanity* (eds A. Marneros & J. Angst). Dordrecht: Kluwer Academic Publishers.

McCreadie, R. G. & Morrison, D. P. (1985) The impact of lithium in South-West Scotland. *British Journal of Psychiatry*, **146**, 70–74.

Milligan, S. & Clare, A. (1993) *Depression and How to Survive It*. London: Ebury Press.

Mitchell, J. E. & MacKenzie, T. B. (1982) Cardiac effects of lithium therapy in man: a review. *Journal of Clinical Psychiatry*, **43**, 47–51.

National Institute for Health and Clinical Excellence (2006) *Bipolar Disorder: The Management of Bipolar Disorder in Adults, Children and Adolescents, in Primary and Secondary Care*. NICE clinical guideline 38. London: NICE.

Okuma, T., Kishimoto, A., Inoue, K., *et al* (1973) Anti-manic and prophylactic effects of carbamazepine (Tegretol) on manic depressive psychosis: a preliminary report. *Folia Psychiatrica Neurology Japan*, **27**, 283–297.

Okuma, T., Inanaga, K., Otsuki, S., *et al* (1981) A preliminary double-blind study of carbamazepine in prophylaxis of manic–depressive illness. *Psychopharmacology*, **73**, 95–96.

Plath, S. & Schober Plath, A. (1992) *Letters Home by Sylvia Plath: Correspondence 1950–1963*. New York: Harper.

Pope, H. G., McElroy, S. L., Keck, P. E., *et al* (1991) Valproate in the treatment of acute mania: a placebo-controlled study. *Archives of General Psychiatry*, **48**, 62–68.

Post, R. M. (1992) Trans-duction of psychosocial stress into the neurobiology of recurrent affective disorder. *American Journal of Psychiatry*, **149**, 999–1010.

Post, R. M., Uhde, T. W., Ballenger, J. C., *et al* (1983) Prophylactic efficacy of carbamazepine in manic–depressive illness. *American Journal of Psychiatry*, **140**, 1602–1604.

Post, R. M., Roy-Byrne, P. P. & Uhde, T. W. (1988) Graphic representation of the life causes of illness in patients with affective disorder. *American Journal of Psychiatry*, **145**, 844–848.

Post, R. M., Rubinow, D. R., Uhde, T. W., *et al* (1989) Dysphoric mania: clinical and biological correlates. *Archives of General Psychiatry*, **46**, 353–358.

Poynton, A., Bridges, P. & Bartlett, J. R. (1988) Resistant bipolar affective disorder treated by stereotactic subcaudate tractotomy. *British Journal of Psychiatry*, **152**, 354–358.

Prien, R. F., Caffey, E. M. Jr & Klett, C. J. (1973) Prophylactic efficacy of lithium carbonate in manic–depressive illness. *Archives of General Psychiatry*, **28**, 337–341.

Reichart, C. G., Nolen, W. A., Wals, M., *et al* (2000) Bipolar disorder in children and adolescents: a clinical reality? *Acta Neuropsychiatrica*, **12**, 132–135.

Rosenthal, N. E., Sack, D. A., Gillin, J. C., *et al* (1984) Seasonal affective disorder. *Archives of General Psychiatry*, **4**, 72–80.

Schou, M. (1979) Artistic productivity and lithium prophylaxis in manic–depressive illness. *British Journal of Psychiatry*, **135**, 97–103.

Schou, M. (1984) Long-lasting neurological sequelae after lithium intoxication. *Acta Psychiatrica Scandinavica*, **70**, 594–602.

Schou, M., Juel-Nielsenn, N., Stromgren E., *et al* (1954) The treatment of manic psychoses by the administration of lithium salts. *Journal of Neurology Neurosurgery and Psychiatry*, **17**, 250–260.

Sclare, P. & Creed, F. (1987) Life events and the onset of mania. *British Journal of Psychiatry*, **156**, 508–514.

Segal, H. (1975) *Introduction to the Works of Melanie Klein*. London: Hogarth Press.

Sellers, J., Tyrer, P., Whiteley, A., *et al* (1982) Neurotoxic effects of lithium with delayed rise in serum lithium levels. *British Journal of Psychiatry*, **140**, 623–625.

Sernetti, A., Rietchel, M., Lattuada, E., *et al* (1999) Factor analysis of mania. *Archives of General Psychiatry*, **56**, 671–672.

Shorter, E. (1997) *A History of Psychiatry: From the Age of the Asylum to the Era of Prozac*. New York: Wiley.

Shukla, S., Godwin, C. D., Long, L. E. B., *et al* (1985) Lithium–carbamazepine neurotoxicity and risk factors. *American Journal of Psychiatry*, **141**, 1604–1606.

Small, J. G., Klapper, M. H., Kellams, J. J., *et al* (1988) Electroconvulsive treatment compared with lithium in the management of manic states. *Archives of General Psychiatry*, **45**, 727–732.

Smith, S. J. M. & Kocen, R. S. (1988) A Creutzfeldt–Jakob like syndrome due to lithium toxicity. *Journal of Neurology, Neurosurgery, and Psychiatry*, **51**, 120–123.

Soames, M. (1993) Life with my father Winston. *The Observer*, 14 February, pp. 49–50.

Spitzer, R. L., Endicott, J. & Robins, E. (1978) Research diagnostic criteria: rationale and reliability. *Archives of General Psychiatry*, **35**, 773–782.

Stokes, P. E., Kocsis, J. H. & Arcuni, O. J. (1976) Relationship of lithium chloride dose to treatment response in acute mania. *Archives of General Psychiatry*, **33**, 1080–1084.

Storr, A. (1969) *Churchill's Black Dog and Other Phenomena of the Human Mind*, pp. 3–51. London: HarperCollins.

Suppes, T., Webb, A., Paul, B., *et al* (1999) Clinical outcome in a randomized 1-year trial of clozapine versus treatment as usual for patients with treatment-resistant illness and a history of mania. *American Journal of Psychiatry*, **156**, 1164–1169.

Tohen, M., Hennen, J., Zarate, C. M. Jr, *et al* (2000) Two-year syndromal and functional recovery in 219 cases of first-episode major affective disorder with psychotic features. *American Journal of Psychiatry*, **157**, 220–228.

Tohen, M., Baker, R. W., Altshuler, L. L., *et al* (2002) Olanzapine versus divalproex in the treatment of acute mania. *American Journal of Psychiatry*, **159**, 1011–1017.

Tohen, M., Zarate, C. A., Hennen, J., *et al* (2003) The McLean–Harvard First-Episode Mania Study: prediction of recovery and first recurrence. *American Journal of Psychiatry*, **160**, 2099–2107.

Tohen, M., Chengappa, K. N. R., Suppes, T., *et al* (2004) Relapse prevention in bipolar I disorder: 18-month comparison of olanzapine plus mood stabiliser v. mood stabiliser alone. *British Journal of Psychiatry*, **184**, 337–345.

Tohen, M., Calabrese, J. R., Sachs, G. S., *et al* (2006) Randomized, placebo-controlled trial of olanzapine as maintenance therapy in patients with bipolar I disorder responding to acute treatment with olanzapine. *American Journal of Psychiatry*, **163**, 247–256.

Turner, T., Cookson, J. C., Wass, J. A. H., *et al* (1984) Psychotic reactions during treatment of pituitary tumours with dopamine agonists. *BMJ*, **289**, 1101–1103.

Tyrer, P., Alexander, M. S., Regan, A., *et al* (1980) An extrapyramidal syndrome after lithium therapy. *British Journal of Psychiatry*, **136**, 191–194.

Viguera, A., Nonacs, R., Cohen, L. S., *et al* (2000) Risk of recurrence of bipolar disorder in pregnant and nonpregnant women after discontinuing lithium maintenance. *American Journal of Psychiatry*, **157**, 179–184.

Von Knorring, L. (1990) Possible mechanisms for the presumed interaction between lithium and neuroleptics. *Human Psychopharmacology*, **5**, 287–292.

Wehr, T. A. & Goodwin, F. K. (1979) Rapid cycling in manic–depressives induced by tricyclic antidepressants. *Archives of General Psychiatry*, **36**, 555–559.

Wehr, T. A., Sack, D. A. & Rosenthal, N. E. (1987) Sleep reduction as a final common pathway in the genesis of mania. *American Journal of Psychiatry*, **144**, 201–204.

Wehr, T. A., Sack, D. A., Rosenthal, N. E., *et al* (1988) Rapid cycling affective disorder: contributing factors and treatment responses in 51 patients. *American Journal of Psychiatry*, **145**, 179–184.

Weisler, R. H., Kalali, A. H., Ketter, T. A., *et al* (2004) A multicentre, randomised, double-blind, placebo-controlled trial of extended-release carbamazepine capsules as monotherapy in bipolar disorder patients with manic or mixed episodes. *Journal of Clinical Psychiatry*, **65**, 478–484.

Weisler, R. H., Keck, P. E., Swann, A. C., *et al* (2005) Extended-release carbamazepine capsules as monotherapy for acute mania in bipolar disorder: a multi-centre, randomised, double-blind, placebo-controlled trial. *Journal of Clinical Psychiatry*, **66**, 323–330.

West, A. P. & Meltzer, H. Y. (1979) Paradoxical lithium neurotoxicity: a report of five cases and a hypothesis about risk for neurotoxicity. *American Journal of Psychiatry*, **136**, 963–966.

World Health Organization (1992) *International Classification of Diseases* (10th revision) (ICD–10). Geneva: WHO.

Young, R. C., Biggs, J. T., Ziegler, V. E., *et al* (1978) A rating scale for mania: reliability, validity and sensitivity. *British Journal of Psychiatry*, **133**, 429–435.

CHAPTER 3

The causes of depression

Kezia Lange and Anne Farmer

Introduction and history

Around one in four women and one in ten men in the UK are likely to suffer a period of depression that requires treatment (National Institute for Clinical Excellence, 2003) and today depression is ranked as the fourth leading cause of burden among all diseases. It is expected to show a rising trend over the next 20 years, so that, according to the predictions of the World Health Organization (WHO), by 2020 depression will be second only to heart disease in the ranking of diseases causing years lived with disability.

In this chapter we highlight the biological, social and psychological hypotheses relating to the causes of depression, as well as their history, and outline current research support for the various theories.

One of the great fascinations of the history of ideas regarding the causes of depression is to see the extent to which our present-day notions of aetiology find their roots in the distant past, even though these earlier formulations lacked any research evidence. Thus, Hippocrates, as early as 400 BC, in his treatise *The Nature of Man*, identified mania as being due to yellow bile and melancholia due to an excess of black bile, a bitter humour produced in the spleen. Later humoral theories included toxic causes, theories of electrolyte imbalance, hormonal causation and most recently theories of monoamine depletion.

Notions of evil and sin associated with depression start in the Old Testament, with the 'evil spirit' that descended on King Saul, but which could be soothed by David, playing on his harp. In the early Christian period a condition known as *acedia*, characterised by dejection and disgust, was described and it was thought to be one of the seven deadly sins. However, in the 5th century Pope Gregory the Great distinguished acedia from the other deadly sins, as he considered it to require medical care, and in so doing made one of the first distinctions between mental disorder and sin. Acedia was still equated with sadness and laziness, and the term continued to be used up until the time of St Thomas Aquinas in the Middle Ages, and the descriptions of acedia provide some insight into how depression was conceived by the early church (Alliez & Huber, 1987).

The modern era of study of both the phenomenology and the aetiology of depression probably starts with Robert Burton's (1577–1640) masterpiece *The Anatomy of Melancholy*, subtitled *'what it is, with all kinds of causes, symptoms and prognosticks and several cures of it'*. Burton was the vicar of Christ Church, Oxford, and his book was an encyclopaedia with more than 1000 citations, but much of it was based on his own experience of depression or, as he put it:

> 'others get their knowledge by books, I mine by melancholizing ... that which others hear or read of, I felt and practised myself.'

Burton was a keen observer of the clinical material he saw and his account of its hereditary origin includes a description of its sporadic yet familial appearance, its similarities across generations, as well as the occasional appearance of depressive equivalents, which he calls symbolising disease:

> 'That other inbred cause of melancholy is our temperature in whole or in part which we receive from our parents ... it being an hereditary disease. Such is the temperature of the father such is the son; and look what the father had when he begot him, such his son will have after him. Now this doth not so much appear in the composition of the body, but in manners and conditions of the mind. And what is more, it skips in some families the father and goes to the son or takes every other and sometimes every third in linear descent and does not always produce the same but some like and symbolising disease.' (Hunter & Macalpine, 1963, pp. 95–97)

Burton favoured no particular theory of causation and wrote extensively only on the clinical material he saw. Thus, following on from his section on hereditary influences he went described the importance of child abuse:

> 'Parents and such as they have the tuition and oversight of children, offend many times in that they are stern, always threatening, brawling, whipping or striking; by means of which their poor children are so disheartened and cowed that they never after have any courage or a merry hour in their lives or take pleasure in anything.'

He also wrote about bereavement, separations and other losses which modern research has termed 'exit events':

> 'A heap of other accidents ... causing melancholy, amongst which loss and death of friends may challenge a first place.... If the parting of friends, and absence can work such violent effects, what shall death do when they must be eternally separated forever never to meet again.... There is another sorrow which arises from the loss of temporal goods and fortunes which equally afflicts; loss of time, loss of honour, loss of office, of good name, of labour, these will frustrate hope and cause much torment.' (Brink, 1979)

Modern genetic research hinges to a great extent on twin studies and the first report of a monozygotic twin pair concordant for 'affective' disorder is thought to have been given in 1812 by Benjamin Rush, Professor of Chemistry and the Practise of Physic at the University of Pennsylvania, and one of the signatories of the American Constitution. He described a pair of identical twins, C and L, who both rose to the level of captain in the American Civil War but who both became deranged in their mid-30s, and then both committed suicide by slitting there throats within 2 years of each other, even though they lived 200 miles apart. Rush went on to state that the mother of the twins and two other sisters were also deranged and had been for many years (Hunter & Macalpine, 1963, pp. 663–669).

An example of one of the many early neuropsychiatric explanations is that credited to Nicholas Robinson (1707–75), a governor of Bethlem, who proposed the nerve fibres were in a convulsive state. He wrote:

> 'as in cases of hypochondriac melancholy, natural melancholy and religious melancholy, the *machinulae* of the Fibres that compose the brain and organs of several senses were disconcerted and set at too great a distance from each other, so in this lunacy, their springs are drawn too near each other, that is the fibres are too much under a convulsive state or violent contraction.' (Hunter & Macalpine, 1963, p. 347)

He went on to describe the cure, which was 'bringing the *machinulae* to their natural standard by bleeding, purging and medicines of the harsher operation'. The later 19th-century literature provided a large number of other neuropsychiatric formulations; these were summarised by Hollander in a paper entitled 'The cerebral localization of melancholia (Hollander, 1901), which placed the locus for melancholia in the central area of the parietal lobe, particularly the angular and supra marginal gyri. A present-day review, which might easily bear a similar title, might place the locus more in the frontal lobes and the limbic system, as well as have some scanning evidence from magnetic resonance imaging (MRI) in its support, but it is of interest to see that theories of cerebral localisation for depression have been around for a very long time. Other 20th-century developments, such as Freud's more exclusive psychological approach, are described later in this chapter, while the discovery of antidepressants and the monoamine theory are described in Chapter 4.

Epidemiological studies

Epidemiological data are not only useful for identifying rates of a given illness, but can also be used for analysing patterns of distribution, and for identifying possible risk factors. Although the discovery of an association of a risk factor with a particular disorder does not establish causation, it may provide a first step in developing illness models and provide an impetus for further research.

Treatment/admission studies

The review by the National Institute of Clinical Excellence (2003) provides some information on the treated prevalence of depression in the UK. Of the estimated 130 cases of depression (including mild cases) per 1000 of the population, only 80 will consult their general practitioner (GP). Of these 80 cases, 49 will not be recognised, mainly because most such patients are consulting for a somatic symptom. The majority of those recognised as depressed are treated in general practice: only 1 in 4 or 5 is referred to secondary care. Only 1–2 per 1000 of the population will have psychotic depression, and around 1 per 1000 will be admitted for depression (Bebbington, 1978). It should be noted that the latter figure is almost 30 years old and so the present admission rate for depression may be lower still. More recently, among a sample of 75 858 people attending their primary care physician in the USA, researchers found an overall prevalence of clinically significant depressive symptoms (as measured on the Zung self-rating depression scale) of 20.9%, although only 1.2% of the sample cited depression as the reason for attending their doctor (Zung *et al*, 1993).

Although hospital studies have largely been superseded by community surveys, treatment/admission reviews confirm the considerable morbidity associated with depression: the median prevalence of chronicity (symptoms persisting for 2 or more years) in those treated for depression in hospital is 16% (Scott, 1988) and 5–15% of new long-stay patients have a primary diagnosis of affective disorder.

Community studies

The first structured diagnostic interview that could be used by lay interviewers to generate diagnoses according to DSM definitions and criteria was the Diagnostic Interview Schedule (DIS). This was first used in the Epidemiologic Catchment Area (ECA) study (Robins & Regier, 1991), which surveyed the prevalence and correlates of a wide range of psychiatric conditions. This important study generated a number of similar surveys around the world, which were brought together by the Cross-National Collaborative Group.

In the mid-1980s the WHO set up a working group which, together with the US Public Health Service, aimed to develop a fully structured research diagnostic interview that could generate reliable and valid diagnoses (including those of the *International Classification of Diseases*) in a variety of languages. The new instrument, the Composite International Diagnostic Interview (CIDI; Robins *et al*, 1989) was released in 1990 and further refined to include DSM-IV criteria in 1997. Versions of the CIDI have been used in a number of large, well-conducted studies, most notably the National Comorbidity Survey in the USA, and the International Consortium in Psychiatric Epidemiology (ICPE) was set up by the WHO to coordinate the analysis of worldwide data (Kessler, 1999). The results of the 10 national ICPE surveys, which had a combined total of approximately 37 000 respondents, demonstrated a wide variation in the estimate of the lifetime prevalence of major depression, from 3% (in Japan) to 16.9% (in the USA), with five surveys reporting prevalence between 5% and 10% (Andrade *et al*, 2003).

This variation between countries is consistent with the earlier results of the Cross-National Collaborative Group, again with the lowest prevalence in Asian communities. This may reflect differences in risk factors

Box 3.1 Clinical implications of epidemiological surveys

Large epidemiological surveys such as those described are not only useful in providing evidence for the clinical burden of disease, but the socio-demographic data collected at the same time provide associations which may identify risk factors for depression. Careful study of the disorder across populations and across time also facilitates understanding of the variability in course and outcome. This has practical implications for the management of individual patients, especially when discussing prognosis. Counting 'cases' across large populations as well as frequency of disorders in specific subgroups also allows health service planners to assess the need for care and facilities.

for depression or methodological failings, such as the cultural validity of DSM criteria.

In the ICPE surveys, the 12-month prevalence estimates for depression ranged from 1.2% in Japan to 10% in the USA and the 30-day prevalence was in the range 0.9–4.6%. These results are in keeping with older studies which reported 12-month prevalence as between one-half and one-third of the lifetime prevalence, suggesting that major depression is a chronic disorder, and a similar ratio of 30-day prevalence to 12-month prevalence, suggesting that major depression is intermittent, with sufferers experiencing recurrent episodes lasting less than 1 year (Andrade *et al*, 2003).

In Britain, 10 108 adults from a random sample of households were interviewed as part of the National Psychiatric Morbidity Survey. Lay interviewers used the Revised Clinical Interview Schedule to estimate the 1-week prevalence of 'neurotic' psychiatric disorder. The overall 1-week prevalence was 16%, with just over 2% suffering from a depressive disorder and over 8% mixed anxiety/depression (Jenkins *et al*, 2003).

A recent major epidemiological survey of depression was the National Comorbidity Survey Replication (NCS-R) (Kessler *et al*, 2003), a nationally representative household survey conducted in 2001–02 of 9090 adults (i.e. aged over 18 years) living in the USA. A revised form of the CIDI, which took into account the increased emphasis on the 'clinical significance' of symptoms in DSM–IV, was used and a proportion of the sample was reappraised with the Structured Clinical Interview for DSM–IV (SCID) (Kessler *et al*, 2003). Despite the prediction that the previous NCS had significantly overestimated the prevalence of depression, due to the inclusion of clinically insignificant mild cases, the NCS-R prevalence estimates for depression were 16.2% for lifetime and 6.6% for the 12 months before the interview, compared with the NCS estimates of 14.9% and 8.6%, respectively.

Socio-demographic risk factors

Gender

One of the most robust socio-demographic associations is the significant female predominance in rates of unipolar disorder (Bebbington, 2003). These differences appear at the time of puberty and most evidence suggests they continue across the age spectrum, including into old age. Since several studies have shown that these differences are similar in community and primary care studies, are mainly consistent across cultures (although there are some exceptions – see Chapter 31, p. 791) and are persistent over time, the results are unlikely to represent biases in help-seeking behaviour (Maier *et al*, 1999). The finding of a gender difference is not adequately explained by genetics and there is conflicting evidence for the role of sex hormones. Sex differences for depression appear only after puberty. Before this developmental milestone, as for most childhood psychiatric disorders, rates in boys usually exceed rates in girls.

Explanations of this gender imbalance have mainly focused on psychosocial and intrapsychic risk factors: women are more likely to experience childhood sexual abuse, poverty, poor education, role overload and a lack of decision-making, all of which have been linked to depression. A recent review suggests that in societies where the role of women is valued similarly to that of men, the sex ratio in depression rates is reduced or eliminated (Piccinelli & Wilkinson, 2000) and in a primary care study the sex ratio was halved when social role inequalities were controlled for (Maier *et al*, 1999). Cognitive hypotheses suggest that women are cognitively more vulnerable to some psychosocial stressors, one example being that women may have a ruminating coping style, which has been linked to depression (Hankin & Abramson, 2001).

Socio-economic status

Previous examinations of a possible association between social class and affective disorders have been hampered by a number of confounding variables, such as treatment biases (those of lower social class are less likely to obtain treatment) and difficulties in accurately defining social class. None the less, community studies of milder depressions and dysthymia have confirmed a relationship between depression and social disadvantage and a review by Smith & Weissman (1992) suggested that a higher level of education, employment and financial independence were associated with lower rates of depression.

A recent meta-analysis of population-based studies of the prevalence of depression demonstrated that the odds of being depressed were nearly doubled among people of low socio-economic status, and that the association was particularly strong with persistent depression (Lorant *et al*, 2003). Most of the studies in this meta-analysis were based on North American populations. The ICPE surveys found that this inverse relationship between family income and the prevalence of major depression existed in the USA and the Netherlands, but no such association was found in the other three countries where family income had been measured. The link between lack of education and depression was found in only 2 out of 10 ICPE countries, indicating that the link between socio-economic factors and depression is far from solid.

Explanations for the association between depression and socio-economic disadvantage include the 'social causation' theory (depression is caused by the stress of poverty, unemployment, etc.) and the 'social selection' theory (social drift in those with a vulnerability to depression) (Johnson *et al*, 1999).

Ethnicity

When socio-economic and education variables are controlled for, there is minimal evidence of racial or ethnic differences in the prevalence of depression (Somervell *et al*, 1989; Jenkins *et al*, 2003). It has been suggested that previously reported differences related more to biases in sample selection or misdiagnosis of individuals from black or other ethnic minorities (Neighbors *et al*, 1989). This topic is further discussed in Chapter 30.

Geography

Trends in the differences in depression rates between urban and rural locations are largely in the expected direction, with several studies in Britain, the USA and other countries (e.g. Puerto Rico) showing significantly higher rates of depression in urban areas. However, the NCS-R study in the USA showed that depressive disorder was largely unrelated to region of country or urbanicity (Kessler *et al*, 2003) and in the ICPE surveys in only one out of the six countries in which rural–urban differences were studied was the urban excess of depression statistically significant (Andrade *et al*, 2003). There is some evidence that areas in transition from rural to more industrialised environments show particularly high morbidity rates.

Genetics

Enough convincing genetic work has been carried out to confirm the hypothesis that genetic factors play an important role in the causation of the affective disorders. The strongest evidence for the role of genes is for bipolar affective disorder (see below) but there is also good evidence for gene involvement in unipolar depression.

There have been many recent advances in our knowledge of genes, their effects and their relationship with brain function. The traditional approach in epidemiological genetics has consisted of twin, family and adoption studies, which offer the prospect of studying the interplay between genes and the environment (see Chapter 10, pages 205–210, for an explanation of these methods). In addition, recombinant DNA technology has produced major advances in psychiatric genetics, as it is now possible to screen chromosomes for susceptible genes. These techniques may be applied to the study of pedigrees, which brings the hope of identifying gene defects at the level of abnormal nucleotide sequencing, which should help to clarify the mechanisms of disease as well as to promote the development of novel or better-targeted treatments.

Family studies

Much of the earlier evidence for the importance of genetic risk factors in the aetiology of affective disorders was derived from family studies. With this method, the morbid risk (adjusted prevalence) of the illness is determined within families and rates of occurrence in the different classes of relative are compared with those of the general population.

An early meta-analysis by McGuffin & Katz (1989) pooled results from a large number of studies and concluded that the risk of developing bipolar illness in the first-degree relatives of bipolar probands is elevated (at approximately 7%), while the first-degree relatives of unipolar probands have a risk for bipolar illness no higher than that of the general population (0.7%). The morbid risk of unipolar depression in the first-degree relatives of bipolar and unipolar probands was 11.5% and 9.1%, respectively.

More recently, Sullivan *et al* (2000) conducted a meta-analysis of genetic epidemiology studies of major depression and found familial aggregation in the rigorously conducted studies, with strong evidence for an association between major depression in the proband and major depression in first-degree relatives: the odds ratio (OR) across five studies was 2.84.

Family studies serve another useful purpose: because large numbers are studied, subgroups and 'risk factors' can be identified. One reasonably consistent finding is the association between early onset of depression and increased morbid risk in relatives (Sullivan *et al*, 2000), although it has been suggested that very early onset depression (prepubertal) is associated with less genetic loading (Harrington *et al*, 1997). Confirming the findings of population-based epidemiological studies, family studies also demonstrate a gender bias, with more women being affected than men (Weissman *et al*, 1984), although the rates of depression among relatives does not appear to be affected by the sex of the proband. Some early family studies suggested an increased risk of depression in families with a history of alcoholism or antisocial behaviour in male members of the family and anxiety disorder in female ones, identifying a 'depressive spectrum' of genetic risk (discussed below, on pages 60–61), but this has not been consistently supported by subsequent studies (Merikangas & Gelernter, 1990).

In the past it has been assumed that depression arising for no apparent reason ('endogenous') is more 'genetic' than that following stress or adverse life events ('reactive'). However, a comparison between the frequency of depression in the relatives of probands who had significant life events compared with those who had none showed no difference (McGuffin & Katz, 1989).

Twin studies

Twin studies have traditionally relied on comparing the concordance rates of diagnosis in twins, both monozygotic (who have 100% of their genes in common) and dizygotic (who share an average of 50% of their genes), thus allowing researchers the possibility of dissecting the role of genes from that of the environment. Early studies simply compared the rate of concordance of disease in monozygotic and dizygotic twins. For example, Bertelsen *et al* (1977) used the Danish Twin Study Register to study bipolar disorder and unipolar depression, and found a concordance rate of 67% for monozygotic twins and 20% for dizygotic twins, which suggests a substantial genetic effect.

Bipolar disease

Studies based on the Maudsley Hospital twin register have recently shown a very high degree of genetic loading for bipolar disorder. Thus, an analysis of concordance rates of 30 monozygotic and 37 dizygotic twin pairs in which the proband had bipolar disorder (that met DSM–IV criteria) gave a proband-wise concordance rate of 40% for monozygotic and only 5% for dizygotic twins, and the hereditability was estimated to be 85%. The authors attempted to fit various models to the data. In the first of these, in which it was proposed that bipolar disorder was a more severe manifestation of unipolar disorder, model fitting was unsuccessful. The second model proposed two separate diseases (bipolar and unipolar disorder) but this model also failed to fit the data, as 29% of the genetic liability for mania was shared with depression. This suggests the appropriate relationship was neither one disease nor two diseases but rather that there were some genetic commonalities (McGuffin *et al*, 2003).

Population-based twin studies yield more accurate information because case ascertainment is free from biases related to treatment. Kieseppä *et al* (2004) have reported a study on the genetics of bipolar disorder, based on the Finnish national twin register ($n = 19\,124$ twin pairs), from which they identified 38 twin pairs (0.2%) where one twin had bipolar I disorder. Concordance in monozygotic twins was 0.43, and in dizygotic twins only 0.06. Statistical model fitting yielded a hereditability of 93%, probably the highest for any functional disorder.

These twin studies suggest that bipolar disorder is a strongly genetically determined condition.

Unipolar depression

The relatively high prevalence of unipolar depression has allowed the use of population-based twin registers which better represent the general population. The method of biometric model fitting has now been used extensively on the data from twin registers, allowing the relative contribution of genetic, familial and unique environmental factors to the aetiology of depression to be examined.

In a meta-analysis by Sullivan *et al* (2000), pooled data gave a heritability for unipolar depression in the range of 31–42%, with a point estimate of 37%, but rates were significantly higher for narrowly defined major depression or subtypes such as recurrent major depression. Analysis of data from the Maudsley Hospital twin register (McGuffin *et al,* 1996), using clinically ascertained probands, estimated the heritability of unipolar disorder to be 48–75%, depending on the estimated population risk. In the study of Kendler *et al* (1995), the heriditability was 66% for female twins who had been reliably diagnosed with depression. Higher estimates of heritability may be due to the nature of proband ascertainment, with preferential selection of those with a more severe form of illness, as well as a more rigorous diagnosis. Several studies have now suggested that genetic risk factors are of equal importance in depression for men and women (McGuffin *et al*, 1996; Kendler *et al*, 2003).

Statistical modelling of the pooled data in the Sullivan meta-analysis indicated a very low contribution for environmental influences common to family members (e.g. general parenting style or socio-economic status) – in the range of only 0–5% of the variance – but there was a substantial contribution from individual environmental effects, of the order of 58–67%. Multivariate twin models using the population-based Virginian twin registry, examining patterns of psychiatric comorbidity, have suggested that common psychiatric disorders may be characterised as 'externalising' (e.g. alcohol dependence, adult antisocial behaviour, etc.) and 'internalising' (e.g. depression, anxiety and phobia) (Kendler *et al,* 2003). Fitting models to the twin data revealed a common genetic factor loading largely on major depression and generalised anxiety disorder, with little evidence of contribution from shared environmental factors (Kendler *et al*, 2003). The authors suggest that exposure to unique environmental experiences may explain why depression, rather than generalised anxiety, may present in vulnerable individuals. Further evidence for this comes from an earlier study of 2164 individuals in a population-based sample of female–female twin pairs, which examined the role of genetics and stressful life events. The best-fitting model for the joint effect of stressful events and genetic liability on the onset of major depression suggested that genetic factors alter the sensitivity of individuals to stressful life events (Kendler *et al*, 1995).

An additional hypothesis to emerge from family and twin studies is that there may be an element of 'genetic control of exposure to the environment' (Kendler, 1993), so that genetically susceptible individuals are more likely to be exposed to life events or environments that increase the risk developing depression. Thus, McGuffin *et al* (1988) found that the relatives of probands with depression had an increased rate of severe life events.

Adoption studies

Adoption studies are advanced as a method of separating biological and environmental factors but few such studies have been undertaken in unipolar depression. Those that have been undertaken have shown a role for genetic factors, and little evidence for family-associated environmental factors (Wender *et al*, 1986). This study showed an eightfold increase in the rate for affective disorder among the relatives of index adoptees with affective disorder (compared with controls), and a 15-fold increase in suicide rates (although the numbers were small).

Mode of transmission

Segregation analyses

Segregation analysis compares the likelihood for the observed frequency of illness in a pedigree containing many cases of affective disorder with those that can be predicted by different modes of transmission. There have been no consistent findings in studies of unipolar depression and a variety of complex genetic mechanisms have been proposed as modes of inheritance in bipolar disorder, such as mitochondrial inheritance, allelic or locus heterogeneity, epistasis, imprinting and dynamic mutation, and these may also apply to unipolar depression (Jones *et al*, 2002). Although there have been some suggestions that a single major gene has influence in depression, most studies have concluded that depression has a multifactorial inheritance – that is, multiple genes, each of small effect size, interact and act together with environmental risk factors.

Susceptibility genes

Genetic linkage studies

Individuals with unipolar depression have been included in large linkage studies of bipolar pedigrees, but there has been little work on unipolar depression in its own right, mainly because the genetic effect size is relatively small, and large samples would have to be examined to provide adequate power to detect linkage. At the time of writing, a number of large, multicentre studies are in the process of collecting DNA from several hundreds (even thousands) of well-defined affected sibling pairs and other relatives (Levinson *et al*, 2003) with unipolar and bipolar disorder in order to perform genome scans. However, linkage analysis of unipolar disorder has been a relatively neglected area and there have been no large-scale systematic genome scans published to date.

Association studies

Association studies allow researchers to follow up regions of interest identified in linkage analyses or to examine candidate genes of *a priori* interest. Initially, the gene of interest is scanned for systematic polymorphisms; this is followed by association studies in disease comparison samples. Smaller sample sizes are required than in linkage studies, although for a variety of reasons spurious associations may sometimes occur (usually due to poorly matched control subjects). Association studies of bipolar disorder have concentrated on the genes encoding for tyrosine hydroxylase (the rate-limiting enzyme in catecholamine synthesis), the serotonin transporter and catechol-o-methyl transferase (COMT), which is involved in monoamine degradation. In addition, recent interest has focused on brain-derived neurotrophic factor (BDNF) and polymorphisms related to the circadian clock. Candidate genes have also been examined in unipolar pedigrees, generally without consistent results (Ogilvie *et al*, 1996), although in a recent prospective longitudinal study of a representative birth cohort, individuals with one or two copies of the short allele of the serotonin transporter gene polymorphism under investigation were more likely to become depressed following stressful life events (Caspi *et al*, 2003). This provides further evidence for mechanisms involved in the gene–environment link in the aetiology of depression.

Conclusions

Genetic risk factors certainly play an important role in the aetiology of depression, although precisely which are the relevant genes and how they act remain uncertain. However, with the rapid pace of technological advance, especially in the automation of molecular genetic methods, and the number of large linkage and association collections currently being built up, there is a real possibility that the key genes will be identified in the next few years. Genes that predispose individuals to be vulnerable to depressogenic environmental factors, or to be exposed to more of these factors, may influence symptom presentation and/or response to antidepressant drugs. However, research into the genetics of affective disorder has shown that, even where genetic factors are strong, environmental influences are also important in terms of whether (and when) illness occurs and the form it takes.

Box 3.2 Clinical implications of genetic studies

A family history of a disorder assists the diagnostic procedure, since psychiatric disorders 'breed true': that is, if the diagnosis in a first-degree relative is bipolar disorder, then it is likely that similar symptoms are indicative of the same disorder in your patient. Patients who have been aware of their own strong family history of affective disorder are generally not surprised to hear that their current episode of depression may have a hereditary component. Those who first become aware of their strong family history through the systematic enquiry of the psychiatrist may experience some relief that a partial cause has been identified, as this may help to diminish guilt and anxiety that they are somehow responsible. Those with families will often follow on with questions about risks to their children. Enquiry about family history can also assist with finding suitable treatment. If a particular drug has helped a close family member with the disorder, it is highly likely that the same drug will benefit to your patient too.

Childhood risk factors

Although earlier research tended to focus on single risk factors during childhood, such as maternal separation or poor attachment, cumulative childhood disadvantage probably poses the most significant risk for depression later in life (see also Chapter 18, page 451).

Parental loss

A major theme in psychoanalytic writings on depression suggested that deficiencies in, or loss of, the early mother–child relationship predisposes to adult depression. Bowlby (1951) suggested that the disruption to bonding caused by maternal loss (rather than the meaning of the event) was critical in predisposing to depression. Rutter (1985) extended the argument, suggesting that the loss may lead to a range of other adverse events, producing a cascade-like effect more pathogenic than the loss itself. The well-documented community studies of Brown & Harris (1978) suggest that loss of mother before the age of 11 years is associated with increased risk of adult depression in the presence of a provoking agent. Refinements of the research have looked at loss as a consequence of parental death, loss due to parent–child separations and the effects of parental style on early development (see below on parenting style).

A critical review of the literature by Birtchnell (1980) found that when the loss was separated into that due to parental death and that due to parent–child separation, there is no evidence that childhood bereavement, as such, specifically predisposed to adult depression. It appears that the negative effects are probably a consequence of the inadequate parental care after the loss (Birtchnell, 1980).

A recent large follow-up study by Gilman *et al* (2003) examined 1104 offspring of mothers enrolled in the National Collaborative Perinatal Project and demonstrated that parental divorce by the age of 7 years was associated with a higher risk of depression. In this study (taking the risks of developing depression after being reared in a two-parent family with non-conflictual relationships as 1) the relative risks for the following subgroups were found: single motherhood 1.32; mother divorced 1.68; conflict with divorce 1.85; remarriage 1.93; remarriage with conflict 3.45; single parenthood perceived as conflictual 3.42. It can be seen that the quality of the parental relationship, especially with regard to conflict, has a major effect on the offspring's subsequent risk for the development of depression, and probably for a variety of other psychopathology as well.

Parenting

Parker hypothesised that parental attitudes and behaviours may have an impact on their children's vulnerability to psychiatric disorder, and developed the Parental Bonding Instrument to examine parenting (Parker *et al*, 1979). This allows participants reliably to rate their parents' attributes on two subscales: 'care' and 'protection'. Low scores on the 'care' scale and high scores on the 'protection' scale (a combination termed 'affectionless overcontrol') are associated with increased risk of development of neurotic disorders, particularly depression, in adult life (Oakley-Browne *et al*, 1995). A recent analysis of data from the US NCS demonstrated that the impact of parenting was not diagnostically specific and had a modest effect, accounting for only 1–5% of the variance in the occurrence of adult psychopathology (Cox *et al*, 2000).

Box 3.3 Clinical implications of childhood experiences

Systematic enquiry into the patient's childhood is an integral part of the psychiatric assessment. Sometimes patients and therapists overestimate its significance, placing excessive blame on earlier events, and in so doing may fail to face present realities. In other cases patients are oblivious to the damage caused by a severely traumatic childhood, which may need further therapeutic exploration. In either case, knowledge of the literature as described here may help clinicians reach a more objective assessment of the likely causal role that earlier losses or conflicts may have had, although their significance for an individual may depend on a variety of other factors, such as resilience, as well as the patient's perception of his or her childhood.

There is also considerable debate regarding the relative contribution of genetics to parental temperament, offspring temperament and attitudes derived from the parent's family of origin, all of which may influence parenting.

There is increasing evidence that having a parent suffering from depression is a risk factor for developing depression. Thus, Lieb *et al* (2002), in a large prospective study ($n = 2427$) of adolescents and young adults, found that those with one parent suffering from depression also had an increased risk of depression (OR = 2.7), with the risk only slightly increased if both parents suffered from depression (OR = 3.0). Although the risk may be largely genetic, there is evidence that depressive symptoms affect parenting ability (Edhborg *et al*, 2003) and this may well further increase the risk of depression in offspring.

Childhood sexual abuse

There is increasing evidence for a relationship between childhood sexual and physical abuse and the later deveĺopment of depression (as well as other types of psychopathology). A study by McCauley *et al* (1997), in which over 2000 women were interviewed, demonstrated that those subjects who had experienced childhood sexual or physical abuse exhibited more symptoms of anxiety and depression and had more frequently attempted suicide than those without a history of abuse. This relationship was confirmed in another large study, which showed a fourfold increase in depression in women exposed to childhood abuse compared with controls (Mullen *et al*, 1996). These studies have also shown that the magnitude of childhood abuse correlates with the severity of depression in adulthood and is associated with earlier onset of depression and an increased rate of chronic depression.

The way in which childhood sexual abuse may produce vulnerability to depression is unclear, but one mechanism may be by causing dysregulation of the hypothalamic–pituitary axis, resulting in a differential response to stresses in adulthood (Weiss *et al*, 1999).

Resilience

The finding that there are large variations in individuals' response to environmental adversity has given rise to the concept of resilience (Rutter, 1985). Some individuals may be very resilient and will therefore experience fewer psychiatric consequences from adversity than those with less resilience. The concept of resilience is multifaceted, comprising mastery of internal and external resources in order to adapt to substantial adversity. Research has suggested that one good relationship with an adult and high intelligence in a child may, in part, protect against the long-term psychiatric effects of childhood adversities (Tiet *et al*, 1998).

The role of adverse life events

Early questionnaire studies of the effects of adverse life events generally focused on common events – those that happen to most people at one time or another. Holmes

& Rahe (1967) believed that if the clustering of events in an individual's life reached a sufficient magnitude, this would provide a necessary if not sufficient cause for the onset of disorder. They explored the events recorded in the life charts of naval ratings who developed physical illness and derived a list of 43 frequently reported life events. To try to measure the magnitude of the effect of an event on an individual, the authors then developed the Social Readjustment Rating Scale (Holmes & Rahe, 1967). This list of events was presented to samples of the general population and each individual was asked to rate the degree of adjustment required, regardless of the desirability of the event. Marriage was chosen as the 'modulus' and individuals then gave quantitative judgements of the amount of change or readjustment required, measured in 'life change units' (LCU) relative to this arbitrary standard. The top five events on this scale (i.e. those considered to be the most stressful) were death of a spouse, divorce, marital separation, jail term and death of a close family member, but some positive experiences were also regarded as stressful, for example pregnancy or gaining a new family member. It was argued that the risk of illness in any individual was directly related to the LCU score.

The deficiencies of this model have been commented on, and questionnaire surveys have lost favour as more sophisticated, interview-based research tools have been developed. Hudgens (1974) suggested that many events listed on questionnaires (29 out of the 43 on the Social Readjustment Rating Scale) could occur as a consequence of illness rather than precede it (and they therefore might represent dependent rather than independent events). Brown & Harris (1978) also noted that there was considerable variability in the LCU ratings obtained from individuals with different social or cultural backgrounds and demonstrated that the use of an interview rather than a questionnaire approach to life events was more accurate. These workers at Bedford College went on to develop a specialised interview, the Life Events and Difficulties Scale (LEDS), which became the accepted 'gold standard' interview for assessing life events. This group also showed that 'contextual threat' (the circumstances surrounding the event and whether they had threatening implications) had an important influence on the impact of the event for the individual (Dew *et al*, 1987).

A large body of research has since explored the potential role of recent stress in precipitating the onset of depressive episodes and the occurrence of highly stressful events in the previous 6 months appears to be associated with a sixfold increased the risk of depression (Paykel & Cooper, 1992). This association does not appear to be coincidental, nor to be a function of 'effort after meaning' (which refers to the patient's retrospective reinterpretation of an event as stressful in an attempt to explain the causes of the depression). When comparisons are made with other groups, only suicide attempters have a higher rate of life events than people with depression.

Paykel (2003) suggests that, overall, there is only weak evidence for a relation between the type of event and the type of psychiatric disorder or category of depression, although there is good evidence for depression to be preceded by loss or humiliation events or separations (Farmer & McGuffin, 2003; Paykel, 2003). A convincing example of this comes from a population-based nested case–control study of 13 006 patients who received a diagnosis of depression at their first ever admission to a psychiatric ward, who were compared with a gender- and age-matched control group ($n = 260\,108$). A recent divorce, recent unemployment and suicide of a first-degree relative were associated with an increased risk of being admitted for the first time to a psychiatric ward with a diagnosis of depression, although death of a relative other than by suicide had no significant effect (Kessing *et al*, 2003).

Tennant & Bebbington (1978) demonstrated an association between the threatfulness of events and the level of emotional distress experienced (as measured on the General Health Questionnaire), but the association was not deemed specific to depression.

Even allowing for the considerable overlap between the symptoms of grief and depressive disorder, bereavement generally shows a high rate of association with depression. A prospective study showed that 42% of recently bereaved spouses met research criteria for depression at 12 months (Clayton & Darvish, 1979). Many studies suggest that loss of a child is the most significant and traumatic form of bereavement.

Although the association between life events and depression is not in question, the magnitude of the overall effect is unclear. Paykel & Cooper (1992), in their review of studies of community depression and life events, found in most studies around 40% of the variance (based on the population attributable fraction) was due to life events, suggesting that stress in the form of life events is probably one of the more significant causes of depression.

Susceptibility to life events

The trend for patients with depression to have experienced more life events in the months before episode onset must be understood in the context of variations in individual susceptibility to the impact of such events. Paykel & Cooper (1992) demonstrated hypothetically that only about 10% of individuals in the community who experienced an 'exit' (loss) life event actually developed a clinical depression. In addition, 30% of those with depression give no history of significant life events, which indicates that they are not a necessary cause for depression.

One interesting body of research has examined the origins of life events themselves (Paykel, 2003), and several studies have confirmed that depression itself can generate stressful life events (Harkness & Luther, 2001). As previously discussed, there may be a genetic contribution to the experience of more adverse life events (McGuffin *et al*, 1988; Plomin, 1994), and Kendler's work on the Virginia twin registry found that genetic influences may alter susceptibility to the depressogenic effects of life events (Kendler *et al*, 1995).

Employment status

Employment and financial independence are associated with lower rates of depression and the risk of depression is three times higher among those who are unemployed. British studies suggest that unemployment is associated

Box 3.4 Clinical implications of life event studies

Patients will often ask their psychiatrist why they became ill or may proffer their own interpretation by saying things like 'I'm depressed because my mother died when I was a child' or 'It's all because I lost my job'. It is important to point out that there is no single reason why someone develops depression and that depression is caused by an interplay of life events and other adversities occurring throughout the life span to an individual with a genetically determined vulnerability. Explaining this ensures that undue emphasis is not given to a single risk factor.

with an increase in psychiatric morbidity, particularly anxiety and depression (Melville *et al*, 1985), and that this trend is reversed by gaining employment outside the home. While the link between unemployment and depression may arise directly because of the adverse influence on socio-economic status, indirect mechanisms may also be relevant. Thus, as well as providing income, employment has several functions, including providing the individual with status, a sense of purposefulness and control, a social network and a structure for daily activity. Research supports the importance of these latent functions, as unemployment has been found to have a strong negative impact on social supports and self-esteem (Scott *et al*, 1992).

Chronic difficulties

Brown & Harris (1978) defined 'life events' as sudden changes in an individual's social world, while 'chronic difficulties' represented problems which last at least 4 weeks without substantial change. In their studies of women in the community, these chronic difficulties included the absence of a close confiding relationship and the presence of three or more children aged under 5 years at home. Chronic difficulties rated as threatening and persistent (>2 years) are independently associated with an increased risk of depression (Paykel & Cooper, 1992). However, an Australian study of elderly people found no association between depression and chronic difficulties (Emmerson *et al*, 1989).

Specific trauma

The aftermath of natural or manmade disasters has provided clear evidence of the impact of extreme stress on the psychological well-being of previously healthy individuals. While such disasters are rare, the study of these situations has provided a theoretical model for investigations of the relationship between life events and psychiatric disturbance.

Following the explosion of the Mount St Helens volcano in Washington in 1980, an increase in the rates of three types of psychiatric disorder was observed: single-episode depression, generalised anxiety disorder and 'St Helens-specific' post-traumatic stress disorder (PTSD) (Shore *et al*, 1986). For those in a high-exposure group (personal losses and property damage but not death), rates of psychiatric disorder were increased 11- to 12-fold compared with controls from the neighbouring state of Oregon. Even subjects with low exposure showed a small increase in psychopathology (2.1% versus 0.9% in controls for men). Most of the new cases had their onset in the first year and there were no new cases 18 months after the explosion, illustrating the temporal relationship between the event and the time of onset of depression. Of those who had someone close to them die as a result of the explosion, 40% experienced psychiatric disorder, compared with 7% of Oregon controls who had experienced bereavement, which suggests that an unexpected and apparently random death may be associated with high rates of psychiatric morbidity.

Interpersonal risk factors

Marriage

Research has suggested that marriage protects men from depression but is detrimental for women (Bebbington, 2003). However, it is difficult retrospectively to disentangle cause and effect: marital status may change as a result of depression rather than being associated with its onset. The ECA study showed that even when controlling for gender and age, continuously married participants demonstrated the lowest rates of depression, while divorced or separated participants had the highest rates, with a threefold increase in risk. The prevalence of depression among those who had never married was closest to that of the continuously married or cohabiting participants.

Combining data from a number of studies has shown that the sex ratio (an excess of female:male sufferers) persists across all marital categories but diminishes slightly in the post-marital category (separated, divorced or widowed), which may suggest a greater impact of marital breakdown for men (Bebbington, 2003). However, a Dutch study that examined the longitudinal trends (1975–96) of depressive symptoms demonstrated that divorced people have become progressively less likely, and never marrieds more likely, to suffer from depressive symptoms over time, compared with married people (Meertens *et al*, 2003).

Presence of a confidant

Of all the vulnerability/protective factors identified by Brown & Harris (1978), the role of a confidant in reducing depression among women experiencing adversity has received the most robust support. Lack of intimacy may also independently increase the rate of adverse events (Champion, 1990) as well as the risk of depression (Tennant & Bebbington, 1978).

Women report more stressful life events relating to proximal relationships, such as loss of a confidant, than men and women are more sensitive to the depressogenic effects of such life events (Kendler *et al*, 2001). Women in a relationship characterised by coldness and indifference have three times the risk of depression following a major life event (35% versus 10%) compared with those in a more positive partnership (Brown *et al*, 1986).

A confiding relationship, particularly one in which reciprocity exists, may protect an individual against recurrence of depression, and it appears that the level of useful support given by the confidant in crisis situations is the critical element that prevents depression. The effect of support from the confidant appears to be highly specific, because other forms of support do not appear to be able to attenuate the effect of being let down by the confidant. The suggestion is that the confidant somehow protects the individual from depression by alleviating the impact of adversity on the subject's self-esteem (Paykel & Cooper, 1992).

Expressed emotion

Expressed emotion (EE) describes the quality of close family relationships. The bulk of the research into EE has been into its role in triggering relapses in schizophrenia. The concept of EE, its separate components and its measurement are described in detail in Chapter 10 (page 228). In studies of depression, it has been the relationship particularly between the patient and the spouse that has been the focus of study.

Vaughn & Leff (1976) found that the level of EE in a key relative at the time of an index depressive episode was a significant predictor of further relapse but also noted that the individuals with depression also had high rates of life events (Leff & Vaughn, 1980). More recently, Hayhurst *et al* (1997) failed to confirm the link between criticism and recovery from depression, but patients with residual symptoms while in remission had more critical partners. They concluded that this criticism was probably the result of the ongoing depressive symptoms. There is a suggestion from a meta-analysis of six studies of EE ratings in affective disorder that a high-EE family may be a more powerful predictor for depressive relapse than for a relapse in schizophrenia. Butzlaff & Hooley (1998) gave an effect size for a high EE rating being associated with a depressive relapse as $r = 0.39$, slightly higher than its effect size for causing relapses in schizophrenia ($r = 0.31$) but not as great as the effect size for relapses in eating disorders ($r = 0.51$).

Box 3.5 Clinical implications of interpersonal risk factors

Many patients, perhaps the majority, describe their depression and its causes in terms of their current interpersonal environment, their close relationships and recent life stress. They usually find it helpful if their therapists continue to explore the same interpersonal themes that they have brought to the consultation. Knowledge of the literature in this area, as described here, may sometimes help to focus the enquiry, for example whether a particular life event carried a high degree of threat to the individual or whether the relationship they were in was cold or non-supportive. In addition, one type of brief psychotherapy, interpersonal psychotherapy, rests on the assumption that the depression has its origins mainly in the interpersonal realm and therapy is directed almost exclusively at exploring the quality of the patient's interpersonal relationships and possible ways of improving them.

Support networks

Cobb (1976) viewed social support as information-giving mechanisms that helped people believe they were cared for, loved, esteemed, valued and belonged to a social network. Current concepts of social support incorporate both structural and functional components (Turner & Turner, 1999): structural aspects relate to the size and interconnectedness of the primary and secondary groups, while functional aspects describe the practical help and emotional support these groups provide. The most robust evidence in relation to the prevention of depression concerns perceived or 'emotional' support (Turner & Turner, 1999). A review by Brugha (2003) suggested that perceived numerical and qualitative deficiencies in close personal relationships predict the onset of depression, but at the same time it appears that individuals prone to developing depression may also have premorbid deficits in both making and sustaining relationships, which highlights the possible confounding role of personality (Lara *et al*, 1997).

Two theories have been proposed to explain the link between the lack of social support and the onset of depression:

- the *buffer theory* suggests that the presence of social support reduces the risk of depression by modifying the impact of adversity
- the *main effect* hypothesis suggests that it is the lack of social support that predisposes to depression.

Longitudinal, prospective studies may shed some light on the relationship between social support and depression. Stansfeld *et al* (1998) reported on a large ($n = 7697$) follow-up study of British civil servants and found no evidence of a buffering effect among men or women who experienced life events or chronic stressors, but that emotional support itself was predictive of good mental health in both women and men. Alloway & Bebbington (1987), reviewing several earlier studies, also found little evidence for the 'buffer theory'. A study of 2163 female twin pairs found some evidence for the main effects model but none for a buffering effect for social support (Kendler *et al*, 2001).

Intrapersonal risk factors

Cognitive factors

There has been increasing interest in the two cognitive–behavioural models of depression: the learned helplessness model (Seligman *et al*, 1978), and Beck's cognitive model (Beck *et al*, 1983). Both are partly supported by empirical data (Twaddle & Scott, 1991). The learned helplessness model was derived from laboratory experiments with animals, while Beck's model originated from his own observations of the thoughts and ideas expressed by patients with depression whom he was seeing at the time for psychoanalytic treatment.

Learned helplessness

Seligman's original learned helplessness model suggested that animals exposed to inescapable shock later failed to learn to avoid escapable stimuli in similar situations. The central issue in this hypothesis is that rewards (or punishments) are non-contingent on actions. The model in its original form was probably an oversimplistic explanation for the laboratory observations and was reformulated by Abramson *et al* (1978) into a more comprehensive theory, with four premises. It was suggested that the 'depression prone' individual:

- perceives that highly aversive outcomes are likely to happen
- believes that these events will be uncontrollable
- possesses a maladaptive attributional style such that negative events are attributed to internal, stable global causes and positive events to external, unstable and specific causes
- experiences greater disruption to affective state and self-esteem the greater the certainty of the aversive state of affairs, its expected uncontrollability and its importance to the individual.

Alloy *et al* (1988) proposed a further modification to Seligman's theory, which requires the matching of a particular stressor with the attributional style relating to that specific domain of functioning (the 'hopelessness model'). For example, a depressive reaction may occur following social rejection in someone with a maladaptive attributional style for interpersonal events.

The cognitive model

In its most succinct form, Beck's model of depression suggests that three elements of psychological functioning are implicated in the development or maintenance of depression: depressogenic schemata (underlying beliefs), negative automatic thoughts and systematic logical errors of reasoning. Those at risk of depression are believed to have developed (as a result of certain types of early negative experiences) dysfunctional cognitive structures (schemata), which determine how the individual interprets subjective reality. These underlying beliefs may be conditional (e.g. 'In order to be happy, I must be successful in everything I do') or unconditional (e.g. 'I am unlovable'). It is hypothesised that these schemata are latent for long periods but become activated when the individual is exposed to negative events in later life.

The reactivation of the schemata leads to the generation of repetitive, unintended and largely uncontrolled 'negative automatic thoughts', characterised by the cognitive triad, which comprises negative thoughts about the self, the world and the future. These negative cognitions are sustained through information-processing biases, or systematic errors in thinking such as overgeneralisation, selective abstraction or catastrophising. A vicious cycle is then generated in which increases in the intensity of depressed mood lead to further negative thinking, exacerbating the severity of mood and behavioural disturbance. Beck *et al* (1983) later clarified components of the model and suggested that while it may represent a causal theory for some unipolar non-biological depressions, in other depressions it had more relevance as a model to explain the maintenance of the disorder (Ferrier & Scott, 1998).

Links to vulnerability

Brown & Harris' (1978) early studies suggested that vulnerability factors are crucial in the development of depression. In their original studies, the key vulnerability factors identified for women in the community predisposing them to depression were: absence of a close confiding relationship, death of mother before the age of 11, and having three or more young children under 5 years at home. Different population groups will have different vulnerability factors, for example among the elderly physical illness may be important. Vulnerability factors act by lowering the threshold for experiencing hopelessness in the face of subsequent stressors.

Both the hopelessness/attributional style model and Beck's model help to explain the vulnerability of some individuals to the effects of stressful life events. In the hopelessness theory, the person with depression makes negative inferences with regard to the causes, implications and consequences of stressful life events, and so engenders a feeling of hopelessness and 'hopelessness depression'. Beck's model operates slightly differently and suggests that negative life events activate the negative schemata, with resulting negative appraisal of the self, world and future, and this is the cause of the depression. Beck *et al* (1983) also suggested that the matching of particular events to certain personality modes may explain why the same experience can have a different effect on different individuals. Thus, for example, 'sociotropic' individuals (those placing high value on positive interchanges with others) may have a strong negative reaction to personal rejection. However, 'autonomous' individuals (who place high value on independent functioning) might be less troubled by personal rejection but would be more likely to become depressed in response to an event such as failure to achieve a personal goal.

Gladstone & Parker (2001) proposed a neat 'lock and key' hypothesis, whereby earlier adverse life circumstances may establish specific vulnerabilities ('locks') which are later activated by mirroring life events ('keys').

Studies of cognitive theories

There have been a considerable number of studies examining cognitive vulnerability to depression. Initially these focused on 'remitted depression', examining the cognitive styles of people who had recovered from depression and comparing them against controls who had never suffered depression. Just *et al* (2001) reviewed such studies and found that when people had recovered from their depression they no longer had depressive cognitive schemata, suggesting such styles may reflect 'state' rather than 'trait' markers.

Retrospective studies of those who have recovered from depression have considerable methodological problems and so prospective studies are now being undertaken (Lewinsohn *et al*, 2001). One example of an ongoing study is the Temple–Wisconsin Cognitive Vulnerability to Depression Project, in which non-depressed university students were followed for up to 5 years and at the start of the project assessed for cognitive style, stressful life events and psychopathology. Participants were categorised as cognitively at 'high risk' using questionnaires assessing cognitive vulnerability according to the hopelessness and Beck's models. A summary of the initial findings (Alloy *et al*, 1999) found that those at high cognitive risk, compared with those at low risk, had a greater lifetime risk of major depression, and a greater likelihood of experiencing a first episode of depression during the study follow-up period. High-risk participants showed preferential self-referring processing for negative material, for example better recall and greater endorsement of material with themes of incompetence and worthlessness (Alloy *et al*, 1999).

Psychodynamic factors

It is difficult to do justice to the huge psychoanalytic literature on depression, partly because of the complexities of the different theories put forward and partly because of the intricacies of the 'metaphoric' language used (Ryle, 1991); only the barest outline can be presented here. Ryle has pointed out that the most important concept to grasp is that intrapsychic structure (which is central to the psychoanalytic model for all disorders) is interpersonally derived. Thus, adult personality bears traces of both the infant and the internalised parent. It is hypothesised that problems in early life lead to defects in development that render the individual vulnerable to depression in later life.

Psychodynamic models of depression have largely developed from the basic paradigm postulated by Freud in his classic work 'Mourning and melancholia' (1917). Freud observed a striking resemblance between grief and psychotic depression and on this basis proposed that melancholia occurred following object loss (either a real loss or the loss of 'some abstraction'). The model also proposed that the hostility experienced towards the lost object (which was largely denied) became directed against the self, explaining some of the classic features of depression. As he wrote in this classic paper:

> 'If one listens patiently to a patient's many and various self-accusations, one cannot in the end avoid the impression that often the most violent of them are hardly applicable to the patient himself, but that with insignificant modifications they do fit someone else, someone who the patient loves, or has loved or should love.' (Freud, 1917)

Freud also believed that the individual's ambivalent relationship with the object (the simultaneous presence of feelings of love and hostility) predisposed him or her to the development of depression.

As highlighted in the excellent review by Mendelson (1990), important modifications or alternatives to Freud's model were proposed by Bibring, Jacobson and object relations theorists (Klein, 1934). Object relations theory, focusing on the mother–infant relationship, describes the 'depressive position' as a developmental phase during which a child learns to modify ambivalence and retain self-esteem during periodic loss of the 'good mother' (Klein, 1934; Mendelson, 1990). It is proposed that if the infant does not acquire confidence that its mother will return and be loving, despite hostile feelings towards the parent during separation, the child becomes fixated at this level of development and will be more prone to depression in adulthood. Bibring's work (1953) highlighted two key concepts related to self-esteem which she considered to be of central importance: first, while loss of self-esteem was frequently experienced in the oral phase, it could also occur in other developmental phases when narcissistic aspirations (such as the desire to be good or to be strong) were frustrated; and second, depression is an ego phenomenon and results from inner system tensions within the ego rather than from inter-system conflicts (between ego and superego, or ego and id).

Although Jacobson (1953) agreed with Bibring on the importance of self-esteem, her model also makes a distinction between the ego (a psychic structure) and the self (one's person as distinct from others). It was suggested that optimal levels of self-esteem were determined by the individuals' self-representations, superego, ego ideal and self-critical ego functions. With a less positive self-image, a more primitive superego, a less attainable ego ideal or more unrealistic expectations and goals, the more vulnerable the self-esteem became, and the greater the risk of depression. Jacobson proposed that in 'regressive identification' there was a loss of the boundaries between self and object representations, which explained why hostility directed at the object was turned inward. Jacobson saw aggression (in the sense of a psychic force, not a behavioural manifestation) as critical to the development of depression, through its impact on self-esteem (Ferrier & Scott, 1998).

Personality factors

The relationship between premorbid personality and vulnerability to depression is complex but a topic of central clinical importance in day-to-day psychiatry. Personality factors may indicate latent vulnerability to the development of depression, may be pathogenetically linked to depressive disorders, or may be a 'diluted antecedent' of depression or form independent comorbid disorder (Sass & Junemann, 2003; see also Chapter 18).

Personality traits

No personality characteristics have been found to be specifically associated with onset of depression (as opposed to any other disorder) but there has been considerable interest in the traits of introversion and neuroticism, traits originally described by Jung. Eysenck's model of temperament (1981) is based on cortical arousal – suggesting that arousability and, concomitantly, the preferred level of stimulation vary across individuals. This gives rise to the primary personality dimension of extroversion–introversion. Introverts have an inherently reactive reticular system and obtain optimum levels of cortical arousal at low levels of stimulation, whereas extroverts tend to prefer more intense and novel forms of stimulation. Eysenck (1981) also proposed a dimension of neuroticism–stability that depends on limbic activation: those with high neuroticism have high limbic reactivity.

Introversion/extroversion and neuroticism can be measured via a number of scales, including the Eysenck and Maudsley Personality Inventories, Myer Briggs Type Indicator and the five-factor Neuroticism, Extroversion,

Openness Personality Inventory. Studies in non-clinical populations have shown that low extroversion and high neuroticism both correlate significantly with depression scores. In clinical populations, increased introversion and neuroticism scores occur in patients with depression (Sauer *et al*, 1997), but there is considerable debate as to whether or not this represents a state or trait correlation. The reliability and validity of measures of personality made during an episode of depression are questionable due to the impact of the mood state on the answers to questions and hence the scores. Similarly, measures made after recovery may also be influenced by the previous episode of depression.

One approach that can circumvent such difficulties is to undertake a prospective longitudinal study. In the psychobiological study run by the US National Institute of Mental Health, a cohort of adult ($n = 438$) first-degree relatives of people with depression were assessed with 17 self-report personality assessment questionnaires before anyone had shown any depression. After 6 years of follow-up there were no significant premorbid differences between the participants who developed depression ($n = 29$) and the remainder ($n = 370$) for those in the 17- to 30-year age group. However, for participants in the 31- to 40-year age group, those who became depressed had higher neuroticism scores, lower levels of emotional stability, less resilience and more interpersonal dependence (Hirschfeld & Shea, 1992). Similarly, Krueger *et al* (1996) found that a higher premorbid neuroticism score was associated with the later development of depression.

Studies based on samples of people whose depression has remitted have been inconclusive, with some showing that introversion/extroversion scores approach those of normal controls (Griens *et al*, 2002; Kool *et al*, 2003) and others showing that patients in remission continue to have decreased extroversion and increased introversion scores (Bagby *et al*, 1997; Kessler *et al*, 2003).

Another approach is to examine the personality characteristics of the healthy siblings or other first-degree relatives of people with depression and compare them to the personality characteristics of healthy controls. This method excludes any present or past effect of depressed mood state influencing the ratings. Any significant differences found between the groups can be attributed to the increased number of depression-related genes in the siblings of the participants with depression (who share on average 50% genes with their brother or sister) compared with the controls (who do not have this increase in depression-related genes). This approach was adopted by Farmer *et al* (2002), who examined probands with depression and their siblings and compared them with healthy probands with no history of depression and their siblings. As expected, the probands with depression scored significantly higher than the other three groups on neuroticism scores and lower on extroversion scores. However, there were no significant differences in scores between the two never-depressed sibling groups (although family studies imply that the siblings of probands with depression should have a higher risk of depression themselves, and a premorbid 'marker', if present, should have been detected in this group). An alternative explanation is that neither scale was measuring a genetically influenced vulnerability trait for depression. However, among the same participants, other personality measures, such as sensation seeking, harm avoidance, novelty seeking and self-directedness, were able to distinguish these groups, which suggests that these may be the relevant trait markers for vulnerability to depression (Farmer *et al*, 2003).

Current theories largely relate to vulnerability models, where certain traits predispose to depression, and spectrum models, which view certain traits as a milder manifestation of the disorder. In the best-known of the former models, Cloninger (1987) proposed a model of personality based on three independent measurements of temperament: novelty seeking, harm avoidance and reward dependence. These are postulated to be independently heritable, manifest early in life and are related to the activity of specific neurotransmitter systems. The theory has evolved into a seven-factor model. The additional temperament factor is 'persistence' and three character dimensions were added: self-directedness, cooperativeness and self-transcendence. Cloninger (1987) suggested that all aspects of personality, as defined by his theory, interact in influencing susceptibility to depression and some studies suggest harm avoidance is a trait characteristic of patients with major depression (Farmer *et al*, 2003) while response to antidepressant medication may correlate with reward dependence and self-directedness (Joffe *et al*, 1993).

Although there has been a large amount of research over the past 50 years into personality traits that might or might not predispose to depression, apart from general agreement that during the depressive episode itself a wide variety of abnormalities can be detected, there do not appear to be any strong associations for particular personality traits and the premorbid state for people who become depressed. This is in contrast to anxiety, where 'trait' anxiety can be reasonably well identified.

Personality disorder

A review of the relationship between depression and personality disorder estimated that 20–30% of in-patients and 50–85% of out-patients with current major depression have an associated personality disorder (Corruble *et al*, 1996). The main comorbid personality disorders were borderline (10–30%), histrionic (2–20%) and antisocial (0–10%). The presence of comorbid 'cluster C' personality disorders (particularly avoidant and dependent) differed widely across studies with the exception of obsessive–compulsive personality disorder, which had a consistently high prevalence (up to 20%). The link probably lies in the high degree of affective dysregulation found in those with personality disorders (see also Chapter 18).

It has been suggested that there exists a 'subaffective' personality disorder, part of a spectrum from temperament to full-blown affective disorder. The great German psychiatrists Kraepelin, Kretschmer and Schneider all proposed continuum theories with severe mental illness at one pole and affective personality subtypes at the milder end of the spectrum. Winokur (1974) suggested that antisocial personality disorder (ASPD) and alcoholism form part of a spectrum with depression. Support for this model came from familial studies which demonstrated an increased prevalence of ASPD and alcoholism in the first-degree relatives of unipolar probands. The latter were regarded as having 'depressive spectrum disease' and often showed

Box 3.6 Clinical implications of personality disorder in depression

Patients who are diagnosed as having a personality disorder are frequently regarded as 'difficult', even by experienced clinical teams. The stigmatising effect of a diagnosis of, for example, 'borderline personality disorder' can be considerable and the individual so labelled may not have sufficient care and attention paid to any other psychopathology. This is particularly true for those with comorbid depression. The same attention to diagnostic accuracy is required when diagnosing personality disorder as when making any other diagnosis in psychiatry. When personality disorder and depression co-occur, both need treatment in their own right. The personality disorder may make the management of depression more difficult, with problems in engagement, in psychological treatment and the possibility of more drug resistance.

some character disturbance along with their affective disorder. Those with no such family history were regarded as having 'pure depressive disease'.

Akiskal *et al* (1997) described a chronic, mild, fluctuating course of affective symptoms as constituting a sub-syndromal affective disorder. Depressive personality disorder was included in the appendix of DSM–IV entitled 'Criteria sets and axes provided for further study' (American Psychiatric Association, 1994). This appendix covers a group of conditions that the DSM–IV task force decided were not sufficiently well delineated to include in the main text but which merited further study, and in this way highlighted their nosological uncertainty. There is also considerable debate as to the distinction between depressive personality disorder and dysthymia (an axis I affective disorder) (Ryder *et al*, 2001). A 3-year follow-up study of women diagnosed with depressive personality disorder found an increased risk for developing dysthymic disorder (in comparison with healthy controls) but not for major depression (Kwon *et al*, 2000).

The role of physical illness

Medical illness is a risk factor for depression; it acts via psychosocial stressors, functional impairment and direct biological mechanisms. The topic is also discussed in Chapter 17 (page 414). Research into the correlations between depression and several physical illnesses are described here in some detail, as they provide insight into the bio-psychosocial models of causation in affective disorder.

Neurological disease

Stroke

Depression is common in patients who have had a stroke, with reported prevalence rates of about 20% (Robinson, 2003). A recent meta-analysis concluded that there is a significant inverse correlation between severity and proximity of the lesion to the frontal pole in people with left-sided lesions, but not right-sided brain injury (Narushima *et al*, 2003). Such findings may have implications for research into the functional and structural neurobiology of depression.

Parkinson's disease

The prevalence of depression in Parkinson's disease is approximately 50% and is associated with significant impairment (Menza & Mark, 1994). The presentation is quite specific and it has been argued that sensitive screening and diagnostic tools are required. Depression may be not only the result of disability and added life stressors, but also a direct consequence of neurodegeneration. The finding that patients with Parkinson's disease suffer more depressive symptoms than those with other chronic, disabling diseases and the absence of any clear correlation between level of disability and severity of symptoms (Menza & Mark, 1994) has been used to argue for a direct physiological effect of the disease process contributing to the development of depression. One study suggests that this depression arises from an illness-related vulnerability of attentional mechanisms to negative emotional stimuli causing cognitive distortions, possibly mediated by common involvement of the anterior cingulate region in both selective attention and mood regulation (Serra-Mestres & Ring, 2002).

Epilepsy

The lifetime prevalence of depression in those with epilepsy ranges from 6% to 30% and there is a 10-fold higher rate of suicidality compared with the general population (Robertson, 1997). There is evidence that depletion of brain monoamines may be implicated in a common pathway for epilepsy and depression (Robertson, 1997).

Persistent pain

Banks & Kerns (1996) found high rates of depression (30–54%) among patients with persistent pain. There is now an emerging consensus that persistent pain is more likely to lead to depression than vice versa (Fishbain *et al*, 1997). Severe pain is associated with significantly higher levels of suicidal ideation, suicidal gestures and completed suicide. Depression seems to be more strongly associated with diseases where the pain is linked to changes in the central nervous system, such as fibromyalgia or irritable bowel syndrome, rather that in peripheral systems such as rheumatoid arthritis or cartilage damage. Similar neurotransmitters appear to be involved in both depression and pain, with some antidepressants, particularly those with both serotonergic and noradrenergic reuptake activity, also showing efficacy in a variety of patients experiencing chronic pain (Fishbain, 2000; Jackson *et al*, 2000). Substance P and corticotrophin-releasing factor have also been implicated in mediating both pain and depression.

Patients with maladaptive coping responses to pain, such as catastrophising, perceived helplessness and low self-efficacy, also report higher pain levels (Covic *et al*, 2002) and such cognitive biases have been shown to increase depression scores and rates of depression in patients with chronic pain (Campbell *et al*, 2003).

Similarly, patients with chronic pain are more likely to develop depression if they have poor family cohesion, high levels of family conflict or report negative responses from their partners.

Other medical illnesses

Cardiovascular disease

As many as 27% of patients with coronary heart disease (CHD) have major depression (Rudisch & Nemeroff, 2003) and depression is a significant risk factor for mortality following myocardial infarction and stroke. A variety of factors have been implicated in the association between CHD and depression, including overlapping risk factors (such as obesity, diabetes, etc.), hypothalamic–pituitary–adrenal axis overactivity, cortisol elevation, platelet activation and psychological stress (Joynt *et al*, 2003).

Endocrine diseases

Cushing's syndrome and hypothyroidism are associated with depression and in severe cases the depression can be psychotic in form (see Chapter 20). Rapid and usually complete resolution of the depression is seen when the underlying disorder is treated. Interestingly, however, a recent large population-based study showed no correlation between thyroid status and depression (Engum *et al*, 2002).

The neurobiology of depression

Neuropathology

Several research groups have now suggested that there are specific neuroanatomical circuits involved in depression, most likely those involving fronto-subcortical structures (Drevets, 2001). Research has focused on circuits involving the prefrontal cortex, basal ganglia, thalamus and hypothalamus, as well as the interconnecting white-matter tracts and projections to the cerebral cortex. Specifically, studies implicate limbic–thalamo–cortical (LTC) circuits, involving the amygdala, medial thalamus, and orbital and medial prefrontal cortex, and limbic–cortical–striatal–pallidal–thalamic circuits, involving the components of the LTC circuit along with related parts of the striatum and pallidum (Drevets, 2001). Mesolimbic dopaminergic circuits are thought to be involved in processing motivation and reward (Spanagel & Weiss, 1999) and may be implicated in depression. Abnormalities in these structures – perhaps caused during brain development or acquired (e.g. by ageing, stroke or other brain disease) – may render an individual more vulnerable to depression.

Much of the current research on the neuropathology in unipolar and bipolar depression has been undertaken using the Stanley Foundation brain collection (Torrey *et al*, 2000). The Neuropathology Consortium funded by the Stanley Foundation has collected (with family permission) brain specimens at post-mortem from individuals who had suffered from a range of mental disorders. The Neuropathology Consortium forms a subset of 60 specimens from the collection and includes 15 well-matched subjects in three major diagnostic categories (as well as normal controls): schizophrenia, bipolar disorder and non-psychotic unipolar disorder. Examination of these brains by Knable *et al* (2001) showed that major depression was associated with relatively few abnormalities, although the same group (Knable *et al*, 2004) have found decreased reelin protein in the molecular layer of a dentate gyrus in schizophrenia, bipolar disorder and depression, which may indicate a dysfunction of inhibitory GABA-ergic inter-neurons in severe mental illness.

Other post-mortem studies of people with major depression and bipolar disorder showed three patterns of abnormality: cell loss (particularly in the subgenual prefrontal cortex), cell atrophy in the dorsolateral prefrontal cortex and orbitofrontal cortex, and an apparent increase in the number of cells in the hypothalamic raphe nucleus (Rajkowska, 2000). It has been suggested that these findings are due to the influence of stress and glucocorticoids on neuronal pathways. Other authors have suggested that the reduced neuronal somal size and increase in neuronal density in cortical layers 5 and 6 of the anterior cingulate cortex may be a general feature of severe mental disorders such as schizophrenia, bipolar disorder and major depression (Chanar *et al*, 2003).

From the above it would seem that the neuropathological changes in major depression are fairly limited and non-specific. More recently attention has turned to abnormalities in glial cells rather than the neurons that they support. Glial cells, particularly astrocytes, have well-recognised roles in neuronal migration and inflammatory processes. However, it is also now recognised that they provide trophic support to neurons, and are involved in neuronal metabolism, in the formation of synapses and in neurotransmission. Astrocytes also provide the energy requirements of neurons. Consequently, deficient astrocyte function could account for both the quantitative post-mortem changes as well as the neuroimaging abnormalities (see below) found in major depression (Cotter *et al*, 2001).

A recent study compared cell pathology in three groups of participants: those with alcohol dependence alone, those with major depression alone, and those with alcohol dependence and major depression. The two groups with depressed participants had significant pathological changes to glial cells in the dorsolateral prefrontal cortex (Miguel-Hidalgo & Rajkowska, 2003).

It has been suggested that elevated glucocorticoid levels (caused by stress or hyperactivity of the hypothalamic–pituitary–adrenal axis) downregulate glial activity, enhancing neurotoxicity and thereby predisposing the person to, or exacerbating, psychiatric disorder. The finding that glial cells may be crucial in the pathogenesis of depression offers an opportunity for the development of agents to upregulate glial activity or normalise glial cell numbers as treatments for psychiatric disorders, including major depression (Cotter *et al*, 2001).

Neuroimaging

Structural imaging

Numerous studies have examined whether structural brain changes are associated with depression. Meta-analysis of a number of studies suggests that, particularly in the elderly, ventricular enlargement and sulcal widening are associated with severe depression (Elkis *et al*, 1995). Similarly, an increase in the number of white-matter hyperintensities on magnetic resonance imaging (MRI) has been found in elderly patients with depression and these were associated with treatment resistance and poor outcome (Hickie *et al*, 1997). Post-mortem investigation of such hyperintensities demonstrate three neuropathological mechanisms – ependymal loss, differing degrees of myelination in adjacent fibre tracts, and cerebral ischaemia with associated demyelination – and an excess of ischaemic lesions has been shown in those with depression compared with controls (Thomas *et al*, 2002).

Studies of younger patients with depression have been less consistent. Reviews of research conclude that unipolar depression is associated with a smaller frontal lobe (particularly the subgenual prefrontal cortex), cerebellum, basal ganglia (most notably the caudate and putamen) and hippocampus/amygdala complex (Beyer & Krishnan, 2002). The authors argue that these changes may involve regions of the brain critical to the pathogenesis of mood disorders. An excess of white-matter and periventricular grey-matter hyperintensities has also been demonstrated in younger patients with depression, although one well designed study spanning the age range found no difference between participants with depression and controls in hyperintensity number or volume (Lenze *et al*, 1999).

Overall, the findings of structural imaging studies must be taken in context and it is unclear whether these changes represent neurodevelopmental or acquired injury, or whether they are due to changes in regional blood flow or neuronal or glial structure, or whether they represent state or trait changes. More recently, the focus has been on region-of-interest analyses, on specific areas of the brain thought to be involved in the pathogenesis of depression, and lateralisation or asymmetry of limbic structures (Lacerda *et al*, 2003). New techniques such as diffusion tensor imaging (see page 217) will, in the future, help researchers to investigate regional microstructures, particularly of white matter (Lim & Helpern, 2002).

Functional imaging

A variety of techniques are able to investigate the functioning of brain regions *in vivo*, using glucose metabolism or oxygen uptake as markers of increased brain activity. Currently available methods include single-photon emission computed tomography (SPECT), positron emission tomography (PET), functional magnetic resonance imaging (fMRI) and magnetic resonance spectroscopy (MRS). Age and gender are significant confounding factors in neuroimaging studies and patient groups are rarely homogeneous in terms of symptom profile, genetic risk, chronicity and so on. Studies are also difficult to compare, as numbers are often small, methods are constantly being refined and there is little standardisation of the way mood changes are initiated or of the induction tasks. Studies of normal participants have demonstrated brain activation in the medial frontal gyrus during the generation of both positive and negative moods, and in the left amygdala, left insula and right ventrolateral prefrontal cortex (VLPFC) when sadness is induced (Posse *et al*, 2003).

The most consistent difference between patients with depression and controls is reduced glucose metabolism and blood flow in some frontal regions, particularly the subgenual prefrontal cortex, the dorsolateral prefrontal cortex (Michael *et al*, 2003), and in the caudate nucleus (Kimbrell *et al*, 2002). Abnormalities in the anterior cingulate gyrus and temporal lobes, with evidence for hippocampal and amygdala hyperarousal, have also been described (Videbech *et al*, 2001). One study found more sustained activity in the amygdala of patients with depression, and exaggerated activity in the left amygdala which resolved with treatment (Sheline *et al*, 2001).

In a recent review, Drevets (2003) concluded that limbic and stress–response systems connected to the amygdala were pathologically activated in depression. Treatment–response studies have shown normalisation of areas with previously reduced or exaggerated activity, suggesting that many of these functional abnormalities are state rather than trait alterations (Goldapple *et al*, 2004).

Neuroendocrine studies

The accumulating evidence for the link between stressful life events and the development of depression has focused interest in those neurobiological pathways that mediate stress responses, and how these contribute to the vulnerability for depression. Heim *et al* (2004) have postulated that corticotrophin-releasing factor (CRF) systems mediate this link. Neurons containing CRF are found in the hypothalamic paraventricular nucleus, the amygdala and throughout the cortex – all regions involved in the cognitive appraisal and modulation of affective responses. In humans, stress activates the hypothalamic–pituitary–adrenal (HPA) axis, resulting in the synthesis and release of CRF, which, in turn, stimulates the production of adrenocorticotrophin hormone (ACTH), which causes the release of glucocorticoids from the adrenal cortex. However, the effects of CRF are more extensive: not only does it mediate this response, it also activates the autonomic system, changes behavioural responses and leads to changes in immune function (Heim *et al*, 2004). In animal models, centrally administered CRF can produce symptoms resembling classical depression and anxiety. Elevated glucocorticoid secretion has been the most consistently found biochemical abnormality in patients with depression and was first noted over 50 years ago. In addition, a proportion of patients fail to suppress cortisol secretion when given the synthetic glucocorticoid dexamethasone (DST non-suppression) (Charlton & Ferrier, 1989). Dexamethasone non-suppression is greatest in patients with severe depression and reverses when the depression is treated. Non-suppression appears to be due to increased hypothalamic CRF release and there is evidence that patients with depression show increased CRF mRNA expression (Raadsheer *et al*, 1995).

The effect of early adverse experiences on the HPA axis has been investigated in animal models. Rodent pups separated from their mothers were shown to have an increased vulnerability to stress later in life associated with an exaggerated HPA axis response to stress, particularly when the stress was psychological rather than physical (Liu *et al*, 2000). Adult survivors of childhood abuse, with or without depression, have also been found to have significantly greater ACTH responses than controls. The responses were particularly high in those with depression and correlated with the level of abuse experienced. Nemeroff and his group have postulated that early adverse experiences sensitise the stress–response system and this confers a vulnerability to the later development of depression and anxiety (Heim *et al*, 2004), while genetic factors may mediate the vulnerability of an individual's HPA axis to adverse experiences (McGuffin & Katz, 1989).

Neurotransmitters and their receptors

During the past 25–40 years, the biogenic amine hypothesis of affective disorders has dominated research in biological psychiatry. Results from neuropsychopharmacological studies have, by and large, provided data to support this hypothesis and an account of the discovery of the first antidepressants and the monoamine theory of depression is given in Chapter 4 (page 72). More recently, the focus of research has moved to receptor sensitivity and second-messenger systems, and attempts to explain why, despite rapid alteration in the central nervous system (CNS) of amine levels, antidepressant action takes several weeks to become clinically evident.

The catecholamine hypothesis of affective disorder

Schildkraut (1965) is credited with formulating the noradrenergic hypothesis of affective disorder, which postulates that depression is due to a deficiency and mania to an excess of brain noradrenaline (NA). Knowledge of the noradrenergic neuronal anatomy also suggests that NA is likely to be important in depression and stress responses: the locus ceruleus and lateral tegmental areas contain the highest concentrations of noradrenergic neurons and projections from these areas connect to key limbic structures, including the amygdala, hippocampus and hypothalamus (Brunello *et al*, 2002).

Attempts to show that urinary levels of the NA metablite 3-methyoxy-4 hydroxy-phenol glycol (MHPG) were brain derived (and therefore reflected central NA metabolism) provided inconsistent results. Studies involving the administration of amino-methyl-para-tyrosine (AMPT), which reversibly inhibits the rate-limiting step in the synthesis of both noradrenaline and dopamine, have proved more consistent. AMPT administration leads to depletion of these neurotransmitters in animal models and to a relapse of symptoms among patients treated for depression, particularly those who had responded to a noradrenaline reuptake inhibitor (Miller *et al*, 1996).

Research into receptor sensitivity has also implicated noradrenaline pathways. Chronic antidepressant treatments affect NA receptor-coupled adenylate cyclase (the second messenger) and induce a decrease in the density of β-receptors in the brain. This downregulation occurs around 2 weeks after the initial receptor blockade and coincides with the onset of the clinical effects of antidepressants. However, chronic SSRI administration has been shown to upregulate β_1-adrenoreceptors in rat brains (Palvimaki *et al*, 1994). Examination of the brains of unmedicated suicide victims has also shown higher densities of β-adrenoreceptors compared with controls, but no difference was shown for those suicide victims who had a history of depression (De Paermentier *et al*, 1991).

There is also evidence that some antidepressants downregulate central α-adrenoreceptors, thus inducing increased NA release because of the reduced α_2-receptor-mediated autoinhibitory control (Garcia-Sevilla *et al*, 1992). A higher density, and upregulation, of α_{2A}-autoreceptors in various brain regions of depressed suicide victims has also been demonstrated (Callado *et al*, 1998). It is thought that inhibition of NA reuptake together with desensitisation of α_2-receptors overrides the downregulation of β-receptors, resulting in an overall increase in postsynaptic NA transmission (Brunello *et al*, 2002).

Further evidence for NA involvement in depression comes from research focusing on the locus ceruleus: significantly raised levels of tyrosine hydroxylase, increased agonist binding to α_{2A}-autoreceptors and reduced NA transporter have been demonstrated in the locus ceruleus of patients with depression (Ordway *et al*, 2003).

The serotonin (5-HT) hypothesis of affective illness

It is known that the 5-HT system has an important role in the regulation of sleep, appetite, sexual function, pain and circadian rhythms, all of which are disrupted in depression. There is an extensive and widespread innervation of the cerebral cortex and limbic system by ascending projections of 5-HT neurons, whose cell bodies are located in brain-stem raphe nuclei and each of which is linked to over half a million terminals within the cerebral cortex. There is now extensive evidence implicating a key role for serotonin in the pathogenesis of depression:

- Although only some antidepressants act as 5-HT reuptake inhibitors, all antidepressants given chronically have been shown to enhance 5-HT neurotransmission.
- The essential amino acid tryptophan is the precursor of serotonin and oral administration of a tryptophan-free amino acid mixture causes rapid depletion of plasma tryptophan, and thus brain serotonin. Studies have shown a relapse of depressive symptoms when tryptophan was removed from the diet of people who had recovered from depression (both those on antidepressant medication and medication-free), while controls with no history of depression remained relatively unaffected (Delgado *et al*, 1994). This effect was most marked in the patients on monoamine oxidase inhibitors and was reversed on replacing L-tryptophan in the diet. A number of patients with severe chronic depression on monoamine oxidase inhibitors or tricyclic antidepressants relapsed when L-tryptophan was withdrawn from the market (Ferrier *et al*, 1990).
- Earlier studies had suggested that depressed patients have lower levels of plasma tryptophan, a lower ratio of plasma tryptophan to neutral amino acids and

lower levels of 5-hydroxy-indole-acetic acid (5-HIAA, the major metabolite of 5-HT) after L-tryptophan infusion, although these findings have not been replicated in recent years.

- Medication-free patients with depression have been shown to have lower levels of 5-HIAA within the cerebrospinal fluid (CSF) and reduced concentrations of both 5-HT and 5-HIAA have been found in post-mortem studies of depression and suicide.
- Neuroendocrine studies show that the prolactin response to L-tryptophan and fenfluramine is blunted when patients are depressed, suggesting that presynaptic 5-HT dysfunction is a state marker in depression (Delgado *et al*, 1994): these changes normalise with antidepressants, which suggests that they reverse the deficit.

An increased density of 5-HT_2 binding sites has been demonstrated in post-mortem studies of depression and suicide, with the strongest evidence being for increased 5-HT_{2A} receptors in the dorsolateral prefrontal cortex, as well as in the platelets of medication-free patients with depression. These post-mortem studies have also demonstrated a reduction in 5-HT_{1A} receptors in several cortical areas (Stockmeier, 2003) and desensitisation of these receptors. Long-term antidepressant treatments have been shown to downregulate 5-HT_2 receptors and may also increase the function of postsynaptic 5-HT_{1A} receptors. However, downregulation of 5-HT_2 receptors occurs faster than the antidepressant action, levels of these receptors are actually increased by electroconvulsive therapy and most direct-acting 5-HT_{1A} receptor agonists are not good antidepressants. It has been suggested that alterations in receptor sensitivity due to antidepressants simply reflect functional changes due to excess monoamines and the actual antidepressant effects may involve intracellular signal transduction pathways, which can be mediated by antidepressants acting on either noradrenergic or serotonergic receptors (Bhalla & Lyengar, 1999).

Other neurotransmitters

The cholinergic, dopaminergic, GABA-ergic and glutaminergic systems have all been implicated in depression and there are a number of circumstantial pieces of evidence to support each of these hypotheses (Meltzer, 1987).

Acetylcholine

Janowsky *et al* (1994) hypothesised that excess cholinergic activity is involved in depression. Evidence for the involvement of acetylcholine in depression includes the findings that some cholinomimetic drugs are associated with depression in normal people, the cholinergic agonist arecholine worsens depressive symptoms in patients with depression, and sleep and neuroendocrine studies suggest a degree of postsynaptic cholinergic supersensitivity in depression. However, there is no evidence that anticholinergic drugs are effective antidepressants.

Dopamine

Randup & Braestrup (1977) first proposed that underactivity of dopamine (DA) plays a role in the aetiology of depression. The psychostimulants amphetamine and methylphenidate, which cause dopamine release, as well as the direct dopamine agonists bromocriptine and peribedil, all have short-lived antidepressant properties. Low CSF homovanillic acid (a measure of dopamine turnover) has also been reported consistently in a proportion of patients with depression (particularly those with retardation) and dopamine is increasingly being understood as crucial in reward and motivation circuits in the brain.

GABA

There is little direct evidence for a disturbance of GABA or GABA binding in depression but increasing evidence that antidepressants affect GABA receptors and that GABA-B agonists enhance monoaminergic neurotransmission. One functional neuroimaging study suggested that patients with depression have reduced cortical GABA levels (Sanacora *et al*, 1999).

Glutamine

There is increasing evidence that glutaminergic transmission is altered in depression. Lamotrigine (Calabrese *et al*, 1999) and lithium, both of which have utility in treating resistant depression, have been shown to reduce glutamine transmission by reducing release or facilitating reuptake, and antidepressants have been shown to reduce N-methyl-D-asparate receptor subunit expression (Petrie *et al*, 2000).

Cellular neurobiology

Recent advances in our understanding of the long-term effects of antidepressants have highlighted the importance of intracellular signalling pathways and how these affect two processes: cellular 'plasticity', and cellular generation and survival. Studies have shown that neurons are 'plastic' – they adapt to stimuli by enhancing synaptic connections, by altering spine density, and by dendrite branching and axonal sprouting (Thoenen, 1995). Reduced adaptation or plasticity may result in an inability to deal with environmental or other stresses. It has also been shown that new cell birth in the brain continues into old age and structural abnormalities associated with depression are now thought to be the result of impairments in cellular survival and neurogenesis. Abnormal cellular plasticity and survival may represent the fundamental pathophysiological mechanisms causing or maintaining depressive disorders (Kempermann & Kronenberg, 2003).

Glucocorticoids

As outlined above, significant stressors increase the risk of developing a major depressive disorder, and this may be modulated by activation of the HPA axis. In animal models, glucocorticoids have been shown to directly cause dendritic atrophy or death in hippocampal CA3 pyramidal neurons (Sapolsky, 2000) and to reduce cellular resilience – making certain neurons more susceptible to other physiological or pathological insults (such as ischaemic events) (Sapolsky, 2000). Reduced resilience is thought to be due to the effects of glucocorticoids on glutaminergic pathways and glucose transport and by stress, which has been shown to reduce the expression of brain-derived neurotrophic factor (BDNF) (Sapolsky, 2000). Neurotrophic factors such as BDNF inhibit cell death and subtle alterations in the balance of such factors may have profound implications for regional cellular survival (Riccio *et al*, 1999). Recently, stress has been shown to reduce neurogenesis and although the implications for neurogenesis have yet to be understood in human brains, regional alterations (e.g. in the hippocampus or dentate gyrus) have been postulated as contributing factors in depression (Kempermann & Kronenberg, 2003).

Antidepressants

Stewart *et al* (2001), investigating the Stanley Foundation brains, found that antidepressants appeared to stimulate components of the cyclic adenosine monophosphate (cAMP) pathway in patients with depression, while mood stabilisers blunt the same pathways in patients with bipolar disorder. Long-term antidepressant use has been shown to upregulate the cAMP cascade (regulated by both serotonin and noradrenaline) – via cAMP-dependent protein kinase (PKA) – causing alterations in cAMP responsive element binding protein (CREB), which is involved in cell survival (Duman *et al*, 2000). The gene encoding for BDNF is regulated by CREB, and upregulation of the CREB pathway, caused by chronic antidepressant use, has been thought to produce neurotrophic effects, inducing regeneration of catecholamine axon terminals in the cerebral cortex, improving synaptic plasticity and protecting against stress-induced hippocampal CA3 pyramidal neuron atrophy (Duman *et al*, 2000) as well as increasing, and protecting, neurogenesis (Jacobs *et al*, 2000). Lithium, which has considerable utility in treating resistant depression, has been shown to increase levels of the cytoprotective protein Bcl-2 in animal and *in vitro* human tissue studies, as well as affecting enzymes involved in neuronal survival (Chen *et al*, 1999). Functional imaging, using SPECT, has demonstrated that several weeks of lithium treatment significantly increased levels of a marker of neuronal viability and function in brain grey matter, and volumetric studies have demonstrated an increase in grey matter volume with lithium treatment (Moore *et al*, 2000). Alterations in the cAMP pathways, resulting in changes in gene expression, may result not only in altered neurogenesis and neuronal survival (Kempermann & Kronenberg, 2003), but also in a change to adaptive responses, for example the metabolism of neurotransmitters and expression of receptors (Brady *et al*, 1992)

Conclusions

A key element in the treatment of any patient with depression is to try to understand the cause for the individual concerned. The first part of this chapter has summarised scientific investigations in the realms of genetics, sociology and psychology, although the findings relate more to groups of patients with depression, rather than to individuals. Nevertheless, this information provides an essential background to enable clinicians to form a more balanced view of the relative contributions of the many different causes of depression in the individual patients they are treating. In this way the wealth of information accrued in these scientific studies may have some direct clinical relevance.

The latter half of this chapter has described more recent advances in our understanding of depression made by the application of modern medical technology and perhaps rests more with an assumption that depression is a mainly neurobiological disease. It is likely that much will change over the next 10 years. Neuroimaging studies should lead to a better understanding of the neural, biochemical and hormonal mechanisms that underlie depression. Advances in cellular neurobiology will improve our understanding of how the brain changes throughout the life span. The spectacular advances in molecular genetics should enable the location of the genes responsible for an increased vulnerability to depression to be found, and it may become possible to identify individuals susceptible to the disorder. With the sequencing of these genes it may also be possible to identify the relevant proteins and explain the key biochemical mechanisms, as well as the way these proteins interact with developmental and other environmental risk factors. There is also the hope that these developments will lead to new treatments for depression, and perhaps even to tailored and targeted treatments for individual patients

References

Abramson, L. Y., Seligman, M. E. & Teasdale, J. D. (1978) Learned helplessness in humans: critique and reformulation. *Journal of Abnormal Psychology*, **87**, 49–74.

Akiskal, H. S., Judd, L. L., Gillin, J. C., *et al* (1997) Subthreshold depressions: clinical and polysomnographic validation of dysthymic, residual and masked forms. *Journal of Affective Disorders*, **45**, 53–63.

Alliez, J. & Huber, J. P. (1987) Acadia, or the depressed between sin and illness. *Annales Medicines et Psychologie (Paris)*, **145**, 393–408.

Alloway, R. & Bebbington, P. (1987) The buffer theory of social support – a review of the literature. *Psychological Medicine*, **17**, 91–108.

Alloy, L. B., Abramson, L. Y., Metalsky, G. I., *et al* (1988) The hopelessness theory of depression: attributional aspects. *British Journal of Clinical Psychology*, **27**, 5–21.

Alloy, L. B., Abramson, L. Y., Wayne, G., *et al* (1999) Depressogenic cognitive styles: predictive validity, information processing and personality characteristics, and developmental origins. *Behavioral Research Therapy*, **37**, 503–531.

American Psychiatric Association (1994) *Diagnostic and Statistical Manual of Mental Disorders* (4th edn) (DSM–IV). Washington, DC: APA.

Andrade, L., Caraveo-Anduaga, J. J., Berglund, P., *et al* (2003) The epidemiology of major depressive episodes: results from the International Consortium of Psychiatric Epidemiology (ICPE) Surveys. *International Journal of Methods in Psychiatric Research*, **12**, 3–21.

Bagby, R. M., Bindseil, K. D., Schuller, D. R., *et al* (1997) Relationship between the five-factor model of personality and unipolar, bipolar and schizophrenic patients. *Psychiatry Research*, **70**, 83–94.

Banks, S. M. & Kerns, R. D. (1996) Explaining high rates of depression in chronic pain: a diathesis–stress framework. *Psychological Bulletin*, **119**, 95–110.

Bebbington, P. E. (1978) The epidemiology of depressive disorders. *Culture, Medicine and Psychiatry*, **2**, 297–341.

Bebbington, P. E. (2003) The origins of sex differences in depressive disorder: bridging the gap. *International Review of Psychiatry*, **8**, 295–332.

Beck, A. T., Epstein, N. & Harrison, R. (1983) Cognitions, attitudes and personality dimensions in depression. *British Journal of Cognitive Psychotherapy*, **1**, 1–16.

Bertelsen, A., Harvald, B. & Hauge, M. (1977) A Danish twin study of manic–depressive disorders. *British Journal of Psychiatry*, **130**, 330–351.

Beyer, J. L. & Krishnan, K. R. (2002) Volumetric brain imaging findings in mood disorders. *Biological Disorders*, **4**, 89–104.

Bhalla, U. S. & Lyengar, R. (1999) Emergent properties of networks of biological signaling pathways. *Science*, **283**, 381–387. (See also comment, pp. 339–340.)

Bibring, E. (1953) The mechanism of depression. In *Affective Disorders* (ed. P. Greenacre), pp. 14–47. New York: International Universities Press.

Birtchnell, J. (1980) Women whose mothers died in childhood: an outcome study. *Psychological Medicine*, **10**, 699–713.

Bowlby, J. (1951) Maternal Care and Mental Health, monograph no. 2. Geneva: WHO.

Brady, L. S., Gold, P. W., Herkenham, M., *et al* (1992) The antidepressants fluoxetine, idazoxan and phenelzine alter corticotropin-releasing hormone and tyrosine hydroxylase mRNA levels in rat brain: therapeutic implications. *Brain Research*, **572**, 117–125.

Brink, A. (1979) Depression and loss: a theme in Burton's *Anatomy of Melancholy*. *Canadian Journal of Psychiatry*, **24**, 767–771.

Brown, G. W. & Harris, T. (1978) *Social Origins of Depression: A Study of Psychiatric Disorder in Women*. London: Tavistock.

Brown, G. W., Andrews, B., Harris, T., *et al* (1986) Social support, self-esteem and depression. *Psychological Medicine*, **16**, 813–831.

Brugha, T. S. (2003) The effects of life events and social relationships on the course of major depression. *Current Psychiatric Reports*, **5**, 431–438.

Brunello, N., Mendlewicz, J., Kasper, S., *et al* (2002) The role of noradrenaline and selective noradrenaline reuptake inhibition in depression. *European Neuropsychopharmacology*, **12**, 461–475.

Butzlaff, R. I. & Hooley, J. M. (1998) Expressed emotion and psychiatric relapse. *Archives of General Psychiatry*, **55**, 547–551.

Calabrese, J. R., Bowden, C. L., McElroy, S. L., *et al* (1999) Spectrum of activity of lamotrigine in treatment-refractory bipolar disorder. *American Journal of Psychiatry*, **156**, 1019–1023.

Callado, L. F., Meana, J. J., Grijalba, B., *et al* (1998) Selective increase of $alpha_{2A}$-adrenoceptor agonist binding sites in brains of depressed suicide victims. *Journal of Neurochemistry*, **70**, 1114–1123.

Campbell, L. C., Clauw, D. J. & Keefe, F. J. (2003) Persistent pain and depression: a biopsychosocial perspective. *Biological Psychiatry*, **54**, 399–409.

Caspi, A., Sugden, K., Moffitt, T., *et al* (2003) Influence of life stress on depression: moderation by a polymorphism in the 5-HTT gene. *Science*, **301**, 386–389.

Champion, L. (1990) The relationship between social vulnerability and the occurrence of severely threatening life events. *Psychological Medicine*, **20**, 157–161.

Chanar, G., Landau, S., Beasley, C., *et al* (2003) Two-dimensional assessment of cyto architecture in the anterior singulate cortex in major depressive disorder, bipolar disorder and schizophrenia: evidence for decreased neuronal somal size and increased neuronal density. *Biological Psychiatry*, **53**, 1086–1098.

Charlton, B. G. & Ferrier, I. N. (1989) Hypothalamo–pituitary–adrenal axis abnormalities in depression: a review and a model. *Psychological Medicine*, **19**, 331–336.

Chen, G., Zeng, W. Z., Yuan, P. X., *et al* (1999) The mood-stabilizing agents lithium and valproate robustly increase the levels of the neuroprotective protein bcl-2 in the CNS. *Journal of Neurochemistry*, **72**, 879–882.

Clayton, P. & Darvish, H. S. (1979) Course of depressive symptoms following the stress of bereavement. In *Stress and Mental Disorder* (eds J. Barret, R. M. Rose & G. L. Klerman), pp. 121–136. New York: Raven Press.

Cloninger, C. R. (1987) A systematic method for clinical description and classification of personality variants. A proposal. *Archives of General Psychiatry*, **44**, 573–588.

Cobb, S. (1976) Presidential address 1976. Social support as a moderator of life stress. *Psychosomatic Medicine*, **38**, 300–314.

Corruble, E., Ginestet, D. & Guelfi, J. D. (1996) Comorbidity of personality disorders and unipolar major depression: a review. *Journal of Affective Disorders*, **37**, 157–170.

Cotter, D. R., Pariante, C. M. & Everall, I. P. (2001) Glial cell abnormalities in major psychiatric disorders: the evidence and implications. *Brain Research Bulletin*, **55**, 585–595.

Covic, T., Adamson, B., Howe, G., *et al* (2002) The role of passive coping and helplessness in rheumatoid arthritis depression and pain. *Journal of Applied Health Behaviour*, **4**, 31–35.

Cox, B. J., Enns, M. W. & Clara, I. P. (2000) The Parental Bonding Instrument: confirmatory evidence for a three-factor model in a psychiatric clinical sample and in the National Comorbidity Survey. *Social Psychiatry and Psychiatric Epidemiology*, **35**, 353–357.

De Paermentier, F., Cheetham, S. C., Crompton, M. R., *et al* (1991) Brain beta-adrenoceptor binding sites in depressed suicide victims: effects of antidepressant treatment. *Psychopharmacology*, **105**, 283–288.

Delgado, P. L., Price, L. H., Miller, H. L., *et al* (1994) Serotonin and the neurobiology of depression. Effects of tryptophan depletion in drug-free depressed patients. *Archives of General Psychiatry*, **51**, 865–874.

Dew, A. M., Bromet, E. J. & Schulberg, H. C. (1987) Mental health effects of the Three Mile Island nuclear reactor restart. *American Journal of Psychiatry*, **144**, 1074–1077.

Drevets, W. C. (2001) Neuroimaging and neuropathological studies of depression: implications for the cognitive–emotional features of mood disorders. *Current Opinion in Neurobiology*, **11**, 240–249.

Drevets, W. C. (2003) Neuroimaging abnormalities in the amygdala in mood disorders. *Annals of the New York Academy of Sciences*, **985**, 420–444.

Duman, R. S., Malberg, J., Nakagawa, S., *et al* (2000) Neuronal plasticity and survival in mood disorders. *Biological Psychiatry*, **48**, 732–739. (See also comment, pp. 713–714.)

Edhborg, M., Lundh, W., Seimyr, L., *et al* (2003) The parent–child relationship in the context of maternal depressive mood. *Archives of Women Mental Health*, **6**, 211–216.

Elkis, H., Friedman, L., Wise, A., *et al* (1995) Meta-analyses of studies of ventricular enlargement and cortical sulcal prominence in mood disorders. Comparisons with controls or patients with schizophrenia. *Archives of General Psychiatry*, **52**, 735–746.

Emmerson, J. P., Burvill, P. W., Finlay-Jones, R., *et al* (1989) Life events, life difficulties and confiding relationships in the depressed elderly. *British Journal of Psychiatry*, **155**, 787–792.

Engum, A., Bjoro, T., Mykletun, A., *et al* (2002) An association between depression, anxiety and thyroid function – a clinical fact or an artefact? *Acta Psychiatrica Scandinavica*, **106**, 27–34.

Eysenck, H. J. (1981) *A Model of Personality*. New York: Springer-Verlag.

Farmer, A. E. & McGuffin, P. (2003) Humiliation, loss and other types of life events and difficulties: a comparison of depressed subjects, healthy controls and their siblings. *Psychological Medicine*, **33**, 1169–1175.

Farmer, A., Redman, K., Harris, T., *et al* (2002) Neuroticism, extraversion, life events and depression. The Cardiff Depression Study. *British Journal of Psychiatry*, **181**, 118–122.

Farmer, A. E., McGuffin, P., Mahmood, A., *et al* (2003) A sib-pair study of the temperament and Character Inventory scales in major depression. *Archives of General Psychiatry*, **60**, 490–496.

Ferrier, I. N. & Scott, J. (1998) Causes of depression. In *Seminars in General Adult Psychiatry* (1st edn) (eds G. Stein & G. Wilkinson), pp. 102–153. London: Gaskell.

Ferrier, I. N., Eccleston, D., Moore, P. B., *et al* (1990) Relapse in chronic depressives on withdrawal of L-tryptophan. *Lancet*, **336**, 380–381.

Fishbain, D. (2000) Evidence-based data on pain relief with antidepressants. *Annals of Medicine*, **32**, 305–316.

Fishbain, D. A., Cutler, R., Rosomoff, H. L., *et al* (1997) Chronic pain-associated depression: antecedent or consequence of chronic pain? A review. *Clinical Journal of Pain*, **13**, 116–137.

Freud, S. (1917) Mourning and melancholia. Reprinted (1953–1974) in *Standard Edition of the Complete Psychological Works of Sigmund Freud* (trans. and ed. J. Strachey), vol. 14, p. 239. London: Hogarth Press.

Garcia-Sevilla, J. A., Meana, J. J., Barturen, F., *et al* (1992) $Alpha_2$-adrenoceptors in the brain of depressed suicide victims. *Clinical Neuropharmacology*, **15**, 321A–322A.

Gilman, S. E., Kawachi, I., Fitzmaurice, G. M., *et al* (2003) Family disruption in childhood and risk of adult depression. *American Journal of Psychiatry*, **160**, 939–946.

Gladstone, G. & Parker, G. (2001) Depressogenic cognitive schemas: enduring beliefs or mood state artefacts? *Australian and New Zealand Journal of Psychiatry*, **35**, 210–216.

Goldapple, K., Segal, Z., Garson, C., *et al* (2004) Modulation of cortical–limbic pathways in major depression: treatment-specific effects of cognitive behavior therapy. *Archives of General Psychiatry*, **61**, 34–41.

Griens, A. M., Jonker, K., Spinhoven, P., *et al* (2002) The influence of depressive state features on trait measurement. *Journal of Affective Disorders*, **70**, 95–99.

Hankin, B. L. & Abramson, L. Y. (2001) Development of gender differences in depression: an elaborated cognitive vulnerability-transactional stress theory. *Psychological Bulletin*, **127**, 773–796.

Harkness, K. L. & Luther, J. (2001) Clinical risk factors for the generation of life events in major depression. *Journal of Abnormal Psychology*, **110**, 564–572.

Harrington, R., Rutter, M., Weissman, M., *et al* (1997) Psychiatric disorders in the relatives of depressed probands. I. Comparison of prepubertal, adolescent and early adult onset cases. *Journal of Affective Disorders*, **42**, 9–22.

Hayhurst, H., Cooper, Z., Paykel, E. S., *et al* (1997) Expressed emotion and depression. A longitudinal study. *British Journal of Psychiatry*, **171**, 439–443.

Heim, C., Plotsky, P. M. & Nemeroff, C. B. (2004) Importance of studying the contributions of early adverse experience to neurobiological findings in depression. *Neuropsychopharmacology*, **29**, 641–648.

Hickie, I., Scott, E., Wilhelm, K., *et al* (1997) Subcortical hyperintensities on magnetic resonance imaging in patients with severe depression – a longitudinal evaluation. *Biological Psychiatry*, **42**, 367–374.

Hirschfeld, R. M. A. & Shea, M. T. (1992) Personality. In *Handbook of Affective Disorders* (ed. E. S. Paykel), pp. 185–194. Edinburgh: Churchill Livingstone.

Hollander, B. (1901) The cerebral localization of melancholia. *Journal of Mental Science*, **47**, 458–485.

Holmes, T. H. & Rahe, R. H. (1967) The Social Readjustment Rating Scale. *Journal of Psychosomatic Research*, **11**, 213–218.

Hudgens, R. W. (1974) Personal catastrophe and depression. In *Stressful Life Events: Their Nature and Effects* (ed. R. A. Depue), pp. 119–134. New York: Academic Press.

Hunter, R. & Macalpine, I. (1963) *Three Hundred Years of Psychiatry 1535–1860*. London: Oxford University Press.

Jackson, J. L., O'Malley, P. G., Tomkins, G., *et al* (2000) Treatment of functional gastrointestinal disorders with antidepressant medications: a meta-analysis. *American Journal of Medicine*, **108**, 65–72.

Jacobs, B. L., Praag, H. & Gage, F. H. (2000) Adult brain neurogenesis and psychiatry: a novel theory of depression. *Molecular Psychiatry*, **5**, 262–269.

Jacobson, E. (1953) Contribution to the meta-psychology of cyclothymic depression. In *Affective Disorders* (ed. P. Greenacre), pp. 49–83. New York: International Universities Press.

Janowsky, D. S., Overstreet, D. H. & Nurnberger, J. I. (1994) Is cholinergic sensitivity a genetic marker for the affective disorders? *American Journal of Medical Genetics*, **54**, 335–344.

Jenkins, R., Lewis, G., Bebbington, P., *et al* (2003) The National Psychiatric Morbidity Surveys of Great Britain – initial findings from the Household Survey. *International Review of Psychiatry*, **15**, 29–42.

Joffe, R. T., Bagby, R. M., Levitt, A. J., *et al* (1993) The Tridimensional Personality Questionnaire in major depression. *American Journal of Psychiatry*, **150**, 959–960.

Johnson, J. G., Cohen, P., Dohrenwend, B. P., *et al* (1999) A longitudinal investigation of social causation and social selection processes involved in the association between socioeconomic status and psychiatric disorders. *Journal of Abnormal Psychology*, **108**, 490–499.

Jones, I., Kent, L. & Craddock, N. (2002) Genetics of affective disorders. In *Psychiatric Genetics and Genomics* (eds P. McGuffin, M. J. Owen & I. I. Gottesman), pp. 211–245. Oxford: Oxford University Press.

Joynt, K. E., Whellan, D. J. & O'Connor, C. M. (2003) Depression and cardiovascular disease: mechanisms of interaction. *Biological Psychiatry*, **54**, 248–261.

Just, N., Abramson, L. Y. & Alloy, L. B. (2001) Remitted depression studies as tests of the cognitive vulnerability hypotheses of depression onset: a critique and conceptual analysis. *Clinical Psychology Review*, **21**, 63–83.

Kempermann, G. & Kronenberg, G. (2003) Depressed new neurons? Adult hippocampal neurogenesis and a cellular plasticity hypothesis of major depression. *Biological Psychiatry*, **54**, 499–503.

Kendler, K. S. (1993) Twin studies of psychiatric illness. Current status and future directions. *Archives of General Psychiatry*, **50**, 905–915.

Kendler, K. S., Kessler, R. C., Walters, E. E., *et al* (1995) Stressful life events, genetic liability, and onset of an episode of major depression in women. *American Journal of Psychiatry*, **152**, 833–842.

Kendler, K. S., Thornton, L. M. & Prescott, C. A. (2001) Gender differences in the rates of exposure to stressful life events and sensitivity to their depressogenic effects. *American Journal of Psychiatry*, **158**, 587–593.

Kendler, K. S., Prescott, C. A., Myers, J., *et al* (2003) The structure of genetic and environmental risk factors for common psychiatric and substance use disorders in men and women. *Archives of General Psychiatry*, **60**, 929–937.

Kessing, L. V., Agerbo, E. & Mortensen, P. B. (2003) Does the impact of major stressful life events on the risk of developing depression change throughout life? *Psychological Medicine*, **33**, 1177–1184.

Kessler, R .C. (1999) The World Health Organization International Consortium in Psychiatric Epidemiology (ICPE): initial work and future directions – the NAPE Lecture 1998. Nordic Association for Psychiatric Epidemiology. *Acta Psychiatrica Scandinavica*, **99**, 2–9.

Kessler, R. C., Berglund, P., Demler, O., *et al* (2003) The epidemiology of major depressive disorder: results from the National Comorbidity Survey Replication (NCS–R). *Journal of the American Medical Association*, **289**, 3095–3105.

Kieseppä, T., Partonen, T., Hanukka, J., *et al* (2004) High concordance of bipolar I disorder in a nationwide sample of twins. *American Journal of Psychiatry*, **161**, 1814–1821.

Kimbrell, T. A., Ketter, T. A., George, M. S., *et al* (2002) Regional cerebral glucose utilization in patients with a range of severities of unipolar depression. *Biological Psychiatry*, **51**, 237–252.

Klein, M. (1934) *Contributions to Psychoanalysis 1921*, pp. 282–310. London: Hogarth Press.

Knable, M. B., Torrey, E. F., Webster, M. J., *et al* (2001) Multi-variant analysis of prefrontal cortical data from the Stanley Foundation Neuropathology Consortium. *Brain Research Bulletin*, **55**, 651–659.

Knable, M. B., Barci, B. M., Webster, M. J., *et al* (2004) Molecular abnormalities of the hippocampus in severe psychiatric illness: post-mortem findings from the Stanley Neuropathology Consortium. *Molecular Psychiatry*, **6**, 544.

Kool, S., Dekker, J., Duijsens, I. J., *et al* (2003) Changes in personality pathology after pharmacotherapy and combined therapy for depressed patients. *Journal of Personality Disorders*, **17**, 60–72.

Krueger, R. F., Caspi, A., Moffitt, T. E., *et al* (1996) Personality traits are differentially linked to mental disorders: a multitrait–multidiagnosis study of an adolescent birth cohort. *Journal of Abnormal Psychology*, **105**, 299–312.

Kwon, J. S., Kim, Y-M., Chang, C. G., *et al* (2000) Three-year follow-up of women with the sole diagnosis of depressive personality disorder: subsequent development of dysthymia and major depression. *American Journal of Psychiatry*, **157**, 1966–1972.

Lacerda, A. L., Nicoletti, M. A., Brambilla, P., *et al* (2003) Anatomical MRI study of basal ganglia in major depressive disorder. *Psychiatry Research*, **124**, 129–140.

Lara, M. E., Leader, J. & Klein, D. N. (1997) The association between social support and course of depression: is it confounded with personality? *Journal of Abnormal Psychology*, **106**, 478–482.

Leff, J. & Vaughn, C. (1980) The interaction of life events and relatives' expressed emotion in schizophrenia and depressive neurosis. *British Journal of Psychiatry*, **136**, 146–153.

Lenze, E., Cross, D., McKeel, D., *et al* (1999) White matter hyperintensities and gray matter lesions in physically healthy depressed subjects. *American Journal of Psychiatry*, **156**, 1602–1607.

Levinson, D. F., Zubenko, G. S., Crowe, R. R., *et al* (2003) Genetics of recurrent early-onset depression (GenRED): design and preliminary clinical characteristics of a repository sample for genetic linkage studies. *American Journal of Medical Genetics*, **119B**, 118–130.

Lewinsohn, P. M., Joiner, T. E. Jr & Rohde, P. (2001) Evaluation of cognitive diathesis–stress models in predicting major depressive disorder in adolescents. *Journal of Abnormal Psychology*, **110**, 203–215.

Lieb, R., Isensee, B., Hofler, M., *et al* (2002) Parental major depression and the risk of depression and other mental disorders in offspring: a prospective-longitudinal community study. *Archives of General Psychiatry*, **59**, 365–374.

Lim, K. O. & Helpern, J. A. (2002) Neuropsychiatric applications of DTI – a review. *NMR in Biomedicine*, **15**, 587–593.

Liu, D., Caldji, C., Sharma, S., *et al* (2000) Influence of neonatal rearing conditions on stress-induced adrenocorticotropin responses and norepinephrine release in the hypothalamic paraventricular nucleus. *Journal of Neuroendocrinology*, **12**, 5–12.

Lorant, V., Deliege, D., Eaton, W., *et al* (2003) Socioeconomic inequalities in depression: a meta-analysis. *American Journal of Epidemiology*, **157**, 98–112.

Maier, W., Gänsicke, M., Gater, R., *et al* (1999) Gender differences in the prevalence of depression: a survey in primary care. *Journal of Affective Disorders*, **53**, 241–252.

McCauley, J., Kern, D. E., Kolodner, K., *et al* (1997) Clinical characteristics of women with a history of childhood abuse: unhealed wounds. *JAMA*, **277**, 1362–1368.

McGuffin, P. & Katz, R. (1989) The genetics of depression and manic–depressive disorder. *British Journal of Psychiatry*, **155**, 294–304.

McGuffin, P., Katz, R. & Bebbington, P. (1988) The Camberwell Collaborative Depression Study. III. Depression and adversity in the relatives of depressed probands. *British Journal of Psychiatry*, **152**, 775–782.

McGuffin, P., Katz, R., Watkins, S., *et al* (1996) A hospital-based twin register of the heritability of DSM–IV unipolar depression. *Archives of General Psychiatry*, **53**, 129–136.

McGuffin, P., Rijsdijk, F., Andrew, M., *et al* (2003) The hereditability of bipolar affective disorder and the genetic relationship to unipolar depression. *Archives of General Psychiatry*, **60**, 497–502.

Meertens, V., Scheepers, P. & Tax, B. (2003) Depressive symptoms in the Netherlands 1975–1996: a theoretical framework and an empirical analysis of socio-demographic characteristics, gender differences and changes over time. *Sociology, Health and Illness*, **25**, 208–231.

Meltzer, H. Y. (1987) *Psychopharmacology. The Third Generation of Progress*. New York: Raven Press.

Melville, D. I., Hope, D., Bennison, D., *et al* (1985) Depression among men made involuntarily redundant. *Psychological Medicine*, **15**, 789–793.

Mendelson, M. (1990) Psychoanalytic views on depression. In *Depressive Disorders* (eds B. B. Wolman & G. Strickler), pp. 22–37. New York: John Wiley.

Menza, M. A. & Mark, M. H. (1994) Parkinson's disease and depression: the relationship to disability and personality. *Journal of Neuropsychiatry and Clinical Neurosciences*, **6**, 165–169.

Merikangas, K. R. & Gelernter, C. S. (1990) Comorbidity for alcoholism and depression. *Psychiatric Clinics of North America*, **13**, 613–632.

Michael, N., Erfurth, A., Ohrmann, P., *et al* (2003) Metabolic changes within the left dorsolateral prefrontal cortex occurring with electroconvulsive therapy in patients with treatment resistant unipolar depression. *Psychological Medicine*, **33**, 1277–1284.

Miguel-Hidalgo, J. J. & Rajkowska, G. (2003) Comparison of prefrontal cell pathology between depression and alcohol dependence. *Journal of Psychiatric Research*, **37**, 411–420.

Miller, H. L., Delgado, P. L., Salomon, R. M., *et al* (1996) Clinical and biochemical effects of catecholamine depletion on antidepressant-induced remission of depression. *Archives of General Psychiatry*, **53**, 117–128.

Moore, G. J., Bebchuk, J. M., Hasanat, K., *et al* (2000) Lithium increases N-acetyl-aspartate in the human brain: in vivo evidence in support of bcl-2's neurotrophic effects? *Biological Psychiatry*, **48**, 1–8.

Mullen, P. E., Martin, J. L., Anderson, J. C., *et al* (1996) The long-term impact of the physical, emotional, and sexual abuse of children: a community study. *Child Abuse and Neglect*, **20**, 7–21.

Narushima, K., Kosier, J. T. & Robinson, R. G. (2003) A reappraisal of poststroke depression, intra- and inter-hemispheric lesion location using meta-analysis. *Journal of Neuropsychiatry and Clinical Neuroscience*, **15**, 422–430.

National Institute for Clinical Excellence (2003) *Depression: The Management of Depression in Primary and Secondary Care*. London: NICE.

Neighbors, H. W., Jackson, J. S., Campbell, L., *et al* (1989) The influence of racial factors on psychiatric diagnosis: a review and suggestions for research. *Community Mental Health Journal*, **25**, 301–311.

Oakley-Browne, M. A., Joyce, P. R., Wells, J. E., *et al* (1995) Adverse parenting and other childhood experience as risk factors for depression in women aged 18–44 years. *Journal of Affective Disorders*, **34**, 13–23.

Ogilvie, A. D., Battersby, S., Bubb, V. J., *et al* (1996) Polymorphism in serotonin transporter gene associated with susceptibility to major depression. *Lancet*, **347**, 731–733.

Ordway, G. A., Schenk, J., Stockmeier, C. A., *et al* (2003) Elevated agonist binding to alpha$_2$-adrenoceptors in the locus coeruleus in major depression. *Biological Psychiatry*, **53**, 315–323.

Palvimaki, E. P., Laakso, A., Kuoppamaki, M., *et al* (1994) Up-regulation of beta$_1$-adrenergic receptors in rat brain after chronic citalopram and fluoxetine treatments. *Psychopharmacology*, **115**, 543–546.

Parker, G., Tupling, H. & Brown, L. B. (1979) Parental Bonding Instrument. *British Journal of Medical Psychology*, **52**, 1–10.

Paykel, E. S. (2003) Life events and affective disorders. *Acta Psychiatrica Scandinavica*, **108**, suppl. 418, 61–66.

Paykel, E. S. & Cooper, Z. C. (1992) Live events and social stress. In *Handbook of Affective Disorders* (ed. E. S. Paykel), pp. 149–170. Edinburgh: Churchill Livingstone.

Petrie, R. X., Reid, I. C. & Stewart, C. A. (2000) The N-methyl-D-aspartate receptor, synaptic plasticity, and depressive disorder. A critical review. *Pharmacology and Therapeutics*, **87**, 11–25.

Piccinelli, M. & Wilkinson, G. (2000) Gender differences in depression. Critical review. *British Journal of Psychiatry*, **177**, 486–492.

Plomin, R. (1994) The Emanuel Miller Memorial Lecture 1993. Genetic research and identification of environmental influences. *Journal of Child Psychology and Psychiatry*, **35**, 817–834.

Posse, S., Fitzgerald, D., Gao, K., *et al* (2003) Real-time fMRI of temporolimbic regions detects amygdala activation during single-trial self-induced sadness. *Neuroimage*, **18**, 760–768.

Raadsheer, F. C., van Heerikhuize, J. J., Lucassen, P. J., *et al* (1995) Corticotropin-releasing hormone mRNA levels in the paraventricular nucleus of patients with Alzheimer's disease and depression. *American Journal of Psychiatry*, **152**, 1372–1376.

Rajkowska, G. (2000) Postmortem studies in mood disorders indicate altered numbers of neurones and glial cells. *Biological Psychiatry*, **48**, 766–777.

Randrup, A. & Braestrup, C. (1977) Uptake inhibition of biogenic amines by newer antidepressant drugs: relevance to the dopamine hypothesis of depression. *Psychopharmacology*, **53**, 309–314.

Riccio, A., Ahn, S., Davenport, C. M., *et al* (1999) Mediation by a CREB family transcription factor of NGF-dependent survival of sympathetic neurons. *Science*, **286**, 2358–2361.

Robertson, M. M. (1997) Suicide, parasuicide and epilepsy. In *Epilepsy: A Comprehensive Textbook* (eds J. Engel & T. A. Pedley), pp. 2141–2151. Philadelphia, PA: Lippincott-Raven.

Robins, L. N. & Regier, D. A. (1991) *Psychiatric disorders in America: The Epidemiological Catchment Area Study*. New York: Free Press.

Robins, L. N., Wing, J., Wittchen, H. U., *et al* (1989) The Composite International Diagnostic Interview. An epidemiologic instrument suitable for use in conjunction with different diagnostic systems and in different cultures. *Archives of General Psychiatry*, **45**, 1069–1077.

Robinson, R. G. (2003) Poststroke depression: prevalence, diagnosis, treatment, and disease progression. *Biological Psychiatry*, **54**, 376–387.

Rudisch, B. & Nemeroff, C. B. (2003) Epidemiology of comorbid coronary artery disease and depression. *Biological Psychiatry*, **54**, 227–240.

Rutter, M. (1985) Resilience in the face of adversity. Protective factors and resistance to psychiatric disorder. *British Journal of Psychiatry*, **147**, 598–611.

Ryder, A. G., Bagby, R. M. & Dion, K. L. (2001) Chronic, low-grade depression in a nonclinical sample: depressive personality or dysthymia? *Journal of Personality Disorder*, **15**, 84–93.

Ryle, A. (1991) Depression. In *Textbook of Psychotherapy in Psychiatric Practice* (ed. J. Holmes), pp. 265–286. Edinburgh: Churchill Livingstone.

Sanacora, G., Mason, G. F., Rothman, D. L., *et al* (1999) Reduced cortical gamma-aminobutyric acid levels in depressed patients determined by proton magnetic resonance spectroscopy. *Archives of General Psychiatry*, **56**, 1043–1047.

Sapolsky, R. M. (2000) Glucocorticoids and hippocampal atrophy in neuropsychiatric disorders. *Archives of General Psychiatry*, **57**, 925–935.

Sass, H. & Junemann, K. (2003) Affective disorders, personality and personality disorders. *Acta Psychiatrica Scandinavica Supplementum*, (418), 34–40.

Sauer, H., Richter, P., Czernik, A., *et al* (1997) Personality differences between patients with major depression and bipolar disorder – the impact of minor symptoms on self-ratings of personality. *Journal of Affective Disorders*, **42**, 169–177.

Schildkraut, J. J. (1965) The catecholamine hypothesis of affective disorders: a review of supporting evidence. *American Journal of Psychiatry*, **122**, 509–522.

Scott, J. (1988) Chronic depression. *British Journal of Psychiatry*, **153**, 287–297.

Scott, J., Eccleston, D. & Boys, R. (1992) Can we predict the persistence of depression? *British Journal of Psychiatry*, **161**, 633–637.

Seligman, M. E. P., Abramson, L. Y. & Semmel, A. (1978) Depressive attributional style. *Journal of Abnormal Psychology*, **88**, 242–247.

Serra-Mestres, J. & Ring, H. A. (2002) Evidence supporting a cognitive model of depression in Parkinson's disease. *Journal of Nervous and Mental Disorders*, **190**, 407–410.

Sheline, Y. I., Barch, D. M., Donnelly, J. M., *et al* (2001) Increased amygdala response to masked emotional faces in depressed subjects resolves with antidepressant treatment: an fMRI study. *Biological Psychiatry*, **50**, 651–658.

Shore, J. H., Tatum, E. L. & Vollmer, W. M. (1986) Psychiatric reactions to disaster: the Mount St Helens experience. *American Journal of Psychiatry*, **143**, 590–595.

Smith, A. L. & Weissman, M. M. (1992) Epidemiology. In *Handbook of Affective Disorders* (ed. E. S. Paykel), pp. 111–130. Edinburgh: Churchill Livingstone.

Somervell, P. D., Leaf, P. J., Weissman, M. M., *et al* (1989) The prevalence of major depression in black and white adults in five United States communities. *American Journal of Epidemiology*, **130**, 725–735.

Spanagel, R. & Weiss, F. (1999) The dopamine hypothesis of reward: past and current status. *Trends in Neurosciences*, **22**, 521–527.

Stansfeld, S. A., Fuhrer, R. & Shipley, M. J. (1998) Types of social support as predictors of psychiatric morbidity in a cohort of British civil servants (Whitehall II Study). *Psychological Medicine*, **28**, 881–892.

Stewart, R. J., Chen, B., Dollatshahi, D., *et al* (2001) Abnormalities in the cAMP signalling pathway in post-mortem brain tissue from the Stanley Neuropathology Consortium. *Brain Research Bulletin*, **55**, 625–629.

Stockmeier, C. A. (2003) Involvement of serotonin in depression: evidence from postmortem and imaging studies of serotonin receptors and the serotonin transporter. *Journal of Psychiatric Research*, **37**, 357–373.

Sullivan, P. F., Neale, M. C. & Kendler, K. S. (2000) Genetic epidemiology of major depression: review and meta-analysis. *American Journal of Psychiatry*, **157**, 1552–1562.

Tennant, C. & Bebbington, P. (1978) The social causation of depression: a critique of the work of Brown and his colleagues. *Psychological Medicine*, **8**, 565–575.

Thoenen, H. (1995) Neurotrophins and neuronal plasticity. *Science* **270**, 593–8.

Thomas, A. J., O'Brien, J. T., Davis, S., *et al* (2002) Ischemic basis for deep white matter hyperintensities in major depression: a neuropathological study. *Archives of General Psychiatry*, **59**, 785–792.

Tiet, Q. Q., Bird, H. R., Davies, M., *et al* (1998) Adverse life events and resilience. *Journal of the American Academy of Child and Adolescent Psychiatry*, **37**, 1191–1200.

Torrey, E. F., Webster, M., Knable, M., *et al* (2000) The Stanley Foundation Brain Collection and Neuropathology Consortium. *Schizophrenia Research*, **44**, 151–155.

Turner, R. J. & Turner, J. B. (1999) Social integration and support. *Handbook of Sociology and Social Research*, 301–319.

Twaddle, V. & Scott, J. (1991) Depression. In *Adult Clinical Problems: A Cognitive–Behavioural Approach* (eds W. Dryden & R. Rentoul), pp. 56–85. New York: Routledge.

Vaughn, C. E. & Leff, J. P. (1976) The influence of family and social factors on the course of psychiatric illness. A comparison of schizophrenic and depressed neurotic patients. *British Journal of Psychiatry*, **129**, 125–137.

Videbech, P., Ravnkilde, B., Pedersen, A. R., *et al* (2001) The Danish PET/depression project: PET findings in patients with major depression. *Psychological Medicine*, **31**, 1147–1158.

Weiss, E. L., Longhurst, J. G. & Mazure, C. M. (1999) Childhood sexual abuse as a risk factor for depression in women: psychosocial and neurobiological correlates. *American Journal of Psychiatry*, **156**, 816–828.

Weissman, M. M., Gershon, E. S., Kidd, K. K., *et al* (1984) Psychiatric disorders in the relatives of probands with affective disorders. The Yale University–National Institute of Mental Health Collaborative Study. *Archives of General Psychiatry*, **41**, 13–21.

Wender, P. H., Kety, S. S., Rosenthal, D., *et al* (1986) Psychiatric disorders in the biological and adoptive families of adopted individuals with affective disorders. *Archives of General Psychiatry*, **43**, 923–929.

Winokur, G. (1974) The division of depressive illness into depression spectrum disease and pure depressive disease. *International Pharmacopsychiatry*, **9**, 5–13.

Zung, W. W., Broadhead, W. E. & Roth, M. E. (1993) Prevalence of depressive symptoms in primary care. *Journal of Family Practice*, **37**, 337–344.

CHAPTER 4

Drug treatment of depression

Morris Bernadt

> Canst thou not minister to a mind diseas'd,
> Pluck from the memory a rooted sorrow,
> Raze out the written troubles of the brain,
> And with some sweet oblivious antidote
> Cleanse the stuff'd bosom of that perilous stuff
> Which weighs upon the heart?
>
> *Macbeth*, Act V, Scene 3

Four fundamental advances in psychopharmacology occurred in the 9 years between 1948 and 1957. These concerned imipramine, iproniazid, chlorpromazine and lithium.

Imipramine was introduced by the Swiss drug company Geigy, which had been investigating antihistamine substances similar to chlorpromazine as potential antipsychotic drugs. Geigy arranged for the Zurich professor of psychiatry Roland Kuhn to test imipramine on patients with schizophrenia. Kuhn treated more than 300 patients suffering from a variety of mental disorders and noticed that a few patients suffering from severe depression showed a pronounced improvement. In his classic paper on imipramine he wrote:

> 'G22355 (imipramine) is a substance with markedly antidepressive properties. Its mode of action remains completely unknown. The effect is striking in patients with depression. The patients get up in the morning of their own accord, speak louder and more rapidly, their facial expression becomes more vivacious, they begin to entertain themselves and take part in games, become more cheerful and are once more able to laugh.' (Kuhn, 1958)

Using a drug as an antidepressant was a momentous development because, as Kuhn pointed out, the only other treatments for depression available at the time were electroconvulsive therapy (ECT) and psychoanalysis.

Serendipity also led to the discovery of the therapeutic effects of iproniazid, chlorpromazine and lithium. The two hydrazine derivatives of isonicotinic acid, isoniazid and iproniazid, had been developed by another Swiss drug company, Hoffman La-Roche, for the treatment of tuberculosis. During clinical trials of these drugs in 1951 and 1952, physicians noted that patients on iproniazid but not isoniazid became cheerful, exuberant and even manic (Bloch *et al*, 1954). The psychiatrists who examined these patients diagnosed the mania, attributed it to the drug and yet failed to follow up on the antidepressant potential of iproniazid. The initial clinical trials in psychiatry were with chronically apathetic patients with schizophrenia, but in 1957 a New York psychiatrist, Nathan Kline, conducted a small open trial of iproniazid with patients with depression and reported that it had a stimulating and clinically beneficial mood-elevating effect. Only later did laboratory studies show that iproniazid was a much more potent inhibitor of monoamine oxidase (MAO) than isoniazid.

In contrast, the development of the more modern antidepressant drugs such as the selective serotonin reuptake inhibitors (SSRIs) was the outcome of planned commercial investment rather than serendipity. With the identification of the critical role of the monoamines serotonin and noradrenaline in the monoamine theory of depression, the major drug companies embarked on targeted programmes. Large numbers of related chemicals were synthesised and screened *in vitro* for blockade of monoamine reuptake activity and *in vivo* in animal models of depression. The more promising compounds were then selected for further stages of drug development, with the role of the psychiatrist being largely confined to the phase of drug trials of efficacy.

Terminology

The first drug to be introduced was iproniazid, which was an irreversible monoamine oxidase inhibitor (MAOI); some time later, reversible inhibitors of monoamine oxidase-A (RIMAs), for example moclobemide, were discovered. Imipramine, which has a three-ring structure, was the first of the tricyclic antidepressant (TCA) group. The older TCAs, including imipramine and amitriptyline, were known as the first-generation TCAs and their use dates from the late 1950s. TCAs with fewer anticholinergic side-effects, such as lofepramine, introduced after 1980, were known as second-generation TCAs. The term 'second generation' or 'novel' has also been applied to drugs with a more selective action, such as the SSRIs (e.g. fluoxetine), as well as drugs that are selective noradrenaline reuptake inhibitors (NARIs) (e.g. reboxetine). The next generation of antidepressant drugs included those that are selective serotonin and noradrenaline reuptake inhibitors (SNRIs), such as venlafaxine. Mirtazapine is included in a group said to be noradrenergic and specific serotonergic antidepressants (with yet another acronym, NaSSAs), although its action is more complex.

The vast literature on antidepressant drugs is summarised in this chapter. The focus is on antidepressant actions and uses (including in special groups), side-effects, drug interactions and treatment resistance. The first part of the chapter provides an account of the basic pharmacology of each of the major groups of antidepressants, and starts with an account of the SSRIs, as these are the most commonly prescribed in the UK today (see Fig. 4.1). The latter part of the chapter describes the treatment of depression, and reports on some of the recently published guidelines, such as those produced by the National Institute for Clinical Excellence (NICE, 2004).

The selective serotonin reuptake inhibitors (SSRIs)

The SSRIs have a common pharmacodynamic mechanism of action: they are all inhibitors of 5-HT reuptake – they all bind with high affinity to the 5-HT transporter and so inhibit the reuptake of the neurotransmitter from the synaptic cleft back into the neuron. Initially, cell body reuptake inhibition with resultant increase in synaptic serotonin activates the inhibitory cell body 5-HT_{1A} autoreceptors and results in reduced cell body firing, with resultant reduced release of serotonin by the axon terminal. The cell body may be in the brain-stem and the axon terminal in the frontal cortex. Chronic administration of the SSRIs results in downregulation of the cell body 5-HT_{1A} autoreceptors, which restores both cell body firing and serotonin release by the axonal terminal. Given the reuptake blockade at the axon terminal synapse, the restoration of 5-HT release results in increased 5-HT concentration at this site.

All current antidepressants have the common action of boosting monoamine transmission. This leads to changes in gene expression in the neurons targeted by the monoamines, resulting not only in receptor downregulation (e.g. of the postsynaptic 5-HT receptor) but also affecting neurotrophic substances such as brain-derived neurotrophic factor (BDNF). This is discussed further in Chapter 3 (page 65). The time course of downregulation of receptors (which occurs over weeks) fits better with the time taken to respond to an antidepressant, whereas 5-HT reuptake blockade occurs within a few hours of ingestion of an SSRI.

The term 'selective' is used because these drugs are selective for the serotonin transporter and have comparatively little effect on noradrenergic reuptake (see Fig. 4.2). They also have low affinities for other neurotransmitter receptor systems, such as α_1 and α_2 adrenergic systems, H_1 histaminic and muscarinic receptors (in contrast to the TCAs, which have high affinities for these receptors), and the relative absence

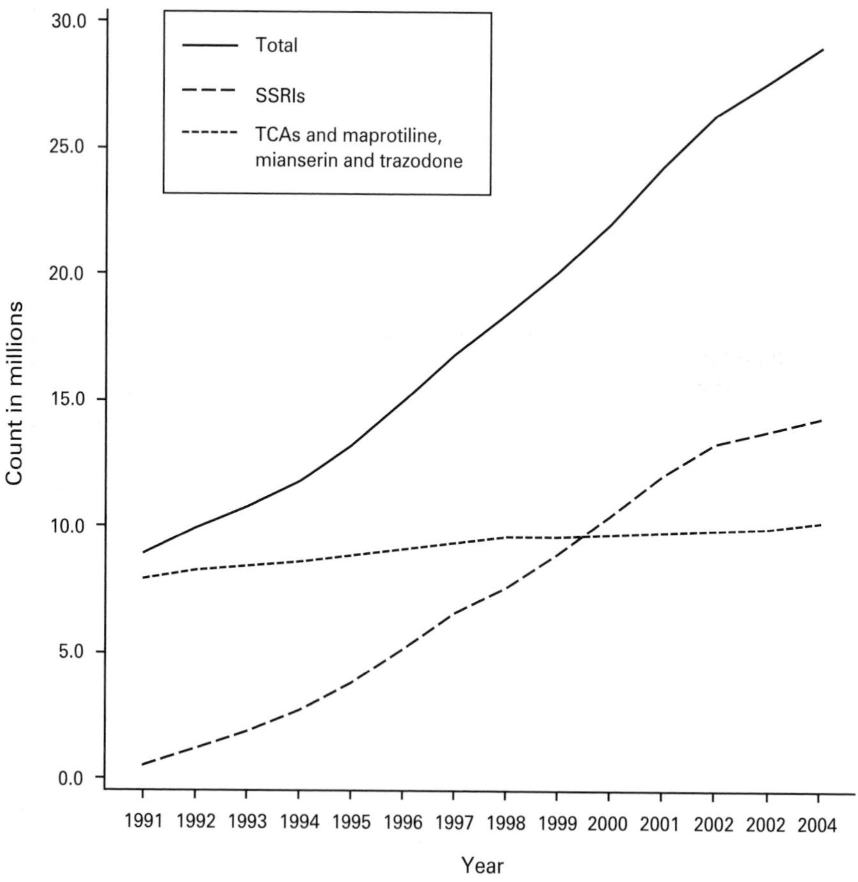

Fig. 4.1 Number of community antidepressant drug prescriptions in England, 1991–2004 (Prescription Cost Analysis data). During the 1990s there was a doubling in the rate of antidepressant drug prescribing in England and Wales, largely accounted for by the rising rate of SSRI prescriptions, though there was also a small rise in TCA prescribing. This dramatic change in the 1990s spread across Europe, the USA and Canada.

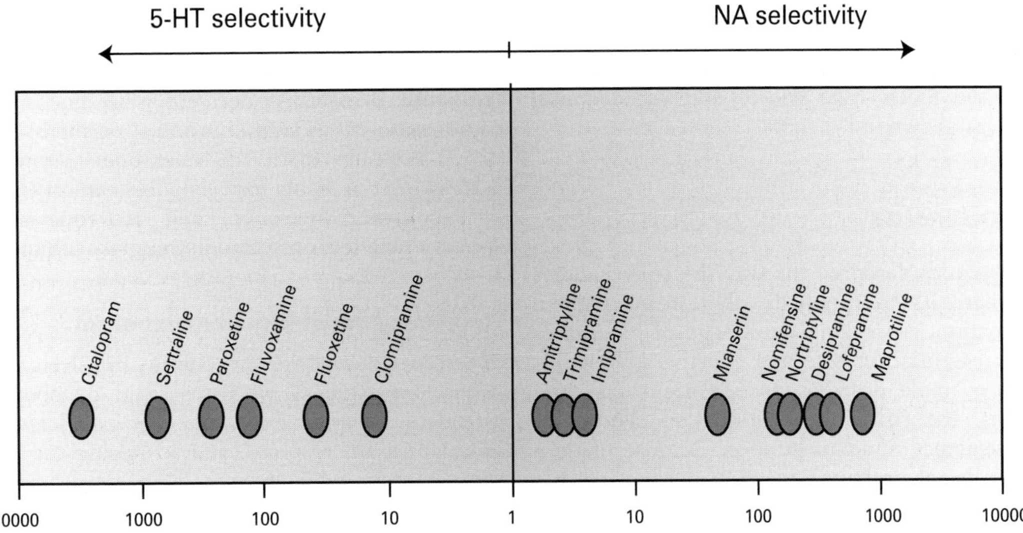

Fig. 4.2 *In vitro* selectivity ratios for parent (non-metabolised) antidepressant compound. On the *x*-axis the measure is a ratio: to the left, IC_{50} NA/IC_{50}5-HT; to the right, IC_{50} 5-HT/IC_{50}NA. IC_{50} represents 50% inhibition of uptake of noradrenaline (NA) or serotonin (5-HT) into rat brain synaptosomes. (The lower the IC_{50} the more potent is the drug effect on uptake.) For further explanation see Hyttel (1994).

of effects on these receptors is thought to confer greater tolerability, lower rates of side-effects and greater safety in overdose.

The first drug in this group, zimelidine, was introduced in 1981, but it was soon withdrawn because of an association with the Guillain–Barré syndrome, a serious neurological complication. Fluvoxamine was introduced in 1983 but had little impact, whereas the arrival of fluoxetine in 1988 led to a great increase in prescribing (the 'Prozac revolution'). Sertraline, citalopram and paroxetine were introduced in the early 1990s. The SSRIs are effective treatments for depression, but it became apparent that they also alleviated a variety of anxiety disorders and they became licensed therapies for panic disorder, social phobia and obsessive–compulsive disorder. Their greater tolerability and wider indications contributed to a huge increase in the amount of antidepressants prescribed (see Fig. 4.1). Isacsson *et al*

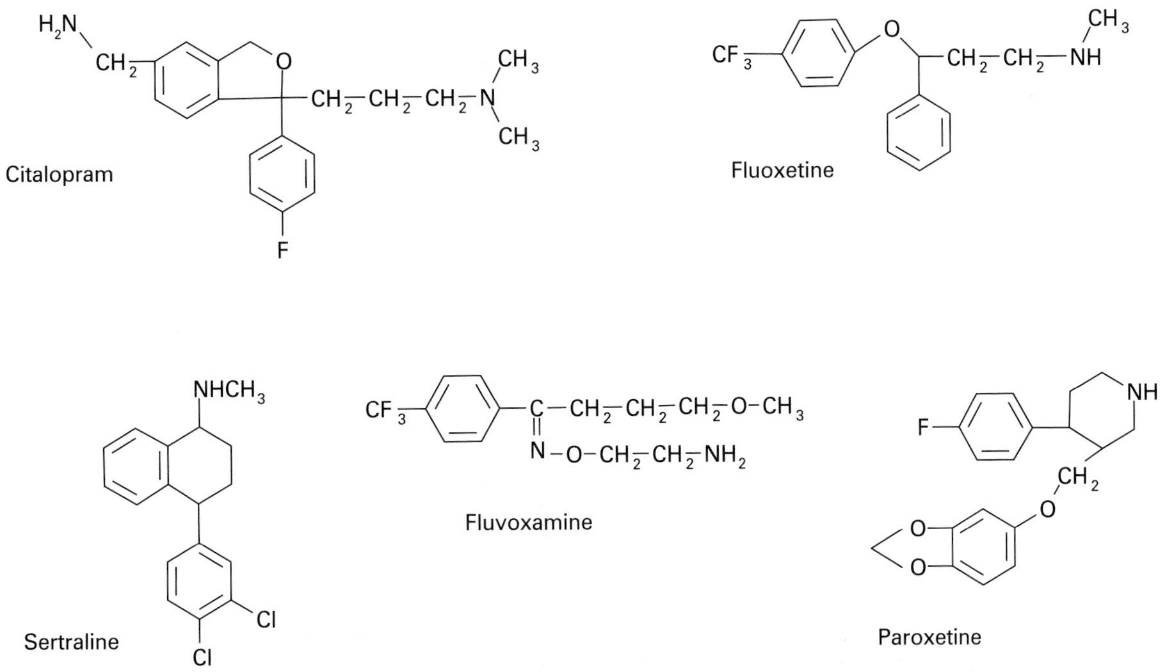

Citalopram

Fluoxetine

Sertraline

Fluvoxamine

Paroxetine

Fig. 4.3 Chemical structure of the SSRIs.

(1999*a*) suggest that around 1995–96 the SSRIs became more frequently prescribed than the TCAs in Sweden.

Unlike the TCAs, which have similarities in chemical structure, the SSRIs have widely different chemical structures, as shown in Fig. 4.3.

Pharmacokinetics

Pharmacokinetics describes the way the body handles the drug, that is its absorption, distribution, metabolism and elimination. A working knowledge of pharmacokinetics is essential for safe and effective practice. It affects, for example, dose–response relationships, drug interactions, the risk of discontinuation syndromes and the frequency of administration. Because of their different chemical structures, the SSRIs have somewhat dissimilar pharmacokinetics. First, features in common are described here, and then individual attributes in the descriptions of each SSRI, below. The topic is reviewed by Heimke & Härther (2000).

Absorption, first-pass metabolism and distribution

All antidepressants are relatively small molecules, with molecular weights of 300–500. They have good intestinal absorption. Because they are highly lipid soluble they readily pass through the blood–brain barrier and are rapidly taken up by the tissues. More than 90% of the orally administered dose reaches the systemic circulation. Fluoxetine, paroxetine and sertraline are more highly protein-bound (> 90%) than citalopram and fluvoxamine (82% and 77%, respectively).

Time to reach peak plasma levels

Because side-effects are usually dose related, they are generally greatest when the drug reaches its peak plasma level. Fluoxetine, fluvoxamine, paroxetine and sertraline reach peak plasma levels after 4–8 hours, whereas citalopram takes 2–4 hours. Apart from paroxetine, which may cause sedation, SSRIs sometimes have a stimulating effect and are therefore usually taken in the morning. Occasionally patients complain of daytime sedation and in these cases the drug may be taken in the evening, as with paroxetine. With sustained treatment and the attainment of plasma steady-state levels, the time to reach peak plasma levels becomes less important. Other side-effects, such as gastrointestinal distress, may come on within 30 minutes of drug ingestion and this is more likely to be due to a direct effect on the intestinal mucosa than to peak plasma levels.

Active metabolites

The SSRIs differ with regard to active metabolites. The two demethylated metabolites of citalopram (demethylcitalopram and didemethylcitalopram) are themselves selective serotonin reuptake inhibitors *in vitro,* but are much less potent than the parent compound. The demethylated metabolite of fluoxetine, norfluoxetine, is three times more selective for serotonin uptake than fluoxetine and is essentially equipotent to fluoxetine in terms of serotonin reuptake inhibition. After a few weeks, plasma levels of norfluoxetine are two to three times higher than fluoxetine levels and so norfluoxetine may be a major determinant of the pharmacological response. By contrast, desmethylsertraline is only one-tenth as potent as sertraline and as desmethylsertraline levels are only about 1.5 times higher than those of sertraline it probably has negligible clinical effects. The metabolites of fluvoxamine and paroxetine are thought to have no effect on serotonin reuptake inhibition.

Individual variability in metabolism

There is wide individual variability in SSRI metabolism. Thus, for patients who are rapid metabolisers the standard effective dose may be insufficient for an antidepressant response and so raising the dose may be necessary, while patients who are deficient in the enzymes involved in drug metabolism may experience severe side-effects at normal dosage.

As might be expected, the metabolism of each of the five SSRIs becomes slower with increasing age. Thus, in the elderly, steady-state plasma levels after a daily dose of 20 mg citalopram were up to four times higher than in younger patients (Baldwin & Johnson, 1995). Compared with younger patients on similar doses, fluoxetine plus norfluoxetine levels may be double in the elderly, paroxetine levels about 70% higher and the clearance of sertraline about 40% less (Wilde *et al*, 1993). The clearances of the SSRIs do not appear to be greatly affected by renal impairment, but as the main site of their breakdown is in the liver their clearance is affected by liver disease, particularly cirrhosis (Heimke & Härther, 2000)

Half-lives

The half-life of a drug is an important pharmacokinetic measure. The half-lives of the different SSRIs are shown in Table 4.1.

Fluoxetine and paroxetine slow their own metabolism by inhibiting the liver enzymes of the cytochrome P450 2D6 group. As dosages increase, the amount of inhibition is also increased and so the half-life is higher at higher dosages. They thus have non-linear pharmacokinetics. This effect is most pronounced for fluoxetine. The increased half-life of fluoxetine and its main metabolite, norfluoxetine, may be responsible for late emergence of dose-dependent side-effects. After fluoxetine has been stopped there may be prolonged carry-over effects because of delayed return of activity

Table 4.1 Half-lives of SSRIs at therapeutic dose ranges

Drug	Approximate half-life (hours)
Citalopram	33
Metabolites (less active)	
Fluoxetine	48–96
Norfluoxetine	168–360
Fluvoxamine	22
11 metabolites largely inactive	
Paroxetine	21
M2 metabolite	< 24
Sertraline	26
Desmethylsertraline	48–96

of the cytochrome P450 2D6. This may also occur with paroxetine, although the prolongation of P450 2D6 inhibition is less than with fluoxetine.

Excretion

The metabolites of the SSRIs are excreted mainly in the urine and to only a small extent in the faeces. For example, 75–80% of ^{14}C-labelled fluoxetine given to volunteers was recovered in the urine and 10% in the faeces. Fluoxetine itself accounted for only 10% of excreted products, the rest having been metabolites. With fluvoxamine 94% of a single dose was recovered in the urine as metabolites and none appeared as the parent compound. Only 2% of paroxetine is excreted unchanged, with metabolites found in both urine and faeces. Both sertraline and desmethylsertraline are metabolised to the ketone and further hydroxylated to the major excretory metabolites, with only a small amount of unchanged sertraline appearing in the urine. For patients who have achieved a steady state on citalopram about 32% of a daily dose is excreted in the urine over 24 hours as citalopram and its metabolites.

Dose–response relationships

None of the SSRIs demonstrates a correlation between steady-state plasma levels and therapeutic response in patients with depression. However, the adverse effects of SSRIs such as nausea, anxiety, restlessness, fatigue and sexual dysfunction are dose dependent, although they tend to lessen with time. The fact that the average antidepressant response rate is achieved regardless of dose escalation and that the dose–response curves tend to be flat is compatible with the presumed mechanism of action. This is because the minimum effective dose of all SSRIs produces approximately 80% inhibition of platelet serotonin uptake in most patients. This may be the degree of inhibition required for an antidepressant response, while higher levels produce more serotonin-mediated adverse effects. The prolonged half-lives of the SSRIs and non-linear pharmacokinetics (i.e. flat dose–response curves) need to be taken into account when prescribing (this is reviewed by Preskorn, 1993).

Drug interactions with the SSRIs

The SSRIs have a large number of interactions but only a few are clinically relevant. To make some sense of this Edwards & Anderson (1999) extracted a list of interactions which the *British National Formulary* (*BNF*) considered to be clinically important (regardless of enzyme mechanism) and this is shown in Table 4.2.

SSRI drug interactions explained by the hepatic cytochrome enzyme system

Most prescribed drugs are metabolised in the liver, initially being oxidised by enzymes of the hepatic cytochrome P450 system (the name derives from the enzymes having an absorption peak at 450 nm on the

Table 4.2 Drug interactions of selective serotonin reuptake inhibitors

SSRIs	Interacting substance		Possible result
	Type	Drug	
All SSRIs		Alcohol	Enhanced effect
	Anticoagulants	Acenocoumarol Warfarin	Enhanced anticoagulant effect
	Antidepressant	MAOIs	CNS toxicity[a]
		Tricyclics	Increased plasma level of some tricyclics
		Trytophan	Agitation, nausea
	Antihistamine	Terfenadine	Increased risk of arrhythmias
	Antimanic	Lithium	CNS toxicity[a]
	Antimigraine	Sumatriptan	CNS toxicity[a]
	Antiviral	Ritonavir	Increased plasma concentration of SSRI
	Dopaminergic	Selegiline	CNS excitation, hypertension
	$5\text{-}HT_1$ agonist	Sumatriptan	CNS toxicity[a]
	Opioid analgesic	Tramodol	Increased risk of convulsions
Fluvoxamine	Anxiolytic/hypnotic	Benzodiazepines	Increased plasma concentration of some benzo-diazepines
	Beta-blocker	Propanolol	Increased plasma concentration of propanolol
	Bronchodilator	Theophylline	Increased plasma concentration of theophylline
Fluvoxamine, fluoxetine	Anticonvulsant	Carbamazepine	Antagonism of anticonvulsant effect (lowering of convulsive threshold)
	Antipsychotic	Clozapine	Increased plasma concentration of clozapine
Fluoxetine	Antiarrhythmic	Flecainide	Increased plasma concentration of flecainide
	Antipsychotic	Haloperidol	Increased plasma concentration of haloperidol
Paroxetine	Anticonvulsant	Phenytoin and possibly others	Increased plasma concentration of anticonvulsant; decreased plasma concentration of paroxetine

[a] Central nervous system (CNS) toxicity is characterised by features of the serotonin syndrome.
Source: Edwards & Anderson (1999) and *BNF* (2005).

Table 4.3 SSRIs, P450 isoenzymes and potential drug interactions

Enzyme system inhibited	Genetic poly-morphism	SSRI[a]	Potential drug interaction	TCA interaction mechanism
1A2	Possible	Fluvoxamine (Paroxetine)	Theophyllin Caffeine Tertiary amine TCAs Haloperidol Clozapine Propranolol	N-demethylation
2C	For 2C19: 3–5% Caucasian 8% African 18% Japanese	Fluoxetine Fluvoxamine Sertraline	Tolbutamide Tertiary amine TCAs Diazepam Phenytoin Warfarin	N-demethylation
2D6	5–10% of Caucasian population	(Citalopram) Fluoxetine (Fluvoxamine) Paroxetine Sertraline	Analgesics Flecainide Propafenone Quinidine Beta blockers Tertiary and secondary amine TCAs Trazodone Antipsychotic drugs including clozapine Antitussives	Ring hydroxylation
3A3	Absent	Fluoxetine	Nifedipine	N-demethylation
3A4	Absent	Fluvoxamine Sertraline	Terfenadine Astemizole Alprazolam Midazolam Triazolam Carbamazepine Tertiary amine TCAs Cyclosporin Ketoconazole	

[a]Those listed in parentheses are relatively weak inhibitors of the enzyme system indicated.
Sources: Popli & Baldessarini (1995); Nemeroff *et al* (1996); Taylor & Lader (1996).

spectrometer). These enzymes are found in the smooth reticulum of the liver cells and contain haem (and so are able to bind oxygen). More than 30 different isoenzymes have been isolated in man, of which six to eight have been shown to have a role in drug oxidation. After oxidation most drugs are usually less active and may be more readily catabolised by the so-called phase 2, or conjugation, enzymes, such as the glucoronyl transferases and sulphate transferases. The conjugated product is then largely inactive, more polar and hence more water soluble, and therefore more readily excreted by the kidney.

A cytochrome-P450-based drug interaction is likely if a drug is eliminated by a single cytochrome enzyme and is coadministered with an inhibitor of that enzyme. The SSRIs are reversible and competitive inhibitors of the cytochrome enzymes, with particular SSRIs inhibiting specific cytochrome enzymes. An example of this type of interaction is the elevation of plasma TCA levels by the SSRIs, which is due to their inhibition of the P450 2D6 enzyme group which normally is responsible for the demethylation and hydroxylation of TCAs. The elevated plasma TCA levels may be toxic and result in delirium, seizures, heart block and sudden death. This mechanism probably contributes to the very high lethality of TCA–SSRI combinations when taken in overdose. However, there is wide variation between different individuals as well as between ethnic groups in the expression of the genes responsible for the enzyme activity. Hence some individuals are more likely to experience such an interaction. Table 4.3 shows drug interactions arranged by P450 isoenzyme involvement. Drug interactions limited to particular SSRIs are mentioned in the description of the individual SSRIs below.

A US pharmaco-epidemiological study (Gregor *et al*, 1997) found that most doctors are co-prescribing drugs which are known to interact with SSRIs. Over a 1-month period more than half a million SSRI prescriptions were processed for the purpose of financial reimbursement and, of these, 25% were found to be co-administered with a drug having a known 2D6 or 3A4 interaction with an SSRI. The main co-prescribed drugs were benzodiazepines (8.9%), calcium channel blockers (6.5%), TCAs (4.8%), beta-blockers (2.8%), antipsychotics (1.9%) and anti-arrhythmics (0.1%). The large number of co-prescriptions suggests that doctors were either rating the risks of significant interactions as low or ignoring them altogether. The SSRIs are a heterogeneous class of chemical compounds, and so drug interactions which occur with one SSRI may not necessarily occur with another.

Efficacy of the SSRIs

Since the introduction of the SSRIs in the late 1980s there has been a large increase in the number of drug trials, often financed by the drug industry. To obtain a product licence a drug must be shown to be superior to placebo. When SSRIs were first introduced, studies comparing them against an established antidepressant usually used imipramine or amitriptyline. Statistical techniques used in meta-analyses allow trial data to be pooled so that the comparison between antidepressant drugs and placebo can be made on the basis of hundreds and sometimes thousands of patients. A comprehensive account of drug trial methodology is given in *Seminars in Clinical Psychopharmacology* (Harrison-Read & Tyrer, 2004), while meta-analysis is explained in Chapter 27 (see page 705). Evaluation of meta-analyses in the NICE (2004) review provides the evidence base for advice about the management of depression.

The first SSRI antidepressant efficacy meta-analysis, by Song *et al* (1993), found no difference between SSRIs and TCAs. A further meta-analysis, by Anderson & Tomenson (1994), based on 90 studies, confirmed these findings but TCAs emerged as superior for in-patient depression (which may represent more severe depression), which is in keeping with earlier studies of an advantage of TCAs for melancholia. The most recent meta-analysis in the NICE (2004) review also confirmed a small advantage for amitriptyline for in-patients only. However, the size of the difference was considered to be too small to be clinically relevant. Otherwise, there were no significant differences between the TCAs (the comparator drugs) and the SSRIs with regard to efficacy.

Placebo effects

In drug trials, patients in the placebo arm have a response rate of 30–40%, whereas there is usually double this rate in those given the active drug. The placebo response may include the response to the combination of the care and counselling patients receive in the trial and spontaneous remission. It is important to note that a sizeable proportion of patients would remit spontaneously without any intervention at all. A placebo response occurs early on and is generally not well sustained (NICE, 2004).

Meta-analysis of side-effects and discontinuation rates

The main advantage of the SSRIs and the other newer drugs to emerge from comparative trials has been their lower frequency of side-effects, and greater tolerability. Patients may stop their drugs because of side-effects, because they think their medication is ineffective, or because they have got better. With appropriate precautions discontinuation rates have been used as a proxy measure of the relative tolerability of different drugs. The NICE review, based on consideration of more than 6000 patients, found a relative advantage for the SSRIs compared with TCAs for discontinuation rates for all reasons, with a relative risk of 0.88, and when side-effects alone were considered the figure was 0.69. Among the SSRIs, fluvoxamine appears to be associated with higher discontinuation rates.

Effectiveness

'Efficacy' indicates whether a particular drug is superior to placebo in a randomised controlled trial (RCT), and such information is required by the licensing authorities. 'Effectiveness' refers to how well treatment works in clinical practice. Many drug trials are conducted on outpatients with depression of mild to moderate severity and exclude patients with, for example, comorbid alcohol and substance misuse, personality disorder and physical illness. Suicidal ideation may be another exclusion criterion. Thus the selection procedure might isolate an unrepresentative sample of patients. The presence of two or more psychiatric disorders in a patient discriminates between those treated in primary and secondary care: that is, those with comorbid conditions are referred to the psychiatrist (Pincus *et al*, 1999).

It can be difficult to measure effectiveness directly. However, it can be inferred from pharmaco-epidemiological data, which provide information on both the pattern and total number of prescriptions in the community and the following have been examined:

- dosages of antidepressants taken
- duration of course of antidepressants
- rates of compliance.

Donoghue & Hylan (2001) reviewed studies of these three measures. They found that most of the older TCA-based studies reported that the majority of patients (around 88%) on TCAs failed to achieve adequate therapeutic dosage (and sub-therapeutic dosing is associated with a poorer outcome). By contrast, SSRIs were often prescribed in full therapeutic dosage from the outset and so sub-therapeutic dosing was much less common.

A retrospective naturalistic study from Sweden (Isacsson *et al*, 1999*a*) showed that patients started on an SSRI were likely to have a longer initial course of therapy, whereas those taking a TCA were twice as likely to seek a second course of antidepressants. On the basis of their own studies of the general practice prescription database, Donoghue & Hylan (2001) estimated that patients started on SSRIs were seven times more likely to take their antidepressants than those started on a TCA. Thompson *et al* (2000), in a randomised trial, compared fluoxetine and dosulepin. They measured compliance with a novel type of drug container: the bottle cap had an electronic chip in it which counted the number of times patients opened the medication container. This 'medication event monitoring system' showed better compliance with fluoxetine than with dosulepin.

From an epidemiological perspective, the increased rate of SSRI prescribing, the better compliance and the more prolonged duration of use would suggest that concerns (e.g. Isacsson *et al*, 1994) that too few depressed patients are treated at all, at too low a dose of antidepressant and for too short a period have now at least partially been addressed.

Antidepressant effectiveness for in-patients

The SSRIs may not be as effective as the TCAs among certain subgroups. Thus, Parker *et al* (2001) followed

Table 4.4 Antidepressant prescribing for in-patients in Germany, 1995 and 2001

1995		2001	
Top five drugs	**% of all**	**Top five drugs**	**% of all**
Dosulepin	22	Mirtazapine	25
Amitriptyline	20	Venlafaxine	13
Paroxetine	14	Sertraline	13
Trimipramine	9	Dosulepin	13
Maprotiline	7	Citalopram	9

Source: Grohmann *et al* (2004).

182 patients with depression (in-patients and out-patients) and interviewed them 12 months after presentation. They found roughly equal response rates for TCAs (34%) and the SSRIs (29%), but for the subgroup with DSM–IV melancholia ($n = 56$) 48% of those on TCAs met the effectiveness criteria of the study compared with only 20% of those receiving an SSRI.

Soon after the SSRIs were introduced, the Danish University Antidepressant Group (1990) showed that they may be less effective than the TCAs for in-patients (who have more severe depression). The NICE (2004) review states that amitriptyline is more effective than the SSRIs for in-patients. Because there are few comparative trials for in-patients, none of the guidelines makes specific recommendations regarding the selection of antidepressants for in-patients.

The German Hospital Survey (AMSP) (Grohmann *et al*, 2004) provided pharmaco-epidemiological data on 52 000 in-patient antidepressant prescriptions (by German psychiatrists at 35 hospitals). Table 4.4 shows the pattern of change that occurred over 6 years. TCAs were the most frequently prescribed group in the mid-1990s but by 2001 the 'third-generation drugs', such as venlafaxine and mirtazapine, were the most commonly used.

The SSRIs have been used less frequently for in-patients than for out-patients.

Individual SSRIs

Citalopram

Citalopram is a substituted phthalane derivative with a tertiary amino group in the side chain (see Fig. 4.3). It and escitalopram (see below) are the most serotonin selective of the SSRIs and TCAs (see Fig. 4.2) but this does not mean that it is the most potent inhibitor of serotonin reuptake. Citalopram also has some affinity for α_1-adrenoreceptors and slight histamine H_1 blocking potency. It is well absorbed and differs from other SSRIs in having a shorter time to reach peak plasma levels, at around 2–4 hours. It has high bioavailability and only 50% is excreted in the urine. Clearance and metabolism by N-demethylation are reduced in the elderly, for whom lower doses may sometimes be necessary. Citalopram is probably the safest SSRI with respect to drug interactions because it is a weak inhibitor of the cytochrome P450 isoenzyme 2D6 and does not inhibit P450 1A2; on present evidence it appears to have only a moderate effect in raising plasma TCA levels, by up to 40–50%. The starting dose, of 20 mg daily, may be increased to 40 mg, but doses of 60 mg per day do not appear to confer any additional advantage (Montgomery & Johnson, 1995). An oral drops formulation of citalopram allows greater flexibility with dose for those patients who develop side-effects at usual doses.

Escitalopram

Citalopram consists of a racemic mixture of the S (+) and R (–) enantiomers (the molecules are mirror images of each other). Escitalopram is the isolated S enantiomer, which has a 5-HT uptake inhibitory potency 100 times greater than the R enantiomer and twice that of citalopram. There are claims for a faster onset of action than with citalopram, but the pharmacokinetics and side-effects closely resemble those of citalopram. A recent review of the efficacy of escitalopram in drug trials in primary care found superiority for remission rates over placebo (49% versus 38%) and over citalopram itself (62% versus 50%), and equivalence to venlafaxine (Einarson, 2004). An RCT comparing escitalopram (20 mg) with venlafaxine (225 mg) in out-patients with major depression found the two drugs to be equally efficacious, but side-effects such as nausea were less (6% versus 24%) and discontinuation rates were lower (4% versus 16%) with escitalopram (Bielski *et al*, 2004). The dose is half that of citalopram (i.e. 10 or 20 mg per day).

Fluoxetine

Fluoxetine also exists as both and S and R enantiomers and is marketed as the racemic mixture. Its structure is shown in Fig. 4.3. The S enantiomer is 1.5 times more active than the R enantiomer, but the S enantiomer of the main metabolite – norfluoxetine – has 20 times the affinity of the corresponding R enantiomer for receptor blockade. Fluoxetine is well absorbed and has a half-life of 1–4 days. Norfluoxetine has a long half-life, of 7–15 days. Both fluoxetine and norfluoxetine have low affinities for muscarinic receptors (and hence low rates of anticholinergic side-effects), dopamine D_2 receptors and β-adrenoreceptors (and hence low rates of cardiovascular side-effects). The oral dose is directly related to side-effects but does not have a linear relationship to plasma levels, or to clinical response. Nausea, emergent anxiety/agitation and insomnia are among the most common side-effects and are more prevalent at higher doses (60 mg) than the recommended dose, of 20 mg daily.

Whether in a minority of patients fluoxetine can initiate intense suicidal thoughts or exacerbate existing suicidal ideation is discussed further below (page 96).

Fluoxetine was the first SSRI for which drug interactions mediated by inhibition of the liver cytochrome P450 2D6 and other P450 isoenzymes were described (see Table 4.3). Because the P450 isoenzymes are involved in the metabolism of the TCAs and antipsychotic drugs, fluoxetine may elevate their blood levels. Elevations of antipsychotic drug levels may worsen extrapyramidal effects.

Fluoxetine is available in liquid form, so treatment can be initiated at much lower doses than the recommended

20 mg daily. For example, a starting dose of 5 mg daily can be used for patients who are particularly liable to suffer side-effects. Subsequent improved tolerability might allow a gradual dose increase.

Fluvoxamine

Fluvoxamine has a monocyclic structure (see Fig. 4.3). Although 90% is absorbed after an oral dose, there is extensive first-pass metabolism and its bioavailability, at around 50–60%, is lower than for other SSRIs. The most common side-effects are nausea, vomiting, agitation, insomnia and somnolence. Nausea is less common if fluvoxamine is given at night and gastrointestinal side-effects diminish after the first 2 weeks (Stimmel *et al*, 1991). The meta-analysis in the NICE (2004) review showed that, compared with other SSRIs, fluvoxamine had the highest discontinuation rates as a result of side-effects. The starting dose is 100 mg at night and the recommended dose is 100–200 mg per day.

Fluvoxamine is a potent inhibitor of cytochrome P450 1A2 (Brosen *et al*, 1993), which is largely unaffected by other SSRIs, whereas it has little effect on the 2D6 isoenzyme. Through its inhibition of the 1A2 isoenzyme there are interactions with clozapine, olanzapine, theophylline, tacrine and caffeine.

Paroxetine

Paroxetine is chemically distinct from other SSRIs in having a piperidine ring (a ring that contains a nitrogen atom – see Fig. 4.3). It is a potent serotonin reuptake inhibitor, second only to sertraline (Hyttel, 1994), but it is not the most selective of the SSRIs. Paroxetine also blocks muscarinic receptors, although typical anticholinergic side-effects usually appear only with higher doses. Its metabolites do not appear to be clinically active.

The most common side-effects are nausea, anxiety, agitation and tremor. There is a wide inter-individual variability in plasma levels for a given dose of paroxetine and elevated levels may occur in the elderly. Of the SSRIs, paroxetine has recently attracted publicity in relation to both the discontinuation syndrome (which may be linked to its short half-life) and the initiation of suicidal thoughts (which was an issue with fluoxetine in the early 1990) and these are discussed on page 96.

Of the SSRIs, paroxetine is the most potent inhibitor of cytochrome P450 2D6 *in vitro* (Crewe *et al*, 1992). Because of this, levels of TCAs and clozapine may be elevated if they are co-administered. However, because of its comparatively short half-life, the inhibition of cytochrome P450 2D6 is usually reversed within 1 week of stopping paroxetine, compared with 1–2 weeks after stopping sertraline and up to 5 weeks after stopping fluoxetine. Paroxetine does not appear to have any significant effect on other isoenzymes, other than a weak interaction with 1A2 (Table 4.3). The usual daily dose is 20 mg, which may be increased to a maximum recommended dose of 50 mg per day. Paroxetine is also available in liquid form.

Sertraline

Sertraline is a naphthalenamine, with a two-ring amine complex (see Fig. 4.3). In respect of serotonin reuptake inhibition, it is the second most potent of the SSRIs (Hyttel, 1994) and in serotonin selectivity it is second only to citalopram (Fig. 4.2). It is relatively slowly absorbed from the gastrointestinal tract, reaching peak plasma levels after 4–8 hours. With a half-life of approximately 26 hours, daily doses reach a steady-state after 1 week. In contrast to fluoxetine, the relationship between dose and plasma level kinetics appears to be linear. The main metabolite, desmethylsertraline, may have 1.5 times the blood level of sertraline, but it has only one-tenth of its potency.

Sertraline (like fluoxetine and paroxetine) is highly protein bound and these SSRIs may displace other protein-bound drugs, such as warfarin, from their binding sites. In addition, warfarin is metabolised by cytochrome P450 2C, which sertraline inhibits (see Table 4.3). Thus, sertraline has two mechanisms by which warfarin's effect on bleeding time may be prolonged. The 2C inhibition may also explain the interaction with tolbutamide: a 16% reduction in tolbutamide clearance occurs in conjunction with sertraline administration. Sertraline also inhibits cytochrome P450 2D6, but not as potently as fluoxetine, norfluoxetine or paroxetine. Sertraline clearance is reduced during co-administration with cimetidine. The prevalence of side-effects is similar to that with fluoxetine.

The manufacturers recommend a starting dose of 50 mg daily; the usual maintenance dose is also 50 mg daily. The dose may be increased over several weeks to a maximum of 200 mg daily.

Adverse responses to SSRIs

An adverse drug reaction (ADR) is defined as 'a noxious and unintended response in man to a drug administered at a dose appropriate for prophylaxis, diagnosis, or therapy' (Karch & Lasagna, 1975). ADRs, used interchangeably with the term 'side-effects', are obviously important. Whenever one prescribes, one has to anticipate likely side-effects, recognise their occurrence, differentiate them from unrelated phenomena such as the depression itself and deal with them effectively. Their prevalence depends on how they are defined. Thus, an arbitrary measure of severity will determine whether an ADR is present or not in a controlled study.

The actions of many neurotransmitters underlie ADRs. In a pharmacogenetic study (Murphy *et al*, 2003) among a group of elderly patients who were treated with either paroxetine or mirtazapine, discontinuation of paroxetine due to side-effects was strongly associated with genetic polymorphisms of the 5-HT_{2A} receptor and not with polymorphisms of the P450 2D6 gene. In the same study, discontinuation of mirtazapine was not associated with polymorphisms of either gene.

The main ADRs of the SSRIs are described below. ADRs which are common to most other antidepressants, such as weight gain and sexual side-effects, are described on pages 93–97.

Gastrointestinal effects

Nausea

Nausea, the most common side-effect of the SSRIs, is usually transient and dose related. Because it is so common all patients should be forewarned about it.

It may be most common with fluvoxamine, at an incidence of 36%; by way of comparison, with imipramine it is 20% and with placebo 16% (Feighner *et al*, 1989). Loss of appetite represents a milder form of this phenomenon, but dyspepsia, diarrhoea and constipation may all occur. Gastrointestinal distress may occasionally be severe, possibly accompanied by vomiting, but usually presents as a feeling of stomach discomfort.

Gastrointestinal bleeding
Case–control and cohort studies show that the use of the SSRIs increases the risk of gastrointestinal bleeding threefold (*Drug and Therapeutics Bulletin*, 2004; Paton & Ferrier, 2005). It is estimated that this represents around one extra hospital admission per 300 patient-years of treatment and is similar to that due to aspirin or other non-steroidal anti-inflammatory drugs (NSAIDs). The mechanism is thought to involve the SSRI inhibition of platelet serotonin uptake. Serotonin is released by platelets in response to vascular injury. Serotonin promotes vasoconstriction and a change in the shape of platelets that leads to aggregation. Platelets cannot themselves synthesise serotonin and so the inhibition of the platelet serotonin transporter reduces platelet release of serotonin, thus impairing the clotting process.

The SSRI risk is increased in those aged over 80 years, those with a history of gastrointestinal bleeding and by the concomitant use of aspirin or other NSAIDs. Aspirin also reduces the effectiveness of the clotting process and directly damages the gastrointestinal mucosa, whereas other NSAIDs affect the mucosa only. With such analgesia an antidepressant with a low affinity for the serotonin transporter should be chosen, such as doxepin, mirtazapine, moclobemide or nortriptyline. If an SSRI is used, it might be combined with gastroprotective measures in the form of an H_2 antagonist, a proton pump inhibitor or misoprostol (the only drug that has been shown to reduce the risk of serious bleeds).

Central nervous system effects

Psychiatric
Nervousness, emergent anxiety, agitation, irritability, dizziness, fatigue, malaise and paraesthesia have been reported with all SSRIs. These side-effects usually appear early in treatment and generally subside after 2–3 weeks. Over time, the SSRIs are as effective as TCAs in reducing anxiety. Associated with this initial nervousness may be racing thoughts, insomnia, headache and tremor. Headache has been reported in 20–30% of patients taking SSRIs but in these studies there was a similar prevalence with placebo (Feighner *et al*, 1989). Although there may be insomnia, SSRIs sometimes cause sedation. Less common psychiatric side-effects include increased aggression, which may present rarely as an 'out of character' episode of violence, confusional states and suicide attempts (see page 96).

A recent meta-analysis of the treatment of bipolar depression (Gijsman *et al*, 2004) suggested that, in the short term (i.e. during the trials), the risk of mania was similar for all antidepressants (3.8%) and for placebo (4.7%). The power to detect a difference was low because there were few manic episodes, which tempers the conclusion that the switch to mania that may occur during the acute treatment of bipolar depression is independent of SSRI treatment. TCAs, in contrast, had a significantly increased risk of mania (10%) compared with non-tricyclics (3.2%).

Neurological
As well as tremor, extrapyramidal features such as akathisia, dystonia and, rarely, an orolingual dyskinesia have been reported. Rarely convulsions may occur, more commonly following an overdose. Giving an SSRI to patients already taking antipsychotic drugs may result in a worsening of extrapyramidal effects. The mechanism is thought to be via brain-stem serotonergic neurons, which have a tonic inhibitory influence on dopamine function and hence alter the acetylcholine–dopamine balance. Through this antidopaminergic effect on the hypothalamus, prolactin secretion may be increased and secondary amenorrhoea may occasionally occur. Perhaps because TCAs are less serotonergic, extrapyramidal side-effects may be less common with TCAs than with SSRIs.

Cardiovascular effects

The only consistent cardiovascular effect of the SSRIs to be reported has been a minor degree of slowing of the pulse rate. The mechanism is unclear and is not the same as with TCAs, which slow cardiac conduction via a quinidine-like effect on the His–Purkinje system (Fisch, 1985). The SSRIs are now usually the preferred drugs for those with cardiovascular disease. Since they do not block adrenergic receptors, postural hypotension does not occur.

The almost complete absence at therapeutic doses of cardiovascular side-effects (especially in comparison with the TCAs) is a major factor contributing to the safety of this group of drugs. The SSRIs are much safer in overdose than the TCAs, although fatalities have been reported with citalopram, which in overdose is associated with bradycardia and arrhythmias.

Anticholinergic effects

The SSRIs have fewer anticholinergic side-effects than the TCAs, although dry mouth, blurred vision and constipation have been reported. Also involved in producing these ADRs are noradrenergic innervation of the salivary glands and serotonergic innervation of the pupil and gut. Urinary retention has not been reported.

Are there differences between the side-effects of the different SSRIs?

The patient event monitoring unit in Southampton monitors cohorts of 10 000 patients given a new drug for the first 2 years after its release, by sending out questionnaires to patients who have been exposed to a new drug as well as their general practitioners. The advantage of this type of data is that they are derived from much larger numbers of patients than is the case in drug trials. The following differences in the frequencies of side-effects between the different SSRIs have been reported by the unit (Mackay *et al*, 1997):

- Nausea and vomiting were more common with fluvoxamine.

- Drowsiness was more common with fluvoxamine and paroxetine.
- Tremor was more common with fluvoxamine and paroxetine.
- Sweating, impotence and ejaculatory failure were more common with paroxetine.
- Withdrawal problems were more common with paroxetine.

The syndrome of inappropriate antidiuretic hormone (SIADH) secretion

This uncommon but potentially fatal condition has been reported with all classes of antidepressant. In a survey of psychotropic medication prescribing in German hospitals, the AMSP programme (Degner *et al*, 2004), the SIADH occurred with an overall prevalence of 0.05% for all antidepressant prescriptions and accounted for 64% of all the 'severe' reactions to SSRIs.

The antidiuretic hormone (ADH) from the posterior pituitary gland promotes water retention by increasing readsorption from nephrons. ADH is normally released in response to a fall in plasma volume or an increase in serum osmolality, which is largely dependent on serum sodium. Osmotically driven ADH secretion is appropriate, but non-osmotically driven ADH secretion in the absence of haemodynamic disturbance is 'inappropriate' and characterises this syndrome.

The biochemical picture is one of hyponatraemia, and low plasma osmolality combined with raised urine osmolality and sodium excretion.

Symptom severity depends on the serum sodium level (normally 135–145 mEq/l) and the speed of onset of hyponatraemia. If serum sodium levels fall to 115–120 mEq/l there may be anorexia, nausea, vomiting, headache, irritability, weakness, myalgia and disorientation. If the level falls below 110 mEq/l the patient may experience tremor, ataxia, seizures, psychosis, delirium, coma, focal neurological signs, myoclonus, hypoactive reflexes and papilloedema.

The syndrome should be considered in any patient on an antidepressant who develops drowsiness, confusion or convulsions. It is more common in the elderly. Diagnosis requires a measurement of serum sodium. The difficulty lies in retaining a reasonably high index of suspicion for a rare complication. Thus, in the AMSP study 6 out of 11 cases first presented with severe neurological disorders (fits, coma, confusional states) before any estimate of the serum sodium had been made (Degner *et al*, 2004).

The risks are increased by older age, female sex, previous hyponatraemia and concomitant administration of another medication known to cause hyponatraemia. Treatment involves stopping the antidepressant drug and, in consultation with a physician, considering water restriction, saline infusions, frusemide and demeclocycline, a tetracycline antibiotic which blocks the effect of ADH on the renal collecting ducts.

The serotonin syndrome

Among patients taking L-tryptophan in the 1960s there were a few reports of drowsiness, nystagmus, hyper-reflexia, ankle clonus and clumsiness. Similar neurological features as well as excessive sweating and an agitated delirium were noted in patients taking MAOIs with L-tryptophan and an MAOI–TCA combination, even in the absence of an elevation in blood pressure. Animal studies suggested that serotonin may be responsible. Thus, rats given the combination of tranylcypromine and L-tryptophan developed hyperactivity (Grahame-Smith, 1971). Tetrabenazine, which inhibits the uptake and storage of serotonin and other amines by intraneuronal vesicles, greatly increases the speed of onset and development of this hyperactivity, while pre-treatment with a decarboxylase inhibitor which blocks the synthesis of serotonin from its precursor, 5-hydroxytryptophan, prevents the development of the syndrome. It is thought to be due to overstimulation of 5-HT receptors.

Sternbach (1991) reviewed reports of 38 patients said to have the 'serotonin syndrome': 16 patients had received a combination of an MAOI with L-tryptophan (with or without lithium); 14 had been treated with fluoxetine and an MAOI; five with fluoxetine and L-tryptophan; and there were three miscellaneous cases. Those who took lithium had blood levels within normal limits. The main clinical features were restlessness (45%), confusion (42%), myoclonus (34%), hyper-reflexia (29%), diaphoresis (26%), shivering (26%), tremor (26%), hypomania (21%), diarrhoea (16%) and incoordination (13%).

The delineation of the syndrome is unclear because of variation in severity and there may be overlap with the neuroleptic malignant syndrome (NMS). In NMS, which occurs in association with treatment with an antipsychotic drug, the onset is slower: progression is over 24–72 hours, whereas the serotonin syndrome makes its appearance over a few hours. NMS is characterised by Parkinsonian motor features, such as akathisia, bradykinesis, leaden rigidity and occasionally stupor. The mechanism is thought to be blockade of dopamine receptors in the nigrostriatal tracts. There is a tonic balance of dopamine and serotonin in many areas of the central nervous system (CNS), such that increased serotonin lowers dopamine activity, and there are case reports of clomipramine causing NMS (Haddow *et al*, 2004).

Usually the serotonin syndrome resolves within 24 hours once the offending drugs are withdrawn. Supportive measures include cooling for hyperthermia, anticonvulsants for seizures and, if required, artificial ventilation for respiratory insufficiency, as well as for further cooling. If supportive measures are ineffective, serotonin receptor blockade by methysergide or cyproheptidine (both non-selective $5\text{-HT}_1/5\text{-HT}_2$ antagonists) or propranolol (which blocks 5-HT_{1A} receptors as well as beta-adrenergic ones) should be considered, although there are no controlled studies of these drugs.

Tricyclic antidepressants

The first-generation of antidepressants include many of the older standard tricyclic antidepressants (TCAs) and the monoamine oxidase inhibitors. In the latter half of the 1970s, newer TCAs and antidepressants with related chemical structures were introduced.

The chemical structures of some tricyclics are shown in Fig. 4.4. Slight modifications in the ring structure and side chain identify the different TCAs and result in

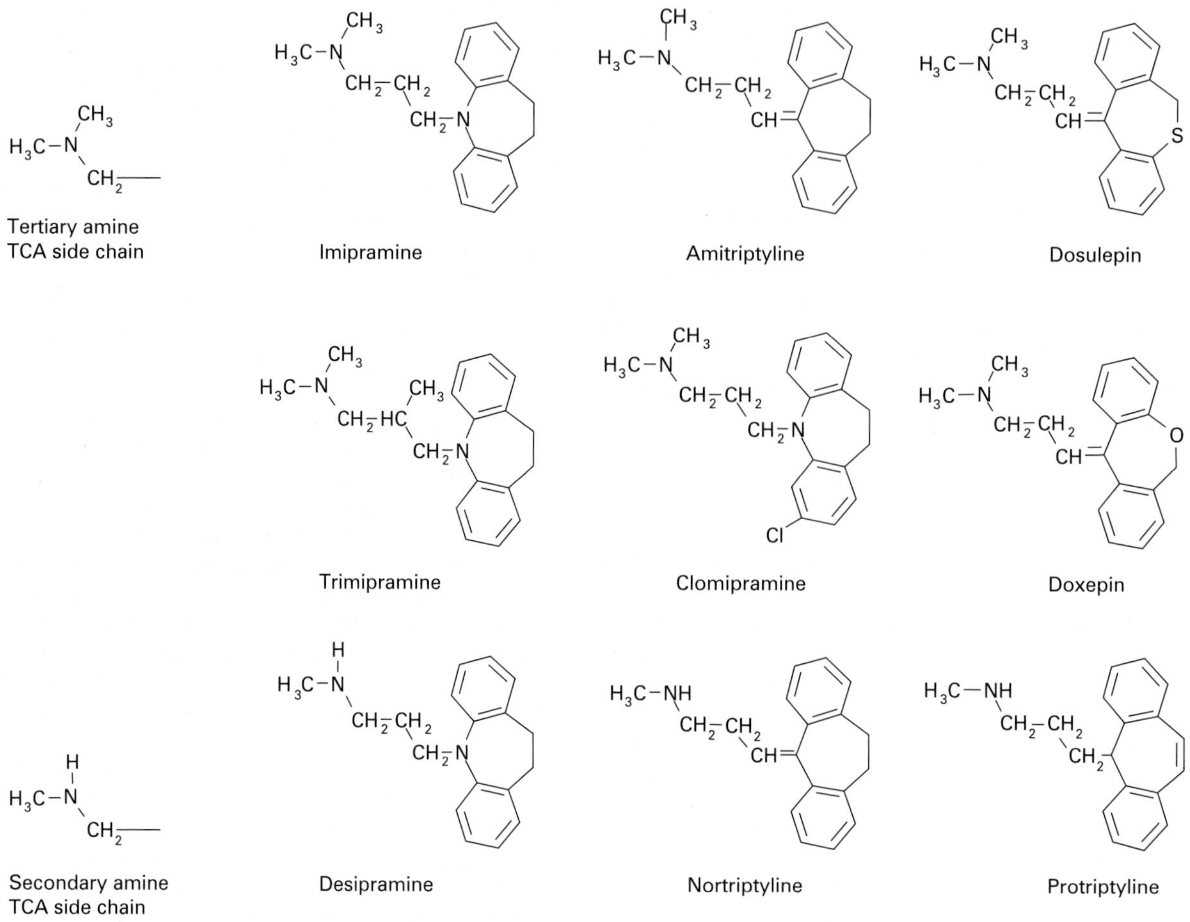

Tertiary amine TCA side chain

Imipramine

Amitriptyline

Dosulepin

Trimipramine

Clomipramine

Doxepin

Secondary amine TCA side chain

Desipramine

Nortriptyline

Protriptyline

Fig. 4.4 Chemical structure of some tricyclic antidepressants.

pharmacological differences. In the first two rows of Fig. 4.4, the nitrogen atoms in the side chains have three carbon atoms attached and these tricyclics are known as tertiary amine TCAs. This group includes imipramine, amitriptyline, dosulepin (formerly dothiepin), doxepin, clomipramine and trimipramine. Drugs with side chains where the nitrogen atom is linked to two carbon atoms are known as secondary amine TCAs and these are shown in the second row of the figure. It is also possible to group the TCAs according to the middle ring structure, where imipramine, desipramine, trimipramine and clopramine, with a nitrogen in the middle ring, could be contrasted with amitriptyline, nortriptyline and protriptyline, with a carbon in that position, and with dosulepin and doxepin.

Pharmacokinetics

Absorption and first-pass metabolism

In contrast to the SSRIs, the TCAs have relatively similar pharmacokinetics. The account below is drawn from Preskorn (1993). TCAs are lipid soluble and therefore well absorbed from the gastrointestinal tract and also readily pass through the blood–brain barrier and across the placenta. Because of first-pass metabolism, only 50–60% of an orally administered TCA dose reaches the systemic circulation.

The extent of first-past metabolism is affected by genetic factors, and is also decreased by liver disease and right heart failure, which causes hepatic congestion. Alcohol has a triphasic effect on the first-pass metabolism of TCAs. Acute ingestion of alcohol through its effect on the liver can substantially impair first-pass metabolism, resulting in a doubling or even a tripling of the amount of the drug that reaches the systemic circulation (Weller & Preskorn, 1984). This may explain why overdoses of TCAs taken in conjunction with alcohol are more likely to be lethal. With more long-term alcohol intake the hepatic isoenzymes are induced and this increases first-pass metabolism. However, once cirrhosis and portacaval shunting have developed, the TCA may pass directly into the systemic circulation and have a more rapid and greater effect, so TCAs should not be used in these patients.

Time to reach maximum plasma concentration

The tertiary amine TCAs reach their maximum plasma concentration 1–3 hours after ingestion. By contrast, the secondary amine TCAs are more slowly absorbed, reaching their peak concentration around 4–8 hours after ingestion. This difference may contribute to the better tolerability and safety of secondary amine TCAs.

The anticholinergic effect of TCAs decreases the rate of gastric emptying and intestinal peristalsis and so delays their own absorption, as well as that of other drugs.

Peak plasma levels of TCAs are associated with sedation, postural hypotension and a quinidine-like effect on the heart. The peak effect can be used to advantage; for example, the patient can obtain a maximum sedative effect at night by taking the total daily dose of a tertiary amine TCA around 2 hours before going to sleep. Plasma drug levels will have fallen substantially by the next morning, so daytime sedation is reduced. During the night it is best if the patient lies flat, so that the risk of postural hypotension is reduced. However, for the elderly who visit the toilet more frequently at night, postural hypotension may occur and result in falls.

Metabolism and excretion

The TCAs are extensively metabolised before their elimination from the body. The initial liver biotransformations are either hydroxylation of the ring structure or demethylation of the side chain terminal nitrogen. Demethylation involves converting a tertiary amine TCA to a secondary amine TCA and then to a primary amine TCA. Thus imipramine becomes desipramine, and amitriptyline is demethylated to nortriptyline (see Fig. 4.4). Some of these secondary amines, but not the primary amine metabolites, are antidepressant in their own right.

The metabolites of the TCAs are generally more polar and therefore more water soluble than the parent compounds. Conjugation with glucuronic acid makes them even more polar, and hence more readily cleared by the kidney. Diseases that lower glomerular filtration as well as the age-related decrease in renal function can result in an accumulation of polar metabolites, causing toxicity in some patients. Thus, with elderly patients plasma levels of 10-hydroxynortriptyline may be three times higher than plasma levels of nortriptyline itself (Young *et al*, 1987). Hospital laboratories measure the main demethylated metabolite but not the plasma level of these polar metabolites. SSRIs are less affected by changes in renal function.

Variability in metabolism

Among physically healthy individuals there can be as much as a 30-fold variation in plasma TCA levels after the administration of the same dose of a TCA. The main rate-limiting step in the elimination of TCAs is the biotransformation mediated mainly by the hepatic cytochrome P450 2D6 isoenzyme (Preskorn, 1993). Some 5–10% of Caucasian populations have an inherited deficiency in the functional integrity of this isoenzyme and other populations carry this deficiency to varying extents. TCA clearance rates in individuals with this deficiency are substantially prolonged and they may have fourfold higher plasma TCA levels. For these individuals conventional doses may result in symptoms of toxicity such as confusion, seizures and cardiac arrhythmias. At the other extreme, a small proportion of patients are 'fast metabolisers', so that apparently therapeutic or even high doses of TCAs have negligible therapeutic effects or side-effects, associated with low plasma levels.

Half-lives

Tertiary amine TCAs have the following half-lives: doxepin 6–8 hours, amitriptyline 9–25 hours and clomipramine 19–37 hours. The demethylated secondary amine TCAs have half-lives of about 24 hours. The half-lives of the TCAs are sufficiently long for once-daily administration to achieve steady-state plasma levels. Assuming a half-life of approximately 24 hours, TCAs will achieve a steady state in about 5 days (i.e. five times the half-life). When the dose is changed the new steady state is reached in a further 5 days. If a drug is discontinued, near complete washout (i.e. to about 3% of the original level) will therefore also take approximately 5 days. This will take longer for slow metabolisers and may need to be taken into account when adding or switching to another antidepressant.

Plasma drug levels

Estimation of antidepressant blood levels is available for most TCAs. Asberg *et al* (1971) reported that there is a curvilinear relationship between nortriptyline plasma levels and therapeutic efficacy, with optimal therapeutic effects at concentrations of 50–150 ng/ml and reduced benefits both above and below this range. Because of wide individual differences in the metabolism of TCAs, a fixed-dose schedule (e.g. amitriptyline 150 mg daily) may not constitute a therapeutic trial. For some patients the dose may be too large and for others too small and in these circumstances monitoring plasma antidepressant concentrations may be helpful. Plasma levels can also be used as a check on compliance; an unexpectedly low plasma level has obvious implications. Non-response to treatment may simply be a consequence of low plasma levels due to rapid metabolism. Similarly, for those who are genetically deficient in the hepatic cytochrome isoenzyme P450 2D6, high plasma levels on an average starting dose of a tricyclic may explain severe side-effects. Most laboratories report the levels of the tertiary and secondary TCAs as well as the sum of the two. Therapeutic total plasma levels for a tertiary TCA range from 100 to 300 ng/ml.

Efficacy of TCAs

An early meta-analysis of placebo-controlled studies of TCAs found that 61 (65%) of 93 studies favoured the TCA (Morris & Beck, 1974). A more recent summary is provided by Davis & Glassman (1989). Imipramine has been the most frequently studied TCA and 30 (68%) of 44 studies have shown it to be better than placebo. In these studies there were 1334 patients, of whom 65% improved substantially on imipramine compared with 30% who improved substantially on a placebo, giving a drug–placebo difference of 35% (Davis & Glassman, 1989). There are no studies reporting that placebo produced more improvement than imipramine, and TCAs provided the mainstay for antidepressant treatment for the decades 1960–90.

Tertiary amine TCAs

Amitriptyline

Before the advent of the SSRIs amitriptyline was a commonly used antidepressant and was often the comparator drug in research trials. Fig. 4.2 shows the selectivity of antidepressants in respect of serotonin and noradrenaline. Amitriptyline lies about midway, appearing to have similarly large effects on both systems, although once metabolites are taken into account the picture becomes more complicated because its main metabolite, nortriptyline, is more noradrenergic. Amitriptyline is one of the most sedative and anticholinergic of the tricyclics. The *BNF*-recommended doses are in the range of 30–200 mg per day.

Clomipramine

Clomipramine has a chemical structure similar to imipramine, but with a chlorine atom attached to one of the benzene rings (see Fig. 4.4). Clomipramine is the most serotonin selective of the TCAs (see Fig. 4.2), but its demethylated metabolite, chlordesipramine, which does have antidepressant activity, has higher affinity for noradrenergic reuptake sites. During its early development clomipramine was approved for intravenous administration, but this had no advantage over oral administration. Clomipramine was the first antidepressant to be shown to have a therapeutic effect in obsessive–compulsive disorder, independent of whether or not there is comorbid depression. The manufacturers advise starting at a low dose, such as 10 mg daily, and gradually titrating the dose up; the *BNF* maximum recommended dose is 250 mg daily.

Dosulepin (formerly called dothiepin) and doxepin

These two antidepressants are identical in chemical structure to amitriptyline except that in the central ring dosulepin has a sulphur substitution and doxepin has an oxygen substitution (see Fig. 4.4). A reputed ranking of anticholinergic side-effects runs, from most to least: amitriptyline, dosulepin, doxepin. The NICE (2004) review reported that, among the TCAs, dosulepin has lower discontinuation rates, but did not recommend its use because of its toxicity in overdose. Dosulepin was the most widely prescribed antidepressant in use in the UK until the mid-1990s and of the TCAs it remains popular (see Table 4.4). For dosulepin, doses range from 50 mg to a maximum of 225 mg per day, while for doxepin the maximum dose is 300 mg daily in divided doses (the manufacturer recommends that no more than 100 mg should be taken as a single dose).

Imipramine

This was the first tricyclic shown to have antidepressant activity, initially in a group of patients with chronic schizophrenia (Kuhn, 1958). Imipramine is demethylated to desipramine, which is an active metabolite. At steady state the amount of desipramine usually exceeds that of the parent compound. Desipramine used to be available as a licensed antidepressant but in the context of its infrequent use the manufacturer discontinued its production. Imipramine blocks reuptake of both noradrenaline and serotonin; desipramine is a more specific noradrenaline reuptake inhibitor (see Fig. 4.2). Imipramine has moderate sedative, anticholinergic and α-adrenoreceptor blocking actions, the latter leading to postural hypotension. The daily dose range is 25–300 mg.

Lofepramine

Although lofepramine is metabolised in the liver to desipramine, there is evidence that lofepramine itself has some antidepressant activity. The mortality from suicide for those prescribed lofepramine is among the lowest for all the antidepressants and this finding has been repeated in diverse studies (Isacsson *et al*, 1994*b*; Henry *et al*, 1995; Jick *et al*, 1995; see also Table 4.7). The mortality figure is in the same range as for the SSRIs, and so if a TCA is selected as the preferred class of drug for a particular patient then the NICE (2004) guidelines suggest that lofepramine should be considered. The recommended dose range is 140–210 mg daily in divided doses, but the elderly may respond to lower doses.

Trimipramine

Trimipramine has a similar structure to imipramine, the only difference being an additional methyl group attached to the side chain (Fig. 4.4). It is the most sedative of the TCAs and its hypnotic properties may be useful in those with depressive sleep disorders. Although MAOI–TCA combinations are rarely used today for resistant depression, when this combination was more popular trimipramine was the preferred TCA. Doses range from 25 mg to a maximum of 300 mg daily and the usual maintenance dose is 75–150 mg daily.

Secondary amine TCAs

Amoxapine

Amoxapine is the N-desmethyl derivative of the antipsychotic drug loxapine and has a tricyclic structure with a fourth ring attached by an -N bond. Some authorities have classified it as a secondary amine TCA, others as a tetracyclic. Amoxapine has weak dopamine-blocking activity and this is associated with occasional extrapyramidal side-effects, menstrual irregularities, breast enlargement and galactorrhoea. The drug is infrequently used and appears to have a high mortality in overdose (Shah *et al*, 2001; Cheeta *et al*, 2004). It has some anticholinergic activity but negligible effect on α_1 and histamine receptors. Doses range from 100 to 300 mg daily.

Nortriptyline

This metabolite of amitriptyline is available for prescription. It is mainly noradrenergic in its effect (see Fig. 4.2) and weakly blocks dopaminergic reuptake. The 10-hydroxy metabolite is more abundant than the parent compound and is probably more selective for noradrenergic neurons, so there is a predominance of noradrenergic effects. Nortriptyline has fewer sedative, α_1-blocking and anticholinergic effects than amitriptyline. The usual dose range is 75–100 mg daily, to a maximum of 150 mg daily.

Table 4.5 Antidepressant affinities for muscarinic acetylcholine receptors of human brain

Drug	Affinity[a]
Amitriptyline	5.5
Protriptyline	4.0
Clomipramine	2.7
Trimipramine	1.7
Doxepin	1.3
Imipramine	1.1
Nortriptyline	0.7
Desipramine	0.5
Maprotiline	0.2
Amoxapine	0.1
Trazodone	0.0003
Atropine[b]	48

[a]Affinity = 10^{-7}/Kb, where Kb is the equilibrium dissociation constant in moles.
[b]Listed for comparison.
Source: El-Fakahany & Richelson (1983).

Side-effects of the TCAs

Anticholinergic effects

Anticholinergic effects include dry mouth, blurred vision, urinary retention, constipation, memory impairment and confusion. Table 4.5 shows *in vitro* affinities of antidepressants for the muscarinic acetylcholine receptors of the human brain. Some tolerance to these effects usually develops after a few days and they then diminish in severity.

Dry mouth
Diminished parasympathetic stimulation decreases salivation. A dry mouth is a common ADR of TCAs and may result in dental caries and stomatitis. Its frequency contributes to the poorer tolerability of the TCAs. A persistently dry mouth is usually treated by a reduction in dose, or switching to a different antidepressant drug.

Blurred vision
This may be caused by mydriasis (pupillary dilatation), a sluggish pupillary reaction to light, cycloplegia (paresis of the ciliary muscle acting on the lens) and presbyopia (disturbed near vision). Narrow-angle glaucoma is a contraindication to TCAs but open-angle glaucoma is not. SSRIs have negligible or weak anticholinergic effects and are therefore usually the antidepressants of choice in patients with glaucoma. For those patients with glaucoma who are maintained on a TCA, regular ophthalmological consultation with tonometry is necessary.

Urinary retention
The detrusor muscle of the bladder serves to propel the stream of urine and is under parasympathetic control. The internal and external bladder sphincters are likewise affected by anticholinergic activity. Anticholinergic side-effects in the bladder may result in urinary slowness, dribbling, decreased flow and retention, and so patients with an enlarged prostate gland are particularly at risk. The absence of this side-effect with the SSRIs means they are the preferred option for those elderly men with benign prostatic hyperplasia. In children with nocturnal enuresis this effect can be turned to advantage and small doses of imipramine are sometimes helpful in the treatment of enuresis.

Constipation
Anticholinergic effects on the gastrointestinal tract lead to decreased intestinal motility, slowing of transit time and hence increased water reabsorption from the bowel contents. In the elderly this may cause faecal impaction and rarely a paralytic ileus. An osmotic or bulk laxative is the preferred option and stimulant laxatives are best avoided.

Memory impairment
Cognitive function has a large cholinergic component and the anticholinergic effect of TCAs is associated with poor memory. Even young adults taking TCAs may notice difficulty in remembering, but this effect is more marked among the elderly. A complaint of poor memory may also be symptomatic of depression itself, for example in depressive pseudo-dementia, and may improve with antidepressant treatment.

Confusional states
This anticholinergic effect of TCAs is more prevalent in the elderly, presenting with evening restlessness, sleep disturbance, disorientation, illogical thoughts and sometimes delusional states, with the risk of delirium being greater with higher plasma TCA levels.

Other neurological ADRs of the TCAs

Tremor
The underlying mechanism of the fine tremor produced by TCAs is uncertain. Blockade of noradrenaline reuptake at post-ganglionic sympathetic receptors may contribute and noradrenaline also has a weak stimulating effect on beta-receptors. Adrenaline may play a role as it stimulates both alpha and beta sympathetic receptors. Propranolol, a beta-blocker, reduces this tremor. There may also be a contribution from serotonergic receptors since 10–13% of patients on SSRIs also develop a fine tremor.

Sedation
Sedation is probably associated with blockade of histamine H_1 receptors. It can be used to advantage in alleviating depressive insomnia. Sedative effects are greatest at the start of TCA therapy or when the dose is increased. Morning drowsiness after a nocturnal TCA dose may pass after a few days. The tertiary amines (amitriptyline, doxepin and trimipramine) are more sedative than the secondary amines (nortriptyline, protriptyline and desipramine). Imipramine is a less sedative tertiary amine.

Convulsions
This serious side-effect of the TCAs has an incidence of between 0.5% and 2.2% (Rouillon *et al*, 1992) and although this effect is dose dependent the mechanism is unknown. The risk is greatest for maprotiline, which accounted for 63% of all reported convulsions in one survey of antidepressant side-effects (Schmidt *et al*, 1986).

Myoclonus
This is defined as an involuntary, irregular contraction of a muscle or a group of muscles. The phenomenon includes jaw-jerking, intermittent arm myoclonus (causing patients to drop objects) and nocturnal myoclonus (a relatively continuous sequence of single myoclonic jerks of various muscles throughout the night). Myoclonus usually develops in the first few weeks of treatment and may be dose related. Garvey & Tollefson (1987) reported that 30% of patients treated with imipramine suffered from a mild degree of myoclonus but in 9% it was sufficiently troublesome to require a medication change.

Extrapyramidal signs
Choreo-athetoid movements are rare and may be related to a TCA-induced hyperdopaminergic state. Depression itself may constitute a risk factor for the onset of tardive dyskinesia. Akathisia has been reported in women taking conjugated oestrogens as oral contraceptives and TCAs. Oestrogens also affect dopamine-sensitive adenylate cyclase and modulate dopamine receptors.

Other CNS side-effects
Sleep disturbance, nightmares, hypnagogic hallucinations and hypnopompic hallucinations may all occur. Reduced sleep time and increased wakefulness may be found in antidepressants acting selectively on serotonin receptors and are more pronounced with SSRIs. Impaired speech may be related to high plasma levels of antidepressants. Speech problems consist of difficulty in finding words, stuttering or increased verbal pauses, and usually respond to a lowering of the dose. Paraesthesia may occur.

Cardiovascular effects of the TCAs

TCAs can affect blood pressure, cardiac conduction and cardiac contractility (reviewed by Warrington *et al*, 1989). Sinus tachycardia is also quite common as a result of a vagolytic (anticholinergic) effect.

Postural hypotension
The most common cardiovascular side-effect of TCAs is postural hypotension, which is due to α-adrenergic blockade. The constriction of veins in the legs is mediated by the α-adrenoceptors. TCAs are α-adrenoreceptor antagonists and block this compensatory mechanism. This results in 'pooling' of blood in the major veins in the legs and postural hypotension. Patients complain of dizziness, unsteadiness, and sometimes falls which may occasionally be complicated by fractures. This is particularly serious in the elderly. Predictive factors for postural hypotension include a large pre-treatment postural drop, being older and having a higher plasma TCA concentration. Amitriptyline causes more postural hypotension than lofepramine

Effects on cardiac conduction
The TCAs can cause abnormalities of cardiac conduction and arrhythmias. These effects are uncommon at therapeutic doses, affecting less than 5% of patients (Warrington *et al*, 1989). The anticholinergic effects of TCAs may cause some degree of tachycardia. However, the most important effect of TCAs is membrane stabilisation via a quinidine-like effect due to inhibition of the enzyme Na^+/K^+-ATPase. This results in slowing of atrial and ventricular depolarisation and prolongation of conduction time in the bundle of His. Manifestations on the electrocardiogram (ECG) include increased PR, QRS and QT intervals and a decrease in T wave amplitude. The changes appear to be dose related; thus, at very high plasma levels, over 350μg/l, around 70% of physically healthy young adults with depression will develop first-degree heart block, compared with only 3% with levels below 350μg/l (Preskorn & Fast, 1991).

The best ECG measure of a quinidine-like effect is the QT interval after it has been corrected for heart rate ($QT_c = QT/\sqrt{RR \text{ interval}}$) and modern ECG machines print out both QT and QT_c values. Long QT_c intervals are thought to predict the onset of potentially fatal ventricular arrhythmias such as *Torsades de pointes*. (This topic is also discussed in Chapter 11, page 257.) A QT_c interval should not be longer than 450 ms and if 500 ms or greater drug doses should be reduced immediately. Some authorities suggest concern leading to action should occur at a level of 440 ms in men and 470 ms in women. Lofepramine has little quinidine-like activity or membrane-stabilising effect (although its main metabolite, desipramine, may have) and this has been proposed as the explanation for its decreased cardiotoxicity and low lethality in overdoses.

Other cardiovascular issues
Hypertension itself does not increase the hazards of treatment with antidepressant drugs, and TCAs may decrease blood pressure. Because of their anticholinergic and quinidine-like effects, TCAs should not be used in patients with angina pectoris, recent myocardial infarction, arrhythmias or cardiac failure. The SSRIs are now the drugs of choice for these patients. The NICE (2004) review recommends the use of sertraline for patients who have had a recent myocardial infarct or who have unstable angina.

TCA overdose

After a TCA overdose, signs of TCA intoxication are seen. In the CNS these include coma, convulsions and respiratory depression, while in the cardiovascular system there is tachycardia, blood pressure changes, conduction disturbance and arrhythmias. Fatalities are associated with ventricular tachycardia because this may progress to ventricular fibrillation or asystole. QRS duration and TCA plasma concentrations are strongly correlated (Petit *et al*, 1977), which suggests there is a linear dose–response relationship for cardiotoxicity. QRS duration has also been evaluated as a predictive measure for the more serious ventricular arrhythmias, which are seen only with a QRS of 160 ms or longer.

Drug interactions

A variety of drugs interact with TCAs. Bernstein (1995*a*) has reviewed the pharmacokinetic and pharmacodynamic mechanisms of these interactions.

Smoking, and most anticonvulsants, may increase TCA metabolism by liver enzyme induction, and this results in a lowering of TCA plasma levels and hence decreased antidepressant effects. Drugs that inhibit

TCA metabolism, such as the SSRIs (of which fluoxetine and paroxetine are the most potent inhibitors of the P450 2D6 isoenzyme), stimulants (dexamphetamine, methylphenidate and cocaine), disulfiram, isoniazid, cimitidene, beta-blockers and calcium channel blockers, may lead to raised levels in the plasma, brain and heart, a greater antidepressant effect and increased toxicity. High levels in the heart may explain the lethality of combinations of drugs when taken in overdose.

Additive sedative interactions may occur with alcohol, barbiturates, benzodiazepines and antipsychotic drugs, causing excessive drowsiness. States of anticholinergic toxicity (with possible agitation and confusion) can result when TCAs are prescribed with some of the older typical antipsychotic drugs which also have significant anticholinergic effects, particularly when anti-Parkinsonian anticholinergic drugs are used, such as benztropine or procyclidine. The elderly are more at risk.

The TCAs also lower seizure threshold and the likelihood of fits is increased. TCAs have dopaminergic effects and in Parkinsonian patients they may sometimes be beneficial, but in combination with L-dopa they may cause agitation, tremor and rigidity.

The TCAs may be inadvertently combined with catecholamines such as adrenaline and noradrenaline in dentistry, and when local anaesthesia at other sites is used. In these instances the TCA inhibition of neuronal uptake of adrenaline and noradrenaline may result in these catecholamines having an enhanced effect, causing acute hypertension. TCAs also inhibit the neuronal uptake of antihypertensive drugs such as guanethidine, bethanidine, clonidine and debrisoquine, and through this mechanism decrease the antihypertensive effect of these drugs.

At the cell membrane level, quinidine-like effects occur and so the co-administration of anti-arrhythmic drugs such as quinidine, procainamide, lidocaine and propranolol may result in ECG changes, arrhythmias and myocardial depression. As mentioned, these effects are less with lofepramine. Occasionally, in patients with diminished cardiac reserve, cardiac failure may occur. General anaesthetics may also interact, leading to an increased risk of arrhythmias and hypotension.

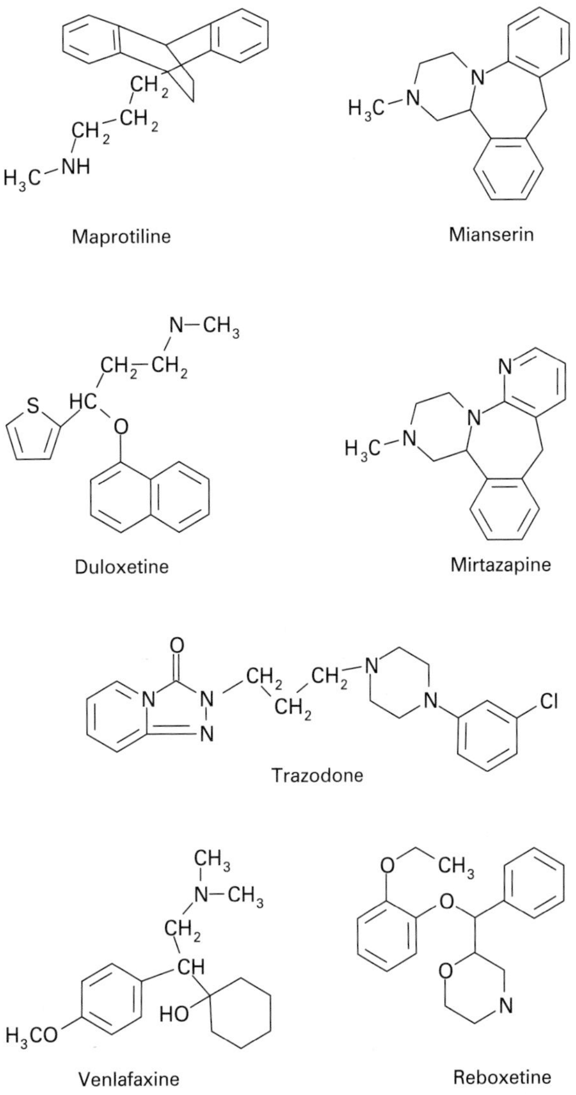

Maprotiline Mianserin Duloxetine Mirtazapine Trazodone Venlafaxine Reboxetine

Fig. 4.5 Chemical structure of some non-tricyclic antidepressants.

Related antidepressant drugs

Tetracyclics and similar antidepressants

Maprotiline

This tetracyclic (Fig. 4.5) was introduced as one of a 'new generation' of antidepressants following the tricyclics. The parent compound is the most noradrenergic of the antidepressant drugs (Fig. 4.2). It seems to have no advantages over the tricyclics and is little used today. It is particularly prone to cause convulsions and appears to have a relatively high lethality in overdose.

Mianserin

Mianserin, another tetracyclic (Fig. 4.5), does not block the reuptake of serotonin, noradrenaline or dopamine. It blocks presynaptic α_2-adrenoreceptors, which are inhibitory, and through this mechanism increases the synaptic availability of noradrenaline. Mianserin also blocks postsynaptic 5-HT_2 receptors. It is quite sedative, which is helpful for the insomnia associated with depression, and also has fewer anticholinergic side-effects than the TCAs. However, several years after its introduction, reports appeared of granulocytopenia and sometimes agranulocytosis as a result of bone marrow suppression. These effects are rare, generally occur in the first 4–6 weeks of treatment, are more common in the elderly and are usually reversible on stopping treatment. If mainserin is used, a full blood count is recommended every 4 weeks for the first 3 months of treatment, and monitoring should continue subsequently.

Trazodone

This antidepressant, which is neither a tricyclic nor a tetracyclic, is chemically related only to nefazodone, an antidepressant withdrawn from the market in 2003. Its pharmacodynamic actions are complex. Its antidepressant actions are thought mainly to relate to increased release of noradrenaline via pre-synaptic α_2 blockade. The compound antagonises the 5-HT_{2A} postsynaptic receptor. Blockade at this site may stimulate other receptor responses to serotonin, in particular the 5-HT_{1A} response. A trazodone metabolite is an agonist for other serotonin receptors. It is also a weak serotonin reuptake inhibitor, having only about 7% of the potency of clomipramine. The half-life is relatively short, at 5–13 hours. It is sedative and so is sometimes chosen for its hypnotic effect in those patients with sleep disturbance and depression. It has little anticholinergic effect. Reported ADRs include sedation, dizziness, headaches, nausea, vomiting and postural hypotension. Priapism, a prolonged painful engorgement of the penis, which may be a surgical emergency, has been reported with an incidence of one per 6000 males treated (Warner *et al*, 1987).

It is sometimes used with SSRIs in small doses (e.g. 50–100 mg) for its sedative effect. It should never be combined with MAOIs. The drug is also available in liquid form, the dose range is 100–600 mg daily and it is usually taken at night because of its sedative effect.

Other non-tricyclic antidepressants

This diverse group of antidepressants was marketed after the SSRIs. The aims were to increase both noradrenaline and serotonin transmission in order to improve efficacy, and to avoid the side-effects and toxicity in overdose associated with the TCAs. Duloxetine, mirtazapine, reboxetine (which increases predominantly noradrenergic transmission) and venlafaxine make up this group.

Duloxetine

Duloxetine is a phenepropylamine. Like venlafaxine it has a dual action in inhibiting the reuptake of both serotonin and noradrenaline (i.e. it is an SNRI); it also inhibits dopamine reuptake, although to a lesser extent. Unlike venlafaxine it exerts a more equal inhibition of both serotonin and noradrenaline, and it is a more potent inhibitor of reuptake of these monoamines than venlafaxine. It has little affinity for acetylcholine and histamine receptors. Because the capsules are enteric coated there is a 2-hour lag before absorption begins and maximum plasma concentrations occur after 6 hours, although food delays this to 10 hours. It is highly protein bound (> 90%). It has a half-life of about 12 hours (range 8–17 hours). Extensive metabolism to numerous metabolites occurs and after administration of ^{14}C-labelled duloxetine, duloxetine itself comprises only 3% of the total radiolabelled material in the plasma. Both P450 2D6 and P450 1A2 catalyse its oxidation. Of its metabolites, 70% appear in the urine and 20% in the faeces. It is not recommended for use in those with severe renal insufficiency where creatinine clearance is < 30 ml/min. Inhibitors of P450 2D6 (such as TCAs, fluoxetine, paroxetine and quinidine) and 1A2 (such as fluvoxamine, cimetidine and ciprofloxacin) raise plasma duloxetine levels, sometimes several-fold. It should not be used with an MAOI because of the risk of the serotonin syndrome.

Its efficacy has been established in the treatment of major depression. The usual dose is 60 mg once daily. There is no evidence that larger doses confer any advantage, although there are safety data for doses up to 120 mg per day. Approximately 10% of 1139 patients who received duloxetine in placebo-controlled trials discontinued it because of an adverse event, whereas the figure was 4% of the 777 patients who received placebo (Sullivan *et al*, 2005). Commonest placebo-adjusted side-effects are nausea, dry mouth, constipation, reduced appetite, dizziness, somnolence, insomnia and fatigue. Weight loss of 0.5–1.1 kg in trials lasting from 9 to 13 weeks has been reported. Because of reports of a discontinuation syndrome, the dose should be tapered off gradually.

Duloxetine has been shown to reduce neuropathic pain in diabetic peripheral neuropathy and to lessen pain in patients with depression. If there is diabetic renal impairment and creatinine clearance is greater than 30 ml/min, a lower dose than 60 mg daily should be used.

Mirtazapine

Mirtazapine has a tetracyclic chemical structure identical to mianserin apart from one nitrogen atom in the first benzene ring (see Fig. 4.5). Mirtazapine is a noradrenaline and specific serotonin antagonist (NaSSA). Like mianserin it blocks presynaptic α_2-adrenoreceptors, which are inhibitory, thereby increasing synaptic noradrenaline. This action also enhances serotonergic transmission by stimulation, via noradrenergic neurons, of α_1-adrenoreceptors located on serotonergic cell bodies, which leads to enhanced serotonergic cell firing. In contrast, on the serotonergic axon terminals there are inhibitory α_2-heteroceptors and mirtazapine itself blocks the inhibitory effect of noradrenaline on these, thereby again increasing the release of serotonin. These two mechanisms of enhancing synaptic serotonin leads to preferential 5-HT_1 stimulation, because mirtazapine in addition blocks 5-HT_2 and 5-HT_3 postsynaptic receptors. Unlike the SSRIs and TCAs, mirtazapine does not block presynaptic monoamine reuptake.

Blockade of 5-HT_2 receptors is thought to result in fewer anxiety, agitation and sexual side-effects, while blockade of 5-HT_3 receptors is thought to be associated with a lesser tendency to nausea. Blockade of H_1 histaminergic receptors is associated with sedation and weight gain, and these side-effects appear at low dosage (e.g. 15 mg). The NICE (2004) review recommends that all patients be forewarned about somnolence, sedation, increased appetite and weight gain. A dry mouth may also occur.

There have also been a few reports of leucopenia and agranulocytosis, but the evidence is less than for mianserin, and apart from being watchful (e.g. by doing a white cell count if there is any fever) no specific guidance has been issued. A single case report has shown that mirtazapine may be helpful in hyperhydrosis (excessive sweating), which is an occasional but troublesome side-effect of other antidepressants (Pasquini *et al*, 2003).

Mirtazapine has linear pharmacokinetics within the usual dose range, and has relatively low non-specific protein binding, with an elimination half-life of 20–40 hours. It is metabolised by hepatic cytochrome P450 2D6, 3A3, 3A4 and 1A2 isoenzymes, but neither induces nor inhibits these isoenzymes and so has much less potential for drug interactions. This means it can be combined rather more safely with other psychotropic medication than the SSRIs. The most common metabolite, desmethylmirtazapine, has only around one-quarter of the activity of mirtazapine.

It has been shown to have comparable antidepressant efficacy to tricyclics and SSRIs. There is some evidence for anxiolytic activity in both depression and primary anxiety states. The NICE (2004) review found a small advantage, in terms of efficacy, for mirtazapine over other antidepressants in depression (relative risk RR = 0.91) but this was not considered to be clinically significant. However, side-effects were fewer and discontinuation rates were lower for mirtazapine (RR = 0.69) than for other antidepressants, which the NICE (2004) review did consider to be significant. Mirtazapine may cause fewer sexual side-effects than the SSRIs, SNRIs or tricyclics, and has been suggested as an alternative antidepressant for those experiencing SSRI-induced sexual difficulties. The dose range is 15–45 mg per day, usually taken as a single dose at night.

Reboxetine

Although the reboxetine molecule bears some resemblance to paroxetine (see Figs 4.3 and 4.5), it is a relatively selective noradrenaline reuptake inhibitor (NARI). In contrast to the other noradrenergic antidepressants such as desipramine, lofepramine, maprotiline and nortriptyline, reboxetine has little anticholinergic, α_1-adrenergic or histaminergic effects and so lacks many of the side-effects of these drugs. The NICE (2004) review concluded it had the same efficacy as other antidepressants but that there was insufficient trial data to comment on whether it was better tolerated or not.

Reboxetine is rapidly absorbed after ingestion, highly protein bound, metabolised in the liver and has a half-life of about 13 hours. Its noradrenergic action has led to suggestions that it may be useful for treating patients with anergia, loss of interest, hypersomnia and psychomotor retardation. Placebo-adjusted side-effects are dry mouth (11%), constipation (9%), insomnia (9%), sweating (7%) and hypotension (2%). There are reports of it lowering the plasma potassium level on prolonged administration in the elderly, for whom it is not recommended for use. As it has a relatively low rate of sexual side-effects (5%) it may be an antidepressant to choose for those liable to develop sexual side-effects or those who have had these while taking other antidepressant drugs. However, it causes more urinary hesitancy in men compared with fluoxetine. As it does not inhibit the P450 liver isoenzymes, interactions are uncommon but it should not be combined with MAOIs. Reboxetine has a relatively low lethality in overdose, although CNS stimulation and convulsions may occur. The usual daily dose is 4–12 mg per day, in divided doses because of the short half-life.

Venlafaxine

The bicyclic structure of this phenylethylamine is shown in Fig. 4.5. It inhibits the reuptake of both serotonin and noradrenaline (i.e. it is an SNRI). Amitriptyline also inhibits the reuptake of serotonin and noradrenaline, but in contrast venlafaxine has little affinity for muscarinic, histaminic or α_1-adrenergic receptors. Venlafaxine is well absorbed from the gastrointestinal tract and little affected by food intake; it undergoes extensive first-pass metabolism to its major metabolite, O-desmethyl-venlafaxine.

The peak serum concentrations of venlafaxine are seen within 2 hours of oral administration, while concentrations of its metabolite rise and fall more slowly. The half-life of venlafaxine is 3–4 hours, while that of its metabolite is around 10 hours. Thus, in most patients plasma levels of the metabolite may be higher than those of venlafaxine. Protein binding of both is low, usually below 30%. This, taken together with little or no inhibition of liver P450 isoenzymes, means that venlafaxine has a low potential for pharmacokinetic drug interactions. Cimetidine inhibits venlafaxine's hepatic first-pass metabolism. Venlafaxine may increase the anticoagulant effect of warfarin and increase plasma levels of clozapine. It should not be used with an MAOI because of the risk of the serotonin syndrome.

In doses below 150 mg daily, venlafaxine is thought to be selectively serotonergic and it is at higher doses that its noradrenergic effects appear. Venlafaxine has been advocated for use in treatment-resistant depression and there are suggestions that it may be more efficacious than the SSRIs.

The NICE (2004) review found no clinically important differences between venlafaxine at any dose and other antidepressants on any efficacy outcome. Statistically significant differences mentioned below are considered to be of a size unlikely to be of clinical importance. Venlafaxine was more efficacious than the SSRIs for in-patients. For out-patients, venlafaxine was superior to TCAs in terms of tolerability as assessed by discontinuation rates (RR = 0.72). It was only marginally better than the SSRIs in terms of efficacy. Because of its increased risk of discontinuation in comparison with SSRIs and reported cardiotoxic effects, NICE (2004) expressed caution over its use in primary care, preferring the SSRIs.

An interesting finding relates to the dual action of venlafaxine at doses of 150 mg and above. Here there was an advantage when compared with other antidepressants (RR = 0.85), but when mirtazapine was excluded from the analysis this effect was sharpened (RR = 0.78). Because venlafaxine acts like an SSRI at lower doses, it has a similar side-effect profile to the SSRIs, with the most common ADR being nausea. Somnolence, sweating, headache, dizziness, asthenia and nervousness may also occur, while insomnia is sometimes the reason for discontinuation. Anticholinergic side-effects, particularly dry mouth, may also occur but less frequently than with the TCAs. Hypertension is dose dependent: its prevalence is 0% at 75 mg per day but this rises to 13% at doses greater than 300 mg per day. It is thought to be due to a sympathomimetic effect resulting from noradrenaline reuptake inhibition. The NICE guidelines (2004) state that before prescribing venlafaxine an ECG and blood pressure measurement should be taken, that blood pressure should be monitored and that consideration should be given to regular monitoring of cardiac function. However, updated prescribing advice from the Commission on Human Medicines (Duff, 2006) is that a pre-treatment ECG is not necessary and that specialist supervision is now required only for initiation of venlafaxine treatment in those patient with severe depression who require doses of 300 mg daily or above.

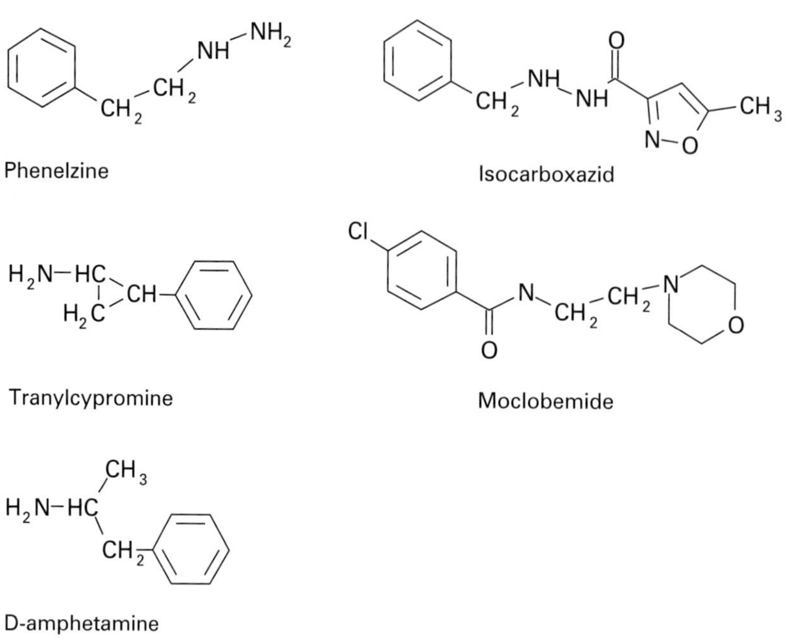

Phenelzine

Isocarboxazid

Tranylcypromine

Moclobemide

D-amphetamine

Fig. 4.6 Chemical structure of some MAOIs and D-amphetamine.

The usual starting dose is 37.5 mg twice daily, and the dose can be increased to the maximum *BNF*-recommended dose of 375 mg per day. Its relatively short half-life may explain a discontinuation syndrome, which usually presents with nausea, dizziness, insomnia and headache. The drug should be gradually tapered when it is withdrawn.

An extended release (XL) formulation with once-daily administration gives the same bioavailability as twice-daily dosing with the immediate-release preparation and is said to be associated with less nausea and fewer symptoms of the discontinuation syndrome between doses. The maximum recommended dose of venlafaxine XL is 225 mg daily.

Monoamine oxidase inhibitors

The MAOIs were among the first antidepressants to be used. Although their use is now less frequent, they are of both historical and theoretical interest.

The enzyme monoamine oxidase (MAO) inactivates the key neurotransmitters serotonin, noradrenaline and dopamine. Thus, inhibition of mitochochondrial MAO in the nerve axon leads to increased presynaptic monoamine storage (in axonal vesicles), turnover and release. The antidepressant effects of the MAOIs are probably mediated through three separate mechanisms:

- an amphetamine-like stimulant effect due to catecholamine release in the case of tranylcypromine, which has a chemical structure similar to D-amphetamine (see Fig. 4.6)
- MAO enzyme inhibition
- blockade of monoamine reuptake.

The cerebral cortex contains approximately 45% MAO-A and 55% MAO-B. These two types of MAO enzyme are distinguished by their affinity for the MAOI clorgyline, which binds selectively to MAO-A. Serotonin and noradrenaline are exclusively catabolised by MAO-A, which is selectively located in serotonergic and adrenergic nerve endings in the CNS and peripheral sympathetic nervous system. Adrenaline, tyramine (an amino acid) and dopamine are catabolised by both MAO-A and MAO-B.

Antidepressant effect is largely confined to the MAO-A inhibitors. The MAO-B inhibitors are not antidepressant in normal dosage, although selegiline, which is an MAO-B inhibitor and which is used in the treatment of parkinsonism (it enhances the effect of L-dopa), may have some antidepressant effects at higher doses.

The MAOIs are also classified on the basis of whether enzyme inhibition is irreversible or reversible (RIMA stands for 'reversible inhibitor of MAO-A'). Because all the older MAOIs cause irreversible inhibition and because they are non-selective, there is the risk of interactions with tyramine-containing foods, resulting in hypertensive reactions (see below). However, moclobemide is reversibly bound to MAO-A and hence is much less likely to be associated with dietary-induced hypertensive reactions.

Pharmacokinetics

All the MAOIs are rapidly absorbed and peak plasma levels occur within 1–3 hours, when the risk of postural hypotension is greatest. Both reversible and irreversible MAOIs have short half-lives, of 2–4 hours, so they should be taken twice a day. Steady-state plasma levels of phenelzine increase over the first 6–8 weeks of treatment, which suggests that the drug may inhibit its own metabolism.

As much as 20% of tranylcypromine may be converted to amphetamine and this may explain its potential for abuse and dependence. Phenelzine is converted to beta-phenylethylamine and phenylacetic acid. The plasma levels of these drugs show considerable variability, with no clear relationship between plasma levels, the degree of MAO inhibition or therapeutic effects, and so plasma drug monitoring is of no value.

The NICE (2004) meta-analysis for the efficacy of phenelzine found it was greater than for the TCAs (RR = 0.66), but they suggested this was probably a consequence of large numbers of patients (71%) with atypical depression (a subgroup known to do better with MAOIs) being included in the RCTs considered.

Side-effects of the MAOIs

Daytime drowsiness and dizziness due to postural hypotension are common at the start of treatment. Anticholinergic side-effects such as blurred vision, dry mouth and constipation also occur but these are less common than with the TCAs. Oedema, hepatocellular jaundice, peripheral neuropathy, bone marrow suppression and acute hypertension have been reported.

Cardiovascular side-effects

The best-known side-effect of the MAOIs is the so-called 'cheese reaction' (an acute hypertensive episode), which is relatively uncommon but occurs when cheese or other tyramine-rich foods are eaten. This occurs because inhibition of MAO in the gut wall (which has 75% MAO-A and 25% MAO-B) leads to tyramine being absorbed instead of catabolised. Tyramine has a sympathomimetic effect (like ephedrine) and releases noradrenaline from the vesicles in peripheral preganglionic sympathetic neurons, resulting in hypertension.

Hypertensive reactions have varying degrees of severity. They usually have an abrupt onset, from within minutes to up to 3 hours after the ingestion of an inappropriate food or medication, starting with an occipital pounding headache which then radiates widely, or with palpitations, nausea or vomiting. A sensation of fear, chills, sweating, restlessness, photophobia, neck stiffness and dilated pupils accompanied by a rise in blood pressure may occur. Typically, during such a reaction, systolic blood pressure may range from 150 to 220 mmHg and diastolic blood pressure from 100 to 130 mmHg. The severity of the headache may diminish after an hour but a dull ache may persist. There may be persistent hypertension, alteration of consciousness, hyperpyrexia, convulsions and cerebral haemorrhage, which may be fatal. The fatality rate has been estimated as 1 in every 8000 hypertensive reactions, or more generally as one per 100 000 patients treated with tranylcypromine (Davidson, 1992).

Treatment is with an α-adrenoceptor-blocking agent, such as phenoxybenzamine or phentolamine. If these are unavailable, chlorpromazine (oral or intramuscular, but never intravenous), which has powerful α-adrenergic blocking effects, can be used in an emergency.

The newer selective MAOIs, such as selegiline, in combination with other drugs have sometimes also been associated with hypertensive reactions (Livingston, 1995). Life-threatening paroxysmal hypertension has also been induced by noradrenaline, a condition known as pseudo-phaeochromocytoma. Symptoms include paroxysmal hypertension, vasoconstriction, confusion, abdominal pain and sweating. Medications known to cause this reaction include those affecting both the catecholamine and the indoleamine systems, for example terbutaline, phenylephrine, fluoxetine and TCAs.

Box 4.1 Tyramine-rich foods to be avoided while taking an MAOI drug

- Cheeses (particularly mature cheese)
- Broad (sava) bean pods (green beans may be eaten)
- Alcohol, especially Chianti, Vermouth, wines, draught beer
- Sausages, pepperoni, salami, liver, spam, canned ham
- Pickled herring, sardines, anchovies
- Any non-fresh or fermented meat, fish or protein product
- Yeast extract (e.g. Marmite), brewers' yeast, meat extracts (e.g. Bovril).
- Sauerkraut, banana peel

Source: Bernstein (1995*b*).

Drug interactions and food restrictions

The MAOIs interact with a variety of drugs and foodstuffs (reviewed by Bernstein, 1995*b*). Box 4.1 shows the tyramine-rich foods which should be avoided. MAOIs are dispensed with an information leaflet which lists foods and medicines to be avoided. Patients should carry this leaflet and show it to any doctor or dentist who treats them. The two most serious reactions are hypertensive crises and the serotonin syndrome. MAOIs are absolutely contraindicated with the SSRIs, although not with certain TCAs. A strategy occasionally used in the past in the treatment of resistant depression was a combination of trimipramine or amitriptyline with phenelzine. Clomipramine should not be used. The TCA was the first treatment, to which the MAOI was added, never the other way around. A 5-week washout period is recommended if an MAOI is to be introduced after fluoxetine and a 2-week washout if other SSRIs are to be used.

Hypertensive reactions may occur with stimulants (e.g. dexamphetamine, methylphenidate and pemoline), diet pills (fenfluramine and diethylpropion), other sympathomimetics (ephedrine and adrenergic-based bronchodilators used in asthma), and over-the-counter cold cures, nose drops, nasal decongestants and cough syrups (many of which contain phentermine, phenylephrine and phenylpropanolamine). Patients with asthma preferably should not take an MAOI, but if they do, only steroid-based inhalers should be used. The possibility of a drug interaction, particularly with the irreversible MAOIs, needs to be considered if the patient is taking any other drug.

Individual MAOIs

Phenelzine

Phenelzine (see Fig. 4.6) was the MAOI used in the Medical Research Council's (1965) study of depression, which found phenelzine to be no more effective than placebo. Since then it has been suggested that higher doses were needed to achieve an antidepressant effect. It has been shown to be superior to imipramine in atypical depression characterised by reactive mood and reversed vegetative symptoms (i.e. hyperphagia, hypersomnolence and weight gain, etc. – see page 101). It is anxiolytic, particularly in phobic anxiety.

The main side-effects include postural hypotension, drowsiness, dizziness, dry mouth and constipation, but it is thought to be among the better tolerated of the MAOIs. Although tolerance does not develop, when the drug is stopped the original anxiety symptoms may reappear. A dose of 30–90 mg per day is used.

Isocarboxazid

Isocarboxazid (Fig. 4.6) is also helpful in atypical depression and is also relatively free of side-effects. The usual dosage is 20–50 mg daily.

Tranylcypromine

Tranylcypromine (Fig. 4.6) is a non-hydrazine and this is thought to increase the risk of the cheese reaction. It has amine-releasing properties similar to amphetamine, as well as some monoamine reuptake inhibition activity. Some regard it as the most potent MAOI and it features in stepwise drug algorithms for in-patients with depression (Adli *et al*, 2002) and treatment-resistant out-patients (McGrath *et al*, 2006). The usual dose is 10–30 mg per day.

Moclobemide: a reversible MAOI

The chemical structure of moclobemide is shown in Fig. 4.6; it resembles isocarboxazid. Because moclobemide is a reversible monoamine oxidase inhibitor (RIMA) it is regarded as safer than the older, irreversible MAOIs. Reversible inhibition permits excess tyramine to displace the drug from its binding site on the enzyme. This enables MAO in the intestinal mucosa to catabolise tyramine while it is being absorbed, making a hypertensive reaction 10 times less likely than with tranylcypromine. In fact, studies with a total of 2300 patients taking moclobemide without dietary restrictions reported no tyramine-related hypertensive reaction (*Drug and Therapeutics Bulletin*, 1994).

Because it has a short half-life, the drug should be prescribed twice daily. Its effects decline rapidly once the drug is stopped. This is in marked contrast to the irreversible MAO inhibition of the traditional MAOIs, because once the enzyme is irreversibly inhibited it may take several weeks to regenerate new enzyme, even after the drug has been stopped.

Although the NICE (2004) review found moclobemide to be just as efficacious in drug trials as other antidepressants and with a comparatively low discontinuation rate, the drug is relatively infrequently prescribed. Among the elderly one study found it to be less efficacious than nortriptyline, but anticholinergic side-effects and postural hypotension were less common (Nair *et al*, 1995). The main side-effects of moclobemide are insomnia and nausea, which occur in about 10% of patients. The incidence of postural hypotension is low, at around 1%, which is much less than with irreversible MAOIs. Moclobemide has no appreciable effect on body weight, it has a low prevalence of sexual side-effects and it lacks the cardiotoxic and stimulant effect of the older MAOIs.

Cimetidine blocks moclobemide metabolism and so reduces the dose requirement of moclobemide by 50%. In therapeutic doses combinations of moclobemide with a tricyclic appear safe, but SSRIs are best avoided because of the risk of the serotonin syndrome. Thus, among patients who took overdoses, of the 13 patients who took moclobemide alone, 12 required no treatment, but there were five fatalities when the moclobemide was taken together with an overdose of clomipramine or citalopram (Neuvonen *et al*, 1993). As moclobemide is short-acting, interactions can be avoided if it is stopped 24 hours before another drug is given. The recommended starting dose is 150 mg twice daily, up to a maximum daily dose of 600 mg.

Other substances used in the treatment of depression

Antipsychotic drugs

Antipsychotic drugs may also be effective antidepressants (reviewed by Robertson & Trimble, 1982; Willner, 1995). Early placebo and TCA comparator trials had shown that chlorpromazine, thioridazine and oral flupenthixol are effective antidepressants. However, typical antipsychotic drugs carried the risk of extrapyramidal effects and they were not used as a first-line treatment.

Atypical and typical sedative antipsychotic drugs are sometimes used in combination with an antidepressant for the management of insomnia, anxiety, worry and agitation, particularly in the early weeks of treatment. In contrast to the benzodiazepines, they are not addictive. Tohen *et al* (2003) showed that, in the treatment of bipolar I depression, the combination of olanzapine plus fluoxetine was more efficacious than olanzapine alone and placebo alone. Olanzapine on its own was significantly better than placebo. There was no fluoxetine-alone group. Side-effects of fluoxetine–olanzapine were similar to those with olanzapine alone, but there was more nausea and diarrhoea in the combined group.

Some patients with ideas of reference may benefit from the addition of a small dose of an antipsychotic drug. Olanzapine or chlorpromazine may be used in severe agitated or psychotic depression (see page 102).

Lithium

In spite of its established value in mania, and as a prophylactic agent in bipolar disorder (see Chapter 2), there is little evidence for a hypothesised acute antidepressant effect. One small placebo-controlled trial showed it to be as effective as imipramine, but antidepressant effects did not appear until the third week (Worral *et al*, 1979). The US Food and Drug Administration (FDA) does not recognise it as an antidepressant and its effect in bipolar depression is disappointing (Goodwin, 2003). Its main use in treatment of depression is as lithium augmentation (see page 106). In a few cases it may play a role in long-term maintenance (see page 104) but the NICE guidelines (2004) state that it should not be used as a sole agent to prevent episodes of recurrent depression.

St John's wort (Hypericum perforatum)

The plant *Hypericum perforatum* has been used in herbal medicine for centuries for a variety of conditions, including depression. Herbal medicines such as hypericum are used much more extensively in Germany than in the UK. One constituent, hypericin, a naphthodianthron, has been suggested as the active ingredient but there are at least 10 others, including flavonoids, biflavonoids and xanthons, which may all contribute to its pharmacological activity. Standardisation of the dose is problematic, as the active ingredients can vary from one hypericum preparation to another. The crude plant extract has been shown to inhibit the reuptake of serotonin, noradrenaline and dopamine, stimulate gamma-aminobutyric acid (GABA) receptors and inhibit monoamine oxidase activity. It is unclear which of these mechanisms is operative.

A large number of RCTs have compared St John's wort with placebo and pharmaceutical antidepressants. The NICE (2004) meta-analysis found superiority over placebo (RR = 0.79), but moderate depression did especially well (RR = 0.64) compared with severe depression (RR = 0.81). There were no differences in efficacy between St John's wort and antidepressants (RR = 1.01) but hypericum had lower overall discontinuation rates (RR = 0.39) and discontinuation rates due to side-effects (RR = 0.65).

St John's wort induces P450 liver isoenzymes, including 3A4, 1A2 and 2C9, causing lowering of blood levels of oral contraceptives, warfarin, digoxin, theophylline, anticonvulsants, cyclosporins, HIV protease inhibitors and HIV non-nucleoside reverse transcriptase inhibitors. If patients switch from one St John's wort preparation to another the degree of liver enzyme induction may change. There have also been case reports of elderly patients developing the serotonin syndrome when taking SSRIs with hypericum.

Because this preparation is available without a prescription, patients presenting with depression should always be questioned whether they are using any over-the-counter remedies. Antidepressant drugs should not be used with St John's wort because of the potential for interaction. In spite of the favourable efficacy data, the NICE (2004) review did not recommend its use because of uncertainty about the appropriate dose, variation in the nature of the preparations available and the potential for serious interactions with other drugs.

Side-effects common to many antidepressants

Cookson (1993) has proposed a classification of ADRs based on the pharmacodynamic action of antidepressants on particular neurotransmitters.

Sexual side-effects

It is thought that the sexual dysfunction associated with antidepressants is mainly due to their serotonergic effect. Stimulation of 5-HT_2 receptors inhibits sexual desire, ejaculation and orgasm. Antidepressant drugs which are 5-HT_2 blockers, such as trazodone and mirtazapine, appear to have lower rates of sexual side-effects. Of course, a general loss of libido occurs in depression. Unless the doctor enquires about sexual side-effects, they may not be reported until the depression has improved. In men, ADRs include loss of libido, erectile dysfunction, delayed orgasm, analgesia and absent ejaculation; in women common complaints include decreased libido, decreased vaginal lubrication and anorgasmia.

Montejo *et al* (2001) list some less common sexual side-effects reported in individual cases and these include: penile and clitoral anaesthesia (fluoxetine); painful orgasm; orgasm associated with yawning (clomipramine, fluoxetine); priapism (trazodone, paroxetine); increased libido (trazodone); spontaneous orgasm (bupropion); and decreased ejaculatory volume (all SSRIs). Some patients tolerate sexual side-effects, but others do not. Montejo *et al* (2001) reported that 27% had good tolerance and 35% were able to accept them, but 38% considered the sexual side-effects to be unacceptable. This is associated with a non-compliance, which is often not disclosed.

One study of antidepressant tolerability found that for men the placebo-adjusted incidence of abnormal ejaculation and orgasm was as follows: paroxetine 13%, sertraline 13%, venlafaxine 12% and nefazodone (now withdrawn) 1%. For paroxetine the placebo-adjusted rates of other sexual dysfunctions, such as erectile impotence, was 10%, and libido was decreased in 3%. SSRI-associated sexual dysfunction in women was under 2% (Preskorn, 1995). Surveys of out-patients with depression have reported much higher rates. Thus, Montejo *et al* (2001) conducted a survey among Spanish out-patients taking antidepressants ($n = 1002$). The rates for reporting of any sexual dysfunction were high: citalopram 73%, paroxetine 70%, sertraline 62%, fluvoxamine 62%, fluoxetine 58%. Venlafaxine, which is predominantly serotonergic except at large doses (see above), was also associated with high rates. Drugs with lower rates for sexual dysfunction were mirtazapine (24%), nefazodone (8%) and moclobemide (4%). In this survey too few patients were on TCAs to provide meaningful figures, but previous surveys have suggested rates of around 30%, with especially high rates for clomipramine, which for men had associated anorgasmia and delayed ejaculation.

A large survey by Clayton *et al* (2002) showed somewhat lower rates of sexual dysfunction; for example, the rate for the SSRIs was 36–43%. However, this study also found a high rate for mirtazapine (40%). Patient risk factors for antidepressant-induced sexual dysfunction were: increasing age, higher daily antidepressant dose, being married, less than college education, employment status other than full time, any comorbid medical illness associated with sexual dysfunction, taking any other medication, and higher tobacco usage. Some of these factors are associated with sexual dysfunction without antidepressant use. Patient perception of sexual dysfunction was twice as high as that perceived by their physicians.

Because sexual side-effects are dose dependent, reducing the dose sometimes helps, and sexual function often returns to normal a few weeks after antidepressant therapy ceases. Switching to an antidepressant with lower rates of sexual side-effects may help: there are reports of switches to mirtazapine, moclobemide and reboxetine leading to improved sexual function. Nefazodone is no longer available and bupropion is not licensed in the UK as an antidepressant. The risk in switching is that there may be a recrudescence of depressive symptoms if the second antidepressant does not suit the patient as well as the first. Sildenafil appears efficacious in drug-induced cases of sexual dysfunction, although there are certain precautions concerning its use (see page 682).

Weight changes

Antidepressant-induced weight changes have been reviewed by Zimmerman *et al* (2003) and Table 4.6 compares the liability of the different antidepressants to produce this. Among some patients with depression, particularly those with atypical depression, weight gain and food craving (a 'sweet tooth') may be a feature of the depression itself, but this may be exacerbated by antidepressants.

Apart from paroxetine, the SSRIs seem not to have an effect on body weight. During the initial phases of treatment they may be associated with a small weight loss. However, more prolonged observations in SSRI trials have shown that weight gain of up to 3 kg may occur; although as this is similar to weight gain on placebo, it may reflect no more than the restoration of the weight lost during the depressive episode. Within the SSRI group, fluoxetine may have a greater tendency to weight loss than either sertraline or paroxetine.

Of the newer antidepressants mirtazapine is associated with significant weight gain, which tends to occur in the first few weeks of treatment and thereafter plateau. In controlled trials the weight gain due to mirtazapine is greater than that with placebo, but less than that associated with amitriptyline.

The mechanism of the weight gain is unknown. Zimmerman *et al* (2003) suggested that one of the cytokines involved in the inflammatory reaction, tumour necrosis factor α (TNF-α), may be involved. This substance is synthesised by fat cells and levels are increased in obesity. Psychotropics that induce considerable weight gain (e.g. clozapine, olanzapine, amitriptyline and mirtazapine) all activate the TNF-α system, whereas drugs that do not cause weight gain (e.g. haloperidol and venlafaxine) have no influence on this system.

Weight gain has important health implications in its own right and is a side-effect that sometimes results in antidepressant discontinuation. Dosage reduction is usually ineffective, because weight gain is not a dose-dependent side-effect. Switching to a weight-neutral drug is a commonly used option, but there is the risk of loss of the therapeutic response. If antidepressant withdrawal is envisaged at a later date (e.g. after an acute episode), patients can be informed that body weight may return to normal once the drug is withdrawn. For those who need to remain on medication, counselling, dietary programmes and behaviour therapy may be tried (Zimmerman *et al*, 2003) but are not easy to implement with patients who are depressed and demoralised.

Table 4.6 Classification of psychotropic drug effects on body weight

Effect on weight	Antidepressants
Marked weight gain	Amitriptyline, doxepin, imipramine, clomipramine, maprotiline, mirtazapine, nortriptyline, trimipramine
Moderate weight gain	Paroxetine,[a] desipramine, isocarboxazid, trazodone
Slight weight gain	Phenelzine
No weight change	Fluoxetine,[a] fluvoxamine,[a] sertraline,[a] citalopram,[a] nefazodone, bupropion, venlafaxine, tianeptine, tranyl-cypromine, moclobemide
Weight loss	SSRI[a] (only initially)
No data available	Reboxetine

[a]SSRIs may cause weight loss during the first weeks of treatment, but often result in weight gain during long-term treatment.
Source: Adapted from Zimmerman *et al* (2003).

Skin reactions

Around 2–4% of patients on antidepressants develop skin reactions, usually in the first 2 weeks of treatment. Of these, the most common are exanthematous (46%) and urticarial (23%). Less commonly, erythema multiforme (5.4%), exfoliative dermatitis (3.7%) and photosensitivity (2.8%) occur. Allergic reactions usually appear soon after the drug is started. No particular antidepressant has been associated with any specific skin reaction.

Discontinuation syndrome

A discontinuation syndrome has been defined as:

> 'a well defined syndrome with predictable onset, duration and cessation of action containing psychological and bodily symptoms not previously complained of by the patient. It can be suppressed by the reinstitution of discontinued medication.' (Lader, 1983)

Individuals reporting symptoms shown in Box 4.2 1–3 days after discontinuing an SSRI are likely to be experiencing this syndrome. Dizziness is a common symptom which may markedly worsen with movement and suggests benign paroxysmal positional vertigo; other conditions which may be mimicked include upper respiratory infection, influenza, pulmonary embolism, stroke and myocardial infarction as well as alcohol and other substance withdrawal states. The return of depressive symptoms after antidepressant withdrawal usually takes longer to manifest (e.g. 2–3 weeks).

Discontinuation symptoms are usually relieved within 24 hours by restarting the antidepressant. Untreated discontinuation symptoms are likely to last 1–3 weeks.

While there are no known associations with gender or diagnosis, the discontinuation syndrome appears to be more common in SSRIs with a short half-life (i.e. paroxetine and fluvoxamine) (Table 4.1), and less common with fluoxetine and sertraline, which

Box 4.2 Features of the SSRI discontinuation syndrome

Psychiatric
- Anxiety
- Crying spells
- Insomnia
- Irritability
- Mood lability
- Vivid dreams

Gastrointestinal
- Nausea
- Vomiting

Neurological
- Dizziness
- Headache
- Paraesthesia

Motor
- Dystonia
- Tremor

Somatic
- Chills
- Fatigue
- Lethargy
- Myalgias
- Rhinorrhea

Source: Ditto (2003).

both have metabolites with longer half-lives. Risks may be increased for those who have been taking antidepressants for 8 weeks or more, those who had increased anxiety at the beginning of treatment, children and adolescents, those who have had previous discontinuation symptoms, and patients who are also taking centrally acting medications (antihypertensives, antihistamines and antipsychotics). Pharmacodynamic factors among the SSRIs that may be important are the potency of inhibition of serotonin reuptake and affinity for anticholinergic blockade, both of which are maximal for paroxetine. Although sometimes called the SSRI discontinuation syndrome, a discontinuation syndrome has been described for TCAs, MAOIs, mirtazapine, trazodone and venlafaxine (Ditto, 2003). According to the NICE (2006) guidelines on bipolar disorder, paroxetine and venlafaxine have a higher risk than other antidepressant drugs of discontinuation symptoms. Thus, the picture for TCA discontinuation is one of flu-like symptoms, myalgia, excessive sweating, headache, nausea, insomnia and excessive dreaming, and, rarely, movement disorders and cardiac arrhythmias.

If the symptoms are mild the patient may be reassured that the condition will improve. If severe, the original antidepressant may be restarted with a view to a slow dose reduction (over weeks). Recurrence of the discontinuation syndrome after a slow taper may be managed by attempting to switch via a cross-taper to a different antidepressant with a view to a slow dose reduction of the second antidepressant. Following the successful routine treatment of an episode of depression, drugs should be withdrawn over 1–2 months by gradual dosage tapering. For long-acting drugs such as fluoxetine, gradually reducing the frequency of administration (e.g. alternate-day dosing) is sometimes advised. The patient's mood needs to be closely monitored. Minor mood swings may occur, but if depression lasts more than a few days then the therapeutic dose of antidepressants may have to be reintroduced and a further attempt at withdrawal made 6–12 months later.

Suicide and antidepressants

Three areas of interest are mentioned here:

1 the relative lethality of different antidepressants when taken in overdose

2 the possibility that antidepressants may trigger suicide, a suicide attempt or suicidal thoughts

3 whether the greatly increased rate of prescribing of antidepressants has resulted in a reduction in suicide rates.

Lethality in overdose

There is no doubt that taken in overdose TCAs are more toxic than the SSRIs (Henry *et al*, 1995). For the years 1993–97 in England and Wales, Shah *et al* (2001) examined fatalities from overdose and poisoning and found that the death rate for TCAs per 100000 prescriptions was 5.3, whereas for the SSRIs the figure was 0.4, which is 13-fold less. Cheeta *et al* (2004) found that for fatal overdoses TCAs featured seven times more commonly in their database than did the SSRIs and this difference was accentuated when each single drug (as opposed to drug combinations) was considered. After an overdose, the membrane-stabilising action of the TCAs with inhibition of the cardiac sodium and potassium channels is considered an important mechanism for cardiac arrhythmias and death. All three studies identified lofepramine as having low lethality in overdose. Venlafaxine was identified as having a similar lethality to the TCAs; an infrequently used TCA, amoxapine, had a high self-poisoning fatality (Henry *et al*, 1995; Shah *et al*, 2001; Cheeta *et al*, 2004).

Cheeta *et al* (2004) provide data about combinations of other drugs with antidepressants used in fatal overdoses. The more common other substances were alcohol, a second antidepressant, antipsychotics and opiates. Around 24% of those who took a fatal SSRI overdose were also taking a TCA. The combination of an SSRI and a TCA may be particularly dangerous because of the possibility of the SSRI inhibiting liver cytochrome P450 enzymes, leading first to elevated TCA levels in all body tissues (including the heart) and second to delayed catabolism, resulting in prolonged toxic exposure.

Fatal self-poisoning with antidepressants has to be considered in the context of all causes of suicide. Thus, the causes of 4025 suicides in a year (Department of Health, 2002) were:

- hanging and strangulation 1900 (47%)
- self-poisoning with any substance 1330 (33%)
- motor vehicle exhaust gas 350 (9%)
- railway deaths 210 (5%)

Table 4.7 Antidepressants by deaths from fatal poisoning and all causes of suicide

Antidepressant	Fatal poisonings per million defined daily doses[a] (95% CI)	Adjusted relative risk for all causes of suicide[b] (95% CI)
Lofepramine	0.08 (0.03–0.11)	0.5 (0.2–1.6)
Amitriptyline	1.64 (1.46–1.74)	0.7 (0.4–1.2)
Imipramine	1.47 (1.2–1.74)	0.7 (0.3–1.7)
Clomipramine	0.38 (0.25–0.54)	0.8 (0.4–1.8)
Dothiepin	1.54 (1.42–1.63)	1.0 (reference drug)
Doxepin	1.40 (0.98–1.88)	1.0 (0.3–3.7)
Trazodone	0.6 (0.21–0.99)	1.2 (0.4–4.0)
Flupenthixol	Not available	1.5 (0.7–3.0)
Mianserin	0.2 (0.22–0.35)	1.6 (0.7–3.3)
Fluoxetine	0.02 (0–0.07)	3.8 (1.7–8.6)

[a]Henry *et al* (1995).
[b]Jick *et al* (1995).

- jumping from a high place 140 (3%)
- use of firearms 95 (2%).

Hawton *et al* (2003) found that, of 15 299 suicides, 4162 (27%) were drug related, of which 309 (2% of the 15 299) were due to TCAs alone. In Sweden, Isacsson *et al* (1999*b*) reported that, among 3400 suicides, antidepressants were detected in 12% of the men and 26% of the women, but that sufficiently high blood levels of antidepressants to indicate that the cause of death was antidepressant poisoning were found in 4% of the sample. Although the study was done before SSRIs were widely prescribed in Sweden, it showed that the newer antidepressants mianserin and moclobemide (which are safer in overdose than TCAs) in fact had significantly higher standardised mortality ratios (SMRs) for suicide (2.0 and 1.8, respectively), while lofepramine had a significantly lower SMR, of 0.14. In a second study based on the UK General Practice Research Database of more than one million prescriptions, there were 143 suicides (Jick *et al*, 1995). The adjusted relative risk of suicide (of all causes) for each antidepressant is shown in Table 4.7 (third column) and these were raised only for fluoxetine. It also shows (second column, from Henry *et al*, 1995) how the various antidepressants compare in relation to risk of fatal poisoning. The difference is due to the fact that fatal antidepressant poisoning constitutes only a small proportion of completed suicides, and patients kill themselves by a variety of other means.

There are several possible biases that could explain these results. Suicidal features at initial assessment may favour the prescription of a non-toxic antidepressant, so that patients are non-randomly allocated to different types of drug. Those at high risk may subsequently kill themselves by other means, such as a paracetamol overdose or by hanging. Alternatively, some of the new antidepressants may be less effective in preventing suicide. Current studies cannot distinguish between these possibilities.

In contrast to the consideration of suicide in the whole population, Henry *et al* (1995) pointed out that, for patients prescribed an antidepressant for depression, the proportion of suicides due to antidepressant overdose is much higher, perhaps as high as 50%, and that in this group TCAs account for most cases. Assuming this to be the case, if the rate of suicide in this group is 200 per 100 000 per annum, one would have to treat 1000 patients with SSRIs to prevent one such death (Hotopf & Lewis, 1997).

Can antidepressants occasionally trigger a suicide?

An early example of a drug associated with suicide was the tranquilliser and antihypertensive drug reserpine, which is derived from the Indian herb *Rauwolfia serpentina*. This was introduced in the 1950s for the treatment of hypertension, but depression became recognised as a side-effect and suicides occurred. Its mechanism of depletion of central monoamines constituted evidence originally used in the formulation of the monoamine theory of depression. In an evaluation of an antidepressant maintenance trial which showed that maprotiline was 'effective' in preventing depression, maprotiline was associated with five suicides and nine suicide attempts, compared with one suicide and no suicide attempts in the placebo arm of the trial (Rouillon *et al*, 1989).

The early phase of treatment of depression with TCAs, ECT and even light therapy has been considered a risk period for suicide. It was thought that, as patients' energy returned, they became more active and hence more able to act on suicidal thoughts.

In the early 1990s, soon after the introduction of fluoxetine, there were several case reports for the first time of intense suicidal ideation or aggression in association with fluoxetine treatment (Teicher *et al*, 1990). In a meta-analysis, Healy & Whitaker (2003) presented evidence for an overall increase in suicide and suicide attempts in those given antidepressant drugs compared with placebo during acute treatment of depression. Among adolescents there were reports of self-destructive behaviour and it was thought that this lay behind the small number of suicides occurring relatively early in the course of SSRI treatment. In 2004 the FDA reported on 24 trials of 4400 children and adolescents, and found that the risk of suicidal thinking and attempts for those given an SSRI was 4%, whereas for placebo the risk was 2%. There were no suicides in the FDA-reported trials and the cause of the increased risk was unclear (FDA, 2004; see also Hammad *et al*, 2006).

In a meta-analysis of Medline-reported RCTs of SSRIs together with the Cochrane Collaboration register of controlled trials (702 trials were included), Fergusson *et al* (2005) found a significant increase in the risk of suicide and suicide attempts in the SSRI group compared with placebo (odds ratio 2.28, 95% CI 1.14 to 4.45). The number needed to treat (NNT) to harm was 684, which means that for every 684 patients treated with an SSRI rather than a placebo, there would be one case of attempted suicide or suicide. There was no difference in the odds ratio when comparing SSRIs with TCAs (0.88, 0.54 to 1.42), whereas there was an increase in the odds ratio of suicide and suicide attempts when SSRIs were compared with therapeutic interventions other than TCAs (1.94, 1.06 to 3.57). The SSRI increase in risk was largely accounted for by episodes of non-fatal self-harm because of the small number of suicides.

In a meta-analysis evaluating suicides, episodes of non-fatal self-harm and suicidal thoughts in 342 placebo-controlled trials of SSRIs derived from the UK Medicine and Healthcare Products Regulatory Agency (MHRA), Gunnell *et al* (2005) found no evidence that SSRIs increase the risk of suicide compared with placebo (odds ratio 0.85, 95% Bayesian credible interval 0.20 to 3.40) and non-significant evidence for an increased risk of self-harm (1.57, 0.99 to 2.55). For suicidal thoughts the findings were not significantly in favour of a protective effect (0.77, 0.37 to 1.55).

Martinez *et al* (2005), utilising the UK General Practice Research Database, compared SSRIs with the TCAs and found no significant difference for non-fatal self-harm (odds ratio 0.99, 95% CI 0.86 to 1.14) or suicide (0.57, 0.26 to 1.25). However, these authors found that, for those aged 18 years or younger, there was a higher risk of non-fatal self-harm for SSRIs than for TCAs (odds ratio 1.59, 1.01 to 2.50). In June 2003 the MHRA withdrew its licence for all antidepressants with the exception of fluoxetine in the treatment of depression in those below 18 years of age. The FDA now requires that a warning about the risk of suicide is placed on the packaging used for dispensing antidepressants.

The mechanism by which antidepressant drugs might increase suicidal thinking, suicidal behaviour and suicide is not established. It has been suggested that emergent anxiety, agitation, panic, insomnia, irritability, hostility, impulsivity and akathisia on starting treatment are risk factors, as such activation could lead to the commission of suicidal acts which would not otherwise have occurred. In keeping with this, Jick *et al* (2004) found that the risk of non-fatal suicidal behaviour in the first 9 days, in comparison with the risk for days 10–90, of a new antidepressant prescription was raised fourfold (odds ratio 4.1, 95% CI 2.9 to 5.7) and there was also an increased relative risk of suicide, although the latter finding was based on small numbers.

A second proposed mechanism is that SSRIs themselves directly promote suicidal thoughts – that patients may develop a round of pervasive and compelling suicidal thoughts after starting treatment. This was described in a few cases shortly after fluoxetine was introduced (Teicher *et al*, 1990).

Weiss & Gorman (2005) have proposed a third mechanism. They have commented that poor treatment adherence often occurs in adolescence and that this is well documented in medical disorders such as asthma and diabetes. Their argument is that inconsistent antidepressant drug compliance may result in the frequent occurrence of acute discontinuation symptoms, to which adolescents may respond impulsively by self-harm. Using FDA data, these authors reported a significant negative correlation (Spearman's rho –0.93, $P < 0.01$) between plasma half-life and the suicide risk, the implication being that antidepressants with a short half-life have a higher propensity to cause both discontinuation symptoms and suicidal acts.

Clinicians, patients and their families should be on the watch for emergent anxiety, akathisia, an increase in suicidal thoughts and poor compliance. These features may require the patient to stop medication or change to another drug.

Has the increased rate of SSRI prescribing reduced the suicide rate?

In a provocatively entitled paper 'Suicide prevention – a medical breakthrough', Isacsson (2000) posed the question of whether the large increase in SSRI prescribing had led to a fall in the suicide rate. In Sweden, population-based antidepressant prescribing rates rose from 1% of the population in 1991 to 3.4% in 1996, which suggested that almost half of all those with depression (base rates of around 5–6%) were being treated and this was paralleled by a fall in the suicide rate of 19%. The study found no association of suicide rates with unemployment or alcoholism rates, both of which are usually linked with suicide. Reports from Norway, Denmark and Finland have also shown associations between increased rates of antidepressant prescribing and falling suicide rates.

In Australia, Hall *et al* (2003) examined the period 1991–2000 and found no overall decrease in suicide rates. There was an increase in the suicide rate in young men but falls in the rates for women and older men, and for these two subgroups there was a negative correlation between the fall in suicide rate and the increased number of antidepressant prescriptions.

Between 1990 and 1997 in Hungary, there was a 25% fall in the suicide rate, while the antidepressant prescribing rate rose from 3.7 to 12.0 per 1000 persons. With the collapse of the communist regime, unemployment rates rose sixfold, divorce rose by 21%, and alcoholism by 25% – all social changes that would be expected to raise the suicide rate (Rihmer *et al*, 2000).

Olfsun *et al* (2003) examined suicide rates among adolescents in 588 'zip code' regional postal districts in the USA and found that a 1% increase in use of antidepressants was significantly associated with a decrease of 0.23 suicides per year per 100 000 adolescents. This applied particularly to males, adolescents aged 15–19 years and regions of the USA with lower median family incomes, and was not accounted for by TCA prescription rates, which showed a small fall over the study period.

Correlation is not causation. Thus, Hall *et al* (2003) in their Australian study pointed out that an increase in antidepressant prescriptions will inevitably be accompanied by more frequent consultations, greater awareness and assessment of suicidal risk and probably more counselling as well. These count against a pharmacological effect as a sole explanation. No previous medical intervention has ever been shown to reduce the suicide rate and so these observations are of considerable interest.

Treatment of a depressive episode

Depressive episodes are common. The prescription of antidepressants is probably the most frequent single intervention made by general adult psychiatrists, and it is also among the more common interventions made by general practitioners. Three important treatment guidelines have recently been published and these make broadly similar recommendations. Those produced by

> **Box 4.3** Grading of the quality of the evidence base and associated recommendations within the NICE system
>
> **Grade A recommendation**
> I Evidence obtained from at least one RCT, or a meta-analysis of several RCTs
>
> **Grade B recommendation**
> IIa Evidence obtained from at least one well-controlled (but not randomised) trial
> IIb Evidence obtained from at least one other well-designed quasi-experimental study
> III Evidence obtained from well-designed non-experimental descriptive studies, such as comparative studies, correlation studies and case studies
>
> **Grade C recommendation**
> IV Evidence obtained from experts or from expert committee reports or opinions and/or clinical experiences of respected authorities or experts
>
> In the rest of this chapter A, B or C refer to these NICE recommendations and are placed after particular forms of intervention.

the American Psychiatric Association (APA), 'Practice guidelines for the treatment of patients with major depressive disorder (revision)' (American Psychiatric Association, 2000), are presented in an easily readable essay form and are comparatively short. The British Association for Psychopharmacology (BAP) publication 'Evidence-based guidelines for treating depressive disorders with antidepressants' (Anderson *et al*, 2000) has a similar approach and is also written in essay form. The set of guidelines published by NICE (2004), *Depression: Management of Depression in Primary and Secondary Care*, is the most authoritative of the three. An earlier, lengthy document gave details of the large number of meta-analyses, with associated statistics, upon which the NICE (2004) recommendations were based. Summary documents of varying length have also been produced.

All three sets of guidelines grade the strength of their recommendations according to the quality of the underlying research data. Recommendations from all three sets of guidelines are mentioned, but the NICE system is shown in Box 4.3. The levels I, II and III refer to the quality of the evidence base and grades A, B and C to the strength of the associated recommendations.

All the guidelines highlight that the overall management of depression will entail using a broad array of psychiatric interventions, which should be available to all patients whatever their primary choice of treatment modality (medication, psychological treatment or ECT) and that overall management consists of more than a simple exercise in psychopharmacology. The APA and NICE guidelines outline the following steps.

Diagnostic evaluation and risk assessment

A standard psychiatric assessment should be made for all patients and in cases of depression this should emphasise specific features of affective disorder, such as a personal or family history of mania or depression, duration of episodes and responsiveness to various treatments. Presenting affective symptoms should be clearly documented because monitoring progress with these symptoms at the patient's return visits will form the basis of deciding whether improvement has occurred and whether the medication should be changed.

Severity should be assessed in terms of the number and severity of symptoms. In the ICD–10 scheme (World Health Organization, 1992) the depression should be classed as:

- mild if there are four symptoms
- moderate if there are five or six symptoms with moderate functional impairment
- severe if there are more than seven symptoms.

In the DSM–IV scheme (American Psychiatric Association, 1994):

- mild depression has five or six symptoms and little functional impairment
- moderate is between mild and severe
- severe has many symptoms and much functional impairment, with or without psychotic features.

It is worth noting that 'mild' ICD–10 depression is below the DSM–IV threshold for 'mild' depression and that antidepressant drug trials use DSM–IV in preference to ICD–10.

Safety and risk assessment comprise a second and distinct dimension from severity. Suicide risks (see Chapter 7) or even occasionally homicidal risks, as may occur in psychotic depression, or risks of infanticide, as in postnatal illnesses (Chapter 25, page 659), will need to be separately assessed.

Assessment of the degree of functional impairment

Major depression is associated with functional impairment in areas of family relationships, academic achievement, work, self-care and other aspects of life. Sometimes this impairment is severe and damaging both to the individual and to family members. In other instances, especially where personal relationships are impaired, it may be difficult (at least initially) to determine whether a deteriorating domestic situation has caused the depression or whether a primary depressive disorder has disturbed family relationships. Either way, the severity of these impairments needs to be identified, documented and addressed as soon as possible. Further deterioration should be prevented, for example by excusing patients temporarily from responsibilities such as work, or counselling other family members on the nature of the illness. The NICE guidelines recommend (grade C) that, when loss of work and other social derangements have occurred, appropriate rehabilitation should be instituted. Depressive episodes may occur during the midst of a major life crisis and in these cases patients should be counselled not to take any important (life-changing) decisions while they have an abnormal mood and are desperately unwell, even though they often feel impelled to do so (APA guidelines).

Table 4.8 The stepped care model

Step	Severity	Personnel responsible	Types of action
1	Mild symptoms	Primary care	Recognition and assessment
2	Mild depression	Primary care	Watchful waiting, brief interventions, medication if no response
3	Moderate or severe	Primary care	Medication, structured psychological interventions, social support
4	Treatment resistant, recurrent, atypical, psychotic or high risk	Mental health specialists, including crisis team	Medication, complex psychological interventions, combined treatments
5	Risk to life, severe self-neglect	In-patient care, crisis teams	Medication, combined treatments, electroconvulsive therapy

The stepped care approach

Both the APA and NICE guidelines discuss the setting and personnel involved in treatment. The approaches are slightly different because primary care is much stronger in the UK than in the USA, where more depression is treated by specialists. In the UK the NICE (2004) review suggests that a stepped care approach should be used, with the first rungs of the ladder for milder depressions, as might be found in general practice settings, and the later steps for the more severe depressions, as might be found in specialist care. The stepped care approach is a useful model for organising services as well as providing an approximate demarcation for the roles of primary and secondary care in the management of depression (Table 4.8).

There are no data concerning the frequency of out-patient visits in the UK but NICE and BAP guidelines suggest that initially patients should be seen after 1–2 weeks. Out-patient visits are used to monitor progress, side-effects, treatment adherence and suicidality as well as to provide a setting for psychotherapeutic intervention. Health professionals should try to contact with patients who miss follow-up appointments (NICE, grade C). Defaulting on contact with psychiatric services is itself a suicide risk factor. The addition of psychological treatments such as counselling or cognitive–behavioural therapy (CBT) improves the prognosis and the APA guidelines refer to this as 'the split model'.

A small proportion of patients with severe depression require immediate admission to hospital. Those with active suicidal or homicidal ideation (NICE, grade C), those who may have harmed themselves in the past, and those with severe psychotic depression, refusal to eat or drink, stupor or comorbid medical and psychiatric disorders may be candidates for hospital admission. The decision will be influenced by a variety of individual and social circumstances; the threshold for admission will be lower for those living alone and without the support of family or others. In general, the need to admit usually depends on a balance between the severity of the depression, the patient's wishes and the perceived risks.

The APA guidelines also recommend the use of 'partial hospitalisation', for example the patient spending the day in a healthcare setting but sleeping at home. The NICE guidelines on reviewing the literature made no particular recommendation in this regard, as no study had demonstrated a therapeutic advantage over intensive home support.

Psycho-education

Most patients appreciate a supportive relationship and education about their depression and their drugs while taking a course of antidepressants, and there is now some objective evidence that psycho-education can improve outcome. Thus, Peveler *et al* (1999) compared the effects of an education programme (4 hours of counselling about depressive illness, lifestyle, antidepressant drugs and their side-effects, and the importance of compliance) with treatment as usual among a group of patients being treated mainly with TCAs in general practice. After 12 weeks, 63% of those who received counselling were still taking their medication, compared with only 39% in the treatment-as-usual group (odds ratio = 2.7; number needed to treat = 4). Beneficial effects in terms of symptom reduction were seen only for those on 75 mg or more of their TCA. Information leaflets did not have any significant effects on compliance.

A meta-analysis of controlled trials of CBT combined with antidepressants compared with antidepressants alone showed that not only did the CBT group do better, but also antidepressant discontinuation rates were significantly lower (13%) in the CBT group, indicating that a psychotherapeutic approach may also tend to improve compliance (Pampallona *et al*, 2004).

It is helpful to explain to the patient at the outset that some guesswork is involved in prescribing and that changes in both the dosage and the drug may be necessary. Patients should be advised to telephone the clinic (NICE, grade B) if they experience unwanted side-effects, as dealing with such problems speedily may diminish the risk of the patient defaulting from treatment.

An essential component of the treatment programme is the communication of four key items of information about antidepressant drugs:

1 *All antidepressants have side-effects*. The patient should be told the common side-effects of the drug that he or she has been prescribed. This is good practice and is also part of the right to information in the Patients' Charter. Advice should be given on how best to manage side-effects (e.g. if they are mild and transient, to persist with the treatment, but if severe or persistant, to contact the service). Patients should be told that side-effects commonly diminish after a few days, but that if they persist a lower dose or

an alternative antidepressant may be used. Patients should be told that there is no need to endure severe side-effects, especially as there is now a wide range of other antidepressants from which to choose.

2 *Improvement in mood and other symptoms is commonly delayed and may be noticed only after 1–3 weeks and may not be maximal until 2 months*. Symptoms tend to improve in a similar order, with mood and sleep improving relatively early, whereas negative cognitions, loss of interest and low energy may take longer to disappear.

3 *Emotional lability is common during improvement and may be distressing*. Patients should be told that during recovery 'bad days' may occur and on these occasions they may feel as depressed as ever. A few patients may report a worsening of suicidal thoughts. These features may make some patients inclined to stop treatment. It is helpful to explain that these bad days gradually become less frequent and will eventually disappear, and that the mood lability is a sign that the drugs are producing changes.

4 *Stopping antidepressants at any time may precipitate symptoms*. For some antidepressants, particularly those with a short half-life such as paroxetine or venlafaxine, stopping for even 1 or 2 days may trigger a discontinuation syndrome and patients need to be forewarned of this. Even well-informed individuals may want to stop their antidepressants as soon as their depression has resolved. Many patients need to be specifically counselled not to stop their antidepressants prematurely and of the need to take their drugs for months after recovery. This advice may have to be given repeatedly.

Non-compliance and reluctance to take antidepressants

The psychiatrist's task is to ensure that patients who agree to take an antidepressant receive an *efficacious* drug, in *sufficient dose* and for an *adequate duration* of time. This may seem obvious, but it is often surprisingly difficult to implement. Many factors may interfere with the administration of a course of antidepressants, and it is essential to seek out information in the follow-up interviews concerning the patient's medication adherence. Patients are usually prepared to discuss their reasons for being reluctant to take medication and the type of non-compliance encountered in depression usually differs from that found in schizophrenia, where a lack of insight may explain refusal to take medication.

Illness factors which contribute to non-compliance with antidepressants include:

- lack of motivation
- feelings of hopelessness
- a mild degree of cognitive impairment leading to forgetfulness.

Drug factors include:

- side-effects – there is considerable variation between the tolerability of drugs, and certain side-effects, notably sexual side-effects, may not be reported yet result in drug discontinuation.
- delay in response, which needs to be explained to the patient.

Patient factors include:

- a distaste for taking any medication
- misinformation, for example the belief that antidepressants are addictive or that taking a drug may lead to a change of personality.

Life events may also contribute. Depressive episodes, whether or not precipitated by recent life events, respond equally well to antidepressants (NICE, 2004), but patients who have experienced a recent life event may find this difficult to understand. They may question how a tablet can help in a social crisis and be sceptical of the role of medication. Time taken in exploring patients' attitudes and anxieties concerning medication is fruitful.

The management of non-compliance requires careful consideration but it is usually possible to help patients negotiate this impasse. The initial assessment interview establishes a relationship that should allow the patient to trust the doctor's advice concerning treatment. Eliciting the reasons for non-compliance or reluctance to take medication, which may include other factors than those described above, is essential. The NICE (2004) review recommends that patients with moderate or severe depression who do not take or refuse to take an antidepressant be offered CBT. Excessive pressure on the patient to take medication may prove counterproductive, as a patient may drop out of treatment altogether. In general it is best to continue to offer reviews in the clinic, as patients who initially refuse medication may later change their mind. Sometimes at an appropriate moment it is helpful to point out that the natural history of depression may be lengthy. For example, Braftos & Haug (1968) stated that the average duration of an untreated depressive episode is about 8 months. The prospect of relief of symptoms in 3–6 weeks may lead some patients to reconsider their earlier decision not to take an antidepressant.

The choice of antidepressant

Treatment of uncomplicated depression

All three sets of guidelines are similar and quite explicit in stating that issues of safety and tolerability are paramount in the choice of the initial antidepressant. The NICE (2004) guideline states: 'for routine care choose an SSRI, because they are as effective as tricyclic antidepressants and their use is less likely to be discontinued due to side effects' (grade A recommendation).

The starting dose of an SSRI may be the full therapeutic dose. Side-effects that are dose dependent may soon appear and are occasionally initially severe. The NICE guidelines state that if agitation appears and persists, a switch to another drug should be considered. If a TCA is selected, the dosage needs to be gradually titrated upwards, as starting at full dosage would result in severe side-effects. The NICE guidelines favour lofepramine, as it is safer in overdose, with the dosage being titrated up at weekly intervals. If amitriptyline or dosulepin are selected, patients can be started on doses of 50 mg, which again can be gradually titrated upwards. For the few patients starting on either an SSRI or a TCA who are especially sensitive to side-effects, liquid preparations are available (e.g. for fluoxetine, paroxetine, citalopram and amitriptyline). These permit smaller than usual doses to be prescribed, which can sometimes then gradually be increased. Given the large number of antidepressants now available, it may be better to become thoroughly acquainted with a few drugs drawn from different classes than to prescribe from the whole range.

Mild depression

The NICE (2004) review suggests that patients with mild depression (four symptoms meeting ICD–10 criteria and where there is little in the way of functional impairment) probably do not merit antidepressant therapy, because the risk–benefit ratio is high (grade C recommendation). Drug trial data have shown that there are no placebo–drug differences for patients with scores below 13 on the Hamilton Rating Scale for Depression, and placebo–drug differences tend to increase as the severity of the depression increases.

Mild depression should be distinguished from dysthymia (a similar presentation, but persisting for 2 or more years), which is a much more disabling condition and which probably does merit drug therapy (see below), as well as from recurrent brief depression, which may be a precursor for episodes of major depression. Mild depression also has a high tendency to remit spontaneously, and may be a reaction to some short-term stress. Instead, NICE (2004) recommends that a variety of non-medical approaches are applied, such as counselling, sleep hygiene, anxiety management, physical exercise, problem solving, guided self-help or 'watchful waiting' (grade C).

Antidepressants may be considered in mild depression if:

- it fails to resolve after a period of observation
- there are associated social or medical problems
- a patient who has previously experienced moderate or severe depression presents with mild depression.

Moderate and severe depression and melancholia

The NICE (2004) guidelines state that 'In moderate to severe depression, medication should be offered to all patients before psychological intervention'. The APA guideline singles out a melancholic subtype, which in DSM–IV is characterised by severe anhedonia, lack of reactivity to pleasurable stimuli, and biological symptoms of depression, such as diurnal mood variation, early morning wakening, psychomotor retardation or agitation, anorexia, weight loss and excessive guilt. It probably corresponds to the older formulation of 'endogenous depression'. The APA guidelines state that it responds well to antidepressant medication in general.

Anxiety, obsessions and atypical depression

The presence of obsessional symptoms or comorbid obsessional disorder may favour a serotonergic TCA such as clomipramine or an SSRI. The use of irreversible MAOIs in the treatment of anxiety, depression, agoraphobia with depression or social phobia has become less common. Panic disorder responds to both TCAs and SSRIs.

Atypical depression, which is characterised by a reactive mood, lability, increased appetite, increased sleep, and sometimes weight gain, and is more common in women, is reported to respond better to MAOIs than to TCAs (NICE, grade B). In practice today, SSRIs are used in atypical depression.

Sedation

Sleep disorder is a cardinal feature of depression. If insomnia is a distressing symptom, a sedative antidepressant taken at night will provide rapid relief of initial insomnia, interrupted sleep and early waking. Although an SSRI will help insomnia once the depression has resolved, during the early weeks of treatment a sedative antidepressant has a definite advantage. Sedative TCAs include amitriptyline, dosulepin, doxepin and trimipramine. However, sleep research indicates that although they help sleep initiation, they do not increase slow-wave sleep. Trazodone and mirtazapine are also strongly sedative and are considered to improve sleep efficiency. In addition to its use as antidepressant monotherapy, trazodone in low dose is sometimes added to a conventional dose of an SSRI.

Gender

The NICE (2004) review commented that the SSRIs are better tolerated by women than by men (women tolerated sertraline better than imipramine, but this difference was not present for men). The NICE guidelines recommend that in cases of chronic depression an SSRI should be preferentially prescribed for women (grade B), but if a man develops side-effects or is intolerant of an SSRI then switching to a TCA may be helpful (grade C).

Dysthymia

Dysthymia is probably an underdiagnosed disorder, with an estimated prevalence of 3% (American Psychiatric Association, 1994). It presents as low mood with at least two other depressive symptoms out of the following: appetite disturbance, sleep disturbances, low energy, low self-esteem and difficulty in making decisions. The most important diagnostic feature is its chronicity: symptoms are virtually continuous for more than 2 years, so they appear to be part of the person's character or personality. The condition does not respond well to CBT alone (Ravidran *et al*, 1999) but does to antidepressant therapy. A trial of CBT combined with sertraline gave response rates for placebo of 33%, CBT 33%, sertraline alone 54%, and sertraline with CBT 71%. The condition is disabling, and sufferers are prone to episodes of superimposed major depression (which is termed 'double depression'). It may respond to the longer-term use of a variety of antidepressants. Evaluation of response should be over prolonged periods because improvement may occur after 6 months or more. If one antidepressant fails, another should be tried.

Psychotic depression

Distinguishing between psychotic and non-psychotic depression has implications for treatment because psychotic depression responds poorly to antidepressant monotherapy. The condition is diagnosed when there are mood-congruent depressive delusions (e.g. 'I am a sinner' or 'I have no brain') or, less commonly, depressive auditory hallucinations. It is also known as delusional depression. The condition is probably a severe variant of major depression and has higher morbidity and mortality. Community surveys suggest that around 15% of those with major depression have psychotic depression. It may present acutely, with patients acting on their delusions requiring immediate action such as hospital admission, but sometimes the delusions are concealed and emerge only as treatment progresses. Psychotic depression should be suspected in any case of severe or resistant depression and among the elderly.

An early study found that 22% of patients with psychotic depression responded to a TCA alone in comparison with 80% of patients with non-delusional depression. An antipsychotic alone gave a response rate of 31%, while a combination of an antipsychotic and a TCA gave a response rate of 68%; for ECT the response rate was 82% (Charney & Nelson, 1981).

A meta-analysis of treatment response in psychotic depression compared 'effect sizes'. Effect size is a standardised score, being the improvement in depression rating score divided by the standard deviation of the initial severity level. Parker *et al* (1992) found that the effect size was highest for ECT, at 2.3 (based on 21 studies), while a combination of an antipsychotic and a TCA had an effect size of 1.6 (based on 12 studies) and a TCA alone had an effect size of 1.2 (28 studies). There was a tendency for bilateral ECT to be superior to unilateral ECT in this meta-analysis.

The NICE (2004) review recommended the use of an antipsychotic with an antidepressant but indicated there was no reliable information on which antipsychotic drug to use, its dosage or the duration of treatment (grade C recommendation). Since then, one good RCT has been published that compared placebo, olanzapine and a combination of olanzapine (5–20 mg) and fluoxetine (20–80 mg daily) in psychotic depression (Dube *et al*, 2002). It found that olanzapine on its own was no better than placebo (with a response rate of 28%), but the combination of olanzapine and fluoxetine gave a significantly higher response rate, of 64%. This is in keeping with observations made with the previous generation of antidepressants and antipsychotics, that one drug of each class was necessary for efficacy in psychotic depression. Price *et al* (1983) also reported that some patients already taking an antidepressant and chlorpromazine responded to lithium augmentation.

Bipolar depression

Although bipolar depression is similar phenomenologically to unipolar depression, it may be more difficult to treat and patients with bipolar depression spend far longer in depressed states than in manic phases. Thus, Judd *et al* (2002) found that patients with bipolar disorder spend almost three times longer in their depressed phases (mean duration 40 weeks) than in their manic episodes (mean duration 15 weeks). A retrospective case-note study comparing the treatment of patients with unipolar and bipolar depression illustrates the types of difficulties encountered when treating bipolar depression (Ghaemi *et al*, 2004). Short-term non-response was more frequent in bipolar (51%) than unipolar disorder (31%). Loss of antidepressant responsiveness was also 3.4 times more frequent for bipolar disorder. For patients with bipolar depression who had been on an antidepressant for more than a year, rapid cycling occurred in 32% and cycle acceleration occurred in 25%. Both rapid cycling and cycle acceleration were non-significantly more frequent among bipolar-I than bipolar-II patients, and were not observed among patients with unipolar depression. However, post-discontinuation relapse into depression was four times more common among patients with unipolar depression than among those with bipolar depression. This study found no difference in rates of post-discontinuation relapse between the older TCAs and a variety of 'newer' antidepressants.

A study by Tohen *et al* (2003) on the use of olanzapine in bipolar depression gave relatively low rates for manic switching: 7% for placebo, 6% for olanzapine and 6% for those on an olanzapine–fluoxetine combination. The response rates in this trial were placebo 24%, olanzapine alone 33%, and the combination of olanzapine and fluoxetine 49%.

A meta-analysis of 12 RCTs, with a total of 1088 patients (Gijsman *et al*, 2004), found that, in the short-term treatment of bipolar depression, antidepressants are effective and switching to mania is not a common early complication of treatment. Thus, 3.8% of patients treated with antidepressants switched to mania, whereas for those on placebo the rate was 4.7%. Here there was a difference between class of antidepressant, the rate for TCAs having been 10% and for all other antidepressants combined 3.2%.

The BAP guidelines similarly suggest that the switching tendency may be greater with TCAs and venlafaxine than with the SSRIs, and that lithium as a sole antidepressant drug is disappointing in the management of bipolar depression

Bipolar depression has a comparatively high suicide rate: between 25% and 50% of these patients attempt suicide at least once in their life, and Goodwin & Jamieson (1990) estimate that 8–19% of these patients die through completed suicide. A study by Slama *et al* (2004) compared patients with bipolar disorder who had attempted suicide at least once, with those who had never attempted suicide. There were increased risks for suicidal behaviour for those with an earlier onset of disorder, more depressive episodes, antidepressant-induced mania, comorbid alcohol use, previous suicide attempts and a family history of suicidal behaviour (but not simply a family history of affective disorder). These important risk features need to be enquired about when treating patients.

The BAP guidelines indicate that there is some evidence that lithium but not sodium valproate may reduce the mortality due to suicide.

It is not established that the anti-epileptic lamotrigine is useful in acute bipolar depression. Whatever antidepressant is used, the BAP guidelines suggest co-administation with a 'mood stabiliser' to prevent a manic switch.

Comorbid medical disorders

Because of their more favourable side-effect profile, the SSRIs are the preferred drug for depression comorbid with some medical disorders. For example, they are relatively non-cardiotoxic and therefore suitable for use by people with cardiovascular disease. In patients with closed-angle glaucoma or prostatic enlargement, in whom anticholinergic side-effects must be avoided, SSRIs are preferred to TCAs. In epilepsy with depression it is thought that the SSRIs are less epileptogenic than the TCAs. Of the few studies comparing different antidepressants in medical disorders, most have been in the area of cardiovascular disease, but there are very few comparative studies (see also Chapter 17 for discussion of treatment of depression in medical disorders).

Driving

Patients frequently ask whether antidepressants will affect their driving. Depression itself, particularly in the presence of impaired concentration or psychomotor retardation, is more likely to impair psychomotor performance than antidepressant drugs. Few studies have attempted to separate out the effects of the depression from those of drugs.

Among healthy volunteers who take a TCA, psychomotor performance is impaired initially but tolerance for the drug soon develops, so that by the seventh day there is no difference from placebo. Tolerance for these effects has been observed for clomipramine, dosulepin, doxepin, mianserin and maprotiline. SSRIs cause less initial sedation and impairment than TCAs on tests of critical flicker fusion, choice reaction time, memory and stimulated car tracking (Edwards, 1995). Older drivers may be at greater risk from TCAs. In road trials in specially instrumented cars driven around closed circuits, single doses of antidepressants such as mianserin, trazodone, amitriptyline and dosulepin may increase the stopping distance of a car travelling at 70 m.p.h. by up to 10 feet (Freeman & O'Hanlon, 1995).

Affective disorder may contribute to road traffic accidents; patients with depression concentrate poorly, those with mania may drive recklessly or at great speed, and patients sometimes commit suicide in fatal accidents. The overall contribution of antidepressant drugs to road traffic accidents is probably small and the adverse effect of alcohol is greater than that of all other drugs combined. Everest *et al* (1989) analysed the body fluids from people in 1273 fatal road traffic accidents and found the following substance prevalence: alcohol 35%, cannabis 2.4%, benzodiazepines 1.6%, anticonvulsants 1.0%, phenothiazines 0.3%, hypnotics 0.3%, antidepressants 0.2%, decongestants 0.2% and other drugs 0.2%.

For most patients with depression, driving can continue, but if patients report feeling impaired in respect of driving (whether due to depression or medication), they should not drive. Among the elderly there should be increased caution while taking antidepressants. Periods of greater risk are when first starting antidepressants and after a dose increase, although sedative effects wear off. Patients should be cautioned about driving long distances or at speed while taking antidepressants.

In the UK, the responsibility for determining fitness to drive rests with the Driving and Vehicle Licensing Authority (DVLA). All drivers have a responsibility to notify the DVLA of a relevant medical condition or any change in it. In most instances of depression drivers of 'group 1' vehicles (private cars and motorcycles) are permitted to continue to drive even if taking antidepressants, and only a small minority whose driving is likely to be affected need to notify the DVLA. However, for drivers of 'group 2' vehicles (lorries, buses and taxis) who have a serious acute mental illness it is obligatory for them to inform the DVLA. The doctor should advise patients to do this and record in the case notes that this advice has been given. It should be noted that section 4 of the Road Traffic Act 1988 states: 'A person who when driving a motor vehicle on a road or other public place is unfit to drive through drink or drugs is guilty of an offence'.

Long-term treatment of depression

Terminology

The natural history of a depressive episode is shown in Fig. 4.7 (solid line), as is response to treatment (dotted line). *Remission* refers to alleviation of symptoms during the natural history of the episode while *recovery* implies that the natural history of the particular episode is past. *Relapse* means a recrudescence of symptoms during the episode; recurrence refers to a different episode. Fig. 4.7 illustrates the three different phases of treatment: acute, continuation and maintenance. Some patients do not fit neatly into these patterns and have a chronic fluctuating and labile course, where they have neither fully remitted nor properly relapsed.

Continuation therapy after an acute episode

Continuation drug therapy reduces the risk of relapse after remission. A meta-analysis of 31 randomised trials with a total of 4410 patients (Geddes *et al*, 2003) showed that there is a halving of the absolute risk of relapse, so that over the 6–36 months of the studies' follow-up, the relapse rate for patients on antidepressant medication was 18%, compared with 41% on placebo. It is not known whether drug treatment shortens the episode or whether it serves only to relieve the symptoms until the episode has completed its natural course. Withdrawal of antidepressants in the 6 months following remission is likely to be associated with relapse, particularly if there are residual depressive symptoms (Mindham *et al*, 1973; Faravelli *et al*, 1986). Individuals who are free of significant symptoms or who have returned to their usual level of inter-episode functioning, both for at least 4 months, have a lower rate of relapse when their continuation therapy is withdrawn than those who have not reached these levels; this highlights the importance of ensuring that residual symptoms have disappeared

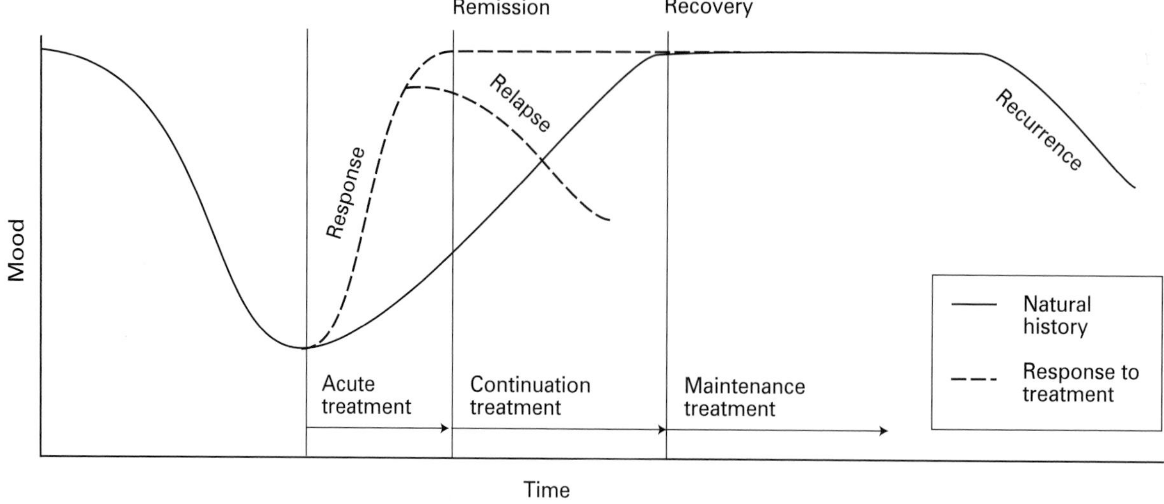

Fig. 4.7 Terms used to describe phases of treatment.

before withdrawal is attempted. Other variables that increase the risk of relapse when antidepressants are withdrawn are: previous episodes of depressive illness, poor social support and the presence of continuing social difficulties, such as unemployment or disharmony in interpersonal relationships (Prien, 1992).

The APA guidelines suggest the continuation phase for an acute depressive episode should last 4–5 months following remission, after which a decision is made as to whether to withdraw the antidepressants or to initiate more longer-term maintenance therapy, while the NICE guidelines state that antidepressants should be continued for at least 6 months (grade A recommendation), or longer if there are concurrent social difficulties or residual symptoms.

Maintenance treatment

Depression is a recurrent and disabling condition. Around 40% of those with an episode of depression will have another episode within 1 year, 60% within 2 years and 75% within 5 years. From the available studies (reviewed by Angst, 1992) the only known predictors of a recurrent course are an early age of onset, a greater number of previous episodes and bipolarity. Angst *et al* (1973) showed that the period between episodes tends to decrease with each successive episode, but then reaches a plateau after four or five bouts. This period drops from 3 years following a first episode to 18 months after the third. A recurrent pattern rarely remits spontaneously. One study (Dawson *et al*, 1998) suggested that for those with less than four previous episodes there is about a 1% risk per week for recurrence; however, for those who have already shown a strongly recurrent pattern (more than five previous episodes) this risk rises to 3.3% per week.

There is now good evidence that taking antidepressants over the long term can reduce the risk of recurrence and substantially improve the quality of lives of people suffering from recurrent depression. In a meta-analysis of these studies, Geddes *et al* (2003) showed that, for patients in the placebo arms of long-term antidepressant trials, the risks of recurrence were 60%, compared with only 19% for those who took antidepressants for 12 months after recovery. These benefits continued in the second and third years (29% recurrence rate for placebo versus 10% for active antidepressant prophylaxis), but there are no reliable data beyond this, although many patients take their antidepressants for a decade or more.

The NICE guidelines also provide a meta-analysis (24 studies) with strong evidence favouring continuation therapy (RR = 0.43), and they recommend that patients with two or more episodes of depression in the recent past should continue their antidepressants for at least a further 2 years (grade B recommendation), after which the regimen should be re-evaluated. The NICE guidelines also state that CBT should be considered for patients with recurrent depression (grade C recommendation). For patients who recovered on a lithium augmentation combination, both drugs should be continued for 6 months and then the lithium stopped in preference to the antidepressant (grade C). Lithium is not recommended as a sole treatment for those with recurrent unipolar depression (grade C), but lithium–antidepressant combinations may be helpful for the prophylaxis of depression in bipolar disorder. It is also widely held that the dose used to treat the acute episode should also be the maintenance dose – 'the dose to treat is the dose to keep' (grade C).

In practice, most patients with recurrent depression have little difficulty in accepting the need for long-term treatment, as they usually dread their depressions. They should remain under occasional surveillance because sometimes dosage adjustments and medication changes need to be made. Post (1993) described a state of lithium refractoriness, a state where patients who once responded well to lithium, after stopping it somehow failed to respond when the drug was reintroduced. The condition of refractoriness to an antidepressant after a period of use probably occurs with most antidepressants but has not been so well documented. It is important to recognise when this has occurred, as sometimes switching drugs can alleviate the situation.

Table 4.9 Staging of treatment-resistant depression

Stage	Previous treatment
0	Has not had a single adequate trial of medication
1	Failure to respond to an adequate trial of one medication
2	Failure to respond to an adequate trial of two medications with different profiles
3	Stage 2 plus one augmentation strategy
4	Stage 2 plus two augmentation strategies
5	Stage 4 plus ECT

Source: Adapted from Thase & Rush (1995).

Treatment-refractory depression

There is no agreed definition of treatment-refractory depression (TRD), yet it is a common and serious problem; it occurs in around 10–20% of people who experience major depression (NICE, 2004). In the first study of lithium augmentation, de Montigny *et al* (1981) gave a definition of TRD as a failure to respond to imipramine (150 mg daily) after 3 weeks. Most would regard such a short duration of treatment as far too brief, and Thase & Rush (1995) pointed out that there is a continuum of resistance, which can be staged according to the degree of previous exposure to antidepressant treatment (Table 4.9).

The term *treatment resistance* is applied to patients who fail to respond to one course of treatment and are *treatment refractory* to several different courses of treatment. The NICE (2004) definition of *refractory depression* is when it has 'failed to respond to two or more antidepressants given sequentially in an adequate dosage and for an adequate period of time'.

There are some predictors of TRD. Keller *et al* (1986) found that delay in recovery from a depressive episode was associated with low family income, other psychiatric comorbidity (e.g. depression with schizophrenia or anorexia nervosa), older age and increased scores for neuroticism on the Eysenck Personality Questionnaire; there are also associations with personality disorder (Black *et al*, 1988). Wilhelm *et al* (1994) confirmed the association with older age, more severe depression, and later age of onset for the first episode, and also showed that psychotic depression was over-represented in their series of TRD cases, at 43% compared with its more usual prevalence of around 15%. Undiagnosed physical illness such as thyroid disorder, early Huntingdon's disease and carcinoma (pancreatic carcinoma particularly) may also present as a 'resistant' depression. Magnetic resonance imaging studies in TRD have shown the presence of white-matter hyperintense regions, which may suggest cortical hypoperfusion, and in the study by Wilhelm *et al* (1994) the number of hyperintensive regions correlated with a worse response to somatic therapy.

Management of TRD

The first step is to reconsider the diagnosis. It is important to confirm that the patient at some stage satisfied diagnostic criteria for a depressive episode, since a partial response to treatment may mean that some key depressive symptoms such as sleep disturbance are no longer present. Does the patient have an undiagnosed medical illness? Physical investigations such as a full blood count, thyroid function and chest radiograph may be indicated. Are covert psychological factors operative? Psychological issues which have not been elicited during the original history taking may emerge later, for example undisclosed sexual abuse, an oppressive marital relationship or work difficulties.

The patient's drug compliance must be assessed. A history from an informant, the presence of side-effects and determination of blood antidepressant level are useful pointers. Admission to hospital may be considered in more severe cases and this will assist in the assessment of drug compliance. Further information may be sought about possible alcohol misuse, personality disorder and undisclosed individual problems.

Spontaneous resolution may occur even in cases of TRD. Stimpson *et al* (2002) reported that 14% of a placebo group recovered during the study period, although this rate is lower than the spontaneous recovery rate for non-resistant depression, of around 30–35%. Improvements may also occur with changes in the patient's life circumstances. The NICE review gives a grade B recommendation for the use of CBT in severe and refractory depression but a grade A recommendation for its use in chronic depression. Social support or 'befriending' should be offered to patients with more long-term depression (grade C). Thus, there should be continued psychosocial support for patients with TRD. The more commonly used drug strategies in TRD are now described: high-dose monotherapy, switching to another antidepressant and augmentation strategies (the addition of psychological therapy is described in Chapter 6, and the use of ECT in TRD is described in Chapter 5).

High-dosage monotherapy

An antidepressant non-responder or a partial responder may be a fast metaboliser and so increasing the dose to the upper end of the *BNF* dosage range is usually the simplest first move when the initial response is poor. In the 1970s and 1980s, when far fewer antidepressants were available, high-dosage monotherapy, sometimes for prolonged periods, was a commonly used strategy for the management of TRD. Thus, Greenhouse *et al* (1987) reported that, after 5 weeks, only 25% of patients taking 150–300 mg of a TCA had responded, but by 17 weeks this had risen to 75%.

As noted previously, the NICE (2004) review found that high-dose venlafaxine (above 150 mg daily) has a definite advantage over SSRIs, and so another strategy for TRD is to use high-dose venlafaxine on its own.

The routine use of high doses of antidepressants is probably unhelpful. Bollini *et al* (1999) conducted a meta-analysis of 27 studies of drug trials that included one arm in which participants were randomised to take a high dose of the antidepressant. The response rate for subjects taking 100–200 mg imipramine or equivalent was 53%, and the response rate for participants taking higher doses was no better, but the adverse drug reaction rate was greater for those on higher doses

(0.48 adverse events per week compared with 0.30 for those on lower doses). Bollini *et al* (1999) also provided data on the therapeutic equivalence of different antidepressants to imipramine 150 mg.

Switching antidepressants

When patients are studied in drug trials or larger groups are considered in meta-analyses, most antidepressants used as first-line treatments have approximately equal efficacy. However, when there is no response to the first drug, the patient may do well on another antidepressant and so switching drugs after an appropriate interval of non-responsiveness (usually 6–8 weeks) is often a useful manoeuvre. Whether it is the action of the second antidepressant or the effect of stopping the first that is beneficial may be unclear. Thus, Licht & Qvitzau (2002) randomised patients who had not responded well to 100 mg doses of sertraline into three groups: sertraline 200 mg, mianserin 30 mg, and placebo. All the patients thought they were being given another antidepressant. The response rates for those given mianserin (67%) and placebo (70%) were equal and significantly better than that achieved with sertraline 200 mg (56%).

Switching antidepressants is not always straightforward and may be associated with certain risks:

- Stopping the first antidepressant too abruptly may lead to a discontinuation syndrome.
- If the drug was partially effective, the withdrawal may cause an exacerbation of the depression.
- Starting a new drug may expose the patient to a new set of side-effects, which the patient may not be able to tolerate.
- If a TCA or venlafaxine is being introduced, dosage titration will be necessary.
- The simultaneous prescription of two antidepressants during a cross-taper, especially if the first drug was prescribed at a high dose, increases the risk of new side-effects such as orthostatic hypotension, or even the serotonin syndrome (grade B NICE recommendation).
- Switches to MAOIs (both reversible and irreversible) may entail prolonged washout periods, which patients may find difficult to cope with. For switches from fluoxetine, a 5-week washout period is recommended, although that for other SSRIs is shorter.

The Maudsley guidelines (Taylor *et al*, 2005) state that if an antidepressant has been taken for 6 weeks or longer it should not be stopped abruptly (unless there has been a serious complication). For switches not involving incompatible combinations such as an MAOI and SSRI, the Maudsley guidelines recommend switching by cross-tapering over 2–4 weeks, that is, increasing the dose of the new antidepressant while reducing to zero the dose of the first drug over this period.

There is limited evidence about which the best switches are, but around 50% of previous non-responders become responders to a second antidepressant. Thus, in a study of imipramine non-responders, around 50% responded when switched to sertraline, and in the same study when imipramine was given to a group of sertraline non-responders a similar response rate was observed (Thase *et al*, 2002).

Thase & Rush (1995) summarise the earlier switching studies in cases of TCA-resistant depression, with a 40–70% response rate for switching to older irreversible MAOIs and a 40–60% response rate for switching to trazodone, fluvoxamine or paroxetine. The NICE guidelines state (assuming the first drug is an SSRI) that a reasonable choice for a second antidepressant would be a second SSRI or mirtazapine, but consideration should also be given to lofepramine, reboxetine or moclobemide (grade B).

There is no evidence that switching to an antidepressant of a different class confers any advantage over a switch to an antidepressant of the same class.

The Texas Medication Algorithm Project, which has attempted to define an optimal sequence of treatments for those with TRD (Adli *et al*, 2002; Trivedi, 2003; Trivedi *et al*, 2004), starts with two sequential stages of monotherapy, assuming there is no response in the first stage. It permits clinicians a choice of antidepressants at each stage, but suggests that TCAs should be restricted to the second stage because of poorer tolerability.

Although switching may occasionally be accompanied by some of the difficulties described above, it is usually an uncomplicated and beneficial manoeuvre.

Augmentation strategies

A patient's failure to respond to adequate doses of different classes of antidepressant drugs, as described above, will sometimes warrant the addition of a second medication to the existing antidepressant drug. Although monotherapy is the preferred option for treating depression, as expressed in all the guidelines, the German antidepressant hospital survey, the AMSP (Grohmann *et al*, 2004), found that less than a quarter of patients were on one drug only. Antidepressants were most commonly combined with atypical antipsychotic drugs (44%), typical neuroleptics (32%), hypnotics (28%), another antidepressant (22%) or lithium (13%).

Lithium augmentation

The NICE (2004) review considered lithium augmentation to be the best-studied augmentation strategy for TRD (grade B). The technique was introduced by de Montigny *et al* (1981), who demonstrated a rapid resolution of symptoms in eight TCA-resistant patients. There have been a number of open studies but few double-blind randomised controlled trials. Stein & Bernadt (1993) found that, of 34 TCA-resistant patients, 44% responded to 750 mg lithium, while 250 mg lithium was no better than placebo. Katona *et al* (1995) first treated a large group of patients with depression ($n = 144$) with either lofepramine or fluoxetine; 62 patients were non-responders, and in the second phase of the study 52% responded to lithium augmentation compared with 25% to placebo augmentation. Side-effects in the lithium–TCA and lithium–SSRI groups were similar.

Price *et al* (1986) studied the effect of lithium augmentation in 84 patients and suggested the response to it lies on a continuum, with 31% of their patients showing a good response, 25% a partial response and the remainder showing no response. Dinan & Barry (1989) found that lithium augmentation was as effective as ECT for TCA-resistant depression and several further RCTs have demonstrated efficacy for lithium.

The mechanism underlying lithium augmentation may be related to lithium's enhancement of serotonergic transmission. Worral *et al* (1979) suggested that lithium itself is an antidepressant, and that patients who responded to the lithium–tricyclic combination represent those who might have responded to lithium alone, but the NICE guidelines state that there is no evidence that lithium on its own is antidepressant. Katona *et al* (1995) found that response to augmentation depends on attaining adequate serum lithium levels, as patients with values below 0.4 mmol/l did not respond.

Lithium augmentation therapy requires close monitoring; symptoms of lithium toxicity may occur even at normal serum lithium levels. Tremor and nausea are more frequent, as lithium and antidepressants may cause each independently. Some patients respond in 1–2 weeks, but a trial should continue for at least 8 weeks because there are late responders. In the case of non-response or severe side-effects, lithium augmentation should be stopped. Some elderly patients cannot tolerate lithium in the usual dose range yet still derive therapeutic benefit, and in these cases lithium augmentation in lower than usual doses may be helpful (Kushnir, 1986).

L-tryptophan

This amino acid, a precursor of serotonin, was previously used as an adjunct to treatment with an MAOI. Because it is mildly sedative it was also taken in a chocolate powder form in milk as a nightcap. It is also used in combination with a tricyclic (e.g. amitrityline or clomipramine).

In April 1990, oral tryptophan preparations were withdrawn following reports of an eosinophilia–myalgia syndrome (EMS). This potentially fatal multi-system disorder is characterised by eosinophilia (more than 2000 eosinophils per mm^3), severe myalgia, arthralgia, oedema and a rash, together with lung and CNS involvement. It was thought that the EMS might have been due to an impurity in the L-tryptophan. The Committee on Safety of Medicines (1994) recommends it should be prescribed only:

- by hospital specialists
- for patients who have severe depressive illness of more than 2 years' duration
- after adequate trials of standard drug treatments have failed
- as an adjunct to other medication
- not with an SSRI.

Patients are prescribed tryptophan on a named-patient basis and are registered with the drug company monitoring service. They require regular eosinophil counts and surveillance for features of EMS.

Thyroid augmentation

In the pre-psychopharmacological era, thyroid extract was sometimes used to treat psychiatric disorder and was shown to have demonstrable benefits for the treatment of period catatonia (Gjessing, 1947). Prange *et al* (1969) added tri-iodothyronine (T3) to imipramine and noted a quicker response to imipramine, a finding later confirmed by Goodwin *et al* (1982). Joffe *et al* (1993) randomly assigned 50 TCA-resistant patients to lithium, T3 or placebo; 53% of the lithium group and 50% of the T3 group responded, compared with 19% in the placebo group. T3 has a short half-life (of 2–4 hours) and therefore needs to be given in divided doses. Joffe *et al* used a three times per day dose regimen. Targum *et al* (1984) found that thyroid augmentation was more useful among a small subgroup of patients who had an exaggerated thyroid stimulating hormone (TSH) response to thyroid releasing hormone (TRH) (suggestive of subclinical hypothyroidism). If thyroid hormones are to be used, they should be introduced slowly, especially in the elderly. There have been no studies on the effect of thyroid augmentation combined with the SSRIs and other newer antidepressants, and the NICE (2004) review did not recommend its use in TRD (NICE B).

All patients with TRD should be routinely screened for hypothyroidism, which may be more common among the elderly, possibly among post-partum cases, as well as some patients on lithium, and in these instances there may be a case for trying thyroxine, even where the biochemical impairment is mild.

Olanzapine

Atypical antipsychotic–antidepressant combinations are a commonly used augmentation strategy in the treatment of TRD. Evidence from RCTs is best for olanzapine and there are trials showing beneficial effects for olanzapine–fluoxetine combinations for psychotic depression, bipolar depression (page 102), TRD and depression in people with borderline personality disorder (Zanarini *et al*, 2004). Usually this combination has been shown to have a similar number of side-effects to each drug used singly. The German hospital antidepressant survey showed that 44% of in-patients (who usually have the most severe and difficult to treat depressions) were taking these combinations.

Shelton *et al* (2001) tested a combination of fluoxetine (mean dose 52 mg daily) plus olanzapine (mean dose 13 mg daily) for 28 patients with TRD (without psychotic features). The combination was superior to either drug singly. On some measures the olanzapine monotherapy group did better than the fluoxetine monotherapy group. Clinical responses were evident by the first week of treatment, with no difference in the prevalence of ADRs, including extrapyramidal side-effects, in the three groups. The most frequently reported ADRs were somnolence, increased appetite, asthenia, weight gain, headache, dry mouth and nervousness. The authors quoted neurochemical studies in support of a possible pharmacodynamic synergy of fluoxetine and olanzapine.

Pindolol

The 5-HT_{1A} receptor is thought to play a crucial role in depression. Blockade of this inhibitory autoreceptor leads to increased neuronal firing and release of more monoamine transmitter into the synapse. The beta-blocker pindolol is an antagonist of the presynaptic 5-HT_{1A} autoreceptor and hence there has been interest in its effect in TRD. A meta-analysis of nine studies of pindolol augmentation of SSRIs (either paroxetine 20 mg or fluoxetine 20 mg daily) showed a superior response of pindolol compared with placebo for the first 2 weeks of treatment, but no difference for weeks 3–6 (Ballesteros & Callado, 2004). The NICE (2004) review did not recommend its use in TRD.

Conclusion

The NICE review makes a number of recommendations concerning augmentation strategies in TRD. It states that only lithium augmentation has grade B evidence to support its use. The augmentation of an antidepressant with thyroid supplementation, pindolol, carbamazepine, valproate, lamotrigine or buspirone is not recommended in the management of resistant depression (grade B).

Use of two antidepressants together

The severe morbidity and increased mortality from suicide arising from TRD warrant consideration of measures that have the potential for benefit albeit with increased risk of ADRs. After the failure of monotherapy, augmentation with a second antidepressant may be a useful option; the response rate is around 60%. The advantages of combining two antidepressants include:

- Two different pharmacodynamic mechanisms are utilised.
- A partial response to a first antidepressant can be built on. In contrast, in switching an antidepressant this may be lost without the patient necessarily showing any improvement on the second drug, so that, overall, the patient deteriorates.
- The patient avoids the risk of a discontinuation syndrome adding on to existing depressive symptoms.

The disadvantages are:

- The evidence base for efficacy is limited.
- There is an increased risk of side-effects, such as slowing of cardiac conduction, seizures or delirium for certain combinations.
- Using two drugs when one might have done as well – when patients improve there is uncertainty as to whether they might have responded to the second antidepressant as monotherapy.
- There are no guidelines on how long to treat with two antidepressants.

The intent to switch antidepressants may be an inadvertent route by which the patient ends up on two antidepressants. That is, in cross-tapering the doses of the first and second antidepressants the patient might get worse on lowering the dose of the first antidepressant and persist with an existing dose while improvement occurs following the increased dose of the second antidepressant.

Among in-patients, combinations of two antidepressants are not uncommonly used. The German hospitals survey (Grohmann *et al*, 2004) found that 59% of their in-patients were on two antidepressants and their survey gave frequencies for particular antidepressant combinations. The non-TCA, non-SSRI antidepressants were called 'other antidepressants' (i.e. mianserin, trazodone, mirtazapine, nefazodone and reboxetine). The most common groupings were TCA–SSRI (20%), TCA–other (18%), TCA–MAOI (3%), TCA–TCA (2%), SSRI–other (9%) and other–other (7%).

The limitations to the evidence base for the use of two antidepressant drugs in combination include small sample sizes and few RCTs. Most studies have not been blind, so placebo effects may have occurred. Variable definitions of treatment resistance, dose ranges, durations of treatment and outcome measures make comparisons between studies difficult if not impossible. There may be a publication bias in favour of those studies with a positive outcome. The NICE (2004) review pooled data from 15 RCTs, where participants had been acute-phase non-responders, and a second antidepressant was added in. The second antidepressant was often mianserin, a drug little used today because of the risk of blood dyscrasias. The meta-analysis showed that two antidepressants were significantly superior to one (RR = 0.81), but as might be expected one antidepressant was better tolerated, and had lower discontinuation rates (RR = 1.69). Lam *et al* (2002) reviewed 27 studies of combinations of two antidepressants and identified 10 different types of combination based on the pairing of different groups of antidepressants.

Combination of a TCA and an MAOI

This was the first published strategy for the use of two antidepressants together and in the 1960s and 1970s was known as 'combined antidepressant therapy', as these were the only available groups of antidepressants. Phenelzine was the most commonly used MAOI, while trimipramine was the most commonly used TCA. Pare *et al* (1982) presented evidence that the risk of a hypertensive reaction is reduced for patients taking combined antidepressants (a TCA and an MAOI) compared with MAOI monotherapy. They suggested that the TCA's mechanism of action, blocking the uptake of a secondary amine such as tyramine into the presynaptic neuron, prevents tyramine from having a pressor effect. Combinations of MAOIs with clomipramine, imipramine, venlafaxine and all five SSRIs must be avoided because of the risk of the serotonin syndrome and fatality. No study has shown that the combination of a TCA and an MAOI is more efficacious than either used separately. TCA–MAOI combinations are rarely used today.

Combination of a TCA and an SSRI

In the first open trial of this combination, Weilburg *et al* (1989) added fluoxetine to the medication of a group of 30 out-patients whose depression had failed to respond to a variety of other antidepressants, mainly TCAs, and reported that 26 (86%) responded. Eight patients relapsed when their TCA was withdrawn, so they were on fluoxetine alone. As these patients had previously failed to respond to a TCA alone, it appeared that the combination was required for the therapeutic response. Lam *et al* (2002) pooled results from later published studies of this combination and reported that 65% of patients (73/112) responded to this combination. However, in studies where plasma TCA levels were also measured, the levels were often elevated (Taylor, 1995), presumably by competitive inhibition of liver P450 isoenzymes. For example, paroxetine and sertraline raised desipramine levels by 400% and 250%, respectively. If the combination is used, there is an increased risk of toxicity and so plasma TCA levels do need to be monitored (Taylor, 1995).

Levitt *et al* (1999) reported that those who did well had higher TCA levels than partial responders, which suggests that beneficial effects may simply be the result of elevating TCA levels.

Other combinations

Zajecka *et al* (1995) found that the response rate to a mianserin–fluoxetine combination was 63%, compared with 49% for mianserin alone, and 37% for fluoxetine alone. An open study of the addition of mirtazapine for 20 patients who had been on high doses of various other antidepressants reported that 55% responded after 4 weeks, although 15% discontinued because of side-effects (Carpenter *et al*, 1999). In an open study, venlafaxine (75–300 mg) was added to the drug regimens of 11 patients who had failed to respond to high doses of a TCA with blood levels greater than 250 mg/ml. Of these 11, 9 (82%) responded, in some cases to the addition of only low doses of venlafaxine (75–150 mg) and the authors reported that the regimen was well tolerated (Gomez & Perramon, 2000).

Other commonly used combinations are mirtazapine with an SSRI or with an SNRI.

Uncertainty in the choice of therapeutic intervention in TRD

Although there is an evidence base in TRD for the efficacy of switching antidepressants, augmentation of them, use of two antidepressants together, addition of psychological treatment (see page 133) and ECT, when a patient has not responded to monotherapy with an antidepressant drug at a sufficient dose and for a sufficient length of time, there is uncertainty about which strategy to choose. That is, these therapeutic interventions have not been compared with each other. In the USA the National Institute of Mental Health is organising, via a coordinating centre at the University of Texas, a multicentre study of 4000 out-patients with non-psychotic major depressive or dysthymic disorder. Six switch or augmentation options are being compared in what is termed the 'STAR*D sequenced treatment alternatives to relieve depression' (Trivedi, 2003). The Texas Medication Algorithm Project currently describes a treatment algorithm based on a consensus statement of experts. A second treatment algorithm based on a consensus statement from a Berlin group (Adli *et al*, 2002) is designed for in-patients. Consensus statements constitute weaker evidence than the results of RCTs but the STAR*D project has the potential to improve on existing algorithms, and provide a more scientific base for decision making in TRD.

Conclusions

Notable advances in the treatment of depression have occurred since the early 1990s, including the introduction of new antidepressant drugs and the development of effective psychological treatments. The newer antidepressants have better tolerability and safety. In the UK, the prescribing of antidepressant drugs more than doubled during this period and it is likely that fewer people are suffering from untreated or inadequately treated depression.

Acknowledgement

I thank Dr Hamish McAllister-Williams for his very helpful comments.

References

Adli, M., Berghofer, A., Linden, M., *et al* (2002) Effectiveness and feasibility of a standardised stepwise drug treatment regimen algorithm for inpatients with depressive disorders: results of a 2-year observational algorithm study. *Journal of Clinical Psychiatry*, **63**, 782–790.

American Psychiatric Association (1994) *Diagnostic and Statistical Manual of Mental Disorders* (4th edn) (DSM–IV). Washington, DC: APA.

American Psychiatric Association (2000) Practice guidelines for the treatment of patients with major depressive disorder (revision). *American Journal of Psychiatry*, **157**, suppl. 4, 1–45.

Anderson, I. & Tomenson, B. (1994) The efficacy of selective serotonin re-uptake inhibitors in depression: a meta-analysis of studies against tricyclic antidepressants. *Journal of Psychopharmacology*, **8**, 238–249.

Anderson, I. M., Nutt, D. J. & Deakin, J. F. W. (2000) Evidence based guidelines for treating depressive disorders with anti-depressants: a revision of the 1993 British Association for Pharmacology guidelines. *Journal of Psychopharmacology*, **14**, 3–20.

Angst, J. (1992) How recurrent and predictable is depressive illness? In *Long-Term Treatment of Depression* (eds S. Montgomery & F. Rouillon). Chichester: Wiley.

Angst, J., Baastrup, P. C., Grof, P., *et al* (1973) The course of monopolar depression and bipolar psychoses. *Psychiatrica Neurologie et Neurochirugie (Amersterdam)*, **76**, 489–500.

Asberg, M., Cronholm, B., Sjoqviost, F., *et al* (1971) Relationships between plasma level and therapeutic effect of nortriptyline. *BMJ*, **iii**, 331–334.

Baldwin, D. & Johnson, F. (1995) Tolerability and safety of citalopram. *Reviews in Contemporary Pharmocotherapy*, **6**, 315–325.

Ballesteros, J. & Callado, L. (2004) Effectiveness of pindolol plus serotonin uptake inhibitors in depression: a meta-analysis of early and late outcomes from randomised controlled trials. *Journal of Affective Disorders*, **79**, 137–147.

Bernstein, J. G. (1995*a*) Tricyclic, heterocyclic and serotonin selective antidepressants. In *Drug Therapy in Psychiatry* (3rd edn). St Louis, MO: Mosby.

Bernstein, J. G. (1995*b*) Monoamine oxidase inhibitors. In *Drug Therapy in Psychiatry* (3rd edn). St Louis, MO: Mosby.

Bielski, R. J., Ventura, D. & Chang, C. C. (2004) A double blind comparison of escitalopram and venlafaxine extended release in the treatment of major depression. *Journal of Clinical Psychiatry*, **65**, 1190–1196.

Black, D., Bell, S., Hulbert, J., *et al* (1988) The importance of personality disorders in major depression: a controlled study. *Journal of Affective Disorders*, **14**, 115–122.

Bloch, R. G., Dooneief, A. S., Buckberg, A. S., *et al* (1954) The clinical effects of isoniazid and iproniazid in the treatment of pulmonary tuberculosis. *Annals of Internal Medicine*, **40**, 881–900.

Bollini, P., Pampallona, S., Tibaldi, G., *et al* (1999) Effectiveness of antidepressant. Meta-analysis of dose–effect relationships in randomised clinical trials. *British Journal of Psychiatry*, **174**, 297–303.

Braftos, O. & Haug, J. O. (1968) The course of manic depressive psychosis: a follow up of 215 patients. *Acta Psychiatrica Scandinavica*, **44**, 89–112.

Brosen, K., Skjelbo, E., Rasmussen, B., *et al* (1993) Fluvoxamine is a potent inhibitor of cytochrome P450-1A2. *Biochemical Pharmacology*, **45**, 1211–1214.

Carpenter, L. L., Jocic, Z., Hall, J. M., *et al* (1999) Mirtazapine augmentation in the treatment of resistant depression. *Journal of Clinical Psychiatry*, **50**, 45–49.

Charney, D. S. & Nelson, J. C. (1981) Delusional and non-delusional unipolar depression: further evidence for distinct subtypes. *American Journal of Psychiatry*, **138**, 328–333.

Cheeta, S., Schifano, F., Oyefeso, A., *et al* (2004) Antidepressant-related deaths and prescriptions in England and Wales 1998–2000. *British Journal of Psychiatry*, **184**, 41–47.

Clayton, A. H., Pradko, J. F., Croft, H. A., *et al* (2002) Prevalence of sexual dysfunction among newer antidepressants. *Journal of Clinical Psychiatry*, **63**, 357–366.

Committee on Safety of Medicines (1994) Fluvoxamine increases plasma theophylline levels. *Current Problems in Pharmacovigilance*, **20**, 12.

Cookson, J. (1993) Side-effects of antidepressants. *British Journal of Psychiatry*, **163**, suppl. 20, 20–24.

Crewe, H., Lennard, M., Tucker, G., *et al* (1992) The effect of selective serotonin re-uptake inhibitors on cytochrome P450-2D6 (CYP2D6) activity in human liver microsomes. *British Journal of Clinical Pharmacology*, **34**, 262–265.

Danish University Antidepressant Group (1990) Paroxetine: a selection serotonin reuptake inhibitor showing better tolerance but weaker antidepressant effect than clomipramine in a controlled multi-centre trial. *Journal of Affective Disorders*, **18**, 289–299.

Davidson, J. (1992) Monoamine oxidase inhibitors. In *Handbook of Affective Disorders* (ed. E. S. Paykel). Edinburgh: Churchill Livingstone.

Davis, J. M. & Glassman, A. H. (1989) Antidepressant drugs. In *Comprehensive Textbook of Psychiatry* (eds H. Kaplan & B. Sadock). Baltimore, MD: Williams & Wilkins.

Dawson, R., Lavori, P. W., Corgell, W. H., *et al* (1998) Maintenance strategies for unipolar depression: an observational study of levels of treatment and recurrence. *Journal of Affective Disorders*, **49**, 31–44.

de Montigny, C., Grunberg, F., Mayer, A., *et al* (1981) Lithium induces rapid relief of depression in tricyclic antidepressant drug non-responders. *British Journal of Psychiatry*, **138**, 252–256.

Degner, D., Grohmann, R., Kropp, S., *et al* (2004) Severe adverse drug reactions of antidepressants: results of the German multicenter drug surveillance program AMSP. *Pharmacopsychiatry*, **37**, suppl. 1, S39–S45.

Department of Health (2002) *National Suicide Prevention Strategy for England*. London: Department of Health Publications.

Dinan, T. G. & Barry, S. (1989) A comparison of electroconvulsive therapy with a combined lithium and tricyclic combination among depressed tricyclic nonresponders. *Acta Psychiatrica Scandinavica*, **80**, 97–100.

Ditto, K. (2003) SSRI discontinuation syndrome. *Postgraduate Medicine*, **114**, 79–84.

Donoghue, J. & Hylan, T. R. (2001) Antidepressant use in clinical practice efficacy versus effectiveness. *British Journal of Psychiatry*, **179**, suppl. 42, s9–s17.

Drug and Therapeutics Bulletin (1994) Moclobemide for depression. *Drug and Therapeutics Bulletin*, **32**, 6–7.

Drug and Therapeutics Bulletin (2004) Do SSRIs cause gastrointestinal bleeding? *Drug and Therapeutics Bulletin*, **42**, 17–18.

Dube, S., Andersen, S., Clemow, T., *et al* (2002) Olanzepine–fluoxetine combination for treatment of psychotic depression. *European Psychiatry*, **17**, suppl. 1, 130.

Duff, G. (2006) *Updated Prescribing Advice for Venlafaxine (Efexor/Efexor XL)*. London: Commission on Human Medicines.

Edwards, J. G. (1995) Depression, antidepressants and accidents. *BMJ*, **311**, 887–888.

Edwards, J. G. & Anderson, I. (1999) Systematic review and guide to selection of selective serotonin reuptake inhibitors. *Drugs*, **57**, 507–533.

Einarson, T. R. (2004) Evidence based review of escitalopram in treating major depression in primary care. *International Clinical Psychopharmacology*, **19**, 305–310.

El-Fakahany, E. & Richelson, E. (1983) Antagonism by antidepressants of muscarinic acetylcholine receptors of human brain. *British Journal of Pharmacology*, **78**, 97–102.

Everest, J., Tunbridge, R. & Widdop, B. (1989) *The Incidence of Drugs in Road Accident Fatalities* (TRL Research Report 202). Crowthorne: Transport Research Laboratory.

Faravelli, C., Ambonetti, A., Pallanti, S., *et al* (1986) Depressive relapses and incomplete recovery from index episode. *American Journal of Psychiatry*, **143**, 888–891.

FDA (2004) Public health advisory: suicidality in children and adolescents being treated with antidepressant medications. http://www.fda.gov/cder/drug/antidepressants/SSRIPHA200410.htm

Feighner, J., Boyer, W., Meredith, C., *et al* (1989) A placebo-controlled inpatient comparison of fluvoxamine maleate and imipramine in major depression. *International Clinical Psychopharmacology*, **4**, 239–244.

Fergusson, D., Douchette, S., Glass, K., *et al* (2005) Association between suicide attempts and selective serotonin reuptake inhibitors: systematic review of randomised controlled trials. *BMJ*, **330**, 390–399.

Fisch, C. (1985) Effect of fluoxetine on the electrocardiogram. *Journal of Clinical Psychiatry*, **46**, 42–44.

Freeman, H. & O'Hanlon, J. (1995) Acute and subacute effects of antidepressants on performance. *Journal of Drug Development and Clinical Practice*, **7**, 7–20.

Garvey, M. & Tollefson, G. (1987) Occurrence of myoclonus in patients treated with tricyclic antidepressants. *Archives of General Psychiatry*, **44**, 269–272.

Geddes, J. R., Carney, S. M., Davies, C. *et al* (2003) Relapse prevention with antidepressant drug treatment in depressive disorders: a systematic review. *Lancet*, **361**, 653–661.

Ghaemi, S. N., Rosenquist, K. J., Ko, J. Y., *et al* (2004) Antidepressant treatment in bipolar versus unipolar depression. *American Journal of Psychiatry*, **161**, 163–165.

Gijsman, H. J., Geddes, J. R., Rendell, J. M., *et al* (2004) Antidepressants for bipolar depression: a systematic review of randomised, controlled trials. *American Journal of Psychiatry*, **161**, 1537–1547.

Gjessing, R. (1947) Biological investigations in endogenous psychoses. *Acta Psychiatrica Neurologica Scandanavica*, suppl. 47, 93.

Gomez, J. M. & Perramon, C. T. (2000) Combined treatment with venlafaxine and tricyclic antidepressants in depressed patients who had partial response to clomipramine or imipramine. *Journal of Clinical Psychiatry*, **61**, 285–289.

Goodwin, F. & Jamieson, K. R. (1990) *Manic–Depressive Illness*. New York: Oxford University Press.

Goodwin, F., Prange, A., Post, R., *et al* (1982) The augmentation of antidepressant effects by L-triiodothyronine in tricyclic non-responders. *American Journal of Psychiatry*, **139**, 34–38.

Goodwin, G. (2003) Evidence-based guidelines for treating bipolar disorder: recommendations from the British Association for Psychopharmacology. *Journal of Psychopharmacology*, **17**, 149–173.

Grahame-Smith, D. (1971) Studies *in vivo* on the relationship between brain tryptophan, brain 5-HT synthesis and hyper-activity in rats treated with a monoamine oxidase inhibitor and L-tryptophan. *Journal of Neurochemistry*, **18**, 1053–1066.

Greenhouse, J. B., Kupfer, D. J., Frank, E., *et al* (1987) Analysis of time to stabilization in the treatment of depression. Biological and clinical correlates. *Journal of Affective Disorders*, **15**, 259–266.

Gregor, K. J., Way, K., Young, C. H., *et al* (1997) Concomitant use of SSRIs with other P450 2D6 or 3A4 metabolized medications: how often does it really happen? *Journal of Affective Disorders*, **46**, 59–67.

Grohmann, R., Engel, R., Geisler, K., *et al* (2004) Psychotropic drug use in psychiatric inpatients. Recent trends and changes over time–data for the AMSP study. *Pharmacopsychiatry*, **37**, suppl. 1, 527–538.

Gunnell, D., Sapeira, J. & Ashby, D. (2005) Selective serotonin reuptake inhibitors (SSRIs) and suicide in adults: meta-analysis of drug company data from placebo controlled, randomised controlled trials submitted to the MHRA's safety review. *BMJ*, **330**, 385–388.

Haddow, A. M., Harris, D., Wilson, M., *et al* (2004) Clomipramine induced neuroleptic malignant syndrome and pyrexia of unknown origin. *BMJ*, **329**, 1333–1335.

Hall, W. D., Mant, A., Mitchell, P. B., *et al* (2003) Association between suicide and antidepressant prescribing in Australia 1991–2000: trend analysis. *BMJ*, **326**, 1008–1011.

Hammad, T., Laughren, T. & Racoosin, J. (2006) Suicidality in pediatric patients treated with antidepressant drugs. *Archives of General Psychiatry*, **63**, 332–339.

Harrison-Read, P. & Tyrer, P. (2004) The application of drug treatment in psychiatric practice. In *Seminars in Clinical Psychopharmacology* (ed. D. King), pp. 92–140. London: Gaskell.

Hawton, K., Simkin, S. & Deeks, J. (2003) Co-proxamol and suicide: a study of national mortality statistics and local non-fatal self poisonings. *BMJ*, **326**, 1006–1008.

Healy, D. & Whitaker, C. (2003) Antidepressants and suicide: risk–benefit conundrums. *Journal of Psychiatry and Neuroscience*, **28**, 331–337.

Heimke, C. & Härther, S. (2000) Pharmacokinetics of selective serotonin reuptake inhibitors. *Pharmacology and Therapeutics*, **85**, 11–28.

Henry, J., Alexander, C. & Sener, E. (1995) Relative mortality from overdose of antidepressants. *BMJ*, **310**, 221–224.

Hotopf, M. & Lewis, G. (1997) Suicide and the cost effectiveness of antidepressants. *British Journal of Psychiatry*, **170**, 88.

Hyttel, J. (1994) Pharmacological characterization of selective serotonin reuptake inhibitors (SSRIs). *International Clinical Psychopharmacology*, **9**, suppl. 1, 19–26.

Isacsson, G. (2000) Suicide prevention – a medical breakthrough. *Acta Psychiatrica Scandinavica*, **102**, 113–117.

Isacsson, G., Holmgren, P., Wasserman, D., *et al* (1994) Suicide and the use of antidepressants. *BMJ*, **308**, 916.

Isacsson, G., Boethims, G., Hendrikson, S., *et al* (1999*a*) Selective serotonin reuptake inhibitors have broadened the utilisation of antidepressant treatment in accordance with recommendations. *Journal of Affective Disorders*, **53**, 15–22.

Isacsson, G., Holmgren, P., Druid, H., *et al* (1999*b*) Psychotropics and suicide prevention. Implication from toxicological screening of 5281 suicides in Sweden 1992–1994. *British Journal of Psychiatry*, **174**, 259–265.

Jick, S., Dean, A. & Jick, H. (1995) Antidepressants and suicide. *BMJ*, **310**, 215–218.

Jick, H., Kaye, J. A. & Jick, S. (2004) Antidepressants and the risk of suicidal behaviour. *JAMA*, **292**, 338–343.

Joffe, R., Singer, W., Levitt, A. J., *et al* (1993) A placebo-controlled comparison of lithium and triiodothyronine augmentation of tricyclic antidepressants in unipolar refractory depression. *Archives of General Psychiatry*, **50**, 387–393.

Judd, L. L., Akiskal, H. S., Schettler, P. J., *et al* (2002) The long term natural history of the weekly symptomatic status of bipolar 1 disorder. *Archives of General Psychiatry*, **59**, 530–537.

Karch, F. & Lasagna, L. (1975) Adverse drug reactions. *JAMA*, **234**, 1236–1241.

Katona, C., Abou-Saleh, M., Harrison, D., *et al* (1995) Placebo-controlled trial of lithium augmentation of fluoxetine and lofepramine. *British Journal of Psychiatry*, **166**, 80–86.

Keller, M. B., Klerman, G. L., Lavori, P. W., *et al* (1986) The persistent risk of chronicity in recurrent episodes of non-bipolar depression: a prospective follow up study. *American Journal of Psychiatry*, **143**, 24–28.

Kuhn, R. (1958) The treatment of depressive states with G-22355 (imipramine hydrochloride). *American Journal of Psychiatry*, **111**, 459–464.

Kushnir, S. L. (1986) Lithium antidepressant combination in the treatment of depressed physically ill geriatric patients. *American Journal of Psychiatry*, **143**, 378–379.

Lader, M. (1983) Benzodiazepine withdrawal states. In *Benzodiazepines Divided* (ed. M. Trimble), pp. 17–31. New York: Wiley.

Lam, R., Wan, D., Cohen, N., *et al* (2002) Combining antidepressants for treatment-resistant depression: a review. *Journal of Clinical Psychiatry*, **63**, 685–693.

Levitt, A., Joffe, R., Kamil, R., *et al* (1999) Do depressed subjects who have failed both fluoxetine and a tricyclic antidepressant respond to the combination? *Journal of Clinical Psychiatry*, **60**, 613–616.

Licht, R. W. & Qvitzau, S. (2002) Treatment strategies in patients with major depression not responding to first line sertraline treatment. A randomised study of extended duration of treatment, dosage increase or mianserin augmentation. *Psychopharmacology*, **161**, 143–151.

Livingston, M. (1995) Interactions with selective MAOIs. *Lancet*, **345**, 533–534.

Mackay, F. R., Dunn, N. R., Wilton, L. V., *et al* (1997) A comparison of fluvoxamine, fluoxetine, sertraline and paroxetine examined by observational cohort studies. *Pharmaco Epidemiology and Drug Safety*, **6**, 235–256.

Martinez, C., Rietbrock S., Wise, L., *et al* (2005) Antidepressant treatment and the risk of fatal and non-fatal self harm in first episode depression: nested case–control study. *BMJ*, **330**, 389–393.

McGrath, P., Stewart, J., Fava, M., *et al* (2006) Tranylcypromine versus venlafaxine plus mirtazapine following three failed antidepressant medication trials for depression: a STAR*D report. *American Journal of Psychiatry*, **163**, 1531–1541.

Medical Research Council (1965) Clinical trial of the treatment of depressive illness. *BMJ*, **i**, 881–886.

Mindham, R. H. S., Howland, C. & Shepherd, M. (1973) An evaluation of continuation therapy with tricyclic antidepressants in depressive illness. *Psychological Medicine*, **3**, 5–17.

Montejo, A., Llorca, G., Izquierdo, J., *et al* (2001) Incidence of sexual dysfunction associated with antidepressant agents: a prospective multicenter study of 1022 outpatients. *Journal of Clinical Psychiatry*, **62**, suppl. 3, 10–21.

Montgomery, D. & Johnson, F. (1995) Citalopram in the treatment of depression. *Reviews in Contemporary Pharmacotherapy*, **6**, 297–306.

Morris, J. B. & Beck, A. T. (1974) The efficacy of antidepressant drugs. *Archives of General Psychiatry*, **30**, 667–674.

Murphy, G. M., Kremer, C., Rodriguez, H., *et al* (2003) Pharmacogenetics of antidepressant medication intolerance. *American Journal of Psychiatry*, **160**, 1830–1835.

Nair, N., Amin, M., Holm, P., *et al* (1995) Moclobemide and nortriptyline in elderly depressed patients. A randomised, multicentre trial against placebo. *Journal of Affective Disorders*, **33**, 1–9.

Nemeroff, C., De Vane, L. & Pollock, B. (1996) Newer antidepressants and the cytochrome P450 system. *American Journal of Psychiatry*, **153**, 311–320.

Neuvonen, P., Pohjola-Sintonen, S., Jacke, U., *et al* (1993) Five fatal cases of serotonin syndrome after moclobemide–citalopram or moclobemide–clomipramine overdoses. *Lancet*, **342**, 1419.

NICE (2004) *Depression: Management of Depression in Primary and Secondary Care*. National Clinical Practice Guideline Number 23. London: National Institute for Clinical Excellence.

NICE (2006) *Bipolar Disorder: The Management of Bipolar Disorder in Adults, Children and Adolescents, in Primary and Secondary Care*. NICE Clinical Guideline Number 38. London: National Institute for Health and Clinical Excellence.

Olfsun, M., Shaffer, D., Marcus, S., *et al* (2003) Relationship between antidepressant medication and suicide in adolescents. *Archives of General Psychiatry*, **60**, 978–982.

Pampallona, S., Bollini, P., Tibaldi, G., *et al* (2004) Combined pharmacotherapy and psychological treatment for depression. *Archives of General Psychiatry*, **61**, 714–719.

Pare, C., Kline, N., Hallstrom, C., *et al* (1982) Will amitriptyline prevent the 'cheese' reaction of monoamine oxidase inhibitors? *Lancet*, **ii**, 183–186.

Parker, G., Roy, K., Hadzi-Pavlovic, D., *et al* (1992) Psychotic (delusional depression): a meta-analysis of physical treatments. *Journal of Affective Disorders*, **24**, 17–24.

Parker, G., Roy, K., Wilhelm, K., *et al* (2001) Assessing the comparative effectiveness of antidepressant therapies: a prospective clinical practice study. *Journal of Clinical Psychiatry*, **62**, 117–125.

Pasquini, M., Trincia, V., Garavini, A., *et al* (2003) Mirtazapine for hyperhydrosis. *Psychosomatics*, **44**, 442.

Paton, C. & Ferrier, N. (2005) SSRIs and gastrointestinal bleeding. *BMJ*, **331**, 529–530.

Petit, J., Spiker, D., Ruwitch, J., *et al* (1977) Tricyclic antidepressant plasma levels and adverse effects after overdosage. *Clinical Pharmacology and Therapeutics*, **21**, 47–51.

Peveler, R., George, C., Kinmonth, A., *et al* (1999) Effect of antidepressant drug counselling and information leaflets on adherence to drug treatment in primary care: randomised controlled trial. *BMJ*, **319**, 612–615.

Pincus, H., Zarin, D., Tanielian, M., *et al* (1999) Psychiatric patients and treatments in 1997. Findings from the American Psychiatric Practice Research Network. *Archives of General Psychiatry*, **56**, 441–449.

Popli, A. & Baldessarini, R. (1995) Interactions of serotonin reuptake inhibitors with tricyclic antidepressants. *Archives of General Psychiatry*, **52**, 784–785.

Post, R. (1993) Issues in the long-term management of bipolar affective illness. *Psychiatric Annals*, **23**, 86–92.

Prange, A. J., Wilson, I. C., Robon, A. M., *et al* (1969) Enhancement of imipramine antidepressant activity by thyroid hormone. *American Journal of Psychiatry*, **126**, 457–469.

Preskorn, S. (1993) Pharmacokinetics of antidepressants: why and how they are relevant to treatment. *Journal of Clinical Psychiatry*, **54**, suppl., 14–34.

Preskorn, S. H. (1995) Comparison of the tolerability of bupropion, fluoxetine, imipramine, nefazodone, paroxetine, sertraline and venlafaxine. *Journal of Clinical Psychiatry*, **56**, suppl. 6, 12–21.

Preskorn, S. H. & Fast, G. (1991) Therapeutic drug monitoring for antidepressants: efficacy, safety, and cost-effectiveness. *Journal of Clinical Psychiatry*, **52**, suppl. 6, 22–33.

Price, L. H., Conwell, Y. & Nelson, J. C. (1983) Lithium augmentation of combined neuroleptic–tricyclic treatment in delusional depression. *American Journal of Psychiatry*, **140**, 318–322.

Price, L. H., Charney, D. S. & Henniger, G. R. (1986) Variability of response to lithium augmentation in refractory depression. *American Journal of Psychiatry*, **143**, 1387–1392.

Prien, R. F. (1992) Maintenance treatment. In *Handbook of Affective Disorders* (ed. E. S. Paykel), pp. 419–435. London: Churchill Livingstone.

Ravindran, A. V., Anisman, H., Merali, Z., *et al* (1999) Treatment of dysthymia with group cognitive therapy and pharmacotherapy. Clinical symptoms and functional impairments. *American Journal of Psychiatry*, **156**, 1608–1617.

Rihmer, Z., Appleby, L., Rihmer, A., *et al* (2000) Decreased suicide in Hungary. *British Journal of Psychiatry*, **177**, 84–89.

Robertson, M. & Trimble, M. (1982) Major tranquillisers used as antidepressants. A review. *Journal of Affective Disorders*, **4**, 173–193.

Rouillon, F., Phillips, R., Serrurier, D., *et al* (1989) Rechutes de dépression unipolaire et efficacité de maprotiline. *Encéphale*, **15**, 527–534.

Rouillon, F., Lejoyeux, M., Filteau, M., *et al* (1992) Unwanted effects of long-term treatment. In *Long-Term Treatment of Depression* (eds S. Montgomery & F. Rouillon). Chichester: Wiley.

Schmidt, L., Grohmann, R., Müller-Oerlinghausen, B., *et al* (1986) Adverse drug reactions to first- and second-generation antidepressants. A critical evaluation of drug surveillance data. *British Journal of Psychiatry*, **148**, 38–43.

Shah, R., Uren, Z., Baker, A., *et al* (2001) Deaths from antidepressants in England and Wales: analysis of a new national database. *Psychological Medicine*, **31**, 1203–1210.

Shelton, R., Tollefson, G., Tohen, M., *et al* (2001) A novel augmentation strategy for treating resistant major depression. *American Journal of Psychiatry*, **158**, 131–134.

Slama, F., Bellivier, F., Henry, C., *et al* (2004) Bipolar patients with suicidal behaviour: towards the identification of a clinical sub group. *Journal of Clinical Psychiatry*, **65**, 1035–1039.

Song, F., Freemantle, N., Sheldon, T., *et al* (1993) Selective serotonin reuptake inhibitors: meta-analysis of efficacy and acceptability. *BMJ*, **306**, 683–687.

Stein, G. & Bernadt, M. (1993) Lithium augmentation therapy in tricyclic-resistant depression. A controlled trial using lithium in low and normal doses. *British Journal of Psychiatry*, **162**, 634–640.

Sternbach, H. (1991) The serotonin syndrome. *American Journal of Psychiatry*, **148**, 705–713.

Stimmel, G., Skowron, D. & Chameides, W. (1991) Focus on fluvoxamine: a serotonin reuptake inhibitor for major depression and obsessive–compulsive disorder. *Hospital Formulary*, **26**, 635–643.

Stimpson, N., Agrural, N. & Lewis, G. (2002) Randomised controlled trials investigating pharmacological and psychological interventions for treatment refractory depression: a systematic review. *British Journal of Psychiatry*, **181**, 284–294.

Sullivan, P., Valuck, R., Brixner, D., *et al* (2005) A pharmacoeconomic model for making value-based decisions about serotonin reuptake inhibitors. *Pharmacy and Therapeutics*, **30**, 96–106.

Targum, S. D., Greenberg, R. D., Harmon, R. L., *et al* (1984) Thyroid hormone and the TRH stimulation test in refractory depression. *Journal of Clinical Psychiatry*, **45**, 345–346.

Taylor, D. (1995) Selective serotonin inhibitors and tricyclic antidepressants in combination. Interactions and therapeutic use. *British Journal of Psychiatry*, **167**, 575–580.

Taylor, D. & Lader, M. (1996) Cytochromes and psychotropic drug interactions. *British Journal of Psychiatry*, **168**, 529–532.

Taylor, D., Paton, C. & Kerwin, R. (2005) *The South London and Maudsley NHS Trust and Oxleas NHS Trust Prescribing Guidelines*. London: Martin Dunitz.

Teicher, M., Glod, C. & Cole, J. (1990) Emergence of intense suicidal preoccupation during fluoxetine treatment. *American Journal of Psychiatry*, **147**, 207–210.

Thase, M. E. & Rush, A. J. (1995) Treatment resistant depression. In *Psychopharmacology: The Fourth Generation of Progress* (eds F. Bloom & D. Kupfer), pp. 1081–1097. New York: Raven Press.

Thase, M. E., Rush, J., Howland, R. H., *et al* (2002) Double blind switch study of imipramine or sertraline treatment of antidepressant-resistant chronic depression. *Archives of General Psychiatry*, **59**, 233–239.

Thompson, C., Peveler, R. C., Stephenson, D., *et al* (2000) Compliance with antidepressant medication in the treatment of major depressive disorder in primary care: a randomised comparison of fluoxetine and a tricyclic antidepressant. *American Journal of Psychiatry*, **157**, 338–343.

Tohen, M., Vieta, E., Calabrese, J., *et al* (2003) Efficacy of olanzapine and olanzapine–fluoxetine combination in the treatment of bipolar I depression. *Archives of General Psychiatry*, **60**, 1079–1088.

Trivedi, M. (2003) Using treatment algorithms to bring patients to remission. *Journal of Clinical Psychiatry*, **64**, suppl. 2, 8–13.

Trivedi, M. M., Rush, A. J. & Crismon, L. (2004) Clinical results for patients with major depressive disorder in the Texas Medication Algorithan Project. *Archives of General Psychiatry*, **61**, 669–680.

Warner, M., Peabody, C., Whiteford, H., *et al* (1987) Trazodone and priapism. *Journal of Clinical Psychiatry*, **50**, 256–261.

Warrington, S., Padgham, C. & Lader, M. (1989) The cardiovascular effects of antidepressants. *Psychological Medicine*, monograph suppl. 16.

Weilburg, J. B., Rosenbaum, J. F., Biederman, J., *et al* (1989) Fluoxetine added to non-MAOI antidepressants converts nonresponders to responders: a preliminary report. *Journal of Clinical Psychiatry*, **50**, 447–449.

Weiss, J. & Gorman, J. (2005) Antidepressant adherence and suicide risk in depressed youth. *American Journal of Psychiatry*, **162**, 1756–1757.

Weller, R. & Preskorn, S. (1984) Psychotropic drugs and alcohol: pharmacokinetic and pharmacodynamic interactions. *Psychosomatics*, **25**, 301–309.

Wilde, M., Plosker, G. & Benfield, P. (1993) Fluvoxamine. An updated review of its pharmacology and therapeutic use in depressive illness. *Drugs*, **46**, 895–924.

Wilhelm, K., Mitchell, P., Sengoz, A., *et al* (1994) Treatment resistant depression. Outcome of a series of patients. *Australian and New Zealand Journal of Psychiatry*, **28**, 23–33.

Willner, P. (1995) Dopaminergic mechanisms in depression and mania. In *Psychopharmacology: The Fourth Generation of Progress* (eds F. Bloom & D. Kupfer), pp. 921–931. New York: Raven Press.

World Health Organization (1992) *The Tenth Revision of the International Classification of Diseases and Related Health Problems* (ICD–10). Geneva: WHO.

Worral, E., Moody, J., Peet, M., *et al* (1979) Controlled studies of the acute antidepressant effects of lithium. *British Journal of Psychiatry*, **35**, 255–262.

Young, R., Alexopoulis, G., Sharmoian, C., *et al* (1987) Plasma 10-hydroxy nortriptyline and renal function in elderly depressives. *Biological Psychiatry*, **22**, 1283–1287.

Zajecka, J. M., Jeffries, H. & Fawcett, J. (1995) The efficacy of fluoxetine combined with a heterocyclic antidepressant in treatment resistant depression: a retrospective analysis. *Journal of Clinical Psychiatry*, **56**, 338–343.

Zanarini, M. C., Frankenburg, F. R. & Parachini, E. A. (2004) A preliminary, randomised trial of fluoxetine, olanzapine and the olanzapine–fluoxetine combination in women with borderline personality disorder. *Journal of Clinical Psychiatry*, **65**, 903–907.

Zimmerman, U., Krans, T., Himmerich, H., *et al* (2003) Epidemiological implications and mechanisms underlying drug-induced weight gain in psychiatric patients. *Journal of Psychiatric Research*, **37**, 193–230.

CHAPTER 5

Electroconvulsive therapy and other physical therapies

Arun Jha

As with other sciences, psychiatry has not progressed in a neat, linear fashion. Every so often, a sudden change of direction or a dramatic breakthrough has occurred. Some speak of the removal of chains in the asylums as the first revolution and of Freud's psychoanalysis as the second. If so, surely the third was the birth of 'shock therapy'.

From 'chemical shock' to 'electroshock' to 'electroconvulsive therapy'

A description of the history of the discovery of convulsive therapy is given by Abrams (1988) and Berrios (1997), from which the account below is taken. Abrams (1988) stresses that even though there are many earlier accounts of 'fits' and 'shocks' being given to psychiatric patients, the story really starts with Meduna's discovery of the beneficial effects of camphor-induced fits. Ladislav Joseph Von Meduna (1896–1964) was a Hungarian psychiatrist who espoused the notion that there is a biological antagonism between schizophrenia and epilepsy. He observed 'an overwhelming and almost crushing growth of glial cells in the brains of epileptics' and this contrasted with an equally evident lack of a glial reaction in the brains of people with schizophrenia. At the time there were also epidemiological studies that had suggested there is a low incidence of epilepsy among those with schizophrenia. Meduna was encouraged by his friend Dr Joseph Nyirö, who had observed that patients with epilepsy had a better prognosis if they also had schizophrenia, and Nyirö even went as far as trying (unsuccessfully) to treat patients with epilepsy with injections of blood from patients who had schizophrenia. Even by the 1940s, the notion that there is an antagonism between schizophrenia and epilepsy had been shown to be quite untrue, but this false hypothesis endured sufficiently long to motivate researchers to see whether induced fits might benefit patients with schizophrenia.

Thus, Meduna sought to induce seizures in his patients. He initially experimented on guinea pigs, on which he tried to induce seizures wiht strychnine, coramine, caffeine, brucine and even absinthe, but without any success. However, he learned from an officer of the International League against Epilepsy that camphor was effective and could induce fits, and he eventually managed to induce fits in his guinea pigs. On 23 January 1935, Meduna gave an injection of camphor in oil to a patient who had been in a catatonic stupor for four years, who never moved, who was incontinent and who never ate (and so required drip feeding). Meduna went on to describe how, after the first fit, the patient improved, but that he himself was so anxious about it that he went into a state of nervous collapse. After a few further convulsions the patient was cured, and in the first series of 26 patients with schizophrenia 10 recovered, 3 were improved and 13 showed no change (Meduna, 1934).

Camphor was switched to cardiazol, as this is water soluble (and therefore safer and easier to inject) and was more reliable, but cardiazol-induced fits had a serious disadvantage in that, during the pre-ictal phase, they produced an extremely unpleasant subjective sensation and this stimulated researchers to seek other methods for inducing the fits.

Ugo Cerletti (1877–1963), Professor of Neuropathology and Psychiatry in Rome, became interested in the problem and sent one of his assistants to see Meduna. Cerletti focused on the use of electricity to induce convulsions. Chauzzi, one of his associates, had been able to produce convulsions in dogs by passing a 50 Hz, 220 V stimulus for 0.25 s between electrodes placed in the mouth and rectum, but unfortunately many of the dogs had died. Lucio Bini (1908–64), who was 30 at the time and not yet a psychiatrist (he later became a prominent psychiatrist and wrote a textbook of psychiatry), joined Cerletti's group and is credited with having the crucial insight that the reason why 50% of the experimental dogs died was because the mouth–rectal electrode placement meant that a large charge of electricity went through the dog's heart. He suggested the electrodes should be placed on the temples of the dogs instead; this indeed produced fits and had a negligible mortality rate. That this was safer was confirmed by Cerletti in a visit to the Rome slaughterhouse, where he had been told the pigs were killed by electricity. In fact, the pigs were first given convulsions by an electrical stimulus to the head and then dispatched while they were comatose. In later years, when Cerletti was reminiscing about the discovery of electroconvulsive therapy (ECT), he wrote that observation that electricity could produce convulsions in pigs had encouraged him to seek out those parameters that might make it safe and effective for human application (see Abrams, 1988).

The first patient to receive ECT was a 39-year-old unidentified man found wandering in a train station without a ticket who was hallucinating and having alternating periods of mutism and neologistic speech. On 14 April 1938 ECT was administered, but the first stimulus (70 V for 0.2 s) proved to be unintentionally sub-convulsive. The patient had a brief myoclonic reaction and began to sing loudly but when he came round said 'not another; it will kill me'. He was nevertheless restimulated at a higher dosage (110 V for 0.5 s) and a grand mal seizure ensued. After awakening he was asked 'What has been happening to you?', to which he replied 'I don't know; perhaps I have been asleep'. After a course of 11 ECTs he was cured. The publication of this case in their famous paper 'Un nuevo metodo di shockterapie: "L'elettro-shock"' (Cerletti & Bini, 1938) marks a major turning point in the history of psychiatry and was to usher in the modern era of useful physical treatments.

The use of ECT spread rapidly in Europe and the USA because it was the first effective, reliable and inexpensive treatment modality for major psychiatric disorder. A wave of enthusiasm then resulted in a period of indiscriminate use and misuse, particularly during the middle decades of the 20th century, resulting in ECT acquiring a bad reputation and a public reaction against it, which to some extent persists today. Early adverse effects such as bitten tongues, fractured bones and broken teeth caused by the induction of generalised seizures made the treatment in the early days a high-risk procedure, but after the introduction of general anaesthesia and the use of muscle relaxants these more severe complications disappeared.

Incremental advances in the method of administering ECT have in recent years permitted refinement of the treatment to the point that most patients can enjoy the full therapeutic benefit of ECT without the cognitive side-effects that were so prominent with the original method. Unilateral ECT, as we know it, was invented in 1949. The risk associated with ECT has been significantly reduced over the years, especially with the introduction of controlled-current ECT machines, optimum use of anaesthetics, muscle relaxants and resuscitation equipment, and an increasing use of monitoring with electroencephalography (EEG) during the application of ECT.

Although ECT is widely used in modern psychiatry, the number of patients reported to be receiving it has been gradually falling. Thus, in 1985 there were 137 940 administrations of ECT in the UK National Health Service, and this figure fell to 105 466 in 1991 and to 65 930 (equivalent to 5.8 patients per 100 000 total population) by 1999. In the period January–March 2002, some 2300 patients received ECT, compared with 2800 in 1999.

ECT is available only in specialist centres in Belgium and Germany, and it is prohibited in some cantons in Switzerland. In Italy, where Cerletti and Bini first introduced ECT, it has almost been abolished, more for political than for scientific reasons. The current decline in the use of ECT has been attributed to the introduction of newer and possibly more effective antidepressants, improved community care and earlier detection of mental illness, as well as an overall better appreciation of the indications for ECT (Eranti & McLoughlin, 2003). However, it still remains a controversial intervention, arousing some fear in members of the public and the profession alike, and this is reflected in the guidelines from the National Institute for Clinical Excellence (NICE) (2003), which seek to curb the use of ECT in the UK.

Practice of ECT in England and Wales

Electroconvulsive therapy involves the passage of an electric current across the brain to induce generalised cerebral seizure activity of an adequate duration. The treatment is administered only to an anaesthetised patient who has also been administered a muscle relaxant. ECT is usually given twice weekly in the UK, as opposed to three times a week in the USA. Six treatment sessions of ECT have been estimated to cost £2475 (this excludes in-patient costs, estimated at £171 per day) (NICE, 2003).

All psychiatrists using ECT should be familiar with the procedure, its indications and potential pitfalls, and should also have a clear idea about the practical issues concerning its clinical administration. The NICE (2003) guidance on the use of electroconvulsive therapy, along with *The ECT Handbook* (Royal College of Psychiatrists, 2005) and the local ECT protocol, should always be followed.

In the UK 20 000 people are given ECT annually, as are perhaps 1 000 000 patients worldwide; ECT is also a commonly used treatment in the developing nations because it is relatively cheap and also quick and effective. Standards for the administration of ECT in the UK were first set by the Royal College of Psychiatrists in 1977. A critical editorial in the *Lancet* in 1981, as well as adverse coverage in the lay media, prompted a national survey of the use of ECT for the first time (Pippard & Ellam, 1981). This found that some centres were still using obsolete machines and that training of psychiatrists in the administration of ECT was generally poor. In response to these findings, the College produced its first ECT handbook in 1989, which was later revised as *The ECT Handbook*, which has now gone to a second edition (Royal College of Psychiatrists, 1995, 2005). A further survey (Duffett & Lelliott, 1998, following up Pippard, 1992) found that many aspects of the organisation and administration of ECT had improved between 1991 and 1996, but two-thirds of the clinics surveyed still fell short of the most recent College standards, particularly in relation to: the frequency of consultant attendance; the training of junior doctors; the way in which information is provided to patients; and the way in which consent is obtained. According to Rose *et al* (2003), half of those undergoing ECT reported that they had not been given an adequate explanation. The standards of ECT in Scotland have been reported to be higher than the UK average (Fergusson *et al*, 2003).

Possibly because there is still considerable anxiety in the community about ECT, NICE (2003) has issued new guidance for England and Wales on the use of ECT, and the Royal College of Psychiatrists has developed a new voluntary quality assurance scheme for ECT clinics, 'the ECT accreditation service' (Royal College of Psychiatrists, 2003). The College will award an accreditation rating to participating ECT clinics that meet essential standards, and this in turn should help to reassure patients that their local ECT clinic not only meets certain standards but that they are also striving to improve them.

Efficacy of ECT

The classic UK Medical Research Council trial (1965) showed a significantly greater improvement in patients with depression receiving ECT compared with other treatments (71% improved with ECT, 52% with imipramine, 30% with phenelzine and 39% with placebo). In a systematic review of 18 trials (with a total of 1144 participants) comparing ECT with drug therapy, the UK ECT Review Group (2003) concluded that ECT is significantly more effective than pharmacotherapy for depressive illness. Similarly, Pagnin *et al* (2004) found a significant superiority for ECT in all comparisons: ECT vs simulated ECT; ECT versus placebo; and ECT vs antidepressants in general. A recent Scottish national ECT audit reported an average clinical improvement of 71% for patients treated for depressive illness (Fergusson *et al*, 2003). Similarly, a rating of 'definite improvement' on the Clinical Global Impression scale was recorded for 72% of patients with depressive disorder and over 60% for other (psychotic) illnesses. Also, of the 636 patients who fully recovered, 342 (54%) did so within 3 weeks of starting ECT. Although the clinical literature establishing the efficacy of ECT in major depression and some other disorders is substantial, its precise mechanism of action and its effect on memory remain elusive.

Which element of the ECT procedure brings about the necessary therapeutic effect: the passage of the electric current, induction of seizure, stimulus intensity, or the repeated treatment spaced out over several weeks? Or is it a combination of these elements? To separate out some of these issues in a clinical setting, the effects of real ECT have been compared with those of simulated (or 'sham') ECT. Simulated ECT involves exactly the same procedure as real ECT except that once the patient is unconscious no electrical stimulation is applied and therefore no seizure is induced.

The seizure of ECT is generated when a quantity of electrons (the charge) flows through the brain with sufficient voltage to depolarise cell membranes synchronously. The therapeutic value of the epileptic seizure in ECT was first realised quite early on, but in the 1980s it became evident that seizure duration itself has little bearing on efficacy. Gregory *et al* (1985), for example, found that patients receiving bilateral ECT responded significantly better than those receiving unilateral ECT, who in turn responded better than those receiving sham treatment. Sackeim *et al* (1987) demonstrated for the first time that generalised seizures produced by bilateral ECT were more effective than those produced by unilateral ECT, even though the seizures were identical in duration and character. The UK ECT Review Group (2003) also confirmed that: ECT is more effective than simulated ECT; bilateral ECT is more effective than unilateral ECT; and high-dose ECT is more effective than low-dose (ECT). The more effective forms tend to cause greater cognitive impairment, however, and in recent years stimulus intensity, seizure threshold and dose titration have gained prominence (see below).

Indications

Electroconvulsive therapy is an important treatment option for major depression, although its use extends to the treatment of mania, schizophrenia and occasionally other conditions, such as catatonia, the neuroleptic malignant syndrome and Parkinsonism. The NICE (2003) guidelines advocate restriction of the use of ECT 'only to achieve rapid and short-term improvement of severe symptoms after an adequate trial of other treatment options has proven ineffective and/or when the condition is considered to be potentially life-threatening'. In the recent Scottish national ECT audit, 87% of patients had a diagnosis of depressive illness, 6.3% schizophrenic illness and 3% manic illness (Fergusson *et al*, 2003).

The indications for ECT recognised by the Royal College of Psychiatrists (2005) and by NICE (2003) are similar, but the latter may be too restrictive (Table 5.1) and have been criticised by the Royal College of Psychiatrists' Special Committee on ECT, as reported by White (2003): 'it is perverse to prevent *moderately* ill patients from freely choosing electroconvulsive therapy until their symptoms deteriorate badly'.

As the longer-term benefits and risks of ECT have not been clearly established, NICE (2003) does *not* recommend ECT as maintenance therapy in depressive illness or the use of ECT in schizophrenia.

The indications for ECT are considered below.

Depression

Electroconvulsive therapy is a widely used and effective treatment for depressive disorders. It provides rapid relief from the more serious immediate life-threatening symptoms of depressive illness (Box 5.1).

Table 5.1 Comparison of three sets of indications for ECT

Royal College of Psychiatrists (2005)	American Psychiatric Association (2001)	National Institute for Clinical Excellence (2003)
Major depressive episode/disorder	Unipolar and bipolar major depression	Severe depressive illness
Mania	Mania	A prolonged or severe manic episode
Acute schizophrenia	Schizophrenia, schizophreniform and schizoaffective disorders	
Catatonia	Catatonic states	Catatonia
	Parkinson's disease	
	Neuroleptic malignant syndrome	
	Intractable seizure disorder	

Box 5.1 Indications for ECT in the treatment of depression

ECT is indicated where:
- the depression is resistant to drug therapy
- the illness is severe
- the patient is suicidal
- the patient is psychotic
- the illness is puerperal.

It is particularly indicated in cases of severe psychomotor retardation in which there are immediate concerns about the patient's physical well-being, for example if fluid intake is poor. It may be used urgently when there is acute risk of harm to the individual or to other people, due to the patient acting on psychotic delusions or hallucinations. However, there is no direct evidence that ECT prevents suicide. Although many of the randomised trials are old, and most were small, the evidence from them has consistently shown that, in the short term (i.e., at the end of a course of treatment), ECT is an effective treatment for adult patients with depressive disorders (UK ECT Review Group, 2003). There is less randomised evidence that the short-term benefits are maintained in the long term.

Remission rates are higher and remission occurs earlier in patients with psychotic as opposed to non-psychotic depression (Petrides *et al*, 2001). Although the bipolar/unipolar distinction has no predictive value in determining the outcome of ECT, patients with a bipolar illness show more rapid clinical improvement than those with a unipolar illness (Daly *et al*, 2001).

While most major depressive episodes are relatively brief, a substantial minority of patients with severe mood disorders respond poorly to available treatments and remain ill for extended periods. Increasingly, ECT is reserved for these difficult-to-treat, medication-refractory patients, although there is limited randomised evidence for the treatment in this group.

The clinical scenario set out in Box 5.2 is a typical example of the use of ECT in day-to-day practice. Clinical practice of this type is not uncommon, at least in the UK, where pharmacological treatment is often tried first, despite the assertion of the American Psychiatric Association (2001) that:

> 'as a major treatment in psychiatry with well-defined indications, electroconvulsive therapy should not be reserved for use only as "last resort". Such practice may deprive patients of an effective treatment, may delay response and prolong suffering, and may possibly contribute to treatment resistance.'

Box 5.2 A clinical scenario for the use of ECT

Mrs X, a 73-year-old married woman, experienced an episode of severe depression that had lasted 12 months. Initially, her family doctor treated her with fluoxetine. Despite a brief period of improvement she remained very worried and depressed. She was therefore referred to the local psychiatric team. Treatment with mirtazapine and venlafaxine, even with lithium augmentation, proved ineffective. Her condition continued to deteriorate. She refused to eat and drink adequately, and neglected her personal hygiene. It was decided to treat her with ECT.

Mania

In recent years there has been some renewed interest in the use of ECT in mania, but the supporting literature is small. In cases of severe manic illness, where there is severe exhaustion, excitement or manic stupor, it has the advantage of producing a rapid response.

In the randomised controlled trial by Sikdar *et al* (1994), two groups each of 15 patients with mania received eight ECT sessions, either real or simulated, and all patients also received 600 mg chlorpromazine daily. Patients receiving the combination of chlorpromazine and real ECT did significantly better than those receiving chlorpromazine with sham ECT. Mukherjee *et al* (1994) reviewed the literature of the past 50 years and concluded that 'ECT is associated with remission or marked clinical improvement in 80% of manic patients and that it was an effective treatment for patients whose manic episodes have responded poorly to pharmacotherapy'.

Electroconvulsive therapy may be especially useful in mixed affective states, where symptoms of depression and mania coexist, as patients in this group tend to respond poorly to drug treatment (Ciapparelli *et al*, 2001).

Catatonia

Electroconvulsive therapy has traditionally been recommended for acute catatonic symptoms associated with both schizophrenia and affective disorders. Classic cases of catatonia have become much less frequent with the introduction of neuroleptic drugs, but cases of catatonia still occur. ECT can be life-saving in acute catatonia, as reported in an interesting case of neuroleptic malignant syndrome (Carey *et al*, 2002).

Schizophrenia and schizoaffective disorder

Electroconvulsive therapy is not traditionally considered as first-line treatment for schizophrenia and the NICE (2003) guidelines state it should no longer be used. It has no place in the management of symptoms of withdrawal, apathy or social incongruence that are associated with the defect state of chronic schizophrenia. However, there is evidence that ECT may be useful for patients with medication-resistant acute schizophrenia. A combination of ECT and neuroleptics may sometimes be more effective than either treatment alone (Chanpattana *et al*, 1999) and ECT is a useful treatment for schizoaffective disorder (American Psychiatric Association, 2001).

Other conditions

Electroconvulsive therapy is highly effective in the management of puerperal psychosis, especially when affective symptoms predominate, although the treatment is not popular with patients (see page 639) and there are no randomised controlled trials of its use for women with psychiatric symptoms associated with pregnancy or recent childbirth.

There is no evidence to suggest that ECT is of benefit in any other psychiatric disorder. It has no therapeutic use in the control of violent or aggressive patients, and should not be prescribed as a last resort, without any clear indication, when other treatments have failed.

Relapse of depression after ECT

The chronic and recurrent nature of the mood disorders constitutes one of the major challenges facing psychiatry. ECT is usually stopped following a response, but relapse of depression after successful treatment with ECT is common, as an acute course of ECT generally confers only transient benefits. There is less evidence from randomised controlled trials that the short-term benefits are maintained over the long term. In fact around half of patients successfully treated with ECT relapse within the first six months (Bourgon & Kellner, 2000).

The question of whether medication-resistant patients do better or worse with ECT has long interested psychiatrists. As early as 1965, the results of the Medical Research Council's trial had indicated that resistance to antidepressant medication may be associated with a reduced rate of response to ECT, because most of the patients who did not respond to pharmacotherapy received subsequent ECT, and their response rate was 52%, while 71% of patients without prior pharmacotherapy responded to ECT.

However, more recent studies have shown that medication resistance does not influence short-term response to subsequent ECT and that it can still be of considerable efficacy. In a prospective Dutch study, van den Broek *et al* (2004) assessed the influence of resistance to antidepressant pharmacotherapy on the short-term response to subsequent ECT. Eighty-five patients who met the DSM–IV criteria for a diagnosis of depression were included for analysis and the results showed that medication-resistant patients were equally likely to respond to subsequent ECT (82.5%) as patients without medication resistance (81.1%).

Patients with prior medication-resistant depression relapse at a high rate, especially in the first few weeks after ECT. It is possible that starting an antidepressant medication early during the course of ECT will help sustain the remission. A randomised trial found that a concurrent tricyclic antidepressant may improve clinical outcome with ECT, but this benefit did not occur with a selective serotonin reuptake inhibitor (Lauritzen *et al*, 1996). It may make more sense to administer an antidepressant of a different class during and after ECT, rather than continuing one to which the patient has already shown resistance.

Sackeim *et al* (2001) have demonstrated that continuation monotherapy with nortriptyline has limited efficacy, but the combination of nortriptyline and lithium was more effective in preventing early relapse after a course of ECT. However, the rate of relapse during the first month of continuation therapy after ECT was still high. Two alternative strategies have been suggested: first, the course of ECT can be tapered off over a few weeks, rather than ended abruptly; second, the antidepressant medication used in continuation therapy may be started during the course of ECT, followed by the post-ECT addition of lithium. A low post-ECT relapse rate had been noted in earlier studies in which patients began taking their antidepressant at the beginning of their course of ECT.

The search for characteristics of the patient or illness that can predict relapse has been disappointing. In a double-blind, randomised controlled study of ECT, 7 of the 17 depressed patients allocated to the right unilateral group failed to respond. The non-responders subsequently responded to bilateral ECT (Delva *et al*, 2001). A comparison of responders and non-responders showed that the responders had substantially lower initial seizure thresholds as well as longer convulsions. These factors may be associated with a good response to lower doses of charge in right unilateral ECT. Avoidance of benzodiazepines may also obviate the need for excessive dosage, which may otherwise cause unnecessary cognitive side-effects (Jha & Stein, 1996).

Continuation and maintenance ECT

Continuation ECT (to prevent early relapse of an index episode of illness) and maintenance ECT (to prevent the recurrence of the illness) have been used since 1943, and appear to be safe and effective. The NICE (2003) guidelines do not recommend the long-term use of ECT for maintenance and state that 'clinical status should be assessed following each ECT session and treatment should be stopped when a response has been achieved', but the guidelines do accept the need for continuation ECT in a few cases.

After a successful course of ECT, continuation therapy with psychotropic drugs is the current practice for the vast majority of patients, but, as indicated by NICE, continuation ECT may also be necessary in a few cases. One study compared two groups of patients with chronic depression (29 in each group) who had responded to an acute course of ECT, and found that only four subjects relapsed in the group who received continuation ECT combined with an antidepressant, whereas 15 patients relapsed in the group who received an antidepressant alone (Gagné *et al*, 2000). During the subsequent follow-up, which lasted more than 5 years, the mean time to relapse was more than twice as long in the ECT continuation group as that in the antidepressant-only group.

Maintenance therapy is defined as the prophylactic use of psychotropics or ECT for longer than 6 months past the end of the index episode, when a decision is made as to whether continuation therapy should be initiated (American Psychiatric Association, 2001). Remissions are usually sustained with progressively fewer ECT treatments, at progressively wider intervals. A common approach is to administer ECT treatments once a week for 3 or 4 weeks, then every two weeks for 4 weeks, and then monthly for 4–6 months (Fox, 2001).

Maintenance ECT is usually given as an out-patient procedure; this may be more cost-effective than in-patient ECT but it demands caution. Patients receiving ambulatory ECT should avoid activities that may be affected by the anticipated adverse cognitive effects of

ECT, particularly on treatment days. The Royal College of Psychiatrists (2003) recommends that day patients or their carers should sign a form which confirms:

- that they will not drive for the next 24 hours (or a longer period if so advised by the anaesthetist concerned)
- that they will be accompanied home
- that they will have appropriate supervision by a responsible adult for the night after each ECT.

Maintenance ECT may sometimes be the only treatment that yields an extended period of euthymia to patients with severe, treatment-resistant depression or mania and it does not appear to have long-term detrimental cognitive effects. Thus, Vothknecht *et al* (2003), in a prospective naturalistic study, compared the effect of 11 sessions of maintenance ECT to maintenance pharmacotherapy alone and found neither a difference in neuropsychological functioning between the two groups nor a decline during the maintenance phase of treatment. In an interesting case report, one patient received a total of 60 brief-pulse unilateral ECT treatments over 5 years, yet no pathological changes could be detected by positron emission tomography (Anghelescu *et al*, 2001).

Contraindications and safety in physical illness

Electroconvulsive therapy is a safe treatment, having a mortality rate no greater than that associated with the administration of a general anaesthetic for minor surgery. No systemic condition bars its use, and there are no absolute contraindications to it: all patients should be individually assessed and the benefits of ECT weighed against its potential hazards.

Central nervous system

Administration of ECT affects the central nervous system (CNS) and although it appears safe in most neurological conditions, patients with space-occupying lesions with increased intracranial pressure, and recent cerebral trauma, are of special concern and these are relative contraindications. Most clinicians also prefer to avoid the use of ECT within 3 months of stroke. In severe cervical spondylosis, there is a risk that neck movement during ECT will cause injury, unless the procedure is used with maximal muscle relaxation and minimum neck manipulation.

Cardiovascular system

The use of ECT in patients with known cardiovascular disease requires caution, because the cardiovascular changes accompanying the procedure may be quite profound. A history of recent myocardial infarction, unstable angina, uncomplicated congestive cardiac failure, severe valvular heart disease, clinically significant cardiac arrhythmias and fragile vascular aneurysms place patients at increased risk with ECT (American Psychiatric Association, 2001).

Box 5.3 A case of unstable blood pressure during ECT

One morning, following routine anaesthesia, oxygenation and muscle relaxation, bilateral ECT was given to Mrs X. A dose of 150 mC produced a very mild fit lasting less than 20 s. The patient took 20 min to recover from the anaesthesia and 1 h 15 min to become fully conscious. During the recovery period her blood pressure initially fell from the normal 130/90 to 84/40 mmHg, and she required intravenous fluid. Gradually, her blood pressure started to rise, and went up to 181/104 mmHg. Because she looked unwell she was transferred to the local general hospital. Her blood pressure continued to rise, to a maximum 200/88 mmHg. However, no further ECT was attempted, despite continued deterioration of her depression.

An initial tachycardia accompanies the induction of anaesthesia. The administration of the ECT itself produces a bradycardia, followed by tachycardia, both of which can lead to marked swings in blood pressure and cardiac output. These may be accompanied by various arrhythmias and electrocardiographic (ECG) changes consistent with myocardial ischaemia. Acute coronary insufficiency leading to myocardial infarction has been reported with status epilepticus and occurs rarely in association with ECT.

The management of these patients during ECT is directed at minimising the swings in blood pressure and heart rate that occur during the treatment. The clinical scenario set out in Box 5.3 illustrates the dilemma of administering ECT to Mrs X, the same 73-year-old patient described in Box 5.2, whose blood pressure became so unstable during the first administration of ECT that further ECT could not be administered.

The presence of a cardiac pacemaker is *not* a contraindication to ECT, but the patient should be isolated from the ground during the procedure. ECT should be delayed for at least 3 months following myocardial infarction. A period of treatment with anticoagulants such as warfarin should be considered for patients thought to be at increased risk of systemic thromboembolism.

Special populations

Electroconvulsive therapy is an effective and relatively safe procedure in high-risk special patient populations (Rabheru, 2001) and may be safer than the alternative treatments. This may apply to those who are medically ill (see above), elderly or pregnant (American Psychiatric Association, 2001). For elderly people, for instance, the ECT clinic is expected to have a protocol which includes reference to cognitive side-effects, seizure threshold and choice of anaesthetic induction agent.

Elderly patients

Age does not necessarily increase the risk of cognitive side-effects from ECT, but this risk is increased by age-associated conditions such as Alzheimer's dementia and cardiovascular disease; there are also age-related risks associated with anaesthesia and other medications. Although evidence from non-randomised studies shows that ECT is both safe and effective in the acute phase of treatment and generally is safe in elderly patients with depression, there is limited evidence of its safety and efficacy in certain in-patient subgroups of elderly patients, such as those with Parkinson's disease.

In spite of having higher levels of physical illness and cognitive impairment, even the oldest patients (75 and older) with severe depression tolerate ECT as well as younger patients and show similar acute response rates. However, older patients are more likely to develop cognitive impairment, especially with bilateral ECT. Older patients who fail to respond to moderate-charge right unilateral ECT (150% above seizure threshold) may benefit from a switch to high-charge right unilateral ECT (450% above threshold) rather than bilateral ECT (Tew *et al*, 2002).

Adolescents

There is a general reluctance to use ECT in adolescents, as information on the indications and effectiveness of ECT in this age group is scarce. ECT has been successfully given to prepubertal children as young as 8 years with major depression and catatonia but this is extremely rare. Thus, in Scotland, no patient under the age of 17 years received ECT during the survey period, August 1997 to July 1999 (Fergusson *et al*, 2003).

Bloch *et al* (2001) reviewed the case notes of 24 Israeli adolescents, and compared the findings with those from 33 adult patients who received their course of ECT over the same period. The remission rate was 58% for both groups of patients. However, the diagnosis for which patients were referred was in the 'psychotic spectrum' for most adolescents compared to the 'affective spectrum' for adults.

Pregnancy

Electroconvulsive therapy is safe and effective in pregnancy, the risk being associated only with anaesthesia. Complications associated with ECT during pregnancy include transient benign foetal arrhythmias, mild vaginal bleeding, abdominal pain and self-limited uterine contractions (Miller, 1994). With appropriate medical care, it is relatively safe in all trimesters of pregnancy, as well as in the post-partum period (Rabheru, 2001).

The treatment of a pregnant woman with severe depression requires skilled assessment, as dangerousness, symptom severity and patient choice all need to be taken into account.

Adverse effects

As stated above, ECT is a safe procedure but it is not free from side-effects (Box 5.4). The most significant of these are cognitive. There are also other immediate but much less common potential complications associated with the procedure, such as status epilepticus, laryngospasm and peripheral nerve palsy, which overall have an estimated incidence of 1 per 1300–1400 treatments (NICE, 2003).

Box 5.4 Common adverse effects associated with ECT

- Headache
- Nausea
- Muscular aches
- Brief confusion
- Prolonged seizure
- Spontaneous seizures
- Cognitive side-effects

Cognitive side-effects

Cognitive impairments associated with ECT mainly reflect changes in memory function. Factors associated with adverse cognitive effects are summarised in Box 5.5. Depressive illness itself may cause memory impairment, and the memory effects of ECT may sometimes be confused with the effects of the illness.

Shortly after a course of ECT, most patients will have gaps in their memory for recent events. These consist of difficulties in retention of both newly learned material (anterograde amnesia) and past events (retrograde amnesia). Immediate or short-term memory impairment during a course of ECT usually returns to pre-treatment levels within a few weeks. The retrograde amnesia associated with ECT is generally thought to cause more difficulties over the longer term than the anterograde amnesia.

Extensive research has shown that the severity of ECT-induced cognitive impairment can be reduced through modification of treatment parameters such as stimulus waveform, stimulus intensity, electrode placement and temporal spacing of the treatments. The UK ECT Review Group (2003) concluded that real ECT causes more memory impairment than simulated ECT or drug therapy, and that the method of ECT may affect the degree of cognitive impairment produced:

- bilateral ECT produces greater impairment than unilateral ECT
- treatment three times a week produces more impairment than treatment twice a week
- high-dose ECT produces more impairment than low-dose ECT.

Box 5.5 Factors associated with adverse cognitive effects of ECT

- Older ECT machines using sine waves
- Bilateral electrode placement
- Unnecessarily high stimulus intensity
- Administration more than twice per week
- Two or more seizures per treatment session
- Concurrent use of some psychotropic drugs
- High doses of anaesthetic agents

There appears to be a positive relationship between the amount of electrical current administered to the dominant hemisphere and both the clinical efficacy and the amount of cognitive impairment caused by ECT. Thus, bilateral ECT is more effective than non-dominant unilateral ECT, high-dose ECT is more effective than low-dose ECT, and these more effective forms tend to cause more memory impairment.

Bilateral versus unilateral ECT

There has been a long-standing debate on the comparative risks and benefits of bilateral versus unilateral ECT. Thus unilateral ECT does not appear to induce persistent amnesia, whereas detectable retrograde amnesia has been found 2–6 months after bilateral ECT. Sackeim *et al* (2000) reported that, in a double-blind trial, right unilateral ECT at a high dosage was as effective as bilateral ECT, but produced less severe and persistent cognitive deficits. In another study, McCall *et al* (2000) used right unilateral ECT and compared the effects of two types of dosing: either titrated to 2.25 times the threshold (mean dose 136 mC), or fixed high dosing (403 mC). Patient receiving fixed high-dose unilateral ECT had a markedly superior therapeutic response, but immediately after the unilateral ECT the high-dose group had significantly more global cognitive disturbance.

Brain damage

There is no evidence that ECT causes brain damage. Use of the most sensitive techniques for detecting cerebral change offers no evidence that ECT leads to acute structural brain changes. Similarly, no biological evidence of neuronal/glial damage or dysfunction of the blood–brain barrier could be demonstrated following a therapeutic course of ECT (Zachrisson *et al*, 2000).

Abrams (2002), citing an extensive literature, refutes the argument that ECT induces brain damage and notes that 'there is simply no evidence, and virtually no chance, that ECT as presently administered is capable of causing brain damage'. Interestingly, he cites reports of increased neurogenesis in hippocampal regions with induced seizures, and suggests that:

> 'if this hypothesis [augmentation of neurogenesis as promoting recovery from depression] is confirmed, it would not only contravene the possibility of ECT-induced brain damage, but would suggest a potential application of ECT – ameliorating the structurally based impairment of memory function [of] Alzheimer's or Parkinson's disease.'

Concurrent use of drugs and ECT

Both pharmacotherapy and ECT are frequently administered concurrently and some medications may increase the risks of ECT. Drugs prescribed for medical conditions are usually continued, although some of them may require an adjustment of dosage. Whenever possible, all psychotropic medication should be withheld until after the treatment course. This is particularly important for lithium, benzodiazepines and anticonvulsants (American Psychiatric Association, 2001).

Jha *et al* (1996) investigated the adverse effects of concomitant use of ECT and lithium, and did not detect any significant risk of delirium compared with ECT without lithium. Benzodiazepines are known to reduce seizure duration, and there are indications that concurrent use of benzodiazepines may diminish the efficacy of ECT. One study found that the therapeutic effect of unilateral ECT was compromised by the concomitant use of benzodiazepines (Jha & Stein, 1996). Similarly, anticonvulsants such as barbiturates, carbamazepine, phenytoin, valproic acid, lamotrigine and gabapentine may inhibit seizure activity by increasing seizure threshold. CNS stimulants, on the other hand, may prolong seizures as well as produce arrhythmias and elevate blood pressure. Calcium channel antagonists may cause significant cardiovascular depression (Naguib & Koorn, 2002). The decision to continue these drugs during ECT should be weighed against the risk of relapse if the drug is discontinued. The ECT psychiatrist and the anaesthetist should remain vigilant at all times, as an untoward response during ECT may occur unpredictably as a result of an interaction between psychotropics, anaesthetic agents and/or ECT.

Assessment and prevention of cognitive impairment

Assessment of cognition should be done before the start of ECT and should be repeated regularly throughout the course of ECT. The Royal College of Psychiatrists' ECT accreditation service (Royal College of Psychiatrists, 2003) has laid down the following standards regarding adverse events:

- The patient's orientation is assessed and recorded between treatment sessions.
- The patient's memory and cognitive functioning are assessed and recorded between treatment sessions.
- The patient is interviewed to determine the extent of retrograde and anterograde amnesia.
- The patient's memory and cognitive functioning are recorded 3 and 6 months after a treatment course is finished.

Non-cognitive side-effects should also be assessed regularly. The patient's subjective experience of treatment side-effects as well as objective cognitive side-effects should be recorded between the treatment sessions as well as 3 and 6 months after treatment. Formal cognitive assessment may be conducted using an instrument such as the Mini-Mental State Examination (Folstein *et al*, 1975).

As suggested above, optimisation of the certain parameters of ECT can minimise the short- and long-term cognitive side-effects. In general, right unilateral electrode placement, brief-pulse waveform, lower electrical intensity, more widely spaced treatments, fewer treatments and lower dosage of barbiturate anaesthesia are each independently associated with less intense cognitive side-effects (American Psychiatric Association, 2001). Abrams (2002), on the other hand,

Box 5.6 Mechanism of action of ECT: hypotheses

- The seizures cause a shift in the body's neuroendocrine system so that the stress hormones are kept in balance.
- Artificially inducing seizures somehow taps into the brain's natural ability to stop seizures, and the endogenous process involved in the termination of seizures are critical to the therapeutic mechanisms of ECT.
- ECT somehow changes the level of neurotransmitters in the brain.
- ECT increases blood flow in certain brain regions, as shown in imaging studies.
- The generation of new neurons in the hippocampus underlies the clinical effects of ECT.

advocates starting every patient with depression referred for unilateral ECT at maximum present-day standard device capacity. Those patients who fail to improve sufficiently after a predetermined number of seizures can then be offered bilateral ECT.

Mode of action

The exact mode of action of ECT is not known; it even remains unclear whether its antidepressant, antimanic and antipsychotic effects all share the same mechanism. However, several different hypotheses have been put forward (see Box 5.6). Recent studies indicate that electrically induced seizures result in a variety of alterations in neurotransmitters, neuropeptides, neuroendocrine function and functional brain activity. Moreover, there is a growing body of literature that indicates that similar alterations occur after treatment with antidepressant drugs.

The monoamine hypothesis postulates that reduced monoaminergic neurotransmission is involved in the pathogenesis of depression, and most antidepressant drugs elevate the concentration of monoamines in the synaptic cleft. However, it is not the enhancement of monoaminergic signalling *per se* that is thought to underlie the therapeutic effect but rather the long-term adaptive changes. Recently, evidence has emerged that remissions induced in patients through the use of lithium or ECT are also accompanied by structural changes in the neuronal network, thereby affecting synaptic plasticity in various regions of the brain (reviewed by Schloss & Henn, 2004).

Clinical administration of ECT

The role of the ECT consultant

Electroconvulsive therapy is a powerful physical treatment and probably the only treatment method uniquely available to psychiatrists. Hence, it is important for those psychiatrists who are responsible for the administration of ECT to master the techniques to maximise its benefits and avoid any untoward events. Observing ECT administered by a senior psychiatrist and personal training and supervision are the necessary first steps. ECT consultants will be providing ECT services for the patients under the care of other psychiatrists, and may need to make an opinion or decision quite quickly regarding some aspect of ECT even though they will not have an extended period of time with the patient. While relying heavily on the opinion of the referring psychiatrist, the ECT consultant will quickly have to reach an accurate second opinion. This opinion should cover:

- an estimation of the potential medical risks during the procedure
- advice on ways to reduce the risks
- deciding whether further medical or surgical consultation is indicated or additional laboratory tests are required
- considering whether the patient has the capacity to understand the risks and benefits of the proposed treatment plan.

The ECT psychiatrist will need detailed knowledge of pharmacology (i.e. not just psychopharmacology), especially concerning the effect of various drugs used in medical disorders on the therapeutic action of ECT and their influence on ECT-related haemodynamics, as well as on ECT-induced cognitive effects. And, twice per week (at least in the UK), ECT requires pushing a button.

The ECT Handbook (Royal College of Psychiatrists, 2005), *The Practice of Electroconvulsive Therapy* (American Psychiatric Association, 2001) and standards produced by the ECT Accreditation Service (Royal College of Psychiatrists, 2003) provide comprehensive practical recommendations and checklists for good practice in ECT. In the sections below some of the more practical aspects of ECT are described.

ECT suite and team

The ECT suite, placed in a designated area, is an integral part of any psychiatric service. The minimum requirement for a treatment centre is three rooms: a pre-ECT waiting area, the treatment room and the post-ECT recovery room. The treatment should be given by a team consisting of a psychiatrist, a registered nurse and a senior anaesthetist. Each ECT suite should have a routine and backup ECT machine, oxygen and a pulse oximeter, a suction machine, an ECG monitor, resuscitation equipment and a complete set of emergency drugs, which should be checked at least every 6 months.

According to guidelines for ECT anaesthesia produced by the Royal College of Psychiatrists (2002), 'for any patient assessed as being ASA3 or above, serious consideration should be given to transferring them to the district general hospital'. ASA (American Society of Anaesthesiologists) grade 3 applies to those patients' medical conditions that may affect their lifestyle (e.g. reduced exercise tolerance).

Before a course of treatments

Pre-ECT evaluation of the patient should be performed as close as possible to the initiation of treatment. A carefully taken general medical history, examination of the case notes and physical examination will identify any medical risks. Enquiry should be made about current medication, drug allergies and pregnancy, and about previous anaesthesia. Although no laboratory tests are mandatory, a local policy should be agreed with the anaesthetic department as to which investigations are needed before the first of a course of treatment. Common practice is to perform a full blood count and measurement of serum urea and electrolyte levels. Patients suffering from cardiovascular disease may require an ECG and chest radiograph.

Before each treatment

It is the responsibility of the psychiatrist and the nursing staff to ensure that patients are adequately prepared before each treatment. Obtaining a valid consent to ECT is essential before and during the entire course of the treatment (discussed later). Nursing staff should make sure that patients have nothing to eat for at least 6 hours or drink for 2 hours before treatment. The ECT psychiatrist should be made aware of any change in medications since the last treatment. Patients should wear loose clothes and not wear excess make-up or jewellery. Patients who normally use contact lenses should wear spectacles, as these can be easily removed immediately before treatment. The ECT nurse should ensure that the patient has voided urine and removed any dentures or hearing aids.

The practical administration of ECT

The basic steps of ECT are described in Box 5.7. The ECT stimulus should be administered only after the patient has been anaesthetised and oxygenated. Regardless of whether unilateral or bilateral ECT is selected, it is best to start treatment at a low setting (i.e. 'dose' of electricity) and if necessary restimulate the patient. The dose of electricity can then be titrated up over the entire course of treatment (see below).

Box 5.7 Basic steps of ECT

- Prepare the patient and the equipment
- Administer drugs
- Insert bite-block
- Deliver stimulus
- Monitor seizure/recovery

Anaesthesia and muscle relaxation

General anaesthesia is needed to produce a brief period of unconsciousness when muscle relaxation can be induced and the electrical stimulus applied. Methohexitone was the drug of choice for ECT until it ceased to be available in the UK in 1999. The Royal College of Psychiatrists (2002) recommends three agents – propofol, etomidate and thiopental sodium – as acceptable alternatives, although there are disadvantages with each.

Both propofol and etomidate are non-barbiturate intravenous induction agents. Propofol (1.0–2.0 mg/kg) has a rapid onset similar to that with methohexitone but has a shorter duration of action. Etomidate (0.15–0.2 mg/kg) produces longer seizures with slower awakening than does propofol or methohexitone; propofol shortens seizure duration but this does not affect the therapeutic efficacy of the ECT (Scott & Boddy, 2002). Many anaesthetists choose propofol because it is a non-barbiturate drug that is metabolised rapidly; however, its injection may be painful. There are indications that cognitive impairment in the early recovery period after ECT is less with propofol than with thiopental anaesthesia (Butterfield *et al*, 2004). Etomidate has minimal myocardial depressant properties and may be a safer choice for patients with cardiac disease.

Relaxant drugs are used to prevent forceful and potentially damaging convulsions. Suxamethonium (0.5 mg/kg), introduced in 1952, remains the muscle relaxant of first choice and is administered as an intravenous bolus immediately after the anaesthetic agent. Its action is terminated by the patient's plasma cholinesterase. Mivacurium is the alternative muscle relaxant to suxamethonium.

ECT device and stimulus waveform

Modern machines, introduced in 1981, provide electrical stimulation in the form of brief (1–2 ms) square-wave pulses, delivering only a fraction of the electrical energy of traditional ECT machines. These machines also estimate the impedance of the patient's head and can be pre-set to give a fixed amount of electrical energy, hence the expression 'constant current'. All modern machines work on the constant-current, brief-pulse principle.

Seizure threshold, stimulus intensity and dose titration

The term 'seizure threshold' refers to the minimum instrument setting required to induce an adequate seizure in a particular patient. The dose of electrical charge, usually delivered in a train of brief pulses by an ECT machine, is called the stimulus intensity. It is measured in units of charge (millicoulombs, mC). *The ECT Handbook* recommends that new ECT machines deliver a dose range of 25–1000 mC (Royal College of Psychiatrists, 2005). There is a 40-fold inter-individual variation in seizure threshold; also, for one individual, it rises by 25% to 200% during a course of ECT. Factors altering seizure threshold are summarised in Box 5.8.

Thus, there is no single electrical dose that will produce an adequate seizure at minimal intensity for all patients. Furthermore, although charge is probably the

Box 5.8 Factors raising the seizure threshold

- Male sex
- Advanced age
- Multiple seizures over the past few weeks
- Administration of bilateral ECT
- Anticonvulsants
- Benzodiazepines
- General anaesthesia

Box 5.9 ECT stimulus dose titration

The Royal College of Psychiatrists (2005) recommends that selection of the electrical dose for an individual patient be contingent upon the patient's seizure threshold. This is an explicit and important change from the practice recommended in the first edition of *The ECT Handbook* (Royal College of Psychiatrists, 1995), in which it was stated that it may be acceptable to select a dose that is known to be appropriate for the majority (i.e. 80% or more of similar patients).

The initial seizure threshold cannot be reliably predicted for individual patients based on demographic or clinical features. The routine empirical measurement of the initial seizure threshold would be good practice in non-urgent treatment. ECT clinics with no experience of this technique may prefer to develop experience by routinely identifying patients with a low initial seizure threshold by using a low electrical dose (25–50 mC) as the first stimulation at the first treatment.

In unilateral ECT:

- The initial electrical dose should be at least 200% above (i.e. three times) the initial seizure threshold.
- If the clinical improvement is definite but slight or temporary after four to six treatments, then doses of up to 500% above (i.e. six times) the seizure threshold are indicated.

In bilateral ECT:

- The initial electrical dose should be at least 50% above (i.e. one-and-a-half times) the initial seizure threshold.
- Where emergency treatment is required (i.e. to save life), the initial electrical dose should be at least 50–100% above the initial seizure threshold.
- If clinical improvement is inadequate after four to six treatments, then doses of up to 150% above (i.e. two-and-a-half times) the seizure threshold are indicated.

best unit of measurement to describe the stimulus, it is not sufficient on its own, and it is good practice to describe the stimulus fully, that is, in terms of frequency, pulse width, duration and current (Kellner *et al*, 1997).

The clinical response is determined not so much by the dose of stimulus as by the degree by which the dose exceeds the seizure threshold. A dose below the seizure threshold will fail to induce a generalised seizure. Missed and partial seizures have no therapeutic effect. A dose just above the seizure threshold may induce a generalised seizure, but the seizure may be of short duration and associated with incomplete generalisation. On the other hand, a dose greatly in excess of the seizure threshold is likely to produce cognitive side-effects without any therapeutic advantage. The best results are obtained with a 'moderately suprathreshold' dose, which is considered to be between 50% and 200% above the seizure threshold (i.e. 1.5–3 times the stimulus dose). An adequate dose tends to be in the lower range for bilateral ECT and higher for unilateral ECT (Sackeim *et al*, 2000).

The most important advance in recent years has been the acceptance of the need to adjust stimulus intensity to the individual patient. Currently, three methods are used to determine stimulus intensity: empirical titration, formula based, and fixed dosage. Empirical titration provides the most precise method for quantifying seizure threshold (American Psychiatric Association, 2001). The Royal College of Psychiatrists (2005) recommends that the titration procedure should be begun at the first treatment session (Box 5.9). It is essential to be familiar with the stimulus parameters of the local ECT device, as different manufacturers have fixed different parameters.

The literature suggests that high stimulus intensity represents adequate treatment, although it may produce short seizures. That is, the therapeutic effect of ECT may be related more to having a stimulus of adequate intensity than to seizure duration (Sackeim *et al*, 2000).

Electrode placement

Electrode placement for conventional bilateral frontotemporal and unilateral ECT is shown in Fig. 5.1, along with that for the less-established bifrontal ECT. The decision whether to use bilateral or unilateral electrode placement should be made by the clinical team responsible for the patient. Although bilateral treatment is more widely used in the UK, efficacy and cognitive side-effects determine the choice of electrode placement. For bilateral ECT, the bifrontotemporal position is commonly used. Electrodes are placed approximately 4 cm above the midpoint of the line joining the external angle of the orbit and the external auditory meatus (just above the hairline – see Fig. 5.1). Recently, a bifrontal placement has been proposed, on the basis that it produces fewer cognitive side-effects and has greater efficacy than the traditional bifrontotemporal placements.

For unilateral ECT, the d'Elia placement has been in common use. The frontotemporal electrode is placed in the same position as in traditional bilateral ECT, while the second electrode is placed on the same side, 10 cm away, vertically above the meatus. Although Sackeim *et al* (1993) have shown that the efficacy of unilateral ECT improves significantly when stimulus intensity is at least 2.5 times the initial threshold, unilateral ECT may still be less effective than bilateral ECT. However, it has been clearly established that non-dominant unilateral ECT (usually right unilateral) induces less memory impairment than bilateral treatment, even when higher levels of electrical stimulation are applied.

Abrams (2002) advocates *left* unilateral ECT in some patients, especially for those whose right hemisphere is very important to them, such as musicians and artists. He also argues that, because left unilateral ECT results in less cognitive disturbance than bilateral ECT while having the same efficacy, it has the potential to replace right unilateral ECT.

Determination of cerebral dominance

Given that the placement of electrodes on the dominant hemisphere may cause a greater disturbance in memory than their placement on the non-dominant hemisphere in unilateral ECT, determination of cerebral dominance

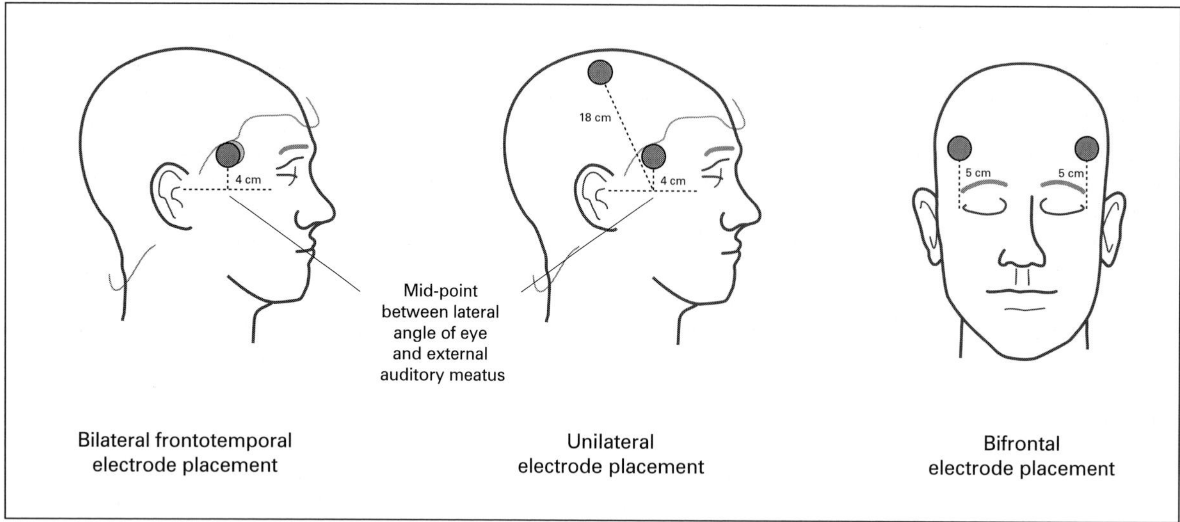

Fig. 5.1 Electrode placement.

becomes crucial. Traditionally, the routine clinical determination of cerebral dominance has been through the assessment of hand, foot and eye dominance, which is an easy but frequently inaccurate method.

Until recently, accurate determination of speech dominance before a course of ECT was possible only through an invasive procedure known as the Wada test, and through the administration of ECT itself – the ECT test. In the Wada test, the patient receives sodium amytal into (usually) the left carotid artery. If this were the dominant hemisphere, language capacity (primarily speech) would be affected. Although accurate, for obvious reasons the Wada test is hardly ever used. The ECT test involves giving left-side and right-side ECT alternately, followed by the administration of a simple verbal performance test and then continuing treatment with the side associated with the better result.

The new and more sophisticated non-invasive techniques now available include functional magnetic resonance imaging and functional transcranial Doppler sonography (fTCD). While fTCD is presently expensive and not in routine use, it can reliably replace the Wada test. Dragovic *et al* (2004) have argued that it should become standard procedure to determine cerebral dominance before unilateral ECT treatment, because this should help to reduce the cognitive side-effects of ECT.

Seizure duration

The aim of ECT is to induce a generalised seizure lasting 20–30 s. Although an adequate seizure duration does not guarantee treatment efficacy, a seizure lasting less than 15 s is considered 'abortive' or 'inadequate' and should usually be followed by restimulation at higher stimulus intensity (Box 5.10).

Although seizure duration usually decreases over the course of treatment, the magnitude of this drop between successive treatments is variable, possibly owing to marginally suprathreshold stimulation or other limiting factors.

Older patients usually have shorter seizures than younger ones. Moderately or markedly suprathreshold treatment may result in motor or EEG manifestations for between 15 and 30 s, but older patients may be receiving fully effective treatment, so further increments in stimulus dosage can cause a decrease in seizure duration accompanied by an accentuation of cognitive side-effects (American Psychiatric Association, 2001).

Seizures lasting longer than 120 s ('prolonged seizures') may cause cerebral hypoxia and cognitive impairment, and should be terminated immediately, either by a further dose of induction agent or by intravenous diazepam (Royal College of Psychiatrists, 2005). Prolonged seizures are quite common; one UK study reported a figure of 19% in courses of ECT (Benbow *et al*, 2003).

Seizure monitoring

The Royal College of Psychiatrists (2005) recommends that the convulsive activity must be timed: that timing starts at the end of the electrical stimulation and stops at the end of convulsive activity. When a higher dose of muscle relaxant is used, convulsive movements are generally mild and may be absent altogether. If seizure duration is in doubt, EEG monitoring will yield more accurate information. At minimum, one channel of EEG activity should be monitored, preferably with a frontal–mastoid montage (American Psychiatric Association, 2001). One lead is placed on the left forehead and the other behind the left ear, over the mastoid

Box 5.10 Procedure for restimulation following missed or abortive seizures

- Notify the anaesthetist.
- Recheck impedance.
- Wait 20–40 s (for possible delayed seizure).
- For abortive seizure (seizure < 15 s), wait 60 s (refractory period).
- Restimulate at 25–100% above previous stimulus.

bone. This lead placement, referred to as left fronto-mastoid, allows monitoring of seizure activity in the left hemisphere; this is appropriate for both bilateral and right unilateral ECT, because with right unilateral ECT it is important to observe that the seizure is generalised to the left hemisphere.

A more accessible but rather less accurate method is the Hamilton 'cuff method', which involves pumping a blood pressure cuff to beyond the systolic blood pressure before the administration of any muscle relaxant. Twitching in the forearm distal to the cuff indicates seizure activity, but the method is little used now.

Summary and guidelines

Different clinical situations will need a different approach to the administration of ECT, because there is a trade-off between making ECT optimally effective and minimising any cognitive impairment. If, for example, there is a need to achieve a rapid clinical response, and this appears to be more important than minimisation of cognitive impairment, then the most effective form of ECT is bilateral high-dose ECT. On the other hand, if there is less urgency about achievement of clinical response, then it is probably most prudent to use non-dominant unilateral ECT, with dose titration according to the seizure threshold to keep side-effects to a minimum.

To make ECT maximally effective, as well as keep side-effects to a minimum, and tailor the treatment to an individual patient, the best results will be achieved in a dedicated service in which the staff keep up to date with emerging evidence and have the necessary practical skills to deliver the appropriate treatment; they will also be well placed to provide information to the patient about the risks and benefits of ECT (UK ECT Review Group, 2003).

Consent and the Mental Health Act

The psychiatrist has a responsibility to ensure that, whenever possible, patients have given their explicit, written consent to ECT. The psychiatrist needs to explain why ECT has been selected as a treatment, the procedure and its side-effects, and that a general anaesthetic is used, as well as the likely consequences of not having ECT. Consent should be clearly documented on a typed consent form. Patients may withdraw their consent at any time during the course of treatment. It is good practice to offer patients a written information sheet about the treatment. It is also sensible to inform the relatives fully of the decision to treat and to explain the potential side-effects.

If a patient seems unable to give consent or refuses treatment in the face of severe or life-threatening illness, then the psychiatrist should use the relevant section of the Mental Health Act. If emergency ECT is administered (under common law), the opinion of a 'second-opinion doctor' is required and the patient will then need to be placed under the Mental Health Act. Currently, ECT is the only treatment requiring a general anaesthetic that can be administered, under the Mental Health Act 1983, without consent to a patient who has mental capacity.

The draft Mental Health Bill for England and Wales (Department of Health, 2004, pp. 46–47) contains the following procedural safeguards relating to ECT: 'when a patient over 16 has capacity they may refuse ECT as well as consent to it', except in emergency situations in order to save life. It is difficult, however, to see how a person who needs ECT as an emergency could have such capacity. In March 2005, the House of Lords and the House of Commons Joint Committee on the Draft Mental Health Bill recommended that, where a course of ECT is prescribed under emergency procedures, the maximum number of treatments be limited to two. The Bill provides for a tribunal to authorise ECT where a patient lacks capacity, following consultations with professionals involved in the care of the patient. Similarly, ECT cannot be given to any child under 16 (whether treated under formal powers or not) without authorisation by a tribunal or a court. To make an application there must be evidence of the views of the child, those with parental responsibility, and at least one second-opinion doctor.

Psychosurgery

In November 1935, Egas Moniz, a Portugues neurologist, directed his neurosurgical colleague, Almeida Lima, to perform a prefrontal leucotomy on a 63-year-old woman with melancholia, acute anxiety and paranoid delusions. They later developed a special instrument called a 'leucotome' to crush discrete cores of white matter in the frontal lobes. They reported the effects of this procedure on nearly 100 patients, and those with depression, anxiety and obsessional neurosis did better than those with schizophrenia. 'Psychosurgery', a term coined by Moniz in 1936, was later defined by the World Health Organization as 'the selective surgical removal or destruction of nerve pathways for the purposes of influencing behaviour'. For his pioneering work Moniz received the Nobel Prize for Physiology or Medicine in 1949.

In 1936 Freeman and Watts modified Moniz's procedure by using a lateral approach. Thus incision and burr holes were made behind the canthus of the eye and the white matter was destroyed in a coronal plane. This closed procedure became known as 'standard leucotomy' and many thousands of patients were operated on. By the mid-1940s severe side-effects were reported, such as apathy, lethargy, placidity, lack of emotional spontaneity, and epilepsy.

With the advent of chlorpromazine in 1950s, leucotomy fell into disrepute and its use in schizophrenia eventually ceased. Psychosurgery is still practised today, but on a much smaller scale and in only a few countries, including the UK. The three operations in use today are stereotactic subcaudate tractotomy, capsulotomy and cingulotomy. These operations have in common the interruption of tracts between the frontal cortex and the limbic system. They are considered only for serious, incapacitating and persistent treatment-resistant non-schizophrenic illnesses. These include depressive illness, anxiety state, phobic anxiety and obsessive–compulsive disorders, as well as persistent suicidal behaviour and self-mutilation. In recent years, there have been signs indicating a renewed interest in what should more adequately be termed 'neurosurgical treatment of mental disorders' instead of the stigmatising term 'psychosurgery'.

In the UK, section 57 of the Mental Health Act 1983 requires an independent doctor and two other persons appointed by the Mental Health Act Commission to have 'certified in writing that the patient is capable of understanding the nature, purpose and likely effects of the treatment in question and has consented to it'. In the Mental Health Bill (Department of Health, 2004) the procedural safeguards relating to psychosurgery for all patients (whether treated under formal powers or not) are broadly similar to those set by the current Act, but the treatment of patients who lack capacity to consent would have to be authorised by the High Court.

Neurosurgery is *not* curative. We must continue to evaluate the efficacy of neurosurgery for mental disorder against a constantly evolving knowledge base. It is also necessary to evaluate 'reversible' alternatives (Matthews & Eljamel, 2003), such as deep brain stimulation (DBS) and vagus nerve stimulation (VNS) (see below).

Other somatic therapies

The past two decades have seen rapid progress in new and less invasive ways to stimulate the brain to study and treat psychiatric disorders. These include repeated transcranial magnetic stimulation (rTMS), deep brain stimulation (DBS) and vagus nerve stimulation (VNS). Unlike ECT, these new methods enable us selectively to influence higher cognitive processes and mood systems by electrically stimulating – directly or indirectly – focal regions of the cortex and subcortical structures in the brain.

Repetitive transcranial magnetic stimulation and magnetic seizure therapy

The rTMS technique uses repeated short bursts of magnetic energy to stimulate nerve cells in the brain. Magnetic seizure therapy (MST) is a higher-dosage, convulsive form of magnetic stimulation. Clinical studies suggest that rTMS may have efficacy in treating mania and depression. Both rTMS and MST induce far less electricity and stimulate more focal regions than ECT, and so have fewer cognitive side-effects.

The clinical results obtained with rTMS have approximated those obtained in similar patient samples when treated with antidepressant drugs or with moderate-dose brief-pulse unilateral ECT, but not those obtained for bilateral or high-dose unilateral ECT. Moreover, it cannot be administered to psychotic, delusional, suicidal or other severely or dangerously ill patients (Abrams, 2002).

Deep brain stimulation

In DBS an electrode is implanted in a location relevant to the illness in question; for example, to treat patients with Parkinson's disease the substantia nigra would be targeted. It involves the implantation of a battery-operated neurotransmitter (a pacemaker-like device) under the clavicle, through a small incision in the chest. Attached to this device is a hair-thin wire with an electrode at the end. This wire is inserted just under the skin and leads along the length of the neck up to the scalp, where it is placed through a small hole in the skull. Once in place, electrical impulses are sent from the neurotransmitter up along the wire to the brain. These impulses interfere with and block the electrical signals generated in the designated area of the brain. DBS does not damage healthy brain tissue; it simply blocks its electrical signals. The neurotransmitter device is easy to adjust without requiring further surgery. It generally needs to be replaced every 3–5 years.

Although it is more invasive than other modalities, it is able to reach deeper structures in a highly focal way, which may be important for illnesses like obsessive–compulsive disorder, whose circuitry relies heavily on subcortical structures (Christmas *et al*, 2004). Some of the risks of DBS include temporary weakness in the limbs, possible changes in cognitive function and infection at the site of implantation. Through a series of computerised tests, the incidence of these risks and others can be minimised significantly when the device is implanted.

Vagus nerve stimulation

Vagus nerve stimulation is less invasive than DBS but more invasive than rTMS. It has become an accepted therapy for the treatment of refractory epilepsy, and there are indications of its usefulness in depression (Christmas *et al*, 2004). In the mid-1980s researchers discovered that internal electrical stimulation of the vagus nerve produces inhibition of certain neural processes which in turn can alter brain electrical activity and so terminate seizures. Since then many thousands of people have had the device implanted for treatment-resistant epilepsy. There are now indications that VNS may have antidepressant effects, especially in treatment-resistant depression, with benefits being maintained for more than 12 months (Marangell *et al*, 2002).

Vagus nerve stimulation has come to mean the electrical stimulation of the cervical portion of the left vagus nerve and this is usually achieved using a specific commercial electronic device – the NeuroCybernetic Prosthesis system, manufactured by Cyberonics Inc. (Houston, Texas, USA). VNS therapy was approved for use in patients with resistant depression in the European Union in March 2001.

Vagus nerve stimulation is not a form of brain surgery, even though it is an invasive surgical procedure that changes the function of the brain. The stimulator is a pacemaker-like device that generates an electrical pulse; it is implanted under the skin in the left chest wall through a small incision. The surgery for VNS involves two small incisions – one in the chest and one at the lowest part of the neck – and it usually takes between 45 minutes and 2 hours to implant the device. Once implanted, the VNS can be turned off and on and its intensity adjusted by the patient through a magnetic device.

Considering that the procedure depends on the surgical implantation of a battery-operated stimulator in the chest wall, the likelihood that it will either clinically or commercially supplant ECT is exceedingly slim.

References

Abrams, R. (1988) History of convulsive therapy. In *Convulsive Therapy*, pp. 3–9. Oxford: Oxford University Press.

Abrams, R. (2002) *Electroconvulsive Therapy* (4th edn). New York: Oxford University Press.

American Psychiatric Association (2001) *The Practice of Electroconvulsive Therapy – Recommendations for Treatment, Training, and Privileging* (2nd edn). Washington, DC: APA.

Anghelescu, I., Klawe, C. J., Bartenstein, P., *et al* (2001) Normal PET after long-term ECT. *American Journal of Psychiatry*, **158**, 1527.

Benbow, S. M., Benbow, J. & Tomenson, B. (2003) Electroconvulsive therapy clinics in the United Kingdom should routinely monitor electroencephalographic seizures. *Journal of ECT*, **19**, 217–220.

Berrios, G. E. (1997) History of ECT. *History of Psychiatry*, **8**, 105–119.

Bloch, Y., Levcovitch, Y., Bloch, A. M., *et al* (2001) Electroconvulsive therapy in adolescents: similarities to and differences from adults. *Journal of the American Academy of Child and Adolescent Psychiatry*, **40**, 1332–1336.

Bourgon, L. N. & Kellner, C. H. (2000) Relapse of depression after ECT: a review. *Journal of ECT*, **16**, 19–31.

Butterfield, N. N., Graf, P., Bernard, A. M., *et al* (2004) Propofol reduces cognitive impairment after electroconvulsive therapy. *Journal of ECT*, **20**, 3–9.

Carey, S. T., Hall, D. J. & Jones, G. A. (2002) Grand round: catatonia. *Psychiatric Bulletin*, **26**, 68–70.

Cerletti, U. & Bini, L. (1938) Un nuevo metodo di shockterapie 'L'elettro-shock'. *Bollettino della Accademia Medica di Roma*, **64**, 136–138.

Chanpattana, W., Chakrabhand, M. L., Kongsakon, R., *et al* (1999) Short-term effects of combined ECT and neuroleptic therapy in treatment-resistant schizophrenia. *Journal of ECT*, **15**, 129–139.

Christmas, D., Morrison, C., Eljamel, M. S., *et al* (2004) Neurosurgery for mental disorder. *Advances in Psychiatric Treatment*, **10**, 189–199.

Ciapparelli, A., Dell'Osso, L., Tundo, A., *et al* (2001) Electroconvulsive therapy in medication-nonresponsive patients with mixed mania and bipolar depression. *Journal of Clinical Psychiatry*, **62**, 552–555.

Daly, J. J., Prudic, J., Devanand, D. P., *et al* (2001) ECT in bipolar and unipolar depression: differences in speed of response. *Bipolar Disorders*, **3**, 95–104.

Delva, N. J., Brunet, D. G., Hawken, E. R., *et al* (2001) Characteristics of responders and nonresponders to brief-pulse right unilateral ECT in a controlled clinical trial. *Journal of ECT*, **17**, 118–123.

Department of Health (2004) *Improving Mental Health Law – Towards a New Mental Health Act*. London: Department of Health.

Dragovic, M., Allet, L. & Janca, A. (2004) Electroconvulsive therapy and determination of cerebral dominance. *Annals of General Hospital Psychiatry*, **3**, 14.

Duffett, R. & Lelliott, P. (1998) Auditing electroconvulsive therapy. *British Journal of Psychiatry*, **172**, 401–405.

Eranti, S. V. & McLoughlin, D. M. (2003) Electroconvulsive therapy – state of the art. *British Journal of Psychiatry*, **182**, 8–9.

Fergusson, G., Hendry, J. & Freeman, C. (2003) Do patients who receive electroconvulsive therapy in Scotland get better? *Psychiatric Bulletin*, **27**, 137–140.

Folstein, M., Folstein, S. & McHugh, P. (1975) Mini-Mental State. *Journal of Psychiatric Research*, **12**, 189–198.

Fox, H. A. (2001) Extended continuation and maintenance ECT for long-lasting episodes of major depression. *Journal of ECT*, **17**, 60–64.

Gagné, G. G., Furman, M. J., Carpenter, L. L., *et al* (2000) Efficacy of continuation ECT and antidepressant drugs compared to long-term antidepressants alone in depressed patients. *American Journal of Psychiatry*, **157**, 1960–1965.

Gregory, S., Shawcross, C. R. & Gill, D. (1985) The Nottingham ECT study. A double-blind comparison of bilateral, unilateral and simulated ECT in depressive illness. *British Journal of Psychiatry*, **146**, 520–554.

Jha, A. & Stein, G. (1996) Decreased efficacy of combined benzodiazepines and unilateral ECT in treatment of depression. *Acta Psychiatrica Scandinavica*, **94**, 101–104.

Jha, A. K., Stein, G. S. & Fenwick, P. (1996) Negative interaction between lithium and electroconvulsive therapy: a case–control study. *British Journal of Psychiatry*, **168**, 241–243.

Kellner, C. H., Pritchett, J. T., Beale, M. D., *et al* (1997) *Handbook of ECT*. Washington, DC: American Psychiatric Press.

Lauritzen, L., Odgaard, K., Clemmesen, L., *et al* (1996) Relapse prevention by means of paroxetine in ECT-treated patients with major depression: a comparison with imipramine and placebo in medium-term continuation therapy. *Acta Psychiatrica Scandinavica*, **94**, 241–251.

Marangell, L. B., Rush, A. J., George, M. S., *et al* (2002) Vagus nerve stimulation (VNS) for major depressive episodes: one year outcomes. *Biological Psychiatry*, **51**, 280–287.

Matthews, K. & Eljamel, M. S. (2003) Status of neurosurgery for mental disorder in Scotland – selective literature review and overview of current clinical activity. *British Journal of Psychiatry*, **182**, 404–411.

McCall, W., Reboussin, D. M., Weiner, R. D., *et al* (2000) Titrated moderately suprathreshold vs fixed high-dose right unilateral electroconvulsive therapy. *Archives of General Psychiatry*, **57**, 438–444.

Medical Research Council (1965) Clinical trial of the treatment of depressive illness. *British Medical Journal*, **i**, 881–886.

Meduna, L. J. (1934) Über experimentelle Campherepilepsie. *European Archives of Psychiatry and Clinical Neuroscience*, **102**, 333–339.

Miller, L. J. (1994) Use of electroconvulsive therapy during pregnancy. *Hospital and Community Psychiatry*, **45**, 444–450.

Mukherjee, S., Sackeim, H. A. & Schnur, D. B. (1994) Electroconvulsive therapy of acute manic episode: a review of 50 years' experience. *American Journal of Psychiatry*, **151**, 169–176.

Naguib, M. & Koorn, R. (2002) Interaction between psychotropics, anaesthetics and electroconvulsive therapy: implications for drug choice and patient management. *CNS Drugs*, **16**, 229–247.

NICE (National Institute for Clinical Excellence) (2003) *Guidance on the Use of Electroconvulsive Therapy*. Technology appraisal 59, April 2003. See www.nice.org.uk.

Pagnin, D., Queiroz, V. D., Pini, S., *et al* (2004) Efficacy of ECT in depression: a meta-analytic review. *Journal of ECT*, **20**, 13–20.

Petrides, G., Fink, M., Hussain, M., *et al* (2001) Electroconvulsive therapy remission rates in psychotic versus nonpsychotic depressed patients: a report from CORE. *Journal of ECT*, **17**, 244–253.

Pippard, J. (1992) Audit of electroconvulsive treatment in two National Health Service regions. *British Journal of Psychiatry*, **160**, 621–637.

Pippard, J. & Ellam, L. (1981) Electroconvulsive therapy in Great Britain: a report to the College. *British Journal of Psychiatry*, **139**, 563–568.

Rabheru, K. (2001) The use of electroconvulsive therapy in special patient populations. *Canadian Journal of Psychiatry*, **46**, 710–719.

Rose, D., Fleischmann, P., Wykes, T., *et al* (2003) Patients' perspective on electroconvulsive therapy: systematic review. *British Medical Journal*, **326**, 1363–1366.

Royal College of Psychiatrists (1995) *The ECT Handbook* (second report of the Royal College of Psychiatrists' Special Committee on ECT). Council Report 39. London: Royal College of Psychiatrists.

Royal College of Psychiatrists (2002) Guidelines for ECT anaesthesia: statement from the Royal College of Psychiatrists' Special Committee on ECT. *Psychiatric Bulletin*, **26**, 237–238.

Royal College of Psychiatrists (2003) *The ECT Accreditation Service (ECTAS) – Standards for the Administration of ECT*. London: Royal College of Psychiatrists. See www.rcpsych.ac.uk/cru.

Royal College of Psychiatrists (2005) *The ECT Handbook* (2nd edn). Council Report CR128. London: Royal College of Psychiatrists.

Sackeim, H. A., Decina, P., Kanzler, M., *et al* (1987) Effects of electrode placement on the efficacy of titrated low-dose ECT. *American Journal of Psychiatry*, **144**, 1449–1455.

Sackeim, H. A., Prudic, J., Devanand, D. P., *et al* (1993) Effects of stimulus intensity and electrode placement on the efficacy and cognitive effects of electroconvulsive therapy. *New England Journal of Medicine*, **328**, 839–846.

Sackeim, H. A., Prudic, J., Devanand, D. P., *et al* (2000) A prospective, randomised, double-blind comparison of bilateral and right unilateral electroconvulsive therapy at different stimulus intensities. *Archives of General Psychiatry*, **57**, 425–434.

Sackeim, H. A., Haskett, R. F., Mulsant, B. H., *et al* (2001) Continuation pharmacotherapy in the prevention of relapse following electroconvulsive therapy: a randomized controlled trial. *Journal of the American Medical Association*, **285**, 1299–1307.

Schloss, P. & Henn, F. A. (2004) New insights into the mechanisms of antidepressant therapy. *Pharmacological Therapy*, **102**, 47–60.

Scott, A. & Boddy, H. (2002) Induction agent in electroconvulsive therapy: a comparison of methohexitone and propofol. *Psychiatric Bulletin*, **26**, 455–457.

Sikdar, S., Kulhara, P., Avasthi, A., *et al* (1994) Combined chlorpromazine and electroconvulsive therapy in mania. *British Journal of Psychiatry*, **164**, 806–810.

Tew, J. D., Jr, Mulsant, B. H., Haskett, R. F., *et al* (2002) A randomized comparison of high-charge right unilateral electroconvulsive therapy and bilateral electroconvulsive therapy in older depressed patients who failed to respond to 5 to 8 moderate-charge right unilateral treatments. *Journal of Clinical Psychiatry*, **63**, 1102–1105.

UK ECT Review Group (2003) Efficacy and safety of electroconvulsive therapy in depressive disorders: a systematic review and meta-analysis. *Lancet*, **361**, 799–808.

van den Broek, W. W., de Lely, A., Mulder, P. G. H., *et al* (2004) Effects of antidepressant medication resistance on short-term response to electroconvulsive therapy. *Journal of Clinical Psychopharmacology*, **24**, 400–403.

Vothknecht, S., Kho, K. H., van Schaick, H. W., *et al* (2003) Effects of maintenance electroconvulsive therapy on cognitive functions. *Journal of ECT*, **19**, 151–157.

White, C. (2003) New guidance on electroconvulsive therapy looks set to curb its use. *BMJ*, **326**, 1003.

Zachrisson, O. C., Balldin, J., Ekman, R., *et al* (2000) No evident neuronal damage after electroconvulsive therapy. *Psychiatry Research*, **96**, 157–165.

CHAPTER 6

Psychological treatment of depression

Stirling Moorey

Psychosocial intervention, in its broadest sense, is a vital component in the management of all types of depression, from mild depressive reactions to psychotic episodes. Even if pharmacological therapy (Chapter 4) or electroconvulsive therapy (Chapter 5) is the main treatment, the way in which the clinician assesses and engages the patient, gives information about the illness and its treatment, and provides support contributes significantly to outcome. In addition to this basic level of supportive work, many patients will benefit from more structured forms of psychotherapy. This chapter considers the psychological therapies available for depression and the evidence for their effectiveness. Some general principles of psychological management of patients with depression are described.

Individual therapies

There are two broad approaches to therapy for patients with depression. First, there are therapies that aim to relieve depressive symptoms directly, such as cognitive, behavioural and interpersonal therapies. These problem-oriented therapies are used during the depressive phase itself, with or without accompanying antidepressants. In addition to relieving distress they also attempt to reduce vulnerability to relapse. The second approach, associated more with therapies derived from psychoanalysis, aims to resolve conflict and modify deeper personality structures. Treatments based on psychoanalytic theory are usually applied after the patient has recovered from the most severe part of the depressive episode.

Cognitive–behavioural therapy

Cognitive–behavioural therapy (CBT) is the psychological treatment for depression with the strongest evidence-base. There are several types of empirically validated CBT for depression, including problem-solving therapy, behaviour therapy, self-control therapy and social skills training, but the most well known is Beck's cognitive therapy (CT). This is based on Beck's cognitive model of depression (Beck *et al*, 1979), which states that depression is characterised by a negative bias in information processing.

Beck's theory is a tripartite one, consisting of cognitive structures (assumptions), which when activated bias cognitive processing (cognitive distortions) and produce depressive cognitions (automatic thoughts). In depression there is a *depressive cognitive triad*: a negative view of the self, the world and the future. Thus patients with depression believe themselves to be inadequate and worthless, their surroundings seem bleak and uninteresting, and the future seems hopeless. Interpretations of current events and predictions about future events are distorted. Beck identifies particular biases in information processing, called *cognitive distortions* or thinking errors (see Box 6.1). These often take the form of faulty inferences. One of the commonest thinking errors is 'overgeneralisation', where a single negative event is seen as the beginning of a never-ending pattern of defeats. For example, a person in a depressive state

Box 6.1 Thinking errors in depression

All-or-nothing thinking
You see things in black and white, missing all the shades of grey in between. If you are depressed you may think 'If I can't do everything I used to do, then there's no point in doing anything'. If you do less well than usual, you may think 'If I don't succeed, I must be a total failure'.

Overgeneralisation
From a single event (and therefore without a real factual basis), you predict an exaggerated, never-ending pattern of loss or defeat.

Magnification and selective attention
You focus on the negative aspects of the problem and selectively attend to them. You tend to filter out or disqualify more positive information. If you face an operation, for example, you neglect the likely benefits and instead dwell on the possible side-effects without remembering that they are extremely rare.

Arbitrary inference
Instead of looking at the evidence available, you jump to conclusions. For instance, if a loved one is late coming home you might conclude 'He's had an accident!'

Labelling
Here the distortion leads to a global, over-generalised negative view of yourself. You label yourself as hopeless, incompetent and invalid, or a victim.

may forget to buy some items at the supermarket, concludes from this that his memory is beginning to fail, and becomes convinced that he is facing an inexorable decline into senility.

The patient's distorted view of the world manifests itself as frequent *negative automatic thoughts*. These are spontaneous, plausible thoughts and images that enter the mind unbidden and are associated with unpleasant emotions. When viewed logically, they appear to be exaggerated and unrealistic. For instance, if criticised for a small mistake at work a patient might have the following negative automatic thoughts:

> Negative view of self: 'I'm stupid. This job's beyond me. I never get anything right.'
>
> Negative view of world: 'Nobody likes me here; I just don't fit in.'
>
> Negative view of future: 'What's the point? It's useless even trying. They'll give me the sack soon.'

Other symptoms of depression are derived from this cognitive bias: behavioural symptoms such as social withdrawal and low activity levels; loss of motivation and interest; and cognitive deficits such as poor concentration. Cognitive factors are not the cause of depression but mediate other factors, such as biological and environmental stressors and depressive symptoms. Two vicious circles maintain depression. First, depressed mood is associated with more depressive thinking, which distorts reality, in that the patient selectively attends to negative aspects of the environment and ignores or disqualifies positive information. This causes further depression and mood spirals downwards. Second, depressive thinking influences behaviour. The future looks hopeless and patients believe they are helpless and inadequate, so they give up trying to solve their problems and disengage from rewarding activities. This behavioural deactivation further depresses their mood and confirms their negative beliefs about themselves. Indeed, the interpersonal consequences of their depressive behaviour (friends being unsure of how to deal with them or partners becoming exasperated and critical) may confirm their negative self-image. Cognitive therapy is aimed at breaking into these vicious circles of negative thinking, depressed mood and maladaptive behaviour.

Vulnerability to depression is explained by the presence of *depressogenic schemas*. These are collections of idiosyncratic beliefs or rules derived from experiences in childhood and later life. At their root are unconditional core beliefs around the themes of helplessness and unlovability (e.g. 'I am inadequate'; 'I am unlovable'). More intermediate beliefs take the form of imperatives such as 'I must always be nice to people', or conditional statements such as 'I can be happy only if I'm a success at everything I do'.

Case example

A woman presenting with depression had experienced her parents' divorce at the age of six. She believed she was responsible for the break-up of the marriage and developed the assumption that she had to have the perfect marriage to make up for it. Whenever she got into a relationship this assumption was activated and she put so much effort into the affair that her partner backed off. She ended up rejected and depressed, feeling her negative beliefs about herself were correct.

Like many assumptions this one remained latent until activated by a critical event (the relationship), when its true maladaptive nature became apparent. It also illustrates the rigid, global and idiosyncratic characteristics of these silent rules. Often the conditional beliefs may protect the person from depression until a major life event occurs.

Case example

A policewoman had a set of beliefs that if she did everything within the rules she would never be criticised and her secret fear that she was inadequate would not be confirmed. When she was accused of wrongful arrest and her seniors did not support her, she became bewildered and deeply depressed because her rule system did not work.

Characteristics of cognitive therapy

Cognitive therapy aims to make patients their own therapist. The emphasis is on teaching patients both to identify problems and strategies for coping with and resolving them. The therapist is therefore more active and directive than in traditional psychotherapy, and the relationship is a collaborative partnership in problem solving. The focus is on how maladaptive thinking is maintaining current problems rather than the origins of these problems.

From the first session patients are told that the therapy is time limited and that it will involve learning and practising self-help skills, which the patient will be able to continue to use after therapy ends. In addressing their problems, patients are encouraged to distance themselves from their thoughts and beliefs and to see them as hypotheses which can be examined and tested, rather than facts set in stone. In challenging these maladaptive beliefs the therapist uses questioning and guided discovery, rather than confrontation. Box 6.2 summarises some of the techniques used in cognitive therapy.

Behavioural techniques in cognitive therapy

In the treatment of depression, behavioural assignments are important in the early stages since they often lead to a rapid improvement in mood. The tasks are set up as experiments for testing negative beliefs and predictions.

Case example

A patient believed his family would be better off without him because he was useless and a burden to them. The therapist was aware that his relatives were very supportive, so he encouraged the patient to test the belief by asking them if they did indeed feel they would be better off if he were dead. The response was a very moving, open display of affection from his grown-up children which they had not been able to show before. This convinced him that he was valued and needed, and led to a marked improvement in his mood.

Activities that give a sense of pleasure or achievement are particularly useful in raising mood. The therapist establishes what activities patients used to find rewarding and then helps them to plan these for each day. A daily activity schedule (Fig. 6.1) is used to log what is actually done and the degree of pleasure and mastery (achievement) are recorded. Sometimes tasks need to

Box 6.2 Cognitive therapy techniques

Behavioural techniques

Activity scheduling
Patients structure time to distract themselves from negative thoughts and to encourage pleasurable and rewarding activities.

Graded task assignment
Large or complex tasks are divided into smaller, readily achievable ones to give graded success experiences.

Mastery and pleasure ratings
Patients rate activities for mastery and pleasure on a 10-point scale. Tasks scoring high are scheduled more frequently over coming weeks.

Behavioural experiments
Homework tasks are assigned to test negative beliefs.

Cognitive techniques

Identifying negative automatic thoughts
Patients learn to monitor negative thoughts associated with exacerbation of depressed mood, and to link external event, thought and affect.

Challenging negative automatic thoughts
Patients keep a mood diary and replace negative thoughts with more realistic alternatives. There are various methods for challenging thoughts:

- labelling distortions
- reality testing
- searching for alternatives
- decatastrophising.

Preventive strategies: challenging assumptions
Underlying assumptions and core beliefs are challenged using a cost–benefit analysis followed by cognitive challenging and experimental behaviour change.

Relapse prevention
Risk factors for future relapses are identified and strategies for coping reviewed before the end of therapy.

be broken down into small, manageable steps so that they are more readily achievable, as many people with depression have very high expectations of themselves even when they are ill, and they set themselves up for failure. For instance, if a patient has a problem with concentration, a graded task programme would involve reading for increasing time spans, reading materials of increasing complexity and gradually increasing the amount of time spent on work-related activities. Success at a homework task helps to build self-esteem.

In grading a task, care must be given to ensuring the task is not too difficult for the patient. However, even if the patient is unable to carry out the assignment it is not considered a failure, but gives valuable information about the patient's negative thoughts.

Case example

A woman who had some difficulty deciding which problems she wanted to tackle in therapy was asked to write down three problems as homework and to fill out the assessment questionnaires. She came back feeling despairing that the therapy could not help her, because she had such difficulty in doing the homework. This gave information about the degree of her problems with concentration and decision making; the therapist used her catastrophic reaction (based on the thought 'If I can't do this homework it means the therapy can't help me') to show her how she was overgeneralising from the failure on one task to conclude that she would never get anything out of cognitive therapy.

Strategies for changing cognition

Cognitive interventions are aimed at helping patients to identify and change the cognitive processes that are at the centre of their depression. This can be seen as a three-step process.

Step 1. Teaching the model

In the early stages of therapy patients are introduced to the cognitive model of emotion, and their problems are conceptualised using this framework. They are shown how their problems are part of the depressive syndrome, and the central role of negative thinking in depression is illustrated. The link between events, cognitions and emotion is described and patients are encouraged to look at how this fits in with their own experiences.

Rate activities (0–10) for mastery and pleasure.							
Time	Monday	Tuesday	Wednesday	Thursday	Friday	Saturday	Sunday
9–10 Activity							
Mastery							
Pleasure							

Fig. 6.1 Weekly activity schedule. (Only the first hour of the morning is shown here, by way of illustration, when in fact the schedule would extend to cover the whole day.)

Situation	Emotions *(rate 0–10)*	Automatic thoughts *(rate 0–10)*	Alternative response *(rate 0–10)*	Action plan *(rate 0–10)*

Fig. 6.2 Dysfunctional thought record.

For instance, patients may be asked to recall a day during the week when the depression was more severe, then asked what events might have triggered this exacerbation. The negative interpretation of the situation will then demonstrate how negative thinking increases depressed mood. If the patient became more depressed after a friend did not return a telephone call, say, a link might be found between this trigger and negative thoughts such as 'She's not interested in me; if I was worth anything people would want to be with me. I must be boring.' The material from behavioural assignments is often used to illustrate the model. For example, when thinking about a task the patient may say 'I won't be able to do it' or 'There's no point in trying'. The link between these negative thoughts and depressed mood and lack of motivation can then be demonstrated. A booklet outlining the model and form of therapy (*Coping with Depression*, by Beck & Greenberg, 1974) is often given at the first session to reinforce the discussion within the session.

Step 2. Identifying negative automatic thoughts

Once patients understand the basic concepts involved, the next step is to identify their repetitive automatic thoughts. Initially the therapist elicits negative automatic thoughts in the session, and then the patient records instances of these as homework. A daily form monitoring upsetting events, associated emotions and intervening thoughts can be used to structure this exercise (Fig. 6.2). Even if the mood disorder is pervasive, there is usually a fluctuation with everyday events, and noticing this change is a step towards gaining control over the mood. Naming the type of distortions in thinking can be helpful at this stage (see Box 6.1) and this can be given as a handout to the patient. Most patients, if they are given clear instructions about how to monitor thoughts, with examples, can catch their thoughts with a little practice. If they have difficulty, their thoughts about the monitoring itself can be examined. This may reveal negative thoughts about the therapist despising them if they reveal themselves, fear of exposing themselves to painful cognitions, or thoughts about the whole exercise being pointless. Once these cognitions are identified they can be challenged with the usual cognitive techniques.

Step 3. Challenging negative automatic thoughts

As the behavioural work helps to lift the patient's mood and he or she becomes familiar with automatic thoughts, the therapy moves into a more cognitive mode. From session 1, the therapist has used cognitive techniques to question the reality of the patient's negative thinking. Now the patient learns to do this, recording the automatic thoughts as they occur and challenging them with rational responses. The aim is not to think positively, but to subject thoughts and beliefs to reality testing, and thus overcome the depressive bias. This is known as cognitive restructuring. Several techniques are commonly used to challenge automatic thoughts. Patients can be taught to ask these as the following types of question:

- *What's the evidence?* This represents one of the core cognitive techniques. It could be argued that the whole of cognitive therapy is about helping the patient to stop accepting thoughts at face value and instead to always ask the question 'What's my evidence?' A simple way of doing this is to draw a line down the centre of a piece of paper and list on one side the evidence for and on the other side the evidence against a particular belief. If you were a psychiatrist with depression you might have the automatic thought 'I'm incompetent: I can't do my job properly'. Table 6.1 sets out the

Table 6.1 Example responses to the negative automatic thought 'I'm incompetent: I can't do my job properly'

Evidence for the thought	Evidence against the thought
I keep putting off writing that court report	I know I'm depressed at the moment, and my concentration and motivation are badly affected by that
I can't concentrate when talking to my patients	Until six months ago I never had any problems with my work
My colleagues seem to look down on me	I know I'm not the only person to procrastinate
I've taken weeks off work lately and I'm letting people down	I've no evidence that my colleagues really look down on me – I'm just making assumptions. In fact, I know they value me for my contributions because they have told me so in the past
	Taking time off work is not a sign of incompetence
	No one has ever criticised my work or complained about my efficiency

possible responses within the framework of cognitive therapy. With practice this questioning of evidence becomes automatic and gradually challenges the ingrained negative bias in the patient's thinking.

- *What alternative views are there?* Alternative interpretations of an event are considered. The depressed person usually chooses the most negative interpretation of an event and automatically assumes this is correct. The therapist teaches the patient to generate alternatives. At first these are also quite negative, but as more and more alternatives are asked for by the therapist the patient is forced to think of more positive ones. This starts to break up the depressive bias in interpretations. After practising in the session patients are able to question their immediate response to situations in the outside world. For instance, if a friend passes the patient in the street, rather than automatically thinking 'He's deliberately ignoring me', the patient starts to consider other explanations, such as 'He's busy and he probably didn't notice me'. The likelihood of these various explanations being correct can then be assessed, and a less biased judgement made about the situation.
- *What are the advantages and disadvantages of this way of thinking?* Even if a negative thought is accurate, it is not necessarily helpful. Looking at the usefulness of a belief or thought can help to change it. In this exercise the patient can list the advantages and disadvantages of the negative belief or thought. Ruminations about real-life problems such as unemployment, loss, or even impending death may be accurate reflections of reality, but in depression they rarely lead to effective problem-solving or emotional working through. In fact, they have the disadvantage of making people feel worse, preventing them from engaging in life and even alienating them from loved ones. Once patients see these disadvantages they are often able to reduce the frequency of these thoughts themselves, or to use distraction techniques.
- *If my interpretation is correct, are things as catastrophic as they seem?* Patients who are anxious and depressed often catastrophise, but rarely think beyond the catastrophe. Facing up to the worst fear often reveals that it is not as terrible as it seems, or that the person has the resources to cope with it. For example, a depressed student convinced he will fail an examination can explore what would actually happen if he did. He may never have even thought about the fact that he would be able to retake them again without any bad effect on his career.

Preventive strategies

These are aimed at changing the underlying assumptions about the world that make people vulnerable to psychological problems. The same cognitive change techniques that are applied to thoughts can be used with assumptions. Evidence for and against the reasonableness of each assumption is sought, the advantages and disadvantages of the assumption explored and its origins plotted. Finally a more flexible, less punitive rule is developed and behavioural assignments set so the patient can experiment with acting differently. The final sessions of therapy usually involve some preparation for the future, with the discussion of relapse prevention strategies.

Case example

A patient had a very negative relationship with her mother, who had been critical and rejecting throughout her childhood. A typical painful memory was of her mother refusing to give her a goodnight kiss. The one way she did get acceptance was through achievement, and the patient developed the rule that she must do things perfectly or she would be rejected. A specific example of this rule applied in her relationship with her partner: she believed completely that if she was not a perfect partner, giving no cause for criticism, her lover would eventually leave her. The reality and usefulness of this assumption was challenged in the session. Then the patient showed her partner the beliefs she had written down. She was astonished to find that her partner did not agree with her at all, and in fact had a more flexible rule that no one was perfect, and it was healthy to have the occasional row about the irritating things the other person did. As a result her belief in this diminished greatly, and with help from the therapist she began gradually to give up her perfectionistic view of relationships.

Efficacy of cognitive–behavioural therapy

Cognitive–behavioural therapy has been compared with no-treatment and waiting-list controls in several studies. The results consistently show a significant advantage of therapy over no treatment. Numerous studies have compared the use of Beck's cognitive therapy with the use of tricyclic antidepressants for out-patients with depression (Box 6.3). All these studies found that cognitive therapy was as effective as drug treatment (for reviews see DeRubeis & Crits Cristoph, 1998; Deckersbach *et al*, 2000). In mild–moderate acute depression the combination of cognitive therapy with antidepressants does not seem to be more effective than giving the treatments individually. For in-patients with more severe depression, however, combined cognitive therapy and medication is more effective than medication alone (Stuart & Bowers, 1995) and this may also be the case for chronic depression (Keller *et al*, 2000).

There is evidence to suggest that cognitive therapy may reduce relapse rates when compared with antidepressant medication when both are withdrawn after

Box 6.3 Cognitive–behavioural therapy and antidepressant medication

- Cognitive–behavioural therapy is as effective as antidepressants in out-patient depression.
- The combination of cognitive–behavioural therapy and antidepressants may be more effective than either alone in severe (in-patient) and chronic depression.
- The combination of cognitive–behavioural therapy and medication in mild–moderate (out-patient) depression is not more effective than either alone.
- When both treatments are withdrawn, relapse rates are lower after cognitive–behavioural therapy than after antidepressants.
- When combined with maintenance medication, cognitive–behavioural therapy further reduces relapse rates.

3 months (26% in the cognitive therapy group versus 64% in the medication condition) and that this effect may persist over a 2-year follow-up (Deckersbach *et al*, 2000). More recent studies have compared cognitive therapy with maintenance medication. For partially recovered out-patients, adding cognitive therapy to maintenance medication leads to a greater reduction in relapse rates than maintenance medication alone (Paykel *et al*, 1999). In recurrent depression, maintenance cognitive therapy has a similar effect to maintenance medication (Blackburn & Moore, 1997).

Comparisons of cognitive therapy with behavioural therapy have not shown one approach to be superior. Jacobson *et al* (1996) dismantled the components of cognitive therapy for depression into: behavioural activation; behavioural activation plus cognitive restructuring; and the full package. Patients were randomly allocated to the three groups and all three types of therapy proved equally effective. They also had similar effects on relapse rates at follow-up.

The National Institute for Clinical Excellence has published guidance on the use of cognitive–behavioural therapy in depression (NICE, 2004) and this is summarised below.

The NICE (2004) recommendations

In parallel with the huge database on antidepressants from randomised controlled trials (RCTs), there has been a substantial increase in the number of psychotherapy trials in depression, mostly focusing on cognitive–behavioural therapy. The NICE (2004) review contains an extensive number of meta-analyses of these studies and it would be quite beyond the scope of this chapter to present anything but a summary of these findings. Box 6.4 lists those recommendations based on level A evidence (at least one RCT or meta-analysis of RCTs) and level B evidence (good controlled studies); the recommendations at level C (expert opinions but not trial data) have not been included. The NICE reviewers point out that studies that compare the different psychotherapies (cognitive–behavioural therapy, interpersonal therapy, dynamic therapy, behavioural therapy) usually fail to show any differences in efficacy and so, although the bulk of the research and recommendations apply specifically to cognitive–behavioural therapy, other types of therapy may be equally useful.

Box 6.4 NICE (2004) recommendations for CBT in depression

Level A recommendations (based on one or more randomised controlled trials or a meta-analysis)

1 For moderate or severe depression, antidepressant medication should be offered to all patients before psychological interventions.
2 Patients with chronic depression should be offered a combination of cognitive–behavioural therapy and antidepressants.

Level B recommendations (based on good controlled studies, but not randomised controlled trials)

3 Patients with moderate or severe depression should be offered 16–20 sessions of cognitive–behavioural therapy extending over 6–9 months.
4 Patients with mild to moderate depression should be considered for 6–8 sessions of cognitive–behavioural therapy, counselling or problem solving extending over 10–12 weeks.
5 Cognitive–behavioural therapy should be offered to patients who express a personal preference for it, who are refractory to antidepressants, who refuse medication or who are especially fearful of the side-effects of medication (e.g. because of a previous bad experience).
6 Cognitive–behavioural therapy may have a role in relapse prevention. Thus, it should be offered to those who relapse after stopping antidepressants. Cognitive–behavioural therapy should also be offered to those who have had three or more previous episodes (even though they may be well at the time) as this may reduce the risk of relapse.
7 Patients whose depression has responded well to cognitive–behavioural therapy should be given a further 2–4 sessions over the next 12 months as maintenance.
8 Where a patient or therapist prefers interpersonal therapy, this may be offered instead of cognitive–behavioural therapy.

Interpersonal therapy

Interpersonal therapy is a treatment that was developed by Weissman and Klerman in the New Haven–Boston Collaborative Depression Project. It is a brief (12–16 weeks) weekly treatment originally devised for out-patients with non-psychotic unipolar depression, and focuses on improving the patient's interpersonal functioning.

Theoretical framework

Interpersonal therapy is based on the assumption that psychosocial and interpersonal factors are of major significance in the development and maintenance of depression, and possibly contribute to vulnerability to further episodes. Two main areas of empirical evidence support the contention that problems with social roles are important in depression. First, there is strong evidence that interpersonal relations are impaired in depression and research shows that people with depression behave in a way that elicits negative responses from others. Although these findings may be a result rather than a cause of the depression, their role in maintenance and relapse may still be significant. Second, research on social stresses and social support has shown that a close confiding relationship with a spouse is a buffer against depression (Brown & Harris, 1978).

Interpersonal therapy sees all roles, in the nuclear and extended family, work, friendship and the community, as having a potential buffering effect against depression. Thus, any disruption of these roles may lead to depression. This psychosocial contribution will interact with the effects of biological factors to produce the final common pathway to depression.

Four main problem areas are defined and become the focus of treatment:

- grief
- role transitions
- interpersonal disputes
- interpersonal deficits.

Clinical application of interpersonal therapy

This section can give only a brief description of the techniques used in interpersonal therapy. A manual describing the therapy in detail has been published (Weissman *et al*, 2000).

Like cognitive therapy, interpersonal therapy is a here-and-now therapy. Current relationships rather than childhood experiences are the focus of attention. The therapeutic techniques are eclectic, incorporating reassurance, clarification of emotional states, improvement of communication and reality testing of perceptions and performance. These methods are used to achieve two main goals: the alleviation of depressive symptoms; and the development of strategies for dealing with the interpersonal problems associated with the depressive episode.

Managing the depressive state

This phase is supportive and educational. Patients are educated about the nature of depression. The therapist reviews all the patient's symptoms and describes how they are all part of a syndrome of depression, which is a well-recognised and treatable condition. Information is then given about the prevalence of the condition. Hopelessness may be directly addressed by informing patients that their belief that they will never recover is part of the depressive syndrome, just like symptoms of weight loss or sleep disturbance. Symptom management is another component of this phase and is similar in many ways to the behavioural techniques used in cognitive therapy. Situations that exacerbate the depression are identified and strategies devised to avoid them or reduce their impact. For instance, if the patient feels worse when alone, measures for increasing social contact can be explored; or if the patient is overwhelmed at work he or she may be helped to reduce expectations and plan essential tasks. Antidepressant medication may be considered in this symptom-reduction phase.

Targeting interpersonal problem areas

Once there has been some reduction in the patient's depressive symptoms, the therapist adopts a more interpersonal focus. The initial assessment will show which of the four interpersonal problem areas are affected, and one or two of these will be dealt with in therapy. If an unresolved grief reaction is part of the problem the therapist will help the patient to mourn by expressing feelings about the lost person, particularly suppressed anger, to reconstruct more realistically the relationship and finally to go on to re-establish interests and new relationships. The last stage may involve the prescription of quite specific tasks, such as joining social organisations. Dealing with role transitions involves a similar approach to handling the loss, plus developing a more positive attitude to the new role. Interpersonal role disputes most frequently occur with the spouse. During treatment the patient is helped to identify the dispute and to make choices about a plan of action, and is then encouraged to modify maladaptive patterns of communication. Interpersonal therapy works individually with the patient to change either the patient's or the spouse's behaviour, or to change the patient's attitude to the problem. Finally, interpersonal deficits may contribute to depression. Social isolation, lack of social skills, or low self-esteem may all be present. Interpersonal therapy reviews past relationship problems and adopts problem solving and role play to develop social skills. The therapeutic relationship is also used as a vehicle for demonstrating and working with interpersonal problems in the session.

Efficacy of interpersonal therapy

There have been fewer outcome studies of interpersonal therapy than of cognitive therapy. In one of the earliest studies (Weissman *et al*, 1974, 1979) women with depression who had responded to 4–6 weeks of treatment with amitriptyline were randomly allocated to maintenance treatment with amitriptyline, placebo or no medication, and then either received once-monthly (i.e. low-contact) or weekly interpersonal therapy. Antidepressant medication reduced the relapse rate and prevented symptom return, but had no impact on social functioning. Interpersonal therapy had little effect on symptoms, but had a significant effect on social functioning. In a second study (DiMascio *et al*, 1979) drugs and interpersonal therapy both had effects on symptoms and the combination produced the greatest improvement. Sequential therapy, in which interpersonal therapy is offered to all patients and then antidepressant medication is added for those who do not recover, leads to a remission rate of 79% (Frank *et al*, 2000).

Comparison of cognitive therapy and interpersonal therapy

The promising results of trials using cognitive and interpersonal therapy encouraged the US National Institute of Mental Health (NIMH) to set up a multicentre project to compare the two treatments with pharmacotherapy (Elkin *et al*, 1989). Two hundred and fifty patients were randomly assigned to four treatments:

1 cognitive–behavioural therapy

2 interpersonal therapy

3 imipramine plus clinical management

4 placebo plus clinical management.

The two psychotherapies were based on manuals and controlled for quality. The clinical management consisted of minimal supportive therapy sessions of 20–30 minutes' duration over 16 weeks. Patients in all groups showed a significant reduction in symptoms over the course of treatment. There were no significant differences between therapies, although there was a consistent ordering of treatments, with the active drug doing best, placebo worst and the two psychotherapies coming somewhere in between. A *post hoc* analysis on subgroups with severe and mild depression found no significant differences for the less severely depressed group, but in the more severely depressed group there was some evidence for the specific effectiveness of imipramine and, to a lesser extent, of interpersonal therapy. Comparison of four randomised trials of cognitive therapy and drugs in severe depression failed to confirm this superiority of antidepressants (DeRubeis *et al*, 1999).

In reviewing the evidence for interpersonal and cognitive therapy as relapse prevention strategies, Paykel (2001) concluded that:

> 'trials of interpersonal therapy in the prevention of recurrence show some benefit, but effects are weaker than those of drug[s] and additional benefit in combination is limited. There is better evidence for effects of cognitive therapy in preventing relapse and an emerging indication for its addition to antidepressants, particularly where residual symptoms are present.'

Psychodynamic therapy

Cognitive therapy and interpersonal therapy were designed to treat the depressive syndrome. They focus on problems and symptoms. In contrast to this, therapies derived from psychoanalysis are not primarily concerned with changing symptoms. They seek to bring about a more radical change of personality or a resolution of unconscious conflicts. Depression is seen as a manifestation of an underlying disturbance, and recovery from depression does not mean that the true underlying disturbance has been modified. A distinction should be made between *psychoanalysis* (a highly specialised form of psychotherapy carried out three to five times weekly for years, where the therapist adopts a deliberately impersonal and passive stance) and *psychoanalytically oriented* therapies (which generally last 3–12 months, with once-weekly sessions and a more active therapeutic stance). While individual psychoanalysis provides many insights and hypotheses about depression, there is no place for it as a treatment in the National Health Service.

There is no single psychodynamic model of depression but rather a corpus of theoretical writings which build on each other to develop and expand various themes (see Karasu, 1990, for a succinct description of psychodynamic models of depression). Freud (1917) was the first to point out the similarities between depressive reactions and grief reactions. He suggested that the patient with depression has high dependency needs for a parental figure, with consequent ambivalent feelings (love mixed with anger and frustration because of the dependency). In depression the loss of a real or imagined object results in an introjection of the lost object (i.e. an internal unconscious representation of the lost person as an attempt to avoid the real loss). The anger towards this object then becomes unleashed on the ego itself, resulting in depression. Freud believed the patient's self-reproaches were not really anger at the self but an indirect attack on the lost loved object. Similar themes can be found in subsequent psychoanalytic theories: loss, internal objects, dependence and ambivalence, and anger directed at the self (see page 59).

Present-day theories (notably object relations theory), influenced by the work of Klein, Bowlby and Winnicott, see depression as primarily an *interpersonal* problem, resulting from conflict, confusion or deficit in the person's internal representations of significant others. Although different metaphors may be used, they share the idea that, as children, we build up working models of ourselves and other people derived from repeated interactions with our carers. If there is an absence of loving, consistent parenting through loss, abandonment or lack of affective response, the child will not develop a sufficiently caring and soothing set of internal representations to call upon in times of crisis. Parental figures may be represented in the internal world as harshly critical, absent or unpredictable and the child's rage against them may be disavowed because of guilt or fear of the consequences of rejection. Adult experiences of loss or failure may evoke these unresolved developmental representations and the conflict can lead to anger being directed at the self, which would explain the self-criticism and self-hatred seen in many depressive states.

For all psychoanalytically oriented treatment, the relationship between the patient and therapist is the major vehicle for change. As treatment progresses the patient becomes dependent on the therapist, recapitulating past relationships. Treatment involves interpreting the links between the patient–therapist relationship and early childhood relationships. Therapy often involves helping the patient to see how this dependence and attachment extends to various ongoing relationships, and to uncover the underlying ambivalence and anger. Patients work through these feelings to a point where they can establish a view of themselves as their own person.

Short-term, focused psychotherapies modify analytic technique. The therapy is brief (15–30 sessions), the therapist is more active and techniques tend to be more confrontational. Therapy often focuses on the defensive manoeuvres used by the patient to evade feelings of anger and disappointment aroused by the therapist not being a perfect replacement for the lost or faulty parental figures of the past (Karasu, 1990).

Evidence for the effectiveness of long-term psychodynamic therapy in depression is scant. Until recently, psychoanalysts generally eschewed objective or symptom-based measurement of their work and randomised trials of psychoanalysis have not been conducted. Short-term dynamic therapy has been set out in manuals and shown to be effective in depression. Direct comparisons between short-term dynamic therapy and cognitive–behavioural therapy have not demonstrated one to be superior to the other (Leichsenring, 2001), but meta-analyses of treatment studies tend to show a greater effect for the latter (DeRubeis & Crits Cristoph, 1998).

Group and systemic therapies

One of the themes running through much depression research is the relevance of interpersonal factors to both an initial vulnerability to depression and its subsequent maintenance. There is therefore a rationale for using group therapy in depression and some empirical evidence to support this contention: in a meta-analysis of group therapy for depression it was found that treated patients were better off than 85% of untreated controls (McDermut *et al*, 2001).

All forms of individual therapy can be applied in groups, which have the advantage of treating more patients for a given input of therapist time. Cognitive–behavioural groups tend to be structured and educational in nature, and little attention is paid to group dynamics. A good example of this psycho-educational model is Lewinsohn's 'Coping with Depression Course' (Antonuccio, 1998). This approach is probably appropriate for out-patients with straightforward depression but may be less easy to apply to chronic depression or patients with personality disorders. Overall, results suggest that cognitive–behavioural therapy is as efficacious when given in groups as it is when given individually (Morrison, 2001).

Skills-based groups (e.g. for social skills and assertiveness training) can be used as an adjunct to other treatments. The indication for these treatments will depend upon the problems identified at assessment. Many people with depression have long-standing difficulties with assertiveness, and tend to suppress their own wishes and try excessively to accommodate and please others. This may predispose them to depression, and assertiveness training can help to make them less vulnerable to depression in the future.

Two other approaches to group work are the psychodynamic group, which applies psychoanalytic principles to the group setting, and the interpersonal approach, pioneered by Yalom (1985), which emphasises 'here and now' experiences. In a group, the members' relationship with the therapist can provide valuable interpersonal learning. The therapist's realistic, supportive and tolerant attitude replaces the patient's harsh self-criticism, and allows the members to treat themselves in a gradually more accepting way (in analytic terms, the members internalise the therapist's more tolerant superego, which replaces the punitive superego of the patient with depression). The group also allows patients to express guilt and hostile feelings in a supportive atmosphere.

The effectiveness of this type of group work in patients with active depression has not been evaluated. An eclectic, interpersonal form of group therapy is often used with hospital in-patients. Ward groups are frequently led by inexperienced therapists, with little supervision. Group psychotherapy with in-patients demands quite specialist skills and modifications of techniques used with out-patients. Because in-patients with depression may show psychomotor retardation, their capacity to engage in group work is limited. In-patient groups need to be less challenging, less demanding and more focused than out-patient groups. Group therapy has more to offer after the resolution of the acute depressive phase. Patients can then explore and change interpersonal patterns that predispose to depression. Groups can also function as vehicles for support for people with chronic depression.

Like group therapy, couples therapy and family therapy are modes of delivery rather than specific models of therapy. Cognitive, behavioural and psychodynamic forms of therapy all exist, but they have as their focus the naturally occurring systems within which the depression develops. They all have in common the assumption that the interactional patterns in the family contribute to depression and can be used as a vehicle for change. Interactional patterns may include complementary role fits between a dependent partner with depression and a controlling caring partner, or problems in distance regulation in the family. Evidence exists for the effectiveness of couples therapy in women with depression with critical spouses (Leff *et al*, 2000).

Principles of psychological management

Two major themes run through the psychological literature on depression and its treatment. One is the cognitive–behavioural axis, on which there is substantial evidence that patients with depression show behavioural deficits and cognitive abnormalities. The other is the interpersonal axis. Critical losses of important relationships or current relationship difficulties are closely related to depression. These two lines of research and the treatment associated with them should inform the psychiatrist's clinical management of the patient. No research has yet been done on the application of these techniques in a traditional out-patient psychiatric consultation. Antidepressant medication is likely to be the main treatment modality used by the psychiatrist for out-patients, but even in a series of 15–30-minute consultations at monthly intervals it is possible to apply psychological understandings and interventions.

Psychological aspects of the assessment process

The process of taking a history and assessing mental state can be therapeutic in its own right if it is done in a sensitive and respectful manner. To be able to tell your story and to have someone empathically listen is helpful. The assessment can challenge beliefs such as 'I'm the only person like this' and 'No one can understand me'.

A problem-oriented assessment can be more beneficial than one that simply focuses on symptoms. Defining problems and drawing up lists of them can help to diminish the idea that depression is overwhelming, and can start to engender hope. Problems that the patient considers important may become the focus of therapeutic work. For instance, if insomnia is particularly worrying for the patient, identifying this as a problem could lead to selection of an appropriate antidepressant or the giving of information and advice about sleep hygiene. Risk assessment is obviously a primary concern at this stage. If a suicide risk is identified, then this should be the primary focus for any psychological work done in the first consultations. At the end of the assessment a diagnostic formulation which both names the disorder as depression and provides some understanding of how biological and psychosocial factors interact to make the person depressed right now can help to give meaning to the patient's experience, and encourage trust.

Engaging the patient and maintaining the therapeutic relationship

Challenging hopelessness

Trust and hope are the most important concerns in establishing a helping relationship with a patient in a depressed state. Hopelessness has been shown to correlate more strongly with suicide risk than severity

Table 6.2 Example of a patient's cost–benefit analysis of suicide

Reasons for dying	Reasons for living
This feeling will never go	My mother would be devastated if I killed myself
No one cares if I live or die	I've been told I'll feel better
I'll never pay off my debts	Once I kill myself it's final
I'm useless and I might as well admit it	I'm trying a new medication, which might work
It will be a way out of the pain	I haven't always felt I'm useless: perhaps this will pass
	I might be able to get help with my debts

of depression, so interventions that engender hope are of particular importance in the early stages of consultation. Traditionally, psychiatrists have used their status as knowledgeable professionals as well as reassurance and the giving of information to instil hope in the patient. In addition to this there are some cognitive techniques which may be of help in this setting:

Cost–benefit analysis of suicide
In actively suicidal patients, considering reasons for dying and reasons for living both gives information about the risk of self-harm and can engender hope. The process involves first asking the patient for all the reasons why life is not worth living. It is important to do this before looking at the reasons for living because otherwise the psychiatrist will be seen as yet another person trying to convince the patient to think positively about a hopeless situation. Asking for more reasons for suicide will eventually take the person to the point at which no more advantages can be listed; this realisation that there is a finite limit to the reasons can be therapeutic. Then a list of reasons for living can be placed alongside the reasons for dying. An example is shown in Table 6.2. By focusing on the benefits of living and establishing whether there are alternative ways out of the apparently hopeless situation, the clinician can often help the patient to feel more hopeful that it is worth holding on.

Review of past depressive episodes and periods of euthymia
People who are depressed and also people who self-harm have deficits in their problem-solving ability and distortions in their autobiographical memory. It is difficult for them to gain access to specific positive memories to dispel their pessimistic view of the future. The psychiatrist can help by asking focused questions about the past, such as the following:

- Have you always felt this way, or were there times when you were not depressed?
- How long did your last depression last?
- Did you feel as hopeless then as you do now?
- What did you do to recover?
- Could the same things work again?
- What would you have said to me about your life last year, before you became depressed?
- What are the strengths you have when well?
- How could we help you find them again?

Time projection
Negative thoughts about the future prevent the patient from thinking beyond the present. Asking what life might be like when the patient recovers from depression gives the message that there is a future and gets the patient thinking about it as a definite possibility. A time projection exercise can help patients elaborate on what life might be like in a year's time or 2 years' time, when their depression has remitted. Identifying possible goals for the future and looking at ways to achieve them can also engender hope.

The therapeutic relationship

The doctor–patient relationship is important in the management of all psychiatric disorders. In depression the doctor needs to achieve a balance between under- and over-involvement with the patient. Too distant a stance will fail to engage the patient and confirm the person's view that he or she is isolated and not understood. Over-involvement can lead the psychiatrist to 'buy into' the negative world view of the person with depression, and see the situation as hopeless and overwhelming. A warm, friendly, supportive and empathic manner is necessary, but this needs to be balanced with objectivity and professionalism. The patient's negative bias may influence the therapeutic relationship. He or she may think, 'He's not interested in me; I'm boring'. These automatic thoughts about the therapist can be checked out periodically and corrected with appropriate information.

Psychodynamic theory can inform the clinician of transference phenomena that may interfere with the supportive relationship. The patient's ambivalence over important relationships means that the psychiatrist is likely to be perceived as both hostile and punishing as well as nurturing at various times. Negative thoughts may be associated with a transference in which the therapist is seen as critical. When a good rapport exists, the therapist may be idealised and a dependent transference may develop. This, and the patient's sensitivity to loss, means that cancellations of appointments, holidays and so on may be particularly difficult.

The psychiatrist should also be aware of how his or her own feelings to the patient may be a sign of 'countertransference', which may be elicited when the therapist is drawn into a reciprocal role, playing unconsciously a real or fantasised relationship from the patient's childhood (e.g. the role of a critical parent). Strong feelings of anger, wanting to punish or get rid of the patient, or alternatively urges to look after or rescue the patient, are indications of possible countertransference reactions. If these occur the clinician should discuss the patient with a colleague or obtain supervision.

Education about depression and medication

Education can be invaluable in giving the patient a sense of hope and trust in the clinician. The negative cognitive bias in depression can lead to misinterpretation of symptoms: lack of motivation and loss of energy are seen as signs of weakness, failure or laziness, and so create a syndrome of 'depression about depression'. Giving the person information about depression can dispel these self-criticisms:

1 depression is a syndrome with characteristic symptoms

2 depression is associated with negative views of the self, experience and the future

3 depression is treatable.

Similarly, education about the side-effects of medication prevents misattribution of symptoms and improves compliance (see Chapter 4). Many patients expect antidepressants to work immediately, and if they are not told otherwise become disillusioned and may give up taking the drugs before they can take effect. The treatment plan should be explained to the patient and the rationale for any intervention given.

Fatigue, poor concentration and a negative bias may all contribute to difficulties in decision making and impairment of work performance. It is therefore wise to advise patients not to make any major life decisions and to delay large, difficult tasks until the depression has lifted.

It is vital to check the patient's understanding of the information given. In severe depression, impairment of concentration may reduce the amount that is taken in, and even in less severe cases misunderstandings can occur. Information leaflets, books and websites can all reinforce the message that depression is a common, treatable disorder that need not carry a stigma. Some self-help books for patients are listed under 'Utilising specific change techniques', below.

Interviewing family members

Partners, friends and relatives can not only give information about the patient and his or her relationships, but can also be directly involved in treatment. Education about the nature of depression can be helpful for them too. If the relationship is good, the partner can be used as a co-therapist. If the relationship is poor, some simple work on communication combined with education about the nature of depression may be helpful. In assessing relationship problems, think of the four problem areas focused on in interpersonal therapy, listed above: grief, role transitions, interpersonal disputes and interpersonal deficits.

Utilising specific change techniques

Cognitive–behavioural techniques

It is obviously not possible to carry out a full course of cognitive–behavioural therapy in a busy out-patient setting where time is limited, but some simple techniques can be used. These are best instituted in conjunction with a self-help programme. There is growing evidence for the effectiveness of cognitive–behavioural therapy delivered through books and computer self-help programmes (Williams, 2001*a*). Psychiatrists should have a supply of these materials for use with out-patients. Some of these books are workbooks which give exercises for patients to follow (e.g. *The Feeling Good Handbook*, Burns 1999; *Mind Over Mood*, Greenberger & Padesky, 1995; *Overcoming Depression*, Williams, 2001*b*). The psychiatrist can select chapters from these books to work on between appointments. Behavioural techniques may be easier for psychiatrists with no formal training in cognitive–behavioural therapy to use in brief out-patient sessions. The self-monitoring, activity scheduling and graded task assignment described above can easily be incorporated into the psychiatric interview, particularly when integrated with a self-help book. Patients can also be taught simple problem-solving skills. *Overcoming Depression* (Williams, 2001*b*) has a good module on this method.

Guidance and advice

Sometimes more direct guidance and advice can be helpful. A good assessment may indicate activities that can be discouraged (e.g. a patient with depression visiting a friend who overloads her with her own problems) and which encouraged.

In the long run, larger environmental changes may be indicated, such as moving house, changing job, divorce or medical retirement. Sometimes it may be clear that environmental stresses are maintaining the depression, and the psychiatrist can contribute by helping to remove them.

Case example

A patient presented one month after a cot death with severe depression and suicidal thoughts. She reported that she was unable to go into the room in which the baby had died. Despite classical biological features of depression she refused antidepressant medication and confided little in her community psychiatric nurse. She insisted that the only thing that would help her would be for the local authority to arrange a move to another flat. The psychiatrist wrote a letter strongly supporting such a move and once the patient had moved she felt considerably better.

The following case of a depressed police officer in a stressful job illustrates the therapeutic role of medical retirement.

Case example

A 47-year-old Flying Squad officer worked in a very stressful job which involved waiting in banks that were thought to be the target of robberies. His teenage daughter had become delinquent because he was away for considerable periods of time, quite unpredictably, as part of his job. He presented with a classical depressive syndrome but once he had been off sick for a month he felt quite unable to return to his previous work. The psychiatrist offered to support retirement on medical grounds, and once this had been arranged his depression cleared completely, indicating that the underlying cause had been great fear associated with his stressful job and the destructive effect it had had on his family's life.

Both the above examples describe social interventions, which are not really psychotherapy but may nevertheless have psychotherapeutic effects. The psychiatrist can and should intervene on the patient's behalf whenever this is appropriate to diminish the external stresses on the patient.

Table 6.3 Indications for different types of psychotherapy in depression

Problem	Therapy
Recurrent depression Depression not responsive to adequate trials of antidepressants Residual depression after severe depressive illness	Cognitive–behavioural therapy
Current problems in marital relationship	Couples therapy
Unresolved grief Maladaptive relationship patterns: role conflicts or role transitions	Interpersonal therapy
Recurrent problems with relationships Unresolved childhood trauma, conflict or deprivation Patient wants exploratory/insight-focused, rather than symptom-focused approach	Psychodynamic psychotherapy
Chronic depressive illness	Supportive psychotherapy

Monitoring change and considering referral for specialist psychological therapy

In considering referral for more specialised psychological treatment, it is useful to distinguish between treatments that are designed to reduce symptoms of depression (such as cognitive therapy) and treatments whose main aim is to treat other aspects of the person (more traditional therapies, such as psychoanalysis). If the depression is a single episode arising in someone with a previously good adjustment to life (e.g. stable relationships and a good work record), psychological therapy is not indicated. If conventional treatment is proving unsuccessful (e.g. only partial response to medication or recurrent depression), a treatment aimed at the symptoms of depression and relapse prevention may be a useful adjunct. Cognitive therapy would seem to be the treatment of choice in this case.

More traditional forms of psychotherapy are indicated when there are other personal problems coexisting with the depression (i.e. vulnerability factors). Current problems within the family are indications for marital or family therapy. Wider-ranging relationship difficulties, particularly if associated with a disturbed early life (e.g. parental loss or family disruption in childhood), suggest a consideration of individual or group psychodynamic therapy. This type of therapy, in contrast to cognitive therapy, may well be more effective once the symptoms of depression have lifted.

Table 6.3 summarises some of these clinical referral criteria. Unfortunately, the limiting factor is often the availability of psychological treatment. While cognitive therapy is becoming more generally available, typically from clinical psychologists and nurse behaviour therapists, interpersonal therapy remains a research therapy. In many districts the length of individual psychodynamic therapy means that only a very small proportion of National Health Service patients can receive it, but group psychotherapy may be more easily accessible.

Conclusions

A variety of psychological therapies for depression are now available, and there is a growing research literature to support their efficacy. Cognitive and behavioural treatments are the most extensively researched, but there is also evidence for the effectiveness of interpersonal psychotherapy and, to a lesser extent, brief focal psychodynamic psychotherapy. Questions remain about which of these therapies, if any, have long-term effects on vulnerability to depression. Some of the clinical insights from those therapies shown to be effective in depression can be used in the psychological management of depression, even if formal psychotherapy is not being undertaken.

References

Antonuccio, D. O. (1998) The coping with depression course: a behavioral treatment for depression. *Clinical Psychologist*, **51**, 3–5.

Beck, A. T. & Greenberg, R. L. (1974) *Coping with Depression*. New York: Institute for Rational Living.

Beck, A. T., Rush, A. J., Shaw, B. F., *et al* (1979) *Cognitive Therapy of Depression*. New York: Guilford Press.

Blackburn, I. M. & Moore, R. G. (1997) Controlled acute and follow-up trial of cognitive therapy and pharmacotherapy in outpatients with recurrent depression. *British Journal of Psychiatry*, **171**, 328–334.

Brown, G. W. & Harris, T. (1978) *Social Origins of Depression: A Study of Psychiatric Disorder in Women*. New York: Free Press.

Burns, D. (1999) *The Feeling Good Handbook*. New York: Plume.

Deckersbach, T., Gershuny, B. & Otto, M. W. (2000) Cognitive behavioral therapy for depression. *Psychiatric Clinics of North America*, **23**, 795–809.

DeRubeis, R. J. & Crits Cristoph, P. (1998) Empirically supported individual and group treatments for adult mental disorders. *Journal of Consulting and Clinical Psychology*, **66**, 37–52.

DeRubeis, R. J., Gelfand, L. A., Tang, T. Z., *et al* (1999) Medications versus cognitive behavior therapy for severely depressed outpatients: mega-analysis of four randomized comparisons. *American Journal of Psychiatry*, **156**, 1007–1013.

DiMascio, A., Weissman, M. M., Prusoff, B. A., *et al* (1979) Differential symptom reduction by drugs and psychotherapy in acute depression. *Archives of General Psychiatry*, **36**, 1450–1456.

Elkin, I., Shea, M. T., Watkins, J. T., *et al* (1989) National Institute of Mental Health treatment of depression collaborative research program. *Archives of General Psychiatry*, **46**, 971–982.

Frank, E., Grochincinski, V. J., Spanier, C. A., *et al* (2000) Interpersonal psychotherapy and antidepressant medication: evaluation of a sequential treatment strategy in women with recurrent major depression. *Journal of Clinical Psychiatry*, **61**, 51–57.

Freud, S. (1917) Mourning and melancholia. In *The Standard Edition of the Complete Psychological Works*, Vol. IV. London: Hogarth Press.

Greenberger, D. & Padesky, C. (1995) *Mind over Mood*. New York: Guilford Press.

Jacobson, N. S., Dobson, K. S., Truax, P. A., *et al* (1996) A component analysis of cognitive–behavioural treatment for depression. *Journal of Consulting and Clinical Psychology*, **64**, 295–304.

Karasu, T. B. (1990) Toward a clinical model of psychotherapy for depression, I: systematic comparison of three psychotherapies. *American Journal of Psychiatry*, **147**, 133–147.

Keller, M. B., McCullough, J. P., Klein, D. L., *et al* (2000) A comparison of nefazodone, the cognitive–behavioral systems analysis system of psychotherapy, and their combination for the treatment of chronic depression. *New England Journal of Medicine*, **342**, 1462–1470.

Leff, J., Vearnals, S., Brewin, C. R., *et al* (2000) The London Depression Intervention Trial. Randomised controlled trial of antidepressants v. couple therapy in the treatment and maintenance of people with depression living with a partner: clinical outcome and costs. *British Journal of Psychiatry*, **177**, 95–100.

Leichsenring, F. (2001) Comparative effects of psychodynamic psychotherapy and cognitive–behavioral therapy in depression: a meta-analytic approach. *Clinical Psychology Review*, **21**, 401–419.

McDermut, W., Miller, I. W. & Brown, R. A. (2001) The efficacy of group psychotherapy for depression: a meta-analysis and review of the empirical research. *Clinical Psychology: Science and Practice*, **8**, 98–116.

Morrison, N. (2001) Group cognitive therapy: treatment of choice or sub-optimal option? *Behavioural and Cognitive Psychotherapy*, **29**, 311–332.

NICE (2004) *Depression. The Management of Depression in Primary and Secondary Care*, pp. 95–140. London: National Institute of Clinical Excellence.

Paykel, E. S. (2001) Continuation and maintenance therapy in depression. *British Medical Bulletin*, **57**, 145–159.

Paykel, E. S., Scott, J., Teasdale, J. D., *et al* (1999) Prevention of relapse in residual depression by cognitive therapy. *Archives of General Psychiatry*, **56**, 829–835.

Stuart, S. & Bowers, W. A. (1995) Cognitive therapy with inpatients: review and meta-analysis. *Journal of Cognitive Psychotherapy*, 9, 85–92.

Weissman, M. M., Klerman, G. L., Paykel, E. S., *et al* (1974) Treatment effects on the psychosocial adjustment of depressed patients. *Archives of General Psychiatry*, **30**, 771–778.

Weissman, M. M., Prusoff, B. A., DiMascio, A., *et al* (1979) The efficacy of drugs and psychotherapy in the treatment of acute depressive episodes. *American Journal of Psychiatry*, **136**, 555–558.

Weissman, M. M., Markowitz, J. C. & Klerman, G. L. (2000) *Comprehensive Guide to Interpersonal Psychotherapy.* New York: Basic Books.

Williams, C. (2001*a*) Use of written cognitive–behavioural therapy self-help materials to treat depression. *Advances in Psychiatric Treatment*, **7**, 233–240.

Williams, C. (2001*b*) *Overcoming Depression: A Five Area Approach.* London: Arnold.

Yalom, I. D. (1985) *The Theory and Practice of Group Psychotherapy* (3rd edn). New York: Basic Books.

CHAPTER 7

Suicide and non-fatal deliberate self-harm

Christopher A. Vassilas, Gethin Morgan, John Owen and George Tadros

Acts of suicide and non-fatal deliberate self-harm (DSH) usually have a complex aetiology. This chapter considers some theoretical issues, particularly the relevance of clinical, psychosocial and biological factors, before setting out the principles of sound clinical practice. Suicide is discussed separately from non-fatal DSH.

Suicide

History of suicide

Suicide is a phenomenon that is unique to humans. It is possible to trace it back into antiquity. Some societies sanctioned it, as in ancient Greece, where the Senate would allow an individual to take hemlock if a case for suicide had been made. The stoic school of philosophy defended suicide in certain situations and the founder of the school, Zenon, hanged himself at the age of 98, when, after breaking a toe, he found that his life was not worth living.

The early Christians also sometimes took their own lives in the face of persecution, but a change in attitude was signalled in a statement by St Augustine (AD 354–430) that suicide was 'a greater sin than any one might avoid by committing it'. By the middle of the 16th century, suicide had become a criminal offence in England, termed *felo de se*, literally a felony against oneself, and was considered equivalent to murder. Punitive attitudes were reflected in the practice of burying the body of a suicide at a crossroads with a stake through the heart and a stone over the face in order to prevent the ghost haunting the survivors. However, if suicide victims were said to be insane at the time of the act they were exempt from religious and legal punishments.

The emperor of China would send a yellow silk scarf to a person of high rank who had lost face through breaking the law. The intention was that the scarf should be used by the 'criminal' to hang himself in order to avoid criminal prosecution and disgrace.

In 18th-century Europe, fear grew that fictional portrayals of suicide might trigger imitation suicides and as a result Goethe's *The Sorrows of Young Werther* was banned in some countries. John Hume, the 18th-century Scottish philosopher, published a book arguing that an individual had a right to take his or her own life. France repealed its laws against suicide after the French Revolution and in Scotland suicide had ceased to be a criminal act by the middle of the 19th century. However, suicide and attempted suicide remained criminal offences in England and Wales until the Suicide Act became law in 1961.

A more detailed historical account can be found in Rosen (1971).

Definition of suicide

There is no universally accepted definition of suicide and defining suicide has caused controversy. Farmer (1988) has stated that the first problem encountered in the study of suicide is its definition in linguistic terms. The word 'suicide' appeared in the English language only in 1635 (Alvarez, 1990, pp. 59–93). The 19th-century French sociologist Durkheim proposed the following definition of suicide:

> 'the term suicide is applied to all cases of death resulting directly or indirectly from a positive or negative act of the victim himself, which he knows will produce this result.'

Of course, any definition has to address the issue of intent and this can be problematic to assess retrospectively. In psychoanalytical terms, suicide is defined as the urge to self-destruction, either as an attack on an introjected object or as a derivative of the death instinct (Rycroft, 1988, p. 160).

Suicide statistics from official figures are derived from what is essentially a legal process. This differs from the way in which a clinical diagnosis is reached. In England and Wales, a coroner brings in a verdict of suicide only when there is explicit evidence of suicidal intent. In the case of self-inflicted death where there is insufficient evidence of an intention to die, the coroner will give either an open verdict or one of accidental death or death by misadventure (legally the last two terms are synonymous). There is no doubt that the majority of cases returned as open verdicts are in fact suicides (Linsley *et al*, 2001). The UK Department of Health's (1999*a*) *Saving Lives: Our Healthier Nation* implicitly recognises this by including all open verdicts with suicides when setting national targets for suicide reduction.

Epidemiology of suicide

Global rates

Suicide is among the top ten causes of deaths worldwide, and one of the three leading causes of death in the

15- to 35-year age group. It accounts for approximately 1% of all deaths. The suicide burden, estimated in terms of disability-adjusted life years, represents 1.8% of the total burden of disease worldwide; that is twice the burden of diabetes. The average global suicide rate is 24.7/100000 for men and 6.9/100000 for women (World Health Organization, 2000).

Sainsbury & Barraclough (1968) suggested that the variation in suicide rates between different countries is due to real differences in social, biological and psychological factors rather than a simple reflection of the different ways of ascertaining suicide. They studied the suicide rates of immigrants to the USA from 11 different countries and found that the rank order of the suicide rates of the immigrant groups was nearly identical to the rank order of the suicide rates of the countries of origin. They concluded that official suicide statistics are valid tools for international comparison. Their findings echoed those of Durkheim a century earlier.

Between 1950 and 1995, global suicide rates increased by approximately 50% for men and 35% for women, and it is predicted that these figures will continue to rise (Bertolote, 2001). Lithuania, Estonia and Latvia are the countries with the highest overall suicide rates in the world. Lithuania has the highest annual rate of suicide in the world for men (79.3/100000) and China has the highest suicide rate for women (17.8/100000). The Middle East is the region with the lowest suicide rate (0.1/100000), but stigma and under-reporting could be contributory factors to this. Recent figures show a large increase in suicide rates for South-East Asia but a slight decrease for the Far East, with Sri Lanka experiencing an eight-fold increase over the past 50 years (Cheng & Lee, 2000).

UK rates

Annual suicide rates in the UK (11/100000 for men and 3.2/100000 for women) lie between the moderately high rates of Scandinavia and the low rates of Southern Europe. In England and Wales, the suicide rate reached a postwar peak in the early 1960s but then between 1963 and 1975 suicide rates for both genders declined. This decline was associated with the detoxification of domestic gas in the UK.

Between 1975 and 1990, the suicide rate for females continued to fall, but that for males increased by 32%. This increase was associated with an increase in unemployment, violence, divorce, debt, the number of homeless people, the number of repossessed houses, and alcohol and substance misuse (McClure, 2000). This was also a time during which women became more economically independent. During this period there were fewer cases of drug overdoses and more cases of hanging and poisoning using car exhaust.

Between 1990 and 1997, overall suicide rates decreased by 14% for men and by 22% for women. Kelly & Bunting (1998) attributed this decrease to a decline in suicides by poisoning with car exhaust, as all new petrol cars sold in the UK since 1992 have had to have catalytic converters, although this cannot entirely account for this phenomenon. The relevance of the availability of lethal agents to suicide rates has been emphasised by Schapira *et al* (2001). Despite these overall declines, there is cause for concern regarding younger adults in England and Wales: Middleton & Gunnell (2000) cite evidence for a 7% increase in suicide by 24- to 34-year-old men and a 6% increase in 15- to 24-year-old women between 1990–92 and 1996–98. Boyle *et al* (2005) examined data from Scotland for the period 1980–2001 and showed increased rates in young adults, especially in men and in deprived areas.

Suicidal thoughts

The National Psychiatric Morbidity Survey gives an overall rate for the annual incidence of suicidal thoughts in the general population in the UK of 2.3%; the rate is highest for women aged 16.2 years. Fewer than 1 in 200 go on to complete suicide, however, and suicidal thoughts resolved in 57% over an 18-month period (Gunnell *et al*, 2004).

Gender

The highest suicide rates are found in males above the age of 75 and females above the age of 65 in England and Wales. However, increased rates in certain younger age groups mean the elderly no longer dominate the scene. Worldwide, suicide rates for men are higher than those for women, with the one exception of China. In Europe and the UK, the male:female suicide ratio is about 3:1. In China, the ratio is about 0.8:1, mainly because of the large number of suicides by young rural women (Phillips *et al*, 2002). The predominance of men among suicides may be due in part to their tendency to use more lethal methods and to have a greater propensity to impulsive violence (Brent & Moritz, 1996). Worldwide, suicide rates increase with age, especially for females, and this trend is even more pronounced in Asia (Yip *et al*, 2000).

Method

The choice of method of suicide depends on availability, ease of use, social acceptability, cost, symbolism, scope for second thoughts and chances for intervention. In England and Wales, self-poisoning is the commonest method of suicide for women but is the second most common method for men, after hanging (Kelly & Bunting, 1998). Between 1979 and 1998 hanging increased threefold in men aged 15–34 years and doubled in young women. This is a cause for concern, particularly as reducing the availability of hanging is not really feasible, except possibly in a restricted environment such as a hospital ward. Hanging is the commonest method used in Asia, and among Asian migrants in the USA.

In the USA, firearms are the chosen method in 60% of suicides (Moscicki, 1997). Also in the USA, Marzuk *et al* (1992*a*) described a positive association between suicide by jumping and the number of tall buildings, as well as between suicide by motor vehicle exhaust and more private garages in the area.

In the Asia Pacific region, death by suicide from the ingestion of pesticides is a major problem (Eddleston & Phillips, 2004), particularly in rural areas of countries such as China, Sri Lanka and the Pacific islands, where there is ready access to these very toxic compounds.

In Hong Kong in 1998 a woman was reported as having killed herself by burning charcoal in her room and dying from carbon monoxide poisoning. The phenomenon was widely reported in the local media and on the internet, and the method became increasingly popular in Hong Kong, Taiwan and southern coastal China (Chan *et al*, 2005).

Seasonal variation

Early reports suggested that deaths by suicide in the UK show a spring peak for males and spring and autumn peaks for females. Yip *et al* (2000) re-examined this seasonal variation in suicide in England and Wales and found that it had diminished.

Aetiology of suicide

Psychiatric illness

Representative samples of suicides have been examined using the so-called 'psychological autopsy' method. This involves interviewing relatives and friends of the deceased as well as scrutinising medical records. Using this method it has been found (in the West at least) that over 90% of those killing themselves by suicide may be judged to have some form of psychiatric illness (Barraclough, 1974; Rich *et al*, 1986). In those few suicides which lacked evidence of such illness, it may have been present but undetected because of the unreliability of retrospective analysis. 'Rational' suicide therefore appears to be rare in Western countries.

All categories of psychiatric illness except for dementia and mental retardation carry an increased risk of suicide. The various diagnostic groups can be ranked in decreasing order of risk, as in Table 7.1. However, some caution needs to be observed since these data are based on patients treated in a hospital setting, and it is probable that patients treated in primary care are at a lower risk of suicide.

Higher lifetime rates of suicide for depression are often quoted, but many of the older studies, from which these high figures are derived, concentrated on high-risk patients admitted to psychiatric hospital (Guze & Robins, 1970).

A recent systematic review of case-controlled and cohort studies of schizophrenia showed that the following features were associated with increased suicide risk: previous depressive disorder; previous suicide attempts; drug misuse; agitation or motor restlessness; fear of mental disintegration; poor adherence to treatment; and recent loss. Reduced risk was associated with hallucinations (Hawton *et al*, 2005).

Table 7.1 Suicide risk for different psychiatric disorders

Disorder	Standardised mortality rate for suicide[a]	Lifetime risk of suicide[b]
Major depression	2035	6%
Schizophrenia	845	4%
Personality disorder	708	
Bipolar disorder	1505	
Substance misuse	574	7% (alcohol addiction)
Anxiety neurosis	629	
Organic disorders	332	

[a] From Harris & Barraclough (1997).
[b] From Inskip *et al* (1998).

Societal factors

Although psychiatric illness is an important aetiological factor, causal mechanisms leading to suicide are usually multifactorial. We know that 94% of people who have suffered a depressive episode will not kill themselves. Adverse aspects of a person's life situation should always be assessed because they often play a central role in the development of suicidal despair, whatever the precise categorisation of psychiatric illness. The importance of social factors can be illustrated by the fact that the incidence of suicide in pregnancy and the puerperium appears to have fallen dramatically in recent years, so that now the incidence is lower than the rate expected in the general population, even though the puerperium is a time of major biological and psychological stress. Such a reduction in morbidity may be due to changes in social attitudes to pregnancy, the availability of contraception and abortion (thereby reducing the likelihood that the pregnancy will be unwanted), and the lessening of stigma attached to an unwanted pregnancy (Appleby, 1991).

The first attempt to produce a sociological theory of suicide was made by Durkheim, who, in the mid-19th century, examined the suicide rates in various European countries (Durkheim, 1897). Finding a remarkable stability in ranked order of national suicide rates over successive 5-year periods, he suggested that suicide results primarily from social factors. Durkheim argued that the society in which people live exerts control over them in two ways: individuals are integrated into the values and norms of their social group; and in turn society regulates their goals and aspirations.

Durkheim proposed four types of suicide: egoistic, altruistic, anomic and fatalistic. Egoistic suicide results from poor integration into society, as a result of the way an individual behaves, for example by virtue of mental illness. In altruistic suicide there is an over-integration into society. An example is the act of *hara-kiri*, in which the customs of feudal Japanese society obliged an individual to commit suicide in certain circumstances. 'Protest' suicide (e.g. political hunger strike) is not easy to categorise under Durkheim's system but presumably reflects an over-identification with a social subgroup or set of ideals. Anomic suicide occurs if the bonds between people have been loosened, as in an inner-city area, and norms regulating behaviour no longer apply, In fatalistic suicide there is an excessive regulation by society, so that individual feel they have no personal freedom and no hope. An example is the suicide of a slave.

Societal attitudes to suicide may themselves be of aetiological importance. Diekstra & Kerkhoff (1989) suggest that the development of more permissive views towards taking one's life have played a part in the trend contributing to increased suicide rates in certain population subgroups.

Imitation

Imitation may be a precipitating factor in some cases of suicide. Despite the methodological problems in studying this area, there is compelling evidence that the portrayal of suicide by the mass media influences subsequent suicide rates (Schmidtke & Hafner, 1988).

It is likely that imitation underlies the phenomenon of cluster suicides, which occur both in the community and in psychiatric hospitals from time to time (see below).

Marital status

Suicide rates in the divorced and single are greater than those in the married (Charlton *et al*, 1993).

Life stress

The relationship between mental illness, suicide and life stress is complex because mental illness itself may predispose an individual to adverse life stress and vice versa. Researching this area in the case of suicide is fraught with difficulties; none the less, adverse life stress had been shown to occur more frequently before suicide than in a control group (Foster *et al*, 1999).

Occupation and unemployment

Relative poverty is associated with an increased risk of suicide. In the UK between 1991 and 1993 the standardised mortality ratio for suicide was four times higher in men aged 20–64 from social class V than in men aged 20–64 from social class I (215 versus 55) (Gunnell *et al*, 1995). The reasons for this are complex but could be mediated through mental illness, the direct effects on mental health of material deprivation, higher levels of unemployment and job insecurity in people of lower socioeconomic position, differences in social support in relation to social class, and downward social migration by people who develop mental illness.

For men, occupational groups that stand out as being particularly vulnerable to suicide include farmers, dentists, veterinary surgeons, sales representatives and medical practitioners; for women they include medical practitioners, housekeepers, vets, waitresses and nurses (Kelly & Bunting, 1998). Clearly, those in the medical and allied professions have both knowledge of and access to drugs. Similarly, farmers have relatively easy access to firearms.

Cognitive ability

Gunnell *et al* (2005*b*) reported that in Swedish male military conscripts during the period 1968–94 the risk of suicide was two to three times higher in those with the lowest compared with the highest scores on intelligence tests. The greatest risks were seen among poorly performing offspring of well-educated parents. This might reflect the importance of cognitive ability in either the aetiology of severe mental illness or in problem solving when dealing with life crises.

Genetics

The tendency to suicide is familial, and twin and adoption studies support the idea of genetic risk factors in suicide. It is still not clear to what extent suicide is inherited directly or whether it is mediated through the liability to develop a psychiatric illness, such as depression. One large community study of twins found that genetic factors accounted for approximately 45% of the variance in suicidal thoughts and behaviour (Statham *et al*, 1998). It has been postulated that at least some of the large variation in suicide rates across Europe is accounted for by genetic factors (Marusic & Farmer, 2001). McGuffin *et al* (2001) review the genetics of suicide.

Cholesterol and serotonin

A few studies have examined the brains of those who have died by suicide. Serotonin transporter sites appear to be reduced in suicide victims when compared with control groups (Arango *et al*, 1995). There is also evidence of a role for serotonin in suicidal behaviour. Low levels of 5-hydroxyindoleacetic acid (5-HIAA) in the cerebrospinal fluid (CSF), which is an index of serotonin release and turnover, are associated with high suicidal intent and to more medically significant episodes of DSH (Mann & Malone, 1997).

In a meta-analysis of studies looking at the relationship between serum cholesterol and suicide, Lester (2002) concluded that follow-up studies showed that those with lower cholesterol levels do have a tiny but statistically significant increased risk of completing suicide. Individuals who had attempted suicide in the past had lower cholesterol levels, especially if had they used violent methods. Again, altered serotonin metabolism may be involved (Hawton *et al*, 1993).

Risk factors

Box 7.1 lists some individual correlates of suicide. However, these 'risk factors' need to be interpreted with some caution. A risk factor should help to predict suicide at an individual level. The low base rate of suicide (which is as low as 2% even in high-risk groups) is just one of many problems that beset the identification of relevant and reliable risk factors. Amsel & Mann (2001) point out that a risk factor with a predictive power as

Box 7.1 Correlates of suicide risk

General

- Male
- Elderly (although high rates may also occur in young adult males)
- Separated > widowed > single > married
- Living alone
- Presence of stressful life events
- Physical disorder

Psychiatric disorder and personality factors

- Major depression
- Substance misuse (particularly alcohol)
- Schizophrenia
- Borderline personality disorder
- History of suicide attempts
- History of other deliberate self-harm
- Family history of suicide

Symptoms associated with suicide

- Hopelessness
- Suicidal ideation
- Depression
- Anhedonia
- Insomnia
- Severe anxiety
- Impaired concentration
- Psychomotor agitation
- Panic attacks

high as 90% would have a positive predictive value of only 16% (i.e. there would be 84% false positives). As yet we cannot quantify risk factors, which in any case vary in significance from one individual to another and according to situation, for example whether in hospital or the community. Ideally, each risk factor would be independent of others, whereas many of the currently identified risk factors cross-correlate and are multifactorial, with unmeasured common causal variables. Although we have some information about risk factors for suicide, we have very little reliable knowledge about the accurate clinical quantification of risk, a prerequisite for effective risk management.

An overall aetiological hypothesis

A hypothetical comprehensive explanation of suicidality has been presented under the term 'the suicidal process' (van Heeringen, 2001*a*). This invokes a mechanism based on personality vulnerability and which focuses on the traits of impulsivity and aggressiveness, which in turn are related to hypo-serotonergic functioning. The stress–diathesis model postulates that in such a vulnerable individual the supervention of stressful events such as adverse life episodes, depression or other mental illness may lead to suicidal behaviour, and in these cases the hypophyso-pituitary axis is the related neurochemical parameter.

Suicide in special groups

Ethnic minorities

In the UK rates of suicide vary considerably between different ethnic groups. In the population from India, for example, women of all ages and in particular young women represent a high-risk group, as do young men. Among Pakistanis and Bangladeshis, rates of suicide are low except for in young women, who have higher than expected rates. Raleigh *et al* (1990) identified suicides among immigrants from the Indian subcontinent for the period 1970–78. The pattern of suicide that emerged was quite different from that of the general population of England and Wales, but it did resemble the picture reported in the subcontinent. The highest rates were found in women, the young and especially young married women. In particular, the level in women aged 15–24 was 80% higher than in the general population. Men from the subcontinent had low overall rates, but an excess of suicides of social class I, a high proportion of whom were doctors and dentists. The authors speculated that the esteem in which the elderly are held in these ethnic groups and the support they receive within their cultures may act as protective factors against suicide, while among young women arranged marriages with a tradition of dowries are common and these may act as a contributory factor in suicides.

East African women of all ages and also young East African men have high suicide rates. Among immigrants from the Caribbean, suicide rates are high for the young (Raleigh, 1996). Among suicides who had been in contact with mental health services within the previous 12 months, more violent methods of suicide were used by those from ethnic minorities than by whites (Hunt *et al*, 2003).

In the USA there are substantially higher rates of suicide among Native Americans than among the majority population and lower rates among African-Americans, Puerto Ricans and Mexican-Americans. The rates for Chinese- and Japanese-Americans are slightly lower than the national figures (Group for the Advancement of Psychiatry, 1989).

McKenzie *et al* (2003) review suicide within ethnic minority groups.

Psychiatric patients

In recent decades several countries have reported an increase in the number of suicides occurring among psychiatric in-patients. A survey into deaths in detained patients in England and Wales reported that during the 24-month period 1993–94 there were 95 suicides among detained patients, but during 36 months of 1998–2000 there were 204 such suicides (Mental Health Act Commission, 2001), suggesting a real increase in the number.

Complex factors need to be taken into account in analysing the statistics involved. The number of patients greatly exceeds the bed complement because of short stays and rapid patient turnover; unless this is allowed for, a spuriously low denominator leads to misleadingly high rates. There may also have been changes in the type of patient admitted to hospital. For example, patients admitted with personality disorder and substance misuse represent individuals at significantly increased risk (Wolfersdorf *et al*, 1988) and these may now constitute a larger proportion of the total number of psychiatric in-patients.

The National Confidential Inquiry into Suicide and Homicide by People with Mental Illness provided data on a comprehensive national sample of 5852 suicides and open verdicts during the 4 years from 1996 in England and Wales, Scotland and Northern Ireland. All had been in contact with mental health services in the year before death (Department of Health, 2001). Some key descriptive findings from the Inquiry's report are set out in Box 7.2. See also a more recent report from the Confidential Inquiry concerning suicides in England and Wales (Meehan *et al*, 2006).

Risk factors for in-patients who killed themselves within a year of discharge have been identified as: not being white, living alone and having a history of DSH (King *et al*, 2001). Discontinuity of care from a significant professional was also associated with an increased risk of suicide.

Maternal suicide

Suicide is the leading cause of maternal death (defined as death following a registered live birth or stillbirth at or more than 24 weeks of gestation) (Oates, 2003). 'Maternal suicide' is defined as suicide either in pregnancy or up to a year later. Suicide rates are generally low in pregnancy (standardised mortality ratio = 0.05) and although elevated in the postnatal period are still relatively low (s.m.r = 0.17). Such suicides are more likely to be through violent methods, in contrast to female suicides in general (Appleby, 1991).

An apparent protective effect of pregnancy on suicide risk (the annual suicide rate is 2/100 000 maternities compared with an overall female suicide rate of

Box 7.2 Suicide among psychiatric patients: key descriptive data

- Among all patients dying by suicide (around 1500 cases/year), approximately one-quarter had been in contact with mental health services in the year before death
- The commonest methods of suicide were hanging and self-poisoning by overdose
- Overdose is most common with psychotropic drugs (only 3% use paracetamol compared with 13% suicides in the general population)
- Males (at 66–69%) outnumbered females. The male:female ratio was highest in the younger age groups (except in Scotland)
- The primary psychiatric diagnosis for 60–72% was major affective disorder or schizophrenia and related disorders. Other common diagnoses were personality disorder and alcohol dependence
- Secondary psychiatric disorders were most commonly depressive illness, personality disorder, alcohol and drug dependence
- Some 62–64% had a history of deliberate self-harm
- In England and Wales younger patients more often had a history of schizophrenia, personality disorder, drug or alcohol misuse and violence
- In England and Wales 33% were less than 34 years of age
- In Scotland and Northern Ireland 50% were aged 39 years or less
- Suicide was most common in males aged 25–34 years (25–44 years in Northern Ireland)
- Some 7–12% were aged over 65 years.

Source: National Confidential Inquiry into Suicide and Homicide by People with Mental Illness (Department of Health, 2001).

3.4/100 000) might mask an elevated risk of suicide in certain subgroups. The incidence of suicide in puerperal psychosis is not known but it is likely that some of the violent suicides that occur in the first post-partum year are related to puerperal psychiatric disorder. The risk of recurrence of the illness (between 1 in 3 and 1 in 2 in subsequent pregnancies) emphasises the need to anticipate this in planning care of women with a history of this illness and who become pregnant again. Adequate specialist services should be readily available. Long-term follow-up studies of those who have been admitted for a post-partum psychiatric disorder show a considerably elevated risk for suicide over the long term (Appleby *et al*, 1998) (see also Chapter 25 on post-partum mental disorders).

Suicide in prison

The number of suicides in UK prisons has increased markedly over recent years (Shaw *et al*, 2004). Overall rates in the 1990s rose by approximately 5% per annum, in spite of a decrease in the incidence of suicide in the general population. Comparison of prison suicide rates with those in the general population is hazardous because it is necessary to match population subgroups precisely to achieve any meaningful findings (Gore, 1999). Furthermore, accurate evaluation of the denominator is again very difficult, given the mobile and rapidly changing nature of much of the prison population.

About 50% of prison suicides are among remand prisoners, even though these make up on only 19% of the prison population. About a third of these occur within the first week of imprisonment. About 75% have a history of substance misuse. The commonest method of prison suicide is hanging using bedclothes and window bars, usually at night. There is often a history of psychiatric treatment and self-harm. Those with convictions for violent or sexual offences and those given life sentences are over-represented and some suicides occur many years after reception into prison (Dooley, 1990).

Suicide among the elderly

Despite the recent rise in suicide rates among young men, in most industrialised countries the group with the highest rates of suicide remains males over the age of 75. There are clear differences between younger and older suicides; for instance, physical illness is a major risk factor for suicide in the elderly (Rubenowitz *et al*, 2001) (although there is no evidence that it is an independent risk factor for suicide, in that physical illnesses are linked to psychiatric disorders, which in turn are linked to suicide). Comparison with younger suicides had suggested that substance misuse was less frequently found in the elderly (Conwell *et al*, 1996), but a more recent Swedish study suggested that it may also be a risk factor for elderly suicide (Waern *et al*, 2002). Harwood *et al* (2001) identified personality factors as well as depression as important factors associated with elderly suicide. In older adults, the difference between suicide rates in men and women is lower than that between younger adults, at 3:2 (men: women). Tadros & Salib (2000) found that overdosing was the most common method of suicide used by the elderly, while hanging was the most common method used by younger adults; drowning and asphyxia were significantly more common among the elderly. Contact with primary care before death is more common among older suicides, which suggests that there may be greater scope for preventive strategies targeted at the elderly (Vassilas & Morgan, 1994; Luoma *et al*, 2002).

People with a physical illness

Physical illness is associated with an increased risk of suicide. In a review of the literature, Harris & Barraclough (1994) reported that those illnesses particularly associated with an increased risk include HIV/AIDS, malignant neoplasms, head and neck cancers, Huntington's disease, multiple sclerosis, peptic ulcer, renal disease, spinal cord injury and systemic lupus erythematosis. They found that pregnancy and the puerperium had a protective value and decreased the risk.

People taking antidepressants

As discussed in Chapter 4, a point of considerable interest is whether antidepressant medications can precipitate suicide.

Suicide rates have fallen in recent years, while the prescribing of antidepressants has increased. This has led some to conclude that there is a causal relationship between the two. None the less, there have been suggestions that antidepressants can actually precipitate suicidal behaviour.

Selective serotonin reuptake inhibitors (SSRIs)

A large meta-analysis concluded that, for adults, while there was no evidence of an increased risk of suicide associated with the prescribing of SSRIs (Gunnell *et al*, 2005*a*), there are insufficient data to rule out the possibility that one exists. Doctors should therefore advise patients of the possible risk of suicidal behaviour and monitor them closely in the early stages of treatment. In contrast, when Hammad *et al* (2006) carried out a meta-analysis of trials of SSRIs prescribed to children, a consistent increase in suicidal behaviour was found across trials. Although the effect was described by the authors as modest, caution must be observed when prescribing these drugs for the young.

Adolescents and young adults

Over the past 30 years there has been a dramatic increase in male youth suicides in developed countries. This was initially reported in the USA and Australia but was later confirmed in other countries, including the UK (McClure, 2000). Charlton *et al* (1993) suggested that this is related to an increased incidence of alcohol and drug misuse and, in those aged under 20 years, the inhalation of volatile substances. These authors also postulated that about half the overall increase might be related to an increased proportion of young adults who are single or divorced. There might in addition be increased vulnerability due to early exposure to parental divorce, which itself increased sharply in incidence in the 1970s and 1980s, although it is difficult to explain why this should affect only male children.

A further possibility is that these trends may represent a shift to more lethal methods of suicide (Gunnell *et al*, 2000).

Suicide clusters

A suicide that occurs in a relatively closed community, such as a hospital, may kindle an intensive preoccupation with suicidal ideas in other vulnerable individuals, and a cluster of suicides within the hospital can follow. Intense local media publicity increases the risk of this happening. Such kindling of suicide risk is poorly understood but is certainly a real hazard and should be taken into account by those who have clinical responsibility for in-patient services. The needs of all other individuals who are at particular risk should be considered without delay whenever a patient commits suicide.

Rarely, family or even mass suicide pacts occur. These usually arise as a response to an overwhelming crisis facing the group. Historical examples of mass suicide include the Jewish Zealots at Masada, and, more recently, the 1978 Jonestown massacre in Guyana. These tragedies have certain common themes: a charismatic leader, strong loyalties and religious belief under threat. Explanatory theories for such episodes include *folie collective* and mass hysteria, but they are difficult to study retrospectively.

Occasionally suicide results from pacts in which two or more people form an agreement to kill themselves. These events are relatively rare and seem to be decreasing in frequency. In the UK they account for about 6 in every 1000 suicides. People who commit suicide in a pact are more likely than those who commit suicide alone to be female, older, married and of a high social class. Such pacts often involve two individuals who are closely interdependent emotionally, one of whom is usually dominant. The potential loss of a partner from ill-health may be a major factor (Brown & Barraclough, 1999). One disturbing trend is that of young people, especially in Japan, meeting via the internet and entering into suicide pacts with one another. What is particularly concerning is that these individuals are unknown to each other beforehand (Rajagopal, 2004; Hitosugi *et al*, 2007).

Suicide terrorism

In recent years the problem of terrorism involving the suicide of a single individual, or groups of them, has become a major global threat. The issues involve political and ideological conflict in the setting of a revival of religious fundamentalism, intense group identification and indoctrination (Salib, 2003).

It is hazardous to assume that the individuals involved can be regarded as psychiatrically ill in the conventional sense. Gordon (2002) comments that the psychiatric terminology is as yet deficient in not having the depth to encompass the emotions and behaviour of groups of people whose levels of hate, low self-esteem, humiliation and alienation are such that it is felt that they can be remedied by the mass destruction of life, including their own.

Homicide-suicide

Murder followed by the suicide of the assailant is a comparatively rare event: in England and Wales on average 60 deaths a year are accounted for by murder-suicide, which represents 0.01% of all deaths, and rates are similar throughout the world (Barraclough *et al*, 2002). They lead to profound distress and disadvantage for survivors, and account for a high proportion of child and adult female homicides.

Such killers are mainly young men with intense sexual jealousy, depressed mothers, or despairing elderly men with ailing spouses. The main victims are female sexual partners or consanguineous relatives, usually young children. Clinical depression, specific motivations such as male sexual possessiveness or maternal salvation fantasies, and a history of previous suicide attempts are considered explanatory psychopathological mechanisms (Marzuk *et al*, 1992*b*).

The findings of the one published study of homicide-suicide in England and Wales were similar to those with smaller samples in other parts of the world (Barraclough *et al*, 2002). The majority of killers were men who had killed their wife or partner (58% of cases). Men also killed their children in 9% of cases. It was comparatively rare for a woman to be the killer (13% of cases) and almost invariably in these cases the victims were the women's children. It was extremely rare for a victim to be unknown to the killer.

Assessment of suicide risk

A full psychiatric history and mental state examination is necessary for every patient. There may be risks other than suicide, for example aggressive behaviour, and appropriate clinical skills are required. The Confidential Inquiry (Department of Health, 2001) advised that staff should attend skills training programmes at least every 3 years. Such clinical skills involve accurate evaluation of the mental state and of current as well as previous risk factors for suicide.

Interviewing

The suicidal state of mind frequently includes despair, a sense of humiliation and ambivalence concerning whether to live or die. The last has been referred to as the 'Janus-faced' quality of suicidality. It explains how suicidal individuals may appear to appeal for help at the same time as feeling true despair and being at high risk. An attitude of hopelessness generated by a sense of defeat, entrapment and inability to escape is another important feature leading to both a disinclination to seek help and loss of hope (Williams & Pollock, 2001).

Forming an understanding, empathic relationship with the individual and promoting mutual trust are essential to generating hope. Listening and allowing discussion of important issues are crucial features in establishing such rapport, though too liberal reassurance may merely confirm a person's fears that others do not understand what it means to have lost hope. Suicidal individuals often declare their intent to die to a number of people before killing themselves, and it is a fallacy to assume that those who talk about such ideas are less likely to commit suicide.

Although suicide risk questionnaires may be a useful adjunct to clinical interview, they cannot replace a full psychiatric assessment. In day-to-day clinical care, careful assessment of an individual's mental state, recent behaviour and relationship with others, against the background of a thorough clinical history, affords the most reliable means of evaluating the immediate degree of risk, to which standardised questionnaires may then add useful back-up data. An interesting study showed that worst-ever degree of suicidal ideation as assessed by questionnaire may be as useful as the current level in predicting risk (Beck *et al*, 1999). This emphasises again the importance of the previous history in clinical assessment.

It is advisable to lead into the topic of suicidal ideation gradually. In this way the interviewer signals sensitivity to the individual's distress. The approach should take the form of a series of open questions, although it may be necessary to ask some leading questions to ensure that all the items are covered. Assessment of suicidal ideation is a very important part of risk evaluation. A case–control study of psychiatric in-patient suicides (Morgan & Stanton, 1997) concluded that attempts to define a clinical stereotype of suicide are unrealistic, and face-to-face evaluation of each patient, particularly with regard to the severity of suicidal ideation, is of paramount importance. Powell *et al* (2000) also suggested that suicidal thoughts or activities are the most important risk factor for suicide in psychiatric patients.

Box 7.3 illustrates an approach based on these principles.

Box 7.3 Recommended interview sequence of topics in assessing suicidal ideation and motivation

- Do you hope that things will turn out well?
- Do you get pleasure out of life?
- Are you able to face each day?
- Do you ever despair about things?
- Do you feel life is a burden?
- Are you feeling entrapped, defeated, hopeless?
- Do you wish you were dead?
- Why do you feel this way (e.g. to be with a person who has died, life bleak, morbid guilt)?
- Do you have thoughts of ending your life? (If so, are they intermittent or more persistent?)
- Have you ever acted on these ideas?
- How strongly are you able to resist them? Is there anything that makes them worse or alleviates them?
- Assess how likely the person is to kill him-/herself (intent, detailed plans made, method considered and available)
- Assess the ability of the patient to give assurance about safety, for example until next appointment if the patient is to remain in the community
- Assess the willingness of the patient to seek help in crisis
- Review sources of help and how to activate them
- Look at options other than suicide
- Assess risk to others (e.g. are others included in the patient's sense of hopelessness; is there aggressive behaviour related to personality difficulties or psychotic mental illness?)

Difficulties in assessment

Difficulties in assessment are summarised in Box 7.4. The degree of risk is sometimes underestimated despite the communication of suicidal ideas (Morgan & Priest, 1991). The Confidential Inquiry reported that in 80% of in-patient suicides, the patients were regarded as being of no or low risk (Department of Health, 2001).

Suicidal patients may exhibit provocative or uncooperative behaviour. As a result others, including

Box 7.4 Difficulties in suicide risk assessment

- Variability in degree of distress (ambivalence towards suicide, removal from stress factors)
- Misleading improvement due to final decision to kill self or removal from stressful situation
- Deliberate denial of suicidal ideas
- Uncooperative and difficult behaviour
- Anger, resentment, sometimes displaced on to staff
- Staff assumptions that talk of suicide is no more than a manipulative threat
- Staff fears that direct discussion of suicide might precipitate it
- Surveillance difficulties
- Physical hazards in hospital ward surroundings
- Malignant alienation
- Setting over-ambitious goals, which foster sense of failure

healthcare professionals, may lose sympathy and become critical of a person at real risk of suicide, who then in turn perceives staff as unhelpful and rejecting. Similarly, recurrent relapse can lead to staff frustration and breakdown of the therapeutic relationship. This process has been termed 'malignant alienation', and deserves consideration when treatment runs into difficulties (Morgan, 1979; Watts & Morgan, 1994).

A further problem worthy of special mention is short-lasting and misleading improvement, which has been reported before 45% of in-patient suicides (Morgan & Priest, 1991). This may be related to temporary disengagement from stressful situational factors, and care should be taken to address such problems adequately before arranging leave or discharge, which might otherwise trigger relapse. Lack of overt distress may also follow a final decision to commit suicide, with a resulting freedom from agonising indecision.

Overall assessment of risk

It has already been emphasised that the known correlates of suicide are imperfect indicators of risk at an individual level, particularly in the short term. They should inform rather than lead the face-to-face clinical assessment, which must encompass the widest possible perspective, including:

- previous history (e.g. previous history of self-harm and level of suicidal ideation)
- personality characteristics (especially traits of aggression and impulsivity)
- evaluation of current mental state, with particular attention to detailed and systematic assessment of suicidal ideation and intent.

Such an approach helps to distinguish between what may be primarily an appeal for help as opposed to an unequivocal wish to die. In most cases both mechanisms apply.

Environmental hazards should also be monitored constantly. The overall approach should take into account the balance between risk and protective factors.

Box 7.5 Management of suicide risk presented by psychiatric in-patients

- Sixty-four per cent of patients dying by suicide are male
- Patients dying by suicide tended to be more morbid than those dying by suicide overall (79% had affective disorders or schizophrenia, with higher rates of previous deliberate self-harm and violence, and multiple previous admissions)
- By far the most frequent method was hanging (42%). Other common methods were jumping from a height or in front of a moving vehicle (27%), drowning (8%) and overdose (11%)
- For hanging, the most common ligature used was a belt, and the most common suspension point was a curtain rail
- Of those suicides that occurred on the ward, 74% were by hanging
- Overall, 31% of patient suicides occurred on the ward, 53% at a distance from the ward, and 14% otherwise in or around the hospital
- Around a third were on agreed leave and a quarter had left the ward without staff agreement
- Of all patients dying by suicide, 28% were detained under the Mental Health Act
- Of all patients dying by suicide, 23% were under non-routine observation (see later for fuller discussion)
- Particularly vulnerable times were the first week after admission (24% of deaths) and when discharge was planned (41% of deaths)
- Though most patients (76%) had been in contact with a staff member in the 24 hours before death, in only 15% were suicidal ideas detected
- Problems identified by staff included the need for close supervision, patient non-compliance, insufficient staff numbers, and the need for better staff training and communication

Source: Data drawn from 754 patients in England and Wales, in the National Confidential Inquiry (Department of Health, 2001; Meehan *et al*, 2006).

Management of suicide risk

The treatment requirements of each individual will be determined by diagnostic considerations and must be dictated by the nature of any psychiatric comorbidity. In particular, great care should be taken to observe the requirements of any mental health legislation under which the patient may have been admitted to hospital.

Psychiatric in-patients

Background data

Selected data concerning the large series of suicides from England and Wales, as reported by the Confidential Inquiry (Department of Health, 2001; Meehan *et al*, 2006) are set out in Box 7.5. Small series from Scotland and Northern Ireland are also described in the report. Overall findings were similar, though in Scotland overdose was the second most common method, and in Northern Ireland it was the commonest.

Thorough admission procedures

The Confidential Inquiry reported that 24% of suicides occurred during the first week after admission. Inadequate admission procedures present serious hazards: policies need to be clear and fully understood by all staff.

Supportive observation

A clear care policy for suicidal patients is imperative, inherent in which should be the principle that increased risk must be matched by more intensive care in terms of relationship with staff, provision of appropriate physical security (including control of exits and removal or at least control of hazards in the ward and wider hospital environment) and provision of adequate numbers of staff. The aim should be to establish a supportive alliance with the patient against suicidal ideas and behaviour. The terminology should be explicit and unambiguous: words such as 'close' or 'special' convey little to newcomers or to those who work in other hospital units, and are a recipe for confusion.

The process should be one of intense support for the patient rather than unwelcome intrusive surveillance. Levels vary from intensive face-to-face supervision at all times for patients at the highest risk (when there is a risk of violence more than one staff member may need to be present), to 'known place' or 'remain on the ward' for low levels of risk. The Confidential Inquiry found that around a quarter of in-patient suicides occurred during non-routine observation (48% of these had left the ward, 11% with staff agreement) and suggests that intermittent observation is of unproven value. However, it is important to stress that regular, face-to-face contact with a patient at risk needs to be a supportive alliance of therapeutic value rather than impersonal policing: the value of such support must surely be hard to gainsay when treating patients who are struggling against being overwhelmed by suicidal ideas.

Working with the suicidal patient

It is necessary to move as quickly as possible towards establishing a close, supportive relationship, one that may even need to be assertive and controlling, especially at times of crisis. Identifying the painful reality of depressive symptoms is a useful early step. Similarly, it can be very helpful to indicate an understanding of feelings of ambivalence and even anger towards others. Isolating the suicidal drive by seeing it as part of an illness, agreeing on ways of minimising it (having identified what may worsen or relieve it), explaining how depressive illness usually resolves with time and the manner in which it can distort ways of thinking all help to regenerate hope.

When relatives become included in morbid depressive thinking concerning the need to die, or in any other form of psychotic ideation, risks to their safety should also be carefully evaluated, as suicides are occasionally accompanied by homicides (see above).

Failure to respond to therapy should lead to a review of medication, as well as a fresh look at how to deal with adverse events and situations that appear intractable. The therapist should be consistent in what is said and done and needs to see the patient regularly and predictably. Even the most despairing patients can derive considerable comfort from another person's willingness to listen and sit with them.

Use of medication

If medication is judged to be necessary it is important to target it carefully. Individuals who proceed to commit suicide often receive inappropriate medication in a low and ineffective dose during the last few weeks of their lives (Barraclough, 1974; Isometsa *et al*, 1994). The state of depression also may not be recognised (Rihmer *et al*, 1990). Liquid medication will prevent patients from holding tablets. The Confidential Inquiry recommended that 'atypical' antipsychotic medication should be made available for all patients with severe mental illness who are not compliant with the use of 'typical' drugs because of side-effects. On discharge, patients with a history of DSH in the previous 3 months should receive supplies of medication covering no more than 2 weeks' use.

Particular hazards

Occasionally the risk is very great yet the patient deceptively claims to feel better. It has been suggested (Shah & Ganesvaran, 1997) that unstable suicidal ideation that varies in severity throughout the day may be strongly associated with a high risk of suicide. Factors liable to complicate risk management have been set out in Box 7.1. If alienation of staff occurs it is wise to discuss this openly so that attitudes of frustration and hostility directed towards the patient can be dealt with objectively. Setting limits to the degree of uncooperative behaviour that will be tolerated is sometimes necessary, particularly for psychiatric in-patients with personality disorders (see below) and adolescents. In the presence of a genuine suicidal risk, limit setting in the face of disturbed behaviour can be one of the most taxing tasks in clinical psychiatry, and the patient's management will require frequent discussions within the whole clinical team.

Control of hazards in the hospital environment is a most important issue. The high proportion of in-patient suicides due to hanging demands regular scrutiny of the ward regarding possible suspension points, and the removal of belts, cords and other potentially dangerous possessions from those at high risk. Among the elderly, plastic bags are a particular hazard. Most obviously curtain rails should be non-weight-bearing. Many so-called hangings by in-patients are more in the nature of strangulation and do not involve bodily suspension from a height (Mental Health Act Commission, 2001). This means that it is necessary to be vigilant about a wide variety of items found on a typical ward (e.g. shoelaces, bed and window frames, door handles, piping) when an individual's suicide risk is high. These findings have implications for observation techniques: so-called 'hanging' can occur in a supine position (25% of suicides of detained patients occurred despite observations every 15 minutes).

With regard to resuscitation, apart from the need to stabilise the neck because of a possible cervical fracture, attempts to restore respiratory and cardiac function after strangulation can be life-saving. The possibility of concomitant self-poisoning should also be kept in mind (Bennewith *et al*, 2005). Resuscitation protocols need to be reviewed in the light of these findings.

Wider environmental hazards should also be addressed: acute wards should ideally be on the ground or first floor, staircases should be safe, windows should open only to a limited degree, and access to motorways or bridges in the immediate vicinity should be limited as far as possible, for example by the use of barriers.

Suicide clusters

Following an in-patient suicide it is important to provide close support for the ward community as a whole and particularly for vulnerable individuals in whom suicidal risk may be kindled or accentuated.

Treating the unwilling patient

When the immediate risk escalates such that it cannot be controlled adequately because the patient is unable to comply with treatment, it may become necessary to act against his or her will, for example by preventing self-discharge and administering medication or other forms of treatment. The prevention of self-harm is given as one of the three reasons for which patients may be detained under the Mental Health Act 1983 (the legislation was specifically devised to cope with this situation).

The review by the Mental Health Act Commission (2001) of 168 suicidal deaths of detained patients found that 41% occurred in a public place while the patient was on approved leave and 28% of the patients had gone absent without leave. For in-patient suicides as a whole the corresponding figures are 31% and 34% in England and Wales (Meehan *et al*, 2006). These findings again draw attention to the need to review observation and leave strategies.

Discharge and leave

The Confidential Inquiry found that 41% of in-patient suicides occurred when discharge was being planned, and another 32% within two weeks of discharge, most commonly in the first week. Decisions concerning leave and discharge clearly need to be made very carefully. For patients who have been detained under the Mental Health Act, great care should be taken to ensure that leave agreements are consistent with the Act's requirements in each instance. In particular, it must be remembered that section 17 of the Act directs that the relevant consultant (i.e. the responsible medical officer) must give specific permission for any leave arrangements. Decisions should be made on a multidisciplinary basis, based on the Care Programme Approach (Kingdon, 1994). The Confidential Inquiry advised that individual care plans should specify action to be taken if a patient is non-compliant or fails to attend. Enlisting the help of relatives and friends is often very beneficial. The Inquiry recommended an appointment within 7 days of discharge from hospital for every patient with severe mental illness or a history of DSH in the previous 3 months. It found that 40% of post-discharge suicides occurred before the first follow-up appointment (Department of Health, 2001).

Patients with personality disorder

There are particular difficulties with regard to patients with personality disorders complicated by depressive symptoms and adverse life events. It may be tempting to withdraw from such a clinical dilemma on the assumption that such patients are not ill and should take full responsibility for what they do. However, such a clinical problem commonly precedes suicide, and any risk of this should be assessed and managed appropriately.

Prisoners

In the UK Her Majesty's Chief Inspector of Prisons (1999) has reported on the management of prison suicide. Assessment and management of suicide risk in prison should follow the same principles as in the wider community. Closer integration with the community mental health team is desirable in order to achieve this, but such a development is unlikely without the provision of adequate resources.

More recently, the first national clinical survey of self-inflicted deaths among prisoners in England and Wales was published (Shaw *et al*, 2004). This report was based on a 2-year sample and included detailed clinical and social information from prison staff. Recommended preventive measures included special attention immediately after reception into prison, provision of dedicated reception wings for prisoners at risk, with cells without bars for those at high risk; the use of bed linen that cannot be used for hanging or self-strangulation; rapid and effective sharing of information with health services; adequate detoxification facilities for alcohol and drug dependence; close follow-up of prisoners discharged from prison in-patient facilities; and good staff training.

Management of suicide risk in the community

The principles of care as already set out apply to patients in the community as much as in hospital. Special attention should be paid to making effective contact with groups such as young adult males or disaffected adolescents, who tend not to seek help. The assertive outreach team approach is particularly helpful in maintaining contact with vulnerable patients who are at high risk.

The Confidential Inquiry has demonstrated that the antecedents and clinical characteristics of individuals who die by suicide within 12 months of contact with services vary according to age and diagnosis. Comprehensive care packages, especially for schizophrenia in younger and depression in older patients may well be useful. Protocols for monitoring and follow-up of patients with a primary diagnosis of drug dependence or personality disorder are also advised (Hunt *et al*, 2006).

Suicide prevention

Research in the area of clinical suicide prevention is difficult for a number of reasons; most suicide studies are epidemiological. Success in suicide prevention will create no data to study. Also, the low suicide rate in the general population and the relatively low rate even in a high-risk group demand very large study samples and very long follow-ups in order to achieve sufficient statistical power (Mortensen, 1999).

Suicide prevention initiatives range from those on a global scale to those made by individual clinicians (Table 7.2).

International initiatives

Both the World Health Organization (WHO) and the United Nations have identified suicide as a priority area for action. In 1989, the WHO produced guidelines and recommended that its member states develop national prevention programmes, where possible linked to other public health policies. The main approach was based on identifying groups at high risk and restricting access to the means of suicide (World Health Organization, 1990), and the website (www.who.int) is a valuable source of information. The United Nations (1996) published a report on suicide which proposed the targeting of background antecedent social factors for suicide and focusing on high-risk groups.

National/governmental initiatives

In the 1990s, the UK government set suicide reduction targets for the general population and also, more specifically, for suicide among people with a serious mental illness as part of the 'Health of the Nation'

Table 7.2 Strategies for suicide prevention

Category	Example
Mental health promotion	Mental illness awareness training in schools
General improvement in psychiatric treatments/ practice, including increased accessibility of services	Effective psychiatric liaison services in accident and emergency departments
Increased accessibility of other services	Increased availability of Samaritans and other crisis telephone lines
General improvement in social welfare/cohesion	Policies on employment, education, social welfare, housing, child welfare
Reduced availability of means of self-harm	Conversion of coal gas to North Sea gas; stricter gun laws; restricted paracetamol sales
Reduced availability of disinhibiting factors	Policies on street drugs and alcohol usage
Improved care of high-risk groups	Improved risk assessment procedures
Addressing negative attitudes to suicide prevention among healthcare professionals	Education to challenge attitudes
Improved clinical practice during high-risk periods for individual patients	Comprehensive practice guidelines for the management of suicidal patients on in-patient units

strategy (Department of Health, 1994). These aims were reinforced by a further strategy document, *Saving Lives: Our Healthier Nation*, which suggested a target of reducing the death rate from suicide and undetermined injury by a sixth (17%) from a baseline of 1996 (Department of Health, 1999*a*). In the National Service Framework for Mental Health (Department of Health, 1999*b*) prison suicides, suicide audit and risk assessment were specifically highlighted. More recently, the Department of Health's National Suicide Prevention Strategy for England (Department of Health, 2002) aims to reduce the death rate from suicide by at least 20% by 2010. There are six stated goals in this document:

1 to reduce risk in key high-risk groups

2 to promote mental well-being in the wider population

3 to reduce the availability and lethality of suicide methods

4 to improve the reporting of suicidal behaviour in the media

5 to promote research on suicide and suicide prevention

6 to improve monitoring of progress towards the *Saving Lives: Our Healthier Nation* target for reducing suicide.

The Scottish Executive (2002) aims to reduce the number of suicides by 20% between 2003 and 2013. People in isolated or rural communities are identified as one priority group. Boyle *et al* (2005) have produced evidence that people in deprived areas, especially young adults, should be prioritised.

Gunnell & Lewis (2005) suggest that prevention should focus on two discrete areas: the prevention of the psychiatric illnesses that precede suicide; and tracking those risk factors particular to suicide, such as media influences (see below), the availability of methods and the medical management of self-harm.

Many countries have instituted national suicide prevention strategies, for example the USA, Scotland and Japan (US Department of Health and Human Services, 2001; Japan Ministry of Health, Labour, and Welfare, 2002; Scottish Executive, 2002). In Finland, the national strategy for suicide prevention has been particularly well developed. It emphasises local implementation and reducing alcohol misuse (Beskow *et al*, 1999) and may have produced a significant reduction in suicide mortality rates over the past decade.

Changes in social policy and society more widely can significantly influence the suicide rate by reducing access to means of self-harm. In the UK, the 30% reduction in suicides during the 1960s may well have been related to the removal of toxic coal gas from the domestic scene at that time, and as catalytic converters fitted to car exhausts are becoming more common a decline in suicides from carbon monoxide poisoning may become apparent, as has already happened in the USA (Clarke & Lester, 1987). Altering the shape of the exhaust pipe to make it harder to attach tubing might also result in a fall in deaths (Hawton, 1992). Another way to reduce the number of deaths is to restrict the sale of analgesics sold over the counter to small quantities. This strategy has been used successfully in France and Ireland and was more recently introduced in the UK, where it seems to have resulted in a reduction in suicide deaths from paracetamol and salicylates by a fifth (Hawton *et al*, 2004).

It is unrealistic to imagine that all lethal methods can be eliminated from the environment and the likelihood is that some substitution by other methods will take place over the long term. Improving social circumstances by, for example, reducing social isolation and unemployment is extremely difficult but may have a significant impact on suicide rates. In the USA, stricter gun control laws have, in certain states, been associated with a fall in the number of suicides using fire arms (Lester & Murrell, 1980) and there is now a convincing body of evidence that controls on gun ownership would significantly reduce suicide rates (Winokur & Black, 1992).

Mass media

There is strong evidence that copycat suicide clusters follow the depiction of suicide on television, radio or in film. This is particularly the case for younger age groups (Schmidtke & Hafner, 1988; Hassan, 1995). There has been considerable debate in this area regarding the balance between the rights to freedom of expression and the mass media's duty to be socially responsible. This has led the WHO to produce guidelines for press and broadcasting media when dealing with the issue of suicide (World Health Organization, 2000) and one of the goals for the suicide prevention strategy in England is to improve reporting in the media of matters related to suicide (Department of Health, 2002).

The role of public education by the media in relation to suicide has been less well validated. A positive example, however, has been reported by Etzersdorfer *et al* (1992), who described the effect of publication of media guidelines by the Austrian Association for Suicide Prevention. Before 1987, dramatic reports of suicide in the Vienna subway appeared in the Austrian media. Following the publication of the guidelines and their adoption by the media, the number of suicides in the subway system appeared to decline abruptly.

Individual clinicians/clinical services

Gunnell & Frankel (1994) concluded that 'no single intervention has been shown, in a well-conducted, randomised trial to reduce suicide rates'. Their review did not encompass the undoubtedly important role of clinical skills in assessing and managing suicidal individuals, and the potential for using proxy intermediate goals as opposed to the final act of suicide in evaluating such skills. At an individual level it is of course impossible to prove that any intervention has actually prevented a suicide, which is the ultimate goal of research in suicide.

None the less, there is some evidence to suggest that changes in practice or policy may reduce the risk of suicide (Table 7.2). Indeed, any improvement of clinical practice is likely to influence suicide rates in a positive direction. Such changes in practice may be led by professional bodies. The Royal College of Psychiatrists has published clinical policy guidelines as a result of the Confidential Inquiry (Appleby *et al*, 1999), as described earlier. Risk assessment training, adequate service resourcing and safe in-patient environments are all important areas that have been highlighted recently, as has safe prescribing of psychotropic medication.

While some have suggested that lithium may have a protective effect against suicide, clear evidence is lacking (Burgess *et al*, 2001). Similarly, it has been suggested that clozapine may have a preventive effect on suicide in schizophrenia (Reid *et al*, 1998). Isacsson (2000) postulated that if there were a fivefold increase in the use of antidepressants this might reduce Swedish suicide rates by 25%. Electroconvulsive therapy has also been claimed to reduce the risk of suicide (Isometsa *et al*, 1996).

Close coordination between primary and secondary care services is essential, and the potential role of general practitioners (GPs) in suicide prevention needs to be exploited to the full. Rutz *et al* (1992) offered a structured education programme to help in the recognition and treatment of depressive disorders for GPs on the island of Gotland in Sweden. The authors claimed that this led to a significant reduction in the number of suicides on the Swedish island. This approach may, of course, not be effective for all target populations; for instance, in one study only a fifth of suicides under the age of 35 had seen their GP in the 4 weeks before death, whereas 68% of those over 65 did so (Vassilas & Morgan, 1993, 1994). If contact with a GP or psychiatric services is taken as the combined index, then 39% of all males and 76% of all females make contact in the last month of their lives (Vassilas & Morgan, 1997). An international review (Luoma *et al*, 2002) concluded that 45% of suicide victims had contact with primary care providers in the month before death and confirmed the higher rates of contact among older adults. Recently, several studies have shown that it is possible to train a wide variety of healthcare professionals, not just doctors, to assess suicide risk, but there is no evidence yet that this strategy can affect suicide rates (Fenwick *et al*, 2004; Morriss *et al*, 2005).

Encouraging findings have been reported on the suicide prevention potential of twice-weekly telephone support with an emergency response service for elderly patients (De Leo *et al*, 2002). The role of telephonic communication in the care of the elderly has been reviewed by Jones (2002).

Managing alcohol and drug misuse and suicide prevention

Along with the example from Finland presented above (Beskow *et al*, 1999), a change in policy on alcohol usage may have led to a reduction in the numbers of suicides in the former USSR (Varnik, 1998), where a strict anti-alcohol policy was introduced as a part of perestroika. Suicide rates dropped in all 15 republics over the period 1984–90. Dhossche *et al* (2001) found that in 40% of a series of 512 suicides in the USA, alcohol, cocaine or cannabis were detected, which suggests that the assessment and management of drug and alcohol misuse at both the individual and the community level are important in the process of suicide prevention.

Making the environment safer

As mentioned above, the conversion from coal gas to North Sea gas for domestic use in the UK in the 1960s, strict gun control laws, limiting the availability of paracetamol and close control of potential hazards in hospital wards are all examples of this approach. Some consider this approach may be more useful than individual risk assessment.

Addressing negative attitudes

Up to a third of healthcare professionals may have equivocal or even negative attitudes concerning the feasibility of suicide prevention, and these probably impede the delivery of effective clinical care. They can be effectively challenged by appropriate factual presentation and discussion (Morgan *et al*, 1996).

The aftermath of suicide

Persons who have had some link with someone who commits suicide may experience considerable difficulty in coming to terms with the death. Problems may be experienced by relatives, friends, healthcare professionals, work colleagues and other patients. Campbell & Fahy (2002) have reviewed such adverse responses and ways of coping with them.

The consequences of suicide are particularly traumatic for the bereaved family because the act is self-inflicted, often unexpected and sometimes violent in nature. It can be especially difficult for relatives to resolve their grief in the face of strong conflicting feelings, which may include guilt, perplexity and anger. If the deceased was receiving psychiatric treatment, anger towards others is probably less likely to develop in those cases where the relatives felt they had previously been involved and kept well informed during treatment.

Routine clinical practice should encompass interviewing relatives soon after a suicide has occurred in order to provide support. In the community, the GP is well placed to recognise the need for such help (Shepherd & Barraclough, 1979). If the person who committed suicide had received help from healthcare services, the staff may also need to support any patients who had contact with the deceased.

Audit of suicide

Morgan & Priest (1991) in their study of unexpected deaths of psychiatric patients showed that it is feasible to incorporate a routine audit-type review into clinical practice. Deaths from suicide can be identified, without any need for specialised research staff, by cross-checking coroner inquest data with hospital admission/discharge registers and recent mortality statistics (King, 1983).

Although suicide audit procedures have never been evaluated systematically, the principles on which they should be based are clear. Within 24 hours of the suicide, an initial meeting of the ward community should be held. This is not strictly for audit because the primary aim of this first meeting should be to provide support for both patients and staff. The key audit meeting is best restricted to the three or four key staff members who were involved in the patient's care. Use of a standard checklist should ensure that the review includes all relevant issues and does not avoid controversial matters which might be difficult to discuss. If such a procedure is to succeed it has to be supportive yet encourage full exchange of information. The utmost tact is required by whoever acts as chairperson.

In a similar way, routine suicide audit should be developed in community services.

Non-fatal DSH

History and definition of DSH

In the UK, before the Suicide Act 1961, any suicide attempt was punishable under the law. Up until that time the number of reported episodes was small, but now it is so large that it represents a major challenge in healthcare.

There is continuing debate about the relative merits of the terms 'deliberate self-harm', 'parasuicide' and 'attempted suicide', which are often used synonymously. The WHO has defined parasuicide usefully as the following:

> 'An act with non-fatal outcome, in which an individual deliberately initiates a non-habitual behaviour that, without intervention from others, will cause self-harm, or on purpose ingests a substance in excess of the prescribed or generally recognized therapeutic dosage, and which is aimed at realizing changes which the subject desired via the actual or expected physical consequences.' (Platt *et al*, 1992)

In this chapter the term deliberate self-harm (DSH) is used for the reason that no suicidal intent is implied by it.

For many years suicide and 'attempted' suicide were regarded as varieties of the same behaviour, and Stengel *et al* (1958) showed that they did indeed overlap. The difficulty in using the term 'attempted suicide' is that it implies an intention that may not be present; some authors have suggested that people who deliberately harm themselves and display significant suicidal intent should be categorised separately as 'suicide attempters'.

Epidemiology of DSH

After the decriminalisation of suicide in 1961, the UK witnessed a sharp increase in the incidence of DSH. The rise continued during the 1970s but rates stabilised during the latter part of the 1980s, only to show another rise in the 1990s (Hawton *et al*, 1997). Many other European countries as well as the USA and Australia showed similar trends. A word of caution is required at this point: it is very difficult to establish accurate figures for DSH, as statistics are usually derived from hospital admission records, for which the definition of what constitutes DSH may vary. These figures also miss out a substantial number of people who either do not seek treatment or who are treated in primary care. DSH research also needs to distinguish rates for persons from rates of number of episodes.

Deliberate self-harm poses a significant financial burden on the healthcare system. In one study in England DSH was the third most frequent reason for acute general hospital admissions (Gunnell *et al*, 1996); 10% of admissions for DSH resulted in psychiatric in-patient care, and 10% of patients were readmitted over the following 12 months with a repeated episode of DSH. A recent systematic review of the literature on hospital-treated DSH indicated a 16% rate for non-fatal repetition, and a 2% suicide rate after 1 year (Owens *et al*, 2002). In a multinational European study organised by the WHO Regional Office for Europe (WHO/EURO) average rates of DSH for females were 193/100 000 and for males were 140/100 000 (Schmidtke *et al*, 1996).

Age and gender

In contrast to the pattern of a male predominance for completed suicide rates, the rates of DSH among females are higher than those among males for all age groups. On average, the rates for females are 1.5–2 times higher than those for males, but the gap is narrowing. The peak for females occurs in the 15- to 24-year age group, and for males is in the 25- to 34-year age group. The average ratio of DSH to suicide in females is 21:1 but this decreases steeply with age, being 61:1 in the 15- to 24-year age group and 5:1 in those aged over 55. For males, the average ratio of DSH to suicide is 6:1, and it similarly decreases with age, from 11:1 in the 15- to 24-year age group to 1.2:1 in those aged over 55 (Pritchard, 1995).

Social factors

Single and divorced people are over-represented among those who attempt suicide (Schmidtke *et al*, 1996). When compared with the general population, people who engage in DSH more often belong to the social categories associated with social destabilisation and poverty, and rates of DSH are higher among people in social class V (Gunnell *et al*, 1995). Hawton *et al* (2001) found that socio-economic deprivation was associated with DSH rates among males ($r = 0.89$) and females ($r = 0.79$).

The literature on unemployment and DSH has been systematically reviewed by Platt & Hawton (2000). Although individual cross-sectional studies point towards an association between DSH and unemployment, aggregated cross-sectional studies have failed to find any evidence of an association. Unemployment is higher in areas of socio-economic deprivation but it is unclear whether it is a causal factor or not.

Methods of DSH

Mostly non-violent methods are used in DSH, as violent methods often lead to death at the first attempt. The ratio of DSH to suicide in the USA is lower than in the UK and it has been suggested that this is because of the more frequent use of firearms in attempting suicide (Spicer & Miller, 2000). The vast majority of DSH episodes in the UK involve self-poisoning by drug overdose. In one Oxford-based study (Townsend *et al*, 2001), around 88% of all the episodes of DSH involved self-poisoning, 8% involved self-injury and 4% involved both; paracetamol overdoses were more common in first-time attempters and young people, whereas overdoses of antidepressants and tranquillisers were more common in repeaters and older people. These differences may reflect the differential availability of the various medications. The WHO/EURO reported similar findings: 64% of males and 80% of females used self-poisoning, whereas self-injury was the method chosen by 17% of males cases and 9% of female cases.

Self-injury

As indicated above, self-injury is the second most common method of DSH. Hawton (1989) classified self-cutting as superficial, deep, or self-mutilation. Superficial self-cutting tends to be associated with less suicidal intent. Deep cutting sometimes involves major blood vessels, nerves and tendons, and is sometimes (although not necessarily) associated with serious suicidal intent; it is, though, usually associated with severe psychiatric disorder. Carving on the skin and picking at a wound are the most commonly reported types of self-mutilation. These occurred in about a third of a sample of US adolescents presenting with DSH. Those with self-mutilation behaviour were more likely to be diagnosed with oppositional defiant disorder, major depression or dysthymia. They also had higher scores on measures of hopelessness, loneliness, anger, risk taking, reckless behaviour and alcohol use (Guertin *et al*, 2001). Self-mutilators appear to have more persistent suicidal ideation and to perceive their behaviour as less lethal than it actually is (Stanley *et al*, 2001). Psychotic self-mutilation is rare, and may affect the eyes, tongue or genitalia.

Attempting suicide by burning is rare. One study reported that DSH by burning constituted 1% of all admissions to a burns unit, and that among these cases there was high incidence of prior psychiatric illness (Krummen *et al*, 1998). People who survive an episode of DSH by jumping from a height are more likely than expected to be single and unemployed and psychotic, whereas those who survive self-shooting are more likely to be male, to misuse alcohol, to have a forensic history and to have an antisocial or borderline personality disorder (De Moore & Robertson, 1999). The relationship between the severity of suicidal intent and the lethality of the method used is not clear. It was observed in one small study that people who made fewer communications beforehand regarding their intended self-damaging behaviour tended to use more lethal methods in their attempts (Handwerk *et al*, 1998).

Aetiology of DSH

Biological factors

The biological aetiological factors in DSH are similar to those related to suicide (see above). Low levels of cholesterol have been reported in patients admitted with an episode of DSH (Kim & Myint, 2004), particularly those who have used violent methods (Alvarez *et al*, 2000), although other studies have failed to replicate these findings (Diesenhammer *et al*, 2004). Sublette *et al* (2006) have postulated that lipid levels are involved in the serotonin-mediated link between lower cholesterol and suicidality. The possible role of serotonin in impulsivity is discussed below.

Psychiatric illness

Comorbid psychiatric disorders are common in samples of people who deliberately harm themselves: up to 80% had a DSM–III–R diagnosis in one Finnish study (Suominen *et al*, 1996). In a more recent UK study, 92% of the sample met ICD–10 criteria for a psychiatric disorder (Haw *et al*, 2001). The commonest diagnosis made is depression, with about 70% meeting diagnostic criteria for a depressive disorder, while 14–17% meet criteria for an anxiety disorder.

Personality

Personality disorders are strongly associated with DSH (Modestin *et al*, 1997). There is a particularly strong relationship with borderline personality disorder, although it should be noted that the definition of this disorder includes recurrent threats or acts of self-harm (Suominem *et al*, 1996). Among people who deliberately harm themselves rates of personality disorder of 41–46% have been reported (Suominen *et al*, 1996; Haw *et al*, 2001).

Alcohol and substance misuse

Alcohol dependence and harmful use are commonly found in association with DSH. Rates of 27% have been reported in the UK (Haw *et al*, 2001) and higher rates have been found in other countries, for example 53% in Finland (Suominen *et al*, 1996). Drug misuse and dependence are also reported in about 10–17% of cases (Ennis *et al*, 1989; Suominen *et al*, 1996; Haw *et al*, 2001).

Psychosocial factors

Motivation

Stengel *et al* (1958) were the first to point out that it is a mistake to regard all 'attempted suicides' as failed suicides. Each episode has a social meaning that has to be addressed in order to understand the reasons for the act. The precise causes of an act of DSH are notoriously difficult to assess and often are unclear even to the patient. Bancroft *et al* (1979) interviewed a sample of patients who had been admitted after an episode of DSH and asked them about the reasons for the episode. The commonest reason – spontaneously expressed by about half the sample – was the 'wish to die'. About a third denied any suicidal intention. Three psychiatrists were asked to evaluate the interviews with the patients and to choose reasons based on 'common-sense criteria' that they thought were important. The four reasons chosen most often were, in order: communicating hostility, influencing others, relieving a state of mind and suicidal intent. The first two were attributed to 71% and 54% of cases, respectively. Interestingly they were the reasons chosen least frequently by the patients themselves. Of 23 patients (56%) who claimed suicidal intent, only 12 (29%) were judged to be suicidal by psychiatrists.

Episodes of DSH are often unplanned. Impulsivity has consistently been found to be a personality trait associated with DSH, especially for those who repeat it (Evans *et al*, 1996). Abnormalities in the serotonergic system correlate with high levels of impulsivity (Oquendo & Mann, 2000) and have been implicated in suicidal behaviour.

Hopelessness and problem-solving ability

Hopelessness and pessimism about the future have been found to be key cognitions preceding DSH. Hopelessness is also associated with repetition of DSH (Petrie *et al*, 1988). Suicidal intent is closely correlated with hopelessness and is one mechanism by which depression is thought to lead to suicidal behaviour (Minkoff *et al*, 1973). A key finding has been that many of those who harm themselves have difficulties in problem solving (Pollock & Williams, 1998). Researchers are now focusing on psychological mechanisms to devise strategies to help.

Life stress

Adverse life events are frequently reported to have occurred before the act of self-harm. When the relative risk of developing various psychiatric illnesses is calculated for the 6 months following a stressful life event, DSH carries the highest risk. In the month following an adverse life event the relative risk of DSH is raised to ten times that of the general population, indicating a strong and immediate relationship (Paykel, 1980). Serious argument with a partner is the single most commonly reported event by the DSH group.

Imitation

As with completed suicide, an imitation effect may occur in DSH and produce clusters. Those involved in psychiatric in-patient units should proceed with caution when several vulnerable individuals are present on the ward at one time. Social influences probably explain the phenomenon of epidemics of self-mutilation, which have been reported as spreading through hospital wards (Rosen & Walsh, 1989).

Fictional portrayals of DSH, for example on a popular television drama, seem to lead to an increase in patients presenting to accident and emergency departments with similar behaviour (Hawton *et al*, 1999).

Physical illness

A consistent finding is that people who deliberately harm themselves have a higher than expected incidence of physical illness and recent admissions to hospital (Stenager *et al*, 1994). Increased rates of self-mutilation have been observed among those who have experienced surgery or hospital treatment before the age of 5 years (Rosenthal *et al*, 1972).

DSH in special groups

Adolescents

Deliberate self-harm is most common in adolescents, among whom the female:male ratio is at its highest. Understandably, developmental factors play an important role in DSH behaviour for this group. In particular, family factors appear to play a crucial role. DSH is associated with lower levels of family support, disturbed relationships with parents, and sexual or physical abuse within the family (Garnefski *et al*, 1992; Wagner, 1997). These factors also correlate with poor self-esteem in the adolescent. Furthermore, individuals in this age group tend to be more impressionable and are therefore more likely to imitate DSH behaviour seen within their family or shown on the mass media.

Adolescents with a more formal psychiatric disorder have also an increased risk of DSH. Diagnoses of particular importance are affective disorders, conduct disorders, drug misuse, early onset of psychotic illness, eating disorders and those with borderline personality disorder (Apter & Freudenstein, 2000).

Ethnic minorities

In the UK, rates of DSH are significantly raised among Asian women: in one London study rates were 1.6 times those in white women (Bhugra *et al*, 1999*a*). Among Asian women aged less than 30 years, the rates were 2.5 times those of white women. However, among black groups rates were found to be lower than expected. A further study in west London (Bhugra *et al*, 1999*b*) compared the characteristics of Asian and white people who presented themselves to hospital services following DSH. It found that white patients were more likely to have mental illness and were more likely to have used alcohol as part of the method of attempted suicide. By contrast, Asian patients had more often experienced adverse life events pertaining to relationships and took fewer tablets.

Merrill & Owens (1986) compared the characteristics of UK-born white DSH patients with those born in India, Pakistan or Bangladesh (Asians) admitted to a regional poisons unit in Birmingham. The rate of self-poisoning for Asian females was higher than for white females, but for Asian males it was lower than for white males. Significantly more Asian females reported marital problems than white females and culture conflict was also more common among the former. The authors reported that the pattern of DSH on the Indian subcontinent (predominately a male activity with low incidence rates) was quite different to what they found among Asians in Birmingham. This contrasts with the pattern of suicide in immigrants from the Indian subcontinent to the UK, which reflect those of the subcontinent (see above). Cultural conflicts were common. These mostly centred around families who expected their teenage daughters to conform to a traditional lifestyle. The adolescent girls themselves were often torn between these family pressures and their own desires for what they perceived as a less restrictive Western lifestyle.

In the USA, as with suicide, rates of DSH in the black community have generally been lower than among whites, although rates among Hispanics are reported as being higher than expected (Moscicki *et al*, 1988).

The elderly

Compared with the general adult population, DSH in the elderly has a greater similarity to the profile of completed suicides. For example, although the behaviour is still more common in women, the gender ratio is much smaller than in younger groups. Similarly, clinical depression has a much higher correlation with DSH compared with the behaviour in younger populations (Draper, 1996). DSH in this group is also a much stronger predictor of eventual suicide (Heppel & Quinton, 1997). Physical illness, bereavement, social isolation and frontal lobe dysfunction are all stronger correlates of DSH in elderly populations than in younger ones (Draper, 1994).

One small study found no clinical difference between a group of elderly people who committed suicide after a series of DSH episodes and a matching group of elderly people who committed suicide without having any history of DSH (Salib *et al*, 2001) and on this basis the authors argued that DSH in the elderly should be taken seriously and be considered as failed suicide. A more recent study found little clinical difference between elderly people with depression who had deliberately self-harmed and those who had not, other than poorly integrated social networks and a greater sense of hopelessness (Denniss *et al*, 2005).

Assessment of DSH

The National Institute for Health and Clinical Excellence (NICE) is responsible for providing guidance on treatment in the National Health Service for England and Wales, and it has issued a guideline on the short-term physical and psychological management and secondary prevention of self-harm in primary and secondary care (NICE, 2004). A quick reference guide is available on the NICE website (www.nice.org.uk) and this is essential reading.

Immediately after an episode of DSH

In hospital practice most patients who present after an episode of DSH are first seen in the accident and emergency department. The urgent task there is to assess and treat any immediate risk and needs, whether physical, psychological or social. Preliminary psychosocial assessment should be carried out at the earliest opportunity (at triage in hospital or at initial assessment in primary care) to determine mental capacity, willingness to remain for further assessment, level of distress and presence of mental illness (NICE, 2004). Admission to hospital can, of course, help to ensure that medical treatment is adequate and this also facilitates full psychosocial assessment once the mental state is clear of any toxic effects of the overdose (Department of Health and Social Security, 1984). The Royal College of Psychiatrists (2004) has published a report which provides excellent practical guidance for some of the dilemmas that can occur in assessing patients in accident and emergency departments.

Although a majority of DSH patients are admitted to a medical ward, there is great variability in hospital practice within England (Bennewith *et al*, 2004). A third or more are discharged directly from the accident and emergency department; sometimes this is because the event is regarded as trivial, but it may also reflect non-availability of beds, or the patient self-discharges (Owens, 1990). The NICE (2004) guideline advises that temporary (including overnight) admission be considered, especially for: people who are very distressed; people in whom psychosocial assessment proves too difficult as a result of drug and/or alcohol intoxication; and people who may be returning to an unsafe or potentially harmful environment. Obviously this also applies to those who have significant continuing physical adverse effects of overdose from drugs or other toxic agents and when significant continuing risk of repeat DSH or suicide is suspected. Before a patient is allowed to leave the accident and emergency department, evaluation of risk (as below) is always necessary, and rapid availability of advice from specialist mental health staff is crucial. It is important to remember that apparent physical risk in DSH may not accurately reflect the suicide risk, if only because patients are often ignorant of the dangers associated with various agents that are used: a small overdose with a minor tranquilliser can be associated with serious suicidal intent, yet a highly lethal overdose of paracetamol might be taken by someone without suicide in mind.

Patients who are uncooperative and demand self-discharge from the accident and emergency department can be at significant risk, as such behaviour tends to be associated with substance misuse and a repetitive pattern of DSH (Crawford & Wessely, 1998). Adolescents who self-discharge may be at particular risk. Whether or not to allow a patient at significant risk to leave against advice can be a difficult decision. The type and quality of social support are very relevant. If mental illness is thought to be present, then consideration should be given to detaining the patient under the Mental Health Act 1983 in order to ensure further assessment and, if necessary, urgent treatment. In situations of high risk it may on occasion be necessary to restrain the patient under common law until the appropriate detention procedures can be completed. In such circumstances, when staff have clearly acted in good faith with the intention of saving life or preventing severe injury, subsequent litigation on grounds of battery or wrongful detention is rare and unlikely to succeed. To cover this eventuality, however, staff should write full contemporaneous notes which set out clearly the reasons for the action taken, and these should be signed and dated at the time. If subsequent additions or clarification to the notes are needed, these should be set out discretely from the original and again signed and dated. The management of these difficult situations is further discussed in Chapter 17 (page 424). In deciding whether urgently needed, potentially life-saving medical treatment can be given without consent, the doctor should take into account the patient's mental competence to understand the situation fully, to believe all information about it, and to weigh up its implications rationally (Hassan *et al*, 1999). Discharges direct from the accident and emergency department require notification to the relevant GP either immediately by telephone when continuing risk demands or in any case within 24 hours.

Full assessment and management

Although the management is based primarily on the interview with the patient, information from other sources such as key informants and the GP may be invaluable. The NICE (2004) guideline emphasises the importance of healthcare professionals acquiring appropriate clinical skills in assessing and managing DSH patients. It advises that the needs assessment should, where possible, be agreed with the patient and should be written into the case notes, and that any disagreement should also be recorded.

Physical

Assessment of any medical risk is one of the first and most urgent tasks and treatment may be needed without delay. Obviously, an unconscious patient needs urgent life support. Paracetamol overdose may require immediate administration of the antidote (N-acetyl cysteine). Respiratory support may be needed to combat the depressant effect of dextropopoxyphene, which is commonly present in paracetamol preparations. The danger of cardiac arrhythmia in tricyclic antidepressant overdose may necessitate treatment in an intensive-care unit. A patient who has survived hanging needs adequate cardiorespiratory resuscitation as well as the management of possible cervical cord injury. Detailed consideration of toxicology and resuscitation is not within the remit of this chapter but the NICE (2004) guideline provides a fuller discussion.

Psychological

It is important first to focus on the episode of DSH, its nature, recent events leading up to it, and the motivation behind it. Then follows the collection of background data, including history of psychiatric disorder and DSH, and previous personality, especially aggressive/impulsive traits. A full mental state assessment will help determine the type and degree of psychological distress, the significance of any ongoing ideation regarding suicide and non-fatal repetition (see below) and whether formal mental illness is present.

A number of studies have identified the following correlates of suicide following DSH (Sakinofsky, 2000):

- age over 45
- either high or low socio-economic class
- currently unemployed
- male
- living alone
- high lethality of episode
- high intent to die
- communication of suicidal intent
- precautions to avoid discovery
- repeated self-harm
- personality disorder (anxiety prone, impulsive)
- mental disorder (axis I psychosis, mood disorder, schizophrenia, alcoholism, substance misuse)
- previous in-patient psychiatric treatment.

Harriss *et al* (2005) have shown that suicidal intent at the time of self-harm is associated with an increased risk of subsequent suicide. Furthermore, a long-term study of a large cohort (11 583) of DSH patients has shown that a history of repeated DSH is associated with an increased risk of subsequent suicide (Zahl & Hawton, 2004). The authors emphasise the importance of including a detailed enquiry into a history of DSH in risk assessment. The severity of self-harm can also be an important predictor of subsequent suicide (Carter *et al*, 2005). To assess the likelihood of repeat non-fatal DSH in the immediate future it is useful to obtain the patient's own view and ascertain whether the relevant stressful events remain unchanged (non-fatal repetition is discussed below, under 'After-care').

Problem-solving ability should also be evaluated because this will provide some idea of what kind of help is likely to be found acceptable and useful.

Social

The hazards faced by others, such as dependent children, should form an integral part of the overall evaluation of risk, as should assessment of whether substantial problems remain, or perhaps have been made worse.

Management of DSH

Following the above assessment it should be possible to set out a full formulation of the problem, which in turn will lead on to a management plan. Treatment of mental illness is initiated in parallel with measures aimed at DSH itself.

Treatment setting

In determining the most appropriate setting for ongoing treatment the patient's preference, for example referral back to a trusted GP, should be taken into account in order to maximise compliance. Around a half of all DSH patients are given a psychiatric out-patient appointment, although about 60% either fail to attend or do not attend after the first appointment. Another 10% are admitted directly into psychiatric in-patient units.

Service provision for DSH in the general hospital

Adequate provision for the assessment and management of DSH (Royal College of Psychiatrists, 1994) is an essential part of any comprehensive suicide prevention strategy. Most services fall well below recommended standards (Hughes *et al*, 1998). Specialised mental illness staff should be dedicated to the assessment and management of DSH, and relevant medical wards should be safe. Admission to one specialised ward is probably better than wide dispersal, if only because such an arrangement fosters more positive staff attitudes. An overall planning and coordinating group is also desirable. Psychosocial assessment of DSH patients can be carried out satisfactorily by a range of health professionals, provided that they have had appropriate training and that close supervision is maintained by the senior psychiatrist responsible for the service.

The special needs of children and young people have been set out in the NICE (2004) guideline. Particularly important is the need for care in a separate children's area of the accident and emergency department by staff who are appropriately trained. Overnight admission should normally be arranged, in a paediatric ward or other specialised facility. Parental consent (or that of whatever adult is legally responsible) should be obtained for mental health assessment. Special attention should be paid to confidentiality, competence, parental consent, child protection, the use of the Mental Health Act in young people and the Children's Act.

After-care

Several well-recognised hazards need to be taken into account in planning ongoing treatment for DSH patients.

Non-fatal repetition

The literature on repeat non-fatal episodes of DSH has been reviewed by Sakinofsky (2000). In cohorts of patients seen because of DSH, slightly more than a half will have a history of DSH. In 1 year 30% repeat at least once, 17% two or more times (Kerkhof, 2000). In devising treatment programmes, 'first timers' should not be ignored, if only to attempt prevention of their recruitment into the 'repeater' group. Such subgroups probably warrant differing therapeutic approaches, and these need to be clarified.

Prevention of repetition is an important element in the management of DSH patients. Although the heterogeneity of DSH makes prediction difficult, and the significance of each factor for an individual probably changes with time, an 11-item prediction scale based on clinical and demographic factors (Kreitman & Foster, 1991) has proved useful. The items are: previous DSH, personality disorder, previous psychiatric treatment, unemployment, social class V, alcohol misuse, drug misuse, criminal record, involvement in violence, age 25–34 years, and being single, divorced or separated. However, probably more than a half of repeaters do not score highly (Kapur & House, 1998) and this poses a dilemma for any approach restricted to high-risk individuals (Kapur *et al*, 2005). Recent advice rightly focuses on needs assessment that aims to identify psychosocial factors that might explain an act of self-harm, leading to the formulation of vulnerability and precipitating factors that require addressing (National Collaborating Centre for Mental Health, 2004). Prediction may be improved by including other factors, such as personality traits (impulsivity, aggression, problem-solving skills) and a motivation for the DSH that involves some form of appeal (Sakinofsky & Roberts, 1990; Corcoran *et al*, 1997; Kerkhof *et al*, 1988). This 'appeal' aspect of DSH has been succinctly summarised as:

> 'the knowledge that the wish to die, made obvious, can be a powerful way of releasing intolerable stresses or generate concern.' (*Lancet*, 1974)

Suicide

The risk of suicide following DSH is far larger than that in the general population (Hawton & Fagg, 1988). The period of greatest risk appears to be in the first 3 years, and particularly in the first 6 months following DSH. Some 1–3% of DSH patients will kill themselves in the first year; this is about 100 times the rate in the general population. A remarkable 37-year follow-up study (Suominen *et al*, 2004) showed that the suicide risk continues at least into the fourth decade, with 13% of DSH patients having killed themselves. Up to 15% of persons who self-mutilate may eventually kill themselves (Nelson & Grunebaum, 1971). Life-threatening episodes should be assumed to indicate high suicide risk in the absence of compelling evidence to the contrary, but even trivial self-harm may sometimes disguise serious risk. In spite of problems related to the low base rate, predictive scales have met with some success (Pierce, 1981; Pallis *et al*, 1984; Beck & Steer, 1989).

Social and family difficulties

An act of DSH often has a dramatic impact upon relationships with others, making them worse or even ending them. In other cases, however, even if probably only transiently, support may be generated that was not previously forthcoming. The likelihood of repetition depends to some degree upon whether such conflicts are resolved or continue unabated, although some patients continue to repeat DSH in spite of improvement in these areas (Sakinofsky *et al*, 1990). Such individuals tend to see their problems as more insuperable, score higher on measures of social deviancy and hostility, and are particularly likely to exhibit low self-esteem (Farmer & Creed, 1989; Joiner & Rudd, 1995).

Poor compliance with treatment

Early repetition is more likely among patients with a previous history of DSH, and for this subgroup compliance with an early appointment (i.e. within days of the index episode) is very important (Gilbody *et al*, 1997). Poor compliance with any offered treatment has long been recognised as a feature of DSH patients (Turner & Morgan, 1979) and 'repeaters' tend to be much less compliant than 'first timers'. Compliance may be improved by offering patients fixed appointments and by ensuring continuity of therapist throughout both in-patient and subsequent out-patient care (Moller, 1989) or by making home visits to patients who default from follow-up appointments (van Heeringen *et al*, 1995).

Treatment options

Basic approaches

All aspects of the clinical problem should be taken into account. Any mental illness should be treated in parallel with measures aimed specifically at DSH. If the prescription of psychotropic medication is considered necessary, care should be taken to ensure that the patient is not given possession of dangerous amounts of medication. Close coordination with the GP and strict control of amounts issued on prescription are essential. A responsible relative may usefully take custody of medication as long as the risk continues. There is some evidence that benzodiazepines may impair cognitive processes and so delay resolution of psychological difficulties following stressful events, and some have advised that they should be avoided in the management of DSH (van Heeringen, 2001*b*). Relationship difficulties may require conjoint therapy, and the needs of family members such as dependent children as well as wider social/situational problems should be addressed adequately.

Problem-solving therapies are useful basic techniques because they focus on the 'here and now' and foster compliance in patients who are often reluctant to engage in self-evaluation. It attempts to clarify the problems faced, sets goals, works out agreed ways to achieve them, and reviews progress regularly (Hawton & Catalan, 1987). Manuals are available for the problem-solving therapies and these approaches can be learnt relatively easily by clinicians (Hawton & Kirk, 1989).

Suicidal patients seem to have difficulties in being able to solve problems and their coping style in the face of problems is described as being passive. Problem-solving therapy seeks to change this coping style by enabling patients to identify problems and then implement appropriate ways of dealing with them. The therapy is divided into two phases. First, the therapist helps the patient identify and define problems; this may involve a detailed behavioural analysis of the sequence of events, thoughts and behaviours that led to a particular episode of maladaptive behaviour. In the second phase the therapist aids the patient in generating several alternative ways of dealing with a problem. This may be an area that suicidal patients find difficult and where they will tend to emphasise the negative side of any solution. None the less, the patient is guided in evaluating potential solutions and choosing the most appropriate solution. The therapist then provides coaching to help the patient implement the chosen solution. Rehearsal of the solution during the therapy session is encouraged so that any potential problems can be identified and dealt with (Heard, 2000).

Evaluation of treatments

A systematic review (Hawton *et al*, 1998) concluded that while some treatments show promise, further randomised intervention trials are needed to confirm their efficacy: nearly all trials were too small to allow reliable statistical interpretation. Other difficulties included failure to specify clearly the nature of standard (control) care and the specific intervention used (e.g. whether it excluded episodes that did not require admission to hospital). The types of intervention that were included in the review were: problem solving, intensive care plus outreach, emergency card, dialectic behavioural therapy, general hospital admission versus discharge, medication with flupenthixol or other antidepressants, and long-term versus short-term therapy. Problem solving, such as that already described, was picked out as a promising approach.

The use of emergency cards, which involve giving patients, on discharge from hospital, a card with a telephone number for 24-hour access to a clinician, also initially appeared to be promising. However, one evaluation of this approach produced some paradoxical results (Evans *et al*, 1999): while there was some success with 'first timers' (i.e. the emergency card led to a reduction in DSH repetition, although larger trials are needed to clarify this), among patients with a previous history of DSH the response was an increase in repetition. So, on the present evidence, the emergency card technique cannot yet be recommended for use among DSH patients, although its potential with 'first timers' warrants further evaluation (Evans *et al*, 2005). Similar paradoxical increases in repetition in various subgroups of DSH patients as a result of various interventions have also been reported in other studies (Moller, 1989; van der Sande *et al*, 1997). They are difficult to explain but may be related to personality difficulties, perceived ineffectiveness of services arising out of previous abortive contacts and alcohol misuse.

Patients suffering from borderline personality who repeatedly harm themselves are particularly difficult to treat. In a randomised controlled trial, Linehan *et al* (1991) evaluated the effects of a variant of cognitive–behavioural therapy (CBT) for this group. Those patients who received the experimental intervention were found to be significantly less likely to repeat DSH, and spent fewer days on a psychiatric ward during the 1-year study period. (See page 479 for a more comprehensive description of dialectical behaviour therapy.)

A randomised controlled trial of brief psychodynamic interpersonal therapy has also produced promising results (Guthrie *et al*, 2001). The intervention, which was delivered on a domiciliary basis, was well defined and of proven cost-effectiveness. Although only a half ($n = 119$) of the eligible individuals agreed to participate, such difficulty is common in most studies of intervention in DSH. Over a follow-up period of 6 months the experimental intervention was associated with more treatment satisfaction, greater symptomatic improvement and fewer repeats of DSH compared with control treatment.

In a trial of manual-assisted CBT (Tyrer *et al*, 2003), in which 480 patients were randomised, there was no reduction in the repetition rate of DSH in individuals given brief CBT (they were offered up to seven sessions). A more recent, although smaller study, in which 120 patients were randomised following an episode of DSH, found a significant reduction in the repetition rate of DSH among those who had undergone ten sessions of CBT compared with those patients who had received treatment as usual (Brown *et al*, 2005).

Primary prevention of DSH

Given its complex aetiology it is not surprising that primary prevention of DSH has not been achieved. Suicide prevention strategies may be relevant to the minority in whom suicidal ideation is clear. In DSH as a whole it is necessary to address a complex web of causal factors both within and outside the individual concerned. Although various aspects of personal vulnerability may set the scene, other factors, such as relationship difficulties and adverse life events, may precipitate and perpetuate situations that lead to DSH. It is particularly important to take into account the 'appeal effect' (see above).

Gender-specific social and cultural changes, as well as increasing levels of alcohol and drug misuse, are likely to be related to the recent increases in DSH rates in younger men. The ease of availability of psychotropic agents also increases the risk of DSH in vulnerable individuals. The importance of scrupulous care in the prescription of such agents is obvious: they may be particularly hazardous if used merely for the purpose of symptom relief without any underlying causes being properly addressed.

References

Alvarez, A. (1990) *The Savage God. A Study of Suicide.* New York & London: Norton.

Alvarez, J. C., Cremniter, D., Gluck, N., *et al* (2000) Low serum cholesterol in violent but not in non-violent suicide attempters. *Psychiatric Research*, **95**, 103–108.

Amsel, L. & Mann, J. J. (2001) Suicide risk assessment and the suicidal process approach. In *Understanding Suicidal Behaviour* (ed. K. van Heeringen), pp. 163–181. Chichester: Wiley.

Appleby, L. (1991) Suicide during pregnancy and in the first postnatal year. *BMJ*, **302**, 137–140.

Appleby, L., Mortensen, P. B. & Faragher, E. B. (1998) Suicide and other causes of mortality after post-partum psychiatric admission. *British Journal of Psychiatry*, **173**, 209–211.

Appleby, L., Shaw, J., Amos, T., *et al* (1999) *Safer Services: Report of the National Confidential Inquiry into Suicide and Homicide by People with Mental Illness*. London: The Stationery Office.

Apter, A. & Freudenstein, O. (2000) Adolescent suicidal behaviour: psychiatric populations. In *The International Handbook of Suicide and Attempted Suicide* (eds K. Hawton & K. van Heeringen), pp. 261–274. Chichester: Wiley.

Arango, V., Underwoood, M. D., Gubbi, A. V., *et al* (1995) Localized alterations in pre- and postsynaptic serotonin binding sites in the ventrolateral prefrontal cortex of suicide victims. *Brain Research*, **688**, 121–133.

Bancroft, J., Hawton, K., Simkin, S., *et al* (1979) The reasons people give for taking overdoses: a further inquiry. *British Journal of Medical Psychology*, **52**, 353–365.

Barraclough, B. M. (1974) A hundred cases of suicide: clinical aspects. *British Journal of Psychiatry*, **125**, 355–373.

Barraclough, B. M., Harris, E. & Clare, E. (2002) Suicide preceded by murder: the epidemiology of homicide-suicide in England and Wales 1988–92. *Psychological Medicine*, **32**, 577–584.

Beck, A. T. & Steer, R. A. (1989) Clinical predictors of eventual suicide: a 5 to 10 year prospective study of suicide attempters. *Journal of Affective Disorders*, **17**, 203–209.

Beck, A. T., Brown, G. K., Steer, R. A., *et al* (1999) Suicide ideation at its worst point: a predictor of eventual suicide in psychiatric patients. *Suicide and Life Threatening Behaviour*, **29**, 1–9.

Bennewith, O., Gunnell, D., Peters, T., *et al* (2004) Variations in the hospital management of self harm in adults in England: observational study. *BMJ*, **328**, 1108–1109.

Bennewith, O., Gunnell, D., Kapur, N., *et al* (2005) Suicide by hanging: multicentre study based on coroners' records in England. *British Journal of Psychiatry*, **186**, 260–261.

Bertolote, J. M. (2001) Suicide in the world: an epidemiological overview 1959–2000. In *Suicide: An Unnecessary Death* (ed. D. Wasserman), pp. 3–10. London: Martin Dunitz.

Beskow, J., Kerkhof, A., Kokkola, A., *et al* (1999) *Suicide Prevention in Finland 1986–1996: External Evaluation by an International Peer Group*. Helsinki: Ministry of Social Affairs and Health.

Bhugra, D., Desai, M. & Baldwin, D. S. (1999*a*) Attempted suicide in west London, I. Rates across ethnic communities. *Psychological Medicine*, **29**, 1125–1130.

Bhugra, D., Baldwin, D. S., Desai, M., *et al* (1999*b*) Attempted suicide in West London, II. Inter-group comparison. *Psychological Medicine*, **29**, 1131–1139.

Boyle, P., Exeter, D., Feng, Z., *et al* (2005) Suicide gap among young adults in Scotland: population study. *BMJ*, **330**, 175–176.

Brent, D. A. & Moritz, G. (1996) Developmental pathways to adolescent suicide. In *Adolescent Opportunities and Challenges* (eds D. Cichetti & S. Toth), pp. 233–258. Rochester, NY: University of Rochester Press.

Brown, G. K., Ten Have, T., Henriques, G. R., *et al* (2005) Cognitive therapy for the prevention of suicide attempts: a randomized controlled trial. *JAMA*, **294**, 563–570.

Brown, M. & Barraclough, B. (1999) Partners in life and in death: the suicide pact in England and Wales 1988–1992. *Psychological Medicine*, **29**, 1299–1306.

Burgess, S., Geddes, J., Hawton, K., *et al* (2001) Lithium for maintenance treatment of mood disorders (Cochrane review). *Cochrane Database Systematic Review*, (**3**), CD003013.

Campbell, C. & Fahy, T. (2002) The role of the doctor when a patient commits suicide. *Psychiatric Bulletin*, **26**, 44–49.

Carter, G., Reith, D. M., Whyte, I. M., *et al* (2005) Repeated self-poisoning: increasing severity of self-harm as a predictor of subsequent suicide. *British Journal of Psychiatry*, **186**, 253–257.

Chan, K. P. M., Yip, P. S. F., Au, J., *et al* (2005) Charcoal-burning suicide in post-transition Hong Kong. *British Journal of Psychiatry*, **185**, 67–73.

Charlton, J., Kelly, S., Dunnell, K., *et al* (1993) Suicide deaths in England and Wales: trend in factors associated with suicide deaths. *Population Trends*, **70**, 34–42.

Cheng, A. T. A. & Lee, C. (2000) Suicide in Asia and the Far East. In *The International Handbook of Suicide and Attempted Suicide* (eds K. Hawton & K. Heeringen), pp. 29–48. Chichester: Wiley.

Clarke, R. U. & Lester, D. (1987) Toxicity of car exhausts and opportunity for suicide. *Social Science and Medicine*, **41**, 114–120.

Conwell, Y., Duberstein, P. R., Cox, C., *et al* (1996) Relationships of age and axis I diagnoses in victims of completed suicide: a psychological autopsy study. *American Journal of Psychiatry*, **153**, 1001–1008.

Corcoran, P., Kelleher, M. J., Keeley, K. S., *et al* (1997) A preliminary statistical model for identifying repeaters of parasuicide. *Archives of Suicide Research*, **3**, 65–74.

Crawford, M. J. & Wessely, S. (1998) Does initial management affect the rate of repetition of deliberate self-harm? Cohort study. *BMJ*, **317**, 985.

De Leo, D., Buono, M. D. & Dwyer, J. (2002) Suicide among the elderly: the long term impact of a telephone support service and assessment intervention in Northern Italy. *British Journal of Psychiatry*, **181**, 226–229.

De Moore, G. M. & Robertson, A. R. (1999) Suicide attempts by firearms and by leaping from heights: a comparative study of survivors. *American Journal of Psychiatry*, **156**, 1425–1431.

Denniss, M., Wakefield, P., Molloy, C., *et al* (2005) Self harm in older people with depression. *British Journal of Psychiatry*, **186**, 538–539.

Department of Health (1994) *Health of the Nation Key Area Handbook*. London: The Stationery Office.

Department of Health (1999*a*) *Saving Lives: Our Healthier Nation*. London: HMSO.

Department of Health (1999*b*) *National Service Framework for Mental Health. Modern Standards Service Models*. London: HMSO.

Department of Health (2001) *Safety First: Five Year Report of the National Confidential Inquiry into Suicide and Homicide by People with Mental Illness*. London: Department of Health.

Department of Health (2002) *National Suicide Prevention Strategy for England*. London: The Stationery Office.

Department of Health and Social Security (1984) *The Management of Deliberate Self-harm*. Health Notice HN(84)25. London: DHSS.

Dhossche, D. M., Rich, C. L. & Isacsson, G. (2001) Psychoactive substances in suicides. Comparison of toxicologic findings in two samples. *American Journal of Forensic Medical Pathology*, **22**, 239–243.

Diekstra, R. F. W. & Kerkhof, A. J. F. M. (1989) Attitudes towards suicide. The development of a suicide attitude questionnaire. In *Suicide and Its Prevention* (eds R. F. W. Diekstra, R. Maris, S. Platt, *et al*), pp. 91–108. Leiden: E. J. Brill.

Diesenhammer, E. A., Kramer-Reinstadler, K., Liensberger, D., *et al* (2004) No evidence for an association between serum cholesterol and the course of depression and suicidality. *Psychiatric Research*, **121**, 253–261.

Dooley, E. (1990) Prison suicide in England and Wales (1962–1987). *British Journal of Psychiatry*, **156**, 40–45.

Draper, B. (1994) Suicidal behaviour in the elderly. *International Journal of Geriatric Psychiatry*, **9**, 655–661.

Draper, B. (1996) Attempted suicide in old age. *International Journal of Geriatric Psychiatry*, **11**, 577–587.

Durkheim, E. (1897) *Le Suicide* (Trans. as *Suicide: A Study in Sociology* by J. A. Spaulding & G. Simpson, 1952). London: Routlegde & Kegan Paul

Eddleston, M. & Phillips, M. R. (2004) Self poisoning with pesticides. *BMJ*, **328**, 42–44.

Ennis, J., Barnes, R. A., Kennedy, S., *et al* (1989) Depression in self-harm patients. *British Journal of Psychiatry*, **154**, 41–47.

Etzersdorfer, E., Sonneck, G. & Nagel-Kuess, S. (1992) Newspaper reports and suicide. *New England Journal of Medicine*, **325**, 502–503.

Evans, J., Platts, H. & Liebenau, A. (1996) Impulsiveness and deliberate self-harm: a comparison of 'first-timers' and 'repeaters'. *Acta Psychiatrica Scandinavica*, **93**, 378–380.

Evans, J., Evans, M., Morgan, H. G., *et al* (2005) Crisis card following self-harm: 12-month follow-up of a randomised controlled trial. *British Journal of Psychiatry*, **187**, 186–187.

Evans, M. O., Morgan, H. G., Hayward, A., *et al* (1999) Crisis telephone consultation for deliberate self harm patients. *British Journal of Psychiatry*, **175**, 23–27.

Farmer, R. D. T. (1988) Assessing the epidemiology of suicide and parasuicide. *British Journal of Psychiatrists*, **153**, 16–20.

Farmer, R. & Creed, F. (1989) Life events and hostility in self-poisoning. *British Journal of Psychiatry*, **154**, 390–395.

Fenwick, C. D., Vassilas, C. A., Carter, H., *et al* (2004) Training health professionals in the recognition, assessment and management of suicide risk. *International Journal of Psychiatry in Clinical Practice*, **8**, 117–121.

Foster, T., Gillespie, K., McClelland, R., *et al* (1999) Risk factors for suicide independent of DSM-III-R axis I disorder. Case–control psychological autopsy study in Northern Ireland. *British Journal of Psychiatry*, **175**, 175–179.

Garnefski, N., Diekstra, R. F. & de Heus, P. (1992) A population-based survey of the characteristics of high school students with and without a history of suicidal behaviour. *Acta Psychiatrica Scandinavica*, **86**, 189–196.

Gilbody, S., House, A. & Owens, D. (1997) The early repetition of deliberate self harm. *Journal of the Royal College of Physicians*, **31**, 171–172.

Gordon, H. (2002) The 'suicide' bomber: is it a psychiatric phenomenon? *Psychiatric Bulletin*, **26**, 285–287.

Gore, S. (1999) Suicide in prisons. Reflection of the community served or exacerbated risk? *British Journal of Psychiatry*, **175**, 50–55.

Group for the Advancement of Psychiatry (1989) *Committee on Cultural Psychiatry. Suicide and Ethnicity in the United States. Report of the Group for the Advancement of Psychiatry*. New York: Brunner/Mazzel.

Guertin, T., Lloyd-Richardson, E., Spirito, A., *et al* (2001) Self-mutilative behaviour in adolescents who attempt suicide by overdose. *Journal of the American Academy of Child and Adolescent Psychiatry*, **40**, 1062–1069.

Gunnell, D. & Frankel, S. (1994) Prevention of suicide: aspirations and evidence. *BMJ*, **308**, 1227–1233.

Gunnell, D. & Lewis, G. (2005) Studying suicide from the life course perspective: implications for prevention. *British Journal of Psychiatry*, **187**, 206–208.

Gunnell, D., Peters, T., Kammerling, M., *et al* (1995) The relation between parasuicide, suicide, psychiatric admissions, and socio-economic deprivation. *BMJ*, **311**, 226–230.

Gunnell, D., Brooks, J. & Peters, T. J. (1996) Epidemiology and patterns of hospital use after parasuicide in the south west of England. *Journal of Epidemiology and Community Health*, **50**, 24–29.

Gunnell, D., Middleton, N. & Frankel, S. (2000) Method availability and the prevention of suicide – a re-analysis of secular trends in England and Wales 1950–1975. *Social Psychiatry and Psychiatric Epidemiology*, **35**, 437–443.

Gunnell, D., Harbord, R., Singleton, N., *et al* (2004) Factors influencing the development and amelioration of suicidal thoughts in the general population. *British Journal of Psychiatry*, **185**, 385–393.

Gunnell, D., Saperia, J. & Ashby, D. (2005*a*) Selective serotonin reuptake inhibitors (SSRIs) and suicide in adults: meta-analysis of drug company data from placebo controlled, randomised controlled trials submitted to the MHRA's safety review. *BMJ*, **330**, 385–340.

Gunnell, D., Magnusson, P. K. E. & Rasmussen, F. (2005*b*) Low intelligence test scores in 15 year old men and risk of suicide: cohort study. *BMJ*, **330**, 167.

Guthrie, E., Kapur, N., Mackway-Jones, K., *et al* (2001) Randomised controlled trial of brief psychological intervention after deliberate self-harm. *BMJ*, **323**, 135–138.

Guze, S. B. & Robins, E. (1970) Suicide and primary affective disorders. *British Journal of Psychiatry*, **117**, 437–438.

Hammad, T. A., Laughren, T. & Racoosin, J. (2006) Suicidality in pediatric patients treated with antidepressant drugs. *Archives of General Psychiatry*, **63**, 332–339.

Handwerk, M. C., Larzelere, R. E., Friman, P. C., *et al* (1998) The relationship between lethality of attempted suicide and prior suicidal communications in a sample of residential youth. *Journal of Adolescence*, **21**, 407–414.

Harris, E. C., & Barraclough, B. M. (1994) Suicide as an outcome for medical disorders. *Medicine (Baltimore)*, **73**, 281–296.

Harris, E. C. & Barraclough, B. (1997) Suicide as an outcome for mental disorders. A meta-analysis. *British Journal of Psychiatry*, **170**, 205–228.

Harriss, L., Hawton, K. & Zahl, D. (2005) Value of measuring suicidal intent in the assessment of people attending hospital following self-poisoning or self-injury. *British Journal of Psychiatry*, **186**, 60–66.

Harwood, D., Hawton, K., Hope, T., *et al* (2001) Psychiatric disorder and personality factors associated with suicide in older people: a descriptive and case-control study. *International Journal of Geriatric Psychiatry*, **16**, 155–165.

Hassan, R. (1995) *Suicide Explained: The Australian Experience*. Melbourne: Melbourne University Press.

Hassan, T. B., MacNamara, A. F., Davy, A., *et al* (1999) Managing patients with deliberate self harm who refuse treatment in the accident and emergency department. *BMJ*, **319**, 107–109.

Haw, C., Hawton, K., Houston, K., *et al* (2001) Psychiatric and personality disorders in deliberate self-harm patients. *British Journal of Psychiatry*, **178**, 48–54.

Hawton, K. (1989) Self-cutting: can it be prevented. In *Dilemmas and Difficulties in the Management of Psychiatric Patients* (eds K. Hawton & P. Cowen), pp. 91–104. Oxford: Oxford Medical.

Hawton, K. (1992) By their own young hand. *BMJ*, **304**, 1000.

Hawton, K. & Catalan, J. (1987) *Attempted Suicide. A Practical Guide to Its Nature and Management* (2nd edn). Oxford: Oxford University Press.

Hawton, K. & Fagg, J. (1988) Suicide, and other causes of death, following attempted suicide. *British Journal of Psychiatry*, **152**, 359–366.

Hawton, K. & Kirk, J. (1989) Problem solving. In *Cognitive Behaviour Therapy for Psychiatric Problems: A Practical Guide* (eds K. Hawton, P. M. Salvkovskis, J. Kirk, *et al*), pp. 406–427. Oxford: Oxford University Press.

Hawton, K., Cowen, P., Owens, D., *et al* (1993) Low serum cholesterol and suicide. *British Journal of Psychiatry*, **162**, 818–825.

Hawton, K., Fagg, J., Simkin, S., *et al* (1997) Trends in deliberate self-harm in Oxford, 1985–1995. *British Journal of Psychiatry*, **171**, 556–560.

Hawton, K., Arensman, E., Townsend, E., *et al* (1998) Deliberate self harm: systematic review of efficacy of psychological and pharmacological treatments in preventing repetition. *BMJ*, **317**, 441–447.

Hawton, K., Simkin, S., Deeks, J. J., *et al* (1999) Effects of a drug overdose in a television drama on presentations to hospital for self poisoning: time series and questionnaire study. *BMJ*, **318**, 972–977.

Hawton, K., Harriss, L., Hodder, K., *et al* (2001) The influence of the economic and social environment on deliberate self-harm and suicide: an ecological and person-based study. *Psychological Medicine*, **31**, 827–836.

Hawton, K., Simkin, S., Deeks, J., *et al* (2004) UK legislation on analgesic packs: before and after study of long term effect on poisonings. *BMJ*, **329**, 1076–1110.

Hawton, K., Sutton, L., Haw, C., *et al* (2005) Schizophrenia and suicide: systematic review of risk factors. *British Journal of Psychiatry*, **187**, 9–20.

Heard, H. L. (2000) Psychotherapeutic approaches to suicidal ideation and behaviour. In *The International Handbook of Suicide and Attempted Suicide* (eds K. Hawton & K. van Heeringen), pp. 503–518. Chichester: Wiley.

Hengeveld, M. W., Kerkhof, A. J. & van der Wal, J. (1988) Evaluation of psychiatric consultations with suicide attempters. *Acta Psychiatrica Scandinavica*, **77**, 283–289.

Heppel, J. & Quinton, C. (1997). One hundred cases of attempted suicide in the elderly. *British Journal of Psychiatry*, **171**, 42–46.

Her Majesty's Chief Inspector of Prisons for England and Wales (1999) *Suicide Is Everyone's Concern: A Thematic Review*. London: Home Office.

Hitosugi, M., Nagaia, T. & Tokudom, S. (2007) A voluntary effort to save the youth suicide via the Internet in Japan. *International Journal of Nursing Studies*, **44**, 157.

Hughes, T., Hampshaw, S., Renvoize, E., *et al* (1998) General hospital services for those who carry out deliberate self-harm. *Psychiatric Bulletin*, **22**, 88–91.

Hunt, I. M., Robinson, J., Bickley, H., *et al* (2003) Suicide in ethnic minorities within 12 months of contact with mental health services. *British Journal of Psychiatry*, **183**, 155–160.

Hunt, I. M., Kapur, N., Robinson, J., *et al* (2006) Suicide within 12 months of mental health service contact in different age and diagnostic groups: national clinical survey. *British Journal of Psychiatry*, **188**, 135–142.

Inskip, H. M., Harris, E. C., & Barraclough, B. (1998) Lifetime risk of suicide for affective disorder, alcoholism and schizophrenia. *British Journal of Psychiatry*, **172**, 35–37.

Isaacsson, G. (2000) Suicide prevention – a medical breakthrough? *Acta Psychiatrica Scandinavica*, **102**, 113–117.

Isometsa, E. T., Aro, H. M., Henriksson, M. M., *et al* (1994) Suicide in major depression in different treatment settings. *Journal of Clinical Psychiatry*, **55**, 523–527.

Isometsa, E. T., Henriksson, M. M., Heikkinen, M .E., *et al* (1996) Completed suicide and recent electroconvulsive therapy in Finland. *Convulsive Therapy*, **12**, 152–155.

Japan Ministry of Health, Labour, and Welfare Special Committee on Prevention of Suicide (2002) *Jisatsu yobou ni mukete no teigen*. Tokyo: JMHLW.

Joiner, T. E. Jr & Rudd, M. D. (1995) Negative attributional styles for interpersonal events and the occurrence of severe interpersonal disruptions as predictors of self-reported suicidal ideation. *Suicide and Life-Threatening Behaviour*, **25**, 297–304.

Jones, B. N. (2002) Suicide among the elderly: the promise of telecommunications. *British Journal of Psychiatry*, **181**, 191–192.

Kapur, N. & House, A. (1998) Against a high risk strategy in the prevention of suicide. *Psychiatric Bulletin*, **22**, 534–536.

Kapur, N., Cooper, J., Rodway, C., *et al* (2005) Predicting the risk of repetition after self harm: cohort study. *BMJ*, **330**, 394–395.

Kelly, S. & Bunting, J. (1998) Trends in suicide in England and Wales, 1982–1996. *Population Trends*, **92**, 29–41.

Kerkhof, A. J. F. M. (2000) Attempted suicide: patterns and trends. In *The International Handbook of Suicide and Attempted Suicide* (eds K. Hawton & K. van Heering). Chichester: Wiley.

Kim, Y. K. & Myint, A. M. (2004) Clinical application of low serum cholesterol as an indicator for suicide risk in major depression. *Journal of Affective Disorders*, **81**, 161–166.

King, E. (1983) Identifying out-patient and ex-patients who have died suddenly. *Bulletin of the Royal College of Psychiatrists*, **7**, 4–7.

King, E., Baldwin, D. S., Sinclair, J. M. A., *et al* (2001) The Wessex Recent In-patient Suicide Study, 1. *British Journal of Psychiatry*, **178**, 531–536.

Kingdon, D. (1994) Care programme approach. *Psychiatric Bulletin*, **18**, 68–70.

Kreitman, N., & Foster, J. (1991) The construction and selection of predictive scales, with special reference to parasuicide. *British Journal of Psychiatry*, **159**, 185–192.

Krummen, D. M., James, K. & Klein, R. L. (1998) Suicide by burning: a retrospective review of the Akron Regional Burn Center. *Burns*, **24**, 147–149.

Lancet (1974) Annotation: self-injury. *Lancet*, *ii*, 936–937.

Lester, D. (2002) Serum cholesterol levels and suicide: a meta-analysis. *Suicide and Life-Threatening Behaviour*, **32**, 333–346.

Lester, D. & Murrell, M. E. (1980) The influence of gun control laws on suicidal behaviour. *American Journal of Psychiatry*, **137**, 121.

Linehan, M. M., Armstrong, H. E., Suarez, A., *et al* (1991) Cognitive–behavioural treatment of chronically parasuicidal borderline patients. *Archives of General Psychiatry*, **48**, 1060–1064.

Linsley, K. R., Schapira, K. & Kelly, T. P. (2001) Open verdict v. suicide – importance to research. *British Journal of Psychiatry*, **178**, 465–468.

Luoma, J. B., Martin, C. E. & Pearson, J. L. (2002) Contact with mental health and primary care providers before suicide: a review of the evidence. *American Journal of Psychiatry*, **159**, 909–916.

Mann, J. J. & Malone, K. M. (1997) Cerebrospinal fluid amines and higher lethality suicide attempts in depressed inpatients. *Biological Psychiatry*, **41**, 162–171.

Marusic, A. & Farmer, A. (2001) Genetic risk factors as possible causes of the variation in European suicide rates. *British Journal of Psychiatry*, **179**, 194–196.

Marzuk, P. M., Leon, A. C., Tardiff, K., *et al* (1992*a*) The effect of access to lethal methods of injury on suicide rate. *Archives of General Psychiatry*, **49**, 451–458.

Marzuk, P. M., Tardiff, K. & Hirsch, C. S. (1992*b*) The epidemiology of murder-suicide. *JAMA*, **267**, 3179–3183.

McClure, G. M. G. (2000) Changes in suicide in England and Wales, 1960–1997. *British Journal of Psychiatry*, **176**, 64–67.

McGuffin, P., Marusic, A. & Farmer, A. (2001) What can psychiatric genetics offer suicidology? *Crisis*, **22**, 61–65.

McKenzie, K., Serfaty M. & Crawford, M. (2003) Suicide in ethnic minority groups. *British Journal of Psychiatry*, **183**, 100–101.

Meehan, J., Kapur, N., Hunt, I. M., *et al* (2006) Suicide in mental health in-patients and within 3 months of discharge. National clinical survey. *British Journal of Psychiatry*, **188**, 129–134.

Mental Health Act Commission (2001) *Deaths of Detained Patients in England and Wales*. Nottingham: Mental Health Act Commission.

Merrill, J. & Owens, J. (1986) Ethnic differences in self-poisoning: a comparison of Asian and white groups. *British Journal of Psychiatry*, **148**, 708–712.

Middleton, N. & Gunnell, D. (2000) Trends in suicide in England and Wales. *British Journal of Psychiatry*, **176**, 263–270.

Minkoff, K., Bergman, E., Beck, A. T., *et al* (1973) Hopelessness, depression, and attempted suicide. *American Journal of Psychiatry*, **130**, 455–459.

Modestin, J., Oberson, B. & Erni, T. (1997) Possible correlates of DSM–III–R personality disorders. *Acta Psychiatrica Scandinavica*, **96**, 424–430.

Moller, H. J. (1989) Efficacy of different strategies of after-care for patients who have attempted suicide. *Journal of the Royal Society of Medicine*, **82**, 643–648.

Morgan, H. G. (1979) *Death Wishes? The Understanding and Management of Deliberate Self-harm*. Chichester: Wiley.

Morgan, H. G. & Priest, P. (1991) Suicide and other unexpected deaths among psychiatric in-patients. *British Journal of Psychiatry*, **158**, 368–374.

Morgan, H. G. & Stanton, R. (1997) Suicide among psychiatric in-patients in a changing clinical scene: suicide ideation as a paramount index of short term risk. *British Journal of Psychiatry*, **171**, 561–563.

Morgan, H. G., Evans, M., Johnson, C., *et al* (1996) Can a lecture influence attitudes to suicide prevention? *Journal of the Royal Society of Medicine*, **89**, 87–90.

Morriss, R., Gask, L., Webb, R., *et al* (2005) The effects on suicide rates of an educational intervention for front-line health professionals with suicidal patients (the STORM Project). *Psychological Medicine*, **35**, 957–960.

Mortensen, P. B. (1999) Can suicide research lead to suicide prevention? *Acta Psychiatrica Scandinavica*, **99**, 397–398.

Moscicki, E. K. (1997) Identification of suicide risk factors using epidemiological studies. *Psychiatric Clinics of North America*, **20**, 1–15.

Moscicki, E. K., O'Carroll, P., Rae, D. S., *et al* (1988) Suicide attempts in the Epidemiologic Catchment Area Study. *Yale Journal of Biology and Medicine*, **61**, 259–268.

National Collaborating Centre for Mental Health (2004) *Self-Harm: The Management and Secondary Prevention of Self-Harm in Primary and Secondary Care (Full Guideline)*. Clinical Practice Guideline 16. Leicester and London: British Psychological Society and Royal College of Psychiatrists.

Nelson, S. H. & Grunebaum, H. (1971) A follow-up study of wrist slashers. *American Journal of Psychiatry*, **127**, 1345–1349.

NICE (2004) *Self Harm. The Short Term Physical and Psychological Management and Secondary Prevention of Self-harm in Primary and Secondary Care*. Clinical Guidelines 16. London: National Institute for Clinical Excellence.

Oates, M. (2003) Suicide: the leading cause of maternal death. *British Journal of Psychiatry*, **183**, 279–281.

Oquendo, M. A. & Mann, J. J. (2000) The biology of impulsivity and suicidality. *Psychiatric Clinics of North America*, **23**, 11–25.

Owens, D. (1990) Self harm patients not admitted to hospital. *Journal of the Royal College of Physicians of London*, **24**, 281–283.

Owens, D., Horrocks, J. & House, A. (2002) Fatal and non-fatal repetition of self-harm. *British Journal of Psychiatry*, **181**, 193–199.

Pallis, D. J., Gibbons, J. S. & Pierce, D. W. (1984) Estimating suicide risk among attempted suicides, ii. Efficacy of predictive scales after the attempt. *British Journal of Psychiatry*, **144**, 139–148.

Paykel, E. S. (1980) Recent life events and attempted suicide. In *The Suicide Syndrome* (eds R. Farmer & S. Hirsch), pp. 105–115. London: Croom Helm.

Petrie, K., Chamberlain, K. & Clarke, D. (1988) Psychological predictors of future suicidal behaviour in hospitalized suicide attempters. *British Journal of Clinical Psychology*, **27**, 247–257.

Phillips, M. R., Li, X. & Zhang, Y. (2002) Suicide rates in China, 1995–99. *Lancet*, **359**, 835–840.

Pierce, D. W. (1981) The predictive value of a suicide intent scale: a five year follow-up. *British Journal of Psychiatry*, **139**, 391–396.

Platt, S. & Hawton, K. (2000) Suicidal behaviour and the labour market. In *The International Handbook of Suicide and Attempted Suicide* (eds K. Hawton & K. V. Heeringen), pp. 309–384. Chichester: Wiley.

Platt, S., Bille-Brahe, U., Kerkhof, A., *et al* (1992) Parasuicide in Europe: the WHO/EURO Multicentre Study on Parasuicide. I. Introduction and preliminary analysis for 1989. *Acta Psychiatrica Scandinavica*, **85**, 97–104.

Pollock, L. R. & Williams, J. M. (1998) Problem solving and suicidal behaviour. *Suicide and Life-Threatening Behaviour*, **28**, 375–387.

Powell, J., Geddes, J., Deeks, J., *et al* (2000) Suicide in psychiatric hospital in-patients. Risk factors and their predictive power. *British Journal of Psychiatry*, **176**, 266–272.

Pritchard, C. (1995) Deliberate self-harm and suicidal behaviour in young adults and adolescents. In *Suicide – The Ultimate Rejection? A Pycho-social Study*, pp. 76–89. Buckingham: Open University Press.

Rajagopal, S. (2004) Suicide pacts and the internet. *BMJ*, **329**, 1298–1299.

Raleigh, V. S. (1996) Suicide patterns and trends in people of Indian subcontinent and Caribbean origin in England and Wales. *Ethnicity and Health*, **1**, 55–63.

Raleigh, V. S., Bulusu, L. & Balarajan, R. (1990) Suicides among immigrants from the Indian subcontinent. *British Journal of Psychiatry*, **156**, 46–50.

Reid, W. H., Mason, M. & Hogan, I. (1998) Suicide prevention effects associated with clozapine therapy in schizophrenia and schizoaffective disorder. *Psychiatric Services*, **49**, 1029–1033.

Rich, C. L., Young, D. & Fowler, R. C. (1986) San Diego suicide study. I. Young vs old subjects. *Archives of General Psychiatry*, **43**, 577–582.

Rihmer, Z., Barsi, J. & Katona, C. L. E. (1990) Suicide rates in Hungary correlate negatively with reported rates of depression. *Journal of Affective Disorders*, **20**, 87–91.

Rosen, G. (1971) History in the study of suicide. *Psychological Medicine*, **1**, 267– 285.

Rosen, P. M. & Walsh, B. W. (1989) Patterns of contagion in self-mutilation epidemics. *American Journal of Psychiatry*, **146**, 656–658.

Rosenthal, R. J., Rinzler, C., Wallsh, R., *et al* (1972) Wrist-cutting syndrome: the meaning of a gesture. *American Journal of Psychiatry*, **128**, 1363–1368.

Royal College of Psychiatrists (1994) *The General Hospital Management of Adult Deliberate Self-harm*. Council Report 32. London: Royal College of Psychiatrists.

Royal College of Psychiatrists (2004) *Assessment Following Self-harm in Adults*. Council Report 122. London: Royal College of Psychiatrists.

Rubenowitz, E., Waern, M., Wilhelmson, K., *et al* (2001) Contact with mental health and primary care providers before suicide: a review of the evidence. *Psychological Medicine*, **31**, 1193–1202.

Rutz ,W., von Knorring, L. & Walinder, L. (1992) Long term effects of an educational programme for general practitioners given by the Swedish Committee for the Prevention and Treatment of Depression. *Acta Psychiatrica Scandinavica*, **85**, 83–88.

Rycroft, C. (1988) *A Critical Dictionary of Psychoanalysis*. London: Penguin.

Sainsbury, P. & Barraclough, B. M., (1968) Difference between suicide rates. *Nature*, **220**, 1252.

Sakinofsky, I. (2000) Repetition of suicidal behaviour. In *The International Handbook of Suicide and Attempted Suicide* (eds K. Hawton & K. van Heeringen), pp. 385–404. Chichester: Wiley.

Sakinofsky, I. & Roberts, R. S. (1990) Why parasuicides repeat despite problem resolution. *British Journal of Psychiatry*, **156**, 399–405.

Sakinofsky, I., Brown, Y., Cumming, C., *et al* (1990) Problem resolution and repetition of parasuicide. A prospective study. *British Journal of Psychiatry*, **156**, 395–399.

Salib, E. (2003) Suicide terrorism: a case of folie a plusieurs? *British Journal of Psychiatry*, **182**, 475–476.

Salib, E., Tadros, G. & Cawley, S. (2001) Elderly suicide and attempted suicide: one syndrome. *Medicine, Science and the Law*, **41**, 250–255.

Schapira, K., Linsley, K. R., Linsley, J. A., *et al* (2001) Relationship of suicide rates to social factors and availability of lethal methods: comparison of suicide in Newcastle upon Tyne 1961–1965 and 1985–1994. *British Journal of Psychiatry*, **178**, 458–464.

Schmidtke, A. & Hafner, H. (1988) The Werther effect after television films: new evidence for an old hypotheses. *Psychological Medicine*, **18**, 665–676.

Schmidtke, A., Bille-Brahe, U., De Leo, D., *et al* (1996) Attempted suicide in Europe: rates, trends and sociodemographic characteristics of suicide attempters during the period 1989–1992. Results of the WHO/EURO Multicentre Study on Parasuicide. *Acta Psychiatrica Scandinavica*, **93**, 327–338.

Scottish Executive (2002) *Choose Life: A National Strategy and Action Plan to Prevent Suicide in Scotland*. Edinburgh: The Stationery Office.

Shah, A. K. & Ganesvaran, T. (1997) In-patient suicides in an Australian mental hospital. *Australian and New Zealand Journal of Psychiatry*, **31**, 291–298.

Shaw, J., Baker, D., Hunt, I. M., *et al* (2004) Suicide by prisoners. National clinical survey. *British Journal of Psychiatry*, **184**, 263–267.

Shepherd, D. M. & Barraclough, B. M. (1979) Help for those bereaved by suicide. *British Journal of Social Work*, **9**, 69–74.

Spicer, R. S. & Miller, T. R. (2000) Suicide acts in 8 states: incidence and case fatality rates by demographics and methods. *American Journal of Public Health*, **90**, 1885–1891.

Stanley, B., Gameroff, M. J., Michalsen, V., *et al* (2001) Are suicide attempters who self-mutilate a unique population? *American Journal of Psychiatry*, **158**, 427–432.

Statham, D. J., Heath, A. C., Madden, P. A., *et al* (1998) Suicidal behaviour: an epidemiological and genetic study. *Psychological Medicine*, **28**, 839–855.

Stenager, E. N., Stenager, E. & Jensen, K. (1994) Attempted suicide, depression and physical diseases: a 1-year follow-up study. *Psychotherapy and Psychosomatics*, **61**, 65–73.

Stengel, E., Cook, N. G. & Kreeger, I. (1958) *Attempted Suicide: Its Social Significance and Effects*. Maudsley Monograph No. 4. London: Chapman & Hall.

Sublette, M. E., Hibbeln, J. R., Galfalvy, H., *et al* (2006) Omega-3 polyunsaturated essential fatty acid status as a predictor of future suicide risk. *American Journal of Psychiatry*, **163**, 1100–1102.

Suominen, K., Henriksson, M., Suokas, J., *et al* (1996) Mental disorders and comorbidity in attempted suicide. *Acta Psychiatrica Scandinavica*, **94**, 234–240.

Suominen, K., Isometsa, E., Suokas, J., *et al* (2004) Completed suicide after a suicide attempt: a 37-year follow-up study. *American Journal of Psychiatry*, **161**, 562–563.

Tadros, G. & Salib, E. (2000) Age and methods of fatal self harm (FSH). Is there a link? *International Journal of Geriatric Psychiatry*, **15**, 848–852.

Townsend, E., Hawton, K., Harriss, L., *et al* (2001) Substances used in deliberate self-poisoning 1985–1997: trends and associations with age, gender, repetition and suicide intent. *Social Psychiatry and Psychiatric Epidemiology*, **36**, 228–234.

Turner, R. J. & Morgan, H. G. (1979) Patterns of health care in non-fatal deliberate self-harm. *Psychological Medicine*, **9**, 487–492.

Tyrer, P., Thompson, S., Schmidt, U., *et al* (2003) Randomized controlled trial of brief cognitive behaviour therapy versus treatment as usual in recurrent deliberate self-harm: the POPMACT study. *Psychological Medicine*, **33**, 969–976.

United Nations (1996) *Prevention of Suicide. Guidelines for the Formulation and Implementation of National Strategies*. New York: United Nations.

US Department of Health and Human Services (2001) *National Strategy for Suicide Prevention: Goals and Objectives for Action*. Rockville, MD: US Department of Health and Human Services, Public Health Service.

van der Sande, R., Van Rooijen, L., Buskens, E., *et al* (1997) Intensive in-patient and community intervention versus routine care after attempted suicide: a randomised controlled intervention study. *British Journal of Psychiatry*, **171**, 35–41.

van Heeringen, K. (2001*a*) The suicidal process and related concepts. In *Understanding Suicidal Behaviour: The Suicidal Process Approach to Research, Treatment and Prevention* (ed. K. van Heeringen), pp. 3–14. Chichester: Wiley.

van Heeringen, K. (2001*b*) The process approach to suicidal behaviour: future directions in research, treatment and prevention. In *Understanding Suicidal Behaviour: The Suicidal Process Approach to Research, Treatment and Prevention* (ed. K. van Heeringen), pp. 288–305. Chichester: Wiley.

van Heeringen, C., Jannes, S., Buylaert, W., *et al* (1995) The management of non-compliance with referral to out-patient after-care among attempted suicide patients: a controlled intervention study. *Psychological Medicine*, **25**, 963–970.

Varnik, A. (1998) Suicide in the former republics of the USSR. *Psychiatrica Fennica*, **29**, 150–162.

Vassilas, C. A. & Morgan, H. G. (1993) General practitioners' contact with victims of suicide. *BMJ*, **307**, 300–301.

Vassilas, C. A. & Morgan, H. G. (1994) Elderly suicides. Contact with their general practitioners before death. *International Journal of Geriatric Psychiatry*, **9**, 1008–1009.

Vassilas, C. A. & Morgan, H. G. (1997) Suicide in Avon: life stress, alcohol misuse and use of services. *British Journal of Psychiatry*, **170**, 453–455.

Waern, M., Runeson, B. S., Allebeck, P., *et al* (2002) Mental disorder in elderly suicides: a case–control study. *American Journal of Psychiatry*, **159**, 450–455.

Wagner, B. M. (1997) Family risk actors for child and adolescent suicidal behaviour. *Psychological Bulletin*, **121**, 246–298.

Watts, D. & Morgan, H. G. (1994) Malignant alienation. Dangers for patients who are hard to like. *British Journal of Psychiatry*, **164**, 11–15.

Williams, J. M. G. & Pollock, L. R. (2001) Psychological aspects of the suicidal process. In *Understanding Suicidal Behaviour: The Suicidal Process Approach to Research, Treatment and Prevention* (ed. K. van Heeringen), pp. 76–93. Chichester: Wiley.

Winokur, G. & Black, D. W. (1992) Suicide – what can be done? *New England Journal of Medicine*, **327**, 190–191.

Wolfersdorf, M. G., Vogel, R., & Hole, G. (1988) Suicide in psychiatric hospitals. In *Current Issues in Suicidology* (eds H. J. Moller, A. Schmidtke & R. Welz), pp. 83–100. Berlin: Springer-Verlag.

World Health Organization (1990) *Consultation on Strategies for Reducing Suicidal Behaviour in the European Region. Summary Report*. Geneva: WHO.

World Health Organization (2000) *Preventing Suicide: A Resource Series. 2 A Resource for Media Professionals*. Geneva: WHO.

Yip, P. S. F., Chao, A. & Chinn, C. W. F. (2000) Seasonal variation in suicides: diminished or vanished. Experience from England and Wales, 1982–1996. *British Journal of Psychiatry*, **177**, 366–369.

Zahl, D. L. & Hawton, K. (2004) Repetition of deliberate self-harm and subsequent suicide risk: long term follow up study of 11 583 patients. *British Journal of Psychiatry*, **185**, 70–75.

CHAPTER 8

Schizophrenia: the clinical picture

Peter F. Liddle

Schizophrenia is a psychotic illness that undermines fundamental aspects of the personality. It erodes the ability to initiate and organise self-directed mental activity and to recognise oneself as the source of such activity. It can produce a diverse array of disturbances within the domains of thought, perception, affect and volition. Typically, the illness follows a course in which acute episodes of hallucinations, delusions and florid disorganisation of thought are superimposed upon more persistent and subtle disorders of the initiation and organisation of thought and behaviour. These persistent disorders can produce profound disruption of occupational activities and social relationships. However, the severity of persisting disorder varies greatly between cases.

The origins of the concept

The concept of schizophrenia emerged from 19th-century attempts to describe the psychotic illnesses of young and middle adult life. At the beginning of that century, the English psychiatrist Haslam (1809) recognised a state of insanity unaccompanied by furious or depressing passions. In 1860, the French psychiatrist Morel described a condition, which he named *demence precoce*, that had its onset in late adolescence with odd behaviour and self-neglect, and a subsequent deterioration in mental function. However, the major developments that led to the concept of schizophrenia occurred in Germany, in the three decades that extended from Griesinger's (1867) formulation of the concept of a unitary psychosis, including both affective psychoses and the condition we now call schizophrenia, to Kraepelin's (1896) conclusion that these two conditions should be separated on the grounds of their tendency to differ in course.

The seminal figure of these four decades was Kahlbaum. He described three chronic psychotic conditions: catatonia, hebephrenia and dementia paranoides. He is best known for his description of catatonia (Kahlbaum, 1874), a condition dominated by disturbances of voluntary motor activity. Kahlbaum emphasised the importance of evaluating not only the current symptoms but also the course of an illness. Catatonia runs a course which includes atonic or stuporous periods of underactivity and periods of excitement and overactivity. In some instances it progresses to a demented state. Kahlbaum also emphasised the association between affective symptoms and catatonic motor symptoms, and thus foreshadowed the notion that, irrespective of whether or not it is appropriate to distinguish schizophrenia from affective psychosis, there are pathophysiological processes common to these two types of psychosis. Kahlbaum's colleague Hecker (1871) provided the classic description of hebephrenia, a condition beginning in young adult life with silly behaviour, inappropriate affect, disordered form of thought and fragmentary delusions. Dementia paranoides is characterised by delusions in a setting of deteriorating personality.

Kahlbaum's seminal ideas came to fruition at the turn of the century, when Emil Kraepelin separated manic–depressive psychosis – which tends to be episodic, with the restoration of virtually normal mental function between episodes – and the chronic psychoses, hebephrenia, catatonia and dementia paranoides – which tend to produce persisting disability. He amalgamated these three chronic psychoses to form a single illness which he named dementia praecox, in recognition of its tendency to begin in early adult life and its propensity to lead to a state of mental enfeeblement. In a later essay (Kraepelin, 1920) which reflected a distillation of his views on psychopathology, he described the essential feature of this illness as:

> 'that destruction of conscious volition ... which is manifest as loss of energy and drive, in disjointed volitional behaviour. This rudderless state leads to impulsive instinctual activity: there is no planned reflection which suppresses impulses as they arise or directs them into proper channels.'

Although Kraepelin regarded impaired volition and loss of unity of mental processes as cardinal features of the illness, he also emphasised the prevalence of auditory hallucinations, especially in the acute phase.

The illness was renamed schizophrenia by Eugen Bleuler in 1911. He wished to discard the name dementia praecox because he recognised that many cases did not show progressive deterioration. Furthermore, in at least some cases, the illness began in mid-adult life. He regarded fragmentation of psychic functions as the hallmark of the illness and chose the name schizophrenia to denote this fragmentation of mental activity. He specified a number of fundamental symptoms that he considered were present in every case, including affective flattening, looseness of associations, ambivalence and autism. He assigned a special prominence to looseness of associations:

> 'Of the thousands of associative threads which guide our thinking, this disease seems to interrupt, quite haphazardly, sometimes such single threads, sometimes a whole group, and sometimes even large segments of them. In this way thinking becomes illogical and often bizarre.' (Bleuler, 1911, p. 14)

He considered than many of the other symptoms arose from looseness of associations

Bleuler regarded hallucinations and delusions as accessory symptoms:

> 'Besides these specific permanent or fundamental symptoms we can find a host of other more accessory manifestations such as delusions, hallucinations or catatonic symptoms. The fundamental symptoms are characteristic of schizophrenia, while the accessory symptoms may also appear in other types of illness.' (Bleuler, 1911)

Thus, in the evolution of the concept of schizophrenia, the emphasis was initially on fragmentation of mental functions and enduring deficits. Delusions and hallucinations were recognised as concomitant of the disorder, but were considered to be a transient though potentially recurring feature. However, as attempts were made to improve the reliability of diagnosis, delusions and hallucinations, especially those identified as 'first-rank symptoms' by Schneider (see below), assumed greater importance, and the emphasis shifted from the enduring deficits to the acute phases of the illness, during which delusions and hallucinations are usually prominent. This shift in emphasis was reinforced in the second half of the 20th century by the development of pharmacological treatments which were relatively successful in alleviating the symptoms of the acute phase. However, these treatments do not cure the illness: the chronic deficits present a persisting challenge.

The phenomena of schizophrenia

The Schneiderian first-rank symptoms

In his attempt to define of set of symptoms that might provide a reliable basis for the diagnosis of schizophrenia, Kurt Schneider identified a group of experiences (Box 8.1) which have become known as 'first-rank symptoms'. Schneider did not give explicit definitions of the first-rank symptoms and clinicians have subsequently employed various definitions that differ in detail. Mellor (1970) formulated a set of strict definitions and reported that 72% of people with schizophrenia exhibit at least one such symptom. The following descriptions of first-rank symptoms are based on Mellor's definitions, although illustrations from Schneider's (1959) account are also given where possible.

Box 8.1 Schneider's first-rank symptoms

- Voices commenting
- Voices discussing or arguing
- Audible thoughts
- Thought insertion
- Thought withdrawal
- Thought broadcast
- Made will
- Made acts
- Made affect
- Somatic passivity
- Delusional perception

Voices commenting

This symptom describes patients hearing a voice describing their actions as they occur. The actions are often quite mundane, although in some instances a special significance might be suspected. Schneider (p. 97) describes a woman with schizophrenia who heard a voice say, whenever she wanted to eat: 'Now she is eating; here she is munching again'.

Voices discussing or arguing

Patients experience hallucinations of voices that discuss them, or argue about them, referring to them in the third person. Schneider (p. 97) refers to a patient who experienced auditory hallucinations night and day, 'like a dialogue, one voice always arguing against the other'.

Audible thoughts (*Gedankenlautwerden; écho de la pensée*)

This is the experience of hearing one's own thoughts aloud. The thoughts might be heard either simultaneously with the act of thinking or after a very brief delay. One of Schneider's patients reported: 'I hear my own thoughts. I can hear them when everything is quiet.' Another complained: 'When I try to think, my head gets full of noise; it's as if my own brain were in an uproar with my thoughts' (p. 97).

Thought insertion

This is the experience that thoughts that are not one's own have been inserted into one's mind. It is not merely a matter of being influenced to think a particular thought: the essence of the symptom includes the experience that the thought is not one's own.

> 'A skilled shirt-maker knew how large the collars should be but when she proceeded to make them there were times when she could not calculate at all. This was not ordinary forgetting, she had to think thoughts she did not want to think, evil thoughts. She attributed all this to being hypnotised by a priest.' (Schneider, p. 101)

Thought withdrawal

This is the experience that thoughts are removed by an alien influence. Schneider (p. 100) gives as an example:

> 'A schizophrenic man stated that his thoughts were "taken from me years ago by the parish council". They had constantly robbed him of all his thoughts.'

The experience that one's thinking has stopped, leaving a state in which all thought is absent (thought blocking), is less specific to schizophrenia and is not regarded as a first-rank symptom.

Thought broadcast

This is the experience that one's thoughts are broadcast so that others might share them. Schneider (p. 101) describes a female patient who was so convinced that the doctor knew exactly what she was thinking that she suggested that she would stop talking and he could just listen. The belief that others can read one's thoughts is not in itself a first-rank symptom: the essential feature is the experience that one's thoughts are in the public domain.

Made will

The patient has an impulsion to act that is experienced as arising from an alien source. The impulse is usually so strong that it is acted upon. The execution of the action itself is not experienced as alien. Mellor (p. 17) gives as an example the account of a patient who had emptied a urine bottle over the dinner trolley: 'The sudden impulse came over me that I must do it. It was not my feeling; it came into me from the X-ray department.' Schneider (p. 119) describes a patient who was unable to respond to suggestions because 'thousands and thousands of wills act against me'.

Made acts

This is the experience of one's actions being executed by an external influence, such that one is a passive observer of one's own actions. Mellor (p. 17) reports a patient who described his fingers moving to pick up objects:

> 'but I don't control them.... I sit there watching them move, and they are quite independent, what they do is nothing to do with me. I am just a puppet ... I am just a puppet who is manipulated by cosmic strings.'

Made affect

Here, affects are experienced as imposed by an alien influence. A young woman described by Mellor (p. 17) complained:

> 'I cry, tears roll down my cheeks and I look unhappy, but inside I have a cold anger because they are using me in this way, and it is not me who is unhappy, but they are projecting unhappiness into my brain.'

Somatic passivity

This is the experience of alien influence over bodily functions. Mellor (p. 18) specifies that there two essential components: a somatic experience, which is usually, but not always, hallucinatory, combined with a delusional belief in alien origin of that experience. The experience is most commonly one of visceral function. He gives the example of a young man's experience:

> 'X-rays [enter] the back of my neck, where the skin tingles and feels warm; they pass down the back in a hot tingling strip about six inches wide to the waist. Then they disappear into the pelvis which feels numb and cold and solid like a block of ice. They stop me from getting an erection.'

Schneider was less strict, and allowed that the symptom might entail *either* a somatic hallucination *or* a belief in strange influences acting on the body. Schneider also points out that the content is frequently sexual in nature. He gives as an illustration a woman who described:

> 'a sort of intercourse as if a man was really there. He was not there of course ... but it was as if a man was with me... That is what I felt.'

In this case, the patient reported a somatic hallucination, but her explanation does not have the conviction of a delusion.

Delusional perception

This describes the attribution of abnormal significance, usually with self-reference, to a genuine perception without any comprehensible rational or emotional justification. Delusional perception is sometimes preceded by a delusional atmosphere, a sense of oddness or strangeness. Mellor (p. 18) describes a young Irishman at breakfast with a fellow lodger who felt a sense of unease, as if something frightening was about to happen. When the lodger pushed the salt cellar towards him he perceived the event and understood his companion's intentions correctly, but suddenly knew he must return home to greet the Pope, who was visiting Ireland to see his family and reward them, 'because Our Lord is going to be born again of one of the women ... and because of this they are all born with their private parts back to front.'

Schneider (p. 113) emphasised that there is sometimes a substantial delay – of hours or even years – between the perception and the development of a delusional belief in its significance. He gives as an example a girl employed in domestic service who 'later on' decided that an earlier visitor to the house was the disguised son of the household who intended to test her out and marry her.

First-rank symptoms in other disorders

Schneider was careful to emphasise that schizophrenia involves not merely first-rank symptoms but also more widespread changes in mental function: 'A psychotic phenomenon is not like a defective stone in an otherwise perfect mosaic' (p. 95).

First-rank symptoms are not unique to schizophrenia: they are reported in approximately 10–15% of patients with manic–depressive psychosis and in patients with overt organic brain conditions. However, clinicians have differed in the interpretation of Schneider's concepts, and no adequate study has established the prevalence of stringently defined first-rank symptoms in conditions other than schizophrenia.

In a small study that addressed the question of whether or not use of narrow definitions increased the specificity for schizophrenia, O'Grady (1990) found that patients with major depression reported symptoms that satisfied broad criteria for first-rank symptoms, yet did not satisfy narrow definitions. (For example, in the case of thought insertion, the broad definition would include thoughts believed to arise from an outside source but experienced as one's own, whereas the narrow definition would demand that the patient experienced the thought as not being his or her own.) The balance of evidence suggests that adherence to stringent definitions of first-rank symptoms enhances their specificity to schizophrenia.

Hallucinations and illusions

Hallucinations in any of the sensory modalities occur in schizophrenia, although auditory hallucinations are the most common. Most characteristic are the three types of auditory hallucination identified as Schneiderian first-rank symptoms: voices commenting; voices discussing or arguing; and hearing one's own thoughts aloud. Second-person auditory hallucinations are also common. In the International Pilot Study of Schizophrenia (IPSS), conducted by the World Health Organization (1973), hallucinations involving voices speaking to the patient were recorded in 65% of cases of acute schizophrenia.

Often the voices are harsh, critical or frightening, although occasionally they are a source of comfort. In contrast to the situation in affective psychosis, hallucinations in schizophrenia are usually mood incongruent in so far as their content cannot readily be understood as a consequence of the patient's mood.

The source of hallucinatory voices seems nearby for some patients and distant for others. Often the patient assumes it is the voice of a neighbour. Such a belief can become incorporated into a more extensive system of delusional beliefs in persecution by the neighbour, together with hallucinations in other sensory modalities. A patient who attributed the voices to neighbours also reported smelling gas which the neighbours had piped into his house. Other patients attribute the hallucinatory voice to God or to organisations such as state intelligence services. The perceived source can be located within the patient's own body. Patients sometimes attribute their experience to a transmitter embedded in their brain, or in some other organ. For example, a young man maintained that a transmitter had been implanted in his teeth.

Behaviour such as whispering or looking around as if seeking the source of the voice can provide a clue to the presence of hallucinations. An elderly man repeatedly denied hearing voices but was observed at times to suffer distraction and then to engage in whispering. When asked about the content of his whispered conversations he described a dialogue with strangers.

The strictest definition of a hallucination is the experience of a sensory perception not based on a sensory stimulus. While the hallucinations of schizophrenia usually satisfy this strict definition, some patients report hearing voices that are triggered by a sensory stimulus. For example, muffled or indistinct sounds, such as the noise of a distant car engine, can trigger the voices. In other instances, the presence or absence of sensory input appears to affect the propensity to suffer auditory hallucinations even though the patient does not recognise any specific trigger. A patient who was frequently observed to sit hunched with his head to one side, so that his right ear was buried in the shoulder pad of his jacket, admitted that this posture diminished the voices. There is some evidence that asymmetry of sensory input influences hallucinations, and use of a unilateral earplug sometimes reduces their intensity. Unfortunately, this strategy is only occasionally successful. When asked why he was no longer using an earplug provided the previous day, a patient replied that the voices had told him to throw it into the lavatory pan, illustrating the tantalising unpredictability of schizophrenic phenomena. In contrast to those who find that blocking external stimuli is helpful, others obtain relief by focusing attention on their surroundings and actively processing environmental information.

When patients with schizophrenia relate their experiences of hearing voices during acute episodes of the illness, they usually describe the perceptions as having the same sensory quality as voices arising from real sources in the external world and heard through the ears. At this stage of the illness it is not uncommon for patients to act on commands issued by the voices.

In contrast, in the chronic stage of the illness it is quite common for patients to describe voices which are recognised as arising from within their own minds. Kraepelin (1919, p. 7) reported:

> 'at other times they do not appear to the patient as sense perceptions at all; they are "voices of conscience"; voices which do not speak with words ... it is thought inwardly within me.'

These experiences resemble pseudo-hallucinations, which are sensory perceptions in the absence of external stimuli that patients clearly recognise as morbid products of their own mind. However, usually patients with chronic schizophrenia who describe the voices as arising in their own mind none the less remain ambivalent about their source. Such hallucinations should be afforded less weight in the process of diagnosis, but can be very intrusive into the patient's mental activities, and should not be ignored in assessing the impact of the patient's condition on his or her life. It is also quite common in the chronic stages of the illness for the patient to be unable to repeat the content of the hallucination. Kraepelin (1919, p. 7) noted that 'in the more advanced stages what the voices say is indifferent or quite nonsensical and incomprehensible'. Auditory hallucinations of sounds other than voices, such as music, can occur in schizophrenia, but have little diagnostic value.

Olfactory hallucinations occur, as do other olfactory disorders, including disturbances of the affective connotations of smells. Sometimes patients become convinced that they themselves are giving off an unpleasant odour. Somatic hallucinations are common and are often associated with delusional interpretations. A man who experienced a strange sensation in his bowels was convinced that a snake had entered through his anus. Another described the experience of being cut with a knife by his parents. While this statement might well have been understood as an expression of his tense relationship with his parents, he was adamant that the experience was real, not merely a metaphor.

Although visual hallucinations are usually regarded as evidence of an overtly organic psychosis, such hallucinations are not uncommon in schizophrenia, especially in cases of severe persistent illness. Sometimes the patients experience them as personal, intended only for themselves, yet they believe in their reality. A patient described the appearance of King George V and Queen Mary regularly at the ward entrance. Both were dressed in full coronation regalia. When asked why others could not see them she replied 'because they have come to see me'.

Rarely, visual hallucinations occur at the onset of an acute episode of illness as a feature of a dream-like (oneiroid) state in which the patient is detached from reality. In this altered state of consciousness, complex vivid visual hallucinations can occur, as can visual illusions, in which perceptions of real stimuli are distorted. Objects can: be surrounded by an aura; have either an unnatural intensity of colour or be muted and grey; be changed in shape; be reduced in size (micropsia); or be enlarged (macropsia). The patient might report the experience that the scene has been encountered before (déjà vu). These specific distortions of reality are not characteristic of schizophrenia, and unless they are accompanied by other clinical features more typical of schizophrenia, some other organic disorder of the brain should be suspected.

Delusions

Virtually all patients with schizophrenia suffer from delusions at some time in their illness, and a wide variety of types of delusions can occur. Especially characteristic of schizophrenia are delusional beliefs that are incomprehensible, either because they arise suddenly and without any foundation in preceding mental processes, or because they refer to fantastic events or circumstances which could not possibly occur. For example, a young woman suddenly knew, with total conviction, that she was a cat. It was not possible to elicit any mental precursor to this notion. Such a belief arising suddenly from unaccountable origins is called a primary or autochthonous delusion.

Also characteristic of schizophrenia are the delusions of alien control of thought, action, will, affect and somatic function that express the disordered experience of autonomy lying at the heart of many of the Schneiderian first-rank symptoms described above. These phenomena are delusions in so far as they entail beliefs based on a faulty evaluation of reality, but they involve disturbance of more than just the process of evaluating reality: they reflect disorder of the mental process that creates awareness of oneself as the source of one's own thoughts, feelings and actions. Although Schneider's primary purpose in identifying the first-rank symptoms was to assemble a group of phenomena of special utility for diagnosis, the fact that the experience of alien control is common to the majority of the first-rank symptoms suggests that a disturbed experience of self is a cardinal feature of schizophrenic psychopathology.

Schneider also drew attention to the phenomenon of delusional mood. This is a scarcely tangible experience that something strange or unusual is happening. It can occur for a period of hours or days before the emergence of more clear-cut delusional beliefs. In Mellor's account of the Irishman who had the delusional perception when his companion pushed the salt cellar towards him (described above) there was evidence of a preceding delusional mood: a sense of unease as if something frightening was about to happen. Sometimes the delusional mood encompasses a sense of exaltation. A young woman woke one morning filled with a sense of cosmic strangeness and power as if she could ride a bicycle (which she had never previously done). She then stabbed herself in the abdomen with a bread-knife, but after her recovery could give no explanation of why she had done this.

Patients with schizophrenia sometimes have delusional memories. These are accounts of fictitious events or circumstances which the patient is convinced he or she has experienced in the past. For example, a young man was convinced that several years previously he had had an operation in which his abdominal organs had been removed. He held tenaciously to this belief despite the absence of a surgical scar.

Delusions of persecution and of reference have little diagnostic specificity but are none the less common in schizophrenia. In the International Pilot Study of Schizophrenia (World Health Organization, 1973) ideas of reference were reported in 70% of cases and suspiciousness in 66%. Patients commonly report that television programmes make special reference to them. Delusions of grandiose identity or grandiose ability also occur in schizophrenia, although they are more typical of mania. In contrast to the situation in mania, however, where grandiose thinking is associated with elated mood, grandiose delusions in schizophrenia are usually not congruent with mood. Similarly, nihilistic delusions, which entail a belief that a part or all of one's own body is non-functioning or even absent, and which are characteristic of depressive psychosis, can occur as mood-incongruent delusions in schizophrenia. For example, a middle-aged man suffering from schizophrenia stated that his head was absent, but apart from accompanying agitation, his concurrent mental state betrayed no underlying feelings or thoughts that might account for this nihilistic delusion.

Delusions can be either fragmentary or part of a system of linked, relatively self-consistent delusions. The man who claimed his head was absent also reported that there was blood all over his face, and showed no awareness of the contradiction implied by these statements. Another patient repeatedly referred to the fact that an axe had split his head but could give no explanation of how this had happened or what consequences it had produced. In contrast, a middle-aged woman, who had been experiencing auditory hallucinations and thought insertion for several months before a real burglary at her house, subsequently developed a relatively self-consistent persecutory delusional system based on the premise that the intelligence services were keeping her under surveillance and placing pressure on her by transmitting messages to her. Such organised delusional systems are most frequently encountered in female patients with onset of illness in middle age.

In acute episodes, patients often act in accordance with their delusions, but in the more chronic phase of the illness it is common to encounter 'double orientation', in which there is a dissociation of affect and behaviour from the implications of the delusion. A man who maintained he was the Duke of Hamilton, and from time to time referred casually to a family member named Liz (Queen Elizabeth II), none the less accepted without demur the rather lowly accommodation and lack of privacy afforded by the hospital ward in which he lived.

Disorders of the form and flow of thought

Form of thought

Despite many attempts to define and classify the disorders of the form of thought that occur in schizophrenia since Bleuler introduced the apt term 'loosening of associations' more than 80 years ago, these disorders remain perhaps the most enigmatic of all schizophrenic phenomena. One of the problems lies in the sheer variety of manifestations of disordered form of thought, and it is difficult to tease out the essential elements. There are at least three distinguishable classes of formal thought disorder in schizophrenia, which tend to differ with regard to the phase of illness in which they are most prominent (see Table 8.1 for definitions of the various phenomena).

1 There are phenomena such as tangentiality, derailment, perseveration and distractibility, which appear to reflect instability of goal in thinking. This class of disorders is most prominent during acute exacerbations of the illness.

   Case example

   A 48-year-old woman who suffered from a sustained florid schizophrenic illness reported having a telephone in her head. When she was asked what she heard on the telephone, she replied: 'Well, it's like meeting people and I [pause] have a jug of hot tea and relax therapy, relaxation, and I can speak to the sinus arrhythmia doctor.' Her reply begins in a slightly tangential manner, and then becomes derailed. At times she has difficulty in finding words. The term 'sinus arrhythmia doctor' appears to be an idiosyncratic use of words to describe a psychologist or psychiatrist. At another point in the interview, in an attempt to delineate suspected ideas of reference, the interviewer asked: 'Has there been anything about you on the TV?' She replied: 'There's been the union jack and the hospital fire alarm and plastic surgery.' Interviewer: 'Did those things have anything to do with you?' Patient: 'The Boer war'. These replies illustrate marked tangentiality and derailment.

2 There are idiosyncrasies of thought and language. These include idiosyncratic use of words, idiosyncratic ideas and idiosyncratic logic. The idiosyncrasies of logic do not usually involve a failure of strict, syllogistic logic. Rather, they appear to reflect unusual lines of thought that, at least in some instances, appear to reflect a private logic that ignores the common knowledge of the world that guides normal thinking. For example, the woman who was asked why only she could see King George and Queen Mary at the doorway and replied 'because they have come to see me' appeared to be following an internally consistent line of thought but ignoring common knowledge of the world. In the past, clinicians might have described this as autistic logic, but it is preferable to avoid that term because this type of thinking is not identical to that characteristic of childhood autism. Idiosyncrasies of thought and language can occur at any phase of the illness. In particular, these disorders are sometimes prominent among the residual symptoms that persist after the resolution of the acute phase of illness. They also occur relatively frequently in some first-degree relatives, which suggests that they may be a marker for a schizophrenic trait.

   Case examples

   When asked about a scene depicting a boat tied to a tree, a patient with persisting stable symptoms replied: 'I'd like to get in the boat, put in on the canal and row it away, 'cos there's a waistline there. The tree here is er ... somebody ... a man or a woman will come there ... they'll sit down because that's there ... they'll feel uneasy and they'll take it and burn it.' His reason for wanting to get in the boat reveals both idiosyncratic logic and idiosyncratic use of the word 'waistline'. The subsequent sentence exhibits derailment. When asked whether he meant that they would burn the boat he said: 'Yes, only for a person in the mind ... you put that up there so it's a Van Gogh, you know, Christ knows. What the hell is the boat doing there, you know you give five million quid for it, he'd change his mind.' The reply begins tangentially and becomes derailed. As a result of the derailment, it is unclear to whom the pronoun 'he' refers. The phrase 'only for a person in the mind' is an idiosyncratically expressed idea whose meaning is difficult to discern.

   The idiosyncrasy of thought and language can be quite subtle. When asked about his daily activities, a 37-year-old man with only slight evidence of residual

Table 8.1 Disorders of the form of thought (synonyms or variants in parentheses)

Category	Symptom	Definition
Unstable goal	Tangentiality	Responses that are off the point
	Derailment	Inappropriate shift to a loosely related or unrelated idea during flow of speech (asyndetic thought)
	Distractability	Shift to an irrelevant idea triggered by an external stimulus
Idiosyncratic thought and language	Idiosyncratic word use	Normal words used in an inappropriate context (word approximations, metonyms) or non-words (neologisms)
	Idiosyncratic ideas	Unusual ideas that appear to reflect peculiar, personal concepts, or ideas expressed in an unusual manner that impedes comprehension
	Idiosyncratic logic	Reasoning that does not follow normal rules of logic
	Incoherence[a]	Incomprehensible speech, apparently reflecting absent or idiosyncratic connections between words ('word salad')
Weakening of goal	Empty speech	Utterances lacking an identifiable goal, and composed mainly of vacuous phrases of the type normally used merely to maintain flow of speech (poverty of content of speech)
	Generalisation	Speech lacks specificity and conveys little information because of over-generalisation
	Unelaborated ideas	Ideas lack normal development; speech contains few adjectives, adverbs or modifying clauses
	Perseveration	Unwarranted repetition of a previously expressed word or idea

[a] Incoherence apparently involves both unstable goal and idiosyncrasy.

Table 8.2 Disorders of the flow of thought

Symptom	Definition
Poverty of speech	Decreased amount of speech: brief replies, lack of spontaneous speech
Pressure of speech	Excessive rate of speech
Blocking	Transient interruptions of speech during which the subject experiences absence of thought

schizophrenic symptoms replied: 'I look at walls and windows and that bothers my life.' In poetry, such a sentence might be accepted as legitimate. Indeed, his reply might be regarded as a poignant description of the impoverishment of life faced by many patients. However, when idiosyncrasy in everyday speech impedes communication substantially, it indicates pathological thought.

3 There are disorders that appear to reflect weakening of the goal of thinking, such as empty speech, uninformative generalisations and lack of elaboration of ideas. Empty speech is characterised by utterances that begin without any identifiable goal and is dominated by vacuous phrases, of the type that are used from time to time in normal speech to maintain flow (e.g. 'you know'). Patients do not seem to be sure of what they are saying, thinking or perceiving. Empty speech is similar in concept to poverty of content of speech as defined by Andreasen (1982), but, unfortunately, ratings of poverty of content according to Andreasen's definition tend to correlate with ratings of derailment, which reflects instability rather than weakening of goal. Weakening of goal may also give rise to perseveration, although it is probable that several different pathological processes can contribute to perseveration. Weakening of goal is occasionally encountered during acute episodes, but is much more common among patients with chronic illness.

Case example

Poverty of speech and lack of elaboration are illustrated in the following response by a chronic patient to an invitation to describe a depiction of an active dock-side scene illuminated by a bright sun: 'Reminds me of some ... um ... er ... sun ... er ... clouds and sun ... [long pause].... That's all.'

There are also some disorders that appear to reflect the coincidence of two different classes of phenomena. For example, the combination of markedly unstable goal with idiosyncratic use of language generates incoherence and, in extreme cases, 'word salad' (verbigeration).

Of these three classes of formal thought disorder, idiosyncrasy of thought and language is perhaps the most specific to schizophrenia, although instances occur occasionally in manic speech. In contrast, instability of goal is commonly encountered in mania. Weakening of goal is not a feature of mania, but can be a prominent feature of speech in a variety of chronic brain disorders other than schizophrenia. The coexistence of all three types of thought disorder is very rarely encountered in any condition other than schizophrenia. It should, however, be noted that occasional instances of all three classes of formal thought disorder occur in the speech of normal individuals; it is the frequency of occurrence and degree of disorder that distinguishes the thought of people with schizophrenia.

Flow of thought

There are also a variety of disorders of the flow of thought (see Table 8.2). During acute phases, the flow of thought can be accelerated, generating pressure of speech. When this is combined with unstable goal, the pattern of speech closely resembles that seen in mania. During any phase of schizophrenic illness, but especially in chronic illness, there can be an impoverishment or slowing of thought, leading to poverty of speech, which is manifest as lack of spontaneous speech and brevity of replies. Slowing of thought also occurs in depression, but it may be that there is only a partial overlap between the mechanism of poverty of speech in depression and that in schizophrenia. Poverty of speech, which refers to the flow of speech averaged over a period of several minutes or more, differs from the phenomenon of blocking, which is manifest as brief interruptions of speech during which the patient has the experience of having no thoughts at all. It is possible that this phenomenon is closely related to the experience of thought withdrawal, but lacks the delusional attribution of alien influence.

Positive and negative thought disorder

The various disorders of form and flow of thought can be grouped into two major divisions:

1 positive thought disorder, comprising unstable goal, idiosyncrasy and pressure of speech

2 negative thought disorder, comprising weakening of goal and poverty of speech.

Such a dichotomy is consistent with the overlap in the nature of unstable goal and idiosyncrasy in so far as both involve a tendency to make connections between words or ideas on the basis of incidental features. However, it scarcely does justice to the variety and temporal course of thought disorders in schizophrenia.

Assessment

The clinical assessment of thought disorder is difficult because the expression of these disorders depends on the extent to which the patient is given the opportunity to exhibit spontaneity and to direct the flow of conversation. Thought disorder can be more overt when the patient is faced with an intellectually challenging task, or when explaining delusional beliefs.

There are several useful rating scales for thought disorder, but none is fully satisfactory. Andreasen (1979) devised a scale for disorders of thought, language and communication (the TLC scale). It provides definitions of 23 items that can be rated with reasonable reliability in a clinical interview. However, the TLC scale is not sensitive to the relatively subtle idiosyncratic uses of language that are perhaps most characteristic of schizophrenia. Holzman *et al* (1986) constructed the Thought Disorder Index (TDI), which is much more sensitive to these subtle idiosyncrasies of schizophrenic thought. However, the procedure devised by Holzman *et al* for assigning TDI scores involves assessment of thinking during the completion of both the Rorschach Test and the verbal subtests of the Wechsler Adult Intelligence Scale, which makes it too cumbersome for use in the setting of a clinical interview.

Disorders of affect

Although disorders of thinking and perception are the most distinctive features of schizophrenia, disorders of affect are also a major component of the condition. Affect can be blunted, incongruous, unstable, irritable, depressed or elevated. Blunted and incongruous affect are characteristic of schizophrenia, and depressed affect is common.

Blunted affect

Blunted affect has long been regarded as a cardinal feature of chronic schizophrenia, but it is also prevalent in acute schizophrenia. For example, in the International Pilot Study it was reported in 66% of cases of acute schizophrenia (World Health Organization, 1973). It is manifest as a failure to express feelings either verbally or non-verbally, even when talking about issues that would normally be expected to engage the emotions. Expressive gestures are rare and there is little animation in facial expression or in vocal inflection.

In some cases, objective evidence of affective blunting is accompanied by subjective awareness of loss of the ability to experience emotion. More commonly, the patient is unaware of having blunted emotions. However, friends and relatives often find the difficulty in establishing emotional contact with the patient a source of frustration and distress.

Incongruous affect

The expression of affect can be markedly inconsistent with the circumstances. A patient may laugh in a hollow and meaningless way for no understandable reason. However, this degree of incongruity of affect is not common in schizophrenia. A shallow, fatuous affect similar to that arising from damage to the frontal lobes of the brain is more common.

Depression

Depression can occur during various phases of schizophrenia. Dysphoric mood is very common in the prodromal phases preceding a psychotic episode. Overt depression is often present during acute psychotic episodes. Knights & Hirsch (1981) found a wide range of depressive features in 65% of a sample of patients with acute schizophrenia. In general, this overt depression shows some evidence of diminution as the psychotic episode resolves, but it is also common to find depression persisting or becoming apparent in the months following an acute episode. Depression also occurs in the chronic, stable phase of the illness. The point prevalence in this phase lies between 15 and 25%.

In both the acute and stable phases of the illness, depressed mood usually occurs as part of a syndrome of depression similar to that occurring in primary depressive illness. In particular, the depressed mood is likely to be accompanied by anhedonia and negative cognitions, such as low self-esteem, pessimism and hopelessness, as well as suicidal ideation. Suicide itself is not rare, although in some instances suicide in schizophrenia occurs when there is no significant evidence of depression, which suggests that factors such as delusional ideation, hallucinatory voices, idiosyncratic judgement and reduced impulse control can play a part. Biological features of depression such as disturbance of sleep and appetite also occur in association with depressed mood.

The observation that depression is a feature of virtually all phases of schizophrenia has prompted various proposals regarding the relationship between depression and schizophrenia. Some of the evidence suggests that a liability to depression is simply one aspect of the diathesis to schizophrenia. However, it appears that there is also a more intimate relationship between psychotic episodes in schizophrenia and depression. The observation that depression tends to resolve as psychotic symptoms respond to medication (Donlon *et al*, 1976) raises the possibility that the neurochemical processes associated with acute episodes of schizophrenia produce both psychotic symptoms and depression. In contrast, there is also evidence that antipsychotic medication can have a depressive effect in addition to inducing Parkinsonian symptoms (Rifkin *et al*, 1975). While at first sight this is inconsistent with the proposal that depression can be an intrinsic part of the pathological process of an acute schizophrenic episode, it is possible that the depressive component of an acute episode actually reflects a compensatory neuronal response. A psychological response to the implications of having schizophrenia may also be a factor in the pathogenesis of depression.

Anhedonia

Anhedonia, which is a loss of the ability to experience pleasure, is a feature of depression in schizophrenia. It also occurs independently of depression, especially in the chronic phase of the illness, when it tends to be associated with flattened affect, poverty of thought and decreased volition. When it occurs as part of a depressive syndrome it often comprises loss of the ability to experience satisfaction in achievement and also loss of consummatory pleasure. When associated with flattened affect, anhedonia usually entails loss of the pleasures of the hunt rather than of the feast.

Disorders of volition

In schizophrenia, volition can be either weakened or disjointed.

Weakened volition

Weakened volition is manifest as a lack of spontaneous motor activity; it is often accompanied by a lack of spontaneity in speech and affect. The patient is inclined to sit inertly in an armchair, or to remain in bed throughout much of the day.

Case example

A 63-year-old woman, who lived alone in a flat provided by the local authority after her discharge from mental hospital several years previously, lay in bed throughout the day, despite attempts by the community nurse, occupational therapist and doctor to engage her in activity. Left to her own devices, she would eat only candy bars bought for her by a friend. Her flat became increasingly squalid and her physical health was at risk. She was readmitted to hospital compulsorily, and after a month of treatment showed some marginal improvement in her level of activity. However, her cooperation was limited by resentment concerning her compulsory admission. After discharge, she returned to her former state.

Disjointed volition

The patient can be overactive in an ill-directed manner. There is a reduced ability to withstand impulses to act.

Case example

An intelligent and artistic young woman who had been unable to re-establish either stable social relationships or regular occupation after her psychotic symptoms abated lived alone in a poorly furnished rented room. One day she felt cold, so she gathered together a pile of paper and lit a fire on the carpet beside her bed. Fortunately, she managed to extinguish it before serious damage was done, but the carpet was ruined. She was quite capable of appreciating the consequences of acts such as lighting a fire. It appeared that she had been unable to suppress the impulse to act despite the ability to appreciate the likely consequences.

Catatonia

Catatonia is a disturbance of voluntary motor activity and hence overlaps with the disorders of volition described above. Catatonia is reflected in abnormalities of the form of motor activity and in the amount of activity (either underactivity or overactivity).

At times, an apparently normal motor act is arrested in mid-flight. For example, a patient might become frozen in the act of reaching out for the door handle to open a door, and stand with an arm extended for many minutes. Catatonic phenomena described in the early years of the 20th century were often more dramatic in character. Patients were more commonly reported to exhibit *flexibilitas cereus* (waxy flexibility), a condition in which the patient adopted a posture which could be adjusted by an examiner, as if the patient were a passively deformable wax model.

Catatonic underactivity can be manifest as an apparently stuporous state, but one in which consciousness is usually maintained.

A catatonic act can appear to reflect abnormal compliance with or resistance to cues for action, resulting in a movement or posture that is inappropriate to the circumstances. For example, the patient might mimic a movement made by the examiner (echopraxia). At times it as if the patient is continually changing his or her mind about whether or not to execute a socially appropriate action such as shaking hands on meeting, and alternates between extending and withdrawing a hand. Such ambivalence when exhibited in the sphere of motor actions is known as ambitendence. Catatonic acts can also be negativistic, such as withdrawing the hand when the interviewer appropriately proffers a hand.

Case example

The wife of a 42-year-old man who had a 14-year history of schizophrenia summoned an ambulance to the house because her husband had collapsed. The ambulance men found him inert on the floor, mute but with his eyes open. In an attempt to establish his level of consciousness, they first rubbed the skin over his sternum and then twisted a handful of the trapezius muscle above his scapula. He did not respond. Several days later in hospital, when he had resumed a normal level of activity, he reported being fully aware of the ambulance men's attempts to elicit a response and was angry at the way they had treated him. He could not account for his failure to respond.

Catatonic overactivity takes the form of apparently pointless activity that is usually repetitive, such as walking rapidly around and around a table for a period of an half an hour or more. In at least some cases, an abrupt switch from a state of underactivity to overactivity can occur.

In the pre-treatment era, a primary catatonic presentation of schizophrenia was relatively common, occurring in up to 20% of new cases. Today, a primary catatonic schizophrenic illness is relatively rare, whereas the syndrome of catatonia is not uncommon. Thus, Taylor & Fink (2003), summarising 14 case series collected between 1919 and 2000, found that 7–20% of all hospitalised in-patients had some catatonic symptoms.

Catatonia has a spectrum of symptoms, ranging from the classical features, such as stupor, automatic obedience, echo phenomena, ambitendency and mutism, to a variety of lesser known symptoms, such as whispered or robotic speech, unexplained foreign accents, tip-toe walking, hopping, rituals and mannerisms.

Catatonia has a multiplicity of causes. Classically it was linked to schizophrenia, but in more recent series up to 25% of cases are associated with mania, and catatonic attacks can also occur during a depressive episode. Catatonia may also be a presenting feature of a wide variety of metabolic and neurological disorders, including tumours, and hence a new case of catatonia always merits a comprehensive medical, psychiatric and neurological assessment, including a brain scan. Rare familial types such as Gjessing's periodic catatonia, with alternating phases of catatonic stupor and catatonic excitement, have also been described.

Violent behaviour

Violent behaviour is usually the product of an interaction between an individual and his or her surroundings. The type and frequency of violent behaviour in schizophrenia are strongly dependent on social circumstances, and any attempt to describe such violence as if it were purely a manifestation of schizophrenia would be misleading. Occasionally, patients do perpetrate serious violence against others. Violence against the self, such as self-mutilation or suicide, is more common. Minor physical violence against people or property and verbal aggression are common, though.

There are several aspects of the mental disturbances in schizophrenia that can contribute to violence.

Delusional misinterpretations can generate fear or anger. Hallucinatory voices sometimes instruct the patient to carry out a violent act. Irritability can arise as a consequence of persistent, intrusive and unpleasant psychotic experiences, or as a direct consequence of the disease process on the level of cerebral arousal. Disturbance of volition can diminish control over impulses that are recognised to be inappropriate. Lack of judgement can result in a faulty evaluation of the consequences of an act or of its ethical implications.

Aggression can be directed against members of the patient's family, against mental health professionals and occasionally against members of the general public. The family of patients living at home, and nursing staff caring for patients in hospital, are quite commonly the target of verbal aggression and minor physical violence. Serious violence driven by delusions or hallucinations, though much rarer, sometimes has a fatal outcome. Again, family and professionals are at greatest risk. Even matricide, an extremely rare crime, can occur in schizophrenia. Therefore careful assessment of the risk of violence is an important aspect of the assessment of acutely disturbed patients. This assessment will take account of any history of violence, current level of arousal and irritability, the content of delusions and hallucinations, and the degree of insight. Preparing in advance for the possibility of violence is an important aspect of a domiciliary visit.

Case example

A patient who was in general considerate and gentle towards others developed grandiose and persecutory delusions, and became irritable and aggressive. The police were summoned, and when a policeman appeared at his front door he shot him with a bolt from a crossbow. After conviction in court, he was detained in a secure unit for treatment under the Mental Health Act. The episode of acute disturbance settled and he was eventually transferred to an unlocked ward. He once again resumed his characteristic gentle and considerate manner in most matters, but continued to maintain that the policeman deserved to be shot and he had been right to do it. In light of this evidence of limited of insight and lack of judgement, he was very closely supervised following discharge to a group home under a Home Office restriction order. After he had been living in the group home for about a year, the community nurse noted that he was again becoming agitated. When the community nurse returned a few days later, the patient was suspicious and angry. An urgent psychiatric assessment confirmed that he was harbouring the delusional belief that the community nurse was part of a conspiracy against him. He was compelled to return to hospital immediately under the terms of the restriction order. The manager of the group home subsequently found a partially assembled crossbow in the patient's room.

Cognitive impairment

Patients with schizophrenia often perform poorly in formal tests of cognitive function, although the patterns of impaired performance vary between cases. Cognitive impairment is of clinical importance because its severity is a more reliable indicator of social and occupational outcome than is the severity of symptoms (Green, 1998). Virtually all aspects of cognitive function have been reported to show impairment in at least some people with schizophrenia. The diversity of cognitive impairments that can occur suggests that some may arise from non-specific abnormalities of brain structure or function that have increased the person's susceptibility to schizophrenia, but that are only incidentally related to the core pathophysiological processes. On the other hand, certain cognitive impairments are especially prevalent, raising the possibility that these have a more specific link to the core processes, as considered below. Impairments of executive functions (characteristic of the role of the frontal lobes), of memory functions (associated with both frontal and temporal lobes) and of various aspects of attention are common.

Executive function

Failure of executive functions is illustrated by the deficit in performance in word-generation tasks in which the patient is asked to generate as many words as possible in a given category in a specified time. Some patients with schizophrenia, like those with Alzheimer's disease, tend to produce few words. However, unlike the situation in Alzheimer's disease, if the patient is asked to perform the same task on numerous occasions, many different words are generated in total, indicating that the store of words is intact: the problem lies in employing strategies to obtain access to the store.

Ability to change strategies in response to changing task demands is another aspect of executive function commonly impaired in schizophrenia. This can be demonstrated by tasks such as the Wisconsin Card Sorting Test, in which the participant is required to discover a rule governing the sorting of cards according to specific features and, when the rule is changed, to discover the new rule. People with schizophrenia, like individuals with frontal lobe lesions, tend to make incorrect perseverative responses.

Memory

Many aspects of memory function can be impaired, especially declarative memories (e.g. recall of events or stories, paired associate learning, visual recall of designs). In the verbal domain it is typical to find a disproportionate impairment of recall compared with recognition. At least in cases that are not too chronic, the deficit in recall can be overcome by preparing the patients with strategies for organising the material to be recalled (Calev *et al*, 1983), which suggests that even in the case of memory, some of the deficit lies in the domain of developing strategies for the task.

Attention

Among the attentional impairments observed in schizophrenia are impairment of both selective attention and the ability to sustain attention.

Selective attention involves the ability to attend to a specific aspect of a situation in the face of competition from other features that tend to intrude. The Stroop task, in which the participant is presented with colour names printed in inks which are not congruent with those colour names, and required to name the colour of the ink, tests selective attention and also ability to select a response. People with schizophrenia, especially those suffering disorganisation of thought, are generally less able to suppress the influence of the irrelevant colour name.

The ability to sustain attention (vigilance) is commonly assessed using the continuous performance test (CPT). In this test, the participant is presented with a long series of varying stimuli, including irrelevant stimuli and designated target stimuli, and is required to respond whenever a target stimulus appears. Again, people with schizophrenia, and also a substantial number of their first-degree relatives, perform poorly.

Studies of nature of the cognitive impairment

In studies of twins discordant for schizophrenia, the twin with the illness usually does worse on such tests than the unaffected twin, even though the affected twin's performance may be within the normal range (Goldberg *et al,* 1993). This suggests that even in cases where there is no marked cognitive impairment, the illness obstructs the realisation of potential cognitive ability. Furthermore, the cognitive impairments are associated with development of overt illness, not merely with the genetic predisposition to the illness. On the other hand, Goldberg *et al* (1993) did find that there was evidence of some impairment, most notably in episodic memory, in the non-affected twins relative to healthy controls, implying that genes play some role.

Longitudinal studies of large cohorts reveal that cognitive impairments can be discerned from early childhood in individuals who subsequently develop schizophrenia (Jones *et al,* 1994). There is substantial evidence that the impairments become more marked around the time of onset of the illness.

The evidence regarding the evolution of cognitive impairment once the illness is established is complex. In a minority of cases, there is progressive decline over many years, leading to levels of impairment comparable to those seen in Alzheimer's disease, but in many cases cognitive performance stabilises and may even improve. None the less, cognitive impairments are usually more persistent than psychotic symptoms.

Indeed, the persistence of cognitive impairments raises the possibility that these impairments reflect the core pathophysiological processes underlying the clinical features of the illness. Various investigators have proposed theoretical accounts based on psychological mechanisms postulated to reflect the core processes of schizophrenia (e.g. Frith, 1992; Hemsley, 1992; Liddle *et al,* 1992). While these various theories are each supported by a substantial body of evidence and potentially offer useful pointers towards the nature of the core processes, the essence of schizophrenia remains elusive.

Neurological signs

Abnormal involuntary movements

In 1926, several decades before the development of antipsychotic medication, Farran-Ridge described a range of abnormal involuntary movements, which he attributed to basal ganglion disorder, in patients with schizophrenia. The movements include tics, twitches and grimaces. After the introduction of antidopaminergic antipsychotic medication in the mid-1950s, abnormal involuntary movements became more prevalent, although the onset of abnormal movements related to treatment is usually seen only after prolonged administration. Furthermore, the movements can be exacerbated by withdrawal of antipsychotic medication, and often persist long after cessation of treatment. Hence, these medication-related dyskinetic movements are called tardive dyskinesia.

Dyskinetic movements in schizophrenia fall into two groups: orofacial dyskinesia, and trunk and limb dyskinesia. While the former are more characteristic of drug-induced dyskinesia, it is probable that aspects of the disease process itself contribute to both types. In particular, core negative symptoms such as poverty of speech and flat affect are associated with both. However, the two types of dyskinesia differ in their relationship to ageing. The prevalence of trunk and limb dyskinesia is virtually independent of age, whereas orofacial dyskinesia is rare in young patients but increases rapidly in late middle age. The age range in which this increase in prevalence occurs is about a decade earlier in patients with marked negative symptoms in comparison with those without negative symptoms, which suggests the pathological process underlying negative symptoms interacts with age-related neuronal degeneration in a way that hastens the onset of orofacial dyskinesia (Liddle *et al,* 1993*a*).

Cortical signs

Both dyspraxia and agnosia are common, at least among chronic patients. Typically, patients are clumsy or hesitant in performing motor sequences, or have impairments of integration of sensory information such as dysgraphaesthesia or impaired two-point discrimination. These neurological signs have limited localising power, but are probably indicative of impaired function of association cortex. They are related to core negative symptoms and, to a lesser extent, to disorganisation of mental activity (Liddle *et al,* 1993*b*).

Abnormal eye-movements

Saccadic intrusions in smooth pursuit eye movements are reported in 50–85% of patients and 40–50% of first-degree relatives (Holtzman *et al,* 1988). The familial pattern prompted Holtzman and colleagues to propose the existence of a heritable neurological characteristic (a latent trait) which can be manifest as either schizophrenia or as an abnormality of smooth pursuit or both disorders. Since eye movements are governed by the cortical frontal eye-fields and by brain-stem nuclei, the relevant deficit in patients with schizophrenia may in principle be at either or both of these two sites. A large body of evidence favours involvement of the frontal eye-fields (Levin, 1980).

In addition to saccadic intrusions in smooth pursuit, other abnormalities of eye movement occur. For example, some patients fail to suppress an automatic saccade towards a stimulus in the periphery when instructed to perform a saccadic movement away from the side of the stimulus (an antisaccade).

Insight

While some impairment of insight is implicit in the classification of schizophrenia as a psychotic illness, the degree to which unrealistic thinking interferes with the patient's understanding of the nature of the illness is quite variable, both over the course of the illness in an individual case and between cases. At its most severe level, impaired insight may lead patients to deny that they are suffering from an illness at all. It is difficult to engage them in any therapeutic programme. At less severe levels, patients may accept that they have an illness, but deny that it is a mental illness. More commonly, patients do accept, at least implicitly, that they have a mental illness, but they have unrealistic ideas that diminish their ability to evaluate issues regarding treatment, or to comprehend the impact of the illness on their lives.

Assessment of the level of insight is especially important where there is a risk of dangerous behaviour.

Case example

A 22-year-old man who had suffered a schizophrenic episode 1 year previously developed a delusional belief that he belonged to the Knights Templar, and had to defend the temple against enemies. He assembled a collection of weapons, including guns and swords. His parents informed his general practitioner, but the man maintained he was not ill and was unwilling to accept medical assessment. When a social worker and psychiatrist came to his house to assess him with a view to compulsory admission to hospital under the Mental Health Act 1983, he threatened them with a shotgun. The police were called and in the ensuing gun battle the patient and two police officers were injured. The patient was admitted to hospital under section 2 of the Act and treated with haloperidol. In the following weeks, he accepted that he required treatment with antipsychotic medication in hospital. None the less, he continued to believe that he was besieged by enemies. In particular, he regarded his parents as enemies, possibly because of their attempts to seek medical help for him. Thus, despite an increase in the level of his insight during treatment, he developed only a partial appreciation of the nature of his condition and remained potentially dangerous.

Subtypes and syndromes of schizophrenia

The classical subtypes

Classically, schizophrenia is divided into four subtypes: hebephrenic, paranoid, catatonic and simple. This reflects the fact that the disease had its origins in Kraepelin's amalgamation of hebephrenia, catatonia and dementia paranoides into a single disease entity, to which Diem had added dementia simplex in 1903. In practice, it is difficult to allocate patients within this classical subdivision because many patients show features of more than one type in the course of their illness.

Dimensions of psychopathology

The limited success of attempts to divide schizophrenia into discrete subtypes vindicates Kraepelin's proposal that hebephrenia, catatonia and dementia paranoides may best be regarded as different manifestations of a single disease. None the less, it is clear that the clinical manifestations are heterogeneous. This heterogeneity suggests that several distinguishable but related psychopathological processes can occur within schizophrenia. In recent years, accumulating evidence has pointed to the existence of various distinct neuropathological processes underlying the disorder. This has led to the proposal that schizophrenia is a disease in which there are a number of dimensions of psychopathology, reflecting distinct but related neuropathological processes, which might or might not occur together in a single case.

The type 1/type 2 dichotomy

The first attempt at such a dimensional model was by Crow (1980). He proposed that there were two independent dimensions, which he designated type 1 and type 2. Type 1 schizophrenia was characterised by positive symptoms, which tend to be acute. Positive symptoms entail the presence of an abnormal mental process, and include delusions, hallucinations and formal thought disorder. Crow proposed that type 1 schizophrenia reflected a biochemical imbalance, such as dopaminergic hyperactivity. Type 2 schizophrenia was characterised by negative symptoms, which tend to be chronic. Negative symptoms reflect the absence of a mental function present in normal individuals, and include poverty of speech and blunted affect. Crow proposed that type 2 schizophrenia arose from structural abnormality of the brain.

As predicted by Crow's hypothesis, a great deal of evidence indicates that negative symptoms are more strongly associated with various indices of brain abnormality than are positive symptoms. However, the structural abnormalities revealed by X-ray computed tomography and magnetic resonance imaging are not associated exclusively with negative symptoms. Furthermore, the efficacy of atypical antipsychotic drugs such as clozapine in treating hitherto persistent negative symptoms, in at least some cases, implies that a biochemical imbalance plays some role in the genesis of these symptoms.

While the type 1/type 2 proposal now appears to be an oversimplification of the relationship between symptoms, chronicity and neuropathology, it was perhaps the first credible attempt to link the symptoms of schizophrenia with underlying neuropathology in a way that accounted for the occurrence episodes of acute disturbance superimposed upon a background of enduring deficits. In particular, it provided a major stimulus to investigation of the enduring deficits.

Three syndromes of characteristic schizophrenic symptoms

Most detailed analyses of the pattern of correlations between schizophrenic symptoms have revealed at least three distinguishable groups of symptoms. In studies limited to patients with persistent, stable symptoms (e.g. Liddle, 1987), three distinguishable groups of symptoms emerge:

1 psychomotor poverty (the core negative symptoms – poverty of speech, blunted affect, decreased spontaneous movement)

2 disorganisation (disorders of the form of thought, inappropriate affect)

3 reality distortion (the core positive symptoms – delusions, hallucinations).

Many other studies have reported a similar segregation of schizophrenic symptoms, even in groups of patients who were more heterogeneous with regard to chronicity of symptoms (e.g. Arndt *et al*, 1991; Frith, 1992; Peralta *et al*, 1992).

In many ways these three syndromes resemble the three principal psychotic illnesses that Kraepelin had amalgamated to form dementia praecox: reality distortion comprises symptoms that were a feature of dementia paranoides; disorganisation is similar to hebephrenia; and psychomotor poverty, which reflects diminished spontaneous activity, resembles the hypoactive phase of catatonia. It is important to emphasise that the syndromes can coexist within an individual patient, and hence reflect distinguishable dimensions of psychopathology within a single illness.

Each of the three syndromes is associated with a distinct pattern of impairment in neuropsychological tests, which suggests that there are three different patterns of underlying brain function. The evidence indicates that psychomotor poverty, disorganisation and reality distortion are, respectively, associated with impairment of the supervisory mental functions responsible for initiation, selection and monitoring of self-generated mental activity. A study of regional cerebral blood flow (rCBF) using positron emission tomography confirmed that each syndrome is associated with a particular pattern of cerebral activity (Liddle *et al*, 1992). For each syndrome, the associated pattern of rCBF embraces anatomically connected regions of association cortex and related subcortical nuclei. Furthermore, for each syndrome, the cerebral regions involved include those areas of cortex implicated in the corresponding supervisory mental function in normal individuals. Thus, the evidence suggests that there are several distinct patterns of brain malfunction in schizophrenia. Subsequent studies have provided support for these patterns, but not all of the data are consistent (see Liddle, 2001).

Box 8.2 Dimensions of psychopathology in schizophrenia

Reality distortion
- Delusions
- Hallucinations

Disorganisation
- (Positive) formal thought disorder
- Inappropriate affect
- Disjointed volition

Psychomotor poverty
- Poverty of speech
- Flat affect
- Motor underactivity

Psychomotor excitation
- Pressure of speech
- Irritability
- Motor overactivity

Depression
- Depressed mood
- Pessimism/hopelessness
- Low self-esteem/guilt
- Anhedonia

Non-specific psychopathology
- Attentional impairment
- Disorientation
- Anxiety
- Sleep disturbance
- Somatic complaints

Five dimensions of psychopathology in schizophrenia

The three characteristic schizophrenic syndromes that emerge from exploration of the relationships between persistent symptoms do not embrace the entire gamut of symptoms in schizophrenia. In particular, there are two additional syndromes, which are usually transient: depression, characterised by low mood and depressive cognitions such as low self-esteem and pessimism; and psychomotor excitation, characterised by motor overactivity and excited, labile affect, which appears to be the polar opposite of psychomotor poverty and resembles the excited phase of catatonia.

Factor analyses of the symptoms assessed using the Positive and Negative Syndrome Scale (PANSS) (Kay, 1991), which covers the symptoms of schizophrenia in a comprehensive manner, reveal a complex pattern with five main factors:

1 core negative symptoms (including social withdrawal, lack of spontaneity, poor flow of conversation, blunted affect, motor retardation)

2 core positive symptoms (delusions and hallucinations)

3 excitement (including poor impulse control, tension, hostility)

4 depressive symptoms (including anxiety, guilty feelings, depression, somatic concern)

5 cognitive disorders (including difficulty in abstract thinking, disorientation and conceptual disorganisation).

The group of cognitive disorders resembles the disorganisation syndrome. Unfortunately, PANSS ratings do not provide a clear delineation of the disorganisation syndrome because several negative symptom items on it are defined in a manner that includes features of the disorganisation syndrome. In particular, the blunted affect item includes inappropriate affect.

With this relatively minor caveat, factor analysis of PANSS ratings confirms that virtually the entire gamut of schizophrenic symptoms can be accounted for by five principal dimensions of psychopathology. Box 8.2 presents these in a manner that reflects the consistent patterns of relationships between symptoms delineated by recent factor analytic studies. If psychomotor poverty and psychomotor excitation are regarded as lying at opposite poles of a bipolar continuum, it would perhaps be more correct to say that there are four independent dimensions, one of which is bipolar. These dimensions apparently reflect five major pathological processes that generate five distinguishable syndromes. Although these five syndromes are distinguishable in so far as they can occur separately, evidence of more than one syndrome is detectable in the majority of patients. Furthermore, the probability of observing a particular combination of syndromes depends on the phase of illness, which suggests that there are various shared features linking these distinguishable syndromes.

Overall, there appears to be a constellation of symptoms, all of which are related, but some of the relationships are closer than others, with the symptoms clustering into five major groups.

The course and prognosis of schizophrenia

Despite the fact that Kraepelin distinguished dementia praecox (schizophrenia) from affective psychosis largely on the basis of time course, with dementia praecox typically beginning in adolescence and persisting throughout adult life, the course of schizophrenia shows substantial variability. There is variability in the mode of onset, in the degree of persistence of symptoms through the mid-stage of the illness and in the long-term outcome.

The onset

At one extreme, the onset can be insidious, with subtle evidence of abnormality beginning in childhood, or even in infancy. In some cases, the patient's mother declares that even in the first year of life the patient differed from siblings in responsiveness. At school, one of several different patterns of behaviour may emerge: in some cases the child is shy and socially awkward, in others cases hostile and disruptive in class. During adolescence these patterns develop further. The shy, awkward child becomes introspective and socially isolated. The more disruptive child may as an adolescent become quite erratic in behaviour. In either case, the developing young adult finds it difficult to form stable intimate relationships, or to establish a consistent work record. Sooner or later, perhaps while still at school, a decline in performance becomes noticeable. In unfavourable circumstances, there may be a drift into a vagrant lifestyle, with marked neglect of personal hygiene. In most cases, the illness eventually declares itself with delusions and hallucinations.

At the other extreme, the onset can be quite abrupt. In such cases patients become unsettled over the course of a few weeks. They may experience dysphoric mood or irritability and a puzzled sense that something odd is happening. They often appear preoccupied. In some instances, obsessional thoughts intrude. Concentration deteriorates and sleep is disturbed. From this unsettled state, delusions or hallucinations emerge and behaviour is likely to become disruptive, even aggressive. There is a rapid deterioration in occupational performance and social activity. Such an onset often follows a stressful experience.

In the majority of cases, the onset of florid symptoms occurs after a prodromal phase lasting many months, which begins with a subtle alteration of behaviour and may progress through a phase of preoccupation and social withdrawal before agitation becomes prominent and overt psychosis appears. Not uncommonly, onset occurs during the first year of a university or college course. The young person may be living away from home for the first time and as pressures build up, perhaps as first-year examinations approach, the breakdown occurs.

The distribution of age of onset of overt symptoms is one of the most characteristic features of schizophrenia. In males, the frequency of onset rises rapidly through adolescence to a peak at about age 22, followed by a steady decrease, such that onset after 40 is rare. In females, the frequency of onset rises through adolescence, but the peak is later, the distribution is somewhat broader and an appreciable risk of onset persists into middle age.

Outcome of the first episode

In a major study conducted at Hillside Hospital, New York, of the course of illness in a cohort of patients who satisfied Research Diagnostic Criteria for schizophrenia or schizoaffective disorder of predominantly schizophrenic type, Robinson *et al* (1999*a*) found that 87% achieved remission within the first year. The median time to achieve remission was 9 weeks.

The medium-term evolution of the illness

In a minority of cases there is complete recovery after the first episode. In a systematic 5-year follow-up study of a comprehensive, representative cohort of patients from a defined catchment area in Buckinghamshire, a relatively affluent rural English county, 16% of patients had only one episode and showed no residual impairment (Watt *et al*, 1983). The patients had been selected according to Present State Examination diagnostic criteria, which place emphasis on the presence of Schneiderian first-rank symptoms, but which do not demand persistence of symptoms. Similarly, in the first-episode study conducted at Hillside Hospital, New York, follow-up of the 87% of patients who had responded to treatment in the first year revealed that only 18% did not have any relapses in the following 5 years (Robinson *et al*, 1999*b*). Thus, approximately 16% of patients recover after a single episode.

A synthesis of findings from the major longitudinal studies (Bleuler, 1974; Huber *et al*, 1975; Ciompi & Muller, 1976; Watt *et al*, 1983) indicates that 20–30% of cases run an episodic course with relatively minor disability between episodes. Even in such relatively good-outcome cases, it is common to find that the patient experiences brief periods of mild dysphoric symptoms and attentional difficulties several times a year. Some of these episodes of mild disturbance prove to be the prodromal phase of florid psychotic relapse.

In the middle range of severity of illness are cases in which an appreciable degree of disability persists between episodes of florid symptoms. Between episodes, the patient typically exhibits abnormal sensitivity to stress, and some oddities of behaviour or lack of initiative, but is able to sustain relationships and may be able to work, albeit at lower level than might have been otherwise expected. The middle range also includes patients who have persisting delusions or hallucinations that interfere minimally with daily life so that occupational and social activities suffer only mild disruption. Some patients who initially exhibit an illness of medium severity appear to suffer a stepwise deterioration after successive episodes, and the rate of remission in later episodes is lower than in first episodes (Robinson *et al*, 1999*b*).

Towards the severe end of the spectrum of illness, about 20–25% of patients achieve at best partial remission of symptoms and suffer from substantial persisting disability. The most severe cases, amounting to perhaps 5–10% of all cases, show severe persistent symptoms and behavioural disorder that seriously disrupts all aspects of life.

Persistent symptoms and the defect state

The features most likely to persist are psychomotor symptoms such as apathy, flat affect and poverty of speech, and signs of disorganised mental activity, such as formal thought disorder and disjointed volition. Occupational and social behaviour disintegrate. Sociable greetings and polite conversation disappear, table manners deteriorate and basic hygiene is neglected. In such cases, there is often overt cognitive impairment.

Delusions and hallucinations tend to be intrinsically more episodic than negative (psychomotor poverty) symptoms and cognitive impairments; furthermore, they usually respond to treatment with conventional dopamine-blocking antipsychotic medication. None the less, they persist in about 20% of cases despite such treatment. In a small proportion of the patients at the severe end of the spectrum, the clinical picture is dominated by persistent active psychotic symptoms and chaotic or aggressive behaviour. The use of the atypical antipsychotic drug clozapine produces substantial improvement in about 40% of hitherto treatment-resistant patients.

Long-term outcome

In contrast to the implication of Kraepelin's original choice of the name dementia praecox, there is a tendency for schizophrenia to resolve eventually in many cases, though the time scale of improvement can be several decades. Pooled data from the major studies that have followed patients for more than 20 years (Bleuler, 1974; Huber *et al*, 1975; Ciompi & Muller, 1976; Harding *et al*, 1987) show that 57% of 1117 patients followed up over a mean of 27 years showed either recovery or significant improvement. Improvement was not confined only to those with mild illness. For example, Harding *et al* (1987) studied 118 patients who satisfied DSM–III criteria for schizophrenia who had been representative of the most impaired third of the Vermont State Hospital in-patient population prior to a programme of active rehabilitation in the mid-1950s. They were resettled in the community and three decades later 68% were judged either to have recovered or to have improved significantly.

Factors predicting outcome

There are no reliable guidelines for predicting outcome in an individual case. However, there are constitutional factors and also features of the onset of illness that indicate an increased likelihood of better outcome.

Box 8.3 Prognostic factors

Factors indicating poor prognosis

- Poor premorbid adjustment
- Insidious onset
- Onset in adolescence
- Marked cognitive impairment
- Enlargement of cerebral ventricles

Factors indicating good prognosis

- Evidence of schizoaffective features:
  - Marked mood disturbance at onset
  - Family history of affective illness
- Female gender

Female gender, good premorbid social adjustment and a family history of affective disorder are associated with better outcome. Abrupt onset associated with major precipitants, onset at a later age and the presence of marked mood disturbance at onset are indicators of a relatively good prognosis (Box 8.3). Some studies have found that long duration of untreated psychosis is a predictor of poor outcome, although more recent studies have cast doubt upon this finding (Robinson *et al*, 1999*a*,*b*).

Among neurobiological features, extent of structural abnormality of the brain is perhaps the one most consistently observed to be associated with poor outcome, although some studies have not confirmed this association. In his review of X-ray computed tomography studies of ventricular size in schizophrenia, Lewis (1990) reported that five of the nine studies that addressed the issue found a significant relationship between increased ventricular size and poorer response to treatment. It should be noted that ventricular enlargement tends to be present from the beginning of the illness, and hence can be regarded as predictive of outcome rather than a consequence of poor outcome.

Standardised assessment and diagnosis

The US–UK diagnostic project (Cooper *et al*, 1972) demonstrated substantial discrepancies between diagnostic practices in the United States, where a relatively broad concept of schizophrenia had evolved from a tradition influenced by Bleuler, and the UK, where the prevailing concept of schizophrenia placed more emphasis on Schneiderian first-rank symptoms. The International Pilot Study of Schizophrenia, conducted by the World Health Organization (1973), demonstrated that consistency across cultures was possible using semi-standardised criteria leaning heavily on Schneiderian symptoms. Shortly after, operational criteria were introduced that took account in a systematic manner of the current symptoms, the time course of illness and other associated features.

One of the first sets of operational criteria was proposed by Feighner and colleagues from St Louis, Missouri. The Feighner criteria specifically demanded that the illness be chronic (i.e. lasting for at least 6 months), without return to premorbid social adjustment. This particular criterion shifted the definition of schizophrenia nearer to Kraepelin's original concept of dementia praecox. The 6-month criterion was also included in the criteria for schizophrenia specified in the third edition of *Diagnostic and Statistical Manual* (DSM–III), published by the American Psychiatric Association in 1980. While DSM–III (and the subsequently revised edition, DSM–III–R, published in 1987) achieved widespread use, the ninth edition of *International Classification of Diseases* (ICD–9; World Health Organization, 1978) remained the official guide to diagnosis in many parts of the world. In the mid-1990s, with the publication of the 10th edition of ICD (World Health Organization, 1992) and the fourth edition of the *Diagnostic and Statistical Manual* (DSM–IV) (American Psychiatric Association, 1994), a reasonable degree of concordance was achieved between the two major sets of operational diagnostic criteria in use worldwide. However, it is important to recognise that these sets of operational criteria reflect the decisions of committees of experts and are to some extent arbitrary. Issues such as the degree of emphasis that should be placed on particular symptoms or on the details of the time course of illness are unlikely to be resolved definitively until the essential nature of the illness has been delineated.

Although features such as time course are crucial for diagnosis, the cornerstone of diagnosis is the assessment of the symptoms characteristic of the illness. Before examining the criteria specified in DSM–IV and ICD–10, we shall therefore review some of the rating scales that have been developed to providing reliable assessment of symptoms for the purpose of diagnosis, or for other purposes, such as monitoring response to treatment.

Symptom assessment

The approach to symptom assessment adopted in the International Pilot Study of Schizophrenia is embodied in the Present State Examination (PSE). The PSE is a semi-standardised clinical interview in which a set of standard questions, augmented by additional questions as required to clarify the nature of the patient's symptoms, is used to detect the presence and determine the severity of designated symptoms, which are defined carefully in a glossary. The Pilot Study employed a modified 380-item version of the eighth edition of the PSE.

The ninth edition of the PSE included 140 symptom items, each scored 0, 1 or 2, focused predominantly on psychotic symptoms, and proved to be a very successful and practical instrument. The tenth edition was expanded to include 299 items, covering all majority of areas of psychopathology, and was incorporated in the Schedules for Clinical Assessment in Psychiatry (SCAN) (World Health Organization, 1994). Most items are scored on a scale ranging from 0 to 4, reflecting increasing degrees of severity. The greater range allows greater sensitivity, but teasing out a sufficiently detailed description of the patient's experience to rate severity on a five-point scale for a substantial number of the items can be very demanding of a patient's attention and cooperation.

The PSE does not lend itself easily to sensitive measurement of change in overall severity of illness. The Brief Psychiatric Rating Scale (BPRS), constructed by Overall & Goreham (1962), allows the scoring of each of 16 items commonly occurring in psychotic illnesses on a seven-point ordered scale, and is potentially suitable to measure change in severity of individual symptoms and of overall severity of illness. It was used in the majority of pharmacological treatment trials in the three decades after its introduction. However, some items embrace a variety of different phenomena, while some particular classes of phenomena are scattered over several different items. For example, delusions contribute to the scores for several different items, which makes it difficult to quantify overall severity of delusions.

In the 1980s, several scales were developed which emphasised the observable deficits of speech, affect and behaviour in schizophrenia. For example, the Scale for the Assessment of Negative Symptoms (SANS) (Andreasen, 1982) comprises five sub-scales concerned with affective flattening, alogia, avolition, anhedonia and attentional impairment. There are 25 individual items, each scored in the range 0–5. It is possible to score the observable behavioural items with acceptable reliability. This scale has been widely used in the exploration of the clinical and neurobiological correlates of negative symptoms of schizophrenia. If the SANS is used in conjunction with Andreasen's Scale for the Assessment of Positive Symptoms (SAPS) (Andreasen, 1986), a comprehensive coverage of the symptoms characteristic of schizophrenia is provided.

Shortly after the development of the SANS, Kay and colleagues produced the Positive and Negative Syndrome Scale (PANSS) (Kay, 1991), which expanded the BPRS so as provide a more comprehensive coverage of the symptoms of schizophrenia, especially the negative symptoms. It contains three sub-scales: positive symptoms (including delusions, hallucinations and positive formal thought disorder); negative symptoms (including lack of spontaneity, blunted affect); and general psychopathology. Although it was designed on the basis of a view of schizophrenic symptoms that afforded special importance to a positive–negative dichotomy, subsequent factor analysis of PANSS symptom scores revealed a more complex pattern of relationships between symptoms, consistent with a five-dimensional model of schizophrenic pathology (see above). Unfortunately, some of the PANSS items embrace differing phenomena, which are not closely related, and, as with the BPRS, delusional thinking is included in several different items in combination with non-delusional phenomena. Because the contamination occurs within items, it is intrinsically difficult to tease apart aspects of psychopathology which probably should be assessed separately.

More recently, the Signs and Symptoms of Psychotic Illness (SSPI) scale has been shown to provide a reliable and sensitive assessment of the five major dimensions of psychotic illness within a brief (20-item) scale (Liddle *et al*, 2002). The SSPI provides an efficient measure of schizophrenic psychopathology, which is suitable for use in serial assessments of the severity of illness, and its administration is usually tolerable even to very disturbed patients.

Unfortunately, there is no single symptom scale that combines the virtues of tolerability, reliability, sensitivity to change in clinical state and coverage of the phenomena of schizophrenia in a comprehensive and well structured manner. It is probably unreasonable to expect all of these qualities in one scale. The PSE provides rigorous assessment but is cumbersome and so unsuitable for monitoring clinical change. SANS when combined with SAPS provides good coverage of schizophrenic phenomena but the original subscale composition differs from current understanding. PANSS offers the possibility of efficient measurement of overall severity of illness and a reasonably adequate estimation of severity of the five major syndromes that occur within schizophrenia, but there are some problems with item composition. SSPI covers the five main dimensions of psychotic illnesses in a brief scale, but by virtue of its brevity does not provide a detailed picture.

The Diagnostic and Statistical Manual

The American Psychiatric Association's DSM–IV (1994) applies relatively rigorous criteria to diagnosis that take account of a variety clinical features in addition to psychiatric symptoms. It does this in two ways. First, it employs a multi-axial description of illness: axis I deals with clinical syndromes; axis II, personality disorders; axis III, physical disorders and conditions; axis IV, severity of psychological stressors; axis V, highest level of adaptive function in the preceding year. Second, axis I diagnosis is based on operational criteria that demand not only the presence of a specified number of items from a list of symptoms or signs considered characteristic of the illness, but also criteria concerning features such as duration of the illness and absence of clinical features sufficient to justify certain alternative diagnoses.

In the case of the axis I diagnosis of schizophrenia, the criteria demand the presence of at least one of the symptoms regarded as most characteristic of the illness (e.g. bizarre delusions or commenting voices) or at least two items from a list of less specific symptoms (other delusions or hallucinations, disorganised speech, disorganised behaviour, negative symptoms). There must be impairment of occupational or social function, and prodromal or residual symptoms must persist for at least 6 months. Illnesses dominated by mood disturbance are excluded, as are conditions attributable to a general medical condition or to drug intoxication or withdrawal.

The International Classification of Diseases

The World Health Organization's ICD–10 (1992) provides criteria very similar to those specified in DSM–IV, although there is less emphasis on chronicity. The ICD–10 criteria are summarised in Box 8.4. The ICD code for schizophrenia is F20.*xy* where *x* denotes the subtype and *y* denotes the course of illness. In making the diagnosis, Schneiderian first-rank symptoms and persistent 'impossible' delusions are given special weight, but other persistent hallucinations, formal thought disorders, catatonic behaviour and negative symptoms, such as apathy, poverty of speech and blunted affect, can contribute to the diagnosis.

Box 8.4 Summary of ICD–10 criteria for schizophrenia

Symptoms and signs

Either one or more of the following specific symptoms:

- thought echo, insertion, withdrawal or broadcast
- delusions of control of the body, thoughts, actions, or sensations; delusional perception
- hallucinatory voices commenting or discussing, or coming from a part of the body
- persistent delusional beliefs that are completely impossible

Or two or more of the following specific symptoms or signs:

- other persistent hallucinations if either occurring daily for many weeks, or accompanied by evidence of delusional thinking or sustained overvalued ideas
- formal thought disorder (incoherent or irrelevant speech, neologisms)
- catatonic behaviour (excitement, posturing, waxy flexibility, negativism, mutism, stupor)
- apathy, paucity of speech, flat or inappropriate affect, usually resulting in social impairment (but not due to neuroleptic medication or depression)

Or (for a diagnosis of simple schizophrenia only)

- a consistent change in behaviour manifest as loss of interest, aimlessness, idleness, a self-absorbed attitude and social withdrawal over a period of at least 1 year.

Duration of symptoms

Symptoms or signs must be clearly present for most of the time for at least 1 month (and at least 1 year for a diagnosis of simple schizophrenia).

Exclusion of affective psychosis

If there are extensive manic or depressive symptoms, the schizophrenic symptoms must antedate the mood disturbance.

Exclusion of overt brain disease

Schizophrenia should not be diagnosed in the presence of overt brain disease or during states of drug intoxication or withdrawal.

This summary is an abbreviation of more expansive clinical criteria which were intended to be a guide to diagnosis rather than to provide rigid rules. In addition to the criteria for clinical use, ICD–10 specifies research criteria, which are more rigid.

Significant consistent change in personal behaviour manifest as loss of interest, aimlessness, self-absorbed attitude or social withdrawal are taken into account in the diagnosis of simple schizophrenia.

The guidelines specify that specific symptoms are clearly present most of the time during a period of 1 month or more, but acknowledge that prodromal symptoms often precede the onset of specific symptoms. In the case of simple schizophrenia, duration of at least 1 year is required.

A diagnosis of schizophrenia should not be made in the presence of extensive depressive or manic symptoms, unless it is clear that schizophrenic symptoms antedated the affective disturbance. When schizophrenic and affective symptoms develop together and are evenly balanced, a diagnosis of schizoaffective disorder should be made.

Disorders presenting with clinical features resembling schizophrenia but arising from overt brain disease are classified as organic disorders, and those occurring during drug intoxication or withdrawal are classified as drug-induced disorders, not schizophrenia. Delusional disorders, in which the delusions are neither Schneiderian nor bizarre, nor accompanied by other characteristic schizophrenic features such as hallucinations, are also classified separately from schizophrenia.

The four classic subtypes – paranoid (F20.0), hebephrenic (F20.1), catatonic (F20.2) and simple schizophrenia (F20.6) – are recognised, but the additional category of undifferentiated schizophrenia (F20.3) is introduced to accommodate cases not fitting the subtypes, or with mixed features without a clear preponderance of the features of any one subtype. In addition, there are categories for post-schizophrenic depression (F20.4) and residual schizophrenia (F20.5) for patients who previously exhibited features sufficient to satisfy criteria for schizophrenia, but for whom the clinical picture is currently dominated by either depression or long-term negative symptoms.

The course of illness is classified into six types: continuous; episodic with progressive deficit; episodic with stable deficit; episodic remittent; incomplete remission; and complete remission. While ICD–10 clearly recognises the possibility of complete remission, the demand that specific symptoms be present for most of the time for at least 1 month defines a concept of schizophrenia that excludes brief, transient psychoses. Illnesses that meet the symptomatic requirements but have a duration less than 1 month are diagnosed as acute schizophrenia-like psychotic disorders.

The retention of simple schizophrenia is perhaps the most controversial aspect of the ICD–10 concept of schizophrenia. Simple schizophrenia is defined as an uncommon disorder in which there is an insidious but progressive development of oddities of conduct, inability to meet the demands of society and decline in overall performance. The characteristic negative features of residual schizophrenia develop without being preceded by any overt psychotic symptoms. The criteria include a marked loss of interest, idleness and social withdrawal over a period of at least 1 year. With increasing social impoverishment, the patient may drift into vagrancy.

While it is clearly important to avoid overuse of this category by including individuals who should simply be regarded as eccentric, a strong case can be made for regarding simple schizophrenia as closely related to other schizophrenic illnesses. First, overt schizophrenia is often preceded by a prolonged prodromal phase, which can resemble simple schizophrenia. Furthermore, at least some cases satisfying criteria for simple schizophrenia would fall within the spectrum of disorders which are genetically related to overt schizophrenia (see below). It is very likely that the cerebral abnormalities that predispose to overt schizophrenia can also produce the clinical picture described by the ICD–10 definition of simple schizophrenia.

The boundaries of schizophrenia

The schizophrenia spectrum

Family studies reveal that there is a range of disorders that have an increased prevalence among the relatives of people with schizophrenia. These disorders include affective psychosis, depression, alcohol misuse and schizotypal personality disorder. It is likely that a heritable cerebral abnormality that plays a part in schizophrenia can contribute to the development of any disorder in this spectrum.

The relationship between schizophrenia and affective psychosis

The observation that depression and excitation occur in schizophrenia, while, conversely, features of the three characteristic schizophrenic syndromes – reality distortion, disorganisation and psychomotor poverty – can occur in affective psychosis suggests that there are common elements in the pathophysiology of these two psychotic conditions. Furthermore, the evidence from family studies indicating at least a degree of familial relationship between schizophrenia and affective illness is consistent with the proposal that there is a continuum of psychotic illnesses, extending from affective psychosis, through schizoaffective disorder, to schizophrenia.

None the less, if we follow Kahlbaum and Kraepelin and examine the overall picture of the illness, there can be little doubt that it is useful to distinguish between schizophrenia and affective psychosis. Although similar clusters of symptoms can occur in the two conditions, there are differences in both the cross-sectional and the longitudinal picture. As emphasised by both Kraepelin and Bleuler, in schizophrenia there is a lack of unity in the mental processes. For example, the delusions and hallucinations are less readily understood on the basis of the prevailing mood. Longitudinally, the impoverishment and fragmentation of mental activity are prone to persist even when the transient mood disturbance has abated.

When an illness presents features characteristic of both disorders, a diagnosis of schizophrenia should be made if the periods of marked depression or elation are brief in comparison with the total duration of discernible illness, whereas a diagnosis of affective psychosis should be made if depression or elation are prominent throughout the period of discernible illness. In the majority of cases, it is possible to distinguish between schizophrenia and affective psychosis on this basis. In a minority, the distinction cannot be made, and a diagnosis of schizoaffective psychosis is appropriate. (ICD–10 specifies that the diagnosis should be affective psychosis if extensive manic or depressive symptoms precede the schizophrenic symptoms.)

Schizophrenia and other organic psychoses

Brain imaging studies reveal that the association cortex of the temporal, frontal and parietal lobes, and the related subcortical nuclei, are all implicated in the pathophysiology of schizophrenia. The symptoms that occur in schizophrenia are associated with disorder of the neural systems linking these brain areas (for a review, see Liddle, 2001). Many different diseases that affect the structure or function of these neural systems can produce symptoms similar to those of schizophrenia. This raises the question of whether or not schizophrenia is a specific disease that should be distinguished from other organic psychoses exhibiting similar symptoms, and has led some clinicians to question the logic of excluding organic psychosis before making a diagnosis of schizophrenia.

While there is little doubt that schizophrenia is an organic psychosis, the observation that, despite the variability in time course, many cases of schizophrenia follow the characteristic pattern of a series of acute episodes beginning in early adult life, superimposed upon a degree of sustained impairment, is consistent with the proposal that schizophrenia is distinct from other organic psychoses. However, until the pathophysiology of the condition is delineated, the principal basis for this distinction will remain the exclusion of those organic conditions whose aetiology or pathophysiology is known. From a practical point of view, in the clinical assessment of a patient presenting the symptomatic picture of schizophrenia, it is necessary to carry out investigations to identify any other organic psychosis that might have a specific treatment. These investigations should include screening tests for the known infectious, metabolic, endocrine and neoplastic diseases that can affect the central nervous system.

What is the essence of schizophrenia?

As details of the neural basis of schizophrenia have begun to emerge, it is pertinent to seek to define the essence of schizophrenia. Which of the various clinical features that we have considered is likely to be most relevant to the identification of the essence of the condition? The overlap between the symptoms of schizophrenia and those of affective psychosis and other organic psychoses indicates that the cross-sectional clinical picture alone is not adequate to define a discrete disease. In general, symptoms reflect the neural systems involved rather than the specific disease process. Course of illness appears more specific, but which features of the course are most relevant? A degree of persistence is probably an essential feature of the condition, although the long-term follow-up studies have provided very little evidence of a tendency to lifelong deterioration in mental function implied by the word 'dementia' in Kraepelin's term dementia praecox. In contrast, the tendency for the disease to become manifest early in adult life, indicated by the word 'praecox', has been repeatedly confirmed.

The characteristic form of the distribution of age of onset in males, with its peak in early adult life, is one of the strongest reasons for proposing that schizophrenia in males is a single disease (or group of closely related diseases). In females, the somewhat broader distribution of age of onset indicates either that female gender can exert a moderating influence on onset, or that schizophrenia in females embraces several different diseases, including the early-onset condition seen in males, but also other conditions with later onset.

Overall, the data on age of onset supports the proposal that the majority of cases currently diagnosed as schizophrenia (including virtually all male cases and a substantial proportion of female cases) represent a single type of disease with a characteristic tendency to have onset in early adult life. This proposal is in accord with recent neurobiological evidence (reviewed by Liddle, 2001) that the essential feature of schizophrenia is disordered connections between association cortical areas and related subcortical nuclei, arising during intra-uterine development and becoming manifest after the highest functions of association cortex come into action in adolescence. Although this hypothesis requires further confirmation, the fact that nearly 100 years of research has produced an evolving clinical definition which, on the one hand, preserves many of the features described by Kraepelin at the beginning of the 20th century and, on the other, fits in a consistent manner with recent neurobiological evidence, offers reasonable hope that the essence of this enigmatic condition may soon be identified.

References

American Psychiatric Association (1980) *Diagnostic and Statistical Manual of Mental Disorders* (3rd edn) (DSM–III). Washington, DC: APA.

American Psychiatric Association (1987) *Diagnostic and Statistical Manual of Mental Disorders* (3rd edn, revised) (DSM–III–R). Washington, DC: APA.

American Psychiatric Association (1994) *Diagnostic and Statistical Manual of Mental Disorders* (4th edn) (DSM–IV). Washington, DC: APA.

Andreasen, N. C. (1979) Thought, language and communication disorders. I. Clinical assessment, definition of terms, and evaluation of their reliability. *Archives of General Psychiatry*, **36**, 1315–1321.

Andreasen, N. C. (1982) Negative symptoms in schizophrenia: definition and reliability. *Archives of General Psychiatry*, **39**, 784–788.

Andreasen, N. C. (1986) *Comprehensive Assessment of Symptoms and History*. Iowa: University of Iowa.

Arndt, S., Alliger, R. J. & Andreasen, N. C. (1991) The distinction of positive and negative symptoms: the failure of a two-dimensional model. *British Journal of Psychiatry*, **158**, 317–322.

Bleuler, E. (1911) *Dementia Praecox or the Group of Schizophrenias* (trans. J. Zinkin, 1950). New York: International Universities Press.

Bleuler, M. (1974) The long term course of the schizophrenic psychoses. *Psychological Medicine*, **4**, 244–254.

Calev, A., Venables, P. H. & Monk, A. F. (1983) Evidence for distinct verbal memory pathologies in severely and mildly disturbed schizophrenics. *Schizophrenia Bulletin*, **9**, 247–263.

Ciompi, L. & Muller, C. (1976) *Lebensweg und Alter der Schizophrenen: Eine karamnertische Langzeitstudie bis ins Senium*. Berlin: Springer-Verlag.

Cooper, J. E., Kendall, R. E., Gurland, B. J., *et al* (1972) *Psychiatric Diagnosis in London and New York*. London: Oxford University Press.

Crow, T. J. (1980) The molecular pathology of schizophrenia. *BMJ*, **280**, 1–9.

Donlon, P. T., Rada, R. T. & Arora, K. K. (1976) Depression and the reintegration phase of acute schizophrenia. *American Journal of Psychiatry*, **133**, 1265–1268.

Frith, C. D. (1992) *The Cognitive Neuropsychology of Schizophrenia*. Hove: Lawrence Erlbaum.

Goldberg, T. E., Torrey, E. F., Gold, J. M., *et al* (1993) Learning and memory in monozygotic twins discordant for schizophrenia. *Psychological Medicine*, **23**, 71–85.

Green, M. F. (1998) *Schizophrenia from a Neurocognitve Perspective*. Boston: Allyn and Bacon.

Griesinger, W. (1867) *Mental Pathology and Therapeutics* (trans. from the German 2nd edn by C. Lockhart Robertson & J. Rutherford). London: Sydenham Society.

Harding, C. M,, Brooks, G. W., Ashikaga, T., *et al* (1987) The Vermont longitudinal study of persons with severe mental illness. *American Journal of Psychiatry*, **144**, 727–734.

Haslam, J. (1809) *Observations on Madness and Melancholy* (2nd edn). London: Hayden.

Hecker, E. (1871) Die hebephrenie. *Virchows Archiv für Pathologische Anatomie und Physiologie und klinische Medizin*, **52**, 394–429.

Hemsley, D. R. (1992) Cognitive abnormalities and schizophrenic symptoms. *Psychological Medicine*, **22**, 839–842.

Holzman, P. S., Shenton, M. E. & Solloway, M. R. (1986) Quality of thought disorder in differential diagnosis. *Schizophrenia Bulletin*, **12**, 360–371.

Holzman, P. S., Kringlen, E. & Matthysse, S. (1988) A single dominant gene can account for eye tracking dysfunctions and schizophrenia in offspring of discordant twins. *Archives of General Psychiatry*, **45**, 641–647.

Huber, G., Gross, G. & Schuttler, R. (1975) A long term follow-up study of schizophrenia: psychiatric course of illness and prognosis. *Acta Psychiatrica Scandinavica*, **52**, 49–57.

Jones, P. B., Rodgers, M., Murray, R. M., *et al* (1994) Child developmental risk factors for adult schizophrenia in the British 1946 birth cohort. *Lancet*, **344**, 1398–1402.

Kahlbaum, K. L. (1874) *Die Katatonie oder das Spannungsirrescien*. Berlin: Hirschwald.

Kay, S. R.(1991) *Positive and Negative Syndromes in Schizophrenia*. New York: Brunner/Mazel.

Knights, A. & Hirsch, S. R. (1981) Revealed depression and drug treatment for schizophrenia. *Archives of General Psychiatry*, **38**, 806–811.

Kraepelin, E. (1896) Dementia praecox. In *The Clinical Roots of the Schizophrenia Concept* (eds J. Cutting & M. Shepherd), pp. 15–24. Cambridge: Cambridge University Press. Trans. from *Lehrbuch der Psychiatrie* (5th edn), pp. 426–441. Leipzig: Barth.

Kraepelin, E. (1919) *Dementia Praecox and Paraphrenia* (trans. R. M. Barclay, ed. G. M. Robertson). Edinburgh: Livingstone.

Kraepelin, E. (1920) *Die Erscheinungsformen des Irresciens*. Trans. H. Marshall, 1974, as Patterns of mental disorder. In *Themes and Variations in European Psychiatry* (eds S. R. Hirsch & M. Shepherd). Bristol: Wright.

Levin, S. (1980) Frontal lobe dysfunction in schizophrenia – 1. Eye movement impairments. *Journal of Psychiatric Research*, **18**, 27–55.

Lewis, S. W. (1990) Computerised tomography in schizophrenia 15 years on. *British Journal of Psychiatry*, **157**, suppl. 9, 16–24.

Liddle, P. F. (1987) The symptoms of chronic schizophrenia: a re-examination of the positive–negative dichotomy. *British Journal of Psychiatry*, **151**, 145–151.

Liddle, P. F. (2001) *Disordered Mind and Brain: The Neural Basis of Mental Symptoms*. London: Gaskell.

Liddle, P. F., Friston, K. J., Frith, C. D., *et al* (1992) Patterns of cerebral blood flow in schizophrenia. *British Journal of Psychiatry*, **160**, 179–186.

Liddle, P. F., Barnes, T. R. E., Speller, J., *et al* (1993*a*) Negative symptoms as a risk factor for tardive dyskinesia in schizophrenia. *British Journal of Psychiatry*, **163**, 776–780.

Liddle, P. F., Haque, S., Morris, D. L., *et al* (1993*b*) Dyspraxia and agnosia in schizophrenia. *Behavioural Neurology*, **6**, 49–54.

Liddle, P. F., Ngan, E. T. N., Duffield, G., *et al* (2002) The Signs and Symptoms of Psychotic Illness: a rating scale. *British Journal of Psychiatry*, **180**, 45–50.

Mellor, C. S. (1970) First rank symptoms of schizophrenia. *British Journal of Psychiatry*, **117**, 15–23.

O'Grady, J. C. (1990) The prevalence and diagnostic significance of Schneiderian first rank symptoms in a random sample of acute psychiatric patients. *British Journal of Psychiatry*, **156**, 496–500.

Overall, J. E. & Goreham, D. R. (1962) The Brief Psychiatric Rating Scale. *Psychological Reports*, **10**, 799–812.

Peralta, V., deLeon, J. & Cuesta, M. J. (1992) Are there more than two syndromes in schizophrenia? A critique of the positive–negative dichotomy. *British Journal of Psychiatry*, **161**, 335–343.

Rifkin, A., Quitkin, K. & Klein, D. F. (1975) Akinesia: a poorly recognised drug-induced extrapyramidal behavioral disorder. *Archives of General Psychiatry*, **32**, 672–674.

Robinson, D. G., Woerner, M. G., Alvir, J. M., *et al* (1999*a*) Predictors of treatment response from a first episode of schizophrenia or schizoaffective disorder. *American Journal of Psychiatry*, **156**, 544–549.

Robinson, D., Woerner, M. G., Alvir, J. M., *et al* (1999*b*) Predictors of relapse following response from a first episode of schizophrenia or schizoaffective disorder. *Archives of General Psychiatry*, **56**, 241–247.

Schneider, K. (1959) *Clinical Psychopathology*. Trans. M. W. Hamilton. New York: Grune Stratton.

Taylor, M. A. & Fink, G. (2003) Catatonia in psychiatric classification: a home of its own. *American Journal of Psychiatry*, **160**, 1233–1241.

Watt, D. C., Katz, K. & Shepherd, M. (1983) The natural history of schizophrenia: a 5-year prospective follow-up of a representative sample of schizophrenics by means of a standardized clinical and social assessment. *Psychological Medicine*, **13**, 663–670.

World Health Organization (1973) *The International Pilot Study of Schizophrenia*. Geneva: WHO.

World Health Organization (1978) *The Ninth Revision of the International Classification of Diseases* (ICD–9). Geneva: WHO.

World Health Organization (1992) *The Tenth Revision of the International Classification of Diseases and Related Health Problems* (ICD–10). Geneva: WHO.

World Health Organization (1994) *Schedules for Clinical Assessment in Psychiatry (SCAN 2.0)*. Geneva: WHO.

CHAPTER 9

Schizoaffective, paranoid and other psychoses

Clive Mellor

This chapter describes a miscellaneous group of non-organic psychoses. The factor common to these conditions is that they do not seem to belong to either of the two major Kraepelinian groups of non-organic psychoses: the schizophrenias and the affective psychoses.

Kraepelin's division of the non-organic psychoses into two major groups attracted criticism at the time. His critics observed that often cases occurred that were not typical of schizophrenia or affective psychosis. These cases of 'atypical' psychosis have continued to pose nosological difficulties that have not been helped by inconsistencies in their nomenclature. At times, dissimilar disorders have been given the same name and almost identical conditions have received different names.

The 'atypical' psychoses fall into two main groups: the schizoaffective and the paranoid (delusional) disorders. In schizoaffective disorder, symptoms of the two major psychoses occur during the same illness. Paranoid disorders are characterised by delusions without other evidence of schizophrenia, or affective psychosis. The 'atypical psychoses' are listed in Table 9.1, together with the authorities principally responsible for defining them. Dissimilar conditions with the same name have more than one entry.

History of the atypical psychoses

The student of psychiatry viewing Table 9.1 might sympathise with the psychiatrist Hoche, who, more than a century ago, was frustrated by his contemporaries' efforts at classification. According to Lewis (1934), he likened them to 'a great number of diligent workmen, most energetically engaged in clarifying a turbid fluid by pouring it busily from one vessel into another'. Present-day attempts to resolve the problem of the atypical psychoses can best be understood from a historical perspective, which in large part is that of the distinctions made between the affective psychoses and schizophrenia.

Kraepelin

The atypical psychoses have a pre-Kraepelinian history that is of academic interest but of little relevance to current thinking. Contemporary classification began with Kraepelin's division of the non-organic psychoses into dementia praecox (schizophrenia) and manic–depressive disorders (affective psychoses). By definition, the atypical psychoses lie outside the diagnostic boundaries he set for these conditions.

Kraepelin (1919), in discussing the diagnostic differentiation of dementia praecox from manic–depressive insanity, stressed the total clinical picture. The diagnosis cannot be based upon a single symptom, or rest solely on a cyclical course. Outcome is the diagnostic arbiter. Complete recovery with good insight after the acute phase of the illness is diagnostic of manic–depressive insanity. Patients with dementia praecox did not recover; he estimated that only 13% were eventually able to lead an independent existence and most of these had residual symptoms and personality changes.

Table 9.1 Non-organic psychoses not typical of schizophrenia or of affective psychosis

Name	Authorities responsible for definitions
Schizoaffective group	
Schizoaffective disorder	Kasanin
Schizoaffective disorder	ICD-10
Schizoaffective disorder	DSM–IV
Schizophreniform disorder	Langfeldt
Schizophreniform disorder	DSM–IV
Psychogenic psychoses	Faegerman
Brief psychotic disorder	DSM–IV
Cycloid psychoses	Kleist, Leonhard
Atypical psychoses	Mitsuda
Periodical psychoses	Hatotani
Bouffée délirante	Mangan
Acute polymorphic psychotic disorder	ICD-10
Non-systematic schizophrenias	Kleist, Leonhard
Paranoid (delusional) disorders	
Paranoia	Kahlbaum, Kraepelin
Acute delusional psychotic discorder	ICD-10
Persistent delusional disorder	ICD-10
Delusional disorder	DSM–IV
erotomania	
grandiose	
jealous	
persecutory	
somatic	
delusional dysmorphophobia	
monosymptomatic hypochondriacal psychosis	
induced delusional disorder (folie à deux)	

Kraepelin believed that most cases could be diagnostically accommodated within these two classifications. The history of the paranoid psychoses, discussed in more detail below, diverges from that of the other atypical psychoses.

Post-Kraepelinian approaches

Four post-Kraepelinian approaches to the atypical psychoses are considered here:

1 the concepts of Jaspers and Schneider, which reinforced Kraepelin's dichotomy

2 the description of schizoaffective disorder by Kasanin and the subsequent development of this concept in the USA

3 the German school, which originated with Meynert and Wernicke, and whose successors, Kleist and Leonhard, identified a number of different non-organic psychoses

4 the Scandinavian concept of psychogenic (or reactive) psychoses, which are produced by psychic stress and have a benign course.

Jaspers and Schneider

Jaspers' (1963) hierarchical classification of psychiatric disorders and Schneider's (1959) identification of first-rank symptoms of schizophrenia reinforced the division of the non-organic psychoses into two groups. Jaspers based his hierarchical classification on the premise that one diagnosis, rather than several, is to be preferred, if all the patient's symptoms can be accounted for by one illness. Although some of a patient's symptoms may occur in other conditions, a second diagnosis should not be made unless the evidence for it is overwhelming. (This is a medical application of Occam's razor – preference should be given to the most economical explanation.)

Jaspers ranked conditions according to the diagnostic specificity of their typical symptoms. Organic mental disorders head this hierarchy, because their typical symptoms are highly specific and do not occur in other disorders. Symptoms typical of other conditions may also occur in the organic disorders, but do not change the diagnosis. Therefore, an organic illness has to be excluded before schizophrenia, affective psychosis and neurosis become diagnostic possibilities. The neuroses lie at the lowest level of this hierarchy because their typical symptoms are also found in affective psychoses, schizophrenia and organic mental disorders. Jaspers, like most of his contemporaries, gave symptoms typical of schizophrenia precedence over those of the affective psychoses. Therefore, when there are typical symptoms of schizophrenia accompanied by typical affective symptoms, the diagnosis, according to Jaspers, is schizophrenia. In summary, his hierarchy of symptom specificity has the following rank order – organic psychoses, schizophrenia, affective psychoses and neuroses.

Schneider, unlike Kraepelin, believed the patient's current mental state, rather than the course of the disorder, should have diagnostic priority. Possibly this was because Schneider used Jaspers' phenomenological method, which had refined the mental examination. Schneider's (1959) promotion of first-rank symptoms of schizophrenia over the symptoms of manic–depressive disorder reflects the Jasperian hierarchy of symptom specificity. Schneider believed that it was usually possible to diagnose schizophrenia or affective psychosis in patients with 'atypical psychoses'. When this was not possible, he used the term '*Zwischen-fallen*' (cases in between) to describe such patients. In spite of criticism, Jaspers' diagnostic hierarchy continued to influence European thinking on psychiatric nosology. However, DSM–III (American Psychiatric Association, 1980) changed Jaspers' rankings by promoting affective disorders over schizophrenia.

Kasanin and subsequent developments in the USA

The revolution against the European hierarchical view of nosology came from the USA. Kasanin (1933) used the term 'schizoaffective psychosis' in a paper that described nine patients who exhibited a mixture of schizophrenic and affective symptoms. Although the patients were diagnosed as having dementia praecox, the outcome was better than expected. They were young, had good premorbid personalities, and had been severely stressed before becoming ill. Unfortunately, it is difficult to determine from Kasanin's descriptions exactly what mental symptoms were present. Kasanin and his contemporaries considered schizoaffective disorder to be a variant of schizophrenia. The American Psychiatric Association (in DSM–II, 1968) continued to define schizoaffective disorder as a subtype of schizophrenia in which elation or depression is prominent.

American thinking about schizoaffective disorder changed in the 1970s. This followed a series of investigations, comprising follow-up and family studies, which concluded that schizoaffective disorder should be included with the affective disorders (see review by Clayton, 1982). The identification of manic and depressive subtypes strengthened this notion. At the same time, the concept of schizophrenia, which had been largely Bleulerian, was narrowed and that of affective disorder widened (see also: Chapter 2, page 24; Chapter 8, page 184). These changes were reflected in DSM–III, in which schizophrenia became an illness of at least six months' duration. Psychoses that were not organic or affective became 'brief reactive psychoses' if they had lasted for less than a month, and 'schizophreniform psychoses' if they had endured for 1–6 months. Before DSM–III, the symptoms associated with these conditions would have justified a diagnosis of schizophrenia. A diagnosis of affective disorder, particularly mania, was not excluded by typical symptoms of schizophrenia, such as Schneider's first-rank symptoms. This made the distinction between affective and schizoaffective disorder more difficult, a topic that is discussed below. DSM–IV (American Psychiatric Association, 1994), in this respect, did not change from DSM–III.

Cerebral localisers: Meynert, Wernicke, Kleist and Leonhard

The great neuropathologist psychiatrists Meynert and Wernicke approached psychiatric disorders from the position that mental illnesses are brain diseases. Their models were hereditary degenerative conditions, such

Table 9.2 Diagnostic criteria for schizoaffective disorder: DSM–IV and ICD–10

	ICD–10	DSM–IV
Symptoms	Schizophrenic and affective, simultaneously present and both prominent	Major depressive, or manic concurrent with 'criteria A' schizophrenic symptoms.[a] At least 2 weeks of delusions and hallucinations *without* prominent mood disorder
Types	Manic,[b] mixed,[b] depressive[b] and also affective type of schizophreniform psychosis	Bipolar and depressive
Course	Recurrent Manic-type episode – residual defect state unusual Depressive-type episode – residual defect state sometimes	Not in the criteria, but mentioned in the preamble Outcome better than in schizophrenia, but worse than in mood disorders. Tends to become chronic
Excluded	Patients with separate episodes of schizophrenia and affective disorder	Patients with schizophrenia, psychotic mood disorders and organic disorders

[a] See Chapter 8 on schizophrenia.
[b] At least one, preferably tow, typical symptoms of schizophrenia.

as Friedreich's ataxia. They believed that if they could precisely define the syndromes of mental illness, this would improve the chances of finding the responsible pathology.

Kraepelin's division of the non-organic psychoses into two groups was too limited for this approach. Kleist, Wernicke's pupil, studied the effects of head wounds in soldiers wounded in the First World War, and drew comparisons between symptoms of schizophrenia and those attributable to specific brain lesions. This work led to Leonhard (1979) developing a detailed classification of the 'endogenous psychoses'. He proposed four major groups, each having several subgroups. The major groups were: systematic schizophrenias; phasic psychoses, which included manic–depressive psychosis; cycloid psychoses; and non-systematic schizophrenias. The last two groups identify specific syndromes that in other diagnostic schema would be atypical psychoses. Beckman *et al* (2000) have reviewed the potential value of pursuing investigations using this approach.

Scandinavian concepts of schizophreniform and reactive psychoses

Scandinavian psychiatry differed from most other psychiatry in its acceptance of two diagnostic concepts – the reactive psychoses and the schizophreniform psychoses. This tradition started with Wimmer, Professor of Psychiatry in Copenhagen, whose work was unknown outside Scandinavia. He described a group of psychoses that he believed were reactions to an 'affective shock'. Subsequent developments of this concept are associated with Faegerman, Stromgren and Retterstol (for a review, see Rettersol, 1978). Langfeldt (1982) used the term 'schizophreniform psychosis' in a series of monographs on the prognosis of schizophrenia. DSM–III introduced 'reactive psychosis' and 'schizophreniform disorder' as diagnostic categories, but these terms identify conditions that differ from their original descriptions. DSM–IV has continued this DSM–III practice.

Summary

The history of the atypical psychoses reflects a variety of nosological approaches. Schneider denied that the proportion of such cases was significant. Leonhard did not believe that schizophrenia and affective psychosis were the only diagnostic entities and provided an elaborate nosological schema that encompassed most forms of atypical psychosis. The Scandinavians focused upon the role of stress in these conditions. DSM–IV, with its Kraepelinian emphasis on outcome, puts most atypical psychoses into the affective disorders group.

Schizoaffective disorder

Definition

Schizoaffective disorder is characterised by symptoms of schizophrenia and affective disorder occurring in the same episode of a patient's illness. Its recognition, therefore, is contingent upon prior definitions of schizophrenia and affective disorder. Not surprisingly, Brockington & Leff (1979) identified 23 different definitions of schizoaffective disorder. When they used eight of these definitions to classify a group of patients with a psychosis, they found a low level of agreement (kappa = 0.19) for this diagnosis, suggesting that these definitions had failed to identify a clinically homogeneous group of disorders.

Both ICD–10 (World Health Organization, 1992) and DSM–IV provide the definitions most commonly used in clinical practice, but there are differences between these two sets of clinical criteria. They are compared in Table 9.2. In research, other definitions are often used, notably those of the Research Diagnostic Criteria (RDC) of Spitzer *et al* (1978) and the St Louis Criteria (Feighner *et al*, 1972). A more recent research strategy uses and compares findings from several sets of diagnostic criteria. This is the OPCRIT approach, 'the polydiagnostic application of operational criteria' (McGuffin *et al*, 1991).

Case example

SB, a married 38-year-old woman, was admitted to psychiatric care after a taking a drug overdose. Two months before admission she had become depressed, with diurnal variation of mood. She had loss of libido and appetite, and had lost 3 kg. She had been in hospital three times during the previous 2 years, with a diagnosis of major depression, and had improved with antidepressants and neuroleptics. However, her husband stated that after the first episode she had never fully regained the interests that she had once enjoyed. Her

> symptoms of depression, including suicidal ideation, were confirmed in hospital and antidepressants were restarted. Five days after admission she became withdrawn and suspicious, and repeatedly looked at herself in the mirror. On mental examination, she had first-rank symptoms of schizophrenia, which included 'made' bodily experiences and auditory hallucinations of voices discussing her and commentating on her activities. The bodily experiences consisted of strange, unpleasant pulling and prickling sensations in the area of the lower jaw, chest and perineum. She believed that her face was changing into that of a dog and her body into that of a man. She could see early signs of these changes in the mirror but could not describe them. These experiences, she believed, were imposed from the outside by the devil and his helpers, who were changing her into a dog-headed man. She failed to improve with antidepressants or with a neuroleptic and the later addition of lithium. But she recovered completely following treatment with electroconvulsive therapy (ECT) combined with a neuroleptic. Her husband confirmed that after discharge she was 'the best she had been for years'.

This case illustrates some of the difficulties in making a diagnosis of schizoaffective disorder. The patient met the inclusion criteria for an ICD–10 diagnosis of a severe depressive episode and the DSM–IV criteria for a major depression. She also had persistent psychotic symptoms typical of schizophrenia. The diagnosis rests upon the answer to the question: 'Did the schizophrenic and depressive symptoms always occur together?' If they did, then the ICD–10 diagnosis is schizoaffective disorder and the DSM–IV diagnosis is major depression with mood-incongruent psychotic features. If she had experienced the schizophrenic symptoms for at least 2 weeks without depressive symptoms, then the DSM–IV diagnosis is schizoaffective disorder and the ICD–10 diagnosis is schizophrenia! In practice, this question was difficult to answer. The patient was depressed when she had the schizophrenic symptoms, but this appeared to be congruent with her experience of being changed by the devil into a dog-headed man. The treatment to which she responded was non-specific and not diagnostically helpful.

Epidemiology

The definitions of schizoaffective disorder have varied so much that data derived from older studies are of limited value. The best estimates point to an annual incidence of 2 per 100 000 (Brockington & Meltzer, 1983), similar to that of mania and a quarter that of schizophrenia. The frequency of the diagnosis of schizoaffective disorder in psychiatric admissions has been variously estimated to be in the range of 2–11% (Levinson & Levitt, 1987). Demographic variables in patients with schizoaffective disorder have values between those for schizophrenia and affective psychosis (Benabarre *et al*, 2001).

Validation of the concept of schizoaffective disorder

Conceptual hypotheses

Various hypotheses have been put forward about the nature of schizoaffective disorder. These include:

1 It is a diagnostic 'waste basket' for patients, with symptom clusters that defy conventional categorisation.

2 It is a subtype of schizophrenia.

3 It is a variant of manic–depressive disorder.

4 It is the third psychosis – a disease entity independent from schizophrenia and affective psychosis.

5 There is only one psychosis, the 'unitary psychosis'. Schizophrenia and manic–depressive psychosis are constructs that lie at opposite ends of the psychosis continuum, with schizoaffective disorder occupying an intermediate position. (For a conceptual history of the unitary psychosis, see Berrios & Beer, 1994.)

6 Schizoaffective disorder is a combination of two inherited diseases, schizophrenia and manic–depressive psychosis.

Methodology

Validating the concept of schizoaffective disorder first requires the condition to be defined according to one, or more, sets of clinical criteria. These are then related to external criteria, such as the course of the illness, response to specific treatments, family studies and biological investigations. If the findings resemble those for another diagnostic group, then they indicate that schizoaffective disorder, as defined, belongs to that group. If there are findings exclusive to the condition, then this suggests that the criteria chosen to diagnose schizoaffective disorder have identified a distinct disorder.

Outcome

Harrow & Grossman (1984) reviewed outcome studies in schizoaffective disorder. In earlier investigations, schizoaffective disorder appeared to be a variant of schizophrenia, but later studies suggested that it was a variant of affective disorder. They concluded that in good prospective studies, schizoaffective disorder occupied a position between the poorer outcome of schizophrenia and the better outcome of affective psychosis. Harrow & Grossman (2000), in a 10-year prospective study using RDC, confirmed their earlier conclusions. The outcome in schizoaffective disorder also varies with the course of the illness, the bipolar type having a good outcome and the depressive type a relatively poor one (Maj & Perris, 1990).

Diagnostic stability

If schizoaffective disorder were a diagnostic entity, then most patients who have been hospitalised with the condition should retain this diagnosis when readmitted. Forrester *et al* (2001) studied diagnostic stability in 204 subjects with multiple admissions for non-organic psychotic illnesses. They used an OPCRIT approach (see above) with six different diagnostic criteria. The diagnostic stability of the schizoaffective group was low for all sets of criteria (5–39%), while that for schizophrenia (58–98%) was high and that for affective disorder was moderate (24–83%). This diagnostic instability does not support the concept that schizoaffective disorder is a distinct and separate category of mental illness.

Family studies

The possibility that schizoaffective disorder results from the combined inheritance of schizophrenia and affective psychosis is small. If these two disorders are genetically independent, then the likelihood of inheriting both sets of genes is about 1 in 10000. Abrams (1984) reviewed early US studies and found no evidence that schizoaffective disorder 'bred true'. However, family studies have shown consistently that the mentally ill first-degree relatives of schizoaffective probands have greater than expected rates of both schizophrenia and affective disorder.

In one of the larger studies, Gershon *et al* (1988) compared the psychiatric diagnoses of the relatives of patients with chronic schizophrenia and chronic schizoaffective disorder. There were few differences; thus, schizophrenia was found among the relatives of patients with schizophrenia and schizoaffective disorder at roughly the same rate, but bipolar I disorder tended to aggregate more among the relatives of schizoaffective probands. An interesting finding of this study was the effect of comorbid drug misuse: the rate of any psychiatric disorder among the relatives of probands with schizophrenia or schizoaffective disorder who were also comorbid for substance misuse was 75%, compared with a rate of 55% when there was no comorbid drug misuse. Much of this difference was accounted for by raised rates of unipolar depression among the relatives of drug-misusing probands with chronic schizophrenia or schizoaffective disorder. Comorbid drug misuse is a serious complicating factor in the treatment of any psychosis and these observations suggest that patients with comorbid substance misuse may have more psychiatrically ill relatives and so may have a higher degree of genetic loading and possibly therefore more severe illnesses (Gershon *et al*, 1988).

It also appears that the first-degree relatives of schizoaffective probands have higher rates of schizophrenia than the families of probands with an affective disorder, and higher rates of affective disorder than the families of schizophrenic probands (see Maj *et al*, 1991; Tsuang 1991). Kendler *et al* (1995) confirmed these findings as part of the Roscommon family study. In addition, this family study found no evidence to support the distinction between bipolar and unipolar schizoaffective disorder.

In one of the few twin studies, Franzek & Beckmann (1998) found that monozygotic and dizygotic twins did not differ significantly in concordance for the atypical psychoses. In discordant pairs the affected twins had suffered significantly more severe birth complications than had the healthy co-twins, which suggests that brain injury played a role in the aetiology.

Biological investigations

Various biological measures have been studied in the hope that they would yield a specific test for schizophrenia or affective disorder. This goal has not so far been realised, although some tests with a modest degree of specificity have been found. These include hormonal, biochemical and neurophysiological investigations. Meltzer *et al* (1984) reviewed the findings from such tests in schizoaffective disorder. Similarities were found between schizoaffective disorder and affective disorder with regard to decreased platelet 5-hydroxytryptamine (5-HT) uptake, shortened rapid eye movement (REM) latency and a blunted growth hormone response to clonidine. However, patients with a schizoaffective disorder were more like the schizophrenic group in that they had increased cerebrospinal fluid levels of noradrenaline and increased platelet 5-HT. Krishnan *et al* (1990) have reviewed the results of the dexamethasone suppression test (DST) and the overall finding was that the proportion of non-suppressors in the schizoaffective group was midway between that for affective disorder and schizophrenia. Wahby *et al* (1990, 1990–91) used two state markers for depression, the DST and the suppression of prolactin by thyrotrophin-releasing hormone (TRH). They concluded that schizoaffective disorder was more like schizophrenia than affective disorder. Sharma *et al* (2001) compared cerebrospinal fluid levels of TRH in patients with schizophrenia, affective disorder and schizoaffective disorder and found the schizoaffective group had significantly higher levels than the other two groups.

Neuropsychological tests

Tests of neuropsychological functions have demonstrated a close resemblance between schizoaffective disorder and schizophrenia. Evans *et al* (1999) used a battery of tests to compare subjects with schizoaffective, schizophrenic and non-psychotic mood disorders, and Gooding & Tallent (2002) compared groups of patients with schizophrenia or schizoaffective disorder and normal subjects on measures of executive functioning.

Specific treatment effects

The use of treatment response as an external validating criterion for a diagnosis requires that the treatment effect is specific. Unfortunately, psychiatric treatments lack such specificity. Claims that lithium prophylaxis in bipolar or manic schizoaffective disorder is similar to that in bipolar disorder now appear doubtful (Levinson *et al*, 1999).

Conclusion

On the present evidence, schizoaffective disorder does not appear to be a distinct disease entity, but rather a heterogeneous group of conditions. It is now thought that there may be more than 50 genes responsible for schizophrenia and a similar number for bipolar disorder. It is possible therefore that schizoaffective disorder and the other atypical psychoses are associated with complex combinations of the genes responsible for both major disorders, and this may explain the mixed clinical picture as well as the wide range of psychiatric disorders found among the first-degree relatives of schizoaffective probands. The diagnostic instability of schizoaffective disorder supports the view that it is a collection of different conditions, in which schizophrenia and manic–depressive disorder play the largest parts. Presumably, patients with these two major conditions are given this diagnosis when their clinical presentation is unusual. If patients with schizophrenia and bipolar disorder could be identified and excluded from the schizoaffective group, then a homogeneous group of cases with true schizoaffective disorder, or the 'third psychosis', might remain. The hypothesis that schizoaffective disorder occupies an intermediate position on a unitary psychosis continuum remains in the psychiatric literature with little available evidence either to prove or to disprove it.

Diagnosis and differential diagnosis

The diagnosis of schizoaffective disorder is made after first excluding an organic mental disorder, schizophrenia and an affective disorder. The presence, at the same time, of equally severe symptoms of both schizophrenia and of a manic, mixed or depressive episode is then sufficient to make the ICD–10 diagnosis. The difficulties that attend the DSM–IV diagnosis have already been discussed. Patients with schizoaffective disorder may be assigned to diagnostic subtypes: manic, mixed or depressive in ICD–10 and bipolar or depressive in DSM–IV.

Differential diagnosis

The disorders that have to be distinguished from schizoaffective disorder are schizophrenia with a depressed or elated mood, affective disorder with psychotic symptoms (mania, psychotic depression) and organic mental disorders. An organic psychosyndrome, due to drugs or other physical causes, superimposed upon a typical non-organic psychosis, can produce an atypical clinical picture.

1 *Schizophrenia with depression*. This condition frequently occurs. It is diagnosed by giving weight to clinical features common in schizophrenia but unusual in schizoaffective disorder. These are negative schizophrenic symptoms, lengthy episodes of illness with slow and incomplete recovery, and extended treatment with neuroleptics.

2 *Schizophrenia with elation*. Heightened mood states in schizophrenia differ from those in schizoaffective disorder. They are usually short-lived and often accompanied by evidence of affective disorganisation, such as incongruity of affect. Schizophrenic elation usually evokes feelings of discomfort in the examiner rather than empathic good humour.

3 *Affective disorder with psychotic symptoms*. When delusions are mood congruent, the differentiation of this condition from schizoaffective disorder is not difficult. Delusions in depressed patients have themes such as guilt, poverty, disease and nihilism. However, affective disorders with mood-incongruent psychotic symptoms have attracted the interest of American psychiatrists and have been given official recognition. DSM–IV notes that these symptoms include 'persecutory delusions (not directly related to depressive themes), thought insertion, thought broadcasting and delusions of control'. These, the text suggests, are associated with a poorer prognosis. Kendler (1991) has provided an extensive review of this concept. Distinguishing between affective disorder with mood-incongruent psychotic symptoms and schizoaffective disorder depends upon the choice of diagnostic criteria, ICD–10 or DSM–IV, not on any symptomatic differences (see the case of SB above).

4 *Organic mental disorders*. These may resemble schizoaffective disorder but should present little diagnostic difficulty, as specific organic symptoms will be evident. However, the misuse of stimulant drugs such as cocaine, amphetamines and methylphenidate may produce paranoid symptoms and elation when the patient is 'high', and depression after drug withdrawal. No evident clouding of consciousness strengthens the resemblance between these states and schizoaffective disorder. Other drugs that can produce schizoaffective-like mental states are phencyclidine, L-dopa and corticosteroids. Therefore, in cases of atypical psychosis, particularly those with an acute onset, suspect drug intoxication. Substance misuse superimposed upon a pre-existing chronic psychosis can pose a particularly difficult diagnostic problem. In such cases, drug screening and a collateral history are needed.

Treatment

Logically, the treatments used in schizoaffective disorder should be a combination of those employed in schizophrenia and affective disorder. The division of schizoaffective disorder into bipolar or depressive subtypes invites the appropriate treatment for that kind of affective disorder. Indeed, the practice of adding lithium to antipsychotic medication in bipolar schizoaffective disorder, and antidepressants to the depressive form of this disorder, is prescribed in the 'Practice guidelines for the treatment of patients with schizophrenia' (American Psychiatric Association, 1997). The use of lithium in this condition has declined, however, and it has been largely replaced by the newer mood stabilisers (Grieger *et al*, 2001).

The therapeutic value of antipsychotic medication for the treatment of schizoaffective disorder is established, but the benefits of mood stabilisers and antidepressants are less certain. Levinson *et al* (1999) reviewed the literature from 1976 onwards but found only 18 acceptable studies. These provided no evidence to support the use of lithium in the acute or long-term management of schizoaffective disorder. Similarly, they found no justification for using antidepressants in the depressed subtype of the disorder, except in post-psychotic depression. The newer mood stabilisers and antidepressants, anecdotally reported to be effective, have not yet been the subject of stringent clinical trials.

Our present knowledge suggests that the best course is optimal antipsychotic treatment without mood stabilisers and to reserve antidepressants for post-psychotic depression. Several controlled trials have found that the newer, atypical antipsychotics are superior to older ones in acute schizoaffective disorder, and clozapine is their superior in maintenance treatment (Hummel *et al*, 2002).

There is good evidence that schizoaffective disorder responds well to ECT, which should therefore be considered when the patient has not responded to medication. The risk of suicide, which is the same as that for affective psychoses, should always be a consideration.

The psychosocial management of schizoaffective disorder uses strategies employed in both major psychoses, with the selection of those that are appropriate for a particular case.

Cycloid psychoses

This group of psychoses, perhaps more than any other, may qualify as the 'third psychosis'. Perris (1988) has made the case for the cycloid psychoses being nosologically distinct from schizophrenia and the affective disorders. This case rests upon their distinctive symptoms, a bipolar form, a recurrent course with complete remissions, and a strong familial tendency. In a Swedish study, cycloid psychoses constituted about 10% of all admissions and 25% of first admissions for functional psychoses (Lindvall *et al*, 1990).

Leonhard (1979) described three types of cycloid psychosis. All have a bipolar form, a cyclical course and a good prognosis. The names identify their predominant symptoms, but any symptom of an affective disorder or schizophrenia may appear during the course of a cycloid psychosis. Leonhard's types of cycloid psychosis are:

1 anxiety–elation psychosis, in which affective symptoms predominate

2 excited–inhibited confusion psychosis, in which thought disorder is dominant

3 hyperkinetic–akinetic psychosis, in which motor disorders are the most conspicuous symptoms.

It is often difficult to assign cases to these subcategories because the patient's symptoms can change so quickly and so frequently. Leonhard later came to acknowledge this difficulty.

Recent neurophysiological studies have supported the view that the cycloid psychoses are a distinct group of disorders. Strik *et al* (1998) have demonstrated that P300 evoked responses on electroencephalography (EEG) are of higher amplitude and more symmetrical than those found in schizophrenia and mania. Subjects with cycloid psychoses, unlike those with schizophrenia, had a generalised increase in hemispheric blood flow, which was also related to symptom intensity (Warkentin *et al*, 1992). A state of generalised cerebral hyperarousal has been proposed to explain these findings.

Diagnosis

Diagnostic guidelines for the cycloid psychoses, published by Perris & Brockington (1981), have found general acceptance and are given below:

1 The condition is an acute psychosis not related to the administration or misuse of any drug, or to brain injury, occurring for the first time in subjects aged 15–50 years.

2 The condition has a sudden onset, with a rapid change from a state of health to a full-blown psychotic condition within a few hours, or at the most a few days.

3 At least four of the following must be present:
   - confusion of some degree, mostly expressed as perplexity or puzzlement
   - mood-incongruent delusions of any kind, mostly with a persecutory content
   - hallucinatory experiences of any kind, often related to themes of death
   - an overwhelming, frightening experience of anxiety, not bound to particular situations or circumstances ('pan anxiety')
   - deep feelings of happiness or ecstasy, most often with a religious colouring
   - motility disturbances of an akinetic or hyperkinetic type, which are mostly expressional
   - a particular concern with death
   - mood swings in the background, and not so pronounced as to justify a diagnosis of affective disorder.

4 There is no fixed combination of symptoms; on the contrary, the symptoms may change frequently during the episode and show bipolar characteristics.

These criteria are similar to those used in ICD–10, but the term 'cycloid psychosis' was replaced with 'acute polymorphic psychotic disorder'. This diagnosis can be further qualified by 'with or without symptoms of schizophrenia'. There is no equivalent DSM–IV category. In making the diagnosis, the polymorphous nature of the symptoms is of greatest value. Schizophrenic and manic–depressive symptoms occur in unusual combinations and can rapidly change. Even within 1 hour, the clinical picture can change completely.

Severe post-partum psychoses closely resemble the acute cycloid psychoses and Pfuhlmann *et al* (1999) have claimed that predominantly these disorders are cycloid psychoses of the motility type. Other conditions that may have a polymorphic unstable clinical picture are rapid-cycling bipolar disorder and cannabis intoxication. Diagnosing cycloid psychoses needs frequently repeated mental examinations if the rapidly changing polymorphous clinical picture is to be recognised.

Case example

EP is a 38-year-old housewife whose first attack of mental illness, at the age of 19 years, led to her compulsory admission to hospital with a diagnosis of schizophrenia. She recovered fully, resumed work, married, and remained well for 7 years. Then, over the next 12 years, she had seven distinct episodes of psychosis, variously diagnosed as manic–depressive illness, schizophrenia and schizoaffective disorder. A complete remission followed each episode. She presented for admission 5 weeks after an uncomplicated hysterectomy with a 5-day history of severe insomnia and anxiety. On admission she had severe psychomotor retardation, but later that day her mutism changed to echolalia. At night she frequently screamed 'They are going to kill me!' and appeared to be having auditory hallucinations. The following day she was active, restless and walked in a bizarre way, on the balls of her feet (manneristic catatonia). Her mood was cheerful and she repeatedly sang an advertising jingle. This behaviour lasted about 2 hours, before anxiety dominated the clinical picture. At various times over the next 2 weeks she had intermittent auditory hallucinations, both complex, such as voices, and simple, such as bangs and whistles. She experienced first-rank symptoms: 'made thoughts', 'made bodily experiences' and 'audible thoughts', all of which occurred episodically. Anxiety remained the dominant symptom, but it fluctuated in severity and was occasionally punctuated with short episodes of disinhibited behaviour. She recovered completely after 4 weeks and remained well for 3 years on treatment with lithium and carbamazepine. She fulfilled the ICD–10 criteria for acute polymorphic psychotic disorder with symptoms of schizophrenia. Although motor symptoms were evident at the onset of this psychosis, affective symptoms predominated and so the diagnosis, according to Leonhard, was anxiety–elation psychosis.

Management

In managing the acute phase of the illness, neuroleptics are the drugs of choice. Perris (1988) advocated rapid neuroleptisation with haloperidol, followed by the addition of lithium. If there is severe persistent anxiety, then the temporary addition of clonazepam may be helpful. Long-term treatment with lithium or depot neuroleptics has been advocated, but the decision to pursue this course depends upon the history of the number and frequency of cycles. The newer mood stabilisers and atypical neuroleptics are probably superior to the older methods of treatment, but substantial evidence for this is not yet available. The cycloid psychoses also resemble acute puerperal psychoses in their dramatic improvement with ECT, when other treatments have failed (Little *et al*, 2000).

Conditions related to the cycloid psychoses

Non-systematic schizophrenias

Leonhard (1979) describes these conditions as the 'evil relatives' of the cycloid psychoses. The symptomatology is also polymorphous, but not as variable over time, the onset is less abrupt, and the outcome worse. The chance of a complete remission is the same as that for schizophrenia. There are three types of non-systematic schizophrenia, which correspond in their dominant symptoms to the cycloid psychoses:

1 *Affect-laden paraphrenia* resembles the anxiety–elation psychosis. Fluctuations in mood between anxiety and ecstasy dominate the clinical picture in the early stages. Ideas of self-reference, illusions and hallucinations appear and are congruent with the affective abnormalities. However, congruency tends to disappear as the patient's condition deteriorates.

2 *Cataphasia (schizophasia)*, like the confusional cycloid psychosis, has excited and inhibited forms of thought disorder as the dominant symptoms, but of greater severity.

3 *Periodic catatonia* resembles the cycloid motility psychosis in that motor symptoms predominate and switch between hyperkinesis and akinesis. Other catatonic symptoms occur, including parakinesia and manneristic behaviour. As the name suggests, this condition usually runs an intermittent course, but without complete remission between episodes. Gjessing's use of thyroid extract as treatment in the 1930s followed extensive metabolic studies of catatonic patients and provided a model for the future development of biological psychiatry (for a review, see Gjessing, 1974).

Boufée délirante

The French psychiatrist Mangan first described these disorders as psychoses with an acute onset, a fluctuating clinical picture, a recurrent course and a tendency to appear in successive generations of the same family. Wernicke and his school acknowledged this work, but renamed these disorders 'cycloid psychoses'. French psychiatry still recognises these conditions, qualifying them as 'reactive' if there is a psychological stressor or 'genuine' in its absence (Pull *et al*, 1985).

Mitsuda's atypical psychoses and Hatotani's periodical psychoses

The Japanese were influenced by German psychiatry and Wernicke's concepts are apparent in the work of Mitsuda and Hatotani. They have described conditions that closely resemble the cycloid psychoses and have supported their clinical observations with genetic and biological evidence. They suggest that these psychoses lie on the border between epilepsy and schizophrenia, or epilepsy and bipolar disorder. See Hatotani (1996) for a review.

Reactive (psychogenic) psychoses

The diagnosis of reactive or psychogenic psychosis, widely employed in Scandinavia, has attracted little research attention in recent times, according to Opjordsmoen (2001). This condition accounts for 15–20% of all first-time admissions for psychotic illness in Denmark (Rettersol, 1978).

Reactive psychoses, also termed 'psychogenic psychoses' by Faegerman (1963), are conceptualised as psychotic reactions to external stresses. Rettersol (1986), in a summary of Scandinavian opinion, stated that the psychic trauma must be of such significance that the psychosis would not have appeared in its absence. In addition, there must be a temporal connection between the trauma and the onset of the psychosis, and the content of the psychotic symptoms must reflect the traumatic experience. In most cases the patient recovers after some weeks or months.

ICD–10 recognises these conditions as 'acute and transient psychotic disorders, with stress', the stress being the only feature that distinguishes it from the other acute and transient psychotic disorders. A similar condition is identified in DSM–IV as a subtype of brief psychotic disorder, 'with marked stressor(s)'. (The other subtypes of brief psychotic disorder are 'without marked stressor(s)' and 'with post-partum onset'.)

Rettersol (1986) pointed out that the Scandinavian diagnostic criteria for reactive psychosis differed from those subsequently employed by DSM–IV and ICD–10. Both major diagnostic systems stipulate that the onset of the psychosis should follow closely upon the stress, within 2 weeks in the case of the ICD–10. A close temporal relationship, in the Scandinavian view, is not critically important. DSM–IV and ICD–10 also define stressors as events stressful to most people of the patient's culture under similar circumstances, but Scandinavians recognise stressors that are specific to a particular individual. This accords with clinical practice but is difficult to define operationally. The duration of the reactive psychosis also is not so critical from the Scandinavian viewpoint as it is in ICD–10 (2–3 months) and DSM–IV (4 weeks). However, all agree that the outcome is good.

Scandinavian psychiatrists recognise three forms of reactive psychosis, which, together with their relative frequencies, are emotional reactions (65%), paranoid reactions (20%) and disorders of consciousness (15%).

Case example

CP, a single, 18-year-old woman, had lived all her life in a small fishing community. She had seven older brothers and was the only child left at home, with middle-aged, indulgent parents. She had left school at age 16 and had never been able to find work. She moved to the city, 1000 miles away, with a new boyfriend, intent on finding employment. She found work on three occasions but left each time because it was too stressful. Two months after leaving home she was admitted to hospital with acute anxiety and confusion. She believed that she was pregnant and could feel an animal moving around inside her abdomen and she could hear its cries. Other auditory hallucinations included voices talking about her pregnancy. No physical cause, including drug misuse, was found. She was treated with neuroleptics and transferred to a hospital closer to her home, where only mild anxiety was observed and the neuroleptics were gradually withdrawn. She then became acutely disturbed and restless, and repeatedly absconded from hospital. Her delusions of pregnancy returned; she felt that people were trying to kill her and that her thoughts were being interfered with. Following reintroduction of treatment her hallucinations slowly diminished, as did her delusions of pregnancy. She remained anxious and convinced that people were trying to kill her. At her parents' insistence she was discharged home. Following this she rapidly improved and 1 month later was asymptomatic and off all medication. Four months later her family reported that she was 'back to her normal self' and 1 year after discharge she was living in the parental home, unemployed and free from symptoms.

This patient's illness conforms to the Scandinavian concept of reactive psychosis of the paranoid type and to the ICD–10 concept of acute and transient psychotic disorder. The temporal relationship between the stressor and the appearance of the psychotic symptoms, about 2 months, was too long to qualify for the diagnosis 'with associated acute stress'. This patient also illustrates the problem of defining stress. The move away from home would not be a major stressor for her peers but was uniquely stressful for her. The duration of the illness is too long for the DSM–IV diagnosis of brief psychotic reaction and fits that of schizophreniform disorder.

Treatment

Treatment of these conditions is symptomatic, since they are by definition self-limiting. If psychotic symptoms predominate, short-term neuroleptic treatment is indicated. In milder cases anxiolytics alone may suffice. The persistence of the condition, or the failure to make a complete recovery when the stressor has gone, suggests the diagnosis of reactive psychosis is wrong.

Schizophreniform disorder

The term 'schizophreniform' was first used by Langfeldt in 1937 to identify those patients with schizophrenic symptoms who had a good prognosis. He proposed that psychoses with typical schizophrenic symptoms should be termed 'schizophreniform disorder' if they had a good prognosis and 'schizophrenia' if the prognosis was poor. He used schizophreniform as a general term and applied it to organic as well as non-organic psychoses. Langfeldt (1982) comments on the DSM–III use of this term (the discussion is also pertinent to DSM–IV).

When Bergem *et al* (1990) reclassified Langfeldt's schizophreniform patients according to ICD–9 and DSM–III criteria, they raised doubts about the value of this concept. One-third of these patients had schizophrenia, most of the remainder had affective or adjustment disorders and only 14% fulfilled the DSM–III criteria for schizophreniform disorder.

DSM–IV followed DSM–III and used schizophreniform disorder for conditions that fulfilled the criteria for schizophrenia but lasted only 1–6 months. This duration included the prodromal, active and recovery phases of the illness. Impairment of social and occupational functioning, required for the diagnosis of schizophrenia, was not obligatory. (ICD–10 does not use the term schizophreniform disorder.) DSM–IV also has diagnostic subtypes – 'with or without good prognostic features'. The 'good prognosis' category requires the patient to have at least two of the following features:

1 psychotic symptoms that appear within 4 weeks of the onset of the illness

2 confusion, disorientation and perplexity

3 good premorbid or social functioning

4 the absence of blunted or flat affect.

Beiser *et al* (1988) have claimed that schizophrenia can be differentiated from schizophreniform disorder before the six-month outcome is known. Relative to patients with schizophrenia, patients with schizophreniform disorder have higher ratings on DSM–III Axis V (their general level of functioning is better), are less ill, do not have a flattened affect, and have a better rapport with the examiner. The confusion, disorientation and perplexity that can occur at the height of the illness may be related to the acuteness of the onset and the experiential difficulty of the sudden psychotic experience.

The majority of patients with DSM–IV schizophreniform disorder eventually have this diagnosis changed to schizophrenia. Zarate *et al* (2000) demonstrated this in a 2-year prospective study of first-episode cases and Iancu *et al* (2002) in a follow-up study of patients given this diagnosis 12 years earlier.

Treatment

The treatment is the same for schizophreniform disorder as that for schizophrenia. When symptoms completely remit and the prognostic features are good, the medication should be gradually reduced. If the symptoms return, then the diagnosis is schizophrenia.

Delusional (paranoid) disorders

Delusional disorders are chronic psychiatric conditions that have delusions as the predominant or often the only symptoms. They have a history that illustrates many of the nosological and semantic problems encountered in psychiatry.

History

Psychiatrists have come to view the term 'paranoia' and its adjective 'paranoid' with suspicion, as they have acquired a variety of meanings. Lewis (1970) wrote a definitive history of the psychiatric use of these terms. The Greeks used the word paranoia, meaning to be 'beside one's self', as a general term for insanity.

The modern use of 'paranoia' started with Kahlbaum, who gave this name to a group of chronic conditions with delusions as the major symptoms. Kraepelin (1921) endorsed this work and defined paranoia as the 'insidious development of a permanent and unshakable delusional system, resulting from internal causes, which is accompanied by perfect preservation of clear and orderly thinking, willing and acting'. Psychiatrists, in general, subscribed to this definition and accepted the diagnosis in clinical practice.

Unfortunately, psychiatrists later applied the terms to other conditions. 'Paranoid' was used to identify the type of schizophrenia in which delusions of any kind predominated. Later, in the Anglo-American literature, 'paranoid' became synonymous with delusions of persecution, as they are the commonest delusions in paranoid schizophrenia. The meaning of the term was further expanded to include non-delusional ideas of persecution and self-reference and it made a nosological appearance, in this guise, as paranoid personality disorder. Finally, the lay public found it too useful a word to be monopolised by psychiatrists and 'paranoid' has entered into everyday language.

This semantic confusion led the authors of DSM–III to replace 'paranoia' and 'paranoid disorder' with the term 'delusional disorder'. DSM–IV continued this practice and defined delusional disorder as 'the presence of a persistent, non-bizarre delusion that is not due to any other mental disorder, such as schizophrenia, schizophreniform disorder, or a mood disorder'. ICD–10 followed suit and the 'paranoia' of ICD–9 became 'persistent delusional disorder'. DSM–IV and ICD–10 differ slightly in their diagnostic criteria for delusional disorder. For example, the minimum duration of the disorder is 1 month for DSM–IV but 3 months for ICD–10, and DSM–IV requires the delusions to be non-bizarre (defined as 'situations that can conceivably occur in real life'), whereas ICD–10 does not stipulate a type of delusion.

Kraepelin identified a separate condition, paraphrenia, that was similar to paranoia but for the presence of persistent hallucinations. Munro (1999), in his monograph *Delusional Disorder: Paranoia and Related Illnesses*, has argued that the following conditions should be included among the delusional disorders: paraphrenia, late paraphrenia, delusional misidentification syndromes and *folie à deux* (see below).

Epidemiology

The figures for the frequency of delusional disorder in the general population are probably underestimates. Those with this disorder rarely acknowledge their illness and come to psychiatric attention only when they behave in a conspicuously abnormal manner. The prevalence in the general population is estimated to be about 0.03% and the lifetime risk 0.05-0.1%. The onset is usually in the age range 40–55 years, but it can occur in adults of any age and has a male:female ratio of 0.85:1.

Theories of causation

There are two basic theories about the cause of delusional disorders. One postulates an abnormal personality development in which the development of delusions is both understandable and inevitable. The second attributes the delusion to a 'process', that is, a pathophysiological change in the brain caused by schizophrenia, or a physical insult to the brain. According to the process theory, the formation of a delusion is not psychologically understandable, but the content, in terms of the patient's personality and life experience, may be understandable.

Theories derived in association with cognitive therapy for delusions postulate that delusional thinking is an abnormality of cognitive functioning, which can be modified using behavioural methods (for a critical review, see Garety & Freeman, 1999). These cognitive abnormalities may be traits predisposing to the development of delusions, or states associated with the presence of delusions.

Kraepelin appears to have preferred the personality development theory, but it was Gaupp and Kretschmer who provided supporting evidence. A famous case, from 1914 and cited as an example of psychologically understandable paranoia, was that of the mass murderer Ernst Wagner (see Gaupp, 1974).

Case example

Gaupp described Wagner as a sensitive, intelligent, self-critical man who, in his youth, was troubled by thoughts of the moral and physical damage he had sustained by masturbating. Later in life, while a schoolmaster in a small village, he committed bestiality. No one else knew of this, but he was convinced that the villagers were aware of this crime and mocked him for it. He then moved, but over the next 7 years plotted the destruction of these villagers. His papers revealed that he waited 4 more years before acting. He first killed his wife and children, then set fire to the village and shot the inhabitants as they fled, killing 8 and seriously wounding 12 others.

Kretschmer's theory of the development of sensitive ideas of reference appeared as a monograph in 1927. He described a particular type of personality, 'the sensitive', who was liable to develop delusions (Kretschmer, 1974). These personalities consciously retain significant emotional complexes, which they continuously work over, and this gives rise to strong feelings that they are unable to discharge. Given a particular set of life experiences, and a 'key experience' to unlock them, such persons develop delusions of self-reference, particularly when they are mentally or physically exhausted.

Case example

JW was a 33-year-old man referred by a urologist, to whom he had repeatedly taken his complaint of a small penis. The patient believed that this was common knowledge and discussed by his neighbours. Changes of residence provided only temporary relief. These beliefs began at the age of 13, when he was taking a communal shower at school. Another lad had laughed at him, saying his genitalia were small and recruited other boys to join in the teasing. This distressed him greatly for a short period, but then he forgot about it. Following conscription into the army, feeling homesick and miserable, he recognised in the barracks the boy who had teased him at school. He was with a group of recruits and suddenly the entire group laughed. (This was the 'key experience'.) He knew immediately that they were laughing about his small penis. From that time on, he knew that he had a small penis and that this was common knowledge. Later, his wife became unable to tolerate his repeated questioning about whether he was too small for her. When she left him for another man, he knew his small penis was the reason. When seen, he lived alone, padded his underwear, and prefaced any sexual encounter with an apology to the prospective partner.

A discussion of the psychogenesis of paranoid disorder would be incomplete without mentioning Freud's analysis of the Schreber memoirs. Daniel Schreber was 51 years old, and President of the Court of Appeals of Saxony, when he developed 'paranoia' and was confined in hospital for the next 9 years. His memoirs, written to secure his release, are a vivid personal account of this illness. Freud concluded that Schreber's paranoia was attributable to his repressed homosexual impulses towards his father. The central conflict in paranoia, for males, was the unacceptable homosexual wish to love another man. Freud explained the principal types of paranoia as contradictions of the repressed wish 'I, a man, love him' (Freud, 1911). Persecutory delusions arose from the contradiction 'I do not love him, I hate him', which by projection became 'He hates me'; in grandiose delusions this same contradiction became 'I love myself'. Delusions of jealousy arose from the contradiction 'I do not love him, she loves him'. In delusions of love the contradiction 'I do not love him, I love her' became by projection 'She loves me'.

The second hypothesis – that delusional disorder is attributable to schizophrenia – found support from Kolle (1931). He followed up cases of paranoia, including those described by Kraepelin, and found that most of them developed schizophrenia. More recently, Osby *et al* (2001) found that first-admission rates for schizophrenia, in Stockholm, from 1974 to 1994 had fallen, but rates for paranoid disorders had risen by an equivalent amount, suggesting that paranoid disorder was a milder form of schizophrenia. Munro (1988) examined a group of 50 subjects with delusional disorder and found that 40% had suffered some form of brain insult. He suggested that delusional disorder might arise in individuals with a weak genetic loading for schizophrenia who had suffered a brain insult before or during adolescence.

Clinical presentation

Patients with delusional disorder rarely complain directly of their delusions. Usually, they have been coerced into seeing a psychiatrist by their family, or by some legal process. The diagnosis of delusional disorder requires an independent account of the illness from someone who knows the patient well, particularly if the delusional content is culturally acceptable, that is, non-bizarre (see below).

The subject of the patient's delusions should be approached circumspectly. Patients with delusional disorder are often hostile, sarcastic and marshal many reasons against cooperating in the psychiatric assessment. Once the area of the delusional belief is touched upon, it is important for the examiner to convey an attitude of open-mindedness and of a sympathetic interest in the patient's concerns. This reduces the patient's distrust and evasiveness and can lead to disclosure of the delusional content. The examiner should not agree or disagree with the patient's delusional beliefs. Delusions should be challenged, and then cautiously, only when the strength of the beliefs has to be assessed for diagnostic or treatment purposes.

Apart from the delusions, the mental examination should be normal. However, both the ICD–10 and the DSM–IV criteria do allow the presence of tactile and olfactory hallucinations related to the delusional theme. A most important part of the assessment, both initial and continuing, is the danger that patients pose to those who feature in their delusions. Expressions of anger towards these subjects, plans for exacting revenge, or using force to stop their 'harmful' activities are indicative of risk and the need for preventive action.

Delusional disorder is usually categorised according to the delusional content. The major subtypes are listed below:

1 *Erotomania,* also known as de Clérambault's syndrome, is characterised by delusions in which patients believe a particular person is in love with them. This person may be a superior at work, a public figure or a celebrity. Less frequently it is someone of equivalent or lower social status. When this 'lover' denies feelings for the patient and rejects all approaches, further delusional elaborations arise. These provide reasons why the 'lover' cannot publicly acknowledge this love and must communicate through secret messages and signs, which the patient can interpret. For example, a patient who believed that a rock star was in love with her knew that the sequence of songs he performed had a secret message meant only for her. More women than men present with erotomania, but men provide the major forensic problems. Legal remedies, including imprisonment, have no effect on their beliefs and do little to modify their behaviour outside the limits of custody. Feelings of love, although still declared, may become mixed with hostile and jealous feelings as the condition deteriorates. When this happens the patient may pose a significant risk to the 'lover' and those close to him or her.

2 *Grandiose.* These patients have erroneous and extravagant delusional beliefs about themselves, which may involve social status, wealth, intellectual powers and spiritual gifts. A patient who believed he was the only legitimate and direct heir of Charles II attributed his considerable financial problems to the machinations of the Royal Family, who knew that they had usurped his throne and were trying to discredit him.

3 *Jealous*. This is characterised by delusions that a partner, usually a spouse, has been unfaithful. It is also known, more dramatically, as the 'Othello syndrome'. 'Morbid jealousy' is a general term for pathological jealousy, which can be a symptom of psychiatric conditions other than delusional disorder (alcoholism is probably the commonest cause). Morbid jealousy is not always delusional and, for example, can be an overvalued idea or a compulsive thought. When jealousy is attributable to a delusional disorder, it appears to develop insidiously in middle life. However, careful enquiry will sometimes reveal episodes of unjustifiable jealousy in the past. The development of jealousy is sometimes associated with erectile impotence in the male and concomitant sexual dysfunction in the female partner. However, these psychosexual difficulties, more often an effect rather than a cause of the disorder, reinforce the delusions of jealousy. Sometimes the jealousy appears to be evoked by a 'key experience', termed the 'jealous flash' by Enoch (1991), in a review. Patients will persistently question their partner as they seek evidence to support the delusion. They often spy on their partners, follow them, set traps, intercept their mail and scrutinise their underwear. Confrontations frequently occur as attempts are made to extort a confession from the partner. Sometimes, worn down by these continuous demands, the partner makes a false confession in the hope that this torment will cease. This hope is not realised. At best, further information about other lovers will be demanded. At worst, physical violence or even murder can result. The condition is difficult to treat and tends to recur with each new partner. Delusional jealousy should be suspected in cases of domestic violence and, if confirmed, measures taken to protect the spouse. On occasions, the 'rival' may also require protection.

4 *Persecutory*. The patient is usually the subject of the persecution, but occasionally it is someone close to the patient. The delusional system is very well organised, much better so than in other psychiatric conditions. Convinced that the evidence supporting their belief is irrefutable and frustrated by the proper authorities, which take no action, patients may attempt to expose their persecutors in a public forum; the law courts and 'letters to the editor' serve this purpose.

5 *Somatic*. Delusions of physical abnormality or of physical disorder characterise this subtype. If the delusional content is concerned with aspects of physical size or form (see the case of JW above) then it may also be termed 'delusional dysmorphophobia'. Another subgroup, monosymptomatic hypochondriacal psychosis, is distinguished by delusions of illness, or infestation, or foul smells and secretions leaking from body orifices.

Differential diagnosis

The diagnosis of delusional disorder requires the recognition of a delusion and the exclusion of other psychotic disorders. Delusions, particularly those that are non-bizarre, may be difficult to distinguish from two non-psychotic phenomena, overvalued ideas and compulsive thoughts.

Overvalued ideas are beliefs that arise comprehensibly from the patient's personality and life experience. The subject's peer group, given the same evidence, might reasonably make the same judgement. However, this reasonable belief is pursued to an unreasonable degree, dominates the personality and becomes a self-righteous quest undertaken without consideration for others. (Terrence Rattigan's play *The Winslow Boy* illustrates such an occurrence.)

The resemblance between obsessive–compulsive and delusional thoughts is superficial. The former, unlike delusions, are unwanted intrusions into the psychic life of the subject, who consciously resists them and knows they are irrational. Another non-psychotic condition, paranoid personality disorder, is also readily distinguished from delusional disorder, because the objects of mistrust and suspicion vary with circumstances and have done so continuously since early adulthood.

Paranoid syndromes can occur in any of the major psychoses, so that schizophrenia and affective and organic psychoses enter into the differential diagnosis.

Schizophrenia

Hallucinations, particularly those in sensory modalities unrelated to the content of the delusion, suggest a diagnosis of schizophrenia. DSM–IV does allow the presence of olfactory and tactile hallucinations in delusional disorder, if they relate to the delusional theme. Patients with delusional disorder may describe delusions of attempted control by others, but exploration of these experiences will distinguish them from the 'made' phenomena reported by patients with schizophrenia: in the former, the delusion of control by others is solely a belief, whereas in the latter there are complex phenomena, characterised by the experience of mental activities made in the external world that pass through the ego boundary and take up an alien existence within the self. These 'made' experiences and the other first-rank symptoms of schizophrenia do not occur in delusional disorder. The diagnosis is probably schizophrenia if any of the following symptoms are undoubtedly present: positive or negative formal thought disorder, affective disorganisation or affective flattening.

Psychotic affective disorder

Patients with delusional states often have mood disorder. The possibility that delusional symptoms are due to depression is greater if the delusions are mood-congruent delusion-like ideas. However, the diagnosis of depression will rest largely on the presence of neurovegetative signs. Manic delusions are grandiose in content. Mania of such severity that it gives rise to delusions will be characterised by obvious psychomotor acceleration.

Organic delusional disorder

Some patients, particularly those with a paranoid personality, may develop delusional disorder when affected by some physical insult to the brain. The commonest physical cause of acute delusional disorder is drug intoxication. Stimulants such as amphetamine, cocaine and methylphenidate are notorious for producing delusional disorders without evident impairment of consciousness.

Therefore, a history of drug use should always be sought in delusional disorder. Alcoholism may be a factor in the development of delusions, particularly those of morbid jealousy. Other drugs particularly associated with organic paranoid disorders are steroid hormones and dopamine agonists such as L-dopa and disulfiram.

The possibility that delusions are secondary to a dementia is always a consideration in older patients. When a patient with a diagnosis of delusional disorder continues to deteriorate, this may be due to the development of dementia or schizophrenia, the delusional state having been the prodrome.

Management

The first goal in treatment is the most difficult: it is to develop a therapeutic relationship with a patient who does not want to participate in psychiatric treatment. Patients do not see why they should enter into such a relationship, because they do not perceive a need for psychiatric treatment. Also militating against this relationship, which requires a large measure of trust, are the suspiciousness and distrust that are part of the illness. Patients are usually angry and hostile towards those responsible for their entry into treatment and these feelings are immediately extended to psychiatric staff.

By the time patients enter into treatment they have come to expect that their beliefs will be met by disbelief and argument. Consequently, they are sullen, resentful and evasive. The approach to eliciting the delusions has already been described and the importance of maintaining an attitude of concerned and sympathetic interest stressed. Because patients are suspicious and distrustful, the psychiatrist should do nothing to reinforce these feelings. It helps to appear open and friendly, maintain eye contact, avoid physical contact and be consistent. It does not help to argue against or agree with the delusion and the psychiatrist should avoid doing anything that patients might interpret as deceptive, hostile or a breech of trust.

Physical treatment (see below) can often be initiated by focusing upon symptoms other than the delusion, particularly anxiety and depression. By keeping the delusion in the background, the patient may be encouraged to accept medication for these associated symptoms. At subsequent interviews to assess progress, the psychiatrist should defer questions about delusions until enquiries have been about the associated symptoms.

Physical treatment

There are obvious difficulties in enrolling patients with delusional disorder in double-blind controlled treatment studies. The number of potential subjects is also relatively small. Therefore, the evidence on which treatment recommendations are made is largely anecdotal.

Pimozide, a piperidine derivative, has long been the treatment of choice for delusional disorders. Following reports of its efficacy in the treatment of monosymptomatic hypochondriasis, other reports of its effectiveness in erotomania and persecutory delusions followed (Munro & Mok, 1995). However, recent evidence that pimozide is one of the antipsychotics associated on EEG with QTc prolongation, *torsades de pointes* and sudden death (Haddad & Anderson, 2002) indicates that it should be reserved for patients who have failed to respond to another and safer antipsychotic. Risperidone is the drug, after pimozide, best supported by anecdotal evidence as being an effective treatment for paranoid disorders. A growing number of reports have favourably described the use of the newer atypical antipsychotic drugs in delusional disorder, but there is insufficient evidence to choose one over another. A few case reports on the use of the selective serotonin reuptake inhibitors (SSRIs) alone, particularly in the somatic form of delusional disorder, suggest that these types of antidepressant may merit a trial.

Psychological treatments

There are two approaches to the psychological treatment of delusional disorder. The first, which is the more traditional, does not challenge the delusional beliefs, but takes a pragmatic approach, which emphasises the benefits patients can derive from changing their behaviour. Examples of such changes, all of which can be achieved without requiring patients to recant their beliefs, are: seeking less socially disruptive remedies for their delusional wrongs, not proselytising, and not expressing hostile or amatory feelings. The underlying presumption is that this behaviour without conviction limits harm until the delusions respond to a physical remedy.

The cognitive theory of delusions was noted above. The associated treatment approach is similar to the cognitive therapy employed in the treatment of delusions in schizophrenia (see page 304). The aim is to moderate delusions using behavioural methods. There are different approaches, but all challenge the intensity of patients' belief in their delusions. The combination of cognitive–behavioural therapy with medication appears promising.

Rare delusional disorders

It is customary to include certain unusual and fascinating delusional syndromes under the heading of delusional disorders. However, the majority of them are secondary to some other cause, such as an organic brain disorder or schizophrenia.

Folie à deux, or shared delusional disorder, is the development in a second person of the delusions already entertained by someone who is a close personal contact. There is no other evidence of mental illness in the second person, who has usually been in a subordinate relationship to the first.

Case example

A patient with paranoid schizophrenia believed that he should go into space, so that he might destroy a satellite that was transmitting thought waves into his mind. His wife, who had a dependent personality and borderline intelligence, but who was otherwise normal, believed in his mission and his capabilities as a 'rocket scientist'. Some time after his discharge from hospital both were apprehended by the police as they attempted to launch a plywood and aluminium foil 'spaceship' 3 metres high. He was sitting in this structure, which she was attempting to ignite.

The other types of rare delusional disorder are those that involve misidentification, namely:

1 Capgras syndrome – the delusion that a familiar person, or persons, have been replaced by an exact double

2 Frégolie syndrome – the delusion that an unfamiliar person, or persons, is believed to be someone very familiar (usually a persecutor), even though their physical appearance is not the same

3 intermetamorphosis syndrome – similar to the Frégolie syndrome except that the stranger is believed to have both the physical and psychological characteristics of the familiar person

4 subjective doubles syndrome – the delusion that other people have the same physical appearance as the patient.

References

Abrams, R. (1984) Genetic studies of the schizoaffective syndrome: a selective review. *Schizophrenia Bulletin*, **10**, 26–29.

American Psychiatric Association (1968) *Diagnostic and Statistical Manual of Mental Disorders* (2nd edn) (DSM–II). Washington, DC: APA.

American Psychiatric Association (1980) *Diagnostic and Statistical Manual of Mental Disorders* (3rd edn) (DSM–III). Washington, DC: APA.

American Psychiatric Association (1994) *Diagnostic and Statistical Manual of Mental Disorders* (4th edn) (DSM–IV). Washington, DC: APA.

American Psychiatric Association (1997) Practice guidelines for the treatment of patients with schizophrenia. *American Journal of Psychiatry*, **154** (April suppl).

Beckman, H., Bartsch, A. J., Neumarker, K., *et al* (2000) Schizophrenia in the Wernicke–Kleist–Leonhard school. *American Journal of Psychiatry*, **157**, 1024–1025.

Beiser, M., Fleming, J. A. E. & Lin, T. (1988) Refining the diagnosis of schizophreniform disorder. *American Journal of Psychiatry*, **145**, 695–700.

Benabarre, A., Vieta, E., Colom, F., *et al* (2001) Bipolar disorder, schizoaffective disorder and schizophrenia: epidemiologic, clinical and prognostic differences. *European Psychiatry*, **16**, 167–172.

Bergem, A. L. M., Dahl, A. A., Guldberg, C., *et al* (1990) Langfeldt's schizophreniform psychoses fifty years later. *British Journal of Psychiatry*, **157**, 351–354.

Berrios, G. E. & Beer, M. D. (1994) The notion of a unitary psychosis: a conceptual history. *History of Psychiatry*, **5**, 13–36.

Brockington, I. F. & Leff, J. P. (1979) Schizoaffective psychosis: definitions and incidence. *Psychological Medicine*, **9**, 91–99.

Brockington, I. F. & Meltzer, H. Y. (1983) The nosology of schizoaffective psychosis. *Psychiatric Developments*, **4**, 317–338.

Clayton, P. J. (1982) Schizoaffective disorders. *Journal of Nervous and Mental Disease*, **11**, 646–650.

Enoch, D. (1991) Delusional jealousy and awareness of reality. *British Journal of Psychiatry*, **159**, 52–56.

Evans, J. D., Heaton, R. K., Paulsen, J. S., *et al* (1999) Schizoaffective disorder: schizophrenia or affective disorder? *Journal of Clinical Psychiatry*, **60**, 874–882.

Faegerman, P. M. (1963) *Psychogenic Psychoses*. London: Butterworths.

Feighner, J. P., Robins, E., Guze, S. B., *et al* (1972) Diagnostic criteria for use in psychiatric research. *Archives of General Psychiatry*, **26**, 57–67.

Forrester, A., Owens, D. G. & Johnstone, E. C. (2001) Diagnostic stability in subjects with multiple admissions for psychiatric illness. *Psychological Medicine*, **31**, 151–158.

Franzek, E. & Beckmann, H. (1998) Different genetic background of schizophrenia spectrum psychoses: a twin study. *American Journal of Psychiatry*, **155**, 76–83.

Freud, S. (1911) Psychoanalytic notes upon an autobiographical account of a case of paranoia (dementia paranoides). In *Collected Papers, Vol. III*. London: Hogarth Press (1950).

Garety, P. A. & Freeman, D. (1999) Cognitive approaches to delusions: a critical review. *British Journal of Clinical Psychology*, **38**, 113–154.

Gaupp, R. (1974) The scientific significance of the case of Ernst Wagner. In *Themes and Variations in European Psychiatry* (eds S. R. Hirsch & M. Shepherd), pp. 121–134. Charlottesville, VA: University Press of Virginia.

Gershon, E. S., DeLisi, M. D., Hamovit, J., *et al* (1988) A controlled family study of chronic psychoses, schizophrenia and schizoaffective disorder. *Archives of General Psychiatry*, **45**, 328–336.

Gjessing, L. R. (1974) A review of periodic catatonia. *Biological Psychiatry*, **8**, 23–45.

Gooding, D. C. & Tallent, K. A. (2002) Spatial working memory performance in patients with schizoaffective psychosis versus schizophrenia: a tale of two disorders? *Schizophrenia Research*, **53**, 209–218.

Grieger, T. A., Benedek, D. M. & Flynn, J. (2001) Pharmacologic treatment of patients hospitalized with the diagnosis of schizoaffective disorder. *Journal of Clinical Psychiatry*, **62**, 59–60.

Haddad, P. M. & Anderson, I. M. (2002) Antipsychotic-related QTc prolongation, torsade de pointes and sudden death. *Drugs*, **62**, 1649–1671.

Harrow, M. & Grossman, H. S. (1984) Outcome in schizoaffective disorders: a critical review of the literature. *Schizophrenia Bulletin*, **10**, 87–108.

Harrow, M. & Grossman, H. S. (2000) Ten year outcome: patients with schizoaffective disorders, schizophrenia, affective disorder and mood-incongruent psychotic symptoms. *British Journal of Psychiatry*, **177**, 421–426.

Hatotani, N. (1996) The concept of 'atypical psychoses': special reference to its development in Japan. *Psychiatry and Clinical Neurosciences*, **50**, 1–10.

Hummel, B., Dittman, S., Fortshoff, A., *et al* (2002) Clozapine as add-on medication in the maintenance of bipolar and affective disorders. *Neuropsychobiology*, **45**, 37–42.

Iancu, I., Dannon, P. N., Ziv, R., *et al* (2002) A follow-up study of patients with DSM–IV schizophreniform disorder. *Canadian Journal of Psychiatry*, **47**, 56–60.

Jaspers, K. (1963) *General Psychopathology* (English translation). Manchester: Manchester University Press.

Kasanin, J. (1933) The acute schizoaffective psychoses. *American Journal of Psychiatry*, **13**, 97–126.

Kendler, K. S. (1991) Mood-incongruent psychotic affective illness. *Archives of General Psychiatry*, **48**, 362–369.

Kendler, K. S., McGuire, M., Gruenberg, A. M., *et al* (1995) Examining the validity of DSM–III–R schizoaffective disorder and its putative subtypes in the Roscommon family study. *American Journal of Psychiatry*, **152**, 755–764.

Kolle, K. (1931) *Die primäre Verrücktheit*. Leipzig: Thieme.

Kraepelin, E. (1919) *Dementia Praecox and Paraphrenia* (trans. R. M. Barclay). Edinburgh: E. & S. Livingstone.

Kraepelin, E. (1921) *Manic Depressive Insanity and Paranoia* (trans. R. M. Barclay). Edinburgh: E. & S. Livingstone.

Kretschmer, E. (1974) The sensitive delusions of reference. In *Themes and Variations in European Psychiatry* (eds S. R. Hirsch & M. Shepherd), pp. 153–196. Charlottesville, VA: University Press of Virginia.

Krishnan, K. R. R., Raysam, K. & Carroll, B. J. (1990) Dexamethasone suppression test in schizoaffective disorders. In *Affective and Schizoaffective Disorders* (eds A. Marneros & M. T. Tsuang), pp. 208–217. London: Springer-Verlag.

Langfeldt, G. (1982) Definition of schizophreniform psychoses. *American Journal of Psychiatry*, **139**, 703.

Leonhard, K. (1979) *The Classification of Endogenous Psychoses* (5th edn). New York: Irvington Publishers.

Levinson, D. F. & Levitt, M. E. M. (1987) Schizoaffective mania reconsidered. *American Journal of Psychiatry*, **144**, 415–425.

Levinson, D. F., Umapathy, C. & Musthaq, M. (1999) Treatment of schizoaffective disorder and schizophrenia with mood symptoms. *American Journal of Psychiatry*, **156**, 1138–1148.

Lewis, A. (1934) Melancholia: a historical review. *Journal of Mental Science*, **80**, 1–42.

Lewis, A. (1970) Paranoia and paranoid: historical perspective. *Psychological Medicine*, **1**, 2–12.

Lindvall, M., Hagnell, O. & Ohman, R. (1990) Epidemiology of cycloid psychosis. *Psychopathology*, **23**, 228–232.

Little, J. D., Ungvari, G. S. & McFarlane, J. (2000) Successful ECT in a case of Leonhard's cycloid psychosis. *Journal of Electroconvulsive Therapy*, **16**, 62–67.

Maj, M. & Perris, C. (1990) Patterns of course in patients with a cross-sectional diagnosis of schizoaffective disorder. *Journal of Affective Disorders*, **20**, 70–77.

Maj, M., Starace, F. & Pinozzi, R. (1991) A family study of schizoaffective disorder depressive type, compared with schizophrenia and psychotic and nonpsychotic major depression. *American Journal of Psychiatry*, **148**, 612–616.

McGuffin, P., Farmer, A. & Harvey, I. (1991) A polydiagnostic application of operational criteria in studies of psychotic illness. *Archives of General Psychiatry*, **48**, 764–770.

Meltzer, H. Y., Arora, R. E. & Metz, J. (1984) Biological studies of schizoaffective disorders. *Schizophrenia Bulletin*, **10**, 49–70.

Munro, A. (1988) Delusional (paranoid) disorder: etiologic and taxonomic considerations. I: The possible significance of organic brain factors in the etiology of delusional disorders. *Canadian Journal of Psychiatry*, **33**, 171–174.

Munro, A. (1999) *Delusional Disorder: Paranoia and Related Illnesses*. New York: Cambridge University Press.

Munro, A. & Mok, H. (1995) An overview of treatment in paranoia/delusional disorder. *Canadian Journal of Psychiatry*, **40**, 616–622.

Opjordsmoen, S. (2001) Reactive psychosis and brief psychotic episodes. *Current Psychiatric Reports*, **3**, 338–341.

Osby, U., Hammar, N., Brandt, L., *et al* (2001) Time trends in first admissions for schizophrenia and paranoid psychosis in Stockholm County, Sweden. *Schizophrenia Research*, **47**, 247–254.

Perris, C. (1988) The concept of cycloid psychotic disorders. *Psychiatric Developments*, **1**, 37–56.

Perris, C. & Brockington, I. F. (1981) Cycloid psychoses and their relation to the major psychoses. In *Biological Psychiatry* (eds C. Perris, *et al*), pp. 447–450. Amsterdam: Elsevier.

Pfuhlmann, B., Stober, G., Franzek, E., *et al* (1999) Cycloid psychoses predominate in severe postpartum psychiatric disorders. *Journal of Affective Disorders*, **50**, 125–134.

Pull, C. B., Pull, M. C. & Pichot, P. (1985) Comparing French and international classification schemes: I Schizophrenia. In *Psychiatry the State of the Art. Vol. I: Clinical Psychopathology Nomenclature and Classification* (eds P. Berner, R. Wolf & K. Thau), pp. 87–92. New York: Plenum Press.

Rettersol, N. (1978) The Scandinavian concept of reactive psychosis, schizophreniform psychosis and schizophrenia. *Psychiatria Clinica*, **11**, 180–187.

Rettersol, N. (1986) Classification of functional psychoses with special reference to follow-up studies. *Psychopathology*, **19**, 5–15.

Schneider, K. (1959) *Clinical Psychopathology* (English translation). New York: Grune and Stratton.

Sharma, R. P., Martis, B., Rosen, C., *et al* (2001) CSF thyrotrophin-releasing hormone concentrations differ in patients with schizoaffective disorder from patients with schizophrenia and mood disorders. *Journal of Psychosomatic Research*, **35**, 287–291.

Spitzer, R. L., Endicott, J. & Robins, E. (1978) *Research Diagnostic Criteria (RDC) for a Selected Group of Functional Disorders* (3rd edn). New York: New York State Psychiatric Institute.

Strik, W. K., Ruchsow, M., Abele, S., *et al* (1998) Distinct neurophysiological mechanisms for manic and cycloid psychoses: evidence from a P300 study on manic patients. *Acta Psychiatrica Scandinavica*, **98**, 459–466.

Tsuang, M. T. (1991) Morbidity risks of schizophrenia and affective disorders among first-degree relatives of patients with schizoaffective disorder. *British Journal of Psychiatry*, **158**, 165–170.

Wahby, V. S., Ibrahim, G. A., Leechuy, I., *et al* (1990) Prolactin response to thyrotrophin-releasing hormone in schizoaffective depressed compared to depressed and schizophrenic men and healthy controls. *Schizophrenia Research*, **3**, 227–281.

Wahby, V. S., Ibrahim, G. A., Giller, E. L., *et al* (1990–91) The dexamethasone suppression test in a group of Research Diagnostic Criteria schizoaffective depressed men. *Neuropsychobiology*, **23**, 129–133.

Warkentin, S., Nilsson, A., Karlson, S., *et al* (1992) Cycloid psychosis: regional cerebral flow studies of a psychotic episode. *Acta Psychiatrica Scandinavica*, **85**, 23–29.

World Health Organization (1992) *Tenth Revision of the International Classification of Diseases* (ICD–10). Geneva: WHO.

Zarate, C. A. Jr, Tohen. M. & Land, M. L. (2000) First-episode schizophreniform disorder: comparisons with first-episode schizophrenia. *Schizophrenia Research*, **46**, 31–34.

CHAPTER 10

The aetiology of schizophrenia

Pak Sham, Peter Woodruff, Michael Hunter and Julian Leff

Elucidating the cause of schizophrenia presents a classic set of methodological challenges to researchers; these are perhaps more daunting than for any other disorder in medicine. The problems begin with case definition. Researchers have developed several detailed sets of operational criteria, but in the absence of pathognomonic biological markers, the validity of these diagnostic criteria is unproven. There may be several types of schizophrenia, and the complexity and heterogeneity of the disorder are likely to reflect multiple and interacting aetiological and pathoplastic influences. Epidemiological research addresses some of these concerns by studying the pattern of morbidity on a broad canvas, examining the interacting and confounding relationships between biological and social factors.

We begin this chapter with a review of the epidemiology of schizophrenia, before examining in detail the robust evidence in support of the genetic contribution to aetiology, including some of the newer exciting findings in molecular genetics. Prenatal risk factors are next examined, followed by the neuroanatomical aspects of schizophrenia. For a long time it has been known that schizophrenia could arise in certain neurological diseases, such as temporal lobe epilepsy, and structural brain imaging has recently provided direct evidence of brain abnormalities in schizophrenia; these are reviewed in detail in this chapter. The importance of social and neuropsychological factors in the onset and course of schizophrenia is considered here, reflecting the increasing interest in non-pharmacological approaches. The way in which antipsychotic drugs work and the resultant neurochemical theories of schizophrenia are reviewed in Chapter 11.

Although the format of this chapter follows a traditional structure in placing the results of research under separate disciplinary headings, the most striking trend is towards interdisciplinary research, which combines perspectives and methods from different approaches, for example epidemiology and genetics, functional neuroimaging and neuropsychology, while over the past few years there have been striking advances in the field of molecular genetics, which in turn have suggested new candidate genes. The chapter takes the form of a review of the present state of knowledge and highlights some key papers, but it is important to note that, despite the huge volume of published research, the key causes of schizophrenia remain elusive and a similar review on this topic in the next decade might read very differently.

Epidemiology

Methodological problems

One of the problems of much of the early research on schizophrenia was a lack of diagnostic uniformity, which made comparison between studies almost impossible. For example, the diagnosis of schizophrenia was much more loosely applied in the USA than in the UK, leading to the quip that the easiest cure for the disease was a transatlantic flight. Indeed, the US/UK diagnostic project (Cooper *et al*, 1972) investigated rates of schizophrenia and manic–depression in the two countries using standardised criteria, and concluded that most of the previously reported difference in rates was due to variations in diagnostic practice.

Lately, the advent of operationalised criteria for schizophrenia, such as DSM–IV and ICD–10, combined with standardised interviews (e.g. PSE, SADS, SAPS, SANS) (see Chapter 8), has resulted in far more consistency in schizophrenia research. However, one difficulty with greater reliance on operationalised criteria is that, while they do show good reliability, they are not all necessarily valid, and their continued widespread use may result in the tacit acceptance that they are. Also, different sets of even well-validated criteria emphasise different aspects of the illness; for example, DSM–IV specifies a 6-month duration, whereas ICD–10 requires only 1 month (see Chapter 8), and this needs to be taken into account when studies are compared.

The second major problem area in studying the epidemiology of schizophrenia is that of case finding. Most designs fall into one of three groups:

1 clinical case detection, for example derived from hospital admission data

2 population surveys, for example conducted door to door, or derived from representative samples

3 follow-up studies of birth cohorts.

The vast majority of studies have been based on hospital admissions, which are themselves subject to variations in service provision and admission policies. Reliance on admission statistics alone also leads to bias from the inclusion of readmissions. For example, more severely affected patients, especially those with positive symptoms, are more likely to be readmitted, and this will confound work in such areas as gender differences, as males tend to have a more severe form of illness, which will result in an exaggerated male:female ratio in hospital samples. The inclusion of only first admissions is methodologically more sound, but biases still arise. For example, more severely affected patients are more likely to be admitted, as are those with a history of violence or disturbed behaviour. By contrast, a small proportion of cases – mainly people with simple schizophrenia – have no hospital contact. Thus, Link & Dohrenwend (1980) found that 17% of patients living in the community in the USA had never presented to the services.

Case registers, which record all first contacts with the psychiatric services for a specified area over a specified time period, are a very useful resource, particularly for the determination of incidence rates for severe mental illness, but case registers require considerable work and special funding, and in the UK today very few are maintained. However, the Scandinavian countries have excellent national case registers, on which all psychiatric admissions are recorded, and some of the studies based on Scandinavian data (often conducted by US and UK researchers) are described in this section.

There is an added problem in countries where a substantial proportion of psychiatric practice is in the private sector. In these circumstances, thorough case finding can be assured only by covering all caring agencies, or by doing population screens. An example of the former strategy was employed in the World Health Organization (WHO) Collaborative Study (Sartorius *et al*, 1986), which ascertained all psychiatric contacts with any caring agency in sites in ten countries. The five-centre Epidemiologic Catchment Area survey (ECA) in the USA is an example of population screening. These studies require enormous financial and organisational input. Also, diagnostic issues remain troublesome. Thus, while the WHO study used the Present State Examination (PSE) administered by trained psychiatrists, the ECA resorted to lay interviewers using the Diagnostic Interview Schedule, which has been shown to be overinclusive with respect to schizophrenia.

The third method of case ascertainment has been following particular birth cohorts. For example, the National Survey of Health and Development followed a 1946 birth cohort, and similar birth cohort studies have been particularly useful in studying early influences such as birth complications, abnormalities in childhood, mild cognitive defects and so forth. The main drawback of using birth cohorts is the very long latency before schizophrenia spectrum disorders develop and the relatively small number of cases that appear and are amenable to study.

Prevalence and incidence

The conclusion of many authors on reviewing incidence studies in schizophrenia is that the disease is fairly evenly distributed around the globe. However, the reported annual incidence rates even for 'core' schizophrenia (PSE nuclear schizophrenia) ranged from 0.7 per 1000 in Aarhus, Denmark, to 1.4 per 1000 in Nottingham, England, in the WHO studies (Sartorius *et al*, 1986). More recently, Jablensky (2003) has tabulated the results of 13 studies on the incidence rates of schizophrenia conducted between 1946 and 1999. He points out that the Scandinavian studies, which adopt a similar methodology and case definition, and also use whole national populations for their denominators, all yield broadly similar annual incidence rates, of 0.20–0.27 per 1000. When a broader definition, based on ICD–9, was used, the figures were rather higher and had a greater range (0.16–0.42 per 1000).

A figure of interest to most people is the risk that a particular individual may have of developing schizophrenia during his or her lifetime and this is known as the morbid risk. By combining data based on annual incidence rates, population census data, and the estimated duration of the entire risk period for developing the disorder (which for schizophrenia is usually taken as a 40-year risk period, covering the age range 15–54 years), it is possible, using formulae such as Weinberg's abridged method, to calculate the lifetime morbid risk (see also page 206). This is a probability estimate, usually expressed as a percentage, and most incidence studies yield morbid risk estimates of between 0.5% and 1.6%, with a figure of around 1% often quoted.

The prevalence of a disorder is defined as the number of cases (per 1000 at risk) at given points in time or over a given time period. Prevalence rates are less sensitive than incidence rates to different causative factors. A point-prevalence survey will miss the large number of cases that are in remission, and hence to be meaningful a prevalence study will need to take into account previous episodes of the disorder. For a disorder with a more or less continuous course, like schizophrenia, the point prevalence and 1-year prevalence rates will tend to approximate towards the lifetime prevalence (assuming past episodes are taken into account). Jablensky (2003), summarising data from 23 prevalence studies conducted between 1931 and 1999, gave a range for prevalence rates of 1.4–4.6 per 1000 of the population at risk.

Outlier populations

Even taking account of the difficulties with case finding and diagnosis, a few small geographical pockets exist with true 'outlier' populations where there is either an excess or a deficit of patients with schizophrenia. Thus, high rates have been described in northern Sweden and some parts of Finland. High rates have also been described in a small area of Croatia (the Istrian peninsula) and this is thought to have been due to high rates of emigration during the 19th and early 20th century. A virtual absence of schizophrenia combined with a moderate to high rate of depression has been observed among the Hutterites of South Dakota. Negative selection for individuals who fail to adjust to the communal lifestyle and eventually emigrate has been suggested as a possible cause. Two surveys in Taiwan separated by 15 years (see Lin *et al*, 1989) found that an already low prevalence rate of 2.1 per 1000 had fallen even further, to 1.4 per 1000. In these studies the native aboriginal Taiwanese were found to have lower rates than the mainland Chinese population who had migrated to Taiwan after the Second World War. Thus, although the general consensus is that the prevalence and incidence rates for schizophrenia are broadly similar across populations, there are a few outlier groups, possibly as a result of a complex interaction between genes, culture and migration (Jablensky, 2003).

Age and sex

Schizophrenia may start at any age, but the vast majority of cases occur in the age range 15–54 years. Neither the childhood-onset nor late-onset cases present with any features that are qualitatively different from those characterising schizophrenia in young adults. Peak onset for males is in the 20- to 24-year age group, and the peak is said to occur around 5 years later for females. However, in women there is a less prominent peak in the 20- to 24-year age group, followed by a gradual increase in inception rates for those over 35; with increasing age, say over 60 years, female onset is more common. The WHO ten-country study (Sartorius *et al*, 1986) found that the cumulative risks for males and females up to age 54 were approximately equal, but there were raised rates of onset for females among older people. Thus, for example, Helgason & Magnusson (1989), who examined cohorts up to 85 years of age, found that females actually had a higher accumulated lifetime risk of schizophrenia. Hormonal theories, for example the stimulant effect of androgens on the brain as compared with the possible protective effects of oestrogens on dopaminergic systems in the brain, have been suggested as possible explanations for the observed sex differences in Western studies.

Although most studies point to a sex difference in the age of onset, a study from India comparing consecutive male and female admissions found no difference between the sexes with regard to age of onset, whether the schizophrenia was diagnosed by DSM–IV or other criteria (Murthy *et al*, 1998). The authors suggested that cultural factors, such as learned gender-assigned roles, may explain these findings, but the absence of any sex difference in this study makes a simple hormonal explanation for the sex differences found in Western studies unlikely. An alternative explanation for the difference in reported rates may be that males are more likely to present to services because they tend to have a more severe disease with an earlier onset, more frequent structural brain disease, worse premorbid adjustment and a lower IQ, a picture more consistent with Kraepelin's dementia praecox.

Geographical and social drift

The pioneering study by Faris & Dunham (1939) in Chicago reported that the prevalence rates for schizophrenia decreased from the city centre outwards, in a zonal pattern. Subsequently, Hare (1956) in Bristol found higher rates of schizophrenia in an area where a high proportion of people were living alone. The clustering of patients with schizophrenia in deprived inner-city areas has been repeatedly confirmed since.

Two hypotheses of social causation were developed to explain this. According to the 'breeder' hypothesis, the socio-economic adversity characteristic of inner-city life precipitates schizophrenia in genetically vulnerable individuals, through a variety of mechanisms (e.g. increased rates of obstetric complications, more viral infections in pregnancy, lower social class, greater stress, as well as more frequent later life stresses). Alternatively, according to the 'social drift' explanation, patients with schizophrenia drift down the social scale and move into inner-city areas. This was supported by a study by Goldberg & Morrison (1963), who found that although patients with established schizophrenia were more likely than controls to be categorised as social class V, their fathers showed the same social class distribution as the general population.

The literature is divided on the question of whether lower socio-economic group is a risk factor for schizophrenia; most of the earlier studies (Silverton & Mednick, 1984) found an effect of lower social class, but a recent study, based on the north Finland 1966 birth cohort, found that the risk of schizophrenia was higher among young persons from social class I (as determined by the father's occupation) at the time of illness onset. Rates were 1.14% among children from social class I as compared with 0.47% among children from lower social classes. Since this study was based on a birth cohort, and not on hospital admission data, which are potentially more biased, it tends to negate previous suggestions of an effect for lower socio-economic status, at least before the onset of the first episode (Makikyro *et al*, 1997).

Urban effects

The current literature emphasises the existence of a true urban effect: that is, a high proportion of patients are born in inner cities or deprived areas and they do not merely drift into them. This has not always been the case. Thus, Hare (1998) quotes Prichard (1835, p. 336): 'The fact that insanity presents so much in agricultural districts is favoured by some of the conditions connected with agricultural life', and Hare also comments on the situation in 19th-century Ireland, where there was little in the way of industrialisation and very few large towns, yet the prevalence of insanity rose even more steeply than it did in England.

None the less, by the latter part of the 19th century an effect of urbanisation on the rates for psychosis was apparent. Thus, Torrey *et al* (1997*a*) reanalysed the 1880 US census data for insanity and, taking baseline rates in purely rural counties as 1, the odds ratio for psychosis in semi-rural counties was 1.46, and for urban residence 1.66. This urban effect seemed to be confined to those born in cities.

In confirmation of the latter point, Mortensen *et al* (1999) conducted a study based on the Danish birth register and the Danish national psychiatric case register and found a relative risk of 2.2–4.2 for those born in the capital, Copenhagen, relative to those with a rural birth. Because urban birth is a common risk factor, the population-attributable fraction for urban birth was 34.3% of all cases of schizophrenia in Denmark. This figure should be contrasted with that associated with a high-risk, low-frequency causal factor, such as having a first-degree relative with schizophrenia. Here the relative risk is high at 9.3, but the population-attributable fraction is only 5.5% of cases.

A study by Marcelis *et al* (1999) also confirmed the increased risk was specifically for those born in urban areas and found no additional effect for later urban residence, while urban residence alone, for those who had not been born in the city, did not increase the risk of schizophrenia. These findings tend to negate earlier suggestions of geographical drift (although not of downward social drift). Castle *et al* (1993) found that, compared with non-psychotic controls, patients with schizophrenia were more likely to have been born in socially deprived households in inner London.

Although no single 'urban factor' has been identified, the urban excess is likely to reflect a complex interaction of factors related to genes, selective migration into and out of cities, possibly over several generations, as well as cultural and socio-economic factors, including higher rates of social deprivation and dysfunctional families within urban areas. There is also a suggestion that much of this interplay occurs early in life, or even *in utero*, rather than at the time of illness onset, since it appears that urban birth rather than simple urban residence is the more relevant variable.

Immigration and ethnicity

Studies from a number of different countries have shown that immigrants tend to have a higher risk of schizophrenia than the general population of either their native or their adopted country. For example, Ødegäard (1932) showed that Norwegian immigrants to Minnesota had higher rates than natives of Minnesota, while more recent studies have shown that Afro-Caribbean immigrants have rates of schizophrenia well above those of the indigenous population and with even higher rates in the second generation; this topic is comprehensively reviewed in Chapter 31, on pages 798–799.

Trends over time

Changes in the incidence of a disease over time can afford useful insights into the aetiology of the condition. It has been suggested that schizophrenia was virtually unknown before the industrial revolution and urbanisation. Thus, Cooper & Sartorius (1977) questioned why descriptions of chronic schizophrenia were quite scarce in the European and earlier literature and suggested that social conditions of living in small village communities with supportive extended families may have had a comparatively benign effect on people with schizophrenia, a pattern still found in some developing nations. These protective effects were lost during the process of industrialisation and urbanisation. Certainly, during the 19th century, which was a period of rapid industrialisation, there was a dramatic rise in hospital admissions for insanity. Hare (1998) showed there was a doubling of the admission rate between 1859 and 1909, with the bulk of these increased admissions due to functional disorder. In part this rise may reflect the harsh conditions of Victorian England, where people with a chronic psychosis had no hope of surviving outside an asylum. The rise may also partly be explained as a consequence of the large increase in the number of hospital beds and the number of asylums. Hare (1998) and others, however, have postulated that there may also have been a real increase in disease frequency and also speculated that an infectious agent, such as a virus, may have been responsible.

More recently, reports from a number of Western countries have suggested that there has been a decline in the treated incidence of schizophrenia in recent decades. Der *et al* (1990) found no reciprocal increase in the rate of other psychiatric disorders, which suggests that the effect was not merely due to changes in diagnostic habit; a similar finding has been reported in a case register study in Oxfordshire (de Alarcon *et al*, 1990) and was also reported in Denmark and New Zealand between 1960 and 1990. Presently, it is unclear whether rates are changing or are stable – a judgement that can be made only retrospectively.

Cannabis use

Cannabis (marijuana) is an ancient drug containing many different chemicals, but the most active substance appears to be tetra-hydro-cannabinol (Δ-9-THC). There is general agreement that cannabis can cause acute psychosis or a relapse of symptoms among patients with an established psychotic illness. Cannabinoid receptors are co-localised within the dopaminergic system in the brain and Δ-9-THC may increase the release of dopamine. This may explain why acute cannabis intoxication worsens the psychotic symptoms.

Another compound present in cannabis, cannabidiol, lacks these psychotogenic effects, and may even be antipsychotic, but certainly has anxiolytic effects. This may explain the frequently reported 'relaxing' effect of smoking cannabis (Atakan, 2004).

Cannabis use is increased among people who develop schizophrenia, but this does not necessarily mean that cannabis is a cause: the increased use may merely be an epiphenomenon. Arseneault *et al* (2004) reviewed five longitudinal studies that had addressed this question. In the first of these studies, Andréasson *et al* (1998) observed a dose–response relationship between cannabis use at age 18 and the development of schizophrenia 15 years later, and found a relative risk of 2.3. However, only 3% of heavy cannabis users went on to develop schizophrenia, or, put another way, 97% of heavy cannabis users do not develop schizophrenia. Two studies from New Zealand also showed that cannabis use preceded the onset of schizophrenia and in one of these a dose-dependent relationship was also shown; cannabis use was more strongly associated with schizophrenia than with other psychiatric disorders. Even after controlling for social class, employment status, IQ and a variety of other socio-demographic variables, cannabis use appeared to double the risk for schizophrenia. Arseneault *et al* (2004) estimated that the population-attributable fraction due to cannabis use is around 8%. They cautioned against assuming that cannabis is a major cause, and suggested that it must interact with other causes, although precise mechanisms are presently unclear.

Genetics

Systematic family studies on schizophrenia began soon after Kraepelin's delineation of dementia praecox from manic–depressive illness at the end of the 19th century. These early studies, summarised by Gottesman & Shields (1982), demonstrated both familial clustering and the lack of simple Mendelian ratios (Table 10.1). The methodology of these studies is described in Box 10.1. The results show that, compared with the general population, in which there is a lifetime risk of schizophrenia of 0.5–1.6%, the siblings and offspring of

Table 10.1 Lifetime expectancy of schizophrenia in the relatives of people with schizophrenia

Type of relative	Number at risk (BZ)	Morbid risk (%)
Parents	8020	5.6
Siblings	9920	10.1
Children	1577	12.9
Half-siblings	499	4.2
Uncles/aunts	2421	2.4
Nephews/nieces	3965	3.0
Grandchildren	739	3.7
First cousins	1600	2.4

BZ: *Bezugsziffer*, the equivalent number of relatives after age adjustment.
From Gottesman & Shields (1982).

people with schizophrenia have a 10- to 20-fold increase in risk. The relatively low risk in the parents compared with the offspring of schizophrenic probands has been attributed to the reduced fecundity of individuals who have developed the disorder. Omitted from Table 10.1 are data on children whose parents both have schizophrenia. Erlenmeyer-Kimling (1968) summarised the relevant data from the literature and found 62 affected out of 194 such offspring, which, after age correction, represents a lifetime risk of 46%.

More recent family studies have employed DSM criteria and included relatives of unaffected individuals; these have found similarly elevated risk ratios in the relatives of affected probands (Kendler *et al*, 1985, 1993; Gershon *et al*, 1988; Maier *et al*, 1993).

Twin studies

Familial aggregation can result from both shared environmental influences and shared genes. Twins offer a 'natural experiment' that allows genetic factors to be untangled from environmental factors. Twin data can be interpreted in the framework of a *liability-threshold model* to estimate *heritability*, an index of the importance of genetic relative to environmental factors for explaining individual differences in vulnerability. The methodology and the underlying assumptions of twin studies are described in Box 10.2, while the liability-threshold model and the interpretation of the often misunderstood concept of heritability is explained in Fig. 10.1.

Gottesman & Shields (1982) summarised the results of earlier and more recent twin studies of schizophrenia. Overall, the earlier studies gave MZ and DZ pairwise concordance rates of 65% and 12%, respectively. More systematic studies were conducted in Finland (Tiernari, 1971), Norway (Kringlen, 1976), Denmark (Fischer *et al*, 1971), the USA (Pollin *et al*, 1969) and the UK (Gottesman & Shields, 1972). Pooled MZ and DZ probandwise concordance rates from these studies were 46% and 14%, respectively.

The first studies to apply modern diagnostic criteria to twins were by McGuffin *et al* (1984) and Farmer *et al* (1987). These used a polydiagnostic approach and found that schizophrenia as defined by DSM–III criteria was more heritable than schizophrenia as defined by broader definitions, such as Schneider's first-rank symptoms. Onstad *et al* (1991) addressed the same issue and found that broadening the diagnosis

Box 10.1 Methods in genetic studies of schizophrenia

The primary aim of family studies is to demonstrate familial aggregation of a disease or trait. The presence of familial aggregation suggests, but does not prove, genetic aetiology. Family studies are also useful for investigating the relationships between different diseases and traits.

Sampling

In order to avoid the overinclusion of families with multiple affected members, families must be systematically ascertained. The standard methodology is to adopt a two-stage sampling scheme:

- In stage 1, a random sample of individuals with the disease is obtained. These affected individuals are called index cases or 'probands'.
- In stage 2, the relatives of the probands are assessed for the presence or absence of the disease (as well as other related traits). Relatives found to have the disease are called 'secondary cases'.

Comparison groups

An ideal study would include a comparison group, in which the probands are individuals from the same population as the index cases but who do not have the disease. Where possible, the diagnoses of both probands and relatives should be made according to operational criteria using information obtained from personal interviews with standardised instruments (e.g. the Diagnostic Interview for Genetic Studies, DIGS). However, some relatives may be deceased or for other reasons unavailable for direct interview. In order to avoid bias it is important to obtain information on these individuals from informants (e.g. their parents, siblings or children) using standardised instruments (e.g. the Family Interview for Genetic Studies, FIGS), supplemented by medical notes. It is also important that the assessment of relatives is blind to the diagnostic status of the proband.

Risk estimation

The risk of disease in a relative of a proband is called 'morbid risk' or 'recurrence risk'. For a disease with variable age at onset, there is the problem of 'censoring', which is that some unaffected relatively young individuals may yet develop the disease in later life. There are two classes of methods for making an 'age-adjustment' in the calculation of morbid risk. The simpler methods, introduced by Weinberg and modified by Stromgren (see Slater & Cowie, 1971), require assumptions to be made about the age-at-onset distribution. The more sophisticated methods use some form of survival analysis (life table or Kaplan–Meier estimators) and do not require prior assumptions to be made about the age-at-onset distribution.

A measure of familial aggregation is the relative risk ratio, often designated λ, which is defined as the ratio of morbid risk among the relatives of cases to that among the relatives of controls, for a specific class of relatives (e.g. parent, sibling, offspring).

Box 10.2 Twin studies

The existence of two types of twin pairs, monozygotic (MZ) and dizygotic (DZ), provides a natural experiment for untangling genetic from environmental factors. MZ twins are developed from the same fertilised ovum and are therefore genetically identical; DZ twins are developed from two separate fertilised ova and share on average 50% of their genes. The validity of the twin design depends on two critical assumptions

- Twins are no different from the general population in terms of the trait in question.
- MZ and DZ twin pairs share their environments to the same extent, with respect to factors relevant to the trait in question (the equal environment assumption).

There are two main types of twin studies: those based on twin pairs ascertained through affected probands, and those based on population twin registers. The inference of a genetic component from proband-ascertained twin pairs is usually based on a difference between MZ and DZ concordance rates. The probandwise concordance rate is defined as the percentage of probands who have an affected co-twin. An earlier measure, called the pairwise concordance rate, is defined as the percentage of twin pairs in which both members are affected. However, this measure cannot be interpreted without knowledge of the intensity of ascertainment, and is therefore obsolete.

A variation of the twin method is the co-twin control method. This method studies differences in MZ twins who are discordant for a particular disorder. The ill and healthy twins are genetically identical, so these pairs can be used to study environmental reasons why some individuals develop the disorder and others do not.

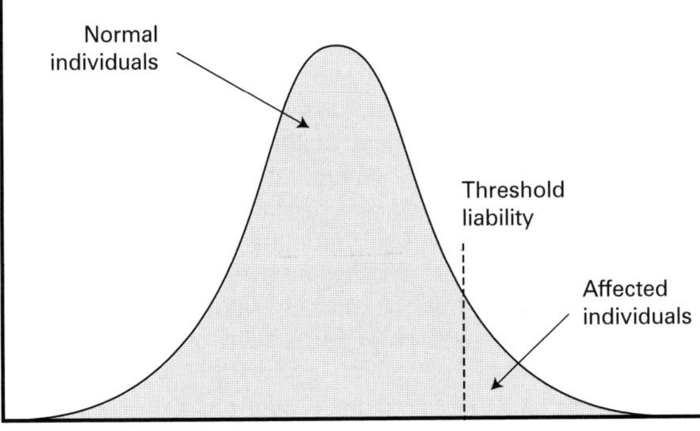

Fig. 10.1 Liability threshold model: heritability. Each individual has an underlying liability which is determined by both genetic and environmental factors. The frequency distribution of liability in the population follows a normal, bell-shaped distribution, reflecting the operation of multiple genetic and environmental factors, each of small or modest effect. There is a threshold value in liability: individuals whose liability is above the threshold develop the disorder, whereas those with lower liability do not (see Falconer, 1965).

to include schizoaffective disorder, atypical psychosis and schizotypal personality increased the MZ:DZ ratio in concordance rates, but broadening out further to include affective disorders and personality disorders lowered the ratio.

The most recent twin studies, which have used ICD–10 or DSM–III–R criteria have been summarised by Cardno & Gottesman (2000): the pooled MZ and DZ probandwise concordance rates were 50% and 4% for DSM–III–R criteria, and 42% and 4% for ICD–10 criteria. Using model-fitting methods, they estimated heritabilities of 88% for DSM–III–R and 83% for ICD–10 criteria, which are quite high and indicate that more than four-fifths of the variance in the cause of schizophrenia is genetically determined.

Further evidence that familial resemblance for schizophrenia is mostly due to genetic factors is provided by data from identical twins reared apart. Gottesman & Shields (1982) identified from the literature 14 pairs of MZ twins in which at one least one member had schizophrenia and found that nine of these were concordant for schizophrenia.

Adoption studies

Adoption provides another method for untangling genetic from environmental influences on disease (see Box 10.3). In the first major adoption study of schizophrenia, conducted in Oregon, USA, Heston (1966) studied 47 adoptees born to mothers with schizophrenia and 50 control adoptees. He reported rates of schizophrenia in the index group that were significantly higher (5/47, 11%) when compared with the control group (0/50, 0%).

In Denmark, Rosenthal *et al* (1971) found that the rate of 'schizophrenia spectrum' disorders among the adoptees with a psychotic biological parent was 14/52

Box 10.3 Adoption studies

Individuals who are adopted at birth receive their genes from their biological parents and their rearing environment from their adoptive parents. Similarities between adoptees and their biological relatives are therefore likely to be due to shared genes, whereas similarities between adoptees and the adoptive family are likely to be due to shared environment.

There are several types of adoption study. The adoptees design compares the adopted children of affected and unaffected biological parents. An improved version of this design incorporates the affection status of the adoptive parents. If the affection status of the biological parents is related to morbid risk in the adoptee, after adjusting for the affection status of the adoptive parents, then genetic factors are implicated.

The adoptee's family design compares morbid risk in the biological and adoptive families of affected adoptees. An improved version of this design includes the biological and adoptive families of unaffected adoptees. A greater morbid risk among biological than among adoptive family members of affected but not unaffected adoptees would implicate genetic factors.

(27%), compared with a rate of 12/67 (18%) among control adoptees. When these data were reanalysed using DSM–II criteria for parents and DSM–III for offspring, the rates of schizophrenia spectrum disorders (defined as schizophrenia and schizotypal and schizoid personality disorders) were 11/39 (28%) among adoptees with an affected biological parent and 4/39 (10%) among control adoptees (Lowing *et al*, 1983).

Conversely, does being reared by ill parents cause schizophrenia among individuals of normal genetic risk? Wender *et al* (1974) examined 21 adoptees of normal biological parents but whose adoptive parent developed schizophrenia, and found only one adoptee with a schizophrenia spectrum disorder.

A more detailed account of the Finnish cross-fostering studies of Tienari *et al* (2004) and the way genes and the environment interact is given towards the end of this chapter on page 229.

Kety *et al* (1976, 1994) conducted further adoption studies in Denmark using the adoptee's family method. They compared the rate of illness among the biological and adoptive relatives of ill and well adoptees. The combined results of the two samples ('Greater Copenhagen' and 'Provincial') gave the rates of schizophrenia spectrum disorders as 46/344 (13%) among the biological relatives of affected adoptees, 9/295 (3%) among the biological relatives of control adoptees, 2/145 (1%) among the adoptive relatives of affected adoptees, and 5/146 (3%) among the adoptive relatives of control adoptees. An independent analysis of these samples, using personal interviews and DSM–III criteria, found the rate of schizophrenia spectrum (defined as mainly schizophrenia, but also schizoaffective disorder, as well as schizotypal and schizoid personality disorders) in the above four classes of relatives to be 9/38, 5/107, 0/30 and 1/102, respectively (Kendler *et al*, 1994).

Mode of inheritance

From the earliest family studies it was clear that schizophrenia does not exhibit simple Mendelian segregation ratios and is therefore genetically complex (Box 10.4). Before the molecular revolution in genetics, many attempts were made to discriminate between different complex genetic models, with limited success (Rao *et al*, 1981; Baron, 1986). Nevertheless, most of the evidence supports the operation of multiple genes. For example, McGue & Gottesman (1989) considered the empirical relative risk ratios of schizophrenia as a function of genetic relationship and excluded a single-locus model. Similarly, Risch (1990) compared the same data with predictions from multi-locus models and concluded that there are at least three loci acting multiplicatively on the risk of illness.

Given that multiple loci are likely to be involved in schizophrenia, an obvious question is whether there is a single locus among these multiple loci that has a disproportionately large effect. Risch (1990) concluded from his analyses that a major gene is unlikely to be present. Similarly, complex segregation analysis of a systematically ascertained sample of 270 pedigrees from Sweden also failed to find evidence for a major locus (Vogler *et al*, 1990). Taken together, these results suggest that most cases of schizophrenia are caused by a combination of multiple genetic and environmental factors, and that genes with a very large effect are either absent or very rare.

Box 10.4 Mode of inheritance

Simple Mendelian modes of inheritance such as autosomal dominant and recessive have predictable patterns of relative risk ratios. For a rare autosomal dominant disease, the ratios are ½ for parents, siblings and offspring, ¼ for second-degree relatives, and so on. For a rare recessive condition, the ratio is ¼ for siblings, and other relatives are rarely affected. Most psychiatric disorders such as schizophrenia do not show such simple Mendelian ratios. Their mode of inheritance is sometimes called non-Mendelian or complex. The complexity refers to the likely involvement of multiple genes and environmental factors.

Although the true complexity of psychosis is likely to be great, attempts have been made to fit data to idealised models that might represent approximations to reality. The two extreme types are the single major locus model and the polygenic model. In the single major locus model, the genetic component is due to a single gene that has a major influence on risk but is nevertheless neither necessary nor sufficient for the disease. Technically, the absence of disease among some genetically predisposed individuals is called incomplete penetrance, while individuals who are affected despite being genetically non-predisposed are called phenocopies. At the other extreme, the polygenic model posits a very large number of genes, each of small effect. The cumulative effects of multiple genes lead to a continuous distribution, which may be related to disease through a liability-threshold model. Between these extremes are oligogenic models, in which a small number of genes are involved, and mixed models, in which a major locus is present in a background of polygenes.

Different genetic models are discriminated by an assessment of their goodness of fit with family data. For schizophrenia, morbid risk data on many classes of relatives from multiple studies have been summarised and tabulated, and provide convenient data for model fitting. When raw pedigree data are available, however, a statistically more powerful approach is complex segregation analysis. The results of such analyses, however, are often inconsistent, with some studies favouring a single major locus model and others favouring a polygenic model. It appears that the analysis of disease phenotypic data alone (without the help of molecular genetic markers) is limited in its ability to resolve different genetic models. Power is more favourable for quantitative traits; a locus that accounts for a substantial proportion (say, over a third) of the phenotypic variance is likely to be detectable by segregation analysis.

Refining the phenotype

The first systematic family study of schizophrenia, conducted by Rüdin in Kraepelin's Psychiatric Institute in Munich in 1916, found that the siblings of patients with schizophrenia had increased rates not only of schizophrenia but also of other potentially related disorders. Similarly, the classic adoption studies by Heston, Rosenthal and Kety, as described above, all showed an increase in the rate of a 'schizophrenia spectrum' of disorders. Furthermore, the twin studies have shown that the MZ:DZ concordance ratio is increased by the inclusion of schizoaffective disorder, atypical psychosis and schizotypal personality disorder, but decreased by the inclusion of affective disorders. These data suggest that what is inherited is a liability to develop not only schizophrenia but also a range of other psychotic conditions and personality disorders.

Early family and twin studies also examined the degree to which the classic schizophrenia subtypes (i.e. hebephrenic, paranoid, catatonic and simple – see Chapter 8) tend to breed true in families. The results indicate only a weak tendency for the subtypes to sort within families, so that the risk of every subtype is increased for the siblings of probands of any subtype (Gottesman & Shields, 1982). Age of onset is another potential variable for classifying schizophrenia but it is only modestly correlated between pairs of affected relatives, and early onset is only moderately predictive of higher familial morbid risk (Kendler & MacLean, 1990; Sham *et al*, 1994).

Another attempt to tease out genetic from environmental cases of schizophrenia is to separate out patients with a family history of the illness from those without (Murray *et al*, 1985). However, the absence of a family history does not necessarily imply the absence of a genetic predisposition. Even for twins with schizophrenia whose MZ co-twin is unaffected, the risk of schizophrenia among their offspring is elevated to a level similar to that observed among offspring of people with schizophrenia in general (Gottesman & Bertelsen, 1989; Kringlen & Cramer, 1989). A similar increase in risk is observed also for the offspring of the well members of these discordant MZ twin pairs, which clearly indicates the non-expression of some high-risk genotypes.

Another issue concerning the phenotypic boundaries of schizophrenia is the relationship with affective disorders. While Kraepelin distinguished dementia praecox from manic–depression, and early family studies appeared to support this distinction, the frequent co-occurrence of symptoms of both disorders in the same patients would suggest the operation of some common aetiological factors. Cardno *et al* (2002) used the Maudsley twin register to examine the relationship between the non-hierarchical syndromes of schizophrenia, schizoaffective disorder and mania, and found evidence of a large common genetic component for all three syndromes, with schizophrenia and mania (but not schizoaffective disorder) also having syndrome-specific genetic components.

Linkage studies

Molecular biology has transformed the study of genetics. Whereas the 'old genetics' was merely concerned with establishing whether there are significant hereditary effects and attempted to quantify them, the 'new genetics' has a very different approach and aims to isolate and discover the actual genes, locate their positions on the various chromosomes and determine their chemical structure. There has been an explosion of research interest in this area. As in any new area of research, exciting findings made by one group fail to be replicated by another team, and effects initially thought to be large are then found virtually to disappear when examined by large multinational groups. The whole area is in a state of flux and the account below provides only a snapshot of the present and rapidly changing picture; it is more than likely that some of the genes that are presently of interest will fade in importance, only to be replaced by other candidate genes.

Box 10.5 Linkage studies

Linkage analysis is based on the principle that the alleles of two or more genetic loci on the same chromosome tend to segregate (i.e. be passed on) together from parent to offspring. This is because they are physically linked to each other on the same strand of DNA. During the process of meiosis (specialised cell division that occurs in the manufacture of sperm or egg cells) chromosome breaks occur and there is a physical exchange of chromosomal material, so that only one part of an old chromosome will be incorporated into the new chromosome; this process is called recombination. The closer two loci are together, the lower is the chance of their being separated by a recombination event during meiosis, and the stronger the observed linkage. This phenomenon can be applied to the detection of loci for genetic diseases. If a marker is close to a disease-causing gene, alleles of the marker will tend to co-segregate with the disorder in families, or be shared between affected relatives.

Until the 1980s, the application of linkage analysis to disease gene mapping was hampered by the lack of suitable genetic markers in many regions of the genome. Then, the discovery of highly polymorphic, short-sequence repeat markers throughout the genome, and the development of high-throughput genotyping technology, made it feasible to scan the entire genome for disease-predisposing loci. This method of mapping disease-related genes does not depend on knowledge of disease pathophysiology and is therefore known as positional cloning.

Classical linkage analysis of Mendelian diseases is usually conducted on large, multigenerational, multiply affected pedigrees. The standard method of analysis is based on log-likelihood ratios (or lod scores) for the alternative hypotheses of linkage and non-linkage at a particular marker or chromosomal location, assuming a specific model of the disease. A lod score of 3 (which corresponds to an odds ratio of 1000:1 in favour of linkage) or more is the standard criterion for declaring linkage, since at this level of evidence the probability of a false positive result is less than 0.05, assuming the specified model to be correct (Morton, 1955; Ott, 1991).

An alternative strategy of linkage analysis that does not require a disease model to be specified is the affected sib pair method. This method simply uses the marker data to estimate the allele sharing between affected sibling pairs at a particular chromosomal location, and then tests whether the level of allele sharing is greater than that expected for sibling pairs in general.

The first generation of linkage studies on schizophrenia targeted chromosomal regions that contain candidate genes (e.g. dopamine receptor genes) or where abnormalities such as translocations or deletions have been associated with schizophrenia. These studies also sought large, multiply affected pedigrees, considered most likely to harbour genes with major effect. Following a report of partial trisomy of the long (q) arm of chromosome 5 resulting from an unbalanced translocation with chromosome 1 (Bassett *et al*, 1988), Sherrington *et al* (1988) analysed seven UK and Icelandic pedigrees and found a lod score of 6.49 in the region 5q11–13. Although this original report was accompanied by a negative study on the same chromosomal region (Kennedy *et al*, 1988), this discrepancy was interpreted as likely to be due to genetic heterogeneity (Lander, 1988). However, numerous attempts at replication failed to find linkage to this region, and reanalyses of the original pedigrees yielded reduced evidence for linkage (Kalsi *et al*, 1999). The reasons for the very high lod score in the original study are unclear, although one factor might be that multiple phenotypic definitions were considered in order to find one that gave the best lod score.

Positive linkage was next reported, at 22q12–13, by Pulver *et al* (1994*a*). These authors established a multicentre collaboration in an attempt to confirm their finding, but the results from the combined sample of 256 families were negative (Pulver *et al*, 1994*b*). Recognising the need for large samples in order to detect linkage to genes with a modest effect size, a further collaborative study was set up that involved the pooling of data from 11 groups (Gill *et al*, 1996). The combined data provided modest but statistically significant evidence for linkage to one of the markers, using an affected sib pair method of analysis.

Positive linkage signals were subsequently reported at 8p22–21 (Pulver *et al*, 1994*c*) and 6p24–22 (Straub *et al*, 1995). Both findings received additional support from the Schizophrenia Linkage Collaborative Group study, which pooled data from 14 groups (Levinson *et al*, 1996).

Linkage to 13q32 markers was first reported by Lin *et al* (1995, 1997). These reports were followed by a strikingly positive study by Blouin *et al* (1998), but no linkage was found in this region by the Schizophrenia Linkage Collaborative Group (Levinson *et al*, 2000). Other regions for which positive linkage findings have been reported include 1q21–22, 6q21–22, 10p11–15, and 15q14 (see review by Sklar, 2002). The finding at 15q14 was intriguing in that the phenotype was P50, an event-related potential that is a possible endophenotype for schizophrenia, and in that the region also contained the alpha-7 nicotinic receptor (Freedman *et al*, 1997).

Two recent meta-analyses of schizophrenia linkage studies have been conducted. The first (Badner & Gershon, 2002) focused on specific regions and found significant results on chromosomes 8p, 13q and 22q. The second (Lewis *et al*, 2003) was genome-wide and identified 2p–q to be the most significant locus, followed by 5q, 3p, 11q, 6p, 1p–q, 22q11–12, 8p, 20p and 14pter–q13. These meta-analyses differed in important respects, including statistical methodology and the choice of studies.

In summary, linkage studies of schizophrenia have produced somewhat inconsistent results. This picture is consistent with multi-locus aetiology where the contribution of each locus to risk is small. Nevertheless, some regions have provided positive findings in multiple studies, and in recent years some of these have been subjected to intensive search for susceptibility alleles by association analysis.

Association studies

Box 10.6 describes the design of association studies. Two major strategies have been adopted in the search for genetic variants that increase the risk of schizophrenia. The first is to focus on genes for which there are

Box 10.6 Association studies

An association between a specific allele and a disease is defined as a greater frequency of the allele among individuals with the disease than among those without. As is well known in epidemiology, association suggests, but does not imply, causation. Aside from direct causation, an allele may be associated with a disease for two main reasons:

- poor matching between cases and controls – either in ethnic origin (population stratification) or age (selection of longevity genes)
- the association of the allele with a causative allele through linkage disequilibrium (LD).

LD is the tendency for very closely linked loci to show allelic association with each other. The reason for LD is that recombination rarely occurs between very closely linked loci during meiosis, so that any allelic association introduced into the population by past mutations or population bottlenecks will be maintained for many generations. Thus, a disease allele that arose through a mutation on a chromosome that happens to contain a particular combination of alleles in close proximity will continue to be associated with this combination of alleles (known as a haplotype) for many generations.

The existence of LD raises the possibility of scanning chromosomal regions or the entire genome by association analysis with only a fraction of all genetic polymorphisms in the regions or in the genome. The discovery and cataloguing of millions of single-nucleotide polymorphisms (SNPs) and the development of economic, high-throughput genotyping technologies are preparing the ground for large-scale association studies. An international effort, called the HapMap project, is currently characterising the whole-genome LD structure in the major human populations, in order to identify SNP sets that are most efficient for large-scale association studies.

The most common design for association studies is the case–control study. Specific alleles or haplotypes are tested for differences in frequency between cases and controls, adjusting for potential confounding factors if necessary. Alternative designs that use related controls, usually parents or siblings of affected individuals, have the advantage that they are robust to false positive association arising from hidden population stratification. Data on affected individuals and their parents are usually analysed using the transmission/disequilibrium test (TDT), which examines heterozygous parents to see whether some alleles are preferentially transmitted to affected offspring.

functional or other reasons for a possible role in the aetiology of schizophrenia. Examples of genes suggested by functional considerations include those involved in the dopaminergic, serotonergic, and glutamatergic and other neurotransmitter pathways, and those involved in neuromodulation and in neurodevelopment. Other genes have been suggested by cytogenetic abnormalities, such as deletions or translocations that are associated with psychotic features, and still others by gene expression studies demonstrating differences between patients and controls. The second major approach is the systematic screening of regions suggested by linkage studies.

The dopaminergic system has been extensively examined for allelic association with schizophrenia. Homozygosity for a Ser9Gly polymorphism in exon 1 of the dopamine D3 receptor gene (DRD3) was reported to be associated with schizophrenia (Crocq *et al*, 1992). Attempted replication studies have produced both positive and negative results, but a more recent meta-analysis of 48 studies, excluding the original report, supported a weak association – an estimated relative risk of only 1.13 (Lohmueller *et al*, 2003).

A similar story has also emerged from the serotonergic system. An initial report of an association between a T to C polymorphism at nucleotide 102 in the 5-HT_{2A} receptor gene and schizophrenia was replicated by a large European consortium (Williams *et al*, 1996) and further supported by a meta-analysis (Williams *et al*, 1997). However, the latest relative risk estimate based on 28 studies, excluding the original report, is only 1.07 (Lohmueller *et al*, 2003).

Cytogenetic studies

Cytogenetic abnormalities associated with psychotic symptoms may provide clues to the locations of susceptibility genes (Bassett *et al*, 2000; MacIntyre *et al*, 2003). For example, balanced reciprocal translocation between chromosomes 1q42 and 11q14.3 was found to co-segregate with schizophrenia, bipolar disorder and recurrent major depression in a large Scottish family (St Clair *et al*, 1990). This translocation disrupts two genes on chromosome 1 called DISC1 and DISC2 (Millar *et al*, 2000), and there is evidence that the DISC1 protein may regulate cytoskeletal function, and that its disruption may affect neuronal migration and neurite architecture (Miyoshi *et al*, 2003). Interestingly, DISC1 is close to regions of the genome with positive linkage findings for schizophrenia from Finland (Hovatta *et al*, 2000).

Another cytogenetic abnormality that may be relevant to schizophrenia is the velo-cardio-facial syndrome (VCFS), also known as DiGeorge or Shprintzen syndrome, which is caused by small interstitial deletions of chromosome 22q11. Individuals with VCFS show characteristic cranial facial dysmorphology, cleft palate and congenital heart disease and learning difficulties, and have an increased risk of psychosis (Pulver *et al*, 1994*c*). These patients have smaller cerebellar and temporal lobes and decreased hippocampal volumes than controls. In a series of 50 patients, 15 (30%) had a psychosis and 12 (24%) met DSM–IV criteria for schizophrenia (Murphy *et al*, 1999). The location of the deletions on chromosome 22 has been implicated by some linkage studies on schizophrenia (Lewis *et al*, 2003). The gene for catechol-o-methyl transferase (COMT), an enzyme involved in dopamine metabolism, is also on chromosome 22 and is deleted in VCFS; this has aroused great interest in the genes on chromosome 22. A valine-to-methionine (Val/Met) polymorphism in COMT was reported to be associated with schizophrenia in Chinese families (Li *et al*, 1996), but not in a more recent study on Ashkenazi Jews, which instead found strong evidence for association with a haplotype containing the Val/Met polymorphism and two other polymorphisms (Shifman *et al*, 2002). Studies have shown the valine allele to be associated with impaired frontal lobe function (Egan *et al*, 2001).

Another gene located in the VCFS region codes for proline dehydrogenase, a mitochondrial enzyme that when inactivated leads to sensorimotor gating deficits in mice. A complex pattern of association between polymorphisms in the proline dehydrogenase gene and schizophrenia has been reported (Liu *et al*, 2002) but so far attempts at replication have been negative (Williams *et al*, 2003).

Anticipation

In contrast to cytogenetic abnormalities, the phenomenon of anticipation has provided possible clues about the nature, but not the locations, of the susceptibility genes for schizophrenia. Anticipation is the tendency, in families with affected individuals in multiple generations, for those affected individuals in the younger generations to have earlier onset and greater severity of the disease than those in the older generations. Anticipation is often observed in diseases caused by expanded trinucleotide repeats (e.g. Huntington's disease), because of the tendency of the number of repeats to increase from one generation to the next.

Anticipation has long been documented in serious mental disorders, and has been reported to occur in schizophrenia in more recent family studies (O'Donovan & Owen, 1996). Although anticipation in mental disorders is often attributed to sampling artefacts (e.g. the relative ease of ascertaining affected parent–offspring pairs whose onsets are close in time compared with those whose onsets are far apart), the discovery that expanded trinucleotide repeats can cause anticipation led to speculation that such mutations may be involved in schizophrenia.

Repeat expansion detection (RED) is a type of analysis that allows for a search for trinucleotide expansion anywhere in the genome. The anticipation hypothesis was supported by two groups who used RED and found that the maximum length of the most common known pathogenic trinucleotide repeat, CAG/CTG, was greater in patients with schizophrenia than in unaffected controls, findings that were later replicated in a European multicentre study (O'Donovan *et al*, 1996). Unfortunately, these early RED studies were followed by a series of unsuccessful attempts to identify the relevant repeat-containing loci by a variety of other methods, as well as by several failures to replicate the RED findings (Laurent *et al*, 1998; Vincent *et al*, 1999), thus casting doubt on the CAG/CTG repeat hypothesis.

Systematic screening

The systematic screening of positive linkage regions for association requires the genotyping of a large number of genetic markers and is therefore an expensive undertaking. Association between polymorphisms in the dysbindin (DTNBP1) gene and schizophrenia was found in a systematic screen of positive linkage regions identified in Irish families (Straub *et al*, 2002). This finding was replicated in a sample of German and Israeli families (Schwab *et al*, 2003), but not in a case–control sample from Dublin (Morris *et al*, 2003). DTNBP1 codes for a protein that binds to dystrobrevin, part of the dystrophin receptor complex involved in muscular dystrophy. The protein is also found in some neurons and may be involved in synaptic formation and maintenance, signal transduction and receptor gene expression via N-methyl-D-aspartate (NMDA) glutamatergic receptor function (Benson *et al*, 2001).

In a systematic screen of a positive linkage region on chromosome 8p, associations were found between schizophrenia and a specific haplotype of several polymorphisms around neuro-regulin 1 (NRG1) (Stefansson *et al*, 2002). The finding was replicated in Scottish and Welsh samples (Stefansson *et al*, 2003; Williams *et al*, 2003). NRG1 modulates the expression and activities of the NMDA glutamatergic receptors, and is an important regulator of glial cells and myelination.

A novel gene called G72 was found to be associated with schizophrenia in a systematic screen of the positive linkage region on chromosome 13 (Chumakov *et al*, 2002). G72 is primate-specific gene expressed in human caudate and amygdala, and its protein product was found to show *in vitro* interaction with D-amino-oxidase (DAAO), an enzyme that may affect NMDA glutamatergic receptor function via modulation of the levels of D-serine. Chumakov *et al* (2002) also found evidence for an association between DAAO and schizophrenia, and an interaction between G72 and DAAO in elevating the risk of schizophrenia. Intriguingly, a subsequent study found a possible association between G72 markers and bipolar disorder (Hattori *et al*, 2003).

Genome-wide expression studies

The results of genome-wide gene expression studies of post-mortem brain tissues using microarray technology have also provided candidate genes for schizophrenia. One study identified the downregulation of six genes, all of which are expressed in oligodendrocytes and implicated in the formation of myelin sheaths (Hakak *et al*, 2001). Remarkably, one of these genes, ERBB3, is a member of the family of neuregulin receptors.

Another genome-wide gene expression study has found that the regulator of G-protein signalling-4 is downregulated in schizophrenia (Mirnics *et al*, 2001). This protein dampens the effects of agonists at G-protein-coupled receptors, including some dopamine and serotonin receptors. Association between polymorphisms of this gene was reported in two US samples but not in a larger Indian sample (Chowdari *et al*, 2002).

Summary

Because schizophrenia is thought to be inherited by polygenetic mechanisms, it is not surprising that a large number of genes have been isolated; it is quite unclear at present which ones will survive more rigorous study and remain of interest. Presently, the evidence is best for neuregulin and dysbindin genes, but almost certainly new genes will be discovered in the coming years. Riley *et al* (2003) conclude their comprehensive review of the topic by expressing the view that, as more key loci are identified, it may be possible for the molecular basis of schizophrenia to be understood in the foreseeable future – a dream that would have been unthinkable a generation ago.

Prenatal risk factors

Time and place of birth

Since the first report of an association between severe psychiatric disorder and season of birth, by Tramer (1929), more than 250 studies from 29 countries in the northern hemisphere and several in the southern hemisphere have been remarkably consistent in showing a 5–8% winter–spring excess of births for both schizophrenia and mania/bipolar disorder (see Hare *et al*, 1974; Bradbury & Miller, 1985; Torrey *et al*, 1997*b*). However, a meta-analysis of 12 studies from the southern hemisphere failed to replicate this, finding only a very small effect (odds ratio = 1.04) for winter births compared with all other births (McGrath & Welham, 1999). It is important to note that 'season of birth' effects are not specific for schizophrenia and have also been described in bipolar affective disorder, autism, attention-deficit hyperactivity disorder, alcoholism, still births, Alzheimer's disease and Down's syndrome, and their cause is poorly understood (Jablensky, 2003). Some of the proposed explanations for the effect – notably that it is a methodological artefact, or represents a seasonal pattern of procreation – have been considered unlikely (Hare, 1976). A currently popular hypothesis is that it may be due to some environmental factor that fluctuates with the seasons, for example a virus, and exerts its effects on the foetus or the newborn (Torrey *et al*, 1997*b*). Such an explanation is also compatible with the more recent data from the southern hemisphere, where possibly the putative environmental factor may be less prevalent or weaker.

Obstetric complications

The presence of obstetric complications (OCs), either during pregnancy or around birth, is one of the most studied risk factors for schizophrenia (reviewed by McNeil *et al*, 2000). The earlier studies mostly compared small numbers of cases and controls, using maternal recall for the assessment of OCs. A meta-analysis of these earlier studies gave a statistically significant pooled odds ratio (OR) of 2.0, although there was some evidence of publication bias (Geddes & Lawrie, 1995). This was followed by an analysis of the data from 12 case–control studies that used the Lewis–Murray scale for OCs (Geddes *et al*, 1999). Schizophrenia was significantly associated with premature rupture of membranes (OR = 3.1), gestational age less than 37 weeks (OR = 2.4) and use of resuscitation or incubator (OR = 2.2). There was an almost significant association with birth weight of less than 2500 g (OR = 1.5).

Recent studies have used population cohorts with contemporaneous obstetric records to circumvent the problem of maternal recall, but suffer from other methodological problems, including the variability of obstetric records and inadequate statistical power due to the rarity of both schizophrenia and particular types of OC (Cannon *et al*, 2000). Nevertheless, a number of these studies have reported significant associations with hypoxia-related OCs (Cannon *et al*, 2000) and with prematurity and low birth weight (Sacker *et al*, 1995; Jones *et al*, 1998; Dalman *et al*, 1999). Although the presence of OCs increases the risk of schizophrenia, the overall contribution (i.e. the population-attributable fraction) is probably quite small. For example, in the study by Dalman *et al* (1999), in which a total of 500 000 births were examined, pre-eclampsia emerged as the strongest risk factor, with the increase being 2–2.5 times; however, out of 238 individuals who subsequently developed schizophrenia, only 11 had a history of pre-eclampsia and of these around five would have been expected to have had it anyway. Figures were also low for extreme prematurity (five cases) and for very low birth weight (two cases). The effect of OCs is probably non-specific, as people are more likely to have abnormalities on magnetic resonance imaging (MRI) in later life and raised rates of OCs have also been described in association with anorexia nervosa (see Chapter 18, page 445) and violent personality disorders (see Chapter 24, page 620).

Prenatal influenza

The occurrence of influenza in well-defined epidemics provides a means of looking for an association between prenatal exposure to influenza and later schizophrenia at the population level. Mednick *et al* (1988) reported an approximately two-fold excess of patients with schizophrenia who were born 3–6 months following the 1957/58 influenza A_2 pandemic in Helsinki, suggesting that second-trimester exposure to influenza infection may increase the risk of the foetus subsequently developing schizophrenia. Many, though not all, subsequent studies of the 1957/58 pandemic replicated this finding (e.g. Kendell & Kemp, 1989; O'Callaghan *et al*, 1991). The evidence was further strengthened by studies that found a significant relationship between influenza epidemics and the birth dates of patients with schizophrenia over a number of years (Sham *et al*, 1992; Adams *et al*, 1993; Takei *et al*, 1994). Two case–control studies also found an association between second-trimester exposure to influenza and later schizophrenia, but suffered from the use of maternal recall (Stöber *et al*, 1992; Wright *et al*, 1995). Two cohort studies did not find an association (Crow & Done, 1992; Cannon *et al*, 1996), but these are inconclusive because of their low statistical power and the questionable reliability of self-reported influenza infection.

Other infections

In the Prenatal Determinants of Schizophrenia Study, Brown *et al* (2000*a*) showed that second-trimester exposure to a wide variety of respiratory infections (including influenza, pneumonia, tuberculosis and acute bronchitis) are associated with a significantly increased risk of schizophrenia spectrum disorders. An association between prenatal infection and adult schizophrenia has been reported also for poliovirus (Suvisaari *et al*, 1999) and rubella (Brown *et al*, 2000*b*). There is also a report of an association between the presence of maternal antibodies to herpes simplex virus (type 2) in serum collected at birth, and the risk of schizophrenia (Buka *et al*, 2000). Childhood infections involving the central nervous system (e.g. meningitis, encephalitis) may also be associated with a modest increased risk of subsequent schizophrenia, as reported by a cohort study in Finland (Rantakallio *et al*, 1997).

Prenatal famine

A twofold increase in the risk of schizophrenia was observed in a cohort of individuals who were subjected to famine during early gestation, by the Nazi blockade of the Netherlands in 1944–45 (Susser & Lin, 1992, 1994; Susser *et al*, 1996). A subsequent study using military conscription data demonstrated that prenatal famine during early gestation was associated with a twofold elevation in risk for schizoid or schizotypal personality disorders (Hoek *et al*, 1996).

Rhesus incompatibility

An elevated risk of schizophrenia among the offspring of women with rhesus-incompatible pregnancies compared with rhesus-compatible pregnancies was found in the Danish Perinatal Cohort (Hollister *et al*, 1996). Rhesus incompatibility can give rise to haemolytic disease of the newborn, which is known to result in childhood neuromotor abnormalities and behavioural disorders such as emotional instability. Schizophrenia may be yet another, remote consequence of rhesus haemolytic disease (Cannon *et al*, 2003).

Prenatal stress

In addition to being a precipitating factor in the onset of schizophrenia (Brown & Birley, 1968), psychosocial stress of mothers during pregnancy may increase predisposition. Huttunen & Niskanen (1978) reported that individuals whose father died before the child's birth have a significantly higher risk of schizophrenia than do those whose father died in the first year after birth. Van Os & Selten (1998) demonstrated a small increased risk of schizophrenia among individuals in Holland who were *in utero* during the Nazi invasion in May 1940. Selten *et al* (1999) found a non-significant increased risk of psychosis among those exposed during gestation to the 1953 Dutch flood disaster. Kinney *et al* (1999) reported a similar effect for prenatal exposure to a tornado in Worcester, Massachusetts. In the 1966 north Finland birth cohort, both maternal depression in late pregnancy (Jones *et al*, 1998) and 'un-wantedness' of a pregnancy by the mother (Myhrman *et al*, 1996) were independently associated with a modest increase in the risk of schizophrenia in the offspring.

Schizophrenia and neurological disorder

The existence of a wide range of neurological disorders that occasionally give rise to schizophrenia provided one of the first tangible clues that the origins of schizophrenia might lie in the brain. These conditions have been reviewed by Hyde & Lewis (2003), from which the account below is drawn.

Brain scanning studies of unselected groups of patients with schizophrenia show that 6–9% have some sort of focal abnormality and in about 3% of cases an underlying neurological condition is thought to be causal. ICD–10 uses the word 'organic' and describes 'organic schizophrenia-like conditions' (World Health Organization, 1992), whereas DSM–IV makes no such causal assumptions in its category of 'psychotic disorder due to a general medical condition' (American Psychiatric Association, 1994).

Secondary schizophrenias

Epilepsy

Davison & Bagley (1969) in their classic study reviewed 150 cases of organically determined psychosis and found evidence for an association between schizophrenia and a wide range of disorders of the central nervous system (CNS). The evidence appeared greatest for epilepsy, particularly temporal lobe epilepsy, but was present also for head injuries and brain tumours.

Slater & Beard (1963) described the development of typical schizophrenia in 69 patients with epilepsy, and the psychoses followed the onset of the fits after a mean interval of 14 years. Most of the participants had temporal lobe epilepsy and the most common psychiatric picture was of paranoid schizophrenia, but a high proportion also had organic personality change before the onset of their schizophrenia (lack of spontaneity, dullness and retardation, concrete and circumstantial thinking, and memory impairment). However, IQs were in the normal range, indicating that cognitive decline could not explain the development of psychosis. A small number (7 of the 69) had centrencephalic epilepsy and this was associated with a hebephrenic rather than a paranoid picture. Subsequent studies have shown that up to 10% of patients with epilepsy may have a lifetime risk of psychotic symptoms and that patients with epilepsy may have a three- to nine-fold increased risk of schizophrenia. At one time it was thought that left-sided temporal lobe lesions were more frequent, but the more recent studies have shown that up to a sixth of patients with schizophrenia have only right-sided temporal lobe involvement, and so the role of laterality is presently uncertain.

An early finding derived from those surgical cases where temporal lobe surgery was used to treat the epilepsy was that, among patients who developed schizophrenia, the congenital lesions such as hamartomas and focal dysplasias (which developed *in utero*) figured more prominently than the acquired lesions such as mesial temporal sclerosis. This implied that some common causative factor that resulted in both the schizophrenia and the epilepsy might have developed *in utero* – and these observations have been used to support the 'neurodevelopmental model of schizophrenia'. An alternative hypothesis postulates that the schizophrenic process arises through a 'kindling mechanism', with sub-threshold electrical activity continuing over a period of many years and eventually leading to the development of schizophrenia.

Head injury

Head injury may also play a small role. Thus, Achté *et al* (1969, 1991) followed a large cohort of Finnish soldiers (n = 10 000) who had experienced a head injury during the Second World War. Around 30% later developed some psychiatric disturbance in the 50-year follow-up period: delusional psychosis in 28%; major depression in 21%; delirium in 18%; and paranoid schizophrenia in 14%. In the first part of the follow-up study, Achté *et al* (1969) reported that temporal lobe injuries were most often associated with psychosis. Delusional psychosis was a later development, with a peak onset 15–20 years after the head injury; paranoid delusions and morbid jealousy were the most common such disorders. The authors suggested that in some cases the morbid jealousy may have been related to comorbid alcoholism. Paranoid schizophrenia tended to come on rather earlier than delusional disorder, with around a quarter of the cases appearing in the first year after the head injury, but most cases appeared after a delayed onset.

Achté *et al* (1969) found that patients with mild injuries developed schizophrenia more frequently than those with severe injury and suggested that factors other than the neurological disturbance must have played a role in the genesis of psychosis. Hyde & Lewis (2003) quote other studies which have suggested that traumatic brain injury increases the risk of psychoses by a factor of 2–5 and cite occasional case reports where schizophrenia has been associated with left temporal gliosis or atrophy, as shown on MRI. Prolonged delay after the initial head injury appears to be a feature of psychosis arising after head injury and remains unexplained, but suggests that the pathogenesis is more complex than simply being the result of 'brain damage'.

Tumours and space-occupying lesions

Tumours and space-occupying lesions may occasionally be associated with schizophrenia. From the larger series there has been a suggestion of an association of temporal lobe tumours with psychosis. Hyde & Lewis (2003) listed many other conditions, including basal ganglia calcification, abnormalities of the septum pellucidum, including its absence, agenesis of the corpus callosum and a variety of other cerebral lesions, as well as many rare disorders of metabolism, which have all been associated with schizophrenia in isolated case reports, but because these conditions are all very rare it has not been possible to establish whether a true association exists or whether these co-occurrences are merely due to chance.

Demyelinating disorders

Certain demyelinating disorders are rather more definitely associated with schizophrenia and the strongest association is with metachromatic leucodystrophy, a rare autosomal recessive disorder due to a deficiency of arylsuphatase-A, which results in progressive demyelination. Hyde *et al* (1992) reviewed the 129 published case reports and found that 50% of the patients had delusions and hallucinations, while 35% had schizophrenia, with a typical picture including motor and negative symptoms. MRI studies suggest that the main focus of pathology is in the periventricular frontal white matter. When the disease presented between the ages of 10 and 30 years, psychoses might occur, but presentations outside this age range were not associated with psychosis. This led Weinberger & Marenco (2003) to postulate that there are age-related genetic influences that promote the manifestation of schizophrenia (as well as a wide variety of the psychiatric disorders) at specific age ranges (mainly young adulthood) but not outside these age ranges.

The most common demyelinating disorder, multiple sclerosis, is probably not associated with schizophrenia, but an MRI comparison of 10 psychotic and 10 non-psychotic patients with multiple sclerosis showed more plaques around the temporal horns bilaterally among those with psychosis (Feinstein *et al*, 1992). Schizophrenia may also occur in around 5–11% of patients with Huntington's disease.

Summary

There is probably a large overlap between the presenting symptoms and clinical features of 'functional' and 'organic' psychosis and much appears to depend on the cause of the organic psychosis. Thus, for head injuries, paranoid and delusional pictures appear to predominate, while catatonic symptoms may be more common in other organic cases. Cutting (1987) found that thought disorder and visual hallucinations were more common in organic cases, while Schneiderian symptoms were uncommon. Delusions, particularly paranoid delusions, were more common and three themes were present: belief of imminent misadventure to others, delusional misidentity of others and other bizarre occurrences in the immediate vicinity. Cutting he related these themes to delusional elaboration of deficits in perception or memory.

Little is known of the effects of treatment, but Johnstone, remarking on the cases she had personally seen, wrote that these patients had a strikingly poor response to antipsychotic medication; although relatives were usually grateful that some underlying cause had been discovered, this very rarely led to a successful treatment (Johnstone *et al*, 1999).

The secondary schizophrenias provided the first evidence that schizophrenia might be a disease of the brain, and also provided some support for the neurodevelopmental hypothesis of causation. However, today, with the advent of sophisticated techniques of brain scanning, research efforts have moved on from possible associations with rare neurological disorders into more direct visualisation of the human brain, mainly using MRI.

Magnetic resonance imaging studies in schizophrenia

The possible role of brain abnormalities in the aetiology of schizophrenia has been a subject of continuous research since Kraepelin's description of dementia praecox. Early research was confined to case reports of associations between gross neuropathological abnormalities and schizophrenia. Pneumoencephalography was the first technique to provide information on brain structure in living patients. These studies showed non-progressive ventricular enlargement in patients with schizophrenia (Huber, 1957; Huber *et al*, 1975). The development of computed tomography (CT) allowed reproduction of these early findings using a non-invasive technique (Johnstone *et al*, 1976; Andreasen *et al*, 1982). Furthermore, using CT, Jaskiw *et al* (1994) confirmed the apparently *non-progressive* nature of ventricular enlargement in schizophrenia. However, both pneumoencephalography and CT are techniques with limited spatial resolution and may, therefore, have been unable to detect subtle abnormalities or progression.

In contrast, the advent and development of magnetic resonance imaging (MRI) in the 1980s and 1990s provided researchers with a high-resolution tool for structural mapping of the human brain in health and disease. Furthermore, *functional* MRI (Ogawa *et al*, 1990) allows inferences to be drawn regarding neural activation in the brain that might subserve normal cognitive and perceptual processes, or abnormalities of these processes, as occur in schizophrenia. The past decade has seen an enormous increase in both structural and functional MRI research in schizophrenia, and MRI is now the standard imaging research modality in the disorder. For this reason, this section focuses on the results of studies that used MRI methods in the investigation of schizophrenia.

Structural MRI and its application to schizophrenia research

Structural MRI is an *in vivo* technique for producing high-resolution anatomical images. The signal results from resonating hydrogen nuclei in a magnetic field. This signal varies according to the relative contribution to it from different tissues, and so can be used to build an anatomical image. MRI does not expose patients to X-ray radiation, and as long as there are no contra-indications to the high magnetic field employed, such as metallic foreign bodies, it is safer than CT.

Many researchers have adopted an approach based upon manually 'counting' the size of selected regions of interest (ROI) in the brains of people with schizophrenia and control subjects (e.g. hippocampus; Pegues *et al*, 2003). Such a method is very time consuming and may be prone to effects of observer bias (if not properly blinded) and variable intra- and inter-rater reliability. More recently, several research groups have sought to improve the efficiency and reliability of the assessment of brain structure in patients and controls by using automated methods (e.g. Anath *et al*, 2002). These automated, or *voxel-based*, approaches are much quicker to carry out and have a significant further advantage in that the *whole brains* of patient and control groups can be compared; there is no restriction to examining pre-specified ROI.

Owing to the large number of structural MRI studies that have been carried out in schizophrenia, many diverse areas of abnormality have been reported. In this section, the intention is to outline the major findings in those brain areas that have *consistently* been reported to be abnormal in schizophrenia.

Ventricular size

Meta-analysis has confirmed the findings of early CT studies that the ventricles of people with schizophrenia are enlarged in comparison with controls (Van Horn & McManus, 1992). The temporofrontal aspect of the lateral ventricles has been most implicated (with differences possibly more pronounced on the left), but some studies have also demonstrated enlargement of the third ventricle. Where this has been the case, the degree of enlargement of the lateral and third ventricles was reported as similar, even when the *absolute* degree of enlargement varied between studies. For example, Kelsoe *et al* (1988) found that the lateral ventricles were enlarged by 62% and the third ventricle was enlarged by 73%, whereas Hulshoff Pol *et al* (2002) demonstrated a 27% increase in the size of the lateral ventricles compared with a 30% increase in the size of the third ventricle. These observations support the general finding, by more recent studies, that differences in ventricular size between patients and controls may not be as large as previously thought and it seems, for the time being at least, that, in common with other brain abnormalities in schizophrenia, the effect may be observable only at the *population* level. This point is well illustrated by the finding (Andreasen *et al*, 1990*a*) that there was much overlap between patient and control groups on CT scan. Specifically, only 6% of patients had a ventricle:brain ratio (VBR) greater than 2 standard deviations from the control mean (use of the VBR corrects for the effect of the size of the whole brain in comparisons between people). Using MRI to address the same question, Andreasen *et al* (1990*b*) also found that most of the effect observed could be accounted for by an increased VBR in some of the male patients in their sample. This suggests that ventricular enlargement occurs only in some patients with schizophrenia, with the remainder being located well within the normal distribution of healthy controls.

Most studies of ventricular size in schizophrenia have used Western samples of patients, but the finding of lateral ventricular enlargement has now been described in a Chinese sample (Chua *et al*, 2002).

Where the ventricular volume is enlarged, it may be correlated with diminished grey matter volume in adjacent brain structures (Suddath *et al*, 1989). The ventricular region is surrounded by structures such as the amygdala, hippocampus and parahippocampal gyrus. These contain neuronal networks concerned with a number of cortical activities, including selection, association and integration of sensory information, memory and control of basic drives and emotions. The structural and functional relationship between enlarged ventricles and surrounding brain regions is currently an area of research. In contrast with the early CT studies, evidence is now mounting for progressive enlargement of ventricles, accompanied by loss of adjacent grey matter, longitudinally, through the course of a schizophrenic illness (Mathalon *et al*, 2001; Cahn *et al*, 2002*a*). Perhaps this progressive effect is observable now because of the improved spatial resolution of MRI.

Why are the ventricles enlarged in schizophrenia? As foetal brain tissue expands, the proportion of ventricle to brain volume decreases. Therefore, increased VBR in schizophrenia may be a marker of incomplete brain maturation. Furthermore, foetal hypoxia has been shown to correlate with the degree of ventricular enlargement in patients with schizophrenia, but not in controls (Cannon *et al*, 2000). This finding suggests a possible interaction between a predisposition and an environmental insult in the pathogenesis of ventricular enlargement.

Whole-brain changes

Many structural imaging studies now support the idea that there is an overall reduction in cerebral size in schizophrenia. In their meta-analysis of 58 studies, with a total of 1588 patients, Wright *et al* (2000) found that the mean cerebral volume of patients with schizophrenia was 98% of that of controls, a small but significant difference. Another study also reported an overall reduction in total brain volume of the same order (97.8% of control brain) (Hulshoff Pol *et al*, 2002). Furthermore, that study also provided some evidence (albeit cross-sectional) of progressive loss of grey matter; the authors estimated that patients lost, on average, 3.43 ml of grey matter per year, but controls lost only 2.74 ml per year.

Automated, voxel-based approaches have also demonstrated global reductions in grey matter volume in schizophrenia (Anath *et al*, 2002). As in the case of ventricular enlargement, foetal hypoxia predicts reduced grey matter throughout the cortex in patients but not in controls (Cannon *et al*, 2000).

It is possible that the relatively small reduction in overall cerebral volume observed in studies (of the order of 2%) arises because of more pronounced, but anatomically discrete, loss of brain tissue in selected areas. This notion will now be further reviewed, with particular reference to frontal and temporolimbic structures.

Frontal lobe

The frontal lobe has been the focus of much interest in schizophrenia. Patients with frontal lobe damage, in common with patients with the negative syndrome of schizophrenia, may exhibit deficits of attention, abstract thinking, judgement, motivation, affect and emotion, and impulse control, as well as decreased spontaneous speech, verbal fluency and voluntary motor behaviour (see Spence *et al*, 2002, for a review of the neuroscience of voluntary behaviour). As outlined elsewhere in this chapter, patients with schizophrenia also perform poorly on neuropsychological tests of frontal lobe function.

Studying 159 patients and 158 controls, Hulshoff Pol *et al* (2002) found that prefrontal grey matter was reduced by 4.4% and prefrontal white matter by 3.3% in the patient group. Anath *et al* (2002) used a voxel-based method to identify grey matter deficits in the medial prefrontal cortex of patients with schizophrenia. Of particular interest was the additional finding of a relationship between amount of grey matter loss and strength of family history for schizophrenia, supporting a hypothesis regarding the genetics of brain development in schizophrenia (Jones & Murray, 1991).

Alcohol misuse may have a particularly deleterious effect on the prefrontal grey matter of people with schizophrenia. Mathalon *et al* (2003) analysed structural MRI scans of patients with schizophrenia, alcohol dependency and both schizophrenia and alcohol dependency. They found grey matter reductions in all three groups, but the comorbid group was most affected, particularly in the prefrontal cortex.

Temporolimbic regions

The temporal lobes are of theoretical and practical importance to our understanding of schizophrenia. Within the dominant temporal lobe are located many of the auditory and language functions that may underlie abnormalities of thought, speech and auditory perception in schizophrenia.

Woodruff (1994) reviewed 13 MRI studies that compared the temporal lobe volume of patients with schizophrenia and that of controls. Twelve studies found reduced volume on the left (statistically significant in seven studies) and nine found reduced volume on the right (significant in three studies). Three studies measured grey and white matter separately; of these, all found reduced temporal lobe grey matter in patients with schizophrenia, one found white matter reduction bilaterally, and another found white matter reduction on the left but increase on the right. It has been argued that lateralisation of pathology to the left side (usually speech and language dominant) is central to the schizophrenic condition (Crow, 1990). Thus, left-sided pathology may lead to a loss of *normal asymmetry* in the brain and, hence, pathological symmetry or even rightward asymmetry in brain regions involved in speech and language processing.

Structures in the medial temporal lobe, the hippocampus, parahippocampal gyrus and amygdala, have also been shown to be reduced in volume in patients with schizophrenia (Wright *et al*, 2000). Another study has shown a specific reduction in the volume of the anterior part of the hippocampus (Pegues *et al*, 2003).

Magnetic resonance spectroscopy (MRS) allows estimation of the concentration of neuronal and neurochemical markers in the brain (and elsewhere), using MR techniques. Kegeles *et al* (2000) used MRS to demonstrate a relative deficit of amino acid neurotransmitters in the left hippocampus and a relative excess of these in the right hippocampus, perhaps reflecting an asymmetric neurochemical abnormality in the medial temporal lobe.

White matter tracts

The largest white matter tract in the human brain is the corpus callosum, which consists of myelinated axons connecting one cerebral hemisphere to the other. Since the 'split brain' experiments of Sperry, the importance of the corpus callosum in providing the major means of hemispheric transfer of conscious and unconscious information has been apparent. Theorists have long been attracted to the idea that, in schizophrenia, one hemisphere might become 'disconnected' from the other. Evidence supporting such an idea comes from observations that patients with schizophrenia perform poorly on neuropsychological tests reliant on intact interhemispheric communication (David, 1987).

The shape of the corpus callosum is extremely variable. Therefore, area measures of the corpus callosum are probably more reliable than linear ones (Woodruff *et al*, 1993). In a meta-analysis of 11 MRI studies, including 313 patients and 281 controls, there was a significant reduction of callosal area in patients (Woodruff *et al*, 1995*a*). However, this difference was not apparent when callosal area was expressed as a proportion of whole-brain size. In another study, reduced callosal area was reported in first-episode, treatment-naive patients with schizophrenia (Keshaven *et al*, 2002). There also appears to be a gender effect in corpus callosum abnormality in schizophrenia. Panizzou *et al* (2003) found that callosal area was reduced in male *and* female patients with schizophrenia, but that the 'effect size' was greater in males, crossing the threshold for statistical significance. The latter observation suggests that larger studies may be required to detect subtle callosal area reductions in females with schizophrenia.

Narr *et al* (2002) examined the genetic contribution to abnormal callosal structure by studying MZ and DZ twins discordant for schizophrenia and pairs of healthy twins. The unaffected MZ twins of schizophrenic co-twins demonstrated significant vertical displacement ('upward bowing') of the corpus callosum. The authors interpreted their result as suggesting that genetic rather than disease-specific or environmental factors contribute to altered callosal morphology in schizophrenia. On the other hand, Chua *et al* (2000) found no abnormality of callosal area in the relatives of patients with schizophrenia.

Overall, evidence favours reduced area of the corpus callosum in schizophrenia, which might be related to a more generalised diminution of brain size. It is possible that neuronal loss, demyelination or failed development could account for abnormal callosal morphology in patients with schizophrenia.

Conventional structural MRI is not able to image the *organisation* of white matter fibres in the brain, a property that is likely to be critical to their efficient functioning. However, a relatively new MRI modality, diffusion tensor imaging (DTI), is able to address this issue. DTI allows the observation of molecular diffusion in tissues *in vivo* and, therefore, the molecular organisation in tissues, such as the direction of white matter tracts. Foong *et al* (2000) used DTI to demonstrate reduced *fractional anisotropy* (a measure of axonal disorganisation) in the splenium of the corpus callosum in patients with schizophrenia. Another study (Hoptman *et al*, 2002) demonstrated that reduced fractional anisotropy in the right inferior frontal region was associated with impulsivity and aggression in men with schizophrenia. The use of DTI in schizophrenia research is at a relatively early stage, but its future application could lead to a better understanding of the anatomical substrate for abnormal *functional* connectivity that has been suggested by the functional neuroimaging literature (see below).

Major clinical themes of research using structural MRI

In addition to a brain region-by-region approach to the application of structural MRI in schizophrenia research, a brief overview is provided below of those clinical areas that have been subject to intense investigation. The field is very large; in this section we focus on: structural abnormalities in first-episode psychosis; findings in unaffected relatives of people with schizophrenia; and the relationship between structural brain pathology and schizophrenic symptoms.

Structural MRI in first-episode psychosis

That structural brain abnormalities exist in schizophrenia is generally accepted to be established to a position that is beyond dispute. However, the *meaning* of these abnormalities, in understanding the pathogenesis of the illness, is far less clear. Questions remain as to whether structural abnormalities *predispose* to the development of schizophrenia, whether acute schizophrenic psychosis can actually damage the brain, *causing* altered structure. There are also questions as to whether abnormal brain structure can be parsimoniously explained in terms of the effects of neuroleptic medication. For all these reasons, the study of patients around the time of a first psychotic episode (including those at high risk *before* they develop an illness) represents an enormous research effort that may help to clarify the extent to which brain abnormalities predispose to schizophrenia, as opposed to being consequent upon its clinical development and treatment.

Pantelis *et al* (2003) studied 75 people with prodromal signs of psychotic illness who had not yet developed a florid disorder. Of these, 23 people did progress to florid psychosis over the follow-up period. Progression to psychosis was associated with premorbid reduction of grey matter in the right temporal cortex, inferior frontal cortex and bilateral cingulate cortex, suggesting the presence of structural abnormalities before the development of florid psychosis – evidence that supports a structural brain predisposition to schizophrenia. In another group of people at high risk of developing psychosis, Lawrie *et al* (2002*a*) found that the presence of psychotic symptoms was also associated with diminished volume of the right temporal lobe.

A 1-year follow-up study of first-episode schizophrenia has shown that reduction in whole brain volume, and enlargement of the ventricular system, occurs in a progressive manner during this early stage of the illness (Cahn *et al*, 2002*a*). Furthermore, in that study, loss of grey matter was positively correlated with cumulative dose of antipsychotic medication. Another study, by the same group, however, found that the third ventricle was enlarged in people with schizophrenia who had received *no* neuroleptic medication (Cahn *et al*, 2002*b*).

On the other hand, Ho *et al* (2003) studied 156 patients with untreated initial psychosis (including schizoaffective disorder and schizophreniform psychoses in addition to schizophrenia) and found that the median duration of untreated illness was not correlated with structural brain abnormality in any region. They interpreted this result as suggesting that untreated psychosis has no direct toxic neural effects.

Based on current investigation into structural brain abnormalities in first-episode illness, it is possible only to draw a broad conclusion that such abnormalities may precede (or even predict) transition from a 'high risk' state to actual schizophrenia, and that the abnormalities may be progressive, not static, in nature.

Structural abnormalities in unaffected relatives of patients with schizophrenia

There is an important interface between genetics (see above) and imaging, namely the MRI investigation of unaffected relatives of patients.

First-degree relatives of patients with schizophrenia have been shown to have smaller hippocampi than controls (Seidman *et al*, 2002). That study also suggested that the effect is more pronounced in families with more than one schizophrenic member ('multiplex families'). McDonald *et al* (2002) sought to quantify the likelihood of an unaffected relative carrying 'schizophrenia genes' and investigated this group using structural MRI. They found that, in unaffected relatives of patients with schizophrenia, the lateral and third ventricles were enlarged in proportion to their presumed likelihood of carrying genes for the disorder.

The siblings of patients with childhood-onset schizophrenia have also been studied with structural MRI. In one study (Gogtay *et al*, 2003), the unaffected siblings had less total brain grey matter than controls.

'Presumed obligate carriers' of schizophrenia are people with an affected parent and an affected child but who are not, themselves, affected by schizophrenia. These people are of great interest to psychiatric researchers because of the presumption that they must carry genes for schizophrenia without exhibiting the phenotype. Steel *et al* (2002) found that patients with schizophrenia and their siblings who were obligate carriers both had a volumetric reduction of the medial temporal lobe compared with their non-affected, non-obligate siblings. Obligate carriers have also been shown to resemble patients with schizophrenia in terms of altered cerebral asymmetry in comparison with healthy controls (Sharma *et al*, 1999).

The presence of structural brain abnormalities in unaffected relatives of patients with schizophrenia suggests that 'schizophrenia genes' are likely to be involved in (abnormal) brain development, but that the expression of the structural brain correlate of the genes is not, in itself, enough to 'cause' schizophrenia.

The relationship between structural abnormalities and schizophrenic symptoms

In order to understand the possible *consequences* of structural brain abnormalities in schizophrenia, researchers have attempted to find correlations between imaging and clinical data. Correlation, in this sense, implies association, not causation, but may still be helpful in furthering our knowledge with respect to the aetiology of schizophrenia. This section focuses on the clinical phenomena of auditory hallucinations, thought disorder and the negative syndrome.

(1) *Auditory hallucinations*. Perhaps the most frequently studied symptoms in relating clinical phenomena to structural imaging data are auditory hallucinations (AHs). One early study used MRI to demonstrate an inverse correlation between severity of AHs and volume of the left superior temporal gyrus, a large region containing auditory association cortex (Barta *et al*, 1990). A more localised reduction in volume of the left *anterior* superior temporal gyrus has also been found to correlate with severity of AHs (Levitan *et al*, 1999).

A specific region of the posterior superior temporal gyrus, the planum temporale, has received much attention. The planum temporale has long been considered an important speech and language 'specialised' area (Shapleske *et al*, 1999) and hence, it has been hypothesised, abnormalities of its structure could relate to the AHs of schizophrenia. Barta *et al* (1997) found that, in schizophrenia, the surface area of the planum temporale was unusually large on the right.

This result has been interpreted as evidence of reversal of *normal asymmetry* in the auditory cortices of people with schizophrenia. However, a more recent study found no such reversal and, indeed, demonstrated normal *leftward* asymmetry in terms of planum temporale volume and surface area (Shapleske *et al*, 2001). In that study, there was no relationship between severity of AHs and planum temporale structure.

Another comparison, between patients with schizophrenia who had a prominent history of AHs and a group, also with schizophrenia, with no such history of AHs, revealed that the hallucinators had a deficit of grey matter in the left insula and adjacent temporal lobe (Shapleske *et al*, 2002). A strength of this study is its use of automated techniques to assess grey matter volume across the entire brain in the groups being studied, avoiding the potential pitfall of failing to detect abnormalities arising in areas outside of specified regions of interest.

Turning to white matter tracts, Rossell *et al* (2001) found that there was no relationship between structural measures of the corpus collosum and the presence or absence of AHs in schizophrenia.

The relationship between structural brain abnormalities in schizophrenia and AHs has not yet been consistently demonstrated, perhaps reflecting the phenomenological diversity of the symptom being studied. Notwithstanding this caveat, it does seem likely that structural abnormalities of the temporal cortex occur in schizophrenia (see above), although further work needs to be done to elucidate the relationship between anatomical abnormalities in the auditory system and auditory hallucinations.

(2) *Thought disorder*. Perhaps because thought disorder is clinically recognisable in terms of disorganised speech, the planum temporale has also been an area of interest to researchers investigating this symptom. Shenton *et al* (1992) studied 15 right-handed men with schizophrenia, and found that the degree of clinical thought disorder was inversely correlated with volume of the left posterior superior temporal gyrus (which contains the planum temporale). Patients with smaller left posterior superior temporal gyri had more prominent thought disorder. The association was replicated by another group (Menon *et al*, 1995). Directly comparing schizophrenic patients with and without thought disorder, Rossi *et al* (1994) found that the thought-disordered group demonstrated reduced (normal left-sided) asymmetry of the planum temporale. Their findings support the idea that structural abnormality of the left planum temporale is related to the presence of thought disorder. This is because it is generally accepted that, normally, the left planum temporale is 'larger' than the right planum temporale.

The issue of laterality/asymmetry has also been addressed, more obliquely, by Holinger *et al* (1999). They studied left-handed men with schizophrenia and found a *positive* correlation between thought disorder and tissue volume in the *right* anterior superior temporal gyrus. Although, normally, left-handers are considered to have less leftward asymmetry of temporal speech and language areas, such as the planum temporale (Shapleske *et al*, 1999), it is possible that the association, in schizophrenia, between thought disorder and reduced leftward asymmetry of language-related regions reflects the relatively greater size of their right-sided homologues. This idea is consistent with notions of lack of 'pruning' in brain development predisposing to schizophrenia (Keshaven *et al*, 1994). Synaptic pruning is a relatively circumscribed process occurring in early adulthood among primates and involves so-called asymmetric synapses, which are presumably excitatory and glutaminergic. GABA-ergic inhibitory connections are not pruned at this time. There is an overall increase in the growth of dendrites and dendritic spines of the pyramidal neurons in early adult life and it has been hypothesised that abnormalities of the pruning process are involved in schizophrenia.

(3) *The negative syndrome of schizophrenia*. Early MRI studies of patients with negative symptoms found that ventricular size (Andreasen *et al*, 1990*b*), VBR (Gur *et al*, 1994) and the ratio of cerebrospinal fluid to cranial volume (Mozley *et al*, 1994) were all enlarged in this group.

As outlined above, the schizophrenic negative syndrome is characterised by dysfunction of a number of *executive* cognitive processes that are likely to be subserved by prefrontal cortex. Turning to this region, Chua *et al* (1997) used MRI and found that patients with higher psychomotor poverty scores had a smaller volume of grey matter in the left ventromedial prefrontal cortex. Using a combined neuropsychology/neuroimaging paradigm, Baare *et al* (1999) found that a smaller volume prefrontal grey matter was associated with the presence of more severe negative symptoms *and* impaired performance on tests of verbal and visual memory, and semantic (category) fluency.

In addition to reductions in grey matter, abnormalities of white matter have also been described in the negative syndrome. Reduced volume of white matter in the prefrontal cortex of people with schizophrenia has been shown to be associated with prominent negative symptoms (Sanfilipo *et al*, 2000; Wible *et al*, 2001). Using DTI, Wolkin *et al* (2003) produced preliminary data that further refine the interpretation of previous work. They found that more severe negative symptoms were associated with reduced fractional anisotropy (a measure of neuronal organisation) in the white matter tracts of the inferior frontal cortex. Moreover, another study demonstrated reduced fractional anisotropy in the uncinate fasciculus, the largest white matter tract, which connects the frontal and temporal lobes. It is increasingly recognised that the establishment of connections between one brain region and another can, via trophic factors, have considerable influence on subsequent neural architecture. With this in mind, Woodruff *et al* (1997*a*) described a structural frontotemporal dissociation in schizophrenia – the normal strong correlation between the volume of the frontal lobes and temporal lobe structures was lost. This observation was interpreted as consistent with lack of early positive trophic influences between the frontal and temporal cortices, due possibly to diminished structural connections, an interpretation that is supported by work that has identified abnormal organisation of frontotemporal white matter tracts in schizophrenia

Thus, the current data suggest that the clinical and neuropsychological features of the negative syndrome are associated with structural abnormalities in prefrontal (executive) brain regions. Furthermore, the identification of possible white matter lesions suggests a hypothesis regarding problems in the prefrontal cortex's connections with other brain areas, a hypothesis that has been tested using functional MRI in schizophrenia research (see below).

The application of functional neuroimaging in schizophrenia research

Until the 1990s, the predominant *functional* neuroimaging modalities in schizophrenia were single-photon emission computed tomography (SPECT) and positron emission tomography (PET). The basic principle in both techniques is that radiolabelled compounds can be administered to participants and their distribution mapped under different conditions (e.g. psychological or pharmacological) in order to draw inferences regarding brain function or metabolism. Although these approaches have been very informative, their dependence on ionising radiation necessarily limits their application and, in the case of PET, the need for an on-site cyclotron makes the technique very expensive.

In contrast, functional magnetic resonance imaging (fMRI) makes use of a physiological contrast, the blood oxygenation level (Ogawa *et al*, 1990), and does not involve ionising radiation. The principle behind fMRI is that neuronal activation results in local changes in blood oxygenation level, specifically decreased deoxyhaemoglobin and increased oxyhaemoglobin concentration. Oxyhaemoglobin has different magnetic properties from deoxyhaemoglobin, which can be detected as changes of signal intensity on T_2-weighted MRI. The advent of fMRI has transformed the application of functional neuroimaging in psychiatry and has led to an exponential increase in the number of published studies investigating putative abnormalities of brain function that may be important in schizophrenia.

Since this field is rapidly expanding and changing, this section aims to provide a broad overview that may stimulate the interested reader to investigate further.

Functional connectivity and disconnectivity in schizophrenia

In functional neuroimaging, 'connectivity' refers to statistical relationships between activation observed in different brain areas. Statistical methods permit various inferences to be drawn from connectivity analyses, including, for example, whether anatomically distinct brain areas could be part of a functional network, and if so, how certain components may influence others within the interconnected system.

Normally, the performance of an orthographic letter fluency task leads to increased regional cerebral blood flow (rCBF) in the prefrontal cortex and decreased rCBF in the temporal cortex: this is evidence of a functional relationship between the two areas, or *connectivity*. Using PET, Frith *et al* (1995) demonstrated that, in a letter fluency task, while showing the normal increase in rCBF in left dorsolateral prefrontal cortex, patients with schizophrenia did not exhibit a decrease in rCBF in the left superior temporal gyrus. Hence, the normal reciprocal relationship between the two regions was disrupted, a result that the authors interpreted in terms of functional *disconnectivity*. Another study has demonstrated, using fMRI, that the severity of auditory hallucinations in schizophrenia is related to a measure of frontotemporal functional disconnectivity during a sentence completion task (Lawrie *et al*, 2002*b*). Meyer-Lindenberg *et al* (2001) used fMRI and a working memory task, and found that the abnormal pattern of functional connectivity in patients with schizophrenia (compared with controls) was able prospectively to classify PET data as either 'schizophrenic' or 'healthy', in an accurate manner. Similarly, Josin & Liddle (2001) 'trained' a computer (using a neural network) to discriminate accurately between healthy controls and patients with schizophrenia on the basis of disordered functional connectivity in PET data. However, Spence *et al* (2000) used PET and found no evidence of functional disconnectivity between frontal and temporal regions, during letter fluency in patients with schizophrenia in remission and their 'obligate carrier' relatives (see above).

Although the findings of functional disconnectivity, during a variety of cognitive tasks, in schizophrenia have not been universally reproduced (and the mathematical models of connectivity are themselves in a state of continuous development), the current data suggest that this approach may be of great help in understanding the relationship between gross structural abnormalities, white matter disorganisation, their functional correlates and clinical consequences.

The functional correlates of schizophrenic symptoms

The discipline of cognitive neuropsychology seeks to explain how psychological mechanisms subserve normal functions of, for example, perception, language and memory. On the other hand, cognitive *neuropsychiatry* is concerned with how abnormalities of these processes, perhaps associated with functional lesions, might explain psychopathology in mental disorders, including schizophrenia. Functional brain imaging has been extensively used in an attempt to 'map' those functional abnormalities in the brains of people with schizophrenia, helping us to understand the mechanisms by which symptoms occur.

Again, the functional anatomy of AHs has been extensively investigated. An early SPECT study showed that the occurrence of AHs was associated with activation in Broca's area, part of the left inferior frontal gyrus that is involved in speech production. Although the finding was suggestive of a hypothesis regarding the mechanism for AHs in terms of generating speech, it has not been replicated (McGuire *et al*, 1993). Silbersweig *et al* (1995) found evidence from PET that AHs were associated with activation in a number of subcortical structures and, in a patient with visual and auditory hallucinations, both visual and auditory association cortices. Those authors suggested that the latter, neocortical regions may affect the perceptual content of hallucinations and, in the case of AHs, this idea has been supported by further work. Using fMRI, Woodruff *et al* (1997*b*) demonstrated that temporal regions normally involved in the perception of real speech showed an attenuated response to such speech during the experience of AHs. This finding was interpreted as suggesting that AHs and real speech compete for common neural resources in the auditory cortex; this is evidence for 'saturation' of the auditory system by hallucinations. Earlier fMRI work by Woodruff *et al* (1995*b*) and subsequent fMRI studies by Dierks *et al* (1999) and Shergill *et al* (2000) also support the notion that AHs are associated with activation in the auditory cortex. Dierks *et al* (1999) found that, in each of three hallucinating patients with schizophrenia, the onset of AHs coincided with significant activation in Heschl's gyrus, part of the temporal lobe that contains the primary auditory cortex. In a case study, Bentaleb *et al* (2002) also used fMRI to show that AHs were associated with activation in primary auditory cortex.

Formal thought disorder has also been shown to be associated with functional abnormalities in the temporal cortex, specifically the superior temporal gyrus. Kircher *et al* (2001) asked participants to speak about Rorschach inkblots in an fMRI paradigm. They found that more severe formal thought disorder was associated with *reduced* activation in the left superior and middle temporal gyri. Furthermore, that group also demonstrated that, in healthy participants, the amount of speech produced in the Rorschach task correlated with activation in the left superior temporal gyrus, whereas in patients with schizophrenia who were thought-disordered, the amount of speech produced correlated with activation in the right superior temporal gyrus (Kircher *et al*, 2002). These data may represent evidence for a functional correlate of the reduced left–right structural asymmetry that has been described in the superior temporal gyri of people with thought disorder in schizophrenia (see above), perhaps reflecting a more general reduction in functional language lateralisation in schizophrenia (Sommer *et al*, 2001).

Finally, efforts are now being made to relate particular genotypes to behavioural performance and brain activation in the functional imaging environment. Catechol-O-methyltransferase (COMT) is an enzyme that is involved in dopamine catabolism in the prefrontal cortex. A specific functional polymorphism in the COMT gene is associated with variation in the catabolic activity of the enzyme. Egan *et al* (2001) have provided a demonstration that the COMT genotype is related to behavioural performance on a neuropsychological test (the Wisconsin Card Sorting Test) and also that the COMT genotype affects the physiological response in prefrontal cortex, measured by fMRI, during a working memory task. Although preliminary, that work may further advance our understanding of the aetiology of schizophrenia by uniting genetics with brain function and neuropsychological performance.

Conclusion

Structural neuroimaging in schizophrenia has been carried out using pneumoencephalography, CT and MRI, with the last now being the predominant modality. Using these techniques, the brains of *populations* of patients with schizophrenia have consistently been shown to be abnormal, by comparison with *populations* of healthy subjects. Reported structural abnormalities have included increased ventricular size, reduced whole brain volume, reduction in volume of frontal and temporal cortices (including medial temporal structures such as the hippocampus), reduced or reversed brain asymmetry, and abnormal size and shape of major white matter tracts. Some abnormalities may exist before the onset of acute psychosis, progress during a schizophrenic illness, occur in unaffected relatives of people with schizophrenia and demonstrate association with specific symptoms of the illness.

Brain function in schizophrenia has also been investigated using SPECT, PET and fMRI. These approaches have indicated that certain symptoms of schizophrenia may result from abnormal activation in brain areas that normally subserve related physiological processes (e.g. activation of auditory cortex during AHs). Structural evidence of disconnection between brain regions (e.g. reduced fractional anisotropy in DTI data) may be associated with functional disconnectivity in the brains of people with schizophrenia (e.g. abnormal statistical relationships between fMRI activations occurring in distinct brain areas).

Through the application of these imaging techniques, neuroimaging continues to improve our knowledge of the aetiology of, and pathophysiological mechanisms in, schizophrenia. It seems likely that, in the future, further integration of structural and functional imaging data with neuropsychology, electrophysiology and genetics will further increase our understanding of this complex disorder.

Neuropathology

There is no well-defined neuropathology of schizophrenia in the sense that there is a neuropathology of Huntington's disease or brain tumours, nor is it likely that the diagnosis of schizophrenia will ever be made by looking down the microscope. However, the repeated evidence from MRI studies that particular areas of the brain have smaller volumes must presumably have a histological basis and ultimately a molecular explanation. Many of the earlier histopathological findings have not been replicated, and even today there is no single well-defined and agreed set of histopathological abnormalities in schizophrenia, but a number of studies point towards subtle histopathological differences between the post-mortem brains of people with schizophrenia and controls, which do not appear to be due to antipsychotic drugs. Interest has focused on the hippocampus, dorsal prefrontal cortex (DPFC) and the thalamus. The account below is drawn mainly from the review by Harrison & Lewis (2003).

Although one or two early studies suggested the presence of gliosis, the general consensus now appears to be that there is an absence of gliosis in schizophrenia, and in cases where gliosis has been found this is thought to be secondary to some other pathology. This observation is of importance, because proliferation of glial cells is usually seen in most of the degenerative brain conditions and encephalopathies that arise after birth, and the absence of gliosis is therefore against schizophrenia being a neurodegenerative disorder, but more in favour of a neurodevelopmental basis. Furthermore, the glial response is said not to occur until after the end of the second trimester, suggesting that the 'putative damaging' agent(s) are operating before then. Also, there are no Alzheimer-like changes in the brains of patients with schizophrenia, even though the cognitive impairment may be quite severe.

The hippocampus

The earlier histopathological studies on the hippocampus reported: a greater neuronal disarray of the pyramidal neurons in Ammon's horn; aberrantly clustered neurons in lamina II (pre-α cells) and lamina III of the entorhinal cortex; and an overall loss of neurons. However, these findings have not been replicated and so their status is uncertain. One finding that is beginning to emerge, and is being replicated, is that neuronal body size is smaller when this is measured objectively by computerised image analysis, and similar observations have also been found in the DPFC. The significance of reduced neuronal size lies in its relationship to the diameter of the axon as well as other aspects of axo-dendritic organisation, and these may therefore also be reduced.

This has led to investigations into proteins that are associated with synaptic activity, such as synaptophysin, synaptic proteins such as SNAP-25, the synapsins and the complexins. Data from studies of the neurodegenerative disorders indicate that decreased synaptic activity is associated with reductions of these proteins, and recent findings indicate they are also lowered in the hippocampus in schizophrenia.

Dendrites can be investigated in a similar fashion using dendritically located proteins, notably microtubule-associated protein-2 (MAP2), and decreased immunoreactivity for MAP-2 has been found in the hippocampus, as well as a reduced density of dendritic spines in subicular neurons in the hippocampus (Rosoklija *et al*, 2000).

The dorsal prefrontal cortex

As outlined in the section on MRI studies (see page 216), there is a small but definite reduction in the thickness of cortical grey matter in schizophrenia. As in the hippocampal studies, many abnormalities have been reported but few have been consistently replicated, and the interest has now shifted away from an expectation of finding some gross neuronal abnormality to finding evidence for decreased or abnormal connectivity between the different regions of the brain.

Thus the total number of prefrontal cortical neurons does not appear to be decreased in schizophrenia, nor is their density any different. However, as in the hippocampal studies, the neuron body size, particularly of the pyramidal cells in deep layer 3 of DPFC area 9, may be smaller, with a corresponding decrease in size of the basilar dendrites, and presumably dendritic spines and axon terminals, and these changes may explain the reduced cortical volume.

Glantz & Lewis (2000) have also produced convincing histological pictures that show decreased dendritic spine density for the pyramidal neurons located in deep layer 3 of the cortex, and whose basilar dendrites extend through the laminar zone of the termination of projections from the thalamus.

Investigations of neuronal functioning with *in vivo* proton spectroscopy have suggested that there are reduced concentrations of N-acetylaspartate, which is also reduced in the hippocampus (Bertolino *et al*, 2000). Observations on never-medicated patients with schizophrenia using phosphorus-31 spectroscopy have found decreased concentrations of phosphomonoesters and increased concentrations of phosphodiesters in the DPFC. This has been interpreted as indicating an increased breakdown of membrane phospholipids and possibly therefore of a decreased number of synapses (Keshaven *et al*, 2000). There is also a suggestion of reduced levels of synaptophysin in the DPFC, as has been found in the hippocampus.

The thalamus

The MRI data suggest there is a reduction in thalamic volume, and this reduction is greatest in the mediodorsal thalamic nucleus, which is reduced by 17–25% in volume and by 27–40% in terms of total neuron number (Young *et al*, 2000). This nucleus is the principal source of projections from the thalamus to the prefrontal cortex, suggesting that thalamic–cortical connectivity may be reduced in schizophrenia. However, these observations should be treated with caution as there has been one negative study (Cullen *et al*, 2000) and the role of possible comorbid alcoholism has not been completely excluded (alcohol may have marked effects on the thalamus).

Molecular biology and histopathology

Modern molecular biological techniques have recently been used in conjunction with conventional histopathology. Thus, Mirnics *et al* (2000) applied complementary DNA microarray profiling for the expression a large number of genes to area 9 of the DPFC in the brains of ten people with schizophrenia and compared the findings with those from ten controls. Only the genes involved in presynaptic function showed decreased expression in the schizophrenic brains and these results appeared to be fairly specific, because no other differences between patients and controls were found for 250 other genes that were also screened.

The distribution of proteins in the brain can now be mapped using molecular biological techniques such as observing the distribution of the messenger RNA that codes for a particular protein. Thus, messenger RNA that encodes for synaptophysin is not reduced in DPFC, whereas it is reduced in the hippocampus (Glantz *et al*, 2000). However, there is decreased expression of the messenger RNA that codes for glutamic acid decarboxylase (GAD_{67}), the synthesising enzyme for gamma-aminobutyric acid (GABA), an important neurotransmitter in the DPFC.

The application of techniques derived from molecular biology to the study of histopathology of the brain in schizophrenia is still in its infancy but seems to be a logical approach, since ultimately the genes responsible for schizophrenia should find their expression in the proteins of the brain.

At present, histopathological research into schizophrenia is concerned mainly with trying to identify consistent differences between the brains of people with schizophrenia and those of controls. The more consistent and generally accepted findings are shown in Box 10.7. It has not yet been possible to establish links between histological findings, clinical symptoms, MRI findings and other brain scan results. However, the application of molecular biological techniques combined with conventional histopathology holds out the

Box 10.7 Key neurohistopathological findings in schizophrenia

General
- Absence of gliosis
- Absence of Alzheimer's disease or other recognised degenerative pathologies

Morphometric findings in hippocampal formation and dorsal prefrontal cortex (DPFC)
- Smaller pyramidal neuronal cell bodies
- Increased neuronal packing density (only replicated in DPFC)
- Decreased presynaptic protein markers (e.g. SNAP-25, synaptophysin)
- Lower density of dendritic spines
- Decreased markers of inhibitory neurons and their synaptic terminals (in DPFC)
- No overall loss of neurons

Other areas
- Mediodorsal thalamic nucleus: decreased volume and neuronal number

After Harrison & Lewis (2003). Reproduced with permission. For more detailed listings and citations, see text and Harrison (1999).

hope that, one day, specific gene proteins and their precise location will be identified.

Is schizophrenia a neurodevelopmental or neurodegenerative disorder?

When Kraepelin first described the condition 'dementia praecox', deterioration was its hallmark. The clinical course suggested a dementing process and the expectation was for the neuropathology to show a neurodegenerative process. The advent of treatment that could sometimes quickly reverse the symptoms and the repeated demonstration that neuropsychological function failed to decline progressively led to an early rejection of Kraepelin's concept of a dementing illness. The first CT brain studies that showed that the ventricular enlargement was present at the outset and that the degree of enlargement showed no correlation with severity of the disorder also suggested that the brain changes must have occurred before the appearance of clinical symptoms. These observations provided the initial impetus for the neurodevelopmental hypothesis for schizophrenia, which is generally credited to Weinberger (1987). It has recently been comprehensively reviewed in Weinberger & Marenco (2003).

The neurodevelopmental hypothesis of schizophrenia proposes that, early in life, subtle abnormalities arise of cortical development, particularly involving limbic and prefrontal cortices and their connections. An additional part of the theory proposes that the triggering of the syndrome depends on an interaction between these developmental abnormalities with normal cerebral maturation in early adult life, especially the maturation of intracortical connections and of the central dopamine system (Weinberger & Marenco, 2003).

This rather general formulation, which was considered to be quite novel in the 1980s, has stimulated a huge amount of research, much of it detailed in the preceding sections of this chapter, and it has now obtained a degree of qualified acceptance. Some of the specific evidence for it is outlined below.

- OCs occur at the time of birth or, in the case of pre-eclampsia, in late pregnancy. The effect is not specific for schizophrenia, as they occur in many other disorders, such as bipolar disorder, eating disorder and personality disorder; nor is the effect size large. The main mechanism proposed is that foetal hypoxia consequent on the OCs results in brain abnormalities which predispose to schizophrenia – but the vast majority of infants born with OCs do not go on to develop schizophrenia.
- Links with antenatal influenzal epidemics, starvation *in utero* and possibly antenatal stress are presumably mediated by their effects on the developing brain.
- The presence of a higher rate of minor, mainly craniofacial abnormalities found in schizophrenia, which have developed presumably *in utero*, has been taken to indicate that minor abnormalities of cerebral development may also have occurred at the same time.
- Altered finger and hand prints have been reported in schizophrenia, and these have aroused some interest because dermatoglyphic patterns are thought to cease development by the third trimester of pregnancy, and hence any abnormality would have developed *in utero* (Fearon *et al*, 2001).
- Subtle defects in cognitive and social function in children (see page 224, this chapter), occurring long before any manifestation of psychotic symptoms, suggests a brain developmental abnormality.
- The early CT studies found ventricular enlargement in schizophrenia. This was probably present at the onset of the disease, and possibly also some time before that as well. The absence of a correlation with disease severity was believed to indicate that the disease was non-progressive, while the positive correlation of ventricular size with both OCs and childhood adjustment indicate that the cerebral changes must have occurred much earlier on. However, these earlier assumptions have been questioned as new and more refined MRI studies are repeatedly demonstrating small annual decrements in grey matter volume in several areas of the brain (see above) and so the brain scanning evidence in favour of a neurodevelopmental rather than a neurodegenerative disorder is now rather less convincing.
- Psychosis itself does not appear to be neurotoxic. Although this is a popular notion in the literature and partly lies behind many of the early intervention treatment programmes, four studies have now shown that the duration of untreated psychosis has no impact on outcome after treatment response to medication, cognition, psychopathology or structured changes on the MRI scan are taken into account (for details and references see Weinberger & Marenco, 2003).
- Histological features of neurodegeneration, such as decreased neuronal numbers and gliosis, which have been repeatedly looked for, are conspicuous by their absence.

Developmental and psychosocial factors

Psychoanalytic theories

Schizophrenia is now rarely regarded by analysts as psychogenic. The position of Rosenfeld (1965) is probably representative. Trauma in infancy, he states, plays an important part:

> 'but similar traumas and problems related to the parents of our patients are known to us from our experience with neurotic patients and are not typical for schizophrenia. The examinations of a large number of parents and families of patients with schizophrenia have shown that the parents of patients with schizophrenia have no character traits which can be regarded as specific. One has to assume that a certain predisposition to the psychosis exists from birth.'

This constitutional vulnerability is cast in psychoanalytic terms – a rudimentary ego with a tendency to fragmentation and splitting. Rosenfeld also comments on the need to consider 'not only the influence of the mother on the child, but the reaction of the mother to a particularly difficult schizoid infant'. This may include a diminished tolerance of the projections of the infant, with the mother feeling disturbed and persecuted and consequently withdrawing feelings from the child. Psychoanalytic methods may thus illuminate understanding of the content of a patient's illness, but not its form – why schizophrenia rather than depression?

Early development

In one of the first studies, Watt (1978) compared the school records of patients who developed schizophrenia to normal control children and found a pattern of greater irritability, disagreeableness and defiance among boys, while girls were more likely to be insecure, inhibited and shy. Abnormalities were more striking among boys.

A study based on children attending a department of child psychiatry (Cannon *et al*, 2001) who were then traced some years later also confirmed that abnormal suspiciousness, sensitivity and difficulties with peers in childhood were good later predictors for the development of schizophrenia in adult life. In this study a model that included two symptom variables, relationship difficulties, two socio-demographic variables, family psychiatric history and past psychiatric contact was able to correctly classify 81% (26/32) of cases correctly, indicating that at least for children attending the child guidance clinic it may be possible to discern some of those at high risk of developing schizophrenia. The childhood pattern for those in this study who subsequently developed an affective psychosis (bipolar disorder or psychotic depression) was different and in these children eating disorders and hysterical presentations were more common.

Although the findings derived from retrospective school records and the observations based on a special population such as child psychiatry attendees are of interest, such studies are likely to be biased, as they are retrospective and only selected populations are examined. One way round this is to examine whole populations prospectively, as in birth cohort studies, which include everyone born at a particular time, who then receive periodic assessments.

Birth cohort studies

Done *et al* (1994) studied the 1958 British Perinatal Mortality Survey cohort, comprising 98% of births in England, Scotland and Wales during a single week. They were able to trace all the adults who were treated in hospital between 1974 and 1986 for psychiatric disorder. Forty were diagnosed with schizophrenia and 35 with affective psychoses. Social adjustment ratings, made at 7 and 11 years, were compared with random normal controls. By the age of 7 years, those who later developed schizophrenia were rated by their teachers as showing more social maladjustment, especially the boys. Boys were more likely to be rated as 'over-reactive', 'anxious for acceptance', hostile to others, and engaging in 'inconsequential behaviours' (e.g. poor concentration, carelessness, lolling about, mischievousness). The 'preschizophrenic' boys showed a similar pattern at 11 years, but the girls at that age had become more 'under-reactive' – withdrawn, unforthcoming and depressed. The pattern in both sexes was quite different from that seen in children who later developed affective disorders.

Jones *et al* (1994) examined a cohort representing a random sample of all births in England, Scotland and Wales during 1 week in 1946 (the Medical Research Council's National Survey of Health and Development). Cases of schizophrenia developing between the ages of 16 and 43 were identified from a variety of sources. Childhood variables collected between the ages of 6 weeks and 16 years were examined and compared with those of a non-schizophrenic cohort. Again, more abnormalities were found in the 'pre-schizophrenic' group. These included: delayed motor milestones; speech problems; low educational test scores at 8, 11 and 15 years; solitary play at 4 and 6 years; less social confidence at 13 years; and greater social anxiety at 15 years. There was no evidence of increased antisocial or aggressive behaviour. When the child was 4 years old, mothers were also more likely to be rated by health visitors as having below-average mothering skills. Thus differences were noted across a range of developmental domains.

Although the UK birth cohort studies have provided useful data, standards of record keeping are probably better in the Scandinavian countries, where there are national psychiatric registers that record the diagnosis of all admissions. In this context, Cannon *et al* (1999) used the Finnish national birth register to conduct a case–control study based on all children born in Helsinki between 1951 and 1960. Using the Finnish national psychiatric register, they identified 400 children who were later diagnosed as having schizophrenia as adults and compared them with 408 controls also born in Helsinki during the same period. They looked at the school records of those children between the ages 7 and 11. The differences between the two groups were modest. There was no difference in academic performance and a wide range of behavioural items also showed no difference. The only differences found between cases and controls were for a 'non-academic factor' that related to abilities at sports and handicrafts, which the authors explained as a 'motor factor'. A second significant difference related to failure to progress to high school, despite similar eligibility, and the authors suggested this may have been related to motivation.

Summary

It can be seen that the well-designed epidemiologically based studies find very much smaller differences than the retrospective studies or those drawn from special populations, and also the actual findings differ between studies. Nevertheless, the fact that even modest differences can be detected in childhood – at least a decade before the appearance of the florid illness – suggests that, at least in some children, there must already be some mild brain abnormality present. This provides some support for the neurodevelopmental model of schizophrenia.

Studies of people at risk

Another strategy has been to examine people deemed to be at high risk of schizophrenia, that is, people who have at least one first-degree relative with the disorder. Thus, by following up a cohort of offspring of parents with schizophrenia, for example with periodic retesting, it is hoped to identify predictors of later illness. Findings to date have been limited. Background factors, including early life events and disturbed family relations, have shown little evidence of specificity for schizophrenia when controls such as offspring of parents with other psychiatric disorders have been studied (Erlenmeyer-Kimling & Cornblatt, 1987). However, a range of bio-behavioural 'markers' or 'traits' have been posited. The most frequently studied has been attentional dysfunction. For example, performance on complex versions of the continuous performance test is impaired in schizophrenia, even during remission; it is also worse in unaffected relatives (including at-risk children) than in controls, is heritable, and is predictive of later behavioural disturbances, such as social isolation, thought to be related to schizophrenia. Also studied have been eye-tracking dysfunction (e.g. smooth pursuit eye movements), electrodermal responsivity (including both hyper- and hypo-responsiveness), and several different types of event-related brain potential. Each has shown promise, but to date there is insufficient evidence that they predict the emergence of schizophrenia, while inconsistencies and non-replication between studies is common. The whole area has been comprehensively reviewed by Egan *et al* (2003).

Premorbid personality

Bleuler (1911) wrote:

> 'there are early character anomalies which can be demonstrated by careful case histories in more than half the individuals who later become schizophrenic: the tendency to seclusion, withdrawal together with moderate or severe degrees of irritability.'

The premorbid personality refers to the few years that precede the onset of the illness, but after the childhood years. In many cases there is a blurring of the premorbid personality and the prodrome of the illness itself. Reviewing studies of premorbid personality in schizophrenia, Cutting (1985) concluded that about a quarter of patients had a 'schizoid' personality and a further one-sixth were abnormal in other respects. Foerster *et al* (1991) interviewed mothers of 73 consecutively admitted patients with schizophrenia or affective psychosis (meeting DSM–III criteria). Men with schizophrenia showed much greater premorbid schizoid and schizotypal traits than either women with the condition or patients with an affective disorder. The same applied to reported adjustment at secondary school age. Late childhood impairments were more predictive of schizophrenia than early impairments, while the poorer the premorbid adjustment was, the earlier was the age at first admission to hospital.

Chapman *et al* (1994) tested several hundred students with a battery of questionnaires designed to measure schizotypy. Students with high scores and those with normal scores were followed up 10 years later. Fourteen of the high scorers had been admitted to hospital with a psychotic illness, compared with only a single person with a normal score. A further study showed that patients with schizophrenia underachieved occupationally compared with their fathers, as did patients with an affective psychosis. However, only in the former was underachievement evident before the illness began. In both groups decline was noted after illness onset (Jones *et al*, 1993). This suggests that subtle cognitive or social difficulties antedate obvious symptoms of the illness by many years.

A prospective cohort study (Malmberg *et al*, 1998) based on a sample of 50087 men conscripted into the Swedish army probably provides the most reliable data. On entry to the army the men received a battery of psychometric tests and questionnaires, and the 193 who subsequently developed schizophrenia were compared with the rest of the conscripts. Although many differences were noted, after controlling for IQ, family history, diagnosis at conscription, and living in a city, only five variables remained significant. These were:

1 having fewer than two close friends

2 preferring to socialise in small groups

3 feeling more sensitive than other people

4 drug taking

5 not having a steady girlfriend.

The first three of these variables probably reflect the schizoid/schizotypal traits identified in the previous studies, while the two other items probably reflect behaviours that are part of the schizophrenia prodrome.

Malmberg *et al* (1998) suggest that a psychological mechanism underlying these traits might reflect difficulty in performing 'theory of mind' tasks, that is, making accurate inferences about other people's mental states. Such a deficit may result in social withdrawal and isolation, with limited interaction and opportunities for reality testing, and so perhaps encourage a paranoid style of thinking; this in itself could predispose to the development of psychosis.

While it is of some theoretical interest, particularly in the context of the neurodevelopmental model, that abnormalities in childhood and in the premorbid personality can be detected, it is important to note that, for the vast majority of people with schizophrenia, the childhood and early adolescent years are essentially normal, and in almost all cases it would be virtually impossible to predict a later schizophrenic denouement.

Social factors

Life events

The role of life events in the causation of schizophrenia has proved difficult to clarify. Cutting (1985) concluded that there was little evidence that catastrophic single events could cause schizophrenia.

Steinberg & Durrell (1968) studied the impact of a specific major life event – recruitment to the US army. The participants were young men aged 20–24 years and included both volunteers and draftees. There was a striking increase in admissions for schizophrenia during the first year after recruitment, especially in the first few months, compared with the second year. This could not be explained by pre-existing symptoms or a choice to join the army as a result of psychiatric illness or its prodrome, since conscription ensured that everyone had to join the army. There was evidence of more schizoid traits in those developing schizophrenia. The authors concluded that the demands for adaptation and hence the levels of stress were greatest in the early months after entry into the army and that the most predisposed broke down first. The pattern of breakdown following immigration, which is also a life event, is very different, with the schizophrenia often appearing many years later; this is further discussed in Chapter 31, on page 797.

The most common approach to studying life events derives from a seminal study by Brown & Birley (1968), which examined the frequency of a range of life events before the onset or relapse of a schizophrenic illness. Around 46% of patients had a significant independent (see below) life event in the 3 weeks prior to onset compared with 12% during other 3-week periods in the study period, and a 14% rate among a group of normal controls during a 3-week period. Relapse was associated with life events especially in patients compliant with neuroleptic medication; those discontinuing medication relapsed without the occurrence of events.

Further studies in this vein have contended with a variety of thorny issues (Norman & Malla, 1993*b*). These include:

1 *Establishing a valid measure of life events.* Each person's experience of events is unique; a similar occurrence may have quite different meanings to different people. However, a patient's personal view about the seriousness of a life event might be exaggerated by an attempt to explain why he or she became ill ('effort after meaning') or might be coloured by being ill. Which dimension of stress should be emphasised is another problem – choices could include threat or the requirement for change. Some life event instruments such as the Life Events and Difficulties Schedule (LEDS; Brown & Harris, 1978) take a semi-objective approach. Each event is assessed by a research panel for the degree of threat it entails for the individual, rated in the context of other information about the person's life history and current situation.

2 *Problems with recall.* Biases due to differential recall may be introduced when two groups, for example patients and normals, are compared. There may be a 'recency effect' where 3 months before the control's interview is compared with 3 months before the onset of illness (which may have been some time ago) in the patients. Similarly, recall of events in a specified period before illness onset may be favoured when compared with similar-length periods in the more distant past.

3 *Independence between the life events and illness.* Suffering from schizophrenia leads to new life events, such as unemployment, failed relationships, loss of home and so on. Results of the illness may thus be erroneously regarded as causes. The LEDS incorporates an added sophistication in that the likelihood that the life event is independent of the illness is also assessed by trained raters. Furthermore, the onset of the illness is treated conservatively by locating it as far back in time as possible.

In reviewing the role of life events in schizophrenia, Norman & Malla (1993*a*) grouped studies to answer three questions:

1 Do patients with schizophrenia have more severe life events before illness onset than those suffering from other psychiatric disorders? Here, the reviewers found that none of the eight relevant studies showed more severe life events for schizophrenia than for other disorders.

2 Do they have more life events than normal controls? Here, 5 out of 14 studies found more life events for patients admitted for schizophrenia than for normal controls.

3 Is there a relationship in patients suffering from schizophrenia between life event stressors and severity of symptoms? Here the authors found 23 out of 30 studies showed a peaking of life events before either illness onset or worsening of symptoms.

Among the last group of studies was a cross-national study by the World Health Organization (Day *et al*, 1987), which found a clustering of events in the 3 weeks before an episode in six of nine countries. The authors concluded:

> 'In general, there is considerably more evidence for variation in stressors being associated with changes in the course of symptoms for patients with schizophrenia than for patients with schizophrenia having been exposed to more external life event stressors than the general population or patients suffering from other psychiatric disorders.'

The interval over which excess events occur is unclear; in some studies this has been 3–4 weeks before onset; in others it has been up to 6 months.

Most studies have focused on major life events. It is possible, however, that an accumulation of apparently trivial difficulties or 'hassles' might also be capable of precipitating the disorder. Certainly, the long-term stress of an environment high in 'expressed emotion' (see below) is associated with relapse even in the absence of a life event. The type of relapse may take the form either of a depressive episode or a psychotic relapse. One longitudinal study found that independent life event(s) were equally likely to cause a depressive episode as a psychotic relapse (Ventura *et al*, 2000).

Most studies of life events in schizophrenia have focused on the early phases of the illness, but the majority of admissions are for recurrences and it is questionable whether these are also associated with new life events. In the early study by Brown & Birley (1968) there was no difference between the rate of life events for first admissions and relapses, but the number of patients who had multiple relapses was small, and it now appears that the effect of life events may attenuate for those with multiple admissions. Thus, Castine *et al* (1998) found that the number of life events experienced by patients who had been admitted four or more times was only a third of the number of life events that preceded the admissions of patients who had had three or fewer admissions, and this difference was statistically significant; there was also a significant negative correlation between the number of life events and the number of admissions. Because the bulk of the admissions to hospital are for recurrent cases (75% in this study), the overall impact of life events on total admissions may not be large, although perhaps greater during the earlier admissions. The authors suggested that recurrence might be related to a kindling effect, as has been suggested in recurrent depression, where an attenuation of the effect of life events has also been found (Ghazuiddin *et al*, 1990), but other reasons for recurrence such as repeated non-compliance with medication are equally likely.

Medication generally protects against relapses due to all causes and one study found that those on medication who relapsed experienced significantly more stressful life events before their relapse than those who were not on medication, which the authors interpreted as meaning a relatively greater degree of stress was required to trigger a relapse for those on medication (Ventura *et al*, 1992).

Family factors

Interest in family aspects of schizophrenia burgeoned after the Second World War. Initially, the influence of psychoanalytic theory was strong, including the notion of the 'schizophrenogenic mother' (since discredited), but the ideas described below (which are usefully summarised by Hirsch & Leff, 1975) are now more of historical interest. Work in the 1950s and 1960s by researchers such as Lidz failed to identify a specific 'schizophrenogenic' pattern. The focus shifted to relationship difficulties between the parents and the way in which the patient was 'ensnared' by them. This could extend to the patient having a role in stabilising the parental relationship. Bowen described problems of individuation in the family, especially due to projective mechanisms, possibly transmitted across several generations.

Bateson and co-workers focused on family communication, both verbal and non-verbal, leading to the idea of the 'double bind', considered by them an important mechanism in the genesis of schizophrenia. The recipient of the bind picks up contradictory messages at verbal and non-verbal levels, but because of dependency on the sender, is not able to comment on this inconsistency nor quit the relationship. It was hypothesised that a response to this situation might be the development of a communication disorder characteristic of schizophrenia. This group was also prominent in developing the idea of family homeostasis, and the ways in which a family may under certain circumstances achieve stability at the expense of the health of its members.

The 1960s saw many observational studies of families with a schizophrenic member, but few consistent findings emerged. Features such as family efficiency, flexibility, conflict, dominance, coalitions and distorted communications, including the 'double bind', were studied. Variations in the overall framework of the research, the kinds of observations made, the measures used and the definitions employed have made interpretation of the results difficult (Doane, 1978).

These studies were reviewed by Hirsch & Leff (1975), who concluded that there was only weak evidence that parents of patients with schizophrenia might be more psychiatrically disturbed than parents of normal children and that much of this could be explained by the following factors:

1 bringing up an abnormal child
2 more marital disharmony than in the parents of normals
3 parents of patients with schizophrenia show more concern and protectiveness than parents of normals.

However, they noted that none of these conclusions was strong and that no study provided evidence that parental abnormalities exerted a specific effect during the patient's formative years. There was evidence that the 'pre-schizophrenic' child frequently manifested physical ill-health or mild disability in early life, so that parental abnormalities might have been a consequence of these. Since their review, more evidence has accumulated for delayed milestones, neurological abnormalities and social inadequacy in the early years of children who later develop schizophrenia (Crow *et al*, 1995). Parental overprotection and concern may therefore easily develop in response to these features. Peculiarities in both parent and child may also of course share a common genetic basis. In the 1970s, research began to focus on two areas which have become subjects of enduring interest: 'communication deviance' (CD) and, particularly, 'expressed emotion' (EE).

Communication deviance (CD)

This concept, developed by Wynne & Singer (1963), refers to a person's fragmented and disorganised communications, including poor ability to maintain a focus. They hypothesised that such communication styles could result in disturbed information processing and thinking in vulnerable offspring. Measures of CD were developed on the basis of parents' interpretation of projective tests. The researchers found it was possible to differentiate between offspring with and without schizophrenia solely on the basis of parental CD.

An attempt to replicate this work was made by Hirsch & Leff (1975), who compared CD in relatives of patients suffering from schizophrenia with relatives of neurotic controls. CD was increased in the former group, but this was largely accounted for by their greater verbosity. Hirsch & Leff concluded that the relationship between CD and schizophrenia was not supported; but it remains possible that increased verbosity might result from communication difficulties. It is also possible that CD is a genetic trait manifesting in parents and offspring, irrespective of any transactional component, or that it is a consequence of living with a youngster with schizophrenia. The concept of CD in schizophrenia is no longer prominent, but it comprises one element which was incorporated into the assessment of family dysfunction in the very thorough and important cross-fostering studies of Tienari *et al* (2004), which are described below (see page 229).

Expressed emotion (EE)

Prompted by a finding that patients with schizophrenia fared worse when discharged to the family home with parents or spouses than to siblings or to lodgings (Brown *et al*, 1958), a series of studies investigating family emotional climate was initiated (Brown *et al*, 1972). From these arose the influential concept of EE. Early work examined the role of both positive and negative features, but later research focused on relatives' negative and intrusive attitudes to the patient, although warmth was significantly associated with a better outcome.

EE is now assessed on the basis of a semi-structured, standardised interview, the Camberwell Family Interview (Brown *et al*, 1972; Vaughn & Leff, 1976), carried out with a relative. Ratings are made from audiotapes and are based on both content and vocal tone. The key ratings are:

1 critical comments – a frequency count of statements of resentment, disapproval or dislike expressed in a critical tone of voice, together with comments of a critical tone irrespective of content

2 hostility – criticism for what the person is rather than for what he or she does, or generalised criticism

3 emotional overinvolvement – unusually marked concern about the patient, such as constant worry over minor matters, overprotective attitudes, intrusive behaviour, or reports of excessive self-sacrifice.

Warmth and positive comments are also rated. A designation of 'high EE' is based on a score above a threshold for critical comments, hostility and emotional overinvolvement. The ability of a high-EE rating to predict relapse was examined by Bebbington & Kuipers (1994), who carried out an aggregate analysis based on 25 studies. Nine months after the initial assessment, 50% of those with families with high EE scores had relapsed, compared with 21% for those from low-EE families.

While frequent contact with a high-EE relative increased the risk of relapse, low-EE homes appeared protective. Medication independently reduced relapse in high-EE families over 9 months and in low-EE families over 2 years. The predictive validity of EE seems to be independent of patient symptom severity and history of illness, although a minority of studies have found that EE is higher when patients' symptoms are worse and their behaviour more disturbed (MacMillan *et al*, 1986).

Most studies have assessed EE at the time of the patient's admission to hospital and then examined its ability to predict relapse over the next year or so. Assessing EE at admission introduces a possible 'reactive' contribution, relating to relatives facing a crisis and the effectiveness with which they handle it, in addition to any ongoing aspect of the relationship it may reflect. In a study in which EE was assessed in stable out-patients with schizophrenia over 5 years, the level of EE was stable in 63% of families (25% high; 38% low) but fluctuated in the remainder (McCreadie *et al*, 1993). Thus EE, though often steady, is not necessarily a 'static' attribute of a relative or a family and may vary with circumstances and treatment interventions.

EE is able to predict relapse across cultures, including British, American (including both Anglo-Americans and Americans of Mexican descent), Spanish, Italian, Czech, Chinese, Japanese and Indian. Although expressions of criticism and emotional overinvolvement are highly culturally determined, apparently they can be reliably rated. A strength of the measure is that rating incorporates standards appropriate to a specific culture. Levels of criticism and overinvolvement, and their relative contributions to high EE, vary across cultures, yet within different ranges they have predictive validity. It has been suggested that cross-cultural differences in family structure and emotional atmosphere indexed by EE may contribute to the variability in outcomes for schizophrenia across the world (Leff *et al*, 1987).

EE and family interactions

Exactly how EE relates to family interaction is only beginning to be explored. The evidence indicates that high EE is associated with a number of negative patterns. High-EE relatives are probably less informed about schizophrenia, and are more likely to attribute difficult behaviour to personal characteristics of the patient rather than the illness, or to believe more control could be exercised (Brewin *et al*, 1991). High-EE relatives are more likely to be unpredictable in their responses to the patient, while low-EE relatives are often described as calm, empathic and respectful of the patient's, often eccentric, needs, although around a quarter of low-EE relatives report high stress levels, burden or impaired coping.

Reciprocal interactions between patient and relatives make the processes more complex. It has been claimed, for example, that problem behaviours may lead to unsuccessful attempts at coping by relatives who respond with 'high EE', which in turn may exacerbate the problem behaviours and symptoms. Smith *et al* (1993) found that high-EE relatives experience more distress and burden, and perceive themselves as coping with life less well than low-EE relatives.

High-EE parents have been shown to be critical in direct interaction with their ill offspring and negative patterns of interaction have been identified. Thus, Hahlweg *et al* (1989) examined verbal and non-verbal sequences between a parent and patient. When discussing emotion-laden family problems, high-EE, critical parents exhibited more criticism, negative affect and negative solution proposals. Low-EE parents made more positive and supportive statements. Patients with critical relatives displayed more negative nonverbal affect and more disagreement, and made more self-justifying statements. Sequential analyses showed sustained negative reciprocal patterns in critical families, while low-EE relatives were able to cut short these developing patterns.

A study of EE in professional carers working in sheltered houses showed that carers who were high EE towards one patient were always low EE towards another, thus substantiating the interactional nature of the measure (Willetts & Leff, 1997).

Although an effect for EE on relapse rates is no longer in doubt, the size of this effect and the overall cause of relapse is unclear. A meta-analysis (Butzlaff & Hooley, 1998) of 27 high-EE outcome studies in schizophrenia gave an estimate of the effect size at $r = 0.31$, which the authors translated into a relapse rate of 65% for high-EE families and 35% for low-EE families, suggesting that the readmission rate might be reduced by up to a third if an intervention could change a high-EE family to a low-EE one. However, as many patients with schizophrenia live on their own and the overall frequency of a high-EE pattern is relatively low – McCreadie *et al* (1993) estimated that it occurred in around 25% of families – the total number of relapses that might be prevented by successfully reducing high levels of EE is correspondingly smaller.

The EE model has also been investigated in anorexia nervosa and affective disorders, and in both conditions a high-EE family is a predictor of relapse or a poorer outcome. Although the number of studies is fewer, the effect is significantly greater than that found for schizophrenia. In their meta-analysis, Butzlaff & Hooley (1998) gave an effect size of $r = 0.51$ for anorexia nervosa (three studies) and $r = 0.39$ for affective disorder (six studies). Thus, a high EE rating is a relatively non-specific predictor for relapse across a wide range of psychiatric disorders, including schizophrenia. Its importance lies in the possibility that it may be amenable to reversal (in contrast to most of the other known environmental triggers, such as obstetric complications, influenza epidemics, urbanicity, etc.), even though the total number of relapses prevented may be small. Research in this area has highlighted the importance of family factors, so that today even the most biologically minded psychiatrists, relying mainly on drug therapy, will usually ensure that they also have a thorough knowledge of the family relationships, particularly for their frequently relapsing patients.

The EE concept has not proved popular with families, nor with some relatives' organisations, particularly in the United States, as it is sometimes perceived as yet another means of blaming relatives for the patient's illness. A focus on the protective aspects of low EE has been urged by some as a counterbalance to the more common emphasis on determining what is detrimental about high EE (Lefley, 1992). Emphasising the fact that high-EE attitudes are found in relatives across a wide range of psychiatric and non-psychiatric conditions helps, as does their detection in professional carers.

Gene–environment interactions

Two models currently in the psychiatric literature aim to integrate the variety of genetic and environmental factors that have been identified as possible causes of psychiatric disorder. The vulnerability–stress model proposes that vulnerability in an individual is determined by genetic and very early influences, but its expression requires some environmental stress factors. The bio-psychosocial model is similar, but probably more sophisticated, and is more comprehensively discussed on page 446. Briefly, this model proposes a hierarchy of causes, starting with the gene and going on to the cell, the brain and various organs in the body, up to the individual. Beyond the individual lies a further hierarchy of environmental causes, such as the early family environment, the patient's social world, the occupational sphere, socio-economic factors and political/historical events. Interactions between genes and any other causes can occur at any level, and there may be interactive and additive effects between any of the identified causes.

Because of the great difficulties in studying a single parameter thoroughly in schizophrenia, few studies have made any attempt to study both genetic and environmental factors simultaneously. One such study, however, is the Finnish cross-adoption study (Tienari, 1971; Tienari *et al*, 2000, 2004), which is not only the largest adoption study in the field but also the most detailed study of the emotional environment of the rearing family. It has found significant interactive effects. Because of the almost heroic proportions of the study and its long duration (over 30 years), as well as the importance of its findings, it is described in some detail below.

To identify all the women with schizophrenia who had their children adopted, the records of every female psychiatric patient admitted in Finland over a 20-year period (1960–79) were scrutinised for a diagnosis of schizophrenia or paranoid psychosis. To confirm that these women had definitely given up their children for adoption, every single parish register in Finland was searched for information on adoption, and once a mother with schizophrenia who had given up a child for adoption was identified, the judicial court files pertaining to that the adoption were checked to confirm that the adoption had occurred and that in all cases the adoptions were to unrelated families. The authors wrote:

> 'In this tedious search across the whole country we identified 264 index schizophrenic/paranoid mothers who had adopted among 291 offspring.' (Tienari *et al*, 2000, p. 434)

This degree of rigour in case finding, which is almost unparalleled in the literature, makes it likely that case ascertainment was complete or at least more compete than in any of the previous studies.

Selecting the control adoptive parents was equally rigorous. Using the national adoption agency, the next listed adoptee and family was selected, and matched on a variety of socio-demographic variables.

Psychiatric case ascertainment of all the adoptees (index and control) was made 12 and 21 years after the start of the study using standard methods and DSM–III–R criteria, while the mean age at the final case ascertainment was 44 years, by which time the bulk of the risk period for schizophrenia and the schizophrenia spectrum disorders had passed.

The results of the genetic part of the study were in the expected direction. The lifetime morbid risks for schizophrenia for adoptees with a biological mother with schizophrenia (the group at high genetic risk) was

5.34%, which was significantly increased over the rate for adoptees at low genetic risk, which was 1.74%. For all the schizophrenia spectrum disorders, the lifetime risk was 22.46% for the high-risk group, compared with 4.36% for the low-risk group.

The more interesting part of the study related to the interaction between dysfunctional families (the environmental component) and a genetic predisposition to schizophrenia. The measurement of family environment was extremely thorough. Thirty-three scales were used to measure family interaction over a wide range of activities, drawn from concepts thought to be relevant to schizophrenia at the start of the project (in the 1970s). These were grouped into three main areas:

1 'critical/conflictual', which roughly corresponds to the high-EE pattern
2 'constricted', which somewhat resembles 'communication deviance'
3 'boundary problems', which were all combined together.

Families were assessed over 2 days, with individual, joint and whole-family interviews. This provided 14–16 hours of taped material, which is very much longer and more thorough than most other types of family assessment.

Adoptees with a low genetic loading (i.e. having a mother without schizophrenia) had low rates of later psychopathology, regardless of family environment. In particular, even adoptees with a high genetic loading (i.e. a biological mother with schizophrenia) did well in healthy, non-dysfunctional families: their rate for schizophrenia spectrum disorders was 5.8%, which was not significantly greater than the rate for the controls, at 4.8%. It was as if a healthy family environment protected against the expression of the schizophrenic genotype.

However, in the dysfunctional families, the rates for schizophrenia were high: for those with high genetic loading it was 36.8%, compared with 5.3% for the controls (those at low genetic risk). Thus, the dysfunctional family environment yielded a much increased risk for those at high genetic risk (OR = 10.0) but had a negligible effect on those at low genetic risk (OR = 1.11).

While the earlier adoption studies were able to demonstrate that having a mother with schizophrenia led to a simple increase in the rate of schizophrenia spectrum disorders, the studies of Tienari *et al* (2004) have been able to offer some explanation as to why some adoptees at high risk will develop the disorder while others do not. It is likely that many of the other environmental triggers for schizophrenia act in a similar way, with disorders developing in response to the environmental cause only where there is already some genetic predisposition, but having little effect in the absence of such a predisposition.

Table 10.2 Risk factors and antecedents of schizophrenia

Risk factor or antecedent	Estimated effect size (odds ratio or relative risk)
Familial (family member with schizophrenia)	
Biological parent	7.0–10.0
Two parents	29.0
Monozygotic twin	40.8
Dizygotic twin	5.3
Non-twin sibling	7.3
Second-degree relative	1.6–2.8
Social and demographic	
Single marital status	3.9
Stressful life events	1.5
Migrant/minority status (e.g. Afro-Caribbeans in UK)	>7.0
Urban birth	2.1–4.2
Winter birth	1.1
Prenatal, perinatal and early postnatal	
Obstetric complications ('non-optimality' summary score)	4.6
Maternal respiratory infection, second trimester	2.1
Birth weight < 2000 g	3.0
Birth weight < 2500 g	2.9
Severe malnutrition during pregnancy	2.6
Gestation < 37 weeks	2.5
Perinatal hypoxic brain damage	4.6–6.9
Neurodevelopmental and neurocognitive	
Early infection of central nervous system	4.8
Epilepsy	11.1
Low IQ (< 74)	8.6
Preference for solitary play, age 4–6 years	2.1
Speech and educational problems, age < 12 years	2.8
Low score on the continuous performance test	3.3

After Jablensky (2003), reproduced with permission. For references see Jablensky (2003). Note that a high relative risk does not necessarily signify a high population-attributable fraction if the frequency of the cause is very low.

Conclusion

No necessary or sufficient cause of schizophrenia has so far been identified. A large number of environmental risk factors have been identified as possible causes, and these are listed in Table 10.2. The genetic studies have consistently shown that most of the cause is inherited, with the most recent estimates suggesting that hereditable factors account for 80% of the variance. This implies that many of the putative environmental causes probably also include significant genetic elements as well.

Many of the identified environmental causes are non-specific and probably apply to the majority of the population. For example, most people live in cities and everyone will experience life events from time to time. A winter–spring birth will apply to around a quarter of the population and many people will be reared by critical parents, yet only a tiny minority will develop schizophrenia. Even though statistical associations between these causes and schizophrenia have been established, they also contribute to a wide variety of other physical and psychiatric disorders and so lack specificity.

The discovery of the antipsychotic drugs and their obvious clinical usefulness (Chapter 11) has led to a huge amount of research into dopamine and other chemicals in the hope of establishing a neurochemical basis for the disorder. Equally, the search for anatomical abnormalities as demonstrated by MRI scans has established that there are abnormalities in the brain, particularly in the ventricles, temporal lobes and hippocampus. Attempts to draw the existing body of knowledge together in global theories such as the neurodevelopmental model or the various stress–diathesis hypotheses have been only partially convincing, because it is obvious that some major causative factor(s) have yet to be identified. Recent hopes now lie with molecular biology and the new genetics, because there has been an explosion in research in this area right across medicine, which has led to the successful identification of many of the specific genes associated with a wide variety of diseases. This has stimulated the hope that the genes responsible for schizophrenia will be identified in a similar way, but it is possible that this will take longer than for the more simple, Mendelian disorders. If schizophrenia is a largely genetic disorder, and its cause lies in the brain, then the critical abnormalities should lie in a few of the many thousands of different proteins found in the brain, but the relevant ones have still to be identified. If the responsible genes can be determined, it will become possible to identify those environmental factors that interact with the inherited vulnerability to produce schizophrenia.

References

Achté, K. A., Hillbom, E. & Aalberg, V. (1969) Psychosis following war brain injuries. *Acta Psychiatrica Scandinavica*, **45**, 1–18.

Achté, K. A., Jarho, L., Kyykka, T., *et al* (1991) Paranoid disorders following war brain damage. *Psychopathology*, **24**, 209–315.

Adams, W., Kendell, R. E. & Hare, E. H. (1993) Epidemiological evidence that maternal influenza contributes to the aetiology of schizophrenia: an analysis of Scottish, English and Danish data. *British Journal of Psychiatry*, **163**, 522–534.

American Psychiatric Association (1994) *Diagnostic and Statistical Manual of Mental Disorders* (4th edn) (DSM–IV). Washington, DC: APA.

Anath, H., Popescu, I., Critchley, H. D., *et al* (2002) Cortical and subcortical grey matter abnormalities in schizophrenia determined through structural magnetic resonance imaging with optimized volumetric voxel-based morphometry. *American Journal of Psychiatry*, **159**, 1497–1505.

Andreasen, N. C., Smith, M. R., Jacoby, C. G., *et al* (1982) Ventricular enlargement in schizophrenia, definition and prevalence. *American Journal of Psychiatry*, **139**, 292–296.

Andreasen, N. C., Swayze, V. W. 2nd, Flaum, M., *et al* (1990*a*) Ventricular enlargement in schizophrenia evaluated with computed tomographic scanning. Effects of gender, age and stage of illness. *Archives of General Psychiatry*, **47**, 1008–1015.

Andreasen, N. C., Ehrhardt, J. C., Swayze, V. W. 2nd, *et al* (1990*b*) Magnetic resonance imaging of the brain in schizophrenia. The pathophysiologic significance of structural abnormalities. *Archives of General Psychiatry*, **47**, 35–44.

Andréasson, S., Allebeck, P., Engstrom, A., *et al* (1988) Cannabis and schizophrenia: a longitudinal study of Swedish conscripts. *Lancet*, **ii**, 1483–1485.

Arseneault, L., Cannon, M., Witton, J., *et al* (2004) Causal associative between cannabis and psychosis: examination of the evidence. *British Journal of Psychiatry*, **184**, 110–117.

Atakan, Z. (2004) Cannabis and psychosis. In *Fast Facts. Psychiatry Highlights 2003–2004* (ed. M. Lader). Oxford: Health Press.

Baare, W. F., Hulshoff Pol, H. E., Hijman, R., *et al* (1999) Volumetric analysis of frontal lobe regions in schizophrenia: relation to cognitive function and symptomatology. *Biological Psychiatry*, **45**, 1597–1605.

Badner, J. & Gershon, E. (2002) Meta-analysis of whole-genome linkage scans of bipolar disorder and schizophrenia. *Molecular Psychiatry*, **7**, 405–411.

Baron, M. (1986) Genetics of schizophrenia. I: Familial patterns and mode of inheritance. *Biological Psychiatry*, **21**, 1051–1066.

Barta, P. E., Pearlson, G. D., Powers, R. E., *et al* (1990) Auditory hallucinations and smaller superior temporal gyral volume in schizophrenia. *American Journal of Psychiatry*, **147**, 1457–1462.

Barta, P. E., Pearlson, G. D., Brill, L. B., *et al* (1997) Planum temporale asymmetry reversal in schizophrenia: replication and relationship to gray matter abnormalities. *American Journal of Psychiatry*, **154**, 661–667.

Bassett, A. S., McGillivray, B. C., Jones, B. D., *et al* (1988) Partial trisomy chromosome 5 cosegregating with schizophrenia. *Lancet*, **i**, 799–801.

Bassett, A. S., Chow, E. W. & Weksberg, R. (2000) Chromosomal abnormalities and schizophrenia. *American Journal of Medical Genetics*, **97**, 45–51.

Bebbington, P. & Kuipers, L. (1994) The predictive utility of expressed emotion in schizophrenia, an aggregate analysis. *Psychological Medicine*, **24**, 707–718.

Benson, M., Newey, S., Martin-Rebdon, E., *et al* (2001) Dysbindin, a novel coiled-coil containing protein that interacts with the dystrobrevins in muscle and brain. *Journal of Biological Chemistry*, **276**, 24232–24241.

Bentaleb, L. A., Beauregard, M., Liddle, P., *et al* (2002) Cerebral activity associated with auditory verbal hallucinations: a functional magnetic resonance imaging *case study. Journal of Psychiatry and Neuroscience*, **27**, 110–115.

Bertolino, A., Esposito, G., Callicott, J. H., *et al* (2000) Specific relationship between prefrontal neuronal N-acetylaspartate and activation of the working memory cortical network in schizophrenia. *American Journal of Psychiatry*, **157**, 26–33.

Bleuler, E. (1911) *Dementia Praecox oder der Gruppe der schizophrenein*. Leipzig: Deuliche. Translated by Zinkin, J. (1950) *Dementia Praecox or the Group of Schizophrenias*. New York: International Universities Press.

Blouin, J. L., Dombroski, B. A., Nath, S. K., *et al* (1998) Schizophrenia susceptibility loci on chromosomes 13q32 and 8p21. *Nature Genetics*, **20**, 70–73.

Bradbury, T. N. & Miller, G. A. (1985) Season of birth in schizophrenia: a review of evidence, methodology, and etiology. *Psychological Bulletin*, **98**, 569–594.

Brewin, C. R., MacCarthy, B., Duda, K., *et al* (1991) Attribution and expressed emotion in the relatives of patients with schizophrenia. *Journal of Abnormal Psychology*, **100**, 546–554.

Brown, A. S., Cohen, P., Greenwald, S., *et al* (2000*a*) Nonaffective psychosis after prenatal exposure to rubella. *American Journal of Psychiatry*, **157**, 438–443.

Brown, A. S., Schaefer, C A., Wyatt, R. J., *et al* (2000*b*) Maternal exposure to respiratory infections and adult schizophrenia spectrum disorders: a prospective birth cohort study. *Schizophrenia Bulletin*, **26**, 287–296.

Brown, G. W. & Birley, J. L. T. (1968) Crises and life changes and the onset of schizophrenia. *Journal of Health and Social Behaviour*, **9**, 203–214.

Brown, G. W. & Harris, T. (1978) *The Social Origins of Depression. A Study of Psychiatric Disorder in Women*. London: Tavistock.

Brown, G. W., Carstairs, G. M. & Topping, G. C. (1958) The post hospital adjustment of chronic mental patients. *Lancet*, **ii**, 685–689.

Brown, G. W., Carstairs, G. M. & Wing, J. K. (1972) The influence of family life on the course of schizophrenic disorders, a replication. *British Journal of Psychiatry*, **121**, 241–258.

Buka, S. L., Tsuang, M. T. & Torrey, E. F. (2000) Maternal prenatal infections and adult psychosis: a forty year prospective study. *Schizophrenia Research*, **41**, 67–68 (abstract).

Butzlaff, R. L. & Hooley, J. M. (1998) Expressed emotion and psychiatric relapse. *Archives of General Psychiatry*, **55**, 547–552.

Cahn, W., Hulshoff Pol, H. E., Lems, E. B., *et al* (2002*a*) Brain volume changes in first-episode schizophrenia: a 1-year follow-up study. *Archives of General Psychiatry*, **59**, 1002–1010.

Cahn, W., Hulshoff Pol, H. E., Bongers, M., *et al* (2002*b*) Brain morphology in antipsychotic-naive schizophrenia: a study of multiple brain structures. *British Journal of Psychiatry*, **181**, suppl. 43, S66–S72.

Cannon, M., Cotter, D., Sham, P. C., *et al* (1996) Schizophrenia in an Irish sample following prenatal exposure to the 1957 influenza epidemic: a case-controlled, prospective follow-up study. *Schizophrenia Research*, **11**, 95.

Cannon, M., Jones, P., Huttunen, O., *et al* (1999) School performance in Finnish children and later development of schizophrenia: a population-based longitudinal study. *Archives of General Psychiatry*, **56**, 457–463.

Cannon, M., Walsh, E., Hollis, C., *et al* (2001) Predictors of later schizophrenia and affective psychosis among attendees at a child psychiatry department. *British Journal of Psychiatry*, **178**, 420–426.

Cannon, M., Jones, P. B. & Murray, R. M. (2003) Obstetric complications and schizophrenia: historical and meta-analytic review. *American Journal of Psychiatry*, **159**, 1080–1092.

Cannon, T. D., Rosso, I. M., Hollister, J. M., *et al* (2000) A prospective cohort study of genetic and perinatal influences in the etiology of schizophrenia. *Schizophrenia Bulletin*, **26**, 351–366.

Cardno, A. G. & Gottesman, I. I. (2000) Twin studies of schizophrenia: from bow-and-arrow concordances to Star Wars Mx and functional genomics. *American Journal of Medical Genetics*, **97**, 12–17.

Cardno, A. G., Rijsdijk, F. V., Sham, P. C., *et al* (2002) A twin study of genetic relationships between psychotic symptoms. *American Journal of Psychiatry*, 159, 539–545.

Castine, M. R., Meador-Woodruff, J. H. & Dalach, G. W. (1998) The role of life events in onset and recurrent episodes of schizophrenia and schizo-affective disorder. *Journal of Psychiatric Research*, **32**, 283–288.

Castle, D. J., Scott, K., Wessely, S., *et al* (1993) Does social deprivation in utero or in early life predispose to schizophrenia? *Social Psychiatry and Psychiatric Epidemiology*, **28**, 1–4.

Chapman, L. J., Chapman, J. P., Kwapil, T. R., *et al* (1994) Putative psychosis prone subjects 10 years later. *Journal of Abnormal Psychology*, **103**, 171–183.

Chowdari, K., Mirnics, K. & Semwall, P. (2002) Association and linkage analysis of RGS4 polymorphisms in schizophrenia. *Molecular Genetics*, **11**, 1373–1380.

Chua, S. E., Wright, I. C., Poline, J. B., *et al* (1997) Grey matter correlates of syndromes in schizophrenia. A semi-automated analysis of structural magnetic resonance images. *British Journal of Psychiatry*, **170**, 406–410.

Chua, S. E., Sharma, T., Takei, N., *et al* (2000) A magnetic resonance imaging study of corpus callosum size in familial schizophrenic subjects, their relatives and normal controls. *Schizophrenia Research*, **41**, 397–403.

Chua, S. E., Lam, I. W., Chen, E. Y., *et al* (2002) Asymmetric lateral ventricular enlargement in Chinese with 1st episode schizophrenia. *Schizophrenia Research*, **57**, 123–124.

Chumakov, I., Blumenfeld, M., Guerassimenko, O., *et al* (2002) Genetic and physiological data implicating the new human gene G72 and the gene for D-amino acid oxidase in schizophrenia. *Proceedings of the National Academy of Sciences, USA*, **99**, 13675–13680.

Cooper, J. E. & Sartorius, N. (1977) Cultural and temporal variations in schizophrenia: a speculation on the importance of industrialisation. *British Journal of Psychiatry*, **130**, 50–55.

Cooper, J. E., Kendell, R. E., Gurland, B. J., *et al* (1972) *Psychiatric Diagnosis in New York and London*. Maudsley monograph no. 20. London: Oxford University Press.

Crocq, M. A., Mant, R., Asherson, P., *et al* (1992) Association between schizophrenia and homozygosity at the dopamine D, receptor gene. *Journal of Medical Genetics*, **29**, 858–860.

Crow, T. J. (1990) Temporal lobe asymmetries as the key to the etiology of schizophrenia. *Schizophrenia Bulletin*, **16**, 433–443.

Crow, T. J. & Done, J. (1992) Prenatal exposure to influenza does not cause schizophrenia. *British Journal of Psychiatry*, **161**, 390–393.

Crow, T. J., Done, D. J. & Sacker, A. (1995) Childhood precursors of psychosis as clues to its evolutionary origin. *European Archives of Psychiatry and Clinical Neuroscience*, **245**, 61–69.

Cullen, T. J., Walker, M. A., Roberts, H., *et al* (2000) The mediodorsal nucleus of the thalamus in schizophrenia: a post-mortem study. *Schizophrenia Research*, **41**, 5.

Cutting, J. (1985) *The Psychology of Schizophrenia*. Edinburgh: Churchill Livingstone.

Cutting, J. (1987) The phenomenology of acute organic psychosis: comparison with acute schizophrenia. *British Journal of Psychiatry*, **151**, 324–332.

Dalman, C., Allebeck, P., Culberg, J., *et al* (1999) Obstetric complications and the risk of schizophrenia: a longitudinal study of a national birth cohort. *Archives of General Psychiatry*, **56**, 234–240.

David, A. S. (1987) Tachistoscopic tests of colour naming and matching in schizophrenia: evidence for posterior callosal dysfunction. *Psychological Medicine*, **17**, 621–630.

Davison, K. & Bagley, C. R. (1969) Schizophrenia-like psychoses associated with organic disorders of the central nervous system. In *Current Problems in Neuropsychiatry: Schizophrenia, Epilepsy, the Temporal Lobe* (ed. R. Herrington). Special publication no. 4, British Journal of Psychiatry, London.

Day, A., Neilsen, J. A., Korten, A., *et al* (1987) Stressful life events preceding the acute onset of schizophrenia: a cross-national study from the World Health Organisation. *Culture, Medicine and Psychiatry*, **2**, 123–205.

de Alarcon, J., Seagroatt, V. & Goldacre, M. (1990) Trends in schizophrenia. *Lancet*, **335**, 852–853.

Der, G., Gupta, S. & Murray, R. M. (1990) Is schizophrenia disappearing? *Lancet*, **335**, 513–516.

Dierks, T., Linden, D. E., Jandl, M., *et al* (1999) Activation of Heschl's gyrus during auditory hallucinations. *Neuron*, **22**, 615–621.

Doane, J. A. (1978) Family interaction and communication deviance in disturbed and normal families: a review of research. *Family Process*, **17**, 357–376.

Done, D. J., Crow, T. J., Johnstone, E. C., *et al* (1994) Childhood antecedents of schizophrenia and affective illness: social adjustment at ages 7 and 11. *BMJ*, **309**, 699–703.

Egan, M. E., Goldberg, T. E., Kolachana, B. S., *et al* (2001) Effect of COMT Val108/158 Met genotype on frontal lobe function and risk for schizophrenia. *Proceedings of the National Academy of Sciences, USA*, **98**, 6917–6922.

Egan, M. F., Leboyer, M. & Weinberger, D. R. (2003) Intermediate phenotypes in genetic studies for schizophrenia. In *Schizophrenia* (2nd edn) (eds S. R. Hirsch & D. R. Weinberger), pp. 277–297. Oxford: Blackwell.

Erlenmeyer-Kimling, L. (1968) Studies of the offspring of two schizophrenic parents. In *The Transmission of Schizophrenia* (eds D. Rosenthal & S. Kety). Oxford: Pergamon Press.

Erlenmeyer-Kimling, L. & Cornblatt, B. (1987) High-risk research in schizophrenia: a summary of what has been learned. *Journal of Psychiatric Research*, **21**, 401–411.

Falconer, D. S. (1965) The inheritance of liability to certain diseases, estimated from the incidence among relatives. *Annals of Human Genetics*, **29**, 51–76.

Faris, R. E. L. & Dunham, H. W. (1939) *Mental Disorders in Urban Areas*. Chicago: Chicago University Press.

Farmer, A. E., McGuffin, P. & Gottesman, I. I. (1987) Twin concordance for DSM–III schizophrenia: scrutinizing the validity of the definition. *Archives of General Psychiatry*, **44**, 634–640.

Fearon, P., Lane, A., Airie, M., *et al* (2001) Is reduced dermatoglyphic abridge count a reliable marker of developmental impairment in schizophrenia? *Schizophrenia Research*, **50**, 151–157.

Feinstein, A., Du Boulay, G. & Ron, M. A. (1992) Psychotic illness in multiple sclerosis: a clinical and magnetic resonance imaging study. *British Journal of Psychiatry*, **161**, 680–685.

Fischer, M., Harvald, B. & Hauge, M. A. (1971) A Danish twin study of schizophrenia. *British Journal of Psychiatry*, **115**, 981–990.

Foerster, A., Lewis, S., Owen, M., *et al* (1991) Premorbid adjustment and personality in psychosis: effects of sex and diagnosis. *British Journal of Psychiatry*, **158**, 171–176.

Foong, J., Maier, M., Clark, C. A., *et al* (2000) Neuropathological abnormalities of the corpus callosum in schizophrenia: a diffusion tensor imaging study. *Journal of Neurology, Neurosurgery and Psychiatry*, **68**, 242–244.

Freedman, R., Coon, H., Myles-Worsley, M., *et al* (1997) Linkage of a neurophysiological deficit in schizophrenia to a chromosome 15 locus. *Proceedings of the National Academy of Sciences, USA*, **94**, 587–592.

Frith, C. D., Friston, K. J., Herold, S., *et al* (1995) Regional brain activity in chronic schizophrenic patients during the performance of a verbal fluency task. *British Journal of Psychiatry*, **167**, 343–349.

Geddes, J. R. & Lawrie, S. M. (1995) Obstetric events in schizophrenia: a meta-analysis. *British Journal of Psychiatry*, **167**, 786–793.

Geddes, J. R., Verdoux, H., Takei, N., *et al* (1999) Schizophrenia and complications of pregnancy and labour. An individual patient meta-analysis. *Schizophrenia Bulletin*, **25**, 413–423.

Gershon, E. S., De Lisi, L. E., Hamovit, J., *et al* (1988) A controlled family study of chronic psychosis: schizophrenia and schizoaffective disorder. *Archives of General Psychiatry*, **45**, 328–336.

Ghazuiddin, M., Ghazuiddin, N. & Stein, G. S. (1990) Life events and the recurrence of depression. *Canadian Journal of Psychiatry*, **5**, 239–242.

Gill, M., Vallada, H., Collier, D., *et al* (1996) A combined analysis of D22S278 marker alleles in affected sib-pairs: support for a susceptibility locus for schizophrenia at chromosome 22q12. *American Journal of Medical Genetics and Neuropsychiatric Genetics*, **67**, 40–45.

Glantz, L. A. & Lewis, D. A. (2000) Decreased dendritic spine density on prefrontal cortical pyramidal neurons in schizophrenia. *Archives of General Psychiatry*, **57**, 65–73.

Glantz, L. A., Austin, M. C. & Lewis, D. A. (2000) Normal cellular levels of synaptophysin mRNA expression in the prefrontal cortex of subjects with schizophrenia. *Biological Psychiatry*, **48**, 389–397.

Gogtay, N., Sporn, A., Clasen, L. S., *et al* (2003) Structural brain MRI abnormalities in healthy siblings of patients with childhood-onset schizophrenia. *American Journal of Psychiatry*, **160**, 569–571.

Goldberg, E. M. & Morrison, S. L. (1963) Schizophrenia and social class. *British Journal of Psychiatry*, **109**, 785–802.

Gottesman, I. I. & Bertelsen, A. (1989) Confirming unexpressed genotypes for schizophrenia. *Archives of General Psychiatry*, **46**, 867–872.

Gottesman, I. I. & Shields, J. (1972) *Schizophrenia and Genetics: A Twin Study Vantage Point*. London: Academic Press.

Gottesman, I. I. & Shields, J. (1982) *Schizophrenia: The Epigenetic Puzzle*. Cambridge: Cambridge University Press.

Gur, R. E., Mozley, P. D., Shtasel, D. L., *et al* (1994) Clinical subtypes of schizophrenia: differences in brain and CSF volume. *American Journal of Psychiatry*, **151**, 343–350.

Hahlweg, K., Goldstein, M. J., Neuchterlein K. H., *et al* (1989) Expressed emotion and patient–relative interaction in families of recent onset schizophrenics. *Journal of Consulting and Clinical Psychology*, **57**, 11–18.

Hakak, Y., Walker, J. & Li, C. (2001) Genome-wide expression analysis reveals dysregulation of myelination-related genes in chronic schizophrenia. *Proceedings of the National Academy of Sciences, USA*, **98**, 4746–4751.

Hare, E. H. (1956) Mental illness and social conditions in Bristol. *Journal of Mental Science*, **102**, 349–357.

Hare, E. H. (1976) The season of birth of siblings of schizophrenic patients. *British Journal of Psychiatry*, **29**, 49–54.

Hare, E. H. (1998) *On the History of Lunacy*. London: Gabbay.

Hare, E. H., Price, J. S. & Slater, E. T. O. (1974) Mental disorder and season of birth: a national sample compared with the general population. *British Journal of Psychiatry*, **124**, 81–86.

Harrison, P. J. (1999) *The Neuropathology of Schizophrenia: A Critical Review of the Data and Their Interpretation. Brain*, **122**, 593–624.

Harrison, P. J. & Lewis, D. A. (2003) Neuropathology of schizophrenia. In *Schizophrenia* (eds D. R. Weinberger & S. R. Hirsch), pp. 310–325. Oxford: Blackwell.

Hattori, E., Lui, C., Badner, J. A., *et al* (2003) Polymorphisms at the G72/G30 gene locus, on 13q33, are associated with bipolar disorder in two independent pedigree series. *American Journal of Human Genetics*, **72**, 1131–1140.

Helgason, T. & Magnusson, H. (1989) The first 80 years of life: a psychiatric epidemiological study. *Acta Psychiatrica Scandinavica*, **79**, suppl. 348, 85–94.

Heston, L. L. (1966) Psychiatric disorders in foster home reared children of schizophrenic mothers. *British Journal of Psychiatry*, **112**, 819–825.

Hirsch, S. R. & Leff, J. P. (1975) *Abnormalities in the Parents of Schizophrenics*. Oxford: Oxford University Press.

Ho, B. C., Alicata, D., Ward, J., *et al* (2003) Untreated initial psychosis: relation to cognitive deficits and brain morphology in first-episode schizophrenia. *American Journal of Psychiatry*, **160**, 142–148.

Hoek, H. W., Susser, E., Buck, K. A., *et al* (1996) Schizoid personality disorder after prenatal exposure to famine. *American Journal of Psychiatry*, **153**, 1637–1639.

Holinger, D. P., Shenton, M. E., Wible, C. G., *et al* (1999) Superior temporal gyrus volume abnormalities and thought disorder in left-handed schizophrenic men. *American Journal of Psychiatry*, **156**, 1730–1735.

Hollister, J. M., Laing, P. & Mednick, S. A. (1996) Rhesus incompatibility as a risk factor for schizophrenia in male adults. *Archives of General Psychiatry*, **53**, 19–24.

Hoptman, M. J., Volavka, J., Johnson, G., *et al* (2002) Frontal white matter microstructure, aggression and impulsivity in men with schizophrenia: a preliminary study. *Biological Psychiatry*, **52**, 9–14.

Hovatta, I., Varilo, T., Suvisaari, J., *et al* (2000) Screen for schizophrenia genes in an isolated Finnish subpopulation, suggesting multiple susceptibility loci. *American Journal of Human Genetics*, **65**, 1114–1125.

Huber, G. (1957) *Pneumoencephalographische and psychopathologische Bilder bei endogen Psychosen*. Berlin: Springer-Verlag.

Huber, G., Gross, G. & Schutter, R. (1975) A long term follow-up study of schizophrenia: psychiatric course of illness and prognosis. *Acta Psychiatrica Scandinavica*, **52**, 49–57.

Hulshoff Pol, H. E., Schnack, H. G., Bertens, M. G., *et al* (2002) Volume changes in gray matter in patients with schizophrenia. *American Journal of Psychiatry*, **159**, 244–250.

Huttunen, M. & Niskanen, P. (1978) Prenatal loss of father and psychiatric disorders. *Archives of General Psychiatry*, **35**, 427–431.

Hyde, T. M. & Lewis, S. (2003) The secondary schizophrenias. In *Schizophrenia* (eds S. R. Hirsch & D. L. Weinberger), pp. 187–202. Oxford: Blackwell.

Hyde, T. M., Ziegler, J. C. & Weinberger, D. R. (1992) Psychiatric disturbances in metachromatic leukodystrophy: insights into the neurobiology of psychosis. *Archives of Neurology*, **49**, 401–406.

Jablensky, A. (2003) The epidemiological horizon. In *Schizophrenia* (eds D. R. Weinberger & S. R. Hirsch), pp. 203–231. Oxford: Blackwell.

Jaskiw, G. E., Juliano, D. M., Goldberg, T. E., *et al* (1994) Cerebral ventricular enlargement in schizophreniform disorder does not progress. A seven year follow-up study. *Schizophrenia Research*, **14**, 23–28.

Johnstone, E. C., Crow, T. J., Frith, C. D., *et al* (1976) Cerebral ventricular size and cognitive impairment in chronic schizophrenia. *Lancet*, **ii**, 924–926.

Johnstone, E., Humphreys, M., Lang, F., *et al* (1999) Diagnostic issues: aspects of differential diagnosis. In *Schizophrenia: Concepts and Management*, pp. 44–59. Cambridge: Cambridge University Press.

Jones, P. B. & Murray, R. M. (1991) The genetics of schizophrenia is the genetics of neurodevelopment. *British Journal of Psychiatry*, **158**, 615–623.

Jones, P. B., Bebbington, P., Foerster, A., *et al* (1993) Premorbid underachievement in schizophrenia: results from the Camberwell Collaborative Psychosis Study. *British Journal of Psychiatry*, **162**, 65–71.

Jones, P. B., Rodgers, B., Murray, R., *et al* (1994) Child developmental risk factors for adult schizophrenia in the British 1946 birth cohort. *Lancet*, **344**, 1398–1402.

Jones, P. B., Rantakallio, P., Hartikainen, A. L., *et al* (1998) Schizophrenia as a long term outcome of pregnancy, delivery and perinatal complications: a 28 year follow up of the 1966 North Finland general population birth cohort. *American Journal of Psychiatry*, **155**, 355–364.

Josin, G. M. & Liddle, P. F. (2001) Neural network analysis of the pattern of functional connectivity between cerebral areas in schizophrenia. *Biological Cybernetics*, **84**, 117–122.

Kalsi, G., Mankoo, B., Curtis, D., *et al* (1999) New DNA markers with increased informativeness show diminished support for a chromosome 5q11–13 schizophrenia susceptibility locus and exclude linkage in two new cohorts of British and Icelandic families. *Annals of Human Genetics*, **63**, 235–247.

Kegeles, L. S., Shungu, D. C., Anjilvel, S., *et al* (2000) Hippocampal pathology in schizophrenia: magnetic resonance imaging and spectroscopy studies. *Psychiatry Research*, **98**, 163–175.

Kelsoe, J. R., Cadet, J. L., Pickar, D., *et al* (1988) Quantitative neuroanatomy in schizophrenia. *Archives of General Psychiatry*, **45**, 533–541.

Kendell, R. E. & Kemp, J. W. (1989) Maternal influenza in the aetiology of schizophrenia. *Archives of General Psychiatry*, **46**, 878–882.

Kendler, K. S. & MacLean, C. J. (1990) Estimating familial effects on age of onset and liability to schizophrenia. I Results of a large sample family study. *Genetic Epidemiology*, **7**, 409–417.

Kendler, K. S., Masterson, C. C. & Davis, K. L. (1985) Psychiatric illness in first-degree relatives of patients with paranoid psychosis, schizophrenia and medical illness. *British Journal of Psychiatry*, **147**, 524–531.

Kendler, K. S., McGuire, M., Gruenberg, A. M., *et al* (1993) The Roscommon family study. I. Methods, diagnosis of probands, and risk of schizophrenia in relatives. *Archives of General Psychiatry*, **50**, 527–540.

Kendler, K. S., Gruenberg, A. M., Kinney, D. K. (1994) Independent diagnoses of adoptees and relatives as defined by DSM-III in the provincial and national samples of the Danish Adoption Study of Schizophrenia. *Archives of General Psychiatry*, **51**, 456–468.

Kennedy, J. L., Giuffra, L. A., Moises, H. W., *et al* (1988) Evidence against linkage of schizophrenia to markers on chromosome in a northern Swedish pedigree. *Nature*, **336**, 167–170.

Keshaven, M. S., Anderson, S. & Pettegrew, J. W. (1994) Is schizophrenia due to excessive synaptic pruning in the prefrontal cortex? The Feinberg hypothesis revisited. *Journal of Psychiatric Research*, **28**, 239–265.

Keshaven, M. S., Stanley, J. A. & Pettegrew, J. W. (2000) Magnetic resonance spectroscopy in schizophrenia: methodological issues and findings – Part II. *Biological Psychiatry*, **48**, 369–380.

Keshaven, M. S., Diwadkar, V. A., Harenski, K., *et al* (2002) Abnormalities of the corpus callosum in first episode, treatment naïve schizophrenia. *Journal of Neurology, Neurosurgery and Psychiatry*, **72**, 757–760.

Kety, S. S., Rosenthal, D., Wender, P. H., *et al* (1976) Studies based on a total sample of adopted individuals and their relatives. Why they were necessary, what they demonstrated and failed to demonstrate. *Schizophrenia Bulletin*, **2**, 413–428.

Kety, S. S., Wender, P. H., Jacobsen, B., *et al* (1994) Mental illness in the biological and adoptive relatives of schizophrenic adoptees. Replication of the Copenhagen Study in the rest of Denmark. *Archives of General Psychiatry*, **51**, 442–455.

Kinney, D. K., Hyman, W., Greetham, C., *et al* (1999) Increased relative risk for schizophrenia and prenatal exposure to a severe tornado. *Schizophrenia Research*, **36**, 45–46 (abstract).

Kircher, T. T., Liddle, P. F., Brammer, M. J., *et al* (2001) Neural correlates of formal thought disorder in schizophrenia: preliminary findings from a functional magnetic resonance imaging study. *Archives of General Psychiatry*, **58**, 769–774.

Kircher, T. T., Liddle, P. F., Brammer, M. J., *et al* (2002) Reversed lateralization of temporal activation during speech production in thought disordered patients with schizophrenia. *Psychological Medicine*, **32**, 439–449.

Kringlen, E. (1976) Twins: still our best method. *Schizophrenia Bulletin*, **2**, 429–433.

Kringlen, E. & Cramer, G. (1989) Offspring of monozygotic twins discordant for schizophrenia. *Archives of General Psychiatry*, **46**, 873–877.

Lander, E. S. (1988) Splitting schizophrenia. *Nature*, **336**, 105–106.

Laurent, C., Zander, C., Thibaut, F., *et al* (1998) Anticipation in schizophrenia: no evidence of expanded CAG/CTG repeat sequences in French families and sporadic cases. *American Journal of Medical Genetics*, **81**, 342–346.

Lawrie, S. M., Whalley, H. C., Abukmeil, S. S., *et al* (2002*a*) Temporal lobe volume changes in people at high risk of schizophrenia with psychotic symptoms. *British Journal of Psychiatry*, **181**, 138–143.

Lawrie, S. M., Buechel, C., Whalley, H. C., *et al* (2002*b*) Reduced frontotemporal functional connectivity in schizophrenia associated with auditory hallucinations. *Biological Psychiatry*, **51**, 1008–1011.

Leff, J., Wig, N. N., Ghosh, A., *et al* (1987) Expressed emotion and schizophrenia in North India. III. Influence of relatives' expressed emotion on the course of schizophrenia in Chandigarh. *British Journal of Psychiatry*, **151**, 166–173.

Lefley, H. P. (1992) Expressed emotion: conceptual, clinical, and social policy issues. *Hospital and Community Psychiatry*, **43**, 591–598.

Levinson, D. F., Wildenauer, D. B., Schwab, S. G., *et al* (1996) Additional support for schizophrenia linkage on chromosomes 6 and 8: a multicenter study. *American Journal of Medical Genetics and Neuropsychiatric Genetics*, **67**, 580–594.

Levinson, D. F., Holmans, P., Straub, R. E., *et al* (2000) Multicenter linkage study of schizophrenia candidate regions on chromosomes 5q, 6q, 10q, and 13q: schizophrenia linkage collaborative group III. *American Journal of Human Genetics*, **67**, 652–663.

Levitan, C., Ward, P. B. & Catts, S. V. (1999) Superior temporal gyral volumes and laterality correlates of auditory hallucinations in schizophrenia. *Biological Psychiatry*, **46**, 955–962.

Lewis, C. M., Levinson, D. F., Wise, L. H., *et al* (2003) Genome scan meta-analysis of schizophrenia and bipolar disorder. Part II. Schizophrenia. *American Journal of Human Genetics*, **73**, 34–48.

Li, T., Sham, P. C., Vallada, H., *et al* (1996) Preferential transmission of the high activity allele of COMT in schizophrenia. *Psychiatric Genetics*, **6**, 131–133.

Lin, M. W., Curtis, D., Williams, N., *et al* (1995) Suggestive evidence for linkage of schizophrenia to markers on chromosome 13q14.1–q32. *Psychiatric Genetics*, **5**, 117–126.

Lin, M. W., Sham, P., Hwu, H. G., *et al* (1997) Suggestive evidence for linkage of schizophrenia to markers on chromosome 13 in Caucasian but not Oriental populations. *Human Genetics*, **99**, 417–420.

Lin, T. Y., Chu, H. M., Rin, H., *et al* (1989) Effects of social change on mental disorders in Taiwan: observations based on a 15-year follow-up survey of general populations in three communities. *Acta Psychiatrica Scandinavica*, **79**, suppl. 348, 11–34.

Link, B. & Dohrenwend, B. P. (1980) Formulation of hypotheses about the ratio of untreated to treated cases in the true prevalence studies of functional psychiatric disorders in adults in the United States. In *Mental Illness in the United States: Epidemiological Estimates* (eds B. P. Dohrenwend, B. N. S. Dohrenwend, M. S. Gould, *et al*), pp. 133–148. New York: Praeger.

Liu, H., Heath, S. C., Sobin, C., *et al* (2002) Genetic variation at the 22q11 PRODH2/DGCR6 locus presents as unusual pattern and increases susceptibility to schizophrenia. *Proceedings of the National Academy of Sciences, USA*, **99**, 3717–3733.

Lohmueller, K. E., Pearce, C. L., Pike, M., *et al* (2003) Meta-analysis of genetic association studies supports a contribution of common variants to susceptibility to common disease. *Nature Genetics*, **33**, 177–182.

Lowing, P. A., Mirsky, A. F. & Pereira, R. (1983) The inheritance of schizophrenia spectrum disorders: a reanalysis of Danish adoptee study data. *American Journal of Psychiatry*, **140**, 1167–1171.

MacIntyre, D. J., Blackwood, D. H., Porteous, D. J., *et al* (2003) Chromosomal abnormalities and mental illness. *Molecular Psychiatry*, **8**, 275–287.

MacMillan, J. F., Gold, A., Crow, T. J., *et al* (1986) Expressed emotion and relapse. *British Journal of Psychiatry*, **148**, 133–143.

Maier, W., Lichtermann, D., Minges, J., *et al* (1993) Continuity and discontinuity of affective disorders and schizophrenia: results of a controlled family study. *Archives of General Psychiatry*, **50**, 871–883.

Makikyro, T., Isohanni, M., Moring, J., *et al* (1997) Is a child's risk early onset schizophrenia increased in the highest social class? *Schizophrenia Research*, **23**, 245–252.

Malmberg, A., Lewis, G., David, A., *et al* (1998) Premorbid adjustment in people with schizophrenia. *British Journal of Psychiatry*, **172**, 308–313.

Marcelis, M., Takei, N. & van Os, J. (1999) Urbanization and risk for schizophrenia: does the effect operate before or around the time of illness onset? *Psychological Medicine*, **29**, 1197–1203.

Mathalon, D. H., Sullivan, E. V., Lim, K. O., *et al* (2001) Progressive brain volume changes and the clinical course of schizophrenia in men: a longitudinal magnetic resonance imaging study. *Archives of General Psychiatry*, **58**, 148–157.

Mathalon, D. H., Pfefferbaum, A., Lim, K. O., *et al* (2003) Compounded brain volume deficits in schizophrenia–alcoholism comorbidity. *Archives of General Psychiatry*, **60**, 245–252.

McCreadie, R. G., Robertson, L. J., Hall, D. J., *et al* (1993) The Nithsdale Schizophrenia Surveys. XI. Relatives' expressed emotion. Stability over five years and its relation to relapse. *British Journal of Psychiatry*, **162**, 393–397.

McDonald, C., Grech, A., Toulopoulou, T., *et al* (2002) Brain volumes in familial and non-familial schizophrenic probands and their unaffected relatives. *American Journal of Medical Genetics*, **114**, 616–625.

McGrath, J. J. & Welham, J. L. (1999) Season of birth and schizophrenia: a systematic review and meta-analysis of data from the southern hemisphere. *Schizophrenia Research*, **35**, 237–242.

McGue, M. & Gottesman, I. I. (1989) A single dominant gene still cannot account for the transmission of schizophrenia. *Archives of General Psychiatry*, **46**, 478–479.

McGuffin, P., Farmer, A. E. & Gottesman, I. I. (1984) Twin concordance for operationally defined schizophrenia: confirmation of familiality and heritability. *Archives of General Psychiatry*, **41**, 541–545.

McGuire, P. K., Shah, G. M. & Murray, R. M. (1993) Increased blood flow in Broca's area during auditory hallucinations in schizophrenia. *Lancet*, **342**, 703–706.

McNeil, T., Cantor-Graae, E. & Ishmail, B. (2000) Obstetric complications and congenital malformations in schizophrenia. *Brain Research Reviews*, **31**, 166–178.

Mednick, S. A., Machon, R. A., Huttunen, M. O., *et al* (1988) Adult schizophrenia following prenatal exposure to an influenza epidemic. *Archives of General Psychiatry*, **45**, 189–192.

Menon, R. R., Barta, P. E., Aylward, E. H., *et al* (1995) Posterior superior temporal gyrus in schizophrenia: grey matter changes and clinical correlates. *Schizophrenia Research*, **16**, 127–135.

Meyer-Lindenberg, A., Poline, J. B., Kohn, P. D., *et al* (2001) Evidence for abnormal cortical functional connectivity during working memory in schizophrenia. *American Journal of Psychiatry*, **158**, 1809–1817.

Millar, J. K., Wilson-Annan, J. C., Anderson, S., *et al* (2000) Disruption of two novel genes by a translocation co-segregating with schizophrenia. *Human Molecular Genetics*, **9**, 1415–1423.

Mirnics, K., Middleton, F. A., Marquez, A., *et al* (2000) Molecular characterisation of schizophrenia viewed by microarray analysis of gene expression in prefrontal cortex. *Neuron*, **28**, 53–67.

Mirnics, K., Middleton, F. A., Stanwood, G. D., *et al* (2001) Disease-specific changes in regulator of G-protein signalling 4 (RGS4) expression in schizophrenia. *Molecular Psychiatry*, **6**, 293–301.

Miyoshi, K., Honda, A., Baba, K., *et al* (2003) Disrupted-in schizophrenia 1, a candidate gene for schizophrenia, participates in neurite outgrowth. *Molecular Psychiatry*, **8**, 685–694.

Morris, D. W., McGhee, K. A., Schwaiger, S., *et al* (2003) No evidence for association of the dysbindin gene (DTNBP1) with schizophrenia in an Irish population-based study. *Schizophrenia Research*, **60**, 167–172.

Morton, N. E. (1955) Sequential tests for the detection of linkage. *American Journal of Human Genetics*, **7**, 277–318.

Mortensen, P. B., Pedersen, C. B., Westergaard, T., *et al* (1999) Effects of family history and place and season of birth on the risk of schizophrenia. *New England Journal of Medicine*, **340**, 603–608.

Mozley, P. D., Gur, R. E., Resnick, S. M., *et al* (1994) Magnetic resonance imaging in schizophrenia: relationship with clinical measures. *Schizophrenia Research*, **12**, 195–203.

Murphy, K. C., Jones, L. A. & Owen, H. J. (1999) High rates of schizophrenia in adults with velocardiofacial syndrome. *Archives of General Psychiatry*, **48**, 643–647.

Murray, R. M., Lewis, S. W., Reveley, A. M. (1985) Towards an aetiological classification of schizophrenia. *Lancet*, **i**, 1023–1026.

Murthy, G. V. S., Janakiramaiah, N., Gangadhar, B. N., *et al* (1998) Sex difference in age at onset of schizophrenia: discrepant findings from India. *Acta Psychiatrica Scandinavica*, **97**, 321–325.

Myhrman, A., Rantakallio, P., Isohanni, M., *et al* (1996) Does unwantedness of a pregnancy predict schizophrenia? *British Journal of Psychiatry*, **169**, 637–640.

Narr, K. L., Cannon, T. D., Woods, R. P., *et al* (2002) Genetic contributions to altered callosal morphology in schizophrenia. *Journal of Neuroscience*, **22**, 3720–3729.

Norman, R. M. G. & Malla, A. K. (1993*a*) Stressful life events and schizophrenia. I: A review of the research. *British Journal of Psychiatry*, **162**, 161–165.

Norman, R. M. G. & Malla, A. K. (1993*b*) Stressful life events and schizophrenia. II: Conceptual and methodological issues. *British Journal of Psychiatry*, **162**, 166–174.

O'Callaghan, E., Sham, P., Takei, N., *et al* (1991) Schizophrenia after prenatal exposure to 1957 A2 influenza epidemic. *Lancet*, **337**, 1248–1250.

O'Donovan, M. C. & Owen, M. J. (1996) Dynamic mutations and psychiatric genetics. *Psychological Medicine*, **28**, 1–6.

O'Donovan, M. C., Guy, C., Craddock, N., *et al* (1996) Confirmation of association between expanded cag/ctg repeats and both schizophrenia and bipolar disorder. *Psychological Medicine*, **26**, 1145–1153.

Ødegäard, O. (1932) Emigration and insanity: a study of mental disease in Norwegian born population in Minnesota. *Acta Psychiatrica et Neurologica Scandinavica*, suppl. 4, 1–206.

Ogawa, S., Lee, T. M., Kay, A. R., *et al* (1990) Brain magnetic resonance imaging with contrast dependent on blood oxygenation. *Proceedings of the National Academy of Sciences, USA*, **87**, 9868–9872.

Onstad, S., Skre, I., Torgersen, S., *et al* (1991) Twin concordance for DSM–III–R schizophrenia. *Acta Psychiatrica Scandinavica*, **83**, 395–401.

Ott, J. (1991) *Analysis of Human Genetic Linkage*. Baltimore, MA: Johns Hopkins University Press.

Panizzou, M. S., Hoff, A. L., Nordahl, T. E., *et al* (2003) Sex differences in the corpus callosum of patients with schizophrenia. *Schizophrenia Research*, **62**, 115–122.

Pantelis, C., Velakoulis, D., McGorry, P. D., *et al* (2003) Neuroanatomical abnormalities before and after onset of psychosis: a cross-sectional and longitudinal MRI comparison. *Lancet*, **361**, 281–288.

Pegues, M. P., Rogers, L. J., Amend, D., *et al* (2003) Anterior hippocampal volume reduction in male patients with schizophrenia. *Schizophrenia Research*, **60**, 105–115.

Pollin, W., Allen, M. G., Hoffer, A., *et al* (1969) Psychopathology in 15,909 pairs of veteran twins. *American Journal of Psychiatry*, **7**, 597–609.

Prichard, J. C. (1835) *A Treatise on Insanity and Other Disorders Affecting the Mind*. London: Sherwood.

Pulver, A. E., Karayiorgou, M., Lasseter, V. K., *et al* (1994*a*) Follow-up of a report of a potential linkage for schizophrenia on chromosome 22q12–q13.1. Part II. *American Journal of Medical Genetics*, **54**, 44–50.

Pulver, A. E., Karayiorgou, M., Wolniec, P. S., *et al* (1994*b*) Sequential strategy to identify a susceptibility gene for schizophrenia: report of potential linkage on chromosome 22q12–q13.1: Part 1. *American Journal of Medical Genetics*, **54**, 36–43.

Pulver, A. E., Nestadt, G., Goldberg, R., *et al* (1994*c*) Psychotic illness in patients diagnosed with velo-cardio-facial syndrome and their relatives. *Journal of Nervous and Mental Disorder*, **182**, 476–478.

Rantakallio, P., Jones, P., Moring, J., *et al* (1997) Association between central nervous system infections during childhood and adult onset schizophrenia and other psychoses: a 28 year follow up. *International Journal of Epidemiology*, **26**, 837–843.

Rao, D. C., Morton, N. E., Gottesman, I. I., *et al* (1981) Path analysis of qualitative data on pairs of relatives: application to schizophrenia. *Human Heredity*, **31**, 325–333.

Riley, B., Ascherson, P. & McGuffin, P. (2003) Genetics and schizophrenia. In *Schizophrenia* (eds S. R. Hirsch & D. Weinberger), pp. 251–276. Oxford: Blackwell.

Risch, N. (1990) Linkage strategies for genetically complex traits. I Multilocus models. *American Journal of Human Genetics*, **46**, 222–228.

Rosenfeld, H. (1965) *Psychotic States: A Psychoanalytical Approach*. London: Karnac.

Rosenthal, D., Wender, P. H., Kety, S. S., *et al* (1971) The adopted-away offspring of schizophrenics. *American Journal of Psychiatry*, **128**, 307–311.

Rosoklija, G., Toomayan, G., Ellis, S. P., *et al* (2000) Structural abnormalities of subicular dendrites in subjects with schizophrenia and mood disorders: preliminary findings. *Archives of General Psychiatry*, **57**, 349–356.

Rossell, S. L., Shapleske, J., Fukuda, R., *et al* (2001) Corpus callosum area and functioning in schizophrenic patients with auditory-verbal hallucinations. *Schizophrenia Research*, **50**, 9–17.

Rossi, A., Serio, A., Stratta, P., *et al* (1994) Planum temporale asymmetry and thought disorder in schizophrenia. *Schizophrenia Research*, **12**, 1–7.

Sacker, A., Done, D. J., Crow, T. J., *et al* (1995) Antecedents of schizophrenia and affective illness: obstetric complications. *British Journal of Psychiatry*, **166**, 734–741.

Sanfilipo, M., Lafargue, T., Rusinek, H., *et al* (2000) Volumetric measure of the frontal and temporal lobe regions in schizophrenia: relationship to negative symptoms. *Archives of General Psychiatry*, **57**, 471–480.

Sartorious, N., Jablensky, A., Korten, A., *et al* (1986) Early manifestations and first-contact incidence of schizophrenia in different cultures: a preliminary report on the initial evaluation phase of the WHO Collaborative Study on Determinants of Outcome of Severe Mental Disorders. *Psychological Medicine*, **16**, 909–928.

Schwab, S. G., Knapp, M., Mondabon, S., *et al* (2003) Support for association of schizophrenia with genetic variation in the 6q22.3 gene, dysbindin, in sib-pair families with linkage and in an additional sample of triad families. *American Journal of Human Genetics*, **72**, 185–190.

Seidman, L. J., Faraone, S. V., Goldstein, J. M., *et al* (2002) Left hippocampal volume as a vulnerability indicator for schizophrenia: a magnetic resonance imaging morphometric study of nonpsychotic first-degree relatives. *Archives of General Psychiatry*, **59**, 839–849.

Selten, J.-P., van der Graaf, Y., van Duursen, R., *et al* (1999) Psychotic illness after prenatal exposure to the 1953 Dutch flood disaster. *Schizophrenia Research*, **35**, 243–245.

Sham, P. C., O'Callaghan, E., Takei, N., *et al* (1992) Schizophrenia following prenatal exposure to influenza epidemics between 1939 and 1960. *British Journal of Psychiatry*, **160**, 461–466.

Sham, P. C., Jones, P. B., Russell, A., *et al* (1994) Age of onset, sex and familial morbidity: report from the Camberwell Collaborative Psychosis Study. *British Journal of Psychiatry*, **165**, 466–473.

Shapleske, J., Rossell, S. L., Woodruff, P. W. R., *et al* (1999) The planum temporale: a systematic, quantitative review of its structural, functional and clinical significance. *Brain Research Reviews*, **29**, 26–49.

Shapleske, J., Rossell, S. L., Simmons, A., *et al* (2001) Are auditory hallucinations the consequence of abnormal cerebral lateralisation? A morphometric MRI study of the sylvian fissure and planum temporale. *Biological Psychiatry*, **49**, 685–693.

Shapleske, J., Rossell, S. L., Chitnis, X. A., *et al* (2002) A computational morphometric MRI study of schizophrenia: effects of hallucinations. *Cerebral Cortex*, **12**, 1331–1341.

Sharma, T., Lancaster, E., Sigmundsson, T., *et al* (1999) Lack of normal pattern of asymmetry in familial schizophrenic patients and their relatives – the Maudsley Family Study. *Schizophrenia Research*, **40**, 111–120.

Shenton, M. E., Kikinis, R., Jolesz, F. A., *et al* (1992) Abnormalities of the left temporal lobe and thought disorder in schizophrenia. A quantitative magnetic resonance imaging study. *New England Journal of Medicine*, **327**, 604–612.

Shergill, S. S., Brammer, M. J., Williams, S. C., *et al* (2000) Mapping auditory hallucinations in schizophrenia using functional magnetic resonance imaging. *Archives of General Psychiatry*, **57**, 1033–1038.

Sherrington, R., Brynjolfsson, J., Petursson, H., *et al* (1988) Localization of a susceptibility locus for schizophrenia on chromosome 5. *Nature*, **336**, 164–167.

Shifman, S., Bronstein, M., Sternfeld, M., *et al* (2002) A highly significant association between a COMT haplotype and schizophrenia. *American Journal of Human Genetics*, **71**, 1296–1302.

Silbersweig, D. A., Stern, E., Frith, C., *et al* (1995) A functional neuroanatomy of hallucinations in schizophrenia. *Nature*, **378**, 176–179.

Silverton, L. & Mednick, S. (1984) Class drift and schizophrenia. *Acta Psychiatrica Scandinavica*, **70**, 304–309.

Sklar, P. (2002) Linkage analysis in psychiatric disorders: the emerging picture. *Annual Review of Genomics and Human Genetics*, **3**, 371–413.

Slater, E. & Beard, A. W. (1963) The schizophrenia-like psychoses of epilepsy. *British Journal of Psychiatry*, **109**, 95–112.

Slater, E. & Cowie, V. (1971) *The Genetics of Mental Disorder*. Oxford: Oxford University Press.

Smith, J., Birchwood, M., Cochrane, R., *et al* (1993) The needs of high and low expressed emotion families: a normative approach. *Social Psychiatry and Psychiatric Epidemiology*, **28**, 11–16.

Sommer, I. E., Ramsey, N. F. & Kahn, R. S. (2001) Language lateralization in schizophrenia, an fMRI study. *Schizophrenia Research*, **52**, 57–67.

Spence, S. A., Liddle, P. F., Stefan, M. D., *et al* (2000) Functional anatomy of verbal fluency in people with schizophrenia and those at genetic risk. Focal dysfunction and distributed disconnectivity reappraised. *British Journal of Psychiatry*, **176**, 52–60.

Spence, S. A., Hunter M. D. & Harpin, G. (2002) Neuroscience and the will. *Current Opinion in Psychiatry*, **15**, 519–526.

St Clair, D., Blackwood, D., Muir, W., *et al* (1990) Association within a family of a balanced autosomal translocation with major mental illness. *Lancet*, **336**, 13–16.

Steel, R. M., Whalley, H. C., Miller, P., *et al* (2002) Structural MRI of the brain in presumed carriers for schizophrenia, their affected and unaffected siblings. *Journal of Neurology, Neurosurgery and Psychiatry*, **72**, 455–458.

Stefansson, H., Sigurdsson, E. & Steinthorsdottir, V. (2002) Neuregulin 1 and susceptibility to schizophrenia. *American Journal of Human Genetics*, **71**, 877–892.

Stefansson, H., Sarginson, J., Kong, A., *et al* (2003) Association of neuregulin 1 with schizophrenia confirmed in a Scottish population. *American Journal of Human Genetics*, **72**, 83–87.

Steinberg, H. R. & Durrell, J. (1968) A stressful social situation as a precipitant of schizophrenic symptoms: an epidemiological study. *British Journal of Psychiatry*, **114**, 1097–1105.

Stöber, G., Franzek, E. & Beckmann, J. (1992) The role of maternal infectious diseases during pregnancy in the aetiology of schizophrenia in offspring. *European Psychiatry*, **7**, 147–152.

Straub, R. E., MacLean, C. J., O'Neill, F. A., *et al* (1995) A potential vulnerability locus for schizophrenia on chromosome 6q24–22: evidence for genetic heterogeneity. *Nature Genetics*, **11**, 287–293.

Straub, R. E., Jiang, Y., MacLean, C. J., *et al* (2002) Genetic variation in the 6q22.3 gene DTNBP1, the human ortholog of the mouse dysbindin gene, is associated with schizophrenia. *American Journal of Human Genetics*, **71**, 337–348.

Suddath, R. L., Casanova, M. F., Goldberg, T. E., *et al* (1989) Temporal lobe pathology in schizophrenia: a quantitative magnetic resonance imaging study. *American Journal of Psychiatry*, **146**, 464–472.

Susser, E. & Lin, S. P. (1992) Schizophrenia after prenatal exposure to the Dutch Hunger Winter of 1944–1945. *Archives of General Psychiatry*, **49**, 983–988.

Susser, E. & Lin, S. P. (1994) Schizophrenia after prenatal exposure to the Dutch hunger winter of 1944–1945. *Archives of General Psychiatry*, **51**, 333–334.

Susser, E., Neugebauer, R., Hoek, H. W., *et al* (1996) Schizophrenia after prenatal famine. *Archives of General Psychiatry*, **53**, 25–31.

Suvisaari, J., Haukka, J., Tanskanen, A., *et al* (1999) Association between prenatal exposure to poliovirus infection and adult schizophrenia. *American Journal of Psychiatry*, **156**, 1100–1102.

Takei, N., Sham, P., O'Callaghan, E., *et al* (1994). Prenatal exposure to influenza and the development of schizophrenia: is the effect confined to females? *American Journal of Psychiatry*, **151**, 117–119.

Tiernari, P. (1971) Schizophrenia and monozygotic twins. *Psychiatria Fennica*, **2**, 97–104.

Tienari, P., Wynne, L. C., Moring, J., *et al* (2000) Finnish adoptive family study: sample selection and adoptee DSM-III-R diagnoses. *Acta Psychiatrica Scandinavica*, **101**, 433–443.

Tienari, P., Wynne, L. C., Sorri, A., *et al* (2004) Genotype–environment interaction in schizophrenia spectrum disorders. Long term follow up of Finnish adoptees. *British Journal of Psychiatry*, **184**, 216–222.

Torrey, E. F., Bowler, A. E. & Clark, K. (1997*a*) Urban birth and residence as risk factors for psychoses: an analysis of 1880 data. *Schizophrenia Research*, **25**, 169–176.

Torrey, E. F., Miller, J., Rawlings, R., *et al* (1997*b*) Seasonality of births in schizophrenia and bipolar disorders: a review of the literature. *Schizophrenia Research*, **28**, 1–38.

Tramer T. (1929) Uber die biologische Bedeutung des Geburtesmonnates für die Psychogerkrankung. Schweizer. *Archiv für Neurologie und Psychiatrie*, **24**, 17–24.

Van Horn, J. D. & McManus, I. C. (1992) Ventricular enlargement in schizophrenia. A meta-analysis of studies of the ventricle: brain ratio (VBR). *British Journal of Psychiatry*, **160**, 687–697.

Van Os, J. & Selten, J.-P. (1998) Prenatal exposure to maternal stress and later schizophrenia: the May 1940 invasion of the Netherlands. *British Journal of Psychiatry*, **172**, 324–326.

Vaughn, C. & Leff, J. P. (1976) The measurement of expressed emotion in families of psychiatric patients. *British Journal of Social and Clinical Psychology*, **15**, 157–165.

Ventura, J., Neuchterlein, K. H., Hardesty, J. P., *et al* (1992) Life events and schizophrenic relapse after withdrawal of medication. *British Journal of Psychiatry*, **161**, 615–620.

Ventura, J., Nuechterlein, K. H., Subotnik, K. L., *et al* (2000) Life events can trigger depressive exacerbation in the early course of schizophrenia. *Journal of Abnormal Psychology*, **109**, 139–144.

Vincent, J. B., Kovacs, M., Krol, R., *et al* (1999) Intergenerational CAG repeat expansion at ERDA1 in a family with childhood-onset depression, schizoaffective disorder, and recurrent major depression. *American Journal of Medical Genetics*, **88**, 79–82.

Vogler, G. P., Gottesman, I. I., McGue, M. K., *et al* (1990) Mixed-model segregation analysis of schizophrenia in the Lindelius Swedish pedigrees. *Behaviour Genetics*, **20**, 461–472.

Watt, N. F. (1978) Patterns of childhood social development in adult schizophrenics. *Archives of General Psychiatry*, **35**, 160–165.

Weinberger, D. R. (1987) Implications of normal brain development for the pathogenesis of schizophrenia. *Archives of General Psychiatry*, **44**, 660–669.

Weinberger, D. R. & Marenco, S. (2003) Schizophrenia as a neurodevelopmental disorder. In *Schizophrenia* (eds S. R. Hirsh & D. R. Weinberger), pp. 326–348. Oxford: Blackwell.

Wender, P. H., Rosenthal, D., Kety, S. S., *et al* (1974) Cross fostering: a research strategy for clarifying the role of genetic and environmental factors in the etiology of schizophrenia. *Archives of General Psychiatry*, **30**, 121–128.

Wible, C. G., Anderson, J., Shenton, M. E., *et al* (2001) Prefrontal cortex, negative symptoms and schizophrenia: an MRI study. *Psychiatry Research*, **108**, 65–78.

Willetts, L. E. & Leff, J. (1997) Expressed emotion and schizophrenia: the efficacy of a staff training programme. *Journal of Advanced Nursing*, **26**, 1125–1133.

Williams, J., Spurlock, G., McGuffin, P., *et al* (1996) Association between schizophrenia and T102C polymorphism of the 5-hydroxytryptamine type 2a-receptor gene. European Multicentre Association Study of Schizophrenia (EMASS) Group. *Lancet*, **347**, 1294–1296.

Williams, J., McGuffin, P., Nothen, M., *et al* (1997) Meta-analysis of association between the 5-HT (2a) receptor T102C polymorphism and schizophrenia. *Lancet*, **349**, 1221.

Williams, N. M., Preece, A., Spurlock, G., *et al* (2003) Support for genetic variation in neuregulin 1 and susceptibility to schizophrenia. *Molecular Psychiatry*, **8**, 485–487.

Wolkin, A., Choi, S. J., Szilagyi, S., *et al* (2003) Inferior frontal white matter anisotropy and negative symptoms of schizophrenia: a diffusion tensor imaging study. *American Journal of Psychiatry*, **160**, 572–574.

Woodruff, P. W. R. (1994) *Structural Magnetic Resonance Imaging in Psychiatry – The Functional Psychoses*. Cambridge Medical Reviews: Neurobiology and Psychiatry 3 (eds R. Kerwin, D. Dawbarn, J. McCullcoh, *et al*). Cambridge: Cambridge University Press.

Woodruff, P. W. R., Pearlson, G. D., Geer, M. J., *et al* (1993) A computerised magnetic resonance imaging study of corpus callosum morphology in schizophrenia. *Psychological Medicine*, **23**, 45–56.

Woodruff, P. W. R., McMannus, I. C. & Davis, A. S. (1995*a*) A meta-analysis of corpus callosum size in schizophrenia. *Journal of Neurology, Neurosurgery and Psychiatry*, **58**, 457–461.

Woodruff, P., Brammer, M., Mellers, J., *et al* (1995*b*) Auditory hallucinations and the perception of external speech. *Lancet*, **346**, 1035.

Woodruff, P. W., Wright, I. C., Shuriquie, N., *et al* (1997*a*) Structural brain abnormalities in male schizophrenics reflect fronto-temporal dissociation. *Psychological Medicine*, **27**, 1257–1266.

Woodruff, P. W., Wright, I. C., Bullmore, E. T., *et al* (1997*b*) Auditory hallucinations and the temporal cortical response to external speech in schizophrenia: a functional magnetic resonance imaging study. *American Journal of Psychiatry*, **154**, 1676–1682.

World Health Organization (1992) *The Tenth Revision of the International Classification of Diseases and Related Health Problems* (ICD–10). Geneva: WHO.

Wright, I. C., Rabe-Hesketh, S., Woodruff, P. W., *et al* (2000) Meta-analysis of regional brain volumes in schizophrenia. *American Journal of Psychiatry*, **157**, 16–25.

Wright, P., Rifkin, L., Takei, N., *et al* (1995) Maternal influenza, obstetric complications and schizophrenia. *American Journal of Psychiatry*, **152**, 1714–1720.

Wynne, L. & Singer, M. (1963) Thought disorder and family relations of schizophrenics. II. A classification of forms of thinking. *Archives of General Psychiatry*, **9**, 199–206.

Young, K. A., Manaye, K. F., Liang, C.-L, *et al* (2000) Reduced number of mediodorsal and anterior thalamic neurons in schizophrenia. *Biological Psychiatry*, **47**, 944–953.

CHAPTER 11

The pharmacological management of schizophrenia

Amlan Basu, Jerson Pereira and Katherine J. Aitchison

This chapter should be regarded as an introductory overview of the field. It opens with a brief outline of the history of antipsychotic drug discovery, which is followed by a discussion on the terminology of antipsychotic drugs and their pharmacology. A section on the neuropharmacology of schizophrenia and the various receptors is followed by overviews of the individual antipsychotic drugs, their pharmacokinetics and their side-effects. The latter part of the chapter is more clinically orientated and covers the evidence for drug efficacy, together with current approaches for acute and long-term treatment. It includes discussion of special clinical situations, such as treatment resistance and rapid tranquillisation. The chapter ends with a brief section on pharmacoeconomics.

History

Two separate pathways led to the development of modern antipsychotic drugs. The first has its origins in the Ayurvedic medicine of ancient India, where roots of the shrub *Rauwolfia serpentina* have been used for almost 3000 years as *pagla-ki-dawa* ('medicine for the insane'), and it was also used to treat a variety of other ailments, including fever, vomiting and snake bites. In the ancient Ayurvedic texts, insanity was defined by the physician Charka (around 1000 BC) as an abnormal condition of mind, wisdom, perception, knowledge, memory, character, conduct and behaviour, which perhaps corresponds to our modern notion of psychosis. The herb's more formal introduction into Western medicine is attributed to two Indian physicians, G. Sen and K. C. Bose, in their 1931 paper '*Rauwolfia serpentina*, a new Indian drug for insanity and high blood pressure', published in an Indian medical journal.

In the 1950s, Swiss scientists working at the Ciba laboratories (now Novartis) isolated *Rauwolfia*'s active ingredient, the alkaloid reserpine, which acts by depleting central monoamine stores. More recently, *Rauwolfia* extract has also been shown to have a high affinity for central adrenergic α_2 and dopaminergic D_2 receptors. The discovery of reserpine was reported in the *New York Times* and noted by Nathan Kline. He went on to conduct a placebo-controlled trial and was able to demonstrate the alkaloid's effectiveness as a tranquilliser, anxiolytic and 'anti-obsessional' drug (Kline, 1954). Reserpine was, therefore, the first tranquilliser and entered clinical use in the early 1950s. For a period it was even more widely prescribed than chlorpromazine. However, it soon became apparent that it could occasionally cause severe depression, and even suicide. As a result, it was rapidly eclipsed by newly emerging drugs, especially chlorpromazine (Bhatara *et al*, 1997).

The introduction of chlorpromazine, which heralded the second pathway in the development of antipsychotics, was a particularly important event in the history of modern psychopharmacology. According to Cunningham Owens (1999), the discovery of chlorpromazine was not purely serendipitous but rather the culmination of two separate strands of research, neither of which had anything to do with psychiatry. The first was in the field of organic chemistry, and was initiated by Heinrich Caro in 1876. Caro was the chief chemist at the German chemical company BASF and he synthesised a new printing dye called methylene blue. Paul Ehrlich, one of the founders of bacteriology, introduced the dye into medicine as a histopathological stain, and it was subsequently discovered to have the structure of a phenothiazine and to possess antimalarial properties. During the Second World War, when the supply of quinine (the established antimalarial at the time) to allied troops was disrupted, an American chemist named A. Gilman synthesised a number of non-oxidised phenothiazines in the hope that they would be less toxic than methylene blue. However, he found them to be ineffective against malaria and published his results in 1944.

At the same time, but quite independently, chemists working at the French pharmaceutical company Rhone-Poulenc (now Aventis) were also searching for non-toxic phenothiazine antimalarial drugs. Although they confirmed Gilman's findings, they also made the new and important observation that some phenothiazines have potent antihistamine effects. The first of these drugs was promethazine (Phenergan), which Rhone-Poulenc released in 1946 and is still in use today, both as a sedative and as an antihistamine. Rhone-Poulenc then embarked on developing more antihistaminic phenothiazines. Their chief chemist, Paul Charpentier, synthesised chlorpromazine itself and, together with his colleague Simone Courvoisier (1956), showed it to have a large number of physiological actions (hence its commercial name, Largactil).

For the next and perhaps most critical phase of the story, the introduction of chlorpromazine into clinical medicine, Cunningham Owens (1999) attributes considerable importance to the astute observations of Henri Laborit, a French surgeon who worked at the Val de Grace Hospital in Paris. Laborit wanted to devise a way of preventing surgical shock, a relatively common yet potentially lethal post-operative complication which he thought might be due to the release of histamine. In the hope of achieving a dampened autonomic state (or 'artificial hibernation') he began to administer various intravenous drug combinations pre-operatively. Together with his colleague, Pierre Huguenard, Laborit devised the first 'lytic cocktail' of drugs that would 'lyse' post-operative autonomic activity. Laborit and Huguenard experimented with promethazine and reported on its sedative effects, which soon came to be more valued than its antihistamine properties. Laborit was the 12th investigator to be sent samples of the newly synthesised RP4560 (chlorpromazine) from Rhone-Poulenc. He added the compound to his pre-operative cocktail, which also comprised meperidene and promethazine, and reported it to produce a 'remarkable twilight state' in his paper 'Une nouveau stabilisateur végétatif le RP4560' (Laborit *et al*, 1952). In his enthusiasm for the drug, Laborit even administered chlorpromazine to a friend and psychiatrist not due for an operation at all, Dr C. Quatri, who reported 'an extreme feeling of detachment in which perception was filtered and muted'.

Chlorpromazine's move from surgery into psychiatry was swift. On 28 December 1951, J. Sigwald administered the drug to a woman with a chronic psychosis and observed some benefit. Then, in March 1952, Hamon and his psychiatric colleagues (also based at the Val de Grace Hospital) gave chlorpromazine to a young man with mania and presented their findings at a local meeting. Jean Delay and Pierre Deniker (of St Anne's Hospital) were the first to conduct a trial of RP4560, with 38 psychotic patients. They presented their findings to the 50th French Congress of Psychiatry and Neurology, in July 1952, and went on to publish 'Utilisative en therapeutic psychiatric d'une phenothiazine d'action centrale elective (4560 RP)' (Delay *et al*, 1952). Soon after this, the use of chlorpromazine spread rapidly across both Europe and America.

For further details on the history of antipsychotic development, see Cunningham Owens (1999) and Healey (2002).

Terminology and the concept of atypicality

Many names have been given to the family of drugs used to treat schizophrenia and other psychotic conditions. Among the earliest was 'ataraxics', which literally meant 'without anxiety', referring to the relaxed and detached state that chlorpromazine produced. The term 'neuroleptic' (from the Greek *neuro*, nerve and *lepsis*, seize) is still in use in some countries, and highlights the link with extrapyramidal side-effects (EPS), while 'major tranquilliser' is now no longer used, as it implies that efficacy is secondary to sedation, now no longer thought to be the primary antipsychotic effect (although sedation can of course be a beneficial side-effect). Therefore the favoured term for this group of drugs is simply 'antipsychotic'.

In the early 1950s, Hans Steck, a psychiatrist working in Lausanne, used chlorpromazine at doses of up to 500 mg daily and found that many patients developed parkinsonism and a variety of other types of EPS. He postulated that antipsychotics worked on the motor midbrain, and gradually it came to be accepted that EPS were an inevitable accompaniment to the therapeutic actions of these drugs. Clinically, it appeared that 'optimum therapeutic dosage' was just below the threshold for EPS. This was later confirmed by imaging studies (Farde & Nordström, 1992).

The first challenge to this concept came in the form of clozapine. Clozapine was in fact first synthesised (by Wander laboratories in Switzerland) and marketed as an antidepressant, but was withdrawn from many European countries and the United States in 1975, owing to deaths in Finland secondary to clozapine-induced agranulocytosis. Interestingly, studies in rats had found it caused marked psychomotor inhibition without catalepsy, characteristics consistent with antipsychotic efficacy *without* tendency to induce EPS in man. In many other countries (e.g. China) it continued to be used, and was found to be very useful in the treatment of schizophrenia. It was the landmark trial by Kane *et al* (1988*a*) that confirmed its efficacy in treatment-resistant schizophrenia, and led to its reintroduction to the US market in the 1990s, with a condition of licence that patients' white cell counts had to be regularly monitored. Studies in the 1990s by several investigators showed that, despite clinical efficacy on both the positive and the negative symptoms of schizophrenia, it had a low liability for inducing EPS, and moreover had a level of dopamine D_2 receptor blockade (see below) lower than had been previously thought to be required for antipsychotic efficacy (Pilowksy *et al*, 1992). This led to an emerging concept of the 'atypical antipsychotic', of which clozapine was the prototype.

Clozapine has a relatively high ratio of serotonin 5-HT_{2A} to dopamine D_2 receptor blockade, a characteristic that was emulated in the synthesis and successful introduction to market of a number of 'second-generation antipsychotics' (SGAs), including risperidone in 1994, olanzapine in 1996 and quetiapine in 1997. Aripiprazole, introduced to the antipsychotic market in the UK in 2004, in contrast was synthesised as a D_2 receptor partial agonist, and is also a serotonin 5-HT_{1A} receptor partial agonist. Another atypical is amisulpride, which is a dopamine D_2 and D_3 receptor antagonist.

Since the mid-1990s the term 'atypical' has been increasingly used and variously defined. In comparison with the older, 'typical drugs', the term now refers to antipsychotics that:

1 do not tend to cause EPS or tardive dyskinesia following chronic administration

2 have a lower or negligible propensity to cause hyperprolactinaemia

3 may have greater beneficial effects on symptom domains other than positive symptoms

4 produce fewer subjective side-effects, such as 'emotional numbing', than 'typical' antipsychotics.

The UK classification of antipsychotics given in the *British National Formulary* (BNF) lists clozapine, risperidone, olanzapine, quetiapine, amisulpride, zotepine, sertindole and aripiprazole as atypical and all other antipsychotics as typical. In this chapter, the term FGA ('first-generation antipsychotic') will be used for 'typical' and the term SGA ('second-generation antipsychotic') for 'atypical'.

Neuropharmacology of schizophrenia

The dopamine hypothesis

The introduction of reserpine and chlorpromazine in the 1950s led to a great deal of research into how antipsychotic drugs worked, and Healey (2002) gives an account of how the evidence for the importance of dopamine gradually developed. While working on the mechanism underlying reserpine-induced sedation, a Swedish scientist named Arvid Carlsson discovered that reserpine depleted brain noradrenaline and serotonin in rabbits. Replacing the noradrenaline and serotonin was not effective in reversing this sedation but giving the rabbits L-dopa did reverse it. There were two possible explanations for this: either L-dopa directly mediated the sedative effects of reserpine or it was the substance (dopamine) that was thought at the time to be merely a biochemical intermediary between L-dopa and the catecholamine noradrenaline that was responsible. It was already known that reserpine could induce Parkinsonian states and Carlsson hypothesised that dopamine might also play a role in Parkinson's disease, implicating it as a neurotransmitter.

Carlsson (1959) demonstrated using ultraviolet microscopy that there were dopaminergic pathways in the brains of many mammalian species. However, while reserpine depleted catecholamines and produced sedation, chlorpromazine and haloperidol produced sedation without such depletion. It was the critical study by Carlsson & Lindquist (1963) which was to solve this puzzle. They showed that the administration of chlorpromazine or haloperidol in mice resulted in the accumulation of dopamine metabolites in dopaminergic regions of the brain, and on this basis proposed that chlorpromazine and haloperidol were postsynaptic dopamine antagonists. Their paper 'Effect of chlorpromazine and haloperidol on 3-methoxytryptamine and normetanephrine in mouse brain', published in a Swedish toxicology journal, was to lay the foundation for the dopaminergic theory of schizophrenia and antipsychotic drug action. It is one of the few papers in psychiatry to be associated with a Nobel Prize, which was awarded to Carlsson in 2000 (Healey, 2002).

In the 1970s another important discovery was made, which was that all known antipsychotics at the time were found to block a particular subtype of dopamine receptor, the D_2 receptor. Seeman *et al* (1976) were able to demonstrate a linear relationship between the *in vitro* potency of an antipsychotic for displacing [^{3}H]-labelled haloperidol from dopamine receptor binding sites and clinical antipsychotic potency. The dopamine hypothesis of schizophrenia also stated that overactivity of the mesolimbic dopamine system correlated with the positive symptoms of schizophrenia. Further evidence pinpointing the D_2 receptor came from an elegant study by Johnstone *et al* (1978), who conducted a double-blind prospective study comparing the α and β isomers of flupentixol. It was demonstrated that the α isomer (which is a D_2 receptor antagonist) was more effective in treating the positive symptoms of schizophrenia than the β isomer (whose affinity for D_2 receptors was 1/1000 of that of the α isomer). (For definitions of affinity, potency and other general pharmacological terms, see Tsapakis & Aitchison, 2006).

Other evidence for dopaminergic involvement in psychosis derived from the observation that certain stimulant drugs that cause dopamine release can produce a clinical state similar to schizophrenia. Connell (1958) was the first to report the development of paranoid psychoses among people who had misused amphetamine. They presented with over-talkativeness, insomnia, hyperarousal, suspiciousness and delusions of persecution. The symptoms were sometimes accompanied by auditory or visual hallucinations and were not due to an acute confusional state. The clinical picture is therefore similar in many ways to an acute paranoid psychosis, but cessation of amphetamines and treatment with an antipsychotic usually leads to resolution of the symptoms within 2 weeks. (Amphetamine causes the release of dopamine from presynaptic terminals, and the induced psychosis responds well to D_2 antagonists.) In animal models, amphetamine also produces stereotyped motor behaviours (again mediated by dopamine); this model has been widely used in antipsychotic drug development to screen for putative antipsychotic drugs, by observing the degree to which a new drug can reduce these amphetamine-induced stereotyped motor behaviours.

Dopaminergic receptors

Dopamine receptors are of five subtypes, D_1–D_5, including two subfamilies: 'D_1-like' (D_1 and D_5) and 'D_2-like' (D_2, D_3 and D_4). The receptor densities of these subtypes vary across brain regions. All dopaminergic receptors are transmembrane proteins, with seven transmembrane domains (see Fig. 11.1), coupled via G-proteins to adenylate cyclase. The D_1-like family increases the levels of cyclic adenosine monophosphate (cAMP) and the D_2-like family decreases the level of cAMP. The D_2 receptor exists as two different splice variants (D_2 'short' and 'long' – see below).

Location of dopamine receptors in the human brain

The location of dopamine receptors in the human brain are indicated in Fig. 11.2. There are four main dopaminergic pathways:

1 mesolimbic, from the ventral tegmental area (A10) of the midbrain projecting to limbic and cortical areas (this pathway is implicated in various psychiatric disorders, including schizophrenia)

2 mesocortical, from the ventral tegmental area to the cortex, particularly the frontal lobes (this pathway is involved in motivation and emotional response and in the negative symptoms of schizophrenia)

3 nigrostriatal, from the substantia nigra (A9) of the brain-stem projecting to the striatum (this pathway is involved in parkinsonism)

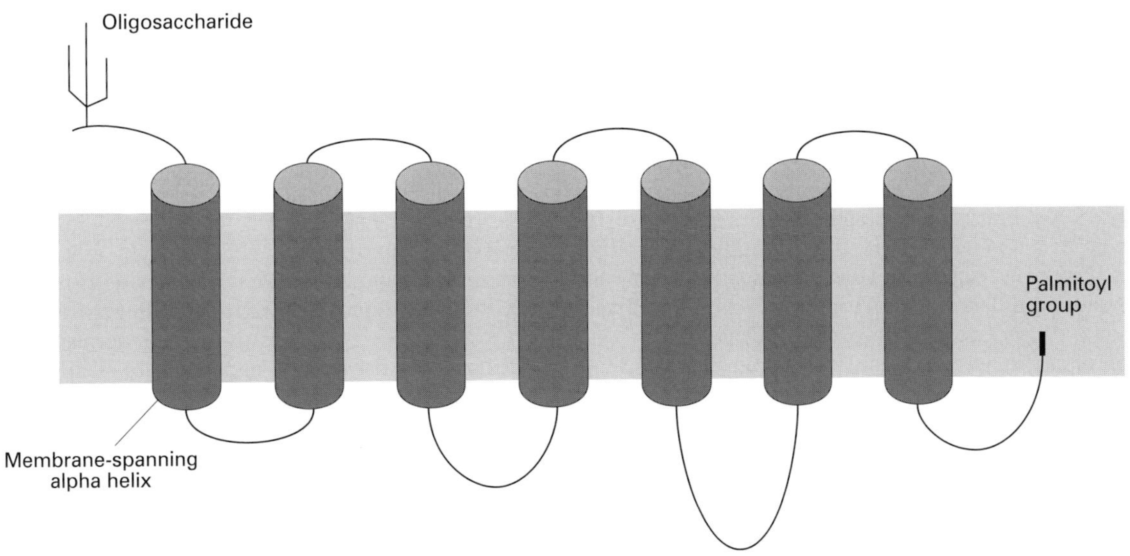

Fig. 11.1 The seven transmembrane domains, coupled via G-proteins to adenylate cyclase. (Taken from 'Dopamine receptors' by Professor P. G. Strange, School of Animal and Microbial Sciences, University of Reading, Whiteknights, Reading RG6 6AJ, UK; published in Tocris Reviews, No. 15, October 2000 by Tocris Cookson Ltd, UK.)

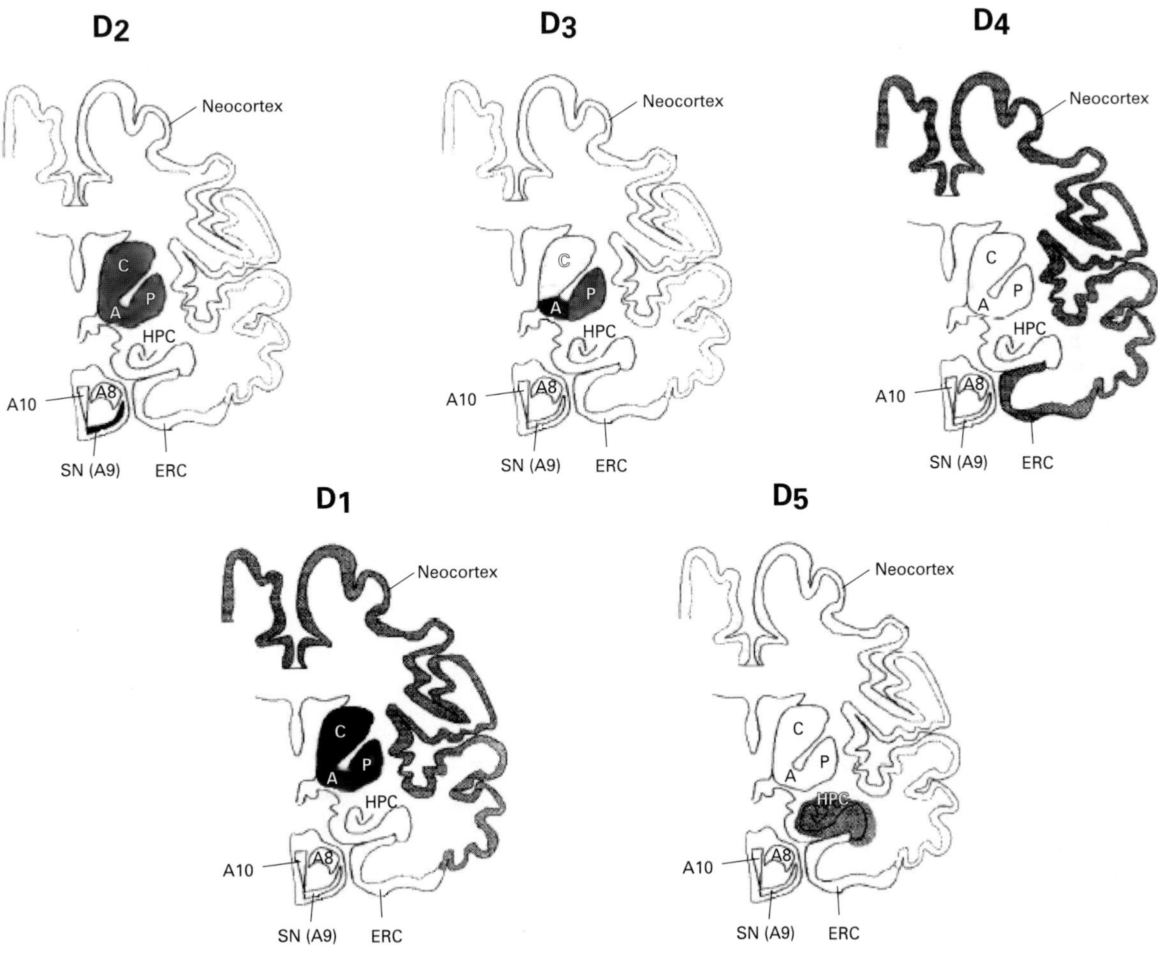

Fig. 11.2 Brain region location of mRNA for human dopamine receptors – grey stippled regions indicate the presence of mRNA. A, nucleus accumbens; C, caudate; P, putamen; HPC, hippocampus (includes dentate gyrus, CA1–CA4 subfields, and subiculum); ERC, entorhinal cortex; A8, retrorubral field; SN (A9), pars compacta of the substantia nigra; A10, ventral tegmental area. From Meador-Woodruff *et al* (1996), reproduced with permission.

4 tuberoinfundibular, from the hypothalamus projecting to the pituitary gland (this pathway mediates the neuroendocrine side-effects of antipsychotics, such as hyperprolactinaemia).

D_1 receptors

The D_1 receptor has been known to exist since the late 1970s, but was not cloned until 1990. It is distributed in a similar pattern to D_2 receptors. Its mRNA expression is higher in the caudate, putamen and nucleus accumbens, and is somewhat lower in the neocortex. As mentioned above, it stimulates the production of cAMP. Some antipsychotics bind significantly to D_1 receptors, an effect that may be relevant to cognition in schizophrenia.

D_2 receptors

The highest concentrations of D_2 receptors are observed in the anterior pituitary, nigrostriatal and mesolimbic dopamine systems; lower concentrations are seen in the cortex. They function both postsynaptically and as presynaptic autoreceptors (stimulation of which inhibits transmitter release and blockade of which increases transmitter release). There are two isoforms (mRNA splice variants), known as 'short' and 'long' forms, which vary in the number of repeats of an amino acid sequence in the third cytoplasmic loop of the receptor, near the guanine nucleotide binding protein (G protein) recognition site. These isoforms may therefore have different mechanisms of intracellular transduction and receptor regulation (Zhang *et al*, 1994).

D_3 receptors

D_3 receptors have 10–100 times the affinity for dopamine than D_2 receptors. They are expressed predominantly in the mesolimbic dopaminergic system and substantially less in the nigrostriatal system, hippocampus and entorhinal cortex. A small amount of D_3 mRNA is also expressed in the motor and parietal cortex (Schmauss *et al*, 1993).

D_4 receptors

Generally, D_4 receptors have a similar or slightly lower affinity for dopamine than D_2 receptors. However, clozapine's D_4 affinity is at least 10 times its affinity for D_2 receptors. This gave rise to interest in the D_4 receptor in the field of drug discovery, but clinical trials of D_4-specific antagonists have been disappointing. There are several variants of the D_4 receptor owing to a hypervariable region (a variable number of tandem repeats or VNTRs) in the DNA sequence, and these variants differ functionally.

Areas of high D_4 mRNA expression include the frontal and entorhinal cortex and hippocampus, with lower expression in the cortex, striatum and nucleus accumbens. This distribution is substantially different to that of the D_2 and the D_3 receptor.

D_5 receptors

The D_5 receptor is homologous to the D_1 receptor (and is in the D_1 family). It has been isolated and cloned from both human and rat tissue. Like the D_1 receptor, it is linked to cAMP production via adenylate cyclase, and has similar affinities for various agonists and antagonists with the notable exception of dopamine itself, which is 10 times more potent at the D_5 receptor. The D_5 receptor is expressed at much lower concentrations than the D_1 receptor, its highest expression being observed in the hippocampus and the entorhinal cortex.

Neuroimaging studies and receptor occupancy

The use of radiolabelled compounds in positron emission tomography (PET) and single-photon emission tomography (SPET) have made it possible to investigate receptor occupancy in patients treated with antipsychotics. These sensitive techniques can measure substances in the brain at nanomolar or even picomolar concentrations; for a more detailed description of these methods see the reviews by Bigliani *et al* (1999) and Talbot & Laruelle (2002).

These imaging techniques have been used to investigate receptor occupancy in the dopamine (DA) and serotonin (5-HT) systems, with studies so far focusing mainly on D_2-like, 5-HT_{2A} and D_1 receptors. A central role for D_2 occupancy in the mechanism of action of antipsychotics is now well established. A 'therapeutic window' has also been defined, with most antipsychotics achieving optimal efficacy at dopamine receptor occupancies of 60–75%, levels above 80% in the striatum being increasingly associated with EPS (Farde & Nordström, 1992; Kapur *et al*, 2000). As mentioned above, clozapine differs from other antipsychotics in having much lower occupancy in the striatum, while still maintaining good clinical efficacy (Pilowsky *et al*, 1992). PET studies show high 5-HT_{2A} receptor occupancy by clozapine at subtherapeutic doses (50 mg per day). The high ratio of 5-HT_2:D_2 binding both in these and in cell culture studies led to the proposition that this might be a feature underlying the 'atypical' profile. Risperidone has a D_2 occupancy of 60% at a dose of 2 mg, with 5-HT_{2A} receptors being saturated at lower doses. Olanzapine also shows high 5-HT_{2A} receptor occupancy at low doses. However, clinical trials with pure 5-HT_2 antagonists have shown them to be ineffective against both positive and negative symptoms of schizophrenia, and SPET studies have shown no relationship between 5-HT_{2A} blockade and the degree of clinical improvement (Travis *et al*, 1997).

D_2 and 5-HT_{2A} receptors and the tendency for EPS

It is now thought that high antipsychotic affinity for 5-HT_{2A} receptors may be associated with a lower propensity for EPS (Travis *et al*, 1997), and it has been suggested that a 5-HT_{2A}:D_2 ratio of at least 1.12 confers atypicality (Meltzer *et al*, 1989). This figure is derived from antipsychotic affinities for cortical 5-HT_{2A} and striatal D_2 receptors and, as such binding affinities (K_i) are expressed as logarithms, apparently small ratios correspond to large differences in affinity (i.e. a ratio of 1.12 corresponds to a 13-fold greater affinity for 5-HT_{2A} than for D_2 receptors). This ratio's relevance to the aetiology of EPS is indirectly supported by the observation that risperidone shows relatively high 5-HT_{2A} binding at low doses, but as its dose is increased and D_2 occupancy rises, so does the risk of EPS. However, there are other possible mechanisms of atypicality. For example, amisulpride achieves 70–80% D_2 occupancy at doses of 600–900 mg per day and has no demonstrable affinity for 5-HT_{2A} receptors, but is a D_2 and D_3 antagonist. It is still classed as an atypical mainly because of other properties, such as its efficacy against negative symptoms.

In vitro studies have demonstrated that antipsychotics dissociate from the D_2 receptor at different rates (the dissocation rate constant is denoted K_{off}). The atypicals as a group have higher dissociation rates than the typicals, but within the atypicals dissociation rates vary (quetiapine>clozapine>olanzapine). It has been proposed that it is the lack of sustained D_2 blockade (conferred by the fast K_{off}) that gives rise to the lower incidence of EPS (Kapur & Seeman, 2001).

Studies have also looked at the regional distributions of antipsychotics in the brain. Pilowsky *et al* (1997) demonstrated higher blockade with atypicals of temporal D_2 and D_3 receptors than of striatal D_2 receptors. However, Talvik *et al* (2001) showed similar receptor occupancies in extrastriatal and striatal regions for both typicals and atypicals. Work in rodents has shown the nucleus accumbens (part of the ventral striatum) to be pivotal in antipsychotic action; because the nucleus accumbens projects to the cortex, this is evidence in support of a role for cortical D_2 and D_3 receptors in the mechanism of action of the atypicals. Further studies in this area are in progress.

Dopamine and the 'attribution of salience' – a neuropsychological theory of dopaminergic action

According to the 'attribution of salience' theory, dopamine mediates the conversion of an external sensory stimulus from an initially neutral cortical representation to one of attraction or aversion, which is then linked to subsequent processes (attention, drive and goal-directed behaviour). 'Salience' in social psychology may be defined as 'the quality or fact being more prominent in a person's awareness or in his memory or past experience'. The mesolimbic dopamine system is hypothesised to be a critical component in this process. In psychosis, it is postulated that dysregulation of this system leads to the decoupling of the release of dopamine from stimuli (Kapur, 2003). This usurps the normal process of 'context-driven salience attribution', and leads instead to the abnormal assignment of salience to external objects and representations. The theory proposes that, in schizophrenia, a delusion is a cognitive ('top-down') explanation by the person of an aberrantly salient experience, while a hallucination is the experience of abnormally salient internal phenomena such as representations of percepts and memories. In this model, antipsychotics dampen salience, that is, reduce stimulus significance and modulate the behavioural impact of positive feedback processes; they do not *erase* the symptoms, but provide the *platform for psychological resolution*. This is consistent with the fact that delusions may persist for years, despite adequate dopamine receptor blockade.

Other neurotransmitter systems

Phencyclidine and the NMDA system

Phencyclidine (Sernyl, PCP) was introduced as a general anaesthetic in the 1950s. It had an advantage over other anaesthetics available at the time in that it lacked depressant effects on the heart. However, post-operatively (and occasionally even intra-operatively) it sometimes caused severe psychotic states (hallucinations), and this phenomenon eventually led to the drug being withdrawn from clinical use. When it had been available, however, some American psychiatrists had become interested in its psychotic-inducing effects among normal volunteers, and termed it a 'schizophreno-mimetic' (Luby *et al*, 1959). The syndrome induced by PCP resembles an acute presentation in schizophrenia, more so than an amphetamine psychosis, since symptoms akin to the 'negative' symptoms of schizophrenia, as well as cognitive dysfunction and social withdrawal may also occur. Further, a single dose of PCP can produce a profound relapse in previously well stabilised patients with schizophrenia. Approximately 20 years after these initial observations were made, a high-affinity binding site for PCP was identified at the N-methyl-D-aspartate (NMDA) subtype of the glutamate receptor. It was discovered that PCP reduced glutamate transmission at this receptor, and hence indicated that the neurotransmitter glutamate might also be involved in the pathogenesis of schizophrenia.

Although PCP is no longer employed as an anaesthetic, one of its derivatives, ketamine, is still commonly used. Ketamine may also induce a schizophrenia-like psychosis and, interestingly, this effect depends on the age of the person taking the drug: it is not usually seen in children but occurs more commonly in adolescents and adults. It can also cause an exacerbation of symptoms in patients with schizophrenia. Like PCP, ketamine acts at the NMDA receptor.

Evidence is now growing that the NMDA receptor also plays a role in the cognitive deficits associated with schizophrenia (Krystal *et al*, 1994; Malhotra *et al*, 1996). Decreased levels of glutamate have been found in the cerebrospinal fluid (CSF) of patients with schizophrenia, as has a reduced expression of NMDA receptor subtypes in the prefrontal cortex. The NMDA receptor (see Fig. 11.3) is known to be involved in synaptic plasticity and long-term potentiation (Tsien *et al*, 1996) as well as in excitotoxic neuronal damage, for example from ischaemia, trauma and epilepsy (Hartnett *et al*, 1997). It is important to note that dopaminergic and glutamatergic systems interact at multiple sites throughout the brain.

Activation of the glycine allosteric site on the NMDA receptor is necessary for its normal functioning. In schizophrenia, if the system is hypofunctional, agonists should theoretically be therapeutic. Javitt *et al* (1994) and Heresco-Levy *et al* (1999) tested glycine (up to 60 g/day) as an adjunct to antipsychotic and anticholinergic medication in schizophrenia, and noted an improvement in negative symptoms. Tsai *et al* (1998) and Coyle *et al* (2002) used D-serine (also an agonist at the glycine site) and saw a significant improvement in positive, negative and cognitive symptom domains. However, this effect was not seen in clozapine-treated participants (Tsai *et al*, 1999), probably because clozapine alone already has a greater influence on glutamatergic neurotransmission than most other antipsychotics (Coyle *et al*, 2002).

A number of genes related to schizophrenia have been identified (including one that encodes D-amino acid oxidase or DAAO, which metabolises D-amino acids, including D-serine) and it has been suggested that one common final pathway by which these genes exert their

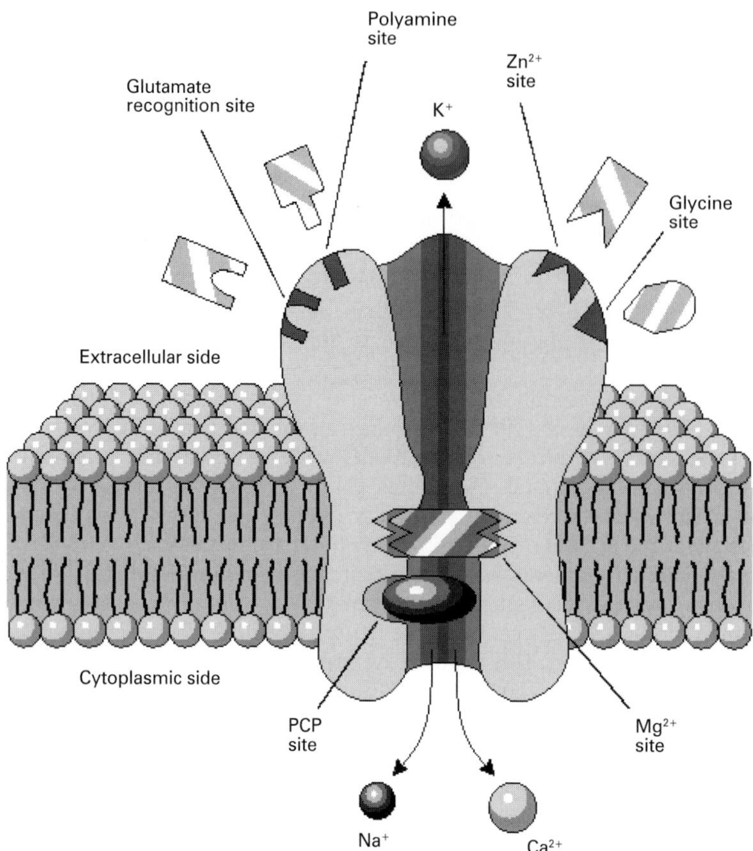

Fig. 11.3 The NMDA receptor. This receptor is likely to be particularly relevant to the pathology, and hence treatment, of schizophrenia. PCP can produce a profound relapse of schizophrenia by reducing glutamate transmission at this receptor, and NMDA agonists have been found to be therapeutically useful. In addition, the NMDA receptor plays a role in the cognitive deficits found in schizophrenia, and genetic findings have also identified this receptor as playing a key role in pathological mechanisms relevant to schizophrenia. See text for further details. From *Fundamentals of Neuropsychopharmacology*, by Robert S. Feldman & Linda F. Quenzer, published by Sinauer Associates Inc. (1984).

effect could be via the glutamate system (Harrison & Owen, 2003). These genetic findings are discussed in Chapter 10 on page 212.

Serotonergic sites

Interest in the role of serotonin in the pathogenesis of psychosis dates from 1943, when a Swiss research chemist, Albert Hoffman, ingested some of the chemical he was working on at the time, lysergic acid diethylamide (LSD). He described his experience as follows:

> 'I lay down and sank into a not unpleasant intoxicated-like condition characterised by an extremely stimulated imagination. In a dream-like state with eyes closed (I found the light to be extremely glaring) I perceived an uninterrupted stream of fantastic pictures, extraordinary shapes with kaleidoscopic play of colours. After some two hours this condition faded away.' (Quoted in Moghaddan & Crystal, 2003, p. 353)

LSD is a 5-HT (especially 5-HT_{2A}) receptor agonist, and also has more complex effects on serotonergic transmission. It has been shown that plant hallucinogens such as mescaline and psilocybin (the latter colloquially known as 'magic mushrooms') produce a dose-dependent psychotic disturbance, including hallucinations, impairments in concentration and attention, depersonalisation, derealisation and thought disorder, but with apparently less blunting of affect and cognitive impairment than the NMDA antagonists. Hallucinogens such as LSD are also likely to interact with a variety of other systems, including the dopaminergic system, owing to the complex interactions between multiple neurotransmitter systems.

Studies using the psychotomimetic drug m-chlorophenylpiperazine (mCPP), which is a serotonergic receptor agonist, offer further support for a serotonergic role in psychosis. Although mCPP does not normally induce psychosis, it causes increased anxiety and agitation in patients with schizophrenia. These effects may be attenuated by clozapine and olanzapine (which are antagonists at 5-HT_{2A} receptors) but not by haloperidol (which has little 5-HT blockade at doses used clinically). Antagonism at the 5-HT_{2A} serotonin receptor, which is part of the spectrum of most atypicals, is thought to contribute both to their efficacy (especially against 'negative' symptoms or comorbid depression) and to their diminished tendency to cause EPS. Thus, there is some evidence for a role of serotonin in the pathophysiology of schizophrenia, but much greater evidence for a primary role of this neurotransmitter in depression (Moghaddan & Crystal, 2003).

In summary, dopamine antagonism is still thought to play the major role in antipsychotic efficacy against 'positive' symptoms. However, it appears that other neurotransmitters, such as glutamate, serotonin and

Table 11.1 Classification of the typical antipsychotics

Chemical group	Antipsychotic	Trade name(s)
Phenothiazines	*Aliphatics (i.e. non-aromatic organic compounds)*	
	Chlorpromazine	Largactil
	Promazine	Sparine
	Piperidines (these are cyclic amines)	
	Thioridazine	Melleril
	Pipotiazine	Piportil
	Piperazines (these are 6-sided organic ring compound containing two opposing nitrogen atoms)	
	Trifluoperazine	Stelazine
	Fluphenazine	Modecate; Moditen
Butyrophenones	Haloperidol	Dozic; Haldol; Serenace
	Benperidol	Benquil
Thioxanthenes	Flupentixol	Depixol; Fluanxol
	Zuclopenthixol	Clopixol; Clopixol Acuphase
Diphenylbutylpiperidines	Pimozide	Orap
Benzamide	Sulpiride (some authors classify this as an atypical)	Dolmatil; Sulpitil; Sulpor

See Fig. 11.4 for the structure of the main typical antipsychotics.

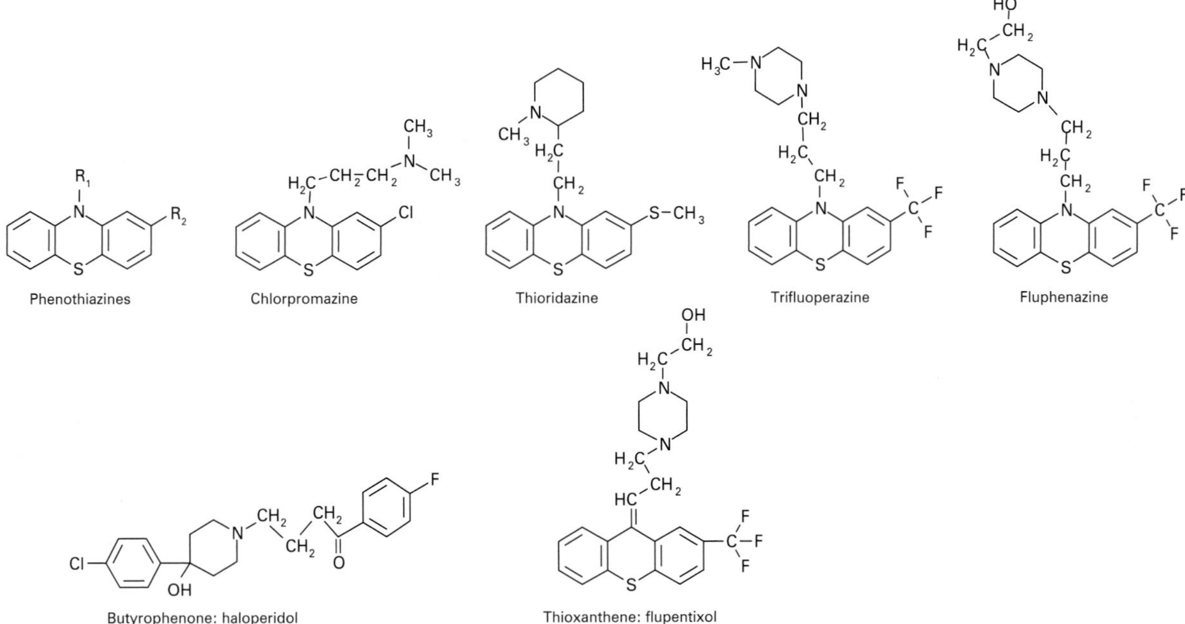

Fig. 11.4 Structure of the main typical antipsychotics.

noradrenaline, are also involved, particularly in other symptom domains (including cognitive and 'negative'), which is not surprising given the multiple interactions between these and the dopamine system.

Antipsychotics

In this section, a number of drugs in common use (both typicals and atypicals) are described. The account is not comprehensive but highlights features of interest about each drug and some of the differences between them. Efficacy is discussed separately on pages 271–274, while side-effects are considered on pages 255–271. Commercial ('trade') names of the drugs have been placed in parentheses after the generic name.

The older, typical drugs dominated the pharmacotherapy of schizophrenia from 1955 to 1990, but they have now been supplanted by the newer, 'atypical' drugs. Nevertheless, several of the older drugs remain in common use, such as haloperidol (e.g. in emergency tranquillisation) and the depot preparations fluphenazine and flupentixol. The major pharmacological classes of the FGAs available in the UK at the time of writing are shown in Table 11.1, along with their structures in Fig. 11.4, while their main disadvantages (as compared with SGAs) are shown in Box 11.1.

Box 11.1 Disadvantages of the first-generation antipsychotics

Limited efficacy
- Residual positive symptoms
- Residual negative symptoms
- Secondary negative symptoms
- Cognitive symptoms
- Secondary depression

Acute pharmacological side-effects
- Extrapyramidal side-effects: parkinsonism, acute dystonia and akathisia
- Postural hypotension
- Anticholinergic side-effects
- Impotence
- Cardiotoxicity

Long-term pharmacological side-effects
- Hyperprolactinaemia, leading to galactorrhoea, amenorrhoea and low libido
- Weight gain
- Tardive dyskinesia
- Tardive dystonia

Idiosyncratic reactions
- Neuroleptic malignant syndrome
- Rash
- Hepatitis
- Agranulocytosis

From Cookson *et al* (2002).

At a pharmacodynamic level, the differences between the various drugs in terms of clinical profile are seen to correlate with their receptor binding profiles, which are shown in Table 11.2. For example, a drug with a strong affinity for histaminic H_1 receptors is likely to be associated with sedation and weight gain.

Typical antipsychotics

The FGAs differ in their propensity to induce sedation, anticholinergic (antimuscarinic) and extrapyramidal side-effects. The differences between the three phenothiazine groups are shown in Table 11.3.

Table 11.3 Side-effect tendencies of the different phenothiazine groups

Type of phenothiazine	Sedation	Anti-muscarinic	EPS
Aliphatic	+++	++	++
Piperidine	++	+++	+
Piperazine	+	+	+++

FGAs of other chemical groups tend to resemble the piperazine phenothiazines.

These differential effects can be understood in terms of their differential affinities (Richelson, 1996):

1 for the histamine H_1 receptor (sedation – chlorpromazine > pipotiazine > fluphenazine)

2 for the muscarinic M_1 receptor (antimuscarinic effects – pipotiazine > chlorpromazine > fluphenazine)

3 in terms of the M_1:D_2 ratio (which contributes to amelioration of EPS – pipotiazine > chlorpromazine > fluphenazine).

A simple mnemonic is that: low-potency, high-milligram compounds (e.g. chlorpromazine, thioridazine) are associated with higher rates of sedation and anticholinergic effects, but lower rates of EPS; on the other hand, high-potency, low-milligram drugs (e.g. haloperidol, pimozide) are less sedative and less anticholinergic, but have higher rates of EPS. It is worth having a good grasp of the pharmacology of FGAs as their use may well be increasing in light of the CATIE study (see page 272).

Chlorpromazine (Largactil)

Chlorpromazine was the mainstay of antipsychotic treatment for a long time. Its chemical structure (Fig. 11.4) is of a standard phenothiazine (a tricyclic structure). The middle ring has an aliphatic side chain. It is said to be a low-potency drug because a relatively large

Table 11.2 Receptor binding affinities of various antipsychotics, data given as K_i (nmol/l)

Receptor	Aripiprazole	Olanzapine	Risperidone	Quetiapine	Ziprasidone	Clozapine	Haloperidol
D_1	265[a]	31	430	455	525	85	210
D_2	0.34[a]	11	4	160	5	126	0.7
D_3	0.8[a]	49	10	340	7	473	2
D_4	44[a]	27	9	1600	32	35	3
5-HT_{1A}	1.7[a]	> 10000	210	2800	3	875	1100
5-HT_{2A}	3.4[a]	4	0.5	295	0.4	16	45
5-HT_{2C}	15[a]	23	25	1500	1	16	> 10000
α_1	57	19	0.7	7	11	7	6
H_1	61[a]	7	20	11	50	6	440
M_1	> 10000	1.9	> 10000	120	> 1000	1.9	> 1500

[a] Data with cloned human receptors.
Note that a lower K_i signifies stronger binding affinity.
Source of data: Arnt & Skarsfeldt (1998); Bymaster *et al* (1996); Seeger *et al* (1995).

dose (in milligrams) is required to produce a therapeutic effect. It has strong sedative properties owing to its antihistaminic effects, and was hence previously often used (intramuscularly) in the management of acute disturbances. However, it is also strongly hypotensive and the intramuscular injection is painful, and no longer recommended. It is now used solely as an oral tablet. In the treatment of acute schizophrenia, it is used in doses of 300–800 mg daily (BNF maximum 1000 mg daily). Sedative effects appear almost immediately, but antipsychotic effects may take longer to appear, with the complete resolution of an acute episode taking at least 4 weeks. Chlorpromazine is well absorbed and has a fairly rapid onset of action (1–3 hours after oral ingestion). It is highly protein bound and hence has a variable plasma half-life, of 8–35 hours, and so is prescribed to be taken twice or three times a day.

Thioridazine (Melleril)

Like chlorpromazine, this low-potency phenothiazine was once very commonly used, particularly for the management of agitation and restlessness. It also has the basic phenothiazine ring structure, but a single nitrogen is incorporated into the side-chain ring (R_1 in Fig. 11.4), placing it in the piperidine subgroup of phenothiazines.

For more than three decades, the drug was thought to be relatively safe. In fact, for a brief period in the late 1980s, following the revelation that benzodiazepines are highly addictive, thioridazine was advocated as a treatment for anxiety in non-psychotic patients. However, although the side-effect profile is similar to that of chlorpromazine, there are two exceptions. First, the use of high doses of thioridazine (600 mg or more for longer than 4 weeks) carries a higher risk of retinal pigmentation than chlorpromazine. A study by Shah *et al* (1998) showed that some patients developed pigmentary changes within 2–8 weeks after initiation of therapy, with acute symptoms including blurred vision, night blindness and colour blindness. Second, it prolongs the QT_c interval and was therefore implicated in a number of sudden unexplained deaths. This may be at least partly due to a cardiotoxic sulphoxide metabolite and the fact that individuals who have low activity in a specific cytochrome P450 enzyme (CYP2D6; see below) have an altered route of metabolism for thioridazine. This resulted in a change in its licence so that it could only be prescribed by specialists under strict conditions. The drug is not used now and it is no longer even listed in the BNF.

Trifluoperazine (Stelazine)

This high-potency phenothiazine (20 times more so than chlorpromazine) has the advantage of causing very little hypotension or sedation. It also has a relatively long half-life (12.5 hours) as the modified release form (Stelazine Spansules), and may hence be administered once daily. It is therefore useful for oral maintenance therapy in compliant patients, and was widely used as such before the introduction of the SGAs. Many patients remain on small doses of trifluoperazine today. However, it is associated with a relatively high risk of EPS, including tardive dyskinesia.

Butyrophenones

These drugs were first synthesised in 1958 by Belgian chemists P. Janssen and H. J. Haase, and were the foundation of the role of Janssen laboratories (now Johnson and Johnson) in schizophrenia drug development.

The butyrophenones are chemically related to pethidine and were discovered when derivatives of norpethidine were screened. Haloperidol was the first butyrophenone to be marketed in the treatment of schizophrenia. As a class of antipsychotic, these drugs have little or no antihistaminic effects (hence little sedation), little anticholinergic activity (and so are less likely to cause autonomic disturbances) and low central anti-adrenergic activity (causing less hypotension). However, because haloperidol is a very potent D_2 blocker, its propensity for EPS is high. In many registration trials (those required by the regulatory authorities) for SGAs it was the standard comparator, and hence it is not surprising that these trials showed a favourable EPS profile for the SGAs. However, haloperidol remains in common use, particularly for states of severe agitation, excitement, aggression and hyperactivity. In small doses, it may also be used in the elderly for the management of restlessness, agitation and acute confusional states. Indeed, its use in the elderly is at present increasing, since the discovery of an increased risk of stroke in this patient group with SGAs, including risperidone and olanzapine. Haloperidol is available in oral form both as a tablet and as a syrup (half-life approximately 2 days), as parental preparations administered both intravenously and intramuscularly (half-life 13–17 hours) and as a long-acting depot preparation, haloperidol decanoate (Haldol) (half-life around 3 weeks). Other butyrophenones include droperidol, which is even more potent than haloperidol but which has been withdrawn in the UK because of its cardiotoxicity, and benperidol, which is long acting and is used occasionally in sex offenders.

Thioxanthenes

Thioxanthenes are structurally very similar to phenothiazines, and this can be seen by comparing flupentixol with fluphenazine in Fig. 11.4. The difference is that thioxanthenes have a carbon atom rather than a nitrogen atom in their middle ring (to which the side chain is attached). Despite their structural similarity, thioxanthenes differ from phenothiazines in that they antagonise both D_1 and D_2 receptors. Zuclopenthixol is used in its depot form (zuclopenthixol acetate); flupentixol, although available as an oral tablet (flupentixol dihydrochloride), is also more commonly used as a depot (flupentixol decanoate). They are therefore discussed later in the chapter, under the heading 'Long-acting depot preparations'.

Diphenylbutylpiperidines

These drugs were derived from the butyrophenones and include pimozide (Orap), which has a particularly high D_2 affinity. The oral preparation of pimozide has a very long half-life (53 hours). In addition to its use in schizophrenia, it has been used in delusional disorders (e.g. monosymptomatic hypochondriacal delusional disorder). However, it was the first antipsychotic to be placed under restriction owing to its cardiotoxicity, and is now rarely used. The BNF recommends an electrocardiogram (ECG) before treatment and annually thereafter, taking note of any prolongation of the QT_c interval. It should not be given in conjunction with any other antipsychotic drugs, tricyclic antidepressants, antimalarials, or antibiotics such as moxifloxacin, because these drugs may also prolong the QT_c (see the BNF interactions appendix).

Benzamides

These drugs are chemically related to the anti-arrhythmic agent procainamide. Modification of its structure initially led to metoclopramide, an anti-emetic that reduces gastric motility and also has weak antipsychotic effects. Further developments from metoclopramide led to sulpiride as well as amisulpride, which is a substituted benzamide and, as already mentioned, is included in the atypical group (see page 250).

Sulpiride is selective for D_2 and D_3 receptors. At low doses it has an activating effect due to the blockade of presynaptic D_2 autoreceptors. It is water soluble and hence less well absorbed orally than other antipsychotics. Up to 27% of the amount ingested may be found unchanged in the faeces, but, more importantly, about 70–90% is excreted in the urine, hence dosage reduction may be required in renal impairment. It has a relatively low propensity for EPS, leading to its initial classification as an atypical. It has less anticholinergic and sedative side-effects than most typicals, and has been used in the treatment of dysthymia as well as obsessive–compulsive disorder (in conjunction with selective serotonin reuptake inhibitors, SSRIs). One trial suggests it may be an effective adjunct in patients with treatment-resistant schizophrenia who have only partially responded to clozapine (Loo *et al*, 1997). Weight gain and hyperprolactinaemia (the latter resulting in galactorrhoea and menstrual dysfunction) are side-effects that tend to limit its use, particularly in women. The usual doses are 200–400 mg twice daily, and the maximum dose 2.4 g daily.

Atypical antipsychotics

The SGAs available at the time of writing in the UK are classified according to their chemical group (Table 11.4).

Table 11.4 Classification of second-generation antipsychotics

Chemical group	Antipsychotic	Trade names
Dibenzodiazepine	Clozapine	Clozaril, Zaponex, Denzapine
Thienobenzodiazepine	Olanzapine	Zyprexa
Dibenzothiazepine	Quetiapine	Seroquel
Benzisoxazole	Risperidone	Risperdal, Risperdal Consta
Dibenzothiepine	Zotepine	Zoleptil
Imidazolidinone	Sertindole	Serdolect
Substituted benzamide	Amisulpride	Solian
Benzothiazylpiperazine	Ziprasidone	Geodon
Dihydrocarbostyril	Aripiprazole	Abilify

Clozapine

In the late 1950s, three German chemists, F. Hunziker, J. Smutz and E. Eichenberger, working at the Wander laboratories in Switzerland, were trying to create tricyclic compounds similar to imipramine. They synthesised clozapine and it was given to clinicians for testing in 1961. It was found to have many adverse side-effects. It was then sent to Pierre Deniker (who first introduced chlorpromazine) in Paris, who gave it to 19 patients. There were four deaths, including one from agranulocytosis and another from malignant hyperthermia. He returned the drug, advising that further work on the compound should cease. It is interesting to note that these days a drug that had had a phase II result of the above kind would certainly not be taken any further. A German psychiatrist named Hans Hippius was the first to notice the very low rate of EPS, and also to observe that it sometimes helped where other antipsychotics had failed. However, the drug was withdrawn from many countries owing to a cluster of deaths secondary to agranulocytosis in the 1970s in Finland. Sandoz (which had taken over the Wander pharmaceutical company) nearly withdrew it altogether but was persuaded not to do so (by Hippius and others). Trials conducted by Honigfeld (working for Sandoz) continued to show that it had unique beneficial effects. In spite of its known toxicity, the US Food and Drug Administration (FDA) continued to take an interest in the drug, with regulators eventually persuading Sandoz to conduct a further study. This was to become the landmark study by Kane *et al* (1988*a*) that confirmed its efficacy in treatment-resistant patients as well as its safety, provided the patient's white cell count was monitored. Clozapine's reintroduction to the US market in the 1990s not only demonstrated its ability to ameliorate both the positive and the negative symptoms of schizophrenia, but also challenged the concept of antipsychotic efficacy being tightly linked to the induction of EPS.

Receptor pharmacology

Clozapine has a unique pattern of receptor binding, with affinities for a wide range of receptor groups, in contrast to the majority of other antipsychotics (Table 11.2). It binds only weakly to D_2 but strongly to D_4 receptors, with the order of binding affinities within the dopaminergic systems being $D_4>D_1>D_2>D_3$. Clozapine's binding to striatal D_2 receptors is only in the range of 20–60%, in contrast to that of most other antipsychotics, for which the binding at therapeutic doses is greater than 60%. Clozapine's low affinity for D_2 receptors leads to a lower tendency to cause hyperprolactinaemia.

Clozapine also has a high affinity for serotonergic receptors (especially 5-HT_{2A} and 5-HT_{2C}). The combination of high 5-HT_{2A} and low D_2 binding may be at least partly responsible for its low tendency to cause EPS. It also binds to several other serotonergic sites, including 5-HT_{2C}, with the latter likely to be at least partly responsible for clozapine-induced weight gain. Its actions at adrenergic receptors have been linked to the side-effect of postural hypotension, and its histamine (H_1) receptor antagonism may be at least partly responsible for the side-effects of weight gain and sedation. It also binds to muscarinic (M_1 and M_4) cholinergic receptors. Its M_1 binding may play a role in its beneficial effects on cognitive function and also in the relatively low EPS induction. It is an agonist at salivary gland M_4 receptors, an effect that contributes to clozapine-induced hypersalivation. Clozapine's combination of high efficacy while binding to multiple receptor sites is unusual. A previously widely held view in pharmacology was that an effective drug should target a single receptor, with minimal binding to other sites, in order to reduce potential side-effects: a so-called 'clean' drug. However, clozapine's 'dirty' profile is now thought to be one of the keys to its greater efficacy and reduced EPS.

Animal studies have revealed three interesting effects. First, in contrast to most other antipsychotics, clozapine does not produce catalepsy in cats. This indicates that it causes little or no depletion of dopamine in the nigrostriatal pathway, and is consistent with its diminished tendency to induce parkinsonism in humans. Second, clozapine inhibits the conditioned avoidance response (CAR) in rodents (another animal test that correlates with antipsychotic activity) at substantially lower doses than those required for the induction of catalepsy. (This separation of dose for CAR versus dose for catalepsy is also seen with olanzapine and risperidone.) Third, in schizophrenia a sensor motor gating phenomenon known as prepulse inhibition is disrupted. This disruption has also been observed in rodents given phencyclidine. Clozapine has been shown to restore the disruption of prepulse inhibition induced by phencyclidine, indicating that some of its effects may be mediated via the NMDA receptor. Further research to identify the pharmacological underpinning of clozapine's superior efficacy is ongoing.

Olanzapine

Olanzapine is a thienobenzodiazepine structurally related to clozapine. It was developed at the Lilly research laboratories in England as part of a strategy to find drugs similar to clozapine but without its tendency to cause agranulocytosis. Like clozapine, it demonstrates greater 5-HT_{2A} than D_2 activity *in vivo*. It binds more strongly to 5-HT_{2A} than to 5-HT_{2C} but also binds to other 5-HT receptors, such as 5-HT_3 and 5-HT_6. At therapeutic doses, olanzapine's D_2 occupancy is greater than that of clozapine. It also has muscarinic cholinergic activity (a feature not shared by risperidone) as well as potent anti-histaminic effects, the latter making it very sedative. There is no significant binding to β-adrenoceptors, GABA or opioid receptors. Electrophysiological studies show it reduces dopamine activity in the mesolimbic (Brodman area A10) pathways thought to mediate psychosis, while being more sparing of striatal (A9) pathways (which mediate EPS). Its main disadvantage is weight gain and related metabolic side-effects (see page 260). Its main advantage in comparison with clozapine is the reduced risk of bone marrow suppression.

Olanzapine has a relatively long half-life (20–55 hours, mean around 30 hours), which enables once-daily administration. Although well absorbed, it undergoes extensive first-pass metabolism, and only 40% of the ingested dose reaches the systemic circulation. Smoking induces cytochrome P450 1A2, which can increase olanzapine's clearance by up to 40%. Although it is possible to measure plasma olanzapine levels, this assay is not widely available. However, plasma levels may be useful for checking compliance, or for determining overdose. For the former purpose, a sample should be taken 12 hours after the last dose, with levels of 20–40 ng/ml being regarded as therapeutic. Elevated levels of liver transaminases may occur, and hence olanzapine should be used with caution in patients with liver disease.

The usual starting dose is 5–10 mg, administered at night as it has sedative properties. Many patients can be maintained at these doses, with the maximum daily dose usually being 20 mg, although doses of greater than 30 mg are used by some clinicians. It is available in tablet, oro-dispersible ('Velotab') and injectable forms, which means that it can be used for rapid tranquillisation (page 282). However, as with other antipsychotics, there have been some reports of sudden death when olanzapine is used in intramuscular form in conjunction with intramuscular lorazepam whilst restraining a patient (page 283). When given intramuscularly, it should not be combined with another intramuscular injection.

Risperidone

Risperidone was discovered during screening for compounds that could reverse the effects of LSD (Colpaert, 2003). It is a potent 5-HT_2 antagonist ($5\text{-HT}_{2A} > 5\text{-HT}_{2C}$), with a high affinity for D_2-like receptors ($D_2 > D_3 = D_4$). It also interacts with histamine H_1, and α_1- and α_2-adrenergic receptors. It produces EPS in a dose-dependent fashion; trials have shown the risk of EPS to be low at doses below 6 mg daily. In addition, it shows a dose-dependent tendency to increase prolactin levels, while its adrenergic antagonism may cause hypotension. The plasma half-life is 3–20 hours. It has an active metabolite (9-hydroxy-risperidone), which is being tested as an antipsychotic in its own right. Side-effects of risperidone that occurred at a frequency of more than 5% and twice that of placebo in the early trials included somnolence and fatigue, orthostatic hypotension, dizziness, tachycardia, nausea, dyspepsia, diarrhoea, weight gain, sexual dysfunction and rhinitis, although discontinuation rates owing to side-effects were low.

Risperidone is available in oral form as tablets and syrup, as well as a rapidly dispersible form ('Risperdal Quicklets') and a long-acting depot preparation (Risperdal Consta; see page 251), but not as a short-acting parenteral injection.

Quetiapine

Quetiapine is structurally related to clozapine and olanzapine. Its greatest affinities are for α_1 and H_1 receptors (see Table 11.2). Its affinities for D_2 and 5-HT_{2A} receptors are moderate. The high affinity for H_1 leads to sedation. It has little or no effect on nigrostriatal dopaminergic neurons (which mediate EPS), and the incidence of EPS at doses of up to 750 mg daily is therefore similar to that with placebo. Quetiapine also has moderate muscarinic cholinergic antagonism, leading to autonomic side-effects. It does not elevate serum prolactin. It has an active metabolite (7-hydroxyquetiapine).

Quetiapine is rapidly absorbed, achieving peak levels 1–3 hours after ingestion. A short half-life (2–4 hours) necessitates twice-daily administration. Because of its α_1-adrenergic effects, it is often started at a dose of only 25 mg twice daily, which is then gradually increased each day up to a therapeutic dose (now regarded as at least 600 mg daily for chronic schizophrenia), while monitoring for hypotension. Quetiapine has a lower potential for weight gain than clozapine or olanzapine, but somnolence and dry mouth are frequent early adverse effects.

Amisulpride

Amisulpride appears to be more potent than sulpiride. It has greater selectivity for pre- rather than post-synaptic dopamine receptors. It is a pure D_2 and D_3 antagonist. The plasma half-life is 12 hours and its excretion is renal, which also distinguishes it from other SGAs, and means that it does not affect liver enzymes. However, lower doses may be needed for those with renal impairment or the elderly. It is recommended to be prescribed at a low dose (50–300 mg) for negative symptoms alone, or at higher doses (600–1200 mg) for positive symptoms. It is, however, associated with dose-related EPS and prolactin elevation, the latter leading to galactorrhoea and menstrual dysfunction in up to 25% of premenopausal women. It may cause insomnia and agitation, and hence may be best prescribed as a single morning dose, especially for daily doses below 300 mg. Amisulpride is classified as an atypical, whereas sulpiride is classed as a typical antipsychotic.

Aripiprazole

Aripiprazole is novel in its mechanism of action – partial agonism at D_2 and 5-HT_{1A} receptors. The D_2 partial agonism means that it is able to act both as an agonist and as an antagonist at D_2 receptors. Its agonist activity (intrinsic activity, or ability to stimulate the receptors) is 25% (in contrast to pure antagonists such as haloperidol, which simply bind to the receptor, blocking the effect of dopamine, and which have zero intrinsic activity). Whether or not aripiprazole acts as an antagonist or as an agonist depends on the extracellular concentration of dopamine, as has been shown in *in vitro* studies (Burris *et al*, 2002). Hence, it is hypothesised that in areas where there is dopaminergic hyperactivity (the mesolimbic pathway, postulated to be associated with positive symptoms), aripiprazole may act as a dopamine antagonist, thus ameliorating symptoms, while in areas in which there is dopaminergic hypoactivity (the mesocortical pathway, postulated to be associated with negative symptoms), aripiprazole may act as a dopamine agonist, also ameliorating these symptoms. This hypothesis is currently being tested using *in vivo* imaging strategies.

Aripiprazole is not associated with EPS other than akathisia, nor elevation of prolactin levels (in fact there is a mean reduction in prolactin, which is *in vivo* evidence of the D_2 agonism; see Casey *et al*, 2003; Mir *et al*, 2006). It is also not associated with glucose dysregulation, and in most studies in adults is weight neutral. The mean half-life for aripiprazole is approximately 85 hours in extensive metabolisers of CYP2D6, and approximately 146 hours in poor metabolisers, which allows for once-daily administration. At a dose of 2 mg, it achieves 90% D_2 occupancy. Aripiprazole is extensively metabolised by the liver and its pharmacokinetics are not significantly affected by gender or smoking, but may be affected by age.

It is a 5-HT_{1A} partial agonist and an antagonist at the 5-HT_{2A} and D_3 receptors, with antagonism to a lesser degree at 5-HT_{2c}, α_1 and H_1 receptors. For the rest of aripiprazole's receptor profile, see Table 11.2. Side-effects such as headache, agitation, akathisia, anxiety, insomnia, dyspepsia and nausea or vomiting occur, especially within the first 3 weeks of therapy. The akathisia may be related to dopaminergic activation. In general, it is otherwise better tolerated than most other SGAs (Mir *et al*, 2006).

Sertindole

Sertindole is an indole derivative with a high affinity for 5-HT_2, D_2 and α_1 receptors. However, soon after its introduction there were reports of fatalities due to arrhythmias associated with a prolonged QT_c interval. In the UK, it can be used only if other drugs have failed, and must be obtained directly from the manufacturer and prescribed on a named-patient basis. Frequent ECGs and electrolyte monitoring are required; because of these risks and restrictions it is very little used.

Zotepine

Zotepine is an antagonist at 5-HT_{2A}, 5-HT_{2C}, D_2-like > D_1-like and H_1 receptors, and has some affinity for NMDA receptors. It is associated with a greater reduction in the seizure threshold than other antipsychotics. It may also prolong the QT_c interval and so ECGs are required before its commencement and at each dose increment. There should also be regular electrolyte monitoring and because of these strict guidelines and the frequency of recommended dosage administration (three times daily, the half-life being 14 hours) the drug is little used. Additional side-effects include insomnia, drowsiness, both hypo- and hyperthermia, blood dyscrasias and raised prolactin levels.

Ziprasidone

Ziprasidone is an indole derivative with a high affinity for 5-HT_2 and D_2-like ($D_2 > D_3 > D_4$) receptors and some affinity for α ($\alpha_1 > \alpha_2$) and H_1 receptors. It also exhibits 5-HT_{1A} antagonism and inhibits the reuptake of noradrenaline and serotonin, the latter effects meaning that it may be particularly useful for the treatment of comorbid depression. Prolongation of the QT_c led to its not obtaining a UK licence, although it is available in the USA, and there may be a further attempt at licensing it in the UK.

Long-acting depot preparations

The history of depot antipsychotic drugs has been described by Simpson (1984). In the early 1950s, the drug company Squibb (now Bristol-Myers Squibb) synthesised the first long-acting hormone preparation, testosterone propionate. In 1957 the company also synthesised fluphenazine, a phenothiazine antipsychotic with a relatively long half-life. Building on their earlier experience with long-acting testosterone, Squibb's researchers esterified the fluphenazine's alcohol side chain with a number of different fatty acids to delay its release into the circulation. Fluphenazine enanthate

(Moditen) was their first long-acting compound (esterified using heptanoic acid). The Squibb scientists soon found that increasing the length of the fatty acid side chain led to further increases in the drug's half-life, but that beyond ten carbon atoms there was no further advantage. Hence they produced fluphenazine decanoate (Modecate). Other manufacturers followed suit and added ten-carbon fatty acid side chains to their antipsychotics, producing flupentixol decanoate (Depixol), zuclopenthixol decanoate (Clopixol) and haloperidol decanoate (Haldol).

These esterified drugs are dissolved in an oil carrier. The choice of oil affects the oil/water partition coefficient, which is one of the factors that determine the speed of release from adipose tissue into the general circulation. Most manufacturers use sesame oil, while flupentixol decanoate and zuclopenthixol decanoate are dissolved in a proprietary low-viscosity trigylceride called Viscoleo, which appears to degrade more rapidly than sesame oil. Once injected, the esters slowly diffuse from the oil and are hydrolysed by esterases, so releasing the active drug. The diffusion of the drug from the oil into the surrounding tissue is the rate-limiting step. The oil is reabsorbed into the lymphatic system; initially this gave rise to fears of pulmonary microembolism, but this complication has not occurred with any significant frequency.

Moditen's successor, fluphenazine decanoate (Modecate), has played an important role in therapy and, until recently, fluphenazine decanoate and haloperidol decanoate were the only depot antipsychotics available in the USA.

The two most common problems with depot preparations are EPS and pain at the site of injection. Nodules, and occasionally abscesses, may also occur. Some patients develop fibrous tissue at injection sites, which may necessitate changing the route of administration. Another important problem is that the persistence of a steady-state drug level once it has been achieved means that a patient experiencing side-effects may do so for some time even after a dose reduction has been undertaken. Issues of patient dignity and autonomy should also be considered; depot preparations are not welcomed by many service users. There is little scientific literature on the relative merits and drawbacks of the various depot agents. Their relevant pharmacokinetic parameters are discussed, below. Most depots require approximately 3 months to attain steady-state levels. Until the arrival of the atypical depot risperidone (Risperdal Consta), flupentixol was by far the most commonly used depot in the UK.

Depot preparations should be given by deep intramuscular injection into the gluteal muscle, taking care to avoid the sciatic nerve. However, patients may find this demeaning, and hence administration into the deltoid muscle, where this is large enough to allow this, has been tried. If the patient has not had a particular depot before, then a test dose should be given (see BNF). Regular injections at the frequency recommended by the BNF can be started, providing the test dose is tolerated.

Fluphenazine decanoate (Modecate)

Fluphenazine is the only depot agent to produce a sharp, though transient, post-injection peak in blood levels, from 2 to 24 hours, which is sometimes associated with side-effects such as acute dystonia. Levels then fall to about one-third of peak levels, with a subsequent slow decline.

Flupentixol decanoate (Depixol)

This drug is a thioxanthene (see Table 11.1) analogue of fluphenazine. Thioxanthenes are different to phenothiazines in that they significantly block D_1 as well as D_2 dopamine receptors. Following a test injection (20 mg), the dose can be gradually titrated upwards until symptoms resolve. Relative to fluphenazine, flupentixol shows a slower rise to peak levels, and so immediate post-injection side-effects are less common. The maximum BNF permitted dose is 400 mg per week, which is 20 times the commonly administered dose of 40 mg per fortnight (i.e. there is a very wide therapeutic range). Depixol normally comes in ampoules of 20 mg/ml but the higher doses are administered as Depixol concentrate (100 mg/ml, or as 200 mg/ml, which is the low-volume version).

In the era before clozapine, high doses of depot preparations were sometimes the only option available for treatment-refractory schizophrenia, but this strategy is little used today. Standard-dose flupentixol is still used for maintenance treatment in the UK, more so than fluphenazine. (Oral flupentixol was previously used as an anxiolytic and antidepressant, but this practice is now rare, owing to the association with agitation and EPS, particularly at higher doses.)

Zuclopenithixol decanoate (Clopixol)

This variant of flupentixol with a chlorine atom in the central ring (see Fig. 11.4) has a reputation in clinical practice for being good for controlling aggression and agitation (especially as a more rapidly acting formulation called Clopixol Acuphase – see page 284). The test dose is 100 mg, the usual maintenance range is 200–400 mg fortnightly and the maximum dose is 600 mg weekly.

Haloperidol decanoate (Haldol)

This is said to be helpful in psychosis with aggression and has been used in the prophylaxis of mania. It has a slightly longer half-life (3 weeks) than the other depot agents, hence some patients can be maintained on injections given every 6–8 weeks. This is advantageous for patients who find an injection painful or demeaning. Its main drawback is EPS, but this may be countered using anticholinergics.

Pipotiazine palmitate (Piportil)

This drug may be given monthly (50 mg) and, as it is a piperidine phenothiazine, it causes less EPS than fluphenazine (a piperazine phenothiazine – see Table 11.3).

Risperidone (Risperdal Consta)

Among the atypicals, only risperidone is currently available as a long-acting preparation (Risperdal Consta). The drug is dispersed in a biodegradable polymer (patented Medisorb microspheres, which have a history of safe use in other extended-release pharmaceuticals, and medical applications such as sutures). Risperdal Consta is supplied as a powder, which must be stored in a refrigerator. However, it should be administered at room temperature, and hence removed from the refrigerator before it is required. It is mixed at the time of injection with a water-based diluent. After deep intramuscular injection (into the gluteal muscle), the polymer is hydrated; the drug diffuses out of the hydrated polymer, with the latter being metabolised to glycolic and lactic acids, releasing risperidone in a sustained manner. The acids are metabolised into carbon dioxide and water, which are of course readily eliminated. After a single injection, less than 1% of the drug is released during the first 3 weeks, with the maximum plasma concentration occurring at approximately 4–5 weeks after the injection. The manufacturer recommends fortnightly administration, with which steady-state levels are achieved after 8 weeks (i.e. four injections). It is therefore essential to co-treat with a therapeutic dose of an oral antipsychotic (ideally, oral risperidone, which should as indicated above be given prior to Risperdal Consta if the patient has not had risperidone before) for 3–8 weeks after the first injection. The test dose is 12.5 mg.

Trials with this formulation of risperidone have demonstrated sustained efficacy over 1 year with no significant difference in benefits or side-effects compared with the oral form (Chue *et al*, 2002). Further trials (e.g. regarding treatment adherence) are ongoing. It may have some advantage over depot preparations in the treatment of negative symptoms, and has been shown to be associated with an improved quality of life. A dose of 25 mg every 2 weeks is considered to offer an optimum risk/benefit profile for maintenance treatment (Kane *et al*, 2003). The pharmcokinetic profile means that it may not be given at a frequency of less than 2 weeks. If symptoms remain after 8 weeks of treatment, the dose may be increased by 12.5 mg, to 37.5 mg every 2 weeks. After two such injections have been given (i.e. after 4 weeks), the patient should be reassessed to see whether or not a further dose increment is required. The most troublesome side-effect is pain at the injection site, especially on administration. After clinical stabilisation for at least 3 months, the dose may be re-evaluated, as the dose required for maintenance of symptom control may be less than the initial starting dose.

Pharmacokinetics

Pharmacokinetics refers to the way the body handles a drug, that is its absorption, first-pass metabolism, plasma binding, and permeability across the blood–brain barrier, as well as the way the drug is eventually metabolised and excreted.

Most antipsychotics are relatively small, highly lipophilic molecules and so are generally well absorbed, with a high bioavailability (e.g. clozapine has a bioavailability of around 50–60%, chlorpromazine 10–40% and trifluoperazine 50–60%). In plasma, antipsychotics are largely protein bound (to albumin or other proteins such as α-1-glycoprotein), but it is the free drug that crosses the blood–brain barrier to reach the brain. CSF drug levels have not been extensively studied, but in the case of chlorpromazine the CSF level is 3–4% that of its plasma levels. However, brain concentrations can be twice as high as plasma concentrations because lipophilic drugs penetrate the blood–brain barrier more easily. The half-life of many antipsychotics permits once-daily dosing (see above). For most antipsychotics a range of plasma levels that is clearly associated with clinical efficacy is not well established, and so therapeutic drug monitoring is not routinely used. An exception is clozapine, for which monitoring is described on page 281.

Principles of antipsychotic drug metabolism

The metabolism of antipsychotics is clinically relevant (e.g. to drug–drug interactions). The lipophilicity of most of these drugs allows them to enter the brain with ease, but this same property makes their excretion difficult. Most must first be metabolised, transforming them into more polar inactive metabolites. This 'biotransformation' occurs throughout the body, most prominently in the liver and gut, and is generally accomplished in two phases.

Phase I reactions are oxidative reactions, such as dealkylation, *O*-dealkylation, hydroxylation, *N*-oxidation and deamination, which increases the polarity of the compound. These reactions are mediated by various enzyme systems, of which the cytochrome P450 (CYP) family is the most important. The CYPs are found in the liver and gut, as well as in other tissues, where they metabolise drugs, dietary constituents and toxins, as well as endogenous substrates such as steroids. The principal CYPs involved in antipsychotic metabolism are: CYP2D6, CYP3A4, CYP1A2 and CYP2C19. Drugs affecting these enzymes may therefore have clinically significant interactions with other drugs. Other phase I enzyme systems involved in antipsychotic metabolism include the flavin mono-oxygenases (FMOs). The mammalian FMOs were discovered in 1964 and are a group of xenobiotic-metabolising enzymes, encoded by the FMO gene family, including *FMOI* and *FMOIII* in man.

Phase II reactions involve conjugation of the phase I product, for example with gluthathione or acetate, to produce a more hydrophilic metabolite. Other reactions include glucuronidation by the enzymes of the family of uridine 5'-diphosphate glucuronosyltransferases (UGTs), and sulphonidation (by sulphotransferases).

Phase I and II metabolism varies considerably between individuals. This may be due to genetic factors, enzyme inhibition or enzyme induction. Drugs that inhibit an enzyme may reduce the metabolism of its substrate, leading to its accumulation in the plasma, with raised plasma levels and possibly an increased risk of side-effects or toxicity. A drug that induces the expression of the particular cytochrome that metabolises it will increase its own metabolism, and is hence termed an auto-inducer; carbamazepine is an example of such a drug. This effect is also seen with chlorpromazine, which means that plasma levels may be lower after some weeks than when the drug was commenced. Altered gastric motility or in some cases reduced absorption due to antacids may also be a factor in lowered plasma drug levels.

It is increasingly important to have an understanding of drug metabolism in order to understand drug–drug interactions (Appendix 1 of the BNF gives mainly major interactions). The possibility of an interaction does not necessarily mean that a clinically significant effect will occur (in fact in most instances it does not – see page 76), nor does it signify that the two drugs are absolutely contraindicated, but it does mean that when both drugs are prescribed the clinician should be aware of the possible increased risks of side-effects, toxicity or therapeutic resistance, and ensure that the patient makes as far as is possible an informed decision in the light of those risks.

Metabolism of the FGAs

Cytochromes CYP2D6, CYP3A4 and CYP1A2 play the major role in the metabolism of most FGAs, although CYP2C19 is also important for some. Numerous metabolites have been found for chlorpromazine, whereas haloperidol has a more clearly defined degradation pathway, including the oxidative *N*-dealkylation and reduction of the ketone group to form an active alcohol hydroxymetabolite, known as reduced haloperidol. This metabolite is less potent as an antipsychotic but may be more potent in inducing EPS (Bareggi *et al*, 1990; Lane *et al*, 1997). The transformation to reduced haloperidol is a reversible reaction, with CYP3A4 and CYP2D6 contributing to the conversion of reduced haloperidol back to haloperidol.

Some FGA metabolites are conjugated by UGTs 1A4 and 1A3 (e.g. in the case of chlorpromazine), whereas others remain unconjugated. Thioridazine is metabolised by CYP2D6 to mesoridazine, a metabolite with antipsychotic activity (von Bahr *et al*, 1991), and also to a cardiotoxic sulphoxide metabolite (sulphoridazine); moreover, thioridazine inhibits its own metabolism by CYP2D6. The BNF now contraindicates it for individuals with reduced CYP2D6 activity, or who are also taking other drugs that inhibit or are metabolised by CYP2D6. Chlorpromazine is metabolised by CYP2D6 to 7-hydroxychlorpromazine (Muralidharan *et al*, 1996), which is also clinically active. With regard to drug–drug interactions with the FGAs, chlorpromazine can potentiate sedative medications, such as antihistamines and hypnotics, and the hypotensive effects of antihypertensives. Jerling *et al* (1996) conducted a study on patients during continuous treatment, and CYP2D6 metaboliser status was shown to predict the oral clearance of perphenazine and zuclopenthixol (CYP2D6 poor metabolisers having a significantly lower clearance than extensive metabolisers – see under 'Pharmacogenetics' below).

However, in general, the metabolism of FGAs, including the contribution that their metabolites make to clinical effects, including side-effects, is relatively understudied.

Metabolism of the SGAs

The major active metabolite of clozapine is norclozapine, and the main enzyme responsible for this transformation is CYP1A2 (Aitchison *et al*, 2000*a*). Interestingly, this enzyme is sometimes deficient in individuals of Asian origin (e.g. Chinese) and blacks. However, other pathways may also be involved (Table 11.5). Olanzapine is metabolised mainly by UGT1A4, CYP1A2 and FMOIII. Risperidone is primarily metabolised by CYP2D6 to 9-hydroxyrisperidone, which has very similar pharmacodynamic properties to the parent compound. Quetiapine is metabolised by CYP3A4 to an inactive sulphoxide metabolite.

By knowing the major route of metabolism of medications that may be co-prescribed with antipsychotics, it is possible to predict which antipsychotics these will interact with (Table 11.5); for example, beta-blockers and codeine-related analgesics are metabolised mainly by CYP2D6, sodium valproate by CYP3A4 (and is an inhibitor of CYP3A4) and carbamazepine by CYP3A4 (and is a potent inducer of CYPs, especially CYP3A4). Carbamazepine may reduce serum haloperidol levels by 40–60%.

Pharmacokinetics of the long-acting depot preparations

The slow release of the active drug contained in depot preparations profoundly affects their pharmacokinetics and they differ from oral drugs in four key respects:

1 Because the drug is given intramuscularly, the first-pass effect (hepatic metabolism via the enterohepatic circulation) is avoided, giving them 100% bioavailability. This may lead to higher circulating levels of the parent drug (as opposed to its metabolites) relative to oral administration of the same drug.

2 For orally administered drugs, the rate-limiting step is metabolism, whereas for depot agents it is their rate of absorption. The absorption rate constant for depot drugs may be less than their elimination rate constant, which is termed a 'flip-flop' pharmacokinetic profile.

3 Drugs delivered as depot preparations take much longer to reach steady state after treatment is begun. They should not be used first line in an antipsychotic-naive individual, both for this reason and because, if the patient has not had the particular drug before, it is advisable to establish that he or she can tolerate it by oral administration first, unless an oral equivalent is not available (e.g. in the case of pipotiazine), in which case a small (test) dose of depot should be given on initiation of maintenance therapy.

4 In addition, their absorption and hence elimination are prolonged, so their effects persist for longer after treatment cessation (up to 3 months), which leads to the phenomenon that relapses may not occur for 3–6 months after drug cessation.

The pharmacokinetic parameters of depot preparations are shown in Table 11.6.

Pharmacogenetics

The term 'pharmacogenetics', coined by Vogel in 1959, refers to the study of the hereditary basis of individual variability in drug effects. Therapeutic doses of drugs are known to show marked inter-individual variation,

Table 11.5 Atypical antipsychotics, metabolising enzymes and drug interactions

Antipsychotic	Metabolising enzymes	Interactions
Clozapine	CYP1A2, CYP3A4 and, to a lesser extent, CYP2D6, CYP2C19, UGT1A4, UGT1A3	Cigarette smoking or caffeine ingestion induces CYP1A2 and may therefore reduce clozapine levels Fluvoxamine inhibits CYP1A2 and CYP2C19, leading to increased clozapine levels Inducers of CYP3A4 (e.g. phenobarbitone, carbamazepine, rifampicin and phenytoin) reduce clozapine levels Erythromycin inhibits CYP3A4 and ciprofloxacin inhibits CYP1A2, hence increasing clozapine levels
Risperidone	CYP2D6, CYP3A4	Clearance of parent drug decreased by CYP2D6 inhibitors (e.g. fluoxetine and paroxetine), but total parent + 9-hydroxyrisperidone level unchanged CYP3A4 inhibitors (e.g. erythromycin and nefazodone) may reduce clearance, but are not thought to produce clinically significant interactions Inducers of CYP3A4 (e.g. carbamazepine) may increase clearance of risperidone by up to 60%
Olanzapine	CYP1A2, CYP2D6, UGT1A4, FMOIII	A major metabolic pathway involves UGT and probenecid, a UGT inhibitor, therefore reduces olanzapine clearance Carbamazepine increases clearance Effects via CYP1A2 and CYP2D6 are similar to those in the case of clozapine
Quetiapine	CYP3A4	CYP3A4 inhibitors (e.g. ketoconazole, erythromycin, nefazodone, diltiazem) increase quetiapine levels CYP3A4 inducers (e.g. carbamazepine) increase clearance
Ziprasidone	Aldehyde oxidase, CYP3A4, CYP1A2	One-third of its clearance is by CYP3A4, aldehyde oxidase being the major metabolic route Clearance is therefore affected by CYP3A4 inducers and inhibitors Can prolong QT_c interval when co-administered with drugs that also prolong QT_c (e.g. anti-arrythmics); Aldehyde oxidase inhibitors (e.g. chlorpromazine, cimetidine and methadone) should be avoided, if possible, as reduced clearance can prolong QT_c interval
Amisulpride	Limited hepatic metabolism; renal clearance >50% in healthy people	Interactions with dopamine agonists, central nervous system depressants and antihypertensives, but these interactions are not based on hepatic enzymes
Aripiprazole	CYP2D6, CYP3A4	Metabolism to some extent affected by CYP3A4 inducers CYP2D6 inhibitors (such as fluoxetine and paroxetine) have the potential to increase plasma levels and so dose reductions of aripiprazole are recommended when the latter are co-administered

Table 11.6 Characteristics of depot antipsychotics

Preparation	Administration frequency	Time to peak plasma level	Approximate elimination half-life	Time to achieve steady-state
Fluphenazine decanoate	2–5 weeks	2–48 hours	6–10 days (single dose); 14–100 days (multiple doses)	6–12 weeks
Pipotiazine palmitate	4 weeks	9–10 days	14–21 days (multiple doses)	10–12 weeks
Flupentixol decanoate	2–4 weeks	4–10 days	8 days (single dose); 17 days (multiple doses)	10–12 weeks
Zuclopenthixol decanoate	1–4 weeks	4–9 days	17–21 days (multiple doses)	10–12 weeks
Haloperidol decanoate	4 weeks	3–9 days	18–21 days (single or multiple doses)	10–12 weeks

with some individuals failing to respond even to high doses, and others showing side-effects at doses well below the usual therapeutic range. There is also inter-ethnic variability (Aitchison *et al*, 2000*b*). In both inter-individual and inter-ethnic variabilities, genetic as well as dietary and other environmental factors play a role (Nebert, 1997).

Alternative forms of the same gene are called alleles. The allele that confers the 'normal' (i.e. most frequent) phenotype is designated the wild type (+). If both alleles in a gene pair are identical, the individual is homozygous for that locus; if they are different, the individual is heterozygous. Genetic variation, or polymorphism, can arise in a number of ways, including single-nucleotide changes, tandem sequence repeats, deletion of an entire coding sequence, and the addition of extra coding sequences.

Pharmacogenetics includes the study of genetic variation in both pharmacokinetic and pharmacodynamic factors. For a more detailed introductory review of pharmacogenetics as applied to psychiatry, see Basu *et al* (2004). An introduction to the role of the broader field of pharmacogenomics (including transcriptomics and proteomics) in psychiatry is given by Tsapakis *et al* (2005).

In this section we cover only some relevant pharmacokinetic genetic considerations. Although more than 40 P450 enzymes have been identified in humans, six of them conduct about 90% of human drug oxidation: CYP1A2, CYP3A4, CYP2C9, CYP2C19, CYP2D6 and CYP2E1. These enzymes are found in the smooth endoplasmic reticulum of hepatocytes. More than 50 alleles of *CYP2D6* (the gene encoding for cytochrome P450 CYP2D6 – the CYP genes are always italicised) have been described (http://www.imm.ki.se/CYPalleles), and these give rise to four main phenotypes:

1 ultrarapid metabolisers (UMs)

2 extensive metabolisers (EMs)

3 intermediate metabolisers (IMs)

4 poor metabolisers (PMs).

Inter-ethnic differences include a low percentage of PMs in Asians, but a relatively high percentage of IMs in Asians and Africans (Aitchison *et al*, 2000*b*).

Pharmacogenetic variation of a pharmacokinetic type is due to genetic variation in drug metabolising enzymes (DMEs). The major CYPs listed above are all encoded by autosomal genes, so a normal diploid individual has two copies of the gene. For example, in the case of *CYP2D6*, if both alleles have a mutation that leads to the absence of functional CYP2D6 enzyme (e.g. by the insertion of a premature stop codon), then the individual is a PM. Such an individual will be less able to metabolise drugs that would be metabolised by CYP2D6 in others, as they would have to rely instead on alternative (lower-efficiency) metabolic routes, and hence may be more vulnerable to side-effects. At the opposite end of this CYP2D6 metabolic spectrum, UMs have extra copies of an active sequence encoding CYP2D6, and hence synthesise more of the enzyme. It appears that in some cases, such individuals may require more CYP2D6-metabolised drug to achieve a therapeutic effect (Bertilsson *et al*, 1993). EMs have at least one functional allele, whereas IMs have more than one reduced allele.

Cytochrome CYP3A4 is encoded on chromosome 7. The genetic basis for inter-individual variation in 3A (CYP3A4 and CYP3A5) expression is only partially understood (Gellner *et al*, 2001). Cytochrome CYP1A2 is the main enzyme responsible for clozapine metabolism (Aitchison *et al*, 2000*a*) and is encoded on chromosome 15. Several allelic variants of *CYP1A2* have been identified, but these do not yet account adequately for the variability in phenotype seen. As with CYP3A, this may be partly due to the influence of other related genetic loci.

Drugs are not necessarily metabolised in a linear fashion. Phase I and II can occur independently of each other and some drugs may undergo solely phase II metabolism. Of the phase II enzymes, the UGTs are the most important and are abundant in the gastrointestinal tract and smooth endoplasmic reticulum of the liver. In this group of enzymes, subfamily 1A is particularly important in psychotropic drug metabolism. Genetic polymorphisms in UGT1A1 can present as congenital hyperbilirubinaemias, since bilirubin is also a substrate of this enzyme.

Adverse effects of antipsychotic drugs

Because the various antipsychotics seem to be of comparable efficacy (Geddes *et al*, 2000; Lieberman *et al*, 2005), their adverse effect profile is increasingly being used to determine which is most appropriate for a given patient. Although they are in general associated with a lower risk of EPS, some SGAs are associated with an increased risk of diabetes, weight gain and cardiovascular disease. Side-effects may be direct or indirect, and are modified by patient characteristics such as age, gender, ethnicity and comorbid physical illness. To some extent, the side-effects of a particular antipsychotic are determined by its receptor binding profile (see Tables 11.2 and 11.7).

Autonomic effects

Anticholinergic effects

Anticholinergic effects are particularly common with aliphatic phenothiazines (Table 11.1), and with other agents with significant M_1 affinity (e.g. olanzapine and

Table 11.7 Putative relationship between pharmacological blockade and adverse effects

Pharmacological effect	Adverse effect
D_2-like blockade	Parkinsonism, dystonia, akathisia, subjective cognitive side-effects, including emotional 'numbing' and reduced drive, hyperprolactinaemia, neuroleptic malignant syndrome, weight gain
Muscarinic (M_1) acetylcholinergic blockade	Dry mouth, constipation, blurred vision, urinary retention, tachycardia, impaired concentration
Cholinergic M_4 agonism	Hypersalivation
H_1 blockade	Sedation, weight gain
Noradrenaline α_1 blockade	Postural hypotension, transient initial sedation, ejaculatory problems
5-HT_{2C} blockade	Weight gain
Blocking cardiac potassium channels	Delayed cardiac repolarisation, prolonged QT_c interval, arrhythmias

Adapted from Cookson *et al* (2002).

clozapine – see Table 11.2). A dry mouth is usually combated by drinking more water, but if severe and accompanied by poor oral hygiene may increase the risk of dental caries and other oral infections. Severe reduction of gastrointestinal motility may result in pseudo-obstruction due to constipation, or paralytic ileus, which requires prompt assessment by a general medical or surgical team.

Sialhorrhoea (or hypersalivation) occurs in 31% of patients treated with clozapine; it develops early in the course of treatment (Safferman *et al*, 1991). The mechanism of this is unclear, as the physiology of saliva production and its regulation is complex, but it may include α_2 adrenergic effects and altered substance P concentration (Kaniucki *et al*, 1984) as well as muscarinic M_4 agonism. Hypersalivation is most pronounced during sleep. Patients should be advised to cover their pillow with a towel each night and, if the hypersalivation is severe, they should use more than one pillow, to reduce the risk of aspiration pneumonia. Although some tolerance appears to occur, the effect may persist even after years of treatment. It may cause such distress that the patient asks to discontinue clozapine.

A variety of drugs have been tried to treat this side-effect but there have been few trials. The most commonly used approaches are drugs with anticholinergic activity, including benzatropine, trihexyphenidyl hydrochloride (also known as benzhexol hydrochloride), hyoscine, atropine, pirenzepine, quetiapine and amitriptyline. Hyoscine hydrobromide may be given orally as 300 μg up to three times daily, or in the form of a hyoscine skin patch (both formulations being available over the counter in the UK). Atropine (0.5% or 1%) eye drops have been tried: one or two drops are mixed with a small volume of water, which the patient keeps next to the bed and sips as needed. However, the safety of this practice has *not* been established. Pirenzepine, a selective antimuscarinic drug, formerly used in the treatment of peptic ulcers, was produced by Boots Pharmaceuticals and tried for this indication, but is no longer marketed. Quetiapine has a moderate affinity for the M_1 receptor (see Table 11.2). A low dose of amitriptyline has also been used, but this is not to be recommended given the potential cardiotoxicity of both clozapine and amitriptyline.

The risk of giving any drug with anticholinergic activity is that the other anticholinergic side-effects of clozapine (as above) may be exacerbated. A number of the above possible different approaches may be tried before alleviation of this troublesome side-effect is achieved, possibly due to pharmacogenetic factors determining the patient's response.

Clonidine (a centrally acting antihypertensive agent via α_2 agonism) has been tried, as its use may be associated with a dry mouth in the early stages of treatment owing to increased vagal tone, but it is not to be recommended as the dry mouth effect tends to wear off, its sudden discontinuation may cause a rebound hypertension, and one of its potential adverse effects is depression. Lofexidine is also an α-adrenergic agonist, which acts centrally to reduce sympathetic tone, and has been tried for sialorrhoea, but again the authors would not recommend its use for this purpose, unless the sialorrhoea is accompanied by clozapine-induced hypertension and the patient will be reliably compliant with lofexidine.

Adrenergic effects

Orthostatic hypotension is one of the commonest side-effects of antipsychotics, secondary to antagonism of postsynaptic α_1 and α_2 adrenoreceptors leading to peripheral vasodilation. It is defined as a:

> 'postural decrease in blood pressure of at least 20 mmHg in systolic or 10 mmHg in diastolic BP, when rising from the supine to a standing position with a gap of at least 2 minutes between measurements after changing position, that is sustained for at least 3 minutes.' (Consensus Committee of the American Autonomic Society and the American Academy of Neurology, 1996)

These criteria differentiate autonomic failure from a sluggish baroreceptor response (seen in the elderly). Symptoms include light-headedness, clouding or narrowing of vision, nausea, sweating, pallor, weakness, fainting and falls (the last especially in the elderly). Concomitant use of certain other medications (e.g. antihypertensives, diuretics, antidepressants or insulin) or comorbid physical illness such as Parkinson's disease or diabetes mellitus can exacerbate this side-effect.

Antipsychotics associated with postural hypotension include chlorpromazine, thioridazine and, among the atypicals, clozapine, risperidone and quetiapine. The risk with ziprasidone and aripiprazole is low. A study of elderly patients on risperidone found a particularly high incidence (symptomatic orthostasis in 10%; Zarate *et al*, 1997), but the use of risperidone in the elderly is now restricted owing to the risk of cerebrovascular accidents (CVAs). The risk of hypotension can be minimised by lowering the starting dose and, once tolerance develops, titrating the dose according to clinical response. Should hypotension develop, a return to the previous effective tolerated dose is advocated. Patients should also be advised to avoid sudden postural changes, alcohol and straining during micturition or defaecation. Support stockings may sometimes be helpful.

In addition to orthostatic hypotension, postsynaptic adrenoreceptor blockade can also cause miosis, nasal congestion and sexual dysfunction (e.g. priapism and ejaculation difficulties). Urinary incontinence may occur with clozapine, and may be more frequent in women, particularly during the first 3 months of treatment, and worse at night. It is thought to be due to decreased bladder detrusor tone secondary to adrenergic blockade, and may be exacerbated by polydipsia secondary to a dry mouth. A fluid chart should be conducted before initiating treatment. Desmopressin may be tried in the tablet form (the nasal spray should be avoided as it may exacerbate nasal congestion), together with fluid restriction as required. Ephedrine nasal drops (used as a nasal decongestant) may help the urinary incontinence as well as the nasal congestion, but excessive or prolonged use should be avoided (excessive use results in tolerance, with diminished effect and rebound congestion).

Another important adrenergic side-effect involves the antagonism of presynaptic α_2 receptors, which leads to the release of noradrenaline, which activates postsynaptic α and β adrenoreceptors, causing vasoconstriction and tachycardia. Tachycardia is common in the initial stages of treatment with clozapine. The risk of this may be reduced by following a slow titration protocol; if it occurs despite this, it may be necessary to reduce the dose back down to the last dose at which tachycardia was not evident. If it persists, a beta-blocker may be tried, provided there are no contraindications to this.

Cardiovascular side-effects

Sudden death

Since the 1960s, antipsychotics have been associated with reports of sudden death, defined as death (excluding by suicide, homicide or accident) within the hour of the initial appearance of symptoms which is both unexpected in relation to the degree of disability before death and unexplained by clinical investigation or autopsy (Jusic & Lader, 1994). A major confounding factor is that psychiatric patients as a group have an excess mortality when compared with the general population.

In a study by Ray *et al* (2001) using the Medicaid database, patients who had been prescribed moderate doses of typical antipsychotics (more than 100 mg of thioridazine per day) had a 2.4-fold increase in sudden death compared with patients not receiving antipsychotic drugs. A case–control study by Reilly *et al* (2002) found unexplained death to be significantly associated with hypertension, ischaemic heart disease and the use of thioridazine, and it was this study that led to the restricted licence for thioridazine in the UK.

Sertindole was withdrawn from the UK market in December 1998 following concerns about serious cardiac events and sudden death. It was reintroduced in 2001 on a restricted basis. Clozapine has also been implicated in sudden death, with suggestions that these cases are associated with myocarditis or cardiomyopathy (both of which are known adverse effects of clozapine). In the case of other antipsychotics, it has been suggested that sudden death might be due to QT_c prolongation (see below).

Cerebrovascular accident (CVA) or 'stroke'

In March 2004, the Medicines and Healthcare Products Regulatory Agency (MHRA) issued a statement declaring that risperidone and olanzapine 'should not be used to treat behavioural problems in older patients with dementia', citing evidence that suggested that there was a threefold higher risk of stroke in this patient group if they took risperidone or olanzapine. The Committee on the Safety of Medicines (CSM) has advised that risperidone may be used to treat psychosis in the elderly, but that this be limited to short-term use under specialist advice. A similar warning about atypical antipsychotics and the risk of CVA in the elderly was issued by the US FDA. Both the MHRA and the FDA were careful to mention that they could not rule out the possibility that there may be a similar risk with other antipsychotics as well, but the trials had not been completed. However, a recent study (Wang *et al*, 2005) found that 'conventional antipsychotic medications were associated with a significantly higher adjusted risk of death than were atypical antipsychotic medications at all intervals studied'. Importantly, this finding was true whether in the presence or absence of dementia.

Prolongation of the QT_c interval

Most antipsychotics currently in use affect cardiac conduction. This action is quinidine-like, appearing to involve blockade of potassium and sodium channels in the cardiac cell membranes, causing a delay in ventricular repolarisation and hence lengthening of the QT_c interval.

The QT interval is measured from the beginning of the QRS complex to the end of the T wave. The interval shortens with increasing heart rate and correcting for this gives the QT_c. Various correction formulae have been proposed. The most commonly used is Bazett's formula:

$$QT_c = QT/\sqrt{RR}$$

where RR is the time in seconds between the two R waves. Most ECG machines now print out a value for the QT_c.

The QT_c interval tends to be longer in females than in males. It also increases in length with age, and may vary with the time of day at which it is measured (known as QT_c dispersion). It is affected by hereditary factors (e.g. long QT syndrome), antipsychotics and many other drugs (e.g. antihypertensives, antiarrhythmics and tricylic antidepressants). Prolongation of the QT_c can predispose some patients to a dangerous ventricular tachycardia known as *torsades de pointes*, where the mean electrical axis of the QRS complex appears to twist around the isoelectric line (Fig. 11.5). Correction of the underlying cause (e.g. stopping the offending drug, or correcting hypokalaemia) may terminate the *torsades de pointes*, or the arrhythmia may be self-limiting. The tachycardia is accompanied by symptoms such as palpitations, dizziness or syncope, and in a small proportion of cases if left untreated may progress to ventricular fibrillation and cardiac arrest. As might be expected, the overall risk is compounded by each additional risk factor.

QT_c intervals above 440 ms in men and 470 ms in women are considered critical and require action (e.g. a dosage reduction, change of drug or specialist opinion). Intervals above 500 ms require the drug to be stopped immediately, as this degree of prolongation is associated with a significantly increased risk of *torsades de pointes*.

Prolonged QT

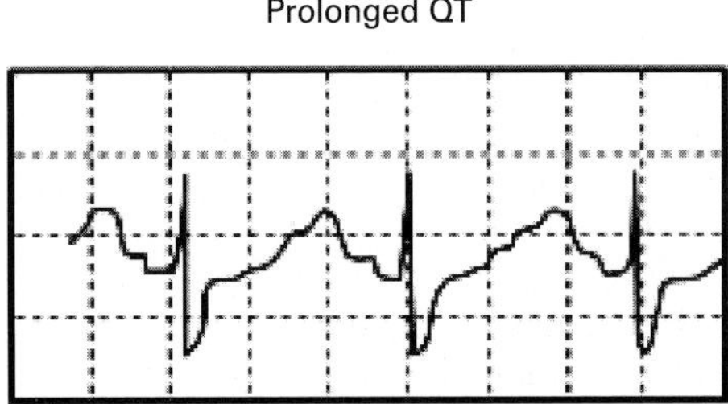

Torsades de pointes

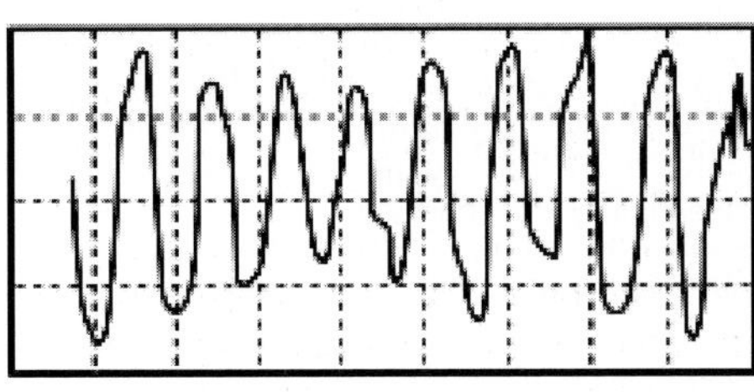

Fig. 11.5 Appearance of prolongation of the QT_c and *torsades de pointes* on the echocardiogram.

The physiological mechanism underlying the effect of antipsychotics on membrane stabilisation is not certain. Cardiac muscle cell repolarisation is initiated by the efflux of potassium ions. This efflux is the sum of two distinct potassium currents, one rapidly acting and the other slowly acting. Blockade of the rapidly acting current leads to QT_c prolongation, and *torsades de pointes*. Calcium channel blockade may reduce this risk. The different propensities of antipsychotics to cause QT_c prolongation reflect their differential effects on cardiac ion channels at therapeutic doses. Haloperidol, droperidol, thioridazine, pimozide and sertindole have all been shown to be high-affinity antagonists and hence potential blockers of the rapidly acting potassium current (Haddad & Anderson, 2002). Thioridazine is now contraindicated in patients with significant cardiovascular disease or known QT_c prolongation, or uncorrected hypokalaemia or hypomagnesaemia.

Box 11.2 gives an overview of the different causes of a long QT interval and Table 11.8 summarises the QT_c changes with different antipsychotics. Box 11.3 gives guidelines on managing the risk of the condition.

Other cardiovascular effects

Studies by Honigfeld *et al* (1998) and Killian *et al* (1999) reported a fivefold increase in myocarditis with the use of clozapine. It is thought to be due to a hypersensitivity reaction, as there is an eosinophilic infiltration of the myocardium. Other drugs such as quetiapine, chlorpromazine, fluphenazine, haloperidol and risperidone have also been associated with a degree of increased risk.

Box 11.2 Causes of long QT interval

Hereditary long QT syndromes

- At least six monogenic disorders have been identified, involving mutations in genes encoding myocardial ion channels

Acquired

- Antiarrhythmics: class Ia with class III properties; class III antiarrhythmics
- Severe bradycardia
- Electrolyte disturbance: hypokalaemia, hypomagnesaemia
- Psychotropics: antipsychotics, tricyclics and tetracyclic antidepressants
- Antimicrobials: tetracycline
- Antifungals: ketoconazole
- Recreational drugs: cocaine, alcohol
- Heart disease, e.g. myocarditis, ventricular tumour
- Endocrine disorders: hypothyroidism, hypoparathyroidism and other rare disorders
- Intracranial subarachnoid haemorrhage, CVA, head injury, encephalitis

Other causes that may be relevant

- Starvation or nutritional deficiency (e.g. in anorexia nervosa)
- Extremes of emotional and physical exertion, as might occur in a restraint procedure

Table 11.8 Propensity of different antipsychotics to prolong the QT_c interval

Antipsychotic	QT_c change	Comments
Chlorpromazine	+	
Thioridazine	+++	Use now restricted to second-line treatment and at lowest possible dose
Haloperidol	Not significant at low doses, ++ thereafter	No effect at doses of 2–5 mg; at higher doses significant QT_c prolongation can occur
Droperidol	+++	Withdrawn by manufacturer after reports of sudden death and known QT_c association
Flupentixol	Not significant	
Pimozide	++	Sudden death in overdose
Clozapine	+	Dose-dependent increase
Risperidone	+	Increase in overdose
Olanzapine	+	Cardiac arrhythmias in less than 2% of overdose cases
Sertindole	+++	>12 mg/day increases QT_c
Quetiapine	+	QT_c prolongation reported in overdose
Amisulpride	Not significant	Dose-dependent QT_c prolongation
Sulpiride	Not significant	Very rare cases of *torsades de pointes* reported
Zotepine	++	Prolongation of QT_c may be dose dependent
Aripiprazole	Not significant	Change in QT_c not significantly different between aripiprazole and placebo
Ziprasidone	++	Not seen with low doses, but concerns led to drug not being licensed in UK

+ = mild change; ++ = moderate elongation; +++ = pronounced elongation.

This condition should be suspected if patients complain of unexplained fatigue, fever, chest pain, palpitations or breathlessness. ECG abnormalities include ST-T wave changes and arrhythmias. Myocarditis usually starts in the first 6–8 weeks of treatment, while cardiomyopathy may occur later. Killian *et al* (1999) identified 15 cases of myocarditis and eight of cardiomyopathy in patients on clozapine, and estimated the rate of these more serious cardiovascular side-effects as 1 per 1300 cases. Six of the cases were fatal, making cardiotoxicity more of a hazard than agranulocytosis. Fatal pulmonary embolism is also described in association with clozapine, with a risk of 1 per 4500 cases.

If suspected, an ECG, chest X-ray and urgent cardiac referral are indicated and the antipsychotic should be discontinued immediately. Tachycardia on its own is common during the first month of clozapine treatment (and also occurs with other drugs, e.g. olanzapine) and should be monitored.

Box 11.3 Managing the risk of QT_c prolongation

1 Use the smallest effective dose, particularly if cardiovascular risk factors are present
2 Concomitant prescribing of other drugs that inhibit the metabolism of antipsychotics associated with QT_c prolongation should be avoided.
3 Check electrolytes regularly (especially potassium and magnesium)
4 For some drugs (e.g. thioridazine, sertindole or pimozide), baseline and serial ECGs are mandatory
5 ECG and electrolyte monitoring should be undertaken if symptoms and signs indicate cardiac arrhythmias. Elderly patients should have baseline ECGs done regardless of drug
6 Polypharmacy should be minimised
7 If using antipsychotics above BNF limits, follow Royal College guidelines, which include baseline ECGs and regular observations
8 In an emergency, if parental administration is required, use intramuscular rather than the intravenous route. Although intravenous administration was once common, there are very few situations where it is specifically indicated
9 Use benzodiazepines, for example in states of acute distress, whenever possible, as they are not cardiotoxic and have an antipsychotic dose-sparing effect

Metabolic side-effects

Diabetes and hyperlipidaemia

Long before the introduction of antipsychotics, there was evidence that individuals with schizophrenia were at an increased risk of metabolic disorders. Investigators in the early 1900s observed that patients with dementia praecox had higher than expected rates of abnormal glucose tolerance and this finding has been replicated several times (Kohen, 2004). Before the introduction of antipsychotics, individuals with schizophrenia had been shown to have an increased risk of developing impaired glucose tolerance, insulin resistance and type II diabetes mellitus, as well as of having a family history of diabetes. The association was shown to occur with established rather than first-onset schizophrenia, and was therefore thought to have been related at least partly to lifestyle – especially the physical inactivity – of many people with prominent negative symptoms. However, more recently, increased visceral fat deposits have been found in antipsychotic-naive first-onset and relapsing antipsychotic-free patients with schizophrenia (Thakore *et al*, 2002).

Schizophrenia is associated with an increased mortality rate (Brown *et al*, 2000) and at least 60% of this excess mortality is attributable to physical illness (Harris & Barraclough, 1998). The commonest cause of death in schizophrenia, as in the general population, is ischaemic heart disease (Herman *et al*, 1983; Newman & Bland, 1991).

Obesity (particularly visceral fat deposition), insulin resistance, hyperinsulinaemia, dyslipidaemia – hypertriglyceridaemia, decreased high-density lipoprotein (HDL) cholesterol and increased low-density lipoprotein (LDL) cholesterol – impaired glucose tolerance or type II diabetes, and hypertension are all commonly present in schizophrenia (Ryan & Thakore, 2002). A group of the above disorders comprise the 'metabolic syndrome', which has been variously defined in recent years, but the core criteria are abdominal obesity (as defined by waist:hip ratio), plus two out of the following four risk factors: elevated triglycerides, reduced HDL cholesterol, raised blood pressure and elevated fasting glucose (International Diabetes Federation, 2005, http://www.idf.org). The underlying causal mechanisms are not clear, though possibilities include increased activity of the hypothalamic–pituitary–adrenal (HPA) axis, alterations of levels of leptin (a satiety hormone), increased visceral fat deposition, inflammatory tissue modulators and low levels of adiponectin (a protein expressed solely in adipocytes and known to be associated with insulin resistance and dyslipidaemia). Other factors may also be involved in the genesis of the 'metabolic syndrome', as patients with schizophrenia have a higher consumption of dietary saturated fat than matched controls (Ryan *et al*, 2003) and also tend to have a higher rate of smoking (Weiser *et al*, 2004).

Although increased rates of diabetes were observed after the introduction of the phenothiazines, it was not recognised as a major clinical problem. Routine testing of blood and urine was rarely advocated. However, the rate of diabetes for patients with schizophrenia on phenothiazines rose from 4.2% in 1956 to 18% in 1968 (Schwarz & Munoz, 1968), and in 1993 the Association of the British Pharmaceutical Industry noted that perphenazine might affect the control of diabetes. Interestingly, this effect was not seen for haloperidol, and as haloperidol has in many ways a different receptor binding profile to the phenothiazines, this may shed some light on the molecular mechanisms underlying antipsychotic-induced diabetes.

The development of new-onset diabetes with treatment by some SGAs has only relatively recently been recognised as a significant problem. After the issue was highlighted, there were many reports of diabetes being either induced or exacerbated by SGAs (Liebzeit *et al*, 2001), particularly with clozapine and olanzapine, with insulin resistance and dyslipidaemia (e.g. elevated triglyceride levels) occurring with both (Melkersson *et al*, 1999, 2000; Henderson *et al*, 2000; Haddad, 2004). Risperidone and quetiapine have also been associated, but to a lesser degree (Melkersson & Dahl, 2004). Whether the association is stronger with SGAs than with FGAs (especially phenothiazines) remains a matter of debate, particularly as monitoring of patients on SGAs is greater in general than it is for patients on FGAs, and dietary and other risk factors may also have changed over the past 50 years.

Of concern are the series of cases that were reported of fatal ketoacidosis occurring among patients on atypicals: Torrey & Swalwell (2003) found reports of 25 deaths of patients on clozapine, of 23 on olanzapine and of 29 on quetiapine. At present there is no comparably large case series of fatal diabetic ketoacidosis reported in association with the FGAs.

A survey of 19 637 patients with schizophrenia drawn from the UK General Practice Research Database compared 451 new incident cases of diabetes with 2696 controls not on antipsychotics, and gave the odds ratios for the risk of diabetes compared with controls as 5.8 for olanzapine (significantly increased) and 2.2 for risperidone, where the increase was non-significant (Koro *et al*, 2002).

There is also an association between prolonged QT_c and altered glucose tolerance, insulin resistance and type II diabetes, as well as the issue of reduced compliance with antipsychotics in obese patients, which increases the risk of psychotic relapse (Olfson *et al*, 2000).

Antipsychotic use in schizophrenia may therefore exacerbate pre-existing or precipitate *de novo* diabetes. Risk factors for type II diabetes include: age over 60 years, family history of diabetes, weight gain (particularly central adiposity), ethnicity (e.g. African or Indian), smoking, lack of exercise, and other diabetogenic medications. These risk factors should be borne in mind when considering the use of agents that have a reported association with diabetes. A healthy lifestyle, including a low-sugar and low-fat diet and physical exercise, should always be advised in patients with schizophrenia on antipsychotics.

Weight gain

Weight gain has always been a problematic side-effect with antipsychotic drugs, both old and new. Allison *et al* (1999) reviewed the relative weight gains made on different antipsychotics and found clozapine to have the greatest effect, with an average of 4.45 kg increase in the first 10 weeks of treatment, followed by a plateau. Corresponding figures for the other antipsychotics were: olanzapine 4.15 kg; thioridazine 3.19 kg; sertindole 2.92 kg; chlorpromazine 2.58 kg; quetiapine 2.18 kg; risperidone 2.10 kg; haloperidol 1.08 kg; fluphenazine 0.43 kg; ziprasidone 0.04 kg; and 0.74 kg for the placebo group (aripiprazole was not included in this study).

Drugs with a relatively low tendency to induce weight gain include: amisulpride, aripiprazole, ziprasidone, haloperidol, fluphenazine and trifluoperazine; these should be considered when weight gain has proved to be a problematic side-effect (Allison *et al*, 1999; Ryan & Thakore, 2002).

Although body weight has been reported in many studies to be an independent risk factor for heart disease, body mass index (BMI) is now thought to be more informative, although the most informative risk factor is central (intra-abdominal) adiposity. For those who are underweight, for example due to poor diet associated with self-neglect, the weight gain may initially be beneficial, but it must be born in mind that individuals with the lowest baseline BMI (including adolescents) are at greatest risk of antipsychotic-induced weight gain (Beasley *et al*, 1997; Findling *et al*, 2005). The risk of weight gain is also greater in females. Fontaine *et al* (2001) estimated that the additional mortality through weight gain (estimated mean 10 kg) associated with taking clozapine for 10 years, with the associated impaired glucose tolerance and hypertension, would be almost equal to the number of suicides the drug could be said to have prevented over that period (through the reduction of suicide risk associated with clozapine treatment). Furthermore, the psychological consequences of weight gain are often very significant.

As with diabetes and dyslipidaemia, the mechanism of antipsychotic-induced weight gain is not well understood. A number of theories have been proposed, including altered regulation of satiety via 5-HT_{2C} and other receptors, histamine H_1 antagonism, dysregulation of hormonal systems (including leptin, adiponectin and prolactin), sedation, poor diet, smoking, and reduced energy expenditure. Reynolds *et al* (2003) reported an association between 5-HT_{2C} receptor polymorphism and antipsychotic-induced weight gain, and there has been some replication of this finding; pharmacogenetic studies in this area are ongoing.

Minimising weight gain, or losing weight once gained, is probably harder for patients with schizophrenia than for the general population, especially if they have negative symptoms or sedation as an additional adverse effect. The rate of weight gain is usually greatest in the first few months of treatment, although body weight may not plateau for 8–12 months (Hennen & Baldessarini, 2005). For a few patients, particularly those on medications associated with the highest risk of weight gain, the degree of weight gain may be extreme and life threatening.

The following interventions are commonly suggested for most patients:

1 Establish baseline weight, BMI and waist:hip ratio at treatment initiation. These indices should be monitored at least every 6 months.

2 Give advice regarding a healthy lifestyle, including regular exercise and a low-sugar, low-fat and high-fibre diet. It may be advisable to refer to an occupational therapist to assess ability to prepare appropriate meals safely.

3 If significant weight gain occurs, referral to a dietician and increasing physical activity (with cardiovascular monitoring as required) should be considered.

4 If there is a risk of non-compliance owing to weight gain, switching to an antipsychotic with a lower risk of inducing weight gain should be considered.

5 Metformin may be used to combat weight gain with diabetes. There are also some reports suggesting that orlistat, topiramate or sibutramine may be useful in combating antipsychotic-induced weight gain. Orlistat is a lipase inhibitor that reduces the absorption of dietary fat. It may be used together with a hypocalorific diet in individuals with a BMI of 30 kg/m^2, or 28 kg/m^2 if metabolic risk factors are present. It is most effective and best tolerated if taken as a single dose of 120 mg 1 hour before the main meal of the day (Aitchison *et al*, unpublished data), and should be continued beyond 6 months only if at least 10% of body weight has been lost since the start of treatment (National Institute for Clinical Excellence, 2001). Topiramate is an anticonvulsant that has weight loss as a side-effect. It should be used with caution in schizophrenia as it has a variety of cognitive side-effects. For sibutramine, psychiatric illness is actually a contraindication, hence the authors do not recommend its use.

Consensus statements on antipsychotic-induced obesity and diabetes

In November 2003 a joint consensus conference convened by four US professional organisations made a statement regarding the risk of diabetes and obesity

Table 11.9 US consensus statement on monitoring for diabetes with antipsychotic treatment

	Baseline	4 weeks	8 weeks	12 weeks	Annually	Every 5 years
Personal or family history	✓				✓	
Weight (BMI)	✓	✓	✓	✓ and quarterly thereafter		
Waist circumference	✓				✓	
Blood pressure	✓			✓	✓	
Fasting plasma glucose	✓			✓	✓	
Fasting lipid profile	✓			✓		✓

with antipsychotic drugs. The differential risks were addressed and a monitoring protocol was suggested, as shown in Table 11.9.

A UK expert consensus meeting was held in Dublin in October 2003. A summary of this meeting was published (Expert Group, 2004) which stated that the prevalence of diabetes and impaired glucose tolerance in schizophrenia could be estimated as 15–18% and 30% respectively, but noted that an increased risk of diabetes was also seen in other severe mental disorders, such as bipolar disorder. A fasting plasma glucose of greater than 6.1 mmol/l but less than 7.0 mmol/l defines fasting plasma glycaemia (impaired fasting glucose, or IFG); diabetes is diagnosable if the fasting glucose is greater than 7.0 mmol/l, or the random plasma glucose greater than 11.1 mmol/l. Where test results indicate impaired glucose tolerance or diabetes, the Expert Group recommended referral to either primary care (if the general practitioner has a good diabetes screening programme) or a diabetes specialist service for a definitive diagnosis and coordination of diabetes follow-up services.

None the less, the recommendations of the US consensus group and the recommendations made in other countries (e.g. Belgium) mean that psychiatrists practising in the UK should ensure that adequate monitoring is conducted by their service and/or primary care and/or a diabetes specialist service or, preferably, by primary care and diabetes specialist care in a shared-care protocol. The minimum acceptable standards for monitoring within psychiatry remain to be defined in the UK, but these may include the use of blood glucose monitoring or urine tests. In addition to the above indices, glycosylated haemoglobin (Hb_{A1c}) may be measured, which is useful for determining disease progression in diabetes (indicative of glycaemic control in the preceding 2 months). Early diagnosis and effective treatment may prevent or reduce the complications of type II diabetes (UK Prospective Diabetes Study Group, 1998). Asking relevant questions (e.g. regarding thirst, polyuria, nocturia, abdominal pain, or infections) in psychiatric follow-up may assist in early detection.

Hyperprolactinaemia

Prolactin is secreted by anterior pituitary lactotrophs. It is tonically inhibited by the action of dopamine in the tuberoinfundibular system on D_2 receptors present on the lactotrophs, and stimulated by thyrotrophin-releasing hormone (TRH), vasoactive intestinal polypeptide and serotonin (the last is particularly relevant to the increased secretion that occurs in stress or breast-feeding). Prolactin in turn inhibits TRH secretion, which may result in a secondary relative hypothalamic hypothyroidism. Prolactin secretion increases during sleep, being related to the *duration* of sleep, regardless of when it occurs during the 24-hour period.

The anterior pituitary is vascularised by a portal circulation connecting the median eminence of the hypothalamus, which is supplied directly from the internal carotid artery. Dopamine antagonists or agonists present in the systemic circulation may therefore reach the lactotrophs without crossing the blood–brain barrier. Antipsychotics with D_2 antagonist activity will rapidly induce hyperprolactinaemia directly in proportion to their potency of D_2 antagonism. Small doses of haloperidol (e.g. 0.5–1.5 mg) may increase prolactin secretion within 1–2 hours, with a return to baseline after 6 hours (Goff & Shader, 2003). Among the SGAs, risperidone, amisulpride and zotepine are the more potent D_2 antagonists and therefore have the highest risks of inducing hyperprolactinaemia. Clinically significant hyperprolactinaemia occurs with a D_2 occupancy of greater than 72% (Kapur *et al*, 2000) and hence using the above antipsychotics at the minimum effective dose for a given patient is advisable. High doses of olanzapine are also associated with elevated prolactin levels, while ziprasidone, clozapine and quetiapine are not usually associated with this side-effect. Aripiprazole is the only antipsychotic currently on the market that reduces a pre-existing elevated prolactin level (owing to its D_2 partial agonism).

Hyperprolactinaemia may be defined as plasma prolactin levels of greater than 20 ng/ml for men and greater than 25 ng/ml for women, or in international units above 480 mIU/l (Smith *et al*, 2002), but the reference range for the local laboratory should be consulted. The associated clinical adverse effects include the following (Halbreich *et al*, 2003):

1 *Sexual dysfunction*. In women, hyperprolactinaemia inhibits the normal pulsatile secretion of luteinising hormone (LH) and follicule-stimulating hormone (FSH) and the mid-cycle LH surge, resulting in anovulation. (Melanocyte-stimulating hormone and antidiuretic hormone secretion are also increased.) There is also inhibition of the positive feedback of oestrogen on gonadotrophin secretion and consequent reduction of oestrogen levels. The resultant gonadal dysfunction includes oligomenorrhoea or amenorrhoea, anovulation (resulting in infertility) and reduced vaginal lubrication. Hirsuitism may also occur. In men, the usual symptoms are of hypogonadism, with the initial symptom being reduced libido, with delayed or absent orgasm, impotence (including azoospermia) and reduced testostorone levels are later effects.

2 *Breast enlargement (gynaecomastia) and galactorrhoea*. These may occur in men and women (although

galactorrhoea is less common in men), and may be accompanied by breast pain and tenderness. With the FGAs, high rates of galactorrhoea have been reported.

3 *Osteoporosis*. Hyperprolactinaemia may be associated with a loss of up to 25% in trabecular bone density; hence, patients taking antipsychotics are at increased risk of osteoporosis (Howes *et al*, 2005). Patients on haloperidol have been found to have a 14% reduction in forearm bone mineral content compared with controls. Uncontrolled studies have found high rates of fractures among patients with chronic schizophrenia (up to 25%), but inadequate exercise, smoking and poor nutrition may be additional risk factors.

4 *Cardiovascular effects*. Oestrogens are protective against atherosclerosis, and hence low oestrogen levels in association with hyperprolactinaemia may increase cardiovascular risk.

5 *Breast cancer*. It has been suggested that hyperprolactinaemia is an independent risk factor for breast cancer because this has been demonstrated in laboratory animal studies. There is evidence of an increased risk of breast cancer in psychiatric patients; however, the relative magnitude of the contribution of other factors (such as smoking and diet) is not clear. The primary care service should therefore be informed of the need to conduct increased screening for breast cancer, especially in postmenopausal women who have been on long-term antipsychotics.

Other symptoms of hyperprolactinaemia include weight gain, fluid retention, irritability, anxiety and depression. The last may be partly due to a relative hypothyroidism.

Hyperprolactinaemia does not require immediate action. However, in patients who may need to take medication over the long term, using a drug that does not elevate prolactin or even reduces prolactin in antipsychotic-induced hyperprolactinaemia should be the first approach to this problem. The use of dopamine agonists such as bromocriptine or cabergoline may be considered with great caution as a short-term treatment of severe hyperprolactinaemia. Bromocriptine is frequently associated with vomiting, but the newer drug cabergoline has fewer side-effects, and is increasingly being used in other settings (e.g. in obstetrics, to suppress lactation by lowering prolactin) and there are reports of its successful use in psychiatric patients as well. However, both drugs may be associated not only with exacerbation of psychosis, but also with pulmonary, retroperitoneal and pericardial fibrotic reactions, and hence it is advisable to measure serum creatinine levels and the erythrocyte sedimentation rate, and to perform chest radiography before treatment is begun, and while the patient is on treatment, to monitor for dyspnoea, persistent cough, chest pain, cardiac failure and abdominal pain or tenderness.

Cavallaro *et al* (2002) reported a successful decrease of prolactin levels to normal values in 11 out of 19 patients with risperidone-induced hyperprolactinaemia. Doses of cabergoline were low (0.125 mg): the usual starting dose for cabergoline for the treatment of hyperprolactinaemia given in the BNF is 0.5 mg daily. At the low dose, exacerbation of psychotic symptoms did not occur.

Other endocrine effects

Haloperidol and perphenazine have both been reported to produce a toxic state resembling a thyroid storm or neuroleptic malignant syndrome (NMS) when administered to patients with thyrotoxicosis. These drugs should therefore be used with caution among patients who are both psychotic and thyrotoxic. In pre-marketing trials, quetiapine was found to elevate TSH levels, but it does not appear to cause clinical thyroid dysfunction. Case reports of the syndrome of inappropriate ADH secretion have been described in association with fluphenazine and trifluoperazine, but they resolved when the drug was discontinued (Goff & Shader, 2003); this syndrome may be secondary to hyperprolactinaemia (see above), and is discussed in Chapter 4 on page 81.

Hepatic side-effects

Chlorpromazine, clozapine and olanzapine may be associated with elevated liver enzyme levels (up to three times the normal upper limit), especially in the first month of exposure. In most patients, the elevated results on liver function tests are transient and asymptomatic, and hence do not require dosage adjustments or discontinuation of the medication. In contrast, about 1–2% of patients treated with chlorpromazine develop cholestatic hepatitis, within 1–5 weeks of starting the drug. This appears to be a hypersensitivity reaction associated with eosinophilia, fever and rash. If this occurs, the antipsychotic should be discontinued, after which liver function usually returns to normal within 8 weeks. Rarely, jaundice may progress to a syndrome resembling primary biliary cirrhosis, although the prognosis for the drug-induced condition is better than for the idiopathic disorder. Switching to another antipsychotic (e.g. haloperidol, which is associated with a relatively low rate of hepatoxicity – 0.2%) is not usually associated with recurrence, and cross-sensitivity between phenothiazines for this particular adverse reaction is rare. For patients with pre-existing hepatic impairment, it is better to choose a drug that is mainly renally excreted (e.g. amisulpride).

Dermatological side-effects

Both allergic and photosensitive drug rashes are described, particularly in association with chlorpromazine and other phenothiazines. Allergic skin rashes occur in 5–10% of those on chlorpromazine. These tend to develop suddenly within 2–10 weeks of starting the drug, and present as an erythematous maculopapular eruption. Occasionally, severe reactions such as exfoliative dermatitis, generalised urticaria and angioneurotic oedema may occur.

An allergic rash is an indication for switching antipsychotic and offering symptomatic treatment (e.g. an oral antihistamine or a topical corticosteroid). Allergic skin rashes are very rare with the atypical drugs.

Seborrhoeic dermatitis has also been described in chronic schizophrenia, particularly in association with antipsychotic-induced parkinsonism. It presents as erythematous plaques with yellow scales; it may require antifungals and topical steroids as well as a dermatological opinion.

Photosensitivity is another problem that has mainly been associated with chlorpromazine and other phenothiazines. This presents as 'sunburn' in exposed areas (with the apparent 'sunburn' occurring at levels and lengths of exposure that would not have caused 'sunburn' if the patient were not on the drug). It is caused by a combination of phototoxicity (chemical injury hypothesised to be due to a reaction that releases free radicals) and photoallergy to UVA light. Patients on chlorpromazine and other phenothiazines should therefore be advised to use an appropriate protective suntan lotion and to avoid prolonged exposure to bright sunshine. Photosensitivity may also occur with the atypicals (e.g. olanzapine).

Long-term exposure to chlorpromazine may also lead to the development of a blue-grey or brown pigmentation in exposed areas, especially in women. This may be associated with generalised pigmentary deposition that may also affect the internal organs, and with a distressing black galactorrhoea.

Kimyai-Asadi *et al* (1999) list other case reports of skin reactions due to antipsychotics and these include:

- for phenothiazines, lupus erythematosus, lichenoid reactions, pigmentary disorders, phototoxicity and seborrhoeic dermatitis
- for fluphenazine, hypopigmentation
- for haloperidol, alopecia and other pigmentary disorders
- for zotepine, alopecia areata.

Ocular side-effects

Impairment of accommodation is a common side-effect of antipsychotics with an anticholinergic profile. Such drugs are contraindicated in closed-angle glaucoma. Long-term use of phenothiazines may be associated with lenticular and corneal deposits related to the dose or total drug intake; these deposits are sometimes associated with generalised pigmentary deposition. If detected early, these appear to be reversible. Pigmentary retinopathy and corneal opacities may occur with chronic administration of chlorpromazine and other phenothiazines, particularly at high doses; as these may impair vision, they are a serious ocular adverse reaction, and hence patients on high doses should have an ophthalmological examination every 6 months.

Haematological side-effects

Neutropenia, thrombocytopenia, agranulocytosis and thrombocytopenic purpura have all been described with antipsychotics. In most cases, the mechanism appears to be either idiosyncratic or allergic, but in some it seems to have been dose dependent (toxic reactions). Haemolytic anaemia is also a rare adverse effect.

Neutropenia and agranulocytosis with clozapine

Agranulocytosis is the most severe adverse reaction to clozapine. However, the risk of neutropenia or agranulocytosis declines over time; 75% of cases of neutropenia or agranulocytosis occur within the first 18 weeks of treatment, with the risk of agranulocytosis being 0.7% in the first year, and fatal in 0.03% of cases; 0.07% of cases occur in the second year of treatment (Atkin *et al*, 1996). Similar rates have been reported from the USA. Agranulocytosis is defined as a granulocyte (neutrophil, basophil and eosinophil) count of less than 500 per mm^3, neutropenia as a neutrophil count of less than 1500 per mm^3 but more than 500 per mm^3, and leucopenia as a white cell count of less than 3500 per mm^3 with granulocytes above 1500 per mm^3. Symptoms include lethargy, weakness, fever and sore throat. Routine monitoring of white cell count (as part of a full blood count with white cell differential) is therefore mandatory in the UK. Clozapine should not be initiated if the white cell count is less than 3500 per mm^3 or the granulocyte count is less than 2000 per mm^3, or if the patient has a history of a myeloproliferative disorder, drug-induced agranulocytosis or granulocytopenia. Lithium may be associated with neutrophilia (i.e. a raised neutrophil count) and has been reported to reverse clozapine-induced neutropenia. However, lithium does not protect against agranulocytosis (Taylor *et al*, 2005).

Following eight deaths associated with clozapine in Finland in 1975, the drug was withdrawn from many countries, and strict haematological monitoring was a requirement of its reintroduction. Regular monitoring of the white cell count may greatly reduce the incidence of haematological adverse effects. Conversely, being female, increasing age and coadministration of other myelosuppressive drugs (e.g. carbamazepine) may increase the risk. A low baseline white cell count is associated with an increased risk of neutropenia but not agranulocytosis. It is important to note that an asymptomatic low white cell count, a condition known as benign ethnic neutropenia, is found in some ethnic groups (e.g. Africans and Caribbeans), in which a lower baseline white cell count and apparent treatment-emergent neutropenia may in fact be due to white cell margination; the rate of agranulocytosis is not elevated. Ashkenazi Jews are also at increased risk of neutropenia and agranulocytosis (Lieberman *et al*, 1990). The pathophysiological mechanism of agranulocytosis remains to be fully elucidated, but some of the facts and hypotheses proposed are outlined below:

- It is not a dose-dependent phenomenon and some cases have occurred after years of use.
- It may be due to a direct toxic effect on neutrophils or their haemopoietic precursors. At high concentrations, clozapine has a toxic effect on both myeloid and erythroid precursors (Gerson *et al*, 1994). The desmethylclozapine:clozapine ratio has been seen to be inversely correlated with neutrophil count in patients treated with clozapine (Mauri *et al*, 1998).
- It may involve the metabolic activation of clozapine, resulting in the formation of free radicals, which are then able to bind covalently to neutrophil or bone marrow proteins. This is then postulated to result in agranulocytosis, either by an effect on the bone marrow or by a similar mechanism to the blood dyscrasias that result from covalent binding of acetaminophen in the liver (Pumford *et al*, 1997).

- The reaction may have an immunological basis with a genetic predisposition (reviewed by Aitchison *et al*, 2000a). Many drug sensitivities are immunologically determined, and preliminary data from a genetic study on clozapine-induced agranulocytosis include genetic associations with three of the human leucocyte antigen (HLA) complex genes (Malhotra *et al*, 2005).
- The reaction may be due to some of the chemically reactive metabolites of clozapine (rather than clozapine itself) formed by neutrophil myeloperoxidase (Gardner *et al*, 1998) or by the various cytochrome P450 enzymes (Pirmohamed *et al*, 1995). Cytochrome P450 isoforms appear to be expressed in neutrophils and bone marrow stem cells (Gonzalez *et al*, 1992) as well as in the liver. There are also studies in progress that aim to identify changes in gene expression that may be associated with agranulocytosis.

A self-remitting mild neutropenia is not uncommon with clozapine therapy; a brief withdrawal of the drug restores the full blood count to normal. If the neutrophil count drops below 1500 per mm^3 (recorded as a 'red' in the UK Clozaril Patient Monitoring System), clozapine must be withdrawn. A haematological opinion should be sought, clozapine and all other myelosuppressive drugs should be stopped, and any infection should be treated vigorously. It has been reported that the use of filgastrim (a haemopoietic growth factor which stimulates granulocyte colonies), or a granulocyte macrophage colony stimulating factor, may reduce the duration of clozapine-induced agranulocytosis by 50%.

After agranulocytosis, clozapine must not be restarted, because the agranulocytosis is likely to recur. Chlorpromazine was previously rarely reported to have an association with fatal leucopenia, but this adverse reaction is now seldom reported (probably because of a combination of better routine monitoring of patients on antipsychotics and a reduced rate of usage of the drug).

Sedation

This is a common side-effect in the initial stages of antipsychotic treatment, and can be useful if the patient is agitated. A rather more unpleasant combination of sedation, drowsiness and an emotional detachment, known as torpor or 'ataraxy', is also sometimes seen. In this state the individual is calm and relatively uninterested in the environment, and patients taking antipsychotics may have a decreased emotional responsiveness (or 'emotional numbing' – Yusufi *et al*, 2005), a feature that may be advantageous in the treatment of an acute paranoid psychosis, but which with chronic treatment may be undesirable. The sedation is partly due to H_1 antagonism, and is greater for the low-potency drugs such as chlorpromazine, including the phenothiazine depot preparations. Clozapine, olanzapine and quetiapine are the most sedative atypicals. The effect is dose dependent and so dosage reduction is helpful, as is administering either the whole dose or the greater part of the dose at night.

The electroencephalogram and seizures

Antipsychotics cause decreased alpha and increased theta and delta activity on the electroencephalogram (EEG). Fast beta activity may be evident but with chronic treatment synchronisation occurs, together with increasing slow-wave activity and amplitude, with superimposed spikes and sharp waves.

Paroxysmal discharge patterns similar to those found in seizure disorders may emerge. Some antipsychotics lower the seizure threshold. The risk of seizures is increased in those with a history of epilepsy, or previous drug-induced fits, head trauma or other cerebral pathology. The evidence suggests the risk is greatest with clozapine and chlorpromazine, intermediate with trifluoperazine and thioridazine, and lowest with pimozide, haloperidol, sulpiride and fluphenazine. This adverse effect is dose dependent and so polypharmacy, high doses and rapid dose escalation should all be avoided whenever possible.

Seizures are not an absolute contraindication to continued antipsychotic treatment: an anticonvulsant (e.g. sodium valproate) may be added and, if appropriate, a gradual switch to an antipsychotic with less potential to lower the seizure threshold may be initiated. Epileptiform EEG abnormalities are more common with clozapine and are dose related, the frequency of seizures at doses below 300 mg/day, between 300 and 600 mg/day and above 600 mg/day being 1%, 2.7% and 4.4%, respectively; patients on clozapine for about 4 years have a 10% risk of developing seizures (Devinsky *et al*, 1991).

Neuroleptic malignant syndrome (NMS)

This is an uncommon adverse effect of antipsychotics, but is potentially life threatening. It is characterised by the sudden development of altered conscious level, fever, rigidity and autonomic instability. The plasma creatinine phosphokinase (CPK, also shortened as CK) level is usually raised. Diagnosis can be missed in atypical or milder forms of the disorder.

Although the condition is rare, for psychiatric inpatients estimates of the annual incidence vary from 0.2% to 3.23%. The range reported may reflect differing diagnostic criteria used in different studies, and possibly varying rates of undetected concurrent physical illness. Although the condition is included in DSM–IV (see Box 11.4), its nosological status is at present uncertain, and it is included only in an appendix (American Psychiatric Association, 1994).

Cases typically start in the first 2 weeks of exposure to a drug, but may occur at any time. The earliest symptom is usually alteration in level of consciousness, which may be confused with neuroleptic-induced sedation. Autonomic instability may include tachycardia, diaphoresis, hypersalivation and incontinence, with labile blood pressure (including hypertension) being a particularly important sign. Parkinsonism unresponsive to anticholinergics is also a sign of NMS, although it is said not to occur among cases associated with atypical antipsychotics. Occasionally opisthotonos, myoclonus, dysphagia or dysarthria may be features. Fever is almost always present and, in a minority, hyperpyrexia (temperature greater than 41°C) may occur. This is associated with a high mortality, as are complications of severe rigidity leading to myoglobinuria and renal failure.

Box 11.4 The DSM–IV criteria for neuroleptic malignant syndrome

A Severe muscle rigidity and elevated temperature associated with neuroleptic medication
B Two or more of the following:
- Diaphoresis tachycardia
- Dysphagia
- Elevated or labile blood pressure
- Tremor
- Leucocytosis
- Incontinence
- Mutism
- Laboratory evidence of muscle injury (elevated CPK level)
- Change in level of consciousness

C Symptoms in groups A and B not due to another substance, neurological or other general medical condition
D Symptoms in groups A and B are not accounted for by a mental disorder (catatonia)

Making the diagnosis of NMS

The key to making a diagnosis of NMS is to retain a high index of suspicion. Daily temperature recording for in-patients is no longer routine in the UK, so a mild fever may go unnoticed unless reported by the patient and, as this and other presenting symptoms are non-specific, in its early phases NMS is frequently missed. However, once the condition has been identified as a possibility, confirming the diagnosis may be relatively straightforward.

Patients on antipsychotics who develop fever should be thoroughly investigated for foci of infection (including chest radiography, white cell count, mid-stream urine sample, etc.) and consideration should be given to stopping the antipsychotic while waiting for the results. Emergence of EPS or dramatic worsening of EPS with fever should trigger prompt further investigations for NMS, including muscle CPK level, which is elevated (may exceed 1000 IU/l, normal being up to 200 IU/l). Intramuscular injections, muscle injury and strenuous exercise may all elevate CPK levels (but in general not above 600 IU/l). Some laboratories unfortunately do not distinguish between the cardiac and muscle CPK isoenzymes. An elevated white cell count is also commonly seen. Lactate dehydrogenase, alkaline phosphatase and transaminases may also be raised and an electrolyte imbalance (hypo- or hypernatraemia) with metabolic acidosis may occur in severe cases. Myoglobinuria due to muscle breakdown may be revealed by dark urine that does not contain red blood cells.

The differential diagnosis of NMS includes:

- malignant hyperthermia (a hypermetabolic state of skeletal muscle associated with anaesthetic agents)
- 'malignant catatonia'
- EPS with intercurrent infection and fever
- heat exhaustion
- atropinism due to anticholinergic overload
- a serotonergic crisis
- thyrotoxicosis
- phaeochromocytoma.

'Malignant catatonia' is difficult to distinguish from NMS, but is characterised by catatonic psychotic excitement followed by other features of NMS occurring in the absence of antipsychotic treatment (see below). Antipsychotics with high D_2 antagonism should be avoided in catatonia, now a relatively rare clinical syndrome.

The pathophysiology of NMS is not wholly understood (Adnet *et al*, 2000). It may involve several neurotransmitter systems, but the primary neurotransmitter mechanism appears to be a sudden increase in central (particularly hypothalamic) dopamine blockade, including in extrapyramidal dopamine regions, with consequent muscle rigidity. Other theories hypothesise that there may be a primary defect in skeletal muscle similar to that seen in malignant hyperthermia; there are a few case reports comparing malignant hyperthermia to NMS, but the muscle biopsy features in NMS do not include the changes characteristically seen in malignant hyperthermia. Gurrera (2002), in a comprehensive review of both disorders, comments on their clinical similarities as well as their differences, and suggests that NMS may belong to a spectrum of disorders caused by inherited defects of intracellular calcium regulation. It may also be that the pathology in skeletal muscle is caused directly by the toxic effects of neuroleptics.

However, the fact that NMS may occur after months or years of treatment with a given antipsychotic may point to a more complex underlying mechanism. It has been reported in association with all antipsychotic drugs, both typicals and atypicals, and prevalence data on each drug are much too sparse to see whether it is more associated with one drug than with another. Taylor & Fink (2003) consider NMS to be a drug-induced variant of malignant catatonia (see above). Malignant catatonia (sometimes a fatal condition, also called lethal catatonia) was well described in the pre-neuroleptic era, indicating that such states may occur as part of dopamine dysregulation related to illness, perhaps only being exacerbated by antipsychotic drugs. NMS is not specific to schizophrenia, cases having been reported with antipsychotic treatment in dementia, Parkinson's disease, Wilson's disease, Huntington's disease and striatonigral degeneration. Risk factors include:

- the use of dopamine-depleting agents
- the abrupt withdrawal of dopamine agonists
- dehydration
- an intramuscular route of administration of antipsychotic
- rapid dose escalation
- the use of physical restraint
- poorly controlled EPS
- alcoholism
- clinical catatonia
- the withdrawal of anti-Parkinsonian medication
- iron deficiency anaemia.

Table 11.10 Atypical antipsychotics and EPS

	Acute EPS	Tardive dyskinesia (TD)	NMS	Akathisia
Clozapine	Very low	Alleviates TD	Very low	Moderate
Quetiapine	Very low	Very low	Very low	Low to moderate
Olanzapine	Low	Low	Low	Low
Ziprasidone	Low	Unknown	Unknown	Moderate
Risperidone	Low to moderate[a]	Low	Low	Low to moderate
Aripiprazole	Low (27% versus 56% for haloperidol)	Uncommon	Rare cases	Common (10% in first few weeks)

[a] Dose dependent, lower doses (< 6 mg/day) being associated with lower risk.

It is possible that the common underlying mechanism is a rapid change in synaptic dopamine availability (e.g. high D_2 antagonism in a state of high synaptic dopamine concentration in acute psychosis).

Management of NMS

Emergence of EPS or dramatic worsening of EPS with fever should prompt investigations for possible NMS. If CPK is elevated, or the patient's condition deteriorates, the antipsychotic should be discontinued. It may also be prudent to discontinue anticholinergics, as these can contribute to increased confusion and to pyrexia by impairment of sweating. All other non-essential medications, especially those with significant anticholinergic activity (e.g. tricyclic antidepressants), should also be stopped. Benzodiazepines may be used as required. Dehydration should be corrected by intravenous infusion if necessary; prompt assessment by a medical team and transfer to a medical ward should be arranged for all but the milder cases. Milder cases include those in which cardiovascular function is not impaired, renal function is normal and the patient is responsive to supportive measures, including antipyretics.

Severe patients will need medical intensive care. Dopamine agonists (e.g. bromocriptine, amantadine, apomorphine, and levodopa with carbidopa) have been tried, with varying results. Dantrolene sodium, a skeletal muscle relaxant, is used in both malignant hyperthermia and NMS. Any associated conditions (e.g. iron deficiency) should also be treated. The psychosis should be conservatively managed and if intervention for this is necessary it should be confined to benzodiazepines and electroconvulsive therapy (ECT). On recovery, it is advisable to switch to an antipsychotic with a lower degree of D_2 antagonism. Gurrera (2002) estimated that a prior episode of NMS increases the risk of recurrence of NMS by a factor of 30. Whichever antipsychotic is chosen, it must be introduced slowly and at a low dose, to reduce the likelihood of a further episode of NMS.

Temperature dysregulation

Antipsychotics can cause a disturbance of thermo-regulation. Benign hyperthermia with temperatures of up to 38^0 C may occur in approximately 5% of patients, and is particularly common in the first few weeks of treatment with clozapine. However, it is essential to exclude neutropenia or agranulocytosis, myocarditis, NMS and infection in the absence of myelo-suppression. In conditions of high ambient temperature and humidity, there is also a risk of heat stroke, which may be further compounded by anticholinergic drugs.

Hypothermia is also a risk with antipsychotics, particularly chlorpromazine. When this drug was more commonly used, patients occasionally died of hypo-thermia in conditions of low ambient temperature.

Box 11.5 The main types of EPS

Acute

These develop within hours to days of exposure, and include the following:

- acute dystonia
- drug-induced parkinsonism (DIP)
- acute akathisia
- acute dyskinesia

Chronic

These develop after months or years of exposure, and include the following:

- tardive dyskinesia
- tardive dystonia
- tardive akathisia

Extrapyramidal side-effects (EPS)

EPS were the most important and 'treatment limiting' side-effects of the FGAs. These side-effects are less frequent with the atypicals, but they still occur (Table 11.10). Among the atypicals, relatively high rates occur with amisulpride, and with risperidone at doses above 6 mg/day. Aripiprazole is associated with akathisia, especially in the first few weeks of treatment, although this may be due to dopaminergic stimulation as opposed to extrastriatal dopamine blockade. The risk of EPS for olanzapine (17 mg/daily) was found to be lower than for risperidone (7 mg) in a double-blind comparison (Tran *et al*, 1998). Higher doses of olanzapine also appear to be associated with increased risk. The risk is lowest for clozapine, which is likely to be due to its low D_2 occupancy, high 5-HT_{2A} blockade and M_1 antagonism (see Table 11.3). Quetiapine, sertindole and zotepine also have a low potential to produce EPS.

The main types of EPS may be classified as shown in Box 11.5.

Acute dystonia

Dystonias are involuntary movements characterised by spastic contraction of discrete muscle groups, in any region of the body.

They have been classified as follows:

- *Focal*. A single body part is affected, as in torticollis.
- *Segmental*. Two or more body parts with the same root innervation are involved.
- *Generalised*. Most of the body is affected.

The head and neck muscles are the most commonly affected, with syndromes including torticollis, laryngospasm, oculogyric crisis and opisthotonos (Box 11.6). Involvement of the laryngeal or pharyngeal muscles may lead to serious problems such as respiratory distress, dysphagia and choking. Mild dystonia may present as stiffness or aching discomfort, without objective signs.

Up to 25–40% of patients on typical drugs experience a dystonic reaction. Among the depot preparations, fluphenazine decanoate has been associated with dystonia within 12 hours of administration, owing to its relatively rapid post-injection peak. Dystonia may be wrongly dismissed as 'behavioural', for example as an attempt to obtain anticholinergics (as these may be euphoric and therefore potentially misused). Alternatively, an apparent dystonia may in fact be muscle spasm associated with hyperventilation, or posturing associated with psychosis (Barnes, 1992). Long before neuroleptics were introduced, both Kraepelin and Bleuler had described spontaneous dyskinesias (grimacing or other facial movements, showing an increasing frequency with age) in psychotic patients. Spontaneous movements such as stereotypies (seemingly purposeless and meaningless actions) and mannerisms (peculiar ways of completing normal actions) also need to be distinguished from dystonias. The natural course of acute dystonia is either persistence over hours or even days, or a waxing and waning, with periods of intense symptoms interspersed with relative relief. The latter should not be taken as evidence of psychogenic aetiology.

Risk factors include: male gender, high doses of high-potency FGAs, history of dystonia, hypothyroidism and hypoparathyroidism. Drug-induced dystonic reactions appear to occur more commonly in those under 40 years of age, who are at most risk from focal and segmental dystonia of the face and neck (Sethi *et al*, 1990). Occasionally, children who are administered antiemetic drugs such as promethazine (related to chlorpromazine) or metoclopramide (related to sulpiride) can develop an acute dystonia. The particularly high incidence of dystonia in young males may in part be due to a tendency to use high doses of antipsychotics and parenteral administration in a crisis. Conversely, acute dystonia is uncommon among the elderly.

The mechanism of acute dystonia appears to include excessive striatal dopamine D_2 antagonism, possibly involving the early adaptive response to dopamine blockade (increased dopamine turnover) and emerging postsynaptic dopamine receptor supersensitivity.

Acute dystonia responds dramatically to prompt administration of an anticholinergic. In severe cases, parenteral administration (intramuscular or intravenous procyclidine 5–10 mg) should be used. Prophylactic use of anticholinergics should be considered for patients on high-potency agents with other risk factors. If dystonia recurs, it may be advisable to switch to an antipsychotic that has a lower risk of dystonia.

Box 11.6 Acute dystonias

Neck
- Retrocollis
- Torticollis
- Laterocollis
- Anterocollis
- Opisthotonos (also affects trunk)

Tongue
- Rotation
- Protrusion
- Retraction
- Lateral deviation

Jaw
- Trismus

Extraocular muscles
- Upward (+/– lateral) deviation of the eye

Trunk
- Scoliosis
- Opisthotonos

Limbs
- Hyperpronation
- Wrist flexion
- Metacarpo-phalangeal flexion/extension, as in fist clenching
- Extension of lower limbs
- Adductor spasm
- Plantar flexion with inversion
- Dorsiflexion with eversion

Anticholinergic drugs

Anticholinergic drugs act by blocking central acetylcholine muscarinic receptors. Dopamine inhibits the release of acetylcholine in the striatum (caudate and putamen), and so by antagonising this effect antipsychotics lead to an increase in striatal acetylcholine release. This disturbs the acetylcholine/dopamine balance, a mechanism that contributes to EPS. Anticholinergics can reverse this imbalance and so alleviate EPS. They also have some antihistaminic effect and may block dopamine reuptake. Common side-effects include drowsiness, dry mouth, delayed gastric emptying, blurred vision and constipation. Less common but potentially more serious side-effects include impaired cognitive functioning, acute confusional states, particularly in the elderly, and urinary retention in men (especially in those with prostatic hypertrophy). They are contraindicated in closed-angle glaucoma. Abrupt cessation may occasionally result in a rebound withdrawal syndrome (with nausea, insomnia and anxiety), while the stimulant or euphoric effects of some of these drugs may lead to their being misused.

Procyclidine is probably the most commonly used anticholinergic for the treatment of acute dystonia, and can be given orally or by intramuscular or intravenous injection. Parenteral administration is very effective, acting within minutes and providing relief for up to 4 hours. The other anticholinergics differ mainly in their side-effect profile. For example, benzhexol is thought to have more of a stimulant effect and hence a greater liability to misuse and dependence; benzatropine has a longer half-life and may be prescribed on a once-daily basis, although the oral formulation is no longer available in the UK; orphenadrine has a lesser tendency to misuse than either benzhexol or procyclidine, but may be more cardiotoxic because it has strong membrane-stabilising activity, increasing the chances of death if taken in overdose (it should therefore be avoided in patients with suicidal intentions or those who have taken overdoses in the past); biperiden is more sedative than the other drugs and was previously used in the UK (Cookson *et al*, 2002).

Drug-induced parkinsonism (DIP)

The core features of the Parkinsonian triad are bradykinesia, tremor and rigidity.

1 *Bradykinesia* is motor slowing. In addition to voluntary actions, speech and facial muscles (a mask-like facies) may also be affected. Some symptoms may be difficult to distinguish from negative symptoms of schizophrenia (e.g. amotivation, affective flattening and poverty of speech), or psychomotor retardation seen in comorbid depression. Bradykinesia is the most common manifestation of DIP.

2 *Tremor* is the regular involuntary oscillation of a body part about a joint. In DIP, two main types of tremor are seen: (i) a postural (or action) tremor of high frequency (15–20 Hz) and low amplitude, usually best seen in the hands with arms outstretched; and (ii) the classical Parkinsonian resting tremor, which is of low frequency (approximately 6 Hz) and high amplitude. In DIP, a postural tremor is a common and early sign, while the resting tremor characteristic of Parkinson's disease is a less frequent and late development. Disturbances of postural reflexes, together with autonomic abnormalities, may also develop.

3 *Rigidity* is an increase in resting muscle tone evident on passive movement. 'Lead pipe' rigidity is uniformly sustained throughout the range of passive movement, whereas 'cog wheeling' is a jerky pattern of resistance that is intermittently broken and re-established throughout the range of passive movement. This is best demonstrated by passive arm movements (rotatory movements for the former, elbow or wrist flexion/extension for the latter) (see Barnes, 1992). Patients experience rigidity subjectively as 'stiffness'. It may require reinforcement to elicit (the patient is asked to move the opposite limb to the one being examined).

DIP often develops within a week of starting the drug. The prevalence of DIP with the FGAs was about 15–20%. DIP is often subjectively highly unpleasant and, in mild or early cases, its symptoms can be difficult to distinguish from negative symptoms (see above).

Different rating scales have been devised to assess DIP. The Simpson–Angus scale was the first to be developed and remains widely used. It contains ten items, each rated on a 5-point scale (0–4), with descriptive definitions. Six of the ten items rate rigidity, one rates gait and the remaining items measure tremor, glabellar tap and salivation (Barnes, 1992).

DIP results from blockade in the nigrostriatal dopaminergic pathway. It is likely that inter-individual susceptibility to DIP is at least partly determined by genotype. The reduced incidence of DIP with atypicals with significant D_2 receptor antagonism may be due to their 5-HT_{2A} antagonism, cholinergic antagonism, relatively fast dissociation from the D_2 receptor, or partial agonist properties.

Before the advent of the atypicals, the usual management of DIP was to lower the dose of the responsible antipsychotic and/or administer an anticholinergic. DIP is now less common, being more prevalent among the elderly or in patients on high-potency FGA depot preparations. Current practice is to switch to an atypical with a lower risk of EPS if possible; if a depot is indicated by the patient's non-compliance, the only atypical long-acting formulation at present is the Consta form of risperidone (see page 251). Long-term or prophylactic anticholinergics are generally avoided, and their use reviewed regularly for up to 3 or 4 months, after which a definitive attempt should be made to discontinue them.

Akathisia

Akathisia means 'an inability to sit still'. Patients experience a most unpleasant subjective sense of inner restlessness and unease (dysphoria), an inability to keep still, and an irresistible urge to move, especially involving the legs, with mounting tension if required to be still. The movements are a voluntary, coordinated, non-goal-directed response to the intensely unpleasant affect that is the cornerstone of this condition. The 'driven' quality of the movements is characteristic. Fidgety movements of the legs when sitting and difficulty standing still are the most common observations. Less commonly experienced symptoms include discomfort, including pulling or drawing sensations of the muscles, as well as paraesthesiae (Barnes, 1992). Akathisia is usually monitored with the Barnes Akathisia Scale.

As with DIP, 80–90% of cases of akathisia are evident in the first 6–10 weeks of treatment. Females are reported to be affected twice as frequently as males. About 25% of patients develop this side-effect on FGAs, and among the atypicals risperidone (especially at doses above 6 mg), amisulpride (over a relatively wide dose range) and aripiprazole (particularly in the first few weeks of treatment) are also associated with it.

Akathisia is distressing and is a major source of treatment non-concordance. The associated dysphoria is so unpleasant that it has been linked to violent behaviour and suicide. Therefore, whenever possible, akathisia should be treated promptly.

The major differential diagnosis is psychomotor agitation, the treatment of which is unfortunately the direct opposite to that of akathisia. Whereas agitation is likely to improve by increasing the dose of the antipsychotic, akathisia is likely to worsen. Dose reduction may therefore help clarify the diagnosis. The frequent coexistence of DIP and akathisia suggests a common mechanism, which is likely to be dopaminergic dysfunction. It is possible, however, that the two conditions are mediated by different dopaminergic pathways; for example, akathisia might result from mesocortical dopaminergic dysfunction (possibly increased receptor activation in this area), and DIP from nigrostriatal antagonism. Indeed, the fact that aripiprazole has a significant association with akathisia, but not with any other EPS, is consistent with the two conditions arising from the dysfunction of different dopaminergic pathways.

Akathisia is more difficult to treat than acute dystonia or DIP. Lowering the dosage or switching to a drug with a lower potential to cause akathisia (e.g. quetiapine) may be tried. Anticholinergics are not helpful in akathisia.

The use of beta-blockers has been supported in open-label studies (e.g. propranolol 30–80 mg/day). Their efficacy in movement disorders was first observed in 'restless legs syndrome' (Ekbom's syndrome), which has features in common with drug-induced akathisia. The main determinant of efficacy for the different beta-blockers appears to be their lipid solubility, and hence their ability to cross the blood–brain barrier. Propranolol is highly lipid soluble and is therefore effective in akathisia, whereas atenolol has low lipid solubility and is ineffective. Low blood pressure is an obvious side-effect of the beta-blockers and hence blood pressure should be monitored if a patient is given propranolol for akathisia, and depression may also occur as a side-effect (Stanilla & Simpson, 2001).

Benzodiazepines may also be effective in the short-term management of akathisia, but their long-term use should be avoided if possible. There are also reports that amantadine and antihistamines, including cyproheptadine, may be helpful.

A high 5-HT_2:D_2 ratio is in general associated with a lower incidence of akathisia and it has been suggested that 5-HT_{2A} antagonists may alleviate akathisia. Mianserin, which is a potent 5-HT_{2A} antagonist, has afforded some improvement in small trials but mianserin affects many other receptor systems as well (see Chapter 4, page 87), and it is therefore possible that its effect on akathisia is related to these (e.g. adrenergic effects).

Tardive dyskinesia (TD)

Chronic or 'tardive' (late-onset) forms of EPS occur after months or years of treatment, often without any recent change in drug or dose. They do not have a clear relationship with dose and may persist or even worsen after the discontinuation of medication. The two main late-onset conditions are tardive dyskinesia and tardive dystonia (discussed below).

Tardive dyskinesia was probably first identified in 1959 by Sigwald and colleagues. The following year it was more clearly described by Uhrbrand and Faurbye in Denmark in 33 diagnostically heterogeneous long-stay patients, all of whom had been treated with a range of physical treatments, including prolonged exposure to antipsychotic medication. The most likely causative factor was considered by the authors to be the prolonged exposure to antipsychotics, and the syndrome of involuntary movements or dyskinesias was subsequently designated *tardive dyskinesia*. In the early descriptions, the terms 'orofacial dyskinesia' and 'tardive dyskinesia' were used interchangeably. However, it soon became clear that orofacial movements could be found in patients never exposed to antipsychotic medication (Waddington *et al*, 1995) and that the involuntary movements could involve any part of the body.

Box 11.7 lists the clinical features of TD. The orofacial area is most commonly affected and the earliest orofacial sign is usually vermicular (worm-like) movements of the tongue. It is important to note that such movements are seen in 5–15% of elderly patients who have never received antipsychotic drugs (Gerlach *et al*, 1996). Tongue movements may be mild, despite pronounced movements elsewhere. Collective involvement of the oral and peri-oral musculature is common, in a 'bucco-linguo-masticatory triad'. Pouting, lip pursing, protrusion of the cheek by the tongue and pseudo-chewing or sucking movements are seen. These movements may lead to oral problems, especially in the elderly, where they can be mistaken for movements associated with ill-fitting dentures. Although these

Box 11.7 Clinical features of tardive dyskinesia

Tongue
- 'Vermicular' movements
- Twisting
- Sweeping of the buccal surface (the 'bonbon' sign)
- Irregular jerky protrusion (the 'fly catcher' sign)
- Displacement, 'tromboning', on voluntary protrusion

Lips
- Puckering
- Pouting
- Puffing
- Smacking
- Lateral retraction ('bridling')

Jaw
- Mouth opening
- Clenching (trismus)
- Grinding (bruxism)
- Forward/lateral protrusion

Facial expression
- Grimacing
- Blepharoclonus
- Blepharospasm
- Irregular eyebrow elevation
- Frowning

Neck
- Torti-/retro-/latero-/antero-collis (kinetic/spasmodic or static)

Trunk
- Unilateral dystonia ('Pisa syndrome')
- Spinal hyperextension
- Axial hyperkinesis ('copulatory' movements)

Upper limbs
- Shoulder tics
- Hyperpronation
- Choreoathetoid finger or wrist movements

Lower limbs
- 'Restless' legs
- Squirming ('out splaying' of toes)
- Ankle rotation
- Eversion/inversion
- Stamping

Oropharynx
- Dysphagia

Diaphragm/intercostals
- Irregular respiration/grunting

movements are designated 'choreoathetoid' in type, they are usually complex, repetitive and coordinated (the opposite of the rudimentary, non-repetitive and uncoordinated movements characteristic of chorea). The individual may initially be unaware of the movements, with family and friends being the first to notice.

In common with many EPS, the emergence of TD is related to mental state. Movements may arise or become more pronounced when the patient is 'aroused' and tend to ease during periods of low anxiety. They can be voluntarily suppressed for variable periods, or disappear altogether while the patient concentrates on a task. Activity in another body part may exacerbate them and this is known as 'activation'; for example, repeatedly touching the thumb to each finger sequentially in both hands may amplify TD in the tongue and face.

Several antipsychotic-related risk factors for TD have been identified. These include: prolonged treatment with antipsychotics, high drug dose, high D_2 receptor potency relative to other receptor potencies, and drug 'holidays' (i.e. stopping the antipsychotic) of more than 3 months followed by reinstatement. The risk with different antipsychotics is estimated to range from 4% to 8% per year of treatment.

TD is seen with some atypicals, although the risks appear to be lower, with olanzapine having a 0.52% annual risk in early reports, compared with an annual risk of 7.45% for haloperidol (Glazer, 2000).

Clozapine is unusual in being associated with clinical alleviation of TD; Lieberman *et al* (1991) reviewed eight uncontrolled studies in which clozapine was used to treat TD, and found that 43% of the cases improved.

Other agents (e.g. metoclopramine, and antidepressants, including paroxetine, fluoxetine and amoxapine) are also associated with a risk of TD. The single most important risk factor appears to be the duration of exposure to a psychotropic agent that is known to bear significant risk. A study by Quinn *et al* (2001) indicated that the prevalence of involuntary movements approaches 100% over a lifetime trajectory for individuals with schizophrenia chronically medicated with FGAs.

Patient risk factors derived from a variety of studies (Muscettola *et al*, 1999; Glazer, 2000) as well as the American Psychiatric Association (1997) and others include: increasing age, a family history of Parkinson's disease, the presence of movement disorder (both subtle movement disorder before treatment and acute EPS, particularly DIP), negative symptoms, cognitive impairment, alcohol or other substance misuse, use of anti-Parkinsonian agents, lithium and diabetes. There is also a relatively high incidence in those with schizophrenia complicated by learning disability (especially in phenylketonuria). Less well replicated risk factors include: gender (female), ethnicity (African) and a diagnosis of mood disorder.

Genetic factors may also be important, and in those presenting with TD there is often a family history of antipsychotic-induced movement disorders, or movement disorders *per se*. Several candidate genes have been investigated for an association with TD, with the most convincing evidence so far for an association with *DRD3*, the gene encoding the dopamine D_3 receptor. An initial report gave an excess of Gly/Gly homozygotes in 24% of patients with chronic TD and in only 4% of those with no or fluctuating TD (Steen *et al*, 1997), a finding that has since been replicated and reviewed in a meta-analysis (Lerer *et al*, 2002). However, a later meta-analysis revealed an association with the Gly allele but no genotypic effect, noting evidence of publication bias and other potentially confounding variables (Bakker *et al*, 2006). *DRD3* has a polymorphic site that gives rise to a serine-to-glycine substitution in the N-terminal extracellular domain of the receptor protein (Ser9Gly). *DRD3* has also been weakly associated with schizophrenia *per se* (Williams *et al*, 1998) and hence the association may reflect a common aetiology for both the drug-induced movement disorder and schizophrenia.

Several mechanisms have been proposed for TD. Carlsson (1985) proposed that postsynaptic dopamine antagonism resulted in the development of supersensitivity of these sites, particularly in the striatum, in a similar manner to the denervation supersensitivity that is known to occur in the peripheral and autonomic nervous systems. Imaging studies have shown a 50% increase in postsynaptic receptor density in the caudate with chronic administration of haloperidol (which can cause TD) but not with clozapine (which is not associated with TD).

Normal motor function depends on a balance between cholinergic and dopaminergic activity in the striatum; and DIP is associated with reduced dopaminergic tone. Anticholinergics restore the balance, and hence alleviate the DIP. Under this model, tardive dyskinesia can be attributed to the eventual development of dopamine supersensitivity, tipping the balance in the opposite direction and so producing hyperkinesis (owing to an exaggerated postsynaptic dopamine receptor response, even to low concentrations of dopamine). It has also been postulated that dysregulation of the balance between D_1- and D_2-mediated effects, resulting in striatal disinhibition of the thalamocortical pathway, may also be involved in the aetiology of TD.

Tardive dyskinesia is difficult to treat and responds to very few agents. Kane *et al* (1988*b*) and subsequently an American taskforce on TD (American Psychiatric Association, 1992) concluded that no effective treatment was available at the time.

The prevalence of TD has probably fallen since the introduction of atypicals. For patients with TD who require continued antipsychotic treatment, clozapine has been recommended (Lieberman *et al*, 1991). Stopping the antipsychotic is an option for only a few patients, and sometimes worsens the movement disorders. Anticholinergics are not helpful and should be discontinued. There are reports that benzodiazepines, particularly clonazepam, may be useful (Thaker *et al*, 1990). Although TD returns on stopping clonazepam, the beneficial effects reappear once it is reinstated. There have also been claims that vitamin E, which may reduce neuronal damage due to free radicals, may alleviate TD. However, a randomised controlled trial (RCT) that compared vitamin E with placebo demonstrated no beneficial effects (Adler *et al*, 1993).

Tetrabenazine is the only drug licensed in the UK for the treatment of TD. It is a benzoquinolizine, originally introduced as an antipsychotic in the early 1960s. It acts like reserpine and depletes central monoamines, but, also like reserpine, it was soon found to cause depression and so its use ceased. However, neurologists found that it was useful for treating hyperkinetic movement disorders. Paleacu *et al* (2004) reported the use of tetrabenazine (median dose 75 mg/daily) in a series of 150 cases with a variety of hyperkinetic movement disorders, some of whom had TD, and they reported a 61% response rate. In this series, side-effects were uncommon; parkinsonism occurred in six cases (4%) and depression in two (1.3%) (the latter responding well to an SSRI).

In the United States, there have been cases of medical negligence in relation to TD. The criticism has been that the physician had not adequately informed the patient of the risk of adverse effects, or had prescribed too high a dose of an antipsychotic for too long without adequate monitoring, or had not recognised or treated TD appropriately when it appeared. Although there have been no such cases as yet in the UK, the US experience highlights the importance of adequately briefing patients on this serious, socially disabling adverse reaction, and of adequate monitoring and management should the condition emerge.

Tardive dystonia

Late-onset, persistent dystonia may be seen in patients on chronic antipsychotic treatment and may be very disabling (Burke *et al*, 1982). Subtypes include focal dystonia (confined to one body site), segmental dystonia (localised to more than one adjacent body region) and unilateral axial dystonia. It tends to present as fixed posturing of the face, neck, extremities or trunk. Unlike TD, tardive dystonia may improve with anticholinergic medication. However, in occasional cases tardive dystonia may be severe and intractable.

There have been reports that botulinum toxin may be helpful. The toxin binds to cholinergic motor terminals, preventing the release of acetylcholine, hence producing a functionally denervated muscle. The effect may last 3–4 months and response rates are high, at around 80% (Stanilla & Simpson, 2001). The injections are usually administered by neurologists, who are familiar with the use of this preparation in the treatment of neuromuscular conditions, including dystonia. There have also been reports of neurosurgical procedures being used to treat severe idiopathic dystonias, such as deep brain stimulation in which electrodes are implanted in the internal globus pallidus (Krauss *et al*, 2004), but no one has advocated this for drug-induced tardive dystonia.

Tardive akathisia

Late-onset, persistent akathisia (tardive akathisia) is usually clinically indistinguishable from acute akathisia other than in its timing in relation to antipsychotic treatment. The accompanying subjective sense of restlessness may be less marked in the tardive form. A similar treatment approach as for acute akathisia should be employed (Barnes, 1992).

Antipsychotic drug efficacy in acute schizophrenia

There is now abundant evidence that antipsychotic drugs are beneficial in the management of acute schizophrenia, although this has not always been the case. Many of the early trials were little more than open case series and there were very few proper RCTs. This is at least partly because the mandatory completion of RCTs by a drug company introducing an antipsychotic to the market is a relatively recent regulatory phenomenon. The only early controlled trials at the time were funded by government agencies, such as the UK Medical Research Council's trial of antidepressants in 1957 and the US National Institute of Mental Health Collaborative Study Group of antipsychotic drugs (Guttmacher, 1964). The latter was a large double-blind placebo-controlled trial that looked at the efficacy of three different phenothiazines (chlorpromazine, thioridazine and fluphenazine) over a 6-week treatment interval. In summary, its findings were:

- Antipsychotics produced a significantly greater improvement in acute symptoms of schizophrenia over the trial period than placebo.
- About 23% of patients showed moderate or marked improvement on a placebo.
- The patient response was variable, with 75% 'much' or 'very much' improved, 20% improved only minimally, and 5% showing no difference from placebo, while 2 patients dropped out because of lack of efficacy.
- Although the trial drugs differed in potency and degree of side-effects, they did not differ in efficacy.

Despite the widespread use of the new drugs in the 1950s, there were claims that the other treatments available, such as ECT and psychoanalysis, were just as effective, particularly as US psychiatry at that time was predominately psychoanalytical in approach. May (1968) then conducted one of the first randomised trials to address these issues. The patients all had a diagnosis of schizophrenia and were first admissions to the Camarillo state hospital in California. Patients were carefully selected by two experienced psychoanalysts to ensure they were in the 'middle third of the prognostic group'; thus, patients who were likely to achieve a spontaneous remission were excluded, as were those thought to have a very poor prognosis, and the resultant group (n = 228) were randomly allocated to one of five treatment groups:

1 'ataraxic drugs' alone – trifluoperazine 3–4 mg daily, maximum dose 120 mg, or chlorpromazine, average dose 500 mg daily

2 individual psychotherapy alone, conducted by residents under the supervision of experienced psychoanalysts, which was a 'social problem based and reality confrontation, not transference based' (7–107 sessions)

3 drugs and individual psychotherapy

4 ECT – males averaged 19 treatments, females 25 treatments (range 7–44), and May (1968) accepted criticism that this might not have been enough ECT to explain the low response rate

5 a 'therapeutic milieu' (i.e. ward environment), featuring hydrotherapy, and occupational and industrial therapy (doctors were free to prescribe as much hydrotherapy and barbiturates as they thought fit).

The results were striking. The percentage of patients released from hospital for each group were: for drugs alone 95.8%; for drugs and psychotherapy 95.1%; for ECT 79%; for milieu 58%; and for psychotherapy alone

55%. The duration of stay for those who were successfully discharged showed a similar effect: drugs alone 130 days, drugs and psychotherapy 135 days, ECT 137 days, milieu therapy 163 days, and psychotherapy alone 185 days. This landmark study established the superiority of the drugs over other therapies, which at the time had been an area of great controversy. This study has in recent years again become important, because follow-up of this cohort showed that the group who received drugs initially did very much better over the longer term (i.e. in the years following the trial) than those receiving psychotherapy and, as these were all first-admission patients, this study represents early support for the importance of initial appropriate intervention for schizophrenia (see Chapter 12, page 300).

Drug trials of the atypicals

In contrast to the era and conditions when the FGAs were introduced, the US FDA now requires drug companies to sponsor standardised trials in accordance with certain strict methodological requirements. Collectively, these trials have involved thousands of patients. Reasons for discontinuing medication, laboratory evaluations (which now include ECGs, prolactin levels, and measures of glucose and lipid control) and a variety of other adverse effects are all monitored. The main instruments used to measure change are described in Chapter 8 (page 182) and include the Brief Psychiatric Rating Scale (BPRS) (Overall & Gorham, 1962), and the Positive and Negative Symptom Scale for schizophrenia (PANSS) (Kay *et al*, 1987). Extrapyramidal symptoms are measured with the Simpson–Angus Rating Scale (Simpson & Angus, 1970), the Abnormal Involuntary Movements Scale (Guy, 1976) and the Barnes Akathisia Scale (Barnes, 1989), as well as by other specialised EPS scales. Antipsychotic non-neurological adverse effects may be measured using the Antipsychotic Non-Neurological Side-Effects Rating Scale (ANNSERS) (Yusufi *et al*, 2005).

The drug is usually compared with placebo as well as another antipsychotic, such as haloperidol (or chlorpromazine), with trials being adequately powered to demonstrate efficacy equal to that of the comparator. The use of haloperidol as the comparator has the disadvantage that it has a very high rate of EPS and hyperprolactinaemia, especially at doses above 10–12 mg, which is likely to reflect advantageously on the new drug being tested. Trials that permit the use of a dose of antipsychotic within a specified dose range have been informative about optimal or effective doses for clinical practice, as well as dose thresholds associated with particular side-effects. The Cochrane Library (http://www.update-software.com/cochrane/) is a useful resource for reviews of RCTs of antipsychotics (summarised in Table 11.11). It should be noted, however, that effects that are not clearly apparent in the RCTs (e.g. glucose dysregulation) may emerge later, during the phase of more widespread clinical use.

Trials sponsored by the pharmaceutical industry have tended to show that atypicals (risperidone, olanzapine, quetiapine and amisulpride) have a broadly similar efficacy, and equivalent to that of haloperidol for the treatment of positive symptoms, with some being possibly superior to haloperidol for negative symptoms (although the effect size for the latter is not large). The most striking advantage in these studies is the lower propensity for EPS, leading to improved tolerability and lower discontinuation rates; this effect, however, is not surprising versus haloperidol, particularly at higher doses of the latter. However, other side-effects, such as weight gain and the metabolic syndrome (e.g. with clozapine and olanzapine), are worse than with haloperidol.

The question of whether the SGAs possess any real advantage over each other or over typical antipsychotics has been addressed in meta-analyses. Geddes *et al* (2000) carried out a meta-analysis aimed at making recommendations on the use of atypicals for patients with schizophrenia. Their results in fact concluded that, using 6–12 mg haloperidol or its equivalent as a comparator, there was no clear evidence that atypicals were more effective or better tolerated than FGAs. The authors therefore recommended the use of FGAs in the first instance, unless the patient had not responded to this class of drugs, or had unacceptable side-effects. This work provides a rational basis for the use of optimal doses of FGAs. In another meta-analysis (Leucht *et al*, 2003), comparing the SGAs with the FGAs, a mean dose of less than 600 mg chlorpromazine or its equivalent had no higher risk of EPS than the SGAs, but as a group the SGAs were moderately more efficacious, irrespective of the comparator drug being used.

The effect sizes for the SGAs versus an FGA comparator for the Geddes *et al* meta-analysis and a subsequent meta-analysis by Davis *et al* (2003) are shown in Table 11.12. (The effect size is a measure of the magnitude of the difference in efficacy between the atypical and the comparator typical(s) used in the drug trials.) Davis *et al* recommended the use of olanzapine, risperidone and amisulpride as first-line antipsychotics. However, one should be cautious about drawing conclusions about other SGAs (whose efficacy was not significantly different from that of FGAs), owing to confounding factors such as smaller total numbers of patients studied, some of these SGAs not being commonly first-line treatments in clinical practice, and different doses of FGA being used as comparator.

The meta-analyses can be criticised on a variety of grounds. For example, at the time of the meta-analysis, there were only three trials of aripiprazole and 31 trials of clozapine. The one clear conclusion that one may draw from the above is that the greatest advantage over haloperidol in terms of efficacy is for clozapine.

Recently, a different approach has been taken. Rather than a meta-analysis of existing clinical trial data, a prospective study of SGAs versus a comparator with a better EPS profile than haloperidol has been undertaken (the Clinical Antipsychotics Trials of Intervention Effectiveness, or CATIE study). The FGA used in this study was perphenazine, and the SGAs were olanzapine, quetiapine, risperidone and ziprasidone (Lieberman *et al*, 2005). In total, 1493 patients were recruited. Interestingly, most (74%) discontinued their assigned treatment due to inefficacy, intolerable side-effects or other reasons. The time to discontinuation was longest with olanzapine, but this drug was associated with more weight gain and metabolic effects. The efficacy of the FGA (perphenazine) was similar to that of quetiapine, risperidone and ziprasidone. The efficacy

Table 11.11 Summary of Cochrane reviews involving the atypical antipsychotics

Drug	Review	Findings
Clozapine	31 studies, 2589 participants (Wahlbeck *et al*, 1999)	Compared with FGAs in treatment-resistant schizophrenia, effective, with fewer relapses, greater reduction in symptoms, fewer drop-outs, high patient satisfaction Side-effect of low neutrophil count more common in children, adolescents and the elderly
Risperidone	9 RCTs, 2368 participants (Hunter *et al*, 2003)	Effective both in the short term and the long term, improving both positive and negative symptoms Fewer drop-outs and EPS on risperidone (at doses of < 6 mg) in comparison with typicals More rhinitis compared with FGAs in some studies, also associated with weight gain
Olanzapine	20 trials (Duggan & Brylewski, 2004)	PANSS ratings favoured olanzapine over 'typical' comparator, but relatively high attrition rates in both groups Less EPS with olanzapine, but more weight gain
Sertindole	(Lewis *et al*, 2005)	Effective antipsychotic, better tolerated than haloperidol but associated with weight gain, rhinitis, erectile dysfunction and cardiac effects (increased QT_c interval)
Ziprasidone[a]	(Bagnall *et al*, 2000)	As effective as haloperidol, with less movement disorder but associated with nausea and vomiting Injectable form noted to cause pain at injection site
Quetiapine	12 RCTs, 3443 patients (Srisurapanont *et al*, 2000)	Effective antipsychotic (equal in efficacy to typicals and to risperidone), low risk of movement disorder but associated with sedation, dry mouth and postural hypotension
Amisulpride	19 RCTs, 2443 participants (Mota Neto *et al*, 2002)	Effective antipsychotic, particularly against negative symptoms at lower doses
Aripiprazole	10 RCTs, 4125 patients (El-Sayeh & Morganti, 2004)	Effective antipsychotic in both acute and maintenance treatment of schizophrenia No glucose dysregulation, weight neutral, low risk of QT_c prolongation, and does not elevate prolactin Associated with insomnia, nausea, vomiting and akathisia in the early stages of treatment
Zotepine	(Fenton *et al*, 2000)	Outcomes were short term (4–12 weeks) with high drop-out in both groups As effective as FGAs, with less movement disorder

[a] Not currently licensed in the UK.

Table 11.12 Effect sizes for atypicals versus FGA comparators: results of two meta-analyses

Drug	Geddes *et al* (2000)	Davis *et al* (2003)
Clozapine	0.68	0.49
Olanzapine	0.22	0.21
Risperidone	0.15	0.25
Amisulpride	0.35	0.29
Quetiapine	0.03	0.003
Zotepine	–	0.146
Ziprasidone	–	0.038
Aripiprazole	–	0.003
Haloperidol vs placebo	–	0.60

of olanzapine was apparently greater, but this may be partly due to the fact that prescribing clinicians were allowed a higher upper dose limit for olanzapine than for the other antipsychotics.

In summary, the available data do not indicate a clear difference in efficacy between atypicals and typicals, except in the case of clozapine. There are possible differences in efficacy between the atypicals but these remain to be clearly elucidated. In clinical practice, therefore, the side-effect profile and other factors (e.g. previous history of response to a particular drug, or medical comorbidity) may be more important in determining the choice of therapeutic regimen.

Drug efficacy for negative symptoms

Core negative symptoms of schizophrenia are described in Chapter 8, page 174. They include: flattening of affect, poverty of speech (alogia), avolition and anhedonia. It is important to try and differentiate between primary negative symptoms and those that are secondary to other factors, such as medication (previously termed the 'neuroleptic deficit state'), depression or social under-stimulation.

Most published trials for the atypical drugs have shown clozapine, olanzapine, risperidone, quetiapine and amisulpride to be moderately more efficacious against negative symptoms (usually measured with the Scale for Assessment of Negative Symptoms, or SANS), than haloperidol. However, it is unclear how much of the improvement is due to an amelioration of *primary* negative symptoms, rather than *secondary* negative symptoms. Statistical procedures such as path analysis have been employed in seeking to answer this question. Moller *et al* (1995) applied path analysis to the data of the North American Risperidone Study and found that, even after controlling for the indirect effects of the drugs on secondary negative symptoms, risperidone appeared to improve negative symptoms to a greater extent than haloperidol (although the analysis may still have been confounded by the dose of haloperidol used).

Loo *et al* (1997) compared low-dose amisulpride (100 mg) with placebo in a group of patients with schizophrenia and predominantly negative symptoms. A greater than 50% reduction in SANS scores was seen in 42% of those treated with amisulpride, in contrast to only 15% of those treated with placebo.

A meta-analysis by Leucht *et al* (2003) found significant reductions in negative symptoms on treatment with olanzapine, risperidone, quetiapine and sertindole, while a second meta-analysis, of 30 RCTs, by Wahlbeck *et al* (1999), showed a small effect in favour of clozapine. (The relatively small effect may at least partly be a reflection of the relatively low numbers of patients in studies of negative symptoms.)

Antidepressant therapy has also been used as an adjunct for treating negative symptoms. However, caution must be exercised, as patients may relapse, especially if they are not consistently compliant with their antipsychotic. Moreover, using an antidepressant together with an antipsychotic may in some cases increase serum levels of antipsychotics, with potential unwanted side-effects, depending on the effect exerted by the antidepressant on drug metabolising enzymes, including cytochrome P450s. The SSRIs have been studied more frequently as adjunctive treatments than the other antidepressants. Studies have shown mixed results, with some showing improvement with fluvoxamine and fluoxetine.

Berk *et al* (2001) studied the use of mirtazapine as an adjunct to haloperidol, and found that PANSS scores in the mirtazapine group were 42% lower than in the placebo group, with no differences in the depression scale scores at end-point. Mirtazapine is a 5-HT_2 and 5-HT_3 receptor antagonist and also affects the 5-HT_{1A} receptor and the noradrenaline α_2 autoreceptor. Data in support of the use of agents that block the α_2 adrenoceptor as adjunctive therapy in the treatment of negative symptoms have been published by Lindström (2000).

Trials for the treatment of negative symptoms have also been undertaken with glycine and other agents that act at the glycine binding site of the NMDA receptor, and have already been mentioned (see under 'Phencyclidine and the NMDA system', on page 243).

The effects of currently available antipsychotics are certainly far greater and more obvious for positive symptoms than for negative symptoms; further research to generate agents effective in treating negative symptoms is therefore indicated.

Effect of antipsychotics on cognitive function

Kraepelin and Bleuler both held that cognitive dysfunction played a central role in schizophrenia – hence Kraepelin's name for the condition, 'dementia praecox'. It appears that there is a premorbid decline in cognitive function that occurs before the onset of positive symptoms. This may then be followed by a further decline during the initial episode, but thereafter cognitive deficits tend to be stable (unlike in true dementias). There is now good evidence that neurocognitive deficits and negative symptoms correlate with functional disability, and so improvements in these areas are of critical importance. A detailed account of the main cognitive deficits found in schizophrenia is given in Chapter 8 on page 176.

While current interest in enhancing cognitive function is focused mainly on the atypicals, Mishara & Goldberg (2004) have summarised the older literature on the neurocognitive benefits of FGAs. Their meta-analysis (based on 208 studies) showed that FGAs did improve cognitive function, with an effect size of 0.22 (95% confidence interval 0.1–0.34). Since the confidence limits did not include zero, the effect size was significant, though modest. Doses in these studies had a wide range and the mean was greater than would be used currently (300–1500 mg chlorpromazine equivalents, mean 685 mg) but there was no correlation between neuropsychological improvement and drug dose. The main areas in which benefits were observed were automatic learning (a large effect size) and perceptual processing (a moderate effect size), while modest benefits were observed for attention, language and memory.

Some atypicals may have a greater effect on improving cognition in schizophrenia. Weickert *et al* (2003) found a median effect size of approximately 0.47 for atypicals and 0.25 for typicals relative to placebo. The meta-analysis of Keefe *et al* (1999) for 'all atypicals' found that they improved attention, verbal fluency, digit-symbol substitution, and fine motor executive functions more than did typical drugs. The advantage of the atypicals in improving fine motor executive functions may be due to the lower propensity to induce EPS. Neuropharmacological mechanisms underlying the possible cognitive benefits associated with the atypicals are unclear, but may include 5-HT_{2A} receptor mechanisms.

In another, more refined meta-analysis, Meltzer & McGurk (2002) attempted to separate out the differential effects of each atypical on cognitive function. Obviously, the database for individual drugs was considerably smaller than the data for 'all atypicals' versus 'all typicals', and there was considerable variation between studies, which should be remembered in the context of the following overall findings:

- for clozapine there was strong evidence for improvement in attention and verbal fluency, moderate evidence for an improvement in executive function, but inconsistent evidence for any improvement in working memory, or secondary verbal or spatial memory
- for risperidone there was a consistent positive effect on working memory, executive function and attention, while effects on verbal learning and memory were inconsistent
- for olanzapine there was good evidence for improvements in verbal learning, verbal fluency, memory and executive function, but not for attention, working memory, visual learning or memory.

Clinical management

Acute episodes

Two important guidelines on the treatment of schizophrenia have been published in recent years. The first was produced by the UK's National Institute for Clinical Excellence in 2002, *Schizophrenia: Core Interventions in the Treatment and Management of Schizophrenia in Primary and Secondary Care*, which will be referred to as the NICE guidelines for the remainder of this chapter. The second was published in 2004 by the American Psychiatric Association, *Practice Guideline for the Treatment of Patients with Schizophrenia* (second edition) and from here on it will be referred to as the APA guidelines. They both describe consensus recommendations for the management of patients with schizophrenia. The APA guidelines are far more detailed and highly referenced but both guidelines make broadly similar recommendations.

Treatment goals

The treatment goals in an acute episode, be it a first admission or a relapse, are to prevent harm, control disturbed behaviour, reduce the severity of the psychosis and manage potentially dangerous behaviours, particularly aggression and suicidality. In addition, every attempt should be made to try to alleviate the fear, anxiety and dysphoria that often accompany an acute psychosis. Pharmacological and social treatments will then need to be optimised to facilitate the next phase of treatment, which in most cases will be discharge back into the community. One of the main challenges is to select an appropriate medication and titrate its dose so that it is efficacious with minimal side-effects.

Assessment

Management of acute episodes will often have to be initiated quickly, when only minimal history on the patient has been obtained. Evaluation will therefore need to be ongoing, with information being collated from various sources to cover the psychiatric and personal as well as the medical background. Effort should be made at every stage to engage the patient and develop a therapeutic relationship, with both the patient and the family, who will often play a major role in the patient's long-term care. Physical examination should be performed on all patients who are admitted to hospital, and this should include the cardiovascular, respiratory, abdominal and neurological systems, a thyroid examination and body weight. In addition, the following investigations are routine in the UK: urine drug screen, full blood count, measures of renal and hepatic function, thyroid stimulating hormone and, for first-episode cases or those for whom no recent results in this regard are available, vitamins B_{12} and folate.

In recent years, with the increasing understanding of the metabolic syndrome in schizophrenia, measures of metabolic dysfunction have been added (e.g. random or fasting blood glucose and lipid profile). Glycosylated haemoglobin (Hb_{A1c}) gives information on glycaemic control in the preceding 2 months in patients with diabetes. Neuroimaging is indicated in patients with focal neurological signs or a history of seizures (who should also be referred to a neurologist). Routine neuroimaging has also been advocated in first-episode cases of acute psychosis, including schizophrenia, as up to 10% may show an abnormality; however, in many National Health Service trusts this is not available for those without focal neurological signs or seizures. Neuroimaging may also be available for patients who have proved refractory to treatment.

Hospital or home treatment?

In recent years in the UK, there has been a trend towards home treatment of acute episodes. The NICE guidelines state that treatment should be 'in the least restrictive setting that is possible'. In taking a decision about whether or not a patient should be admitted, the following factors should be considered:

- degree of risk
- need for particular treatments
- family factors (carer in distress or high in expressed emotion)
- availability of social supports
- availability of home treatment or an early intervention in psychosis or assertive community outreach service.

A more extensive description of the indications for admission and of the psychosocial aspects of in-patient treatment is given in Chapter 12.

The APA recommends that the professional carer–client relationship should be 'tolerant, non-demanding and supportive' during the in-patient stay. None the less, some patients will require a compulsory admission (in the UK, under the Mental Health Act 1983).

Discussing medication with the patient

Both the APA and NICE guidelines recommend that a clinician should discuss the choice of medication with the patient. The NICE guidelines further suggest the patient should take an active role in the decision making. The section on consent to treatment in the Mental Health Act 1983 requires doctors to sign a statement to the effect that they have discussed the medication with the patient and whether or not the patient has consented to taking it.

The days when the doctor decided on medication that patients were expected to take without question are over. The level of the discussion should be appropriate for the patient's level of understanding, while the content should cover the likely benefits, side-effects and what may be done about side-effects if they occur. In due course, the possibility that the drug(s) may have to be taken in the long term may well need to be discussed, and advice given not to discontinue it abruptly.

Clinicians may be reluctant to discuss medication with individuals with schizophrenia who are acutely unwell, for example if psychotic symptoms or cognitive deficits make communication challenging. However, it is important to overcome these challenges, as a patient who is acutely psychotic may understand information of a factual nature (especially if explained in lay terms), even though he or she may have difficulty with abstract concepts. Moreover, a failure to discuss and communicate about medication adequately may feed into a patient's paranoia, whereas adequate discussion and explanation (especially with regard to side-effects) may alleviate a patient's anxiety, and may increase the likelihood of the patient seeking help for side-effects should these occur. Where possible, the individual's carer(s) should also be consulted; this is essential for patients under 18 years and those with significant cognitive impairment.

An entry must always be made in the case notes to indicate that such a discussion has taken place, regardless of the outcome; not only is this good practice but the absence of warnings about side-effects has become an important source of litigation in psychiatry, as it has across the rest of medicine.

Which drug?

The NICE and APA guidelines both recommend that an atypical should be considered in the choice of first-line treatments. Both guidelines also accept the use of FGAs, particularly in cases where the patient has responded well to them in the past and this is their preference. However, the NICE guideline recommends moving from a typical to an atypical if the former is associated with significant side-effects, particularly EPS. Initial stabilisation should be with an oral as opposed to a depot or long-acting preparation, unless one is treating a relapsing individual who has responded well to a particular long-acting preparation in the past and has difficulty in taking oral medication, or is reluctant to do so.

Drug doses and dose equivalents

Both the APA and NICE guidelines recommend that doses should be gradually titrated up to an equivalent of 300–900 mg chlorpromazine daily, as most patients will respond at this range. Treatment should be with the minimum effective dose. The equivalent doses of antipsychotics to 100 mg of chlorpromazine are shown in Table 11.13. These equivalents are fairly well established for typical drugs and relate to D_2 receptor occupancy as well as to drug trial data. Although they are in some cases less accurate for atypicals, they are probably still the best guide for comparing drug potencies; the NICE guidelines state that it may be helpful to use such tables when switching antipsychotic drugs.

Although it can be tempting to escalate the dose very rapidly for severely disturbed patients, there is little evidence that this will hasten the response. It will, however, almost certainly increase the likelihood of side-effects, particularly dose-dependent effects. The BNF maximal dosage of 1000 mg chlorpromazine equivalents should not be exceeded (according to the NICE guidelines) unless there are exceptional circumstances (see below).

Monitoring progress

During the early phases of drug treatment, NICE recommends that the prescribing clinician and keyworker monitor the mental state and side-effects on at least a weekly basis. If florid and dangerous symptoms are not adequately controlled, an adjuvant such as a benzodiazepine (e.g. clonazepam or lorazepam) may be added to the treatment regimen. Side-effects should be treated appropriately. Some (e.g. nausea) may reduce with time, and the addition of an appropriate agent (e.g. an anti-emetic) as required and reassurance that the side-effect will diminish with time may suffice. Patients with orthostatic hypotension should be given appropriate advice (see section on the treatment of the adverse effects of clozapine). If tachycardia occurs, this should be monitored and an ECG done; dosage reduction or even cessation of medication may be required.

Table 11.13 Antipsychotic dose equivalences to 100 mg of chlorpromazine (CPZ)

Drug	**Therapeutically equivalent dose to chlorpromazine 100 mg/day**	
Typicals		*Range*[a]
Promazine	200	100–250
Thioridazine[b]	100	50–120
Pericyazine	18	10–20
Fluphenazine	2	1–5
Perphenazine	10	6.5–20
Trifluoperazine	5	3.5–7
Flupentixol	3	1.25–5
Haloperidol	2.5	1.5–5
Pimozide	2	1.25–2
Sulpiride	200	200–350
Atypicals		*Minimum effective dose in chronic schizophrenia*
Clozapine[c]	50	Dependent on therapeutic plasma level
Risperidone	1	4
Olanzapine	5	10
Amisulpride	100–150	150
Quetiapine	150	350–600
Ziprasidone	60	120
Aripiprazole	5	10–15

[a] Range for therapeutically equivalent dose, as estimated by different sources.

[b] Largely discontinued in the UK. From Rey *et al* (1989), Foster (1989), American Psychiatric Association (1997), Woods (2003) and Aitchison *et al* (1999).

[c] Method to estimate equivalence is based on fixed-dose studies but no fixed-dose studies have been reported for clozapine.

Failure to improve and treatment non-compliance

Failure to improve or only partial response occurs in 40–60% of cases, and may have a number of explanations. For example, the patient may be a late responder, may not have had a trial of the drug in an adequate dosage (up to the BNF maximum) for long enough, or may actually not be taking the medication at all (termed non-compliance, non-concordance or non-adherence – see below). The patient may also be a rapid or ultra-rapid metaboliser, which should be suspected if there are no beneficial effects or side-effects even on high doses, although in the absence of plasma antipsychotic levels or a definitive test of enzyme activity, this can only be suspected. There is also often 'resistance' to the first prescribed drug (i.e. it is not efficacious or adequately tolerated), in which case a switch to another drug is indicated.

Approximately 50% of patients do not take their medication (Bebbington, 1995). The term 'compliance' was used to describe this issue, but terms more recently introduced are 'concordance', which refers to agreement of view between patient and clinician, and 'treatment adherence'.

Schizophrenia is often associated with poor insight and reduced motivation, which may be part of the negative syndrome or cognitive impairment. It may be tempting to think that compliance is often a bigger problem for people with schizophrenia than for those with other chronic illnesses. However, studies have shown that rates of non-compliance are about the same (approximately 50%) as in other chronic illnesses (e.g. rheumatoid arthritis, diabetes, epilepsy and hypertension).

The terms 'overt' (declared) and 'covert' (hidden) non-compliance have been proposed; reports from staff or carers or the use of medication dispensing aids that count pills may assist in making the distinction between these. Covert non-compliance is frequently associated with side-effects, while overt non-compliance tends to be related to the illness (limited insight, poor planning, memory and motivation). In the latter, provision of support, structure and the use of injectable antipsychotics may be more useful, whereas in the former a change to an agent with a more favourable adverse effect profile may be indicated.

If a patient relapses following suspected non-adherence, then the same antipsychotic should be restarted unless there were issues of poor tolerability. If the relapse occurs despite definite and documented adherence (e.g. depot management or monitored in-patient oral drug administration), then the dose and type of drug should be reviewed and the possibility of emerging treatment resistance should be considered.

The stabilisation phase

Although the psychosis may continue to improve over the months following discharge, other difficulties such as depression or deterioration in the social environment may develop, and require close monitoring. NICE recommends using oral atypicals or long-acting injectable antipsychotics (in those with poor adherence) for treatment maintenance and the prevention of relapse.

Clinicians should be wary of premature antipsychotic dose reduction, for example at the first tentative signs of improvement, and should carefully consider the rate at which any dose reduction is undertaken. Owing to the pharmacokinetics of antipsychotics, there may be a delay before any potential deterioration in mental state or alleviation or change in side-effects becomes apparent following a dose reduction. It is important therefore to monitor for the appearance of non-specific symptoms (e.g. anxiety, agitation, irritability or change in sleep pattern), which may be a more sensitive index of incipient deterioration. If such features do emerge, the medication should be increased back to the previous level, as this may be the long-term optimal dosage.

A range of non-medical services and the Care Programme Approach are described in Chapters 12 and 28, while the role of the general practitioner in monitoring the physical health of patients with schizophrenia is described in Chapter 30.

Can the drugs be stopped?

In general, the research literature is not optimistic about the prognosis for a patient who stops antipsychotic medication, even after a first episode of schizophrenia. Nevertheless, a few patients do have only one episode. In a study of the natural history of cases admitted to hospital between 1872 and 1893, Ciompi (1980) identified about 25% as having an acute onset with complete inter-episode remission. Approximately 10% of these never had another attack, and among the rest who had an illness with an acute onset there was often a long gap between relapses.

Unfortunately, the data are still emerging on clinical predictors of which patients will have a benign long-term picture and which will not. Johnson *et al* (1983) asked a group of consultant psychiatrists to identify a group of 'good prognosis patients' who they considered would be less likely to relapse on stopping their medication. However, when their medication was stopped, the relapse rate was no better than when patients themselves decided to stop their medication. Most patients will try omitting their medication at some point during the course of their illness, and most will relapse on so doing, but up to 25% will manage without medication for some time, perhaps years, before they require it again.

Recommendations

Both the APA and NICE suggest that at about 1–2 years after a first episode of schizophrenia, a trial of very gradual drug withdrawal (e.g. over 6 months) may be attempted, but that patients should still continue to be monitored over the next 2 years. Sometimes this is successful, especially if substance misuse (e.g. cannabis) was an important trigger for the presenting episode and the patient abstains from the substance. Drug withdrawal should not be attempted when the initial presentation has been dangerous or remission has been very difficult to achieve. The rate of reduction should be slow; an international consensus conference (Kissling, 1991) recommended that the antipsychotic dose should be reduced by 20% every 6 months until a minimum maintenance dose is reached, considered to be as low as 50 mg haloperidol decanoate monthly.

The 1997 APA guidelines suggested that patients with two or more psychotic episodes should be advised that they will require medication for 5 years before the need for an antipsychotic is reviewed. However, the 2004 guidelines now recommend that patients with multiple episodes or at least two episodes over the past 5 years should be placed on lifetime antipsychotic medication.

Maintenance treatment

Maintaining well-being and preventing further relapses in patients with psychotic illnesses is a significant component of the work of many community mental health teams. A 15-year follow-up study of 82 patients in the Netherlands illustrates this (Wiersma *et al*, 1998). Only a quarter of patients experienced complete remission, even though they complied with medication between episodes. The most common pattern was of two or more episodes leading to admission, related to positive symptoms, followed by a prolonged period with negative symptoms. About 17% had episodes followed by anxiety, depression or other symptoms, 11% were chronically psychotic and 10% committed suicide. Much of the relapse prevention literature is concerned solely with reporting readmission rates, but the study of Wiersma *et al* (1998) illustrates that there is considerable subthreshold morbidity, falling short of severity criteria required for admission. For this reason, Marder & Wirshing (2003) define maintenance treatment broadly, to include patients who are stable as well as those with persistent symptoms. In this section of the chapter, the role of medication is discussed, while psychosocial interventions that should accompany drug therapy are considered in Chapter 12.

Do the drugs help?

Although atypical drugs are now widely used in the long-term treatment of schizophrenia, the scientific basis for using antipsychotics was developed in the period from the 1960s to the early 1990s, when only the typical drugs were available. Davis & Andriukaitis (1986) reviewed placebo-controlled maintenance studies (with a total of 3720 patients) and reported that 55% of those on placebo relapsed over 1 year, compared with 21% on an antipsychotic, while Baldessarini *et al* (1988) gave a similar figure of 55% relapsing on placebo, but only 14% on the active drug. However, both studies suggested that a significant number of patients will relapse even while on medication, indicating that there is considerable room for improvement for both drug efficacy and psychosocial management.

Stopping an antipsychotic that appears to be working is also likely to result in relapse. Kane (1987) pooled six studies of patients who had been well for between 1 and 5 years and who stopped their medication. They reported a relapse rate of 75% 6–24 months after drug cessation, with the greatest risk period being within 5–7 months. It has also been suggested that relapses associated with drug cessation are more severe than those that occur while patients are still on medication. Johnson *et al* (1983) made this comparison, and found that drug cessation relapses were associated with more violent episodes, more overdoses and more compulsory admissions, indicating that rebound phenomena may play a significant role.

Treatment with atypicals may be better tolerated in the longer term, if the side-effect profile is favourable. However, there are very few direct comparisons between drugs in long-term maintenance treatment, because such trials are difficult to conduct. The CATIE study (Lieberman *et al*, 2005) was mentioned above and this showed that time to discontinuation was longer with olanzapine, while perphanazine did not differ in efficacy from the atypicals tested.

Tran *et al* (1998) pooled data from three trials of olanzapine versus haloperidol and reported 1-year relapse rates of 19.7% for olanzapine and 28% for haloperidol. Essock *et al* (2000) found that, over 1 year, 83% of patients on clozapine remained well, compared with 57% on FGAs.

Depot preparations have a definite advantage for non-compliant patients and are recommended for this group (NICE level A recommendation). Glazer & Kane (1992) pooled data from six RCTs comparing oral drugs with depot preparations and found a 15% advantage for the latter in long-term maintenance. Although atypicals are now preferred over typicals for maintenance, there is no particular drug of choice for long-term maintenance. Patients are often continued on the drug that was used to stabilise them in the acute phase.

For the majority of patients, the same maintenance dose may be appropriate before and after each relapse, but an adjustment should always be considered, especially as partial efficacy or side-effects, with resulting reduced compliance, may have contributed to the relapse. There is also a minority of patients with recurrent episodes of schizophrenia who show a pattern of decreasing responsiveness, with longer recovery times with each progressive episode, who appear to develop tolerance to their antipsychotic, but there are few systematic studies of this (Marder & Wirshing, 2003) and few studies have taken into account factors such as enzyme inducers, including dietary factors.

High doses

Before the introduction of clozapine, the only strategy available for treating refractory schizophrenia was gradually to increase the dose of drug. Baldessarini *et al* (1988) reviewed the results of 33 RCTs in which patients on a mean daily dose of 5200 mg chlorpromazine were compared with those on a mean dose of 400 mg daily. Moderate doses were more effective in two-thirds of the trials, while more severe side-effects were reported in 95% of the high-dose studies. Furthermore, in the 1970s and 1980s it was reported that high doses were occasionally associated with arrhythmias and sudden death, particularly in the acute phase of treatment.

The Royal College of Psychiatrists (2006) has published a consensus statement on high-dose antipsychotic medication, updating its previous statement (published in 1993). The statement makes a total of 22 recommendations, including four concerning aggression with psychosis and rapid tranquillisation and four concerning treatment-resistant psychosis. Of note, the statement defines a 'high dose' as a 'total daily dose of a single antipsychotic which exceeds the upper limit stated in the *British National Formulary* … or a total daily dose of two or more antipsychotics which exceeds the *BNF* maximum using the percentage method'. Briefly, the percentage method is used when more than one antipsychotic is being prescribed, and is calculated by 'converting the dose of each drug into a percentage of the BNF maximum dose for that drug and adding these together (where a cumulative dose of more than 100% is a "high dose")'. The main points of this statement are summarised in Box 11.8.

The Maudsley guidelines (Taylor *et al*, 2005) suggest that high doses should be restricted to patients who:

1 have failed on two antipsychotics, one of which is an atypical

2 have either failed to respond to clozapine or are intolerant of it

3 are without doubt compliant

4 have failed to respond to other measures (e.g. antidepressants and cognitive–behavioural therapy).

Box 11.8 Summary of the consensus statement on the use of high-dose antipsychotics by the Royal College of Psychiatrists (2006)

- High doses should be used only after evidence-based strategies have failed, as current evidence does not justify their routine use
- possible contraindications and drug interactions should be considered before a prescription is made
- The decision to prescribe high doses should be taken explicitly in conjunction with the patient and the wider clinical team, and documented in the case notes
- ECG monitoring (particularly of the QT interval) should be carried out before a high dose is prescribed, after a few days of administration, and then every 1–3 months in the early stages
- Dose increases should be in relatively small increments
- High doses used for treatment-resistant schizophrenia should be time limited; if the risk:benefit ratio is unfavourable after 3 months, the dose should be reduced back to conventional levels

In these circumstances, Taylor *et al* (2005) suggest that it is permissible for the specialist to prescribe outside the BNF recommended range. Maximum BNF doses have come down drastically for most oral drugs, but the BNF still permits high doses of depot drugs to be used; for example, the standard dose of flupentixol is 40 mg intramuscularly every 2 weeks, but in exceptional cases the BNF permits up to 400 mg per week to be used (a 20-fold increase). Although cardiovascular monitoring is not mandatory on high doses of this drug, the prescriber would none the less be wise to do this, in the authors' opinion.

Low doses

Early trials had shown higher relapse rates for low-dose regimens at 2 years, although not at 1 year. However, subsequent studies comparing low doses (e.g. 5–10 mg fluphenazine decanoate fortnightly) with standard doses (25–50 mg fluphenazine decanoate fortnightly) indicate that low-dose regimens may be just as effective, and are associated with greater improvements in instrumental and interpersonal role performances at 2 years and fewer EPS, including early-phase TD (Hogarty *et al*, 1988). More recently, Carpenter *et al* (1999) randomised 50 patients stabilised on 25 mg fluphenazine into two groups, one receiving it at 6-weekly intervals and the other group continuing at 2-weekly intervals, and found no difference in relapse rates over the subsequent year. The authors commented that the patients benefited by receiving a lower cumulative dosage of antipsychotic and that lower injection frequency might favour improved long-term compliance, consistent with previous work (Bollini *et al*, 1994). However, in other studies of fluphenazine at doses below the lower dose above, there were much higher relapse rates, indicating a dose threshold effect for the prevention of relapses.

Most patients on long-acting preparations would welcome a reduction in injection frequency (which may also help to spare local side-effects at injection sites). With the typical depot preparations, this is possible to a varying extent, depending on their half-lives (see above), but an injection interval of greater than 2 weeks is not recommended for the atypical depot Risperdal Consta.

Attempts have also been made to test the usefulness of 'drug holidays' and intermittent treatment. Schooler (1991) reviewed four studies and found that, over the course of a year, the relapse rate among patients receiving continuous treatment was 17%, compared with 37% in those taking 'drug holidays'; as a consequence, intermittent treatment regimens are no longer advocated.

Special situations

Antipsychotics are used in schizophrenia in a variety of special situations. For reasons of space only a limited number of these situations are described here: treatment resistance, rapid tranquillisation, catatonia and the management of depression in schizophrenia. The management of first episodes is considered in Chapter 12 and the use of antipsychotics in pregnancy in Chapter 25, page 654. This chapter ends with a short section on pharmacoeconomics.

Treatment-resistant schizophrenia

Around 10–30% of patients do not initially respond to antipsychotics, while a further 30% have only a partial response (Meltzer, 1997; American Psychiatric Association, 2004). A large multicentre trial found that as many as 40% of patients were poorly stabilised after 6 months of treatment (Schooler *et al*, 1997). Treatment resistance may have a variety of causes, including pharmacokinetic factors, inadequate dosage or excessive dosage resulting in significant side-effects, comorbid substance misuse, physical illness, or factors related to the illness subtype. It is not usually possible to predict on clinical grounds alone which patients will be treatment resistant.

There are various definitions of treatment resistance; NICE (2002) gives a relatively narrow definition:

> 'lack of satisfactory clinical improvement despite the sequential use of the recommended doses for 6 to 8 weeks of at least two antipsychotics, at least one of which should be an atypical.'

The literature on differences in drug responsiveness between the classical types of hebephrenic, paranoid, catatonic and simple schizophrenia is relatively sparse, but there are suggestions that patients presenting with mainly negative symptoms or a deficit picture may be more likely to be treatment resistant (Kirkpatrick *et al*, 2001). Cases with onset in childhood or adolescence may have a poorer prognosis; Meltzer (1997) found that the average age of onset was 5 years earlier in refractory cases.

The landmark study by Kane *et al* (1988*a*) led to the reintroduction of clozapine in the management of treatment-resistant schizophrenia. Because of the known risk of agranulocytosis, the study was confined to a group of very treatment-resistant patients, with poor premorbid functioning for at least 5 years, positive symptoms with high scores on the BPRS, and no response to three different typical antipsychotic drug regimens, including a course of haloperidol 60 mg daily. Clozapine (up to 900 mg daily) was compared with chlorpromazine (up to 1800 mg daily). Around 30% of the patients treated with clozapine responded, compared with only 4% of those treated with chlorpromazine, with significant differences emerging as early as the first week of the study. A significant advantage for clozapine was also found in the treatment of negative symptoms. Subsequent studies have confirmed that clozapine is unrivalled in the management of treatment-resistant schizophrenia. There are also suggestions in the literature that treatment with clozapine may be associated with decreased hospital bed usage, improved quality of life, improved cognition and also decreased risk of violence and suicide.

Clozapine

Indications

NICE (2002) recommends clozapine as the treatment of choice for treatment-resistant schizophrenia. The degree of treatment resistance required today is much less than that required by Kane *et al* (1988*a*), because regular monitoring has since been introduced, which has reduced the risk of agranulocytosis (see above, page 263). Many clinicians will none the less wait considerably longer than two courses of antipsychotics of only 6–8 weeks as recommended by NICE, because of issues such as weight gain and the metabolic syndrome. However, despite this, the trend in the UK is now to initiate clozapine earlier, for younger patients with shorter illness histories. This may help to reduce the number of years lost to an intractable psychosis, but the potential benefit of this has to be weighed against the potential disadvantages of the range of adverse effects. Clozapine is also recommended for patients who develop intolerable EPS and have not done well on other atypicals, and is the only antipsychotic that is associated with alleviation of tardive dyskinesia.

Prescribing clozapine

The dose of clozapine has to be titrated up slowly (in daily increments of 12.5–25 mg). Early side-effects, such as postural hypotension and sedation, usually abate with time. If tolerability of early side-effects is an issue, the titration should be slowed down accordingly. A blood test to monitor the white cell count is undertaken weekly for the first 18 weeks, then fortnightly until week 52 (i.e. after 1 year of treatment) and then monthly thereafter. In most cases, clozapine should be commenced on an in-patient basis to allow close monitoring for side-effects, but it is now accepted that this can also be conducted in a day hospital, or in the community (guidelines have been developed by Novartis for starting clozapine in the community).

The patient's pulse, temperature and blood pressure are measured both before and for up to 3 hours after each dose of clozapine has been taken. Close monitoring of this type needs to continue for around 2 weeks. A rise in temperature above 38°C, heart rate above 100 beats per minute, a postural drop in blood pressure greater than 30 mmHg, the presence of over-sedation or any other untoward side-effect should be reported to the prescriber, and a decision made as to whether to continue with clozapine, and whether monitoring in hospital is required (Taylor *et al*, 2005).

Managing the side-effects of clozapine

The following section provides some suggestions for managing the more common side-effects of clozapine, so that treatment cessation can be avoided. This is particularly relevant for clozapine, as it is usually a treatment of last resort. For more detailed coverage of each effect, see the section on the adverse effects of antipsychotics, above.

During treatment initiation, sedation is very frequent; this can be reduced by introducing the drug more slowly, in smaller increments, or by combating daytime sedation by administering the greater part of the dose at night. Hypersalivation, which many patients find very distressing, should be treated as described on page 256. Constipation may be persistent over the long term, and should be treated with a high-fibre diet and bulk-forming laxatives; stimulant laxatives may also be required. Weight gain may be considerable on clozapine; body weight should be monitored regularly during the treatment initiation phase, with the provision of dietary advice and referral to a dietician as appropriate. A benign low-grade pyrexia is common in the first 3 weeks of therapy and may be treated with standard antipyretics, but neutropenia, agranulocytosis, myocarditis, NMS and infection not due to myelosuppression should be excluded.

Hypotension is also common, for which dosage reduction is usually helpful, with the patient being advised to get up slowly. Hypertension is less common and may respond to a beta-blocker. Tachycardia is common in the initial stages of treatment with clozapine. The risk of this may be reduced by following a slow-titration protocol; if it occurs despite this, an ECG should be done, and it may be necessary to reduce the dose back down to the last dose at which tachycardia was not evident. If it persists, further investigations, including chest radiography, should be conducted; referral to a cardiologist to exclude myocarditis or developing cardiomyopathy should be considered (especially if other symptoms such as shortness of breath are present), and a beta-blocker may be tried, provided there are no contraindications to this. Nausea may respond to any standard anti-emetic, but if metoclopramide is used there is a risk of inducing EPS. Although seizures are dose dependent (see below), they may occur at unexpectedly low doses (e.g. if the individual is a poor metaboliser; Aitchison *et al*, 2000*a*). Nocturnal enuresis is a troublesome side-effect, and may lead to treatment cessation; various agents may be tried. Side-effects that require immediate drug cessation include: agranulocytosis, myocarditis, cardiomyopathy, heat stroke, and an acute confusional state. Haematological monitoring may also reveal neutropenia, eosinophilia, or thrombocytopaenia, which all require close monitoring and consultation with a haematologist. Elevation of hepatic enzyme levels is frequent and usually transient, but rarely pancreatitis and hepatitis can occur, also necessitating drug cessation.

Most patients who are going to respond to clozapine will show some improvement by 12 weeks, at a plasma level of clozapine of 300–350 ng/ml (see below), corresponding to daily doses usually within the range of 300–600 mg. About 90% of those who respond will do so by 18 weeks. The risk of seizures is dose dependent; at doses of 600 mg or above, the use of a prophylactic anticonvulsant such as valproate is recommended (carbamazepine being contraindicated owing to its own risk of causing myelosuppression, and phenytoin also being contraindicated).

Other medications taken with clozapine may present specific hazards. Other antipsychotics (especially some FGAs) also have a risk of myelosuppression, and so may increase the risk of agranulocytosis. There have been reports of respiratory and cardiac arrest in association with concomitant benzodiazepine use. Valproate and SSRIs (fluoxetine and paroxetine) may increase plasma clozapine levels, so monitoring of levels should be conducted with concomitant use of these medications.

Plasma clozapine levels

Although measuring plasma levels is not routinely conducted in the UK for most antipsychotic drugs, in the case of clozapine therapeutic drug monitoring is useful in optimising treatment and monitoring compliance. There is wide inter-individual variation (approximately 10- to 50-fold) in the plasma levels of clozapine for a given dose, and several studies indicate that clozapine concentrations of at least 350–420 ng/ml are associated with clinical response. The first of these was conducted by Perry *et al* (1991), with Hasegawa *et al* (1993) later reporting that a level of 370 ng/ml identified responders with a sensitivity of 67%.

The higher response rate to clozapine in women may be partly due to a plasma-level phenomenon, as oestrogens inhibit CYP1A2 (see above, page 255).

Studies have also shown that side-effects are twice as common when levels of clozapine exceed 350 ng/ml. However, a study of patients on the maximum permitted dose of clozapine, 900 mg/daily, found that some patients had high plasma levels (including greater than 1000 ng/ml), while others had lower levels, with no apparent difference in therapeutic response, which the authors felt was not consistent with a clear therapeutic window for clozapine (Buckley *et al*, 2001). None the less, in the authors' opinion, partial responders and non-responders should have their clozapine and norclozapine levels measured; where the blood level is lower than would be expected for a given dose, the possibility of the patient being either non-compliant or a rapid metaboliser should be considered. Similarly, some patients who are experiencing severe side-effects while on a modest dose may be found to have very high clozapine levels; such patients may be poor metabolisers. In either case, it is suggested that the clozapine dose be adjusted to achieve a plasma level ideally in the range 300–350 ng/ml.

Stopping clozapine

Clozapine should not be stopped abruptly (except in cases such as agranulocytosis, mentioned above), owing to the risk of rebound phenomena, including an exacerbation of the psychosis. A study of 28 patients who were abruptly withdrawn from clozapine (mean dosage 200 mg daily) found that 11 had no withdrawal symptoms and 12 had mild symptoms, but in 4 cases the symptoms were severe (including agitation, headache, nausea, vomiting and diarrhoea), which the authors attributed to cholinergic rebound; of note, this could be readily treated with an anticholinergic drug. Only one case showed a rebound psychosis requiring rehospitalisation (Shiovitz *et al*, 1996). There are several other case reports describing rebound psychosis, akathisia and an acute confusional state, and a failure to respond to other antipsychotics following clozapine withdrawal (Shore, 1995).

What if clozapine fails?

Barnes *et al* (1996) considered some of the pharmacological and psychosocial interventions available for clozapine-resistant schizophrenia; none of the studies reviewed at that time demonstrated any major therapeutic benefits. A common approach in this situation is to try augmentation with other antipsychotics. For example, in Denmark, around a third of patients on clozapine are given an additional antipsychotic. Open studies and case reports for these augmentation strategies have been reported for pimozide, sulpiride, loxapine, olanzapine, risperidone, amisulpride, aripiprazole, quetiapine and lamotrigine; the subject has been reviewed by Taylor *et al* (2005). Most of the reports are positive about using these combinations, but there have been few RCTs. A notable exception to the latter is the RCT of augmentation of clozapine with sulpiride conducted by Shiloh *et al* (1997), who found a 20% reduction in the BPRS score for the sulpiride–clozapine-treated group, compared with placebo augmentation.

On the currently available data, it is not possible to make any specific recommendations, although it is legitimate to try to augment with another antipsychotic (despite a small increased risk of exposure to myelosuppressive agents). With an augmentation strategy, it is important to be aware of potential drug interactions due to CYP450 pathways common to the two antipsychotics (see Table 11.5) and to monitor clozapine levels. SSRI augmentation (e.g. with fluoxetine or paroxetine) of clozapine may also be of benefit, partly by increasing the plasma clozapine level (which should hence be monitored) and also by treating comorbid depressive symptoms. Cognitive–behavioural therapy for psychosis, compliance therapy and family work are also indicated for treatment-resistant patients (and ideally for all patients with schizophrenia if appropriate and available).

The use of ECT in schizophrenia

Before the introduction of chlorpromazine, ECT was used commonly in the management of acute schizophrenia. Its use has since declined, to the extent that NICE (2003) allows the use of ECT in only three conditions: catatonia, a prolonged or severe manic episode, and severe depressive illness. Its use may also be justifiable in NMS, treatment-resistant schizoaffective disorder (where clozapine has been tried and failed), or in patients who are completely unable to tolerate antipsychotics (e.g. for medical reasons). ECT has little or no beneficial effect in chronic schizophrenia but it may be helpful in a small number of acute cases that fail to respond to antipsychotic medication. In the pre-clozapine era, ECT was sometimes used on its own or in combination with antipsychotics and a number of studies (but not RCTs) showed that the combination of ECT with typical drugs was sometimes more effective than either treatment alone (Sackeim, 2003). There has also been interest in the use of ECT combined with clozapine in treatment-resistant patients, some of whom had been resistant to

Box 11.9 Predictors of violence in patients with schizophrenia

Fixed risk factors
- Male gender
- Age (late teens, early twenties)
- Low intelligence
- Head trauma or neurological impairment

In-patient factors
- Nursing staff issues
- Other patients instigating violence
- A large number of detained patients
- A high concentration of very ill patients (with severe psychotic symptoms)

Source: Atakan & Davies (1997); Buckley *et al* (2003).

clozapine alone or ECT alone. These case reports have been summarised by Kupchik *et al* (2000), who found that 67% of the patients improved, although 16% suffered a complication due to either the clozapine or the ECT, such as fits or arrhythmias; despite this, the authors concluded that in certain profoundly treatment-resistant cases, an ECT–clozapine combination might be justifiable. The administration of ECT may, however, result in cognitive impairment and patients should be advised of this during the consent process (NICE, 2003; Royal College of Psychiatrists, 2005).

Rapid tranquillisation

The aims of rapid tranquillisation (RT) are to reduce suffering for the patient (psychological or physical, through self-harm or accidents) and to reduce the risk of harm to others (Box 11.9) by achieving a safe environment (Taylor *et al*, 2005). It is also essential to do no harm (by prescribing safe regimens and monitoring physical health). The intention is to achieve rapid and safe sedation; its primary aim is not to treat the underlying psychosis. Schizophrenia complicated by substance misuse, substance withdrawal or personality disorder may increase the likelihood of having to perform RT. In a survey of 46 emergency services in the USA, restraint was required for 8.4% of all patients (Allen, 2000). However, there is a risk of sudden death with RT (usually due to arrhythmias). During the period in which high doses of intravenous drugs were used in RT, the New York State Commission on Quality of Care reported 110 fatalities over the preceding 10 years (Sundram, 1994). Recent UK figures are not available; however, although intravenous injections are rarely used now and drug doses are generally lower, RT is still associated with risks to the patient, and hence it is essential to adhere to guidelines, including appropriate monitoring (Taylor *et al*, 2005).

Risks to staff administering RT are also high and include assault, personal injury, time off work and post-traumatic stress disorder. In the same US report, the average number of serious assaults per year at each site was eight, of which over 50% resulted in time off work. Nurses were six times more likely to be assaulted than doctors, with most incidents occurring during the restraint procedure (Currier, 2000). Again, comparable UK data are not available, but Dowson *et al* (1999) found that while only 7% of RT episodes were associated with injury to a patient, as many as 40% were associated with injury to a staff member (usually minor, although more severe injuries may occur). Repeated staff training, especially in control and restraint and 'breakaway' techniques, the presence of well-designed facilities with good patient observation areas, adequate numbers of staff and personal security alarms may all help to minimise these risks. A recent trend in the UK has been the development of psychiatric intensive care units (PICUs). Staff in these units are more likely to be adequately trained in RT, and are more likely to use a well-coordinated team approach.

Pharmacological aspects

The Maudsley prescribing guidelines (Taylor *et al*, 2005) for acutely disturbed or violent behaviour provide very useful guidance on the use of drugs in RT, and state that, before resorting to pharmacological management, behavioural approaches (e.g. time out and de-escalation, see below) should be employed. Recent naturalistic data indicate that the majority of interventions for agitated patients with a psychosis in a PICU setting do not require the use of medication (Mantua *et al*, 2006*a*).

Oral drugs

Oral treatment should be offered first. The options include haloperidol 5 mg, or olanzapine 10 mg, or risperidone 1–2 mg. Haloperidol and risperidone are available as syrups, and doses up to 10 mg and 4 mg respectively may be administered, although at higher doses EPS are more likely to be induced, and co-administration of an oral anticholinergic (especially to an antipsychotic-naive patient) is therefore advisable. Olanzapine and risperidone may also be given as orodispersible tablets ('Velotabs' and 'Quicklets' respectively), which are more rapidly absorbed than ordinary tablets. Oral lorazepam 1–2 mg (tablets) may also be used (but should not be combined with intramuscular olanzapine – see below), or promethazine in benzodiazepine-tolerant patients. The NICE (2002) guidelines stipulate that two or more antipsychotics should not be used together but that a benzodiazepine and an antipsychotic may be usefully combined. Oral treatment tends to take longer to bring disturbed behaviour under control, but the potentially dangerous arrhythmias and respiratory depression associated with parenteral treatment are far less likely to occur. Oral administration is also more dignified for patients and will incur much less resentment towards staff, which may have significant long-term implications.

Parenteral drugs

The NICE (2002) guidelines and a review of RT from the same period (McAllister-Williams & Ferrier, 2002) recommended only three drugs for intramuscular injection: haloperidol, olanzapine and lorazepam. Other drugs have since become available in the USA (see Box 11.10). Midazolam 7.5–15 mg has been found to be more rapidly sedating than a combination of haloperidol 5–10 mg and promethazine 50 mg (TREC

Collaborative Group, 2003), but it is rarely used in the UK. Flumazenil must be available if midazolam is given, and administered if the respiratory rate falls below 10 per minute.

Haloperidol

Of the three drugs used in the UK in intramuscular form in RT, experience is greatest with haloperidol, as it has been in clinical use the longest. Its principal drawback in RT is the frequent occurrence of EPS (most often acute dystonia and to a lesser extent acute akathisia). This may be very distressing at the time and may also have a long-term effect on patient compliance. Because of this, the NICE guidelines recommend the routine use of prophylactic anti-Parkinsonian drugs, such as 5–10 mg intramuscular procyclidine, given at the same time or shortly afterwards.

Haloperidol is less cardiotoxic than most other antipsychotics, but can still prolong the QT_c interval. In a study by Reilly *et al* (2000), which demonstrated the association of an increased QT_c interval with thioridazine and droperidol that led to their withdrawal, haloperidol was also shown to increase the QT_c interval, although to a lesser degree. It is also important to note that behavioural disturbance, which is common at the time of RT, may be associated with a prolongation of the QT_c interval by around 50 ms. At one time haloperidol was commonly given intravenously, but this route is now thought to carry an increased risk of cardiotoxicity, because the heart may be abruptly exposed to a bolus of the drug, which may increase the risk of arrhythmias. Thus if intravenous haloperidol is used, it should be administered slowly and through a butterfly needle. The NICE guidelines indicate that intravenous haloperidol should be used only 'in exceptional circumstances', while the Maudsley guidelines (Taylor *et al*, 2005) no longer recommend intravenous haloperidol.

Olanzapine

Intramuscular olanzapine has been available in the UK since 2000. It is contraindicated in the presence of cardiovascular disease, including unstable angina, severe hypotension or bradycardia, as well as narrow-angle glaucoma, and NICE recommends intramuscular olanzapine only for moderate behavioural disturbance. The maximum plasma concentration (C_{max}) produced by intramuscular olanzapine is five times that of the corresponding oral dose (Eli Lilly information leaflet on www.fda.gov). An RCT (sponsored by Eli Lilly) of behaviourally disturbed patients suffering from schizophrenia compared 10 mg intramuscular olanzapine and 7.5 mg intramuscular haloperidol with placebo; it showed that both achieved useful and equal degrees of tranquillisation at 2 and 24 hours, but that olanzapine had a significant advantage in the first 45 minutes. The main advantage of olanzapine in this trial was that no patient developed dystonia, an acutely distressing symptom, whereas this occurred in 7% of the haloperidol-treated participants. EPS occurred with both drugs, but rates were lower for intramuscular olanzapine, as indicated by the frequency of anticholinergic use (20% for intramuscular haloperidol versus 5% for intramuscular olanzapine). Changes in the QT_c interval for olanzapine did not differ significantly from placebo (Wright *et al*, 2001). The results of a later trial were also published (Breier *et al*, 2002) and further data are emerging from a more naturalistic study of the use of intramuscular medications in PICU settings (Mantua *et al*, 2006*b*).

An initial dose of 5–10 mg olanzapine is recommended in the BNF; a total of three injections may be given in 24 hours, with a minimum of 2 hours between the first and second injection, up to a maximum cumulative dose (including any oral olanzapine) of 20 mg. In those with renal or hepatic impairment, the dose should be reduced to 5 mg, and to 2.5–5 mg in the elderly. Lower doses should also be considered in the presence of one or more factors that slow metabolism (e.g. females of relatively low body weight, females taking oral contraceptives, or female non-smokers). It is contraindicated in those with narrow-angle glaucoma and those with an unstable cardiovascular condition. The more common side-effects include dizziness (most often due to postural hypotension), bradycardia or tachycardia, and less commonly sinus pause and hypoventilation.

Olanzapine is highly sedative, having 160 times the antihistaminic potency of a standard antihistamine such as diphenhydramine (Currier, 2000). This means that an adequate level of sedation may usually be achieved without the need for additional sedatives; in fact, the simultaneous injection of olanzapine with parenteral benzodiazepines is *not* recommended because of the risk of over-sedation. If parenteral benzodiazepines are considered to be essential, the benzodiazepine injection should be given a minimum of 1 hour after the olanzapine; similarly, if intramuscular olanzapine is to be given after the administration of a parenteral benzodiazepine, the level of sedation should be carefully evaluated before the injection of olanzapine is given and then vital signs closely monitored afterwards.

Benzodiazepines

Benzodiazepines are sedative, anxiolytic and anti-epileptic. Importantly, they are non-cardiotoxic and have a wide therapeutic index. Their main risks are over-sedation and respiratory depression, but such effects may be reversed with the antagonist flumazenil. Other risks include behavioural disinhibition (a 'paradoxical reaction' particularly relevant in the context of violent patients) and, with prolonged use, dependence.

The use of diazepam in RT has declined, with intramuscular lorazepam becoming the benzodiazepine of choice in this setting. Intramuscular diazepam (solution, 5 mg/ml) is slower acting than intramuscular haloperidol, reaching peak plasma levels 1–3 hours after injection. Intravenous diazepam is associated with a high risk of venous thrombophlebitis, which may be reduced by using the emulsion formulation (Diazemuls), but this route should be used only if a very rapid effect is required, and it is essential to monitor vital signs and have flumazenil and resuscitation equipment available.

Benzodiazepines may be administered alone but are generally given in conjunction with haloperidol during RT. A trial by Garza-Trevino *et al* (1989) found that adequate tranquillisation was achieved within 30 minutes by 33% of patients given 5 mg intramuscular haloperidol alone, by 39% given 4 mg intramuscular lorazepam alone, and by 75% of patients given both drugs and without any increase in adverse effects. For many years, a common combination used in RT has been haloperidol 5–10 mg together with lorazepam 1–2 mg.

A retrospective analysis (Salzman *et al*, 1986) found that the mean dose of haloperidol used when given in combination with lorazepam was half that used when haloperidol was given alone. Benzodiazepines may also help counter akathisia (which can worsen agitation) as well as countering the reduction of seizure threshold caused by antipsychotics. However, the risk of over-sedation or a cardiorespiratory event is increased when these drugs are used in combination.

Zuclophenthixol

Zuclopenthixol acetate (Clopixol Acuphase) is indicated for the short-term management of acute psychosis in situations in which repeated injections of shorter-acting intramuscular drugs, as above, have already been required (Taylor *et al*, 2005) and when enough time has elapsed to assess the full response to previously injected drugs. It is *not* recommended as a first-line agent in RT. The antipsychotic effect persists for 2–3 days. Zuclopenthixol should never be used in adolescents or neuroleptic-naive patients because of its prolonged action, nor with other parenteral antipsychotics, depot drugs or benzodiazepines. Dosage is 50–150 mg (in the elderly 50–100 mg) and should be repeated only after 2–3 days (with one additional dose being permitted 1–2 days after the first injection). Up to four injections can be given over 2 weeks but the cumulative dose should not exceed 400 mg (BNF).

Box 11.10 Strategies for rapid tranquillisation

Offer oral medication

- Haloperidol (5–10 mg) or
- Olanzapine (Velotab, e.g. 10 mg) or
- Risperidone (orodispersible or liquid, e.g. 2 mg)
- All of the above may be given with or without lorazepam 1–2 mg

Consider intramuscular treatment (and consider consultation with a senior colleague)

- Lorazepam (1–2 mg)[a] or
- Haloperidol (5 mg) or
- Olanzapine (5–10 mg or less in certain patient groups)[b]
- Ziprasidone 10–20 mg intramuscular or aripiprazole 10 mg intramuscular[c]
- Promethazine 50 mg intramuscular is an alternative to lorazepam in benzodiazepine-tolerant patients; it has a slower onset of action.

Consider intravenous treatment

- Intravenous midazolam injected slowly
- Intravenous diazepam (up to 10 mg, titrated slowly against clinical response over at least 5 minutes)
- Both the above drugs should be used only in exceptional circumstances, when a rapid effect is desired
- Intravenous antipsychotics are no longer recommended
- Expert advice must be sought if intravenous midazolam or diazepam fails to sedate

[a] Post-administration monitoring of vital signs is essential after intramuscular or intravenous benzodiazepine, with flumazenil available and given if the respiratory rate drops below 10 per minute.
[b] Relatively low risk of dystonia or prolongation of the QT_c interval.
[c] Available in the USA but not in the UK.
After Taylor *et al* (2005).

Algorithms and special situations

Trusts publish guidelines on RT, which usually include an algorithm on drug selection; an example from the Maudsley prescribing guidelines (Taylor *et al*, 2005) is shown in Box 11.10. A frequent problem with algorithms is that many patients have some 'special circumstances' that complicate the protocol, which requires clinicians to use their own judgement in addition. A common example is drug or alcohol misuse (which may not be known at the time, although the increasing use of urine dipsticks that can identify drugs of misuse may lead to better recognition of this problem), in which circumstances the use of antipsychotics is preferable to benzodiazepines. In the elderly, low doses of benzodiazepines are preferred, owing to the risk of EPS with FGAs and cerebrovascular accidents with some SGAs. Younger patients with learning difficulties, head injury or other neurological disorders are also at high risk of EPS and so in these an atypical may be preferred, and a benzodiazepine contraindicated owing to the increased risk of disinhibition. The NICE (2002) guidelines specifically recommend that atypicals should be used for RT in new cases of schizophrenia.

Non-pharmacological aspects of managing acute disturbance

It is essential to collate the relevant information, such as precipitants of the crisis that led to the need for RT, previous incidents and the presence of any immediate risks such as a weapon. Of particular importance to the doctor will be the medical history, including history of violence, previous reactions to psychotropic drugs and whether or not alcohol or other drugs (illicit or prescribed) have been taken. Behavioural approaches such as time-out and de-escalation by dialogue and negotiation should be tried initially, and then oral medication should be offered if necessary.

Administration of an intramuscular antipsychotic for acute disturbance

For the more disturbed patient, physical restraint and parenteral medication may be required. Strictly this is a nursing procedure, but junior doctors will usually be summoned and may need to be 'hands on', so it is helpful if they understand the protocol. Each trust will have its own procedure. Table 11.14, adapted from Ritter (1989), sets out an example protocol for the administration of an injection without the patient's consent, and the rationale underlying each step.

Monitoring patients after the injection

The overall rate of serious medical complications following RT is relatively low. Pilowsky *et al* (1992) gave a figure of 2–3%. Nevertheless, most mental health trusts require nursing staff to monitor patients closely after RT, for example by recording pulse and respiration rate and blood pressure at 5-minute intervals for the first hour and at a decreased frequency

Table 11.14 Administering an injection without the patient's consent

Steps	Rationale
1. The nurse in charge of the ward or unit directs the procedure	Only one person only gives the instructions, which are immediately followed
2. If there are fewer than 8 members of staff present, staff should be summoned from other wards	A minimum of 6 people are required for the injection: 4 to restrain the patient, 1 to draw up and check the injection and 1 to administer it. Two nurses are required to look after the rest of the ward
3. The nurse in charge outlines the situation that has led up to the present crisis, including information about the size and likely strength of the patient	Everyone should have some acquaintance with the patient and should be aware of the particular risks involved
4. Members of staff remove all personal jewellery, badges, pens, etc.	This reduces the likelihood of personal injury
5. The nurse in charge assigns roles for each nurse in the restraint procedure	All nurses should be fully trained in 'control and restraint' procedures. One nurse should be assigned for each arm, one for the body, and one for both legs. For larger male patients more nurses may be required to restrain the patient. A pillow or soft rug is placed under the patient's head and a nurse seeks to maintain the patient's head still during the procedure
6. The nurse in charge carries an oral preparation, e.g. a syrup, and approaches the patient followed by the nurse responsible for administering the injection	In a non-confrontational manner it is made clear to the patient that he or she will be receiving medication (it is assumed that the patient has previously refused)
7. The nurse in charge asks the patient to take the oral medication	This offers the patient another opportunity to take control of the situation
8. If the patient refuses, at an agreed signal, the whole team move quickly to restrain and immobilise the patient	Immobilisation will reduce the risk of injury to both patient and staff
9. If a struggle ensues, it may be best to wait until the patient is still before administering an injection	Giving an injection during a struggle may be hazardous and lead to arterial or nerve damage
10. The injection may have to be given through the patient's clothes	It may not be possible to remove the patient's clothing without jeopardising the team's effort at immobilisation
11. The injection is administered intramuscularly to the upper outer quadrant of the buttock or the middle third of the outer aspect of the thigh	These regions have relatively few major nerves or arteries
12. While the injection is being given, the nurse in charge continues to talk to the patient in an attempt to explain the procedure to them and in a calming manner	Every effort should be made to continue to calm the patient down. Very high anxiety levels may prolong the QT_c intervals and have been associated with sudden death
13. After the injection, the team remain in position until it is confirmed that the patient is calm enough to be released	Intramuscular administration may take 10–30 minutes to be effective. Premature release of an irritable psychotic patient may lead to a recurrence of disturbed behaviour
14. At least one nurse should remain with the patient afterwards	To monitor vital signs and in case the patient becomes disturbed again
15. The procedure should be carried out while the patient is detained under the Mental Health Act 1983	To avoid a later charge of assault. Section 141 of the Act offers some legal protection as it allows staff 'to maintain good order in the running of the hospital'
16. Rarely, in dire circumstances, it is possible to carry out the procedure under common law (see page 425), but if this is done, steps should immediately be taken to institute the Mental Health Act	To comply with the law
17. An incident form is completed and an appropriate entry made in the medical notes	The Mental Health Commission will inspect all reports of such incidents to ensure that current best practice has been observed

After Ritter (1989).

thereafter. Continuous recordings are facilitated by pulse oximetry, and temperature measurements may also be indicated.

The main potential medical complications of RT are as follows:

- *Cardiac rhythm effects – bradycardia, tachycardia, prolonged QT_c interval or other arrhythmias.* Anti-arrhythmics should be available and if cardiovascular complications occur then a general medical opinion should be urgently sought.
- *Acute hypotension.* The patient should be laid flat and the legs elevated. Acute hypotension was quite common when chlorpromazine was widely used, but is now less common.

- *Respiratory depression.* This is more likely when parenteral benzodiazepines are used and where alcohol, opiates or other drugs have been taken but not declared to the team at the time of the RT. If the respiratory rate falls below 10 per minute, the benzodiazepine antagonist flumazenil should be administered in small doses (200 μg) followed by 100 μg doses at 60-second intervals if required. Resuscitation equipment and staff trained to administer this must be available.
- *Acute dystonia.* If haloperidol is given intramuscularly, the risk of acute dystonia may be reduced by concomitant administration of an anticholinergic, such as procyclidine 10 mg intramuscularly or benzatropine 1–2 mg intramuscularly. Oral procyclidine should also be started as the parenteral dose will wear off after 4–6 hours.
- *Epileptic seizures.* Patients with epilepsy may default on both their antipsychotics and anti-epileptics, and their drug status may not be known at the time of the emergency restraint. Haloperidol reduces the seizure threshold, while benzodiazepines have anti-epileptic effects. Intravenous Diazemuls should be administered but an intravenous infusion may be indicated if fits recur or status epilepticus develops.
- *Local complications.* Pain, bruising and extravasation are common. Once the patient is settled the injection site should be inspected.
- *Fever.* This is rare but if present may indicate the onset of NMS or, more commonly, an undiagnosed infection, which may in itself have contributed to the behavioural disturbance (e.g. in cases of acute confusional states).

Catatonia

The main clinical features of catatonia are outlined in Chapter 8 on page 175. Antipsychotics (especially those with significant D_2 antagonism) should be avoided in any type of catatonia. Kahlbaum's original description of catatonia was made in 1873, before Kraepelin and Bleuler had developed the concept of schizophrenia, but the condition figured prominently in Kraepelin's descriptions of dementia praecox. Kahlbaum characterised catatonia as a progressive motor disorder typically with phases of mania, depression or psychosis which led on to dementia. In the pre-treatment era, a primary catatonic illness was relatively common, occurring in up to 20% of new cases of psychosis. Today, such presentations are relatively rare.

In more recent series, up to 25% of patients presenting with catatonia have had mania. Catatonia can also be a presenting feature of a wide variety of metabolic and neurological disorders (e.g. tumours). Therefore a new case of catatonia merits a comprehensive physical as well as psychiatric assessment, including neuroimaging. Rare familial types, such as Gjessing's periodic catatonia (alternating phases of catatonic stupor and catatonic excitement), have also been described.

There are case reports of catatonic states associated with exposure to or cessation of certain drugs, including amantadine (a dopaminergic agonist), illicit drugs, opiates and some antipsychotics. Catatonia may therefore be related to rapid changes in dopaminergic neurotransmission.

Malignant catatonia (or 'lethal catatonia') is a rare but potentially fatal condition that was more commonly seen prior to the advent of ECT. It is characterised by catatonic psychotic excitement followed by features similar to NMS, occurring in the absence of antipsychotic treatment.

Catatonic stupors were sometimes fatal, as a result of starvation or infection. 'Catatonic schizophrenia' is now rarely seen in the UK, but catatonia may be seen in other subtypes of schizophrenia as well as in other psychiatric and organic conditions as listed above. The management of malignant catatonia is similar to that of NMS. Mild cases usually respond to a benzodiazepine such as lorazepam given either orally or parenterally, while more severe cases may also require ECT. Antipsychotics must be avoided.

Depression in schizophrenia

Depression is very common in all phases of schizophrenia; proportions of patients affected range from 7% to 75%, with the modal rate of depression in schizophrenia being reported as 25% (Siris *et al*, 2000). The majority of patients are likely to be affected with significant depressive features at some point, whether related to the illness itself or 'pharmacogenic' (e.g. antipsychotic induced). Concurrent substance misuse or sudden withdrawal of substances such as cannabis, cocaine, opiates, alcohol and tobacco may also lead to depression. Other causes of depressive symptoms include 'post-psychotic depression', induced by patients becoming distressed on gaining insight that they have a psychotic illness, with its associated loss issues. Although adverse life events are more likely to trigger a psychotic relapse in schizophrenia, they may also trigger a depressive episode.

However, it is now thought that the most common reason for depressive symptoms in schizophrenia is that they are an integral part of the illness itself. Sax *et al* (1996) examined a group of first-episode patients with schizophrenia who had not been exposed to any psychotropic medication. They found a strong correlation between the presence of depressive and positive symptoms, particularly persecutory delusions and auditory hallucinations. This is not surprising, owing to the intense distress generated by delusions and hallucinations of a persecutory nature. Negative symptoms were also correlated, but this association is more difficult to interpret, owing to the significant overlap between negative and depressive symptoms.

Treatment studies with both FGAs and SGAs have shown that depressive symptoms tend to improve in parallel with improvements in psychotic symptoms. Some atypical antipsychotics appear to have a greater antidepressant effect than the typical drugs. For example, in an olanzapine registration trial (Tollefson *et al*, 1997) at baseline 55% of the patients had a score on the Montgomery–Asberg Depression Rating Scale (MADRS) of more than 16, signifying moderate depression. A greater than 50% reduction in the MADRS score occurred in 48% of the olanzapine-treated group compared with 37% of the haloperidol-treated group.

Levinson *et al* (1999) reviewed studies of the use of antidepressants and lithium in schizoaffective disorder ($n = 15$) and schizophrenia ($n = 18$); their principal conclusion was that there was no evidence from RCTs that antidepressants were effective against depressive symptoms in either schizophrenia or schizoaffective disorder, whereas antipsychotics were. Their main recommendation therefore was to optimise the antipsychotic treatment regimen. They further commented that atypicals appeared to be more useful than typicals in the treatment of depressive symptoms in schizophrenia and this has now been incorporated into the NICE (2002) recommendations. They also reviewed some studies in which tricyclic antidepressants had resulted in a worsening of schizophrenic symptoms, such as increased agitation.

However, diagnostic issues and the recognition of certain subgroups may be important. For example, a subgroup of patients already established on an antipsychotic who *de novo* develop an episode of major depression may benefit from a course of antidepressants. In schizoaffective disorder, mood stabilisers are often helpful, and in schizoaffective disorder, depressive type, antidepressants may in addition be indicated. An open study suggested that clozapine was particularly useful among those patients with treatment-resistant schizophrenia who were also depressed (McElroy *et al*, 1991). In recent years there have also been numerous open studies of SSRIs and venlafaxine in patients with schizophrenia with depression. All of these studies report some benefit, but it is important to note that as yet there have been no reported RCTs in this area. This is partly owing to the difficulty of measuring depressive symptoms in schizophrenia. The consensus now is that the Calgary Depression Scale is better for measuring depression in schizophrenia than rating scales that were designed to measure symptom severity in depression (such as the MADRS).

Despite the lack of robust evidence, most clinicians will still prescribe an antidepressant, usually an SSRI, when they observe depression in patients with schizophrenia. It is important to monitor the patient closely, in case the antidepressant results in destabilisation or side-effects, which may be due to both pharmacodynamic and pharmacokinetic effects. It is wise to start with a low dose of an antidepressant, and increase this only gradually, if tolerated. Moreover, psychosocial approaches should be tried before psychopharmacological ones, and continued after commencement of an antidepressant should that prove necessary.

Can antipsychotics prevent suicide?

It is estimated that around 10% of patients with schizophrenia commit suicide, which corresponds to an annual rate of 0.4–0.8%. Clozapine may substantially reduce this risk. Novartis, the manufacturer of clozapine, reported an annual suicide rate of 34 out of 51 333 treated patients (0.06% per year), which is a tenth of the above rate. In the InterSept trial (Meltzer *et al*, 2003), a 2-year study that compared clozapine with olanzapine in 980 patients with schizophrenia, there was a lower rate of suicidal behaviour in the clozapine group (20.8%) than in the olanzapine group (28.8%). This apparent 'anti-suicide' effect has not yet been found for any other antipsychotic. Moreover, the effect may be even larger than it appears to be, as clozapine is prescribed in the UK and USA only for treatment-resistant, more severe cases, which untreated would probably have a risk of suicide higher than average in schizophrenia.

Pharmacoeconomics of antipsychotics

Like the more recent introduction of the atypicals, the introduction of chlorpromazine 50 years ago was associated with difficulties in gaining permission from budget holders to fund the use of the drug. Duval & Goldman, in a 1956 article entitled 'The new drugs (chlorpromazine and reserpine): administrative aspects', wrote:

> 'we are all aware there is a huge rumble to be heard concerning the budgetary aspects. An ordinary modest drug budget of a state hospital of say 3,000 patients is suddenly increased from its normal $15,000 a year to twenty times that figure! Instead of giving drugs to two or three hundred patients in small doses we find ourselves giving massive doses to one thousand or fifteen hundred: we would like to expand it to two thousand or more because we feel they would benefit. Yet at the same time we are asking money for additional staff….' (Duval & Goldman, 2000)

While the introduction of any new and potentially successful drug is a source of hope for both patients and medical staff, it also tends to cause conflict between healthcare commissioners and the pharmaceutical industry. The costs of developing an unsuccessful drug are borne entirely by the pharmaceutical industry and it is only with the launch of a successful product that pharmaceutical companies recoup some of their development costs. Owing to the costs of drug development, the initial list price of newly introduced drugs tends to be high and, in order to minimise expenditure, healthcare commissioners and governments may discourage the use of these. For example, the NICE (2002) guidelines on schizophrenia state 'where more than one atypical is appropriate, the drug with the lowest purchase price should be prescribed'.

In the field of pharmacoeconomics, the clinical benefits versus costs of treatment with a specific drug may be studied using various methods (e.g. cost-effectiveness analysis). This is an increasingly important field in healthcare. For example, following the introduction of the SSRIs, the UK government continued to recommend the first-line use of tricyclics, mainly on the grounds of cost. However, industry-sponsored pharmacoeconomic studies of the SSRIs at the time demonstrated that SSRIs were no more costly than tricyclic antidepressants when total costs associated with administering a particular drug were considered, especially after the high costs of treating fractured hips in the elderly due to medication-induced falls was included. Similarly, after the introduction of atypicals between 1995 and 2000, editorials in prominent journals and official recommendations were not clear as to whether their high cost (see Table 11.15) could be justified by their apparently more benign side-effect profile, since there was no clear advantage in terms of efficacy. The meta-analysis by Geddes *et al* (2000) concluded that 'typical drugs should

Table 11.15 Comparison of prescription costs of atypical antipsychotics and haloperidol

Antipsychotic	Mean dose (mg)[a]	Cost per year per patient (£)	Ratio of cost to haloperidol
Haloperidol	18.7	19	1:1
Clozapine	469.8	710	37:1
Olanzapine	13.8	1860	98:1
Risperidone	4.4	917	48:1
Quetiapine	430.3	1460	77:1
Amisulpride	592.6	1118	59:1
Aripiprazole	20.0	2076	109:1

[a] Mean dose obtained from an audit of prescribing practice in the South London and Maudsley NHS Trust (Dr David Taylor, personal communication); these costs were calculated on the basis of 2005 drug tariff and purchase price for this London mental health trust.

remain first line treatment and atypicals should be used only when EPS is a problem'. Two years later the NICE (2002) guidelines recommended that 'atypical drugs should be considered among first-line treatments'. Pharmacoeconomic studies of SGAs (usually industry sponsored) have tended to 'prove' that, although these drugs are more expensive than FGAs, once the total aspects of disease costs (including hospital admission) have been taken into account, they are cost-effective.

Pharmacoeconomic issues play a significant role in determining whether or not a drug is allowed in a hospital or primary care drug formulary. In developing countries, the high initial cost of the atypicals precludes their use and so the FGAs continue to be the mainstay of treatment.

Can the cost of schizophrenia be measured?

Although the point prevalence of schizophrenia has been estimated at approximately 1% (Eaton, 1991), 2.76% of the National Health Service budget is spent on the care of patients with schizophrenia (Knapp, 1997). This can be explained by its chronic nature and the high cost of hospitalisation, with the drug budget comprising only 5% of the total cost (NICE, 2002). Studies indicate that between 10% and 40% of individuals with a first episode of schizophrenia never experience a readmission. In addition, the rate of relapse within the first 2 years is 40–60%, and most readmissions occur within the first 5 years of the illness (Engelhardt *et al*, 1982; Ram *et al*, 1992; van Os *et al*, 1996). Differences in outcome should be borne in mind, as at least some of the pharmacoeconomic studies have been performed on 'treatment-resistant patients'. Davies & Drummond (1994), in a modelling study, estimated that approximately 10% of patients incurred about 90% of the direct costs of schizophrenia. A medication that is cost-effective in this group of patients would therefore have the potential to result in highly significant savings overall. Costs include those that are direct (e.g. hospitalisation, residential care, day care and medication) and those that are indirect (e.g. lost employment and earnings by the sufferers and family members caring for them). Many studies look only at the direct costs of the illness and ignore the substantial burden placed on the sufferer and family in terms of lost productivity. Indirect costs at a 'conservative estimate' account for up to 75% of the total lifetime costs (Davies & Drummond, 1994). Some costs of schizophrenia cannot be readily expressed in monetary terms but are arguably much more significant. These include the psychological impact of symptoms, and the psychological and social sequelae for carers. These are important facets of 'quality of life'. There is also the grave impact of early mortality in schizophrenia, including death by suicide (Brown *et al*, 2000).

Examples of pharmacoeconomic studies

Rosenheck *et al* (1997) conducted a year-long, randomised, double-blind trial of clozapine and haloperidol in the US, targeting treatment-refractory patients with high levels of hospitalisation. The mean (SD) daily dose of haloperidol was high, at 28 (5.3) mg. In the intention-to-treat analysis, there was no statistical difference in symptom reduction at 1 year. However, if the crossovers are excluded, including the 22% of patients in the haloperidol group who received 4 weeks or more of clozapine, then clozapine was found to be significantly more effective than haloperidol. Although there was no significant difference in the overall costs, there was a trend for lower total costs in the clozapine group. Rosenheck *et al* (1999) then reanalysed their data by looking at the impact of clozapine in the highest tertile of hospital users (mean 215 bed-days) compared with those in the lowest two tertiles (mean 58 bed-days); they found that cost savings were seen in high bed users but these did not generalise to low bed users, indicating that clozapine was more cost-effective with the more severely affected patients. Essock *et al* (2000) performed a 2-year, open-label, double-blind, RCT comparing the cost-effectiveness of clozapine with usual care. On an intention-to-treat analysis, there were no significant differences in symptom reduction or costs. However, the clozapine group cost US$1112 more than usual care in year 1 but US$7149 less in year 2.

'Mirror image' design studies that compared the pre- and post-initiation costs of clozapine treatment have also been performed (Aitchison & Kerwin, 1997; Meltzer, 1997). The former was a UK-based study of 26 patients that compared the costs in the 3 years before and the 3 years after initiation of clozapine. Clozapine was found to be significantly more cost-effective than the prior treatment regimen, with a mean cost saving of £3768 per patient per year. One difficulty with this type of study is its vulnerability to cohort effects, unless it also includes a contemporaneous rather than a historical control group, to control for longitudinal changes, for example in admission policy or drug prices. However, in this study, the mean length of hospitalisation increased after the introduction of clozapine (i.e. in the opposite direction to that which would be required if the reduced costs with clozapine were due merely to a change in admission policy).

Similar pharmacoeconomic studies have been conducted for many other atypicals (Tandon & Aitchison, 2002), which become more cost-effective as they become generic (e.g. now that clozapine is generic, the mean annual cost per patient has fallen from about £33,000 to about £1000, as above). The cost-effectivenes of Risperdal Consta has been the subject of a number of studies, for review and commentary on which see Haycox (2005) and Annemans (2005).

Clearly, where an antipsychotic is effective and tolerated in schizophrenia, it is cost-effective to prescribe it. The challenge, then, for clinicians, in the absence of widely available pharmacogenetic testing, is to negotiate with their patients with schizophrenia and their carers to identify the most appropriate pharmacological regimen to prescribe in each case. It is our hope that this chapter will have provided information to assist clinicians in this process.

Declaration of interest

Dr Katherine J. Aitchison is on the UK Core Steering Group for Abilify, and has received research grant funding and consultancy payments from both Bristol-Myers Squibb Pharmaceuticals Limited and Johnson and Johnson Pharmaceutical Research and Development. She has also been the recipient of a Lilly Travelling Fellowship from the Royal College of Psychiatrists, conference attendance support from Sanofi-Synthelabo, and medication for a research study from Lundbeck Limited. In addition, she has support for research and consultancy fees from Roche Diagnostics Limited.

Acknowledgements

We thank Dr J. Cookson, Dr S. Frangou, Dr S. Mahli and Mr C. Holvey for comments on the manuscript. We also thank Dr G. Stein for his assistance with this chapter, and Dr V. D. M. McAllister for her contributions.

References

Adler, L. A., Peselow, E., Rotrosen, J., *et al* (1993) Vitamin E treatment of tardive dyskinesia. *American Journal of Psychiatry*, **150**, 1405–1407.

Adnet, P., Lestavel, P. & Krivosic-Horber, R. (2000) Neuroleptic malignant syndrome. *British Journal of Anaesthesia*, **85**, 129–135.

Aitchison, K. J. & Kerwin, R. W. (1997) Cost-effectiveness of clozapine. A UK clinic-based study. *British Journal of Psychiatry*, **171**, 125–130.

Aitchison, K. J., Meehan K. & Murray R. M. (1999) *First Episode Psychosis*. London: Martin Dunitz.

Aitchison, K. J., Jann, M. W., Zhao, J. H., *et al* (2000*a*) Clozapine pharmacokinetics and pharmacodynamics studied with CYP1A2-null mice. *Journal of Psychopharmacology*, **14**, 353–359.

Aitchison, K. J., Jordan, B. D. & Sharma, T. (2000*b*) The relevance of ethnic influences on pharma-cogenetics to the treatment of psychosis. *Drug Metabolism and Drug Interactions*, **16**, 15–38.

Allen, M. H. (2000) Managing the agitated psychotic patient: a reappraisal of the evidence. *Journal of Clinical Psychiatry*, **61**, suppl. 14, 11–20.

Allison, D. B., Mentore, J. L., Heo, M., *et al* (1999) Antipsychotic-induced weight gain: a comprehensive research synthesis. *American Journal of Psychiatry*, **156**, 1686–1696.

American Diabetes Association; American Psychiatric Association; American Association of Clinical Endocrinologists & North American Association for the Study of Obesity (2004) Consensus development conference on antipsychotic drugs and obesity and diabetes. *Diabetes Care*, **27**, 596–601.

American Psychiatric Association (1992) *Tardive Dyskinesia: A Task Force Report of the American Psychiatric Association*. Washington, DC: APA.

American Psychiatric Association (1994) *Diagnostic and Statistical Manual of Mental Disorders* (4th edn) (DSM–IV). Washington, DC: APA.

American Psychiatric Association (1997) Practice guideline for the treatment of patients with schizophrenia. *American Journal of Psychiatry*, **154**, 1–63.

American Psychiatric Association (2000) *Diagnostic and Statistical Manual of Mental Disorders* (4th edn, text revision) (DSM–IV–TR). Washington, DC: APA.

American Psychiatric Association (2004) *Practice Guideline for the Treatment of Patients with Schizophrenia* (2nd edn). Washington, DC: APA.

Annemans, L. (2005) Cost effectiveness of long-acting risperidone: what can pharmacoeconomic models teach us? *Pharmacoeconomics*, **23**, suppl. 1, 1–2.

Arnt, J. & Skarsfeldt, T. (1998) Do novel antipsychotics have similar pharmacological characteristics? A review of the evidence. *Neuropsychopharmacology*, **18**, 63–101.

Atakan, Z. & Davies, T. (1997) ABC of mental health. Mental health emergencies. *BMJ*, **314**, 1740–1742.

Atkin, K., Kendall, F., Gould, D., *et al* (1996) Neutropenia and agranulocytosis in patients receiving clozapine in the UK and Ireland. *British Journal of Psychiatry*, **169**, 483–488.

Bagnall, A., Lewis, R. A., Leitner, M. L., *et al* (2000) Ziprasidone for schizophrenia and severe mental illness. *Cochrane Database of Systematic Reviews*, (**2**), CD001945.

Bakker, P. R., van Harten, P. N. & van Os, J. (2006) Antipsychotic-induced tardive dyskinesia and the Ser9Gly polymorphism in the DRD3 gene: a meta analysis. *Schizophrenia Research*, **83**, 185–192.

Baldessarini, R. J., Cohen, B. M. & Teicher, M. H. (1988) Significance of neuroleptic dose and plasma level in the pharmacological treatment of psychoses. *Archives of General Psychiatry*, **45**, 79–91.

Bareggi, S. R., Mauri, M., Cavallaro, R., *et al* (1990) Factors affecting the clinical response to haloperidol therapy in schizophrenia. *Clinical Neuropharmacology*, **13**, suppl. 1, S29–S34.

Barnes, T. R. (1989) A rating scale for drug-induced akathisia. *British Journal of Psychiatry*, **154**, 672–676.

Barnes, T. R. (1992) Clinical assessment of the extrapyramidal side effects of antipsychotic drugs. *Journal of Psychopharmacology*, **6**, 214–221.

Barnes, T. R. E., McEvedy, C. J. B. & Nelson, H. E. (1996) Management of treatment resistant schizophrenia unresponsive to clozapine. *British Journal of Psychiatry*, **169**, suppl. 31, 31–40.

Basu, A., Tsapakis, E. M., Aitchison, K. J. (2004) Pharmacogenetics and psychiatry. *Current Psychiatry Reports*, **6**, 134–142.

Beasley, C. M. Jr, Tollefson, G. D. & Tran, P. V. (1997) Safety of olanzapine. *Journal of Clinical Psychiatry*, **58**, suppl. 10, 13–17.

Bebbington, P. E. (1995) The content and context of compliance. *International Clinical Psychopharmacology*, **9**, 41–50.

Berk, M., Ichim, C. & Brook, S. (2001) Efficacy of mirtazapine add on therapy to haloperidol in the treatment of the negative symptoms of schizophrenia: a double-blind randomized placebo-controlled study. *International Clinical Psychopharmacology*, **16**, 87–92.

Bertilsson, L., Meese, C. O., Yue, Q. Y., *et al* (1993) Quinidine inhibition of debrisoquine S(+)-4- and 7-hydroxylations in Chinese of different CYP2D6 genotypes. *Pharmacogenetics*, **3**, 94–100.

Bhatara, V. S., Sharma, J. N., Gupta, S., *et al* (1997) Images in psychiatry. *Rauwolfia serpentia*: the first herbal antipsychotic. *American Journal of Psychiatry*, **154**, 894.

Bigliani, V., Mulligan, R. S., Acton, P. D., *et al* (1999) In vivo occupancy of striatal and temporal cortical D_2/D_3 dopamine receptors by typical antipsychotic drugs. [^{123}I]epidepride single photon emission tomography (SPET) study. *British Journal of Psychiatry*, **175**, 231–238.

Bollini, P., Pampallona, S., Orza, M. J., *et al* (1994) Antipsychotic drugs: is more worse? A meta-analysis of the published randomized control trials. *Psychological Medicine*, **24**, 307–316.

Breier, A., Meehan, K., Birkett M., *et al* (2002) A double-blind, placebo-controlled dose–response comparison of intramuscular olanzapine and haloperidol in the treatment of acute agitation in schizophrenia. *Archives of General Psychiatry*, **59**, 441–448.

British National Formulary (*BNF*) (bi-annual publication) London: British Medical Association and the Royal Pharmaceutical Society of Great Britain.

Brown, S., Inskip, H. & Barraclough, B. (2000) Causes of the excess mortality of schizophrenia. *British Journal of Psychiatry*, **177**, 212–217.

Buckley, P. F., Friedman, L., Krowinski, A. C., *et al* (2001) Clinical and biochemical correlates of 'high-dose' clozapine therapy for treatment-refractory schizophrenia. *Schizophrenia Research*, **49**, 225–227.

Buckley, P. F., Noffsinger, S. G., Smith, D. A., *et al* (2003) Treatment of the psychotic patient who is violent. *Psychiatric Clinics of North America*, **26**, 231–272.

Burke, R. E., Fahn, S., Jankovic, J., *et al* (1982) Tardive dystonia: late-onset and persistent dystonia caused by antipsychotic drugs. *Neurology*, **32**, 1335–1346.

Burris, K. D., Molski, T. F., Xu, C., *et al* (2002) Aripiprazole, a novel antipsychotic, is a high-affinity partial agonist at human dopamine D2 receptors. *Journal of Pharmacology and Experimental Therapeutics*, **302**, 381–389.

Bymaster, F. P., Calligaro, D. O., Falcone, J. F., *et al* (1996) Radioreceptor binding profile of the atypical antipsychotic olanzapine. *Neuropsychopharmacology*, **14**, 87–96.

Carlsson, A. (1959) The occurrence, distribution and physiological role of catecholamines in the nervous system. *Pharmacological Reviews*, **11**, 490–493.

Carlsson, A. (1985) Pharmacological properties of presynaptic dopamine receptor agonists. *Psychopharmacology Supplementum*, **2**, 31–38.

Carlsson, A. & Lindquist, M. (1963) Effect of chlorpromazine and haloperidol on 3-methoxytryptamine and normetanephrine in mouse brain. *Acta Pharmacologica Toxicology*, **20**, 140–144.

Carpenter, W. T. Jr, Buchanan, R. W., Kirkpatrick, B., *et al* (1999) Comparative effectiveness of fluphenazine decanoate injections every 2 weeks versus every 6 weeks. *American Journal of Psychiatry*, **156**, 412–418.

Casey, D. E., Carson, W. H., Saha, A. R., *et al* (2003) Switching patients to aripiprazole from other antipsychotic agents: a multicenter randomized study. *Psychopharmacology (Berlin)*, **166**, 391–399.

Cavallaro, R., Cocchi, F., Angelone, M. D., *et al* (2002) Cabergoline treatment of risperidone-induced hyperprolactinemia: a pilot study. *Journal of Clinical Psychiatry*, **65**, 187–190.

Chue, P., Eerdekens, M., Augustyns, I., *et al* (2002) Efficacy and safety of long-acting risperidone microspheres and risperidone oral tablets. *Schizophrenia Research*, **53**, suppl. 3, 174–175 (abstract B165).

Ciompi, L. (1980) The natural history of schizophrenia in the long term. *British Journal of Psychiatry*, **136**, 413–420.

Colpaert, L. (2003) Discovering risperidone: the LSD model of psychopathology. *Nature Review Drug Discovery*, **2**, 315–320.

Connell, P. (1958) *Amphetamine Psychosis*. London: Chapman & Hall.

Consensus Committee of the American Autonomic Society and the American Academy of Neurology (1996) Consensus statement on the definition of orthostatic hypotension, pure autonomic failure, and multiple system atrophy. *Neurology*, **46**, 1470.

Cookson, J., Taylor, D. & Katona, C. (2002) *The Use of Drugs in Psychiatry*. London: Gaskell.

Courvoisier, S. (1956) Pharmacodynamic basis for the use of chlorpromazine in psychiatry. *Journal of Clinical and Experimental Psychopathology*, **17**, 25–37.

Coyle, J. T., Tsai, G. & Goff, D. C. (2002) Ionotropic glutamate receptors as therapeutic targets in schizophrenia. *Current Drug Targets. CNS and Neurological Disorders*, **1**, 183–189.

Cunningham Owens, D. G. (1999) *A Guide to the Extra-pyramidal Effects of Antipsychotic Drugs*. Cambridge: Cambridge University Press.

Currier, G. W. (2000) Atypical antipsychotic medications in the psychiatric emergency service. *Journal of Clinical Psychiatry*, **61**, suppl. 14, 21–26.

Davies, L. M. & Drummond, M. F. (1994) Economics and schizophrenia: the real cost. *British Journal of Psychiatry*, **165**, suppl. 25, 18–21.

Davis, J. M. & Andriukaitis, S. (1986) The natural course of schizophrenia and effective maintenance drug treatment. *Journal of Clinical Psychopharmacology*, **6**, 2S–10S.

Davis, J. M., Chen, N. & Glick, I. D. (2003) A meta-analysis of the efficacy of second-generation antipsychotics. *Archives of General Psychiatry*, **60**, 553–564.

Delay, J., Deniker, P. & Harl, J. M. (1952) Utilisative en therapeutic psychiatric d'une phenothiazine d'action centrale elective (4560 RP). *Annales Medicales et Psychologique (Paris)*, **110**, 112–117.

Devinsky, O., Honigfeld, G. & Patin, J. (1991) Clozapine-related seizures. *Neurology*, **41**, 369–371.

Dowson, J. H., Butler, J. & Williams, O. (1999) Management of psychiatric inpatient violence in the East Anglia region. *Psychiatric Bulletin*, **23**, 486–489.

Duggan, L. & Brylewski, J. (2004) Antipsychotic medication versus placebo for people with both schizophrenia and learning disability. *Cochrane Database of Systematic Reviews*, **(3)**, CD000377.

Duval, A. M. & Goldman, D. (2000) The new drugs (chlorpromazine and reserpine): administrative aspects. 1956. *Psychiatric Services*, **51**, 327–331.

Eaton, W. W. (1991) Update on the epidemiology of schizophrenia. *Epidemiological Reveiws*, **13**, 320–328.

El-Sayeh, H. G. & Morganti, C. (2004) Aripiprazole for schizophrenia. *Cochrane Database of Systematic Reviews*, **(2)**, CD004578.

Engelhardt, D. M., Rosen, B., Feldman, J., *et al* (1982) A 15-year follow-up of 646 schizophrenic outpatients. *Schizophrenia Bulletin*, **8**, 493–503.

Essock, S. M., Frisman, L. K., Covell, N. H., *et al* (2000) Cost-effectiveness of clozapine compared with conventional antipsychotic medication for patients in state hospitals. *Archives of General Psychiatry*, **57**, 987–994.

Expert Group (2004) Schizophrenia and Diabetes 2003. Expert Consensus Meeting, Dublin, 3–4 October 2003: consensus summary. *British Journal of Psychiatry*, **47**, suppl., S112–S114.

Farde, L. & Nordström, A.-L. (1992) PET analysis indicates atypical central dopamine receptor occupancy in clozapine-treated patients. *British Journal of Psychiatry*, **160**, suppl. 17, 30–33.

Fenton, M., Morris, S., De-Silva, P., *et al* (2000) Zotepine for schizophrenia. *Cochrane Database of Systematic Reviews*, **(2)**, CD001948.

Findling, R. L., Steiner, H. & Weller, E. B. (2005) Use of antipsychotics in children and adolescents. *Journal of Clinical Psychiatry*, **66**, suppl. 7, 29–40.

Fontaine, K. R., Heo, M., Harrigan, E. P., *et al* (2001) Estimating the consequences of anti-psychotic induced weight gain on health and mortality rate. *Psychiatry Research*, **101**, 277–288.

Foster, P. (1989) Neuroleptic equivalence. *Pharmaceutical Journal*, **30**, 431–432.

Gardner, I., Zahid, N., MacCrimmon, D., *et al* (1998) A comparison of the oxidation of clozapine and olanzapine to reactive metabolites and the toxicity of these metabolites to human leukocytes. *Molecular Pharmacology*, **53**, 991–998.

Garza-Trevino, E. S., Hollister, L. E., Overall, J. E., *et al* (1989) Efficacy of combinations of intramuscular antipsychotics and sedative-hypnotics for control of psychotic agitation. *American Journal of Psychiatry*, **146**, 1598–1601.

Geddes, J., Freemantle, N., Harrison, P., *et al* (2000) Atypical antipsychotics in the treatment of schizophrenia: systematic overview and meta-regression analysis. *BMJ*, **321**, 1371–1376.

Gellner, K., Eiselt, R., Hustert, E., *et al* (2001) Genomic organization of the human CYP3A locus: identification of a new, inducible CYP3A gene. *Pharmacogenetics*, **11**, 111–121.

Gerlach, J., Lublin, H. & Peacock, L. (1996) Extrapyramidal symptoms during long-term treatment with antipsychotics: special focus on clozapine and D_1 and D_2 dopamine antagonists. *Neuropsychopharmacology*, **14**, 35S–39S.

Gerson, S. L., Arce, C. & Meltzer, H. Y. (1994) N-desmethylclozapine: a clozapine metabolite that suppresses haemopoiesis. *British Journal of Haematology*, **86**, 555–561.

Glazer, W. M. (2000) Expected incidence of tardive dyskinesia associated with atypical antipsychotics. *Journal of Clinical Psychiatry*, **61**, suppl. 4, 21–26.

Glazer, W. M. & Kane, J. M. (1992) Depot neuroleptic therapy: an underutilized treatment option. *Journal of Clinical Psychiatry*, **53**, 426–433.

Goff, D. C. & Shader, R. I. (2003) Non-neurological side effects of antipsychotic drugs. In *Schizophrenia* (eds D. R. Weinberger & S. R. Hirsch), pp. 573–588. Oxford: Blackwell.

Gonzalez, F. J., Crespi, C. L., Czerwinski, M., *et al* (1992) Analysis of human cytochrome P450 catalytic activities and expression. *Tohoku Journal of Experimental Medicine*, **168**, 67–72.

Gurrera, R. J. (2002) Is neuroleptic realignment syndrome a neurogenic form of malignant hyperthermia? *Clinical Neuropharmacology*, **25**, 183–193.

Guttmacher, M. S. (1964) Phenothiazine treatment in acute schizophrenia: effectiveness. The National Institute of Mental Health Psychopharmacology Service Center Collaborative Study Group. *Archives of General Psychiatry*, **10**, 246–261.

Guy, W. (1976) *ECDEU Assessment Manual for Psychopharmacology*. Washington, DC: US Department of Health, Education and Welfare.

Haddad, P. M. (2004) Antipsychotics and diabetes: review of non-prospective data. *British Journal of Psychiatry*, **184**, suppl., S80–S86.

Haddad, P. M. & Anderson, I. M. (2002) Antipsychotic-related QT_c prolongation, torsade de pointes and sudden death. *Drugs*, **62**, 1649–1671.

Halbreich, U., Kinon, B. J., Gilmore, J. A., *et al* (2003) Elevated prolactin levels in patients with schizophrenia: mechanisms and related adverse effects. *Psychoneuroendocrinology*, **28**, suppl. 1, 53–67.

Harris, E. C. & Barraclough, B. (1998) Excess mortality of mental disorder. *British Journal of Psychiatry*, **173**, 11–53.

Harrison, P. J. & Owen, M. J. (2003) Genes for schizophrenia? Recent findings and their pathophysiological implications. *Lancet*, **361**, 417–419.

Hartnett, K. A., Stout, A. K., Rajdev, S., *et al* (1997) NMDA receptor-mediated neurotoxicity: a paradoxical requirement for extracellular Mg^{2+} in Na^{+}/Ca^{2+}-free solutions in rat cortical neurons in vitro. *Journal of Neurochemistry*, **68**, 1836–1845.

Hasegawa, M., Gutierrez-Esteinou, R., Way, L., *et al* (1993) Relationship between clinical efficacy and clozapine concentrations in plasma in schizophrenia: effect of smoking. *Journal of Clinical Psychopharmacology*, **13**, 383–390.

Haycox, A. (2005) Pharmacoeconomics of long-acting risperidone: results and validity of cost-effectiveness models. *Pharmacoeconomics*, **23**, suppl. 1, 3–16.

Healey, D. (2002) *The Creation of Psychopharmacology*. Cambridge, MA: Harvard University Press.

Henderson, D. C., Cagliero, E., Gray, C., *et al* (2000) Clozapine, diabetes mellitus, weight gain, and lipid abnormalities: a five year naturalistic study. *American Journal of Psychiatry*, **157**, 975–981.

Hennen, J. & Baldessarini, R. (2005) Suicidal risk during treatment with clozapine: a meta-analysis. *Schizophrenia Research*, **73**, 139–145.

Heresco-Levy, U., Javitt, D. C., Ermilov, M., *et al* (1999) Efficacy of high-dose glycine in the treatment of enduring negative symptoms of schizophrenia. *Archives of General Psychiatry*, **56**, 29–36.

Herman, H. E., Baldwin, J. A. & Christie, D. (1983) A record-linkage study of mortality and general hospital discharge in patients diagnosed as schizophrenic. *Psychological Medicine*, **13**, 581–593.

Hogarty, G. E., McEvoy, J. P., Munetz, M., *et al* (1988) Dose of fluphenazine, familial expressed emotion, and outcome in schizophrenia. Results of a two-year controlled study. *Archives of General Psychiatry*, **45**, 797–805.

Honigfeld, G., Arellano, F., Sethi, J., *et al* (1998) Reducing clozapine-related morbidity and mortality: 5 years of experience with the Clozaril National Registry. *Journal of Clinical Psychiatry*, **59**, suppl. 3, 3–7.

Howes, O. D., Wheeler, M. J., Meaney, A. M., *et al* (2005) Bone mineral density and its relationship to prolactin levels in patients taking antipsychotic treatment. *Journal of Clinical Psychopharmacology*, **25**, 259–263.

Hunter, R. H., Joy, C. B., Kennedy, E., *et al* (2003) Risperidone versus typical antipsychotic medication for schizophrenia. *Cochrane Database of Systematic Reviews*, **(2)**, CD000440.

Javitt, D. C., Zylberman, I., Zukin, S. R., *et al* (1994) Amelioration of negative symptoms in schizophrenia by glycine. *American Journal of Psychiatry*, **151**, 1234–1236.

Jerling, M., Dahl, M.-L., Åberg-Wistedt, A., *et al* (1996) The CYP2D6 genotype predicts the oral clearance of the neuroleptic agents perphenazine and zuclopenthixol. *Clinical Pharmacology and Therapeutics*, **59**, 423–428.

Johnson, D. A., Pasterski, G., Ludlow, J. M., *et al* (1983) The discontinuance of maintenance neuroleptic therapy in chronic schizophrenic patients: drug and social consequences. *Acta Psychiatrica Scandinavica*, **67**, 339–352.

Johnstone, E. C., Crow, T. J., Frith, C. D., *et al* (1978) Mechanism of the antipsychotic effect in the treatment of acute schizophrenia. *Lancet*, *i*, 848–851.

Jusic, N. & Lader, M. (1994) Post-mortem antipsychotic drug concentrations and unexplained deaths. *British Journal of Psychiatry*, **165**, 787–791.

Kane, J. M. (1987) Treatment of schizophrenia. *Schizophrenia Bulletin*, **13**, 133–156.

Kane, J. M., Honigfeld, G., Singer, J., *et al* (1988*a*) Clozapine for the treatment-resistant schizophrenic. A double-blind comparison with chlorpromazine. *Archives of General Psychiatry*, **45**, 789–796.

Kane, J. M., Woerner, M. & Lieberman, J. (1988*b*) Tardive dyskinesia: prevalence, incidence, and risk factors. *Journal of Clinical Psychopharmacology*, **8**, suppl. 4, 52S–56S.

Kane, J. M., Eerdekens, M., Lindenmayer, J. P., *et al* (2003) Long-acting injectable risperidone: efficacy and safety of the first long-acting atypical antipsychotic. *American Journal of Psychiatry*, **160**, 1125–1132.

Kaniucki, M. D., Stafano, F. J. G. & Pevec, C. J. (1984) Clonidine inhibits salivary secretion by activation of postsynaptic α_2 receptors. *Naunyn–Schmiedeberg's Archives of Pharmacology*, **326**, 313–316.

Kapur, S. (2003) Psychosis as a state of aberrant salience: a framework linking biology, phenomenology, and pharmacology in schizophrenia. *American Journal of Psychiatry*, **160**, 13–23.

Kapur, S. & Seeman, P. (2001) Does fast dissociation from the dopamine D(2) receptor explain the action of atypical antipsychotics? A new hypothesis. *American Journal of Psychiatry*, **158**, 360–369.

Kapur, S., Zipursky, R., Jones, C., *et al* (2000) Relationship between dopamine D(2) occupancy, clinical response and side effects: a double-blind PET study of first-episode schizophrenia. *American Journal of Psychiatry*, **157**, 514–520.

Kay, S. R., Fiszbein, A. & Opler, L. A. (1987) The Positive and Negative Syndrome Scale (PANSS) for schizophrenia. *Schizophrenia Bulletin*, **13**, 261–276.

Keefe, R. S., Silva, S. G., Perkins, D. O., *et al* (1999) The effects of atypical antipsychotic drugs on neurocognitive impairment in schizophrenia: a review and meta-analysis. *Schizophrenia Bulletin*, **25**, 201–222.

Killian, J. G., Kerr, K., Lawrence, C., *et al* (1999) Myocarditis and cardiomyopathy associated with clozapine. *Lancet*, **354**, 1841–1845.

Kimyai-Asadi, A., Harris, J. C. & Noussari, H. C. (1999) Critical overview: adverse cutaneous reactions to psychotropic medications. *Journal of Clinical Psychiatry*, **60**, 714–725.

Kirkpatrick, B., Buchanan, R. W., Ross, D. E., *et al* (2001) A separate disease within the syndrome of schizophrenia. *Archives of General Psychiatry*, **58**, 165–171.

Kissling, W. (1991) The current unsatisfactory state of relapse prevention in schizophrenic psychoses – suggestions for improvement. *Clinical Neuropharmacology*, **14**, suppl. 2, S33–S44.

Kline, N. S. (1954) Use of *Rauwolfia serpentina* Benth. in neuropsychiatric conditions. *Annals of the New York Academy of Sciences*, **59**, 107–132.

Knapp, M. (1997) Costs of schizophrenia. *British Journal of Psychiatry*, **171**, 509–518.

Kohen, D. (2004) Diabetes mellitus and schizophrenia: historical perspective. *British Journal of Psychiatry*, **47**, suppl., S64–S66.

Koro, C. E., Fedder, D. O., L'Italien, G. J., *et al* (2002) Assessment of independent effect of olanzapine and risperidone on risk of diabetes among patients with schizophrenia: population based nested case–control study. *BMJ*, **325**, 243.

Krauss, J. K., Yianni, J., Loher, T. J., *et al* (2004) Deep brain stimulation for dystonia. *Journal of Clinical Neurophysiology*, **21**, 18–30.

Krystal, J. H., Karper, L. P., Seibyl, J. P., *et al* (1994) Subanesthetic effects of the noncompetitive NMDA antagonist, ketamine, in humans. Psychotomimetic, perceptual, cognitive, and neuroendocrine responses. *Archives of General Psychiatry*, **51**, 199–214.

Kupchik, M., Spivak, B., Mester, R., *et al* (2000) Combined electroconvulsive–clozapine therapy. *Clinical Neuropharmacology*, **23**, 14–16.

Laborit, H., Huguenard, P. & Allaume, R. (1952) Un nouveau stabilisateur végétatif, le 4560 RP. *Presse Medicale*, **60**, 206–208.

Lane, H.-Y., Hu, O. Y.-P., Jann, M.W., *et al* (1997) Dextromethorphan phenotyping and haloperidol disposition in schizophrenic patients. *Psychiatry Research*, **69**, 105–111.

Lerer, B., Segman, R. H., Fangerau, H., *et al* (2002) Pharmacogenetics of tardive dyskinesia: combined analysis of 780 patients supports association with dopamine D_3 receptor gene Ser9Gly polymorphism. *Neuropsychopharmacology*, **27**, 105–119.

Leucht, S., Wahlbeck, K., Hamann, J., *et al* (2003) New generation antipsychotics versus low-potency conventional antipsychotics: a systematic review and meta-analysis. *Lancet*, **361**, 1581–1589.

Levinson, D. F., Umapathy, C. & Musthaq, M. (1999) Treatment of schizoaffective disorder and schizophrenia with mood symptoms. *American Journal of Psychiatry*, **156**, 1138–1148.

Lewis, R., Bagnall, A. M. & Leitner, M. (2005) Sertindole for schizophrenia. *Cochrane Database of Systematic Reviews*, **(2)**, CD001715.

Lieberman, J. A., Yunis, J., Egea, E., *et al* (1990) HLA-B38, DR4, DQw3 and clozapine-induced agranulocytosis in Jewish patients with schizophrenia. *Archives of General Psychiatry*, **47**, 945–948.

Lieberman, J. A., Saltz, B. L., Johns, C. A., *et al* (1991) The effects of clozapine on tardive dyskinesia. *British Journal of Psychiatry*, **158**, 503–510.

Lieberman, J. A., Stroup, T. S., McEvoy, J. P., *et al* (2005) Effectiveness of antipsychotic drugs in patients with chronic schizophrenia. *New England Journal of Medicine*, **353**, 1209–1223.

Liebzeit, K. A., Markowitz, J. S. & Caley, C. F. (2001) New onset diabetes and atypical antipsychotics. *European Neuropsychopharmacology*, **11**, 25–32.

Lindström, L. H. (2000) Schizophrenia, the dopamine hypothesis and alpha$_2$-adrenoceptor antagonists. *Trends in Pharmacological Sciences*, **21**, 198–199.

Loo, H., Poirier-Littre, M. F., Theron, M., *et al* (1997) Amisulpride versus placebo in the medium-term treatment of the negative symptoms of schizophrenia. *British Journal of Psychiatry*, **170**, 18–22.

Luby, E., Cohen, B. & Rosenbaum, G. (1959) Study of a new schizophrenomimetic drug – Sernyl. *Archives of Neurology and Psychiatry*, **81**, 363–369.

Malhotra, A. K., Pinals, D. A., Weingartner, H., *et al* (1996) NMDA receptor function and human cognition: the effects of ketamine in healthy volunteers. *Neuropsychopharmacology*, **14**, 301–307.

Malhotra, A. K., Athanasiou, M., Reed, C. R., *et al* (2005) Discovery of genetic markers associated with clozapine induced agranulocytosis. *American Journal of Medical Genetics Part B (Neuropsychiatric Genetics)*, **138B**, 22.

Mantua, V., Travis, M. J., Isaac, M. B., *et al* (2006*a*) Preliminary descriptive data from the South London and Maudsley Intensive Care Units Trial Evaluation (SLAMICUTE) Study. *Schizophrenia Research*, **81**, suppl., 282–283.

Mantua, V., Travis, M. J., Isaac, M. B., *et al* (2006*b*) Preliminary outcome data from the South London and Maudsley Intensive Care Units Trial Evaluation (SLAMICUTE) Study. *Schizophrenia Research*, **81**, suppl., 282.

Marder, S. R. & Wirshing, D. A. (2003) Maintenance treatment. In *Schizophrenia* (eds D. A. Weinberger & S. R. Hirsch), pp. 474–488. Oxford: Blackwell.

Mauri, M. C., Rudelli, R., Bravin, S., *et al* (1998) Clozapine metabolism rate as a possible index of drug-induced granulocytopenia. *Psychopharmacology (Berlin)*, **137**, 341–344.

May, P. R. A. (1968) *Treatment of Schizophrenia: A Comparative Study of Five Treatment Methods*. New York: Science House.

McAllister-Williams, R. H. & Ferrier, I. N. (2002) Rapid tranquillisation: time for a reappraisal of options for parenteral therapy. *British Journal of Psychiatry*, **180**, 485–489.

McElroy, S. L., Dessain, E. C., Pope, H. G., Jr, *et al* (1991) Clozapine in the treatment of psychotic mood disorders, schizoaffective disorder, and schizophrenia. *Journal of Clinical Psychiatry*, **52**, 411–414.

Meador-Woodruff, J. H., Damask, S. P., Wang, J., *et al* (1996) Dopamine receptor mRNA expression in human striatum and neocortex. *Neuropsychopharmacology*, **15**, 17–29.

Melkersson, K. & Dahl, M. L. (2004) Adverse metabolic effects associated with atypical antipsychotics: literature review and clinical implications. *Drugs*, **64**, 701–723.

Melkersson, K. I., Hulting, A. L. & Brismar, K. E. (1999) Different influences of classical antipsychotics and clozapine on glucose–insulin homeostasis in patients with schizophrenia or related psychoses. *Journal of Clinical Psychiatry*, **60**, 783–791.

Melkersson, K. I., Hunting, A. L. & Brismar, K. E. (2000) Elevated levels of insulin, leptin and blood lipids in olanzapine-treated patients with schizophrenia or related psychoses. *Journal of Clinical Psychiatry*, **61**, 742–749.

Meltzer, H. Y. (1997) Treatment-resistant schizophrenia – the role of clozapine. *Current Medical Research Opinion*, **14**, 1–20.

Meltzer, H. Y. & McGurk, S. (2002) The effects of clozapine, risperidone and olanzapine on cognitive function in schizophrenia. *Schizophrenia Bulletin*, **25**, 233–255.

Meltzer, H. Y., Matsubara, S. & Lee, J. C. (1989) The ratios of serotonin$_2$ and dopamine$_2$ affinities differentiate atypical and typical antipsychotic drugs. *Psychopharmacology Bulletin*, **25**, 390–392.

Meltzer, H. Y., Alphs, L., Green, A. I., *et al* (2003) Clozapine treatment for suicidality in schizophrenia: International Suicide Prevention Trial (InterSePT). *Archives of General Psychiatry*, **60**, 82–91.

Mir, A., Shivakumar, K., McAllister, V., *et al* (2006) Change in sexual dysfunction on switching to aripiprazole. *Schizophrenia Research*, **81**, suppl., 137–138.

Mishara, A. L. & Goldberg, T. E. (2004) A meta-analysis and critical review of the effects of conventional neuroleptic treatment on cognition in schizophrenia: opening a closed book. *Biological Psychiatry*, **55**, 1013–1022.

Moghaddan, B. & Crystal, J. H. (2003) The neurochemistry of schizophrenia. In *Schizophrenia* (eds S. R. Hirsch & D. Weinberger), pp. 349–364. Oxford: Blackwell.

Moller, H. J., Muller, H., Borison, R. L., *et al* (1995) A path-analytical approach to differentiate between direct and indirect drug effects on negative symptoms in schizophrenic patients. A re-evaluation of the North American risperidone study. *European Archives of Psychiatry and Clinical Neuroscience*, **245**, 45–49.

Mota Neto, J. I. S., Lima, M. S. & Soares, B. G. O. (2002) Amisulpride for schizophrenia. *Cochrane Database of Systematic Reviews*, **(2)**, CD001357.

Muralidharan, G., Cooper, J.K., Hawes, E.M., *et al* (1996) Quinidine inhibits the 7-hydroxylation of chlorpromazine in extensive metabolisers of debrisoquine. *European Journal of Clinical Pharmacology*, **50**, 121–128.

Muscettola, G., Barbato, G., Pampallona, S., *et al* (1999) Extrapyramidal syndromes in neuroleptic-treated patients: prevalence, risk factors, and association with tardive dyskinesia. *Journal of Clinical Psychopharmacology*, **19**, 203–208.

National Institute for Clinical Excellence (2001) *Orlistat for Treatment of Obesity in Adults – Full Guidance*. London: NICE.

National Institute for Clinical Excellence (2002) *Schizophrenia: Core Interventions in the Treatment and Management of Schizophrenia in Primary and Secondary Care*. London: NICE.

National Institute for Clinical Excellence (2003) *Guidance on the Use of Electroconvulsive Therapy* (Technology Appraisal 59). London: NICE.

Nebert, D. W. (1997) Polymorphisms in drug-metabolizing enzymes: what is their clinical relevance and why do they exist? *American Journal of Human Genetics*, **60**, 265–271.

Newman, S. C. & Bland, R. C. (1991) Mortality in a cohort of patients with schizophrenia: a record linkage study. *Canadian Journal of Psychiatry*, **36**, 239–245.

Olfson, M., Mechanic, D., Hansell, S., *et al* (2000) Predicting medication noncompliance after hospital discharge among patients with schizophrenia. *Psychiatric Services*, **51**, 216–222.

Overall, J. E. & Gorham, D. R. (1962) The Brief Psychiatric Rating Scale. *Psychological Reports*, **10**, 237–246.

Paleacu, D., Giladi, N., Moore, O., *et al* (2004) Tetrabenazine treatment in movement disorders. *Clinical Neuropharmacology*, **27**, 230–233.

Perry, P. J., Miller, D. D., Arndt, S. V., *et al* (1991) Clozapine and norclozapine plasma concentrations and clinical response of treatment-refractory schizophrenic patients. *American Journal of Psychiatry*, **148**, 231–235.

Pilowsky, L. S., Costa, D. C., Ell, P. J., *et al* (1992) Clozapine, single photon emission tomography, and the D_2 dopamine receptor blockade hypothesis of schizophrenia. *Lancet*, **340**, 199–202.

Pilowsky, L. S., O'Connell, P., Davies, N., *et al* (1997) In vivo effects on striatal dopamine D_2 receptor binding by the novel atypical antipsychotic drug sertindole – a ^{123}I IBZM single photon emission tomography (SPET) study. *Psychopharmacology (Berlin)*, **130**, 152–158.

Pirmohamed, M., Williams, D., Madden, S., *et al* (1995) Metabolism and bioactivation of clozapine by human liver in vitro. *Journal of Pharmacology and Experimental Therapeutics*, **272**, 984–990.

Pumford, N. R., Halmes, N. C., Martin, B. M., *et al* (1997) Covalent binding of acetaminophen to N-10-formyltetrahydrofolate dehydrogenase in mice. *Journal of Pharmacology and Experimental Therapeutics*, **280**, 501–505.

Quinn, J., Meagher, D., Murphy, P., *et al* (2001) Vulnerability to involuntary movements over a lifetime trajectory of schizophrenia approaches 100%, in association with executive (frontal) dysfunction. *Schizophrenia Research*, **49**, 79–87.

Ram, R., Bromet, E. J., Eaton, W. W., *et al* (1992) The natural course of schizophrenia: a review of first-admission studies. *Schizophrenia Bulletin*, **18**, 185–207.

Ray, W. A., Meredith, S., Thapa, P. B., *et al* (2001) Antipsychotics and the risk of sudden cardiac death. *Archives of General Psychiatry*, **58**, 1161–1167.

Reilly, J. G., Ayis, S. A., Ferrier, I. N., *et al* (2000) QT_c-interval abnormalities and psychotropic drug therapy in psychiatric patients. *Lancet*, **355**, 1048–1052.

Reilly, J. G., Ayis, S. A., Ferrier, I. N., *et al* (2002) Thioridazine and sudden unexplained death in psychiatric in-patients. *British Journal of Psychiatry*, **180**, 515–522.

Rey, M. J., Schulz, P., Costa, C., *et al* (1989) Guidelines for the dosage of neuroleptics. I: Chlorpromazine equivalents of orally administered neuroleptics. *International Clinical Psychopharmacology*, **4**, 95–104.

Reynolds, G. P., Zhang, Z. & Zhang, X. (2003) Polymorphism of the promoter region of the serotonin 5-HT(2C) receptor gene and clozapine-induced weight gain. *American Journal of Psychiatry*, **160**, 677–679.

Richelson, E. (1996) Preclinical pharmacology of neuroleptics: focus on new generation compounds. *Journal of Clinical Psychiatry*, **57**, suppl. 11, 4–11.

Ritter, S. (1989) Administering an injection without a patient's consent. In *Bethlem Royal and Maudsley Hospital Manual of Clinical Psychiatric Nursing Principles and Procedures*. London: Harper-Collins.

Rosenheck, R., Cramer, J., Xu, W., *et al* (1997) A comparison of clozapine and haloperidol in hospitalized patients with refractory schizophrenia. Department of Veterans Affairs Cooperative Study Group on Clozapine in Refractory Schizophrenia. *New England Journal of Medicine*, **337**, 809–815.

Rosenheck, R., Cramer, J., Allan, E., *et al* (1999) Cost-effectiveness of clozapine in patients with high and low levels of hospital use. Department of Veterans Affairs Cooperative Study Group on Clozapine in Refractory Schizophrenia. *Archives of General Psychiatry*, **56**, 565–572.

Royal College of Psychiatrists (1993) *Consensus Statement on High Dose Antipsychotics*. London: Gaskell.

Royal College of Psychiatrists (2005) *The ECT Handbook* (2nd edn) (Council Report CR128). London: Royal College of Psychiatrists.

Royal College of Psychiatrists (2006) *Consensus Statement on High-Dose Antipsychotic Medication* (CR138). London: Royal College of Psychiatrists.

Ryan, M. C. & Thakore, J. H. (2002) Physical consequences of schizophrenia and its treatment: the metabolic syndrome. *Life Science*, **71**, 239–257.

Ryan, M. C., Collins, P. & Thakore, J. H. (2003) Impaired fasting glucose tolerance in first-episode, drug-naive patients with schizophrenia. *American Journal of Psychiatry*, **160**, 284–289.

Sackeim, H. A. (2003) Electroconvulsive therapy and schizophrenia. In *Schizophrenia* (eds S. R. Hirsch & D. Weinberger), pp. 517–551. Oxford: Blackwell.

Safferman, A., Lieberman, J., Kane, J. M., *et al* (1991) Update on the clinical efficacy and side effects of clozapine. *Schizophrenia Bulletin*, **17**, 247–260.

Salzman, C., Green, A. I., Rodriguez-Villa, F., *et al* (1986) Benzodiazepines combined with neuroleptics for management of severe disruptive behavior. *Psychosomatics*, **27**, 17–22.

Sax, K. W., Strakowski, S. M., Keck, P. E., Jr, *et al* (1996) Relationships among negative, positive, and depressive symptoms in schizophrenia and psychotic depression. *British Journal of Psychiatry*, **168**, 68–71.

Schmauss, C., Haroutunian, V., Davis, K. L., *et al* (1993) Selective loss of dopamine D_3-type receptor mRNA expression in parietal and motor cortices of patients with chronic schizophrenia. *Proceedings of the National Academy of Sciences, USA*, **90**, 8942–8946.

Schooler, N. R. (1991) Maintenance medication for schizophrenia: strategies for dose reduction. *Schizophrenia Bulletin*, **17**, 311–324.

Schooler, N. R., Keith, S. J., Severe, J. B., *et al* (1997) Relapse and rehospitalization during maintenance treatment of schizophrenia. The effects of dose reduction and family treatment. *Archives of General Psychiatry*, **54**, 453–463.

Schwarz, L. & Munoz, R. (1968) Blood sugar levels in patients treated with chlorpromazine. *American Journal of Psychiatry*, **125**, 253–255.

Seeger, T. F., Seymour, P. A., Schmidt, A. W., *et al* (1995) Ziprasidone (CP-88,059): a new antipsychotic with combined dopamine and serotonin receptor antagonist activity. *Journal of Pharmacology and Experimental Therapeutics*, **275**, 101–113.

Seeman, P., Lee, T., Chau-Wong, M., *et al* (1976) Antipsychotic drug doses and neuroleptic/dopamine receptors. *Nature*, **261**, 717–719.

Sen, G. & Bose, K. C. (1931) *Rauwolfia serpentina*, a new Indian drug for insanity and high blood pressure. *Indian Medical Worlds*, **2**, 194.

Sethi, K. D., Hess, D. C. & Harp, R. J. (1990) Prevalence of dystonia in veterans on chronic antipsychotic therapy. *Movement Disorders*, **5**, 319–321.

Shah, G. K., Aurback, D. B., Augsburger, J. J., *et al* (1998) Acute thioridazine retinopathy. *Archives in Ophthalmology*, **116**, 826–827.

Shiloh, R., Zemishlany, Z., Aizenberg, D., *et al* (1997) Sulpiride augmentation in people with schizophrenia partially responsive to clozapine. A double-blind, placebo-controlled study. *British Journal of Psychiatry*, **171**, 569–573.

Shiovitz, T. M., Welke, T. L., Tigel, P. D., *et al* (1996) Cholinergic rebound and rapid onset psychosis following abrupt clozapine withdrawal. *Schizophrenia Bulletin*, **22**, 591–595.

Shore, D. (1995) Clinical implications of clozapine discontinuation: report of an NIMH workshop. *Schizophrenia Bulletin*, **21**, 333–338.

Simpson, G. M. (1984) A brief history of depot neuroleptics. *Journal of Clinical Psychiatry*, **45**, 3–4.

Simpson, G. M. & Angus, J. W. (1970) A rating scale for extrapyramidal side effects. *Acta Psychiatrica Scandinavica Supplementum*, **212**, 11–19.

Siris, S., Pollack, S., Bermanzohn, P., *et al* (2000) Adjunctive imipramine for a broader group of post-psychotic depressions in schizophrenia. *Schizophrenia Research*, **44**, 187–192.

Smith, S., Wheeler, M. J., Murray, R., *et al* (2002) The effects of antipsychotic-induced hyperprolactinaemia on the hypothalamic–pituitary–gonadal axis. *Journal of Clinical Psychopharmacology*, **22**, 109–114.

Srisurapanont, M., Disayavanish, C. & Taimkaew, K. (2000) Quetiapine for schizophrenia. *Cochrane Database of Systematic Reviews*, **(3)**, CD000967.

Stanilla, J. K. & Simpson, G. M. (2001) Treatment of extrapyramidal side effects. In *Essentials of Clinical Psychopharmacology* (eds A. F. Schatzberg & C. B. Nemeroff), pp. 155–177. Washington, DC: American Psychiatric Association.

Steen, V. M., Lovlie, R., MacEwan, T., *et al* (1997) Dopamine D_3-receptor gene variant and susceptibility to tardive dyskinesia in schizophrenic patients. *Molecular Psychiatry*, **2**, 139–145.

Sundram, C. J. (1994) Quality assurance in an era of consumer empowerment and choice. *Mental Retardation*, **32**, 371–374.

Talbot, P. S. & Laruelle, M. (2002) The role of in vivo molecular imaging with PET and SPECT in the elucidation of psychiatric drug action and new drug development. *European Neuropsychopharmacology*, **12**, 503–511.

Talvik, M., Nordstrom, A. L., Nyberg, S., *et al* (2001) No support for regional selectivity in clozapine-treated patients: a PET study with [(11)C]raclopride and [(11)C]FLB 457. *American Journal of Psychiatry*, **158**, 926–930.

Tandon, K. & Aitchison, K. J. (2002) The cost-effectiveness of atypical versus typical antipsychotics. *Psychiatry*, **1**(10), 66–69.

Taylor, D., Paton, C. & Kerwin, R. (2005) *The Maudsley 2005/6 Prescribing Guidelines*. London: Taylor & Francis.

Taylor, M. A. & Fink, M. (2003) Catatonia in psychiatric classification: a home of its own. *American Journal of Psychiatry*, **160**, 1233–1241.

Thaker, G. K., Nguyen, J. A., Strauss, M. E., *et al* (1990) Clonazepam treatment of tardive dyskinesia: a practical GABAmimetic strategy. *American Journal of Psychiatry*, **147**, 445–451.

Thakore, J. H., Mann, J. N., Vlahos, I., *et al* (2002) Increased visceral fat distribution in drug-naive and drug-free patients with schizophrenia. *International Journal of Obesity and Related Metabolic Disorders*, **26**, 137–141.

Tollefson, G. D., Beasley, C. M., Jr., Tran, P. V., *et al* (1997) Olanzapine versus haloperidol in the treatment of schizophrenia and schizoaffective and schizophreniform disorders: results of an international collaborative trial. *American Journal of Psychiatry*, **154**, 457–465.

Torrey, E. F. & Swalwell, C. I. (2003) Fatal olanzapine-induced ketoacidosis. *American Journal of Psychiatry*, **160**, 2241.

Tran, P. V., Dellva, M. A., Tollefson, G. D., *et al* (1998) Oral olanzapine versus oral haloperidol in the maintenance treatment of schizophrenia and related psychoses. *British Journal of Psychiatry*, **172**, 499–505.

Travis, M. J., Busatto, G. F., Pilowsky, L. S., *et al* (1997) Serotonin: 5-HT_{2A} receptor occupancy in vivo and response to the new antipsychotics olanzapine and sertindole. *British Journal of Psychiatry*, **171**, 290–291.

TREC Collaborative group (2003) Rapid tranquillization for agitated patients in emergency psychiatric rooms : a randomised controlled trial of midazolam versus haloperidol plus promethazine. *BMJ*, **327**, 708–713.

Tsai, G., Yang, P., Chung, L. C., *et al* (1998) D-serine added to antipsychotics for the treatment of schizophrenia. *Biological Psychiatry*, **44**, 1081–1089.

Tsai, G. E., Yang, P., Chung, L. C., *et al* (1999) D-serine added to clozapine for the treatment of schizophrenia. *American Journal of Psychiatry*, **156**, 1822–1825.

Tsapakis, E. M. & Aitchison, K. J. (2006) Biological treatments: general considerations. In *Essentials of Psychiatry* (eds R. Murray, K. S. Kendler, P. McGuffin, *et al*). Cambridge: Cambridge University Press.

Tsapakis, E. M., Basu, A. & Aitchison, K. J. (2005) Transcriptomics and proteomics: advancing the understanding of psychiatric pharmacogenetics. *Clinical Neuropsychiatry*, issue 2 (special issue on pharmacogenetics), **1**, 117–124.

Tsien, J. Z., Huerta, P. T. & Tonegawa, S. (1996) The essential role of hippocampal CA1 NMDA receptor-dependent synaptic plasticity in spatial memory. *Cell*, **87**, 1327–1338.

UK Prospective Diabetes Study Group (1998) Intensive blood-glucose control with sulphonylureas or insulin compared with conventional treatment and risk of complications in patients with type II diabetes (UKPDS 33). *Lancet*, **352**, 837–853.

van Os, J., Fahy, T. A., Jones, P., *et al* (1996) Psychopathological syndromes in the functional psychoses: associations with course and outcome. *Psychological Medicine*, **26**, 161–176.

Vogel F. (1959) Moderne Probleme der Humangenetik. *Ergebnisse der inneren Medizin und Kinderheilkunde*, **12**, 52-125.

von Bahr, C., Movin, G., Nordin, C., *et al* (1991) Plasma levels of thioridazine and metabolites are influenced by the debrisoquine hydroxylation phenotype. *Clinical Pharmacology and Therapeutics*, **49**, 234–240.

Waddington, J. L., O'Callaghan, E., Buckley, P., *et al* (1995) Tardive dyskinesia in schizophrenia. Relationship to minor physical anomalies, frontal lobe dysfunction and cerebral structure on magnetic resonance imaging. *British Journal of Psychiatry*, **167**, 41–44.

Wahlbeck, K., Cheine, M. V. & Essali, A. (1999) Clozapine versus typical neuroleptic medication for schizophrenia. *Cochrane Database of Systematic Reviews*, Issue 4. Art. No.: CD000059. DOI: 10.1002/14651858.CD000059.

Wang, P. S., Schneeweiss, S., Avorn, J., *et al* (2005) Risk of death in elderly users of conventional vs. atypical antipsychotic medications. *New England Journal of Medicine*, **353**, 2335–2341.

Weickert, T. W., Goldberg, T. E., Marenco, S., *et al* (2003) Comparison of cognitive performances during a placebo period and an atypical antipsychotic treatment period in schizophrenia: critical examination of confounds. *Neuropsychopharmacology*, **28**, 1491–1500.

Weiser, M., Reichenberg, A., Grotto, I., *et al* (2004) Higher rates of cigarette smoking in male adolescents before the onset of schizophrenia: a historical-prospective cohort study. *American Journal of Psychiatry*, **161**, 1219–1223.

Wiersma, D., Nienhuis, F. J., Slooff, C. J., *et al* (1998) Natural course of schizophrenic disorders: a 15-year followup of a Dutch incidence cohort. *Schizophrenia Bulletin*, **24**, 75–85.

Williams, J., Spurlock, G., Holmans, P., *et al* (1998) A meta-analysis and transmission disequilibrium study of association between the dopamine D_3 receptor gene and schizophrenia. *Molecular Psychiatry*, **3**, 141–149.

Woods, S. W. (2003) Chlorpromazine equivalent doses for the newer atypical antipsychotics. *Journal of Clinical Psychiatry*, **64**, 663–667.

Wright, P., Birkett, M., David, S. R., *et al* (2001) Double-blind, placebo-controlled comparison of intramuscular olanzapine and intramuscular haloperidol in the treatment of acute agitation in schizophrenia. *American Journal of Psychiatry*, **158**, 1149–1151.

Yusufi, B. Z., Mukherjee, S., Aitchison, K. J., *et al* (2005) Reliability of the Antipsychotic Non-Neurological Side-Effects Rating Scale (ANNSERS). *Journal of Psychopharmacology*, **19**, suppl., A10.

Zarate, C. A., Jr, Baldessarini, R. J., Siegel, A. J., *et al* (1997) Risperidone in the elderly: a pharmacoepidemiologic study. *Journal of Clinical Psychiatry*, **58**, 311–317.

Zhang, L. J., Lachowicz, J. E. & Sibley, D. R. (1994) The D2S and D2L dopamine receptor isoforms are differentially regulated in Chinese hamster ovary cells. *Molecular Pharmacology*, **45**, 878–889.

CHAPTER 12

Schizophrenia: psychological and social approaches to treatment and care

Frank Holloway and George Stein

Introduction

Progress in treatment and care

In the years since the publication of the first edition of this book (in 1998) there has been a revolution in the treatment of people with schizophrenia. We have seen impressive advances in the neurobiological understanding of schizophrenia that have followed from technological developments in structural and functional neuroimaging, psychopharmacology and genomics. These have been more than matched by an explosion of interest in psychological approaches to understanding the illness and its treatment, which has resulted in a renewed focus on what patients and their carers experience and in the development of effective therapies. The rights of patients (also called 'service users' and on occasion 'survivors') and carers to full and accurate information about the illness and available treatments and the need to engage them in treatment and care have received increasing recognition. At the policy level, the National Institute for Mental Health in England has been very actively promoting psychosocial interventions (PSI) for psychosis. PSI is an inclusive term that implies a 'holistic' approach towards the treatment of people with schizophrenia, a focus on the possibilities of 'recovery' from psychosis (in a sense elaborated at the end of this chapter) and the routine use of psychological treatments (Brooker & Brabban, 2005).

There have also been spectacular advances in medical informatics. Practitioners now have ready access to good evidence on diagnosis and treatment, summarised in publications such as the quarterly *Evidence Based Mental Health* and meta-analytic reviews, such as those collected in the Cochrane Collaboration (available through the website of the National electronic Library for Health, http://www.nelh.nhs.uk).

Perhaps less impressive have been advances in our understanding of how to organise services to deliver effective treatment and how to translate research findings into routine clinical practice. The evidence base supporting social care practices is also very poorly developed. Readers need to be aware that the evidence base for psychological approaches to the treatment of schizophrenia is developing rapidly.

NICE guideline on schizophrenia

Contemporary best practice is summarised in the first clinical guideline on schizophrenia published by the National Institute for Clinical Excellence (NICE) (2002*a*), which is due to be revised by 2007. It was published in three versions:

1 as guidance for professionals, with recommendations graded according to the strength and nature of the evidence base

2 as guidance designed for users and carers

3 as a full technical appraisal of the evidence base (drawn from relevant randomised controlled trials).

The full appraisal is available from the NICE website (http://www.nice.org.uk), the National electronic Library for Health and in book form (National Institute for Clinical Excellence, 2003). The guideline provides recommendations on the prescribing of psychotropic medication, based on an earlier technology appraisal of atypical antipsychotics (National Institute for Clinical Excellence, 2002*b*). Significantly, the guideline includes very specific statements on the quality of the information to be offered to patients and carers about medication, emphasises respecting patient choice and demands audit of adherence to the guideline. There are very clear recommendations on the provision of cognitive–behavioural therapy (CBT) and family interventions. Reflecting the large gaps that exist in the evidence base, the most frequent recommendations are not, in fact, drawn from the literature reporting randomised controlled trials but reflect expert opinion or good practice as identified by the group drawing up the guideline.

Structure of the chapter

This chapter provides an overview of the social and psychological effects of schizophrenia on the sufferer. The bio-psychosocial model of schizophrenia is presented as a basis for understanding psychological and social approaches to treatment and care. We explore elaborations of this model, in terms of the nature of disability and the psychological underpinnings of positive psychotic symptoms. Approaches to early intervention in psychosis, a current focus of intense research and service activity, are discussed. We review the current status of specific psychological treatments for schizophrenia, which are based on a large and growing number of good-quality randomised controlled trials. Guidelines are offered for the practical management of the acute episode of illness. Mental health policy and practice currently emphasise the risks that people with a mental illness, particularly schizophrenia, may present to themselves and others. This concern is briefly and critically examined. Comorbid substance misuse is a common problem, which brings with it increased risks of violence, self-harm and contact with the criminal justice system and is linked with poorer clinical outcomes. Some potential responses to the problem are presented. Basic issues in the rehabilitation and long-term community care of people with schizophrenia are discussed (mental health services are reviewed in detail in Chapter 29). Finally, the humanistic 'recovery' paradigm is explored; this paradigm is about how individuals seek to transcend, or at least come to terms with, the effects of a psychotic illness and possibly extract personal meaning from it.

The social and psychological impact of schizophrenia

Understanding the psychosocial consequences of schizophrenia

In the past, psychiatrists have tended to focus their attention on issues of mental state, to the exclusion of patients' experiences of their life and their social functioning. Schizophrenia is commonly seen as an illness that results in symptoms that can be characterised along two or three dimensions or symptom clusters: 'positive' and 'negative' psychotic symptoms for the two-factor model; and 'disorganisation', 'psychomotor poverty' and 'reality distortion', in Liddle's terminology, for the three-factor model (Liddle, 1987). Schizophrenia is also characterised by a great deal of distressing and disabling neurotic symptoms, a markedly increased risk of suicide and an increased death rate from other causes.

Equally striking as the occurrence of specific symptoms is the effect of schizophrenia on the sufferers' social networks, intimate relationships, employment, finances and housing (Hafner & an der Heiden, 2003). Social networks are smaller and more commonly non-reciprocal (meaning that the network consists of people providing care and support rather than mutually supportive relationships) than in the general population. People with schizophrenia are much less likely to be married or cohabiting, although women, whose onset of illness tends to be later than that of men and whose social outcomes are typically better, are more often married or cohabiting at onset than men. Unemployment and homelessness are also very much more common than in the general population and, as a consequence of unemployment, income is on average much lower. There is a tendency for social deficits, which are apparent but generally not marked at the onset of the illness, to worsen over the first few years of illness and then stabilise. Poor premorbid social functioning and earlier age of onset predict poorer social outcomes: the more emotional, intellectual and social capital a person has before the illness, the better is the outcome.

Neurocognitive consequences of schizophrenia

A further, much neglected, issue is the effect of schizophrenia on cognitive functioning. People with schizophrenia show significant neurocognitive deficits compared with normal controls. These deficits appear to be manifest very early in the illness and then be fairly stable (Goldberg *et al*, 2003). There is evidence of diffuse impairment of cognitive functioning with more marked impairments in attention, executive functioning and memory. Patients with more deficits have poorer outcomes. Cognitive deficits interfere with or limit the rate of recovery and lead directly to behavioural problems, such as failure to recognise and act on social and affective cues.

Specific cognitive deficits have specific effects on outcomes. For example, patients with verbal memory problems have more difficulty in taking advantage of social skills training than those with normal verbal memory, although they can still learn skills, albeit at a slower pace than those without this cognitive impairment. Negative symptoms appear to be related to generalised brain dysfunction and disorganised symptoms to verbal processing abnormalities, while psychotic symptoms have no particular relationship to cognitive impairment.

The experience of schizophrenia

There is a large and expanding literature of first-person accounts of the experience of psychosis and the processes associated with social and symptomatic recovery (e.g. Chadwick *et al*, 2003). This literature, which can be described as narrative based, is quite separate from the traditional focus of evidence-based medicine on the randomised controlled trial.

The symptoms experienced by someone with a psychotic illness are, by definition, disturbing and socially disruptive. Even where symptoms have remitted and there are no obvious neuropsychological sequelae of the illness, the experience of having been psychotic can leave a residue of deep personal unease. This unease is compounded by the stigma and discrimination associated with mental illness (Hayward & Bright, 1997). It is, for some service users, further compounded by the language used by professionals, which emphasises impairment and disability as opposed to personal strengths and opportunities for recovery.

Patients often also experience treatment very negatively. Medication, which may control symptoms effectively, produces side-effects that can be both highly distressing and utterly unacknowledged by the treatment team. People with schizophrenia are routinely subject to compulsory treatment. The experience of coercion during compulsory treatment is strongly associated with the degree of 'procedural justice' perceived by the patient. In other words patients need to be clear that what is being done to them is for clear reasons and through a due process that allows them a voice and treats them with respect. Perhaps unsurprisingly, patients prefer positive pressures to comply with treatment (persuasion, inducements) to negative pressures (threats or force) (Lidz *et al*, 1998). Less dramatic are the routine perceptions by patients that they are devalued by the services, which are ostensibly there to help them, by casual lack of courtesy, lack of time, poor premises and inefficiency.

An important study explored in detail the experiences of patients who had shown evidence of marked recovery from their illness, even in the face of persistent symptoms (Davidson & Strauss, 1992). The narratives revealed that recovery was associated with rediscovering and reconstructing the individual's sense of self or personal value. The corollary of this finding is that a feeling of engulfment of the individual's identity by psychosis (i.e. a loss of a sense of self) is associated with the later emergence of depression and suicidal ideation (Birchwood & Spencer, 2001). It follows that treatment should incorporate the patient as an active collaborator in treatment and rehabilitation, and include interventions that instil hope, foster positive appraisals of the self, encourage the patient to monitor and manage symptoms and enhance self-esteem.

Psychological and social models of schizophrenia

Psychological and social approaches to the treatment and care of people with schizophrenia flow logically from social and psychological understanding of the illness and its effects on people's lives. Four conceptual models are presented, which all have implications for treatment and service design. The first is a broad bio-psychosocial model of schizophrenia. The second, applicable to all chronic disorders, is a model of impairment, disability and handicap. The third is more general still, and explores the needs of people with a mental illness. Finally, a contemporary cognitive model of schizophrenia, which draws from and enriches psychological therapies for the illness, is briefly presented.

The bio-psychosocial model of schizophrenia

The bio-psychosocial approach to schizophrenia is based on the assumption that the onset, course and outcome of major mental disorders result from an interaction between biological, environmental and behavioural factors. The 'vulnerability interactionist' model of schizophrenia hypothesises an intrinsic vulnerability to the development of schizophrenic symptoms, which itself represents the interaction of genetics and environment. An example of an environmental factor contributing to vulnerability is the strikingly increased incidence of schizophrenia among first- and second-generation African–Caribbean immigrants to the UK, which is not reflected in their country of origin (Bhugra *et al*, 1999). Acute episodes of psychosis can, in vulnerable individuals, be precipitated by a wide range of factors, which include adverse life events, psychosocial stress and illicit drug use (Bebbington & Kuipers, 2003). One well-validated form of stress is the family emotional environment. Numerous studies have confirmed that high 'expressed emotion' in families is a robust predictor of relapse (see Box 12.1).

A psychotic episode will have a range of adverse social and psychological effects on the sufferer, the family and other carers. These adverse effects will in turn make relapse more likely by increasing the stresses experienced by the patient. The model predicts that improving the coping ability and competence of the sufferer, the family and other carers will reduce the capacity of stressors to precipitate relapse and will also result in a decrease in stressors. Interventions aimed at minimising the adverse consequences of the illness by environmental manipulation (e.g. by providing supportive housing, employment, day activities and ready access to welfare benefits) should also reduce stressors. Continuing adherence to antipsychotic treatment will buffer the effects of life stress on relapse (Bebbington & Kuipers, 2003). Given optimal care, the likelihood of relapse should accordingly decrease, and what might be a vicious cycle could be broken.

This model does not deny the biological basis of schizophrenia, and it can comfortably accommodate 'medical' approaches to treatment. However, the

Box 12.1 Components of expressed emotion: the Camberwell Family Interview

Critical comments
Statements of resentment, disapproval or dislike. Statements made with critical intonation.

Hostility
Remarks indicating personal criticism for what a person is rather than what he or she does, or excessive generalised criticism (e.g. 'He's the worst in the world'.)

Emotional overinvolvement
Unusually marked concern for the person, overprotective attitudes and intrusive behaviour.

Warmth
Expressions of warmth in terms of positive comments and voice tone during the interview.

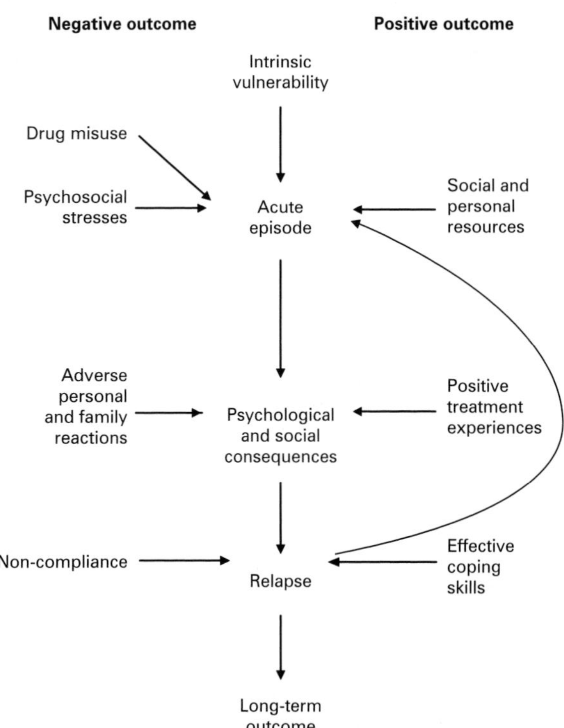

Fig. 12.1 The bio-psychosocial model: positive and negative factors in the outcome of schizophrenia.

'vulnerability interactionist' model provides a heuristic basis for psychosocial interventions and offers hope for sufferers, family members and staff that help is possible even when medication is incompletely effective.

A simplified model of the factors that may impinge on the illness career of someone with schizophrenia is presented in Fig. 12.1. Apart from the intrinsic vulnerability of the individual, all the factors shown are potentially modifiable, and even vulnerability may be tackled if our understanding of the social and biological factors contributing to it improves.

Impairment, disadvantage, disability and handicap

Wing (1993) described the consequences of severe mental illness (and other highly stigmatised conditions, such as leprosy and deafness) in terms of:

1 intrinsic *impairments*

2 consequent or pre-existing *social disadvantages*

3 functional *disability*

4 societally determined *handicap*.

Impairment, disability and handicap defined in Box 12.2. The basic *impairments* of schizophrenia are manifested clinically as symptoms and the abnormalities in cognitive functioning already described. Typical *disabilities* that are encountered include poor interpersonal skills, difficulty coping with finances and inability to carry out domestic chores. Chronic mental illness often results in social *handicaps*, for example poverty, unemployment and homelessness. These handicaps may be compounded by poor premorbid social adjustment and adverse personal reactions to the illness by the sufferer.

Adverse reactions to the illness, sometimes termed 'secondary handicaps', include depression, despair and loss of motivation for self-help. Secondary handicaps may be exacerbated by despair among professional and lay carers.

By definition, the treatments available for the underlying impairments of chronic mental illness are unsatisfactory. Management strategies must therefore also directly address issues of disability and primary and secondary handicaps. Social adaptation is encouraged both by treatment aimed at improving functioning and by providing appropriately supportive environments.

Box 12.2 Impairment, disability and handicap

Impairment
Any loss or abnormality of psychological, physiological or anatomical structure or function

Disability
A restriction in functioning or lack of ability to perform normal activities

Handicap
A disadvantage for a given individual (resulting from impairment or disability) that limits or prevents the fulfilment of a role that is normal for that individual

What mental health services should be providing (meeting needs)

There is no generally accepted view of the needs of people with a severe mental illness. Numerous competing models of need have been developed. These include the often quoted hierarchy of needs described by Maslow (1954), which extends from basic physiological needs through needs for safety, love and self-esteem to 'self-actualisation' needs. Brewin *et al* (1987) adopted a narrowly clinical view of need in the Medical Research Council's Needs for Care Schedule, in which need is defined as a problem requiring specific psychiatric treatment or care.

The normalisation/social role valorisation perspective (Wolfensberger, 1983) has been extremely influential on the development of community-based services for people with all kinds of disability. Key themes to normalisation include:

- the role of the unconscious in human services (societal denial of the unpleasant realities of disability)
- the importance of labelling in the development of deviancy
- the role of social learning in overcoming disability
- the significance of social imagery in promoting or overcoming disability.

Wolfensberger (1983) identified the central goal of services as 'the creation, support and defense of valued social roles'.

The psychodynamic approach to the needs of people with a chronic mental illness stresses their intrapsychic needs and the practitioners' potential role in meeting them (Harris & Bergman, 1987).

Although in general healthcare and social care needs tend to be defined by experts, that is, are 'normative', there is increasing interest in addressing the needs ('wants') identified by the patient or client. The Camberwell Assessment of Need (Slade *et al*, 1999) allows parallel assessment of needs as rated by users, carers and staff.

An alternative approach is provided by Lehman *et al* (1982), who described eight 'quality of life' domains:

1 living situation

2 finances

3 personal safety

4 family relationships

5 general social relationships

6 work

7 leisure activities

8 health.

These domains are relevant to both the general population and people with a chronic mental illness. The majority of people with schizophrenia are unemployed and dependent on welfare benefits. Impoverishment may be extreme: patients may leave hospital after decades with no personal possessions at all. Homelessness or grossly unsatisfactory housing conditions are common, particularly those provided by inner-city psychiatric services. Victimisation is not uncommon and patients may have realistic fears for their personal safety and the security of their property. Chronic mental illness often results in alienation from family and progressive shrinkage of social networks: loneliness, isolation and sexual frustration may result.

Stein & Test (1980) based their 'assertive community treatment' model – now incorporated into UK practice as 'assertive outreach' (Department of Health, 2001) – on an analysis of what would enable patients disabled by a functional psychosis to remain out of hospital in the face of their disability. Patients require:

- material resources (food, shelter, clothing)
- general and psychiatric medical care
- coping skills to meet the demands of community living
- motivation to persevere in the face of life difficulties
- an assertive support system that follows patients up when they cease contact and that acts rapidly and effectively when a crisis occurs.

A synthesis of these multiple perspectives on need allows us to identify the components of a comprehensive system of treatment and support for people with a severe mental illness. As the schizophrenia guideline produced by the National Institute of Clinical Excellence (2002*a*) states:

> 'The assessment of needs for health and social care ... should ... be comprehensive and address medical, social, psychological, occupational, economic, physical and cultural issues.' (1.1.3.1)

Box 12.3 presents some priorities for psychiatric services. The Care Programme Approach (CPA), under which mental health services in England operate, sets out very clearly the issues to be included in a comprehensive care plan (Box 12.4; see also Chapter 29 for a more detailed discussion of the CPA).

Box 12.3 What mental health services should be providing

- Identification of people in need
- Easy access to psychiatric treatment
- Control of psychiatric symptoms (using pharmacological, social and psychological treatments)
- Strategies for relapse prevention
- General healthcare
- Promotion of independent living skills
- Support and education of carers
- Intervention in crisis
- Welfare rights advice
- Appropriately supportive accommodation (including hospitals)
- Opportunities for work and other structured day activities
- Opportunities for leisure activities
- Development of supportive social networks
- Case management/care coordination

Box 12.4 Care Programme Approach: elements of the care plan

- Mental health needs
- Psychological needs
- Physical health needs
- Relationships
- Housing
- Finances
- Occupation/activity
- Risk behaviours/risk management plan
- Relapse indicators
- Contingency plans
- Crisis plans

Adapted from the South London and Maudsley NHS Trust Care Programme Approach policy.

A cognitive model of schizophrenia

The onset of schizophrenia is associated with marked emotional changes and disruptions in cognitive processes of attention, perception and judgement. At onset the most striking symptoms are positive psychotic symptoms (delusions and hallucinations).

Garety *et al* (2001) proposed a cognitive model for the development and maintenance of positive psychotic symptoms. Vulnerability to developing psychotic symptoms may be increased by the person's pre-existing sociocultural background and cognitive style. Social adversity and deprivation, social marginalisation, childhood trauma and loss are all associated with negative schematic models of the self and the world, resulting in low self-esteem and externalised attributions.

Garety *et al* (2001) hypothesise that, in a predisposed person, an event triggers a disruption in cognitive processes, resulting in turn in anomalous conscious experiences (e.g. heightened perceptions, thoughts appearing to be racing, unconnected events appearing to be causally linked). These *prodromal experiences*, which imply a disturbed sense of self, frequently predate the onset of frank psychotic symptoms. Emotional changes will also occur as a result of any triggering event and in response to the anomalous experiences, in turn raising arousal and feeding into the content of hallucinations when they occur. The content of abnormal experiences, when they develop, is contributed to by the individual's pre-existing negative schemas and the current social context. A further link in the causal chain is the attempt by the individual to find meaning for the anomalous experiences, with the possibility of biased appraisal resulting in confirmation that internal experiences are externally caused. People who are socially isolated or who otherwise lack confiding relationships may be more likely to accept psychotic appraisals of the prepsychotic experiences, because they have reduced access to normalising explanations. The core assertion of the cognitive model is that people with anomalous, quasi-psychotic experiences will not become psychotic if they are able to reject the hypothesis that these experiences are externally caused (e.g. if they accept that their mind has been playing tricks on them).

Rarely, in delusional disorder, the triggering event is not associated with a basic information processing disruption and consequent abnormal experiences. In these cases the triggering event results in disturbed affect, which directly results in biased appraisal processes and the activation of biased schemas, which lead in turn to an externalising appraisal (delusion) without the development of hallucinations or other psychotic phenomena.

The cognitive model provides explanations for why psychotic experiences and beliefs are maintained or recur, despite lack of intrinsic plausibility and lack of confirmatory evidence. These are found in continuing biased reasoning processes, such as a tendency to jump to conclusions, an externalising attributional style and a rigidity in thinking that results in a lack of willingness to consider alternatives. They are also contributed to by the dysfunctional schemas held by people who have a psychotic illness, often linked to low self-esteem and adverse social environments, which can feed into the dysfunctional schemas. Ongoing emotional distress, characterised by depression, hopelessness and anxiety, may further contribute to the maintenance of psychotic symptoms. Anxiety has a very specific role in preventing the receipt of disconfirmatory evidence about delusions through the deployment of safety behaviours, and, clinically, anxiety often triggers exacerbations in psychotic symptoms. Cognitive factors are also clearly important to how people appraise their illness ('insight'), and this appraisal will in turn affect adherence to treatment and, to a degree, subsequent illness career.

The model does not provide a complete explanation for the phenomena of psychosis, notably the more florid elements of the 'disorganisation' syndrome, primary 'negative' symptoms (i.e. those that cannot be explained as a reaction to positive symptoms) and the more severe cognitive deficits seen in some people with schizophrenia. The importance of the cognitive model of psychosis, which is both evolving and not in any way incompatible with a neurobiological understanding of symptoms, is that it provides an agenda for psychological treatment approaches and a rationale for social interventions.

Early intervention in psychosis

Schizophrenia strikes at an age when personal, occupational and academic development is usually incomplete. It can have a devastating effect because the psychosis may permit little further personal growth and, indeed, often leads to an initial decline in personal functioning, as well as great disruption of social networks. The aim of early intervention is to minimise the destructive effect of the psychosis and to do everything possible to maintain personal development, as well as to provide patients and their carers with an optimistic view regarding treatment, in the hope of preventing later alienation from psychiatric services.

Traditional practice

The events surrounding first contact with services, the diagnosis of schizophrenia and the initiation of treatment will have a profound effect on the relationship between the patient and carers and services for years to come. Despite its importance, the process of engagement with treatment is poorly understood. The general practitioner (GP) is the major provider of psychiatric care in Britain, and usually the point of first contact with services. However, in inner-city areas in particular, patients often receive treatment after dramatic presentations to emergency departments, the courts or the police. Some patients, particularly those with paranoid states who function well socially, never become engaged with services. Treatment may be postponed until the death or incapacity of a carer.

Obtaining treatment is often a painful process for the patient and carers. Front-line services, notably the GP and the local authority social services department (which has a statutory duty to undertake mental health assessments), frequently prove unhelpful. A message that 'nothing can be done' may be transmitted by primary care workers and first contact with the psychiatrist and community mental health team (CMHT) is often therefore delayed until crisis point is reached. A prolonged delay in the provision of help reflects the inaccessibility of many psychiatric services. Delay in presentation will also be contributed to by patient characteristics such as lack of insight, poor premorbid social adjustment and an insidious onset. Negative family attitudes to mental illness as the explanation for their relative's problems ('He's not one of those loonies') may be a barrier to treatment. Difficulty in accessing services at times of crisis is a major source of frustration for carers, who often do not know whom to turn to, even when the patient has had a long psychiatric career.

It is important that, at the initial presentation to a psychiatrist, a thorough assessment is made of the patient's psychiatric and social history, current social situation and premorbid level of functioning. This information may be vital in later years, when, as the patient's psychiatric career develops, the history becomes a catalogue of contacts with the services and the phenomenology is obscured by repetition to a host of doctors. During the initial assessment, both patients and carers will value information on what is happening and what the care plan is.

Information for distressed relatives and patients whose information-processing capacities are impaired must be presented simply and repeatedly. Hand-outs explaining the rationale for and side-effects of medication can be particularly helpful. Staff should take into account the illness beliefs held by the patient and family, and enter into a dialogue rather than adopt a didactic stance. The aim should be that, from the outset, there is an atmosphere of cooperation between the patient, carers and the services. This can be very difficult to achieve in practice.

The rationale for early intervention

Traditional mental health services were reactive to demand and focused their efforts on the most obviously needy individuals, that is, those who were severely handicapped by the effects of their illnesses. Even today much of the spending on psychiatric services is devoted to the minority of people who are in-patients. Services have not systematically sought to become more accessible to people who are becoming or who have just become psychotic. One consequence has been that presentation to services of people with psychosis is often very delayed indeed, and considerable importance is now attached to the concept and effects of the 'duration of untreated psychosis' (DUP).

The significance of the duration of the untreated psychosis

There is good evidence that a prolonged DUP is associated with a poorer prognosis for schizophrenia (Marshall *et al*, 2005). However, the mechanism of this association is presently unclear. A useful starting point is to consider the natural history of schizophrenia as described in the pre-treatment era. In a study of the long-term prognosis of patients with untreated schizophrenia presenting in the late 19th century, Ciompi (1980) described eight different lifetime trajectories. The most common pattern was of an acute episode with a rapid onset and complete resolution (25% of cases). In around 10% of cases there was only one acute episode but even for those who had two or three acute episodes over their lifetime, there was complete inter-episode remission. The group with the worst outcome (6% of cases) also had an acute onset (and had what Bleuler called 'catastrophic schizophrenia') but then proceeded directly to an end state of 'deteriorated schizophrenia'. Two groups (39% of the total) had an insidious onset (and hence a prolonged DUP) and both had a chronic course, one group having acute exacerbations, the other having a more continuous pattern, extending over many years. These observations suggest that, to a certain extent at least, the dichotomy between 'acute onset, short DUP, good prognosis' and 'insidious onset, prolonged DUP, poor prognosis' may have its origins in the natural history of the disease.

Wyatt (1991), in his review, sought to determine whether treatment (with neuroleptics) had altered the natural history of schizophrenia and found that rates for 'never discharged' patients and rates for those with a more malignant outcome were more frequent in the pre-treatment era than after the introduction of neuroleptics, although, interestingly, relapse rates were about the same. A large German study by Huber *et al* (1975) following up patients who first became ill at around the time the antipsychotics were being introduced found some two decades later that 28% of those who had received either electroconvulsive therapy (ECT) or a neuroleptic drug during their first episode of illness were in complete remission, compared with only 14% of those who received neither treatment, suggesting that early treatment might have conferred some beneficial long-term effects.

Wyatt (1991) also reanalysed the data from Philip May's randomised study of drug therapy versus psychotherapy and milieu therapy (as described in Chapter 11, page 271) and found that, for the 3 years after the end of the trial, patients who had been randomly allocated to drug treatment spent twice as much time in remunerative employment as did those initially allocated to psychotherapy or milieu treatment, even though the latter patients were subsequently treated with antipsychotics.

Crow *et al* (1986) found that patients who received their first antipsychotic treatment less than 1 year from the start of symptoms spent 54% of the time in the next 2 years in remission, as compared with only 18% for those who had a DUP of more than 1 year.

Thus, all the above studies appeared to suggest that early intervention and shortening the DUP may be helpful. However, more recent studies have questioned the role of the DUP and suggested that a prolonged DUP may not play a causal role in poor prognosis; instead, they may simply be a marker of cases with such a prognosis. The argument that a prolonged DUP is causal – through a neurotoxic mechanism, say – would be supported if it correlated with other markers of illness severity, such as changes evident on magnetic resonance imaging (MRI) or the severity of neuropsychological deficits, but studies have shown no link between the DUP and these findings (Craig *et al*, 2000). In addition, Verdoux *et al* (2001) found a strong association between a prolonged DUP and poor premorbid function (a known illness-related factor) and these workers suggested that the association between the DUP and poor prognosis may be an epiphenomenon rather than a true causal link.

Today, the mean DUP is characteristically between 1 and 2 years, even in countries with highly developed systems of healthcare (Larsen *et al*, 2000). The median is typically much shorter because of outliers with very prolonged DUPs. As noted above, the DUP will be determined by a variety of factors, such as the nature of the onset of the illness, the help-seeking behaviour of the patient and relatives, and the availability of care. Although an increased DUP is associated with a poorer prognosis, it remains unclear whether this reflects the differing intrinsic characteristics of those with short DUP, who tend to present with florid and affectively laden symptoms, which have a better outcome, and those with a long DUP, who tend to be characterised by negative symptoms, or some form of neural toxicity associated with being actively psychotic.

Only relatively recently has attention focused on the possibilities of early intervention in psychosis. The rationale is threefold:

1 Untreated psychosis is distressing and damaging to both sufferers and those around them. Effective early treatment should result in decreasing this distress and damage, whatever its cause.

2 Birchwood *et al* (1997) introduced the concept of the 'critical period' of illness. In the first 3–5 years following illness onset there may be considerable decline in social and cognitive function, and this may be may be a critical period for intervention. However, after this the clinical picture and associated deficits tend to stabilise and at this later stage changes may be rather more difficult to reverse. In principle, therefore, active early treatment should arrest the decline that typically occurs in people with schizophrenia and allow them to resume their life trajectory. This may occur either by arresting toxic neurobiological processes or by limiting the psychological and social damage caused by having schizophrenia, and in particular the experience of repeated relapses.

3 The early years after the onset of psychosis is associated with a greatly increased risk of suicide for young people with schizophrenia.

Reduction in duration of untreated psychosis

Reduction in DUP is a current target for mental health services in England. The aim is to connect the individual who is experiencing psychotic symptoms with a professional who can offer accurate assessment and effective treatment. Reduction in DUP has been reported in a study from Melbourne, Australia, and Rogaland County, Stavanger, Norway (Larsen *et al*, 2000). A variety of measures were employed to achieve this goal. These include:

- public education about the symptoms of psychosis, coupled with attempts to address the stigma associated with severe mental illness
- outreach programmes to local schools
- work with front-line education, healthcare and social care staff to inform them of the symptoms of psychosis and the importance of referral
- intensive educational work with GPs
- the provision of rapid-access assessment in non-stigmatised settings.

The study in Rogaland, which had a low baseline incidence of psychosis, demonstrated a reduction of mean (median) DUP from 114 (26) weeks to 17 (12) weeks following the introduction of a comprehensive intervention programme (Larsen *et al*, 2000).

Intervention in 'at risk' mental states

People may be identified as being at high risk because of biological loading for schizophrenia or the emergence of fleeting but not diagnostic psychotic symptoms. The key problem for designing effective interventions targeted at this stage is the lack of specificity of prodromal symptoms and biological risk factors (McGorry, 2000). The prodrome refers to a period before the onset of a frank illness, when patients present with a variety of non-specific symptoms that are often compatible with a depressive picture, and associated with social withdrawal and deteriorated mental function. Initial symptoms include poor concentration, reduced interest in activities, social withdrawal and school or occupational difficulties, which are non-specific and clearly overlap with depression and adolescent behavioural difficulties. However, as the prodrome progresses, negative symptoms and withdrawal begin to appear, as well as some features suggesting positive psychotic symptoms, such as increased sensitivity. Some people do not progress beyond the prodrome and detection of prodromal cases is therefore problematic; some studies have relied on cases self-presenting ('help seeking'), others on reports from informants (e.g. family). Instruments have been devised in an attempt to screen for the prodrome but presently these lack sensitivity and specificity.

McGorry and his colleagues from Melbourne describe what they call 'at risk' mental states, which include three clinical presentations (McGorry *et al*, 2002):

1 patients with non-specific anxiety or depression, a deterioration in global function, and a first-degree relative with a DSM–IV schizophrenia spectrum disorder
2 patients with attenuated psychotic symptoms, as may be found in schizotypal personality disorder (e.g. ideas of reference, magical thinking, perceptual disturbances or paranoid ideation)
3 patients with transient psychotic symptoms (defined as lasting less than 1 week).

Using these criteria McGorry *et al* (2002) found that after 1 year around 40% of people identified as having an 'at risk' mental state became psychotic.

Treating patients in the prodrome is presently controversial and can be recommended only in the context of a research programme.

Early intervention services

Policy in England requires the development of dedicated services for people between the ages of 16 and 35 who have recently developed a psychotic illness (Department of Health, 2001) (see also Chapter 29). These teams build on the traditional good practice offered by well-organised CMHTs. Based on pioneering work in Melbourne, north Birmingham and a number of other sites across the developed world, early intervention services should deploy the range of treatments that can be offered to people with schizophrenia, following the National of Institute for Clinical Excellence (2002*a*) guideline, as well as other psychotic illnesses. These include the psychological and social interventions reviewed in this chapter.

The enhanced staffing of an early intervention service compared with the generic CMHT allows more assertive follow-up and more active support of patients and their carers. This support is equivalent to that offered within assertive outreach teams to people with chronic psychosis and heavy service use (Department of Health, 2001), and requires similar practices and skills, including engagement, assertive outreach and work with comorbid substance misuse.

There are specific challenges that an early intervention service must overcome:

1 *Diagnostic ambiguity*. An initial psychotic episode cannot always be confidently ascribed to a diagnostic category.
2 *Prognostic uncertainty*. Patients and carers will want to know the likely future course of the illness, which is extremely unclear at first presentation.
3 *The provision of developmentally appropriate interventions*. The patient may be an adolescent or, because of the effect of the prodrome, may have missed out on significant adolescent experiences. An important emphasis within early intervention service is the attainment of appropriate educational or occupational roles.
4 *Sensitivity*. Services must be sensitive to the psychological adjustments that patients and their families make to the onset of psychosis.

Family interventions, discussed below, may be both highly relevant and difficult to provide, since there is a typical family response to a first episode, 'sealing over', that seeks to deny the existence of a problem. This reaction will result in difficulty in engaging the individual and the family in treatment. Alternatively, the patient may be traumatised by the experience of being psychotic or appraise the illness in terms of loss, humiliation and entrapment, with potentially disastrous consequences for self-esteem and a risk of depression and self-harm.

Relapse prevention

Relapse of schizophrenia is associated with a further decline in functioning and a decrease in the probability of response to antipsychotic treatment, particularly in the early stages of the illness (Hafner & an der Heiden, 2003). Antipsychotic medication, psychological treatments and appropriate social manipulations will all decrease the probability of relapse. Relapse prevention strategies involve the elaboration with the patient and carers of early warning signs of relapse characteristic for the individual, called a 'relapse signature'. Typically these warning signs are rather non-specific, involving depressed mood, social withdrawal, anxiety and sleep disturbance (Birchwood & Spencer, 2001).

It is possible to develop a relapse plan that sets out actions to be taken by the patient and carer should these signs be manifest. Such a plan may abort a full-blown episode of psychosis or may lead to rapid access to effective treatment for an established episode of illness. Specific treatment programmes for relapse prevention are discussed below.

Outcome studies of early intervention services

Few relevant studies have been published. There is encouraging evidence that intervention in individuals in 'at risk' mental states, with very high risk of subsequent transition to overt psychosis, can reduce the rates of transition into psychosis, at least in the short term (McGorry *et al*, 2002; Morrison *et al*, 2004). There is also some evidence that admission and relapse rates can be reduced by a dedicated early intervention service (Craig *et al*, 2004) and that outcomes, in terms of psychopathology (Petersen *et al*, 2005) or social and vocational functioning are improved (Garety *et al*, 2006). It is clear that, in common with assertive outreach or intensive case management, the low case loads and the person-centred approach of a dedicated early intervention service result in both fewer drop-outs from care and increased user satisfaction, but it has yet to be shown that such services will have a major impact on an individual's long-term illness career.

Psychological treatments for schizophrenia

The range of approaches

Contemporary psychological treatments for psychosis encompass a wide variety of approaches and techniques (Martindale *et al*, 2003). Their development has been driven by increased understanding of the coping strategies that have always been adopted by people with psychotic symptoms, evidence of the impact of family expressed emotion on outcome, the impressive results of early family intervention studies and the remarkable successes of the CBT approach to other psychiatric illnesses. The evidence base for psychological treatments is evolving rapidly.

Perhaps the most familiar approach is psycho-education, which involves the structured presentation of information about the illness and its treatment to patients and their carers. This is now incorporated into guidelines on good clinical practice (National Institute for Clinical Excellence, 2002*a*). There is, however, no firm evidence that psycho-education can reduce either relapse or readmission rates (National Institute for Clinical Excellence, 2003), although family interventions with a psycho-educational component have shown positive outcomes. The sensitivity of meta-analyses to the choice of included studies is demonstrated by the conflicting conclusions of the Cochrane Collaboration meta-analysis on psycho-education (Pekkala & Merinder, 2002) and that of the National Institute for Clinical Excellence (2003). The former concluded that psycho-education *did* reduce relapse and readmission rates, while the latter, which excluded a number of studies included by Pekkala & Merinder on methodological grounds and included additional studies, concluded that it did not.

Without doubt the two treatment modalities that have the firmest evidence base are CBT and family interventions (Pilling *et al*, 2002*a*), and these are discussed in more detail below.

Psychodynamic therapies were extensively employed in the past in the treatment of schizophrenia. Their current role is controversial and the National Institute for Clinical Excellence (2002*a*) guideline recommends a psychodynamic approach only for helping staff manage the often extreme stresses inherent in supporting people with severe disabilities.

A meta-analytic review of controlled trials of social skills training, much favoured in the United States, showed no clear evidence of efficacy in terms of relapse rate, social functioning, quality of life or treatment adherence (Pilling *et al*, 2002*b*). The problem appears to be with the generalisation of skills outside the artificial treatment environment: *in vivo* interaction with staff and peers is likely to be equally or more effective.

A central feature of most rehabilitation programmes is the provision of training in life skills, which is intended to overcome the performance deficits experienced by people handicapped by their severe mental illness. Surprisingly, there is very little literature reporting controlled trials of this form of treatment and further studies are urgently required (Nichol *et al*, 2000). One promising rehabilitative approach, drawn from the literature on the management of head injury and applicable to people with severe functional deficits, is cognitive adaptation training (Velligan *et al*, 2000). Compensatory strategies to overcome cognitive deficits are employed. For behaviours reflecting apathy, for example, prompting and cueing are provided by means of checklists for complex tasks, the use of labels, and the use of electronic devices to cue and sequence behaviour. For behaviours reflecting disinhibition, for example bizarre and inappropriate dressing, supplies can be organised to minimise inappropriate use.

Cognitive remediation is a novel approach aimed at addressing specific cognitive deficits in schizophrenia, such as attention, visual and verbal memory and executive functioning, by structured training in tasks that use these modalities. A meta-analytic review of the few studies undertaken to date found no overall evidence of efficacy, despite promising results in some studies (Pilling *et al*, 2002*b*).

An important specific technique to improve adherence to medication, compliance therapy, combines

Box 12.5 The key elements of compliance therapy

- The symptoms or problems reported by the patient are used as treatment targets.
- The therapist openly predicts common misgivings about treatment, such as fears of addiction, loss of control, loss of personality. If an untoward fear is elicited, a cognitive approach is used to address it.
- Confusion between illness symptoms is discussed.
- Any other meanings attached to medication are explored.
- Discussion of the natural tendency to stop medication if the patient is feeling well is combined with exploration of the patient's views of the consequences.
- The indirect benefits of medication are highlighted (e.g. 'getting on better with people').
- The therapist aims to instil a feeling that poor compliance works against the patient's long-term goals (e.g. sustaining work, avoiding hospital, looking after the children).
- Certain metaphors are used, including 'medication offers a protective layer' and 'medication is an insurance policy'.

After Kemp *et al* (1998).

features of motivational interviewing and CBT in a brief structured approach that has been shown in an influential study both to increase duration of survival in the community before readmission and to improve clinical outcome (Kemp *et al*, 1998), although a negative trial has been reported (O'Donnell *et al*, 2003). (See Box 12.5 for an outline of this treatment approach.)

Relapse prevention, using the monitoring of early signs of illness and the development of a relapse plan in a collaborative approach between care coordinator and patient, has now been incorporated into routine clinical practice under the CPA.

Trials using a CBT approach that specifically focuses on relapse prevention have been reported, with positive results (Tarrier *et al*, 1998; Herz *et al*, 2000; Gumley *et al*, 2003). The most successful (Herz *et al*, 2000) represented a far greater investment in resources than could be managed within routine clinical practice. A similarly complex psychosocial package combining family interventions, motivational interviewing and CBT has been shown to be effective in improving the outcome of patients with a dual diagnosis (i.e. those with comorbid substance misuse) (Barrowclough *et al*, 2001).

There is a considerable overlap between the various psychological treatments. CBT principles influence psycho-education, family interventions, compliance therapy, relapse prevention and dual-diagnosis therapy. Family interventions are used under the rubric of psycho-education, relapse prevention and dual-diagnosis therapy. Many psychological treatments make use of basic problem-solving techniques (Box 12.6). Most forms of psychological treatment are 'manualised', the manual providing clear guidance to inexperienced practitioners about how to carry out treatment. All psychological treatments must be provided with

Box 12.6 Elements of problem solving

- Identification of the problem(s)
- Identification of assets and supports
- Agreement of target problems
- Generation of potential solutions
- Evaluation of each solution
- Selection of the best solution
- Planning of implementation
- Review of progress – modifying tasks and goals

adequate supervision of the therapists. The interventions that have been found to be effective in terms of symptomatic and social functioning tend to decrease rates of relapse (variously defined) or readmission to hospital (see Table 12.1). However, it is clear that relapse and readmission continue to be common even in the face of the best psychological intervention. It is also important to emphasise that, at their present stage of development, these interventions complement rather than replace optimal drug treatment, with evidence suggesting synergy between the two.

Cognitive–behavioural therapy

CBT was originally developed in the 1970s for the treatment of depression but has since been successfully applied to a wide range of conditions. Its application to psychosis is relatively recent, but a variety of treatment approaches have now been applied to early-onset, recently relapsed and continually symptomatic patients. Treatment manuals are available (e.g. Kingdon & Turkington, 1994; Fowler *et al*, 1995). The literature reporting randomised controlled trials has provided convincing evidence of efficacy (improvement in outcomes in selected populations under experimental conditions), although there remain formidable problems in providing the treatment in routine clinical practice as is required by the guideline from the National Institute for Clinical Excellence (2002*a*).

CBT for psychosis can be defined as a structured and time-limited approach to the management of the problems of people with psychosis. Three main goals can be identified (Fowler *et al*, 1995):

1 to reduce the distress and disability associated with psychotic symptoms

2 to reduce emotional disturbance

3 to promote the active participation of the patient in the reduction of the risk of relapse and social disability.

As in all forms of therapy engagement, detailed assessment and the development of a therapeutic alliance are crucial. Other elements of treatment include:

- facilitating self-regulation of psychotic symptoms (utilising coping strategies to reduce symptoms)
- revising the patient's model of symptoms, by offering a normalising rationale for them (such as 'tricks of the mind' that may occur in everyday life)
- carefully and respectfully challenging beliefs held about delusions and hallucinations

Table 12.1 The effects on relapse and readmission of various psychological treatments for schizophrenia

Treatment	Comment	NNT for relapse prevention
Psycho-education	Equivocal support from reports of controlled trials. Reflects good clinical practice. Manuals available	N/A[a]
Cognitive–behavioural therapy	Strongly supported by reports of controlled trials. Manuals available	17[b]
Family interventions	Strongly supported by reports of controlled trials. Manuals available. Engagement issues problematical	11[c]
Social skills training	Not supported by reports of controlled trials. Many manuals available. Popular in the USA	N/A[a]
Cognitive remediation	Not supported by reports of controlled trials. Studies vary in approach, quality and outcome	N/A[a]
Life skills training	Not supported by reports of controlled trials. Key element of rehabilitation programmes	N/A
Cognitive adaptation training	Single report of a randomised controlled trial. Manualised approach	5[d]
Compliance therapy	Two reports of randomised controlled trials (one cited as a study of behavioural therapy by Pilling *et al*, 2002*a*). Manual available	N/A[e]
Relapse prevention	Aspects incorporated into routine clinical practice (controlled trials cited as cognitive–behavioural therapy by Pilling *et al*, 2002*a*)	6[f], 7[g], 9[h]
Dual-diagnosis treatment	Single report of a randomised controlled trial. Complex intervention. Very resource intensive	3[i]
Psychodynamic therapies	Not supported by reports of controlled trials	N/A[a]

NNT: number needed to treat to avoid one relapse or readmission during follow-up.
N/A: no evidence of efficacy in terms of reducing relapse or readmission
[a] National Institute for Clinical Excellence (2003, chapter 6, Psychological interventions in the treatment and management of schizophrenia).
[b] Relapse or readmission, duration of follow-up not specified (Pilling *et al*, 2002*a*).
[c] Relapse with readmission at 2-year follow-up (Pilling *et al*, 2002*a*).
[d] Relapse at 1-year follow-up compared with a group receiving treatment as usual (Velligan *et al*, 2000).
[e] No significant difference in readmission rates at 18 months (study lacked power), although time to readmission significantly longer in treatment group (Kemp *et al*, 1998). O'Donnell *et al* (2003) found no significant difference in outcome.
[f] Readmission at 18 months compared with high-contact control group (Herz *et al*, 2000).
[g] Readmission at 1-year follow-up compared with control group receiving routine care (Tarrier *et al*, 1998).
[h] Readmission at 1-year follow-up compared with control group receiving routine care (Gumley *et al*, 2003).
[i] Relapse at 1-year follow-up compared with controls (Barrowclough *et al*, 2001).

- addressing the dysfunctional assumptions (or schemas) held by patients, which typically reflect worthlessness and helplessness.

The development of CBT is largely credited to Aaron Beck, who originally worked as a psychoanalyst. One of his earliest papers, entitled 'Successful outpatient psychotherapy of a chronic schizophrenic with a delusion based on borrowed guilt' (Beck, 1952), used psychoanalytic language and theory but it also described how he used reality testing to treat a patient with chronic schizophrenia and paranoid delusions. He encouraged him to scrutinise the appearance and behaviour of all the alleged FBI agents who were supposedly visiting his shop in order to test his belief that these persons had him under surveillance. The patient succeeded in narrowing down his original group of 50 possible suspects to two or three possibilities and reported that he would soon be able to eliminate them completely, even though he had held these beliefs as a fixed delusion for 7 years. Nearly three decades later, Beck, together with two other colleagues, had adopted a more formal cognitive approach and they reported on the successful treatment of a further eight patients with schizophrenia and delusions in a paper entitled 'A cognitive investigation of schizophrenic delusions' (Hole *et al*, 1979). The authors commented:

> 'The combination of tracing the antecedents of the delusion and helping the patient to test his conclusions systematically helped him to recognise and to gradually do away with the irrational and rigid belief system.'

One approach to CBT for psychosis

Kingdon & Turkington (1994) describe a cognitive approach that most general psychiatrists would find acceptable and be able to learn. They start by stating the three prerequisites for engaging in CBT for schizophrenia.

- Therapists should have a broad clinical experience of working with patients with a psychosis.
- Therapists should have a sound practical knowledge of CBT for anxiety and depression. This is because the main techniques used in schizophrenia are similar to those employed for anxiety and depression and also because these symptoms are common in schizophrenia.
- CBT is only part of a wider pharmacological, social and rehabilitative programme for the treatment of schizophrenia and therapists should be familiar with all the other elements of the treatment programme which the CBT may complement.

All patients who have a psychosis need a comprehensive assessment, but from the point of view of CBT certain areas may need extra attention. These include specific areas such as:

- the origin and onset of the target symptoms, such as delusions and hallucinations, which the CBT aims to resolve or at least weaken
- the prodromal period of the illness ('how did this come about?'), even if this was many years ago
- the role of stress
- particular 'pressure points' that the patient believes caused the illness
- family values and tensions that may have contributed.

Some of this information may later be used in the CBT to offer alternative explanations to those the patient uses to account for symptoms and distress, which will be grounded in the psychotic beliefs of the patient. The formulation given at the end of the assessment should be expressed in a holistic way rather than in medical terminology.

Explanation

Explanation of the symptoms is one of the key components of CBT for depression, and has been adapted for treating the symptoms of schizophrenia. Explanation in CBT is a much more complex and psychotherapeutic exercise than simple factual explanation. It involves a joint therapist–patient investigation, weighing up 'evidence' that might explain the experiences of the patient. Kingdon & Turkington offer the following types of explanation that can sometimes be usefully explored in a 'Socratic' manner with patients who have schizophrenia.

- *Scientific explanation of phenomena.* Some psychotic phenomena are a part of a continuum of normal functioning. Thus, a thought becomes an idea, then an over-valued idea, then a delusion; a normal perception becomes an illusion, a pseudo-hallucination, and then a true hallucination. The therapist offers an explanation in terms of an exaggeration of normal function, perhaps caused by stress or social isolation or sleep deprivation, as an alternative to the psychotic explanation believed by the patient.

Case example

A patient held the belief that the full moon would fall on his house. The therapist engaged the patient in an explanation of simple physics and the laws of gravity, the rotation of the planets, and was able to sow doubts in the patient's mind, that maybe it just was not possible for the moon to fall on his house.

- *Explanation in terms of cultural beliefs.* Delusional beliefs and passivity phenomena often bear a close resemblance to some commonly held cultural belief, such as the power of the supernatural, magic, religious forces and so on, and an alternative explanation is offered and debated in these terms with the aim of weakening the psychotic beliefs.
- *Explanation in terms of 'normal experience'.* Hallucinations can occur normally in fever, or with sleep deprivation or stress, for example.
- *Use of the vulnerability–stress model.* The therapist offers a stress–vulnerability explanation for the distress as an alternative to a psychotic explanation.

Case example

A man believed that beams from a satellite were destroying his life. The therapist elicited the history. The initial breakdown had occurred 10 years previously, when the patient failed to achieve an expected promotion, and the therapist offered the explanation that the stress arising from the failed promotion had made the patient feel unwell and suggested this as an alternative to the patient's view, that the satellite beams were destroying him.

The patient may agree or disagree with the therapist's alternative explanations for the experiences, but the time spent in the discussion may help lower anxiety levels, weaken the intensity of the psychotic beliefs and improve rapport. This may be of critical importance in otherwise inaccessible, drug-refusing or drug-resistant patients.

Tackling delusions

Delusions cannot and should not be tackled by direct confrontation, because of the degree of emotional involvement in them; confrontation will lead to loss of rapport and a likely termination of the relationship. Although the core belief may be difficult to tackle, the use of inferential questioning (with less brittle patients) may lead to the discovery of cognitive distortions (e.g. 'life is unfair'). These thoughts can be tackled in the same way as the 'automatic thoughts' occurring in depression, with the use of evidence, percentage belief and so on (see Chapter 6, page 132).

Among those with chronic delusional beliefs whose emotional involvement in them may be less, the content can be questioned more directly.

Case example

A patient had for 20 years held the belief that the Chinese triads were persecuting him. His therapist asked him to write a detailed account of every encounter he had with a triad member or every time he thought he saw one, for their next session. When he arrived at the session with a blank piece of paper even the patient began to question his long-standing beliefs.

Some delusional patients cannot tolerate any sort of questioning of their beliefs, and in these instances a 'tactical withdrawal' is advisable, to avoid needless confrontation, while another useful technique is 'an agreement to differ', to avoid getting bogged down in repetitive discussion.

Tackling hallucinations

From the outset, the therapist must accept the clarity of the hallucinations but can sometimes cautiously question their basis in reality. Here, the example considered is the common one of the patient hearing voices. An exercise in joint patient–therapist testing of reality sometimes works or weakens convictions concerning the voices. If the voices come from some external source (which the patient usually believes), then asking others such as family and friends may help – when others say they cannot hear the voices the patient may be puzzled. The therapist then offers alternative explanations and debates these with the patient.

- Most commonly, patients believe that the voice is directed specifically at them, so others cannot hear it. The therapist then asks 'Why are just you selected?

How do you think they were able to target just you? What sort of mechanism is being used?'

- Where patients believe they have been lied to by relatives denying hearing the voices, the therapist might ask 'Why would your mother lie to you? Has she lied to you before?'
- The therapist supplements this with an alternative explanation: 'The voice comes from the mind, not an external source. Stress can cause this. Are you stressed? Any sleep deprivation?'

Even when debates on the presence or absence of hallucinations do not prove not profitable, the content of the hallucination may still be amenable to discussion. Content often revolves around issues of control, identity, violence and sexuality, and these ideas can be treated like the automatic thoughts of the patient with depression, using standard cognitive techniques such as weighing evidence, percentage strength of belief and so on.

Differentiating between thoughts and actions, and other cognitive techniques

Many patients are very disturbed by their strange and sometimes violent or sexual thoughts. Here, the therapist tries to point out that many people – 'you and me' – can transiently have such thoughts but that actions are quite separate from thoughts. The therapist highlights that the patient can exercise control over actions, even if he or she cannot control the thoughts.

The symptoms of anxiety and depression, which are common in schizophrenia, can also be usefully dealt with by CBT. Cognitive techniques are described for dealing with thought disorder, negative symptoms and communication difficulties, but it is uncertain whether these methods are helpful for these rather more difficult symptoms.

Coping strategies

Patients often develop their own strategies for coping with the symptoms and the therapist offers knowledge of how other patients (as described in the literature) have coped with similar experiences. Following a survey, Carr (1988) found that the main coping strategies were as follows:

- *Behaviour control.* This might include distraction by listening to music, the radio or television, or a more active diversion, such as gardening or playing a musical instrument. Sometimes a change in physical activity is helpful, such as becoming passive, taking a rest, relaxing or going to sleep; others report that increasing activity is more helpful, for example taking a walk or going for a run.
- *Self-indulgence.* Many patients cope with symptoms through an indulgence such as eating, smoking or drinking.
- *Socialisation.* Meeting family or friends sometimes enables patients to switch out of psychotic thoughts. This may lie behind the popularity of day hospital and day centre programmes with patients whose isolation (imposed by the illness) results in an excessive preoccupation with psychotic thoughts; this is diminished by the socialisation.
- *Suppression or compartmentalisation.* Some patients have developed their own cognitive strategies to suppress or compartmentalise unwanted thoughts or psychotic experiences: 'I ignore them', 'It's that rubbish again'.
- *Shift of attention.* Some try to shift their attention to more comforting ideas and a few set up specific diversionary projects (e.g. hobbies, self-improvement, shopping trips).
- *Medical help.* Only a small number seek medical help, for example in the form of changing medication, altering the dosage or seeing a mental health worker.
- *Symptomatic behaviours.* As a tension-reducing exercise some patients go along with the voices, for example by telling them to shut up, or to go along to the police station for protection. Some manifest such illness behaviours knowing that they are irrational, but in those who lack such insight it indicates that they are not coping effectively.

It can be useful to eliciting which coping strategies the patient has learned are helpful and any of the above strategies can be offered to the patient as additional ways of coping.

Effectiveness

CBT for schizophrenia is a skilled therapy requiring training, support and supervision from a CBT specialist, but it may be modestly effective. Turkington *et al* (2002) trained a group of community psychiatric nurses (CPNs) in a 10-day intensive CBT course based on methods outlined in their book, and then conducted a controlled trial of CPN-administered CBT under routine (National Health Service) conditions. While the results were not as striking as those reported by specialist psychologists operating with selected patients, they did show modest benefits. Compared with a 'treatment as usual' group, there were significant benefits in the realms of overall symptoms, insight and depression, but not for psychotic symptoms. The number needed to treat (NNT) to achieve insight was 10, and for overall symptomatic improvement the NNT was 13.

Family interventions

The onset of schizophrenia typically occurs in people in their late teens and early 20s, when the sufferer is likely to be living with or to be in close contact with the family of origin. Research has shown that aspects of the family emotional environment, characterised as 'high expressed emotion' (see Box 12.1), predict relapse in those who return to live with their families after an episode of illness. It is also clear that families experience very considerable burden in providing care and support to a person with schizophrenia and are deeply dissatisfied with the traditional response of services (Martindale *et al*, 2003). These observations have resulted in a considerable body of research into family interventions that might improve the outcome of the illness.

Controlled trials have repeatedly demonstrated that family interventions, particularly those that are relatively long term, are effective in improving outcome (Pilling *et al*, 2002*a*). A variety of models – behavioural, cognitive–behavioural, supportive and psychoeducational – have been developed and researched. Therapy may be with individual families or with groups of families. There are a number of commonalities of approach. These include:

- the development of a positive working relationship between the family and therapist
- a structured approach to therapy that offers the opportunity for additional contact with the therapist as necessary
- a focus on current stresses and problems and the elaboration of coping strategies
- encouragement of respect within the family unit
- provision of information about the illness to reduce blame attached to the patient and family guilt
- use of behavioural techniques, such as breaking down problems into manageable steps
- improvement of communication within the family.

The solid research evidence in favour of family interventions has led to a firm recommendation within the guideline from the National Institute for Clinical Excellence (2002*a*) that formal family interventions should be readily available both in the acute episode and to promote recovery. However, many questions remain about their incorporation into routine clinical practice. Problems have been encountered in getting staff who have been trained in family interventions to use their skills. Many families are simply unwilling to engage in formal family treatment, particularly early in a person's psychiatric career. It is, however, clear that services must be more assertive in their engagement with families, provide better information about the illness and available treatments, be more responsive to the concerns of family members and work more closely with them.

Managing the acute episode

Acute episodes of psychosis occur at first presentation and when the patient relapses. The guideline from the National Institute for Clinical Excellence (2002*a*) provides detailed, evidence-based advice on the pharmacological management of the acute episode. Less clear cut are the psychological and social aspects of managing the acutely ill patient and supporting carers.

The traditional approach to an acute presentation or relapse was to arrange hospital admission, if necessary under compulsion. We are now in an era where effective alternatives to in-patient care are readily available and severe bed shortages have raised the threshold for admission. Crisis resolution/home treatment teams can provide intensive community support to patients who are relapsing. Despite these developments, most patients with schizophrenia are admitted to hospital at some stage, often compulsorily.

It is important to recognise that the hospital–community dichotomy is unhelpful. The in-patient unit remains a key component of the comprehensive mental health service, not a last resort when all else has failed (see Chapter 29 for a general discussion of in-patient care).

Indications for hospital admission

Admission generally occurs as a result of a breakdown in social support following a deterioration in mental state, which may in turn be due to a failure of compliance with medication or a psychosocial stressor. There are a number of indications for admission, beyond compulsory treatment (which at the time of writing can occur in England and Wales only in hospital). These include (Stein & Test, 1980):

- the management of dangerous or suicidal behaviour
- the management of a physical illness
- the assessment or reassessment of diagnosis, level of functioning and social circumstances
- refinements of drug management
- the implementation of treatment programmes that are impossible outside hospital.

Admission often occurs when the burden of caring becomes too great for families and community support systems, although non-hospital respite care may well offer a feasible (and less stigmatising and cheaper) alternative in these circumstances. Where the patient is well known to the service, the referring doctor and the ward team should identify clear reasons for hospital admission, the goals that the admission are intended to achieve and some plans if these goals are not achieved. Home treatment/crisis resolution teams are specifically tasked with providing an alternative to admission, which can also be provided by crisis houses (which offer support in non-hospital settings).

In-patient care in schizophrenia

The development of a therapeutic milieu within the in-patient unit owes much to the application to general psychiatry of the principles of the therapeutic community. The aim is to provide a 'stable and coherent social organisation that facilitates the development and application of an individual comprehensive treatment plan', to set limits on disturbed behaviour and to foster the development of psychosocial skills (Leeman, 1986).

In classic 'milieu therapy', the unit was sustained by a variety of meetings: a daily ward report; a community meeting involving all staff and patients; a series of patient discussion and activity groups; ward rounds and discharge planning conferences; regular staff meetings; and educational meetings. The unit aimed to offer containment, structure and support for patients while attempting to involve them in their care.

Regular staff–patient meetings, a keyworker system and good communication within staff hierarchies were required for effective rehabilitation within the mental hospital (Wing & Brown, 1970). Wing & Brown (1970) described the ideal therapeutic environment for patients with chronic schizophrenia as one where, as far as possible, patients do things for themselves. They also emphasised the importance of high staff morale and positive staff attitudes towards patients. Psychiatric in-patient units for both acute and long-stay patients should provide a supportive and low-key environment. A cohesive staff team should be working consistently to a care plan that is negotiated with the patient and that focuses on real-life difficulties. Increasingly nursing teams are organised so that a primary nurse takes overall responsibility for the care planning of an individual patient, in collaboration with nursing colleagues and the multidisciplinary team, utilising the framework of a care pathway. The trust that develops between a skilled staff team and even the most suspicious patient can be of great therapeutic value.

Acutely psychotic patients should not be overstimulated, although prolonged under-stimulation must also be avoided since it may encourage the development of negative psychotic symptoms (Wing & Brown, 1970). Intrusive psychotherapeutic groups and individual psychotherapy are contraindicated. However, there should be clear expectations on the patient to maintain a degree of social competence, and the care plan should address the patient's social functioning and personal relationships. The ward should be equipped to allow patients to look after themselves as much as is feasible, with ready access to a kitchen and washing machine. The ward routine should provide structure without the imposition of institutional practices. Occupational therapy, both on the ward and in the occupational therapy department, can provide a graded range of structured activities as well as the opportunity to assess social and interpersonal functioning.

Until recently little was known about in-patient admission from the patient's perspective. Relationships with hospital staff and other patients are subjectively important in the process of recovery (Lieberman & Strauss, 1986). There is evidence that patients discharged from acute wards in the inner city are overwhelmingly glad to have left hospital despite evident dissatisfaction with the community supports available after discharge. One consumer study (McKintyre *et al*, 1989) found that the most valued aspect of hospitalisation was being free to leave the ward!

The management of disturbed behaviour

Violence, and the threat of violence, is ever present in many in-patient units (Royal College of Psychiatrists, 1998). Recently, particular concern has been expressed over sexual harassment of women on mixed-sex wards. Violent incidents are related to both patient characteristics and environmental factors. Perpetrators are younger, more commonly suffer from schizophrenia and have more commonly previously exhibited verbally aggressive and threatening behaviour compared with non-violent patients. Violent acts are generally preceded by behavioural changes, and assaults tend to be repetitive. The best predictor of future violence is past violence, although psychiatrists are poor predictors of dangerousness. Nursing staff are the commonest reported victims of violence, although this is an artefact, since incidents involving patient victims are much less likely to be recognised and reported.

Among patients with schizophrenia, violence will be more likely if there is evidence of an antisocial premorbid personality and coexisting drug misuse. Violent behaviour may be psychotically motivated (e.g. attacking the perceived source of auditory hallucinations and passivity experiences) or reflect disinhibition, when interpersonal difficulties flare up into physical attacks. The seriousness of the index incident, lack of provocation, lack of remorse, evidence of premeditation, poor response to medication and a negative attitude to treatment are all indicators of a high risk of recurrence of dangerous behaviour.

Behavioural disturbance is clearly and importantly related to environmental factors. Violence is much commoner in inner-city psychiatric units, presumably mirroring the pattern in the local community. Disturbed behaviour tends to occur when the unit is under particular strain. Disturbance will be minimised where there is a well-trained staff group who work together as a cohesive team that adopts a consistent approach to patients, sets clear limits on behaviour and aims to interact positively and respectfully with patients. There is some evidence that bored patients are more likely to be verbally and physically aggressive and provocative to others. Aggression can also be a means of gaining attention when staff otherwise interact little with their patients. Expectations of violence may become a self-fulfilling prophecy: particular concern has been expressed over the stereotyping of patients from ethnic minorities as being prone to act violently. Occasionally, staff members may provoke violence by their attitudes towards a patient.

Overcrowding, design that makes observation difficult and other aspects of the geography of a ward may serve to encourage violence. Also on a practical level, it is important for in-patient units to have clear policies governing the prevention and management of violence and for all staff to be aware of them. Training in the management of threatened violence is now mandatory for staff working within mental health services. Staff working in out-patient settings and the community must also be aware of the risks of violence, particularly when the patient is unknown to services or has a history of dangerous behaviour. Simple measures include telling colleagues when you go to talk to someone who is potentially violent, being accompanied during an interview by a team member who knows the patient, standing between the patient and the door, maintaining a safe distance and adopting non-threatening body language and a measured tone of voice. Personal alarms and panic buttons are invaluable in some settings.

If an incident occurs, help will be vital. An emergency team, led by the nurse in charge of the ward, may be summoned if the incident is serious. Physical restraint, which will require adequate numbers of trained staff working to the unit's policy, may be necessary, although current guidance stresses the importance of de-escalation techniques. If the patient has a weapon, people should run away and the police should be called. Emergency sedation may be required and the use of medication in such emergencies is discussed in the guideline from the National Institute for Clinical Excellence (2002*a*) (see also Chapter 11, page 282). There is increasing awareness of the psychologically traumatic effects of violence on both victims and the perpetrator. Guidance from the National Institute for Health and Clinical Excellence on the short-term management of disturbed behaviour in psychiatric in-patient settings is, at the time of writing, in preparation; the document will build on existing published guidance (Royal College of Psychiatrists, 1998).

Seclusion and time out

Some units have a seclusion room, in which patients may be isolated from the rest of the ward without risk of harm to themselves or others. According to the *Code of Practice to the Mental Health Act 1983* (section 19.16), seclusion is 'the supervised confinement of a patient alone in a room which may be locked' (Department of Health, 1999). There is a lack of research evidence on the efficacy of seclusion, which must:

1 follow locally agreed policies

2 be strictly time limited

3 be reviewed regularly by nursing and medical staff.

An outline seclusion procedure is contained in the Department of Health's *Code of Practice*. Patients in seclusion must be checked regularly, particularly if they have been heavily medicated; a number of deaths have occurred in these circumstances. Precise regulations governing the use of seclusion must be drawn up locally.

Clinical experience suggests that seclusion may bring disturbed behaviour rapidly under control, although its long-term effects on the ward environment and the attitudes of patients towards their treatment may be less desirable.

It is important to distinguish seclusion, which by definition is an unplanned response to an emergency, from time out, which is a psychological technique for managing disruptive behaviour. In essence, time out is the brief (15 minutes at most) exclusion of the patient from positive reinforcement following inappropriate behaviour, generally by moving the patient to a quiet room. Time out is one of a range of behavioural techniques to manage 'challenging behaviours'. Success demands persistence since programmes that involve withdrawing reinforcements for problematical behaviours will often result in an initial increase in the frequency, severity and duration of those behaviours.

Following a serious incident, the staff team should get together for a debriefing session, to facilitate the ventilation of feelings, allow a critical review of the way that policies were implemented and consider a revision of the patient's care plan. Debriefing of the patient may also facilitate emotional processing of distressing events (in the past, patients were rarely talked through their experiences, other than in the sense of being told off). Cognitive–behavioural assessment of the antecedents and consequences of problematical behaviours may be valuable, medication may be have to be reviewed and on occasion the involvement of the police or the forensic psychiatric services may be necessary. The needs of the victim of an assault should never be forgotten, and appropriate counselling should be offered if necessary.

Discharge planning

> 'Planning for discharge is probably the most important process in the inpatient hospitalization of persons suffering from chronic illness. It involves planning the management of the patient's illness over a lifetime.' (Talbott & Glick, 1986)

The CPA provides a structure for the discharge planning process in England. It extends the duty on health and social services set out in section 117 of the Mental Health Act 1983 to provide appropriate after-care for patients who have been detained in hospital under sections 3 and 37. Under the CPA, discharge arrangements should be discussed at a pre-discharge meeting that involves all relevant agencies, the patient and carers. Because of evidence that the incidence of suicide peaks in the period just after discharge from in-patient care there is also a requirement in England for direct, face-to-face follow-up of all vulnerable patients within 7 days of discharge.

Discharge planning should begin soon after admission. Plans should address the needs already described in this chapter, focusing particularly on practical issues such as income maintenance, appropriate accommodation and arrangements to continue physical and psychological treatments.

Long-term planning and the continued involvement of the treatment team are equally important for patients whose acute episodes are managed in the community (Stein & Test, 1980).

Schizophrenia and risk

We live in an era obsessed with risk, and risk assessment is now seen as one of the core activities of mental health professionals. People with schizophrenia present a range of risks, to themselves and others. Schizophrenia is associated with increased all-cause mortality (standardised mortality ratio 260) (Brown *et al*, 2000). Less than half this increased mortality is due to deaths from unnatural causes (injury, suicide, homicide and undetermined cause). Care plans need to address physical health needs, including obvious risk factors such as smoking, obesity and hypertension, either directly or, preferably, through liaison with primary care. People with schizophrenia have a grossly elevated suicide rate (standardised mortality ratio 820), with suicide being commonest among current in-patients and people who have recently been discharged from hospital. Self-neglect is a significant risk, as is violent victimisation and financial exploitation.

There is also, in the era of community care, a clear if complex relationship between schizophrenia and violence (Taylor & Estroff, 2003). There is a very extensive literature on the topic. Epidemiological studies suggest that there is an overall low rate of violence among people with schizophrenia, which is, however, significantly higher than in the general population. It has been calculated from US data (Swanson *et al*, 1990) that people with schizophrenia are responsible for 3% of violent acts in society and, according to the UK National Confidential Inquiry for Suicide and Homicide, between 3% and 5% of homicides (see http://www.national-confidential-inquiry.ac.uk). However, rates of violence and risk factors reflect the propensity to violence of the local population. Much of the violence associated with schizophrenia occurs in people with comorbid substance misuse (substance misuse being separately associated with a high proportion of societal violence).

One other important risk area is that of the person with schizophrenia as a parent: the welfare of the children of people with severe mental illness is a source of increasing concern for mental health services.

It is important to place these risks in context. An average CMHT catchment area in England will experience on average approximately one suicide a year, out of some 700 people in contact with the service that year, and one homicide every 40 years. Prediction of serious adverse events that occur rarely is extremely difficult, if not impossible, unless there are clear risk indicators, such as previous very serious violence in the context of psychosis. Prevention should logically focus on:

- ameliorating underlying risk factors, such as depressed mood, psychotic symptoms, substance misuse and impulsivity
- triggering psychosocial issues
- strong therapeutic relationships with patients and families
- having a clear understanding of each patient's mental state.

Substance misuse

Substance misuse is common among people with schizophrenia and other psychoses: the reported 6-month or 12-month prevalence rates among treated populations range from 22% to 34% (Maslin, 2003). Alcohol misuse and dependence are commoner than misuse of cannabis and stimulants, although the latter substances often have more dramatic effects on mental state. Opiate misuse is both uncommon and clinically not particularly problematical.

Comorbid substance misuse (sometimes termed 'dual diagnosis') is associated with a variety of negative outcomes that include high rates of relapse, more frequent and prolonged hospitalisation, violence (much of the violence associated with schizophrenia relates to 'dual diagnosis' patients), poverty, offending behaviour, imprisonment, homelessness and serious infections such as HIV and hepatitis.

Until recent years there were few serious attempts to tackle the problem, with some professionals adopting an almost moral stance to 'dual diagnosis' patients. They have been habitually rejected from both the mental illness and the drug dependence services. Thus, at the first sign of drinking or substance misuse patients would be discharged from acute admission wards, while current drug treatment programmes do not accept patients with severe functional disorder such as schizophrenia because they would be quite unable to cope with the rigours of groups or intensive psychotherapy. One barrier to joint working between substance misuse and adult mental health services is their conflicting paradigms: at least until recently, all substance misuse treatment was predicated on the willingness of the sufferer to seek change, while adult mental health services frequently work with people within an explicitly coercive framework. (The situation has changed somewhat in recent years as substance misuse services have received more funding from the criminal justice system.)

The problem has until recently received much greater attention in the USA than in the UK. The American experience was reviewed by Drake *et al* (2001). In the early 1980s, attempts were made to apply to patients with schizophrenia traditional substance misuse programmes, such as the 12 steps (the Alcoholics Anonymous programme), but these did not work because they failed to take into account the complex cognitive difficulties experienced by many patients with schizophrenia. It soon became apparent that the counselling needed to go very much more slowly in 'dual diagnosis' patients; it would also have to take into account their negative symptoms, their neurocognitive deficits and their very much greater vulnerability to confrontation (confrontation is a key and frequently used therapeutic technique in many substance misuse programmes). In addition, patients with schizophrenia have a much greater need for support of all types (emotional, financial, social and housing, etc.).

Substance misuse programmes commonly aim for complete abstinence but few patients with schizophrenia will contemplate this goal, as they commonly enjoy taking their substance of misuse, sometimes even deriving symptomatic benefit from it. Motivational interviewing may sometimes help achieve a modest degree of engagement. Traditional substance misuse programmes are usually both intensive and time limited but for patients with a chronic disease this model may be inappropriate. According to Drake *et al* (2001) the recent US experience suggests that benefits, if they come, are achieved only slowly and then often over a period of months or even years, and such programmes need to offer continued support.

US programmes vary, but a good example is provided by Ho *et al* (1999). In that programme, patients attended the day hospital for 6 months and staffing levels were high, with three psychiatrists and three care managers being responsible for 60 patients. A 35-session social skills programme specifically tailored to take into account cognitive and motivational deficits was directed at generally improving social skills, while there were additional psycho-educational modules covering relapse prevention of illness, relapse prevention of substance misuse, stress management, relaxation and exercise groups. The case managers attended to the patient's every need, such as housing, finance and family matters, and patients continued with their antipsychotic drugs, usually haloperidol or fluphenazine. Patients were paid $1.50 for every group they attended and also had to provide twice-weekly urine samples, for which they were also paid $1.50. Benefits of the programme were modest, with 30% maintaining sobriety 3 months after the programme, compared with 5% of those who had only minimal exposure to the treatment.

A programme of this type would not occur in contemporary National Health Service drug and alcohol services, where the model is more of encouraging patients to assume individual responsibility for their addictive behaviours, with confrontation and soul searching in the face of substance misuse relapse. It would be almost unthinkable to pay patients to attend group therapy sessions or to pay for their urine samples, yet a new philosophical and more generous approach may be required to treat dual-diagnosis patients, bearing in mind their neurocognitive and motivational deficits. Many mental health services have appointed 'dual diagnosis' workers, who both work directly with individual substance misusers and, more importantly, provide training, advice and consultancy to their colleagues within mental health teams. Current policy requires staff within adult mental health services to develop skills in working with comorbid substance misuse, 'mainstreaming' these skills (Department of Health, 2002). Although, given the extent of the problem, this makes pragmatic sense, the current literature contains only trials of rather intensive interventions carried out by experts, generally adopting cognitive–behavioural or family intervention paradigms (for an example see Barrowclough *et al*, 2001; for a recent review see Graham *et al*, 2003).

As well as a psychosocial approach to the problem of 'dual diagnosis', there has been considerable interest in optimising the drug treatment of the underlying schizophrenia with the use of atypical antipsychotics, especially clozapine. Drake *et al* (2000) screened a large cohort of patients with schizophrenia for substance misuse and followed them up. A total of 36 patients subsequently went on to take clozapine because of presumed treatment resistance. In the 6 months before they went on to clozapine, these patients averaged 54 days of drinking, compared with only 12 days per 6 months while on clozapine. At the end of their study, 79% of the clozapine-treated patients were in remission from their substance misuse, compared with only 34% of those who were on other typicals or atypicals. Drake *et al* (2000) suggested that there is now sufficient data to justify further proper randomised controlled trials of clozapine among dual-diagnoses patients, with the underlying implication that if such trials showed positive benefits then dual diagnosis might become an additional and licensed indication for clozapine.

Rehabilitation and long-term care

Rehabilitation and long-term care are not fashionable. The word 'rehabilitation' rarely appears in UK mental health policy documents. Despite a long-standing policy focus on severe mental illness, awareness of the impact of mental illness in producing social exclusion in sufferers and the large proportion of mental health spending that still goes on long-term care, few UK mental health professionals specialise in rehabilitation. This current low profile reflects the history of rehabilitation services (which flourished in the traditional mental hospital), shows the continuing ambiguities over the meaning of the term, and reveals a long-standing difficulty in acknowledging the realities of continuing disability in an era of community mental healthcare.

Historically, rehabilitation services were based in the mental hospital. The aim was to enable patients, most of whom suffered from schizophrenia, to move out of hospital, either back to their home or to a supported care setting. Long-stay patients moved down and then up a ladder from the acute ward to the back ward, on to the rehabilitation unit, and eventually out of hospital or to a poorly staffed continuing-care ward, where they might live out the rest of their lives.

Rehabilitation as a process of resettlement proved spectacularly successful, to the extent that the majority of the large mental hospitals in England closed in the last 15 years of the 20th century. The hospital closure and reprovision programme that took place in England during the late 1980s and 1990s was carefully evaluated. However, less is known about the fate of the many thousands who left the declining hospitals in the decades before the closure programme – anecdotally often with only the price of a railway ticket and the address of a boarding home in a seaside town. The development of specialist rehabilitation services is very patchy and, following the hospital closure programme, there is a much larger *de facto* system of continuing care within generic mental health and social care services. Each locality has a substantial number of people with severe mental illnesses receiving supportive care in what might be termed a 'virtual mental hospital'. This comprises largely an uncoordinated network of residential provision with both the private and voluntary sectors, family care and *ad hoc* support from CMHTs.

The rehabilitation approach involves a number of key principles:

- a holistic and detailed approach to assessment and treatment
- a focus on the individual's skills and abilities as well as on symptoms and disabilities
- an explicit aim of fostering social inclusion and individual recovery in the face of continuing illness and disability
- a focus on a working alliance with the patient and carers.

Above all, rehabilitation services take a long-term as opposed to an episodic approach to care. These principles are relevant across the diagnostic spectrum and will be incorporated within well-functioning assertive outreach and early intervention services.

Currently, rehabilitation services tend to comprise two elements (Killaspy *et al*, 2005): the community rehabilitation team and in-patient units. The community rehabilitation team provides support to people who are living outside hospital, either independently or in supported housing. It adopts an assertive outreach style of working, but is also prepared to provide or arrange for the practical support required by people with very severe functional deficits. One or more local in-patient units will offer medium-term and continuing care. Both the community team and the in-patient units will make use of the full range of evidence-based treatments set out in the guideline from the National Institute for Clinical Excellence (2002*a*), together with the practical approaches developed within social work, nursing and occupational therapy that encourage people to engage in appropriate social functioning. If necessary, environmental manipulations are made that allow people with continuing disabilities to function as independently as possible (e.g. in supported housing projects and, where money management is problematical, using appointeeship).

One further important, and evidence-based, aspect of a rehabilitation service is vocational rehabilitation, which is considered in Chapter 29.

Recovery

Recovery, in contrast to rehabilitation, is both fashionable and a word much used within contemporary policy documents relating to mental health, both in the USA and in the UK (Roberts & Wolfson, 2003). Its intellectual underpinnings lie in the first-person accounts of patients with psychoses who have achieved either full functional recovery or a positive accommodation of their illness, so that they regain a sense of themselves (Davidson & Strauss, 1992). Keywords in the recovery literature are 'hope', 'self-esteem', 'self-respect', 'control', 'empowerment' and 'connection' (to the wider social world) (Jacobson & Greenley, 2001). These are obvious targets for psychological interventions, although first-person accounts detail the very idiosyncratic ways in which individuals have experienced recovery. For some, active membership of a user-led consumer or survivor group has been an important element in recovery.

To foster recovery, services need to be provided by people who can develop an effective therapeutic alliance with patients and carers, in a service context that recognises the human rights of users and carers and is appropriately respectful. Above all, mental health services need to move away from a stance of 'doing to' patients, through 'doing with' and towards a facilitative role that allows patients full control over their care and their lives.

This vision must be balanced, of course, with a realistic and honest appraisal of the disabilities and disadvantages that so often accompany schizophrenia. Mental health practitioners are faced with a continual dilemma between, on the one hand, fostering individual autonomy and the taking of clinical risk and, on the other hand, exercising their duty of care in prompting, persuading and if necessary coercing patients to ensure minimal standards of social functioning, treatment adherence and personal safety.

References

Barrowclough, C., Haddock, G., Tarrier, N., *et al* (2001) Randomized controlled trial of motivational interviewing, cognitive–behaviour therapy and family intervention for patients with comorbid schizophrenia and substance use disorders. *American Journal of Psychiatry*, **158**, 1706–1713.

Beck, A. T. (1952) Successful outpatient psychotherapy in a chronic schizophrenic with a delusion based on borrowed guilt. *Psychiatry*, **15**, 303–312.

Bebbington, P. & Kuipers, E. (2003) Schizophrenia and psychosocial stresses. In *Schizophrenia* (eds S. R. Hirsch & D. Weinberger), pp. 613–636. Oxford: Blackwell.

Bhugra, D., Mallett, R. & Leff, J. (1999) Schizophrenia and African-Caribbeans: a conceptual model of aetiology. *International Review of Psychiatry*, **11**, 145–152.

Birchwood, M. & Spencer, E. (2001) Early intervention in psychotic relapse. *Clinical Psychology Review*, **21**, 1211–1226.

Birchwood, M., McGrorry, P. & Jackson, H. (1997) Early intervention in schizophrenia. *British Journal of Psychiatry*, **170**, 2–5.

Brewin, C. R., Wing, J. K., Mangen, S. P., *et al* (1987) Principles and practice of measuring needs in the long-term mentally ill: the MRC needs for care assessment. *Psychological Medicine*, **17**, 955–971.

Brooker, C. & Brabban, A. (2005) *Measured Success: A Scoping Review of Evaluated Psychosocial Interventions Training for Work with People with Serious Mental Health Problems*. Mansfield: National Institute for Mental Health in England/Trent Workforce Development Confederation.

Brown, S., Barraclough, B. & Inskip, H. (2000) Causes of the excess mortality of schizophrenia. *British Journal of Psychiatry*, **177**, 212–217.

Carr, V. (1988) Patient's techniques for coping with schizophrenia: an exploratory study. *British Journal of Medical Psychology*, **61**, 339–352.

Chadwick, P., Lundin, R., Brown, G., *et al* (2003) Psychosis and recovery: some patients' perspectives. In *Schizophrenia* (eds S. R. Hirsch & D. Weinberger), pp. 701–712. Oxford: Blackwell.

Ciompi, L. (1980) The natural history of schizophrenia in the long term. *British Journal of Psychiatry*, **136**, 413–420.

Craig, T. J., Bromet, E. J., Fennig, S., *et al* (2000) Is there an association between duration of untreated psychosis and 24 month clinical outcome in a first admission series. *American Journal of Psychiatry*, **157**, 60–66.

Craig, T. K., Garety, P., Power, P., *et al* (2004) The Lambeth Early Onset (LEO) Team: randomised controlled trial of the effectiveness of specialised care for early psychosis. *BMJ*, **329**, 1067–1069.

Crow, T. J., Macmillan, J. F., Johnson, A. L., *et al* (1986) A randomised controlled study of prophylactic neuroleptic treatment. *British Journal of Psychiatry*, **148**, 120–127.

Davidson, L. & Strauss, J. S. (1992) Sense of self in recovery from severe mental illness. *British Journal of Medical Psychology*, **65**, 131–145.

Department of Health (1999) *Code of Practice to the Mental Health Act 1983*. London: Department of Health.

Department of Health (2001) *Mental Health Policy Implementation Guide*. London: Department of Health.

Department of Health (2002) *Mental Health Policy Implementation Guide: Dual Diagnosis Good Practice Guide*. London: Department of Health.

Drake, R. E., Xie, H., McHugo, G. J., *et al* (2000) The effects of clozapine on alcohol and drug use disorders among patients with schizophrenia. *Schizophrenia Bulletin*, **26**, 441–449.

Drake, R. E., Essock, S. M., Shaner, A., *et al* (2001) Implementing dual diagnosis services for clients with severe mental illness. *Psychiatric Services*, **52**, 469–476.

Fowler, D., Garety, P. & Kuipers, E. (1995) *Cognitive Behaviour Therapy for Psychosis*. Chichester: Wiley.

Garety, P. A., Kuipers, E., Fowler, D., *et al* (2001) A cognitive model of the positive symptoms of psychosis. *Psychological Medicine*, **31**, 189–195.

Garety, P. A., Craig, T. K., Dunn, G., *et al* (2006) Specialised care for early psychosis: symptoms, social functioning and patient satisfaction: randomised controlled trial. *British Journal of Psychiatry*, **188**, 37–45.

Goldberg, T. E., David, A. & Gold, J. M. (2003) Neurocognitive deficits in schizophrenia. In *Schizophrenia* (eds S. R. Hirsch & D. Weinberger), pp. 168–184. Oxford: Blackwell.

Graham, H. L., Copello, A., Birchwood, M. J., *et al* (2003) *Substance Misuse in Psychosis. Approaches to Treatment and Service Delivery*. Chichester: Wiley.

Gumley, A., O'Grady, M., McNay, L., *et al* (2003) Early intervention for relapse in schizophrenia: results of a 12-month randomized controlled trial of cognitive behavioural therapy. *Psychological Medicine*, **33**, 419–431.

Hafner, A. & an der Heiden, W. (2003) Course and outcome of schizophrenia. In *Schizophrenia* (eds S. R. Hirsch & D. Weinberger), pp. 101–141. Oxford: Blackwell.

Harris, M. & Bergman, H. C. (1987) Case management with the chronically mentally ill: a clinical perspective. *American Journal of Orthopsychiatry*, **57**, 296–302.

Hayward, P. & Bright, J. (1997) Stigma and mental illness: a review and critique. *Journal of Mental Health*, **6**, 345–354.

Herz, M. I., Lamberti, J. S., Mintz, J., *et al* (2000) A program for relapse prevention in schizophrenia: a controlled study. *Archives of General Psychiatry*, **57**, 277–283.

Ho, A., Tsuang, J. & Liberman, R. P. (1999) Achieving effective treatment of patients with chronic psychotic illness and comorbid substance dependence. *American Journal of Psychiatry*, **156**, 1765–1770.

Hole, R..W., Rush, A. J. & Beck, A. T. (1979) A cognitive investigation into schizophrenic delusions. *Psychiatry*, **42**, 312–319.

Huber, G., Gross, G. & Schuttler, R. (1975) A long term follow up study of schizophrenia: psychiatric course of illness and prognosis. *Acta Psychiatrica Scandinavica*, **52**, 49–57.

Jacobson, N. & Greenley, D. (2001) What is recovery? A conceptual model and explication. *Psychiatric Services*, **52**, 482–485.

Kemp, R., Kirov, G., Everitt, B., *et al* (1998) Randomised controlled trial of compliance therapy. 18 month follow-up. *British Journal of Psychiatry*, **172**, 413–419.

Killaspy, H., Harden, C., Holloway, F., *et al* (2005) What do mental health rehabilitation services do and what are they for? A national survey in England. *Journal of Mental Health*, **14**, 157–165.

Kingdon, D. G. & Turkington, D. (1994) *Cognitive–Behavioural Therapy of Schizophrenia*. Hove: Psychology Press.

Larsen, T. K., Johannessen, J. O., McGlashan, T., *et al* (2000) Can duration of untreated psychosis be reduced? In *Early Intervention in Psychosis* (eds M. Birchwood, D. Fowler & C. Jackson), pp. 143–165. Chichester: Wiley.

Leeman, C. P. (1986) The therapeutic milieu. In *Inpatient Psychiatry. Diagnosis and Treatment* (ed. L. I. Sederer), pp. 222–233. Baltimore, MD: Williams and Wilkins.

Lehman, A. F., Reed, S. K. & Possidente, S. M. (1982) Priorities for long-term care: comments from board-and-care residents. *Psychiatric Quarterly*, **54**, 181–189.

Liddle, P. F. (1987) The symptoms of chronic schizophrenia: a re-examination of the positive–negative dichotomy. *British Journal of Psychiatry*, **151**, 145–151.

Lidz, C. W., Mulvey, E. P., Hoge, S. K., *et al* (1998) Factual sources of psychiatric patients' perceptions of coercion in the hospital admission process. *American Journal of Psychiatry*, **155**, 1254–1260.

Lieberman, P. B. & Strauss, J. S. (1986) Brief psychiatric hospitalization: what are its effects? *American Journal of Psychiatry*, **143**, 1557–1562.

Marshall, M., Lewis, S., Lockwood, A., *et al* (2005) Association between duration of untreated psychosis and outcome in cohorts of first-episode patients: a systematic review. *Archives of General Psychiatry*, **62**, 975–983.

Martindale, B. V., Mueser, K., Kuipers, E., *et al* (2003) Psychological treatments for schizophrenia. In *Schizophrenia* (eds S. R. Hirsch & D. Weinberger), pp. 657–687. Oxford: Blackwell.

Maslin, J. (2003) Substance misuse in psychosis: contextual issues. In *Substance Misuse in Psychosis. Approaches to Treatment and Service Delivery* (eds H. L. Graham, A. Copello, M. J. Birchwood & K. T. Mueser), pp. 3–23. Chichester: Wiley.

Maslow, A. (1954) *Motivation and Personality*. New York: Harper and Row.

McGorry, P. D. (2000) The scope for preventive strategies in early psychosis: logic, evidence and momentum. In *Early Intervention in Psychosis* (eds M. Birchwood, D. Fowler & C. Jackson), pp. 3–27. Chichester: Wiley.

McGorry, P. D., Yung, A. R., Phillips, L. J., *et al* (2002) Randomized controlled trial of interventions designed to reduce the risk of progression to first-episode psychosis in a clinical sample with subthreshold symptoms. *Archives of General Psychiatry*, **59**, 921–928.

McKintyre, K., Farrell, M. & David, A. (1989) Inpatient psychiatric care: the patient's views. *British Journal of Medical Psychology*, **62**, 249–255.

Morrison, A. P., French, P., Walford, L., *et al* (2004) Cognitive therapy for the prevention of psychosis in people at ultra high risk: randomised controlled trial. *British Journal of Psychiatry*, **185**, 291–297.

National Institute for Clinical Excellence (2002*a*) *Schizophrenia. Core Interventions in the Treatment and Management of Schizophrenia in Primary and Secondary Care. Clinical Guideline 1*. London: NICE.

National Institute for Clinical Excellence (2002*b*) *Guidance on the Use of Newer (Atypical) Antipsychotic Drugs for the Treatment of Schizophrenia*. NICE Technology Appraisal Guidance No. 43. London: NICE.

National Institute for Clinical Excellence (2003) *Schizophrenia. Core Interventions in the Treatment and Management of Schizophrenia in Primary and Secondary Care. National Clinical Practice Guideline*. London: NICE.

Nichol, M. M., Robertson, L. & Connaughton, J. A. (2000) Life skills programmes for chronic mental illnesses. *Cochrane Database of Systematic Reviews*, (**2**), CD000381.

O'Donnell, C., Donohoe, G., Sharkey, L., *et al* (2003) Compliance therapy: a randomised controlled trial in schizophrenia. *British Medical Journal*, **327**, 834–837.

Pekkala, E. & Merinder, L. (2002) Psychoeducation for schizophrenia. *Cochrane Database of Systematic Reviews*, (**4**), CD002831.

Petersen, L., Jeppesen, P., Thorup, A., *et al* (2005) A randomised multicentre trial of integrated versus standard treatment for patients with a first episode of psychotic illness. *BMJ*, **331**, 602–605.

Pilling, S., Bebbington, P., Kuipers, E., *et al* (2002*a*) Psychological treatments in schizophrenia: I Meta-analyses of family intervention and cognitive behaviour therapy. *Psychological Medicine*, **32**, 763–782.

Pilling, S., Bebbington, P., Kuipers, E., *et al* (2002*b*) Psychological treatments in schizophrenia: II Meta-analyses of randomized controlled trials of social skills training and cognitive remediation. *Psychological Medicine*, **32**, 783–791.

Roberts, G. & Wolfson, P. (2003) The rediscovery of recovery: open to all. *Advances in Psychiatric Treatment*, **10**, 37–49.

Royal College of Psychiatrists (1998) *Management of Imminent Violence: Clinical Practice Guidelines to Support Mental Health Services*. Occasional Paper 41. London: Royal College of Psychiatrists.

Slade, M., Thornicroft, G., Loftus, L., *et al* (1999) *Camberwell Assessment of Need*. London: Gaskell.

Stein, L. I. & Test, M. A. (1980) Alternative to mental hospital treatment. *Archives of General Psychiatry*, **37**, 392–397.

Swanson, J. W., Holzer, C. E., Ganju, V. K., *et al* (1990) Violence and psychiatric disorder in the community: evidence from the Epidemiologic Catchment Area Surveys. *Hospital and Community Psychiatry*, **41**, 761–770.

Talbott, J. A. & Glick, I. D. (1986) The inpatient care of the chronically mentally ill. *Schizophrenia Bulletin*, **37**, 392–397.

Tarrier, N., Yusupoff, L., Kinsey, C., *et al* (1998) Randomised controlled trial of intensive cognitive behaviour therapy for patients with chronic schizophrenia. *BMJ*, **347**, 303–307.

Taylor, P. J. & Estroff, S. E. (2003) Schizophrenia and violence. In *Schizophrenia* (eds S. R. Hirsch & D. Weinberger), pp. 591–612. Oxford: Blackwell.

Turkington, D., Kingdon, D. & Turner, T. (2002) Effectiveness of a brief cognitive behaviour therapy intervention in the treatment of schizophrenia. *British Journal of Psychiatry*, **180**, 523–527.

Velligan, D. I., Bow-Thomas, C. C., Huntzinger, C., *et al* (2000) Randomized controlled trial of the use of compensatory strategies to enhance adaptive functioning in outpatients with schizophrenia. *American Journal of Psychiatry*, **157**, 1317–1328.

Verdoux, H., Lirand, F., Bergey, C., *et al* (2001) Is the association between duration of untreated psychosis confounded? A two year follow up study of first admitted patients. *Schizophrenia Research*, **49**, 231–241.

Wing, J. K. (1993) Social consequences of severe mental illness. In *Social Psychiatry* (eds D. Bhugra & J. Leff), pp. 400–412. Oxford: Blackwell.

Wing, J. K. & Brown, G. W. (1970) *Institutionalism and Schizophrenia*. London: Cambridge University Press.

Wolfensberger, W. (1983) Social role valorization: a proposed new term for the principle of normalization. *Mental Retardation*, **21**, 234–239.

Wyatt, R. (1991) Early intervention with neuroleptics may decrease the long term morbidity of schizophrenia. *Schizophrenia Research*, **5**, 201–219.

CHAPTER 13

Anxiety disorders

Spilios Argyropoulos, Adam Campbell and George Stein

A brief history of the neuroses

The term 'neurosis' has been in use for more than a century to describe the anxieties, phobias, obsessions, hysteria, hypochondriasis and a few other non-psychotic conditions, and although it has now finally been abandoned as an official category in both ICD-10 (World Health Organization, 1992) and DSM–IV (American Psychiatric Association, 1994), it still remains in common usage. The word was originally derived from a Greek root meaning 'nerve' and was first introduced into the English language by Lovell in 1661, as 'neurotick', which was a herbal medicine made from rose syrup or vegetables that, it was claimed, had a bracing effect on the nervous system (*Oxford English Dictionary*, 1989). Cullen, the leading Scottish physician of the 18th century, was the first to apply the term 'neurosis' to a class of illnesses:

> 'In a certain view, almost the whole of the diseases of the human body might be called nervous ... in this place I propose to comprehend the title neurosis to all those preternatural affections of sense and motion which are without pyrexia as part of the primary disease and which do not depend on a topical affection of the organs but upon a more general affectation of the nervous system.' (Cullen, 1784)

Cullen distinguished 'local diseases' from 'general diseases' and the neuroses were general disorders that lacked fever. At the beginning of the 19th century, Pinel translated Cullen's work into French, but at the same time criticised his view that the neuroses are physical disorders. He argued that the neuroses are disorders of sense and movement without any neuropathological basis and put forward an explanation of moral or 'sympathetic' causes. The moral element was explained in terms of the 'passions' or 'affections of the soul', while 'the sympathetic cause' described influences arising from the stomach, the reproductive organs or other parts of the body and their effect on the brain (Pinel, 1801). Georget (1840) developed Pinel's ideas and was the first to formulate the modern concept of neuroses as non-fatal, non-psychotic disorders and he included in this group hysteria, asthma, nervous palpitations, gastralgia with or without vomiting and the neuralgias. In England a more mechanistic view prevailed and the terms 'spinal irritation' and 'reflex functional nervous disease' came into use.

Throughout this period, the mental experience of anxiety was seen as part of the melancholic (depressive) state. It was Darwin, in the *Origin of Species* (1859), who differentiated anxiety from depression and observed that the former refers to future experiences and the latter to past ones. At the same time, in mainland Europe the idea arose that these mental and somatic symptoms are the diverse manifestations of a unitary syndrome. Thus, Feuchtersleben, in 1847, re-established the link between mind and body, by viewing anxiety as a cause of organic problems, notably of the heart and digestive system. Morel, in 1866, finally linked the mental symptoms with the then new concept of the autonomic nervous system, and proposed that it is the physical changes that generate the mental anxiety (see Berrios & Link, 1995). In 1894 Freud gathered the clinical manifestations of anxiety under the umbrella of 'anxiety neurosis' (Freud, 1894). This unitary concept dominated discussion and practice during the 20th century, at least up to the 1960s, although individual syndromes reminiscent of the current classification had already been delineated (Berrios & Link, 1995).

Two American physicians also made important contributions. Thus, during the American Civil War, Da Costa (1871) saw cases of severe chest pain and panic in otherwise healthy young men who suffered from a condition he called the 'irritable heart'. This was caused by:

> 'quick long marches producing the affection or even slight exertion in those whose constitution had been impaired by insufficient or indigestible food.... It seems to me most likely that the heart has become irritable from its overactive and frequent excitement and disordered innervation keeps it so.'

Da Costa recognised that the symptoms could also occur in peacetime. During Second World War, Da Costa's syndrome once more assumed importance and the British army had an official category known as 'disordered action of the heart', which was diagnosed in over 60000 British soldiers. In peacetime this was renamed as the 'effort syndrome' by the cardiologist Sir Thomas Lewis.

The second American contribution came from George Beard (1869), who proposed the term 'neurasthenia' to describe a group of severe fatigue and mood disorders that seem to defy other explanations. Beard considered it to be mainly a hereditary disorder. It became a fashionable diagnosis in the latter part of the 19th century and then fell into disrepute, but more recently it has experienced a revival and is now included in ICD–10. A variant of neurasthenia that combined features of

Beard's neurasthenia with those of Da Costa's irritable heart was labelled 'neurocirculatory asthenia' (Oppenheimer & Rothschild, 1918). This disorder comprised cardiovascular symptoms combined with anxiety, and most cases would nowadays be diagnosed as panic disorder (thus, panic disorder has probably been at least partly recognised for a long time).

The separation of the neuroses from the psychoses is officially attributed to Huxley in 1871 (*Oxford English Dictionary*, 1989) and this distinction had until recently assumed rather more importance than the facts warranted. According to ICD–9 (World Health Organization, 1978) the neuroses are disorders characterised by unimpaired 'reality testing', with preservation of insight and an absence of any demonstrable organic basis. By contrast, people with a psychosis lack insight and their mental function is so impaired that contact with reality is lost and even the ordinary demands of life can not be met. Thus, the people with a psychosis are extremely ill but fail to recognise it, while those with a neurosis are much less ill but realise only too well how ill they are (Tyrer, 1989*a*). This old, somewhat arbitrary distinction has little validity in clinical practice because the majority of those who suffer from psychoses are all too painfully aware of their disabilities. Also, many patients who have a neurosis experience severe and lifelong incapacity, and may not be particularly insightful, for example patients with severe hypochondriasis, and so the presence or absence of insight is not a particularly useful diagnostic pointer.

No historical overview would be complete without mentioning the work of Pavlov, the Russian physiologist who described the conditioned reflex (Pavlov, 1927). His ideas were later taken up and extensively modified by Skinner, Wolpe, Marks and others. Although the idea of simple conditioned reflexes and faulty learning as the main cause of neuroses has long since been discarded, the notion that the treatment of neurotic disorders should involve new learning and that this should take place in the 'here and now' rather than through exploration of the distant past has been widely influential.

Definitions, symptoms of anxiety and their differential diagnosis

Lewis (1970) traced the etymology of the word 'anxiety' back to its Indo-European root *angh*, which gave rise to the Greek verb *angho* (to squeeze the throat or constrict the chest), the Latin noun *anxietas* (literally painful mind) and the German *angst* (anguish or dread). While these are all fairly specific concepts, he considered the current use of the word to be somewhat ambiguous and outlined what he believed were its main features:

- anxiety is an unpleasant emotional state with the subjective experience of fear
- the emotion may be accompanied by a feeling of impending death
- anxiety is directed to the future, with the feeling of some kind of threat
- there may be no recognisable threat or it may be one that, by reasonable standards, is insufficient to provoke the degree of anxiety
- there may be subjective bodily discomfort and manifest bodily disturbance.

A more comprehensive definition was given by Barlow (1991), who considered that anxiety can best be characterised as a diffuse cognitive–affective structure. At the heart of this structure is high negative affect, composed of various levels and combinations of activation or arousal, perceptions of lack of control over future events, and shifts in attention to self-evaluative concerns. This structure is described as diffuse because it can be associated with any number of situations or events and may be expressed somewhat differently from one individual to another or even within a given individual over time.

Anxiety is a ubiquitous and normal phenomenon. The biological function of fear and anxiety is adaptive: to alert the organism to threats to its survival, so that appropriate action may be taken. In more primitive animals this is manifest as the 'fight or flight' reaction described by Cannon (1929), an American physiologist.

Hoehn-Saric & McLeod (1986) considered that anxiety becomes abnormal when it is excessively intense or disproportionate to the stimulus, or continues beyond the exposure to danger, or when it is triggered by situations known to be harmless, or occurs without cause. For many psychiatric disorders, the distinction between a pathological symptom and normality is made on the grounds of 'a significant impairment of function', as exemplified by the inclusion of this dimension in the diagnostic criteria of DSM–IV. In the case of anxiety the relationship between functional performance and anxiety levels has the shape of an inverted U. Thus, mild degrees of anxiety improve function but high levels can have an inhibiting effect. This is known as the Yerkes–Dodson law (Yerkes, 1921). For example, a student begins to worry a few months before his finals and this anxiety serves him well, as it motivates him to study, but in the week immediately before the examination he becomes so paralysed with anxiety that he can no longer concentrate or take in any of the material.

Symptoms of anxiety

The symptoms attributed to anxiety are numerous and may include both psychological and somatic manifestations; however, they are not unique to anxiety and may occur in a wide variety of other medical and psychiatric disorders (Table 13.1). It is important to note that several of these symptoms should be present before a clinical anxiety state or disorder is diagnosed. The clusters of symptoms are not rigid in their composition, and almost any combination of symptoms can occur in a given individual, but there is a tendency for a person to display more or less the same characteristic, even stereotyped pattern in different episodes, even when the external stressors have varied. Usually, it is the particular profile of the cognitive symptoms, as well as the specific temporal and situational manifestations, that inform the diagnosis for a particular anxiety disorder.

The mood of anxiety is one of fearful apprehension that some calamity is about to occur. Sometimes the person can name the feared event, but often the apprehension cannot be attributed to any particular cues. Thoughts are dominated by the possibility of

Table 13.1 Manifestations of anxiety

Type of symptom	Examples
Increased arousal	Restlessness, increased startle response, initial insomnia, night-time wakefulness
Mood	Fearfulness, apprehension, worries
Thoughts	Unrealistic appraisal of danger to self or others, belief in personal inability to cope with stress, cognitions specific to syndromes (e.g. fear of impending death, having a heart attack, going crazy, being humiliated)
Behaviour	Constriction of purposeful activity, restless purposeless activity, avoidance of situations that increase feelings of insecurity
Somatic	Sense of retrosternal constriction, hyperventilation, faintness, paraesthesias, carpopedal spasm, muscular tension, fatigue, pain, stiffness, tremor
Overactivity of autonomic nervous system	Tachycardia, hot and cold flushes, dry mouth, diarrhoea, frequency of micturition, sweating
Associated mental symptoms	Depersonalisation, irritability

mishap or failure. Typically, the thoughts centre upon the possibility of failure to cope with some eventuality or appearing foolish or incompetent, or there are themes of serious illness or death (involving oneself or others). Increased arousal leads to restless behaviour and if this is combined with muscular tension there may be futile attempts to divert anxiety-laden thoughts into some trivial activity. Other patients develop avoidant behaviour and make strenuous attempts to stay away from places or situations known to trigger anxiety. In extreme cases, there may be little evidence of the original anxiety disorder. For example, a socially phobic person may lead a hermit-like existence, thus avoiding any exposure to anxiogenic situations, or manage to control anxiety by misusing alcohol. A detailed history of the antecedents to a particular behaviour or secondary condition will lead to the correct diagnosis and appropriate treatment.

A common manifestation of anxiety is a sense of retrosternal constriction, often accompanied by a feeling that sufficient air cannot be breathed in. This leads to an increase in the respiratory rate, with consequent hyperventilation. At a chronic, low-grade level, hypocapnia and hypocalcaemia may result in feelings of faintness, paraesthesia and, in extreme cases, the characteristic carpopedal spasms of tetany. Palpitations, as well as an excessive awareness of the normal heart beat, perceived as either very fast or too slow, are also common. Tachycardia may occur during panic attacks, but its presence should also alert the clinician to exclude possible organic causes.

Muscle tension is usually described by patients as an unpleasant feeling in one or more groups of muscles, coupled with an inability to relax these muscles voluntarily. If the muscle tension is severe, there may be muscle pain, most commonly in the back of the neck, the shoulders and the lower back. Tension pains in the head should be carefully distinguished from other causes of headache, such as migraine. In some cases, the muscle tension, if severe, leads to fidgeting, restlessness and pacing up and down. Two types of tremor may also present in anxiety states: a rather gross irregular tremor and a fine tremor resembling the tremor of thyrotoxicosis.

Some of the somatic manifestations of temporal lobe epilepsy may also occur in acute anxiety states, even though no organic lesion can be found. These include sensations of epigastric nausea and the experience of 'movement' up from the stomach, which patients describe as warmth or a feeling of a swelling rising up through the body. This particular symptom is the basis of the ancient theory of the migration of the womb, which gave rise to the term 'hysteria' and the subsequent causal links with female reproductive and sexual behaviour.

Sleep disturbance is a common feature of anxiety and there is typically difficulty in getting off to sleep and intermittent waking during the night; early morning wakening is not uncommon either. Dreaming is frequent, with the dreams having a threatening quality, often with themes of disaster, and in more severe cases there are repeated nightmares. Appetite is usually decreased but a few patients take comfort in over-eating, while interest in sex is generally diminished.

Differential diagnosis of anxiety

The differential diagnoses of the specific anxiety disorders are covered later in this chapter but because anxiety is such a ubiquitous symptom its differential diagnosis is wide and one of the most important in medicine. The clinician must always entertain alternative diagnoses, apart from simple anxiety (or any of the anxiety disorders), but in the vast majority of cases a few additional questions, a physical examination and simple laboratory tests will soon clarify the diagnosis. Cardiac, endocrine and neurological diseases figure prominently but almost any organ system may be involved. Although a few patients may present with the complete list of anxiety symptoms, which renders a psychiatric diagnosis more likely, the majority present with only a few anxiety symptoms, generally confined to one organ system. Thus, a symptom-based approach to differential diagnosis may be more helpful and the account that follows is drawn largely from the work of Jacob & Lilienfeld (1991).

Cardiovascular symptoms are perhaps the most common. Organic cardiac disorders tend to be more common with increasing age, whereas the anxiety disorders presenting with cardiac symptoms occur more often in younger age groups. The presence of palpitations should suggest the possibility of supraventricular tachycardias, extrasystoles and other arrhythmias. Dyspnoea and hyperventilation indicate the possibility of congestive heart failure, mitral valve disease, chest infections and chronic lung disease. In asthma, which is also common among young people, the breathing difficulty is greater during expiration than during inspiration. The distinction from asthma is particularly important because some of the drugs used to treat panic disorder, such as propranolol, may worsen asthma.

Over-breathing may also be a feature of alcohol withdrawal states. Among the middle aged, chest pain is a cardinal feature of myocardial infarction and angina pectoris. Retrosternal pain also occurs in anxiety but in these cases the patient usually looks physically well. In pleuritic conditions, the pain is confined to coughing and expiration. Chest pain of psychological origin may resemble costal chondritis, which itself may also be associated with retrosternal tenderness.

The symptoms of tremor and sweating should alert the clinician to the possibility of hypoglycaemia, which may be due to diabetes or oral hypoglycaemics or, very rarely, an insulinoma. Dizziness is commonly due to orthostatic hypotension and occurs in anaemia, but in psychiatric patients is most commonly a result of the side-effects of drugs such as the tricyclics or sedative anti-psychotics. Sometimes people with Ménière's disease, who are also anxious, complain of dizziness, but closer questioning reveals a rotational component of the vertigo, which is not a feature of the anxiety disorders. Depersonalisation and feelings of unreality, particularly if intermittent, should suggest temporal lobe epilepsy. Complaints of weakness may indicate neurological disorder such as multiple sclerosis, transient ischaemic attacks and myasthenia gravis. Some patients report feelings of being hot and cold, which is also common during the menopause. The same symptom may also occur in the rare carcinoid syndrome.

Assessment of anxiety

Further to the usual clinical evaluation, many interview schedules and scales have been developed to assess either global anxiety or specific syndromes. Comprehensive diagnostic interviews such as the Structured Clinical Interview for DSM–IV (SCID) (First *et al*, 1997) and the Mini-International Neuropsychiatric Interview (MINI) (Sheehan *et al*, 1998) include sub-sections that measure anxiety disorders and yield either a DSM–IV or an ICD–10 diagnosis. The structured approach of these instruments is particularly useful when the evaluation of comorbidity is of clinical or epidemiological interest, but they are mostly used in research or specialist clinics rather than routine clinical practice.

The most widely used observer-rated scale is the Hamilton Anxiety Scale (Hamilton, 1959). It comprises 14 items, each rated from 0 to 4. This instrument has well-documented limitations. It was designed to measure the old concept of anxiety neurosis and does not distinguish between specific anxiety disorders and anxious depression. It is heavily biased towards somatic symptoms, thus making it unreliable in the presence of physical illness. Further, its psychometric properties have been questioned (Maier *et al*, 1988). However, its use in clinical trials of anxiolytics is a requirement of the American and European regulatory authorities and so it is still widely used. A derivative of this scale, which is shorter and places less emphasis on somatic symptoms, is the Clinical Anxiety Scale (Snaith *et al*, 1982).

Among the general self-rated questionnaires is the Spielberger State–Trait Anxiety Inventory (Spielberger *et al*, 1983), which provides two measures: the present 'state' of anxiety and a 'trait' part, which purports to measure the underlying proneness to anxiety. The Beck Anxiety Inventory (Beck *et al*, 1988) is also a popular general scale.

Many other specific questionnaires exist for the individual disorders, such as the Penn State Worry Questionnaire (Behar *et al*, 2003) for generalised anxiety disorder and the Panic and Agoraphobia Scale (PAS) (Bandelow, 1995) for panic disorder. There are several scales for measuring post-traumatic stress disorder (PTSD); the more popular ones are the Impact of Events Scale (Horowitz *et al*, 1979), the Clinician Administered PTSD Scale (CAPS) (Blake *et al*, 1995) and the Davidson Trauma Scale (Davidson *et al*, 1997).

Cognitive–behavioural therapists use an array of instruments to monitor progress during treatment.

Finally, physiological measures such as the galvanic skin response, heart rate variability, breathing depth and rate, blood pressure and electromyography are mainly used in research.

Classification

The main categories of anxiety in the two classificatory schemes, and the correspondence of the terms used, are shown in Table 13.2. In ICD–10, anxiety disorders form subgroups and then are subsumed under the overarching category of 'Neurotic, stress-related and somatoform disorders', which also includes subgroups for conversion and somatoform disorders, as well as some older conditions such as neurasthenia. In DSM–IV, the separation of anxiety disorders from these other conditions is much clearer and they are dealt with in different chapters. A minor difference between

Table 13.2 Comparison of the categorisation of anxiety disorder within the two main schemes

ICD–10	DSM–IV
F40 Phobic anxiety disorders	
Agoraphobia (with or without panic)	Agoraphobia without history of panic
Social phobia	Social phobia
Specific (isolated) phobias	Specific phobia
F41 Other anxiety disorders	
Panic disorder	Panic disorder with agoraphobia
Generalised anxiety disorder	Generalised anxiety disorder
Mixed anxiety and depressive disorder	Anxiety disorder not otherwise specified (includes mixed anxiety–depressive disorder)
F42 Obsessive–compulsive disorder	Obsessive–compulsive disorder
F43 Reaction to severe stress, and adjustment disorders	
Acute stress reaction	Acute stress disorder
Post-traumatic stress disorder	Post-traumatic stress disorder
Adjustment disorders	Adjustment disorder
	Anxiety disorder due to a general medical condition
	Substance-induced anxiety disorder

the two schemes is the inclusion of a distinct mixed anxiety and depressive disorder in ICD–10 but not in DSM–IV, in which this condition is included only in the section 'Anxiety disorders not otherwise specified'. Finally, with the shift in classification described above, in the DSM system some classical neuroses have been reassigned to groups other than anxiety disorders; thus, depressive neurosis became dysthymic disorder and is now grouped with the mood disorders, while hypochondriasis and conversion are placed in the section on somatoform disorders.

Epidemiology and comorbidity of anxiety

Symptoms of anxiety may be very common, but they are often mild and transient. Still, a substantial proportion of the general population experience persistent and severe symptoms that lead to considerable distress and impairment of their social and occupational functioning. Well-conducted epidemiological studies, using modern criteria and instruments for the identification and diagnosis of anxiety syndromes, have helped to uncover the extent of the problem in the community, as well as in primary and secondary care, where people with anxiety are over-represented.

A European Union-wide task force, commissioned by the European College of Neuropsychopharmacology (ECNP), has performed a reanalysis of 27 community epidemiological studies covering 150 000 people, and reported on the frequency and burden of the mental disorders in Europe (Wittchen & Jacobi, 2005). The 12-month prevalence for all DSM–IV anxiety disorders was estimated to be about 15%, while the lifetime prevalence rose to approximately 21%. Individual disorders were, of course, less frequent. These are reported in Table 13.3.

If all anxiety disorders are taken together and considered across the whole age range, the overall female:male ratio is 2:1. However, variations exist both between disorders and within age groups. For example, panic disorder is 3.4 times more common in women than in men before the age of 34, while the prevalence is roughly the same between the sexes after the age of 50. On the other hand, agoraphobia (without panic), social phobia and specific phobias are consistently much more common in women than in men, across all age bands (Wittchen & Jacobi, 2005).

Table 13.3 Prevalence of individual anxiety disorder in the ECNP survey

Disorder	Prevalence
Twelve-month prevalence	
Panic disorder (with or without agoraphobia)	2.3%
Agoraphobia without panic	2.0%
Generalised anxiety disorder	1.5%
Social phobia	2.0%
Specific phobias	7.6%
Obsessive–compulsive disorder	0.7%
Post-traumatic stress disorder	1.2%
Lifetime prevalence	
Panic disorder (with or without agoraphobia)	3.8%
Agoraphobia without panic	3.8%
Generalised anxiety disorder	5.1%
Social phobia	5.8%
Specific phobias	13.2%
Obsessive–compulsive disorder	0.8%

A lifetime estimate for post-traumatic stress disorder could not be established in this survey.
Source: Wittchen & Jacobi (2005).

In the USA, a large replication study of the National Comorbidity Survey has been conducted, with over 9000 participants interviewed (Kessler *et al*, 2005). The lifetime prevalence of all anxiety disorders was 28.8%. The rates of some specific disorders differed somewhat from the European samples, most likely because of methodological differences in the ascertainment of cases. For example, social phobia in the US sample was reported to have a lifetime prevalence of 12.1% as compared with the 5.8% reported from Europe, but the rates of specific phobias were similar: 12.5% in the US sample versus 13.2% reported from Europe, and the rates for panic disorder, generalised anxiety disorder (GAD) and obsessive–compulsive disorder (OCD) were also comparable. In this study, the lifetime prevalence of PTSD was estimated to be 6.8%.

This US study produced some striking results regarding age of onset. The median age of onset for anxiety disorders was 11 years, which contrasted with the median age of onset for substance misuse (20 years) and mood disorders (30 years). Specific phobias tended to start earlier in life (median 7 years), followed by social phobia (13 years). The other anxiety disorders started much later (medians ranging from 19 to 31 years).

The prevalence rates presented above imply that anxiety disorders tend to run a chronic course. Primary care studies indicate that, although improvement over time is common, complete recovery is rare (Ronalds *et al*, 1997).

Comorbidity of the anxiety disorders

Comorbidity of anxiety with other disorders is the rule rather than the exception. For example, one study found that 69% of a community sample and 95% of a clinical sample of people with an anxiety disorder had more than one diagnosis (Wittchen *et al*, 1986). Depression, substance misuse and personality disorders often occur with anxiety syndromes. The comorbidity of bipolar mood disorder with anxiety disorders is also extensive (Freeman *et al*, 2002).

The relationship of depression to panic disorder has attracted great attention. The point prevalence of the two conditions presenting together is especially high (at least 30%), suggesting a common underlying aetiological mechanism (Bandelow, 2003). However, rates of depression are equally high, if not higher, in patients with GAD and social phobia (Wittchen & Jacobi, 2005).

Comorbidity of the individual anxiety disorders between themselves is also very high, although the majority of patients do not have a second anxiety disorder, thus making the lumping together of anxiety syndromes into one entity, as was the case with the older formulation of 'anxiety neurosis', difficult to justify. The excessive comorbidity of GAD with various other conditions, rising to 90% in some studies, has led to arguments against the independent existence of this syndrome (Bandelow, 2003). As might be expected, patients with more than one diagnosis tend to have more severe symptoms and a poorer response to treatment.

Alcohol misuse

The comorbidity of anxiety disorders and alcohol misuse/dependence is important in clinical populations. The presence of alcohol misuse and/or dependence significantly increases the chances that the same person will also suffer from an anxiety disorder (Swendsen *et al*, 1998). Furthermore, family studies reveal increased rates of alcoholism among first-degree relatives of probands with panic disorder, agoraphobia and PTSD, and vice versa (Maier *et al*, 1993; Nurnberger *et al*, 2004; Goodwin *et al*, 2006).

The notion that alcohol may help reduce anxiety dates back to antiquity. Hippocrates is quoted as saying that 'wine, drunk with an equal quantity of water, puts away anxiety and terrors' (Aphorisms, section VII, 56). Alcohol is probably the most widely used anxiolytic (typically as a means of self-medication to decrease social tension).

In clinical practice, it is important to try to work out whether the alcoholism is the primary problem or whether it has followed from a previously established anxiety condition. Schuckit & Monteiro (1988) suggested that the chronology of symptoms, that is, which disorder came first, as well as the symptom pattern during periods of abstinence may provide useful clues, although disentangling the order of events in the life story of a chronic misuser of alcohol is not always easy.

Kushnir *et al* (1990) suggested that if the anxiety disorder is either agoraphobia or social phobia, then the increased alcohol consumption is probably a form of self-medication, while panic disorder or GAD are more likely to follow from pathological drinking. In either case both the drinking and anxiety disorder may require independent treatment.

George *et al* (1990) pointed out that alcohol withdrawal and panic disorder share some clinical features (sweating, non-directed fear, palpitations, tremor, etc.) and may also have an overlapping neurobiological substrate, notably the hippocampus (see later in this chapter). This may explain both the comorbidity and the recurrent nature of the two disorders.

Suicidality

Lepine *et al* (1993) found that 42% of a series of 100 consecutive out-patients with panic disorder had made a suicide attempt and this was most common at around the time of the onset of panic disorder. Rates were higher (52%) for those who also had other psychiatric disorders (mainly alcoholism, major depression and personality disorder), whereas only 17% of those with pure panic disorder had made suicide attempts.

While other anxiety disorders also appear to be associated with increased rates of suicidal ideation and attempts, some have suggested this may be due to the high comorbidity of anxiety with other mental disorders. However, a recent prospective epidemiological survey showed convincingly that any pre-existing anxiety disorder is an independent risk factor for subsequent suicidality (Sareen *et al*, 2005).

Panic disorder

The ancient Greek god Pan resided in the countryside in Arcadia. Pan did not fit the popular image of a god: he was short and ugly, with legs resembling those of a goat. He had a habit of napping in a small cave or thicket near the road, but when disturbed from his sleep by a passerby he would let out a blood-curdling scream that was said to make one's hair stand on end. Pan's scream was so intense that many a terrified traveller died. This sudden overwhelming terror or fright came to be known as 'panic' and Pan would use his unique talent to vanquish his foes and even frighten the other gods (Barlow, 1988).

The delineation of panic disorder, and its detachment from the all-encompassing anxiety neurosis, owes much to the observation made by Klein & Fink (1962) that administration of the antidepressant imipramine led to a complete resolution of the symptoms of non-situational panic attacks but had little effect on anticipatory anxiety or more generalised anxiety. The significance of this finding was not immediately obvious. Gradually, however, it became clear that people with panic attacks were not simply suffering from depression but had a distinct, very severe and disabling type of anxiety. The presence of reasonably clear-cut phenomenology and specific therapy led to its inclusion as a separate disorder initially in DSM–III (American Psychiatric Association, 1980) and it has remained so in all classificatory systems since. As we discuss later in this chapter, panic disorder also became popular among researchers, because it is possible to produce experimental panic attacks in laboratory conditions.

Clinical features

The core feature of panic disorder is the experience of panic attacks. These are sudden episodes of intense fear or discomfort, accompanied by physical and cognitive symptoms. Panic attacks may be seen in other anxiety disorders as well as conditions like major depression, and in medical conditions such as hypoglycaemia. However, spontaneous attacks 'out of the blue' are unique to panic disorder and usually mark the onset of the condition. The spontaneous attacks may even occur at night and wake the patient up. As the disorder progresses, cue-triggered attacks also occur and may become the norm.

Typical panic attacks have an onset starting within a few seconds, are often overwhelming, and reach their peak intensity within about 10 minutes. Some symptoms may last for up to half an hour, after which they fade. Commonly described physical (somatic) symptoms during an attack include palpitations, sweating, tremor, shortness of breath or choking, chest discomfort, stomach upset or butterflies, light-headedness, tingling sensations and hot or cold flushes. Hyperventilation and hypertension may be seen if the patient is monitored during a panic attack. After the attack is over, the person may continue to feel tense, shaky or exhausted for several hours.

A specific respiratory panic disorder subtype has been described that shows a distinct symptom profile and possibly a different response to treatment (Nardi *et al*, 2003).

Persons with panic disorder are often very aware of bodily sensations, and may be especially sensitive to the physical symptoms listed above. It is usually the physical symptoms that drive people with panic disorder to seek help from their family doctor or the casualty department. Unfortunately, a significant proportion of sufferers are undiagnosed and remain untreated; their condition may not be revealed until they present with other (comorbid) disorders.

During panic attacks there is usually an intense fear of dying, losing control or 'going mad'. Even after the patient has survived many previous panic attacks it can be difficult to shake off these thoughts. Some patients try to terminate the attack by taking some drastic avoiding action. For example, when feeling breathless they may rush outside for air, or when experiencing an attack in a crowded bus get off as soon as possible. Sufferers begin to avoid being in places from which escape would be difficult or uncomfortable should an attack occur. This is known as agoraphobic avoidance, and cinemas, shopping centres and public transport are commonly avoided. In its most severe form, agoraphobia limits sufferers to their homes. Between attacks patients often develop anticipatory anxiety, in which they worry about having further attacks or about their consequences.

The frequency of attacks, intensity of symptoms and level of functioning between attacks are key measures of the severity of panic disorder and markers of improvement with treatment.

The DSM–IV definition of a panic attack is shown in Box 13.1. 'Limited symptom' episodes (fewer than four symptoms) may also occur and can still result in significant functional impairment.

It should be noted that panic attacks are very common in the general population but do not always lead to panic disorder. For example, Norton *et al* (1985) found that 35% of young adults reported at least one panic attack in the previous year, while 17% described experiencing a panic attack in the previous 3 weeks. Interestingly, these respondents also reported a high frequency of panic attacks in their first-degree relatives.

Box 13.1 DSM–IV criteria for a panic attack

A discrete period of intense fear/discomfort in which four (or more) of the following symptoms develop abruptly and reach a peak within 10 minutes:

1. palpitations
2. sweating
3. trembling
4. sensation of shortness of breath
5. feeling of choking
6. chest pain or discomfort
7. nausea or abdominal distress
8. dizzy or faint
9. derealisation or depersonalisation
10. fear of losing control or going crazy
11. fear of dying
12. paraesthesias
13. chills or hot flushes

Diagnosis

The diagnostic requirements for panic disorder in DSM–IV and ICD–10 are similar: recurrent unexpected panic attacks ('several episodes' in ICD–10), of which at least one has been followed by a month or more of persistent concerns about having further attacks, worries about the implications of attacks or significant change in behaviour. General medical and substance misuse causes must first be excluded (see later).

In DSM–IV, the disorder is classified as panic disorder with agoraphobia or panic disorder without agoraphobia, and there is also a third category, of agoraphobia without history of panic disorder. The reverse approach applies in ICD–10, which uses the classifications of agoraphobia with panic disorder, agoraphobia without panic disorder, and the diagnosis of panic disorder alone. These approaches reflect the fact that, despite the very close relationship, panic attacks are unlikely to be the whole explanation for agoraphobia, because agoraphobia consists of more complex fears, such as fears of being alone, fears of travel and fears of crowds, rather than simply the avoidance of more panic attacks. Furthermore, agoraphobia may develop even in the absence of panic.

Differential diagnosis

Panic attacks occurring as part of another anxiety disorder may be difficult to discern from pure panic disorder. A useful clue is to determine the presence of spontaneous attacks that are not situationally bound or situationally predisposed. While the physical symptoms may be indistinguishable, asking about the sufferer's cognitions, thoughts and fears at the time is also helpful. Someone with social phobia may have a panic attack in a public-speaking situation, where the fear is that of embarrassment. In OCD the fear is of loss of control over the repetitive obsession or compulsive act. Patients with PTSD have intense fears related to the past traumatic event, which may lead to a paroxysm of anxiety if they find themselves in a situation reminiscent of the original trauma. In simple phobia (such as fear of spiders) an excessive fear of the specific object or situation occurs with the knowledge (in adults) that this fear is unreasonable. In separation anxiety disorder of childhood the focus is on separation concerns. Only in panic disorder do completely spontaneous panic attacks occur.

Similarly, agoraphobic avoidance can be explored by asking the patient why he or she avoids a particular place or situation. Fear of difficulty in obtaining (physical) help should a panic attack occur is characteristic of panic disorder. Specific fears can point to another anxiety disorder; apathy and world weariness might indicate a depressive illness. In a psychotic disorder a bizarre explanation might be elicited.

Waking from sleep with a panic attack is highly suggestive of panic disorder, but this can also occur in certain sleep disorders, such as night terrors. Asking if panic attacks also occur during the day helps to distinguish these conditions.

Chronic heavy use or intoxication with stimulants (including caffeine) and withdrawal from drugs such as benzodiazepines or alcohol can also trigger panic attacks. Rarely, general medical conditions such as hyperthyroidism and cardiac arrhythmias can produce apparently spontaneous panic attacks. Both hypo- and hyperparathyroidism and other disorders causing hypocalcaemia can present with anxiety and tetany, which confusingly may be worsened by hyperventilation. Episodic attacks of fear sometimes associated with headache and sweating may be a presenting feature of the rare condition of phaeochromocytoma and a variety of drugs can precipitate attacks of anxiety in porphyria. A detailed medical history, a focused physical assessment and limited laboratory tests may be necessary to exclude these causes.

Course and comorbidity

The natural history of untreated panic disorder is typically episodic, with the panic attacks clustering for a few weeks or months at a time, followed by phases of spontaneous remission, with recurrences following new stresses. Regular cycles, as sometimes occurs in bipolar disorder, have not been observed, but the course of panic disorder may extend over many years.

About two-thirds of patients with panic disorder will eventually experience a major depressive episode. Comorbid anxiety disorders are also frequent, with 40% of patients who have panic disorder also meeting criteria for social phobia. Concomitant substance misuse (such as alcohol) is not unusual. Comorbidity results in more severe symptoms and a poorer prognosis than either condition alone (Bruce *et al*, 2005).

Generalised anxiety disorder (GAD)

In DSM–III, GAD was a residual category, describing mainly those patients with non-phobic anxiety who did not experience panic attacks. The condition then comprised feelings of anxiety combined with three out of four categories of somatic symptoms: motor tension, autonomic hyperactivity, apprehensive expectation, vigilance and scanning. The minimum duration of the symptoms was 1 month. This first definition proved to be unworkable and had a low inter-rater reliability (Barlow, 1988). It was modified in DSM–III–R (American Psychiatric Association, 1987) and again in DSM–IV, in four important ways:

1 the new definition specified that the worry and concern should focus on a number of different areas, to show that the anxiety was 'generalised'

2 the duration was increased from 1 month to at least 6 months (although not necessarily continuously)

3 there should be at least three out of six symptoms (see Box 13.2)

4 the hierarchical rule that excluded the diagnosis of GAD in the presence of another disorder such as depression or panic was dropped.

ICD–10 has a less restrictive definition of GAD. The text refers to anxiety that is generalised and persistent but not restricted to particular cues; that is, it is free-floating. It requires the presence of the symptoms for 'several months' and it does not specify how many somatic symptoms should be present for the diagnosis to be made.

Box 13.2 DSM–IV criteria for generalised anxiety disorder

- Excessive anxiety or worry occurring on more days than not for at least 6 months about a number of events or activities
- Difficult to control the worry
- Three or more of the following symptoms
  1 restlessness
  2 easily fatigued
  3 difficulty concentrating or mind going blank
  4 irritability
  5 muscle tension
  6 sleep disorder
- The focus of the worry is not some other axis I disorder
- Significant distress or impairment of function
- Not drug induced or due to a general medical condition

Although the concept in DSM–IV and ICD–10 is essentially the same, ICD–10 still provides an extensive list of potential somatic symptoms, while DSM–IV focuses on fewer symptoms, which are considered to be the core features of GAD.

Clinical features

The central feature of GAD is the presence of one or more persistent worries focusing on everyday events or activities, such as work, academic performance or the welfare of family members. Although the topics of the worries may be apparently quite reasonable, they take the form of anxious anticipation of an impending catastrophe, they are out of proportion with the issues worried about and they cannot be stopped voluntarily (i.e. they are uncontrollable). Associated psychological symptoms include a feeling of restlessness or being on edge, difficulty in concentrating, a feeling that one's mind is going blank, irritability, depersonalisation and derealisation. The sufferer, having retired to bed for the night, tends to be unable to stop worrying and so finds it difficult to fall asleep. The resulting tiredness the following day only serves to reinforce the worries, thus leading to the establishment of a vicious circle.

In addition to the fatigability, people with GAD often complain about muscle tension, autonomic arousal (palpitations, sweating, trembling or shaking), respiratory and abdominal symptoms (chest discomfort, difficulty in breathing, nausea or diarrhoea, churning of the stomach), dry mouth, urinary frequency, paraesthesias, dizziness, light-headedness and so on. Because somatic symptoms may be prominent, patients often seek medical rather than psychological help. As a result, they are more likely to present in specialist medical clinics with unexplained physical symptoms than for an out-patient psychiatric opinion. Even though GAD constitutes up to 10% of all those attending primary care with a mental disorder, its recognition rate remains rather low (Lieb *et al*, 2005).

Differential diagnosis

Patients with other anxiety disorders may worry excessively in relation to the main symptom of their condition, such as having another panic attack (panic disorder), being humiliated in public (social phobia), something terrible happening if certain rituals are not performed (OCD) or being seriously ill (hypochondriasis, somatisation disorder). If the worry is restricted to these themes, then the diagnosis of GAD does not apply. Generalised anxiety is a common feature in the course of an affective or psychotic illness. Patients with an anxiety disorder comorbid with depression are commonly seen in clinical practice. The diagnosis of GAD can be then applied if the criteria were fulfilled at some time when the patient did not qualify for the diagnosis of depression.

Worries are sometimes difficult to distinguish from obsessions, and this topic has attracted the interest of psychologists in recent years. Both are characterised by repetitive cognitive intrusions that are difficult for the person to dismiss and both are accompanied by negative emotions (Langlois *et al*, 2000). However, they also differ in certain key aspects. Subjective reports tend to characterise obsessions as more bizarre in content, more unacceptable and more unrealistic than worries. Obsessions are more likely to occur as impulses, urges or images. By contrast, worries are more likely to occur in a verbalised form, as doubtful thoughts or apprehensions, and they are characterised by greater awareness of their presence and of their triggers (Lee *et al*, 2005*a*). Obsessions are more ego-dystonic than worries (Langlois *et al*, 2000). Worries are more frequent and tend to last longer. From a more theoretical perspective, the cognitive process of 'thought–action fusion' appears to be more strongly related to obsessions than to worries (Coles *et al*, 2001).

The symptoms of GAD may be the consequence of a general medical condition (Box 13.3). For example, endocrine or metabolic disorders may mimic the complete picture of GAD. The most important of these is thyrotoxicosis, which is readily excluded once considered: the anxious person usually sweats with cold clammy hands, in contrast to the warm sweaty palms of the thyrotoxic patient. Less commonly hypothyroidism may present with anxiety, although the mood is more characteristically one of lethargy and depression. In such cases, history, physical examination and laboratory testing clarifies the diagnosis.

Similarly, a GAD-like picture may be due to a medication or other substance (Box 13.4). Care should be also taken to distinguish GAD from normal, everyday anxiety. The usual everyday life worries are thought of as being under control and they can be postponed for a more convenient time in the face of other (voluntary or involuntary) mental and physical activities. They do not interfere significantly with the person's functioning and usually are not accompanied by pronounced physical symptoms. Pathological worries, on the other hand, are pervasive, very distressing and assume control of the person's life.

Box 13.3 Some medical conditions causing symptoms of anxiety

Endocrine
- Hyperthyroidism/thyrotoxicosis
- Hypercalcaemia
- Carcinoid
- Phaeochromocytoma

Respiratory
- Asthma
- Chronic obstructive airways disease
- Pulmonary embolism

Cardiovascular
- Angina pectoris
- Arrhythmia
- Vascular disease

Neurological
- Akathisia
- Mass lesion
- Epilepsy

Metabolic
- Hyperkalaemia
- Hypoglycaemia
- Hyponatraemia
- Hypoxia
- Porphyria

Course and comorbidity of GAD

A number of prospective studies have shown that GAD tends to run a chronic course and may persist for over a decade (Angst & Vollrath, 1991). A large naturalistic study of more than 700 individuals in Boston, USA, indicated that only 25% had achieved full remission 2 years later (Yonkers *et al*, 1996).

The distinction between panic disorder and GAD is blurred and may also be artificial. Thus, in one large series 25% of those with GAD concurrently suffered from panic disorder as a secondary diagnosis, but more significantly 73% had previously experienced at least one panic attack during the past year (Sanderson & Barlow, 1990). Also, the life charts of those with panic disorder suggest that its onset is often preceded by a prolonged period of GAD (Uhde *et al*, 1985). Breier *et al* (1985) commented on the lack of any temporal

Box 13.4 Some substances and medications causing symptoms of anxiety

- Alcohol
- Amphetamines
- Anticholinergics
- Antihypertensives (reserpine, hydralazine)
- Antituberculosis drugs (isoniazid)
- Caffeine
- Digitalis (in toxicity)
- Sympathomimetics (ephedrine, pseudoephedrine)
- Levo-dopa
- Neuroleptics (in akathisia)
- Bronchodilators (salbutamol, theophylline)
- Thyroid hormones
- Non-steroidal anti-inflammatory drugs
- Selective serotonin reuptake inhibitors (at the onset of treatment and when withdrawn)

separation for panic disorder and GAD, and suggested that the separation may be artificial and that GAD may be 'a prodromal, incomplete, or residual manifestation of other psychiatric disorders'. The very high comorbidity of GAD with depression, reported to be up to 80% for lifetime diagnosis, has generated considerable discussion about common underlying mechanisms and possible shared aetiology (Gorwood, 2004) and this is further discussed on page 328.

Acute stress reactions and adjustment disorder

Acute stress reactions and adjustment disorder are relatively common in the community and in general practice settings but rarely reach the attention of the specialist. In these disorders even though the anxiety is directly related to specific situations and particular circumstances and is 'understandable', its experience becomes unusual and alarming, even overwhelming, and its manifestations are easily misattributed to some other cause, such as somatic illness. The clinician must therefore be clear about precisely what are the symptoms of this type of anxiety, what constitutes a stressful event within the patient's specific cultural context, and how this may vary from one person to another, taking into account the constitutional predisposition, cultural background and life experience of the individual. The formulation of such an explanation and conveying it to the patient in an easily understood and empathic manner will often comprise a major part of the treatment of stress reactions and adjustment disorder.

Acute stress reactions

An acute stress reaction is a transient disorder that develops in someone who has no other apparent mental disorder and in response to some exceptional physical or mental stress. Usually, it subsides within hours or days.

People vary considerably in their capacity to cope with adversity and this variation plays a role in the occurrence and severity of acute stress reactions. The accompanying symptoms also vary widely but, typically, they include an initial state of 'daze', with some constriction of the field of consciousness and narrowing of attention, an inability to comprehend stimuli and some apparent disorientation (WHO, 1992). This state may be followed either by withdrawal or by agitation and overactivity. Autonomic signs such as tachycardia, sweating or flushing are commonly present. The diagnosis should not be made if the symptoms are simply an exacerbation of a previous mental disorder.

Typically, the syndrome described in ICD–10 starts at the time of the traumatic event and is self-limited, usually lasting up to 3 days. DSM–IV describes a somewhat different entity, which can encompass typical symptoms of PTSD, but the picture may be dominated by dissociative symptoms, including amnesia for the episode, depersonalisation, derealisation and subjective numbing, and at least three of these symptoms need to be present for the diagnosis to be made. The inclusion of acute stress reaction in DSM–IV aims, to an extent, to aid the differentiation between the early normal responses to trauma from the pathological ones, and to predict the development of PTSD. Our understanding of the underlying processes of an acute stress reaction, and the reasons why in some cases it may remit while in others it persists and progresses into an adjustment disorder or PTSD, is rather limited at present (Bryant, 2003). The overall usefulness of the entity or whether any particular symptoms are clinical predictors has also been questioned (Marshall *et al*, 1999).

Adjustment disorder

Adjustment disorder is a more prolonged disturbance than an acute stress reaction. This state of subjective distress and emotional disturbance, which may interfere with normal everyday functioning, arises during the period of adaptation to a life change or life event. However, the stressor is usually much less severe than is the case with PTSD and may not be out of the ordinary (e.g. a change of job or school, or a house move). Individual predisposition or vulnerability (e.g. low IQ or immature personality) may play an important role in the development of an adjustment disorder. Symptoms usually include depressed mood, anxiety and a feeling of being unable to cope, to plan ahead or to continue in the present situation; there is usually some interference with the performance of the daily routine. Some individuals may be liable to dramatic behaviour, or outbursts of violence, although this is rare. Among adolescents, transient aggressive or antisocial behaviour may occur.

ICD–10 specifies that the onset of the adjustment reaction should be within 1 month of the stressful event, while DSM–IV imposes a 3-month limit. Further, the duration of the disorder should not exceed 6 months after the stressor has terminated (if the condition lasts more than 6 months then PTSD should be considered); nor should the symptoms be sufficiently severe to justify a more specific diagnosis. The diagnosis should be made only in the presence of a stressor, and then only if the symptoms would not have occurred without the stressor. Further, DSM–IV specifically excludes bereavement, which should be classified separately. Finally, the severity of the reaction should be disproportionate to the severity of the stressor.

Specifiers of an adjustment disorder relate to the most prominent symptoms: with depressed mood, with anxiety, with mixed anxiety–depression, with disturbances of conduct, and with mixed disturbance of emotions and conduct.

Variants of an adjustment disorder are common in the community and among general practice attendees, but are less frequent among those presenting to psychiatric clinics. Although the diagnosis may be common in some settings, and the resultant morbidity quite significant, the very concept of adjustment disorder has been criticised as vague (Gur *et al*, 2005), thus rendering interventions more difficult to research or implement.

Post-traumatic stress disorder (PTSD)

Kraepelin described the *Schreck-neurosis* (in German, *Schreck* = terror), a nervous disorder that occurred after shocks or accidents, while English authors of the same period wrote of a condition called 'railway spine', caused by concussion of the spine following railway collisions. Shell shock, battle fatigue and combat neuroses were all terms used in the First World War. The early history of PTSD is reviewed by Trimble (1981).

The modern concept of PTSD was first formulated by Kardiner (1941), who considered it to be a physioneurosis, a mental disorder with both physiological and psychological components. He outlined five principal features of the syndrome which, as noted below, still form the core of the condition:

1 the persistence of the startle response and irritability
2 a tendency to explosive outbursts of aggression
3 fixation on the trauma
4 constriction of the general level of the personality functioning
5 typical dream life.

More recently the Vietnam War, with around half a million psychiatric casualties, brought the disorder again into prominence, and led American psychiatrists to press for its inclusion in DSM–III. Conflicts in the 1990s (notably in Rwanda and Yugoslavia) and the attention given to disasters affecting whole societies or individuals (earthquakes, personal injuries, etc.) raised the profile of PTSD in the media and gave impetus for more research into its aetiology and treatment.

Unlike the other anxiety syndromes, at the heart of PTSD lies the experience of a clear triggering factor, that of a trauma. According to ICD–10, this trauma should be of 'an exceptionally threatening or catastrophic nature which is likely to cause pervasive distress in anyone'. The types of possible trauma are listed in ICD–10 and include natural and man-made disasters, combat, serious accidents, witnessing the violent death of others, or being the victim of torture, terrorism, rape or other serious crime. Witnessing any of these events is also included.

DSM–III–R (APA, 1987) had an added clause: 'that the stress should be outside the range of the usual human experience'. DSM–IV, however, has a different approach and provides a symptom-based definition (Box 13.5) that requires only that the patient should have 'experienced, witnessed or confronted life-threatening events and the patient's response involved intense fear, helplessness or horror'. The reason for this change, and the removal of the stipulation that the trauma should be outside the range of the usual human experience, was that in the field trials involved in the development of DSM–IV stressors of this type proved to be quite common as well as being difficult to define, thus making this item unreliable. DSM–IV, in addition to the above, includes traumas that have been witnessed as well as traumas that others close to the patient have experienced, and the patient has learnt about. For children, it also includes inappropriate sexual experiences, not necessarily with threatened or actual violence. Cases with 6 months or more separating the onset of symptoms from the original trauma are classified in DSM–IV as 'with delayed onset'. ICD–10 specifies that the onset should be within 6 months of the trauma; cases with a later onset should be given a diagnosis of probable PTSD and the more chronic cases should be classified under the category of enduring personality change.

Box 13.5 DSM–IV criteria for post-traumatic stress disorder

A:
- the person experienced, witnessed, or was confronted with an event or events that involved actual or threatened death or serious injury, or a threat to the physical integrity of the self or others *and*
- the person's response involves intense fear, helplessness or horror

B. Re-experiencing symptoms (one of the following):
- recurrent intrusive recollections
- recurrent distressing dreams
- acting or feeling as if the event were still occurring
- distress on exposure to cues that recall the event
- physiological reactivity on exposure to cues

C. Persistent avoidance of stimuli associated with the trauma (three or more of the following):
- efforts to avoid thoughts, feelings or conversations associated with the trauma
- avoidance of activity or places associated with the trauma
- diminished interest or participation in activities
- detachment or estrangement from others
- restricted range of affects (e.g. unable to have loving feelings)
- sense of foreshortened future

D. Symptoms of increased arousal (not present before the trauma) – at least two of the following:
- insomnia
- increased anger
- poor concentration
- hypervigilance
- exaggerated startle response

E. Criteria B, C, D have lasted more than 1 month

F. Clinically significant distress or impairment of function

DSM–IV recognises an acute type of PTSD when the duration of symptoms is less than 3 months, a chronic type when the symptoms last for more than 3 months, and a type with delayed onset starting at least 6 months after the trauma. Separate but broadly similar criteria are given for children.

The nature of the trauma is one of the prime aetiological factors. Figley (1985) suggests that the trauma should be sudden (so there is no time for psychological preparation), dangerous (with a life-threatening potential) and overwhelming (leaving the survivor with at least a temporary sense of helplessness and being out of control). The effects of stress may be cumulative. Thus, among Vietnam veterans the intensity and length of contact exposure were critical variables in the development of PTSD. Kulha *et al* (1990) found that 38.5% of those with high battle exposure developed PTSD compared with 8.5% who had low exposure.

The severity of the trauma is also a factor in the aetiology of PTSD during peacetime. For example,

Kilpatrick & Resnick (1993) in a large follow-up study of the victims of crime found the following rates for DSM–III PTSD: rape, 57%; physical assault, 37%; other sexual assault, 16–33%; and robbery, 18–28%. The risk of PTSD among victims who had experienced a threat to life was 35% and if physical injury occurred 43%; if both were present the rate rose to 59%. The inference from these figures is that both objective injury and subjective fear may contribute to PTSD. Even following a civilian disaster such as the Beverly Hills Club fire, 60% of the variance of PTSD was associated with the disaster itself.

Public attitudes to war can also be important for the development and the severity of PTSD. The soldiers returning from the Second World War to the USA were welcomed home as war heroes but those returning from Vietnam, an unpopular war, were sometimes subjected to abuse and so the rates for PTSD were higher.

There are other risk factors for PTSD. Women are much more likely to develop the condition than men exposed to similar trauma. Some other factors are related to the nature and the characteristics of the trauma. For example, rape victims who were also physically injured during the attack are much more likely to develop PTSD than those who did not suffer injury during the assault. Further, witnesses of a volcanic eruption are more likely to be traumatised the closer they were to the area surrounding the volcano.

Beyond the trauma itself, various pre-trauma factors have been investigated, and there is strong evidence that pre-existing anxiety or depression, earlier trauma history (such as childhood abuse), low socio-economic status, genetic predisposition (see page 328) and personality problems all contribute to a significantly increased likelihood of PTSD after exposure to trauma. Finally, the continuing presence of stressors after the trauma and a lack of social support and resources also contribute to higher rates of PTSD (Fairbank *et al*, 2000).

The concept of PTSD at times has been seen as highly political. For example, Ramsay (1990) pointed out that the DSM system has waxed and waned in its enthusiasm for incorporating PTSD according to whether or not the United States was at war. DSM–I (APA, 1952) was published soon after the Second World War, and included a category of 'gross stress reaction', but DSM–II (1968), formulated at the time of the controversial Vietnam War, dropped this category. The catastrophic ramifications of the Vietnam War on the veterans led to the first formal inclusion of PTSD in DSM–III (1980) and later DSM–III–R (1987). Some have gone as far as arguing that this is a way of absolving the guilt of the perpetrators of war. As there have only been a few military casualties since then, DSM–IV (1994) has switched its emphasis back to civilian and childhood trauma, although the condition of PTSD has been retained.

Clinical features

The re-experiencing of the trauma in the form of intrusive or unwanted memories is the most characteristic symptom of PTSD. Intrusive memories may be triggered by relatively minor stimuli; for example, for some of the Vietnam veterans even a rainy day (the monsoon lasts for months in Vietnam), the noise of a helicopter or any loud discharge could evoke traumatic wartime memories. The intrusive memories tend to be of short duration and the patient remains in touch with reality. Sometimes there are flashbacks, when the person feels she or he is reliving the events, and in severe cases there may be dissociative states and the person acts as if the original trauma is occurring at the present time. Intrusive memories may be troublesome for many years after the original trauma or, as one Vietnam veteran put it, 'It was bad enough that I had to go to Vietnam in the first place, but to live through it over and over again is just too much' (Southwick *et al*, 1994).

Sufferers complain of difficulty sleeping, usually initial insomnia associated with a fear of disturbing dreams and nightmares during which the trauma is often vividly and repeatedly recalled in detail. There may be recurrent dreams of specific traumatic episodes, such as (among the military cases) being shot, running away or witnessing the death of friends in battle. The dream content tends to be repetitious and is all too easily recalled, in contrast to the variable pattern found in normal dreaming, when recall is more remote or absent. Sometimes alcohol is used to treat the insomnia, or other symptoms, and this may complicate the picture.

Avoidance behaviour is also a core symptom of PTSD and is particularly marked among those with strong re-experiencing symptoms as they try to escape from troublesome memories and dreams. Horowitz (1986) describes an avoidance/denial phase of the disorder, when there is a tendency either to deny or to play down any connection between the traumatic event in the past and present psychological problems. There may be excessive pointless activity or the use of fantasy to avoid reality; accompanying this denial there may be a general lack of emotional responsiveness and a constriction of thinking and affect which results in a lack of experience of either pleasure or pain, causing detachment from friends and family and, ultimately, isolation. Some theoreticians considered this to be the most malignant feature of PTSD because it may explain the severe social and psychiatric decline sometimes seen (Titchener, 1985).

An increased startle response may be characteristic, with flinching, grimacing or even shouting when stimuli reminiscent of the original trauma occur. Hypervigilance is shown by excessive alertness and preparation for flight or other forms of self-protection in situations that most would consider innocuous but which the individual views as dangerous. Occasionally this hypervigilance may approach the bizarre and even affect whole communities. For example, after the Buffalo Creek flood in West Virginia:

> 'the community leader and his wife never slept at the same times so that at least one of them could always remain alert. On rainy nights he would be deluged with phone call rumours that another dam might break. He would then spend the night sitting on the dam with a rifle. Other community members stayed on shore nearby in order to protect him from attack.' (Titchener & Kapp, 1976)

Various other symptoms are associated with PTSD and these may depend on the particular nature of the trauma, the individual and the circumstance. Among war veterans, for example, survivor guilt is common. Paramedics who served in war zones and witnessed many deaths are particularly susceptible to survivor guilt and for years afterwards may castigate themselves for being responsible for the deaths of their fellow soldiers, because they were either too slow or incompetent. Victims of assault or rape are prone to feelings of anger or rage, fears of loss of control, uncontrollable crying, and feelings of shame. Following natural disasters, fears of the elements are common. For example, after the Buffalo Creek disaster, mentioned above, many people developed obsessions and phobias about water and rain and other reminders of the disaster.

Differential diagnosis

An acute stress reaction should resolve within 4 weeks, while PTSD is a more prolonged condition and may not even start immediately after the trauma. An adjustment disorder may be associated with a stressor of any severity, but it is of shorter duration, less severe and has a different symptom pattern, usually revolving around anxiety or depressive symptoms, without prominent flashbacks or reliving of the incident. Recurrent intrusive thoughts are also a feature of OCD, but in OCD, even if the obsessions started after some life event, their content is usually unrelated to the trauma. Flashbacks may occur in dissociative disorders or occasionally in brief psychosis. Malingering should always be excluded if financial gain is a possibility or when forensic considerations are present.

Course and comorbidity

The natural history of trauma exposure and PTSD has yet to be clarified fully but most individuals appear to recover from the acute effects of trauma. A series of studies on the effects of rape showed a fairly rapid attenuation of symptom severity in the first few months. Thus, at 2 weeks, 94% of the victims fulfilled criteria for PTSD; this figure fell to 65% at 4 weeks, 58% at 8 weeks, 52% at 12 weeks, 46% at 16 weeks and 40% at 12 months (Rothbaum & Foa, 1993). In general, prospective studies of different populations show that the majority recover in the long term but a substantial minority still experience symptoms many years later (Shalev, 2000). A recrudescence of symptoms can sometimes occur. For example, after the Enniskillen bombing most survivors were thought to have recovered after 6 months but then experienced renewed symptoms at the first anniversary of the event (Curran *et al*, 1990).

Traumas due to interpersonal violence or of human design (e.g. torture) are generally more potent in causing a lifelong damaging effect than the stress caused by natural disasters. Thus, among American prisoners of war (POWs) the degree of maltreatment given by their captors appeared to determine subsequent rates of PTSD: 11% of those incarcerated in Europe during the Second World War developed PTSD, compared with 28% of those in Japanese camps (Langer, 1987). A long-term follow-up study of the POW survivors of the Korean War (where the prisoners had been subjected to a particularly cruel regime, including mock executions, brain-washing and exposure to the elements for months on end) found that 86% still fulfilled criteria for PTSD or another anxiety disorder 30 years after their release, and they continued to be suspicious, confused, isolated and guilt ridden even a generation later (Sulker *et al*, 1991).

Most people who have PTSD also meet the criteria for at least one other psychiatric disorder as well (Fairbank *et al*, 2000). For example, a population of Vietnam veterans with PTSD showed high comorbidity rates for major depression (34%), GAD (45%), alcohol misuse (70%) and drug misuse (25%) (Centers for Disease Control, 1988). Alcohol and drug misuse are particularly prominent in men, while women tend to suffer more depression and other anxiety disorders, although they may also have high rates of alcoholism (Fairbank *et al*, 2000).

Mixed anxiety and depression

ICD–10 included a new category, 'mixed anxiety and depression'. It is important to note that this category refers to patients who have symptoms of anxiety and depression that are not severe enough to justify a separate diagnosis for either major depression or any of the anxiety disorders. This category should be considered if there is a relatively mild depression, some anxiety and perhaps a few autonomic symptoms such as tremor or palpitations. Individuals with this condition are commonly found in the community and may sometimes attend their general practitioner but rarely reach specialist attention. The inclusion of the category was meant to stimulate research into this numerically quite large group of people, and should also help to clarify the stability and autonomy of the diagnosis. DSM–IV does not have a special category for this type of disorder but subsumes it under 'anxiety disorder not otherwise specified'.

If the symptoms are associated with a stressful event, a diagnosis of adjustment disorder should be made; if the symptoms are prolonged, a diagnosis of dysthymia is probably more appropriate.

It is too early to decide whether this diagnosis is useful or valid. Opponents argue that it may become a 'waste basket' category and that it overlaps significantly with adjustment disorder (Liebowitz, 1993). It could well be that some of these patients present with residual symptoms of partially treated depressive or anxiety disorders. However, the significant functional impairment of this under-studied group of patients requires closer investigation and the development of treatments; the presence of this diagnostic category should promote this cause (Boulenger *et al*, 1997).

Aetiological theories of anxiety

The symptoms of anxiety are thought to represent the end-point of several diverse multifactorial processes: genetic, social and neurobiological. All these may influence clinical anxiety syndromes and the contribution of each is reviewed below.

Genetic aspects

The genetics of anxiety has attracted much attention recently and there are now a number of well-conducted family and twin studies, although no adoption studies.

Soon after their delineation, it became clear that panic disorder and GAD are influenced by genetic factors. For example, in one of the first studies using modern diagnostic criteria, Noyes *et al* (1978) compared the first-degree relatives of probands with anxiety disorders with surgical controls, and found a much higher rate (18% *v.* 3%) of anxiety disorders among the relatives of the anxiety probands. Female relatives had an even higher risk for the anxiety disorders, possibly because the prevalence of anxiety is greater among women. An additive effect for genetic loading was also observed in this study. Thus, if only the proband and no other family member had an anxiety disorder, then the risk for the siblings was 9%; however, if one parent as well as the proband had anxiety disorder, this risk rose to 26%, and if both parents and the proband had an anxiety disorder this risk to rose 44%.

A number of authoritative reviews (e.g. Lesch, 2003; Maier, 2003) and a meta-analysis (Hettema *et al*, 2001) on the genetic contribution to anxiety disorders are now available. Family data are best for panic disorder (from five studies) and these show an increased odds ratio of around 5 for the presence of panic disorder in the first-degree relatives of probands with panic disorder. Pooling the results of five twin studies, Hettema *et al* (2001) estimated the hereditability of panic disorder to be 0.43. There are only two family studies of GAD and they produced an elevated odds ratio of 6 for first-degree relatives to have an anxiety disorder in families where the proband had an anxiety disorder, while three twin studies of GAD suggested a hereditability of 0.32 (Hettema *et al*, 2001).

These results strongly support familial aggregation and a genetic contribution to panic disorder and GAD. There was no difference in genetic variance between men and women, which makes it likely that the same genes predispose both men and women to anxiety disorders. However, the non-genetic component showed some differences between the sexes. Thus, for panic disorder (in both men and women) as well as for GAD in men, the remaining variance could be mainly attributed to non-shared environment, but for women with GAD there was a significant contribution from the common familial environment. While the exact mode of familial transmission remains unclear, it is reasonable to assume that the phenotypes are produced by a complex interaction of multiple genes and environmental factors.

In PTSD, the exposure to a traumatic event is a necessary but not a sufficient condition for the syndrome to develop. Thus, many people who are exposed to trauma do not develop PTSD, indicating that for the minority who become symptomatic there must also be some individual vulnerability.

It now appears that the genetic contribution to PTSD is broadly similar in magnitude to that found for the other anxiety disorders. Thus, a large twin study of Vietnam veterans found heritabilities of 0.13–0.30 for the 're-experiencing' cluster (painful memories, nightmares), 0.30 for the 'avoidant' cluster and 0.30 for the 'arousal' cluster (insomnia, irritability, being easily startled) of PTSD symptoms (True *et al*, 1993).

The genetic research into anxiety disorders has rekindled the discussion about how discrete the specific phenotypes/syndromes are. Some investigators have preferred to focus on the heritability of specific symptoms and various anxiety traits, assuming that these are the basic immutable and possibly heritable building blocks of anxiety disorders. This approach further assumes that these symptoms and traits will combine with environmental factors to produce the individual phenotype. While the research on specific symptoms has not proved very fruitful so far, traits such as neuroticism and anxiety sensitivity in twin studies have shown substantial heritability – almost 50% (Martin *et al*, 1988; Stein *et al*, 1999). For example, a Swedish study of 13 000 twin pairs who were given the short form of the Eysenck Personality Questionnaire (EPQ) (Eysenck, 1959) found the hereditability of neuroticism was 0.50 for men and 0.58 for women, and for extraversion the figures were 0.54 and 0.66, respectively (Floderus-Myrhed *et al*, 1980). In that sense, these traits could be seen as potential endo-phenotypes (Maier, 2003).

However, this approach is not without problems. When the inheritance of the symptoms of anxiety and depression was examined in a large Australian twin study, heritability figures of 0.34–0.46 were reported (Kendler *et al*, 1986). Analysis of the same twin data by Jardine *et al* (1984) revealed a high genetic correlation between the EPQ scores for neuroticism and measures of the symptoms of anxiety and depression, indicating that they were probably measuring the same underlying factor. On this basis, Kendler *et al* (1986) suggested that, at least in the case of anxiety, the distinction between personality traits and symptoms is not clear cut. Several earlier studies had shown that existing psychiatric disorder, particularly depression, may have large effects on neuroticism scores (Ingham, 1966).

Comorbidity and genetics

When specific disorders were studied, it became clear that they do not always 'breed true'. For example, GAD shares the same genetic factors with depression (Kendler, 1996), while panic was thought to be genetically discrete from them but linked with specific phobias instead (Kendler *et al*, 1999). Family and twin studies have tended to show a lack of genetic correlation between panic disorder and depression (Maier, 2003). For example, in an elegant study utilising three groups of probands – those with pure panic disorder, those with pure major depression and those with combined panic disorder and major depression – Weissman *et al* (1993) showed that the first-degree relatives of probands with panic disorder (only) had a 20-fold increased risk of panic disorder but had little or no increased risk of major depression. Relatives of probands with major depression had only a threefold increased risk of panic disorder, but a sixfold increased risk of major depression, while relatives of probands with combined disorders had increased risks for both disorders. These results support the hypothesis that panic disorder is genetically distinct from major depression. Where it exists, the genetic commonality between GAD and depression may explain the high comorbidity between the two disorders, but in the absence of a substantial genetic correlation the established high comorbidity between panic and depression is somewhat puzzling.

A twin study of GAD and panic disorder suggested that the genetic factors of panic overlap with those of GAD by about 50% (Scherrer *et al*, 2000). There is also a close genetic relationship between GAD and depression, and this has been confirmed by a number of twin studies (Maier, 2003). Indeed, the two disorders appear to share the same genetic vulnerability factors and the difference in phenotype is thought to be partly the result of distinct environmental stressors or some other factor. Loss and humiliation are thought to predispose to depression, whereas high-threat events constitute a risk factor for GAD (Kendler *et al*, 2003). Another possible explanation is that different phenotypes are preferentially expressed at different ages, with anxiety starting earlier in life than depression.

The search for candidate genes for the anxiety disorders

Research into predisposing genes through genome-wide linkage studies has so far been limited to panic disorder and the results have been inconclusive. Three small samples of families with more than one member afflicted by panic disorder produced linkage signals with modest effects but these results were not replicated between the studies and there was no consensus finding. This suggests that the phenotype for panic disorder is under the influence of multiple susceptibility genes, each of which exerts only a small effect. Loci on chromosomes 7p and 1 showed some suggestive linkage in two out of three studies. Two more candidate loci, on chromosomes 13 and 15q respectively, have been proposed from studies investigating families with panic and comorbid physical conditions, but these results need to be replicated (see Maier, 2003).

Association studies have also investigated candidate genes related to the neurochemistry of anxiety and/or the vulnerability to anxiety-provoking agents. Hence, the serotonin transporter gene attracted a lot of attention, but again the results have been mixed. A polymorphism in the promoter region of this gene became a prime candidate, but replication of the original results has been patchy. However, a polymorphism of the serotonin transporter promoter gene appeared to be related to a susceptibility to develop PTSD (Lee *et al*, 2005*b*). Glucocorticoid receptor polymorphisms were not associated with PTSD (Bachman *et al*, 2005), and susceptibility genes for this condition have not yet been identified with any degree of certainty (Segman & Shalev, 2003).

There are also a few studies, although with equally inconsistent results, on polymorphisms of the 5-HT_{2C} receptor, the 5-HT_{1A} receptor, serotonin metabolising enzymes such as monoamine oxidase inhibitor (MAO) and catechol-O-methyl-transferase (COMT), as well as the receptor subunits for gamma-aminobutyric acid (GABA). Finally, equivocal results have been produced in studies of polymorphisms of genes regulating the cholecystokinin (CCK) and adenosine receptors, prime targets of pentagastrin and caffeine respectively, both substances that reliably provoke anxiety (Maier, 2003).

Thus, the presence of a significant genetic contribution to the anxiety disorders is not in dispute, but the identification of the actual candidate genes has so far proved to be elusive.

Social (and ethological) aspects

Dramatic changes in social conditions over the past 250 years may explain the rising prominence of anxiety and panic. Before the industrial revolution, the universal threats of incessant warfare, famine and epidemics of disease were ever present. The fear generated by these catastrophes sometimes presented as mass psychological expressions of panic, manifesting with bizarre, contagious, short-lived reactions, without significant long-lasting effects (see also Chapter 16, page 391). Literature through the ages provides detailed descriptions of such outbreaks (e.g. the reaction of the Florentines to the Black Death in 1347, as described in the *Decameron* of Boccaccio). By contrast, the anxiety of the individual was given much less attention and became the prerogative of theologians and other moralists at least as much as it was dealt with by physicians (Clark, 1995).

The rise of industrialisation is credited with the eradication of some and minimisation of other traditional risks from the lives of an ever-increasing portion of humanity. Anxiety and panic no longer appeared as a continuous feature in their lives but rather an exceptional circumstance. However, new reasons for anxiety emerged. The 'age of progress' turned also into an 'age of anxiety' by adding new pressures, through the creation of a climate of individuality, the fostering of ambitions and the attribution of great importance to personal attractiveness and success (Zeldin, 1977).

The evolution of the concept of PTSD can also be seen in the same context. The traumatic effects of warfare were always recognised and shell shock became an all too familiar term during the First World War. The frequent original panic reactions in battle (i.e. freezing and desertion) are easily understood from the point of view of the individual, but they were regarded as a grave dereliction of duty, usually leading to summary and exemplary punishment at dawn. This attitude gradually changed over the 20th century, with much greater importance being placed on the suffering of the individual rather than on themes of collective duty to the state. It is plausible to argue that PTSD was acknowledged in DSM–III mainly as a result of the huge influx of sufferers returning from the Vietnam War. Nowadays, there is also an increasing trend to award retrospective pardons to the deserters from the First World War, on the grounds that they were suffering from the recognised medical condition of PTSD, which legitimised their reaction to trauma.

Evolutionary theory sees the capacity of the organism to develop normal anxiety as a very helpful defensive mechanism against a variety of threats, which has been shaped by natural selection. Anxiety disorders are disorders of regulation of this defence system. Subtypes of anxiety may be related to particular kinds of threats or cues that shape behaviour differentially. The four major defensive strategies employed in anxiety disorders (escape, aggression, freezing and submission) are deployed to varying combinations and degrees in accordance with their utility. Ethologists argue that we need to know more about the function of these defence mechanisms if we are to understand the nature and origin of anxiety, as well as its usefulness, and this may aid the development of better treatments (Marks & Nesse, 1994). Others, such as Lorenz, on the basis of their observations on the attachment behaviour of young ducklings, have suggested that much anxiety, particularly separation anxiety, can be traced to problems in attachment. The psychoanalyst

Bowlby is credited with first applying ethology to the study of human anxiety and a brief summary of his work is given below.

The contribution of Bowlby

Bowlby's theory of attachment draws heavily from ethology and animal work. In his scheme, anxiety is viewed as a direct, innately based response to separation or the threat of separation from a primary carer. Holmes (1993), in a lucid account, considered the implications of attachment theory for psychotherapy.

Bowlby (1969) postulated that there is a primary attachment relationship. This appears in the human infant at around 7 months and its original main function was protection from predators. Animal work by Lorenz in ducks and Harlow in monkeys has shown that attachment and bonding behaviours are of central importance and are separate from feeding behaviours. Attachment is also fundamental to all types of psychotherapy. The universality of attachment may explain the paradox of why all types of psychotherapy are equally efficacious, despite wide differences in underlying philosophies and methods of treatment (Frank, 1971).

Attachment is characterised by proximity-seeking behaviour, which is activated in young children by separation from the carer. On separation there is initially increased anxiety and a protest reaction such as a temper tantrum or crying. This is an adaptive response, termed *separation anxiety*, and its aim is to reunite the infant with the carer. Darwin observed that primates may also show separation anxiety, while Freud believed that anxiety in children represented the feeling of loss for the person they love. In later life, threats of separation, losses, illnesses and other catastrophes may trigger this earlier separation anxiety.

Attachment results in the 'secure base phenomenon'. When infants feel securely attached and physically close to their attachment figure, they feel safe and engage in exploratory behaviour. An analogy is made with attachment in psychotherapy, in which one aim is to help patients explore new and better ways of coping with the environment as well as their own internal affects. To facilitate this, the therapist needs to provide a secure environment that is consistent, predictable and has warmth – all of which are also clearly the requirements for good mothering as well. In the absence of secure feelings, 'anxious attachments' may develop, manifested as clinging, dependent behaviour, with little in the way of exploratory behaviour, as well as a constant fear of separation and a proneness to separation anxiety. Bowlby (1969) suggested that school phobia may at least in part be explained in terms of anxious attachments and separation anxiety.

People carry an internal working model, or a map, that represents the relationship patterns that exist between themselves and their attachment figures. The 'map' consists of self-images, core affective states and cognitive schemata which describe the expectations people have of both themselves and the external world. Analysts have tended to focus on the unconscious schemata. More recently cognitive therapists have shown the value of exploring the patient's conscious schemata in psychotherapy.

The attachment dynamic is essential for physical and mental well-being and protection in childhood but it continues throughout life. The same attachment dynamic is found in all later psychosocial relationships, such as work or marriage, and also provides the dynamic for attachment in psychotherapy.

Bowlby's theory of attachment has derived some support from the experimental work of Mary Ainsworth (1969), a colleague of Bowlby. She devised the 'strange situation' test, which can reliably measure the security of a 1-year-old's attachment to a parent. In this test the parent leaves the room, while the infant remains alone with the investigator. There are four patterns of response:

1 around 65% of 1-year-olds display a *secure* pattern, where they make an initial protest but are easily pacified

2 some 20% show an *insecure avoidant* pattern, where there is little protest on the initial separation but on the parents' return the infant hovers warily nearby, unable to play freely

3 around 15% have an *insecure ambivalent* pattern, where they protest at the separation and cannot be pacified, and they cling tenaciously to the mother on her return

4 around 5% seem to freeze and are described as *insecure disorganised*.

These patterns appear to be both innate and persistent. Thus, an avoidant pattern shown at 1 year is also found when the child is 5, and again at 10 years of age.

Neurobiological aspects

Neuroanatomy

Cannon (1929), based on his extensive clinical, experimental and pharmacological observations, proposed that the thalamus plays a central role in the experience of emotions, including anxiety, and that these reactions follow on from the interpretation of the situation at the cortex. The role of a neuronal system or 'circuit' subserving the experience of emotion was first put forward by Papez (1937). Based on animal studies, Gray (1981, 1982) later proposed that the septohippocampal system is the central substrate of anxiety in the brain. He suggested that the hippocampus is crucial in that it operates as a comparator of actual and expected stimuli. The anxiety loop he proposed overlapped to a significant extent with the Papez circuit, but it also incorporated the locus ceruleus. Descending pathways from this structure of the floor of the fourth ventricle affect the sympathetic division of the autonomic nervous system and appear to play an important role in generating the experience of anxiety.

Gorman *et al* (2000) developed a neuroanatomical model for panic attacks which proposed that a panic attack is initiated from the nuclei responsible for noradrenaline transmission (i.e. the locus ceruleus) and respiratory control (i.e. the parabrachial nucleus) in the brain-stem. Following repeated attacks, kindling occurs in various limbic structures, such as the amygdala and the temporal lobes, and this leads to anticipatory anxiety between attacks. Finally, the phobic avoidance, evident in an extreme form in agoraphobia, is the result of activation of specific cortical areas, such as the medial prefrontal cortex, which do not allow extinction to occur.

How is this circuitry put in motion in the first place? Current thinking focuses on the idea that a panic attack, which would be a normal anxiety response within the context of a sudden threat, is allowed to start and progress out of context because there is an absence of the normal suppression of a minor anxiety response, or that some other homeostatic imbalance is at work. Another possible explanation is the development of panic attacks by external cues which the person remains unaware of but which still stimulate the amygdala (Cannistraro & Rauch, 2003).

Structural magnetic resonance imaging (MRI) studies of patients with panic disorder have shown a reduction of temporal lobe volumes compared with controls, but no change in hippocampal volume, which is in contrast to the pattern found with depression and PTSD (Vythilingam *et al*, 2000). Resting-state studies using positron emission tomography (PET) have also confirmed temporal lobe abnormalities and shown that the regional cerebral rate of glucose metabolism in the left hippocampus and parahippocampal area of women is elevated compared with controls, but reduced in the superior temporal regions of the right hemisphere (Bisaga *et al*, 1998). However, functional MRI studies with provocation of panic symptoms tend to implicate cortical regions and the insula. Increases or decreases of regional cerebral blood flow (rCBF) relative to controls have been reported for a number of cortical areas, such as bilateral frontal cortices, including the inferior frontal and orbitofrontal regions, and the cingulate (Woods *et al*, 1988; Bystritsky *et al*, 2001).

Reduced frontal activity during a panic attack may represent a failure of top-down control, consistent with one of the models outlined above by Cannistraro & Rauch (2003). The involvement of the insula probably relates to the autonomic responses in panic, while the temporal/hippocampal areas are involved in the information processing occurring during a panic attack.

Very few functional neuroanatomy studies of GAD have been performed. At rest, the rCBF is normal, but during states of stress it is reported to be decreased in most brain regions (Brawman-Mintzer & Lydiard, 1997). Treatment with benzodiazepines leads to a global decrease in the rate of metabolism, more prominent in areas with a high density of GABA binding sites (Buchsbaum *et al*, 1987). In children with this condition, in comparison with controls, larger bilateral amygdala volumes have been reported (De Bellis *et al*, 2001). The picture of the relevant circuitry for GAD remains unclear, but Nutt (2001) has suggested that different brain regions may be involved in the different symptom complexes that make up GAD. For example, the frontal cortex may account for worries, the thalamus for hypervigilance, the insula for autonomic symptoms, and the basal ganglia for the motor tension that is prominent in this type of anxiety

A number of studies in the 1990s showed that victims of war or childhood abuse with PTSD had a reduced volume of the hippocampus but no changes in the temporal lobes, the amygdala or the caudate nucleus (Gurvits *et al*, 1996; Bremner *et al*, 1997). This led to the neuroanatomical model for PTSD, which proposes that activation of the amygdala mediates chronic hyperarousal, causing stimulation of the hypothalamic–pituitary–adrenal (HPA) axis, and the resulting chronic hypersecretion of glucocorticoids leads to hippocampal atrophy (Sapolsky, 1996). The nodal point for the development of the pathophysiology may be the amygdala, which is thought to be hyperresponsive in PTSD (Rauch *et al*, 1998).

There is now some experimental evidence to support this model. Thus, symptom provocation studies comparing the effect of trauma among people who have developed PTSD and those who have not found that the PTSD patients show greater activation of the amygdala and decreased activation of the medial frontal and the anterior cingulate regions. Further, the level of amygdala activation appears to correlate with the intensity of the PTSD symptoms. The neuroanatomical finding of reduced hippocampal volume mentioned above is complemented by reduced activation of this structure in the functional imaging paradigms (Cannistraro & Rauch, 2003).

Neurochemistry

Panic attacks are one of the very few psychiatric phenomena that can be reliably induced in the laboratory. The original observation by Pitts & McClure (1967) that infusion of sodium lactate provoked panic in susceptible people led to investigation of the neurochemistry of panic, which was later extended to other anxiety states. The inhibitory transmitter GABA and the monoamines noradrenaline, serotonin (5-HT) and, to a lesser extent, dopamine and their role in anxiety disorders has been reviewed by Argyropoulos & Nutt (2003) and a brief overview is presented below.

The GABA–benzodiazepine receptor complex

For more than 2000 years, alcohol has been the most widely used and misused anxiolytic. Following the clinical introduction of the benzodiazepines in the 1960s, it was discovered that the members of this class of drugs bind to a specific high-affinity benzodiazepine site of the $GABA_A$ receptor, and that this site modulates allosterically the GABA–chloride ionophore complex (Braestrup & Squires, 1978). Alcohol, on the other hand, directly opens the chloride channel of the receptor. Since the benzodiazepines exercise their effect by augmenting the function of the endogenous transmitter (GABA), the properties of the $GABA_A$ receptors have been extensively investigated for their role in anxiety.

The $GABA_A$ receptor shows unique bi-directional agonism. Agonists, like the benzodiazepines, increase the effects of the endogenous transmitter (GABA) and are anxiolytic. Another group of drugs, known as the inverse agonists, such as the β-carboline FG 7142 and the benzodiazepine Ro 15-3505, also bind strongly to the $GABA_A$ receptor but they have an opposite effect: they reduce GABA function and they are anxiogenic in humans (Sandford *et al*, 2000). Antagonists of the $GABA_A$ receptor, like flumazenil, have little action of their own but block the actions of both agonists and inverse agonists. Among normal people, a flumazenil challenge has little anxiogenic effect, but untreated patients with panic disorder will experience a marked increase in anxiety (Nutt *et al*, 1990). This finding pointed to an aetiological role for an endogenous agonist or some receptor abnormality, rather than a significant role for inverse agonists. This also led to the formulation of the hypothesis that patients with panic disorder, in particular, may display a shift in the 'set point' of their benzodiazepine receptors, which could be a state or trait phenomenon leading to anxiety.

Further evidence of abnormal benzodiazepine receptor function in panic disorder comes from neuro-imaging studies of patients, which have shown that global benzodiazepine binding is significantly reduced compared with controls. This reduction is more pronounced in the orbitofrontal cortex and the insula (Malizia *et al*, 1998). These observations are consistent with the possibility that downregulation of the $GABA_A$ benzodiazepine receptor results in decreased function of the endogenous transmitter, and this may be the mechanism underlying clinical anxiety.

Interest in the endogenous agonists has also focused on the neurosteroids. These substances act on the $GABA_A$ receptor but at a different site from the benzodiazepines. Among their other actions, they also modulate allosterically the GABA receptor complex. Indirect evidence for the importance of these compounds in the regulation of anxiety comes from the observation that the pronounced natural fluctuations of the gonadal steroids, particularly progesterone, during the menstrual cycle, pregnancy and the postpartum period appears to affect anxiety levels. Animal studies indicate that progesterone is metabolised to a neurosteroid that augments the function of GABA. However, the other important gonadal steroids, the oestrogens, do not appear to affect GABA function (Wilson, 1996). Neurosteroids are produced either from cholesterol in the central nervous system or from precursors in the periphery, while their putative effects make them potential targets for the future development of anxiolytic drugs (Strous *et al*, 2006).

Noradrenaline

Since the middle of the 19th century, malfunction of the sympathetic autonomic system has been linked to behavioural arousal and anxiety symptoms (Berrios & Link, 1995). Much later, it was discovered that this is mediated by the catecholamines, adrenaline in the periphery and noradrenaline in the central nervous system. A number of observations led to the theory that excessive sympathetic activation may produce dysfunctional arousal and anxiety, through increased catecholamine transmission. For example, when Da Costa (1871) described the 'irritable heart syndrome' (a constellation of symptoms that would now fall under the rubric of panic disorder), he postulated an increased function of the cardiac nerve centres. Somatic symptoms of acute anxiety, such as tachycardia, palpitations, tachypnoea, sweating, dry mouth and epigastric discomfort are similar to the peripheral effects of the sympathetic system at times of arousal and stress, when the organism is preparing to fight or flee.

In their seminal study, Klein & Fink (1962) reported that the tricyclic antidepressant imipramine, which acts partly by blocking the reuptake of noradrenaline, is effective in controlling panic attacks. Drugs that lead to an acute increase in central noradrenaline availability, like amphetamines and cocaine, can also have an anxiogenic effect.

The level of sympathetic activity induced during various neurochemical challenges has often been found to correlate with the levels of anxiety that these challenges elicit (Ko *et al*, 1983). In rats, stressful events produce a marked elevation of noradrenaline release in a variety of brain regions, including the hypothalamus, the amygdala and the locus ceruleus (Tanaka *et al*, 2000). However, studies of plasma noradrenaline levels in anxious patients at rest have been mostly negative. Starkman *et al* (1990) found no difference between patients with panic disorder and healthy controls, and the same was true for a group of patients with GAD (Munjack *et al*, 1990) and for a sample with mixed panic and GAD (Cameron *et al*, 1990).

However, the sympathetic system may show no sign of dysfunction at rest, but when the organism comes under stress its reaction may be abnormal. A number of neurochemical challenges that act upon the central or peripheral noradrenaline receptors have been used to study the functional integrity of noradrenaline reaction to stress. Thus, adrenaline and isoprenaline, both selective agonists of β-postsynaptic receptors, induce somatic symptoms as well as mental anxiety, and can provoke panic in patients with panic disorder, although they do not cross the blood–brain barrier. It is of interest that in patients with social phobia, following the ingestion of these two substances the expected peripheral physiological effects are not accompanied by central effects (Argyropoulos & Nutt, 2003). These findings led to speculation that peripheral β-receptors may be hypersensitive, at least in panic (Rainey *et al*, 1984). On the other hand, there is also evidence of downregulation of β-receptors in patients with panic disorder (Nesse *et al*, 1984), presumably secondary to paroxysms of increased noradrenaline activity.

Cognitive or environmental cues will also affect the interpretation of the physiological/somatic sequelae of peripherally acting catecholamines. A study that compared responses to an intramuscular injection of adrenaline between patients who had GAD and normal controls found that both groups had a similar increase in plasma levels of adrenaline and noradrenaline after the injection. However, the patient group showed a substantially increased heart rate and anxiety response compared with the controls, which suggests the possibility of cognitive misinterpretation of the peripheral effects of catecholamines among some people predisposed to anxiety (Mathew *et al*, 1982).

The role of central α_2 autoreceptors in anxiety

Much of the research work in anxiety has focused on the regulatory role of α_2 autoreceptors in the locus ceruleus. Yohimbine is an antagonist to the α_2 presynaptic receptors in this nucleus and can cause anxiety in normal people (Goldberg *et al*, 1983). This antagonism results in disruption of the normal negative feedback loop from the synapse to the cell, leading to increased firing of the cell bodies in the locus ceruleus, and increased synaptic availability of noradrenaline. Yohimbine given to patients with panic disorder leads to an increase in anxiety and panic frequency, as well as a significant increase in plasma catecholamine metabolites, compared with controls (Charney *et al*, 1984*a*). This response of patients with panic disorder to yohimbine can be blocked by diazepam (Charney *et al*, 1984*a*) and is normalised after successful treatment with tricyclic antidepressants, but not after cognitive therapy (Middleton, 1990). Patients with PTSD show a similar anxiogenic response to yohimbine associated with the characteristic flashbacks of the condition, as well as panic attacks (Southwick *et al*, 1993). On the other hand, yohimbine was not more anxiogenic in patients with GAD than in controls, indicating that individual anxiety syndromes may not share the same pathophysiology of the adrenergic system (Charney *et al*, 1989).

If the mechanism whereby yohimbine increases anxiety is by antagonising α_2 presynaptic autoreceptors, then one would expect that an α_2 agonist should have an anxiolytic effect. Clonidine is such a centrally acting α_2 receptor partial agonist, which is efficacious against both spontaneous and lactate-induced panic attacks, although its use in clinical populations is restricted by its hypotensive and sedative side-effects (Argyropoulos *et al*, 2000). Beneficial therapeutic effects have also been obtained in small studies with patients suffering PTSD, but the effect is short-lived, owing to the development of tolerance (Friedman, 1998). Clonidine has also been used as a challenge test in patients with panic disorder who, in comparison with controls, showed a significantly greater decrease in plasma noradrenaline metabolites, as well as an exaggerated hypotensive response, although these results have not been universally replicated (Argyropoulos & Nutt, 2003).

Overall, the above findings of the yohimbine and clonidine studies point towards an abnormal supersensitivity of presynaptic α_2 autoreceptors to both antagonists and agonists, at least in some forms of anxiety. The exaggerated responsiveness of presynaptic α_2 autoreceptors in panic led Nutt (1989) to propose a failure of control of the locus ceruleus as the neurochemical basis of pathological acute anxiety. Animal studies show that α_2 receptors may also be altered by stress and conditioning. This, in turn, could explain the association between life events and anxiety. Further, the system appears to be under the influence of corticotropin-releasing factor (CRF) neurons in the locus ceruleus, thus indicating a putative neuroanatomical link between stress experiences and central catecholamine activity. The sensitivity of the postsynaptic α_2 receptors may also be measured by the growth hormone (GH) response to a clonidine challenge, which is blunted in patients with panic disorder, as also occurs in depression, thus indicating a hyposensitivity of the postsynaptic receptors in these patients. This blunting has also been demonstrated both before and after successful treatment (Coplan *et al*, 1995), as well as in patients with GAD (Abelson *et al*, 1991). The more recent developments in this field have been comprehensively reviewed elsewhere (Argyropoulos & Nutt, 2003).

Serotonin (5-hydroxytryptamine, 5-HT)

The selective serotonin reuptake inhibitors (SSRIs), which block the reuptake of 5-HT from the synaptic cleft back to the nerve terminal, have demonstrated clear efficacy across the full range of anxiety disorders and this clinical observation has led to a resurgence of research interest in the role of serotonin in the pathophysiology of anxiety. A whole host of serotonin receptors have been identified in animal studies in recent years. While the function of many of these is still unclear, there is substantial evidence for the involvement of some of them in anxiety. These include the G-protein-linked pre- and postsynaptic 5-HT_{1A} (Olivier *et al*, 1999), the phosphoinositol (PI)-linked 5-HT_2 (Roth *et al*, 1998) and the sodium-channel-linked 5-HT_3 receptor classes (Olivier *et al*, 2000). Animal studies have also implicated the terminal 5-$HT_{1B/D}$ autoreceptor (Moret & Briley, 2000).

In humans, preliminary evidence from neuroimaging studies using radioligands, such as the [carbonyl-^{11}C] Way-100635 compound, which selectively binds to 5-HT_{1A} receptors, has shown that these receptors mainly localise in the limbic forebrain. This supports the long-held view that they are implicated in the modulation of emotions (Passchier & van Waarde, 2001). Most of the studies on 5-HT systems and their receptors in the brain have focused on depression, but one study in patients treated for panic disorder has reported a decrease in 5-HT_{1A} receptor density, similar to that seen in depression (Sargent *et al*, 2000).

Although the case for the involvement of 5-HT in anxiety is strong, it is still unclear whether anxiety results from an excess or deficiency of central serotonin function. Challenge paradigms that increase central 5-HT transmission have produced mixed results. The 5-HT agonist m-chlorophenylpiperizine (mCPP) is anxiogenic in patients with panic disorder (Charney *et al*, 1987), GAD (Germine *et al*, 1992) and in normal controls at high enough doses (Charney *et al*, 1987). Fenfluramine, a drug that releases 5-HT, is also anxiogenic in people with panic disorder (Targum, 1990), as is intravenously administered clomipramine, a tricyclic antidepressant with a strong degree of serotonin reuptake inhibition (George *et al*, 1995). On the other hand, L-tryptophan and 5-hydroxytryptophan (5-HTP), the precursors of 5-HT, are known to cause sedation and anxiolysis or to have no effect on anxiety (van Vliet *et al*, 1996). Further, the SSRIs are traditionally thought to exert their action by increasing the availability of the transmitter in the synaptic cleft.

A possible explanation for the neuroendocrine activation by fenfluramine and mCPP is that the postsynaptic 5-HT receptors (especially 5-HT_2) become hypersensitive in anxiety. This may also account for the exacerbation of anxiety sometimes observed at the initial stages of treatment with SSRIs, before their therapeutic effect becomes evident a few weeks into administration. Kahn *et al* (1988) proposed that this is the result of initial stimulation of hypersensitive postsynaptic 5-HT receptors by an excess of the transmitter, which is followed somewhat later by downregulation of these receptors in response to the chronic bombardment. If this theory is correct, it suggests that the SSRIs exert their action by reducing central 5-HT transmission, and so by implication anxiety may be considered to be a state of increased global serotonin function.

However, animal studies using microdialysis, a technique that makes it possible to measure the overflow of 5-HT into the extracellular space, show that 5-HT is not increased in the synapse during acute treatment with SSRIs, but only after there is downregulation of the presynaptic 5-HT_{1A} autoreceptors (Blier *et al*, 1990). This causes a reduction of the negative feedback to the 5-HT cell and then a subsequent increase in cell firing and serotonin release. Buspirone, a drug that is effective in GAD, is thought to exert its action through these autoreceptors (Taylor *et al*, 1985).

Tryptophan depletion is a technique that uses a combination of a special diet and consumption of an amino-acid drink that makes it possible to reduce plasma tryptophan levels by up to 80% acutely (see also Chapter 3, page 64). On the day of the tryptophan depletion, patients with panic disorder treated with SSRIs when challenged with flumenazil experience a significant increase in their anxiety (Bell *et al*, 2002). Although these results are still preliminary, they provide an indication that increased, rather than decreased, 5-HT is a necessary condition for the SSRIs to exert their anxiolytic effects.

Central 5-HT pathways in anxiety

The answer to the conundrum of whether there is too much or too little serotonin in anxiety may lie in the complex anatomy of central 5-HT pathways. There are two major serotonergic systems implicated in anxiety. One originates from the medial raphe nuclei (MRN) and the other from the dorsal raphe nuclei (DRN). The two systems are morphologically distinct, and have different afferent and efferent projections (Azmitia & Whitaker, 1995), but they function in parallel (Tork & Hornung, 1990). It may be that each system mediates distinct aspects of anxiety. According to Grove *et al* (1997), the MRN projection is crucial for the modulation of fear and anticipatory anxiety, while the DRN projection modulates cognitive processes related to anxiety. Other authors have suggested that the pathway from the MRN to the dorsal hippocampus mediates resistance to chronic unavoidable stress. The failure of any one of these subsystems may be responsible for the phenomenologically different clinical syndromes of anxiety and depression (Deakin & Graeff, 1991).

While an excess of serotonin may precipitate anxiety in one subsystem, it may be anxiolytic in another. According to Deakin & Graeff (1991), the role of 5-HT in the ascending pathway from DRN to the amygdala and the frontal cortex facilitates anxiety, and more specifically conditioned fear. On the other hand, the 5-HT in the pathway from the DRN to the peri-aqueductal grey matter (PAG) may inhibit unconditioned fear, inborn fight/flight reactions to impending danger and panic. In support of this, animal work suggests that a specific 5-HT_{2C} agonist exerts its anti-panic effect through the PAG (Jenck *et al*, 1998).

Some support for this anatomical/functional diversity of 5-HT systems in relation to anxiety is derived from experiments showing that 5-HT-promoting agents (e.g. fenfluramine and mCPP) increase skin conductance in a paradigm of an aversive conditioned stimulus (loud tone) in healthy volunteers, while fenfluramine decreased the subjective anxiety induced by a paradigm of an unconditioned stimulus (public speaking). On the other hand, a 5-HT-blocking agent (ritanserin) had exactly the opposite effect in the above paradigms (Graeff *et al*, 1996; Guimaraes *et al*, 1997).

Finally, evidence for the molecular/genetic processes involved in the regulation of the central 5-HT system, and their significance for anxiety, is now beginning to emerge. A polymorphism of the 5-HT transporter (5-HTT) gene has been associated with anxiety personality traits (Lesch & Mossner, 1998), while it is also thought that early environmental experiences may modulate the 5-HT system sensitivity to stress (Chaouloff, 2000).

Although some data on the pathophysiology of 5-HT in anxiety are now beginning to emerge, there is so far no comprehensive, unitary theory to explain its role, but the suggestion is that the combination of the specific functional/anatomical pathways and different 5-HT receptor subtypes may ultimately be responsible for the clinical expression of the distinct forms of anxiety.

Other putative neurochemical mechanisms of anxiety

The most widely used natural substance that provokes anxiety is caffeine. In experimental conditions, it can elicit panic attacks in predisposed individuals, while it raises the anxiety levels of healthy volunteers as well (Charney *et al*, 1984*b*). Caffeine interacts weakly with the benzodiazepine receptor, and its central effect is thought to be via the adenosine receptor site (Boulenger *et al*, 1982). Large doses produce an anxiety state including insomnia, headache, tremor, nausea and diarrhoea. Instant coffee contains 80–100 mg caffeine per cup and percolated, filtered or boiled coffee rather higher concentrations. Tea contains rather lower concentrations and caffeine is a constituent of certain carbonated preparations, such as cola drinks. An estimate of caffeine consumption is important in all people presenting with anxiety states and an amount greater than 600 mg/day may contribute to the state of caffeinism (see Chapter 22, page 568).

A number of neuropeptides have been implicated in the pathophysiology of anxiety, including CRF, cholecystokinin, substance P, neuropeptide Y and galanin. Although there is ample evidence for their involvement in circuits subserving the anxiety disorders, the exact nature of their dysfunction and interplay with other neurochemical systems remains undetermined (Gutman *et al*, 2003). The therapeutic role of these peptides and their analogues has been actively investigated but clinical benefits have yet to be seen (Griebel, 1999; Argyropoulos *et al*, 2000).

Neuroendocrinology

The general neuroendocrine response to stress triggers an immediate sympathetic discharge that prepares the organism to fight or flee (Cannon, 1929), and this is followed by a lengthier response of the HPA axis. The latter is generated by neuropeptides that stimulate the paraventricular nucleus of the hypothalamus and result in the release of CRF, cascading further down to the release of adrenocorticotrophic hormone (ACTH) from the pituitary and finally the release of cortisol from the adrenals. With the end of stress activation, cortisol provides the negative feedback that shuts down the HPA axis, via structures that are both very rich in glucocorticoid receptors and central to the stress experience, mainly the pituitary, the hypothalamus, the amygdala and the hippocampus (Chrousos & Gold, 1992).

It has not been possible to trace this chain of events consistently during panic attacks in the laboratory, as some of the panicogenic agents (e.g. sodium lactate) do not increase the levels of cortisol, while others (e.g. pentagastrin) do. Further, spontaneous attacks in the laboratory are not accompanied by cortisol elevation, although there is still an assumption that in a natural environment the situation may be different. On the few occasions when it has been possible to examine the function of the HPA axis during panic attacks in a natural environment, these were followed by cortisol elevation. The dexamethasone suppression test in patients with panic disorder is normal, and evidence that the circulating levels of ACTH and cortisol may be elevated is equivocal (Strohle & Holsboer, 2003).

In PTSD, changes in the HPA axis differ from those found in other anxiety disorders or depression. A number of studies have now shown that while CRF levels are elevated in PTSD, cortisol levels are not higher than among controls and sometimes are even reported to be lower. This appears to be true also for people who later develop PTSD when they are studied shortly after their exposure to trauma (Yehuda, 2000). It has been hypothesised that the low cortisol levels may be the result of an oversensitive negative feedback mechanism. The implication is that not enough cortisol is available to restrain catecholamine actions when acute stress occurs, as in a trauma situation, and this may lead to abnormal 'over-consolidation' of traumatic memories in some predisposed individuals, a phenomenon that appears to be central to the PTSD experience (Yehuda, 2000).

Treatment

Most patients with anxiety disorders are expected to be diagnosed and treated at the primary care level. Referral to specialist mental health services usually follows incomplete recovery and aims at comprehensive assessment, especially of risks and comorbidity, as well as the delivery of more specialised care, such as psychological treatment with an experienced therapist, full exploration of pharmacological options, or a combination of the two.

Lifestyle changes

Simple advice may help alleviate anxiety in some cases. For example, anxious patients may not be aware of the number of cups of coffee and tea they consume during their usual day, and the effect caffeine has on their condition, unless they are specifically asked to monitor this. Similarly, people who panic in the morning or become very anxious in the face of their stressful job may have failed to make any connection between their morning anxiety and their heavy drinking session the night before.

On the other hand, the obvious solutions are not always easy to implement. It may be reasonable to point out to a very busy but permanently exhausted and worried professional that his or her diary reveals an unrelenting time pressure and a schedule in which every moment of the week and weekend is taken up with work or some work-related activity. It may also be pointed out that such a lifestyle leads to the abandonment of hobbies or simple leisure and social activities. People often underestimate how much such activities contribute to a sense of worth and feelings of control over their environment, as well as to the restoration of mental strength and sanity following prolonged periods of pressure. Unfortunately, doctors' recommendations are not always sufficient to lead to a sustained change of lifestyle.

Drug treatments

Alcohol has been the most widely used 'anxiolytic' for over 2000 years. Since the 19th century, people have also used opiates and bromides. Later, the barbiturates were introduced and misused extensively, until the marketing in the 1960s of a safer alternative, the benzodiazepines. At the same time, evidence was accumulating that tricyclic antidepressants were equally if not more effective than benzodiazepines for the treatment of anxiety. It was not until the adverse publicity surrounding the benzodiazepines and the advent of the SSRIs that antidepressants became the first-line pharmacological option for anxiety disorders.

The usual rules for good prescribing apply. The benefits and risks of the specific drug regimens should be discussed with the patient before the start of treatment. There should also be specific discussion about the monitoring of possible side-effects and adverse events. In anxiety disorders, this is particularly relevant at the start and termination of treatment, since there may be an initial worsening of symptoms with antidepressants or a discontinuation syndrome with either benzodiazepines or antidepressants. Benzodiazepines may also cause dependence after prolonged use, and explicit information to this effect should be given to patients before they start taking the drug.

A number of august bodies and panels of experts, such as the International Consensus Group on Depression and Anxiety (Ballenger *et al*, 1998*a*), the World Federation of Societies of Biological Psychiatry (Bandelow *et al*, 2002), the World Council on Anxiety (Allgulander *et al*, 2003; Pollack *et al*, 2003*a*; Stein *et al*, 2003), the British Association for Psychopharmacology (BAP) (Baldwin *et al*, 2005) and the National Institute for Health and Clinical Excellence (NICE) (2004, 2005) have produced guidelines for the use of drugs in anxiety disorders and some of their main recommendations are discussed below.

Antidepressants

Randomised controlled trials (RCTs) of all the SSRIs (escitalopram, citalopram, fluoxetine, fluvoxamine, paroxetine and sertraline) and the dual uptake inhibitor venlafaxine have shown that they are effective in the acute short-term treatment of panic disorder. Long-term treatment and relapse prevention RCT data also exist for fluoxetine, paroxetine, sertraline and citalopram (Baldwin *et al*, 2005). There have been fewer RCTs of tricyclic antidepressants in panic but substantial evidence is available that imipramine and clomipramine are effective, in both the short and the long term. Of the other antidepressants, there is some evidence for the short-term efficacy of phenelzine, mirtazapine and reboxetine (Baldwin *et al*, 2005). There is also some evidence that serotonergic antidepressants are more effective anti-panic agents than purely noradrenergic compounds (den Boer & Westenberg, 1988).

Meta-analytic studies have shown that SSRIs and tricyclic antidepressants are equally effective in panic disorder, but the drop-out rate is higher with the tricyclics (31% *v.* 18%), strengthening the clinical impression that the SSRIs are better tolerated (Bakker *et al*, 2002).

Similarly, a meta-analysis comparing antidepressants with benzodiazepines in panic disorder found no significant differences in efficacy between the treatments (Wilkinson *et al*, 1991), but the overall side-effect burden appeared to favour the SSRIs over the benzodiazepines (Bakker *et al*, 2002).

The BAP guidelines (Baldwin *et al*, 2005) recommend that for patients with panic disorder, an SSRI should be the first pharmacological choice, with imipramine being the second choice; for those who have responded by 12 weeks, treatment should be continued for a further 6 months.

In GAD, short- and long-term RCTs, and relapse prevention studies, have shown that escitalopram, paroxetine and venlafaxine are effective, and these drugs are licensed in the UK for the treatment of the condition. Further, short-term data also exist for sertraline and imipramine (Baldwin & Polkinghorn, 2005). There is some evidence that antidepressants may be more effective for the cognitive symptoms of GAD, while the benzodiazepines may have an advantage for the somatic symptoms (Meoni *et al*, 2004). Higher doses of an SSRI or venlafaxine may be associated with greater response rates, so increasing the dose may be a useful strategy after a poor initial response. As with panic disorder, for GAD responders the BAP guidelines recommend a continuation of maintenance treatment for a further 6 months (Baldwin *et al*, 2005).

The SSRIs are also the pharmacological treatment of choice for PTSD. Fluoxetine, paroxetine and sertraline have shown acute efficacy in RCTs. For sertraline, long-term data are available, while for both sertraline and fluoxetine relapse prevention studies have also been conducted. Both short- and long-term trials have also shown efficacy for venlafaxine (Baldwin *et al*, 2005). Short-term trials have suggested that amitriptyline and imipramine are also helpful in PTSD, but long-term data for the tricyclic antidepressants is lacking (Davidson *et al*, 1990; Kosten *et al*, 1991). Of the other antidepressants, there is evidence that mirtazapine has acute efficacy in PTSD (Davidson *et al*, 2003) and the same applies to the older compound phenelzine, although this drug is little used now (Kosten *et al*, 1991). As with panic disorder and GAD, an initial period of 12 weeks is recommended before its efficacy can be properly assessed. For those who respond, a further 12 months of treatment with the same agent at the same dose is then recommended, with regular monitoring of efficacy and tolerability during this period (Baldwin *et al*, 2005).

Some patients with panic disorder may be very sensitive to a worsening effect early in treatment. This can be manifested by increased agitation and/or exacerbation of the symptoms, such as an increase in panic attacks. This so-called 'jitteriness syndrome' (Ramos *et al*, 1993) tends to be self-limited to up to 2 weeks and the usual approach is to initiate treatment at a lower dose (e.g. 10 mg paroxetine or equivalent) and then titrate upwards after 7–10 days. Sometimes short-term cover with a high-potency benzodiazepine such as lorazepam or clonazepam for 2 weeks may be needed to help establish the longer-term treatment with the antidepressant (Goddard *et al*, 2001). Since most of the new antidepressants are not sedative, alternative measures, psychological or pharmacological, to improve sleep at the beginning of the treatment may be required.

The antidepressants are not fast-acting anxiolytics and patients need to be warned that it may take weeks for the full benefit to emerge. They are useful in all aspects of panic disorder and GAD, although the progression of symptom relief may be variable and behavioural aspects like agoraphobia may take months to resolve. Relapse prevention studies of patients who respond to acute treatment with antidepressants show a significant advantage for those who stay on long-term medication. The evidence for a dose–response relationship in panic disorder is limited (Baldwin *et al*, 2005), but in one study a dosage of 40 mg/day paroxetine produced a better result than 20 mg/day (Ballenger *et al*, 1998*b*). There is a well-recognised discontinuation syndrome from the antidepressants (Haddad, 1998) and so the drug dosage should be gradually tapered off over a period that in some cases extends to 3 months (Baldwin *et al*, 2005).

Benzodiazepines

The RCTs of the high-potency benzodiazepine compounds (alprazolam, clonazepam, lorazepam) and diazepam have shown that they are effective in the acute treatment of panic disorder (Baldwin *et al*, 2005). RCT data are also available for the long-term efficacy of alprazolam, which show significant improvement in all the major symptom areas of panic disorder (i.e. number of panic attacks, avoidance behaviour and residual anxiety between attacks) (Schweizer *et al*, 1993).

Benzodiazepines have been extensively used for the treatment of GAD, for which they are effective (Mitte *et al*, 2005). They have a rapid onset of action and are well tolerated. Diazepam has been the favoured drug in this class for many years. Initiation of treatment with a small dose (e.g. 2 mg three times a day or 5 mg twice a day) allows tolerance to the psychomotor and sedative effects to develop.

Although there is good RCT evidence for the use of benzodiazepines in panic disorder, UK guidelines do not make uniform recommendations. Thus, NICE (2004) does not recommend their use in the treatment of panic disorder, whereas the BAP guidelines suggested that any of the four benzodiazepines mentioned above could be used in the acute treatment of panic disorder, although they make no comment on their longer-term use for panic disorder (Baldwin *et al*, 2005).

For PTSD one RCT, of alprazolam versus placebo, reported no significant improvement in the core PTSD symptoms, although there was a positive effect in subjective well-being, as well as reductions in anxiety, insomnia and irritability (Braun *et al*, 1990). Open trials with alprazolam and clonazepam had similar findings, but withdrawal symptoms were particularly severe (Friedman, 1998). It therefore appears that benzodiazepines have little to offer in PTSD since the intrusion and avoidant/numbing symptoms were unresponsive. In addition, as PTSD has substantial comorbidity with alcohol and drug misuse, the use of benzodiazepines in these patients may lead to iatrogenic dependence.

Despite their near demonisation in the 1980s and 1990s (Lader, 1978; Kraupl Taylor, 1989), the benzodiazepines are still very widely prescribed across all the major psychiatric diagnoses. For example, in a series of consecutive admissions to a Spanish psychiatric hospital, 82.9% of anxious patients with an anxiety disorder, 76.6% of patients with a mood disorder and 68.1% of patients with a psychosis were taking benzodiazepines (de las Cuevas & Sanz, 2005). The secret of their enduring popularity must lie in a number of factors. They provide rapid relief for very prevalent and distressing symptoms, they are generally well tolerated, they are non-cardiotoxic and anti-epileptic, they can be used on an 'as required' basis, they are generally safe in overdose when ingested alone, and they reduce the activation induced by other drugs, such as the antidepressants.

All these advantages need to be weighed against the well-known disadvantages of the benzodiazepines, such as excessive sedation and psychomotor impairment, the discontinuation/withdrawal symptoms, their liability to misuse, alcohol potentiation, disinhibition and lack of efficacy in comorbid depression (Argyropoulos & Nutt, 1999). Further, a host of subtle cognitive effects are also reported, such as visuospatial deficits, a decrease in problem-solving ability, and decline in general intelligence, verbal reasoning, sensory processing and verbal, non-verbal and working memory (Barker *et al*, 2004*a*). However, closer inspection of these disadvantages in recent years has cast some doubt on the wisdom of the wholesale rejection of this class of drugs. Dependence on the benzodiazepines rarely occurs alone; personality disorders are a very prominent comorbidity (Martinez-Cano *et al*, 1999), with up to 83% of the participants in one study manifesting dependence on at least one more drug (Busto *et al*, 1996). Further, physical dependence does not necessarily imply misuse or loss of therapeutic benefit. Long-term naturalistic studies, mainly with patients suffering from panic disorder, do not support the uniform idea of the development of tolerance to the therapeutic effect (e.g. Nagy *et al*, 1989; Worthington *et al*, 1998). The studies on cognition have been criticised on methodological grounds, and the withdrawal of the drugs leads to at least partial recovery of any recorded cognitive deficits (Barker *et al*, 2004*b*).

Disinhibition (a rare phenomenon in itself) does not appear to be more prevalent among benzodiazepine users in the general population than when placebo is administered. However, some groups of patients may be particularly at risk of developing this reaction: those with conditions associated with reduced impulse control (personality disorders, neurological diseases and learning difficulties), the young (i.e. under 18 years) or older patients (above 65), as well as those who have received high doses of benzodiazepines acutely for sedation (Rothschild *et al*, 2000; Paton, 2002).

The severity of the discontinuation syndrome is increased by a number of factors, including: residual anxiety and/or depression; a primary diagnosis of panic disorder; personality psychopathology (neuroticism, dependency); higher levels of education; and female sex (Schweizer & Rickels, 1998).

At first it was thought that the symptoms that appeared when a benzodiazepine was stopped reflected no more than a return of the patient's original anxiety. However, it later became clear that there is a specific benzodiazepine withdrawal syndrome. Petursson & Lader (1981) demonstrated that withdrawal symptoms could occur after taking the drug for as little as 6 weeks. The withdrawal symptoms are of two types: first, more general anxiety symptoms, which are common; and secondly, some more specific sensory symptoms (see Box 13.6). The onset is usually 1–10 days after stopping the drug or after dosage reduction; the withdrawal state usually lasts 5–25 days but may last up to 12 weeks. More severe withdrawal states occur with drugs that have shorter half-lives, such as lorazepam and triazolam.

Box 13.6 Specific and non-specific symptoms of benzodiazepine withdrawal

Specific symptoms/reactions (but uncommon)
- Increased intensity of sensations
- Hyperacusis, tinnitus
- Photophobia
- Blurred vision
- Abnormal perception of motion
- Muscle twitching
- Hyper-reflexia
- Depression
- Confusion
- Psychosis
- Seizures
- Delirium

Non-specific symptoms (common)
- Anxiety
- Insomnia
- Irritability
- Nausea
- Palpitations
- Headache and muscle tension
- Tremor

The management of withdrawal states usually entails switching from a drug with a short half-life to one with a longer half-life, such as from lorazepam to diazepam, and this is accomplished slowly over a period of weeks and then gradually tapering off the diazepam. During the period of withdrawal there should be adequate psychological support. The withdrawal should always be supervised because sometimes a severe depression may supervene. Some patients find anxiety management or group support helpful during drug withdrawal. There are reports that clonidine, propranolol, carbamazepine and tricyclic antidepressants may reduce the severity of withdrawal symptoms, but in practice experience with these drugs is often disappointing. Most patients who have decided to come off one drug to which they have become inadvertently dependent are a little wary of starting another one.

Finally, most countries have either guidelines or legislation that impose some restrictions on the use of benzodiazepines. The Royal College of Psychiatrists' (1997) guidelines, echoed by NICE (2004), suggest short-term use (2–4 weeks) and only when other treatments have failed. It has long been argued that in the light of the current evidence, the guidance of the College is ripe for revision (Williams & McBride, 1998), but even so a degree of caution, careful patient selection and a clear follow-up plan should be applied whenever these drugs are prescribed (Tyrer, 1989*b*).

Other drugs used in anxiety

Buspirone, a partial 5-HT_{1A} agonist, is an effective alternative in GAD in doses of up to 60 mg/day (Rickels *et al*, 1982). This drug is neither fast acting nor sedative but may induce insomnia at the onset of treatment or in high doses. It is not associated with tolerance, dependence or withdrawal, and does not interact with alcohol. However, it is not useful in anxiety disorders other than GAD (Argyropoulos *et al*, 2000). The antihistamine hydroxyzine is also a fast-acting anxiolytic that is effective in GAD, even at lower doses (50–100 mg/day), which do not cause sedation (Ferreri & Hantouche, 1998). As with buspirone, hydroxyzine is not indicated for any other anxiety disorder.

Against the widespread belief that beta-blockers are effective anxiolytics because they control the peripheral symptoms of anxiety, RCTs have not supported the use of these drugs in panic disorder or GAD (Argyropoulos *et al*, 2000). If anything, the resultant bradycardia is reported by some patients to be anxiogenic in itself. An open trial has suggested that propranolol may be helpful in PTSD. High doses of this drug (120–160 mg/day) led to improvement in sleep, hyperarousal, startle responses and even reduced nightmares and intrusive phenomena in 11 out of 12 Vietnam veterans (Kolb *et al*, 1984). Propanolol has not been properly tested in PTSD, although there is evidence for its use prophylactically after exposure to trauma (Pitman *et al*, 2002).

The antihypertensive α_2 partial agonist clonidine has also shown some anxiolytic potential, especially in PTSD, but its effect appears to be transient, probably because of the development of tolerance (Friedman, 1998).

Finally, the classical antipsychotics became popular drugs for treating anxiety when the benzodiazepines fell out of favour, but, given the side-effect profile of these drugs, the benefit:risk ratio is probably very low and their use is no longer supported (El-Khayat & Baldwin, 1998). Studies with atypical agents in anxiety are ongoing, but so far most information derives from augmentation trials (see below).

A number of other potentially useful treatments have emerged in recent years, although they have not yet reached the stage of licensing for clinical use for the anxiety disorders. Those that are supported by positive placebo-controlled trials include pregabalin, a structural analogue of GABA, in GAD, and the anticonvulsant lamotrigine in PTSD (Baldwin *et al*, 2005). In a small study, the α_1 adrenergic antagonist prazosin was found to be superior to placebo in a number of core symptom measures of combat-related PTSD, including a reduction of nightmares (Raskind *et al*, 2003). There is interest in partial agonists of the GABA–benzodiazepine receptor complex, various drugs that act on serotonin receptors and compounds that affect neuropeptide transmitters, but these agents are still in development (Hood *et al*, 2003).

Augmentation strategies

There is limited information about the choice of treatment strategies to adopt when no response has appeared after an initial treatment lasting around 12 weeks. Most clinicians tend to switch to a different drug class or treatment modality, or augment a psychological therapy with a drug treatment or vice versa. There is a small amount of evidence to support such a strategy. For example, the addition of paroxetine (up to 40 mg/day) to cognitive–behavioural therapy (CBT) in patients with panic disorder proved to be more effective than placebo over 8 weeks (Kampman *et al*, 2002). The addition of olanzapine or risperidone to other psychotropic medication in patients with PTSD was also beneficial (Stein *et al*, 2002; Bartzokis *et al*, 2005). Similar positive results were obtained with the addition of olanzapine (at an average dose of just below 10mg/day) to fluoxetine in partially responding GAD, although some weight gain was noted (Pollack *et al*, 2006). Finally, for patients with panic disorder, concurrent treatment with clonazepam and an SSRI gave a faster response than if the SSRI was used alone (Pollack *et al*, 2003*b*).

Combined psychological and pharmacological treatments

The routine combination of therapeutic approaches in panic disorder is not generally recommended from the start of treatment, because the evidence for an enhanced synergistic effect is not consistent (Baldwin *et al*, 2005). However, the combination is a reasonable next step when either treatment modality fails to deliver acceptable results when used alone. A large meta-analysis, representing more than 5000 patients, concluded that the combination of antidepressants with exposure *in vivo* was particularly effective in panic disorder with agoraphobia, more so than the individual treatments administered alone (van Balkom *et al*, 1997) and this finding has been replicated in a more recent systematic review of the acute treatment of panic with or without agoraphobia (Furukawa *et al*, 2006).

Further well-conducted trials in panic disorder have pointed to specific advantages of combined treatments even in the absence of an overall synergistic effect. For example, the combination of paroxetine with a psychoeducation booklet produced more rapid improvement (Dannon *et al*, 2002), while the combination of imipramine with CBT produced fewer relapses in long-term treatment (Barlow *et al*, 2000). However, for PTSD, there is so far no evidence of enhanced efficacy to support the combination of treatments.

Psychological treatments

There are two broad psychological approaches to the treatment of anxiety disorders: the cognitive–behavioural and the psychoanalytic. The essential difference between these two important bodies of theory is that the cognitive–behavioural model attends mainly to people's conscious thinking, their behaviour and the forces that seem to be working for and against them in terms of maintaining the problem. The psychoanalytic model lays its emphasis on anxiety being a symptom of deeper difficulties. These are in the form of internal (unconscious) mental conflict, in which basic desires and instincts are met with resistance from other parts of the mind, in particular those concerned with adjustment to external reality. The contrast, therefore, can be organised around the extent to which the focus is placed on the 'here and now' or the repetition (in the present) of past interpersonal difficulties (often from the long distant past, particularly childhood) that in large part lies outside the conscious awareness of the individual. What is accepted by both approaches, however, is that anxiety is a fundamental state of mind that has both primitive and sophisticated elements to it – subcortical, cortical and neocortical – and that it dates back to our early evolution.

At its most general level, the psychological model of anxiety proposes that humans (and other mammals) experience an increase in arousal when they feel threatened. This response of autonomic arousal is viewed as involuntary and self-protective. Self-protection, in the wider scheme of things, is, of course, adaptive. When frightened by someone or something, the individual prepares psychologically and physiologically either to run away or, if running is not sensible or possible, to engage the enemy. Not surprisingly, the capacity to make appropriate fight or flight decisions fits neatly with the theory of natural selection. Those better at 'knowing what to do' are more likely to survive for longer. It may be argued that, as a group, humans now (i.e. in the early 21st century) experience a significant genetic loading in favour of a response to threat that entails the prompt arousal of anxiety, against a backdrop of living in an arguably safer world. We have this defensive stance in abundance and one view is that we may have too much of it.

Clinically, we find that a subset of the population either become anxious too readily or, once they have experienced 'legitimate' anxiety, are too slow to relinquish it, and these are interrelated. Learning theory is relevant to this: individuals learn from experience that the world can be dangerous and their response, with a significant involuntary component, is to hold on to that lesson. The underlying, at least partly unconscious, idea is that it is better to be on the safe side and not drop to one's guard. This uncomfortable psychological and physiological experience keeps the providers of psychological treatments very busy.

The cognitive–behavioural model of anxiety

The development of the cognitive–behavioural model is based on an extensive body of psychological experimentation and treatment studies which were conducted during the first six or seven decades of the 20th century under the well-known heading of 'behaviourism'. At the centre of behaviourism is learning theory. Learning theory proposes that we think and behave in ways that we acquire as a result of experience, in combination with instinct. We develop trust when we encounter trustworthiness, and we fear when we have been attacked, let down or criticised.

The earliest experiments in behaviourism, Pavlov's dogs, showed that a mammal can learn quickly and efficiently. Pavlov paired the presentation of food with the ringing of a bell in such a way that, subsequently, the ringing of the bell triggered in the dogs their response to food (i.e. salivation). Models of paired learning can apply to frightening or painful stimuli, and this is of relevance to human psychopathology. Following an appropriate number of trials in animal studies, pairing an electric shock with a yellow light was observed to lead to fear responses with the presentation of the yellow light only.

Behaviourism was a rigorous approach to the study and prediction of what could be externally observed, but it paid little attention to what individuals might be thinking in relation to their observable behaviour. This disinclination to focus on thinking was based on a view that it would lack scientific rigour to ask people what they were thinking or feeling, and so would not meet acceptable standards of objectivity. Gradually it came to be realised that the mediation of thinking was likely to be of central importance in understanding psychopathology. This led to a new emphasis being placed on the cognitions (i.e. the thoughts) of people in relation to their problems. In behavioural experiments it had long been observed that there were wide individual differences in responses to the same stimuli, and this required some explanation.

The cognitive–behavioural approach is systematic and attempts to be very specific about treatment models with respect to the separate anxiety disorders. For example, GAD, panic disorder and PTSD all have condition-specific treatments (they are outlined below).

The essence of CBT is for the patient and therapist to work together to identify the thinking patterns that are maladaptive and therefore probably maintaining the patient in an unhappy frame of mind. Negative automatic thoughts often play a significant part in this. These lie at the core of the patient's thinking but frequently the patient hardly knows about them; they are often instantaneous, virtually unconscious and very powerful. It may sometimes take considerable time and therapeutic work to elicit these, but once they have been accurately identified, alternative thinking approaches can be developed and tried out by the patient.

Cognitive–behavioural therapy for generalised anxiety disorder

Case example

Alice was 41 and for a number of years would have considered herself robust and one for coping with life's vicissitudes. Over recent years this had gradually changed but it took some time for her to become conscious of it. She found herself worrying about things that before would not have affected her. For example, if she had to go food shopping after work she would become stressed in anticipation. But the main problem was thinking about work. She found herself waking at night, thinking about assignment deadlines at work, and found it difficult to get back to sleep. For what felt like the first time she was abrupt at work with one of her junior colleagues, placing demands on him that she later thought were unreasonable. She was irritable waiting for the train. She worried about her health, her husband's health, as well as the state of the economy. Eventually things came to a head one Thursday at work when she could not stay at her desk: she had to get out of the office and go for a walk. But she could not understand why this was, and her thinking just went round in circles. Two weeks later she visited her general practitioner and got herself signed off work. She could not stop worrying and the list of things that made her worry got longer and longer.

In DSM–IV the diagnostic criteria for GAD include excessive worry that is hard to control, as well as symptoms such as restlessness, being easily fatigued, poor concentration, irritability, muscle tension and disturbances of sleep. People who complain of persistent and pervasive anxiety often feel it has always been with them. This suggests a comparatively early and possibly non-contingent onset, and there are those who propose that it has some elements consistent with personality disorder. This is based on the lack of obvious contingency (i.e. it is difficult to identify what the anxiety might be in response to). Barlow (1988) places 'anxious apprehension' at the centre of his conceptual model and delineates it as a mood state of negative emotion, consistent over-arousal, feeling out of control, and over-awareness and over-sensitivity to environmental threats.

The aims of treatments based on the cognitive–behavioural model centre on the pervasive and often rampant worry that exists over a wide range of domains, and on the often painful over-arousal and sensitivity to stimulation. Treatment takes the form of an in-depth clinical interview with the goal of gathering together as full a picture as possible of the elements described above. How much worry? About what? How pervasive? What makes it worse and what might alleviate it? Is there a family history of worry? Did the patient's parents worry (i.e. did the patient witness excessive worry during childhood?) and what effect might that have had?

The components of CBT for GAD include cognitive therapy, exposure to worry, relaxation training (see page 342), worry behaviour prevention, time management and problem solving.

- *Cognitive therapy* concerns educating patients with respect to the range of their cognitions that might engender or reinforce pervasive and persistent anxiety. A key aim is to psychologise the problem, that is, to help patients to see that much of their difficulty is not necessarily real in the external, 'real world' sense, but rather a phenomenon of their mind. This is not to reduce the significance of their distress nor undermine the legitimacy of their desire for, or the possibility of, assistance.
- *Exposure to worry* involves documenting in detail the two or three main domains in which worry figures significantly and then planning for patients to expose themselves to it in the cognitive sense. In this technique, patients are helped to visit their worry domains systematically, using guided imagery, and then are asked to stay in that mental space for some time (e.g. half an hour). They should be encouraged and helped to go fairly deeply into the details of what they see and feel in association with their worries, so as to make the experience 'real'. Following this period of exposure, the next step is to encourage patients to formulate alternative views of what has been up to now the dominant and very negative themes that have been so consistently anxiogenic.
- *Worry behaviour prevention* concerns patients' attempts to alleviate their anxiety by means of behaviours that address one or more anxieties. These behaviours are usually reinforcing, as they prevent or reduce the anxiety early in an anxiety cycle and thereby block the possibility of the individual managing to 'survive' the anxiety or to see that a terrible event will not follow. Such behaviours therefore tend to maintain the anxiety as a fear to be avoided rather than overcome and left behind. The actual intervention is to encourage or direct patients not to carry out the identified behaviour but to experiment with an alternative and more benign behaviour instead.
- *Time management* aims to address the general sense that 'everything is too much' for patients, which heightens their levels of arousal. The core techniques are helping patients to structure their time and to set boundaries around it, which includes not taking things on, following a predetermined structure within a given period of time, and requesting help to do things (in an appropriate manner).
- *Problem solving*, as the name suggests, concerns bringing structure and thought to situations that feel overwhelming but often are not. The first task is to try to bring the problems to within manageable proportions, unless this is not possible. Often problems are seen as being 'out of control', but a closer examination often shows that an ill-defined if not amorphous problem area can be broken down into smaller and more discrete elements, which can be more readily understood. The second task is to explore alternative views and pathways from the problem to solutions. This can be formulated in many steps, the size of which depends on patients' current coping skills and, of course, the problems they feel they have.

Cognitive–behavioural treatment sample from 'Alice', the patient with GAD

The initial steps in CBT that apply to most interventions are first to educate the patient about the cognitive model, then to normalise the patient's difficulties and instil some hopeful thinking, elicit what the patient is expecting of therapy, and work towards drawing up a list of goals. It is important not to embark on therapy unless the therapist has a good sense the patient is 'on board' and has a reasonable understanding of why the therapist is proposing the intervention and is able to agree with it. All sessions begin with agenda setting, so that both parties are clear what the plan is for that particular appointment.

> 'Alice, I understand that you experience worry and anxiety in all sorts of ways. I would like to build up a detailed picture of what you go through. This includes drawing up a list of what you worry about, your understanding of why you worry, how long, what you do to try to cope, and how this all affects your life, relationships and work or other responsibilities. It would be useful to put your list of worries into a hierarchy, with what affects you most at the top.'

The worries/anxieties are very likely to fall into a number of domains: relationships, home, work, health (to be differentiated from hypochondriasis) and so on. Alice does focus on work and her concerns are relatively few but very significant. She is worried about: being sacked for incompetence; keeping up her mortgage payments, given that she noticed interest rates were set to rise; and her health and that of her husband (anxiety about ageing rather than a specific illness).

Putting the difficulties into their hierarchy is important as it tells the therapist what the patient feels is the worst thing and provides some idea as to the overall severity of the problem. Once the hierarchy is explicit, the therapist can focus on the most difficult two or three problems.

> 'We've put them into your order of importance. First, I would like to talk about your fear that you are seen as incompetent and sooner or later you're going to be sacked. Tell me what you go through, what you think about your competence. When does the worry typically occur?'

While gathering some detail of patients' experiences (which patients often find therapeutic in itself), the therapist can enquire how much it bothers them, that is, the effects in terms of distress and whether they can be distracted from the worries or whether the anxious thoughts are dominant and all pervasive. It may also be possible to ask about the evidence on which they base their beliefs.

During this phase the therapist is gradually building up a more detailed and empathic understanding of patients' anxieties, to permit the move to the next and more crucial phase of the treatment, which is gradually to expose patients to their worry domains. This must be done very gradually and at a pace that is appropriate. Specifically, you are seeking to elicit what underpins their particular anxieties. This underpinning consists of negative automatic thoughts and, deeper still, other underlying assumptions.

For Alice, it emerges that she has harboured deep insecurities about her abilities ever since failing her 11-plus examination some 30 years earlier. Her academic career recovered as she was a 'late bloomer', but the experience instilled in her a permanently niggling question about her true abilities.

The therapist reached this specific event and its associated distress by asking more generally about fear of failure and incompetence at any point in her life, and whether there were any memories that stood out. Alice had remembered her 11-plus result, but it took some peeling back the layers to uncover her long-term interpretation that it meant she felt she was always incompetent and that it was only a matter of time before this would come out. Alice was helped to identify alternative evidence, that is, evidence of her considerable ability, including the recognition by others at her current place of work, where her abilities were held in high esteem.

The second anxiety, fear about the economy and the impact this would have on her real financial future, had a pervasive and catastrophic feeling to it. Alice's cognitions were that interest rates would lead both to her being made redundant as the business climate changed and to her losing her house owing to rising interest rates making her mortgage repayments unaffordable. In the relevant sessions negative automatic thoughts emerged that her personal financial situation would deteriorate beyond salvation. She found it difficult to think realistically about this. Her automatic thinking more or less blocked her thinking about the facts that her personal finances were healthy and that her employer was very much in a thriving sector of the economy that many believed to be inflation proof. Unhelpfully, these facts were not impinging on her thinking, which was increasingly constrained and 'blinkered'. This was the principal maintaining factor in her predicament, which saw this normally intelligent and adaptive woman become slowed down almost to a point of paralysis by her anxiety.

Alice's concern about her own and her husband's ageing was not entirely unnatural or pathological. What she was doing, however, was more frequently falling into states of mind where she would begin to think about the fact that she was no longer as young as she was, and then 'jump' to thinking that she was in a dreadful terminal decline, and finally blocking it out mentally while bordering on a state of panic. Her difficulty was that she could not think about her ageing, but rather reacted to notions of it, and this included involuntary and unpleasant imagery entering her mind, and she became distressed accordingly.

With respect to her fear for her own finances and her ageing, the therapist identified that Alice would benefit from worry behaviour prevention to address the power of these negative automatic thoughts. (Here we focus on her fear of ageing, as it was the most distressing and the least open to the influences of credible evidence.)

Her worry behaviour consisted of worry about ageing without being able to be calm or to think about the evidence relevant to her and her husband's reality. This was, briefly, that they were both fit and well. The therapist correctly identified that it was important to normalise fear of ageing and death, while at the same time keeping it in proportion.

During one session, Alice was helped to think about her ageing fears and to become a little anxious. Being anxious *in vivo* was important, as it would foster a true life example that could, in turn, bring about cognitive and affective change. Alice's worry about ageing raised her anxiety levels very quickly and she would try to get rid of the thoughts by forcing herself to do or think about something else. She had intuitively discovered guided imagery and imagined herself somewhere pleasant, whereas she was in fact lying in bed awake or on a train going home from work. Blocking out painful cognitions seems to be adaptive at the time, but it does not allow for new learning or examination of the evidence that may genuinely alleviate or resolve the problem. Alice did not want to go too deeply into the 'ageing' domain, as for her this was a terrible place. As stated above, she could not think, but rather only react. The therapist's task was to help her to think about her own ageing, to say what came to mind, to seek the basis for these beliefs, and then to challenge those thoughts for which there was little or no evidence. It was a struggle to elicit Alice's cognitions as she became virtually frozen with anxiety at points during the sessions.

Alice's fears centred on the sudden onset of illness, which would then almost certainly be followed by rapid decline and death. The therapeutic concern was to distinguish reasonable fear of illness and death from its exaggerated counterpart. Alice was slowly able to think about the evidence, which was that ageing happens to all of us, but life expectancy has improved (both her parents were still alive and well, and both she and her husband had very good health records). Alice was trained to slow her thinking down and to be mindful of the things she needed to think about when contemplating her mortality. These included respecting evidence and being sensitive to her own actual reality rather than rapidly descending mentally into a frightening place based on thoughtlessness in the true sense of the word.

Cognitive–behavioural therapy for panic disorder

Case example

Colin was on his way to work, taking the usual bus and trains. He had changed jobs 4 months previously and, while the change also amounted to a promotion, it meant a considerable increase in pressure and responsibility. Colin was a good planner and problem solver but he wondered more than once whether taking this new job might prove to be a mistake. One day while on the bus, traffic was particularly heavy and the bus felt especially crowded. Colin became sweaty and as he was standing far from the door he felt trapped. He knew he could get out if he had to but this somehow also seemed impossible. He noticed his heart beating in his chest and remarked to himself that this was not how it usually was. Then he became flushed and perspired even more. He found it increasingly hard to catch his breath and holding on to the passenger handle left his hand with a feeling of pins and needles. He then could not stop himself focusing on his heart and felt it pounding with great speed and force. He had never experienced anything like this before and could not understand it. It then occurred to him that he might be having a heart attack. This was very frightening, as he knew heart attacks can strike the most unlikely people. He felt panicky, out of control and trapped. He then abruptly pushed his way to the door and opened it himself, using the emergency switch. He found a nearby bench and sat there trying to catch his breath and used his mobile phone to call an ambulance. At hospital, tests revealed no cardiac problems, but his nervousness was noted, and he overheard a nurse speculating that he was probably having a panic attack.

Clark's (1986, 1988) model of panic and panic disorder suggests that the sequence of events in panic attacks starts with certain external stimuli being interpreted as a sign of danger being near, either in place or in time. This generates nervous apprehension, which triggers autonomic responses. The individual who is susceptible to panic will tend to interpret these signs and symptoms in the worst possible way. In a circular fashion, these catastrophic cognitions will reinforce the interpretation of threat and impending danger, to create a vicious circle. Thus, the core difficulty for those susceptible to panic is their tendency to pessimistic interpretations, especially of bodily events. Panicky feelings and the experience of having only one panic attack are relatively common in the general population. Those who experience recurrent panic attacks are comparatively rare (Wittchen & Essau, 1991) but panic disorder can be debilitating.

The cognitive approach to treating panic disorder consists of a number of components. A typical treatment can take between 8 and 15 sessions, depending on the severity of the problem and other factors relating to the client's capacity to engage and personality factors. The overall evidence for the effectiveness of these treatments is good (Craske & Barlow, 2001).

Cognitive restructuring focuses on addressing the misappraisals of bodily sensations. Clients are systematically taken through their thinking patterns in relation to their appraisals of bodily events and the evidence for the conclusions they reach are examined and challenged, as appropriate. This can take some time, especially if the panic attacks have become established or even entrenched.

Breathing retraining is aimed at addressing the physiological side of panic attacks. The retraining focuses on helping patients to manage their breathing as well as countering the effects of hyperventilation. Panic that is associated with hyperventilation is particularly suitable for breathing retraining. The interaction of catastrophic interpretation and autonomic arousal can in some instances be especially malignant in terms of the distress patients feel. Individuals can be convinced they are having a heart attack and in some instances the symptoms of PTSD may also occur.

Applied relaxation involves progressive muscle relaxation. Patients are helped to become skilled in calming themselves down through reconnecting with their bodies and allowing their sensitivity to what is actually happening physically to them in the here and now to assist their coping mechanisms. It serves as a countermeasure to the muscular tension that is commonly generated in association with panic. It also allows for a sense of mastery over the body to be regained, as this is commonly lost during a panic attack.

Interoceptive exposure entails helping patients gradually to work through exercises that induce panic-type sensations in a safe and controlled manner. Examples are aerobic exercise, hyperventilation, inhaling carbon dioxide and movements that induce dizziness. The aim is for patients to have the experience of panic-like symptoms while maintaining control and 'enjoying' the possibility of non-catastrophic responses. *In vivo* exposure, as the name suggests, consists of real-life exposure. It can be therapist directed or client directed, and there are degrees of intensity, from graduated exposure to flooding (full intensity from the outset).

Cognitive–behavioural treatment sample from 'Colin', the patient with panic disorder

First, the therapist sets the agenda.

> 'Colin, I want us to go through one of your recent panic attacks, a typical one, in considerable detail so we can build up a good picture of what happens. This way we can learn more, and discover things that perhaps we don't already know, and identify what we might need to focus on. Patterns emerge that can be difficult to see if you're not looking for them. Can you take a moment to think about a recent panic attack that you feel is typical?'

Patients are given about 30 seconds (more if necessary) to think about this and then once they have confirmed they have a real panic attack in mind, the therapist moves on to gather a detailed 'anatomy' of a typical panic attack.

> 'Let's go through what happens to you, what you feel, what you think, and how your body feels. I also want to know what happens next, what you do to try to cope, how long it lasts.'

Then the therapist will work through the symptoms list, eliciting yes or no answers as well as details about the severity, duration and so forth. Typical questions to ask along the way are:

> 'Can you recall what you were thinking at that very moment?'
>
> 'What did you think was happening to you?'
>
> 'What did you do next?'
>
> 'Can you remember why you did that?'

These questions should reveal the underlying fears, however irrational they seem to be at the time.

Of particular importance, especially if working with the Clark model of CBT for panic disorder, are the patients' misappraisals of bodily sensations. Patients who, in the heat of the moment, believe they are genuinely in the early stages of a heart attack will be very distressed (not unnaturally). Phenomenologically, this can be like a mini-trauma, with the patient vulnerable to phobic responses. Treatment requires a careful working through of the experiences so that patients can unlearn self-protective responses that maintain high anxiety levels and avoidant behaviours. These self-protective responses stand in the way of the development of new cognitions and so need to be challenged. One example is 'If then' thinking: 'If I go on a bus I will be overwhelmed and then I will have a panic attack.' The therapist should gently attempt to explore the evidence supporting this type of logic so that the patient will not hold the link so strongly.

The essence of a panic attack is the person feeling out of control and genuinely in danger, for example of having a heart attack. This fear significantly diminishes people's capacity to think adaptively and their main aim is to calm down, regain control and feel less absolutely hopeless in the crucial moment. The 'heat of the moment' intervention is to help control breathing and to take time out to allow for focusing on calming down, in part by removing other pressures and distractions. Relaxation training provides the background for avoiding further panic attacks.

Cognitive–behavioural therapy for post-traumatic stress disorder

Case example

Ahmed was driving back to Manchester on a Sunday evening when he was involved in a crash. His car was struck from behind while stationary at a red light and he sustained minor whiplash but fortunately no other physical injuries. He was also very shaken mentally and left feeling anxious. At the time of the accident he had accumulated 21 years of driving experience and felt confident as a driver. This was his first accident in which he was 'properly' injured. His physical injuries resolved fairly quickly but it was 4 months before he could get behind the wheel again and even after 2 years he was still driving with much more caution, usually below the speed limit. He was especially anxious when stopped at traffic lights. He knew that the roads were no more dangerous than they had been before, but this logical thinking had little effect on his anxiety. He also experienced frequent flashbacks and nightmares for the first 8 weeks or so, but these diminished to about one per a month.

Ahmed now found that being in a car was frightening. He had not had that reaction before his crash. Involuntarily, Ahmed was pairing driving with fear. He had learned this in the specific context of his car crash. He was not frightened to the same extent in taxis, buses or on the train. He was frightened when he was a passenger in a car, but less so than if he were the driver. At the centre of his fear was being a car driver, and as the situation resembled less and less the fear-producing situation, his fear diminished accordingly.

Any type of incident can induce trauma and it is the individual's interpretation of the event(s) that is now recognised as crucial. In the DSM–IV criteria for PTSD there are three areas of symptoms: re-experiencing symptoms (often in the form of flashbacks), numbing and avoidance, and susceptibility to physiological arousal. Flashbacks can occur while the individual is awake or during sleep. The sufferer can lead a very restricted life if reminder cues are numerous (i.e. if the traumatic event took place within normal life circumstances). For example, someone involved in a road traffic accident can hardly avoid cars in most Western countries. A key dimension to bear in mind when assessing patients is the degree of distress, as there are wide individual differences in resilience for a given trauma.

The treatment of PTSD reflects the disorder: it is complex. The cognitive–behavioural approach combines stress inoculation training (four components), exposure techniques and cognitive therapy. There can be other elements but these are not covered here.

Stress inoculation training starts with an educative process, during which the therapist helps patients understand what they have been going through, with a view to making sense of and validating their own often very distressing experiences. Their experience can be 'organised' into three broad domains (see Resick & Calhoun, 2001), namely the physical or autonomic channel, the behavioural or motor channel, and the cognitive channel. Coping with the PTSD is the essence of the stress inoculation training and its four components. Relaxation training, with a focus on physical relaxation, attends to all the major muscle groups and is included in treatment from the beginning. Often a tape is given so that the tasks can be done at home. Closely linked to this is controlling breathing. The third component is guided or imagined modelling, in which patients expose themselves visually and cognitively to frightening situations (which should be labelled 'anxiety provoking'), the aim being for patients to imagine managing the situation successfully, and holding on to the mastery of the situation rather than being overwhelmed by it. This is intentionally contrasted with their previous trauma experience. The final component is role play, during which patient and therapist may act out some elements of the original traumatic situation.

The use of exposure techniques in PTSD is a controversial area and the outcomes are seen as mixed. Very gentle exposure, carefully tailored to the needs of the patient, is recommended. For some, exposure may not be indicated, or at least not until much later in the therapy.

Treatment sample from 'Ahmed', the patient with post-traumatic stress disorder

At the beginning of each session the therapist should set the agenda.

People with PTSD who are suitable for treatment can be especially fragile; when this is the case it is often readily discernible. The pace may have to be very gentle, with the therapist consistently evaluating the patient's capacity to tolerate treatment.

After identifying the traumatic events, the next step is to get a picture of what the patient has made of these events. What meaning does the event have? What particular difficulties were triggered by it? Which problems have endured and which have now resolved? How has the patient's life changed? What has been the effect on relationships?

In the first session, the therapist explains the proposed approach.

> 'Ahmed, I would like us to talk about what has happened to you. This may be difficult for you, and I understand that, so we need to go at a pace that suits you. Please feel free to tell me when it feels too difficult and you would like to stop. I also want to outline a number of tasks and exercises that people who have had shocks to the system, like you have had, have sometimes found helpful. For example, there is relaxation training, controlling your breathing, then trying to imagine and model in your head how you would achieve mastery over situations, and if it is appropriate, we can also try some role play.'

In the first session the therapist should ask the patient to say, if possible, what happened. The therapist works through the patient's story, finding out more and filling in gaps, while always mindful of what is happening to the patient during the session. Afterwards the therapist should validate patients' experiences, especially their distress, for example by saying something like 'It's not at all surprising you're feeling that way, given what happened to you.'

> Ahmed talks about his car crash, running through it in an attempt to be detailed. He is surprised by the effect it has had on him. You find there is quite a lot you still do not know. You ask him further questions.

In the second session the therapist will seek to find out more about the meaning of events. The meaning of events will inform the therapist's understanding of the intensity of the distress.

> 'Ahmed, you told me last time that the crash left you with particular fears, which you very helpfully outlined. Are you able to recall what it was that went through your mind at the time?'

Ahmed may say something like 'I thought for a second that I was going to die, and that this was the end.' The therapist then asks further questions to determine the intensity of that fear, how real it felt at the time.

> 'Ahmed, you say you thought for a moment that you were about to die. Were these thoughts accompanied by any visual imagery? Did you imagine what would happen?'

It may also be informative to learn more about Ahmed's premorbid anxiety and susceptibility to fear.

> 'Before this accident, how were you in fearful situations? How much did you fear the worst in life, say, when crossing the road, flying in an airplane, and so on?'

Such questioning may tell the therapist a lot about patients' underlying resilience and why they have reacted the way they have.

> Following session 2, when Ahmed is observed getting upset and revealing how his distress remains a live issue, it seems important to help him with his distress. 'Ahmed, I saw last time how distressing it can be for you at points and so I suggest I go through some relaxation training and controlling breathing exercises.'
>
> The treatment continues, with Ahmed working his way through events, and the therapist giving him diary sheets in order for him to record his mental life in relation to therapy while at the same time working on the trauma. The aim is, over time, to try to help him to make sense of his thoughts and identify the negative automatic thoughts, and to follow this up by putting into practice alternative interpretations and responses.
>
> The therapist uses the diary sheets to begin the task of identifying, by means of further questions if necessary, what Ahmed's automatic thoughts are. The point of identifying negative automatic thoughts is to challenge them and this usually reveals faulty thinking, which can then be a trigger for finding alternative thoughts. This process, recursive in nature, forms the basis of the remainder of treatment.

The psychoanalytic model of anxiety

The founder of psychoanalysis, Sigmund Freud (1856-1939), proposed that anxiety is the product of affect that had not been mastered. Significantly, anxiety as an idea and its treatment cannot easily be separated. From a psychoanalytic perspective, anxiety is not a phenomenon that can be singled out as a circumscribed disorder needing treatment; rather, anxiety is a sign or symptom of some deeper distress. Learning what this is will entail careful and consistent exploration using the main therapeutic technique in psychoanalysis, which is to allow the patient to become anxious in a safe therapeutic space. In this brief overview, for reasons of space it is not possible to provide a comprehensive account of the psychoanalytic treatment of anxiety; the intention is merely to give the reader a flavour of the psychoanalytic approach. For a more detailed account the interested reader is referred to the *Textbook of Psychotherapy in Psychiatric Practice* by Holmes (1991) or the rather lengthier account in *The Techniques and Practice of Psychoanalysis* by Greenson (1967).

Case example:

Bruce had been married for 9 years and had two children. Subjectively, he felt settled in life. If asked, he would have described himself as happy and as having got things more or less the way he would like them. He was confident that he loved his wife and children, and on the whole his career was working out well. He felt reassured that he was doing a good job of parenting, considering all the conflicting demands in modern life. Bruce was also a religious man and was guided by a quiet faith. However, one day at work he found himself agitated in a way that was unusual for him. A month earlier, his long-term colleague, Eric, left to work elsewhere and Eric's replacement, Susan, arrived. Susan was a little younger than Bruce and his first reaction to her was to see that she was an attractive and likeable woman. He had been on the selection panel that had chosen her. But it was not long before he was tense around her, despite her not having changed, and he did not know why.

The therapist could see that Bruce was experiencing something in relation to Susan. First, he knew he started out positively disposed towards her. Second, he saw allusions to attraction. And, third, he learnt of a change in his state of mind, triggered by something to do with Susan. The inference he began to draw, and which he wanted to explore in some detail, was that Bruce was attracted to Susan and that that troubled him. The therapist assumed that Bruce had been attracted in passing to other women and that he had negotiated these moments within himself. With Susan, however, more was happening and Bruce was unable to negotiate his feelings of attraction. His feelings were not going away and this was a source of conflict with other feelings and values he held dear, mainly in terms of his wife and children. This lack of mastery was generating anxiety.

Anxiety is the product of one set of feelings in effect coming up against another, and there is no easy intrapsychic answer. Freud called this 'signal anxiety', as the anxiety signalled a conflict, at the centre of which were powerful affects that did not agree.

Psychoanalytic treatment of anxiety

The psychoanalytic approach to the treatment of anxiety disorders is very different from that proposed by cognitive–behavioural techniques. Psychoanalytic thinking is much less concerned with addressing symptoms in a circumscribed and possibly linear way, and as a result there are no treatments for specific presentations. The approach focuses instead on the personality of the individual and how he or she relates to others in a much more global sense (Lemma, 2003). As stated above, anxiety is viewed as the result of conflict within the mind, at both conscious and unconscious levels, in an often complex configuration. As with GAD, the psychoanalytic model also views anxiety as a fundamental state of mind that arises in a very wide range of contexts, almost as if it were a common currency for the emotional disorders.

Psychoanalytic psychotherapy is often a high-frequency and long-term treatment and can entail up to three sessions each week (sometimes more). It is an intensive therapeutic experience in which working to understand the individual's relationship to the therapist forms a central part of the technique. This therapeutic relationship is seen not just as a 'here and now' relationship, but also as a repetition/re-enactment of earlier relationships. This is known as the transference and it can be very powerful and highly informative for both therapist and patient. The general aim is to explore and examine the signs of these unconscious conflicts in terms of feeling, emotion and fantasy, which are held to be the basis of the symptoms and other, wider problems.

Within the psychoanalytic model, there is the view that more than genetic and constitutional elements constitute the personality. The experience of birth, early relationships with parents and other attachments, intimacy and sexuality, as well as strong and often uncomfortable states of mind such as the dichotomies of love and hate and unavoidable life events such as loss and death may all generate anxiety. For some people anxiety is very intense and can be overwhelming, while the presence of raised levels of anxiety is taken as a sign that an internal conflict is both active and highly troubling for the individual.

References

Abelson, J. L., Glitz, D., Cameron, O. G., *et al* (1991) Blunted growth hormone response to clonidine in patients with generalised anxiety disorder. *Archives of General Psychiatry*, **48**, 157–162.

Ainsworth, M. (1969) Object relations dependency and attachment. A theoretical review of the mother infant relationship. *Child Development*, **40**, 969–1025.

Allgulander, C., Bandelow, B., Hollander, E., *et al* (2003) World Council on Anxiety (WCA) recommendations for the long-term treatment of generalized anxiety disorder. *CNS Spectrums*, **8**, suppl. 1, 53–61.

American Psychiatric Association (1952) *Diagnostic and Statistical Manual of Mental Disorders* (1st edn). Washington, DC: APA.

American Psychiatric Association (1968) *Diagnostic and Statistical Manual of Mental Disorders* (2nd edn) (DSM–II). Washington, DC: APA.

American Psychiatric Association (1980) *Diagnostic and Statistical Manual of Mental Disorders* (3rd edn) (DSM–III). Washington, DC: APA.

American Psychiatric Association (1987) *Diagnostic and Statistical Manual of Mental Disorders* (3rd edn, revised) (DSM–III–R). Washington, DC: APA.

American Psychiatric Association (1994) *Diagnostic and Statistical Manual of Mental Disorders* (4th edn) (DSM–IV). Washington, DC: APA.

American Psychiatric Association (2000) *Diagnostic and Statistical Manual of Mental Disorders* (4th edn, text revision) (DSM–IV–TR). Washington, DC: APA.

Angst, J. & Vollrath, M. (1991) The natural history of anxiety disorders. *Acta Psychiatrica Scandinavica*, **84**, 446–452.

Argyropoulos, S. V. & Nutt, D. J. (1999) The use of benzodiazepines in anxiety and other disorders. *European Neuropsychopharmacology*, **9**, suppl. 6, S407–S412.

Argyropoulos, S. V. & Nutt, D. J. (2003) Neurochemical aspects of anxiety. In *Anxiety Disorders* (eds D. J. Nutt & J. C. Ballenger), pp. 183–199. Oxford: Blackwell.

Argyropoulos, S. V., Sandford, J. J. & Nutt, D. J. (2000) The psychobiology of anxiolytic drugs. Part 2: Pharmacological treatments of anxiety. *Pharmacology and Therapeutics*, **88**, 213–227.

Azmitia, E. C. & Whitaker, P. M. (1995) Anatomy, cell biology and plasticity of the serotonergic system. Neuropsychopharmacological implications for the actions of psychotropic drugs. In *Psychopharmacology: The Fourth Generation of Progress* (eds F. E. Bloom & D. J. Kupfer), pp. 443–490. New York: Raven Press.

Bachman, A. W., Sedgley, T. L., Jackson, R. V., *et al* (2005) Glucocorticoid receptor polymorphisms and post-traumatic stress disorder. *Psychoneuroendocrinology*, **30**, 297–306.

Bakker, A., Van Balkom, A. J. & Spinhoven, P. (2002) SSRIs vs. TCAs in the treatment of panic disorder: a meta-analysis. *Acta Psychiatrica Scandinavica*, **106**, 163–167.

Baldwin, D. S. & Polkinghorn, C. (2005) Evidence-based pharmacotherapy of generalized anxiety disorder. *International Journal of Neuropsychopharmacology*, **8**, 293–302.

Baldwin, D. S., Anderon, I. M., Nutt, D. J., *et al* (2005) Evidence-based guidelines for the pharmacological treatment of anxiety disorders: recommendations from the British Association for Psychopharmacology. *Journal of Psychopharmacology*, **19**, 567–596.

Ballenger, J. C., Davidson, J. R. T., Lecrubier, Y., *et al* (1998*a*) Consensus statement on panic disorder from the International Consensus Group on Depression and Anxiety. *Journal of Clinical Psychiatry*, **59**, suppl. 8, 47–54.

Ballenger, J. C., Wheadon, D. E., Steiner, M., *et al* (1998*b*) Double-blind, fixed-dose, placebo-controlled study of paroxetine in the treatment of panic disorder. *American Journal of Psychiatry*, **155**, 36–42.

Bandelow, B. (1995) Assessing the efficacy of treatments for panic disorder and agoraphobia. II. The Panic and Agoraphobia Scale. *International Clinical Psychopharmacology*, **10**, 73–81.

Bandelow, B. (2003) Epidemiology of depression and anxiety. In *Handbook of Depression and Anxiety* (2nd edn, revised and expanded) (eds S. Kasper, J. A. den Boer & J. M. Ad Sitsen), pp. 49–68. New York: Marcel Dekker.

Bandelow, B., Zohar, J., Hollander, E., *et al* (2002) World Federation of Societies of Biological Psychiatry (WFSBP) guidelines for the pharmacological treatment of anxiety, obsessive–compulsive and posttraumatic stress disorders. *World Journal of Biological Psychiatry*, **3**, 171–199.

Barker, M. J., Greenwood, K. M., Jackson, M., *et al* (2004*a*) Cognitive effects of long-term benzodiazepine use: a meta-analysis. *CNS Drugs*, **18**, 37–48.

Barker, M. J., Greenwood, K. M., Jackson, M., *et al* (2004*b*) Persistence of cognitive effects after withdrawal from long-term benzodiazepine use: a meta-analysis. *Archives of Clinical Neuropsychology*, **19**, 437–454.

Barlow, D. H. (1988) Generalised anxiety disorder. In *Anxiety and Its Disorders* (eds D. H. Barlow), pp. 566–597. New York: Guilford Press.

Barlow, D. H. (1991) Disorders of emotion. *Psychological Inquiry*, **2**, 58–105.

Barlow, D. H., Gorman, J. M., Shear, M. K., *et al* (2000) Cognitive–behavioral therapy, imipramine, or their combination for panic disorder. A randomized controlled trial. *JAMA*, **283**, 2529–2536.

Bartzokis, G., Lu, P. H., Turner, J., *et al* (2005) Adjunctive risperidone in the treatment of chronic combat-realted posttraumatic stress disorder. *Biological Psychiatry*, **57**, 474–479.

Beard, G. (1869) Neurasthenia or nervous exhaustion. *Boston Medical and Surgical Journal*, **80**, 217–221.

Beck, A. T., Epstein, N., Brown, G., *et al* (1988) An inventory for measuring clinical anxiety: psychometric properties. *Journal of Consulting and Clinical Psychology*, **56**, 893–897.

Behar, E., Alcaine, O., Zuellig, A. R., *et al* (2003) Screening for generalized anxiety disorder using the Penn State Worry Questionnaire: a receiver operating characteristic analysis. *Journal of Behaviour Therapy and Experimental Psychiatry*, **34**, 25–43.

Bell, C., Forshall, S., Adrover, M., *et al* (2002) Does 5-HT restrain panic? A tryptophan depletion study on panic patients recovered on paroxetine. *Journal of Psychopharmacology*, **16**, 5–14.

Berrios, G. E. & Link, C. (1995) Anxiety disorders: clinical section. In *A History of Clinical Psychiatry* (eds G. Berrios & R. Porter), pp. 545–562. London: Athlone Press.

Bisaga, A., Katz, J. L., Antonini, A., *et al* (1998) Cerebral glucose metabolism in women with panic disorder. *American Journal of Psychiatry*, **155**, 1178–1183.

Blake, D. D., Weathers, F. W., Nagy, L. M., *et al* (1995) The development of a clinician-administered PTSD scale. *Journal of Trauma and Stress*, **8**, 75–90.

Blier, P., De Montigny, C. & Chaput, Y. (1990) A role for the serotonergic system in the mechanism of action of antidepressant treatments; preclinical evidence. *Journal of Clinical Psychiatry*, **6**, suppl. 5, 5–12.

Boulenger, J. P., Patel, J. & Marangos, P. J. (1982) Effects of caffeine and theophylline on adenosine and benzodiazepine receptors in human brain. *Neuroscience Letters*, **30**, 161–166.

Boulenger, J. P., Fournier, M., Rosales, D., *et al* (1997) Mixed anxiety and depression: from theory to practice. *Journal of Clinical Psychiatry*, **58**, suppl. 8, 27–34.

Bowlby, J. (1969) Attachment. In *Attachment and Loss. Vol. 1*. London: Hogarth Press.

Braestrup, C. & Squires, R. F. (1978) Brain specific benzodiazepine receptors. *British Journal of Psychiatry*, **133**, 249–260.

Braun, P., Greenberg, D., Dasberg, H., *et al* (1990) Core symptoms of posttraumatic stress disorder unimproved by alprazolam treatment. *Journal of Clinical Psychiatry*, **51**, 236–238.

Brawman-Mintzer, O. & Lydiard, R. B. (1997) Biological basis of generalized anxiety disorder. *Journal of Clinical Psychiatry*, **58**, suppl. 3, 16–25.

Breier, A., Charney, D. & Heninger, G. R. (1985) The diagnostic validity of anxiety disorders and their relationship to depressive illness. *American Journal of Psychiatry*, **142**, 787–797.

Bremner, J. D., Randall, P., Vermetten, E., *et al* (1997) Magnetic resonance imaging-based measurement of hippocampal volume in posttraumatic stress disorder related to childhood physical and sexual abuse – a preliminary report. *Biological Psychiatry*, **41**, 23–32.

Bruce, S. E., Yonkers, K. A., Otto, M. W., *et al* (2005) Influence of psychiatric comorbidity on recovery and recurrence in generalized anxiety disorder, social phobia, and panic disorder: a 12-year prospective study. *American Journal of Psychiatry*, **162**, 1179–1187.

Bryant, R. A. (2003) Acute stress reactions: can biological responses predict posttraumatic stress disorder? *CNS Spectrums*, **8**, 668–674.

Buchsbaum, M. S., Wu, J., Haier, R., *et al* (1987) Positron emission tomography of effects of benzodiazepines on regional glucose metabolic rate in patients with anxiety disorders. *Life Sciences*, **40**, 2393–2400.

Busto, U. E., Romach, M. K. & Sellers, E. M. (1996) Multiple drug use and psychiatric comorbidity in patients admitted to the hospital with severe benzodiazepine dependence. *Journal of Clinical Psychopharmacology*, **16**, 51–57.

Bystritsky, A., Pontillo, D., Powers, M., *et al* (2001) Functional MRI changes during panic anticipation and imagery exposure. *Neuroreport*, **12**, 3953–3957.

Cameron, O. G., Smith, C. B., Lee, M. A., *et al* (1990) Adrenergic status in anxiety disorders: platelet alpha-2-adrenergic receptor binding, blood pressure, pulse and plasma catecholamines in panic and generalised anxiety disorder patients and normal subjects. *Biological Psychiatry*, **28**, 3–20.

Cannistraro, P. A. & Rauch, S. L. (2003) Neural circuitry of anxiety: evidence from structural and functional neuroimaging studies. *Psychopharmacology Bulletin*, **37**, 8–25.

Cannon, W. B. (1929) *Bodily Changes in Pain, Hunger, Fear and Rage: An Account of Recent Researches into the Function of Emotional Excitement* (2nd edn). New York: D. Appleton.

Centers for Disease Control (1988) Health status of Vietnam veterans psycho-social characteristics. *JAMA*, **249**, 2701–2707.

Chaouloff, F. (2000) Serotonin, stress and corticoids. *Journal of Psychopharmacology*, **14**, 139–151.

Charney, D. S., Heninger, G. R. & Breier, A. (1984*a*) Noradrenergic function in panic anxiety: effects of yohimbine in healthy subjects and patients with agoraphobia and panic disorder. *Archives of General Psychiatry*, **41**, 751–776.

Charney, D. S., Galloway, M. P. & Heninger, G. R. (1984*b*) The effects of caffeine on plasma MHPG, subjective anxiety, autonomic symptoms and blood pressure in healthy humans. *Life Sciences*, **35**, 135–144.

Charney, D. S., Woods, S. W., Goodman, W. K., *et al* (1987) Serotonin function in anxiety: II. Effects of the serotonin agonist mCPP in panic disorder patients and healthy subjects. *Psychopharmacology*, **92**, 14–24.

Charney, D. S., Woods, S. W. & Heninger, G. R. (1989) Noradrenergic function in generalized anxiety disorder: effects of yohimbine in healthy subjects and patients with generalized anxiety disorder. *Psychiatry Research*, **27**, 173–182.

Chrousos, G. P. & Gold, P. W. (1992) The concepts of stress and stress system disorders: overview of physical and behavioural homeostasis. *JAMA*, **267**, 475–494.

Clark, D. M. (1986) A cognitive model of panic. *Behaviour Research and Therapy*, **24**, 461–470.

Clark, D. M. (1988) A cognitive approach to panic. In *Panic: Psychological Perspectives* (eds S. Rachman & J. Masters). Hillsdale, NJ: Erlbaum.

Clark, M. J. (1995) Anxiety disorders. Social section. In *A History of Clinical Psychiatry* (eds G. Berrios & R. Porter), pp. 563–572. London: Athlone Press.

Coles, M. E., Mennin, D. S. & Heimberg, R. G. (2001) Distinguishing obsessive features and worries: the role of thought–action fusion. *Behaviour Research and Therapy*, **39**, 947–959.

Coplan, J. D., Papp, L. A. Martinez, J., *et al* (1995) Persistence of blunted human hormone response to clonidine in fluoxetine-treated patients with panic disorder. *American Journal of Psychiatry*, **152**, 619–622.

Craske, M. G. & Barlow, D. H. (2001) Panic disorder and agoraphobia. In *Clinical Handbook of Psychological Disorders: A Step-by-Step Treatment Manual* (3rd edn) (ed. D. Barlow), pp. 1–59. London: Guilford Press.

Cullen, W. (1784) *First Lines in the Practice of Physic*. Edinburgh: Elliott.

Curran, P. S., Bell, P., Murray, A., *et al* (1990) Psychological consequences of the Enniskillen bombing. *British Journal of Psychiatry*, **156**, 479–482.

Da Costa, J. M. (1871) On irritable heart: a clinical study of a functional cardiac disorder and its consequences. *American Journal of Medical Science*, **61**, 17–52.

Dannon, P. N., Iancu, I. & Grunhaus, L. (2002) Psychoeducation in panic disorder patients: effect of a self-information booklet in a randomized masked-rater study. *Depression and Anxiety*, **16**, 71–76.

Davidson, J. R. T., Kudler, H. S., Smith, R. D., *et al* (1990) Treatment of posttraumatic stress disorder with amitriptyline and placebo. *Archives of General Psychiatry*, **47**, 259–266.

Davidson, J. R. T., Book, S. W., Colket, J. T., *et al* (1997) Assessment of a new self-rating scale for post-traumatic stress disorder. *Psychological Medicine*, **27**, 153–160.

Davidson, J. R. T., Weisler, R. H., Butterfield, M. I., *et al* (2003) Mirtazapine vs. placebo in posttraumatic stress disorder: a pilot study. *Biological Psychiatry*, **53**, 188–191.

Deakin, J. F. W. & Graeff, F. G. (1991) 5-HT and mechanisms of defence. *Journal of Psychopharmacology*, **5**, 305–315.

De Bellis, M. D., Keshavan, M. S., Shifflett, H., *et al* (2001) Superior temporal gyrus volumes in pediatric generalized anxiety disorder. *Biological Psychiatry*, **51**, 553–562.

de las Cuevas, C. & Sanz, E. (2005) Polypsychopharmacy: a frequent and debatable practice in psychiatric inpatients. *Journal of Clinical Psychopharmacology*, **25**, 510–512.

den Boer, J. A. & Westenberg, H. G. M. (1988) Effect of serotonin and noradrenaline reuptake inhibitor in panic disorder: a double-blind comparative study with fluvoxamine and maprotiline. *International Clinical Psychopharmacology*, **3**, 59–74.

El-Khayat, R. & Baldwin, D. S. (1998) Antipsychotic drugs for non-psychotic patients: assessment of the benefit/risk ratio in generalized anxiety disorder. *Journal of Psychopharmacology*, **12**, 323–329.

Eysenck, H. J. (1959) *The Maudsley Personality Inventory*. London: University of London Press.

Fairbank, J. A., Ebert, L. & Costello, E. J. (2000) Epidemiology of traumatic events and post-traumatic stress disorder. In *Post-traumatic Stress Disorder: Diagnosis, Management and Treatment* (eds D. J. Nutt, J. R. T. Davidson & J. Zohar), pp. 17–27. London: Martin Dunitz.

Ferreri, M. & Hantouche, E.-G. (1998) Recent clinical trials of hydroxyzine in generalised anxiety disorder. *Acta Psychiatrica Scandinavica*, **98**, suppl. 393, 102–108.

Figley, C. R. (1985) Traumatic stress: the role of the family and social support system. In *Trauma and Its Wake. The Study of Post-traumatic Stress Disorder* (ed. C. R. Figley), pp. 39–56. New York: Brunner/Mazel.

First, M. B., Spitzer, R.L., Gibbon, M., *et al* (1997) *Structured Clinical Interview for DSM–IV Axis I Disorders, Research Version, Patient Edition (SCID–P)*. New York: New York State Psychiatric Institute, Biometrics Research.

Floderus-Myrhed, B., Pedersen, N. & Rasmuson, I. (1980) Assessment of heritability for personality, based on a short form of the Eysenck Personality Inventory: a study of 12,898 twin pairs. *Behaviour Genetics*, **10**, 153–162.

Frank, J. D. (1971) Therapeutic factors in psychotherapy. *American Journal of Psychotherapy*, **25**, 350–361.

Freeman, M. P., Freeman, S. A. & McElroy, S. L. (2002) The comorbidity of bipolar and anxiety disorders: prevalence, psychobiology, and treatment issues. *Journal of Affective Disorders*, **68**, 1–23.

Freud, S. (1894) The justification for detaching from neurasthenia a particular syndrome: the anxiety neurosis. In *The Standard Edition of the Complete Psychological Works*, vol. I, pp. 76–106. London: Hogarth Press.

Friedman, M. J. (1998) Current and future drug treatment for posttraumatic stress disorder patients. *Psychiatry Annals*, **28**, 461–468.

Furukawa, T. A., Watanabe, N. & Churchill, R. (2006) Psychotherapy plus antidepressant for panic disorder with or without agoraphobia. *British Journal of Psychiatry*, **188**, 305–312.

George, D. T., Nutt, D. J., Dwyer, B. A., *et al* (1990) Alcoholism and panic disorder: is the comorbidity more than coincidence? *Acta Psychiatrica Scandinavica*, **81**, 97–107.

George, D. T., Nutt, D. J., Rawlings, R. R., *et al* (1995) Behavioural and endocrine responses to clomipramine in panic disorder patients with and without alcoholism. *Biological Psychiatry*, **37**, 112–119.

Georget, E. J. (1840) Nevroses. In *Dictionnairre de Medicine, Vol. XXV*, pp. 27–41. Paris: Bechet.

Germine, M., Goddard, A. W., Woods, S. W., *et al* (1992) Anger and anxiety responses to m-chlorophenylpiperazine in generalised anxiety disorder. *Biological Psychiatry*, **32**, 457–461.

Goddard, A. W., Brouette, T., Almai, A., *et al* (2001) Early coadministration of clonazepam with sertraline for panic disorder. *Archives of General Psychiatry*, **58**, 681–686.

Goldberg, M. R., Hollister, A. S. & Robertson, D. (1983) Influence of yohimbine on blood pressure, autonomic reflexes and plasma catecholamines in humans. *Hypertension*, **5**, 772–778.

Goodwin, R. D., Lipsitz, J. D., Chapman, T. F., *et al* (2006) Alcohol use disorders in patients with panic disorder. *Comprehensive Psychiatry*, **47**, 88–90.

Gorman, J. M., Kent, J. M., Sullivan, G. M., *et al* (2000) Neuroanatomical hypothesis of panic disorder, revised. *American Journal of Psychiatry*, **157**, 493–505.

Gorwood, P. (2004) Generalized anxiety disorder and major depressive disorder comorbidity: an example of genetic pleiotropy? *European Psychiatry*, **19**, 27–33.

Graeff, F. G., Guimaraes, F. S., de Andrade, T. G., *et al* (1996) Role of 5-HT in stress, anxiety and depression. *Pharmacology Biochemistry and Behaviour*, **86**, 334–338.

Gray, J. A. (1981) Anxiety as a paradigm case of emotion. *British Medical Bulletin*, **37**, 193–197.

Gray, J. A. (1982) *The Neuropsychology of Anxiety: An Enquiry into the Functions of the Septohippocampal System*. Oxford: Oxford University Press.

Greenson R. R. (1967) *The Technique and Practice of Psychoanalysis*. New York: International University Press.

Griebel, G. (1999) Is there a future for neuropeptide receptor ligands in the treatment of anxiety disorders? *Pharmacology and Therapeutics*, **82**, 1–61.

Grove, G., Coplan, J. D. & Hollander, E. (1997) The neuroanatomy of 5-HT dysregulation and panic disorder. *Journal of Neuropsychiatry and Clinical Neuroscience*, **9**, 198–207.

Guimaraes, F. S., Mbaya, P. S. & Deakin, J. F. W. (1997) Ritanserin facilitates anxiety in a simulated public-speaking paradigm. *Journal of Psychopharmacology*, **11**, 225–231.

Gur, S., Hermesh, H., Laufer, N., *et al* (2005) Adjustment disorder: a review of diagnostic pitfalls. *Israeli Medical Association Journal*, **7**, 726–731.

Gurvits, T. V., Sheaton, M. E., Hokama, H., *et al* (1996) Magnetic resonance imaging study of hippocampal volume in chronic, combat-related posttraumatic stress disorder. *Biological Psychiatry*, **40**, 1091–1099.

Gutman, D. A., Musselman, D. L. & Nemeroff, C. B. (2003) Neuropeptide alterations in depression and anxiety disorders. In *Handbook of Depression and Anxiety* (2nd edn, revised and expanded) (eds S. Kasper, J. A. den Boer & J. M. Ad Sitsen), pp. 229–265. New York: Marcel Dekker.

Haddad, P. (1998) The SSRI discontinuation syndrome. *Journal of Psychopharmacology*, **12**, 305–313.

Hamilton, M. (1959) The assessment of anxiety states by rating scale. *British Journal of Medical Psychology*, **32**, 50–55.

Hettema, J. M., Neale, M. C. & Kendler, K. C. (2001) A review and meta-analysis of the genetic epidemiology of anxiety disorders. *American Journal of Psychiatry*, **158**, 1568–1578.

Hoehn-Saric, R. & McLeod, D. R. (1986) Panic and generalised anxiety disorders. In *Handbook of Anxiety Disorders* (eds C. G. Last & M. Hersen), pp. 109–127. New York: Pergamon Press.

Holmes J. (1991) *Textbook of Psychotherapy in Psychiatric Practice*. Edinburgh: Churchill Livingstone.

Holmes, J. (1993) Attachment theory: a biological basis for psychotherapy. *British Journal of Psychiatry*, **163**, 430–438.

Hood, S. D., Argyropoulos, S. V. & Nutt, D. J. (2003) New directions in the treatment of anxiety disorders. *Expert Opinion in Therapeutic Patents*, **13**, 401–423.

Horowitz, M. J. (1986) *Stress Response Syndrome. General Treatment Principles* (2nd edn), pp. 111–146. Northvale, NY: Jason Aronson.

Horowitz, M. J., Wilmer, N. & Alvarez, W. (1979) Impact of Events Scale: a measure of subjective stress. *Psychosomatic Stress*, **41**, 209–218.

Ingham, J. G. (1966) Changes in MPI scores of neurotic patients: a three year follow up. *British Journal of Psychiatry*, **112**, 931–939.

Jacob, R. G. & Lilienfeldt, S. O. (1991) Panic disorder: diagnosis, medical assessment, and psychological assessment. In *Panic Disorder and Agoraphobia* (eds J. Walker, O. R. Norton & C. A. Ross), pp. 16–102. Pacific Grove, CA: Brooks/Cole.

Jardine, R., Martin, N. G. & Henderson, A. S. (1984) Genetic covariation between neuroticism and the symptoms of anxiety and depression. *Genetic Epidemiology*, **1**, 89–107.

Jenck, F., Moreau, J. L., Berendsen, H. H., *et al* (1998) Antiaversive effects of $5HT_{2C}$ receptor agonists and fluoxetine in a model of panic-like anxiety in rats. *European Neuropsychopharmacology*, **8**, 161–168.

Kahn, R. S., Wetzler, S., Van Praag, H. M., *et al* (1988) Behavioural indications for receptor hypersensitivity in panic disorder. *Psychiatry Research*, **25**, 101–104.

Kampman, M., Keijsers, G. P., Hoodguin, C. A., *et al* (2002) A randomized, double-blind, placebo-controlled study of adjunctive paroxetine in panic disorder patients unsuccessfully treated with cognitive–behavioral therapy alone. *Journal of Clinical Psychiatry*, **63**, 772–777.

Kardiner, A. (1941) *The Traumatic Neurosis of War.* Psychological Medicine Monograph (I–II). Washington, DC: National Research Council.

Kendler, K. S. (1996) Major depression and generalised anxiety disorder. Same genes, (partly) different environments – revisited. *British Journal of Psychiatry*, **168**, suppl. 30, 68–75.

Kendler, K. S., Heath, A., Martin, N. G., *et al* (1986) Symptoms of anxiety and depression in a volunteer twin population: the aetiologic role of genetic and environmental factors. *Archives of General Psychiatry*, **43**, 213–221.

Kendler, K. S., Karkowski, L. M. & Prescott, C. A. (1999) Fears and phobias: reliability and heritability. *Psychological Medicine*, **29**, 539–553.

Kendler, K. S., Hettema, J. M., Butera, F., *et al* (2003) Life event dimensions of loss, humiliation, entrapment, and danger in the prediction of onsets of major depression and generalized anxiety. *Archives of General Psychiatry*, **60**, 789–796.

Kessler, R. C., Berglund, P., Demler, O., *et al* (2005) Lifetime prevalence and age-of-onset distributions of DSM–IV disorders in the National Comorbidity Survey Replication. *Archives of General Psychiatry*, **62**, 593–602.

Kilpatrick, D. G. & Resnick, H. S. (1993) Posttraumatic stress disorder associated with exposure to criminal victimization in a clinical and a community population. In *Posttraumatic Stress Disorder: DSM–IV and Beyond* (eds J. R. T. Davidson & E. B. Foa), pp. 113–146. Washington, DC: American Psychiatric Association Press.

Klein, D. F. & Fink, M. (1962) Psychiatric reaction patterns to imipramine. *American Journal of Psychiatry*, **119**, 432–438.

Ko, G. N., Elsworth, J. D., Roth, R. H., *et al* (1983) Panic-induced elevation of plasma MHPG levels in phobic-anxious patients, effects of clonidine and imipramine. *Archives of General Psychiatry*, **40**, 425–430.

Kolb, L. C., Burris, B. C. & Griffiths, S. (1984) Propranolol and clonidine in the treatment of post-traumatic stress disorder of war. In *Post Traumatic Stress Disorders: Psychological and Biological Sequelae* (ed. B. A. van der Kolk), pp. 98–107. Washington, DC: American Psychiatric Press.

Kosten, T. R., Frank, J. B., Dan, E., *et al* (1991) Pharmacotherapy for posttraumatic stress disorder using phenelzine or imipramine. *Journal of Nervous and Mental Disease*, **179**, 366–370.

Kraupl Taylor, F. (1989) The damnation of benzodiazepines. *British Journal of Psychiatry*, **154**, 697–704.

Kulha, R. A., Schlenger, W. E. & Fairbank, R. L. (1990) *Trauma and the Vietnam War Generation: Report of findings from the National Vietnam Veterans Readjustment Study*. New York: Brunner/Mazel.

Kushnir, M. G., Sher, K. J. & Beitman, B. D. (1990) The relation between alcohol problems and the anxiety disorders. *American Journal of Psychiatry*, **147**, 685–695.

Lader, M. (1978) Benzodiazepines – the opium of the masses? *Neuroscience*, **3**, 159–165.

Langer, R. (1987) Post traumatic stress disorder in former POWs. In *Post Traumatic Stress Disorders: A Handbook for Clinicians* (ed. T. Williams), pp. 35–51. Cincinnati, OH: Disabled American Veterans.

Langlois, F., Freeston, M. H. & Ladouceur, R. (2000) Differences and similarities between obsessive intrusive thoughts and worry in a non-clinical population: study 1. *Behaviour Research and Therapy*, **38**, 157–173.

Lee, H. J., Lee, S. H., Kim, H. S., *et al* (2005*a*) A comparison of autogenous/reactive obsessions and worry in a nonclinical population: a test of the continuum hypothesis. *Behaviour Research and Therapy*, **43**, 999–1010.

Lee, H. J., Lee, M. S., Kang, R. H., *et al* (2005*b*) Influence of the serotonin transporter promoter gene polymorphism on susceptibility to posttraumatic stress disorder. *Depression and Anxiety*, **21**, 135–139.

Lemma, A. (2003) *Introduction to the Practice of Psychoanalytic Psychotherapy*, pp. 355–364 Chichester: Wiley.

Lepine, J. P., Chignon, J. M. & Teherani, M. (1993) Suicide attempts in patients with panic disorder. *Archives of General Psychiatry*, **50**, 144–149.

Lesch, K. P. (2003) Genetic dissection of anxiety and related disorders. In *Anxiety Disorders* (eds D. J. Nutt & J. C. Ballenger), pp. 229–250. Oxford: Blackwell Science.

Lesch, K. P. & Mossner, R. (1998) Genetically driven variation of serotonin uptake: is there a link to affective spectrum, neurodevelopmental, and neurodegenerative disorders? *Biological Psychiatry*, **44**, 179–192.

Lewis, A. (1970) The ambiguous word 'anxiety'. *International Journal of Psychiatry*, **9**, 62–79.

Lieb, R., Becker, E. & Altamura, C. (2005) The epidemiology of generalized anxiety disorder in Europe. *European Neuropsychopharmacology*, **15**, 445–452.

Liebowitz, M. R. (1993) Mixed anxiety and depression: should it be included in DSM–IV? *Journal of Clinical Psychiatry*, **54**, suppl., 4–7.

Maier, W. (2003) Genetics of anxiety. In *Handbook of Depression and Anxiety* (2nd edn, revised and expanded) (eds S. Kasper, J. A. den Boer & J. M. Ad Sitsen), pp. 189–205. New York: Marcel Dekker.

Maier, W., Buller, R., Philipp, M., *et al* (1988) The Hamilton Anxiety Scale: reliability, validity and sensitivity to change in anxiety and depressive disorders. *Journal of Affective Disorders*, **14**, 61–68.

Maier, W., Minges, J. & Lichtermann, D. (1993) Alcoholism and panic disorder: co-occurrence and co-transmission in families. *European Archives of Psychiatry and Clinical Neuroscience*, **243**, 205–211.

Malizia, A. L., Cunningham, V. J., Bell, C. J., *et al* (1998) Decreased brain GABA(A)–benzodiazepine receptor binding in panic disorder: preliminary results from a quantitative PET study. *Archives of General Psychiatry*, **55**, 715–720.

Marks, I. M. & Nesse, R. M. (1994) Fear and fitness: an evolutionary analysis of anxiety disorders. *Ethology and Sociobiology*, **15**, 247–261.

Marshall, R. D., Spitzer, R. & Liebowitz, M. R. (1999) Review and critique of the new DSM–IV diagnosis of acute stress disorder. *American Journal of Psychiatry*, **156**, 1677–1685.

Martin, N. G., Jardine, R., Andrews, G., *et al* (1988) Anxiety disorders and neuroticism: are there genetic factors specific to panic? *Acta Psychiatrica Scandinavica*, **77**, 698–706.

Martinez-Cano, H., de Iceta Ibanez de Gauna, M., Vela-Bueno, A., *et al* (1999) DSM–III–R comorbidity in benzodiazepine dependence. *Addiction*, **94**, 97–107.

Mathew, R. J., Ho, B. T., Francis, D. J., *et al* (1982) Catecholamines and anxiety. *Acta Psychiatrica Scandinavica*, **65**, 142–147.

Meoni, P., Hackett, D. & Lader, M. (2004) Pooled analysis of venlafaxine WXR efficacy on somatic and psychic symptoms of anxiety in generalized anxiety disorder. *Depression and Anxiety*, **19**, 127–132.

Middleton, H. C. (1990) Cardiovascular dystonia in recovered panic patients. *Journal of Affective Disorders*, **19**, 229–236.

Mitte, K., Noack, P., Steil, R., *et al* (2005) A meta-analytic review of the efficacy of drug treatment in generalized anxiety disorder. *Journal of Clinical Psychopharmacology*, **25**, 141–150.

Moret, C. & Briley, M. (2000) The possible role of 5-$HT_{(1B/D)}$ receptors in psychiatric disorders and their potential as a target for therapy. *European Journal of Pharmacology*, **404**, 1–12.

Munjack, D. J., Baltazaar, P. L., de Quatro, V., *et al* (1990) Generalised anxiety disorder: some biochemical aspects. *Psychiatry Research*, **32**, 35–43.

Nagy, L. M., Krystal, J. H., Woods, S. W., *et al* (1989) Clinical and medication outcome after short-term alprazolam and behaviour group treatment in panic disorder: 2.5 year naturalistic follow-up study. *Archives of General Psychiatry*, **46**, 993–999.

Nardi, A. E., Nascimento, I., Valenca, A. M., *et al* (2003) Respiratory panic disorder subtype: acute and long-term response to nortriptyline, a noradrenergic tricyclic antidepressant. *Psychiatry Research*, **120**, 283–293.

National Institute for Health and Clinical Excellence (2004) *The Management of Panic Disorder and Generalised Anxiety Disorder in Primary and Secondary Care*. London: National Collaborating Centre for Mental Health.

National Institute for Health and Clinical Excellence (2005) *Post-traumatic Stress Disorder. The Management of PTSD in Adults and Children in Primary and Secondary Care*. National Practice Guideline Number 26. London: Royal College of Psychiatrists and British Psychological Society.

Nesse, R. M., Cameron, O. G., Curtis, G. C., *et al* (1984) Adrenergic function in patients with panic anxiety. *Archives of General Psychiatry*, **41**, 771–776.

Norton, G. R., Harrison, B., Hauch, J., *et al* (1985) Characteristics of people with infrequent panic attacks. *Journal of Abnormal Psychology*, **94**, 216–221.

Noyes, R. Jr, Clancy, J., Crowe, R., *et al* (1978) The familial prevalence of anxiety neurosis. *Archives of General Psychiatry*, **35**, 1057–1074.

Nurnberger, J. I. Jr, Wiegeland, R., Bucholz, K., *et al* (2004) A family study of alcohol dependence: coaggregation of multiple disorders in relatives of alcohol dependent probands. *Archives of General Psychiatry*, **61**, 1246–1256.

Nutt, D. J. (1989) Altered alpha-2-adrenoceptor sensitivity in panic disorder. *Archives of General Psychiatry*, **46**, 165–169.

Nutt, D. J. (2001) Neurobiological mechanisms in generalized anxiety disorder. *Journal of Clinical Psychiatry*, **62**, suppl. 11, 22–27.

Nutt, D. J., Glue, P., Lawson, C., *et al* (1990) Evidence for altered benzodiazepine receptor sensitivity in panic disorder: effects of the benzodiazepine receptor antagonist flumazenil. *Archives of General Psychiatry*, **47**, 917–925.

Olivier, B., Soudijn, W. & van Wijngaarden, I. (1999) The 5-HT_{1A} receptor and its ligands: structure and function. *Progress in Drug Research*, **52**, 103–165.

Olivier, B., van Wijngaarden, I. & Soudijn, W. (2000) 5-$HT_{(3)}$ receptor antagonists and anxiety: a preclinical and clinical review. *European Neuropsychopharmacology*, **10**, 77–95.

Oppenheimer, B. S. & Rothschild, M. A. (1918) The psychoneurotic factor in the 'irritable heart' of soldiers. *British Medical Journal, ii*, 29–31.

Oxford English Dictionary (1989) 2nd edition. Oxford: Clarendon Press.

Papez, J. W. (1937) A proposed mechanism of emotion. *Archives of Neurology and Psychiatry*, **38**, 724–743. (Reprinted in *Journal of Neuropsychiatry and Clinical Neuroscience*, 1995, **7**, 103–112.)

Passchier, J. & van Waarde, A. (2001) Visualisation of serotonin-1A (5-HT_{1A}) receptors in the central nervous system. *European Journal of Nuclear Medicine*, **28**, 113–129.

Paton, C. (2002) Benzodiazepines and disinhibition: a review. *Psychiatric Bulletin*, **26**, 460–462.

Pavlov, I. P. (1927) *Conditioned Reflexes*. London: Oxford University Press.

Petursson, H. & Lader, M. H. (1981) Benzodiazepine dependence. *British Journal of Addiction*, **76**, 133–145.

Pinel, P. (1801) *A Treatise on Insanity* (trans. D. D. Davis, 1962). New York: Hagner,

Pitman, P. K., Sanders, K. M., Zusman, R. M., *et al* (2002) Pilot study of secondary prevention of posttraumatic stress disorder with propranolol. *Biological Psychiatry*, **51**, 189–192.

Pitts, F. N. & McClure, J. N. (1967) Lactate metabolism in anxiety neurosis. *New England Journal of Medicine*, **277**, 1329–1336.

Pollack, M. H., Allgulander, C., Bandelow, B., *et al* (2003*a*) World Council on Anxiety (WCA) recommendations for the long-term treatment of panic disorder. *CNS Spectrums*, **8**, suppl. 1, 17–30.

Pollack, M. H., Simon, N. M., Worthington, J. J., *et al* (2003*b*) Combined paroxetine and clonazepam treatment strategies compared to paroxetine monotherapy for panic disorder. *Journal of Psychopharmacology*, **17**, 276–282.

Pollack, M. H., Simon, N. M., Zalta, A. K., *et al* (2006) Olanzapine augmentation of fluoxetine for refractory generalized anxiety disorder. *Biological Psychiatry*, **59**, 211–215.

Rainey, J. M., Pohl, R. B., Williams-Knitter, E., *et al* (1984) A comparison of lactate and isoprotenerol anxiety states. *Psychopathology*, **17**, suppl. 1, 74–82.

Ramos, R. T., Gentil, V. & Gorenstein, C. (1993) Clomipramine and initial worsening in panic disorder: beyond the 'jitteriness syndrome'. *Journal of Psychopharmacology*, **7**, 265–269.

Ramsay, R. (1990) Post-traumatic stress disorder: a new clinical entity? *Journal of Psychosomatic Research*, **34**, 355–365.

Raskind, M. A., Peskind, E. R., Kanter, E. D., *et al* (2003) Reduction of nightmares and other PTSD symptoms in combat veterans by prazosin: a placebo-controlled study. *American Journal of Psychiatry*, **160**, 371–373.

Rauch, S. L., Shin, L. M., Whalen, P. J., *et al* (1998) Neuroimaging and the neuroanatomy of PTSD. *CNS Spectrums*, **3**, suppl. 2, 30–41.

Resick, P. A. & Calhoun, K. S. (2001) Post-traumatic stress disorder. In *Clinical Handbook of Psychological Disorders: A Step-by-Step Treatment Manual* (3rd edn) (ed. D. Barlow). London: Guilford Press.

Rickels, K., Weisman, K., Norstad, N., *et al* (1982) Buspirone and diazepam in the treatment of anxiety: a controlled study. *Journal of Clinical Psychiatry*, **43**, 81–86.

Ronalds, C., Creed, F., Stone, K., *et al* (1997) Outcome of anxiety and depressive disorders in primary care. *British Journal of Psychiatry*, **171**, 427–433.

Roth, B. L., Willins, D. L., Kristiansen, K., *et al* (1998) 5-Hydroxytryptamine2-family receptors (5-hydroxytryptamine2A, 5-hydroxytryptamine2B, 5-hydroxytryptamine2C): where structure meets function. *Pharmacology and Therapeutics*, **79**, 231–257.

Rothbaum, B. O. & Foa, E. B. (1993) Subtypes of posttraumatic stress disorder and duration of symptoms. In *Posttraumatic Stress Disorder: DSM–IV and Beyond* (eds J. R. T. Davidson & E. B. Foa), pp. 23–36. Washington, DC: American Psychiatric Association.

Rothschild, A. J., Shindul-Rothschild, J., Viguera, A., *et al* (2000) Comparison of the frequency of behavioural disinhibition on alprazolam, clonazepam, or no benzodiazepine in hospitalised psychiatric patients. *Journal of Clinical Psychopharmacology*, **20**, 7–11.

Royal College of Psychiatrists (1997) *Benzodiazepines: Risks, Benefits or Dependence – A Re-evaluation*. Council Report 59. London: Royal College of Psychiatrists.

Sanderson, W. C. & Barlow, D. H. (1990) A description of patients diagnosed with DSM–IIIR generalised anxiety disorder. *Journal of Nervous and Mental Disease*, **178**, 588–591.

Sandford, J. J., Argyropoulos, S. V. & Nutt, D. J. (2000) The psychobiology of anxiolytic drugs. Part 1: Basic neurobiology. *Pharmacology and Therapeutics*, **88**, 197–212.

Sapolsky, R. M. (1996) Why stress is bad for your brain. *Science*, **273**, 749–750.

Sareen, J., Cox, B. J., Afifi, T. O., *et al* (2005) Anxiety disorders and risk for suicidal ideation and suicide attempts. A population-based longitudinal study of adults. *Archives of General Psychiatry*, **62**, 1249–1257.

Sargent, P. A., Nash, J., Hood, S., *et al* (2000) 5-HT_{1A} receptor binding in panic disorder: comparison with depressive disorder and healthy volunteers using PET and [^{11}C]WAY-100635. *Neuroimage*, **11**, 189.

Scherrer, J. F., True, W. R., Xian, H., *et al* (2000) Evidence for genetic influences common and specific to symptoms of generalised anxiety disorder and panic. *Journal of Affective Disorders*, *57*, 25–35.

Schuckit, M. A. & Monteiro, M. G. (1988) Alcoholism, anxiety and depression. *British Journal of Addiction*, **83**, 1373–1380.

Schweizer, E. & Rickels, K. (1998) Benzodiazepine dependence and withdrawal: a review of the syndrome and its clinical management. *Acta Psychiatrica Scandinavica*, suppl. 393, 95–101.

Schweizer, E., Rickels, K., Weiss, S., *et al* (1993) Maintenance drug treatment for panic disorder: II. Short- and long-term outcome after drug taper. *Archives of General Psychiatry*, **50**, 61–68.

Segman, R. H. & Shalev, A. Y. (2003) Genetics of posttraumatic stress disorder. *CNS Spectrums*, **8**, 693–698.

Shalev, A. Y. (2000) Post-traumatic stress disorder: diagnosis, history and life course. In *Post-traumatic Stress Disorder: Diagnosis, Management and Treatment* (eds D. J. Nutt, J. R. T. Davidson & J. Zohar), pp. 1–15. London: Martin Dunitz.

Sheehan, D. V., Lecrubier, Y., Sheehan, K. E., *et al* (1998) The Mini-International Neuropsychiatric Interview (MINI): the development and validation of a structured diagnostic psychiatric interview for DSM–IV and ICD–10. *Journal of Clinical Psychiatry*, **59**, suppl. 20, 22–33.

Snaith, R. P., Baugh, S. J., Clayden, A. D., *et al* (1982) The Clinical Anxiety Scale: an instrument derived from the Hamilton Anxiety Scale. *British Journal of Psychiatry*, **141**, 518–523.

Southwick, S. M., Krystal, J. H., Morgan, A., *et al* (1993) Abnormal noradrenergic function in post traumatic stress disorder. *Archives of General Psychiatry*, **50**, 266–274.

Southwick, S. M., Bremner, D., Krystal, J. H., *et al* (1994) Psychobiological research in post-traumatic stress disorder. *Psychiatric Clinics of North America*, **17**, 251–264.

Spielberger, C. D., Gorsuch, R. L., Lushene, R., *et al* (1983) *Manual for the State–Trait Anxiety Inventory*. Palo Alto, CA: Consulting Psychologists Press.

Starkman, M. N., Cameron, O. G., Nesse, R. M., *et al* (1990) Peripheral catecholamine levels and the symptoms of anxiety with and without phaeochromocytoma. *Psychosomatic Medicine*, **652**, 129–142.

Stein, M. B., Jang, K. L. & Livesley, W. J. (1999) Heritability of anxiety sensitivity: a twin study. *American Journal of Psychiatry*, **156**, 246–251.

Stein, M. B., Klein, N. A. & Matlof, J. L. (2002) Adjunctive olanzapine for SSRI resistant combat-related PTSD: a double-blind placebo-controlled study. *American Journal of Psychiatry*, **159**, 1777–1779.

Stein, D. J., Bandelow, B., Hollander, E., *et al* (2003) World Council on Anxiety (WCA) recommendations for the long-term treatment of posttraumatic stress disorder. *CNS Spectrums*, **8**, suppl. 1, 31–39.

Strohle, A. & Holsboer, F. (2003) Stress-responsive neurohormones in depression and anxiety. In *Handbook of Depression and Anxiety* (2nd edn, revised and expanded) (eds S. Kasper, J. A. den Boer & J. M. Ad Sitsen), pp. 207–228. New York: Marcel Dekker.

Strous, R. D., Maayan, R. & Weizman, A. (2006) The relevance of neurosteroids to clinical psychiatry: from the laboratory to the bedside. *European Neuropsychopharmacology*, **16**, 155–169.

Sulker, P. B., Winstead, D. K., Galine, Z. H., *et al* (1991) Cognitive deficit and psychopathology among former prisoners of war and combat veterans of the Korean conflict. *American Journal of Psychiatry*, **148**, 67–72.

Swendsen, J. D., Merikangas, K. R., Canino, G. J., *et al* (1998) The comorbidity of alcoholism with anxiety and depressive disorders in four geographic communities. *Comprehensive Psychiatry*, **39**, 176–184.

Tanaka, M., Yoshida, M., Emoto, H., *et al* (2000) Noradrenaline systems in the hypothalamus, amygdala and locus coeruleus are involved in the provocation of anxiety: basic studies. *European Journal of Pharmacology*, **405**, 397–406.

Targum, S. (1990) Differential responses to anxiogenic challenge studies in patients with major depressive disorder and panic disorder. *Biological Psychiatry*, **28**, 21–34.

Taylor, D. P., Eison, M. S., Riblet, L. S., *et al* (1985) Pharmacological and clinical effects of buspirone. *Pharmacology, Biochemistry and Behaviour*, **23**, 687–694.

Titchener, J. L. (1985) Post traumatic decline: a consequence of unresolved destructive drives. In *Trauma and Its Wake, Vol. II: Traumatic Stress Theory, Research and Intervention* (ed. C. R. Figley), pp. 5–19. New York: Brunner/Mazel.

Titchener, J. L. & Kapp, F. T. (1976) Family and character change at Buffalo Creek. *American Journal of Psychiatry*, **153**, 295–299.

Tork, I. & Hornung, J. P. (1990) Raphe nuclei and the serotonergic system. In *The Human Nervous System* (eds G. Paxinos & F. L. Orlando), pp. 1001–1022. London: Academic Press.

Trimble, M. (1981) *Post-Traumatic Neurosis*. Chichester: Wiley.

True, W. R., Rice, J., Eisen, S. A., *et al* (1993) A twin study of genetic and environmental contributions to liability for post traumatic stress symptoms. *Archives of General Psychiatry*, **50**, 257–264.

Tyrer, P. (1989*a*) *Classification of Neurosis*. Chichester: Wiley.

Tyrer, P. (1989*b*) Risks of dependence on benzodiazepine drugs: the importance of patient selection. *BMJ*, **298**, 102–105.

Uhde, T. W., Boulenger, J. P., Roy-Byrne, P. P., *et al* (1985) Longitudinal course of panic disorder: clinical and biological considerations. *Progress in Neuropharmacology and Biological Psychiatry*, **9**, 39–51.

van Balkom, A. J., Bakker, A., Spinhoven, P., *et al* (1997) A meta-analysis of the treatment of panic disorder with or without agoraphobia: a comparison of psychopharmacological, cognitive–behavioral, and combination treatments. *Journal of Nervous and Mental Disease*, **185**, 510–516.

van Vliet, I. M., Slaap, B. R., Westenberg, H. G., *et al* (1996) Behavioral, neuroendocrine and biochemical effects of different doses of 5-HTP in panic disorder. *European Neuropsychopharmacology*, **6**, 103–110.

Vythilingam, M., Anderson, E. R., Goddard, A., *et al* (2000) Temporal lobe volume in panic disorder – a quantitative magnetic resonance imaging study. *Psychiatry Research*, **99**, 75–82.

Weissman, M. M., Wichramanaratne, P., Adams, P. B., *et al* (1993) The relationship between panic disorder and major depression. *Archives of General Psychiatry*, **50**, 767–780.

Wilkinson, G., Balestrieri, M., Ruggeri, M., *et al* (1991) Meta-analysis of double-blind placebo-controlled trials of antidepressants and benzodiazepines for patients with panic disorder. *Psychological Medicine*, **21**, 991–998.

Williams, D. D. R. & McBride, A. (1998) Benzodiazepines: time for reassessment. *British Journal of Psychiatry*, **173**, 361–362.

Wilson, M. A. (1996) GABA physiology: modulation by benzodiazepines and hormones. *Critical Reviews in Neurobiology*, **10**, 1–37.

Wittchen, H. U. & Essau, C. A. (1991) The epidemiology of panic attacks, panic disorder and agoraphobia. In *Panic Disorder and Agoraphobia* (eds J. Walker, G. Norton & C. Ross), pp. 103–142. Monterey, CA: Brooks Cole.

Wittchen, H.-U. & Jacobi, F. (2005) Size and burden of mental disorders in Europe – a critical review and appraisal of 27 studies. *European Neuropsychopharmacology*, **15**, 357–376.

Wittchen, H.-U., Semler, G. & von Zerssen, D. (1986) Diagnostic reliability of anxiety disorders. In *Panic and Phobias, Vol. I* (eds I. Hand & H.-U. Wittchen). Heidelberg: Springer-Verlag.

Woods, S. W., Koster, K., Krystal, J. K., *et al* (1988) Yohimbine alters regional cerebral blood flow in panic disorder. *Lancet*, *ii*, 678.

World Health Organization (1978) *The ICD–9 Classification of Mental and Behavioural Disorders*. Geneva: WHO.

World Health Organization (1992) *The ICD–10 Classification of Mental and Behavioural Disorders*. Geneva: WHO.

Worthington, J. J. III, Pollack, M. H., Otto, M. W., *et al* (1998) Long-term experience with clonazepam in patients with a primary diagnosis of panic disorder. *Psychopharmacology Bulletin*, **34**, 199–205.

Yehuda, R. (2000) Neuroendocrinology. In *Post-traumatic Stress Disorder: Diagnosis, Management and Treatment* (eds D. J. Nutt, J. R. T. Davidson & J. Zohar), pp. 53–67. London: Martin Dunitz.

Yerkes, R. M. (1921) Psychological examining in the United States army. *Memoirs of the National Academy of Sciences*, **15**, 1–16.

Yonkers, K. A., Massion, A., Warshaw, M., *et al* (1996) Phenomenology and course of generalised anxiety disorder. *British Journal of Psychiatry*, **168**, 308–313.

Zeldin, T. (1977) *France 1848–1945: Anxiety and Hypocrisy*. Oxford: Clarendon Press.

CHAPTER 14

Phobias

Lynne M. Drummond and Naomi A. Fineberg

Background

Fear is a universal and essential emotion. Without it the human race would have fallen over cliffs and failed to run from sabre-toothed tigers until we became extinct. Individuals differ in their background level of fear (trait anxiety) and the situations that provoke fear (state anxiety). Not all fear is rational and based on a threat to survival.

We all have morbid fears that we know to be irrational but which we cannot stop. These fears may be embarrassing but do not lead us to change our lifestyle in any major way. They lie on a continuum with phobic disorders.

Phobias have been defined as morbid fears that are involuntary, cannot be reasoned away and lead to avoidance of the feared object or situation (Marks, 1969). Clearly, they overlap with morbid fears. Most patients with phobic disorder, however, have made major adjustments to their lifestyle to avoid the phobic stimulus. For example, a lady with spider phobia was so fearful of even hearing the word 'spider' that she had left a well-paid job and avoided all parties.

Working definitions of the most commonly seen types of phobic disorder are given in Table 14.1, along with their relative prevalence, age at onset and sex incidence.

Diagnosis

The diagnosis of phobic disorder depends on a history of fear being provoked by specific objects or situations. The anticipation of fear leads to avoidance of these stimuli.

The World Health Organization (1992) defines phobic anxiety disorders in ICD–10 as a group of disorders where anxiety is provoked only, or predominantly, by defined objects or situations that are external to the individual and that would not generally be considered dangerous. As a result, the specified objects or situations are either avoided or endured with dread. Panic may occur, and in such cases the phobia is given diagnostic precedence over the panic symptoms. Subcategories of phobic anxiety disorder defined in ICD–10 are agoraphobia, social phobia, specific (isolated) phobia and 'other' phobic anxiety disorders.

DSM–IV–TR (American Psychiatric Association, 2000) takes a different approach to the definition of phobias. In the case of panic occurring with a phobia, the panic disorder is given precedence. Thus, the categories of phobic disorder are defined as panic disorder with agoraphobia, agoraphobia without history of panic disorder, specific phobia (including animal, natural environment, blood/injection/injury and situational types) and social phobia.

Areas of controversy

The relative importance of panic in the classification of phobic disorders is controversial. Panic may be viewed as very high levels of anxiety. During exposure to fear-provoking situations, some patients suffer from incapacitating panic. This panic may also result from anticipation of a future fear-provoking event. Thus, panic can be seen as a secondary reaction to the feared situation.

However, other workers have argued that the panic attack is the primary event, with the phobic anxiety developing as a secondary phenomenon. According to this view, panic has a separate biological basis to its genesis and should take precedence over the phobic anxiety in terms of classification and treatment. This controversy is demonstrated by the difference in the ICD and DSM views on classification.

In recent years the debate has focused on the nosological position of panic disorder and its links to agoraphobia. While some psychiatrists have been inclined to accept that the apprehension of going out causes the panic, others have viewed the experience of panic as the core problem, which causes the fear of going out and having a panic attack away from the security of the home.

There are persuasive arguments in favour of both positions, and it is possible that an intermediate model may obtain, one with interconnecting biological and environmental factors that act through hypersensitivity of the autonomic nervous system (Faravelli & Paionni, 1999).

In clinical samples, almost all individuals presenting with symptoms of agoraphobia also have a history of panic disorder. In contrast, agoraphobia without a history of panic disorder is consistently reported in community samples, although the rates may have been exaggerated, and the disorder lacks strong support as a separate entity (Andrews & Slade, 2002). Some 35–50% of those with panic disorder in community settings also suffer from agoraphobia (Baldwin & Birtwistle, 1998). Individuals with panic and agoraphobia report more

Table 14.1 Types of phobias

Disorder	Prevalence	Onset	Sex incidence	Feared situation	Comments
Agoraphobia	One of the commonest and most handicapping phobias in psychiatric practice	Early adult life	Females more frequently affected than males	Fear of crowded places. Travelling by public transport, supermarkets, enclosed spaces	Can present with or without panic disorder
Social anxiety disorder	The next most common phobia seen in psychiatric clinics after agoraphobia	Adolescence	Equal	Can be generally fearful of all social situations or specific (e.g. eating, drinking, blushing, vomiting)	Psychological therapy will depend on whether it is general or specific. This phobia is the most studied from the psychopharmacological standpoint
Specific animal phobia	Rarely seen in psychiatric practice and more likely in general practice	Early childhood (usually before the age of 7 years)	More common in adult women but equal sex incidence in childhood	Dogs, cats, spiders, insects and so on	Specificity to the animal. Self-help packages are popular with these patients
Miscellaneous specific phobias	May present in a variety of ways	Varies	Overall equal	Heights, enclosed places, flying, thunder, and so on	
Blood and injury phobia	Possibly more common than is ever recorded as these patients tend to avoid all clinical situations	Often starts in adolescence and may improve in middle age	Equal	Medical or dental procedures, blood	Parasympathetically mediated fainting response rather than sympathetically mediated fight, flight or freeze reaction

comorbid disorders and are more disabled than are those with uncomplicated agoraphobia.

Differentiating between social anxiety disorder and agoraphobia

Social anxiety disorder can easily be confused with agoraphobia, because panic attacks occur in both syndromes. Identifying the reason behind the fear (i.e. fear of social interaction rather than fear of anxiety symptoms) will help the clinician differentiate. In the case of social anxiety disorder, the sufferer experiences intense, excessive or unreasonable, distressing social anxiety, which leads to avoidance of social situations.

In order to distinguish social anxiety disorder from agoraphobia, it can be helpful to enquire, for example, about what kinds of shops cause fear. For the socially anxious person it will be small shops, where they will have to ask for what they want, whereas for the agoraphobic patient large supermarkets with crowds of people will drive the fear. Patients with social anxiety disorder are more likely to experience anxiety in the supermarket queue, because they fear having to talk to the checkout clerk, whereas agoraphobic patients will fear feeling trapped in the queue.

Social phobia or social anxiety disorder?

Some patient groups in the USA have lobbied for the name to change from social phobia to social anxiety disorder, because they think the former trivialises the illness. DSM–IV (American Psychiatric Association, 1994) already recognises both terms, on the basis that the experience of social anxiety may be the primary element, with phobic avoidance occurring as a secondary phenomenon (analogous to panic disorder with or without agoraphobia). Indeed, some individuals simply endure the social anxiety, albeit with distress. For the purposes of this chapter, the term social anxiety disorder is used throughout.

Subtypes of social anxiety disorder

Both DSM–IV and ICD–10 have attempted to distinguish social anxiety disorder from normal shyness. The ICD–10 criteria are more stringent, by excluding anxiety related to public speaking, which is considered to be within normal parameters. ICD–10 also has the advantage of recognising the importance of a range of somatic manifestations of anxiety, such as blushing, tremor and nausea, while DSM–IV focuses on induced panic. Indeed, blushing has been proposed as a specific physical symptom that distinguishes social fear from other anxiety disorders (Ballenger *et al*, 1998*a*; Westenberg, 1998).

Typical anxiety-evoking situations include being introduced, initiating a conversation with the opposite sex, dating, using the telephone, meeting with authority figures, being watched while working and speaking or eating in public. Most sufferers experience up to five specific feared situations, but some fear almost all forms of social engagement, while others fear only a single situation, such as public speaking.

This has led to the suggestion that different subtypes of illness exist. Both DSM–IV and ICD–10 recognise this possibility and specify generalised versus discrete forms of the disorder. Those with generalised illness are more likely to have affected family members (Stein *et al*, 1998), are themselves affected earlier (often in childhood), are more impaired and are less likely to respond positively to treatment (Heimberg *et al*, 1990). Some experts have suggested that fear of public speaking is a separate entity (Westenberg, 1998).

Phobias: differential diagnosis and comorbidity

As with the other anxiety disorders, the problem of comorbidity often confounds the diagnostician, as up to 80% patients with a phobia also fulfil criteria for other anxiety disorders, to the extent that it can be impossible to determine a single, primary source of anxiety (Magee *et al*, 1996). The presence of comorbidity has the effect of increasing the burden of the disorder. For example, suicidality increases from an estimated rate of 1% for uncomplicated social phobia to 16% for comorbid disease.

Obsessive–compulsive disorder

Obsessive–compulsive disorder can be easily mistaken for phobic disorder. There are important similarities and differences between the two conditions. These are highlighted in Table 15.1 on page 365.

Generalised anxiety disorder

Generalised anxiety disorder (GAD) is manifested as symptoms of worry and anxiety that occur in a generalised and persistent manner, and are not related to specific cues. Results from community surveys suggest that the onset of phobic disorders, such as agoraphobia and specific phobias, may predict the later onset of GAD (Kessler & Wittchen, 2002).

In comorbid cases, it may be hard to distinguish the phobia, in which case a behavioural test, where the therapist observes the patient in a variety of situations, can be diagnostic.

Panic disorder

This condition has already been discussed in relation to agoraphobia. The essential features of panic disorder are recurrent attacks of severe anxiety that are not restricted to any specific situation and, therefore, occur unpredictably.

Depression

Patients with depression often experience symptoms of anxiety. In more severe cases anxiety combined with inertia can lead to symptoms almost identical to agoraphobia or social anxiety disorder.

On the other hand, the restricted life of the patient with agoraphobia or socially anxiety disorder can lead to depression. Indeed, depression occurs in roughly 50% of patients with panic, agoraphobia or social anxiety disorder during their lifetime, and there is considerable cross-sectional and longitudinal comorbidity with dysthymia. Often the phobia precedes the onset of depression, which may be considered a secondary reaction associated with the demoralising effect of chronic anxiety (Goodwin, 2002).

In cases of doubt, it is usually advisable to treat the depression first and then to examine the residual symptoms

Post-traumatic stress disorder (PTSD)

This condition can mimic phobic disorder and there can be overlap in these diagnoses as well. A few patients develop phobia after a traumatic event that leads to heightened arousal and other symptoms of PTSD.

Anxious/avoidant personality disorder

This is a controversial diagnosis, characterised by severe social avoidance, low self-esteem, sensitivity to rejection and avoidance of risks, and an early age of onset (see Chapter 18, page 452). It appears to respond to treatments that are effective for social anxiety disorder, and may therefore be regarded as a pervasive form of social anxiety disorder rather than a true disorder of personality (Ballenger *et al*, 1998*a*).

Substance misuse

Alcoholism and misuse of illicit substances also commonly complicate social anxiety disorder, and are particularly problematic in younger patients. For example, in one study, 40% of a cohort of 43 adolescents hospitalised for alcoholism were found to have social anxiety disorder (Clark *et al*, 1996). It is likely that some patients turn to alcohol and drugs in an attempt to relieve anxiety symptoms and because of their powerful disinhibitory effects.

The associated problems of tolerance and dependence also serve to confound the clinical picture. Anyone who has ever experienced a 'hangover' after an alcoholic binge will recognise that the symptoms of dry mouth, palpitation, headache and nausea are all very similar to those of high anxiety.

Physical disorders

Physical conditions such as phaeochromocytoma, thryotoxicosis, hypoglycaemia, mitral valve regurgitation, Parkinson's disease, variant Creutzfeldt–Jakob disease and AIDS can all present with features similar to anxiety and panic and may be mistaken for phobic anxiety disorder. Physical disorders can be excluded by careful history taking followed by relevant physical examination.

Compared with individuals without or with other forms of psychiatric illness, patients with agoraphobia and panic disorder show an increased risk of medically unexplained symptoms, are associated with a high use of medical services, and experience increased mortality from both cardiovascular and cerebrovascular disease (Baldwin & Birtwistle, 1998). A survey of 86 asthma patients revealed a high prevalence of phobic anxiety disorders, with agoraphobia, panic disorder with or without agoraphobia and social anxiety disorder occurring in 26.8%, 13.9% and 9.3%, respectively (Nascimento *et al*, 2002).

Epidemiology

Prevalence

Agras *et al* (1969) found a total prevalence of phobic disorder in the general population of Vermont, USA, of 77 per 1000. However, severely disabling phobias were found in only 2.2 per 1000 of the population, and only 1 person per 1000 was actively receiving treatment. Half the clinical cases involved agoraphobia, but less than 10% of the total phobic population had that condition. This early study showed that clinical populations are not a good guide to the prevalence of a condition in the community.

One of the many problems in epidemiological research involves deciding where the cut-off between annoying, minor personal difficulty and clinically relevant phobic anxiety should be. The choice of diagnostic instrument also influences the outcome. For example, modern studies employing the less stringent DSM criteria for social anxiety disorder have tended to produce higher prevalence rates than those using ICD criteria.

It is generally acknowledged that phobic disorders are extremely common. The US National Comorbidity Survey (Magee *et al*, 1996) examined a range of demographic parameters in 8098 non-institutionalised respondents, aged 15–54 years. DSM–III–R diagnoses were established and the results showed lifetime (and 30-day) prevalence rates of 13.3% (4.5%) for social phobia, 11.3% (5.5%) for specific phobia and 6.7% (2.3%) for agoraphobia. Other studies in America and Europe (e.g. Kessler *et al*, 1994; Lepine & Lellouch, 1995) support high frequencies of disorder. Interestingly, although individuals with agoraphobia perceived themselves to be less impaired, a higher proportion of this group sought professional help than those with social anxiety disorder or specific phobia (Magee *et al*, 1996).

Gender

Women suffer from agoraphobia and specific phobias (animal and blood/injection/injury phobias) up to three times more commonly than men. Social phobia has an approximately equal sex ratio (Degonda & Angst, 1994).

Onset and course of phobic disorders

Specific phobias usually start early in childhood and, although many continue into adolescence, the majority naturally improve with time.

Social anxiety disorder usually starts in adolescence (mean age of onset between 14 and 16 years), at a time when social interactions are exquisitely important for educational, occupational and emotional development. Childhood onset is also common, and if earlier than 11 years predicts a poorer outcome.

Some very young children show excessive fear of unfamiliar situations, people or objects. This has been termed 'behavioural inhibition', and can be identified usually from 4 months to 2.5 years of age. Children with behavioural inhibition have a family risk of anxiety disorders, such as panic disorder and agoraphobia, and often go on to develop social anxiety disorder in adolescence (Kagan, 1997). However, not all patients with social anxiety disorder show behavioural inhibition during childhood.

Untreated social anxiety disorder typically runs a chronic, lifelong course, rarely remitting spontaneously. It is responsible for considerable morbidity, with substantial socio-economic cost (Wittchen & Beloch, 1996). For example, sufferers are less likely to marry, and more likely to be divorced and unemployed. Yet individuals with social anxiety disorder often mistake their problem as mere shyness, and only a small proportion, estimated at around 5%, come forward for treatment (Magee *et al*, 1996).

Agoraphobia usually occurs later than social anxiety disorder, in the late teens or early twenties, and is rarely seen in childhood. It is also observed to run a chronic, enduring course and is responsible for considerable impairment (Noyes *et al*, 1990; Andrews & Slade, 2002).

Aetiology

The two conditions that have been the most studied from a biological viewpoint are social anxiety disorder and agoraphobia with panic disorder. Genetic and behavioural theories have been proposed, and both genes and learning may contribute to the development of the disorders, with maladaptive cognitions and avoidance acting as maintaining factors.

The biological basis of agoraphobia is intimately linked to that of panic disorder, and is covered mainly in Chapter 13, on anxiety disorders.

Genetic theories

The genetic epidemiology of phobias, investigating the interrelationship of agoraphobia, social anxiety disorder, animal phobias and situational phobias, has been examined separately in females and males in two recent large twin studies (Kendler *et al*, 1992, 2001).

The results for females showed that agoraphobia had the highest rates of comorbidity. Greater concordance in the monozygotic twins than in the dizygotic twins supported the importance of genetic mechanisms. A statistical analysis indicated that a third of the variance in liability to phobias was attributable to genetic factors, whereas the remainder was linked to environmental influences, such as parental attitudes and issues around upbringing. Model fitting suggested that for all except animal phobias, familial aggregation was better explained by genetic than specific environmental factors (Kendler *et al*, 1992).

In the second study, which looked at male twins, agoraphobia, social anxiety disorder, animal phobias, situational and blood/injection/injury phobias were all found to aggregate within twin pairs. The aggregation was again thought largely to result from genetic factors, with the heritability ranging from 25% to 37%. Multivariate analysis revealed a genetic factor common to all phobias tested, as well as other genetic factors specific to each phobia, and a common familial–environmental factor (Kendler *et al*, 2001). The authors concluded that genetic risk factors are partially common to all phobias and partially specific to particular subtypes, and also that they play a moderate role in the aetiology of phobias. Family environment also plays a role in the origin of social and agoraphobia.

Stein *et al* (1998) demonstrated that the risk of developing generalised social anxiety disorder, but not a discrete disorder, is ten-fold higher among the first-degree relatives of sufferers than among a control population.

Neurotransmitters and social anxiety disorder

Several neurotransmitter pathways are involved in the generation of the social anxiety, which itself lies at the heart of social anxiety disorder (Nutt *et al*, 1998). Research is under way to identify these mechanisms, using a range of neurobiological techniques, but the area remains poorly understood.

The observations that beta-blockers are useful for controlling the physical manifestations of social anxiety, such as sweating, blushing and tremor, and that the alpha-2 antagonist clonidine, which inhibits the release of noradrenaline, may control axillary sweating, suggest adrenergic involvement in social anxiety disorder. Preliminary results suggest sufferers show enhanced cardiovascular sensivity, compared with normal controls, in certain experimental situations. However, there have been no consistent findings regarding plasma levels of adrenaline or noradrenaline (Nutt *et al*, 1998).

The efficacy of agents that promote gamma-aminobutyric acid (GABA), such as benzodiazepines and alcohol, hints at the involvement of GABA-ergic systems in the disorder. Indirect evidence also points to abnormalities in dopaminergic function, for example the observation of high rates of social anxiety in Parkinson's disease (Berrios *et al*, 1995) and the possible clinical effectiveness of dopamine-enhancing drugs such as buproprion (Emmanuel *et al*, 1991). Reduced striatal dopamine reuptake compared with controls has been reported in a study of a small group of socially anxious individuals using single-photon emission computed tomography (SPECT) (Tiihonen *et al*, 1997).

Robust evidence supporting the efficacy of selective serotonin reuptake inhibitors (SSRIs) in the treatment of social anxiety disorder points to a role for serotonin, although the mediating mechanisms remain poorly understood. People with social anxiety disorder experience heightened anxiogenic responses to challenge with the serotonin-releasing agent fenfluramine (Tancer, 1993) and the serotonin agonist m-CPP (Hollander *et al*, 1991), relative to controls, which implies increased serotonin receptor sensitivity associated with the anxiety response. Fenfluramine and m-CPP have also been shown to increase anxiety linked to public speaking, in non-clinical volunteers, whereas the serotonin antagonist ritanserin decreased public speaking anxiety (Graeff *et al*, 1996). Altogether, these results are consistent with the hypothesis that activating different serotonin systems in the human brain can either increase or decrease anxiety.

Anxiogenic challenge tests

Various anxiogenic challenge agents have been applied in social anxiety disorder, as with other anxiety disorders, in the hope of identifying a physiological sensitivity to situations that mimic naturally occurring stressors, such as suffocation. The studies have focused on the induction of panic symptoms, rather than phobic avoidance. The administration of lactate and carbon dioxide in controlled paradigms allowed a discrimination between social anxiety disorder, panic disorder and normal controls. Individuals with social anxiety disorder showed somewhat enhanced chemoreceptor sensitivity, midway between panic disorder patients and normal controls. However, caffeine challenge produced a similar level of enhanced anxiety among those with panic disorder and those with social anxiety disorder, whereas the results from cholecystokinin challenge studies have been inconsistent (reviewed by Nutt *et al*, 1998).

Neuroimaging in social anxiety disorder

Positron emission tomography has identified increased cerebral metabolic activity in the right dorsolateral prefrontal cortex and left parietal cortex in individuals with social anxiety disorder undergoing a specific anxiogenic challenge (Price & Friston, 1997). These areas are thought to be involved in planning emotional responses and awareness of body position, both of which are relevant to social anxiety disorder.

Psychological theories

Psychoanalytic theories

The original and classic account of a child with phobic disorder is Freud's description of a young boy with a specific fear of horses. The boy, Hans, became frightened of horses after he witnessed an accident involving a horse while he was out walking with his father. Freud believed that this fear of horses was a substitute for his unconscious hatred and fear of his father. Thus, phobias were viewed by Freud as resulting from unresolved Oedipal conflicts.

More modern psychoanalytic views of phobic disorder still tend to concentrate on the theory that anxiety is displaced from one feared object to an associated one, that is, from an unconscious feared object or situation to a conscious, and therefore avoidable, object or situation (Hughes, 1999).

Behavioural theories

The reproduction of phobic-like reactions in the laboratory led to the popularity of conditioning theories for the development of phobias. In their famous case of 'Albert', Watson & Rayner (1920) demonstrated that an 11-month-old child with a positive interest in furry animals developed a fear of rats after a steel bar was struck, making a loud noise, whenever he put out his hand towards a white rat. This case was not replicated, however, and the theory of a straightforward relationship between the genesis of phobias and classical conditioning was modified by other workers, who commented on individual differences in the susceptibility to aversive stimuli (e.g. Pavlov, 1927). Eysenck (1957) suggested that individuals who condition easily are more likely to develop phobias. Other workers emphasised that the intensity and amount of reinforcement following any action also has an effect on the degree of conditioning that takes place (Spence *et al*, 1958).

Early in the development of behavioural treatments for phobias, Mowrer's (1950) view of fear acquisition was widely accepted as the model for the development of clinical phobias. According to this view, classically conditioned fear leads to avoidance behaviour. Avoidance leads to a reduction of fear and thus the avoidance behaviour is reinforced by a reduction in anxiety.

This model, however, was soon to be challenged. First, it was acknowledged that phobic patients are often unable to recall traumatic experiences relating to the onset of their phobia (Buglass *et al*, 1977; Goldstein & Chambless, 1978). Second, several workers had failed to replicate Watson & Rayner's (1920) experiment (English, 1929; Thorndike, 1935). Third, the model did not fit with the gradual onset of phobias usually seen in clinical practice (Emmelkamp, 1985). Finally, it did not explain the common stereotyped patterns of fear-provoking objects and situations.

In a series of laboratory-based experiments with adult volunteers, Ohman *et al* (1984) demonstrated that humans are much more likely to be aversively conditioned to phylogenetically old, fear-relevant stimuli (e.g. snakes and spiders) than to neutral stimuli (e.g. flowers and mushrooms). This led Marks (1969) to propose the concept of 'prepotency'. Prepotency is the tendency for a particular species to attend preferentially to certain stimuli of evolutionary importance rather than to other, evolutionary unimportant stimuli, even when encountered for the first time. Seligman's concept of preparedness extended this evolutionary model further. Preparedness refers to the idea that certain stimuli are more likely to be associated with each other and with certain responses (Seligman, 1971).

Is blood/injection/injury phobia separate from other phobias?

Blood/injection/injury phobia is one of the most interesting phobias. Not only is it difficult to judge the prevalence of the condition (as people who have it tend, by definition, to avoid medical personnel) but the autonomic response to the phobic stimulus is different from that in other phobias. Whereas many phobic patients fear that they may faint in their phobic situation, this actually rarely happens, as the sympathetic response and increased cardiac output prevents fainting. In blood/injection/injury phobia, however, the vaso-vagal reaction frequently does cause fainting (Bienvenu & Eaton, 1998). Presumably this makes sense in evolutionary terms because, whereas with most threatening situations a fight or flight reaction is necessary for survival, once injury is realised, or at least inevitable, a reduction in cardiac output is more likely to be life-saving. Patients with blood/injection/injury phobia demonstrate this response in an exaggerated form. It is therefore important to ensure that any patient with this condition is exposed to phobic stimuli only when lying down, otherwise injury from falling could occur.

Behavioural overview

Overall, the behavioural view of the genesis of phobic disorder is that individuals vary in trait anxiety and susceptibility to conditioning. Phobias are an almost universal experience in childhood but generally pass with age. In some individuals these fears persist. Many sufferers have a family history of phobic disorder, and genetic factors as well as modelling by close family members may be implicated in the development of the phobia. Once a phobia has developed, the patient will tend to escape from the fear-provoking situation. This escape causes the anxiety to abate. Because high anxiety is extremely unpleasant, the reduction in anxiety resulting from escape is like a reward and reinforces the escape behaviour. Thus, every episode of short-lived exposure followed by escape serves to strengthen the phobic escape and avoidance behaviour.

In the case of social anxiety disorder, if children are unduly restricted (e.g. by anxious parents) and are not given the opportunity to engage in social interactions, they may not acquire the necessary skills for later life. Thus, family attitudes may reinforce avoidant behaviours and make the disorder worse (Beidel, 1998).

Cognitive theories

In the cognitive model of phobic anxiety developed by Aaron T. Beck in the USA, it is not the stimulus or the situation that causes the anxiety but the patient's expectations and interpretation of the situation (Beck & Emery, 1985). Clark (1988) developed this model further with the cognitive model of panic. In this model, once patients feel anxious they may focus on specific physical symptoms of anxiety. If these symptoms are interpreted as evidence of a bad event, the anxiety is further increased. This, in turn, leads to exacerbation of the anxiety symptoms.

Case example

A 50-year-old man had a fear that he might drop dead from a myocardial infarct. While standing in a supermarket queue, he noticed that his pulse was rapid. He viewed this as evidence that something was wrong with his heart and that he may experience a myocardial infarct at any moment. Unsurprisingly, this thought led to heightened anxiety and an even faster pulse, and thus a vicious circle of anxiety was established. It is easy to see how this unpleasant experience led to the man fleeing homeward and subsequently avoiding situations linked to the anxiety.

Patients with social anxiety disorder experience social situations as threatening, and this activates the brain mechanisms involved in generating anxiety. The negative cognitions associated with social exposure, including feelings of self-consciousness, humiliation and failure, may also feed into the anxiety mechanism. Anxiety results in cortisol release and stimulates the autonomic nervous system, producing the characteristic somatic symptoms of blushing, sweating and tremor. These physical symptoms serve to reinforce the discomfort even further. Thus, a positive feedback loop develops that may amplify the level of anxiety to such unbearable levels that the individual flees from the situation and learns to avoid similar situations in the future.

Sociological theories

The nature versus nurture debate depends on whether it is believed that children inherit their phobias from a parent or whether they are learned. There are no adoption studies of parents with phobic disorder to answer this question. However, it seems to many clinicians working with phobic patients that trait anxiety levels and ease of conditioning are inherited. The type and the extent of the fear are probably linked directly to environmental factors.

Treatment of phobias

Behavioural psychotherapy

The behavioural treatment of phobic disorders is prolonged, graduated exposure in real life to the feared situation. It is based on the understanding that patients with phobias have learned to escape or avoid fear-provoking phobic situations. This avoidance and escape behaviour strengthens the association between the stimulus and anxiety. In therapeutic exposure, the patient is asked to stay in a previously agreed fear-provoking situation until the anxiety engendered by the stimulus reduces by at least half. This process takes approximately 1 hour and the reduction in anxiety is called habituation.

Most patients with handicapping phobias are not willing or able to engage immediately with the most feared object or situation. For this reason, the patient and the therapist need to work out a hierarchy of different exposure situations. For example, a woman with a severe spider phobia may find that sitting in a room with a spider would cause maximal anxiety – scoring 8 on a 0–8 scale of anxiety. Saying the word 'spider' may be given an anxiety rating of 2 on the same scale. A drawing of a spider may be rated 4, a photograph of a spider 5, a moving film image of a spider 6 and a spider in an enclosed jar 7. Once this has been established the patient and therapist need to agree an initial exposure task that will cause the patient to experience anxiety, but at a level that he or she feels able to tolerate.

Once the patient has performed the first exposure task and experienced habituation of the anxiety, the same task needs to be repeated regularly by the patient as self-exposure homework. This should ideally be performed three times a day but at least daily. The patient should find that, on repeated exposure, the anxiety is progressively lessened and also lasts for progressively shorter periods. Once the first stage has been conquered, the patient is moved on to the next task in the hierarchy.

The most effective exposure has been shown to be:

1 prolonged rather than of short duration (Stern & Marks, 1973)

2 in real life rather than in fantasy (Emmelkamp & Wessels, 1975)

3 regularly practised, with self-exposure homework tasks (McDonald *et al*, 1978).

Although exposure treatment sounds time-consuming, it can be cost efficient, as patients perform much of the therapy themselves. In a study of the treatment of agoraphobia by Mathews *et al* (1981) the total therapist time used was only 7 hours.

Many patients with mild to moderate phobias can treat themselves using self-exposure and regular monitoring by either a therapist or even a specially written computer program (Ghosh *et al*, 1988). Examples of self-help manuals include the time-tested *Living with Fear* (Marks, 1979).

Therapists can easily learn the skills required to administer an exposure programme or to advise patients on self-exposure by reading one of the practical guides to therapy (e.g. Stern & Drummond, 1991) and by obtaining supervision from a registered behavioural psychotherapist.

Behavioural treatment of social anxiety disorder

The type of exposure therapy described above may not be effective for all cases of social anxiety.

Exposure therapy should be effective in cases of discrete social anxiety, where individuals are fearful of only a small component of social activity (e.g. public speaking or eating in public), and where they have otherwise developed appropriate social skills.

In cases of generalised fear of all social situations, however, the patient may have avoided social contact for many years, to the extent that normal adult social skills have not been developed. For these socially maladroit individuals, if exposure therapy is used alone, the feedback from other people may be so discouraging that it reinforces the patient's fear and promotes further avoidance. In these cases it is helpful to include social skills training before attempting real-life exposure to social situations.

Social skills training

Social skills training may be undertaken individually or in a group. If group treatment is offered, it is important that all members of the group have approximately similar levels of skill or else it can be disheartening for those with less or more skill. Social skills training involves:

1 identifying a new skill to be learned

2 watching the skill being performed by someone else

3 practising the new skill

4 receiving feedback on performance

5 trying out the new skill in real life.

An excellent account of the treatment of social anxiety disorder, including the development of new social skills, is given on the website of the Clinical Research Unit for Anxiety and Depression of the University of New South Wales (http://www.crufad.com).

Cognitive therapy

Exposure therapy is successful for most patients with anxiety disorders. However, cognitive therapy may have a place in treating those patients who have failed to respond to exposure therapy or who cannot or are unwilling to enter exposure situations because of their extreme fear.

Cognitive therapy requires more therapist training than exposure therapy.

The type of cognitive therapy that has been described for use with phobic patients is that developed by Beck & Emery (1985). Faulty negative automatic thoughts that cause the patient to feel anxious are identified and challenged by the patient and therapist working collaboratively.

Patients with social anxiety disorder may benefit more from cognitive therapy than those with other phobic disorders. They often learn a number of safety behaviours, designed to guard against the feared situation.

Case example

A young woman is concerned that she may faint in a public place. She has developed a pattern of continually flexing her calf muscles in social situations. Normal exposure to social situations will not result in habituation because this safety behaviour is a form of avoidance. In cognitive therapy she is encouraged to face social situations without performing the safety behaviour.

With some patients it is necessary to use cognitive techniques to encourage an individual to abandon safety behaviours (Wells & Papageorgiou, 1995).

Safety behaviours are also found in some agoraphobic patients.

Case example

An agoraphobic woman would travel on a bus only when carrying her handbag. This bag always contained smelling salts in case she felt faint, mint sweets in case she felt sick, sunglasses in case she found it too bright and a bottle of unopened diazepam tablets which had been prescribed 2 years earlier in case she panicked.

Again, explanation of the maintaining role of such safety behaviour may be sufficient for such patients to instigate effective exposure, or they may need some initial cognitive work.

Comparing outcomes of psychotherapy

Exposure treatment has been shown to be effective in 66% of patients with agoraphobia (Mathews *et al*, 1981) and highly effective for patients with a variety of specific and social phobias (Marks, 1981). A naturalistic study of patients with agoraphobia failed to show any benefit of cognitive sessions in addition to exposure therapy (Burke *et al*, 1997).

A study in the Netherlands examined patients with generalised social anxiety disorder and compared social skills training with cognitive therapy, both given in a group setting (van Dam-Baggen & Kraaimaat, 2000). Both treatments resulted in improvement, but the authors concluded that group social skills training was easier to manage.

Targeted cognitive techniques probably have a role in overcoming specific problems for individual patients. For example, cognitive therapy can be used to alter faulty beliefs and self-judgement in social anxiety (Marks, 1995; Coupland, 2001). Clark's (1988) model of panic and treatment using hyperventilation and cognitive therapy can be used for some patients with agoraphobia and panic.

Nowadays, few psychoanalytically trained therapists would advocate their treatment for patients with a phobia. There are therefore no outcome studies on this type of intervention.

Although the treatment literature for cognitive and behavioural forms of treatment is encouraging, with follow-up studies suggesting sustained improvement in the majority of cases, longitudinal evaluation has revealed a typical clinical course characterised by episodes of well-being interspersed with periods of setback (Burns *et al*, 1986).

Pharmacological treatments

The goals of pharmacotherapy are (Davidson, 1998):

1 to reduce symptoms (i.e. fearful cognitions, anticipatory anxiety and apprehension)

2 to reduce avoidance behaviour

3 to reduce the autonomic and physiological symptoms of anxiety

4 to produce improved social, occupational and emotional function

5 to lessen impairment

6 to produce a concomitant improvement in quality of life.

The considerable literature on the drug treatment of the phobic disorders is almost exclusively confined to the treatment of social anxiety disorder and also agoraphobia with panic. This is because these are the most handicapping and common of the phobic disorders, which are also less reliably responsive to psychological treatments.

Drug treatment of panic disorder and agoraphobia

Most of the data relating to the drug treatment of agoraphobia derives from studies of panic disorder and agoraphobia. As early as 1964, Donald Klein, in his seminal studies, demonstrated the benefit of imipramine in reducing panic attacks (Klein, 1964), while the positive effects of monoamine oxidase inhibitors (MAOIs) were observed in a series of studies from 1959 to 1981 (reviewed by Rosenberg, 1999). In 1980, Sheehan *et al* reported improvements in patients with agoraphobia and panic attacks on treatment with the classical MAOI phenelzine (Sheehan *et al*, 1980).

According to the influential theory of Klein, the core symptom of panic disorder is the recurrent panic attack, which may be either spontaneous or triggered by phobic stimuli. Anticipatory anxiety and agoraphobia are considered secondary phenomena, following the experience of panic attacks. It is easy to understand, therefore, that while pharmacological studies provide substantial information on the effects of drug treatments of panic, the differential effects on other symptoms in the cluster, such as the agoraphobia, are less well defined.

In view of the large placebo effect associated with treating panic and agoraphobia, only data derived from randomised controlled studies stand up to scrutiny. Outcome measures need to include ratings of anticipatory anxiety, phobic avoidance and global improvement, as well as panic attacks.

Tricyclic antidepressants, MAOIs, benzodiazepines and SSRIs have all been subjected to controlled study and found to be effective in reducing panic and agoraphobia in well-defined patient groups.

Tricyclic antidepressants

Among the tricyclic antidepressants, imipramine and clomipramine have been studied the most. Both appear to be effective at improving the whole range of symptoms, including panic attacks, agoraphobia and anticipatory anxiety, independently of their antidepressant effects (e.g. Cross National Collaborative Panic Study; Klerman, 1988). Agoraphobia was noted to accompany the more severe cases of panic disorder, and these cases responded better to drug treatment than cases of uncomplicated panic, which suggests that the ICD–10 classification separating agoraphobia with panic attacks from simple panic disorder may be correct (Maier *et al*, 1991). Meta-analyses (e.g. Wilkinson *et al*, 1991) have demonstrated a moderate but clinically meaningful effect size for tricyclics, with a larger response observed for clomipramine in many studies, suggesting that drugs with serotonergic effects may be more effective.

An early drug-induced exacerbation of panic has been observed in up to 20% of cases, and is thought to be dose related. One way of minimising this problem is to warn the patient and to start at the lowest available daily dose for the first week of treatment, thereafter titrating up gradually over several weeks to the therapeutic level.

MAOIs

The MAOIs are claimed to be effective, but the evidence from controlled studies supporting either the classical compounds or the newer, reversible MAOIs is slim. Their main mode of action may be on agoraphobia, rather than panic. Unfortunately, a large study on moclobemide was compromised by an excessively large placebo response (reviewed by Rosenberg, 1999).

Benzodiazepines

Benzodiazepines were once regarded as ineffective in panic disorder, but studies using higher daily doses, equivalent to 50 mg diazepam, have demonstrated efficacy in the short and long term. Most evidence exists for the triazolobenzodiazepine alprazolam, but positive findings have also been reported for clonazepam and diazepam (reviewed by Burrows *et al*, 1990, 1991).

In the Cross National Collaborative Panic Study (Klerman, 1988), alprazolam was seen to act rapidly in alleviating anxiety, with half the eventual improvement occurring within the first week of treatment. This contrasted with the slower, more gradual response seen with antidepressants. Moreover, alprazolam was seen to maintain its efficacy for the whole range of symptoms in a subgroup of individuals treated over 32 weeks under double-blind conditions, without evidence of therapeutic tolerance to the drug (Burrows *et al*, 1992). However, side-effects included sedation, ataxia and fatigue, and even when drugs are tapered slowly, many patients experience a withdrawal syndrome when the drugs are discontinued (Burrows *et al*, 1991).

These factors preclude their use as first-line treatments. They may be best utilised as adjuncts to SSRIs for a short period (e.g. during the first 2–4 weeks of SSRI treatment), as an antidote to SSRI-induced anxiety and insomnia (see below).

SSRIs

An extensive body of evidence supports SSRIs as the first-line pharmacological treatment for panic disorder and agoraphobia (reviewed by Ballenger, 1999). They are as effective as tricyclics but are not associated with the same burden of side-effects and show very good safety in overdosage.

Like the other antidepressants, SSRIs produce their positive effects slowly, that is, over several weeks, and may temporarily aggravate panic and anxiety in the first 1–2 weeks of treatment. The mechanism underlying this effect is intriguing but still poorly understood. It is recommended, therefore, to warn patients and start treatment at lower doses (e.g. half the minimum recommended dose for the first week) and gradually to titrate upwards thereafter.

Paroxetine has been the most extensively studied of this class of agents, and the results confirm that it continues to improve panic attacks, anticipatory anxiety, agoraphobia and functional disability over a whole year of treatment (LeCrubier *et al*, 1997). A relapse-prevention study investigated treatment responders on paroxetine using a double-blind drug-discontinuation design (Judge *et al*, 1996). The results showed that, over 3 months, only 5% (2/43) relapsed if they remained on paroxetine, compared with 30% (11/37) of those randomised to placebo. A fixed-dose study has established 40 mg as the optimum daily dose (Ballenger *et al*, 1998*b*).

Convincing data for the efficacy of sertraline, fluvoxamine and citalopram in the treatment of panic and agoraphobia also exist, implying efficacy for SSRIs as a class.

Long-term treatment

Panic disorder with or without agoraphobia is recognised as a chronic, enduring illness, and treatment needs to be long term in many cases. Roy-Byrne & Cowley (1994) reviewed the outcome of modern treatments and concluded that, whereas most patients improve, few are cured. Long-term treatment does not appear to lead to loss of efficacy, but after drug discontinuation high rates of relapse are encountered, suggesting medication needs to continue long term. If the drug is to be discontinued, gradual dose tapering over several weeks may be preferable, in order to minimise withdrawal effects and observe for signs of relapse.

Drug treatment of social anxiety disorder

As there is no single scale that measures all the relevant parameters for social anxiety, treatment studies have combined measures, such as the clinician-evaluated Liebowitz Social Anxiety Scale for symptoms (Liebowitz, 1997), the patient-evaluated Sheehan Disability Scale for Functionality (Sheehan, 1983), and a Clinical Global Impression/Improvement scale for general well-being. Most of the pharmacological studies have focused on the more severe forms of generalised social anxiety.

SSRIs

A substantial body of controlled data supports the efficacy of SSRIs, including paroxetine, sertraline and fluvoxamine. Extensive evidence, derived from large-scale randomised controlled studies, including long-term studies, is available on the treatment of generalised social anxiety disorder (Davidson, 1998). Paroxetine, for example, has been shown to reduce fear and anxiety over a 12-week treatment period, to the extent that 45–65% of patients reported being 'much' or 'very much improved'. A positive improvement in social functioning was also reported, representing significantly improved quality of life. On the strength of these data, SSRIs are now recommended as the first-line treatment for social anxiety (Ballenger *et al*, 1998*a*; Nutt *et al*, 1999*a*).

Treatment response may occur within 4 weeks of starting treatment, but in some cases may be delayed for several months before the full benefit is realised, and doses may need to be titrated up to the maximum for optimal efficacy.

Discontinuation studies show that patients who have responded to treatment are more likely to relapse if they are switched to placebo than if they are allowed to remain on active treatment. It is recommended, therefore, that patients continue taking treatment, as long as it is effective, for at least 12 months. Longer-term treatment is advisable if the patient remains symptomatic, or if there is a history of relapse or early onset of the disorder (Ballenger *et al*, 1998*a*).

MAOIs

The earliest placebo-controlled evidence for MAOIs was obtained for phenelzine, but the side-effect profile associated with this agent precludes its regular use as a first-line treatment. Placebo-controlled studies of moclobemide have also shown efficacy for this compound (reviewed by Nutt *et al*, 1999*b*), although its clinical effects may be rather weak and doses may need to be increased to the upper ranges for optimum effect.

Benzodiazepines

Limited but well-controlled data support the efficacy of clonazepam, but the only controlled study, of alprazolam, suggested its efficacy is modest (reviewed by Davidson, 1998). In view of their side-effect profile and dependence-producing actions when used in the long term, they are not recommended as a first-line intervention for social anxiety disorder.

Beta-blockers

Although beta-blockers are frequently used by performance artists to attenuate autonomic symptoms of anxiety, such as tachycardia and tremor, there is no evidence that this class of drugs has efficacy in generalised forms of social anxiety disorder. For example, in one study of 72 patients, atenolol was no different from placebo (Turner *et al*, 1994).

Other medications

There are no controlled studies supporting the efficacy of tricyclic antidepressants in social anxiety disorder, and this serves to distinguish the disorder from panic disorder. Neither is there evidence for buspirone.

Combination treatment for phobic disorders

Both psychological and pharmacological treatments have their benefits and drawbacks. Psychotherapy may be more challenging for the patient and more difficult to come by; its effects may develop more slowly but are likely to endure, and there are no major safety concerns. On the other hand, pharmacotherapy is easily obtained, acts quickly and, in the case of the newer drugs, is also safe and well tolerated, but probably needs to be taken long term to ensure sustained effectiveness (Nutt *et al*, 1999*a*).

In general, patients and therapists find that combining treatments works best in clinical practice, although formal examination of the outcome of this approach is only just being undertaken. Key elements in the psychological approach, including explanation, education and engaging the patient in the therapeutic alliance, are prerequisites for optimising the clinical effect of drug treatment.

Recommended reading

Journal of Clinical Psychiatry (1998) *Focus on Social Anxiety Disorder*. Vol. 59, suppl, 17.

Marks, I. M. (1987) *Fears, Phobias and Rituals*. New York: Oxford University Press.

Nutt, D. J., Ballenger, J. C. & Lepine, J. P. (eds) (1999) *Panic Disorder. Clinical Diagnosis, Management and Mechanisms*. London: Martin Dunitz.

Stern, R. S. & Drummond, L. M. (1991) *The Practice of Behavioural and Cognitive Psychotherapy*. Cambridge: Cambridge University Press.

References

Agras, S., Sylvester, D. & Oliveau, D. (1969) The epidemiology of common fears and phobias. *Comprehensive Psychiatry*, **10**, 151–156.

American Psychiatric Association (1994) *Diagnostic and Statistical Manual of Mental Disorders* (4th edn) (DSM–IV). Washington, DC: APA.

American Psychiatric Association (2000) *Diagnostic and Statistical Manual for Psychiatric Disorders* (4th edn, text revision) (DSM–IV–TR). Washington DC: APA.

Andrews, G. & Slade, T. (2002) Agoraphobia without a history of panic disorder may be part of the panic disorder syndrome. *Journal of Nervous and Mental Disease*, **190**, 624–630.

Baldwin, D. S. & Birtwistle, J. (1998) The side-effect burden with drug treatment of panic disorder. *Journal of Clinical Psychiatry*, **59**, suppl. 8, 39–44.

Ballenger, J. C. (1999) Selective serotonin reuptake inhibitors (SSRIs) in panic disorder. In *Panic Disorder. Clinical Diagnosis, Management and Mechanisms* (eds D. J. Nutt, J. C. Ballenger & J. P. Lepine), pp. 159–178. London: Martin Dunitz.

Ballenger, J. C., Davidson, J. R. T., Lecrubier, Y., *et al* (1998*a*) Consensus statement on social anxiety disorder from the International Consensus Group on Depression and Anxiety. *Journal of Clinical Psychiatry*, **59**, suppl. 17, 54–60.

Ballenger, J. C., Steiner, M., Bushnell, W., *et al* (1998*b*) Double-blind fixed-dose, placebo-controlled study of paroxetine in the treatment of panic disorder. *American Journal of Psychiatry*, **155**, 36–42.

Beck, A. T. & Emery, G. (1985) *Anxiety Disorders and Phobias: A Cognitive Perspective*. New York: Basic Books.

Beidel, D. C. (1998) Social anxiety disorder: etiology and clinical presentation. *Journal of Clinical Psychiatry*, **59**, suppl. 17, 27–31.

Berrios, G. E., Campbell, C., Politynska, B. E., *et al* (1995) Autonomic failure, depression and anxiety in Parkinson's disease. *British Journal of Psychiatry*, **166**, 789–792.

Bienvenu, O. & Eaton, W. W. (1998) The epidemiology of blood-injection-injury phobia. *Psychological Medicine*, **28**, 1129–1136.

Buglass, D., Clarke, J., Henderson, A. S., *et al* (1977) A study of agoraphobic housewives. *Psychological Medicine*, **7**, 73–86.

Burke, M., Drummond, L. M. & Johnson, D. W. (1997) Treatment choice for agoraphobic women: exposure or cognitive–behaviour therapy? *British Journal of Clinical Psychology*, **36**, 409–420.

Burns, L. E., Thorpe, G. L. & Cavallaro, L. A. (1986) Agoraphobia 8 years after behavioral treatment: a follow-up study with interview, self-report, and behavioral data. *Behavior Therapy*, **17**, 580–591.

Burrows, G. D., Norman, T. R., Judd, F. K., *et al* (1990) Short-acting versus long-acting benzodiazepines: discontinuation effects in panic disorders. *Journal of Psychiatric Research*, **24**, suppl. 2, 65–72.

Burrows, G. D., Norman, T. R. & Judd, F. K. (1991) Panic disorder: a treatment update. *Journal of Clinical Psychiatry*, **52**, suppl., 24–26.

Burrows, G. D., Judd, F. K. & Norman, T. R. (1992) Long term drug treatment of panic disorder. *Journal of Psychiatric Research*, **27**, suppl. 1, 111–125.

Clark, D. B., Bukstein, O. G., Smith, M. G., *et al* (1996) Identifying anxiety disorders in adolescents hospitalised for alcohol abuse or dependence. *Psychiatric Services*, **46**, 618–620.

Clark, D. M. (1988) A cognitive model of panic attacks. In *Panic: Psychological Perspectives* (ed. S. Rachman & J. Maser). Hillsdale, NJ: Erlbaum.

Coupland, N. J. (2001) Social phobia: etiology, neurobiology and treatment. *Journal of Clinical Psychiatry*, **62**, suppl. 1, 25–35.

Davidson, J. (1998) Pharmacotherapy of social phobia. *Journal of Clinical Psychiatry*, **59**, suppl. 17, 47–51.

Degonda, M. & Angst, J. (1994) The Zurich study: XX. Social phobia and agoraphobia. *European Archives of Psychiatry and Clinical Neuroscience*, **243**, 95–102.

Emmanuel, N. P., Lydiard, R. P. & Ballenger, J. C. (1991) Treatment of social phobia with buproprion (letter). *Journal of Clinical Psychopharmacology*, **11**, 276–277.

Emmelkamp, P. M. G. (1985) Anxiety and fear. In *International Handbook of Behavior Modification and Therapy* (eds A. S. Bellack, M. Hersen & A. E. Kazdin). New York: Plenum Press.

Emmelkamp, P. M. G. & Wessels, H. (1975) Flooding in imagination v flooding in vivo in agoraphobics. *Behaviour Research and Therapy*, **13**, 7.

English, H. B. (1929) Three cases of the 'conditioned fear response'. *Journal of Abnormal and Social Psychiatry*, **34**, 221–225.

Eysenck, H. J. (1957) *Dynamics of Anxiety and Hysteria*. London: Routledge and Kegan Paul.

Faravelli, C. & Paionni, A. (1999) Panic disorder: clinical course, etiology and prognosis. In *Panic Disorder. Clinical Diagnosis, Management and Mechanisms* (eds D. J. Nutt, J. C. Ballenger & J. P. Lepine), pp. 25–44. London: Martin Dunitz.

Ghosh, A., Marks, I. M. & Carr, A. C. (1988) Therapist contact and outcome of self-exposure treatment for phobias: a controlled study. *British Journal of Psychiatry*, **152**, 234–238.

Goldstein, A. J. & Chambless, D. (1978) A reanalysis of agoraphobia. *Behavior Therapy*, **9**, 47–59.

Goodwin, R. D. (2002) Anxiety disorders and the onset of depression among adults in the community. *Psychological Medicine*, **32**, 1121–1124.

Graeff, F. G., Guimeras, T. S. & De Andrade, T. G. (1996) Role of 5HT in stress, anxiety and depression. *Pharmacology, Biochemistry and Behavior*, **54**, 129–141.

Heimberg, R. G., Hope, D. A., Dodge, C. S., *et al* (1990) DSM–IIIR subtypes of social phobia: comparison of generalised social phobics and public speaking phobics. *Journal of Nervous and Mental Disease*, **178**, 172–179.

Hollander, E., Decaria, C. M., Trungold, S., *et al* (1991) 5HT function and neurology of social phobia. In *New Research Program and Abstracts of the 144th Annual Meeting of the American Psychiatric Association, May 14th, 1991. New Orleans, LA*. Abstract no. 350.

Hughes, P. (1999) *Dynamic Psychotherapy Explained*. Abingdon: Radcliffe Medical Press.

Judge, R., Burnham, D., Steiner, M., *et al* (1996) Paroxetine long-term safety and efficacy in panic disorder and prevention of relapse: a double-blind study. *European Neuropsychopharmacology*, **6**, 26.

Kagan, J. (1997) Temperament and the reactions to unfamiliarity. *Child Development*, **68**, 139–143.

Kendler, K. S., Neale, M. C., Kessler, R. C., *et al* (1992) The genetic epidemiology of phobias in women: the interrelationship of agoraphobia, social phobia, situational phobia and simple phobia. *Archives of General Psychiatry*, **49**, 273–281.

Kendler, K. S., Myers, J., Prescott, C. A., *et al* (2001) The genetic epidemiology of irrational fears and phobias in men. *Archives of General Psychiatry*, **58**, 257–265.

Kessler, R. C. & Wittchen, H. U. (2002) Patterns and correlates of generalized anxiety disorder in community samples. *Journal of Clinical Psychiatry*, **63**, suppl. 8, 4–10.

Kessler, R. C., McGonagle, K. A., Zhao, S., *et al* (1994) Lifetime and 12-month prevalence of DSM–III–R psychiatric disorders in the United States. Results of the Comorbidity Survey. *Archives of General Psychiatry*, **51**, 8–19.

Klein, D. F. (1964) Delineation of two drug-responsive anxiety syndromes. *Psychopharmacologia*, **5**, 397–408.

Klerman, G. L. (1988) Overview of the Cross National Collaborative Panic Study. *Archives of General Psychiatry*, **45**, 407–412.

LeCrubier, Y., Bakker, A., Judge, R., *et al* (1997) A comparison of paroxetine, clomipramine and placebo in the treatment of panic disorder. *Acta Psychiatrica Scandinavica*, **95**, 145–152.

Lepine, J. P. & Lellouch, J. (1995) Diagnosis and epidemiology of agoraphobia and social phobia. *Clinical Neuropharmacology*, **18**, suppl. 2, s15–s26.

Liebowitz, M. R. (1997) Social phobia. *Modern Problems of Pharmacopsychiatry*, **22**, 141–173.

Magee, W. J., Eaton, W. W., Wittchen, H. U., *et al* (1996) Agoraphobia, simple phobia and social phobia in the National Comorbidity Survey. *Archives of General Psychiatry*, **53**, 159–168.

Maier, W., Rosenberg, R., Argyle, N., *et al* (1991) Subtyping panic disorder by major depression and avoidance behaviour and the response to active treatment. *European Archives of Psychiatry and Clinical Neuroscience*, **241**, 22–30.

Marks, I. M. (1969) *Fears and Phobias*. New York: Academic Press.

Marks, I. M. (1979) *Living with Fear*. New York: McGraw-Hill.

Marks, I. M. (1981) *Cure and Care of Neurosis: Theory and Practice of Behavioural Psychotherapy*. New York: Wiley.

Marks, I. M. (1995) Advances in behavioural–cognitive therapy of social phobia. *Journal of Clinical Psychiatry*, **56**, suppl. 5, 25–31.

Mathews, A. M., Gelder, M. G. & Johnston, D. W. (1981) *Agoraphobia: Nature and Treatment*. New York: Guilford Press.

McDonald, R., Sartory, G., Grey, S. J., *et al* (1978) Effects of self-exposure instructions on agoraphobic outpatients. *Behaviour Research and Therapy*, **17**, 83–85.

Mowrer, O. H. (1950) *Learning Theory and Personality Dynamics*. New York: Arnold Press.

Nascimento, I., Nardi, A. E., Valenca, A. M., *et al* (2002) Psychiatric disorders in asthmatic outpatients. *Psychiatry Research*, **110**, 73–80.

Noyes, R., Reich, J., Christiansen, J., *et al* (1990) Outcome of panic disorder. Relationship to diagnostic subtypes and comorbidity. *Archives of General Psychiatry*, **47**, 809–818.

Nutt, D. J., Bell, C. J. & Malizia, A. L. (1998) Brain mechanisms of social anxiety disorder. *Journal of Clinical Psychiatry*, **59**, suppl. 17, 4–9.

Nutt, D. J., Ballenger, J. C. & Lepine, J. P. (1999*a*) Overview and future prospects. In *Panic Disorder. Clinical Diagnosis, Management and Mechanisms* (eds D. J. Nutt, J. C. Ballenger & J. P. Lepine), pp. 221–228. London: Martin Dunitz.

Nutt, D., Baldwin, D., Beaumont, G., *et al* (1999*b*) Guidelines for the management of social phobia/social anxiety disorder. *Primary Care Psychiatry*, **5**, 147–155.

Ohman, A., Dimberg, U. & Ost, L.-G. (1984) Animal and social phobias: biological constraints on learned fear responses. In *Theoretical Issues in Behavior Therapy* (eds S. Reiss & R. R. Bootzin). New York: Academic Press.

Pavlov, I. P. (1927) *Conditioned Reflexes*. London: Academic Press.

Price, C. J. & Friston, K. J. (1997) Cognitive conjunction: a new approach to brain activation experiments. *Neuroimage*, **5**, 261–270.

Rosenberg, R. (1999) Treatment of panic disorder with tricyclics and MAOIs. In *Panic Disorder. Clinical Diagnosis, Management and Mechanisms* (eds D. J. Nutt, J. C. Ballenger & J. P. Lepine), pp. 125–144. London: Martin Dunitz.

Roy-Byrne, P. P. & Cowley, D. S. (1994) Course and outcome in panic disorder: a review of recent follow-up studies. *Anxiety*, **1**, 151–160.

Seligman, M. E. P. (1971) Phobias and preparedness. *Behavior Therapy*, **2**, 307–320.

Sheehan, D. V. (1983) *The Anxiety Disease*. New York: Schreiber.

Sheehan, D. V., Ballenger, J. C., Jacobsen, G., *et al* (1980) Treatment of endogenous anxiety with phobic, hysterical and hypochondriacal symptoms. *Archives of General Psychiatry*, **37**, 51–59.

Spence, K. G., Haggard, P. F. & Ross, L. G. (1958) UCS intensity and the associated (habit) strength of the eyelid CR. *Journal of Experimental Psychology*, **95**, 404–411.

Stein, M. B., Chartier, M. J., Hazen, A. L., *et al* (1998) A direct-interview family study of generalised social phobia. *American Journal of Psychiatry*, **155**, 90–97.

Stern, R. S. & Drummond, L. M. (1991) *The Practice of Behavioural and Cognitive Psychotherapy*. Cambridge: Cambridge University Press.

Stern, R. S. & Marks, I. M. (1973) Brief and prolonged flooding: a comparison in agoraphobic patients. *Archives of General Psychiatry*, **28**, 270–276.

Tancer, M. E. (1993) Neurobiology of social phobia. *Journal of Clinical Psychiatry*, **54**, suppl. 12, 26–30.

Thorndike, E. L. (1935) *The Psychology of Wants, Interests and Attitudes*. London: Appleton-Century.

Tiihonen, J., Kuikka, J., Bergstrom, K., *et al* (1997) Dopamine reuptake site densities in patients with social phobia. *American Journal of Psychiatry*, **154**, 239–242.

Turner, S. M., Beidel, D. C. & Jacob, R. G. (1994) Social phobia: a comparison of behaviour therapy and atenolol. *Journal of Consulting and Clinical Psychology*, **62**, 350–358.

van Dam-Baggen, R. & Kraaimaat, F. (2000) Group social skills training or cognitive group therapy as the clinical treatment of choice for generalised social phobia. *Journal of Anxiety Disorders*, **14**, 437–451.

Watson, J. B. & Rayner, R. (1920) Conditioned emotional reactions. *Journal of Experimental Psychology*, **3**, 1–14.

Wells, A. & Papageorgiou, C. (1995) Worry and the incubation of intrusive images following stress. *Behavioural Research and Therapy*, **33**, 579–583.

Westenberg, H. M. (1998) The nature of social anxiety disorder. *Journal of Clinical Psychiatry*, **59**, suppl. 17, 20–24.

Wilkinson, G., Balestrieri, M., Ruggeri, M., *et al* (1991) Meta-analysis of double-blind placebo-controlled trials of antidepressants and benzodiazepines for patients with panic disorders. *Psychological Medicine*, **21**, 991–998.

Wittchen, H. U. & Beloch, E. (1996) The impact of social phobia on quality of life. *International Clinical Psychopharmacology*, **11**, suppl, 3, 15–23.

World Health Organization (1992) *Tenth Revision of the International Classification of Diseases and Related Health Problems* (ICD–10). Geneva: WHO.

CHAPTER 15

Obsessive–compulsive disorder

Lynne M. Drummond and Naomi A. Fineberg

Historical perspective

Our conceptualisation of obsessive–compulsive disorder (OCD), alongside that of other common mental disorders, has developed throughout history according to prevailing attitudes. Medieval religious explanations for obsessive blasphemous thoughts, based on demoniacal possession, had been superseded by a more humane understanding by the time of Shakespeare, whose description of Lady Macbeth trying to purge guilty memories by compulsive hand-washing remains one of the most compelling descriptions of the syndrome to date.

In the 19th century, recognisable descriptions of OCD began to appear in the European medical literature, initially linking the disorder with 'melancholia'. By the beginning of the 20th century, with the development of psychoanalysis, the focus shifted onto unconscious conflicts as an explanation (see below), but this approach did not prove useful for treatment, and OCD gained a reputation as a particularly treatment-refractory condition.

One of the first full descriptive accounts of OCD in the British medical literature was by Professor Sir Aubrey Lewis, in which he emphasised the importance of unwanted thoughts that came into the patient's mind but were actively resisted by the patient (Lewis, 1935).

The introduction of learning theory in the 1960s and 1970s provided a practical strategy for treating individuals with OCD that seemed to work. The concurrent development of effective medical treatments triggered a dramatic expansion of scientific interest in OCD in the last two decades of the 20th century, which continues today. Burgeoning research into the epidemiology, psychopharmacology, neurobiology, neuropsychology and genetics of OCD has redefined OCD as a common, treatable, major mental disorder.

Diagnosis

Current classification

DSM–IV (American Psychiatric Association, 1994) approaches the definition of OCD by dividing it into obsessions and compulsions.

Obsessions are intrusive and unwanted thoughts, images or impulses which cause anxiety or distress and which the patient tries, at least in the early stages of the illness, to resist. These emotionally charged thoughts are recognised as being a product of the patient's own mind but are seen as contrary to his or her wishes or personality (i.e. they are 'egodystonic'). Examples include a parent thinking of harming a loved child or a religious person having blasphemous thoughts.

The sufferer may try very hard not to have the obsession. This in itself can lead to an increased frequency and intensity of the thought. The reader can try this out by carrying out a simple experiment of self-observation: put this book down and try to think about anything at all *except* a pink hippopotamus. Most people will immediately have the visual image of a pink hippopotamus when attempting this exercise, illustrating how hard it is to dismiss a 'forbidden' thought. Obsessional thoughts have a much greater persistency and are thus much more difficult to dismiss.

Compulsions may be either overt actions or covert 'neutralising' thoughts. These are activities designed to reduce the anxiety caused by the obsessional thought or to 'put the thought right' in some way. For example, a person with an obsession that he or she has been contaminated by a dreaded disease may compulsively wash to 'undo' the contamination; a minister plagued by blasphemous obsessions may have to repeat a stereotyped prayer to 'undo' or neutralise the obsession. These activities, however, are either not in reality linked with the fear (e.g. a spinster with thoughts of having sex with strangers in a shop may have the compulsion to wash her hands repeatedly) or they are clearly excessive. For example, a man with the obsession that his home may be burgled may check that he has locked the front door 25 times.

ICD–10 (World Health Organization, 1992) also divides the problem into obsessions, defined as thoughts, ideas or images, and compulsions. It states that although the compulsive urge is alien to the patient's personality, it is perceived as originating from the mind of the patient, not from outside. It also emphasises that carrying out the obsessive thought or compulsive act is not, itself, pleasurable.

DSM–IV prioritises anxiety as a core symptom, and classifies OCD together with the anxiety disorders, even though OCD shares few features with the other disorders in this group. ICD–10, in contrast, has followed a European tradition by defining OCD as a 'stand-alone' disorder, and has placed it in the category of neurotic, stress-related and somatoform disorders. Further separation of OCD may well occur in the future, as more neurobiological and epidemiological evidence places the disorder at the core of a spectrum of so-called 'OCD-related' disorders, such as hypochondriasis, body dysmorphic disorder, depersonalisation disorder and tic disorders.

In both DSM–IV and ICD–10, having either disabling obsessions or compulsions (or both) will satisfy the criteria for a diagnosis. ICD–10 applies a more rigorous threshold, requiring the symptoms to be present for most days over a 2-week period. Resistance to the symptoms need not always be present, and in chronic cases patients sometimes find that active resistance makes the symptoms worse.

Common symptoms

Most patients with OCD experience a mixture of different obsessions and compulsions. Excessive or unrealistic fears about contamination are consistently reported as the commonest form of obsession, and are usually accompanied by washing or cleaning compulsions and avoidance of situations that might lead to contamination. These patients may, for example, find it difficult to attend the hospital out-patient clinic. Other common obsessions include the irrational fear that harm will befall oneself or one's loved one, obsessions relating to aspects of the body being diseased or disfigured, and pathological doubts (see below). These obsessions are commonly linked to repetitive checking behaviours, which may extend to asking family members or doctors for help or reassurance. An overwhelming need for orderliness or symmetry is another common symptom that links itself to tidying and arranging compulsions. Unwelcome or perverse sexual obsessions can be particularly distressing and embarrassing, to the extent that sufferers may be reluctant to divulge these symptoms for fear of being labelled as a sexual deviant. Key themes have been identified that underlie most obsessions. These include abnormal assessment of risk, excessive doubt and the need for completeness.

Obsessions without compulsions may occur, but careful examination in most cases identifies some form of compulsion, possibly performed covertly (Salkovskis, 1985).

Case example

A 40-year-old man presented with a 20-year history of incapacitating ruminations concerning homosexuality. He spent roughly 10 hours a day ruminating and had been unable to work or socialise because of his problem. Although initially reluctant to discuss his ruminations, he eventually admitted that he had worries that he might have touched men's bottoms. This had led him to worry that he was homosexual, despite the fact that he had been married for 15 years and had no homosexual fantasies or experience. Whenever he was near another man he would think that he might have touched him on the bottom. This made him feel anxious. He would then have the urge to try to relive in his mind every movement he had made since first seeing the man to check that he had not touched the man's bottom. Although this checking reduced his anxiety a little, he would soon doubt his recall and repeat the checking activity several times.

From this example it can be seen that the obsessional thought was 'I have touched his bottom', which was followed by repeated covert checking compulsions. Because these compulsions took the form of mentally visualising his own actions, they could easily have been overlooked if the patient had not been asked to report exactly what went through his mind.

Some obsessions take the form of obsessional images. In the previous example, another man might have the mental image of himself actually touching another man's bottom.

Compulsions without obsessions have also been described. Many of these patients have suffered from OCD for several decades and it appears that the original obsession, or reason for performing the compulsion, has been lost over time. The compulsions, therefore, seem to persist as a form of habit.

Patients with obsessional slowness appear to have pure compulsive activity without a history of obsessions (Rachman, 1976). These patients take several hours to get up, get dressed or have a bath. They deny any clear obsessional thoughts that lead to this extreme difficulty.

Case example

A 24-year-old man had a 10-year history of slowness. Washing and shaving in the morning took between 2 and 5 hours to complete, so that he felt unable even to attempt to get up and dressed. Initially he would spend an hour going over in his mind the activities he was going to perform. Following this he set out all the objects he was going to use in advance. He would put his razor on the shelf and then stand and stare at it for several minutes before picking it up and putting it down again. This placing of objects and repetition could continue for as much as an hour. Once this was completed, the actual actions of shaving and washing were similarly methodically performed, with each action being followed by close scrutiny, prolonged periods of thought and repetition.

Although patients with obsessional slowness deny obsessional thoughts, the motivation for their slowness is usually an effort to ensure that everything they do is performed perfectly. By aiming at perfection, they constantly fail and thus have to try harder, which takes increasingly longer.

A frequent experience is that of obsessional doubt. This is the subjective feeling of doubt that an action has been performed, even though the person knows that he or she has done it.

Case example

A man had obsessions that his house might burn down. On leaving the house he would check all the electrical switches and gas taps. Immediately after the compulsive checking, he had doubts that he had checked everything properly and therefore repeated the checks many times. On one level he knew that he had checked everything but he felt he could not trust his memory. Such repetition can be understood in terms of the temporary anxiety-reducing effect of compulsive rituals.

OCD with poor insight

Patients with OCD usually retain full insight into their symptoms, but this is not always the case. DSM–IV singles out a small group, comprising roughly 5% of patients, with poor insight, as a meaningful subgroup. These cases have a more complex symptom pattern, which can make diagnosis more difficult, and tend to be more severely disabled. They harbour overvalued ideation (Foa, 1979) and have a limited understanding of the irrationality or excessiveness of their behaviour, which makes them difficult to engage in treatment. They may appear to be deluded and hence receive inappropriate antipsychotic treatment, but longitudinal studies show that they do not usually go on to develop schizophrenia.

Differential diagnosis and comorbidity

Mild forms of obsessional behaviour, such as repetitive checking or superstitious acts are common in everyday life, and the diagnosis of OCD should only be made if the symptoms are time-consuming, or associated with impairment or distress.

The diagnostic criteria for OCD carefully specify that the intrusive thoughts associated with the disorder need to be experienced as coming from within the individual's own mind, not imposed from outside, as in cases of schizophrenia.

Recurrent intrusive thoughts, impulses or images also occur in other mental disorders that are thought to share a relationship with OCD, such the preoccupation with bodily appearance in body dysmorphic disorder, with illness in hypochondriasis, or with hair pulling in trichotillomania. The diagnosis of OCD should be made only if there are additional, unrelated obsessions or compulsions, whereupon more than one diagnosis may be warranted.

Other preoccupations, such as with sex, shopping, eating or gambling, are not considered true obsessions or compulsions because they are in keeping with the individual's belief system and may even be enjoyed, any regret being associated with the adverse consequences of the behaviour.

Depression

OCD shares comorbidity with a range of mental disorders, of which depression is the commonest. Its strong association with depression has been noted for many years (Lewis, 1934; Kendell & DiScipio, 1970). A diagnosis of OCD can be made in the presence of comorbid depression as long as the ruminations are not exclusively restricted to depressive themes. In the large US Epidemiologic Catchment Area studies (see below) (Myers *et al*, 1984; Robins *et al*, 1984), one-third of adults with OCD also met DSM criteria for major depression at the time of interview, and three-quarters reported a history of depression at some time during their illness. Moreover, 12% of individuals diagnosed with depression also had a history of OCD. A study of childhood OCD showed that the depression was equally likely to pre-date as to follow the obsessional illness (Swedo *et al*, 1989*a*).

The link between OCD and depression remains poorly understood, and some symptoms usually associated with depression, such as anxiety, lack of pleasure, concentration difficulties and lack of drive, may also be part of OCD. It is thought that some individuals have a vulnerability to both disorders. Given that OCD can be severely disabling, it is not surprising that sufferers become dysphoric to the extent of developing depression. In these cases treatment of the OCD leads to an improvement of both conditions.

Table 15.1 Comparison of obsessive–compulsive disorder (OCD) and phobias

Similarities	Differences
Fear is a core feature	Unlike in phobias, in OCD the fear is not of the situation itself but of its consequences
Avoidance of situations that provoke thoughts, anxiety or rituals	Unlike in phobias, in OCD elaborate belief systems develop around the rituals

Further, many patients are secretive about their OCD and cope for years despite severe obsessional symptoms, and choose to present to their doctor for treatment only when depression supervenes. In these cases it is important that the OCD is not missed, because the depression will respond only if the OCD is treated as well.

OCD and phobic disorder

Phobic disorders can easily be confused with OCD. Important similarities and differences between the two conditions are highlighted in Table 15.1.

Spider phobia is an example of a specific animal phobia where the fear is purely related to the presence of spiders in the vicinity. Contrast this with the following case of OCD.

Case example

Eleanor had a 10-year history of fear of contamination by household dirt with the concern that she might catch diseases which could then be passed on to others and which would result in her feeling responsible for this plague. She viewed spiders as evidence that a place was dusty and 'unclean'. This made her avoid any situations where she had seen spiders in the past. Even if she saw a spider in her garden through the window, she would feel anxious and resort to cleaning rituals, which consisted of stripping off all her clothes, which she considered contaminated, and repeatedly washing them in multiples of four, which she considered a good number.

A spider phobic has an extreme fear of spiders and will avoid any situation that causes him or her to think about spiders. Eleanor's problem is different. Her fear is not of spiders themselves but of the *consequences* that may result from contact with spiders and dust. The development of *elaborate belief systems* in people with OCD is also demonstrated in Eleanor's case, where she performed her stereotyped washing rituals in multiples of four.

Tourette's syndrome

People with Tourette's syndrome (TS) commonly also have OCD (Montgomery *et al*, 1982); estimates range from 35% to 50%. Also, the families of TS sufferers have a raised incidence of OCD (as well as of TS, tics and agoraphobia) (Eapen *et al*, 1997). The incidence of TS in OCD is lower (5–7%), although tics are reported in 20–30% of individuals with OCD. Patients with TS often turn out to be more resistant to conventional treatments.

It can sometimes be difficult to distinguish between compulsive rituals and tics: close questioning about the reasons why movements are performed is required. Compulsions are performed to reduce the anxiety associated with an obsessional idea, whereas tics are performed to reduce discomfort or tension, which is worsened by stress and anxiety.

Obsessive–compulsive (anankastic) and other personality disorders

A colleague once decided to examine the residual personality attributes and symptoms of patients successfully treated by behavioural psychotherapy for OCD. He then made a fatal mistake: for his control group he used medical and psychology students. His findings were that the control group had far more obsessional personalities and more florid obsessive–compulsive symptoms than his patient group.

On reflection, this finding is not surprising. Anankastic or obsessive–compulsive personality disorder (OCPD) is described in DSM–IV as leading to excessive conscientiousness, checking, stubbornness, parsimony and caution, combined with perfectionism and meticulous accuracy. These personality traits can obviously have an advantage in certain careers, and people with an obsessive–compulsive personality are frequently high achievers, entering professions such as medicine, law, accountancy and insurance, as well as the world of the media. Unlike OCD, however, OCPD is compatible with the individual's wishes and temperament, and unacceptable obsessions and compulsions are lacking.

It was traditionally thought that OCD tended to develop in those with pre-existing obsessional personalities. Systematic studies, however, have identified OCPD in only a minority of cases of OCD, with other forms of personality disorder occurring more commonly.

Several famous historical and contemporary personalities are thought to demonstrate not only OCPD but at times florid OCD. John Bunyan, Samuel Johnson, Hans Christian Andersen and Woody Allen have all been suggested to exhibit evidence of OCD (Toates, 1990). Howard Hughes is perhaps the most widely publicised contemporary example. He was a famous film producer, aircraft manufacturer and playboy. However, obsessions about his health and fear of death led him ultimately to live the life of a recluse, living in a bare room with no clothes, eating at starvation levels. Ironically, his obsessional personality had previously contributed to his success in the film and engineering worlds.

Up to 5% of individuals with OCD have a schizotypal personality disorder, which tends to confer a poor prognosis characterised by inadequate social function, poor treatment compliance and poor insight.

Schizophrenia and other psychoses

It is exceptionally rare for patients to present with an apparent OCD that eventually develops into schizophrenia (Black, 1974). These patients are usually young and have previously exhibited schizotypal tendencies, including isolated lifestyles and bizarre fantasies.

A significant minority, estimated at 10–25%, of patients with schizophrenia or other psychoses experience distressing obsessions or compulsions, and these are often the most challenging and severe cases.

Case example

A young, male long-stay in-patient made himself exceedingly unpopular on his ward because of his compulsion to use excessive amounts of toilet paper, which continually blocked the toilets.

Preliminary evidence suggests that the comorbid OCD needs separate treatment, since antipsychotic treatments on their own are generally ineffective.

Anorexia nervosa and bulimia nervosa

The link between obsessive–compulsive symptoms and eating disorders has been recognised for well over 50 years (Palmer & Jones, 1939; DuBois, 1949). Studies looking at people with OCD have reported a high lifetime prevalence of anorexia nervosa and bulimia nervosa, reaching 6–12% (Thiel *et al*, 1995). A review of this subject by Steinhousen & Glanville (1983) showed that obsessive–compulsive traits or symptoms had been reported variously in between 3% and 83% of anorexic patients.

Of course, intrusive thoughts and forced behaviours relating specifically to weight, body size and food intake are integral to the eating disorder, and do not constitute OCD. However, many individuals also have obsessions and compulsions unrelated to food. Thiel *et al* (1995), using standardised rating instruments, showed that 37% of a cohort of 93 anorexic or bulimic females concurrently fulfilled DSM criteria for OCD. Comorbidity correlated positively with the severity of the eating disorder.

Stammering and stuttering

Some individuals have to perform rituals that result in disordered speech patterns. Common examples are patients who need to check that every word they say is totally accurate or patients who may count the number of words in their sentence or letters in their words before uttering them. Careful assessment may be needed to reveal the problem, and patients with speech abnormalities should be screened for obsessional psychopathology.

Epidemiology

The traditional view that OCD is a rare condition (Nemiah, 1985) has been overturned by several recent large-scale epidemiological surveys that have shown a much higher prevalence of the condition worldwide (Weissman *et al*, 1994): a 6-month prevalence of between 1.3% and 2% (Myers *et al*, 1984) and a lifetime prevalence of 1.9% to 3.3% (Karno *et al*, 1988). These surprisingly high rates of disorder could be related to the fact that many people with OCD do not seek medical help but battle alone in the community. Alternatively, high rates for the community survey may be due to the inclusion of some normal people with obsessional symptoms rather than the full-blown syndrome.

Community prevalence studies identify a female: male ratio of around 1.5:1, whereas males predominate in surveys of OCD referrals, reflecting, perhaps, greater severity in males. Women more commonly suffer from compulsive washing and avoidance, whereas men more frequently have checking rituals or ruminations (Noshirvani *et al*, 1991; Drummond, 1993).

The mean age at onset of OCD is earlier than that of depression, at around 20 years. Males tend to develop the illness earlier, with incidence rates peaking in the early teens for males and in the early twenties for females (Rasmussen & Eisen, 1990).

Until recently, OCD was thought to be rare in children, but we now know that it is in fact one of the commonest mental disorders, affecting 1–5% of children and adolescents in community samples (Flament & Cohen, 2001). The clinical pattern mirrors that in adults, and boys tend to develop symptoms earlier than girls.

The course of OCD can vary from a relatively benign form, in which the sufferer experiences occasional, discrete episodes interspersed between symptom-free periods, to a malignant form with unremitting symptoms and substantial social impairment. A remarkable 40-year follow-up study looked at a cohort of 144 individuals who had been treated in hospital for OCD by the investigators, although this was before the development of modern, effective treatments (Skoog & Skoog, 1999). The study found that 60% showed signs of improvement within the first 10 years of hospital admission, rising to 80% by the end of the study, but only 20% achieved full remission: another 60% continued to experience significant symptoms, 10% showed no improvement whatsoever, and 10% had deteriorated. In 60% of cases the type of symptoms had changed over the course of the illness, and 20% of those whose symptoms initially improved subsequently relapsed, sometimes after as long as 20 years of being free of symptoms (and so early recovery does not appear to rule out the possibility of relapse).

In spite of the early onset and chronic, unremitting course of the untreated illness, people with OCD do not usually present for treatment until many years have elapsed, often when they are in early middle age. Poor recognition of the disorder and fear of stigma are likely reasons. Approximately half of all OCD patients who present for treatment are unmarried (Noshirvani *et al*, 1991).

OCD is seen in cultures as diverse as India (Khanna *et al*, 1986) and Hong Kong (Lo, 1967), as well as the Western countries. Religion is thought to play a part in the genesis of some cases; studies have suggested that it is more common in people who have had a strict religious upbringing, although it does not appear to be related to any particular denomination (Rasmussen & Tsuang, 1986; Raphael *et al*, 1996).

Aetiology

There are many theories for the aetiology of OCD. Most of these are not mutually exclusive and a multifactorial aetiology is likely.

Genetics

A genetic component to OCD has been recognised from the earliest descriptions of the disorder. Evidence for the role of genetic factors has come from family aggregation and twin studies.

Familial aggregation

A number of family studies have been performed in OCD (reviewed by Pauls, 2001) and their results demonstrate that OCD runs closely in families. There is a high rate of various types of psychiatric abnormality in the relatives of probands (McGuffin & Reich, 1984) and OCD itself occurs in roughly 10% of the first-degree relatives of patients, compared with 1.9% in controls (Pauls *et al*, 1995).

Familial aggregation of a disorder is a prerequisite for genetic transmission, but it does not prove genetic transmission because the family unit also transmits environmental and cultural influences that shape human development. Twin studies to some extent control for the cultural effects of shared sibship, and give a better indication of heritability.

Twin studies

The twin method involves comparing the rate of concordance for OCD among monozygotic twins with that among dizygotic twins. If the concordance among monozygotic twins is higher, it is taken as evidence of a genetic contribution to the expression of the disorder. Several twin studies have looked at anxiety and 'neuroticism'. They showed a strong likelihood of heritability. Few studies, however, have looked specifically at OCD. Carey & Gottesman (1981) carefully examined 15 pairs of monozygotic and dizygotic twins with OCD and found that 87% of the monozygotic and 47% of the dizygotic twins were concordant for obsessive symptoms or traits, supporting the view that genetic components are implicated.

Further genetic study

Once a genetic basis has been postulated, the next step is to identify the model of genetic transmission, using techniques such as segregation analysis. Three such studies have been applied to OCD (Nicolini *et al*, 1991; Cavallini *et al*, 1998; Alsobrook *et al*, 1999). The results showed that if you take the OCD population altogether, inheritance patterns are hard to model and do not fit any simple Mendelian rule. However, if you select out those families who have many members affected (i.e. that are clearly familial), a pattern of 'mixed model' transmission emerges. This mixed model implies a gene of major effect combined with a multigenic background. Thus, it is likely that there are several genes involved in OCD, and individuals may be more or less affected by a variety of different genetic mechanisms.

Future work, using genetic linkage studies to elucidate the link between particular genes and their products, will allow us to define more clearly the role of genetic factors in the origin of the disorder.

Neurotransmitters

OCD and the serotonin hypothesis

The evidence for an abnormality in serotonin neurotransmission in patients with OCD rests mainly on the results of drug treatment studies, which have consistently shown that drugs with potent inhibitory effects on the neuronal reuptake of serotonin (5-HT) are effective, while anxiolytic and antidepressant agents acting predominantly on other neurotransmitter systems are not.

Clomipramine is a tricyclic antidepressant which acts predominantly by reducing the reuptake of serotonin into the presynaptic neurons following its release into the synaptic cleft. It has only weak actions on noradrenergic neurons, although one of its metabolites is noradrenergic. Many trials have compared clomipramine with placebo as well as other tricyclic drugs, and have consistently shown superiority for clomipramine. For example, clomipramine has been shown to be more effective in OCD than the noradrenergic antidepressants desipramine (Zohar & Insel, 1987) and nortriptyline (Thoren *et al*, 1980).

Since the discovery of clomipramine's efficacy, more selective serotonin reuptake inhibitors (SSRIs), such as fluvoxamine, fluoxetine, paroxetine, sertraline and citalopram, have been extensively investigated and also found to be effective in patients with OCD (see below). Moreover, direct comparison of SSRIs (e.g. fluvoxamine) and noradrenergic drugs (e.g. desipramine) (Goodman *et al*, 1990) also showed superiority for the serotonergic drug.

While these findings point to serotonin being important for recovery, and provide a rationale for further investigation of serotonergic neurotransmission in OCD, we need to be cautious about extrapolating too far from these data. In spite of extensive investigation, the 'serotonin hypothesis' for OCD, which proposes that OCD results from a specific dysfunction in the 5-HT system, remains speculative.

Platelet studies

Platelets have been used as an accessible model for intracerebral neurons *vis-à-vis* reuptake of serotonin, since they possess very similar serotonin transporter and reuptake machinery. Several studies have investigated the platelet serotonin transporter using a variety of radiolabelled ligands. The most recent studies have identified a reduction in the numbers of transporter sites in OCD patients compared with controls. These reductions appear to be state dependent, and are reversed after successful treatment with SSRIs (reviewed by Marazitti, 2001). While we cannot necessarily infer that the same process is occurring in the brain, these findings provide further support for a link between OCD and serotonin neurotransmission.

Pharmacological responses

More than 17 subtypes of serotonin receptor have been identified, and the question of which receptors might be implicated in OCD has been raised.

Besides blocking the serotonin transporter, clomipramine enhances the responsiveness of the postsynaptic 5-HT_{1A} receptor and desensitises the 5-HT_{2C} receptor, whereas SSRIs reduce somatodendritic and terminal autoreceptor responsiveness. These changes are associated with gradually increasing serotonergic neurotransmission across the synapse. The effects are particularly marked in the orbitofrontal cortex, an area strongly implicated in OCD from neuroimaging studies (see below). The anti-obsessional effect of SSRIs has been linked to increasing activation of 5-HT_2 receptors in the orbitofrontal cortex; these effects can be reversed by coadministration of 5-HT antagonists such as metergoline and ritanserin (Benkelfat *et al*, 1989; Ergovesi *et al*, 1992). The preliminary finding in a small number of resistant patients that sumatriptan, an agonist at the 5-$HT_{1B/D}$ autoreceptor, has an anti-obsessional effect hints that this receptor may also play a role in the treatment response.

Pharmacological challenge tests in OCD

This dynamic approach can be used to probe specific neurotransmitter function in OCD. However, to date, the lack of suitably specific agents that are clinically safe has limited its application.

The most frequently employed challenge involves administration of the non-selective 5-HT partial agonist m-chlorophenylpiperazine (m-CPP), which worsened obsessive–compulsive symptoms in some studies (Hollander *et al*, 1988) but not others (Charney *et al*, 1988). In contrast, another non-selective 5-HT agonist, MK212, produced no behavioural effect. The main pharmacological difference between m-CPP and MK212 rests in the latter having no affinity for the 5-$HT_{1B/D}$ receptor, again pointing to a possible role for this receptor in the origin of obsessive–compulsive symptoms.

Neuroendocrine challenge studies, where the endocrinological effects of specific serotonergic agents are calculated as a measure of receptor sensitivity, have also failed to reveal consistent abnormalities in OCD. Reports of enhanced neuroendocrine responses to the 5-HT precursor l-tryptophan and the non-selective agonist d-fenfluramine in untreated people with OCD but no concurrent depression contrast with the blunted responses usually seen in depression, and highlight the neurochemical differences between these disorders (Fineberg *et al*, 1997). These changes could represent a state of heightened serotonin drive underpinning a neurochemical 'coping' mechanism in the face of prevailing obsessions and compulsions, rather than a causative factor for OCD symptoms themselves.

Overall, the data suggest the involvement of the 5-HT_{2A}, 5-HT_{2C} and 5-$HT_{1B/D}$ receptors in the pathophysiology of OCD. Although we cannot rule out the involvement of other subtypes, future studies of these receptors and the intracellular mechanisms they regulate, using more specific ligands, are warranted.

Other neurotransmitters and OCD

Although the evidence linking OCD with serotonin is converging from different avenues of research, it seems unlikely that OCD results exclusively from a dysregulation of serotonin. For example, one-third of cases fail to respond to treatment with SSRIs. Some authorities believe that the disorder is pathophysiologically heterogeneous. McDougle & Goodman (1991), for example, have argued that OCD is mediated by serotonin neurons in most cases, but that for some patients there is an additional pathology in the dopamine system. They cite evidence from studies of combination drug treatments as well as recent neuroimaging studies (see below). A small amount of supportive neurochemical data links OCD with dysfunction in noradrenaline systems and certain neuropeptides such as arginine, vasopressin and oxytocin (Leckman *et al*, 1995).

Neuropsychiatric factors in OCD

Some of the earliest accounts associated OCD with movement disorders and neurological conditions. Although most cases of OCD are not associated with gross cerebral damage, more subtle signs of neurological dysfunction, involving fine motor coordination, visuospatial errors and involuntary movements, are commonly identified (Hollander *et al*, 1991). Moreover, obsessional symptoms are commonly reported by patients with movement disorders involving basal ganglia pathology, such as post-encephalitic parkinsonism, Sydenham's chorea and Tourette's syndrome. OCD has been shown to be a rare complication of severe head injury (Lishman, 1968); however, for some patients head injury of even a minor degree seems to be the precipitating factor (McKeon *et al*, 1984*a*; Drummond & Gravestock, 1988).

As with the other anxiety neuroses, many of the past theories about the brain pathology underlying OCD have focused on the limbic system and its frontal connections. Animal studies have shown that stimulation of certain parts of the limbic system results in behaviour reminiscent of OCD (Pitman, 1982). The apparent success of a variety of neurosurgical treatments for severe resistant OCD that, in one way or another, separate the limbic system from its frontal connections further supports the neuroanatomical localisation of OCD in frontal and limbic circuitry (Kelly *et al*, 1973) (see below).

Case examples

A famous example was that of Phineas P. Gage, who was employed in building a railway in 1848. He was a hard-working, conscientious foreman with a mildly obsessional personality. While he was working an explosion occurred which drove an iron bar through his frontal lobes. Surprisingly, he survived, but his personality changed. He became unreliable, impulsive and child-like.

More recently, a Canadian student with OCD decided to commit suicide. He shot himself through the mouth. He survived the accident and 6 years later his psychiatrist described how he was free of all obsessive–compulsive symptoms following the shooting.

Difficulties in understanding the repetitive nature of obsessive–compulsive symptoms have led to models of the disorder in which failure of a feedback mechanism is proposed. For example, hand-washing may not be stopped after a reasonable length of time if the central feedback mechanism fails to perceive that the goal of cleanliness has been achieved.

Gray's (1971, 1982) model of septohippocampal function is one such model. He suggested that the septo-hippocampal system functions as a checking system to filter aversive, non-rewarding or novel stimuli. It continually compares stimuli and events perceived by the organism in its surroundings with expected or predicted stimuli and events. According to this model, OCD arises if the septohippocampal system becomes oversensitive and reacts to too many stimuli. For example, a person may become oversensitive to stimuli connected with dirt. The slightest stimulus suggestive of dirt may cause the septohippocampal system to go into a checking mode and leads to excessive and repetitive washing.

Also proposed has been involvement of the amygdala, which mediates anxiety and conditioned fear, the hippocampus, which, if lesioned, results in repetitive behaviours in certain animals, and the cingulate gyrus, which is a major target in neurosurgery for OCD.

While these hypotheses sound plausible, there remains little evidence to link these structures directly to OCD.

Corticostriatal circuits, radio-imaging and OCD

The orbitofrontal cortex is connected to the corpus striatum, globus pallidus and thalamus in a functional loop that underpins switching between behaviours (Alexander *et al*, 1990). The corticostriatal hypothesis for OCD is based on imaging data from several studies that have linked overactivity in this circuitry with OCD.

Computed tomography and magnetic resonance imaging have identified structural abnormalities compatible with this theory, including reduced caudate volume, but the results tend to be inconsistent. More modern brain imaging techniques, such as positron emission tomography (PET), single photon emission computed tomography (SPECT) and functional magnetic resonance imaging (fMRI) allow dynamic assessment of neuronal activity, and have been applied with some success in the investigation of OCD.

In a landmark PET study, Baxter *et al* (1987) identified significant increases in regional cerebral metabolic activity localised in the left orbitofrontal gyrus and bilateral caudate nucleus of 14 patients with OCD, compared with depressed and healthy controls. The investigators replicated these results among ten non-depressed obsessional patients (Baxter *et al*, 1998). The increased metabolic activity in the OCD cases contrasted with reduced activity in the depressive controls.

Increased orbitofrontal activity was confirmed in two subsequent studies using the same techniques, but the caudate changes were not replicated (Nordahl *et al*, 1989; Swedo *et al*, 1989*b*). A third study, which gave a negative result, may have been confounded by the abnormally high levels of regional cerebral metabolic activity observed in the control group (Martinot *et al*, 1990).

After successful treatment – whether pharmacological or psychological – relative reductions were observed in the rates of cerebral metabolism in the caudate nucleus (Benkelfat *et al*, 1990), orbitofrontal cortex (Swedo *et al*, 1992) and cingulate cortex (Perani *et al*, 1995). Further, these reductions were shown to correlate with the degree of improvement in OCD symptoms (Baxter *et al*, 1992; Schwartz *et al*, 1996).

In order to focus on the mechanisms directly underlying the disorder, researchers have attempted to visualise the effects of challenging patients with stimuli that temporarily increase their symptoms. In an early study using SPECT, *in vivo* exposure was used to increase obsessions and anxiety in ten patients. A global reduction of regional cortical blood flow was seen (Zohar *et al*, 1989). It is not clear how far these changes reflected core OCD symptoms, or associated anxiety. A subsequent, smaller, PET study linked the 'provoked' state with a relative increase in blood flow bilaterally in the orbitofrontal cortex, in the right caudate nucleus and the left anterior cingulate cortex. Detailed examination of four patients showed a positive correlation between the severity of the induced obsessional symptoms and the increased neural activity in orbitofrontal cortex, neostriatum, globus pallidus and thalamus. Hippocampal and cingulate changes were thought to be linked to the induced anxiety (McGuire *et al*, 1994).

Functional MRI appears well suited to explore dynamic changes in OCD. Provocation of OCD in ten cases found enhanced activity in orbitofrontal and anterior cingulate cortex, caudate and lenticular nuclei, as well as lateral frontal cortex, insular cortex and the amygdala (reviewed by Lucey, 2001).

Overall, these studies suggest overactivity in the frontal lobe/basal ganglia system in OCD. Alteration of striatal activity seems to be linked to recovery from OCD, regardless of whether the treatment is primarily pharmacological or psychological.

How might these neurological changes produce OCD symptoms? It is widely believed that corticostriatal circuits have a role in organising thinking and motor activities. Procedural knowledge (i.e. non-conscious, automatic knowledge such as how to ride a bicycle, how to wash, how to attack or how to escape harm) is thought to be encoded in the striatum. Experiments showing that individuals with OCD do not activate the normal neural mechanisms while performing a variety of procedural tasks implicate irregularities in striatal processing in OCD. It is postulated that once a trigger – say a speck of dirt – has been identified, an internal process involving ineffective striatal processing leads to an exaggeration of harm avoidance behaviour.

Rapoport & Wise (1988) suggested that the basal ganglia contain an innate stimulus-recognition and behaviour-releasing mechanism that is usually triggered by sensory information passing from the sensory apparatus, through the sensory cortex, to the striatum. In OCD, neuronal activity driving obsessions and compulsions might be originating internally in the 'overactive' orbitofrontal or anterior cingulate cortex, which goes on to generate behavioural responses, through its connections with the striatum, in the absence of the appropriate sensory stimulus.

On the other hand, there is growing evidence that the observed 'orbitofrontal activation' seen in scanning studies embodies a secondary reaction to subcortical dysfunction, perhaps as an attempt to suppress striatally mediated harm exaggeration in OCD. The finding that individuals with low orbitofrontal activity are less likely to respond favourably to treatment is in line with this hypothesis (Stein *et al*, 2001).

Immunological processes and OCD

Similarities between OCD and obsessions occurring in children with Sydenham's chorea led to the investigation of immunological processes in childhood OCD. Sydenham's chorea is a manifestation of rheumatic fever caused by infection with group A beta-haemolytic streptococci. Antibodies directed at the bacteria react with neurons in the basal ganglia and cause damage to neuronal structures, leading to characteristic movement disorders and, in over 80% cases, obsessions and compulsions. Moreover, one-third of children with early-onset OCD also show signs of choreiform movements. This has led to the hypothesis that infection with group A beta-haemolytic streptococci can produce conditions grouped together under the acronym PANDAS (paediatric autoimmune neuropsychiatric disorders associated with streptococci), including subgroups of paediatric OCD and tics. Patients with rheumatic fever show high levels of circulating anti-caudate antibodies, and a specific B-lymphocyte antigen, labelled D8/17. This antigen also appears to be over-represented in children with OCD, Tourette's syndrome and chronic tic disorder, and has been proposed as an immunological marker of susceptibility to rheumatic fever or motor consequences of infection.

The literature on immunological markers in adult OCD remains limited, and no consistent pattern has emerged so far. The suggestion of an immunological aetiology points to other biological methods for treatment, such as antibiotics or immune modulation. However, a pilot study using penicillin prophylaxis in children with PANDAS did not produce a positive result (Garvey *et al*, 1999).

Psychological theories

Psychoanalytic

Freud (1907, 1908) proposed that the symptoms of OCD arise as a compromise between conflicting forces in the mind. For Freud, at the heart of obsessional neurosis are unconscious, aggressive instincts. Unacceptable urges, particularly hostile urges, are admitted into awareness because of incomplete repression, necessitating defensive responses in the form of compulsive rituals to reduce guilt and anxiety.

According to Freud, individuals with OCD show a constitutional predisposition to overvalue anal eroticism and a corresponding weakness in the capacity to confront and integrate the anxieties and realities of the Oedipus complex. Incomplete repression of forbidden sexual impulses, and the resulting compulsive symptoms, were both a reaction formation and a disguised gratification of these wishes. Reaction formation means that behaviour contradicts underlying impulses; for example, a mother who has unconscious violent thoughts towards her children may be unable to discipline them.

In a later discussion, Freud (1926) drew attention to the diphasic form of many compulsive rituals and introduced the notion of 'undoing', whereby 'negative magic', in the form of motor activity, is used to 'blow away' not merely the consequences of an event but the event itself; for example, a man with guilt about masturbation would repeatedly wash himself and his bedding following an episode in order to recreate himself and his environment as if masturbation had never occurred. Undoing relates to the notion of omnipotence of thought or magical thinking, in which the thought is as dangerous as and equivalent to the action.

'Isolation' is another term Freud coined, to describe the mental mechanism whereby an event or thought significant to the obsessional neurosis is not forgotten but is stripped of its associative links and emotional resonance.

Freud opened the way to the development of an object-relations theory of the mind and described OCD in terms of a relationship between an over-severe superego and an ego struggling to balance the demands of id, reality and superego. In OCD, reality is only weakly able to counteract powerful unconscious fantasies or repressed instinctual wishes. This accounts for the only transient value of perception of reality as a reassurance.

Freud's formulation reminds one of the psychobiological hypotheses presented in the previous section. In OCD there may be a non-conscious, striatally mediated process embodying impulsive/disinhibited harm-related activities. This leads to conscious attempts to compensate and turn this mechanism off, using the frontal lobes. Epidemiological data showing an association between OCD and childhood impulsivity and aggression, and observation of higher than expected levels of impulsive behaviour in clinical samples, support this paradigm.

Klein (1932) developed Freud's postulation of conflicting instinctual forces in the mind: libidinal and destructive. Through her work with severely ill children, she concluded that obsessional symptoms develop in relation to both paranoid and depressive anxieties arising from destructive impulses and their confusion with libidinal ones. She regarded the recognition and resolution of paranoid anxieties (i.e. those that threaten the survival of the self) as important in effecting a lasting cure, although she recognised that puberty, with the tremendous upsurge in the strength of libidinal impulses, could be a time of renewed symptoms.

Bion (1984) has further developed the theory concerning the defence of isolation, relating it to psychotic patterns of thought.

Behavioural

Obsessions can be viewed as learned responses to specific situations.

> **Case example**
>
> A 42-year-old man gave a 5-year history of blasphemous thoughts, which were provoked by the sight of churches, crosses or religious personnel. These obsessions started following the death of his mother. It could be postulated that her death caused an agitated and aroused state. At this time, previously neutral stimuli, such as churches, produced aversive blasphemous thoughts. Instead of ignoring these thoughts, which would have allowed his anxiety to habituate, he made efforts to suppress the thoughts and avoid situations that might provoke them. Because anxiety is an aversive experience, anything that reduces anxiety can be viewed as a positive reinforcer. Thus, the man's behaviour in avoiding situations and trying to suppress his anxiety-provoking thoughts was reinforced. This reinforcement served to strengthen the association between the previously neutral stimuli, the thoughts and his avoidance behaviour.

Compulsive behaviours or rituals are inefficient ways of reducing anxiety, as they cause only a small amount of relief and their effect is short lived before anxiety increases again, which leads to a repetition of the ritual.

> **Case example**
>
> A 30-year-old secretary had a 10-year history of fear that she might contaminate her children with toxocara from dog faeces. Upon returning to her house, she would strip off all her clothes and engage in washing rituals, in a set routine from the head downwards. This activity reduced her anxiety and was thus reinforced. Every time she performed washing rituals the association between the thoughts and the washing rituals was strengthened. However, once she had finished washing she would be plagued by doubt that she had performed the ritual totally correctly, and so would start the washing ritual again. This sequence of anxiety followed by washing ritual was repeated 20–30 times before she gave up in a state of exhaustion and continued anxiety. It can be seen that she spent most of her time with high levels of anxiety, with only partial and temporary relief from her rituals. These rituals themselves served to increase the problem by not allowing her anxiety to habituate naturally.

It seems difficult to understand why the individual does not habituate to an obsessional thought after hours spent every day thinking about it. Careful analysis of the content of the thought will generally reveal that there is an anxiety-provoking obsession followed by an anxiety-reducing ritualistic thought, which acts in the same way as covert rituals in temporarily reducing the anxiety and reinforcing the process.

Most people with OCD also use reassurance as an attempt to reduce the anxiety associated with their obsessional thoughts (Warwick & Salkovskis, 1985).

> **Case example**
>
> A man with a fear that he might cause an inferno by leaving the gas on would perform repeated checking rituals. After this he would repeatedly seek reassurance from his wife that everything had been switched off. This reassurance seeking resembled a ritual, as it temporarily reduced his anxiety, but the effect was short-lived and then further reassurance was required.

Evolutionary

The question arises as to why the themes of obsessions are so remarkably similar. Obsessions can usually be divided into one of the following categories:

- fear of contamination with harm to self
- fear of contamination with harm to others
- acts of omission with harm to self
- acts of omission with harm to others
- acts of commission with harm to self
- acts of commission with harm to others
- loss of objects
- perfectionism.

A limited degree of obsessionality can be an advantage in life, for example over hygiene. Thus, obsessional symptoms can be viewed as being selectively maintained within our genetic make-up. The theory of prepotency (Marks, 1969) proposes that members of a species are likely to respond more to stimuli with evolutionary significance. In other words, it is easy for a child to learn fear of spiders, whereas fear of trees rarely occurs and would be expected to be preceded by an aversive event associated with a tree. It does seem that most obsessional fears are of situations that might be prepotent to our species.

Cognitive

Cognitive theories of OCD are compatible with the behavioural theories proposed above. In fact, they can be viewed as an elaboration or extension of behavioural theory. Cognitive theories stem from the idea that faulty thinking patterns are learned as a result of early childhood experiences. These maladaptive patterns or schemata may lie dormant for many years until activated by a later traumatic event or experience.

One of the earliest attempts at using cognitive therapy for OCD and studying it in a scientific way was made by Emmelkamp *et al* (1988). Believing that the irrational thoughts and beliefs were insufficiently challenged by the patient, they advocated the use of a form of cognitive treatment called rational emotive therapy (Ellis, 1962).

Rachman (1976) proposed that compulsive behaviours would be reduced if the patient had less feeling of responsibility for a disastrous outcome. This concept was developed by Salkovskis (1985, 1989), who hypothesised that the basic fault in OCD might be an overinflated idea of personal responsibility, and that this needs to be modified if a successful outcome is to be achieved. He suggested that intrusive thoughts, images and doubts are erroneously interpreted and believed; that is, the individual believes that failure to perform compulsions really will lead to harm to self or others, even when most people would not see themselves as responsible. For example, someone with cognitions of inflated responsibility may telephone the police several times every day to report the slightest suspicious behaviour. Salkovskis (1999) argued that interpretations of heightened responsibility may lead to increased neutralising behaviour, increased selective attention to any perceived threat and a depressed or negative mood, thereby creating a vicious circle involving feelings of excessive responsibility and guilt.

Menzies and his co-workers in Australia focused on an alternative cognitive mediator, 'danger expectancies' (Jones & Menzies, 1997*a*, 1998*a*; Menzies *et al*, 2000). They examined whether belief in the danger of an obsessional thought is related to the performance of compulsive rituals in OCD. Danger ideation was more highly correlated with rituals than measures of responsibility, self-efficacy, perfectionism or anticipated anxiety (Jones & Menzies, 1997*a*,*b*). Experimentally increasing danger expectancies also led to an increase in symptoms in obsessive–compulsive washers (Jones & Menzies, 1998*a*,*b*).

A review by Rachman (2002) examined the various cognitive theories of OCD and suggested that both an overinflated sense of personal responsibility as well as overestimation of danger may have a role to play, at least in compulsive checkers.

Sociological theories

There are obvious problems in separating the effects of genetics and environment. It is perhaps surprising that the majority of children who have a parent with OCD grow up normally. However, a minority do exhibit obsessive–compulsive symptoms, which may be similar to or completely different from those of the parent. Most experts believe that the influence of genetics outweighs that of social learning (or modelling, to use a behavioural term), although more research in this area is needed.

Although the onset of OCD can be insidious or sudden, studies have shown that people with the condition have more life events in the year preceding onset than do matched controls (McKeon *et al*, 1984*b*). OCD resembled schizophrenia to the extent that the life events varied from losses, such as bereavement, redundancy and head injury, to those that would on the surface appear more positive.

This finding links behavioural theories with neurobiological hypotheses. Life events causing increased arousal, if aversive, could be linked to a previously neutral stimulus (e.g. electrical plugs). According to classical conditioning theory, the patient may become conditioned to respond with fear and high arousal to electric plugs. The repetitive checking could then be explained by a model such as Jeffrey Gray's theory of the septohippocampal system (Gray, 1982) (see above) so that the individual is constantly checking for the danger of electrical plugs and ensuring they are safe (Drummond & Matthews, 1988).

Treatment

Psychological treatment

Behavioural psychotherapy

For patients with obsessions and overt compulsions the treatment is prolonged, graduated exposure in real life to the feared situation together with self-imposed response prevention. Other variations on this treatment have been used in the past but this is the combination that has been demonstrated to be effective (see below on outcome).

Exposure works on the observation that a patient who has an intense fear of a situation, when confronted with the situation will either escape or perform activities (compulsions or rituals) to reduce or prevent the harm he or she fears will result. High anxiety is extremely unpleasant. Escape and compulsive behaviours reduce the anxiety. Therefore the escape behaviours are reinforced by the reduction of the anxiety. Consequently, the conditions are worsened by each episode of brief exposure and escape.

In exposure treatment, the aim is to produce prolonged periods of contact with the feared situation until the anxiety naturally reduces (habituation). Compulsions reduce the anxiety and this serves to reinforce the ritual. However, the reduction in anxiety produced by a compulsive ritual tends to be small and the effect temporary. Instead, rituals prevent therapeutic exposure and increase the tendency to ritualise further.

With treatment, patients are asked to expose themselves to the fear-provoking situation and remain in that situation until the anxiety has substantially reduced. This usually takes between 60 and 90 minutes. Although this is a simple technique, the skill lies in the therapist accurately assessing the correct fear-provoking cues, educating the patient about the therapy and helping the patient to agree on a level of exposure that will cause a degree of anxiety that can be tolerated.

Although exposure is the cornerstone of the treatment of OCD it needs to be combined with response prevention, that is, with encouragement not to perform compulsions, either physical or mental. This can usually be achieved by demonstrating to the patient how they interfere with exposure.

The same exposure tasks are then repeated by the patient at least daily (preferably three times a day) until there is little anxiety even at the commencement of the exposure. A more anxiety-provoking situation can then be tackled until the patient has completed the tasks on the 'anxiety hierarchy' devised with the therapist.

Graduated exposure and response prevention is a quick and cost-efficient treatment which can be easily applied in many general practice and hospital settings, and it remains perplexing as to why it is often unavailable outside specialist services. Although some basic training is required, this can easily be obtained by reading about clinical techniques (e.g. Hawton *et al*, 1989) and by obtaining supervision from a trained behavioural psychotherapist. It has been found that instruction in self-exposure techniques may be all that is required for many patients (Ghosh *et al*, 1988; Marks *et al*, 1988). For more intransigent cases, individual therapist-aided exposure rarely involves more than 10–15 hours of therapist time.

The efficacy of self-exposure has led to the development of self-help manuals. However, few patients can successfully complete a treatment programme without some professional guidance. The patient should be seen initially for education about anxiety and its treatment, and for help in devising treatment targets. Subsequent meetings are required to monitor progress, give encouragement and advise on any difficulties that may arise. Investigation of group-based behaviour therapy is still undergoing evaluation as a cost-effective alternative (e.g. Fals-Stewart & Lucente, 1994).

The most effective exposure has been shown to be:

1 prolonged rather than of short duration (Stern & Marks, 1973)

2 in real life rather than in fantasy (Emmelkamp & Wessels, 1975)

3 regularly practised, with self-exposure homework tasks (McDonald *et al*, 1978).

Patients with pure obsessional ruminations have always been considered difficult to treat. This may partly have been because therapists have not identified the associated covert, anxiety-reducing compulsions (as discussed above). The cornerstone of treatment for obsessions is exposure to the anxiety-provoking thought and resistance to the covert mental ritual.

One way of maintaining exposure to the anxiety-provoking thoughts involves the use of a personal stereo. The aim is to use an audiotape to prolong exposure without allowing the patient time to perform mental rituals. The literature has mainly case studies illustrating this treatment (Salkovskis, 1983; Headland & McDonald, 1987) but there has also been one pilot controlled study (Richards *et al*, 1994).

Cognitive–behavioural therapy

The outcome of treatment is fully discussed in the next section. Although cognitive–behavioural therapy has been advocated for OCD, there is no clear evidence that, in general, it produces any better results than simple exposure and response prevention (James & Blackburn 1995; Cottraux *et al*, 2001; McLean *et al*, 2001).

There is more evidence in favour of using targeted cognitive techniques to overcome specific problems in exposure therapy. For example, cognitive therapy may be helpful in reducing the strength of belief in irrational obsessions (Salkovskis & Warwick, 1985) or the erroneous sense of responsibility that may characterise some patients with OCD (Salkovskis, 1999).

A new treatment based on cognitive therapy is being pioneered for patients with contamination fears who refuse to undertake or who fail in exposure therapy. This treatment, called danger ideation reduction therapy (DIRT) (Jones & Menzies, 1998*b*; Krochmalik *et al*, 2001), is radically different from previous exposure and cognitive treatments because it does not encourage the patient to confront the feared contaminant. Indeed, in many of the studies anti-exposure instructions were given. The treatment consists of the following components:

1 cognitive restructuring

2 filmed interviews

3 corrective information

4 microbiological experiment

5 probability of catastrophe

6 attentional focusing.

Cognitive restructuring

With the techniques of rational emotive therapy (Ellis, 1962), the patient is taught to identify unrealistic thoughts about contamination and then to re-evaluate these. Once the patient has developed appropriate thoughts about the feared contaminants, these are recorded. The patient is then asked to rote learn the responses and to repeat them at least daily.

Filmed interviews

These consist of a number of filmed interviews with people who work in situations commonly feared by obsessive–compulsive patients. Examples would be bank tellers who handle money or cleaners who handle cleaning fluids and clean other people's dirt.

Corrective information

The patient is asked to view a list of facts about the feared contaminant. One example would be the number of healthcare workers who have contracted HIV through their work. Another would be the deleterious effects of overzealous hand-washing (e.g. how it can break the skin's natural barrier to infection).

Microbiological experiments

Results of microbiological experiments that were undertaken at the University of Sydney are discussed with the patient. In these experiments participants were asked to touch frequently feared contaminants such as money, dog hair or toilet door handles with one hand while keeping the other hand 'clean'. Fingerprints from both hands were then imprinted on blood agar plates. Normal, commensal flora were found after culture and no pathogens were found.

Probability of catastrophe

Patients are asked to estimate the probability of catastrophe occurring in different situations. They are then asked to break down this scenario into its component parts and estimate the likelihood of the feared consequence at each stage. This is then computed and compared with the original probability estimate.

Case example

A woman who feared touching rubbish bins for fear of contracting salmonella originally estimated this risk as 90%. When asked how often rubbish contained salmonella, she estimated this as 50% of the time. She was then asked to estimate the risk of this salmonella getting on to the outside of the bin, which she said was 50%. The risk of this travelling from the bin to her fingers was estimated at 80%, and then being ingested into her body from her hand she claimed was 80%. The chance of her immune defences not coping with the ingested salmonella she estimated as 60%. This gives a likelihood of contracting salmonella from touching a rubbish bin of 9%, and not the 90% she first believed.

Attentional focusing

This is a form of meditation. Patients are taught to focus the mind away from the danger-related intrusive thoughts and onto benign, non-threatening stimuli.

Outcome of behavioural and cognitive treatments

The treatment of OCD using straightforward graduated exposure and self-imposed response prevention has been shown, by controlled trials, to be effective in the majority of patients who complete the treatment. However, the absence of 'intent to treat' data diminishes the reported success rates of from 75% (Marks *et al*, 1975) to 85% of patients (Foa & Goldstein, 1978). Therapist modelling was not shown to alter the response to exposure treatment but the involvement of the family in the treatment could be helpful (Emmelkamp, 1982). The value of adding specifically targeted cognitive therapy has yet to be evaluated in controlled clinical trials. There has been no evidence of symptom substitution in patients with OCD treated by behavioural psychotherapy (Marks, 1981). Indeed, studies have shown that the gains made in therapy are maintained for at least 4 years (see Marks, 1981).

Despite these good results, many patients fail to engage in exposure treatments, while others relapse and require booster sessions. It is advisable to follow patients up to ensure that their gains are maintained and that if signs of relapse develop, they can be dealt with promptly before the patient has reverted to pre-treatment levels of disability. The usual practice is to see patients 1, 3, 6 and 12 months after treatment.

The outcome of behavioural psychotherapy with patients with obsessional ruminations is less reliably favourable (Emmelkamp & Kwee, 1977). The outcome of audiotaped habituation for this group has not yet been adequately evaluated, although preliminary studies appear promising (Richards *et al*, 1994). Reports of success using cognitive therapy based on issues of responsibility (Salkovskis *et al*, 1998) need to be substantiated in a large, controlled trial.

Despite its superficial attractiveness in this disorder, there is little work to suggest that cognitive therapy has any advantage over exposure therapy in the treatment of OCD. The few trials of rational emotive therapy (Emmelkamp *et al*, 1988; Emmelkamp & Beens, 1991) and of cognitive therapy targeting a heightened sense of responsibility have failed to show convincing evidence of a clinical advantage (James & Blackburn, 1995; van Oppen *et al*, 1995; McLean *et al*, 2001).

Poorly applied cognitive therapy may make some patients with OCD worse. This is because the process of looking for evidence to confirm or refute the obsessions can become incorporated into rituals. More generally, cognitive therapy may not be cost-efficient, as it requires specialist training and supervision for the therapist and therapy can be of relatively long duration.

The new treatment of DIRT appears promising for those patients who have contamination fears and who either refuse to engage with or who have failed to benefit from exposure therapy (Jones & Menzies, 1997*b*; Jones & Menzies, 1998*b*; Menzies *et al*, 2000). Bearing in mind that many of the DIRT techniques seem to be contrary to the exposure principle (e.g. much of the therapy could be viewed as providing reassurance), it is important that therapy in its entirety is carefully evaluated in controlled trials before it is universally accepted. If successful, it will call into question many of the hypotheses currently underpinning cognitive–behavioural treatments. Until recently, this treatment was available only in Australia, but it has now been piloted in the UK (Govender *et al*, 2006).

Overall, it would seem that the most pragmatic approach is to consider the role of cognitive therapy for those patients who fail to improve with exposure therapy. Exposure therapy has stood the test of time, is easy to learn and apply, and is effective for the majority of patients with OCD.

Psychodynamic psychotherapy

Although some psychoanalysts do still recommend psychodynamic psychotherapy for patients with OCD, most would agree with Cawley's (1974) view that 'there is no evidence to support or refute the proposition that formal psychotherapy helps patients with obsessional disorders'.

Biological treatments

Pharmacotherapy

Which drugs are effective in OCD?

The selectivity of the pharmacological response to drugs that act as potent inhibitors of the synaptic reuptake of serotonin (serotonin reuptake inhibitors, SRIs) distinguishes OCD from the other anxiety disorders and from depression, in which both noradrenergic and serotonergic medications appear equally effective. Drugs lacking these properties, such as the tricyclic antidepressants amitriptyline, nortriptyline and desipramine, and the monoamine oxidase inhibitors phenelzine and clorgyline, have been found to be ineffective in controlled trials. Benzodiazepines, lithium and electroconvulsive therapy also appear ineffective (Zohar *et al*, 2000), as do antipsychotics when used alone, although they may have a role in augmenting SRIs in treatment-refractory cases.

The discovery that clomipramine is an effective treatment for OCD was an important breakthrough. The seminal study by Montgomery (1980) specifically excluded patients with comorbid depression, and demonstrated efficacy against placebo at a relatively modest daily dose of 75 mg. Later, larger studies confirmed that does of up to 300 mg daily are effective in adults and children, in the presence as well as in the absence of comorbid depression (Zohar *et al*, 2000). It is established beyond doubt that the anti-obsessional actions of clomipramine do not depend on an anti-depressant effect.

The treatment response in OCD is slow. Incremental improvement occurs over weeks and months, to the extent that a 40–45% improvement was measured by the 10-week end-point of a large multicentre study of clomipramine (De Veaugh-Geiss *et al*, 1989) and gains continue to be made for up to 2 years as long as treatment is continued. Patients may need to be persuaded to continue with treatment in the early stages, if progress seems frustratingly slow.

More recently, the selective SRIs (SSRIs) fluvoxamine, fluoxetine, paroxetine, sertraline and citalopram have been found to be effective in large-scale randomised controlled trials (reviewed by Fineberg, 1999). Claims that clomipramine is more effective have been challenged by the results of a number of controlled comparator studies, which, taken together, imply equivalent efficacy for the SSRIs and clomipramine (Zohar & Judge, 1996; Bisserbe *et al*, 1997).

In the face of equivalent efficacy, the choice of SRI depends to a large extent on the side-effect profile. Clomipramine is associated with unpleasant and potentially dangerous side-effects, such as convulsions (seen in up to 2% of patients on clomipramine, compared with 0.05–0.1% of patients on SSRIs), cardiotoxicity and cognitive impairment. Sexual dysfunction has been reported in up to 80% of patients on clomipramine, compared with 30% of those on SSRIs, and drop-out rates due to side-effects are considerably lower for SSRIs (*c*. 9%) than for clomipramine (*c*. 17%). Improved safety and tolerability indicate that SSRIs should be used as the treatment of first choice, with clomipramine reserved for those who cannot tolerate SSRIs or who have failed to respond to them.

Choosing between SSRIs is difficult because their side-effects are so similar. Occasionally, the possibility of a potential drug interaction directs the choice. In these circumstances sertraline and citalopram may be preferred because they are relatively weak inhibitors of hepatic cytochrome P450 metabolising enzymes. Fluoxetine and its active metabolite have long half-lives, resulting in fewer withdrawal reactions and advantages for patients who frequently forget their medication.

What is the most effective dose?

Fixed-dose studies have been performed with paroxetine, fluoxetine, sertraline and citalopram. The results for paroxetine showed a positive dose–response relationship, with the 40 mg and 60 mg dose levels showing efficacy but the 20 mg dose no different from placebo. Similar results were obtained for fluoxetine; whereas all three dosages were significantly superior to placebo, there was a trend towards superiority for the 60 mg dose, which became significant when data from more than one study centre were pooled. Preliminary results for citalopram also showed efficacy for 20 mg, 40 mg and 60 mg doses, with an advantage for the higher doses. The results for sertraline, however, are less clear, possibly owing to lack of statistical power in the dose-ranging study (reviewed by Zohar & Fineberg 2001).

These results have been interpreted as showing greater efficacy for the higher dosages in OCD. Given that improvements in OCD take several weeks to establish, irrespective of the dose, it is advisable to start SSRIs at the lower end of their dose range to help minimise early side-effects, and titrate upwards slowly, if necessary, while measuring clinical response with standardised rating instruments such as the Yale–Brown Obsessive Compulsive Scale (YBOCS) (Goodman *et al*, 1984).

Is pharmacotherapy effective in the long term?

Because OCD is a chronic illness, we need to be confident that the treatment continues to be effective over the longer term. Some studies have followed treatment responders for up to 1 year under double-blind, placebo-controlled conditions, and have demonstrated that the treatment effect was sustained. Patients on active treatment continued to improve, whereas those on placebo did not. In a large extension study by Greist *et al* (1995), 118 patients were followed up for 40 weeks under double-blind conditions, after 12 weeks of acute treatment with sertraline or placebo. Patients remaining on active sertraline showed ongoing improvements. Side-effects also improved over time and compliance was good, with only 13% of sertraline-treated patients discontinuing treatment prematurely during the extension phase. Fifty-nine patients who completed the study were followed up for a further year on open-label sertraline and showed additional clinical improvement (Rasmussen *et al*, 1997). These results suggest that the treatment continues to be effective in the longer term.

For how long should pharmacotherapy continue?

In order to answer this question, we may attend to the results of a small number of controlled studies that looked at the effects of discontinuing treatment in SSRI responders, under double-blind conditions. The results show unequivocally that discontinuing the drug, irrespective of the length of the treatment course (up to 2 years), is associated with a gradual worsening of OCD, which is unlikely to represent a temporary withdrawal effect. These findings suggest that medication maintains well-being for as long as it is continued, but that discontinuation is likely to result in an eventual relapse. In the study by Romano *et al* (1998) a 60 mg dose of fluoxetine appeared the most effective at preventing relapse over a 24-week extension phase. These findings imply that treatment needs to be continued indefinitely, and that dose reductions below the effective dose are not recommended. The adage 'the dose that gets you well, keeps you well' probably applies.

Treatment of SRI-refractory OCD

Most studies have defined treatment response as a 25–35% improvement in baseline scores on the YBOCS. Although SRIs are impressively effective in OCD, a substantial minority of patients, estimated at around 30%, fail to respond. Results from various controlled and uncontrolled studies looking at strategies for these patients have identified four main approaches.

1 *A higher dose of SRI*. Doses exceeding those recommended by the *British National Formulary* have not been investigated under controlled conditions. Case reports of two treatment-refractory patients who

responded to 300 mg/day sertraline and 160 mg/day citalopram suggest that this area merits further exploration. Owing to the increased risk of convulsions and cardiotoxicity, the use of higher doses of clomipramine cannot be recommended without additional safeguards such as monitoring of plasma drug levels, or electrocardiography.

2 *Intravenous clomipramine*. This has been hypothesised to be more effective than oral clomipramine, owing to improved bioavailability, and some patients have benefited from this route of administration. For example, a double-blind study showed a significant advantage for 14 daily intravenous infusions of clomipramine in 29 otherwise treatment-refractory patients, compared with 25 cases given matched placebo (Fallon *et al*, 1998).

3 *Drug combination strategies*. These have proved popular for treating refractory OCD. While the addition of drugs that enhance serotonin neurotransmission, such as lithium, buspirone, pindolol and L-tryptophan, have not proved useful, there is increasing evidence that adding low doses of antipsychotic agents may be helpful in some cases. Dopamine-receptor blocking drugs do not appear effective on their own in OCD, although they are the treatment of choice for Tourette's syndrome. However, the conventional antpsychotic haloperidol (McDougle *et al*, 1994) and the atypical antipsychotic risperidone (McDougle *et al*, 2000) have each been found to be effective when added to ongoing SSRI treatment in a placebo-controlled study investigating SRI-refractory cases. Patients with comorbid tic disorders had a preferential response to haloperidol augmentation, but not to risperidone augmentation. Uncontrolled studies looking at olanzapine augmentation also appear promising. Atypical antipsychotics are associated with lower rates of extrapyramidal side-effects, and further exploration of this group of compounds is warranted.

4 *Novel compounds*. Drugs such as inositol, sumatriptan and tramadol have not yet been sufficiently investigated for their use to be recommended.

Neurosurgery

Although extensively used in the middle of the 20th century, neurosurgery is rarely advocated today. However, for a tiny percentage of patients with severe OCD who have failed to respond to all other forms of treatment, modern stereotactic surgery is sometimes recommended (see review by Jenicke, 1998). Four surgical procedures have been used for OCD: cingulotomy, capsulotomy, limbic leucotomy and subcaudate tractotomy. They each serve to disconnect areas of frontal cortex from subcortical structures, and no definitive conclusions may be drawn as to the most effective technique. Following stereotactic limbic leucotomy, 84% of patients with OCD were reported to have improved (Mitchell-Heggs *et al*, 1976). Preliminary results using 'gamma-knife surgery' have also shown benefits (Rasmussen & Eisen, 1997). However, no controlled trial has been performed to verify these results and so it is difficult to assess the specific effect of the brain lesions compared with the placebo effect of the drama of brain surgery.

Acknowledgements

We are grateful to Cambridge University Press for allowing us to reproduce some of the material and case histories from Stern, R. S. & Drummond, L. M. (1991) *The Practice of Behavioural and Cognitive Psychotherapy*. Cambridge: Cambridge University Press.

We are also grateful to Dr Sue Davison, who advised and contributed to the section on psychodynamic theory.

Further reading

Fineberg, N. A., Marazitti, D. & Stein, D. (eds) (2001) *Obsessive Compulsive Disorder: A Practical Guide*. London: Martin Dunitz.

Goodman, W., Rudorfer, M. V. & Maser, J. D. (eds) (1999) *Obsessive–Compulsive Disorder*. Rahwah, NJ: Erlbaum.

Koran, L. M. (1999) *Obsessive Compulsive and Related Disorders in Adults*. Cambridge: Cambridge University Press.

Marks, I. M. (1981) *Cure and Care of Neurosis: Theory and Practice of Behavioural Psychotherapy*. New York: Wiley.

Marks, I. M. (1987) *Fears, Phobias and Rituals*. New York: Oxford University Press.

Salkovskis, P. M. & Kirk, J. (1989) Obsessional disorders. In *Cognitive Behaviour Therapy for Psychiatric Problems: A Practical Guide* (eds K. Hawton, P. M. Salkovskis, J. Kirk, *et al*). Oxford: Oxford University Press.

Stern, R. S. & Drummond, L. M. (1991) *The Practice of Behavioural and Cognitive Psychotherapy*. Cambridge: Cambridge University Press.

Swinson, R. P., Antony, M., Rachman, S., *et al* (eds) (2002) *Obsessive–Compulsive Disorder*. New York: Guilford Press.

References

Alexander, G. E., Crutcher, M. D. & DeLong, M. R. (1990) Basal ganglia thalamocortical circuits: parallel substrates for motor, occulomotor, prefrontal and limbic functions. In *Progress in Brain Research* (eds H. B. M. Uylings, C. G. Van Eden, J. P. C. DeBruin, *et al*), pp. 119–146. Elsevier: Amsterdam.

Alsobrook, J. P., Leckman, J. F., Goodman, W. K., *et al* (1999) Segregation analysis of obsessive compulsive disorder using symptom-based factors. *American Journal of Medical Genetics (Neuropsychiatry Genetics)*, **88**, 669–675.

American Psychiatric Association (1994) *Diagnostic and Statistical Manual of Psychiatric Disorders* (4th edn) (DSM–IV). Washington, DC: APA.

Baxter, L. R., Phelps, M. E., Mazziotta, J. C., *et al* (1987) Local cerebral glucose metabolic rates in obsessive compulsive disoder: a comparison with unipolar depression and normal controls. *Archives of General Psychiatry*, **44**, 211–218.

Baxter, L. R., Schwartz, J. M., Bergman, K. S., *et al* (1992) Caudate glucose metabolic rate changes with both drug and behaviour therapy for obsessive–compulsive disorder. *Archives of General Psychiatry*, **49**, 681–689.

Baxter, L. R., Schwartz, J. M., Mazziotta, J. C., *et al* (1998) Cerebral glucose metabolic rates in non-depressed obsessive compulsive disorder. *American Journal of Psychiatry*, **145**, 1560–1563.

Benkelfat, C., Murphy, D. L. & Zohar, J. (1989) Clomipramine in obsessive compulsive disorder, further evidence for a serotonergic mechanism of action. *Archives of General Psychiatry*, **46**, 23–28.

Benkelfat, C., Nordahl, T. H. E., Semple, W.,E., *et al* (1990) local cerebral glucose metabolic rates in obsessive compulsive disorder: patients treated with clomipramine. *Archives of General Psychiatry*, **47**, 840–848.

Bion, W. R. (1984) *Second Thoughts*. London: Karnac.

Bisserbe, J. C., Lane, R. M., Flament, M. F., *et al* (1997) A double-blind comparison of sertraline and clomipramine in outpatients with obsessive compulsive disorder. *European Psychiatry*, **153**, 1450–1454.

Black, A. (1974) The natural history of neurosis. In *Obsessional States* (ed. H. R. Beech), pp. 19–54. London: Methuen.

Carey, G. & Gottesman, I. I. (1981) Twin and family studies of anxiety, phobic and obsessive disorders. In *Anxiety: New Research and Changing Concepts* (eds D. F. Klein & J. Rabkin), pp. 117–136. New York: Raven Press.

Cavallini, M. C., De Bella, D., Pasquale, L., *et al* (1998) $5HT_{2C}$ CYS23/SER23 polymorphism is not associated with obsessive compulsive disorder. *Psychiatric Research*, **77**, 97–104.

Cawley, R. (1974) Psychotherapy and obsessional disorders. In *Obsessional States* (ed. H. R. Beech), pp. 259–290. London: Methuen.

Charney, D. S., Goodman, W. K., Price, L. H., *et al* (1988) Serotonin function in obsessive–compulsive disorder. *Archives of General Psychiatry*, **45**, 177–185.

Cottraux, J., Note, I., Yao, S. N., *et al* (2001) A randomized controlled trial of cognitive therapy versus intensive behaviour therapy in obsessive–compulsive disorder. *Psychotherapy and Psychosomatics*, **70**, 288–297.

De Veaugh-Geiss, J., Landau, P. & Katz, R. (1989) Treatment of obsessive compulsive disorder with clomipramine. *Psychiatry Annals*, **19**, 97–101.

Drummond, L. M. (1993) The treatment of severe, chronic, resistant obsessive–compulsive disorder: an evaluation of an inpatient programme using behavioural psychotherapy in combination with other treatments. *British Journal of Psychiatry*, **163**, 223–229.

Drummond, L. M. & Gravestock, S. (1988) Delayed emergence of obsessive–compulsive neurosis following head injury: case report and review of its theoretical implications. *British Journal of Psychiatry*, **153**, 839–842.

Drummond, L. M. & Matthews, H. P. (1988) Obsessive–compulsive disorder arising as a complication of benzodiazepine withdrawal. *Journal of Nervous and Mental Disease*, **176**, 688–691.

DuBois, F. S. (1949) Compulsion neurosis with cachexia. *American Journal of Psychiatry*, **106**, 107–115.

Eapen, V., Robertson, M. M., Alsobrook, J. P., *et al* (1997) Obsessive compulsive symptoms in Gilles de la Tourette syndrome and obsessive compulsive disorder: differences by diagnosis and family history. *American Journal of Medical Genetics*, **74**, 432–438.

Ellis, A. (1962) *Reason and Emotion in Psychotherapy*. New York: Lyle-Stuart.

Emmelkamp, P. M. G. (1982) *Phobic and Obsessive–Compulsive Disorders: Theory, Research and Practice*. New York: Plenum.

Emmelkamp, P. M. G. & Beens, H. (1991) Cognitive therapy with obsessive–compulsive disorder: a comparative evaluation. *Behaviour Research and Therapy*, **29**, 293–300.

Emmelkamp, P. M. & Kwee, K. G. (1977) Obsessional ruminations: a comparison between thought-stopping and prolonged exposure in imagination. *Behavioural Research Therapy*, **15**, 441–444.

Emmelkamp, P. M. G. & Wessels, H. (1975) Flooding in imagination v flooding in vivo in agoraphobics. *Behaviour Research and Therapy*, **13**, 7.

Emmelkamp, P. M. G., Visser, S. & Hoekstra, R. J. (1988) Cognitive therapy v. exposure in vivo in the treatment of obsessive–compulsives. *Cognitive Therapy and Research*, **12**, 103–114.

Ergovesi, S., Ronchi, P. & Smeraldi, E. (1992) $5\text{-}HT_2$ receptor and fluvoxamine in obsessive compulsive disorder. *Human Psychopharmacology*, **7**, 287–289.

Fallon, B. A., Liebowitz, M. R., Campeas, R., *et al* (1998) Intravenous clomipramine for obsessive compulsive disorder refractory to oral clomipramine: a placebo-controlled study. *Archives of General Psychiatry*, **55**, 918–924.

Fals-Stewart, W. & Lucente, S. (1994) Behavioural group therapy with obsessive compulsives: an overview. *International Journal of Group Psychotherapy*, **44**, 35–51.

Fineberg, N. A. (1999) Evidence-based pharmacotherapy for obsessive compulsive disorder. *Advances in Psychiatric Treatment*, **5**, 357–365.

Fineberg, N. A., Roberts, A., Montgomery, S. A., *et al* (1997). Brain 5-HT function in obsessive compulsive disorder. Prolactin responses to d-fenfluramine. *British Journal of Psychiatry*, **171**, 280–282.

Flament, M. & Cohen, D. (2001) OCD in children and adolescents. In *Obsessive Compulsive Disorder: A Practical Guide* (eds N. A. Fineberg, D. Marazitti & D. Stein), pp. 153–166. London: Martin Dunitz.

Foa, E. B. (1979) Failures in treating obsessive–compulsives. *Behaviour Research and Therapy*, **17**, 169–176.

Foa, E. B. & Goldstein, A. (1978) Continuous exposure and complete response prevention in the treatment of obsessive–compulsive neurosis. *Behavior Therapy*, **9**, 821–829.

Freud, S. (1907) Obsessions and religion. In *The Complete Psychological Works of Sigmund Freud* (standard edn) (ed. J. Strachey), vol. 9, pp. 115–127. London: Hogarth Press.

Freud, S. (1908) Character and anal eroticism. In *The Complete Psychological Works of Sigmund Freud* (standard edn) (ed. J. Strachey), vol. 9, pp. 167–175. London: Hogarth Press.

Freud, S. (1926) Inhibitions, symptoms and anxieties. In *The Complete Psychological Works of Sigmund Freud* (standard edn) (ed. J. Strachey), vol. 20, pp. 75–115. London: Hogarth Press.

Garvey, M. A., Perlmutter, S. J., Allen, A. J., *et al* (1999) A pilot study of penicillin prophylaxis for neuropsychiatric exacerbation triggered by streptococcal infections. *Biological Psychiatry*, **45**, 1564–1571.

Ghosh, A., Marks, I. M. & Carr, A. C. (1988) Therapist contact and outcome of self-exposure treatment for phobias: a controlled study. *British Journal of Psychiatry*, **152**, 234–238.

Goodman, W. K., Price, L. H., Rasmussen, S. A., *et al* (1984) The Yale–Brown Obsessive Compulsive Scale 1: development, use and reliability. *Archives of General Psychiatry*, **46**, 1006–1011.

Goodman, W. K., Price, L. H., Delgado, P. L., *et al* (1990) Specificity of serotonin reuptake inhibitors in the treatment of obsessive disorder: comparison of fluvoxamine and desipramine. *Archives of General Psychiatry*, **47**, 277–285.

Govender, S., Drummond, L. M. & Menzies, R. G. (2006) Danger ideation reduction therapy for the treatment of severe, chronic and resistant obsessive–compulsive disorder. *Behavioural and Cognitive Psychotherapy*, **34**, 1–4.

Gray, J. (1971) *The Psychology of Fear and Stress*. London: Weidenfeld and Nicholson.

Gray, J. A. (1982) *The Neuropsychology of Anxiety: An Enquiry into the Functioning of the Septohippocampal System*. New York: Oxford University Press.

Greist, J., Jefferson, J., Kobak, K., *et al* (1995) A one year double-blind placebo controlled fixed-dose study of sertraline in the treatment of obsessive compulsive disorder. *International Clinical Psychopharmacology*, **10**, 57–65.

Hawton, K., Salkovskis, P. M., Kirk, J., *et al* (1989) *Cognitive Behaviour Therapy for Psychiatric Problems: A Practical Guide*. New York: Oxford University Press.

Headland, K. & McDonald, R. (1987) Rapid audiotaped treatment of obsesssional ruminations. *Behavioural Psychotherapy*, **15**, 188–192.

Hollander, E., Fay, M., Cohen, B., *et al* (1988) Serotonergic and noradrenergic sensitivity in obsessive–compulsive disorder: behavioral findings. *American Journal of Psychiatry*, **145**, 1015–1017.

Hollander, E., Schiffman, E., Cohen, B., *et al* (1991) Neurological soft signs in obsessive compulsive disorder. *Archives of General Psychiatry*, **48**, 278–279.

James, I. A. & Blackburn, I. M. (1995) Cognitive therapy with obsessive–compulsive disorder. *British Journal of Psychiatry*, **166**, 444–450.

Jenicke, M. A. (1998) Neurosurgical treatment of obsessive compulsive disorder. *British Journal of Psychiatry*, **173**, suppl. 35, 79–90.

Jones, M. K. & Menzies, R. G. (1997*a*) The cognitive mediation of obsessive–compulsive handwashing. *Behaviour Research and Therapy*, **36**, 959–970.

Jones, M. K. & Menzies, R. G. (1997*b*) Danger ideation therapy (DIRT): preliminary findings with three obsessive–compulsive washers. *Behaviour Research and Therapy*, **35**, 955–960.

Jones, M. K. & Menzies, R. G. (1998*a*) The role of perceived danger in the mediation of obsessive–compulsive washing. *Depression and Anxiety*, **8**, 121–125.

Jones, M. K. & Menzies, R. G. (1998*b*) Danger ideation reduction therapy (DIRT) for obsessive–compulsive washers. A controlled trial. *Behaviour Research and Therapy*, **8**, 121–125.

Karno, M., Golding, J. M., Sorenson, S. B., *et al* (1988) The epidemiology of obsessive–compulsive disorder in five U.S. communities. *Archives of General Psychiatry*, **45**, 1095–1099.

Kelly, D. H. W., Richardson, A. & Mitchell-Heggs, N. (1973) Stereotactic limbic leucotomy: neurophysiological and operative technique. *British Journal of Psychiatry*, **123**, 133–140.

Kendell, R. E. & DiScipio, W. J. (1970) Obsessional symptoms and obsessional personality traits in patients with depressive illness. *Psychological Medicine*, **1**, 65–72.

Khanna, S., Rajendra, P. N. & Channabasacvanna, S. M. (1986) Sociodemographic variables in obsessive–compulsive disorder in India. *International Journal of Social Psychiatry*, **32**, 47–54.

Klein, M. (1932) *The Psychoanalysis of Children*. London: Hogarth Press.

Krochmalik, A., Jones, M. K. & Menzies, R. G. (2001) Danger ideation reduction therapy (DIRT) for treatment resistant compulsive washing. *Behaviour Research and Therapy*, **39**, 897–912.

Leckman, J. F., Goodman, W. K., Anderson, G. M., *et al* (1995) Cerebrospinal fluid biogenic amines in obsessive–compulsive disorder, Tourette syndrome and healthy controls. *Neuropsychopharmacology*, **12**, 73–86.

Lewis, A. J. (1934) Melancholia: a clinical survey of depressive states. *Journal of Mental Science*, **80**, 277–378.

Lewis, A. J. (1935) Problems of obsessional illness. *Proceedings of the Royal Society of Medicine*, **29**, 325–336.

Lishman, W. A. (1968) Brain damage in relation to psychiatric disability after head injury. *British Journal of Psychiatry*, **144**, 373–410.

Lo, W. H. (1967) A follow-up study of obsessional neurotics in Hong Kong Chinese. *British Journal of Psychiatry*, **113**, 823–832.

Lucey, J. V. (2001) The neuroanatomy of OCD. In *Obsessive Compulsive Disorder: A Practical Guide* (eds N. A. Fineberg, D. Marazitti & D. Stein), pp. 77–87. London: Martin Dunitz.

Marazitti, D. (2001) Integrated pathophysiology. In *Obsessive Compulsive Disorder: A Practical Guide* (eds N. A. Fineberg, D. Marazitti & D. Stein), pp. 89–102. London: Martin Dunitz.

Marks, I. M. (1969) *Fears and Phobias*. New York: Academic Press.

Marks, I. M. (1981) *Cure and Care of Neurosis: Theory and Practice of Behavioural Psychotherapy*. New York: Wiley.

Marks, I. M., Hodgson, R. & Rachman, S. (1975) Treatment of chronic obsessive–compulsive disorder by *in vivo* exposure. *British Journal of Psychiatry*, **127**, 349–364.

Marks, I. M., Lelliot, P., Basoglu, M., *et al* (1988) Clomipramine, self-exposure and therapist-aided exposure for obsessive–compulsive rituals. *British Journal of Psychiatry*, **152**, 522–534.

Martinot, J. L., Allaire, J. F., Mazoyer, B. M., *et al* (1990) Obsessive compulsive disorder: a clinical, neuropsychological and positron emission study. *Acta Psychiatrica Scandinavica*, **82**, 233–242.

McDonald, R., Sartory, G., Grey, S. J., *et al* (1978) Effects of self-exposure instructions on agoraphobic outpatients. *Behaviour Research and Therapy*, 17, 83–85.

McDougle, C. J. & Goodman, W. K. (1991) Obsessive–compulsive disorder: pharmacotherapy and pathophysiology. *Current Opinion in Psychiatry*, **4**, 267–272.

McDougle, C. J., Goodman, W. K., Leckman, J. F., *et al* (1994) Haloperidol addition in fluvoxamine-refractory obsessive compulsive disorder: a double-blind placebo-controlled study in patients with and without tics. *Archives of General Psychiatry*, **51**, 302–308.

McDougle, C. J., Epperson, C. N., Pelton, G. H., *et al* (2000) A double-blind placebo-controlled study of risperidone addition in serotonin reuptake inhibitor-refractory obsessive compulsive disorder. *Archives of General Psychiatry*, **57**, 794–801.

McGuffin, P. & Reich, T. (1984) Psychopathology and genetics. In *Comprehensive Handbook of Psychpathology* (eds H. E. Adams & P. B. Sutker), pp. 47–75. New York: Plenum.

McGuire, P. K., Bench, C. J., Frith, C. D., *et al* (1994) Functional anatomy of obsessive compulsive phenomena. *British Journal of Psychiatry*, **164**, 459–468.

McKeon, J. P., McGuffin, P. & Robinson, P. H. (1984*a*) Obsessive–compulsive neurosis following head injury: a report of four cases. *British Journal of Psychiatry*, **144**, 190–192.

McKeon, J. P., Roa, B. & Mann, A. (1984*b*) Life events and personality traits in obsessive–compulsive neurosis. *British Journal of Psychiatry*, **144**, 185–188.

McLean, P. D., Whittal, M. L., Thordarson, D. S., *et al* (2001) Cognitive versus behaviour therapy in group treatment to obsessive–compulsive disorder. *Consulting and Clinical Psychology*, **69**, 205–214.

Menzies, R. G., Harris, L. M., Cumming, S. R., *et al* (2000) The relationship between inflated personal responsibility and exaggerated danger expectancies in obsessive–compulsive concerns. *Behaviour Research and Therapy*, **38**, 1029–1037.

Mitchell-Heggs, N., Kelly, D. & Richardson, A. (1976) Stereotactic limbic leucotomy: a follow-up at 16 months. *British Journal of Psychiatry*, **128**, 226.

Montgomery, M. A., Clayton, P. J. & Friedhoff, A. J. (1982) Psychiatric illness in Tourette syndrome patients and first degree relatives. In *Gilles de la Tourette Syndrome* (eds A. J. Friedhoff & T. N. Chase), pp. 335–339. New York: Raven.

Montgomery, S. A. (1980) Clomipramine in obsessional neurosis: a placebo-controlled trial. *Pharmacological Medicine*, **1**, 189–192.

Myers, J. K., Weissman, M. M., Tischler, G. L., *et al* (1984) Six-month prevalence of psychiatric disorders in three communities. *Archives of General Psychiatry*, **41**, 959–967.

Nemiah, J. C. (1985) Obsessive–compulsive disorder (obsessive–compulsive neurosis). In *Comprehensive Textbook of Psychiatry* (4th edn) (eds H. I. Kaplan & B. J. Sadock), p. 906. Baltimore, MD: Williams and Wilkins.

Nicolini, H., Hanna, G., Baxter, L., *et al* (1991) Segregation analysis of obsessive compulsive and associated disorders: preliminary results. *Ursus Medicus*, **1**, 25–28.

Nordahl, T. E., Benkelfat, C., Semple, W. E., *et al* (1989) Cerebral glucose metabolic rates in obsessive compulsive disorder. *Neuropsychopharmacology*, **2**, 23–28.

Noshirvani, H. F., Kasviskis, Y., Marks, I. M., *et al* (1991) Gender-divergent aetiological factors in obsessive–compulsive disorder. *British Journal of Psychiatry*, **158**, 260–263.

Palmer, H. D. & Jones, M. S. (1939) Anorexia nervosa as a manifestation of compulsion neurosis. *Archives of Neurology and Psychiatry*, **41**, 856–858.

Pauls, D. L. (2001) The role of genetic factors in OCD. In *Obsessive Compulsive Disorder: A Practical Guide* (eds N. A. Fineberg, D. Marazitti & D. Stein), pp. 61–76. London: Martin Dunitz.

Pauls, D. L., Alsobrook, J. P., Goodman, W., *et al* (1995) A family study of obsessive compulsive disorder. *American Journal of Psychiatry*, **152**, 76–84.

Perani, D., Colombo, C., Bressi, S., *et al* (1995) [^{18}F]FDG PET study in obsessive–compulsive disorder. A clinical/metabolic correlation study after treatment. *British Journal of Psychiatry*, **166**, 244–250.

Pitman, R. K. (1982) Neurological aetiology of obsessive compulsive disorders? *American Journal of Psychiatry*, **139**, 139–140.

Rachman, S. (1976) Obsessional–compulsive checking. *Behaviour Research and Therapy*, **14**, 269–277.

Rachman, S. (2002) A cognitive theory of checking. *Behaviour Research and Therapy*, **40**, 625–639.

Raphael, F. J., Rani, S., Bale, R., *et al* (1996) Religion, ethnicity and obsessive–compulsive disorder. *International Journal of Social Psychiatry*, **42**, 38–44.

Rapoport, J. L. & Wise, S. P. (1988) Obsessive–compulsive disorder: evidence for basal ganglia dysfunction. *Psychopharmacology Bulletin*, **24**, 380–384.

Rasmussen, S. A. & Eisen, J. L. (1990) The epidemiology of obsessive compulsive disorder. *Journal of Clinical Psychiatry*, **51**, suppl., 10–13.

Rasmussen, S. A. & Eisen, J. L. (1997) Treatment strategies for chronic and refractory obsessive compulsive disorder. *Journal of Clinical Psychiatry*, **58**, suppl. 13, 9–13.

Rasmussen, S. A. & Tsuang, M. T. (1986) Clinical characteristics and family history in DSM-III obsessive–compulsive disorder. *American Journal of Psychiatry*, **143**, 317–322.

Rasmussen, S., Hackett, E., DuBoff, E., *et al* (1997) A 2-year study of sertraline in the treatment of obsessive compulsive disorder. *International Clinical Psychopharmacology*, **12**, 309–316.

Richards, D. A., Lovell, K. & Marks, T. M. (1994) Post-traumatic stress disorder: evaluation of behavioural treatment program. *Journal of Traumatic Stress*, **7**, 669–80.

Robins, L. N., Holzer, J. E., Weissman, M. M., *et al* (1984) Lifetime prevalence of specific psychiatric disorders in three sites. *Archives of General Psychiatry*, **41**, 949–958.

Romano, S., Goodman, W. K., Tamura, T., *et al* (1998) Long-term treatment of obsessive compulsive disorder following acute response: a comparison of fluoxetine versus placebo. *European Neuropsychopharmacology*, **8**, suppl. 2, 261.

Salkovskis, P. M. (1983) Treatment of an obsessional patient using habituation to audiotaped ruminations. *British Journal of Clinical Psychology*, **22**, 311–313.

Salkovskis, P. M. (1985) Obsessional–compulsive problems: a cognitive–behavioural analysis. *Behaviour Research and Therapy*, **25**, 571–583.

Salkovskis, P. M. (1989) Cognitive–behavioural factors and the persistence of intrusive thoughts in obsessional problems. *Behaviour Research and Therapy*, **27**, 677–682.

Salkovskis, P. M. (1999) Understanding and treating obsessive–compulsive disorder. *Behaviour Research and Therapy*, **37**, suppl. 1, 29–52.

Salkovskis, P. M. & Warwick, H. M. C. (1985) Cognitive therapy of obsessive–compulsive disorder: treating treatment failures. *Behavioural Psychotherapy*, **13**, 243–255.

Salkovskis, P. M., Forrester, E. & Richards, C. (1998) Cognitive–behavioural approach to understanding obsessional thinking. *British Journal of Psychiatry*, **35**, suppl., 53–63.

Schwartz, J. M., Stoessel, P. W., Baxter, L. R., *et al* (1996) Systematic changes in cerebral glucose metabolic rate after successful behaviour modification treatment of obsessive compulsive disorder. *Archives of General Psychiatry*, **53**, 109–113.

Skoog, G. & Skoog, I. (1999) A 40-year follow-up of patients with obsessive compulsive disorder. *Archives of General Psychiatry*, **56**, 121–127.

Stein, D., Fineberg, N. & Seedat, S. (2001) An integrated approach to the treatment of OCD. In *Obsessive Compulsive Disorder: A Practical Guide* (eds N. A. Fineberg, D. Marazitti & D. Stein), pp. 167–176. London: Martin Dunitz.

Steinhousen, C. H. & Glanville, K. (1983) Follow-up studies of anorexia nervosa: a review of research findings. *Psychological Medicine*, **13**, 239–249.

Stern, R. S. & Marks, I. M. (1973) Brief and prolonged flooding: a comparison in agoraphobic patients. *Archives of General Psychiatry*, **28**, 270–276.

Swedo, S., Rapoport, S., Leonard, H., *et al* (1989*a*) Obsessive compulsive disorder in children and adolescents. *Archives of General Psychiatry*, **46**, 335–341.

Swedo, S., Shapiro, M. B., Grady, C. L., *et al* (1989*b*) Cerebral glucose metabolism in childhood onset obsessive compulsive disorder. *Archives of General Psychiatry*, **46**, 518–523.

Swedo, S., Pitrini, P., Leonard, H., *et al* (1992) Cerebral glucose metabolism in childhood onset obsessive compulsive disorder: revisualisation after pharmacotherapy. *Archives of General Psychiatry*, **49**, 690–694.

Thiel, A., Broocks, A., Ohlmeier, M., *et al* (1995) Obsessive compulsive disorder among patients with anorexia nervosa and bulimia nervosa. *American Journal of Psychiatry*, **152**, 72–75.

Thoren, P., Asberg, M., Cronholm, B., *et al* (1980) Clomipramine treatment of obsessive–compulsive disorders: 1. *Archives of General Psychiatry*, **37**, 1281–1285.

Toates, F. (1990) *Obsessional Thoughts and Behaviour: Help for Obsessive–Compulsive Disorder*. Wellingborough: Thorsons.

van Oppen, P., de Haan, E., van Balkom, A. J., *et al* (1995) Cognitive therapy and exposure in vivo in the treatment of obsessive–compulsive disorder. *Behaviour Research and Therapy*, **33**, 379–390.

Warwick, H. M. C. & Salkovskis, P. M. (1985) Reassurance. *BMJ*, **290**, 1028.

Weissman, M. M., Bland, R. C., Canino, G. L., *et al* (1994) The cross national epidemiology of obsessive compulsive disorder. *Journal of Clinical Psychiatry*, **55**, 5–10.

World Health Organization (1992) *The Tenth Revision of the International Classification of Diseases and Related Health Problems* (ICD–10). Geneva: WHO.

Zohar, J. & Fineberg, N. A. (2001) Practical pharmacotherapy. In *Obsessive Compulsive Disorder: A Practical Guide* (eds N. A. Fineberg, D. Marazitti & D. Stein), pp. 103–117. London: Martin Dunitz.

Zohar, J. & Insel, T. R. (1987) Obsessive-compulsive disorder: psychobiological approaches to diagnosis, treatment, and pathophysiology. *Biological Psychiatry*, **22**, 667–687.

Zohar, J. & Judge, R. (1996) Paroxetine versus clomipramine in the treatment of obsessive compulsive disorder. *British Journal of Psychiatry*, **169**, 468–474.

Zohar, J., Insel, T. R., Berman, K. F., *et al* (1989) Anxiety and cerebral blood flow during behavioural challenge. Dissociation of central from peripheral and subjective measures. *Archives of General Psychiatry*, **46**, 505–510.

Zohar, J., Chopra, M., Sasson, Y., *et al* (2000) Psychopharmacology of obsessive compulsive disorder? *World Journal of Biological Psychiatry*, **1**, 92–100.

CHAPTER 16

Conversion and dissociative disorders, hypochondriasis and chronic pain

Tom Brown and Harold Merskey

This chapter describes a group of complex disorders of uncertain cause. Some, like the somatoform and conversion disorders, resemble a physical illness, while others, such as the dissociative disorders, affect psychological function and are suggestive of a mental disorder. In most of these disorders there is an underlying assumption, which is not necessarily correct, that psychological and social factors always play a significant causal role, although in most cases the underlying mechanisms are still unclear. Conversion and dissociative disorders used to be called 'hysteria', but, after a lengthy history, as well as the acquisition of multiple and sometimes pejorative meanings, the term is no longer used in any of the official glossaries. *Conversion* refers to a loss or alteration of function which is *presumed* to be psychological in origin. *Dissociation* refers to disturbances in the normally integrative functions of the mind, especially in the realms of identity, memory and consciousness.

The somatoform disorders include somatisation disorder and hypochondriasis. They present with physical symptoms and sufferers have a strong belief that they have a physical disorder, with a biological cause, but medical examination fails to establish a link with any known physical disease. The term 'medically unexplained symptoms' or a variation such as 'medically unexplained physical symptoms' or 'incompletely explained symptoms' is often now applied to this situation. These are less contentious in medical circles but are of limited use in communicating with patients. Older terms such as hysteria and hypochondriasis are completely unacceptable to patients. An interesting contribution to the debate on terminology is the study of Stone *et al* (2002*a*), who found that the old term 'functional disorder' is surprisingly acceptable to most patients. This group of conditions is particularly sensitive to external sociocultural factors, especially to prevailing notions of illness within both the medical profession and the wider community, and to the way the welfare state operates. This in no way negates the potential importance of biological factors in these disorders, as highlighted below.

The literature in this area of medicine often begins from a point of view that separates so-called mental illness from physical illness – a dichotomy that some have questioned. A full discussion of this debate is beyond the scope of this chapter and we comment on it only briefly.

Modern psychiatry routinely accepts the notion of a bio-psychosocial understanding and management of various disorders, whether anxiety, schizophrenia or chronic pain. This is held to be a monistic approach, that is, one that is unitary in terms of body–mind relationships and therefore 'good'. So-called dualistic approaches are often condemned. This misunderstands and sometimes mistakenly applies the features of a psychosocial approach to *explanatory* statements about what causes different conditions. Properly understood, the end-point of any illness should be considered to be a unitary phenomenon in which we are looking at the internal experience of the individual, whether that experience reflects pain or a lump in the body, a hallucination or a feeling of sadness. We do not discriminate, for example, between organic and psychological causes of pain subjectively. Pain is pain. It is a subjective experience whatever its cause. However, in understanding pain, and the so-called somatoform disorders, it is important for practical purposes, and theoretically logical, to treat the patient's experience in a monistic fashion and the causes in a dualistic fashion. Thus, we should always be prepared to specify to our colleagues and to patients themselves the specific physical, psychological and social factors that are causing or promoting the illness, and also, at least in broad terms, and where possible, where each starts and ends. Carefully applied, this approach mollifies everyone and prevents doctor and patient from taking one-sided actions. In this respect risk factors should be treated with care, as they are sometimes signs of a problem and not necessarily causes.

Conversion and dissociation disorders

History

It has often been thought that the Greeks believed that the symptoms of hysteria were caused by the womb moving about the body and blocking 'the channels of respiration' (Greek *hystera*, womb). If the womb was displaced upwards, there would be difficulties in swallowing and dyspnoea (Merskey & Merskey, 1993). So far as we can determine, these ideas were never strongly held by the Greeks, but they received a lot of emphasis in medieval times and for a period thereafter.

Typical conversion and dissociative symptoms are relatively rare in developed societies. Sydenham (1697) recognised the effects of mental trauma on bodily function as hysteria but also included much of what we would now regard as organic disease.

> 'When the Mind is disturbed by some grevious [*sic*] Accident, the animal Spirits run into disorderly motions; the Urine appears limpid, and in great quantity; the sick persons cast off all hope of recovery.... the Apoplexy, which ends in a Palsy of one half of the Body, comes presently after Child-bearing; sometimes they are seized with Convulsions, that very much resemble the Epilepsy, and are commonly called the Suffocation of the Womb, in which the Belly and Entrails rise upwards towards the Throat; At other times they are miserably tormented with the Hysterical Clavus [nail], in which there is a most vehement pain in the Head, which you may cover with your Thumb, the sick person in the mean time vomiting up green Matter like to that sort of Choler that has its name from Leeks.' (Sydenham, 1697)

This extract tells us that severe stress may produce both emotional and physical changes. Some of these are observable alterations in bodily functions, such as changes in the urine, apoplexy or hemiplegia, but others are changes that we would consider hysterical, such as non-epileptic fits. In a section that followed the above extract, Sydenham also included some other pains, diarrhoea, dropsy, tears and laughter. Since the 19th century, either an emotional conflict or a brain disorder has been considered to be the commonest cause.

Brodie (1837) appears to have been the first to make the modern distinction between effects that could be explained by structural lesions of the nervous system and effects that could not, and he attributed the latter to the influence of the patient's will.

Romberg (1851) believed hysteria was 'a reflex sexual neurosis', a notion that persisted in the European literature up to the end of the century. However, in France both Georget (1821) and Brachet (1847) formulated hysteria as a 'neurosis', meaning that the seat of the affliction resided within the brain. Although it remained an 'organic concept' caused by a disturbance of brain function, it could still be triggered by stress, business setbacks, unhappy love affairs and ill treatment by parents. In essence it was thought that brain function was disturbed by an unknown cause, possibly related to excessive stimulation. A parallel idea developed, particularly from the 19th century onwards, to the effect that a weakness of personality or constitution promoted 'hysteria' (Alam & Merskey, 1992).

Reynolds (1869) wrote an article on three cases of paralysis 'dependent upon idea'. Following this, Charcot (1889) demonstrated that hypnosis could be used to implant an idea into the patient's thoughts and that this could later cause a symptom such as a paralysis or loss of vision. He demonstrated that when the mind caused the disorder, the symptom pattern corresponded with the patient's views, rather than conforming with anatomical and physiological knowledge, an observation that remains relevant when making the diagnosis today. Janet (1894) suggested that conversion might take place in the patient's mind 'below consciousness', an idea that was taken up and expanded by Freud. By the time Breuer and Freud came to study hysteria, it was viewed as a disorder of brain function but without specific localisation (see Hirschmuller, 1989).

Problems of diagnosis have always beset the recognition of apparent conversion disorder symptoms. For example, 'Anna O', one of Freud's most famous patients, in whom the psychodynamic mechanisms of repression and conversion were said to have been discovered, appears to have suffered from a severe fluctuating depressive illness, complicated by heavy sedation and possibly an iatrogenic dependence on morphine and chloral hydrate (Merskey, 1992*b*).

The origins of the concept of the so-called 'hysterical personality' are less ancient. At one time it was thought to be a well-defined entity, strongly associated with conversion or dissociative symptoms. Carter (1853) recognised the main characteristics, such as emotional lability, intense emotion, reactive sensitivity, liveliness and vivacity, impressionability and an 'affective' temperament. Kraepelin (1904) provided an impressive description of a patient with dependent traits and dramatic skill. By the 1930s the concept of hysterical personality was well established; it comprised a collection of qualities, mostly unfavourable, such as labile with shallow emotions, manipulativeness, seductiveness with frigidity, histrionic behaviour, self-centredness, vanity, exhibitionism, attention seeking, and suggestibility, and this is further discussed in Chapter 18 on page 451.

Shell shock and post-traumatic stress disorder

Conditions were so bad during the First World War, and the risk of death so great, that it was thought that large numbers of men would have deserted if the punishment of death for cowardice had not been employed. Serious breakdowns in morale occurred, but there was often the possibility of an escape into illness. The military authorities could not reject this escape because many men of proven courage gave way to uncontrollable fear after protracted stress. It was not acceptable to call them cowards or to suggest their behaviour was dishonourable, much less to punish them. The British army (but not the Continental armies) accepted a condition called 'shell shock'. The disorder was thought to be the result of changes in the nervous system caused by concussion from nearby explosions but without any evidence of external injury. The main symptoms of shell shock included tremors, blindness, deafness, a bent back, paralyses and anaesthesias, as well as virtually any other complaint. This wide variety of symptoms in the soldiers demonstrated that mental and somatic symptoms could result from severe stress, and that sexual trauma in childhood was far from essential in their production (Merskey, 1991). In later wars and civilian catastrophes the occurrence of post-traumatic stress disorder came to be recognised as an anxiety phenomenon that merited attention in its own right, and without it being necessary to reject the reality of patients' suffering because of the context.

Does the term 'hysteria' still have a place?

The term 'hysteria' is (and has been) used in many different ways. First, the popular use generally denotes noisy, excited or uncontrolled behaviour. Second, clinicians use the term to describe a conversion or a dissociative symptom. (As indicated above, traditionally, dissociative symptoms that affect the body are called *conversion* symptoms, while the term *dissociation* is reserved for disturbances of mental function.) Third, hysteria is used to denote a certain type of personality, the 'hysterical (or histrionic) personality' (histrionic personality disorder is described in Chapter 18, page 451). Not surprisingly, because of the many uses (and abuses) of the word 'hysteria', ICD–10 uses the term 'conversion hysteria' to describe the mechanism, and no ICD–10 syndrome definition contains the word 'hysteria' (World Health Organization, 1992). DSM–IV (American Psychiatric Association, 1994) adopts an even more extreme position and the word appears only once in the text, in association with Briquet's syndrome, and because of its pejorative connotations probably should not be used when making any official diagnosis. The word is not acceptable to patients (Stone *et al*, 2002*a*).

Similarities and differences between the ICD–10 and DSM–IV classifications

These disorders are classified in different ways in the DSM–IV and ICD–10 schemes. The principal difference is that ICD–10 classifies the conversion and dissociative disorders under one umbrella, the dissociative disorders, and dissociation is viewed as the primary phenomenon. DSM–IV has a separate chapter for dissociation, but conversion is classified as a subtype of somatisation (see below), and not of dissociation. Chronic pain, which remains in the DSM–IV system under the heading 'Pain disorder', underwent the deliberate removal of the word 'somatoform' from the title. Both ICD–10 and DSM–IV refer to the term 'somatoform disorders' and under this umbrella describe a number of syndromes (see Table 16.1). Many of the differences between ICD–10 and DSM–IV are trivial and only a question of semantics, but others reflect difficult clinical realities or are long-standing, indeed insoluble dilemmas for which there are obvious solutions, and are therefore worth discussing.

The ICD–10 scheme groups the dissociative and somatoform disorders together with all the anxiety disorders in a chapter entitled 'Neurotic, stress-related and somatoform disorders', and explains the decision to group these disorders together on the basis of their historical link to the concept of neurosis and because a substantial (though uncertain) proportion of the people with these disorders have some element of psychological causation. No attempt is made to justify the use of the term 'neurosis', which DSM–IV has completely eliminated from its text.

As can be seen from Table 16.1, there are some important differences in the categories of disorder that DSM–IV and ICD–10 include. The most obvious difference is that ICD–10 classifies conversion disorder with dissociative disorders and the text states:

> 'The common theme shared by dissociative or conversion disorders is a partial or complete loss of the normal integration between memories of the past, awareness of identity and immediate sensations, and control of bodily movements.... In the dissociative disorders it is presumed that ... [the] ... ability to exercise a conscious and selective control is impaired.'

ICD–10 then goes on to provide brief clinical descriptions of the following traditional dissociative disorders: dissociative amnesia, fugue, stupor, trance and possession disorder and a miscellaneous group that includes Ganser's syndrome and the alleged multiple personality disorder, about which it is sceptical.

Table 16.1 Classification of 'unexplained' symptoms

DSM–IV	ICD–10
Somatisation disorder	Somatisation disorder
Undifferentiated somatoform disorder	Undifferentiated somatoform disorder
Conversion disorder	Dissociative [conversion] disorders
Dissociative disorder	
Pain disorder	Persistent somatoform pain disorder
Somatoform autonomic dysfunction	
Hypochondriasis	Hypochondriacal disorder (including body dysmorphic disorder)
Body dysmorphic disorder	
Somatoform disorder not otherwise specified	Other somatoform disorders

The term 'conversion' implies that an unpleasant affect, engendered by the problems and conflicts that the patient cannot solve, is somehow transformed into the symptoms. The DSM–IV criteria for conversion are shown in Box 16.1. ICD–10 describes the following types of dissociative disorder, which were formerly called conversion disorders: motor disorders, which include aphonias and various types of paralysis, convulsions, anaesthesia and sensory loss (most commonly loss of vision but also deafness and other sensory losses). Somatisation disorder and other somatoform disorders, including pain disorder and hypochondriasis, are presented in a section adjoining that on dissociative disorders.

In the DSM–IV scheme, a completely separate chapter is given over solely to the dissociative disorders. The text states that the essential feature of a dissociative disorder is:

> 'a disruption in the usually integrated functions of consciousness, memory, identity, or perception of the environment. The disturbance may be sudden or gradual, transient or chronic.'

Categories of dissociative disorder include: psychogenic amnesia, fugue, dissociative identity disorder (formerly multiple personality disorder), as well as depersonalisation disorder, and a group of disorders not otherwise specified. DSM–IV gives clear operational criteria (as well as a clinical description) for each disorder. The introduction to the chapter on dissociation points out that cross-cultural factors should also be taken into account when evaluating these disorders and that dissociation on its own is not necessarily pathological, does not always lead to help-seeking behaviours, and can occur as a normal feature of certain cultural and religious activities.

Box 16.1 DSM–IV criteria for conversion disorder

A One or more symptoms or deficits affecting voluntary motor or sensory function that suggest a neurological or other general medical condition.
B Psychological factors are judged to be associated with the symptom or deficit because the initiation or exacerbation of the symptom or deficit is preceded by conflicts or other stressors.
C The symptom or deficit is not intentionally produced or feigned (as in factitious disorder or malingering).
D The symptom or deficit cannot, after appropriate investigation, be fully explained by a general medical condition, or by the direct effects of a substance, or as a culturally sanctioned behaviour or experience.
E The symptom or deficit causes clinically significant distress or impairment in social, occupational or other important areas of functioning, or warrants medical evaluation.
F The symptom or deficit is not limited to pain or sexual dysfunction, does not occur exclusively during the course of somatisation disorder, and is not better accounted for by another mental disorder.

Specify type of symptom or deficit:
- with motor symptom or deficit
- with sensory symptom or deficit
- with seizures or convulsions
- with mixed presentation.

Adapted with permission from DSM-IV-TR. Copyright 2000 American Psychiatric Association.

The classification of somatoform disorders

The DSM–IV concept of the somatoform disorders is of a group of conditions where the presenting features are physical symptoms and suggest a general medical condition. However, these symptoms cannot be fully explained by a general medical condition or by the effects of substances, or by another mental disorder (e.g. panic disorder). The symptoms should also cause 'clinically significant distress or impairment in social, occupational or other areas of functioning'. This is a ubiquitous clause appearing throughout DSM–IV and provides the guide to the degree of severity that will enable a 'condition' to qualify as a 'disorder'. DSM–IV also emphasises that the grouping of these disorders in a single section is made only on the grounds of clinical utility, by which is meant the need to exclude general medical conditions or substance misuse aetiologies. The text makes an explicit statement that the grouping together of these disorders does not imply any assumptions concerning a shared or common aetiology.

ICD–10 emphasises the notion that in somatoform disorders there is a repeated presentation with physical symptoms, with persistent requests for investigation in spite of negative findings and despite reassurance that the symptoms have no physical basis. ICD–10 lists five main categories: somatisation disorder, undifferentiated somatoform disorder, hypochondriacal disorder, somatoform autonomic dysfunction and persistent somatoform pain disorder. ICD–10 also highlights the patient's resistance to discussing the possibility of psychological causation, even when this appears obvious, and that histrionic attention-seeking behaviours may also be present.

Both DSM–IV and ICD–10 invite the doctor to engage in a degree of value judgement. For example, DSM–IV states that in somatoform disorders (in contrast to factitious disorders and malingering) 'the physical symptoms are not intentional i.e. under voluntary control', and ICD–10 invites clinicians to exclude 'histrionic attention seeking behaviour'. In practice, working out whether symptoms are intentional or not, or whether histrionic elaboration is present, is a difficult clinical distinction to make.

A more minor difference relates to the way body dysmorphic disorder is classified. Thus, ICD–10 includes body dysmorphic disorder under the heading of hypochondriacal disorder, whereas DSM–IV considers it to be a separate disorder (i.e. not a subtype of hypochondriasis).

Undifferentiated somatoform (DSM–IV and ICD–10) and somatic autonomic dysfunction (ICD–10 only)

The category 'undifferentiated somatoform disorder' is not commonly used in clinical work but is epidemiologically important and has a different meaning in DSM–IV and ICD–10. The ICD–10 condition is diagnosed when there are multiple and varied physical complaints but the picture is not severe enough to make a diagnosis of somatisation disorder. For example, there may be little or no impairment in social function, and the main differential diagnosis is from the full somatisation syndrome. This picture is common in community settings.

The DSM–IV concept of 'undifferentiated somatoform disorder' includes the syndrome described above (i.e. a lesser version of somatisation disorder) but it also includes symptoms from systems such as the gastrointestinal or genito-urinary, whereas ICD–10 includes these latter symptoms under the category of 'somatoform autonomic dysfunction'. DSM–IV also includes neurasthenia (chronic fatigue syndrome) as one of the undifferentiated somatoform disorders, whereas ICD–10 has a quite separate category for neurasthenia and places it in the section entitled 'Other neurotic disorders'.

Somatic autonomic dysfunction is a category only present in ICD–10 and is not included in DSM–IV. It refers to the wide variety of what were previously considered to be 'psychosomatic syndromes'. These include: in the cardiovascular system, cardiac neurosis, Da Costa's syndrome, and neurocirculatory asthenia; in the gastrointestinal system, dyspepsia, pylorospasm, irritable bowel syndrome and psychogenic flatulence; in the respiratory system, psychogenic cough and hyperventilation; and in the genito-urinary system, psychogenic frequency and dysuria, as well as less common psychosomatic disorders.

Epidemiological studies suggest these syndromes as a group are common (see page 401), and they are mainly encountered in primary care. Indeed, they are far more common than the well-defined traditional somatic syndromes (Lieb *et al*, 2000).

Criticisms of the present schemes of classification

In an editorial entitled 'Somatoform disorders in DSM–V', Mayou *et al* (2003) offer the following criticisms of present classification schemes, which they believe are widely backed by liaison psychiatrists, and suggest these factors should be taken into account when DSM–V is drafted. They make the following points

- The classification is essentially dualist, couched in terms of alternative physical or psychological aetiologies. It has therefore been difficult to apply in many cultures that do not share the Western dualistic view of mind and body causes as alternatives, and the dualistic model has been challenged even in Western cultures.
- Not all the specific categories have good validity or reliability.
- Some categories depend on counting the number of physical symptoms (e.g. somatisation disorder and undifferentiated somatoform disorder) or the type of symptom (pain disorder) that in the real world lacks threshold, yet arbitrary severity and duration thresholds are given in DSM–IV.
- The separation of dissociative from conversion disorders seems arbitrary.
- From a technical recording perspective there is some illogicality, in that physical symptoms can be classified either as a part of an axis I disorder (i.e. a psychiatric condition) and/or an axis III disorder (general medical conditions).

No one knows yet how DSM–V will organise and classify these disorders, but Mayou *et al* (2003) suggest that one solution might be much greater use of the category 'psychological factors affecting a medical condition'. Because none of the conditions in this group is very well defined, it is likely that any classification system will be liable to be criticised the moment it is proposed.

Merskey (2000) has also argued that the classification of somatoform disorders has been unduly influenced by experience derived from secondary and tertiary care. In essence, specialists whose work has been influential in shaping classification usually work in areas where they see highly selected patients, who are often beset with psychological and personality difficulties, and this gives them the misleading impression that a majority of patients with 'medically unexplained symptoms' have mainly psychological difficulties, and this bias favours psychogenesis as the explanation for the somatisation disorders, to the exclusion of other possible causes.

Clinical presentation of conversion disorders

Motor symptoms

One of the commonest motor presentations is loss of speech, or hysterical aphonia. Head (1922) described how these patients may become completely mute while writing voluble accounts of their condition. The patient cannot whisper, yet can cough loudly because 'from a psychological point of view, the resonant sound of a cough has nothing to do with articulated speech'. In the larynx, the vocal cords remain apart on phonation, although during a cough they close normally.

A recent report of 24 cases from India found that: most of the cases had an onset within the previous 2 weeks; there was a 2:1 female:male preponderance; and most patients were young (mean age 18.4 years for females, 21.2 years for males). The most common precipitating factors were examination stress or failure, followed by quarrels with peers or a spouse. Comorbid psychiatric disorder was found in 80% of the cases, most commonly mixed anxiety and depressive disorder (Bhatia & Vaid, 2000).

Aphonia is a good example of what Head called 'positive signs'. The positive signs were said to be: a history of hypochondriasis, secondary gain, *la belle indifference*, non-anatomical sensory loss with a split of the midline by pain or vibration stimulation, changing boundaries of hypalgesia, and give-way weakness. He emphasised that in order to diagnose hysteria it was necessary to demonstrate two phenomena:

1 there should be an absence of relevant organic disease, or at least proportionate organic disease

2 there should be proof of the positive signs.

A third condition is also necessary for the psychiatrist: the demonstration of a psychological aetiology, often confirmed by the patient, or of psychiatric illness that is of sufficient proportion to the symptom.

Gould *et al* (1986) demonstrated in a consecutive series of neurological patients with proven structural central nervous system (CNS) disorder (mainly stroke) that all patients had at least one 'positive sign' and many had three or four, and cautioned against relying too heavily on them. A diagnosis of conversion disorder should not be made on the basis of any of these signs, nor should they be used to distinguish conversion disorders from organic disease, as evidenced from the results of this and other studies. Modern brain scanning has placed diagnosis on a much sounder basis because it is now much easier to exclude structural brain disease. More recently, Stone *et al* (2002*b*) have described signs that may help in diagnosing functional weakness or sensory loss (see below).

Flaccid paralysis may affect one or more limbs, or one side of the face. In a *hysterical spasm* on the same side of the body both the arm and leg are contracted, the hand closed tightly, the knee flexed, and perhaps the leg and the foot drawn up. Sometimes, as Head observed, spasm of the muscle at the knee or other joint actually resists the movement of the limb in the direction in which the contraction is supposed to be occurring. Traditionally these phenomena have been taken as evidence of hysteria, but a pathophysiological cause, such as a joint pain or noxious irritation in a relevant part of the body, is also possible.

If flaccid paralysis or spasms persist, contractures may develop. However, most contractures seen in either physical medicine or psychiatry follow from temporary failure of use of a part due to local pain, or occur after some other major illness, such as myocardial infarction. Paralysis with contractures due to conversion symptoms is now very rare. 'Frozen shoulder' was a once common example but a partially frozen shoulder, or arm that is limited in movement, is usually related to a physical cause. Thus a few patients who were thought to have 'psychogenic' limitation of arm movements were found to have evidence on magnetic resonance imaging (MRI) of tears of one or more tendons in the rotator cuff.

Hysterical tremor is a repeated positive movement of a voluntary type, but varying in rapidity. It ceases if the patient can be persuaded unwittingly to perform some other movement with the same limb. Tremor due to simple anxiety or a physical cause should be excluded before making a diagnosis of hysterical tremor. Difficulties in walking are sometimes due to conversion disorder, as in astasia–abasia. This is an unsteadiness of gait or ataxia, as well as an inability to walk or stand still, characterised by incoordination, which can be quite striking, even though all leg movements can function normally when the patient is sitting or lying down. Some patients appear to be able to perform movements that many normal individuals would find difficult to achieve even with full muscular control.

Three reported series offer different frequencies for the occurrence of motor and other symptoms. Symptoms vary with local cultures, but in Carter's (1949) British series aphonia was the commonest (29%), followed by paralysis (23%), amnesia (23%) and tremor (10%). In Stockholm, astasia (47%) and fits (20%) were the most common (Ljungberg, 1957). In a developing country, Sudan (Hafeiz, 1980), dyspnoea and aphonia were equally common, at 20% each (although not all observers would have classified dyspnoea as hysterical, some might have related it to anxiety when it does not have a physical cause).

Certain abnormal movements such as facial tics, blepharospasm, dyskinesias and the tardive dyskinesias, which were once thought to be psychological in origin, have crossed the porous boundary separating psychiatry from neurology and are now considered to be neurological in origin. The same also substantially applies to Gilles de la Tourette's syndrome. The facial dyskinesias and blepharospasm also changed category after the introduction of L-dopa (Lloyd & Hornykiewicz, 1973). A small excess of L-dopa could result in a switch from a Parkinsonian state to an overt facial dyskinesia that was indistinguishable from conditions that were once diagnosed as hysterical facial abnormalities. Since then, it has generally been assumed that most, if not all, of the blepharospasms and dyskinesias found in clinical practice are of neurological origin. Occasionally a blepharospasm may emerge with a depressive illness, or other emotional changes, and remit with them.

Distinguishing conversion symptoms from physical pathology is by no means straightforward and has been the subject of heated debate over the centuries. As noted above, the old 'positive signs' of hysteria are extremely unreliable. Stone *et al* (2003) attempted to revisit this age-old controversy. They emphasised that functional weakness can be more confidently diagnosed than can functional sensory symptoms and signs, and highlighted the utility of the following:

1 *Evidence of inconsistency* (e.g. in weakness or sensory loss).

2 *Hoover's sign*. This is the most scientifically validated sign of functional weakness in the leg (Ziv *et al*, 1998). It demonstrates a discrepancy between voluntary hip extension (which is weak) and involuntary hip extension when the other hip is being flexed against resistance. This is assessed by the examiner placing a hand under the heel of the 'bad' leg while asking the patient to flex the other hip against resistance. A similar test has been described for arm weakness. Stone *et al* point out that even this test can give both false positives and false negatives.

3 *Collapsing weakness*.

4 *Co-contraction (of antagonist muscles)*.

5 *The arm-drop test*. In this test a paralysed arm is dropped over a patient's face to see if the patient protects him- or herself.

Although these signs are more reliable than the older 'positive signs' of hysteria, Stone *et al* (2003) caution that they must be in the context of the overall presentation and again remind us that patients may have both a functional and an organic disorder at the same time.

Non-epileptic (hysterical) fits or seizures

Non-epileptic (hysterical) seizures occur only in the presence of an audience or when one is close at hand. They may be precipitated by stress, but more often they occur by virtue of the social setting. The patients tend not to fall hard or quickly to the ground, but rather gradually. Crying may occur, but vocalisation is limited to a few words. Movements usually follow the fall, often with dramatic clutching, and sometimes there may be opisthotonos, but there is never the regular tonic–clonic sequence of epilepsy. Tongue biting and incontinence of urine are rare in hysterical fits, while the corneal reflex is preserved and the plantar response is flexor (unless previously abnormal). Firm handling and pressure over the supra-orbital nerves (which may be painful) may arouse the patient.

In contrast, epileptic patients may have a brief aura or cry, particularly with the onset of a tonic convulsion, and are liable to hurt themselves in the fall to the floor. They generally go through regular tonic and clonic phases of muscular contraction, with tongue biting and incontinence of urine. In practice, however, the diagnosis is not so easy because anticonvulsant drugs may modify epileptic fits, and also people with genuine epilepsy can develop hysterical fits. In drug-treated epilepsy, the falls may be rather less abrupt, the characteristic pattern of tonic and clonic movements, tongue biting and incontinence much less obvious, and sometimes, particularly with temporal lobe epilepsy, ictal behaviour is confined to a few smacking movements of the lips or face. Following an epileptic fit there may be a drug-modified automatism, which can resemble dissociative behaviour. Patients who have brief, barely noticeable partial tonic–clonic fits may afterwards have poorly organised behaviour, appearing to be partly in touch with the environment and acting purposively.

Non-epileptic seizures are more common among patients with epilepsy than others, particularly if there are emotional problems or if they have toxic levels of anticonvulsant medication. A few patients with epilepsy learn how to induce ictal discharges, and are able to induce extra fits, while others may consciously or unconsciously demonstrate an increased falling tendency.

Certain tests may be of diagnostic value. The classic Hippocratic diagnostic test between epilepsy and hysteria was to pinch the skin of the abdomen, which would have no effect in the unconscious person with epilepsy. The electroencephalogram (EEG), if available, is abnormal during an epileptic fit but normal during non-epileptic fits. The serum prolactin level is elevated after an epileptic seizure, and this may also be a useful discriminating measure – if the prolactin level is normal it is unlikely that an epileptic seizure has occurred (Trimble, 1978).

Anxious patients sometimes develop phenomena that resemble fits. In the face of severe anxiety, blood pressure may fall, and this is associated with feelings of faintness, or feelings of loss of awareness of the surroundings. There is usually a brief warning before a fainting episode, which allows the patient enough time to subside more gently. Fainting has numerous causes apart from anxiety, and it is important always to exclude cardiovascular disease, which can cause fainting through a variety of different disorders. Neurological conditions such as cataplexy (see page 608) and transient ischaemic attacks should be considered in older people. However, in psychiatric practice, postural hypotension as a result of drug side-effects is the most common cause. Occasionally, patients hurt themselves after a fainting episode, but they usually come around quite rapidly, with the initial pallor soon returning to normal.

Anxious patients, particularly those with phobias and panic disorders, may also *hyperventilate*. In situations such as assemblies, small spaces and underground railway stations, these individuals feel uneasy that they cannot get their breath and as a consequence hyperventilate. Carpopedal spasms, loss of consciousness and (rarely) epileptiform convulsions may result from the fall in carbon dioxide because too much has been breathed off and this results in alkalosis and hypocalcaemia. Although hyperventilation has been termed hysterical, the symptom is most commonly associated with panic disorder and phobias. It can be relieved by demonstrating to the patient how the symptom is caused (i.e. by over-breathing) and cured by re-breathing into a paper bag, or even by holding the breath.

Dizziness is also a common complaint. Such a subjective feeling of unsteadiness has often been called hysterical, but this is probably not the best label. Feelings of unsteadiness and falling are part of the syndrome of astasia–abasia mentioned above, but also occur commonly with anxiety. They should be distinguished from vertigo, in which the patient feels that the environment is rotating.

A further differential diagnosis of a non-epileptic seizure is from an automatism occurring in response to lowered blood sugar levels or other metabolic disorders; these may also mimic an epileptic automatism.

Swallowing difficulties – globus hystericus

Traditionally, the sensation of a ball (globus) in the throat almost always occurred in women, hence the description 'suffocation of the mother'. The idea of a hysterical symptom in the throat was linked with the notion that the wandering uterus blocked the channels of respiration. It is uncertain whether the early writers were describing an anxious dyspnoea or an anxious difficulty in swallowing.

Physiological clinical techniques have suggested that the majority of patients presenting with difficulty in swallowing do have some underlying physical problem. Malcolmson (1966, 1968) found that only 21% of patients with a complaint of difficulty in swallowing had a completely negative physical and radiological examination. Others found evidence of reflux oesophagitis in most patients, or elevated resting pressures in the cricopharyngeal sphincter in patients with gastric reflux. These pressures fell to normal after successful treatment. Lehtinen & Puhakka (1976) described two different types of globus pharyngis (i.e. globus hystericus), one in which the cause was mainly somatic and the other in which the cause was primarily psychological, but even among the latter it would be wrong to label all cases of 'globus' as 'hystericus'.

Other symptoms

Vomiting and diarrhoea, which may be psychogenic, have previously been regarded as hysterical but are now rarely classified in this way. Induced vomiting such as occurs in bulimia nervosa is a deliberate disability, but there may be some overlap because other conversion symptoms are quite common in bulimia. Traumatic experiences during childhood may be a common aetiological factor for both disorders.

Repeated spontaneous vomiting from intestinal obstruction is also sometimes misdiagnosed as hysterical, even to the point of a fatality. Other disorders of bowel control such as diarrhoea or constipation are sometimes caused by the misuse of laxatives, and by underlying physical disorders. Irritable bowel syndrome should not be attributed to psychological motivation even if psychological measures may be helpful. Dyspnoea, which can be psychogenic, is usually due to anxiety rather than being seen as a conversion symptom. Retention of urine has traditionally been regarded as a hysterical symptom, but it is questionable whether retention occurs at all or to an appreciable extent for psychological reasons. Simulation of retention has also been reported.

As noted above, ICD–10 subsumes all these syndromes under the general category 'somatoform autonomic dysfunction', whereas DSM–IV does not mention them specifically as syndromes, but if they are sufficiently severe to qualify as a 'disorder' (i.e. they last more than 6 months and significantly impair function), they are placed in the category of 'undifferentiated somatoform disorders'.

Sensory symptoms

Deafness

Deafness as a conversion symptom is quite rare in civilian clinical practice, but was common among soldiers exposed to blast injury and was then sometimes associated with hysterical paralysis and blindness. A few people who have had their eardrums ruptured, or suffered from industrial deafness, may also prolong or magnify an original injury, particularly where compensation is an issue. Deafness as a conversion disorder can be detected during sleep, because noise may waken the patient. A more subtle method of demonstrating the presence of intact hearing is to take a sleep EEG recording and then speak the patient's name during it. This may produce the characteristic K complex in the EEG that indicates a response to familiar material, although the response tends to extinguish upon repetition. Studies of evoked potentials can also be used to demonstrate intact auditory pathways. Deafness as a conversion symptom may be incomplete. This is rather more difficult to diagnose but may be inferred from inconsistent responses on audiological testing.

Blindness

Blindness as a conversion symptom is common in ophthalmological practice (Kathol *et al*, 1983*a*,*b*; Weller & Wiedemann, 1989) and is often partial rather than complete. It usually presents either as a blurring of vision or as a difficulty in reading in adolescents, particularly when facing examinations.

Difficulty in vision is often thought to be a conversion symptom if the patient shows tubular spiral visual fields. The measurement of the visual fields by perimetry involves moving a small spot systematically from the margin to the centre, and asking the patient to detect the spot. With normal vision the fields should be wider at a distance than close to the eye. If the size of the visual field stays the same on testing, regardless of the distance from the eye, the patient has tubular vision. A spiral change in the visual fields is obtained when the examiner, starting at one point, obtains a visual field of a given magnitude that then gradually decreases as he or she moves around the field in a circle. By the time the test spot has been returned to the starting point, it may be visualised only on the axis where it started, in a position much closer to the centre than was originally found.

In a review of the literature, Kathol *et al* (1983*a*) noted that many as 60% of patients with functional visual loss had no evidence of psychiatric disease either at the time of testing or at follow-up. Inconsistent spiral fields, like tubular vision, may often be due to the persuasive skill of the examiner or to high suggestibility. Stress may make the patient give inconsistent replies, but these are not in themselves disabling or sufficient proof of conversion disorder.

Disabling blindness is a more troublesome problem. Evoked potentials may help to demonstrate intact visual pathways. Other evidence on the processing of visual information may be obtained by using colour filters, and by finding discrepancies in reading different sizes of print at different distances. There may also be discrepancies in what the patient reports when looking at polaroid projector slides and when using polaroid goggles. A further test is to produce opto-kinetic nystagmus, which should not occur in the genuinely blind. Blepharospasm, which may effectively cause blindness, is usually due to anxiety or extrapyramidal dyskinesia.

Hallucinations that are well formed, often visual, and generally of people, can occur in the context of dissociation. La Barre (1975) described numerous reports and instances of hallucinations associated with dissociative behaviour. Hallucinations that occur without evidence of psychological illness are not clinically important; for example, the bereaved often see or hear relatives. Profuse visual images (e.g. of trains of people passing before the eyes) were called *phantasmagoria* and are a normal phenomenon or may occur with retinal damage. Other types of hallucinations, especially at night, may result from anxiety, sensory deprivation, partly impaired consciousness before or after sleep (hypnagogic and hypnopompic hallucinations), or a combination of these causes.

Anaesthesias

A dissociative loss of sensation can involve half the entire body from top to toe, or from right to left. It may also involve the whole of the limb and characteristically has a glove or stocking distribution on the arms or legs, or both. In such cases, the patient may not feel a light touch, firm pressure, pin pricks or vibration. To qualify for a diagnosis of conversion disorder, the distribution of the sensory loss must fail to fit in with known anatomical boundaries, but conform more with the patient's concept of physiology and anatomy. Thus, sensory loss in conversion disorder is likely to stop sharply at the midline, but approaches the midline only if it is organic, since at this point segmental nerves overlap by 1–2 cm on each side. Similarly, vibration ought to be felt on both sides when a tuning fork is placed on the bone near the midline, because the vibration will be transmitted across the midline. As noted above, these classical signs are often unreliable, because they sometimes occur in patients with organic disease such as an acute stroke (Gould *et al*, 1986). In regional pain syndromes the existence of pain in one area of the body may elicit a regional effect that overlaps anatomical boundaries, but is still nevertheless physiological (Merskey, 1988).

Clinical presentation of dissociative disorders

Amnesia

Dissociative amnesia is characterised by a loss of the knowledge of personal identity combined with the preservation of environmental information and often complex learned information or skills. For example, a patient may claim he does not know who he is, and be oblivious to his own past, yet at the same time can play chess. It is usually of sudden onset and there may be evidence of recent psychological stress. Dissociative amnesia most commonly presents to accident and emergency departments and then to neurologists, but is relatively rare in psychiatric clinics. One neurologist observed that, in his experience, patients with hysterical amnesia and fugues had some awareness of counterfeiting their symptoms. Others find that it is wholly genuine, in the sense that some patients appear truly lost, and on recovery give evidence of troublesome personal problems which explain their condition.

Dissociative amnesia may be more frequent among criminals or soldiers in distress. A history of head injury or brain damage is often present in civilian cases. In all cases it is important to exclude neurological disorders, but the specificity of the memory loss for personal information with the retention of complex learnt skills (see above) usually indicates a dissociative disorder and contrasts with the pattern found in organic memory loss.

Fugue states

Amnesic patients with an impulse to wander are said to be in a *fugue* state. The predominant disturbance is sudden, unexpected travel away from home or a customary place of work. There is an inability to recall the past and sometimes the assumption of a partial or completely new identity. Memory for recent events, which may be of a traumatic or stressful nature, is lost, although these aspects may change when other informants are available. In contrast to organic fugue states, basic self-care such as eating or washing, and simple social interactions with strangers – say, buying a ticket, asking directions or ordering a meal – are preserved. Stengel (1941) described 25 patients with fugues, of whom ten had epilepsy, one had schizophrenia and several others had depression. Traumatic childhood experiences are also common in these patients and organic brain disease, particularly head injury, may also play a role.

Dissociative fugue may be differentiated from post-ictal fugue because the latter usually occurs in the presence of a history of epilepsy, without stressful events or problems, and the activities and travels of the epileptic patient are less purposeful and more fragmented.

ICD–10 and DSM–IV provide similar descriptions and require the exclusion of both multiple personality disorder and organic mental disorder. ICD–10 also requires the exclusion of excessive fatigue and intoxication.

Hacking (1998) has shown that purported cases of fugue first described in the 19th-century French literature were often men who were required to serve in the army under conscription in Germany or France and had taken absence without leave.

In summary, it appears that dissociative amnesias and fugues sometimes have an organic factor as a complication or cause, in addition to psychological contributions from depression, early childhood disturbances and current stress.

Stupor

Dissociative stupor is diagnosed on the basis of a profound diminution or absence of voluntary movement and normal responsiveness to external stimuli such as light, noise and touch. However, although there is a disturbance of consciousness, the patient is neither asleep nor unconscious.

Dissociative stupor needs to be differentiated from the more serious causes of stupor such as catatonia, depressive stupor or stupor due to some neurological condition. The presence of other indicators of psychiatric or neurological disease may be helpful pointers. Dissociative stupor is more likely to occur in the context of recent stressful events or current interpersonal difficulties. Dissociative stupor is rare and is included in ICD–10 but not in DSM–IV.

The Ganser syndrome

Ganser (1898) described three prisoner patients who showed the central feature of talking past the point:

> 'The most obvious sign which they present consists of their inability to answer correctly the simplest questions which are asked of them, even though by many of their answers they indicate that they have grasped, in a large part, the sense of the question, and in their answers they betray a baffling ignorance and a surprising lack of knowledge which they most assuredly once possessed, or still possess.... We cannot fail to recognise how in the choice of answers the patient appears to pass over deliberately the indicated correct answer and to select a false one, which any child could easily recognise as such.' (Ganser, 1898)

Ganser wrote of *vorbeigehen*, meaning 'passing by'. The word *vorbeireden*, meaning 'talking past the point', has also been used. Both words essentially signify that a question is answered by deliberately neglecting the correct answer in favour of a related nonsensical response. The term 'approximate answers' has also been used. Thus, the colour of the sky on a fine day may be grey, a cow may have five legs, or two and two add up to five.

The Ganser symptoms reflect a specific memory defect and this should be distinguished from the complete Ganser syndrome (Scott, 1965). Ganser syndrome patients have clouding of consciousness with impairment of attention and concentration. There may also be a memory defect, anxiety, perplexity, hallucinations (often of a frightening visual type), as well as hysterical motor and sensory symptoms.

Whitlock (1967*a*) found that while Ganser symptoms were common, the complete syndrome itself was rare. The syndrome has been found in individuals awaiting trial, particularly for murder charges, in those in prison when under considerable stress. It also occurs in patients with organic brain disease such as strokes and head injury. In other cases individuals were seeking financial benefits, or had depression. Patients with chronic schizophrenia may also give Ganser-like answers to questions, leading to the term the 'fatuous syndrome' (Bleuler, 1950).

Dissociative identity disorder

People with this diagnosis (formerly termed 'multiple personality disorder') are said to have at least two personalities, of which only one is dominant at a given time. The number of cases reported in the literature, particularly in the USA, has grown enormously since the publication of the book *The Three Faces of Eve* (Thigpen & Cleckley, 1957), which received widespread publicity and was made into a film. The book describes the transformation from 'Eve White' to 'Eve Black', and only mentions briefly a little later that the new name was the patient's original one. In her autobiography (Sizemore & Pittillo, 1977), the patient describes the transition from being Chris White to Chris Costner. Costner was her maiden name and she was unhappy in her marriage. The obvious psychodynamic explanation for the second 'personality' is that she resumed her maiden name and this symbolised the denial of her marriage.

The DSM–IV criteria for dissociative identity disorder are:

1 the presence of two or more distinct identities or personality states (each with its own relatively enduring pattern of perceiving, relating to and thinking about the environment and self)

2 at least two of these identities or personality states recurrently take full control of the person's behaviour

3 the inability to recall important personal information that is too extensive to be explained by ordinary forgetfulness

4 the disturbance is not due to the direct physiological effects of a substance or a general medical condition.

The condition is reported most commonly in the USA and is rarely if ever seen in the UK. Those who find the condition common have noted a high frequency of extreme abuse in childhood as a common feature (Ross, 1989). Bliss (1984) suggested that multiple personality disorder is caused by autohypnosis. Much doubt has been cast on the quality of the literature describing the syndrome (Fahy, 1988), to the point where the existence of the syndrome itself has been attributed to iatrogenesis and social encouragement (Merskey, 1992*a*). One of the more bizarre features of this disorder was that DSM–III included a statement that a patient might have more than 100 personalities or fragments of personality (and DSM–IV still does) (American Psychiatric Association, 1980, 1994).

Epidemiology

The incidence and prevalence of conversion and dissociative symptoms has varied across time, place and culture. For example, very high rates were observed among soldiers in the trenches during the First World War. Akagi & House (2001) reviewed all the earlier studies and, although there was no uniformity of methodology or case definition, they estimated the incidence rate for conversion hysteria (i.e. where there was some loss or change in motor or sensory function) to lie somewhere in the range 5–10/100 000 cases per year. Their estimate for the prevalence was 50–100/100 000 cases over a 1- to 2-year period, but they admitted that some approximation was involved because of the variable times used in the prevalence studies.

Higher rates of conversion symptoms are seen in psychiatric liaison practice, especially in neurology clinics (as might be expected for a motor or sensory disorder). Thus, one study gave a figure of 3.8% for neurology out-patients in London, although a German study gave a much higher figure, of 9%, in a German neurology clinic. Rates may also be high in accident and emergency departments (for references see Akagi & House, 2001).

A large epidemiological study of somatoform symptoms (i.e. not disorders) revealed that conversion symptoms are quite common in the community. In that study, of over 3000 people aged 14–24 (Lieb *et al*, 2000), 6.9% reported conversion symptoms, with aphonia being the most common (3.7%), and 7.5% reported dissociative symptoms, with weakness and fainting (5.5%) being the most common. However, the rates for the more severe DSM–IV 'somatic disorders' in this study were much lower and more in line with previously reported figures. Thus, the 12-month rate for conversion disorder was 0.2% (20/100 000) and for dissociative disorder 0.4% (40/100 000). The higher rates in this study may reflect the younger population studied.

Almost all studies show a greater preponderance of women. Akagi & House (2001) reject the notion that hysteria is a rare and disappearing condition and suggest that it remains frequent and often disabling, although it now presents mainly to general medical clinics (especially neurology departments) and hence to liaison psychiatrists rather than to the general psychiatric services. In some developing countries rather higher rates are reported presenting to psychiatric out-patient departments; for example, Hafeiz (1980) found rates of up to 10% in the Sudan.

Aetiology

Genetics

Briquet (1859), who carried out one of the first family history studies in psychiatry, reported a strong familial trend for his patients with hysteria. However, this finding may be partly explained by the fact that his case material included many women with multiple somatic complaints and others with classical affective disorders. The twin study by Shields (1982) failed to demonstrate any significant genetic contribution. However, Inouye (1972) summarised data from the two available twin studies and other case reports and found 9 concordant and 33 discordant monozygotic (MZ) pairs, but among dizygotic (DZ) twins there were no concordant and 43 discordant pairs and this MZ/DZ difference suggests that there may be a heritable component. The lack of any DZ concordant pairs suggests that environmental familial effects cannot play much of a role (see page 206 for explanation). The data are, though, too sparse to draw any conclusions on the heritability of conversion and there have been no new studies in recent years.

Depression and organic brain disease

McKegney (1967) found that 58% of those with hysteria had some depression. Organic brain disease is another contributory factor to hysteria. In one series, around two-thirds of the cases had an accompanying cerebral disorder or preceding organic brain disease (Whitlock, 1967*b*), although in the Maudsley series only 4% had a history of organic brain disease (Lewis, 1975). An intermediate figure was given by Standage (1975), who noted that 32% of patients with hysteria had a history of neurological disease, particularly epilepsy. Slater & Glithero (1965) postulated that organic disease may bring about a general disturbance of the personality 'which results in modes of behaviour such as exaggeration, attention seeking, etc., which we naturally think of as manifestations of hysterical personality'. Whatever the underlying mechanism, an organic cause must always be excluded in anyone aged over 40 years presenting with 'hysterical' symptoms for the first time.

Possible pathogenic mechanisms

Consideration of the literature suggests that there are probably five ways in which physical illness relates to conversion symptoms.

1 The occurrence of previous or intermittent physical symptoms, as in epilepsy, provides a model for the conversion symptom. A psychological stress would then more easily produce a form of illness of which the patient had some knowledge. Past illness in a relative or a close acquaintance may serve the same function.

2 An independent emotional stress may make a patient elaborate the distressing effects of an organic lesion that has already disturbed normal functioning. Thus the weak hand may become paralysed. This mechanism appeared to operate in at least 12 out of 89 cases in one series (Merskey & Buhrich, 1975). It may also explain the long-standing nature of the symptoms, as found in the 12-year follow-up study by Stone *et al* (2003).

3 The unpleasant psychological implications of a physical illness, such as the discomfort and fear attached to it, may make the patient elaborate an existing symptom, or produce a fresh one.

4 The unpleasant psychological implications of a physical illness, such as pain and fear, can lead to the receiving of get-well cards, gifts of fruit and flowers, to relief from painful responsibilities and other intra-psychic dilemmas. This is also known as secondary gain. It should be noted that secondary gain is a frequent accompaniment of physical illness and, although its presence is highly relevant to the assessment and management of conversion disorders, it should in no way be regarded as pathognomonic of conversion disorder.

5 In an unknown way, cerebral damage may operate more specifically to produce conversion symptoms. The relationship between physical and mental disorders more generally is considered in Chapter 17, on page 409.

Brain imaging studies

Brodie (1837) observed 'It is not the muscles which refuse to obey the will but the will itself which has ceased to work', suggesting the pathology lay more in the mind or brain than in the muscles.

Marshall and his colleagues reported the first patient with chronic motor conversion – left leg weakness of non-organic cause – studied dynamically with positron emission tomography (PET) (Marshall *et al*, 1997; Athwal *et al*, 2001). In this patient, *preparation* to move the left leg (relative to the passive control state) activated the lateral premotor cortex and both cerebellar hemispheres, indicating the patient's 'readiness' to move the paralysed leg when touched. When the patient was asked to attempt to *move* the paralysed left leg, a qualitatively different pattern of action from that observed for the right leg appeared. As expected, no activation was seen in the right primary sensory motor cortex; this was consistent with the absence of movement in muscle innervation shown on the electromyelogram (EMG). Instead, there were significant activations in the left dorsolateral prefrontal cortex the right anterior cingulate cortex and the cerebellum bilaterally, as well as in some midbrain and upper brain-stem structures. Significant activations (relative to the baseline) of the left dorsolateral prefrontal cortex and cerebellum were considered evidence against faking and in support of the patient's attempt to comply with the instructions given. In this important experiment the right anterior cingulate region and the medial orbitofrontal cortex significant activation and were the only two areas that were differentially involved in the comparison. It is also of interest that, in a hypnotically induced paralysis of the left leg, increased activation was seen in exactly the same areas – the left orbitofrontal cortex and the right anterior cingulate cortex (Halligan *et al*, 2000).

One can only speculate why these areas were involved. Cingulate lesions following stroke can result in a variety of voluntary movement disorders, such as akinetic mutism, impairments in movement initiation or motor neglect, while the orbitofrontal cortex is involved in learning the regulation of behaviour related to external functioning (Athwal *et al*, 2001). Marshall *et al* (1997) and Athwal *et al* (2001) suggest that hysterical paralysis is associated with a malfunction between those regions of the brain concerned with intention and those concerned with the execution of movement.

Vuilleumier *et al* (2001) in a study employing single photon emission tomography (SPET) examined seven patients with unilateral sensorimotor loss. In four patients they demonstrated reduced levels of regional blood flow in the thalamus and basal ganglia contralateral to the deficit limb in response to bilateral vibratory stimuli to the limbs; 4 months later, when they were asymptomatic, the brain hypo-activation had resolved.

These studies are of some preliminary interest as they suggest there may be detectable cerebral changes among patients with so-called 'functional disorders'.

Outcome studies

In an early, well-known series of 85 cases (Slater & Glithero, 1965), a large number of cases of 'hysteria' later turned out to be structural brain disease, but this finding no longer seems to apply. Indeed, Stone *et al* (2005), in a review, showed that few cases are now misdiagnosed. At one time it was thought that hysteria might be a precursor of the more serious functional psychoses, but this was not really borne out. Thus, Lewis (1975) traced 98 patients with hysteria from the Maudsley Hospital, of whom two developed schizophrenia, and of those who had not recovered eight had depression. Ciompi (1969) traced 38 patients surviving an average of 34 years after their first admission with hysteria, and found two with schizophrenia and two with epilepsy. In Ljungberg's (1957) series the morbidity risk was 2% for psychogenic psychosis, 3.1% for schizophrenia, and 2.4% for manic–depressive psychoses, suggesting only small possible associations.

In a study by Crimlisk *et al* (1998) of medically unexplained symptoms presenting in a neurological clinic, psychiatric disorders were comorbid in 75% of cases at the time of presentation. These were mainly affective disorders, but personality disorder was present in 45% of the cases. Interestingly, the presence of comorbid psychiatric disorder at the time of presentation was a good prognostic sign, as were a briefer duration of symptoms before presentation and a change in marital status (in either direction), suggesting the importance of relationships and environmental factors. New psychiatric disorder was uncommon in this follow-up series and there was no dramatic revelation of new cases of serious physical disorder during the follow-up period.

In the study by Stone *et al* (2003) no new cases of neurological disease appeared during a 12-year follow-up, indicating that the initial diagnosis was generally sound, and these authors suggested that brain scanning has made the exclusion of structural neurological disorder a much easier and more accurate exercise. These workers found a rather worse long-term outcome for unilateral functional weakness and sensory loss. Thus, at the 12-year follow-up, 83% of the patients continued to report weakness or sensory loss, and over half of those initially reporting sensory loss had gone on to develop weakness. Around 29% of the patients in this series had taken early medical retirement at a rather young age – a median of 44 years. In many areas of functioning this group were on the same level as patients with multiple sclerosis, while a follow-up questionnaire completed by their general practitioners indicated that up to 30% also had other medically unexplained symptoms.

Epidemic hysteria

Hysterical symptoms communicated by social contact can affect large numbers of people. This is usually known as mass or epidemic hysteria (Merskey, 1995). Common symptoms include convulsive jerks, headaches, sore throats, abdominal pain, belief in food-poisoning, dizziness and weakness. The syndrome is more frequent in girls, but both sexes may be affected. Factory workers, nurses and other health personnel have also been involved. Moss & McEvedy (1966) described criteria indicating that hysteria was the most likely cause for an epidemic. The epidemic disseminates most rapidly when the social group is large, and in a place where social contact is maximum. During the outbreak new cases tend to start in places of high social contact, such as the school hall, the playground and the corridors, rather than the classroom. Younger girls (in the 11- to 15-year age group) are more susceptible, and the incidence of new cases tends to move to the lower end of the school as the epidemic progresses.

Epidemic hysteria has a long history, particularly in Europe. St John's dance appeared in Germany soon after the Black Death in 1374. Men and women formed circles and danced for hours in a wild delirium and appeared to have lost control of their senses, until at length they fell to the ground exhausted. Another dancing plague, known as St Vitus' dance, appeared in Strasbourg in 1418, although this term was later applied to cases of chorea. Comparable outbreaks in Italy were described as 'tarantism', being attributed to the bite of the tarantula spider, which was alleged to continue its effects indefinitely. Groups of 18th-century Cornish Methodists had attacks of leaping around in frenzied states and were known as 'Jumpers'. An equivalent French group were known as the '*convulsionnaires*', while another group who took to moving on all fours and growling were known as the 'Barkers'. All these outbreaks probably occurred during periods of social upheaval among the affected populations, and the behaviour received popular sanction at the time.

Bartholomew & Wessely (2002) have reviewed the literature on epidemic hysteria and describe its modern equivalent, which they call 'mass sociogenic illness'. Presentations in the 20th century were dominated by environmental concerns over food, air and water quality, or imaginary fears concerning mysterious odours. In the 21st century, with the psychological impact of terrorism, the triggers for episodes relate to fears of mass poisoning, anthrax or poison gas, but the symptomatic picture is usually similar, with outbreaks of acute anxiety, chills, headaches, difficulties in breathing or fainting episodes, or other anxiety-related symptoms, while the precipitant usually reflects the current social and political anxieties of the day .

Chronic pain

Recognising that pain may be much influenced by emotional factors and that sometimes it arises in the context of purely psychological illness, there have been many attempts to define pain in a way that takes account both its physical causes, which are normally recognised, and of the possible psychological contributions. The International Association for the Study of Pain adopted the following definition of pain in 1979, revised slightly in 1994 as follows:

> 'An unpleasant sensory and emotional experience associated with actual or potential tissue damage or described in terms of such damage.' (Merskey & Bogduk, 1994)

The purpose of this definition is to direct attention away from the notion that we cannot define pain in somebody who does not have any physical problem. Pain is understood to be the unpleasant experience that we usually attribute to some physical event.

In the pain literature, a distinction is made between nociception and pain itself, to explain the highly variable and frequently unpredictable relationship between tissue damage and pain. Nociception refers to the activity in the CNS produced by potentially tissue damaging stimuli such as thermal, mechanical or chemical agents. Pain is the perception of nociception and is an entirely subjective experience. A wide variety of influences – including psychiatric disorder, cultural influences, childhood experiences and so on – may influence the degree of pain a person develops for a given nociceptive experience. The clinician may judge that the pain perceived by the patient is disproportionate to the extent of the tissue damage in the course of the clinical assessment, but this does not necessarily mean the pain is of psychogenic origin.

Non-nociceptive pain can still arise from a definite organic cause, such as trigeminal neuralgia, or from some organic cause yet to be identified, a psychological cause or some combination of these causes. It is also important to realise that the vast majority of non-nociceptive pains, including those thought to be psychological, are not factitious or due to malingering but are experienced as very real by the patient (Cheville *et al*, 2000).

Jones *et al* (2003) have reviewed the mechanisms involved in nociception processing, which include some important findings from functional MRI (fMRI) and PET scan studies. It is now clear that the stimulus in terms of anticipation of pain is almost as important as the pain stimulus itself, and anticipation can activate most of the central nociceptive system, particularly areas like the medial prefrontal cortex and the anterior cingulate gyrus, with the only difference being the magnitude of the response. This anticipatory response can be blocked by benzodiazepines, which indicates the importance of anxiety as a mediator. Attention alone can also alter nociceptive responses and the beneficial effects of distraction in pain control are well known. Bantick *et al* (2002) have shown that psychological distraction will diminish fMRI responses to painful stimuli, particularly in the orbitofrontal cortex, and selective attention probably plays some (as yet undefined) role in the somatic pain syndromes, where pain seems to be associated with very much heightened degrees of distress. Patients with chronic atypical facial pain also show changes on PET scanning. They show an enhanced response in the anterior cingulate cortex and other parts of the central pain systems to thermal stimulation in comparison with controls (Derbyshire *et al*, 1994). For a further discussion of pain overall, see McMahon & Koltzenburg (2005).

Classification of pain disorders

DSM–IV made considerable changes from the DSM–III–R definition; the term for the condition changed to 'pain disorder'. The definition has been broadened to include two types of pain disorder, but in neither case are there any inferences about cause. The first is called 'pain disorder associated with psychological factors', and the second 'pain disorder associated with both psychological factors and a general medical condition'. In addition, acute and chronic specifiers are provided for both categories of pain, with 6 months being taken as the dividing line. The diagnosis should not be made if the pain is better accounted for by a mood, anxiety or psychotic disorder. Pain resulting from general medical conditions in which psychological factors are judged to have either no role or a minimal role may form part of the differential diagnosis but are not considered to be a mental disorder and should be coded on axis III (general medical conditions).

ICD–10 provides a somewhat more vague definition of 'persistent somatoform pain disorder'. This is severe and distressing pain that cannot be explained by a physiological process or physical disorder. It includes psychalgia, psychogenic backache and headache.

Both DSM–IV and ICD–10 grapple with the difficult notion of psychological causation in different ways, but ICD–10 appears to come down rather more firmly in favour of psychogenic causation – and furthermore holds out the hope that clinical examination can establish this. Thus, the text states:

> 'pain occurs in association with emotional conflict or psychosocial problems that are sufficient to allow the conclusion that they are the main causative influences.'

DSM–IV is rather more reticent in this respect and does not use the word 'cause', but states that:

> 'psychological factors are judged to have an important role in the onset, severity, exacerbation or maintenance of the pain.'

Perhaps this more modest terminology reflects the many decades of fruitless argument and controversy concerning the aetiology of these pains.

Patients with pain disorders are certainly not a homogeneous group and many do not have psychiatric illness. Conversion mechanisms are not found to be common in chronic pain syndromes (Merskey, 1999).

Some psychiatric illness can cause pain as part of the illness, for example headaches with depression – as the depression resolves these headaches sometimes improve as well. Low back pain and neck pain, which are the commonest types of chronic pain, generally have a physical initiating event, and as information increases have more often been found to have continuing physical causes.

Bizarre pains can sometimes occur in both depression and schizophrenia and these may be intractable. They should not be classified as pain disorder but rather as a symptom of the primary psychiatric condition. In addition, those who suffer from a chronic physical illness associated with pain may be liable to develop secondary emotional changes – social withdrawal, situational disorders, reactive depressions and occasionally major depressive disorder.

Management of pain disorders

Modern pain management (at least for severe pain) is now mainly undertaken in the pain clinic, run by anaesthetists, but the psychiatrist can help the multidisciplinary team in many different ways. In some cases, particularly those of recent onset with distressing circumstances, there may be obvious psychogenesis, but these cases are unusual. More commonly there is comorbid anxiety or depression, but the emphasis now is less on the search for causative links and more on treatment and ways of trying to alleviate the pain and to treat any comorbid psychiatric disorders. Clarifying more subtle issues, such as the identification of personality disorder or Briquet's syndrome, may form part of the unique contribution of the psychiatrist, because non-psychiatrists may be reluctant to make such a diagnosis, but an authoritative confirmation of its presence may come as a relief to other members of the team. Secondary depressions can be usefully treated with drugs. Furthermore, a number of cognitive–behavioural therapy (CBT) programmes for the management of chronic pain have been developed, although these are usually conducted by psychologists.

Individual pain syndromes

For reasons of space it is not possible to describe all the numerous pain syndromes and the interested reader should consult McMahon & Koltzenburg (2005) for a comprehensive account (there are 32 key syndromes, each with many subtypes) and that reference work includes details of all the associated psychological studies as well. Here, only two somatic pain syndromes are briefly discussed, with the emphasis being on the psychological and social aspects of each.

Neck pain associated with whiplash injury

An account of whiplash is included here because its very high frequency makes it almost a public health problem and because psychiatrists often become involved in associated medico-legal consultations.

When a person is sitting in a car and hit from behind the body trunk will accelerate forward but the neck and head do not move because the neck muscles do not have the time to make the necessary adjustments and an abrupt hyperextension of the neck occurs, with only the head-rest of the car being able to stop this. About one in seven rear-end collisions actually results in a whiplash.

The main symptoms often appear during the next 48 hours and comprise severe pain in the mid-cervical spine radiating up to the occiput and laterally into the trapezoid muscles. There may also be shoulder aches and pains (referred to the scapula). Paraesthesia or aching pains in one or both limbs are also described, while headaches, dizziness, tinnitus, and visual and mood disturbance may all be associated features.

Mayou & Bryant (2002) found that around 23% of all road traffic accidents were associated with a whiplash injury and they compared the psychiatric sequelae of whiplash with those of other road traffic accidents. They found that whiplash and other traffic accidents were equally associated with early pain, travel phobias, anxiety and depression, as well as a high rate of post-traumatic stress disorder. They concluded that there was no specific psychiatry of whiplash injury. The only difference found for whiplash was that pain at 1 year was significantly associated with litigation, which increased the risk of pain by a factor of four.

The high rates of litigation associated with whiplash are probably not due to increased rates of people with feigned symptoms (which are always present in a small proportion of insurance claims) but rather, as Mayou & Bryant (2002) point out, probably relate to the cognitive perception of anger at being an innocent victim in this particular type of accident. None the less, the litigation in turn seems to be associated with a prolongation of the pain and other forms of symptomatic distress.

Atypical facial and oral pain

Atypical facial pain provides a good illustration of the different aetiological theories used to explain these conditions over the past 50 years. The presentation is one of chronic pain of a burning quality, which has a constant intensity and is sometimes throbbing. The pain may be intensified by stimulating the painful area itself, suggesting hyperalgesia. In some cases the pain is in the mouth, but in others it is in the face; it may be unilateral or bilateral. Curiously, this pain does not usually interrupt sleep, eating, talking or facial grooming, as do the shooting pains of trigeminal neuralgia, which is the main differential diagnosis. There are numerous dental conditions such as atypical odontalgia as well as different types of temporal mandibular joint dysfunction that may all cause orofacial pain. The diagnosis therefore is one of exclusion and has to be made by a dentist after a thorough examination and sometimes the services of a neurologist are required to exclude a neurological condition. Accurate diagnosis is important because many patients with this disorder end up having unnecessary dental or other surgical procedures, which are usually ineffective and may be damaging.

De Jongh (2003) studied the prevalence of what he called 'inexplicable dental symptoms', which is presumably the dental equivalent of 'medically unexplained symptoms' in dental practice. He found that 8.7% of the patients attending a dental clinic fulfilled one or more criteria for somatisation specific behaviours, most commonly high attendance rates (6.8% of the total dental attendances), and there was a 3:1 female:male predominance.

The history of theories concerning the cause of atypical facial pain is of interest and shows how such inexplicable conditions are made to conform with predominant psychopathological formulations. Thus, Engel (1951), writing at a time when the influence of psychoanalysis in America was at its peak, thought that patients with facial pain were often dejected and had experienced much suffering and misfortune in their lives. He wrote 'in many a diagnosis of psychic masochism seems justified' and he was also firmly of the opinion that the psychiatric disturbance was primary. He proposed that the underlying mechanism was one of conversion hysteria, which, at the time, was the usual explanation for most psychosomatic syndromes.

Soon after the introduction of the monoamine oxidase inhibitors (MAOIs), Lascelles (1966) conducted a double-blind trial of phenelzine (an MAOI) combined with chlordiazepoxide among patients recruited from a special face pain clinic. He found great benefits on both mood and pain for most patients and wrote that he saw little evidence for hysteria. To explain these findings he proposed that atypical facial pain was a presentation of depression, and to get round the issue of why these patients lacked any of the somatic symptoms of depression (sleep disorder, weight loss and other biological symptoms of depression) he argued that it was a form of 'atypical depression', a category that was fashionable from about 1960 to 1980, and the pain was explained as a 'depression variant'. A later trial of a tricyclic antidepressant by Feinmann *et al* (1984) established that the pain relief was independent of the antidepressant effects of the drug and was probably the result of a direct analgesic effect.

More recent studies have indicated that atypical facial pain is similar to all the other functional somatic syndromes, and the present bio-psychosocial model (more fully explained on page 446) is used to explain these syndromes. It is curious that this model was also proposed by Engel (1980), one of the fathers of modern consulting liaison psychiatry, although he proposed this much wider and more embracing model at a much later stage in his life. The depression variant and conversion hysteria, as explanations, have now faded into history and although currently the bio-psychosocial model is in fashion, it is unclear how long this vogue will last.

Hypochondriasis

History

The word 'hypochondriasis' literally means 'below the cartilage' and was first used by Smollius in 1610 (Veith, 1965). It was applied to various mental states that were thought to be caused by changes in the organs of the hypochondrial region, particularly the liver and the spleen (Kenyon, 1976). Burton (1651) and James Boswell (1777–83) used the word to describe a subdivision of melancholia or depression. Thomas Willis (1684) is credited with being the first to make the distinction between hypochondriasis and hysteria. He regarded the latter as an organic brain disease and challenged the uterine view of hysteria, which had prevailed for many centuries.

George Cheyne (1733) wrote an important treatise on hypochondriasis, hysteria and melancholy entitled

The English Malady. He described his own depressive and hypochondriacal symptoms and wrote in the preface of the book that it was 'intended as a legacy and dying speech only to my fellow sufferers'. He attributed these disorders to the pressures of modern living (in the 18th century), by which he meant the influences of mechanisation, city dwelling and affluence.

Robert Whytt recognised nervous disorders, hypochondriacal symptoms and hysterical ones. Some think that he was describing depression, hypochondriasis and hysteria. It seems rather that he recognised the occurrence of anxiety and depression and the somatic complaints related to them. At the beginning of his book (Whytt, 1751, p. iii) he wrote 'physicians have bestowed the character of *nervous* on all those disorders, whose nature and causes they were ignorant of', a comment which remains apposite. He later wrote:

> 'To wipe off this reproach, and, at the same time to throw some light on nervous hypochondriac and hysteric complaints, is the design of the following observations.'

At the end of his book he wrote about low spirits: 'Hypochondriac and hysteric patients are commonly affected with this complaint in a greater or less degree' and he later refers to 'low spirits or melancholy'. His diagnostic concerns remain of interest, including his concern about diagnosis by exclusion. Whytt also gave sensible advice on management, which included the wise counsel not to promise cure, plus the prescription of exercise, dietary change and, for severe cases, opium.

The recent concept of hypochondriasis as a morbid preoccupation with health emerged only in the 19th century, when Falret (1822) referred to abnormal beliefs about one's health as 'hypochondria'. The description of hypochondriasis by Gillespie (1928) paved the way for the DSM–III and DSM–IV concepts of hypochondriasis as a syndrome with disease phobia and disease conviction at its heart.

Since the late 1970s the dominant terminology in this field has been 'somatisation' (from the Greek word *soma*, for body). It was first used early in the 20th century by Stekel, who described a group of neuroses that presented with physical symptoms (Hinsie & Campbell, 1960). In the latter half of the 20th century the term was championed by Lipowski (1988), who defined it as:

> 'a tendency to experience and communicate somatic distress and symptoms which are unaccounted for by pathological findings and to attribute them to physical illness and to seek medical help for them.'

The term 'somatisation' is a generic one and is not to be equated with any one of the DSM/ICD somatoform disorders. It, too, has been criticised recently and the debate over nomenclature in this area seems no nearer to satisfactory resolution (Sharpe & Carson, 2001; Stone *et al*, 2002*a*).

With specific reference to the term 'hypochondriasis', recent literature has preferred the less offensive term 'health anxiety', which is much easier to use with patients, who see 'hypochondriasis' as an accusation rather than a diagnosis. Health anxiety refers to attitudes, fears and beliefs about health, based on appraisals of bodily symptoms and signs. Some degree of health anxiety is virtually universal. It lies on a continuum from mild to severe and disabling. Severe clinically and socially significant health anxiety would meet DSM/ICD criteria for hypochondriasis. See Asmundson *et al* (2001) for a full discussion of health anxiety.

Clinical features

The DSM–IV criteria for hypochondriasis are outlined in Box 16.2. The core features are disease phobia and disease conviction, and preoccupation with the disease that persists despite medical investigation and reassurance. Sufferers are often preoccupied with intrusive thoughts around the themes of having an actual disease or fear of developing an actual disease. Disturbing, frightening images and fear of death are also common. The thoughts have the quality of over-valued ideas, are held with some conviction and rarely respond to reassurance for any length of time. Misinterpretation of normal sensations is extremely common, as is a tendency to self-examine. These patients often engage in checking behaviours, such as monitoring pulse rate and blood pressure, or examining minor skin lesions and body parts (e.g. breasts or testes). Sometimes checking behaviours can produce or exacerbate the very symptoms the patient fears; for example, patients with globus sensation who fear cancer of the oesophagus or larynx often check by repeated swallowing, an action that itself leads to globus sensation. In contrast to patients with somatisation disorder, these patients often have a narrow symptom focus, being preoccupied with a specific organ or specific disease (although this can change and move from system to system).

Box 16.2 DSM–IV diagnostic criteria for hypochondriasis

A Preoccupation with fears of having, or the idea that one has, a serious disease based on the person's misinterpretation of bodily symptoms.
B The preoccupation persists despite appropriate medical evaluation and reassurance.
C The belief in criterion A is not of delusional intensity (as in delusional disorder, somatic type) and is not restricted to a circumscribed concern about appearance (as in body dysmorphic disorder).
D The preoccupation causes clinically significant distress or impairment in social, occupational or other important areas of functioning.
E The disturbance has lasted for at least 6 months.
F The preoccupation is not better accounted for by obsessive–compulsive disorder, generalised anxiety disorder, panic disorder, a major depressive episode, separation anxiety or another somatoform disorder.

Specify 'with poor insight' if, for most of the time during the current episode, the person does not recognise that the concern about having a serious illness is excessive or unreasonable.

Any body area may be involved, although symptoms relating to the chest, abdomen, head and neck are particularly common (Kenyon, 1964). Most patients are in some pain.

Medical assessment and examination do not reveal any evidence of disease, despite which the patient's preoccupation and concerns persists. It is of course the case that physical and psychiatric disorder may coexist and inevitably patients with hypochondriasis will at some point develop physical disorders. This highlights one of the great difficulties in managing patients with hypochondriasis. In clinical practice, what usually happens is that, in the early stages of the patient's presentation, there is a phase of zealous over-investigation on the part of professionals in the hunt for organic disease. When none is found, there can follow a policy of under-investigation and non-investigation, even in the presence of ominous symptoms indicative of organic disorder.

The doctor–patient relationship in hypochondriasis and other somatoform disorders

Many authors on hypochondriasis and other somatoform disorders comment on the difficult nature of the doctor–patient relationship (Ford, 1983; Pilowsky, 1983; Stoudemire, 1988). Doctors commonly become angry and frustrated in their dealings with these patients. Pilowsky (1983) asserted that 'medical writers appear to have been more intemperate in their description of these patients than any other'. Their unwillingness to accept reassurance or medical advice and frequent criticism of their medical investigation and treatment often alienate doctors and certainly present them with a considerable test of their clinical skills. Recognition of these difficulties in the professional relationship is of crucial importance in the management of these patients. If patients are simply told there is nothing wrong with them, they will usually react with fury and merely seek alternative medical opinions. As with other patients with unexplained symptoms, these patients need to feel validated and taken seriously. Reassuring them that you understand the symptoms are real and not imagined and that you accept the reality of their suffering is essential to engaging these patients in useful treatment. Another difficulty in engaging patients with hypochondriasis is the very word itself; in this regard, the term 'health anxiety' is much more useful (see above).

Epidemiology

Estimates of the prevalence of hypochondriasis have been fairly wide ranging. It is probably higher among medical patients than in the general population (Speckens *et al*, 1996) and particular medical specialties have even higher prevalences, with a figure as high as 10% being described in an ear, nose and throat clinic (Schmidt *et al*, 1993).

The demographic risk factors for hypochondriasis are somewhat different from those for other somatoform disorders. The sex incidence appears to be equal (in contrast, for somatisation disorder the female:male ratio is 2:1 – see below). No convincing relationships between age, education and occupational status have been found (Barsky *et al*, 1991; Kirmayer & Robbins, 1991).

Aetiology

Barsky *et al* (1992) reported higher levels of personality disorder in patients with hypochondriasis than among controls. Indeed, in their study, two-thirds of the patients were diagnosed as suffering from personality disorder. This is in keeping with previous observations of obsessional and anxious personality traits as well as self-absorption in patients with hypochondriasis. Pennebaker & Watson (1991) made a major contribution to our understanding of the psychology of physical symptoms; they noted the relationship between hypochondriasis, neuroticism and marked negative affectivity, characterised by high levels of anxiety, distress and dissatisfaction (including dissatisfaction with medical care).

There is considerable interest in the role of early childhood environment. In patients with medically unexplained symptoms, including those with hypochondriasis, a number of studies have shown that an adverse childhood environment can predispose to adult somatisation and hypochondriasis (e.g. Mechanic, 1964; Barsky *et al*, 1994). The traumas described are many and varied – they include sexual trauma, violence and exposure to illness in childhood. Some studies have also found, in contrast to neglect, over-protectiveness and over-concern on the part of parents can also lead to hypochondriasis. For example, Parker & Lipscome (1980) found patients who scored highly for hypochondriasis rated their fathers as more over-protective and their mothers as more highly caring than did those without hypochondriasis. Baker (1989) also provided evidence linking hypochondriasis to maternal over-protection.

A number of other aetiological factors have been linked to hypochondriasis, including the following:

- life events, including medical life events such as myocardial infraction
- somatosensory amplification (Barsky & Wyshak, 1990)
- cognitive factors involving problematic appraisals of body sensations (Salkovskis & Warwick, 1986)
- sociocultural factors (see Chapter 31, page 790).

These are discussed by Noyes (2000).

Differential diagnosis

Kenyon (1964) disputed the existence of a primary hypochondriasis syndrome, claiming that it would 'always be part of another syndrome, commonly an affective one'. Although the concept of primary hypochondriasis is no longer in serious dispute (Appleby, 1987), it remains the case that hypochondriasis symptoms frequently accompany other psychiatric disorders, notably depression and anxiety disorder, including specific illness phobias, obsessive–compulsive disorder and panic disorder. Occasionally hypochondriacal delusions are also a feature of schizophrenia. It is certainly the case that a careful search for other underlying psychiatric syndromes needs to be carried out. Similarly, a small minority of patients do have missed physical illness, especially neurological and endocrine disorders. The need to be vigilant about these is ever present.

DSM–IV makes it clear that a diagnosis of hypochondriasis should not be made if one of the other psychiatric syndromes better accounts for the symptoms. Clarification of the order of onset of symptoms and the longitudinal course of the disorder often resolves diagnostic doubt.

Some patients with specific illness phobias fear illnesses that they have not yet even encountered, for example HIV, in contrast to patients with hypochondriasis who are preoccupied with diseases they believe they have. Similarly, patients with panic disorder present with symptoms such as fear of dying or having a heart attack, which can lead to confusion with hypochondriasis. The obsessional nature of intrusive thoughts and images in hypochondriasis can lead to confusion with obsessive–compulsive disorder. Patients with the latter have obsessions and compulsions across a whole range of areas and not just disease and illness. Careful assessment usually clarifies this. Again, patients who present with hypochondriacal delusions in the context of psychosis will invariably have other features of a psychotic illness. In delusional disorder itself, a somatic delusion may be the only main manifestation of the disorder.

Finally, transient hypochondriacal symptoms can occur after serious medical disorders as highlighted above (e.g. cancer or ischaemic heart disease). Following such illnesses some patients become preoccupied with any ache or pain and misinterpret this as signs of ongoing disease. Appropriate medical evaluation, explanation and reassurance in these cases usually help to resolve the symptoms.

Box 16.3 The Whiteley Index

- Do you often worry about the possibility that you have a serious illness?
- Are you bothered by many pains and aches?
- Do you find that you are often aware of various things happening in your body?
- Do you worry a lot about your health?
- Do you often have the symptoms of very serious illnesses?
- If a disease is brought to your attention (through the radio, television, newspaper or someone you know) do you worry about getting it yourself?
- If you feel ill and someone tells you that you are looking better, do you become annoyed?
- Do you find that you are bothered by many different symptoms?
- Is it easy for you to forget about yourself, and think about all sorts of other things?
- Is it hard for you to believe the doctor when he or she tells you there is nothing for you to worry about?
- Do you get the feeling that people are not taking your illness seriously enough?
- Do you think that you worry about your health more than most people?
- Do you think there is something seriously wrong with your body?
- Are you afraid of illness?

Measurement of hypochondriasis

Two scales generally used in both clinical practice and research to measure hypochondriasis are the Whiteley Index (Pilowsky, 1967) (Box 16.3) and the Illness Attitude Test (Kellner, 1986), both of which are of acceptable reliability and validity. The scales attempt to measure three core elements of the DSM–IV concept of hypochondriasis: disease phobia, disease conviction and lack of response to medical reassurance. The Illness Attitude Test is a 29-item questionnaire with nine sub-scales, including hypochondriacal beliefs, worry over illness, disease phobia and bodily preoccupation. Although the scale was not originally intended as a diagnostic one, Kellner claims that it is a sensitive instrument for detecting hypochondriasis. These scales have been criticised by Kirmayer & Robbins (1991), who claim they sample a limited range of patients' symptoms, mood and attitude and tell us little about behaviour. These authors argue that the scales measure mainly illness worry and fail to address behavioural or interpersonal communicative aspects of patients' response to illness. One scale that attempts to do this is the Illness Behaviour Inventory (Turkat & Pettigrew, 1983). More recently Lucock & Morley (1996) have developed a self-report questionnaire known as a Health Anxiety Questionnaire. This is a 21-item scale dealing with health preoccupation, illness phobia, reassurance seeking, and interference with day-to-day living. Barsky *et al* (1992) developed a diagnostic interview for hypochondriasis.

Management

The key to successful management is a comprehensive assessment that has medical, psychiatric and social aspects to it (Kellner, 1986; Lipowski, 1988). It is important that, from the outset, one doctor, preferably the patient's general practitioner, takes control of the patient's management, as these patients are adept at 'splitting' healthcare professionals. In the early stages, a thorough medical assessment and all appropriate investigations should be carried out. The doctor needs to give the patient the results of the physical examination and investigations in a clear and unambiguous way, supplementing verbal with written information. If no disease is found, the mainstay of management needs to be psychosocial. Doctors often handle the shift from the phase of investigation to the psychosocial management phase in a clumsy way. In order to engage the patient in psychological treatment, the patient will need to feel listened to and taken seriously. The reality of the symptoms will need to be constantly validated and the patient given the impression that the doctor takes his or her suffering seriously. A sudden change of tack from carrying out physical investigations to the discussion of psychological treatment can result in patients becoming angry and defensive. From the outset the patient needs to be made aware that the assessment and management of any problem have physical, psychological, behavioural, cognitive and social aspects.

One issue that often arises in the early stages of treatment is the role of reassurance. Opinions differ about this. Kellner (1986) and Kirmayer & Robbins (1991) state that explanation and reassurance given in the context of an adequate medical assessment for a patient with whom one has a good therapeutic relationship can constitute adequate treatment in themselves. On the other hand, Warwick & Salkovskis (1985) draw attention to the dangers of providing reassurance at the wrong time and in the wrong way. They emphasise that reassurance should be accompanied by an explanation of the nature of symptoms and caution against repeatedly reassuring patients, especially if that involves simply ordering more and more tests or examining them too often. These authors argue that such manoeuvres may reinforce abnormal illness behaviours in a manner similar to reinforcing rituals in obsessive–compulsive disorder: while it can lead to a short-term reduction in anxiety, fear and anxiety will return, along with an increased urge to seek further reassurance.

Reassurance should not be given prematurely, that is, before the results of investigations and evaluations are known or before patients have had a good opportunity to ventilate adequately. In this regard, Pilowsky (1983) notes that many patients who are given the freedom to describe their physical complaints at length will sooner or later start to talk about psychosocial issues. With some patients, functional improvement rather than total symptom relief needs to be the goal of care. Patients need to be reassured that symptoms are not 'all in your head' or 'in your imagination', as they often claim doctors have said to them. Although this is often their interpretation of events rather than what actually happened, it is none the less important to emphasise this.

The treatment of hypochondriasis had no particular evidence base until Warwick *et al* (1996) published a randomised controlled trial of CBT in patients with hypochondriasis. This study had a 16-session programme involving the use of both cognitive and behavioural procedures and patients were compared with a waiting-list control group. The treatment group did considerably better than the control group. The trial seems to have established the efficacy of CBT in patients with hypochondriasis. Clarke *et al* (1998) showed that CBT and a purely behavioural approach produced similar outcomes, both approaches leading to better outcomes than that of waiting-list controls. A larger randomised controlled trial has recently been published (Barsky & Ahern, 2004) in which patients who received six sessions of CBT did better than controls at 1 year on a range of outcome measures. As is often the case with CBT studies, cost–efficacy questions have been raised. In this regard, Stern & Fernandez (1991) demonstrated the efficacy of a group CBT programme for patients with hypochondriasis.

The evidence for pharmacological therapies in hypochondriasis is less strong, as only open studies have been published (e.g. Fallon *et al*, 1993). Patients with secondary hypochondriacal symptoms will respond to drug treatment of the primary syndrome.

Somatisation disorder (chronic multiple functional somatic symptoms)

Somatisation disorder, as defined by both DSM–IV and ICD–10, is found at the severe end of the spectrum of patients with medically unexplained symptoms. It refers to the small group of patients with unexplained symptoms who have chronic multiple somatic complaints extending over a period of years. Some older psychiatric texts confused this syndrome with that characterising the patients studied by Briquet, and the notable contribution of this 19th-century French physician in describing this group of patients has been summarised by Mai & Merskey (1980). Briquet's work corresponded with 19th-century views of hysteria as an illness with prominent episodic manifestations and a 'quieter' (although possibly abnormal) period in between. He rejected the then prevailing view that hysteria was associated with sexual frustration. In Briquet's large study he found the condition occurred in prostitutes, married women, virgins and widows. Interestingly, in his study it appeared less frequently in nuns than in other groups.

Of all the DSM somatoform disorders, it is likely that somatisation disorder is the entity with the highest diagnostic reliability, validity and stability (Hyler & Sussmann, 1984). This notwithstanding, it is still best seen as a disorder lying at the end of a continuum of syndromes in which patients present with medically unexplained symptoms. Changes in the criteria from DSM–III to DSM–IV seem to have shown that the condition is less reliably defined when attempts are made to diagnose it with revised criteria, especially in primary care. Indeed, there are studies that highlight the arbitrary nature of the cut-off (patients must have had at least eight unexplained symptoms) in terms of the number of symptoms required to meet the diagnostic criteria in DSM–IV or ICD–10. Escobar *et al* (1989) suggest there are many patients who have fewer than the required number of symptoms and whose day-to-day consulting behaviour and functioning are similar to those of patients who meet the full diagnostic criteria.

In view of the debate about the use of the word 'somatisation', these patients are sometimes referred to as patients with 'chronic multiple functional somatic symptoms' (e.g. Bass & May, 2002).

Clinical features

Typically, the patient with somatisation disorder will present with a multiplicity of symptoms occurring over a long period of time in different body systems. The symptoms will be unaccounted for by underlying physical disorder, although they will continue to be attributed to medical problems by the patient. Most commonly the symptoms are very subjective and difficult to verify, for example pain and fatigue. Occasionally, however, patients will present with more objective symptoms, such as melaena. Typically patients begin to present in their teens or 20s and, indeed, to meet current diagnostic criteria the onset of the disorder must be before the age of 30. Diagnosis is, however, frequently delayed and thought about only after multiple referrals and multiple investigations, and sometimes even surgical exploration or intervention. It is not uncommon for these patients to have had numerous non-diseased organs removed before diagnosis is made and referral for psychiatric assessment considered. The commonest organs removed are appendix, gall bladder and uterus.

Doctors should be aware of numerous clues to the detection of the condition. Patients often present with complex histories, having seen numerous specialists and having voluminous case notes (they have been regularly referred to in pejorative terms as 'fat-file patients', as well as 'heart-sink patients'). The early age of onset of unexplained symptoms should be apparent from searching the case notes and general practitioner's records and, indeed, a diagnosis of somatisation disorder in someone presenting for the first time over the age of 40 with unexplained symptoms should rarely, if ever, be made. Although patients with somatisation disorder often deny or minimise emotional problems, they have high lifetime rates of depression and anxiety disorders. Deliberate self-harm is common but completed suicide unusual. A variety of personality traits is associated with somatisation disorder (Bass, 1993) and may colour the way the patient presents. Bass has gone so far as to suggest that somatisation disorder is perhaps best seen as a personality disorder.

There is frequently difficulty or confusion about the overlap between somatisation disorder and both malingering and factitious disorder. In practice, this distinction can be extraordinarily difficult. Malingerers usually deliberately feign illness to avoid something difficult or unpleasant or to gain personal advantage. Patients with factitious disorder also intentionally feign symptoms or indeed self-induce disease or injury, to mimic disease. Although it has been stated that in somatisation disorder the motive is unconscious and that this distinguishes it from malingering, in clinical practice the conscious/unconscious distinction is difficult to make (as discussed elsewhere in this chapter). It is likely, particularly with the passage of time, that both factitious and malingering symptoms may sometimes mix with somatisation disorder.

Epidemiology and aetiology

Community studies carried out in the DSM–III era suggested a community prevalence of 0.4% for strictly defined somatisation disorder (Swartz *et al*, 1986). A primary care study found a slightly higher prevalence, of 1–2% (Faravelli *et al*, 1997). As previously stated, modifying the criteria by reducing the large number of symptoms required by ICD–10 and DSM–IV leads to the prevalence rising considerably. Bass & May (2002) claimed that 4% of the general population and 9% of patients admitted to tertiary care have chronic multiple functional somatic symptoms. It is certainly the case that prevalence is higher in tertiary care settings.

Somatisation disorder is commoner in women, with a sex ratio of 2:1. It is found across a range of cultures (Simon *et al*, 1996). Its aetiology is unknown but likely to be multifactorial. An association with both physical and sexual abuse and with exposure to parents with complaints of poor physical health has been found. A history of unexplained symptoms during childhood is also associated with an adult diagnosis of somatisation disorder (Hotopf *et al*, 1998).

Numerous psychological theories attempt to account for the origins of medically unexplained symptoms. These vary from psychodynamic theories to cognitive theories, but there is as yet insufficient evidence by which to judge them. The role of biological function in somatisation disorder has been considerably less studied, although there is some evidence for a problem in filtering out irrelevant bodily stimuli and for limbic hypersensitivity to body stimuli. These notions are discussed by Miller (1984).

Treatment

There is only modest evidence for the efficacy of any treatment for patients with somatisation disorder or chronic multiple unexplained symptoms. Only two randomised controlled trials have been reported, both from one group in the USA (Smith *et al*, 1986, 1995). In the first of these studies, a standardised, largely behavioural intervention and advice given to primary care physicians reduced healthcare costs in the intervention group, although without any improvement in function of the patients. In the second study care costs were again reduced but with no reduction in the patients' satisfaction with their care.

The treatment of somatisation disorder is therefore based on clinical experience and clinical wisdom rather than being evidence based. Mai (2004) has provided a useful review. The following principles are widely held to be useful:

1 One doctor, probably the general practitioner, should be identified as the patient's main carer and should coordinate the patient's care and in particular communicate with any other healthcare professionals who become involved with the patient.

2 Time spent carrying out an initial comprehensive assessment is worthwhile. Patients need to be allowed to talk about their physical symptoms (even when they are seeing psychiatrists). Their views on the aetiology of their symptoms should be actively sought (but not initially actively challenged, especially during the engagement phase with the patient). Any concerns expressed about psychosocial factors should be encouraged and the doctor and the patient should negotiate an agreed problem list to be tackled.

3 The validity of the patient's physical symptoms needs to be strongly acknowledged. Patients will often be anxious that doctors think their symptoms are 'all in my mind' or 'imaginary'. Accepting the symptoms as real and empathising with the patient's suffering is extremely helpful in engaging the patient in a sensible management plan. Physical examination can be a useful part of this, although clear limits have to be set on investigation and referral to specialists.

4 After the initial engagement phase, the doctor should attempt to broaden the agenda and facilitate discussion of relevant psychosocial problems. The goals of management should be clearly negotiated. Functional improvement and damage limitation rather than cure should be the aim. The patient

should be encouraged to think in terms of coping with symptoms rather than in terms of total symptom relief.

Interview skills

A number of writers have highlighted the importance of developing appropriate interview skills for doctors attempting to manage patients with multiple unexplained symptoms (e.g. Salmon *et al*, 1999). Doctors need to pay careful attention to the kind of language they use. Words associated with psychiatry (e.g. depression or anxiety) at the early stages of engagement with these patients will often serve only to confirm the patient's suspicion that the doctor thinks it is simply a psychiatric problem or that the patient is exaggerating symptoms. Patients should be reminded that physical and emotional symptoms commonly coexist, but this is best done after the doctor has spent time engaging the patient and taking an adequate history, especially a history of the physical symptoms.

The explanation given to patients about their symptoms can be crucially important (Salmon *et al*, 1999). It is very useful to give the patient an explanation of the symptoms that embraces physiological factors (e.g. hyperventilation, over-activity of the autonomic nervous system,) behavioural factors (e.g. checking, selective attention to particular body parts) and emotional factors (e.g. relationship of symptoms to stress or fear).

Contracts with high service users

Patients who attend very frequently, including those who often attend out-of-hours services in a variety of settings, can often be contained by the use of a contract. The contract would stipulate the frequency of the patient's visits to the general practitioner and place limits on out-of-hours contact, as well as on who can be expected to prescribe for the patient. The contract may also state that the patient will be physically examined regularly. A contract could, for example, agree to the patient being seen twice weekly for a month, then weekly for a month, then fortnightly for two months. It could include an agreement to examine the patient once monthly and contain limits on out-of-hours contact, as well as on referral to other specialists. These contracts do not always work, but sometimes do at least limit deterioration.

Psychiatric referral

Patients with chronic unexplained symptoms are usually reluctant to engage with psychiatrists, although referral can be helpful, particularly when the psychiatrist (usually a liaison psychiatrist) has a particular interest in these patients and is prepared to carry out an assessment and advise on management. Preparation of the patient for referral is crucial and should emphasise the need to learn to cope with chronic symptoms rather than merely representing a hunt for undiagnosed underlying psychiatric or physical problems. Joint consultations involving a combination of general practitioner, physician and psychiatrist can be very useful and help the patient feel he or she is not merely being 'dumped' on to the psychiatric services.

Body dysmorphic disorder

Body dysmorphic disorder (BDD) was formerly known as dysmorphophobia. That term derives from the Greek word *dysmorfia*, which means ugliness, and according to Philoppopoulos (1979) first appeared in the *Histories* of Herodotus in reference to the myth of the 'ugliest girl in Sparta', who was taken to a shrine each day by her nurse so that she might be delivered from her homeliness.

Body dysmorphic disorder was first described by Morselli (1891) and referred to a subjective feeling of ugliness or physical defect in spite of a normal physical appearance. DSM–IV classifies BDD as a separate somatoform disorder, whereas ICD–10 subsumes it under the heading of 'Hypochondriacal disorder'.

Clinical features

These patients are preoccupied with the belief that an aspect of their appearance is in some way deformed, defective or ugly. Sometimes they are quite specific about what they think is wrong (e.g. 'my nose is too broad') but sometimes they describe only a vague notion that something is not right. The preoccupation may be with a wide variety of perceived bodily abnormalities, but the face, hair and genitalia are particularly common foci of attention. Some people describe dissatisfaction with their overall appearance or concerns about symmetry of body parts. These concerns lead to considerable distress and are often accompanied by time-consuming rituals, including checking behaviours, looking in mirrors (although some patients avoid this), attempting to 'camouflage' the perceived defect and reassurance seeking. The intrusive nature of the thoughts and the checking rituals can lead to this disorder being mistaken for obsessive–compulsive disorder. The patient's preoccupation with a belief in a bodily deformity is the most useful distinguishing feature.

BDD may be comorbid with depression, social phobia, substance misuse or obsessive–compulsive disorder (Veale *et al*, 1996). At its most severe BDD is a far from trivial disorder, as many sufferers are too distressed to function normally at work or in social relationships. Phillips *et al* (1994) highlighted the high level of social impairment in this disorder, the distress, time-consuming BDD-related behaviours, self-consciousness and poor concentration. In their study half the patients had been psychiatric in-patients and one-third had attempted suicide.

The boundary between BDD and its delusional variant (now known as delusional disorder) is extremely blurred. In the study by Phillips *et al* (1994) the two disorders appeared very similar and the authors suggested that they may constitute the same disorder, with the delusional type being the more severe and with the spectrum of insight on the patient's part being much less or almost nonexistent.

Epidemiology

BDD is relatively common. It tends to be under-diagnosed, for two main reasons. The first is ignorance of its existence on the part of doctors. The second is reluctance on the patient's part to consult, often owing to embarrassment. Phillips (1996) reported a 1-year prevalence of 0.77%, with higher rates in cosmetic surgery and dermatology clinics, and in patients with other psychiatric disorders. Phillips & Diaz (1997) reported an almost equal sex incidence.

Treatment

There is a paucity of evidence from randomised controlled trials for both pharmacological and psychological treatments in BDD. Case reports and open-label studies provide some evidence for the efficacy of selective serotonin reuptake inhibitors in BDD (e.g. Hollander *et al*, 1989). Phillips (1996), based on her enormous clinical experience in this area, suggested augmentation of SSRIs with buspirone or neuroleptics when SSRIs alone are not effective, although she acknowledged that this and other pharmacological strategies required further research. Clinical experience suggests that long-term drug treatment is required, as relapse rates are high when drugs are discontinued.

There is preliminary evidence for the efficacy of CBT in BDD. Veale *et al* (1996), in a small randomised controlled trial, demonstrated that CBT (using exposure and response prevention plus some cognitive restructuring) is more effective than a waiting-list control condition for BDD.

Patients with a more severe condition should receive both an SSRI and CBT. It should be noted that, as in obsessive–compulsive disorder, it can take 3–4 months for patients to respond to drug treatment. It is important to emphasise this to both doctors and patients, lest treatment be abandoned prematurely.

Functional somatic syndromes

In the previous edition of this book, a number of disorders were separately described and their treatment outlined. These included irritable bowel syndrome, functional chest pain and chronic fatigue syndrome. Since the first edition was published, the concept of functional somatic symptoms and syndromes has been developed and it now seems sensible to discuss these various syndromes together, for reasons that we will discuss.

These syndromes constitute a huge clinical burden both in primary care and in specialist hospital clinics. Every hospital specialty has its own syndrome (see Table 16.2) and patients with these syndromes account for 30–40% of new out-patient referrals in hospital clinics (Hamilton *et al*, 1996).

Table 16.2 Functional somatic symptom syndrome in hospital clinics

Specialty	Syndrome
Infectious diseases	Chronic fatigue syndrome
Gastroenterology	Irritable bowel syndrome
Cardiology	Atypical chest pain
Respiratory medicine	Hyperventilation syndrome
Rheumatology	Fibromyalgia
Neurology	Tension headache
Gynaecology	Chronic pelvic pain
	Premenstrual syndrome

Concern about physical symptoms is the usual reason for patients to consult doctors. Doctors are trained to diagnose diseases and treat them, yet in only a minority of cases do doctors identify disease to account for the patient's symptoms, at least in primary care (Kroenke & Mangelsdorff, 1989). Most symptoms therefore remain unexplained even after medical assessment.

Classification

Traditionally there have been two approaches to the classification of patients with medically unexplained symptoms. The first highlights a number of symptomatic medical syndromes, such as irritable bowel syndrome and chronic fatigue syndrome. The alternative approach has been to look for underlying psychiatric disorder, for example depression or anxiety, both of which commonly present somatically, or to assign a diagnosis of somatoform disorder.

Both approaches have their limitations. First, it is common for patients with functional somatic syndromes also to have an underlying psychiatric disorder, usually depression or an anxiety disorder. It should, however, be noted that by no means do all patients with these syndromes have underlying or coexisting psychiatric disorder. A significant proportion do not – they are genuinely unexplained (either medically or in terms of 'somatised' psychiatric disorder). It is important for doctors to retain a degree of humility about this, particularly in view of the often acrimonious debate about the nature of some of these syndromes, such as chronic fatigue syndrome (see Wessely *et al*, 1998, for a review of this).

Second, there is increasing evidence that significant overlap exists between syndromes. Wessely *et al* (1999) have postulated that the existence of distinct somatic syndromes is an artefact of medical specialisation. In other words, which particular syndrome(s) are diagnosed depends on which type of medical specialist the patient sees. Their literature review revealed the following:

- The diagnostic criteria for the 12 syndromes they reviewed overlap hugely. For example, fatigue was part of the diagnostic definition of six, headache was mentioned in eight and abdominal bloating in eight syndromes.
- Patients who have one somatic syndrome also met criteria for one or more others. For example, patients with fibromyalgia had raised rates of chronic fatigue, irritable bowel syndrome and chemical sensitivities. There are numerous references in the literature to these disorders being associated with each other.
- There are similarities across these syndromes in terms of sex incidence, prevalence of coexisting psychiatric disorder, prognosis and response to treatment.
- The literature on the treatment of these disorders shows a remarkable degree of concordance, usually comprising three elements:
  1. general advice emphasising good rapport with the patient, an educational component explaining the

symptoms, the need to avoid pointless or invasive investigations and an emphasis on rehabilitation rather than complete cure

2 the use of antidepressants

3 some form of psychotherapy – today CBT is the preferred option.

In summary, these syndromes have more in common than they have differences, and Wessely *et al* (1999) challenged the presently accepted wisdom of a multiplicity of different syndromes, although they did not go so far as to propose a unitary syndrome. They also noted that a previous (pre-war) generation of physicians had also observed a high degree of overlap and commonality and wrote of 'psychosomatic affections' and 'psychosomatic syndromes'.

These findings have considerable implications for classification and for treatment (see below). Wessely *et al* suggested a multi-axial approach to classification, with axes including number of symptoms and their duration, associated psychiatric disorder, patient's attributions for the symptoms and any identifiable physiological processes.

Epidemiology

These syndromes constitute a significant public health problem. They are common in both primary and secondary care. Although in many patients they are self-limiting, they frequently persist, cause distress and disability, and result in frequent consultations, with attendant medical and social costs.

It is poorly understood why these disorders are so common. An epidemiological survey found that the symptoms that comprise these disorders are extremely common in the community (i.e. in non-clinical samples). Lieb *et al* (2000) interviewed 3021 adolescents and young adults using the Munich adaptation of the Composite International Diagnostic Interview (CIDI), which included 46 somatosensory symptoms, all derived from DSM–IV. Interviewers cross-checked that a reported symptom, for it to be counted, was not part of an existing known condition or due to a drug or alcohol, and that it was also clinically significant (a visit to the doctor, medication taken, or some functional impairment). Just over half the population had a lifetime experience of at least one of these symptoms. The 12-month prevalence of these symptoms was also very high. Thus, 33% reported a pain symptom – including 11% headache, 9% abdominal pain, 4% back pain and 4% joint pain – even though the sample was young. A functional gastrointestinal symptom was reported by 13%, pseudo-neurological symptoms by 9% and conversion symptoms by around 7%. The high frequency of these symptoms in the general population may go some way to explaining why the functional somatosensory symptoms may very often be a presenting feature of personal distress, not only in developed nations where this survey was conducted, but also in the poorer developing nations, where somatic presentations tend to be even more common.

What is poorly understood is why these particular symptoms are so strongly linked with extremely high rates of treatment-seeking behaviours resulting in consultation with a wide variety of different medical specialists and the diagnoses of a variety of different syndromes, which in their turn become extremely common.

In the UK the prevalence of these syndromes in primary care is around 20% (Pender *et al*, 1997), and studies by the World Health Organization suggest similar proportions in other countries. Hamilton *et al* (1996) suggest a prevalence of 35% in medical out-patient departments. This is even higher in some specialist clinics, such as gastroenterology and neurology. About half the patients with a functional somatic syndrome (and more in specialist settings) have symptoms persisting for over 1 year.

Aetiology

The aetiology of these syndromes is poorly understood and at present it is wise to keep an open mind on this subject. The historical debate over whether these symptoms should principally be seen as 'organic' or 'psychological' has been sterile and it is a source of great disappointment that this debate lingers on. This is best illustrated by the highly charged politicised debate on chronic fatigue syndrome. Despite attempting to maintain a stance of 'neutrality' with regard to aetiology, psychiatrists who have played a prominent part in this debate (e.g. Wessely *et al*, 1998) have been vilified by some media and self-help groups and caricatured as 'psychologising' what these groups see as an organic disorder (a dispassionate reading of Wessely's work shows this not to be the case). It is in this climate that discussion of the aetiology of these syndromes has taken place.

At present it appears that these syndromes are multifactorial in origin, with biological, psychological and social factors all playing a part in both precipitating and perpetuating symptoms and disability. There has, for example, been considerable research into the biology of chronic fatigue syndrome and fibromyalgia (Komaroff, 2000; Parker *et al*, 2001; Mehendale & Goldman, 2002). The most enduring findings are of central down-regulation of the hypothalamo–pituitary–adrenal axis and hypocortisolism, and problems in central pain processing. These abnormalities, however, affect only some of the patients who meet the criteria for these syndromes. Psychological stress resulting from the disorder, such as depression and anxiety, and the stress of other physical illness or injury may both precipitate unexplained physical symptoms and act as perpetuating factors.

The role of doctors and the healthcare system in causing and perpetuating functional symptoms is significant. Inappropriate reassurance, over-investigation, spurious diagnoses and treatments, and reinforcing disability are all major contributions to chronicity in these syndromes. Family factors of relevance include lack of parental care and childhood experience of severe and/or prolonged illness (Craig *et al*, 1993).

The patient's own knowledge and beliefs about symptoms and the behaviours engaged in when symptomatic are also highly relevant to the aetiology of these syndromes.

A summary of the precipitating, predisposing and perpetuating factors is presented in Box 16.4.

Box 16.4 Aetiology of medically unexplained symptoms

Predisposing factors
- Genetic
- Personality factors (e.g. temperament, health consciousness)
- Learnt illness beliefs
- Childhood experience of illness
- Physical illness

Precipitating factors
- Physical illness
- Psychiatric illness
- Trauma
- Recent change in social support
- Stressful life events

Perpetuating factors
- Physiological (e.g. hyperventilation, inactivity and unfitness, diet, drugs, alcohol)
- Response to others (e.g. doctors, relatives, other therapists, including complementary therapists)
- Financial benefits
- Psychiatric illness
- Illness beliefs and anxieties

Management

Many patients with functional somatic symptoms do not present to doctors at all but deal with the symptoms themselves. Of those who present to doctors, most are treated in primary care. For some, symptoms are self-limiting and brief explanation and reassurance are all that is required. Some, usually those with more persistent or disabling symptoms, reach hospital clinics. In this section on management we emphasise a tiered approach to care, and outline a general approach to managing these patients in primary care settings, before describing the more specialist care that patients will require (see Sharpe *et al*, 1997, for an overview).

Primary care

General practitioners play a critical role in the management of patients with functional somatic symptoms. Their role has been summarised by Sharpe *et al* (1997) thus:

1 to provide simple advice, explanation and reassurance

2 to detect psychiatric disorders that present somatically

3 to deal with obvious cognitive and behavioural factors that exacerbate disability (e.g. disease conviction, avoidance behaviours, checking behaviours)

4 to give simple advice on psychological management (e.g. of anxiety) and on rehabilitation

5 to prescribe appropriately

6 to act as gatekeeper for secondary care services

7 to provide care for patients with more chronic symptoms.

At the initial assessment the general practitioner should identify and acknowledge the patient's concerns. A thorough history needs to be taken and a physical examination carried out, keeping an open mind on both disease and functional diagnoses. The effect of the symptoms on the patient's daily functioning should be assessed. Underlying psychiatric disorders and social problems should be looked for but, as stated above, are by no means omnipresent.

Treatment should follow the principles outlined above and promote self-help and resumption of normal activities. Specific illness fears and beliefs may need to be addressed and appropriate reassurance given. It should be noted, however, that for the small group of patients with marked health anxiety (hypochondriasis) repeated reassurance may make matters worse.

A meta-analysis by O'Malley *et al* (1999) has provided evidence for the efficacy of antidepressants even in the absence of clear-cut depression or anxiety. Antidepressants had a greater effect on physical symptoms than on psychological symptoms. The evidence was greater for tricyclic antidepressants than for SSRIs, although there was evidence of efficacy for both.

Finally, there may be significant social or interpersonal issues which may need to be managed to permit functional improvement; this may require involving significant others in the patient's management.

Specialist treatment

A minority of patients will require specialist psychiatric treatment. Patients in this group are more likely to have problems engaging with psychiatric services and the principles outlined in relation to the management of somatisation disorder (see page 398) are equally relevant here. Psychiatric services based in general hospitals or primary care are more acceptable to most of the patients than services based in psychiatric hospitals. Liaison psychiatrists have particular expertise and experience in organising and delivering these services. Unfortunately, these services are still not uniformly available in the UK and even where they do exist liaison services cannot provide a comprehensive service for all these patients. Part of the role of the liaison psychiatrist therefore is to help educate and advise colleagues in the appropriate management of such patients.

The basis of specialist treatment is a comprehensive assessment aimed at a formulation that makes sense of the patient's problems and about which the patient and doctor can broadly agree. It is critical that doctor and patient have a shared understanding of the problem, in particular regarding its maintaining factors (cognitive, behavioural, physiological, emotional, social), which become the focus of interventions.

Most evidence is for CBT (Kroenke & Swindle, 2000), although other psychological and somatic interventions are effective in some patients. These include interpersonal and brief dynamic psychotherapy (e.g. for irritable bowel syndrome), antidepressants and analgesics. CBT has been shown to be effective in a whole range of functional symptom syndromes (e.g. non-cardiac chest pain, chronic fatigue, irritable bowel syndrome and chronic pain).

Factitious disorders

In the factitious disorders symptoms are intentionally induced or feigned so that the patient can assume the sick role. In malingering (discussed below) the individual will also produce symptoms intentionally but there is usually an obvious external purpose, such as to avoid military service, to obtain a hospital bed for the night or to evade the police.

Factitious disorders in DSM–IV are of two main types:

1 with predominantly physical signs and symptoms

2 with predominantly psychological signs and symptoms.

The text also states that mixed types may occur. The liaison psychiatrist working in a general hospital is likely to encounter those presenting with mainly physical symptoms, and they usually provoke strong negative reactions in the physicians and surgeons who 'expose' them. As a group they are elusive and difficult to study, but a recent large series demonstrates most of the key features. Krahn *et al* (2003) collected 93 cases diagnosed over 21 years from the Mayo Clinic in Minnesota, a clinic renowned for its excellence and high diagnostic standards. The diagnostic criteria in DSM–IV states there should be some evidence of fabrication and Box 16.5 tabulates the specific categories of evidence used to confirm the diagnosis in this study. Most of the 93 patients were women (72%) and just under half (47%) were women with either a training in or practical experience of health work. These patients have both the knowledge and skill to simulate a physical illness. Hospital wandering was more common among men and the Munchausen subtype is said to consist of pathological wandering from one hospital to another, pathological lying and a presentation with dramatic complaints. Pain was present in 85% of the patients and known substance misuse in around 30%. The authors stressed that an important differential diagnosis is to work out whether the patient is only seeking analgesics or whether the main aim is to assume the sick role. The differential diagnosis between factitious disorders, malingering and somatisation disorder is also very difficult to make and is discussed below (see page 404).

Box 16.5 Specific categories of evidence used to confirm the diagnosis of factitious disorders

1 Inexplicable laboratory results (e.g. foreign material in a biopsy sample or body fluid)
2 Obvious inconsistency between history and results of physical examinations and tests
3 Patient admission of self-induced illness
4 Records from other institutions showing similar evaluations or contradictory information
5 Criminal conviction for Munchausen by proxy
6 Observed tampering with wounds (e.g. removal of dressing, interfering with drips)
7 Surreptitious use of medications

Criteria used in the study by Krahn *et al* (2003).

Krahn *et al* (2003) attempted to conduct a follow-up but found this was impossible because too many patients had no permanent address or had changed their names; most of these were in fact untraceable. Of the 28 patients traced, 22 were residing in an institution, which suggests there was a high degree of handicap, but this high rate may reflect the greater ease of tracing people who are in an institution.

Krahn *et al* (2003) decided not to use pseudologia phantastica as a diagnostic feature because they could not operationalise it, but Bass (2001) noted that this is probably the most reliable sign, and is almost always associated with factitious disorders. He stated that the following features are associated with pseudologia phantastica:

- it is not determined by situational factors, whereas in malingering the lying is
- there may be a kernel of truth
- it is often fantastic, with self-aggrandisement
- it may be compulsive and recurring (i.e. the patient cannot seem to stop lying)
- the underlying motive is attention seeking
- it may be very destructive.

Examination of the patients' case notes from several sources and the demonstration of inconsistencies between the patient's case notes from other hospitals and the current history usually provides the first clue of the pathological lying in a patient with a factitious disorders. Bass (2001) suggests that subtle types of brain damage, particularly to the frontal lobes, may be important and quotes cases where lesions in the prefrontal cortex occurring during infancy resulted in chronic persistent motiveless lying later in life.

The traditional management of factitious disorders once the diagnosis is made usually involves confrontation, which is generally followed by dismissal or self-discharge. The usefulness of such an approach has been questioned by Eisendrath *et al* (1996) on the grounds that it does little to prevent further episodes. He advocates a non-confrontational approach that includes the use of 'inexact interpretations' to explain inconsistencies and the link between past stresses and present symptoms, as well as using face-saving manoeuvres in the hope that the patient will remain sufficiently long to be able to engage with psychiatric services in a more meaningful way. There are no trials on treating these conditions, which may be severely disabling.

Malingering

The essential feature of malingering is the intentional production of false or grossly exaggerated physical or psychological symptoms (according to DSM–IV). The motivation is generally external and obvious: classically, in military settings to avoid active military service, in forensic practice to avoid criminal proceedings, and in civilian practice to avoid work, to obtain drugs or to gain financial compensation. Although the condition is described in DSM–IV, it is not included in the main body of the text of accepted psychiatric disorders but is instead relegated to an appendix entitled 'Other conditions that may be the focus of clinical attention'.

Similarly, in the ICD–10 chapter on mental disorders, malingering is described as 'a person feigning an illness', and it is not coded as a mental illness but instead is placed in an obscure category of 'Persons encountering health services in other circumstances'. Possibly this failure officially to include this common yet aberrant form of human behaviour as a mental disorder is a reflection of our continued ignorance of its causes and serious difficulties with its management, as well as a degree of stigma and rejection.

Malingering needs to be distinguished from factitious disorder and conversion hysteria and other somatising disorders. In factitious disorder, simulation of illness also occurs, but the patient is said to be less aware of the deception and the intended gain is the assumption of the sick role, for example to obtain admission to hospital. In practice the distinction between malingering and factitious disorder may be difficult. In conversion hysteria, the patient is said to be not conscious of any deception – the simulation all occurs at an unconscious level, while the gain is said to be intra-psychic (e.g. in reducing intolerable anxiety). Again, the distinction between conscious and unconscious motivation can be difficult to make, because both conscious and unconscious intention tend to work in the same way, resulting in the mimicry of an illness in accordance with the patient's own concept of that particular illness. Malingering commonly is superimposed on a genuine physical or psychiatric disorder. In addition, most psychiatrists try to take their patient's statements on trust and usually do not entertain the possibility of malingering until lying or some inconsistency in the patient's story begins to raise suspicion.

The grosser types of malingering are uncommon nowadays. Hurst (1940) gave two criteria for detecting such malingering: 'detection in *flagrante delicto*' and an unforced confession. Both criteria remain useful today. Few malingerers are as helpful as the soldier who wrote a letter on lined paper without a heading purporting to be signed by the matron of the hospital to the effect that 'Private X is unfit to return to duty because he has a broken ankle'. Equally, some patients will admit that they bring on their symptoms; for example, an epileptic patient who produced 'hysterical' fits was diagnosed as attention seeking, but she later indicated that she was partially aware of what she was doing and had produced the hysterical fits to try to get her 'proper fits' treated better.

People with a genuine disability or even hysterical disability will be disabled on a continuous basis. However, those who are feigning illness are generally unable to maintain their act for the whole time and when they are off guard may drop the pretence and act normally. Insurance companies take advantage of these lapses and claimants seeking large damages for personal injuries are sometimes video-taped by insurance investigators and then found to have capacities that they solemnly swore to the doctor they were lacking. In one case a patient presented with an apparent organic paralysis, but investigators succeeded in installing a camera in a hotel bedroom and filmed the claimant walking around unaided. He was later charged with fraud, although in most cases the detection leads only to an invalidation of the claim.

Today, the vast majority of cases of feigned illness or feigned symptoms are encountered in medico-legal practice, but for obvious reasons it is very difficult to measure the true prevalence of this phenomenon. Rodgers et al (1994) tried to assess this indirectly by surveying forensic assessors and then pooled their estimates for the prevalence of malingering and found an average figure of 15% for malingering in forensic assessments and around 7% for civilian cases.

The degree of malingering is sometimes only partial. Resnick (1997) classified malingering into three groups:

1 'Pure malingering', or complete fabrication of symptoms. This is comparatively rare today.

2 Partial malingering, in which existing symptoms are over-reported or remitted symptoms are reported as ongoing. This is much more common.

3 'False imputation', where symptoms are intentionally misattributed to a traumatic event. This is especially common in medico-legal settings.

Although feigning symptoms can occur with any psychiatric disorder, three conditions are particularly associated with feigned symptoms: PTSD; the cognitive symptoms of head injury; and work-related 'stress'. Possibly this is because the symptoms of these conditions are entirely subjective and hence relatively easily feigned, and also because genuine claimants with these disorders can sometimes receive large sums in compensation. A number of sophisticated psychological tests, mainly based on the Minnesota Multidimensional Personality Inventory, have been devised to try to differentiate genuine PTSD from 'malingering PTSD' (for a review, see Guriel & Fremouw, 2003), while similarly there are several psychometric tests with associated indices that aim to distinguish 'non-credible cognitive symptoms' from more genuine cognitive disabilities (Soumanti *et al*, 2006).

Conclusion

Patients with medically unexplained physical symptoms represent a significant public health burden. Problems in classification/nosology continue to bedevil this area and these difficulties, along with the use of the language of psychiatric classification, which most patients find unacceptable, has led to the present DSM/ICD terms being little used in day-to-day clinical practice, including liaison psychiatry. It is likely that future classifications will make significant changes to the current position. It is important to see these patients as a heterogeneous group of individuals and not to equate 'medically unexplained' with 'psychiatric'. Biological, psychological and social factors are relevant to both the aetiology and the maintenance of these syndromes, as well as to their treatment. In recent years a variety of biological and psychosocial approaches to treatment have been developed and doctors should no longer view these patients as a group for whom medicine has nothing to offer.

References

Akagi, H. & House, A. (2001) The epidemiology of hysteria conversion. In *Contemporary Approaches to the Study of Hysteria* (eds P. W. Halligan, C. Bass & J. C. Marshall), pp. 73–87. Oxford: Oxford University Press.

Alam, C. N. & Merskey, H. (1992) The development of the hysterical personality. *History of Psychiatry*, **3**, 135–165.

American Psychiatric Association (1980) *Diagnostic and Statistical Manual of Mental Disorders* (3rd edn) (DSM–III). Washington, DC: APA.

American Psychiatric Association (1994) *Diagnostic and Statistical Manual of Mental Disorders* (4th edn) (DSM–IV). Washington, DC: APA.

American Psychiatric Association (2000) *Diagnostic and Statistical Manual of Mental Disorders* (4th edn, text revision) (DSM–IV–TR). Washington, DC: APA.

Appleby, L. (1987) Hypochondriasis: an acceptable diagnosis? *BMJ*, **294**, 8857.

Asmundson, G. J. G., Taylor, S. & Cox, B. (2001) *Health Anxiety: Clinical and Research Perspectives on Hypochondriasis and Related Conditions*. Bristol: Wiley.

Athwal, B. S., Halligan, P. W., Fink, G. R., *et al* (2001) Imaging hysterical paralysis. In *Contemporary Approaches to the Study of Hysteria: Clinical and Theoretical Perspectives* (eds P. W. Halligan, C. Bass & J. C. Marshall), ch. 18. Oxford: Oxford University Press.

Baker, G. H. B. (1989) Backache. In *Psychological Management of the Physically Ill* (eds J. H. Lacey & T. Burns), pp. 229–246. Edinburgh: Churchill Livingstone.

Bantick, S. J., Wise, R. G., Ploghaus, A., *et al* (2002) Imaging how attention modulates pain in humans using functional MRI. *Brain*, **125**, 310–319.

Barsky, A. J. & Ahern, D. K. (2004) Cognitive behavior therapy for hypochondriasis: a randomized controlled trial. *JAMA*, **291**, 1464–1470.

Barsky, A. J. & Wyshak, G. (1990) Hypochondriasis and somatosensory amplification. *British Journal of Psychiatry*, **157**, 404–409.

Barsky, A. J., Frank, C. B., Cleary, P. D., *et al* (1991) The relation between hypochondriasis and age. *American Journal of Psychiatry*, **148**, 923–928.

Barsky, A. J., Cleary, P. D., Wyshak, G., *et al* (1992) A structural diagnostic interview for hypochondriasis: a proposed criterion standard. *Journal of Nervous and Mental Disease*, **180**, 20–27.

Barsky, A. J., Wool, C., Barnett, M. C., *et al* (1994) Histories of childhood trauma in adult hypochondriacal patients. *American Journal of Psychiatry*, **151**, 397–401.

Bartholomew, R. E. & Wessely, S. (2002) Protean nature of mass sociogenic illness. *British Journal of Psychiatry*, **180**, 300–306.

Bass, C. (1993) Somatoform disorders: aspects of liaison psychiatry. *Current Opinion in Psychiatry*, **6**, 210–215.

Bass, C. (2001) Factitious disorders and malingering. In *Contemporary Approaches to the Study of Hysteria* (eds P. W. Halligan, C. Bass & J. C. Marshall), pp. 127–142. Oxford: Oxford University Press.

Bass, C. & May, S. (2002) ABC of psychological medicine: chronic multiple somatic symptoms. *BMJ*, **325**, 323–326.

Bhatia, M. S. & Vaid, I. (2000) Hysterical aponia – an analysis of 25 cases. *Indian Journal of Medical Sciences*, **54**, 335–338.

Bleuler, E. P. (1950) *The Group of Schizophrenias*. New York: International Universities Press.

Bliss, E. L. (1984) A symptom profile of patients with multiple personalities, including MMPI results. *Journal of Nervous and Mental Disease*, **172**, 197–202.

Boswell, J. (1777–83) On hypochondria. In *Boswell's Column* (ed. M. Bailey, 1951). London: William Kimber.

Brachet, J. L. (1847) *Traité de l'hystérie*. Paris: J. B. Baillière.

Briquet, P. (1859) *Traité clinique et thérapeutique de l'hystérie*. Paris: Baillière et Fils.

Brodie, B. C. (1837) *Lectures Illustrative of Certain Nervous Affections*. London: Longman.

Burton, R. (1651) *The Anatomy of Melancholy* (eds L. Dell & P. Jordon-Smith, 1948). New York: Tudor Publishing.

Carter, A. B. (1949) The prognosis of certain hysterical symptoms. *BMJ*, *i*, 1076–1079.

Carter, R. B. (1853) *On the Pathology and Treatment of Hysteria*. London: Churchill.

Charcot, J. M. (1889) *Clinical Lectures on Diseases of the Nervous System. Vol. III* (trans. T. Savill). London: New Sydenham Society.

Cheville, A., Caraceni, A. & Portenoy, R. K. (2000) Pain, definition and assessment. In *Pain: What Psychiatrists Need to Know* (ed. M. J. Massia), pp. 1–22. Washington, DC: American Psychiatric Association.

Cheyne, G. (1733) *The English Malady: or, a Treatise of Nervous Diseases of all Kind; as Spleen, Vapours, Lowness of Spirit, Hypochondriacal and Hysterical Distempers* (4th edn). London: G. Strachan.

Ciompi, L. (1969) Follow-up studies on the evolution of former neurotic and depressive states in old age. Clinical and psychodynamic aspects. *Journal of Geriatric Psychiatry*, **3**, 90–106.

Clarke, D. M., Salkovskis, P. M., Hackmann, A., *et al* (1998) Two psychological treatments for hypochondriasis. A randomised controlled trial. *British Journal of Psychiatry*, **173**, 218–225.

Craig, T. K., Boardman, A. P., Mills, K., *et al* (1993) The South London Somatisation Study – I. Longitudinal course and the influence of early life experiences. *British Journal of Psychiatry*, **163**, 570–588.

Crimlisk, H., Bhatia, K., Cope, C., *et al* (1998) Slater revisited: 6 year follow up study of patients with medically unexplained motor symptoms. *BMJ*, **316**, 582–586.

De Jongh, A. (2003) Clinical characteristics of somatisation in dental practice. *British Dental Journal*, **195**, 151–154.

Derbyshire, S. W. G., Jones, A. K. P., Devani, P., *et al* (1994) Cerebral responses to pain in patients with atypical facial pain measured with positron emission tomography. *Journal of Neurology, Neurosurgery and Psychiatry*, **57**, 1166–1172.

Eisendrath, S. J., Rand, D. C. & Feldman, M. D. (1996) Factitious disorders and litigation. In *The Spectrum of Factitious Disorders* (eds M. D. Feldman & S. J. Eisendrath). Washington, DC: American Psychiatric Press.

Engel, G. L. (1951) Primary atypical facial neuralgia. An hysterical conversion symptom. *Psychosomatic Medicine*, **13**, 375.

Engel, G. L. (1980) The clinical application of the biopsychosocial model. *American Journal of Psychiatry*, **137**, 437–446.

Escobar, J. L., Rubiostipec, M., Canino, G., *et al* (1989) Somatic Symptoms Index (SSI) – a new and abridged somatization construct. Prevalence and epidemiological correlates in two large community samples. *Journal of Nervous and Mental Disease*, **177**, 1490–1496.

Fahy, T. A. (1988) The diagnosis of multiple personality disorder: a critical review. *British Journal of Psychiatry*, **153**, 597–606.

Fallon, B. A., Liebowitz, M. R., Salman, E., *et al* (1993) Fluoxetine for hypochondriacal patients without major depression. *Journal of Clinical Psychopharmacology*, **13**, 438–441.

Falret, J. P. (1822) *De l'hypochondrie et du Suicide*. Paris.

Faravelli, C., Salvatori, S., Galassi, F., *et al* (1997) Epidemiology of somatoform disorders: community survey in Florence. *Social Psychiatry and Psychiatric Epidemiology*, **32**, 24–29.

Feinmann, C., Harris, M. & Crawley, R. (1984) Psychogenic facial pain: presentation and treatment. *BMJ*, **288**, 436–439.

Ford, C. V. (1983) *The Somatising Disorders: Illness as a Way of Life*. New York: Elsevier Biomedical.

Ganser, S. (1898) A peculiar hysterical state. *Archiv für Psychiatrie und Nervenkrankheit*, **30**, 633. (Trans. C. E. Schorer, 1989. *British Journal of Criminology*, **5**, 120–126.)

Georget, M. (1821) *De la physiologie de la système nerveux*. Vol. 2, pp. 261–262 and 265–284. Paris: J. B. Baillière.

Gillespie, R. (1928) Hypochondria: its definition, nosology and psycholopathology. *Guy's Hospital Report*, **78**, 308–460.

Gould, R., Miller, B. L., Goldberg, M. A., *et al* (1986) The validity of hysterical signs and symptoms. *Journal of Nervous and Mental Disease*, **174**, 593–598.

Guriel, J. & Fremouw, W. (2003) Assessing malingered post traumatic stress disorder: a critical review. *Clinical Psychology Review*, **23**, 881–894.

Hacking, I. (1998) *Mad Travelers: Reflections on the Reality of Transient Mental Illness*. Charlottesville, VA: University Press of Virginia.

Hafeiz, H. B. (1980) Hysterical conversion: a prognosis study. *British Journal of Psychiatry*, **136**, 548–551.

Halligan, P. W., Athwal, B. S., Oakley, D. A., *et al* (2000) Imaging hypnotic paralysis: implications for conversion hysteria. *Lancet*, **355**, 986–987.

Hamilton, J., Campos, R. & Creed, F. (1996) Anxiety, depression and management of medically unexplained symptoms in medical clinics. *Journal of the Royal College of Physicians*, **30**, 18–21.

Head, H. (1922) An address on the diagnosis of hysteria. *BMJ*, *i*, 827–829.

Hinsie, L. E. & Campbell, R. J. (1960) *Psychiatric Dictionary* (3rd edn). Oxford: Oxford University Press.

Hirschmuller, A. (1989) *The Life and Work of Josef Breuer: Physiology and Psychoanalysis*. New York: New York University Press.

Hollander, E., Liebowitz, M. R., Winchel, R., *et al* (1989) Treatment of body dysmorphic disorder with serotonin re-uptake blockers. *American Journal of Psychiatry*, **146**, 768–770.

Hotopf, M., Carr, S., Mayou, R., *et al* (1998) Why do children have chronic abdominal pain and what happens to them when they grow up? Population based cohort study. *BMJ*, **316**, 1196–1200.

Hurst, A. F. (1940) *Medical Diseases of War.* London: Edward Arnold. (Hurst modified his views with each edition.)

Hyler, S. E. & Sussmann, N. (1984) Somatoform disorder after DSM–III. *Hospital and Community Psychiatry*, **34**, 469–478.

Inouye, E. (1972) Genetic aspects of neurosis. *International Journal of Mental Health*, **1**, 176–189.

Janet, P. (1894) *L'État mental des hystériques*. Paris: Rueff.

Jones, A. K., Kulkarni, B. & Derbyshire, S. W. (2003) Pain mechanisms and their disorders. *British Medical Bulletin*, **65**, 83–93.

Kathol, R. G., Cox, T. A., Corbett, J. J., *et al* (1983*a*) Functional visual loss: I. A true psychiatric disorder? *Psychological Medicine*, **13**, 307–314.

Kathol, R. G., Cox, T. A., Corbett, J. J., *et al* (1983*b*) Functional visual loss: II. Psychiatric aspects in 42 patients followed for 4 years. *Psychological Medicine*, **13**, 315–324.

Kellner, R. (1986) *Somatization and Hypochondriasis*. Westport, CT: Praeger.

Kenyon, F. (1964) Hypochondriasis: a clinical study. *British Journal of Psychiatry*, **110**, 478–488.

Kenyon, F. (1976) Hypochondriacal states. *British Journal of Psychiatry*, **129**, 1–14.

Kirmayer, L. J. & Robbins, J. M. (1991) Three forms of somatization in primary care: prevalence, co-occurrence and sociodemographic characteristics. *Journal of Nervous and Mental Disease*, **179**, 647–655.

Komaroff, A. L. (2000) The biology of chronic fatigue syndrome. *American Journal of Medicine*, **108**, 169–171.

Kraepelin, E. (1904) Hysterical insanity. In *Lectures on Clinical Psychiatry* (trans. T. Johnstone). New York: William Wood.

Krahn, L. E., Hongzhe, L. & O'Connor, M. K. (2003) Patients who strive to be ill. Factitious disorder with physical symptoms. *American Journal of Psychiatry*, **160**, 1163–1168.

Kroenke, K. & Mangelsdorff, D. (1989) Common symptoms in ambulatory care: incidence, evaluation, therapy and outcome. *American Journal of Medicine*, **86**, 262–266.

Kroenke, K. & Swindle, R. (2000) Cognitive behavioural therapy for somatization and symptom syndromes: a critical review of controlled trials. *Psychotherapy and Psychosomatics*, **69**, 205–215.

La Barre, W. (1975) Anthropological perspectives on hallucinations and hallucinogens. In *Hallucinations: Experience and Theory* (eds R. K. Siegel & L. J. West). New York: Wiley.

Lascelles, R. G. (1966) Atypical facial pain and depression. *British Journal of Psychiatry*, **112**, 651–659.

Lehtinen, V. & Puhakka, H. (1976) A psychosomatic approach to the globus hystericus syndrome. *Acta Psychiatrica Neurologica Scandinavica*, **53**, 21–28.

Lewis, A. J. (1975) The survival of hysteria. *Psychological Medicine*, **5**, 9–12.

Lieb, R., Pfister, H., Mastaler, M., *et al* (2000) Somatoform syndromes and disorders in a representative population sample of adolescents and young adults: prevalence, comorbidity and impairments. *Acta Psychiatrica Scandinavica*, **101**, 194–208.

Lipowski, Z. J. (1988) Somatisation: the concept and its clinical application. *American Journal of Psychiatry*, **145**, 1358–1368.

Ljungberg, L. (1957) Hysteria. *Acta Psychiatrica Scandinavica*, suppl. 112.

Lloyd, K. G. & Hornykiewicz, O. (1973) L-glutamic acid decarboxylase in Parkinson's disease: effect of L-dopa therapy. *Nature*, **243**, 521–523.

Lucock, M. P. & Morley, S. (1996) The Health Anxiety Questionnaire. *British Journal of Health Psychology*, **1**, 137–150.

Mai, F. (2004) Somatization disorder: a practical review. *Canadian Journal of Psychiatry*, **49**, 652–662.

Mai, F. M. & Merskey, H. (1980) Briquet's treatise on hysteria: a synopsis and commentary. *Archives of Internal Medicine*, **148**, 2213–2217.

Malcolmson, K. G. (1966) Radiological findings in globus hystericus. *British Journal of Radiology*, **39**, 583–586.

Malcolmson, K. G. (1968) Globus hystericus vel pharyngis: a reconnaissance of proximal vagal modalities. *Journal of Laryngology and Otology*, **82**, 219–230.

Marshall, J. C., Halligan, P. W., Fink, G. R., *et al* (1997) The functional anatomy of a hysterical paralysis. *Cognition*, **64**, B1–B8.

Mayou, R. & Bryant, B. (2002) Psychiatry of whiplash injury. *British Journal of Psychiatry*, **180**, 441–448.

Mayou, R., Levenson, J. & Sharpe, M. (2003) Somatoform disorders in DSM–V. *Psychosomatics*, **44**(B), 449–451.

McKegney, F. P. (1967) The incidence and characteristics of patients with conversion reactions. I: A general hospital consultation service sample. *American Journal of Psychiatry*, **124**, 542–545.

McMahon, S. & Koltzenburg, M. (2005) *Melzack and Wall's Textbook of Pain* (5th edn). London: Elsevier.

Mechanic, D. (1964) The influence of mothers on their children's health, attitudes and behaviour. *Paediatrics*, **33**, 444–453.

Mehendale, A. W. & Goldman, M. P. (2002) Fibromyalgia syndrome, idiopathic widespread pain or myalgic encephalomyelopathy (SME). What is its nature? *Pain Practice*, **2**, 35–46.

Merskey, H. (1988) Regional pain is rarely hysterical. *Archives of Neurology*, **45**, 915–918.

Merskey, H. (1991) Shell shock. In *150 Years of British Psychiatry. 1841–1991* (eds G. E. Berrios & H. L. Freeman), pp. 245–267. London: Gaskell.

Merskey, H. (1992*a*) The manufacture of personalities. The production of multiple personality disorder. *British Journal of Psychiatry*, **160**, 327–340.

Merskey, H. (1992*b*) Anna O. had a severe depressive illness. *British Journal of Psychiatry*, **161**, 185–194.

Merskey, H. (1995) *The Analysis of Hysteria: Understanding Conversion and Dissociation* (2nd edn). London: Gaskell.

Merskey, H. (1999) Pain and psychological medicine. In *Textbook of Pain* (4th edn) (ed. P. D. Wall & R. Melzack), pp. 929–949. Edinburgh: Churchill Livingstone.

Merskey, H. (2000) Beware somatisation. *European Journal of Pain*, **4**, 3–4.

Merskey, H. & Bogduk, N. (eds) (1994) *Classification of Chronic Pain: Descriptions of Chronic Pain Syndromes and Definitions of Pain Terms* (2nd edn). Seattle, WA: International Association for the Study of Pain.

Merskey, H. & Buhrich, N. A. (1975) Hysteria and organic brain disease. *British Journal of Medical Psychology*, **48**, 359–366.

Merskey, H. & Merskey, S. J. (1993) Hysteria or the suffocation of the mother. *Canadian Medical Association Journal*, **148**, 399–405.

Miller, L. (1984) Neuropsychological concept of somatoform disorders. *International Journal of Psychiatry and Medicine*, **14**, 31–46.

Morselli, E. (1891) Sulla dismorfofobia e sulla tafefobia. *Bolletina della R accademia di Genova*, **6**, 110–119.

Moss, P. D. & McEvedy, C. P. (1966) An epidemic of overbreathing among schoolgirls. *BMJ*, *ii*, 1295–1300.

Noyes, R. (2000) Hypochondriasis. In *New Oxford Textbook of Psychiatry* (eds M. Gelder, J. J. Lopez-Ibor & N. Andreasen), pp. 1098–1106. Oxford: Oxford University Press.

O'Malley, P. G., Jackson, J. L., Santoro, J., *et al* (1999) Antidepressant therapy for unexplained symptoms and symptom syndromes. *Journal of Family Practice*, **48**, 980–990.

Parker, A. J. R., Wessely, S. & Cleare, A. J. (2001) The neuroendocrinology of chronic fatigue syndrome and fibromyalgia. *Psychological Medicine*, **31**, 1331–1345.

Parker, G. & Lipscome, P. (1980) The relevance of early parental experiences to adult dependency, hypochondriasis and utilization of primary physicians. *British Journal of Medical Psychology*, **53**, 355–363.

Pender, R., Kilkenny, L. & Kinmonth, A. (1997) Medically unexplained physical symptoms in primary care: a comparison of self report screening questionnaires and clinical opinion. *Journal of Psychosomatic Research*, **4**, 245–253.

Pennebaker, J. N. & Watson, D. (1991) The psychology of somatic symptoms. In *Current Concepts of Somatization: Research and Clinical Perspectives* (ed. L. J. Karmayer & J. M. Robbins), pp. 21–35. Washington, DC: American Psychiatric Press.

Phillips, K. A. (1996) *The Broken Mirror: Understanding and Treating Body Dysmorphic Disorder*. Oxford: Oxford University Press.

Phillips, K. A. & Diaz, S. (1997) Gender differences in body dysmorphic disorder. *Journal of Nervous and Mental Disease*, **185**, 570–577.

Phillips, K. A., McElroy, S. L., Keck, P. E., *et al* (1994) A comparison of delusional and non-delusional body dysmorphic disorder in 100 cases. *Psychopharmacology Bulletin*, 30, 179–186.

Philoppopoluos, G. S. (1979) The analysis of a case of dysmorfophobia. *Canadian Journal of Psychiatry*, **24**, 397–401.

Pilowsky, I. (1967) Dimensions of hypochondriasis. *British Journal of Psychiatry*, **131**, 89–93.

Pilowsky, I. (1983) Hypochondriasis. In *Handbook of Psychiatry 4 – The Neuroses and Personality Disorders* (eds G. Russell & L. Hoersov). Cambridge: Cambridge University Press.

Resnick, P. J. (1997) Malingering and post traumatic disorders. In *Clinical Assessment of Malingering and Deception* (2nd edn) (ed. R. Rodgers), pp. 130–152. New York: Guilford Press.

Reynolds, J. R. (1869) Remarks on paralysis and other disorders of motion and sensation, dependent on idea. *BMJ*, *ii*, 483–485. Discussion, 378–379.

Rodgers, R., Sewell, K. W. & Goldstein, A. (1994) Explanatory models of malingering. *Law and Human Behavior*, **22**, 273–285.

Romberg, M. H. (1851) *A Manual of the Nervous Diseases of Man* (2nd edn) (trans. E. H. Sieveking, 1853). London: New Sydenham Society.

Ross, C. A. (1989) *Multiple Personality*. New York: Wiley.

Salkovskis, P. M. & Warwick, H. M. C. (1986) Morbid preoccupations, health anxiety and reassurance: a cognitive–behavioral approach to hypochondriasis. *Behavior Research and Therapy*, **24**, 597–602.

Salmon, P., Peters, S. & Stanley, I. (1999) Patients' perceptions of medical explanations for somatisation disorders: a qualitative analysis. *BMJ*, **318**, 372–376.

Schmidt, A. J. M., Van Roosmalen, R., Van Der Beek, J. M. H., *et al* (1993) Hypochondriasis in ENT practice. *Clinical Otolaryngology*, **18**, 508–511.

Scott, P. D. (1965) Commentary on a peculiar hysterical state by S. J. M. Ganser. *British Journal of Criminology*, **5**, 120–126.

Sharpe, M. & Carson, A. (2001) Unexplained somatic symptoms, functional syndromes and somatization: do we need a paradigm shift? *Annals of Internal Medicine*, **134**, 926–930.

Sharpe, M., Bass, C. & Mayou, R. (1997) An overview of the treatment of functional somatic symptoms. In *Treatment of Functional Somatic Symptoms* (eds M. Sharpe, C. Bass & R. Mayou). Oxford: Oxford University Press.

Shields, J. (1982) General studies of hysterical disorders. In *Hysteria* (ed. A. Roy), pp. 41–56. Chichester: Wiley.

Simon, G., Gayter, R., Kiseley, S., *et al* (1996) Somatic symptoms of distress: an international primary care study. *Psychosomatic Medicine*, **58**, 481–488.

Sizemore, C. S. & Pittillo, E. S. (1977) *I'm Eve*. New York: Doubleday.

Slater, E. & Glithero, E. (1965) A follow-up of patients diagnosed as suffering from 'hysteria'. *Journal of Psychosomatic Research*, **9**, 9–11.

Smith, G. R., Monson, R. A. & Ray, D. C. (1986) Psychiatric consultation in somatization disorders. A randomized controlled study. *New England Journal of Medicine*, **314**, 1407–1413.

Smith, G. R., Rost, K. & Kashner, T. M. (1995) A trial of the effect of standardized psychiatric consultation and health outcomes and costs in somatizing patients. *Archives of General Psychiatry*, **52**, 236–243.

Soumanti, M., Boone, K. B., Savodnik, I., *et al* (2006) Non-credible psychiatric and cognitive symptoms in a workers compensation 'stress' claim sample. *Clinical Neuropsychology*, **20**, 754–765.

Speckens, A. E. M., Spinhoven, P., Sloekers, P. P. A., *et al* (1996) A validation study of the Whiteley Index, the Illness Attitude Scales, and the Somatosensory Amplification Scale in general medical and general practice patients. *Journal of Psychosomatic Research*, **40**, 95–104.

Standage, K. E. (1975) The etiology of hysterical seizures. *Canadian Psychiatric Association Journal*, **20**, 67–73.

Stengel, E. (1941) On the aetiology of fugue states. *Journal of Mental Science*, **87**, 572–599.

Stern, R. & Fernandez, M. (1991) Group cognitive and behavioral treatment of hypochondriasis. *BMJ*, **303**, 1229–1230.

Stone, J., Wojcik, W., Durrance, D., *et al* (2002*a*) What should we say to patients with symptoms unexplained by disease? The number needed to offend. *BMJ*, **325**, 1449–1456.

Stone, J., Zeman, A. & Carson, A. (2002*b*) Functional weakness and sensory disturbance. *Journal of Neurology, Neurosurgery and Psychiatry*, **73**, 241–245.

Stone, J., Sharpe, M., Rothwell, P. M., *et al* (2003) The twelve year prognosis of unilateral functional weakness and sensory disturbances. *Journal of Neurology, Neurosurgery and Psychiatry*, **74**, 591–596.

Stone, J., Smyth, R., Carson, A., *et al* (2005) Systematic review of conversion symptoms and 'hysteria'. *BMJ*, **331**, 989.

Stoudemire, G. A. (1988) Somatoform disorders, factitious disorders and malingering. In *Textbook of Psychiatry* (eds J. A. Talbott, R. E. Hales & S. C. Yudofsky). Washington, DC: APA.

Swartz, M., Blazer, D., Wodbury, M., *et al* (1986) Somatization disorder in a US southern community: use of a new procedure for analysis of medical classification. *Psychological Medicine*, **16**, 1403–1408.

Sydenham, T. (1697) Discourse concerning hysterical and hypochondriacal distempers. In *Dr. Sydenham's Compleat Method of Curing Almost All Diseases, and Description of Their Symptoms, to Which Are Now Added Five Discourses of the Same Author Concerning Pleurisy, Gout, Hysterical Passion, Dropsy and Rheumatism* (3rd edn). London: Newman & Parker.

Thigpen, C. H. & Cleckley, H. M. (1957) *The Three Faces of Eve*. New York: McGraw-Hill.

Trimble, M. R. (1978) Serum prolactin in epilepsy and hysteria. *BMJ*, *ii*, 1682.

Turkat, I. D. & Pettigrew, I. S. (1983) Development and validation of the Illness Behaviour Inventory. *Journal of Behavioural Assessment*, **5**, 35–47.

Veale, D., Gournay, K., Dryden, W., *et al* (1996) Body dysmorphic disorder: a cognitive behavioural model and pilot randomised controlled trial. *Behaviour Research and Therapy*, **34**, 717–729.

Veith, I. (1965) *Hysteria: The History of a Disease*. Chicago, IL: University of Chicago Press.

Vuilleumier, P., Chicherio, C., Assal, F., *et al* (2001) Functional neuroanatomical correlates associated with hysterical sensorimotor loss. *Brain*, **124**, 1065–1066.

Warwick, H. M. & Salkovskis, P. M. (1985) Reassurance. *BMJ*, **290**, 1028.

Warwick, H. M. C., Clark, D. M., Cobb, A. M., *et al* (1996) A controlled trial of cognitive behavioural treatment in hypochondriasis. *British Journal of Psychiatry*, **169**, 189–195.

Weller, M. P. I. & Wiedemann, P. (1989) Hysterical symptoms in ophthalmology. *Documenta Ophthalmologica*, **73**, 1–33.

Wessely, S., Hotopf, M. & Sharpe, M. (1998) *Chronic Fatigue and Its Syndromes*. Oxford: Oxford University Press.

Wessely, S., Nimnuan, C. & Sharpe, M. (1999) Functional somatic syndromes: one or many? *Lancet*, **354**, 936–939.

Whitlock, F. A. (1967*a*) The Ganser syndrome. *British Journal of Psychiatry*, **113**, 19–30.

Whitlock, F.A. (1967*b*) The aetiology of hysteria. *Acta Psychiatrica Scandinavica*, **43**, 144–162.

Whytt, T. (1751) Observations on the nature, causes and cure of those disorders which are commonly called nervous, hypochondriac, or hysteric: to which are prefixed some remarks on the sympathy of the nerves. In *The Works of Robert Whytt* (3rd edn, 1767). London: Beckett & du Hondt; Edinburgh: Balfour.

Willis, T. (1684) *An Essay of Pathology of the Brain and Nervous Shock in Which Convulsive Diseases Are Treated Of.* London: Dring Lee & Harper.

World Health Organization (1992) *The ICD-10 Classification of Diseases*. Geneva: WHO.

Ziv, I., Djaldetti, R., Zoldan, Y., *et al* (1998) Diagnosis of 'non organic' limb paresis by a novel motor assessment: the quantitative Hoover's test. *Journal of Neurology*, **245**, 797–802.

CHAPTER 17

Psychiatry in the general hospital

Hiroko Akagi and Allan House

Consultation–liaison (CL) psychiatry is one of the newer sub-specialties of adult psychiatry and is concerned with the practice of psychiatry in non-psychiatric settings. Typically this means in general hospital wards and out-patient clinics, although in some countries it also includes liaison with primary care. This chapter provides an outline of the nature and the practice of CL psychiatry, as well as some illustrative examples.

History

Exactly when the sub-specialty started is difficult to define, but the need for psychiatric expertise to assess patients who could not easily fit into a straightforward single medical diagnosis was already recognised towards the end of the 19th century, when J. J. Putnam, a Harvard neurologist working at the Massachusetts General Hospital, was assigned the task of 'evaluating medical patients whose complaints defied diagnoses' (Kornfeld, 1996). From the 1930s onwards general hospital psychiatry became established in the USA, and Edward Billings at the Colorado General Hospital first coined the term 'liaison psychiatry'. The history of CL psychiatry can be traced through three separate strands: the emergence of ideas and models concerning the interaction between mind and body, the need for education and research, and most recently the provision of psychiatric services in general hospitals.

Since the late 19th century, psychoanalytic theory has been influential in formulating ideas about the relation between psychological and physical symptoms. In Sigmund Freud's early work with patients who had hysterical disorders he introduced the concept of unconscious conflict manifesting as physical symptoms. Franz Alexander proposed that psychosomatic disease might be caused by emotional factors (Creed, 1991), while Flanders Dunbar argued for an association of specific personality types with specific medical disorders (Dunbar, 1954). However, this earlier analytically based psychosomatic theory was not substantiated by empirical research and fell out of favour. The First World War also influenced the understanding and treatment of physical symptoms arising from psychological traumas – such as 'shell shock' and 'soldier's heart' – as described in Chapter 13. More recently, thinking about the relationship has concentrated on health-related behaviours and the study of the physiological mediators of the interactions between body and mind, for instance between depression and heart disease.

As CL services gradually developed during the 20th century it became clear that psychiatrists working in a general hospital had an important educational role, teaching a holistic approach to medical students and other healthcare workers, training primary healthcare workers to identify and manage psychiatric disorders as well as establishing close links between medicine and psychiatry.

The first edition of the *Massachusetts General Hospital Handbook of General Hospital Psychiatry* (Hackett & Cassem, 1978) was a landmark text that established the practice of psychiatry in the general hospital in a variety of settings. This was because it was written not only for psychiatrists but also for physicians, surgeons and professionals in other disciplines who worked in the general hospital. A more detailed account of the history of the influence of CL psychiatry on medical practice and its different specialties is given by Kornfeld (1996). Weissman & Hackett (1958) observed that the delirium following cataract surgery was related to the sensory deprivation caused by the use of bilateral eye patches and was therefore due to the surgical procedure itself. Work on the delirium that sometimes occurred after open-heart surgery (Kornfeld *et al*, 1965) influenced the subsequent patient management and design of intensive-care units. The psychological effect of cancer surgery was first pointed out by Sutherland *et al* (1952) and there is now a whole sub-specialty of psycho-oncology (Holland, 1998), with consideration given to the psychological impact of the different cancer treatments, identification of clinical depression in cancer patients, and improved communication between staff and patients. There are numerous other examples of the contribution of CL psychiatry, in the fields of nephrology, transplantation, cardiology, neurology, HIV and pain management for example, but it would be beyond the scope of this brief review to cover all of these areas.

The care of patients with psychiatric disorder in general hospitals in England and Wales can be traced back to the late 18th and early 19th centuries, when several voluntary hospitals provided separate wards for 'lunatics', although none of these survived beyond the middle of the 19th century, when care was taken over by the county asylums (see also Chapter 29, page 754) (Mayou, 1989). The first psychiatric out-patient clinics and wards in Britain were established in a few general hospitals before the First World War, and a new specialty of psychological medicine developed, mainly within neurology departments, during the first half of the 20th century.

The Suicide Act 1961 decreed that suicide was no longer a crime, and this was soon followed by a recommendation by the Ministry of Health (following the Hill report) that all cases of attempted suicide brought to a hospital should have a psychiatric assessment before discharge. This resulted in a rapid increase in the amount of contact between psychiatrists and general hospital departments.

In 1983, the UK Liaison Psychiatry Special Interest Group was established at the Royal College of Psychiatrists in response to the growing interest in and need for psychiatric services in general hospitals. More recently, the importance of the joint working between physicians/surgeons and psychiatrists has been highlighted in joint reports of the Royal Colleges (Royal College of Surgeons & Royal College of Psychiatrists, 1997; Royal College of Physicians & Royal College of Psychiatrists, 2003). These reports highlight the need for doctors and nurses in general hospitals to possess adequate skills in psychological care, as well as the need for general hospitals to have a specialised CL psychiatry service. The manner in which CL psychiatrists, physicians and surgeons work jointly in in-patient, out-patient and emergency settings varies from a free-standing psychiatric service for the general hospital (consultation model) to a fully integrated medical–psychiatric service (Sharpe *et al*, 2000).

The UK Department of Health is publishing a series of National Service Frameworks, which lay out standards of care for patients with different medical conditions; these seek to ensure there is adequate psychological care for general hospital patients. For example, the National Service Framework for Coronary Heart Disease recognises that assessment and management of the psychological needs of the patient are integral to an effective cardiac rehabilitation programme and the National Service Framework for Diabetes recommends regular surveillance and effective management for conditions such as depression and erectile dysfunction. The NHS Cancer Plan 2000 recommends access to counselling and other forms of psychological help in cancer units.

Box 17.1 Physical diseases causing mental disorder

Structural brain disease
- focal – cerebral tumour, abscess, stroke, subdural haemorrhage
- diffuse – degenerative disorders, infections, multiple sclerosis, hydrocephalus

Systemic disturbances
- infection
- endocrine disorders
- metabolic disorders
- paraneoplastic manifestation of cancer

Relation between physical disease and mental disorder

The biomedical versus the bio-psychosocial model of illness

The biomedical model of disease, the dominant model in which medicine came to be practised during the 20th century, assumes that disease can be understood in terms of deviation of a biological variable from the norm. Such a model has the advantage of simplicity and of facilitating scientific investigation into disease. However, the assumption that the nature and extent of biological disease alone will determine illness, and the subjective experience of the disease, ignores the way that social, psychological and behavioural factors influence susceptibility to disease, differences in help-seeking behaviour, and the manner in which symptoms are reported, as well as the response to treatment. A patient's experience of a disease will rarely correlate directly with underlying pathophysiological processes.

Engel (1977) proposed an alternative, bio-psychosocial model, which takes into account how biological, psychological and social factors contribute to illness; a more comprehensive account of this model is given in Chapter 18 (see page 446). Here, we examine each factor that should be considered in patients with comorbid physical and mental disorders.

Biological factors contributing to psychological change in physical disease

Mental function can be disturbed by physical disease either as a direct result of structural brain damage or as a consequence of brain dysfunction from systemic causes (Box 17.1). The structural brain damage could be focal (cerebral tumour, stroke) or diffuse (degenerative disorders, infections, multiple sclerosis); these disorders are more extensively described in Chapter 21. The systemic causes can include infection, endocrine disorders and metabolic disorders, and can lead to psychiatric symptoms (see also Chapter 22). Mood disorders may also be a paraneoplastic manifestation of cancer. Delirium is a common but often under-diagnosed mental complication of a wide variety of physical diseases.

An organic cause should always be suspected in people presenting with a new-onset mental disorder who are already known to have a premorbid coexisting physical disorder. In these instances, comparing the timing of the onset of the mental symptoms with the nature of the physical disease, its onset and treatment may provide valuable clues. If the underlying physical condition can be treated or ameliorated, then the mental disorder may also show some improvement. However, it is not always clear whether the presenting mental symptoms are the result of the underlying physical disease or are a consequence of treatment, such as steroid treatment in systemic lupus erythematosis where there is cerebral involvement. Correlating measures of physical disease activity (where these are available) with the course of the mental disorder may help to clarify whether the disease process or the treatment is the likely cause.

Mental disorder as a direct side-effect of medical treatment

Many drugs have been reported to cause mood disorder or cognitive impairment. Some examples are listed in Box 17.2.

Box 17.2 Drugs associated with mental disorders

Drugs that can cause depression
- Beta-blockers
- Calcium channel blockers
- H_2 receptor antagonists
- Proton pump inhibitors
- Anti-Parkinsonian drugs
- Corticosteroids
- Cancer chemotherapeutic drugs
- Interferon
- Roaccutane

Drugs that can cause psychosis or delirium
- Anti-Parkinsonian drugs
- Digoxin
- Beta-blockers
- Anticholinergic drugs
- Anticonvulsants
- Corticosteroids
- Thyroxine
- Opiates
- Hypnotics

The assessment of a mental disorder in a medically ill patient should always include a comprehensive recent drug history, and drug-induced disorders should be considered in the differential diagnosis. As with physical disease, the temporal relation between the drug therapy and the onset of mental symptoms should be noted.

Non-pharmacological treatments that may affect mood or cognitive function include cranial irradiation and renal dialysis.

Psychological factors in physical disease

Psychiatric illness has been shown to predispose individuals to some physical disorders. A recent systematic review of all the English-language reports of studies on the mortality of patients with depression concluded that depression may increase the risk of death by cardiovascular disease, especially for men (Wulsin *et al*, 1999). In a cohort study of male university students who were followed for over 35 years, major depression was found to increase the risk of coronary artery disease with a mean lag phase of 10 years between the report of depression and the first report of cardiovascular disease (Ford *et al*, 1998). The Baltimore Epidemiologic Catchment Area study also identified major depression as a risk factor for myocardial infarction, even after controlling for other factors (Pratt *et al*, 1996). Women with a current or past history of major depression have been found to have significantly reduced bone mineral density, which would put them at greater risk of hip fractures (Michelson *et al*, 1996).

These studies suggest that the psychiatric illness predisposes to physical disease, such as cardiovascular disease, some years later and may not necessarily result in comorbidity. However, as patients with cardiovascular disease *and* a psychiatric history will have a greater likelihood of further cardiovascular episodes, psychiatric history will be an important risk factor to consider in the assessment, especially as comorbidity is likely to affect prognosis, as discussed below.

Lloyd (1977) categorised the factors influencing psychological response to physical disease in three ways: those related to the patient, those related to the nature of the illness, and those related to the social environment. Patient factors include premorbid attitudes or personality, age and life experiences before and at the onset of the illness. In terms of illness factors, the psychological meaning the condition has for the patient appears to matter more than its objective severity. However, the chronicity of physical illness may be a major influence on the persistence of the psychiatric disturbance. Social factors may include significant people around the patient, the life stage the person is at, and the presence or absence of litigation, as well as background cultural factors, and these are further discussed in Chapter 31, on transcultural psychiatry (see page 789).

There are three main theoretical approaches to understanding a person's psychological reaction to a physical disease; the first has its focus on the cognitive approach, the second on psychodynamic mechanisms and the third weighs the influence of social and behavioural factors.

The cognitive approach

Understanding the cognitive approach is important if cognitive–behavioural methods are to be used in treatment. The key factors influencing patients' reactions to illness are their thoughts, attitudes and beliefs about the illness (Sensky, 1990), that is, the way people come to make sense and give meaning to their experiences. This concept is of central importance in CL psychiatry. Sociologists have also tried to analyse the reasons that lie behind the difference in people's responses to their symptoms and also used the concept of patient attribution processes to explain important phenomena such as 'illness behaviour' (Mechanic, 1978).

A valid explanation of the diversity of the psychological reactions to illness will need to encompass a broad range of cognitions and patient beliefs and then to link them to coping behaviours and functional outcome, as well as to the patient's emotional response to the illness (Horne & Weinman, 1994). The self-regulatory model of illness as described by Leventhal *et al* (1984, 1992) is useful in this respect. It views illness as 'a problem' and the patient's behaviour or reaction to it as an attempt to 'solve the problem'. In response to a health threat, this model postulates that individuals will pass through three stages: first, they generate a representation in their mind (patients' own interpretation of the physical problem) and this representation will be linked to their emotional response; second, these will then determine patients' coping strategy; and, third, they will appraise the outcome of their strategy. This process goes on in parallel at both a cognitive and an emotional level and these may also interact. Thus, the initial representation or emotional reaction is crucial in determining the type of coping strategy, but the way the patient appraises the outcome may also feedback onto the illness representation and so modify it (Fig. 17.1).

The model hypothesises that there are three processes influencing the way individuals form illness representations or react emotionally, which coping

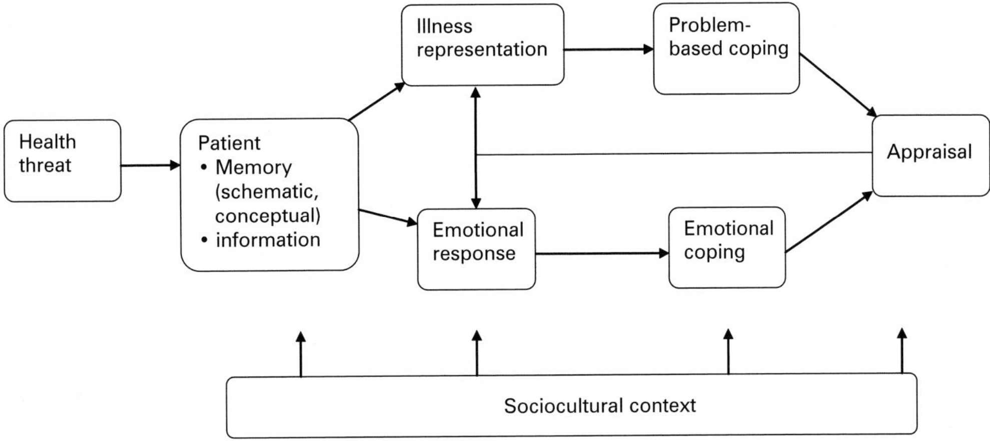

Fig. 17.1 Cognitive model of reaction to illness (adapted from Leventhal *et al*, 1992).

strategy they employ and how they interpret (appraise) the outcome. First, there are memories of previous illness episodes, which may provoke emotional reactions or physical symptoms (schematic memory); second, there are memories about other illness episodes, which will determine how the individual will label emotions and illness (conceptual memory); and third, there is the information the individual receives about the illness, which may come from health professionals or other sources, such as family, the media and so on.

Illness representation has at least five attributes (Leventhal *et al*, 1992):

1 identity (the disease label and its symptom indicator)

2 time line (acute, cyclic or chronic)

3 consequences (physical, social and economic)

4 antecedent causes (e.g. injury, infection, genetic weaknesses)

5 potential for cure and control.

This model provides a useful framework for understanding the patient's cognitive, behavioural and emotional response to disease and hence a good guide to planning psychological interventions. Patients should be questioned in the five areas suggested in the model above to gain a picture of their internal model of the illness. These illness models shape people's health-protective behaviour, how they recover and their perceptions of disability. In a study of patients with a first episode of myocardial infarction, the patient's initial perceptions of the illness were important determinants of attendance at cardiac rehabilitation, return to work, functional disability and sexual dysfunction (Petrie *et al*, 1996). Among patients with rheumatoid arthritis, chronic obstructive pulmonary disease or psoriasis, illness perceptions, coping variables and the expected medical variables were all significantly related to functional outcome (Scharloo *et al*, 1998). For women who had had a mastectomy, those with an avoidant style of coping tended to have more long-lasting depression as well as a greater loss of libido (Maguire & Parkes, 1998). A patient belief system will also influence compliance. Thus medication beliefs were more powerful predictors of reported adherence than clinical sociodemographic factors (Horne & Weinman, 1999).

The psychodynamic approach

The psychodynamic concept of defence mechanisms provides another way of making sense of the ways in which patients react to their illness. In response to a physical illness, patients may use a defence mechanism to deal with the difficult emotions provoked by the diagnosis or the prognosis. Psychiatric referrals may then be made for patients who seem to the clinical team to be reacting to their illness in an unusual or inappropriate way.

- Denial is a common defence mechanism, and patients in denial may not take in a serious diagnosis, or not deal with it appropriately, and this may lead to a referral from the medical team. However, denial can also serve as a short-term adaptive mechanism, enabling the patient to continue to function. Where it leads to delay in seeking medical help, or interferes with treatment adherence or establishing therapeutic relationships, it becomes maladaptive.
- Regression refers to the patient adopting a pattern of behaviour appropriate to an earlier stage of development. Some patients exhibit a child-like dependency on staff, which may be adaptive if it permits them to accept the care and help they need, but equally can interfere with processes that require more active patient involvement, such as rehabilitation.
- Displacement refers to the transfer of powerful emotions from situations or objects with which they are normally associated to other objects which will give rise to less distress. In tandem with projective mechanisms this may result in the distress being directed at clinical staff rather than at the illness itself. This may take the form of patients becoming angry or hostile with the staff caring for them for no apparent or logical reason. Staff understandably feel bewildered by such strange and hostile responses and may seek guidance.

Social factors

Social factors influencing morbidity

In a bio-psychosocial model of understanding illness, factors beyond the individual – principally family, community and societal influences – also need to be taken into account. At its broadest, the relation between health and social circumstances is well established. The

Whitehall study of British civil servants highlighted the relation of both morbidity and mortality to socio-economic status (Marmot *et al*, 1991). The association between socio-economic status and mortality is observed where the former has been measured in a variety of different ways, such as occupation, income, material assets, education or composite indices of deprivation (Carroll & Sheffield, 1998). The relationship is also observed for a range of health outcomes and holds for both sexes. The reasons underlying this association are complex and multifactorial: social factors correlate with health-risk behaviours such as smoking; there may be differences in investment in healthcare; social circumstances determine availability of social support; and adverse social conditions are likely to increase exposure to psychosocial stressors. Feldman *et al* (1987) found that mood disorders in medically ill in-patients were associated with several different social problems: financial troubles, dissatisfaction with social life, housing problems, dissatisfaction with being out of work and dissatisfaction with living alone.

Of particular interest to a liaison psychiatrist are the relation between social factors and help-seeking behaviour, and the relation between psychosocial stressors and psychiatric and physical morbidity.

Social factors influencing help-seeking behaviour

Mechanic proposed the term 'illness behaviour', which he defined as 'the ways in which given symptoms may be differently perceived, evaluated and acted (or not acted) upon by different kinds of persons'. He studied how attentive the subjects were to pain and symptoms, which processes affected the way pain and symptoms were defined, what meaning was given to the symptom, how it was labelled socially, the extent to which help was sought, how it changed the patient's lifestyle and what demands were made on others (Mechanic, 1978). He was among the first to recognise that illness and illness experience are shaped by sociocultural and social–psychological factors (Mechanic, 1986).

Key social factors that may influence a patient's reaction to a medical condition are: emotional responses of significant people around the patient (usually the family); the timing of the illness in relation to stages of life; the quality of the doctor–patient relationship; and the possibility of litigation (Lloyd, 1977). Sociocultural factors may also influence illness representation, and this in turn will affect the way the illness presents, health-seeking behaviours and treatment (Leventhal *et al*, 1992). In particular, strife, emotional turmoil and family disorganisation increase the risk of treatment non-adherence, while a good doctor–patient relationship can improve adherence (Stoudemire & Thompson, 1983).

The emotional response of the key people in the patient's life would have been shaped by their own personal experiences or illness beliefs, or as a consequence of the patient's current illness and the effect the present episode is having on the mental health of the family and carers. The way in which the illness behaviours are conceptualised in wider society may also have some bearing on how the patient is perceived by the community (Mechanic, 1978). Society sanctions or expects certain behaviours in an ill person. Parsons (1951) termed this the 'sick role' and suggested that it has four components:

1 exemption from normal social responsibilities
2 the right to care and help from others
3 an expectation that the sick person will want to recover
4 an obligation to seek and cooperate with appropriate treatment.

Conflict in patient–staff or patient–family relationships may arise when patients are not perceived to be acting in accordance with their expected role. On the one hand, there may be denial of the medical condition and associated non-adherence; on the other, conflict can arise when clinical staff or the family perceive that the patient is exaggerating the sick role by becoming overly dependent and demanding. A perceived lack of will to recover is another issue that can strain patient–staff relationships. An example of role conflict can be seen in patients in end-stage renal failure who are undergoing chronic haemodialysis. The patient is wholly dependent on the dialysis for survival and must comply with fluid and dietary restriction, yet is theoretically restored to normality between treatments. This creates uncertainty over whether the patient is sick or healthy and results in a mismatch in the expectation of roles between patients and carers. Role confusion of this type can lead to conflicts over issues of compliance and autonomy in patients undergoing haemodialysis (Pritchard, 1982).

Relation between psychosocial stressors and morbidity

There has been a great deal of research into the role of life events as a possible causal factor for physical disease as well as psychiatric disorder. An association between a traumatic or stressful life event and an onset of serious illness is a common enough observation, but establishing a causal link between the two can be a challenge: what is a significant life event, how does one capture chronic stressors as well as discrete events, how can these events be identified and recorded, are there different degrees of seriousness, what would be the time lag between the life event and the onset of illness? The first scale developed to measure life events was the Schedule of Recent Experience (SRE; Holmes & Rahe, 1967), while a second and more sophisticated interview – the Life Events and Difficulties Schedule (LEDS; Brown & Harris, 1978) was developed mainly to remove any bias that ill people might have in attributing a reason for their illness retrospectively (termed 'effort after meaning') (see also Chapter 10, page 229).

There is reasonable evidence for an association between life events and vascular episodes such as myocardial infarction (MI) or stroke. Thus, Neilson *et al* (1989) applied the LEDS to a group of men with a recent admission with MI and compared the results with those from a group of civil servants selected at random from a larger ongoing enquiry into heart disease and a general population sample matched for age. The enquiry extended to 10 years before the MI or the interview, except in a subset of the civil servant group, and stressors were categorised as being related to work or not. There was no significant difference between the two groups for the presence of a severe event or major difficulty when individual 1-year periods were compared. However, when the cumulative effect of stressors over time was compared, the MI group had experienced significantly more cumulative stress, especially stress related to work, than the control group, suggesting that length of exposure to stress was of aetiological importance. The authors found that the odds ratio for MI was 4.00 for those who had work stress for more than 70% of the time period covered by the LEDS interview before the MI, compared with only 1.89 for those who had only non-work stress. However, the risk as expressed by the odds ratio nearly doubled, to 7.36, when work and non-work stress occurred together, indicating an additive effect.

House *et al* (1990) investigated the frequency of life events using the LEDS in a case–control study of first-time stroke patients. The interview covered life events for the 12 months that preceded the stroke and the interview was repeated 12 months later, to cover life events for the 12 months following the stroke. The stroke patients reported fewer non-threatening events and fewer events with only a short-term threat, but severely threatening life events were more common in the stroke patients (odds ratio 2.3). The number of severe events reported by the stroke patients was similar to that of the control group in the 12 months following the stroke. Therefore, there was a clear association of severe life events preceding the onset of the stroke when compared with an age- and sex-matched control group.

Since the nature of these life events preceding the onset of vascular events is essentially the same as that associated with the onset of mood disorder, it would not be surprising to find psychiatric comorbidity in the form of mood disorder in both MI and stroke, as a result of their common antecedents.

The role of life events in the onset of cancer has also attracted interest, but the findings of case–control studies comparing women with malignant and benign breast lumps have been conflicting (Chen *et al*, 1995; Protheroe *et al*, 1999).

The epidemiology of physical and psychiatric comorbidity

The burden of physical and psychiatric comorbidity to the health service and society as a whole is very large. The prevalence of psychiatric disorders in different medical populations may vary, but the methodological problems of epidemiological studies are the same. These difficulties arise in the realms of case definition, agreed diagnostic criteria, assessment measures, population bias and heterogeneity, as well as the absence of appropriate controls, because suitable control groups are difficult to identify (Rodin & Daneman, 1991). The psychological response to a physical illness is rarely static: different problems emerge at different phases of the illness. Delirium and anxiety may be seen early in response to an acute illness, whereas depression may appear only at a later stage. Mood may improve with recovery from acute illness, but there may be persistent psychological problems in chronic illness.

Case definition

The continuous distribution of emotional distress means that there will always be a grey area between the normal reaction to an illness and depressive disorder. A diagnosis of depression itself will cover different degrees of severity and epidemiological studies vary in the case definitions and severity thresholds used. In addition, conditions that fail to reach a diagnostic threshold for psychiatric disorder may still be clinically significant in a medical setting. These subclinical disorders may impair quality of life, lead to inappropriate or excessive consultation, result in poor adherence to treatment or an unnecessarily poor physical outcome, and have a destructive effect on family or other relationships (Mayou, 1995). Thus, it may not always be helpful to categorise the psychological problems of medical patients solely in terms of a standard axis I psychiatric diagnosis.

The use of a multi-axial system is one way of capturing the complexity of psychological problems encountered in a medical setting. DSM–IV (American Psychiatric Association, 1994) enables the diagnoses of psychiatric disorder, developmental and personality disorders, and physical disorders, as well as psychosocial stressors and global assessment of functioning, to be documented on separate axes. In addition, it is possible to document psychological influences on a physical disorder using the category '316 Psychological factor affecting a medical condition', which should be coded on axis I. This particular category allows the recording of mental disorders, psychological symptoms, personality traits or coping styles, maladaptive health behaviours, stress-related physiological responses and other or unspecified factors that may affect a medical condition and so represents a useful nosological advance over the simple recording of the presence or absence of a diagnosable psychiatric condition.

Similarly, ICD–10 (World Health Organization, 1992) makes provision for multi-axial assessment, although the axes are classified differently. It has 'F54.0 The presence of psychological or behavioural influences thought to have influenced the manifestation, or affected the course, of physical disorders that can be classified using other chapters of ICD–10', which allows recording of psychological influence on conditions such as asthma, dermatitis, gastric ulcer, mucous colitis, ulcerative colitis and urticaria. Other chapters in ICD–10 allow for coding of physical diseases, intentional self-harm, adverse effects of therapeutic drugs, and psychosocial factors affecting health.

However, in practice it is the psychiatric formulation (which should incorporate all the key psychological, physical, behavioural and social dimensions) that forms the cornerstone of the psychiatric assessment, rather than the formal diagnosis. This formulation should describe the way all the key causal factors interact, as well as provide some sort of an estimate of their relative weighting and so provide an accurate description of psychiatric and physical comorbidity, especially if it is to form the basis of the treatment plan.

Epidemiological studies are not well suited to the description of the complex and multifactorial diagnostic problems encountered in CL psychiatry. The most common psychiatric disorders encountered among people with a physical illness in the general hospital are adjustment disorders, dysthymia, major depression, anxiety and delirium. Other common problems include dementia, panic disorder, phobic anxiety, eating disorders, sexual dysfunction, body image disorders and post-traumatic stress disorders, while mania and other psychotic disorders are rather less frequent but also occur. Substance misuse and other behavioural disorders are also commonly seen, especially in accident and emergency departments.

Case ascertainment

Psychiatric cases can be identified in the general hospital by monitoring referrals to the liaison psychiatry service. However, as discussed below, clinicians usually tend to underestimate psychological and psychiatric morbidity, and any measure of morbidity based solely on referrals will therefore underestimate the true prevalence. Screening of the whole study population at risk is an alternative option; assessment tools include either screening questionnaires or standardised psychiatric interviews. Screening questionnaires are not diagnostic tools in themselves and in most studies a two-stage design is adopted, where patients who reach scores at a predetermined cut-off level on the screening questionnaire are then interviewed with a standardised psychiatric interview. The prevalence figures for psychiatric morbidity based on data from screening instruments alone are much higher than those derived from a two-stage process of screening incorporating a psychiatric interview. This method appears to be both a reliable and a practical option for case ascertainment (see also page 702 in Chapter 27, on epidemiology).

Rates in different populations

The prevalence of comorbid psychiatric disorder appears to be highest among in-patients, followed by out-patients (Mayou & Hawton, 1986). A population-based study of the frequency of psychiatric care before and then again after acute medical admissions found that the numbers receiving psychiatric care increased in the year following admission for a wide range of medical conditions. This suggests that psychiatric disorder is often a late consequence of a medical episode (Mayou *et al*, 1991). These differences reached statistical significance for those who were admitted for acute MI, cancer, diabetes mellitus and chest pain.

In the community setting, the Epidemiologic Catchment Area study found that 34% of the respondents had chronic medical conditions, the most common of which were arthritis and hypertension. The presence of a chronic medical condition was associated with a 41% higher prevalence of recent psychiatric disorder and a 28% increased prevalence of lifetime psychiatric disorder relative to those without a chronic medical condition (Wells *et al*, 1988). Arthritis, neurological disorders, chronic lung disease and heart disease were especially strongly associated with psychiatric disorder.

Individual psychiatric conditions in the medical setting

Affective disorder

The combination of depression and physical illness is the commonest comorbid problem facing the liaison psychiatrist (Robertson & Katona, 1997). A review of the literature by Mayou & Hawton (1986) provided a range of rates of affective disorder in general hospitals: among in-patients it was 13–61%, and in out-patient clinics 15–51%. The commonest pattern was adjustment disorder; a small minority suffered from more specific psychiatric disorders. Using a structured psychiatric interview, Feldman *et al* (1987) found that 14.6% of patients admitted with a medical condition had a diagnosable affective disorder, most commonly anxiety or depression. This contrasts with a general population 1-week prevalence of 1.8–2.7% in the British National Psychiatric Morbidity Surveys (Jenkins *et al*, 1997). The presence of affective disorder in the hospital population was associated with a previous psychiatric history and current social problems, while persistence of the disorder at 4 months was linked to chronic psychosocial difficulties and continuing poor physical health.

The somatic symptoms of depression are a common source of confusion. Thus, three of the nine listed key symptoms (weight changes, insomnia and fatigue) for the diagnosis of DSM–IV major depression are somatic symptoms, and they all commonly occur in people who are medically ill. Perry & Cella (1987) point out that there is consequently a risk of over-diagnosing major depression in these populations. A similar difficulty encountered in the assessment of postnatal depression led Cox *et al* (1987) to drop the somatic symptoms of depression from the Edinburgh Post Natal Depression Scale.

None the less, somatic symptoms may still be a helpful pointer to depressive disorder in physically ill patients, because they may arise from both physical and psychological reasons. Therefore, there does not appear to be any advantage to removing all the somatic symptoms from the diagnostic criteria for depression in medical patients (Craven & Rodin, 1990).

Other sources of confusion may be an associated grief reaction or the behavioural manifestation of a serious medical condition, both of which may be incorrectly attributed to affective disorder.

A study comparing the symptoms of depression between those with and without medical illness found that depressed people with medical illness had more evidence of hopelessness, helplessness, anxiety, a distinct quality to the depression different to normal experience, psychomotor retardation, agitation and self-pity, but less frequent suicidal thoughts (Moffic & Paykel, 1975). However, Hawton *et al* (1990) found little difference between the two groups. In the latter study, only three symptoms were significantly more common in the medical patients: anergia/retardation, early-morning waking and specific phobias. The first two may have been due to the physical disorder itself, while the increased rate of phobias is unexplained and may have been a chance finding. The same study also compared the prevalence of symptoms that met the criteria of the Present State Examination (PSE) in medical patients with and without affective disorder, to identify which were the most useful for distinguishing those with an affective disorder in the medical population. Depressed mood, morning depression and hopelessness provided a reasonable discrimination for depression; nervous tension, free-floating anxiety and panic attacks, and simple phobias provided almost perfect discrimination for anxiety disorder (Hawton *et al*, 1990).

Adjustment disorders

Both anxiety and depressive symptoms in response to a physical illness are very common, but they are usually transient and do not constitute a psychiatric disorder. The diagnosis of adjustment disorder may be made if there is marked distress or impairment in social and occupational function. DSM–IV subdivides this category into depression, anxiety, mixed anxiety and depressed mood, disturbance of conduct, and mixed disturbance of emotions and conduct. For maladaptive reactions that do not fit into any of these categories, the diagnosis is of 'unspecified type'. ICD–10 has similar categories under F43.2. The duration of adjustment disorder can be specified as acute or chronic, with a symptom duration of 6 months taken as the cut-off.

Phobic anxiety disorder

Specific phobias may develop in the course of a medical illness or their treatment and may persist beyond the illness. Some phobias may be serious enough to interfere with medical investigations or treatment, such as needle phobia, or claustrophobia in patients undergoing magnetic resonance imaging or computerised tomography. Conditioned phobic responses may sometimes develop during courses of chemotherapy or radiotherapy and so compromise these treatments.

Organic mental disorder

The prevalence of organic disorders as defined by the Mini-Mental State Examination (Folstein *et al*, 1975) in general medical wards across all ages has been reported to be between a quarter and a third (Mayou & Hawton, 1986). This is far in excess of rates found in the general population, where cognitive dysfunction is rare below 65 years of age. Structured psychiatric interviews identify cognitive dysfunction in 12% of medical admissions of all ages, with acute organic mental disorder being the commonest, followed by dementia or a combination of both. Not surprisingly, organic mental disorders were especially common among older subjects and those seen in a neurology setting, especially those with cerebral rather than peripheral disorders (DePaulo & Folstein, 1978). Patients with delirium had a higher mortality rate than those with dementia (Rabins & Folsteirn, 1982).

Eating disorders

Significant eating disorder may result in physical problems requiring medical admission from malnutrition or metabolic disturbance from vomiting or purgative and diuretic abuse; these complications are described in more detail in Chapter 24 (page 620). Excessive eating due to psychological problems may result in obesity and other health problems. An abnormal eating pattern may also complicate the management of diabetes mellitus, especially among those who are insulin dependent.

Significantly increased rates of eating disorders (15%) and intentional insulin under-treatment (12%) have been reported in young females with diabetes (Rodin & Daneman, 1991). However, when appropriate non-diabetic control populations were included in an interview-based study of young females with diabetes, the latter did not have a higher prevalence of clinical eating disorders (Fairburn *et al*, 1991). Nevertheless, the comorbidity of an eating disorder with insulin-dependent diabetes mellitus poses a major therapeutic challenge, as there will be difficulties in obtaining good glycaemic control and dangers of either diabetic ketoacidosis or hypoglycaemia. Indeed, the same study confirmed that disordered eating was common and the under-use of insulin with an intention to control weight was widespread, even among those without an obvious eating disorder.

Post-traumatic stress disorder

The hospital admission itself may have been caused by an incident that was both physically and psychologically traumatic, for example a serious accident, an assault or a natural disaster, or the trauma may have occurred during the course of hospital treatment, such as a traumatic obstetric delivery or the memory of a frightening episode of delirium.

One prospective follow-up study of a consecutive series of in-patients on a burns unit (Perry *et al*, 1992) found a prevalence of 35.3% for post-traumatic stress disorder meeting DSM–III–R criteria at 2 months, with higher rates at 6 and 12 months. The development of the disorder did not correlate with the severity of the burns but with less perceived emotional support, and with greater emotional distress immediately after admission. This suggests that the individual's psychological state immediately following the event may be more predictive of the outcome than the degree of trauma.

Alcohol-related disorders

Between 20% and 25% of males who are admitted to medical wards and between 5% and 10% of females have alcohol problems (Mayou & Hawton, 1986), which is well in excess of the 1-week population prevalence rates of 7.5% for men and 2.1% for women as found in the British National Psychiatric Morbidity Surveys (Jenkins *et al*, 1997). Alcohol misuse and dependence may lead to a variety of health problems, including heart, liver, pancreatic, cerebral and vascular diseases, accidents and suicide. Also, the complications of alcoholism may cause management difficulties in the general hospital, especially behavioural problems as a result of intoxication and alcohol withdrawal. The latter sometimes goes unrecognised and untreated because staff are unaware of the extent of the patient's dependence or the degree of cognitive impairment, and these patients may present with an apparently unexplained confusional state of acute onset. Lack of a satisfactory classification of problem drinking and its complications has made it difficult to establish a more reliable epidemiology base in this area.

The impact of physical and psychiatric comorbidity

Psychological and physical comorbidity may increase the burden on the individual, the family and the health-care system, as well as influence the outcome of the physical condition itself (see Box 17.3).

Box 17.3 Impact of physical and psychological comorbidity

Patient
- Survival and disease outcome
- Functional disability
- Quality of life
- Suicide

Family
- Relationships
- Mental health
- Financial/occupational status

Healthcare use
- Medication non-adherence
- Length of hospital stay
- Frequency of consultations

Survival and disease outcome

There has been increasing interest in whether psychological factors influence the outcome of a variety of physical diseases, such as cancer and MI. Psychological factors studied have ranged from diagnosable psychiatric disorder to psychological responses to the disease, such as coping strategies or adjustment to illness. A prospective cohort study of women with early-stage breast cancer indicated that a high score on the Hospital Anxiety and Depression (HAD) scale and the helplessness/hopelessness score on the Mental Adjustment to Cancer (MAC) scale had quite a large detrimental effect on 5-year survival rates (Watson *et al*, 1999). Helplessness/hopelessness as defined by the MAC scale affected event-free survival at 5 years with a hazard ratio of 1.55, and HAD-defined depression (score equal to or over 11) influenced 5-year survival with a hazard ratio of 3.59.

In a study of patients with MI, those who had mild to moderate depression, as determined by a score on the Beck Depression Inventory (BDI) equal to or above 10, and those who had a diagnosable major depressive illness assessed 7 days after the MI, had a significantly raised 18-month cardiac mortality rate (odds ratios 3.64 and 7.82, respectively) (Frasure-Smith *et al*, 1995). The study also suggested that sub-threshold psychiatric disturbance (as seen by raised BDI scores in the absence of definitive diagnosis) may also have a significant influence on the outcome of MI. The risk associated with depression was greatest in patients with frequent premature ventricular contractions, which suggests that an arrhythmic mechanism may be the link between psychological factors and sudden cardiac death. A more recent study of patients who developed depression after MI found that high levels of social support, through an alleviation of depressive symptoms, may protect patients from the negative cardiovascular consequences of a depressive episode (Frasure-Smith *et al*, 2000).

Mayou *et al* (1988) studied the influence of psychiatric comorbidity on the outcome of a group of randomly selected patients who had had either an emergency or an elective admission to a general hospital. Patients who had a diagnosable affective disorder at the time of their medical admission suffered more medical, psychiatric and social problems during their index admission as well as over the next 4 months. Compared with controls without affective disorder, they were less likely to show improvement in or to recover from their physical disorder, and more likely to be readmitted. Those who had the combination of affective disorder and pre-existing cognitive disorder did particularly badly and for this subgroup there was also a non-significant trend towards a raised mortality.

Both DSM–IV and ICD–10 recognise the importance that psychological factors have on the outcome of physical disease, as seen by the provision of special diagnostic codes that allow for the documentation of psychological factors affecting physical disease, as described above.

Functional disability and quality of life

Psychiatric comorbidity can influence perceived health status as well as functional ability, and may also impair social and occupational function. A prospective follow-up study of patients with MI in Oxfordshire found that initial emotional distress (as defined by a HAD score of over 19) predicted poor symptomatic, psychological and social outcome at 3 and 12 months after MI (Mayou *et al*, 2000) as assessed by the 36-item Medical Outcomes Study short form (SF-36) and HAD scales.

Functional ability and quality of life are particularly relevant in patients with chronic medical conditions. A large cross-sectional study of patients enrolled in a study funded by the US Veterans Administration looked at the relation between depressive symptoms and scores on the Health Related Quality of Life (HRQoL) scale (Felker *et al*, 2001). Among 1252 patients who completed relevant questionnaires, 59% had significant depressive symptoms as determined by Hopkins Symptoms Checklist 20 (SCL-20) using a cut-off of 1.75. Those with depressive symptoms had worse scores on both general health measures (SF-36) and disease-specific measures (Seattle Obstructive Lung Disease Questionnaire – SOLDQ), which were both statistically and clinically significant. Linear regression analysis indicated that 11–18% of the variance in physical functioning could be attributed to depressive symptoms alone. The contribution of depression to the variance in HRQoL score was greater than those due to age, educational level, marital status, smoking history or the number of comorbid medical conditions. The results were compatible with previous observations that the correlation between objective measures of pulmonary function such as spirometry and quality of life as measured by the HRQoL was weak and that depression or anxiety (or both) accounted for a significant amount of the variance of the HRQoL scores.

Psychological factors, cognitive responses and coping style may have an important influence on outcome. Scharloo *et al* (1998) looked at the influence of coping strategies and illness perceptions on the levels of daily functioning in patients with rheumatoid arthritis, chronic obstructive pulmonary disease or psoriasis in a cross-sectional study of 244 patients. Coping strategies were assessed using the Utrecht Coping List and illness perceptions by an interview and the Illness Perception Questionnaire. They found that a strong illness identity, passive coping, a belief in a long illness duration, a belief in strong consequences and an unfavourable score on medical variables were associated with worse outcomes in the areas of physical and social function. In contrast, coping behaviours involving seeking social support, and beliefs in controllability/curability of the disease, were significantly associated with better functioning. In a prospective study of the initial perception of MI, belief that the illness could be controlled or cured was a factor influencing attendance at a cardiac rehabilitation course, whereas the perception that the illness would last a long time and have serious consequences was associated with a delay in return to work (Petrie *et al*, 1996). These findings emphasise that the way patients think and feel about their physical disorder may have a profound influence on outcome, and therefore needs to be taken into account in the treatment plan.

Suicide

Compared with patients with depression being cared for within the psychiatric services, physically ill patients who experience depression are less likely to report suicidal feelings (Moffic & Paykel, 1975), but they have a slightly higher (but non-significant) increase in the frequency of suicidal plans (Hawton *et al*, 1990). A critical review of suicide in neurological patients found an increased risk among patients suffering from multiple sclerosis (MS), spinal cord lesions and selected groups of patients with epilepsy; the evidence for other neurological disorders is uncertain (Stenager & Stenager, 1992; Feinstein, 1997). Among those with MS, the standard mortality rate of suicide was highest for males, for patients with onset of MS before the age of 30 years and for those diagnosed before the age of 40; it was also higher during the first 5 years after diagnosis.

The risk of suicide in cancer patients has been found to be twice that of the general population. Factors associated with increased risk of suicide in this group of patients are: advanced illness and poor prognosis, depression and hopelessness, delirium, loss of control and helplessness, exhaustion and fatigue, pain, pre-existing psychopathology, a history of suicide attempts and a family history of suicide (Breitbart & Krivo, 1998).

Medication non-adherence

Liaison psychiatric referrals are sometimes made when there is non-adherence to treatment that could have serious consequences. The problem is widespread. In one study based at a university hospital, more than a third of the patients in a medical clinic took less than the prescribed amount of one or more medication (Brody, 1980).

Stoudemire & Thompson (1983) have reviewed the literature on the multiplicity of factors influencing adherence. They found no consistent correlation between the severity of the illness and socio-demographic factors with adherence. Lack of basic knowledge about their medication, more complex regimens and unpleasant side-effects all increased the risk of non-adherence. Certain side-effects, in particular excessive sedation, gastrointestinal distress, anticholinergic symptoms, sexual dysfunction and changes of physical appearance, were found to be much more likely to lead to a complete discontinuation of medication.

Patients' beliefs about their illness, the attitudes of other family members and the quality of the doctor–patient relationship may also influence treatment adherence. This was better: if patients felt susceptible to the illness or its complications; if they believed the illness might have severe consequences for their life; when they also believed that the prescribed medication would probably be effective; and they saw no major obstacle in engaging with the treatment. However, simple attempts at patient education about their illness as a sole measure were not effective. Adherence was better when the doctor and patient agreed on the treatment approach, the doctor–patient relationship was good, and there was good communication between the two. Strife, emotional turmoil and family disorganisation increased the risk of non-adherence, whereas a close and stable family or other social support facilitated it. Serious psychiatric disorders (major depression, bipolar disorder, schizophrenia, dementia/delirium and alcoholism), personality disorders and the maladaptive defence mechanism of denial were the main psychiatric factors associated with poor adherence, through a variety of different mechanisms.

The cause of unstable control in cases of brittle diabetes and brittle asthma is probably multifactorial but variable treatment adherence may be responsible for some of the fluctuations in these conditions and may even trigger acute medical emergencies

Healthcare use

The addition of psychiatric comorbidity to a physical illness increases health service utilisation; this has been confirmed on both sides of the Atlantic. A retrospective study of all medical/surgical patients discharged in 1984 from two hospitals in the USA found that the mean length of stay was much longer for those who had psychiatric comorbidity than for those who did not (19.8 versus 9.2 days and 13.7 versus 8.3 days in two hospitals) (Fulop *et al*, 1987). In a case–control study of medical admissions to a teaching hospital, those who had a comorbid affective disorder on admission had a significantly higher rate of hospital readmission than their age- and sex-matched controls, with a mean of 1.8 readmissions (versus 0.7) for those without affective disorder and staying 12.3 days (versus 3.7 days) (Mayou *et al*, 1988). A critical review of the effect of psychiatric comorbidity on length of stay for medical and surgical in-patients confirmed that psychiatric comorbidity significantly increased costs by extending hospital length of stay as well as leading to greater hospital use following discharge from the index admission (Saravay & Lavin, 1994).

Psychiatric assessment in the general hospital setting

Assessment by non-psychiatrists

Most depression in the community, especially of mild to moderate severity, is now routinely diagnosed and treated by general practitioners. For episodes occurring in the medical setting, it is the physicians, surgeons, nursing and other clinical staff who are in the best position to recognise the signs of possible comorbidity and respond to the patient's psychological needs. However, research suggests that over half of all medical patients who have a diagnosable psychiatric disorder will have the latter undetected by the medical or nursing staff caring for them (Moffic & Paykel, 1975; Bridges & Goldberg, 1984; Feldman *et al*, 1987; Seltzer, 1989). There are several reasons for this: patients may not give any clues suggestive of a psychological disorder; attention may focus exclusively on the somatic disorder during a medical interview; lack of privacy may inhibit patients from admitting to psychological difficulties; there is commonly also a lack of awareness that a psychiatric disorder may exacerbate a patient's physical symptoms; and, finally, some clinicians lack the confidence to assess a patient's mental state (Goldberg, 1985).

Maguire (1985) identified a number of 'distancing tactics' when observing doctors and nurses who were talking to real or simulated patients suffering from a terminal illness. Medical staff may not enquire directly about emotional difficulties, on the assumption that patients would disclose them if they were present. They may try to alleviate distress by explaining that it is understandable or likely to be experienced by anybody in the same predicament. False reassurances may be made by making more positive statements than are warranted by the circumstances. On those occasions when a patient mentions both physical and psychological difficulties, the doctor may follow up only on the physical symptoms, or deflect difficult questions by advising the patient to seek advice from someone else. Doctors and nurses tend to spend less time with patients who are dying and may even avoid them altogether. Clinical staff are usually unaware that they have adopted such strategies, yet they will tend to discourage patients from disclosing their inner anxieties and so create a barrier to effective psychological care.

Screening and standardised tests

Screening tests have been suggested as one way to help clinicians identify those with a psychiatric disorder. Instruments used to screen for affective disorders include the General Health Questionnaire (GHQ), which has versions of different lengths (Goldberg *et al*, 1988), the Hospital Anxiety and Depression scale (HAD; Zigmund & Snaith, 1983), the Beck Depression Inventory (BDI; Beck & Steer, 1987), the Zung depression scale (Zung *et al*, 1965), the Wakefield Self-assessment Depression Inventory (Snaith *et al*, 1976) and the Geriatric Depression Scale (Sheikh & Yesavage, 1986).

There are, however, a number of difficulties in using these screening instruments. First, some patients may have difficulty in completing a questionnaire. Second, the sensitivity and specificity will depend on the cut-off scores used and the prevalence of the condition in the population will determine the positive predictive value of the test (House, 1988). The positive predictive value (the proportion of those tested positive who have the condition) of screening instruments in different medical conditions can vary very widely; Meakin (1992) gave the range as 19–92%, with a median figure of around 60%. This means that between a third to a half of the patients scoring above the cut-off may not actually have the psychiatric condition identified by the screening instrument. Positive results should prompt the clinician not only to make further enquiries about other symptoms of mood disorder and attempt to make a psychiatric diagnosis, but also to assess whether any of the items contributing to the raised score could be explained by the medical condition itself, and whether the distress was only of a transient nature. It should also be borne in mind that because the specificity of a screening test rarely reaches 100%, some patients with a definite psychiatric disorder will score below the cut-off and therefore be missed.

Despite a huge amount of effort in devising these screening instruments and considerable research enthusiasm aimed at detecting psychiatric disorder, it appears that the routine administration of anxiety and depression questionnaires in non-psychiatric settings does not increase the overall rate of recognition of mental disorders. The selective feedback of high scores on these scales has been shown to increase the rate of recognition – but this does not translate into an increased rate of intervention (Gilbody *et al*, 2001).

Most screening questionnaires are designed for one specific problem and so multiple questionnaires would be necessary to screen general hospital patients for all mental disorders. The need for a multiplicity of questionnaires (in different formats and requiring the handling of many sheets of paper) would make it difficult, if not impossible, to implement routine screening in a busy general medical setting. Incorporating these questionnaires on to computer terminals with touch screens may be a better option, but this approach has yet to be explored in routine medical practice.

Two-stage screening procedures (see page 414 in this chapter and page 702 in Chapter 27) might be of use for patients at higher risk of mental disorder in the general hospital setting. Thus, patients with frequent admissions, longer length of stay, poor disease control, intolerance to drugs and poor pain control probably should be screened, because in these groups it may be important not to miss cases of psychiatric disorder. Another approach is to use a simplified interview based on a series of set questions that screen for psychiatric problems. This method has been effective in screening for alcoholism (the CAGE questionnaire – see Box 17.4) and for cognitive impairment in the elderly (the Abbreviated Mental Test Score – see Box 17.5).

Referrals to liaison psychiatry

Referrals to liaison psychiatry generally come from clinicians in other medical specialties, usually from a member of the medical or nursing staff, or occasionally from other disciplines, such as physiotherapy or occupational therapy. Because the patient is already under clinical care for a physical problem, which some patients will strongly believe to be entirely physically caused, there will sometimes be a reluctance to accept a psychiatric referral. Some patients may interpret these referrals as 'They don't believe me', or 'They think this is all in the mind', or 'They think I am being a nuisance', or 'I am being palmed off', and so forth. This makes it all the more important for the general hospital clinician making the referral to allow adequate

Box 17.4 The CAGE questionnaire

- Have you ever felt you should **C**ut down on your drinking?
- Have people **A**nnoyed you by criticising your drinking?
- Have you ever felt bad or **G**uilty about your drinking?
- Have you ever had a drink first thing in the morning or to get rid of a hangover (**E**ye-opener)?

Scoring: one point for yes to each question.

The original paper (Ewing, 1984) suggested that one positive response should lead to further enquiry. Generally, a score of two or more is considered to be clinically significant and found to have good sensitivity and specificity for alcohol misuse or dependence (Hearne *et al*, 2002).

Box 17.5 The Abbreviated Mental Test Score (Hodkinson, 1972)

- Age
- Time [correct to nearest hour]
- Three-item address (e.g. 42 West Street) [registration and recall at end of test]
- Month
- Year
- Name of place [If not in hospital, ask type of place or area of town]
- Date of birth
- Start of First World War
- Name of present monarch
- Count from 20 to 1 (backwards)

Score: abnormal when six or less.

time to explain the reasons for the referral and why a psychological approach may help the patient. If the referral is for a suspected somatoform disorder, for example, it is important to emphasise to the patient that the referral does not negate the reality of the symptoms in question, but its purpose is more to widen the scope for understanding how the symptom(s) came about and/or to find better ways of managing them. The liaison psychiatrist must also be quite clear about the reasons for the referral (Box 17.6) and this may necessitate a discussion with the referrer before the assessment. Seeking the views of the nursing staff who care for the patient and access to the medical notes will also provide important additional information.

Liaison psychiatry assessment

Psychiatric assessments of hospital in-patients are often conducted on general wards, which are usually very busy places. It is better practice to find a private room where the assessment can take place without risk of interruption or being overheard. The patient's medical needs will also have to be taken into account, and this may mean fitting in the assessment between investigations or treatment sessions. A few patients cannot tolerate a full interview, and in these cases more than one visit may be required.

Box 17.7 outlines the elements of the assessment. It is often helpful to open the liaison psychiatry interview by enquiring how the patient felt about the referral, as this will elicit any fears or misunderstandings surrounding a psychiatric referral. It is important to address these issues from the outset, and engage the patient in the interview and generally clear the air. Starting with the medical problem will often entail initially taking an extended physical history and this may be especially helpful when engaging patients with suspected somatoform disorders, who will appreciate the time spent eliciting and understanding their physical symptoms. This may also facilitate moving on to other aspects of the history. In cases where it seems that the physical illness has led to the psychiatric disorder, the time course of the mental symptoms should be clearly noted in relation to other events, such as the development of the physical problems, their investigation and treatment. If medication is suspected as a cause of the mental symptoms, it is important to record the present medication(s), as well as when they were

Box 17.6 Reasons for referral to consultation–liaison psychiatry

- Suspected mental illness and/or advice on treatment
- Assessment of risk, especially in relation to a patient who has suicidal or paranoid ideas, or who is aggressive towards others
- Disturbed or disruptive behaviour from suspected mental disorder
- Refusing treatment or erratic adherence to treatment
- Assessment of capacity to consent to or refuse treatment
- Non-organic symptoms
- Request for transfer to a psychiatric unit

Box 17.7 Consultation–liaison psychiatry assessment

1. Understand the purpose of the referral from the referrer
2. Engage the patient, and allow time to discuss the purpose and nature of the assessment
3. Assess the patient:
   - history of the physical problems
   - nature, time course, treatments, impact of the physical condition
   - psychiatric history, including relationship between life events, physical problems and psychological symptoms
   - assessment of coping styles, risk factors
   - patient's understanding of physical/psychological difficulties
4. Interview significant others
5. Review medical notes/medication chart
6. Formulate a management plan
7. Feedback to patient and referrer

started or stopped. Looking at the current drug chart can also help tell whether the patient is following the prescribed drug regimen.

The main part of the assessment should then continue, covering the usual items in a standard psychiatric interview. The family and previous psychiatric history are important, as a biological predisposition to recurrent psychiatric disorder would increase the risk of a relapse during periods of physical disease. There is a strong association between a history of psychiatric illness and affective disorder in general medical in-patients (Feldman *et al*, 1987). The personal and social history as well as premorbid personality also contribute to the assessment of personality, and it is useful to know the coping style the patient has shown during previous stressful points in life.

The presenting psychiatric problems may not always fit into a neat psychiatric category and significant psychological morbidity may still be present in the absence of a conventionally diagnosable mental disorder. It is important to explore patients' beliefs concerning their symptoms, diagnosis and treatment, their reaction to the illness, their understanding of the prognosis and how they feel they have been dealt with by the medical profession. A similar range of issues should be covered with the patient's family or carers. In cases where cognitive impairment is suspected, a history from an informant is essential. It may also be helpful to obtain further information from the general practitioner, especially where there is complicated or extensive medical or psychiatric history.

Diagnosis

As previously discussed, it is usually neither possible nor useful to categorise the patient's problem under a single diagnosis, and it may be preferable to use a multi-axial system. A formulation that covers the biological, individual psychological and social factors that have contributed to the presenting problem helps to make sense of the patient's current problems and should be recorded in the medical notes (Fig. 17.2). If this can then be shared with the patient and the referrer, it will help to establish a good therapeutic relationship.

In formulating a management plan, the patient's medical needs and the reason for the referral need to be taken into account. The plan may include suggestions for psychological input, psychotropic medication or whether there is any need for further follow-up by the psychiatrist. There should also be guidance to the ward staff on how to manage difficult behaviours or how to meet the patient's emotional needs. There may also be recommendations for family support or social input, which may involve professionals or other voluntary agencies outside the medical and liaison psychiatry team.

It is essential to let the referrer know precisely what information has been given to the patient. The written plan should also clarify who is expected to take responsibility for each item in it. For out-patient assessments, the summary letter should include the formulation, the management plan and an outline of the patient's perspective, and this should be forwarded to the relevant clinical team(s) as well as the patient's general practitioner.

Management of liaison psychiatry patients

Correct diagnosis and correct weighting of the various aetiological factors are essential in preparing a useful formulation in CL psychiatry and this is a major part of

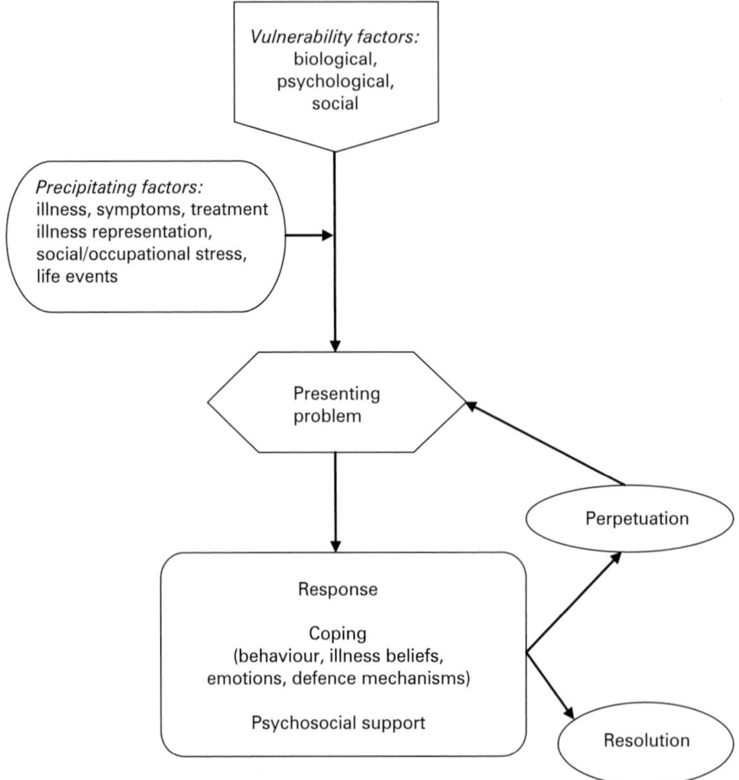

Fig. 17.2 Diagnostic formulation in consultation–liaison psychiatry.

the skill of the liaison psychiatrist. The other important skill is the ability to carry the hospital clinical staff along with the treatment plan. This will entail spending time with the medical and nursing team and discussing the psychiatric and psychosocial aspects of the case with them, and in some cases involving the family as well.

Psychotropic medication

Psychotropic medication will be considered where there is immediate significant risk to the patient or others; this may be suicidal risk or result from behavioural disturbance or severity of the mental illness. In a physically ill patient, it is particularly important to pay attention to the potential of medication to exacerbate particular physical symptoms, and to drug interactions and the potential for drug toxicity. Therefore, it is important to take a full medical and drug history, paying particular attention to any history of cardiovascular disease, hepatic and renal dysfunction, epilepsy or cognitive dysfunction. Any proposed drug should be cross-checked for its use in the presence of organ dysfunction as well as the patient's existing medication, with, for example, the current *British National Formulary* or the *Psychotropic Drug Directory* (Bazire, 2003) (Box 17.8). The starting dose of psychotropic drugs may need to be reduced in medically ill patients as they are especially likely to be sensitive to the side-effects of psychotropic drugs.

Box 17.8 Use of psychotropic medication in the medical setting

Consider existing physical disease
Will the psychotropic medication exacerbate existing problems, such as:
- cardiac dysfunction
- hypertension/postural hypotension
- glycaemic control in diabetes mellitus
- weight gain/loss
- gastrointestinal bleeds
- neurological disorders, including epilepsy?

Are there conditions that require dose adjustment?
- reduced absorption (intestinal disease or surgery, malabsorption)
- altered distribution (hypoproteinaemia)
- reduced metabolism/excretion (hepatic/renal dysfunction)

Guidance on prescribing in specific physical illnesses
- *British National Formulary* (especially appendices on liver disease, renal impairment, pregnancy and breast-feeding)
- *Psychotropic Drug Directory* (Bazire, 2003)

Consider drug interactions
- *British National Formulary*'s appendix on interactions

Antidepressants

In a patient with mild depression of recent onset, the first course of action will be watchful waiting with a review after a couple of weeks, rather than proceeding directly to psychotropic medication. It is helpful to address any other psychosocial factors identified at the first assessment, such as ensuring a good understanding of the medical condition, assisting adjustment to the illness, or coming to terms with the consequences of treatment, such as loss or disfigurement, encouraging helpful coping behaviour, and so on, while also monitoring the mood.

Antidepressants need to be considered for patients who present with major depression where a psychotherapeutic approach may be inappropriate or insufficient. When used appropriately, they significantly increase the chance of recovery from depression, with possible associated improvements in the physical condition (Series, 1992). The principles of the use of antidepressants for the medical population is not as different from that for other psychiatric patients (see Chapter 4) as non-liaison psychiatrists might imagine, especially for those patients in whom the underlying medical condition is well controlled. However, it is important to pay attention to medical cautions and contraindications and the frequent need for dose adjustment, in response to either side-effects or impaired drug metabolism in medical patients. It is a good idea to become familiar with these aspects for one or two selective serotonin reuptake inhibitors (SSRIs) and tricyclic antidepressants that are in common usage. The prescribing of antidepressants for patients with specific physical disorders is reviewed and summarised by MacHale (2002).

Generally, SSRIs are used as first-line antidepressants, as the older tricyclic antidepressants are often poorly tolerated because of their higher incidence of side-effects, especially anticholinergic ones. However, SSRIs should be avoided if possible, or used with caution, in patients aged over 80 years, those with prior upper gastrointestinal bleeding, or in those also taking aspirin or another non-steroidal anti-inflammatory drug (*Drugs and Therapeutic Bulletin*, 2004). SSRIs vary in their effect on the hepatic cytochrome P450 system and may affect metabolism of other drugs prescribed at the same time (Anderson & Edwards, 2001). Citalopram and sertraline have the least problems in this respect. It is also important to be aware of the possibility of serotonin syndrome with other serotonergic medications (e.g. pethidine/pentazocine perioperatively, and 5-HT$_1$ agonists – triptans – for migraine).

It is important to ensure close follow-up over the first few weeks of patients started on antidepressants, to monitor any side-effects and address any other concerns the patient may have, in order to facilitate adherence. Some patients are anxious about starting and staying on antidepressant medication, as they may believe their problems are 'physical' and either do not understand or have difficulty accepting their need for psychotropic medication. If the patient started on the medication as an in-patient, it is important to clarify the follow-up arrangements, whether the general practitioner will be expected to monitor the antidepressant treatment, or whether the patient will be followed up in the liaison psychiatry out-patient clinic. There may also be a need for other clinicians (both hospital and primary care) to be made aware of any medical consequences of introducing the antidepressant medication. For instance, patients on high-dose venlafaxine may need their blood pressure to be monitored, while those with non-insulin-dependent diabetes who have been prescribed fluoxetine need to be made aware of their increased risk of hypoglycaemia. These issues should be communicated clearly to both the treating clinician and the patient's general practitioner.

Intolerance of side-effects is common in medical patients. For patients who are already experiencing physical discomfort from their medical condition or treatment, additional problems due to the introduction of antidepressants may be especially distressing. Some patients become hypervigilant of physiological changes, and they may mistakenly report these as side-effects. It is all too easy then to become caught in multiple changes of antidepressants in response. If it is anticipated that side-effects may become a problem, it may be best start patients on low doses and gradually increase the dosage. Several antidepressants are now available in a liquid form (e.g. fluoxetine, citalopram, lofepramine), which makes it easier to introduce them at sub-therapeutic doses and to make gradual dose adjustments. The fact that these can be diluted in a glass of liquid appears to help patients feel that they are in greater control of how the antidepressant is taken, and this is useful for those who are anxious about taking medication because of previous side-effects. Liquid formulations are also useful when the final dose needs to be reduced or adjusted because of hepatic or renal dysfunction.

Treatment resistance is also commonly observed and, as with any patients, the first steps to take are to check the dose, medication adherence and the duration of treatment. Among liaison patients it is also prudent to list all the other medications the patient is currently taking, in case they are taking a drug known to worsen depression (see Box 17.2, page 410). In these instances it may be helpful to liaise with the treating clinician to see whether there is any scope for a change in the medication prescribed for the physical condition. It is also important to explore whether there are any unaddressed psychosocial factors which may be perpetuating the disorder, as antidepressants are rarely sufficient on their own to treat depression in medical patients. Rarely, augmentation with lithium or other mood stabilisers may be needed. Lithium is contraindicated in patients with impaired renal function, and if it is used among those with hypothyroidism closer monitoring of thyroid function is indicated.

Antipsychotics

Antipsychotics may be required in the medical setting for the treatment of delirium, mania and other psychotic states and in controlling acute behavioural disturbance.

For patients who are behaviourally disturbed, the initial priority is to try to defuse the situation by creating a safe and calm environment, ensuring safety for both the patient and others. As soon as this is achieved, it is essential to look for medical causes for the disturbed behaviour, such as a reaction to medication or the presence of infection, and deal with them. However, medication is required to contain acute and serious disturbance and the most commonly used medications in these situations are short-acting benzodiazepines (e.g. lorazepam) and haloperidol. In cases of delirium tremens, benzodiazepines such as chlordiazepoxide are indicated. Where antipsychotics are required in addition to benzodiazepines, haloperidol is the preferred drug in the short term, especially if an intramuscular injection is required, as it is less likely to cause hypotension or respiratory depression. Longer-acting depot preparations, such as Acuphase, should not be used in the acute management of behavioural disturbance on a medical ward. The clinical state of disturbed and physically ill patients may fluctuate rapidly and require regular adjustment of psychotropic dose, which is not possible with these preparations.

Anxiolytics

As indicated above, short-acting benzodiazepines may be used in controlling acute behavioural disturbance on the ward if non-pharmacological strategies have failed. They may also be helpful when severe or phobic anxiety (e.g. needle phobia) has resulted in non-compliance with key investigations or treatments and non-pharmacological anxiety management methods are not possible. When benzodiazepines are given parenterally, vital signs should be monitored closely, and flumazenil, a competitive benzodiazepine antagonist, should be available on the ward in case significant respiratory depression should occur. Whenever benzodiazepines are recommended by the liaison psychiatry team, it is essential that the recommendation should include their indications, and guidance on the frequency and total duration of their use. This is because prescriptions are sometimes started on the medical ward and then repeated without clear instructions, leading to long-term use and dependence. Care should be taken in the use of benzodiazepines in the presence of significant respiratory illness, owing to the risk of compromising respiratory function even further.

Patients often request night sedation in hospital. It is important to find out whether any worries or physical discomfort is interfering with sleep; sometimes the short-term use of hypnotic medication may be necessary.

Electroconvulsive therapy

Electroconvulsive therapy (ECT) may be required in depressed medical patients for the same indications as for psychiatric patients with depression, which include immediate high risk of suicide, severe psychomotor retardation and risk of dehydration due to limited oral intake, any other condition where a rapid relief of severe depressive symptoms is required. Special attention should be paid to any relative contraindications, such as raised intracranial pressure, recent myocardial infarction or cerebrovascular accident, acute respiratory infection, retinal detachment and phaeochromocytoma. The risks and benefits of the general anaesthetic and ECT should be weighed carefully in discussion with the medical team, anaesthetist, patient and family, and clearly documented in the notes. The topic is discussed at length in Chapter 5.

Alcohol detoxification

Alcohol detoxification may be required on the medical ward when a patient with known alcohol dependence is admitted. However, in a minority of patients the alcoholism is unknown and when these patients are admitted as an emergency, or on the day of their elective surgery, they may abruptly show behavioural disorders apparently occurring without any obvious precipitant, consistent with delirium tremens (DTs). This is a dangerous condition and a comprehensive account of detoxification regimens and the DTs is given in Chapter 22 (see page 560). Because of the high frequency of alcohol problems it is important for the medical and psychiatric liaison teams to agree on the protocol for the management of alcohol withdrawal; this protocol should clearly delineate the responsibilities of each team.

Psychological treatments

A high proportion of affective disorders identified in an acute medical setting are of a mild and transient nature (Feldman *et al*, 1987). For these patients formal referral to psychiatrists or psychologists is inappropriate and first-line psychological support is best provided by the doctors and nurses who are presently caring for them. However, general hospital staff often have difficulty in identifying psychological problems and more importantly in handling them. Therefore the liaison psychiatry team will play an important role in training and supporting the clinical staff, helping them manage minor affective disorders more effectively and with greater confidence.

Ramirez & House (1997) have listed the basic psychological skills general hospital clinicians should possess in order to facilitate the psychological care of their patients. These comprise the following abilities:

- to communicate clearly with patients, discuss their concerns, elicit any misapprehensions and correct them
- to break bad news
- to facilitate the grieving process by patients and their relatives
- to discuss psychological symptoms and distress without embarrassment
- to discuss the need for specialist psychiatric help without seeming dismissive
- to use antidepressants rationally.

Brody (1980) conducted a controlled trial of providing primary care physicians with feedback about the patient's mental health status as determined by the GHQ and scores on a questionnaire regarding recent stressors, and found that those in the feedback group expressed greater satisfaction. Specific workshops can also help to improve the counselling skills of clinical staff (Maguire & Faulkner, 1988).

There are additional constraints to the delivery of psychotherapy in a general hospital setting, or where patients are significantly ill, cognitively impaired or have difficulty attending sessions regularly, for physical reasons, and so treatment should be tailored to needs of the individual patients and delivered more flexibly. Otherwise the whole gamut of psychological therapies available to psychiatric patients should also be available to liaison patients. Some more specialised therapies are shown in Box 17.9.

Box 17.9 Psychological treatments in consultation–liaison psychiatry

- Problem-solving therapy (Wood & Mynors-Wallis, 1997)
- Cognitive–behavioural therapy (White, 2001)
- Motivational interviewing (Miller & Rollnick, 2002)
- Interpersonal psychotherapy (Klerman *et al*, 1984; Markowitz *et al*, 1992)
- Psychodynamic interpersonal therapy (Hardy *et al*, 2003)
- Couples therapy
- Family therapy
- Group therapy

Psychological intervention may be aimed at improving mood, addressing the psychosocial stressors that are maintaining the mental disorder, addressing cognitive or motivational factors that are interfering with medical treatment or dealing with any interpersonal difficulties that have arisen as a consequence of the illness.

Does psychological intervention influence the course of emotional or physical outcome?

Guthrie (1996) reviewed some of the psychotherapeutic interventions for emotional disorder in physical illness, but found that the number of good studies was limited. However, there was an indication that brief psychological intervention in acute physical illness may facilitate the patient's adjustment to illness. Thus, among patients with a first-time MI, counselling by coronary care nurses led to significantly lower levels of anxiety when compared with controls both immediately following the infarction and at 6 months; patients experienced less anxiety about returning to work and their spouses also reported lower levels of anxiety (Thompson & Meddis, 1990). Pre-operative psychological assessment of patients awaiting mastectomy for breast cancer (Burton *et al*, 1991) was found to have a lasting protective effect against body image distress, and was associated with lower anxiety ratings at 3 months and 1 year after surgery. It appears that self-disclosure and exploration of emotional issues may improve the longer-term psychological outcome. Support of this type is also helpful for patients who are facing or who have already had surgery where loss of body parts is involved (Maguire & Parkes, 1998).

Group approaches have also been tried for patients with cancer. These programmes help in a variety of ways: the instillation of hope, problem solving together with others, and ventilating painful feelings, as well as providing medical staff with a greater insight into their patients' needs. A randomised prospective outcome study of a weekly supportive group for women with metastatic carcinoma found that those who attended the group had significantly less mood disturbance and fewer maladaptive coping responses, and were also less phobic than the control group (Spiegel *et al*, 1981). Once-weekly supportive group therapy combined with self-hypnosis for pain relief over a period of 1 year significantly improved the survival time of women with metastatic breast cancer compared with controls (Spiegel *et al*, 1989).

There have also been attempts to improve the prognosis of physical disorders either by modifying risk factors or by improving treatment adherence. An example of this is the modification of 'type A behaviour', which is a complex combination of emotional responses and behaviours that includes impatience, aggressiveness, intense achievement drive, a sense of time urgency and a desire for recognition and advancement, and which was at one time thought to be associated with coronary heart disease. Attempts have been made to modify type A behaviours in the hope of reducing reinfarction rates, but controversy remains as to whether this approach is effective (Friedman *et al*, 1984).

In chronic diseases, the aims of medical treatment are to control and manage the illness rather than cure it. The use of psychological therapies to improve the management of illness over the long term has been explored but the number of controlled studies is limited and results are conflicting (Guthrie, 1996). However, liaison psychiatrists are sometimes asked to help patients and physicians in the management of their chronic illness in a more collaborative manner. Such an approach, developed on the basis of social learning and self-regulation theories and to some extent using methods developed to manage long-term mental illness, aims to define the patient's problems collaboratively, to set goals and targets, and to plan action. Patients are encouraged to acquire skills to manage their own illness but at the same time receive emotional support; and they are then followed up to help them sustain progress (Von Korff *et al*, 1997).

Consent, capacity and the Mental Health Act in the general hospital

Assessment of capacity to consent to medical treatment

Any procedure carried out in the medical setting from examination, investigation to treatment requires consent by the patient. Consent is:

> 'the voluntary and continuing permission of the patient to receive a particular treatment, based on an adequate knowledge of the purpose, nature, likely effects and risks of that treatment including the likelihood of its success and any alternatives to it.' (Mental Health Act 1983; see also the *Mental Health Act 1983 Code of Practice*, Department of Health & Welsh Office, 1999)

The presumption is that adult patients have the capacity to decide whether to consent to or refuse the proposed medical intervention, even where a refusal may result in harm to themselves or even in their own death. A patient with capacity to decide is also free to withdraw consent at any stage. Under current law in England and Wales, no other person can give or withhold consent to treatment on behalf of another adult (see 'Patients who lack capacity', below). This will change when the Mental Capacity Act 2005 comes into force in April 2007, as there is a provision for proxy decision-making powers which will allow consent for medical treatment to be given on behalf of a person deemed to lack capacity.

A child under 16 may give valid consent to medical treatment if he or she is assessed to be 'Gillick competent'; that is, he or she has the capacity to make the decision to have the proposed treatment and is of sufficient understanding and intelligence to be capable of making up his or her own mind. Children of 16 or over may give consent to treatment and it is not necessary to obtain parental consent. However, if a patient under 18 lacks capacity, those with parental responsibility may give consent on that patient's behalf.

It is the responsibility of each clinician to ensure that valid consent is obtained for any treatment proposed (this may be written or otherwise, non-verbal or verbal) (Box 17.10). Informed consent requires a clinician: to give information about the treatment; to be satisfied that the patient has the capacity to make the decision; and to allow the patient to make a voluntary choice without undue influence from others. It is essential for the practice of medicine that all clinicians are able adequately to assess a patient's capacity to consent to treatment. A patient lacks capacity only if some impairment or disturbance of mental functioning renders the person unable to decide whether to consent to or refuse treatment.

The patient has the capacity to decide on the treatment if he or she:

- understands the nature, purpose and reason for the treatment
- understands its principal benefits, risks and alternatives
- understands the consequences of not receiving the treatment
- is able to retain the information for long enough to use it and weigh it in the balance in order to arrive at a decision (British Medical Association & Law Society, 2004).

Box 17.10 Consent and capacity

Valid consent is that which is:

- based on adequate knowledge of –
  - the nature of the treatment
  - the risks associated with the treatment
  - the consequences of not having the treatment
- voluntary – the patient was not under undue influence of others
- given by a patient who has the capacity (see below) to decide.

Assessment of capacity (British Medical Association & Law Society, 2004)

To be deemed to have capacity, the patient should be able:

- to understand the nature, purpose and reason for the treatment
- to understand the principal benefits, risks and alternatives
- to understand the consequences of not receiving the treatment
- to retain the information for long enough to use it and weigh it in the balance in order to arrive at a decision.

When there has been any doubt as to the capacity of the patient to consent to treatment, the patient should be questioned on each of the above items. It is important to record the verbatim responses of such an assessment in the medical notes, as the question of capacity may sometimes later become a legal issue or even a matter for the courts.

The presence or absence of capacity is not an all-or-none matter. Patients may temporarily become incapable of giving consent due to lost or impaired consciousness, fear, fatigue, shock, pain, drugs or alcohol. Some may have longer-term impairment from learning disability or dementia. In either case, a patient may have the capacity to consent to some treatments and not others, and it is important that the presence or absence of capacity is considered on each relevant issue.

Although all clinicians are expected to be able to assess a patient's capacity to make treatment decisions, a psychiatrist may be asked to assist in such an assessment. It will be important to discuss with the referrer the reasons for the request, the nature of the treatment proposed and the consequences of both acceptance and refusal. With the patient, it is important to clarify whether he or she has been given adequate information about the proposed treatment, whether the patient's stated decision is his or her own and has not been made under undue influence from others, and to assess the person's capacity on the points discussed above. In particular, the psychiatrist may be better placed to assess whether a mental disorder is present, and if so, to make a judgement as to whether it has any bearing on the patient's ability to comprehend the information given, believe it, retain it and weigh up the options needed to come to a decision.

Where patients are refusing treatment, especially where this may have serious consequences for their health, it is vital that their capacity to make treatment decisions is assessed carefully, and that senior clinicians should be involved in this type of assessment. Discussion of the reasons for refusal may sometimes reveal some small practical or interpersonal issue that has made the selected treatment unacceptable to the patient. In these instances it may be possible to make alternative arrangements or select a different but equally effective treatment which the patient can accept. Even when the patient is assessed as being capable of refusing a treatment, it is important that there is ongoing discussion and negotiation about management where possible, involving family (if the patient allows this), while respecting the patient's autonomous decision, as he or she may change the decision with time.

Overdose

Psychiatrists covering the emergency department or medical wards are sometimes consulted about patients who have taken an overdose and are refusing treatment. This is a complex legal issue over which there has been considerable debate (Hassan *et al*, 1999; Hewson, 1999; Hull & Haut, 1999). The initial action in this situation should be to assess the patient's capacity to make treatment decisions and there should also be an attempt to lower levels of emotional arousal, to permit further discussion with the aim of persuading the patient to accept treatment. If the patient lacks capacity to consent to treatment, the decision to treat should be taken in the patient's best interest under the common law *doctrine of necessity* (see below). Capacity in these patients may be impaired for a variety of reasons, such as alcohol intoxication, direct effect of drugs taken in overdose affecting the levels of consciousness, or a very high degree of distress which impairs concentration and the ability to weigh up options.

If the patient has been detained under the Mental Health Act for a mental disorder and the overdose is considered to be due to the underlying mental disorder, then the medical treatment for the overdose can be given as an ancillary treatment under section 63. Under the Act this treatment should be under the direction of the responsible medical officer. However, where the patient is not detained under the Act and has been assessed to have capacity to make treatment decisions, the patient's wish cannot be overridden. As with any other significant treatment refusal, senior clinicians should be involved in the assessment of the patient. Even in such circumstances, the patient may accept admission for further observation or may permit clinicians to contact the family, which will facilitate the monitoring of the patient's physical condition and leave open the possibility of a change of mind in due course. In this, as in all medical situations, the clinician's overriding duty is to make decisions that promote the safety and well-being of the patient while upholding any decisions made by a patient who has capacity.

Patients who lack capacity

The Incapacity (Scotland) Act 2000 now covers decision making for adults who lack capacity in Scotland. The Mental Capacity Act 2005 received royal assent in April 2006 and will come into force on 1 April 2007 in England and Wales (see http://www.dca.gov.uk/menincap/legis.htm). Until this Act is enforced, the treatment of patients lacking capacity is covered under the common law. In patients lacking capacity, no other person can give or withhold consent on their behalf at present, but the treating clinician will have the responsibility to make medical decisions that are in the best interest of the patient. For a treatment to be allowed under common law, the doctrine of necessity should be applied. This states: that a treatment given to a patient who lacks capacity should be necessary to save life, or alleviate or prevent deterioration in the patient's physical or mental health; that the benefit of the treatment should outweigh the burden; and that the decision would be supported by a responsible body of medical opinion in the field. In making the decision of 'best interest', there is a strong presumption of preservation of life, although the best interest may be framed in terms of medical, emotional or other welfare issues. It is also good practice in these fraught situations to consult close relatives to clarify the patient's best interest, although any such enquiry should be mindful of the duty of confidentiality owed to the patient (British Medical Association & Law Society, 2004). Where there is a need to restrain a patient who lacks capacity in the general medical setting, this may be permitted under common law, provided the action taken is necessary, reasonable and in the patient's best interest.

If the patient had a valid advance statement (a 'living will') while he or she had capacity to make it, this should be respected, provided the decision is applicable to the procedure in question and there is no reason to believe that the patient had changed his or her mind.

Questions about capacity also arise in situations where a patient is refusing to go to hospital for a physical disorder. If the patient lacks capacity to make a decision about going into hospital and it is in the person's best interest to receive the treatment for that medical condition in hospital, the common law doctrine of necessity allows conveyance to hospital.

The Mental Capacity Act 2005 provides a legal framework for England and Wales, which enshrines these common law principles, sets out a test for assessing capacity and provides a checklist for decisions in the best interest for those who lack capacity. It makes provisions for those having lasting powers of attorney (LPA) or for court-appointed deputies to act on behalf of those who lack capacity. A new Court of Protection will be the final arbiter for capacity matters, while a 'public guardian' will be the registering authority for LPAs and deputies. The Act also makes provision for an 'independent mental capacity advocate' (IMCA) to support those who lack capacity, allows for advance decisions to refuse treatment to be formalised, introduces a new criminal offence of ill treatment or neglect of a person who lacks capacity and sets parameters for research involving such persons. The Mental Capacity Act Code of Practice will provide practical guidance in the application of the Act.

In October 2004, the European Court of Human Rights ruled in the Bournewood case that detention in hospital of a patient lacking capacity, under the common law doctrine of necessity, 'where the patient is under continuous supervision and control', infringed Article 5 of the European Convention of Human Rights. This has come to be known as the 'Bournewood gap' and the UK government intends to close this gap by amending the Mental Capacity Act 2005 (see Department of Health, 2006). The ruling refers to the issue of detention alone and not to medical treatment of incapacitated patients.

Non-therapeutic or controversial treatments (e.g. non-therapeutic sterilisation, organ donation, withdrawal of nutrition in patients in a persistent vegetative state, bone marrow donation) in patients lacking capacity should be referred to court.

Mental Health Act 1983 in the general hospital

The Mental Health Act 1983 in England and Wales allows compulsory detention and treatment of mental disorder where it is in the interest of the patient's health, safety or the safety of other persons and where voluntary admission is not possible. The Act also allows treatment of physical disorder where it has given rise to mental disorder and it is necessary to treat the physical disorder in order to treat the mental disorder (e.g. treatment of thyroid disease that has given rise to severe depression or psychotic illness, or refeeding of patients with severe anorexia nervosa). However, where there is a temporary mental disorder, such as delirium arising from an underlying physical disorder, which results in the patient temporarily losing capacity to consent to treatment, it is more appropriate to consider treatment under common law/the Mental Capacity Act 2005.

The procedure for application for detention of a patient under the Mental Health Act is the same in the general hospital setting as it is in the mental health setting. If an in-patient needs to be held on the ward in an emergency under the Act, the medical holding power of section 5(2) may be considered. The consultant with medical responsibility may use the power to detain the patient for up to 72 hours while awaiting a full assessment under the Act. The Act allows the consultant to nominate a deputy to carry out the detention, but this person must be a fully registered medical practitioner (thus a pre-registration house officer cannot take on this role). Any medical team using the section 5(2) holding power should be advised to contact the psychiatric services as soon as possible. Patients detained under the temporary holding power cannot be moved to another hospital under this power.

As section 5(2) is applicable only to in-patients, patients in the accident and emergency department usually cannot be held under it, as they will not have been formally admitted. Patients who lack capacity to consent to remain will need to be held under the common law doctrine of necessity/Mental Capacity Act 2005 once it has been established it is in their best interest to remain in the emergency department to receive treatment (see above). The nurses' holding power (section 5(4)) can be used only by appropriately registered nurses, with training in mental health or learning disabilities, on informal in-patients already being treated for mental illness, and would not normally be applicable in a general hospital setting. The liaison consultant psychiatrist will be perceived by the rest of the hospital staff as the most knowledgeable concerning these medico-legal conundrums and his or her opinion will often be sought. Thus, whenever a patient is being treated without consent it is important for the liaison psychiatrist to know exactly under which Act, doctrine or law such treatments are taking place.

The provision of consultation liaison psychiatry services

Recent joint reports from the Royal Colleges of Physicians (2003) and Surgeons (1997) with the Royal College of Psychiatrists have recognised the need for the clinical staff in general hospitals to possess basic psychological skills as well as the need for wards to have facilities in which staff can see patients privately and safely. These reports also advocate that CL psychiatry services should become an integral part of acute medical services. There should also be special services for alcohol counselling and for patients who have deliberately harmed themselves. In practice, however, there is wide variation in the provision of CL psychiatry services in general hospitals and well-developed services are found mainly in the larger teaching hospitals in urban areas. In today's National Health Service, CL services are commissioned locally; if they are to develop, a robust case for their need and value needs to be made in the commissioning process.

Models of service

The consultation model

In this model the general hospital clinician refers the patient to a mental health professional, who provides a psychosocial or psychiatric assessment and gives advice to the patient and the clinical team regarding management. A service of this type relies on clinical staff for the detection of potential mental disorders. The effectiveness of the consultation model is also influenced by the quality of the communication between the referrer and mental health professionals.

There are four models of consultation (Lipowski, 1986):

1 *A patient-oriented consultation*, in which the patient is the direct focus. The consultation should incorporate a diagnostic interview and evaluation of the patient's personality, reaction to illness and other psychological aspects.

2 *A crisis-oriented therapeutic consultation*, in which there is a rapid assessment of the presenting problem and coping style as well as active therapeutic intervention, as might occur following an episode of parasuicide. The therapist may give guidance on techniques such as active problem solving or other cognitive methods to help the patient through the crisis.

3 *A referrer-oriented consultation*, which focuses on the referrer's problem with a given patient, for example where the clinicians may be left feeling very anxious or angry, for example in cases of treatment refusal.

4 *A situation-oriented consultation*, which looks at the interaction between the patient (and sometimes the family) and the clinical team, as may occur in cases where conflicts or disagreements arise over the treatment plan.

The liaison model

In this model the psychiatrist meets with the general clinicians in ward rounds or joint clinics. This gives an opportunity to discuss individual patients as well as more general topics, such as the psychosocial contribution and the psychological care of patients, and this provides a forum for educating and training the clinical team. The pure liaison model is very demanding in terms of the consultant psychiatrist's time and most services work with a mixture of the two models. Thus, individual consultations will follow on referral from a clinician but there may also be specific links with medical clinical teams to facilitate liaison work.

Service needs

A liaison psychiatric service will be needed for the accident and emergency department, as well as the in-patient and out-patient departments. Referrals are predominantly for physical and psychological comorbidity, for medically unexplained symptoms, and for problems arising in patient management as a result of psychosocial factors, as well as for deliberate self-harm, which is usually dealt with in the accident and emergency department. Annual referral rates in these settings have been estimated from both published and unpublished reports for a district general hospital of 600 beds serving a population of 250 000: self-harm, 500 per annum; accident and emergency, 150 per annum; ward referrals, 150 per annum; and out-patient contacts, new 50–100, follow-up 500 per annum. However, these figures may vary depending on the type and size of the hospital and the availability and popularity of the liaison service (House & Hodgson, 1994).

The type of CL service that can be offered will depend on a number of factors:

1 *The consultation time available.* This will depend on the composition of the team providing the service (as will the range of disciplines and skills available within it). This can range from a single general adult psychiatrist whose primary responsibility is a community sector but who provides a few liaison sessions, through to a full consultant-led multidisciplinary team.

2 *Any other established services provided to the hospital.* There may be pre-existing services provided by the psychiatric or psychology departments, covering areas such as psychiatry for the elderly, substance misuse, eating disorders, sexual dysfunction, HIV-related disorders, and neuropsychiatry/rehabilitation. The CL service may work independently of the other services without overlap, or work in conjunction with them.

3 *Expectations of other professionals.* Clinical staff in the general hospital and psychiatrists working in the community will have different expectations about exactly what the CL services should be providing. General hospital staff want easy and rapid access, an expectation of a single referral point with a quick response, and an efficient parasuicide assessment service. General psychiatrists working in the community live in the hope that the CL service will deal with all the general hospital referrals, so that the sector teams can be free to concentrate their resources on their patients in the community sector. Good liaison with both groups is important, and the support of general hospital clinicians and psychiatric colleagues will be essential when seeking resources for a new or expanded CL service. The views and needs of the service users and carers should also be taken into account in service planning.

The standard requirements for a CL service

The CL psychiatry service should be led by a consultant who specialises in liaison psychiatry. This person should have responsibilities for: direct clinical work (consultation and liaison); clinical supervision of psychiatric trainees and those from other disciplines; and the administrative and organisational work. A district general hospital (600 beds serving a population of 250 000) would be expected to generate a psychiatric workload equivalent to half a community-based sector (House & Hodgson, 1994). Therefore a minimum of five sessions of consultant time are required, but additional sessions should be allocated for the training and education of staff, both in the CL team and in the general hospital.

A consultant psychiatrist working alone would find it difficult to deliver a good service and an effective CL service today requires a multidisciplinary team

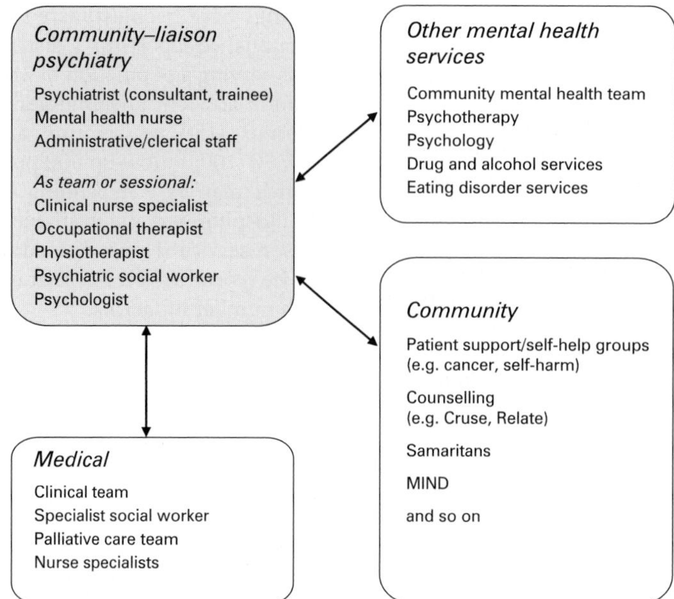

Fig. 17.3 Links between a consultation–liaison psychiatry service and other services.

with nurses, social workers, clinical psychologists, occupational therapists and physiotherapists. Skill mix is probably more important than the professional background of individual members. Skills in interviewing, assessment and short-term psychological therapies are particularly useful. Last but not least, adequate administrative/clerical back-up is essential for effective communication, and accessibility to referrers will also be a crucial aspect of coordinating the CL services.

Some CL services have dedicated in-patient wards in a medical setting, where patients with complex physical and psychiatric needs may be assessed and managed. This may be the best setting for managing those with severe chronic somatisation disorders, who are often reluctant to engage in psychiatric services, or too disabled for out-patient care, and who need all the skills of a multidisciplinary team for the assessment and management of their condition.

Links with other services

Consultation–liaison psychiatry services will need to have links with other services within the mental health field, such as psychodynamic therapy, cognitive–behavioural therapy, the drug and alcohol services, eating disorder services and perinatal psychiatry. In some cases, psychological care can more appropriately be provided by those working in the hospital, such as the clinical team, the palliative care team or specialist nurse counsellors. Links with the voluntary sector may also facilitate referrals to services in this sector, such as self-help groups and patient organisations (Fig. 17.3).

Specialty-based services

As mentioned under the liaison model, CL psychiatric teams may develop specific services for a particular medical specialty, such as oncology, diabetes, neurology, renal dialysis, transplantation, intensive care, a pain clinic or a fatigue clinic. The liaison aspect of this link may take the form of:

- a joint service, joint clinic or joint ward round
- a case review meeting or case conference with the multidisciplinary staff on the ward/clinical area
- psychological supervision or training for medical and paramedical staff in the specialist unit.

It is beyond the scope of this brief overview to give an account of services in the many different specialist settings, but these are described in detail in the book by Peveler *et al* (2000).

Conclusions

In recent years there have been important changes in general medicine relevant to CL psychiatry. There is now a much wider recognition of the high prevalence of psychiatric and physical comorbidity and how this influences consultation frequency, service utilisation, treatment adherence, the physical prognosis and probably the overall cost as well. There has also been recognition of the high prevalence of non-organic complaints among general medical patients, and an awareness of the high costs of investigating these patients, which has led on to a search for better ways to manage this group of patients (Creed, 1991). This means that a liaison psychiatrist should be an integral part of any medical service, from the viewpoint of both quality of care and cost. Making a clear case for the need and providing a realistic service model that meets these needs will prove to be important in sustaining and developing CL services.

Acknowledgements

We would like to thank our colleagues Peter Trigwell, David Protheroe and Manoj Kumar for their helpful comments on earlier drafts of this chapter.

References

American Psychiatric Association (1994) *Diagnostic and Statistical Manual of Mental Disorders* (4th edn) (DSM–IV). Washington, DC: APA.

Anderson, I. M. & Edwards, J. G. (2001) Guidance for choice of selective serotonin reuptake inhibitor in depressive illness. *Advances in Psychiatric Treatment*, **7**, 170–180.

Bazire, S. (2003) *Psychotropic Drug Directory 2003/2004: The Professional's Pocket Handbook and Aide Memoire*. Salisbury: Five Pin Publishing.

Beck, A. T. & Steer, R. A. (1987) *The Beck Depression Inventory Manual*. San Antonio, CA: Psychological Corporation, Harcourt Brace Jovanovich.

Breitbart, W. & Krivo, S. (1998) Suicide. In *Psycho-oncology* (eds J. C. Holland, *et al*), pp. 541–547. New York: Oxford University Press.

Bridges, K. W. & Goldberg, D. P. (1984) Psychiatric illness in inpatients with neurological disorders: patients' views on discussion of emotional problems with neurologists. *BMJ (Clinical Research Edition)*, **289**, 656–658.

British Medical Association & Law Society (2004) *Assessment of Mental Capacity* (2nd edn). London: BMJ Books.

Brody, D. S. (1980) Physician recognition of behavioural, psychological, and social aspects of medical care. *Archives of Internal Medicine*, **140**, 1286–1289.

Brown, G. W. & Harris, T. (1978) *The Social Origins of Depression: A Study of Psychiatric Disorder in Women*. London: Tavistock.

Burton, M., Parker, R. W. & Woliner, J. M. (1991) The psychotherapeutic value of a 'chat': a verbal response modes study of a placebo attention control with breast cancer patients. *Psychotherapy Research*, **1**, 39–61.

Carroll, D. & Sheffield, D. (1998) Social psychophysiology, social circumstances, and health. *Annals of Behavioural Medicine*, **20**, 333–337.

Chen, C. C., David, A. S., Nunnerley, H., *et al* (1995) Adverse life events and breast cancer: case–control study. *BMJ*, **311**, 1527–1530.

Cox, J. L., Holden, J. M. & Sagovsky, R. (1987) Detection of post natal depression. Development of the 10-item Edinburgh Post Natal Depression Scale. *British Journal of Psychiatry*, **150**, 782–786.

Craven, J. L. & Rodin, G. (1990) Somatic symptoms and the diagnosis of depression in medically ill patients. *American Journal of Psychiatry*, **147**, 814–815.

Creed, F. (1991) Liaison psychiatry for the 21st century: a review. *Journal of the Royal Society of Medicine*, **84**, 414–417.

Department of Health (2006) *Bournewood Briefing Sheet*. London: Department of Health. Available at http://www.dh.gov.uk/assetRoot/04/13/68/45/04136845.pdf

Department of Health & Welsh Office (1999) *Mental Health Act 1983 Code of Practice*. London: HMSO.

DePaulo, J. R. Jr & Folstein, M. F. (1978) Psychiatric disturbances in neurological patients: detection, recognition and hospital course. *Annals of Neurology*, **4**, 225–228.

Drugs and Therapeutic Bulletin (2004) Do SSRIs cause gastrointestinal bleeding? *Drug and Therapeutics Bulletin*, **42**, 17–18.

Dunbar, F. (1954) *Emotion and Bodily Changes* (4th edn). New York: Columbia University Press.

Engel, G. L. (1977) The need for a new medical model: a challenge for biomedicine. *Science*, **196**, 129–136.

Ewing, J. A. (1984) Detecting alcoholism. The CAGE questionnaire. *Journal of the American Medical Association*, **252**, 1905–1907.

Fairburn, C. G., Peveler, R. C., Davies, B., *et al* (1991) Eating disorders in young adults with insulin-dependent diabetes mellitus: a controlled study. *BMJ* **303**, 17–20.

Feinstein, A. (1997) Multiple sclerosis, depression and suicide. *BMJ*, **315**, 691–692.

Feldman, E., Mayou, R., Hawton, K., *et al* (1987) Psychiatric disorder in medical inpatients. *Quarterly Journal of Medicine*, **63**, 405–412.

Felker, B., Katon, W., Hedrick, S. C., *et al* (2001) The association between depressive symptoms and health status in patients with chronic pulmonary disease. *General Hospital Psychiatry*, **23**, 56–61.

Folstein, M. F., Folstein, S. E. & McHugh, P. R. (1975) 'Mini-mental state'. A practical method for grading the cognitive state of patients for the clinician. *Journal of Psychiatric Research*, **12**, 189–198.

Ford, D. E., Mead, L. A., Chang, P. P., *et al* (1998) Depression is a risk factor for coronary artery disease in men: the precursors study. *Archives of Internal Medicine*, **158**, 1422–1426.

Frasure-Smith, N., Lesperance, F. & Talajic, M. (1995) Depression and 18-month prognosis after myocardial infarction. *Circulation*, **91**, 999–1005.

Frasure-Smith, N., Lesperance, F., Gravel, G., *et al* (2000) Social support, depression, and mortality during the first year after myocardial infarction. *Circulation*, **101**, 1919–1924.

Friedman, M., Thoresen, C. E., Gill, J. J., *et al* (1984) Alteration of type A behaviour and reduction in cardiac recurrences in post-myocardial infarction patients. *American Heart Journal*, **108**, 237–248.

Fulop, G., Strain, J. J., Vita, J., *et al* (1987) Impact of psychiatric comorbidity on length of hospital stay for medical/surgical patients: a preliminary report. *American Journal of Psychiatry*, **144**, 878–882.

Gilbody, S. M., House, A. O. & Sheldon, T. A. (2001) Routinely administered questionnaires for depression and anxiety: systematic review. *BMJ*, **322**, 406–409.

Goldberg, D. (1985) Identifying psychiatric illness among general medical patients. *BMJ (Clinical Research Edition)*, **291**, 161–162.

Goldberg, D., Bridges, K., Duncan-Jones, P., *et al* (1988) Detecting anxiety and depression in general medical settings. *BMJ*, **297**, 897–899.

Guthrie, E. (1996) Emotional disorder in chronic illness: psychotherapeutic interventions. *British Journal of Psychiatry*, **168**, 265–273.

Hackett, T. P. & Cassem, N. H. (1978) *Massachusetts General Hospital Handbook of General Hospital Psychiatry*. St Louis, MO: C. V. Mosby.

Hardy, G., Barkham, M. E., Shapiro, D., *et al* (eds) (2003) *Psychodynamic–Interpersonal Therapy*. Thousand Oaks, CA: Sage.

Hassan, T. B., MacNamara, A. F., Davy, A., *et al* (1999) Lesson of the week: managing patients with deliberate self harm who refuse treatment in the accident and emergency department. *BMJ*, **319**, 107–109.

Hawton, K., Mayou, R. & Feldman, E. (1990) Significance of psychiatric symptoms in general medical patients with mood disorders. *General Hospital Psychiatry*, **12**, 296–302.

Hearne, R., Connolly, A. & Sheehan, J. (2002) Alcohol abuse: prevalence and detection in a general hospital. *Journal of the Royal Society of Medicine*, **95**, 84–87.

Hewson, B. (1999) The law on managing patients who deliberately harm themselves and refuse treatment. *BMJ*, **319**, 905–907.

Hodkinson, H. M. (1972) Evaluation of a mental test score for assessment of mental impairment in the elderly. *Age and Ageing*, **1**, 233–238.

Holland, J. C. (ed.) (1998) *Psycho-oncology*. Oxford: Oxford University Press.

Holmes, T. H. & Rahe, R. H. (1967) The social readjustment rating scale. *Journal of Psychosomatic Research*, **11**, 213–218.

Horne, R. & Weinman, J. (1994) Illness cognitions: implications for the treatment of renal disease. In *Quality of Life Following Renal Failure: Psychological Challenges Accompanying High Technology Medicine* (eds H. M. McGee & C. Bradley), pp. 113–132. London: Psychology Press.

Horne, R. & Weinman, J. (1999) Patients' beliefs about prescribed medicines and their role in adherence to treatment in chronic physical illness. *Journal of Psychosomatic Research*, **47**, 555–567.

House, A. (1988) Mood disorders in the physically ill – problems of definition and measurement. *Journal of Psychosomatic Research*, **32**, 345–353.

House, A. & Hodgson, G. (1994) Estimating needs and meeting demands. In *Liaison Psychiatry. Defining Needs and Planning Services* (eds S. Benjamin, A. House & P. Jenkins), pp. 3–15. London: Gaskell.

House, A., Dennis, M., Mogridge, L., *et al* (1990) Life events and difficulties preceding stroke. *Journal of Neurology, Neurosurgery and Psychiatry*, **53**, 1024–1028.

Hull, A. & Haut, F. (1999) Managing patients with deliberate self harm who refuse treatment in accident and emergency departments. (Letter.) *BMJ*, **319**, 916 (author reply 917).

Jenkins, R., Lewis, G., Bebbington, P., *et al* (1997) The National Psychiatric Morbidity Surveys of Great Britain – initial findings from the household survey. *Psychological Medicine*, **27**, 775–789.

Klerman, G. L., Weissman, M. M. & Rounsaville, B. J. (1984) *Interpersonal Psychotherapy of Depression*. New York: Basic Books.

Kornfeld, D. S. (1996) Consultation–liaison psychiatry and the practice of medicine. The Thomas P. Hackett Award lecture given at the 42nd annual meeting of the Academy of Psychosomatic Medicine, 1995. *Psychosomatics*, **37**, 236–248.

Kornfeld, D., Zimberg, S. & Malm, J. R. (1965) Psychiatric complications of open-heart surgery. *New England Journal of Medicine*, **273**, 287–292.

Leventhal, H., Nerenz, D. R. & Steele, D. J. (1984) Illness representations and coping with health threats. In *Handbook of Psychology and Health. Social Psychological Aspects of Heath* (ed. A. Baum), vol. IV, pp. 219–252. Hillsdale, NJ: Lawrence Erlbaum Associates.

Leventhal, H., Diefenbach, M. & Leventhal, E. A. (1992) Illness cognition: using common sense to understand treatment adherence and affect cognition interactions. *Cognitive Therapy and Research*, **16**, 143–163.

Lipowski, Z. J. (1986) Consultation–liaison psychiatry: the first half century *General Hospital Psychiatry*, **8**, 305–315.

Lloyd, G. G. (1977) Psychological reactions to physical illness. *British Journal of Hospital Medicine*, **18**, 352, 355–358.

MacHale, S. (2002) Managing depression in physical illness. *Advances in Psychiatric Treatment*, **8**, 297–306.

Maguire, P. (1985) Barriers to psychological care of the dying. *BMJ (Clinical Research Edition)*, **291**, 1711–1713.

Maguire, P. & Faulkner, A. (1988) Improve the counselling skills of doctors and nurses in cancer care. *BMJ*, **297**, 847–849.

Maguire, P. & Parkes, C. M. (1998) Surgery and loss of body parts. *BMJ*, **316**, 1086–1088.

Markowitz, J. C., Klerman, G. L. & Perry, S. W. (1992) Interpersonal psychotherapy of depressed HIV-positive outpatients. *Hospital Community Psychiatry*, **43**, 885–890.

Marmot, M. G., Smith, G. D., Stansfeld, S., *et al* (1991) Health inequalities among British civil servants: the Whitehall II study. *Lancet*, **337**, 1387–1393.

Mayou, R. (1989) The history of general hospital psychiatry. *British Journal of Psychiatry*, **155**, 764–776.

Mayou, R. (1995) Introduction: the relationship between physical and psychiatric pathology. In *Psychiatric Aspects of Physical Disease* (ed. C. Mallinson), pp. 3–7. London: Royal College of Physicians.

Mayou, R. & Hawton, K. (1986) Psychiatric disorder in the general hospital. *British Journal of Psychiatry*, **149**, 172–190.

Mayou, R., Hawton, K. & Feldman, E. (1988) What happens to medical patients with psychiatric disorder? *Journal of Psychosomatic Research*, **32**, 541–549.

Mayou, R., Seagroatt, V. & Goldacre, M. (1991) Use of psychiatric services by patients in a general hospital. *BMJ*, **303**, 1029–1032.

Mayou, R. A., Gill, D., Thompson, D. R., *et al* (2000) Depression and anxiety as predictors of outcome after myocardial infarction. *Psychosomatic Medicine*, **62**, 212–219.

Meakin, C. J. (1992) Screening for depression in the medically ill. The future of paper and pencil tests. *British Journal of Psychiatry*, **160**, 212–216.

Mechanic, D. (1978) Illness behaviour. In *Medical Sociology*, pp. 249–289. New York: Free Press.

Mechanic, D. (1986) The concept of illness behaviour: culture, situation and personal predisposition. *Psychological Medicine*, **16**, 1–7.

Michelson, D., Stratakis, C., Hill, L., *et al* (1996) Bone mineral density in women with depression. *New England Journal of Medicine*, **335**, 1176–1181.

Miller, W. & Rollnick, S. (2002) *Motivational Interviewing: Preparing People for Change* (2nd edn). New York: Guilford Press.

Moffic, H. S. & Paykel, E. S. (1975) Depression in medical inpatients. *British Journal of Psychiatry*, **126**, 346–353.

Neilson, E., Brown, G. W. & Marmot, M. (1989) Myocardial infarction. In *Life Events and Illness* (eds G. W. Brown & T. O. Harris), pp. 313–342. London: Guilford Press.

Parsons, T. (1951) *The Social System*. London: Routledge and Kegan Paul.

Perry, S. W. & Cella, D. F. (1987) Over-diagnosis of depression in the medically ill. *American Journal of Psychiatry*, **144**, 125–126.

Perry, S., Difede, J., Musngi, G., *et al* (1992) Predictors of post traumatic stress disorder after burn injury. *American Journal of Psychiatry*, **149**, 931–935.

Petrie, K. J., Weinman, J., Sharpe, N., *et al* (1996) Role of patients' view of their illness in predicting return to work and functioning after myocardial infarction: longitudinal study. *BMJ*, **312**, 1191–1194.

Peveler, R., Feldman, E. & Friedman, T. (eds) (2000) *Liaison Psychiatry. Planning Services for Specialist Settings*. London: Gaskell.

Pratt, L. A., Ford, D. E., Crum, R. M., *et al* (1996) Depression, psychotropic medication, and risk of myocardial infarction. Prospective data from the Baltimore ECA follow up. *Circulation*, **94**, 3123–3129.

Pritchard, M. (1982) Psychological pressure in a renal unit. *British Journal of Hospital Medicine*, **27**, 512–516.

Protheroe, D., Turvey, K., Horgan, K., *et al* (1999) Stressful life events and difficulties and onset of breast cancer: case control study. *BMJ*, **319**, 1027–1030.

Rabins, P. V. & Folstein, M. F. (1982) Delirium and dementia: diagnostic criteria and fatality rates. *British Journal of Psychiatry*, **140**, 149–153.

Ramirez, A. & House, A. (1997) ABC of mental health. Common mental health problems in hospital. *BMJ*, **314**, 1679–1681.

Robertson, M. M. & Katona, C. L. E. (eds) (1997) *Depression and Physical Illness. Perspectives in Psychiatry*. Chichester: Wiley.

Rodin, G. & Daneman, D. (1991) Eating disorders in patients with diabetes. *American Journal of Psychiatry*, **148**, 957.

Royal College of Physicians & Royal College of Psychiatrists (2003) *The Psychological Care of Medical Patients* (Council Report CR108). London: Royal College of Psychiatrists.

Royal College of Surgeons of England & Royal College of Psychiatrists (1997) *Report of the Working Party on the Psychological Care of Surgical Patients* (Council Report CR55). London: Royal College of Psychiatrists.

Saravay, S. M. & Lavin, M. (1994) Psychiatric comorbidity and length of stay in the general hospital: a critical review of outcome studies. *Psychosomatics*, **35**, 233–252.

Scharloo, M., Kaptein, A. A., Weinman, J., *et al* (1998) Illness perceptions, coping and functioning in patients with rheumatoid arthritis, chronic obstructive pulmonary disease and psoriasis. *Journal of Psychosomatic Research*, **44**, 573–585.

Seltzer, A. (1989) Prevalence, detection and referral of psychiatric morbidity in general medical patients. *Journal of Royal Society of Medicine*, **82**, 410–412.

Sensky, T. (1990) Patients' reactions to illness. *BMJ*, **300**, 622–623.

Series, H. G. (1992) Drug treatment of depression in medically ill patients. *Journal of Psychosomatic Research*, **36**, 1–16.

Sharpe, M., Protheroe, D. & House, A. (2000) Joint working with physicians and surgeons. In *Liaison Psychiatry. Planning Services for Specialist Settings* (eds R. Peveler, E. Feldman & T. Friedman), pp. 195–206. London: Gaskell.

Sheikh, J. I. & Yesavage, J. A. (1986) Geriatric Depression Scale (GDS): recent evidence and development of a shorter version. *Clinical Gerontology*, **5**, 165–173.

Snaith, R. P., Bridge, G. W. & Hamilton, M. (1976) The Leeds scale for the self-assessment of anxiety and depression. *British Journal of Psychiatry*, **128**, 156–165.

Spiegel, D., Bloom, J. R. & Yalom, I. (1981) Group support for patients with metastatic cancer. A randomised outcome study. *Archives of General Psychiatry*, **38**, 527–533.

Spiegel, D., Bloom, J. R., Kraemer, H., *et al* (1989) Psychological support for cancer patients. *Lancet*, **ii**, 1447.

Stenager, E. N. & Stenager, E. (1992) Suicide and patients with neurologic diseases. Methodologic problems. *Archives of Neurology*, **49**, 1296–1303.

Stoudemire, A. & Thompson, T. L. (1983) Medication non-compliance: systematic approaches to evaluation and intervention. *General Hospital Psychiatry*, **5**, 233–239.

Sutherland, A. M., Orbach, C. E., Dyk, R. B., *et al* (1952) The psychological impact of cancer and cancer surgery. I. Adaptation to the dry colostomy; preliminary report and summary of findings. *Cancer*, **5**, 857–872.

Thompson, D. R. & Meddis, R. (1990) A prospective evaluation of in-hospital counselling for first time myocardial infarction in men. *Journal of Psychosomatic Research*, **34**, 237–248.

Von Korff, M., Gruman, J., Schaefer, J., *et al* (1997) Collaborative management of chronic illness. *Annals of Internal Medicine*, **127**, 1097–1102.

Watson, M., Haviland, J. S., Greer, S., *et al* (1999) Influence of psychological response on survival in breast cancer: a population-based cohort study. *Lancet*, **354**, 1331–1336.

Weissman, A. D. & Hackett, T. P. (1958) Psychosis after eye surgery: establishment of a specific doctor–patient relationship in prevention and treatment of black patch delirium. *New England Journal of Medicine*, **258**, 1284–1289.

Wells, K. B., Golding, J. M., Burnam, M. A., *et al* (1988) Psychiatric disorder in a sample of the general population with and without chronic medical conditions. *American Journal of Psychiatry*, **145**, 976–981.

White, C. A. (2001) *Cognitive Behaviour Therapy for Chronic Medical Problems: A Guide to Assessment and Treatment in Practice*. Chichester: Wiley.

Wood, B. C. & Mynors-Wallis, L. M. (1997) Problem solving therapy in palliative care. *Palliative Medicine*, **11**, 49–54.

World Health Organization (1992) *The ICD-10 Classification of Mental and Behavioural Disorders*. Geneva: WHO.

Wulsin, L. R., Vaillant, G. E. & Wells, V. E. (1999) Systematic review of the mortality of depression. *Psychosomatic Medicine*, **61**, 6–17.

Zigmund, A. S. & Snaith, R. P. (1983) The Hospital Anxiety and Depression Scale. *Acta Psychiatrica Scandinavica*, **67**, 361–370.

Zung, W. W., Richards, C. B. & Short, M. J. (1965) Self-rating depression scale in an outpatient clinic. Further validation of the SDS. *Archives of General Psychiatry*, **13**, 508–515.

CHAPTER 18

Clinical features of the personality and impulse control disorders

Patricia Casey

This chapter describes the main clinical and diagnostic features of the classical personality disorders, but also includes at the end a short section on the impulse control disorders. The next chapter reviews the management and outcome of the personality disorders.

History

The history of the personality disorders is among the lengthiest in psychiatry, going back to Hippocrates. It is a tale of ever-changing approaches to classifying these conditions and, until recently, with very little in the way of scientific enquiry.

The theory of Hippocrates, that disorders of personality stem from an excess or imbalance of the four humours, held sway for more than two millennia. The humours consisted of yellow bile from the liver, which corresponded to the choleric humours; black bile from the spleen, secreted under the influence of the planet Saturn, which corresponded to the melancholic; blood, which corresponded to the sanguine; and phlegm, which corresponded to the phlegmatic. According to the Greek philosopher Empedocles, the humours themselves were the embodiments of the four basic elements of the universe: earth, water, fire and air. Theophrastus, a pupil of Hippocrates, went on to describe systematically some 30 or more different personality types, some of which show a resemblance to those outlined in modern schemes; for example, the 'reckless man' of Theophrastus appears to have antisocial personality disorder.

The idea that the shape of the brain and body is responsible for various character types was promulgated by Franz Joseph Gall in the late 18th century and from this he developed the science of phrenology. He started to map in detail the shapes of people's skulls, in turn linking them with the shape of the brain, and ultimately with the person's character. The vision of Gall is now beginning to be realised, as modern radiological techniques have augmented our knowledge of the brain changes associated, in particular, with psychopathy.

Kretschmer (1922) provided an early description of personality *types*, which he associated with different bodily physiques: stocky individuals were described as pyknic, and prone to manic depression, while thin ('asthenic') individuals were more liable to schizophrenia. His American disciple, Sheldon (1940), tried to correlate three bodily types with different temperaments. Endomorphy (predominance of body roundness and softness) was associated with a 'viscerotonic' temperament, characterised by gregariousness, the love of comfort, relaxation and avoidance of pain. Mesomorphy (muscular and connective tissue dominance) was associated with a 'somatotonic temperament', which amounted to being assertive, physical, energetic, indifferent to pain and callous. Ectomorphy (linearity and fragility of structure) had a 'cerebrotonic temperament', characterised by a tendency to restraint, introversion, social awkwardness and a desire for solitude. However, this schema, like many others, is little used and has passed into history.

Personality, character, temperament and traits

The origins of the word 'personality' come from the amphitheatres of ancient Greece and Rome. *Persona* is the Latin word for mask. The Romans took the word from the Greek theatre, where the actors wore masks and used a megaphone, through (*per*) which the sound (*sona*) was magnified. *Personality* therefore represented an amplification of the voice and individual features that the actor was trying to portray (Stone, 1993). The word 'character' is derived from the Greek word *charasso*, which means to dig in or engrave, and refers to those characteristics that have been acquired early in life.

More innate or constitutional aspects of behaviour are sometimes referred to as the person's 'temperament' (Latin *temperare* = mixture, due measure; *mens* = mind). The term is more often used in child psychiatry to describe the manner in which a child behaves rather than the specific behaviours themselves.

The term 'trait' also describes the manner of behaviour but is applied in adult psychiatry to describe more specific features of the personality, and the modern concept of personality disorder is firmly rooted in trait psychology. The best known of these 'trait' approaches is that of Jung (1921), who described introversion and extroversion, traits that were later extensively studied by Eysenck in his description of extroversion–introversion, neuroticism–stability and the psychoticism dimensions (Eysenck & Eysenck, 1964). This formulation has generated a huge amount of research in psychology, but has had a much lesser impact in the clinical world. Other trait formulations are reviewed by Millon (1981).

Kraepelin (1913), attempting to trace the origins of severe mental illness, described cyclothymia, which he believed predisposed to manic–depression, and the autistic temperament, which he thought predisposed to schizophrenia. He also distinguished 'psychopathic inferiority' from other psychiatric disorders, and provided clinical descriptions of the personality disorders; his classification would include individuals who were shiftless, liars, swindlers and trouble-makers.

The modern era of the systematic study of personality disorders begins with Schneider, who published *Psychopathic Personalities for Modern Classificatory Schemes* in 1923, which was translated into English only in 1950. He stressed that a personality disorder must always be judged by its effects on other people, whether they are friends, relations, colleagues or society as a whole. He defined clinically abnormal personalities as 'those who suffer or make society suffer on account of their abnormality', and he called them 'psychopathic'. Most modern definitions of personality disorders are ultimately based on Schneider's concept. His types included the hyperthymic, depressive, explosive, insecure, insensitive, anankastic, fanatic, attention-seeking, labile and affectionless. With some modification, most of these types have appeared in all the various DSM and ICD schemes, and also form the basis for the current DSM–IV and ICD–10 classifications (discussed below).

Psychoanalytical contributions

The analytical contribution has been especially important in the USA, and this is reflected in DSM–IV (American Psychiatric Association, 1994). The early analysts, such as Freud, linked the different character types to the oral, anal and phallic phases of development. The oral phase is divided in two. The first is an oral sucking phase, in which all food is accepted indiscriminately. Excessive indulgence during this phase was said to result in an oral dependent type: excessively dependent, gullible and 'able to swallow anything'. Later there is an oral biting phase, when food is sometimes aggressively chewed or rejected and then spat out. Frustration at this phase was said to lead to oral sadistic character formation, a pattern of pessimistic distrust, sarcasm and a tendency to be cantankerous. The anal phase was concerned with the acquisition of sphincter control, and frustration during this phase was thought to lead to later difficulties in areas of control and authority, as well as obsessional features. Difficulties during the phallic phase were thought to result in sexual impulses being excessively self-orientated, rather than directed towards others of the opposite sex, resulting in phallic narcissistic character formation, and traits of being vain, brash or arrogant. Hysterical and masochistic types may also fail to mature appropriately through the genital phase of development.

Alexander (1930) believed that people with abnormal personalities often suffered from neuroses and advanced the concept of the neurotic character, which has been echoed more recently in the 'general neurotic syndrome' of Tyrer (1989).

Vaillant (1977) suggested that identification of the psychoanalytic defence mechanism typically used by a patient might form a basis for the classification of abnormal personality. The notion that a subject's defence mechanism may be of diagnostic importance is more widely accepted in the USA than elsewhere but it has been partially incorporated in DSM–IV. Thus a new scale and possibly a new axis, the 'Defense functioning scale', is included as 'proposed axes for further study' in DSM–IV, where the individual's defence mechanisms and coping styles are recorded.

Millon (1981) argued that the personality serves as a host mechanism, comparable to the immune system, offering protection against the many psychological and interpersonal stresses of living, and preventing symptom formation and breakdown. In common parlance the terms 'thin-skinned' and 'thick-skinned' neatly describe this aspect of a person's sensitivity to external stress. Stone (1993) has also emphasised the role of the *facade*, a false self outside the true personality that enhances survival in a potentially hostile world, and includes the ability to say nothing or to be tactful, and so forth.

Other analysts have emphasised 'ego psychology': the notion that the unconscious and the id are rather less important than the patient's ego and the experience of reality. Sullivan (1947) emphasised the role of anxiety and the need for security as well as the style of interpersonal relationships. Character types were described almost exclusively in terms of their relationships with others; for example, 'ambition-ridden' personalities were noted for their exploitativeness, competitiveness and unscrupulous manipulations. Adler (1964) emphasised 'over-compensation': an inborn tendency to counteract deficiencies and inadequacies through reparative striving. Undoing this over-compensation played a key role in therapy. Horney's (1939) typology had three groups: those who 'move towards people' in their relationships and who are compliant and self-effacing, with their self-esteem being determined by others (dependent types); those who 'move against others' in relationships and who are aggressive, see life as a struggle, seek power and exploit others (sociopathic types); and those who 'move away' from other people and who become detached and so avoid relationships and consequently lead restricted lives (avoidant and schizoid types).

More recently, Kernberg (1967) broke away from the former rigid adherence to the psychosexual developmental model and suggested a different structural model, based on the level of functioning. At the lowest and most primitive level are the antisocial characters, who have little or no concept of the existence or needs of other people. At an intermediate level are those who function at an infantile level, mainly borderline and narcissistic types. At a higher level are hysterical, obsessive–compulsive and depressive types, who are able to relate to others but not quite at the mature level.

The concept of personality disorder

The topic of personality disorders does not lend itself easily to the medical model. Everyone has a personality, and defining precisely where, on a continuum, normal personality changes into a personality problem and then into a personality disorder is necessarily arbitrary. Schneider's concept of a degree of suffering by the individual and by society is central here. Thus the dividing line is usually taken as where the personality disturbance results in impaired relationships and impaired social or occupational functioning (Schneider, 1923). The idea of functional impairment remains the cornerstone of modern understanding of personality disorder (Skodol *et al*, 2002).

Livesley (2001) lists five diverse concepts of personality disorder:

1 *As a forme fruste of major mental illness*. This particularly applies to schizotypal personality disorder, which appears to be part of the schizophrenia spectrum. This view has implications for whether personality disorders are invariably related to axis I disorders (i.e. clinical syndromes within the DSM system) or whether they should be classified on a separate axis (DSM axis II, which relates to developmental and personality disorders).

2 *As a failure to develop certain key components of the normal adult personality*. Personality disorders are therefore seen as a type of immaturity, with deficits in learning to control impulses, show remorse and other functions usually associated with the super-ego.

3 *As a particular form of personality structure*. An example would be Kernberg's (1967) concept of borderline personality organisation, which is defined in terms of identity diffusion, primitive defences and reality testing.

4 *As social deviance*. A prime example would be the sociopath.

5 *As an abnormality in the statistical sense*. This represents personality disorder as a deviation from normal personality structure. This was Schneider's approach, but for Schneider the statistical abnormality, to be clinically meaningful, had to be associated with 'suffering to themselves or to other people'.

Trait psychology and ICD and DSM

Personality disorder can also be defined on the basis of trait psychology. According to DSM–IV, personality traits are enduring patterns of perceiving, relating and thinking about the environment and oneself, and are exhibited in a wide range of social and personal contexts. They describe the underpinnings of the behaviour pattern, but not specific behaviours themselves. Maladaptive traits can combine to form a limited number of categories of personality disorder, defined in the ICD–10 and DSM–IV schemes (see Table 18.1, below). The limited number of categories fails to do justice to the rich tapestry of morbid human personality, but they probably give the best available scheme in the light of present knowledge. Disorders of personality are usually recognisable in adolescence or early adult life, and persist until middle age, when at least some, particularly the 'dramatic' (see Table 18.1), seem to wane. ICD–10 provides a lucid statement of what constitutes personality disorder, encompassing most of the main features:

> 'These types of condition comprise deeply ingrained and enduring behavior patterns manifesting themselves as inflexible responses to a broad range of personal and social situations. They represent either extreme or significant deviations from the way the average individual in a given culture perceives, thinks, feels and particularly relates to others. Such behavior patterns tend to be stable and become multiple domains of behavior and social functioning. They are frequently, but not always, associated with various degrees of subjective distress and problems in social functioning and performance.' (World Health Organization, 1992)

Dimensions versus categories

Classification systems in psychiatry are based on categorical diagnosis and the underpinning principle in both the DSM and ICD is that the various categories constitute discrete entities that can be distinguished from other disorders. For personality disorders this model suggests that the specific categories are distinct from each other and that personality disorders represent a distinct constellation of features that distinguish them from 'normal' personality.

This oversimplification has the advantage of facilitating easy communication between professionals. However, it is clear that this categorical model has no empirical basis when applied to personality disorder, since most maladaptive traits merge imperceptibly into normality: they are continuously distributed in both the personality-disordered and non-personality-disordered populations, rather than displaying a bimodal distribution.

Although there is little difficulty in distinguishing those with and without the broad diagnosis of personality disorder, agreement in relation to specific categories is notoriously unreliable. Overall reliability is high when structured interviews are used (see below) and is highest for antisocial personality disorder (Zimmerman, 1994). In addition, there is considerable overlap between the individual categories, and one study found that 34 subjects received a total of 92 axis II diagnoses (Sara *et al*, 1996). The lack of specificity for the individual categories is particularly evident for the 'dramatic' cluster of personality disorder.

There is now a sizeable body of evidence that the dimensional approach to measuring personality has greater validity than the categorical one (Livesley *et al*, 1994). A further advantage of the dimensional system is that it allows for the measurement of shades of personality abnormality, in contrast to the dichotomous approach used in making categorical diagnoses. A dimensional system allows for the measurement of personality in everybody and not just those labelled as having a personality disorder. However, a dimensional approach, although more accurate, is just not amenable to the clinical situation, and so the categorical system remains deeply embedded in clinical practice.

There are at least four dimensional models:

1 Eysenck's three-dimensional model, in which the three dimensions are extroversion, neuroticism and psychoticism (although Eysenck's psychoticism refers more to psychopathic tendencies than to the functional psychoses) (Eysenck & Eysenck, 1964).

2 Costa & McRea's (1992) five-factor model, which is based on general population studies of personality, spanning more than half a century. The five factors are: neuroticism, extroversion, openness to experience, agreeableness and conscientiousness.

3 Livesley's (2001) four-dimensional model, also based mainly on general population studies, but using the items in the DSM–III personality description as a starting point. His four factors are: emotional dysregulation, dissocial behaviour, inhibitedness, and compulsivity.

4 Cloninger's (1987) three-factor model, in which each dimension is linked with a biological substrate. Thus novelty seeking is linked to dopamine, harm avoidance to serotonin, and reward dependence to noradrenaline.

Again, while dimensional approaches have dominated psychological thinking and research in personality disorder, they have not had a similar impact in the clinical world.

Differences between ICD–10 and DSM–IV

Although there are considerable areas of agreement between the schemes, there are some differences. The main difference lies in the type and number of categories included in each classification, as shown in Table 18.1. DSM–IV describes criteria for narcissistic personality disorder, which is not represented in ICD–10. This reflects the ongoing influence of psychodynamic schools in the USA. Because of its close genetic connection with schizophrenia, schizotypal disorder is classified with schizophrenic disorders in ICD–10, but remains within the personality disorder section in DSM–IV. Both schemes have removed cyclothymic personality from the personality disorders section and included it within the affective disorders. Borderline personality disorder, which has an extensive section in DSM–IV, has been incorporated as a subtype of emotionally unstable personality in ICD–10.

For diagnostic assessment, DSM–IV tends to favour the clinician's interview with the patient, while ICD–10 emphasises the role of informants as well as of subjects themselves, although data from informants may also be used in making a DSM–IV diagnosis.

DSM–IV groups the personality disorders into three groups. The first group, cluster A, or the eccentric disorders, includes paranoid, schizoid and schizotypal disorder. Cluster B, the dramatic group, includes antisocial, borderline, histrionic and narcissistic personality disorders. Cluster C includes the avoidant, dependent and obsessive–compulsive personality disorders. Individuals with these disorders often appear anxious or fearful and so both the terms 'anxious' and 'fearful' have been used in the literature to describe the personality disorders in the cluster C group. ICD–10 does not have corresponding clusters.

A final difference is the way in which the two schemes meet the problem of patients who cannot be easily placed into the existing categories. Some patients meet the criteria for several categories of personality disorder, and DSM–IV directs the clinician to record all the possible diagnoses; thus, if borderline *and* schizotypal criteria are met, then both conditions should be diagnosed, while ICD–10 has a category called 'mixed personality disorder'.

DSM–IV also has a category 'personality disorder not otherwise specified'. It includes people who are socially impaired with relationship difficulties yet who fail to meet the diagnostic criteria of any one subtype. This category is also used to include other subtypes, such as impulsive or immature types. Finally, ICD–10 includes a category of 'enduring personality changes', in which the personality changes are regarded as being permanent following catastrophic experiences or psychiatric illness. Although revisions of the ICD and DSM schemes are planned, it is premature to speculate on what the new features of ICD–11 and DSM–V are likely to be.

Table 18.1 DSM–IV and ICD–10 personality disorders

DSM–IV	ICD-10	Main features
Cluster A: Paranoid ('eccentric')		
	Paranoid	Suspicious, feelings of perception
Schizoid	Schizoid[a]	Cold, detached, isolated
Schizotypal		Isolated, eccentric ideas
Cluster B: Antisocial ('dramatic')		
	Dissocial	Behaviour disorder, callous, antisocial acts
	Emotionally unstable (impulsive[b] and borderline)	Instability of mood, behaviour, unstable relationships
Histrionic	Histrionic	Shallow, dramatic, egocentric
Narcissistic[c]		Self-centred, grandiosity, entitlement
Cluster C: Avoidant ('fearful')		
Avoidant	Anxious	Hypersensitive, timid, self-conscious
Dependent	Dependent	Submissive, helpless
Obsessive–compulsive		Doubt, caution, obsessional
	Anankastic	
Additional personality disorder not otherwise specified	Mixed and other personality disorders	No predominant pattern of any categories of the above, but still impaired

[a] Schizotypal disorder is classified in the section on schizophrenia.
[b] Impulsive personality disorder is in ICD–10 but not DSM–IV, which instead includes intermittent explosive disorder, in the 'Habit and impulsive disorders' section.
[c] Narcissistic personality disorder is not included in ICD–10.

A critique of the concept

Many criticisms have been levelled at the concept of personality disorder, from sources as varied as philosophy and psychology, as well as from psychiatry itself. These have been enumerated by Westen & Shedler (1999) and include the following concerns:

- The categories are not empirically based and they often disagree with established findings from factor and cluster analysis.
- The comorbidity between categories is high and patients often receive several personality disorder diagnoses out of a possible 10, which tends to invalidate the concept of diagnosis (which is meant to assign only one 'name' to a particular condition or patient).
- The criteria for each diagnosis are not weighted between those of differing diagnostic importance. For example, in making an overall assessment of an antisocial personality disorder, callousness may be a more important trait than failing to learn from experience, or may at least have far graver implications (e.g. in a forensic setting).
- The current concepts fail to consider personality strengths, which protect against personality disorder. For instance, a patient with narcissistic traits may not have full-blown narcissistic personality if there also is a capacity for warmth and empathy, yet by counting only the negative traits such a diagnosis might be made.
- The current system fails to address the wide range of personality pathologies for which patients seek help. For example, many subjects fall short of personality disorder as presently diagnosed yet lead quite impaired lives, with problems such as recurring dysfunctional relationships and low self-esteem.
- The categories fail to recognise the continuum from no personality disorder to moderate or severe personality disorder.
- The categories are not as clinically useful as they might be. Thus, assigning an axis II diagnosis tells the clinician little about the best treatment to apply or even which personality processes to target for treatment.
- The schedules for assessing personality show poor test–retest reliability and there is poor concordance between schedules (see below). This creates problems, since personality disorder is by definition stable over time and the poor agreement between schedules raises questions about the validity of the diagnoses.

Are personality disorders illnesses or not?

Disorders that are almost impossible to define, which may have no actual symptoms, which are of unknown cause and which also lack any specific treatment barely fit into the medical concept of disease. On the other hand, personality disorders can cause a considerable amount of damage and are associated with an elevated mortality and morbidity. There is usually a worse outcome for any comorbid axis I disorder when it is complicated by an axis II disorder than when the axis I disorder occurs on its own.

It is argued that doctors who diagnose and treat personality disorders are arguably positing themselves as arbiters of social behaviour and as implicitly accepting that these are illnesses. This can result in legal conundrums such as the 'irresistible impulse', which has been used to explain the behaviour of some violent psychopathic individuals in forensic settings.

Lewis & Appleby (1988) pointed to the hazard of separating the personality disorders from the mental illnesses, in that it results in therapeutic neglect of those assigned a diagnosis of personality disorder, and they suggested the term should be abandoned. As Gunn (1988) pointed out, being 'ill' entitles a patient to certain types of medical care, hospitalisation and degrees of tolerance not normally accorded to other people. On the other hand, not being ill means 'being well', which implies responsibility for one's actions, and if those with personality disorders are simply viewed as having a behavioural problem it is tantamount to being 'bad', and such a formulation will often lead to the person being rejected by the healthcare system.

Another concern within the profession is that whatever term is used, it eventually becomes a term of opprobrium and the diagnosis is also often made on inadequate grounds. For example, Thompson & Goldberg (1987) found that over half of those diagnosed with histrionic personality disorder actually had none of the DSM–III features of this disorder; the term was being used rather indiscriminately to describe a group of manipulative and difficult individuals.

While all of the above criticisms may be valid, there can be little doubt that a diagnosis of personality disorder is associated not only 'with harm done to others' but also with a considerable degree of functional impairment. The latter has in fact recently been quantified: Skodol *et al* (2002) compared 668 people with personality disorders against a group of patients with major depression and found the former were only half as likely to be employed and also had significantly worse relationships with their parents and siblings. Scores on the DSM–IV axis V scale – the global assessment of function – for those with depression and those with personality disorder were similar, although over time many of the former will improve, whereas those with personality disorders will have lifelong impairment.

Even though the application of the illness model to the problem of personality disorder is of limited usefulness, these disorders are likely to remain conditions of medical concern for the foreseeable future, if only because of their high morbidity and mortality.

Epidemiology

Community samples

The early studies of community samples had serious flaws in their methods. The classification of personality disorder was vague, the disorder was generally equated with psychopathy, and non-clinicians were used to make the psychiatric assessments, which gives the possibility of misdiagnoses and over-reporting. One of the earliest community studies in psychiatry was when Essen-Möller (1956) somewhat heroically personally interviewed 2550 people in the community and applied predetermined clinical criteria to make the diagnoses and estimate the prevalence of psychiatric disorder. This study was a landmark as it was one of the first to incorporate both axis I and axis II diagnoses. He found that 29% of men and 19% of women had a definite or probable personality disorder; a further 13% and 38% respectively had asthenic (dependent) personalities, while 14% and 2% had 'asociality'.

Casey & Tyrer (1986), using the Personality Assessment Schedule (PAS; Tyrer & Alexander, 1979), found that 13% of subjects drawn from the community had a personality disorder. Explosive and anankastic types were most common, with the explosive type being more common in men, and the asthenic (dependent) type in women.

Zimmerman & Coryell (1990) interviewed 687 relatives of psychiatric patients and healthy controls using a structured interview and a self-report questionnaire. A higher prevalence was found using the structured interview (13.5%) than with the self-report questionnaire (10.3%) but there was no agreement between the schedules on the most common category, confirming the poor concordance between these two approaches to the diagnosis of personality disorder.

Maier *et al* (1992) applied DSM–III–R criteria to a German community sample and found a prevalence of personality disorder of 10.3%.

Studies have shown a trend for individuals with personality disorders to congregate in inner cities, particularly in disintegrated areas, and this probably explains urban/rural differences in reported prevalence rates. The natural history of most personality disorders, particularly the dramatic types, is to attenuate with advancing years (most subjects of those who fulfil the diagnostic criteria are under 45 years of age).

A large Australian community survey found that people with a personality disorder were about twice as likely to have days out of their usual role function (school, work, etc.) and that the degree of functional impairment was correlated in a linear fashion with the severity of the personality disorder as measured by the total number of diagnoses given to the individual (Jackson & Burgess, 2002).

Special populations

Parasuicide population

The parasuicide population has a high rate of personality disorder. Using the PAS, Casey (1989) found that 75–83% of men and 54–64% of women had a personality disorder, mainly of the explosive type, but suicide intent was independent of the diagnosis of personality disorder. Haw *et al* (2001), using a structured interview for DSM–IV, found that personality disorders, especially the anxious, anankastic and paranoid types, were present in 46% of patients who had deliberately harmed themselves.

There is a risk that an assumption may be made that when parasuicide occurs together with a diagnosis of personality disorder the episode will be less serious than in other patients. However, such an assumption is probably false, as both Casey (1989) and Suominen *et al* (2000) found that factors normally associated with completed suicide, such as lethality, hopelessness (a known predictor of subsequent suicide), suicide intent and impulsiveness, did not distinguish the two groups at the time of the episode. Parasuicide patients who have personality disorders will more frequently have a history of previous episodes and of psychiatric treatment than patients without a personality disorder. Great care must therefore be taken to avoid contaminating the assessment and management of parasuicide cases by the diagnosis of personality disorder.

Completed suicide

The development of the psychological autopsy as a method for evaluating the psychiatric status of those dying by suicide has facilitated the evaluation of personality disorder as well as axis I disorders in terms of their contributions to this outcome. A study from Taiwan of three ethnic groups (Cheng *et al*, 1997) showed that a high proportion of people dying by suicide had a personality disorder, of which the ICD–10 category of emotionally unstable was the most common (diagnosed in 27–57% of the samples). While comorbidity with severe depression was prominent, a diagnosis of emotionally unstable personality disorder was also an independent risk factor (Cheng *et al*, 2000).

Personality disorder was also a significant risk factor for suicide in the study by Foster *et al* (1997) in a Northern Ireland population. These authors found that having axis I and axis II (especially antisocial, avoidant or dependent) comorbidity increased the risk of suicide associated with an axis I disorder on its own. Overall, at least one axis II disorder was found in 44% of those dying by suicide and a current axis I disorder in 88%.

In another study, the occurrence of life events, especially those dependent on the victim's own behaviour, was shown to increase the risk of suicide among those with personality disorder relative to those suicide completers without personality disorder (Heikkinen *et al*, 1997).

General practice populations

Shepherd *et al* (1966) found that 5% of primary care attendees were assessed by their general practitioners (GPs) as having abnormal personalities. According to Casey *et al* (1984), of those identified by their GP as having 'conspicuous morbidity', the GP diagnosed 9% as having a personality disorder, while 6% were given this diagnosis by the research psychiatrist. When personality was assessed independently of mental state diagnosis using the PAS, 34% had an axis II diagnosis, of which the explosive type was the most common.

Patience *et al* (1995), using similar methods, found a prevalence of 26% for any personality disorder and those with such disorder were more often symptomatic, a factor that may explain the adverse effect of personality disorder on symptom and social outcome in depressive illness.

Using more recent diagnostic criteria, Moran *et al* (2000) confirmed a prevalence of 24% among consecutive general practice attenders for any personality disorder, and those in the DSM–IV cluster B group were particularly associated with psychiatric morbidity and also with unplanned surgery attendance. GPs identified 27% of attenders as having a personality disorder, but in this study those identified by the GPs were generally not the same as those identified by the research psychiatrist, which suggests that different constructs were being used by them to identify personality disorder.

Schafer & Nowlis (1998) found that patients identified as 'difficult' by family practitioners more often had unrecognised personality disorder than did control patients and that dependent rather than antisocial or borderline type predominated in this group.

In summary, then, it can at least be said that personality disorder may have a significant impact on the workload of GPs.

Psychiatric out-patients

High rates of personality disorder have been found among psychiatric out-patients. For example, Tyrer *et al* (1983), using the PAS and applying ICD–9 criteria, found that 39% of non-psychotic out-patients had a personality disorder. These high rates have been replicated in more recent studies. For new out-patients in the USA, Jackson *et al* (1991) gave a figure of 67% and Kass *et al* (1985) of 51%, with borderline type being the most frequent. An exception was the study by Fabrega *et al* (1993), who reported a much lower figure – of 13% with DSM–III criteria – which may be due to the problem of making a diagnosis of personality disorder after a single intake assessment.

Psychiatric in-patients

The publication of multi-axial diagnostic schemes such as DSM–III, which have explicit definitions, led to a substantial increase in the frequency with which the diagnosis of personality disorder was made among in-patients. Loranger (1990) compared the last 5 years of the DSM–II era (1975–80) with the first 5 years of the DSM–III era (1980–85) and showed that the rate of personality disorder diagnoses rose from 19% to 49%, with no change in admission policy for the unit studied.

Table 18.2 Frequency of different DSM–III personality disorders among psychiatric in-patients[a]

Personality disorder type	%
Paranoid	2.4
Schizoid	3.3
Schizotypal	4.1
Compulsive	2.9
Histrionic	2.3
Dependent	9.1
Antisocial	4.6
Narcissistic	5.9
Avoidant	2.4
Borderline	26.7
Passive aggressive	3.5
Atypical/mixed/other	32.6

After Loranger (1990).

[a] Of 10 914 admissions screened, 2916 fulfilled criteria for personality disorder. Note the residual category of atypical/mixed/other accounts for more cases than any specific type, but borderline personality disorder accounts for more than a quarter of the cases.

By far the most common categories were the borderline and 'mixed group', as shown in Table 18.2. This may be a reflection of the high comorbidity between borderline personality disorder and depression, since depression is one of the most common reasons for psychiatric admission.

Among in-patients receiving electroconvulsive therapy, 45% met the criteria for personality disorder when assessed using a combined informant/subject schedule (Casey & Butler, 1995), of which anankastic and avoidant were the most common. Among consecutive first-ever admissions, 26% of patients met the criteria for an axis II disorder, when the diagnosis was based on an informant schedule (Cooney *et al*, 1996).

Prison populations

Evaluating personality disorder in a prison population runs the risk of assuming that, because of antisocial behaviour, personality disorder is inevitably present. This leads to a circular argument that the behaviour is indicative of the disorder and the disorder explains the behaviour. Separating the criminal behaviour from underlying traits (e.g. callousness) is crucial if personality disorder is to be meaningfully evaluated in this population. In particular, high rates of antisocial personality disorder as defined by DSM–IV are present in prison populations (Singleton *et al*, 1998), but rather lower rates of 'psychopathic personality disorder' as defined by Hare's psychopathic checklist are found (Hare, 1991).

Overall, studies in prison have shown a high prevalence (39–76%) of antisocial personality disorder. The variation may be due to differences in the concentration of hardened career criminals in the various prisons. One study of a randomly selected sample of British prisoners (Singleton *et al*, 1998), using the Structured Clinical Interview for DSM–III–R (SCID–II), found that three-quarters of that population had a personality disorder, and antisocial personality disorder was identified in 63% of male remand prisoners, 49% of sentenced prisoners and 31% of female prisoners. Paranoid personality was the second most common category in male prisoners and borderline personality in female prisoners. Not surprisingly, other categories of personality disorder are seldom found among the prison population.

In an impressively large meta-analysis of 62 studies, from 12 countries and over 22 000 prisoners, Fazel & Danesh (2002) found very high rates of psychopathology, including personality disorder, in 65% of men, of whom 47% belonged to the antisocial category, while psychotic illnesses were present in 3.7% and major depression in 10%. Among women, 42% had a personality disorder, of whom half were diagnosed with the antisocial type; psychotic illness was diagnosed in 4% and major depression in 12%.

These findings demonstrate that prisoners, whether detained or sentenced, are approximately 10 times more likely to have antisocial personality disorder than their counterparts in the general population. A small but related group are those who are legally detained on the grounds of psychopathic behaviour and they comprise 0.24% of the general psychiatric hospital population but as many as 25% of the population of the special hospitals (Coid, 1993).

Categories of personality disorder

The individual disorders outlined in ICD–10 will be described first, and differences, if any, from the DSM–IV scheme mentioned. Descriptions are largely drawn from the account given by Millon (1981). Two categories of personality disorder, borderline and dissocial types, have been given some prominence in this account because people with these disorders have a high frequency of contact with medical, psychiatric and forensic services. The boxes that follow use ICD–10 criteria, and any differences from DSM–IV are noted. Prevalence data are taken from the review by Mattia & Zimmerman (2001), which pooled the results from the available studies, and heritabilities are taken from the large twin study of Torgersen *et al* (2000), except for antisocial personality disorder, where heritability data are taken from the large meta-analysis of Rhee & Waldman (2002).

Torgersen *et al* (2000) matched the Norwegian in-patient register with the Norwegian twin register and applied SCID-II interviews to isolate 221 same-sexed twin pairs (92 monozygotic and 129 dizygotic) where one twin had a definite personality disorder according to DSM–III–R criteria. Using this strict and epidemiologically sound methodology (i.e. the use of a national community sample, rather than a potentially biased clinical sample) they showed that the heritability for personality disorders as a whole (when assigned a DSM–III–R categorical diagnosis) was 0.60. This finding is compatible with much previous genetic research on the personality traits, which indicated heritabilities in the range 0.45–0.65. The findings for each cluster were: for the eccentric group (cluster A) 0.37; for the dramatic group (cluster B) 0.60; and for the anxious/fearful group (cluster C) 0.62. The heritabilities for individual personality disorders derived from this study are given in the relevant sections for each disorder.

Anankastic personality disorder (DSM–IV obsessive–compulsive personality disorder)

The obsessional or anankastic personality was first clearly described by Freud (1908). It is characterised by perfectionism, punctiliousness, indecisiveness, reluctance to take risks, rigidity and orderliness. People with an anankastic personality have difficulty with uncertainty and a great need to be in control. Chance has to be reduced to a minimum, and any unplanned situation is avoided. They like routine and may have a timetable for each day, which is not permitted to vary from week to week. They may be rigid in their views, lack spontaneity and in extreme cases insist on others adhering to their views and timetables, leading to disagreements.

They present as neat, stiff and formal, although they are rarely referred for this reason alone since these traits, in a milder form, may be valued by society. Minor degrees of obsessionality are not only commonplace but may even be desirable, when they underpin reliability and competence, a pattern that should not be classified as personality disorder. The ICD–10 diagnostic criteria are given in Box 18.1; those for DSM–IV are similar.

Box 18.1 ICD–10 criteria for anankastic personality disorder

1 Feelings of doubt and caution.
2 Preoccupation with details, rules, lists, etc.
3 Perfectionism that interferes with task completion.
4 Excessive conscientiousness and undue preoccupation with productivity to the exclusion of pleasure and interpersonal relationships.
5 Excessive pedantry and adherence to social conventions.
6 Unreasonable insistence by the patient that others submit exactly to his or her way of doing things; or unreasonable reluctance to allow others to do things.
7 Intrusion of insistence and unwelcome thoughts or impulses.

Three out of seven items are required for the diagnosis. DSM–IV describes 'obsessive–compulsive personality disorder', and the diagnosis is based on four out of eight items. These include items 1–6 above, but item 7 is excluded. The additional two items in DSM–IV are: a miserly spending style towards both self and others; and an inability to discard worthless objects, even when they have no sentimental value.

The median prevalence rate with DSM–III–R criteria was fairly high, at 3.7% (Mattia & Zimmerman, 2001); the personality type may be more common in rural than in urban areas (Casey & Tyrer, 1990).

Obsessional personalities may present with any axis I disorder. There is disagreement about whether obsessional personality forms the basis for obsessional symptoms, although there may be an association with obsessive–compulsive disorder (Tyrer *et al*, 1983). The belief that this type of personality is associated with endogenous depression is probably incorrect and stems from the error of assessing personality only when the patient is ill, when obsessional symptoms may be greatly exaggerated by the presence of depression (see also Chapter 15).

Hereditary factors may be aetiologically relevant; of all the categories of personality disorder studied by Torgersen *et al* (2000), obsessional personality disorder had the highest heritability – of 0.78. Clifford *et al* (1984) showed that obsessional traits and obsessional symptoms had heritability factors of 0.4 and 0.47, respectively.

Paranoid personality

Kretschmer (1918) described a condition he called paranoia sensitiva: an extraordinary sensitivity to rejection by others, and a consequent tendency to resist social contacts because of difficulty in trusting others and suspiciousness. These patients have a constant feeling of threat from others and are always on the alert for perceived dangers, and may even misinterpret common well-meaning gestures of courtesy as ploys to be used against them. Advice from friends that they are not under siege is not accepted, and others describe

Box 18.2 ICD–10 criteria for paranoid personality disorder

1 Excessive sensitivity to setbacks and rebuffs.
2 Tendency to bear grudges.
3 Suspiciousness, misconstrues neutral or friendly actions as hostile.
4 Combative sense of personal rights.
5 Recurrent suspicion, without justification, of sexual partners.
6 Excess in self-importance, self-referential attitude.
7 Preoccupied with unsubstantiated conspiratorial explanations.

Three out of the seven items are required for the diagnosis. DSM–IV excludes item 6 and instead has an item 'reluctant to confide in others because of unwarranted fear that the information will be used maliciously against him or her'.

them as touchy because they take offence easily. Sometimes they may be insensitive to the feelings of others, and fail to trust even those whom they should trust, such as parents or spouses. Not surprisingly, they are often disliked by colleagues, further heightening their sense of mistrust. They rarely seek help, owing to their lack of insight, blaming others instead for their behaviour. As a result of their mistrust of authority figures such as doctors, they rarely present for help.

Because paranoid personalities also have a high degree of anxiety associated with almost any type of attachment, they tend to become isolated and this leads to a gradual impairment of reality testing. These subjects maintain their self-esteem by projecting their malevolence onto others, by denying any personal weakness, and by self-aggrandisement through grandiose and persecutory fantasies. They may decompensate into fantasy, delusion or depression. Morbid jealousy of a non-delusional type sometimes occurs. A small number are querulous litigants, who may sue other people, often repeatedly, usually over trivial issues. The median prevalence rate is 1.0%; the heritability, according to Torgersen *et al* (2000), is lower than for other personality disorders, at 0.28.

An unusual complication of paranoid personality in old age is the so-called senile squalor or Diogenes syndrome. These people neglect themselves to a severe extent so that they end up living in extreme squalor. Macmillan & Shaw (1966) found that while half their cases were psychotic, the remainder had lifelong premorbid severe personality traits of being independent, suspicious, unfriendly, obstinate, secretive and quarrelsome, a pattern suggestive of paranoid personality disorder.

The ICD–10 criteria are shown in Box 18.2, and DSM–IV criteria differ little from these.

Differential diagnosis

Paranoia is a ubiquitous symptom and may be present in schizophrenia (particularly paranoid schizophrenia), organic disorders and affective disorders (both mania and depression). The main differential is from delusional disorder, in which the paranoia is of a psychotic type but, as with paranoid personality disorder, may also be very longstanding. Schizoid personalities share the aloofness of the paranoid personality but lack paranoid ideation. Some people with antisocial personality disorder are also paranoid, but apart from an occasional outburst those with paranoid personalities rarely commit antisocial acts.

Schizoid personality disorder

Bleuler (1922) first coined the term 'schizoidie' to describe a trait he believed was present in everyone, varying only in its degree of biological penetrance. In its full-blown form he suggested it led to schizophrenia, but in milder cases he thought it resulted in schizoid personality. The modern concept has at its core a profound lack of emotion, warmth or any concept of the normal give-and-take of human relationships. This prevents the patient from making or sustaining close relationships. Even in a mandatory situation such as work, communication tends to be formal or perfunctory.

Jobs involving the expenditure of physical or mental energy are generally shunned, and activities such as reading or watching television are preferred by people with a schizoid personality disorder. They rarely present with symptomatic complaints, and to others seem to be introspective and vague. Introspection about philosophy, science and religion are commonplace and may become the sole concern. The ICD–10 definition of schizoid personality disorder is shown in Box 18.3 and there are some minor differences from DSM–IV criteria. Prevalence is low and Mattia & Zimmerman (2001) gave a pooled median prevalence figure of 0.3%; the heritability is also low, at 0.29, which is much less than for schizotypal disorder (Torgersen *et al*, 2000).

Differential diagnosis

The condition is distinguished from schizophrenia by the absence of psychotic symptoms, although a

Box 18.3 ICD–10 criteria for schizoid personality disorder

1 Few, if any, activities provide pleasure.
2 Emotional coldness, detachment or flattened activity.
3 Limited capacity to express warmth, tender feelings or anger.
4 Apparent indifference to praise or criticism.
5 Little interest in sexual experience.
6 Preference for solitary activities.
7 Excessive preoccupation with fantasy and introspection.
8 Lack of close friends (or only one).
9 Insensitivity to social norms and conventions.

Three criteria must be met to make the diagnosis; onset is in early adulthood or before. DSM–IV stipulates four out of seven similar criteria, but excludes items 7 and 9 and includes another item 'neither desires nor enjoys close relationships including being part of a family'.

picture resembling schizoid personality can occur in the prodromal phase of schizophrenia. The distinction from simple schizophrenia is more difficult to make, but in simple schizophrenia the onset is usually later (18 or older), the premorbid personality may have been completely normal or even high functioning, and negative symptoms and social deterioration are rather more severe. Schizotypal disorder is associated with a greater degree of eccentric thought and behaviour, but the two disorders are often comorbid.

Isolation is also present in avoidant personalities, but they are fearful of rejection rather than simply uninterested and they are capable of warm and normal relationships within the family. A rare differential diagnosis is chronic depersonalisation syndrome, in which sufferers complain that they feel 'cut off' or 'outside themselves', but still maintain good human relationships and not the cold, isolated stance of those with schizoid personality disorder.

Autistic disorder is much more severe than the personality disorder and is usually diagnosed in early childhood; it is readily distinguished by the severe language disorder and very early onset.

Asperger's syndrome also enters into the differential diagnosis. This condition, first described by the Austrian psychiatrist Hans Asperger in 1944, is often mistaken for schizoid personality disorder. Although conceptualised by him as a variant of autism, some believe it is related to schizoid personality disorder, while others believe it overlaps with other developmental disorders. The condition has been reviewed by Rhinehart *et al* (2002). Unfortunately, little is known about its aetiology to justify its classification other than as a descriptive syndrome, but the concept has sufficient validity to be included in both ICD–10 and DSM–IV, where Asperger's syndrome is considered as one of the pervasive developmental disorders. Patients with Asperger's may present to adult psychiatric departments because of repeated social failure, eccentricities or other comorbid psychiatric disorders, especially obsessive–compulsive disorder, or to forensic psychiatrists because their peculiar lack of empathy may predispose a small minority of them to serious crimes. Although the condition is usually first diagnosed in childhood, it should always be considered before making a diagnosis of schizoid or schizotypal personality disorder. An excellent overview is provided by Wing (1981), and recent psychometric findings, which are complex, are reviewed by Rhinehart *et al* (2002).

Schizotypal personality disorder

This is not classified as a personality disorder in ICD–10, where it is instead is included with the schizophrenic disorders, as befits its genetic association with this condition. The term 'schizotypal' was first coined by the analyst Rado (1956) as an abbreviation of the 'schizophrenic phenotype'.

Clinical description

Like those with schizoid personalities, people with a schizotypal personality disorder are aloof and isolated, but their inner world is not so barren. There may be referential ideas, odd beliefs, magical thinking and suspiciousness, but these are not of delusional intensity. Unlike those with schizoid personalities, people with a schizotypal personality disorder have some degree of relatedness to others and a feeling of being part of the world. None the less, sometimes individuals complain of feelings of estrangement and depersonalisation, and they may socially isolate themselves for long periods. During these phases, there may be inappropriate affect, paranoid ideation, and communication in odd and circumstantial ways. The DSM–IV criteria are shown in Box 18.4. Prevalence is low: a median prevalence of 0.3% (based on 11 studies) was given by Mattia & Zimmerman (2001). Torgersen *et al* (2000) found a heritability of 0.57 for schizotypal personality disorder, but there has been a much greater interest in the possible genetic relationship with schizophrenia. Almost all family studies of schizophrenia have found an excess of both schizophrenia and schizotypal personality disorder among first-degree relatives. The inclusion of schizotypal personality for the twins of schizophrenic probands gives a higher concordance ratio for monozygotic:dizygotic twins than when the diagnosis is restricted to DSM–III schizophrenia alone (Farmer *et al*, 1987). Although the earlier family studies of schizotypal probands found only an excess of schizotypal but not schizophrenic relatives (Baron *et al*, 1983), others (Battaglia *et al*, 1991) have demonstrated a morbid risk for schizophrenia of around 5%. Miller *et al* (2002) confirmed that schizotypal personality disorder, but not isolated traits, may be a precursor of schizophrenia, especially when all the components of schizotypy were present, including social withdrawal, psychotic symptoms, socio-economic dysfunction and odd behaviour. These findings lend further weight to the view of schizotypy as a part of the schizophrenia spectrum of disorders.

Box 18.4 DSM–IV criteria for schizotypal personality disorder

1 Ideas of reference (not delusions of reference).
2 Excessive social anxiety.
3 Odd beliefs or magical thinking.
4 Unusual perceptual experiences (e.g. illusions).
5 Odd or eccentric behaviour or appearance.
6 No close friends or confidants (or only one), other than first-degree relatives.
7 Odd speech.
8 Inappropriate or constricted affect (e.g. silly or aloof).
9 Suspiciousness or paranoid ideation.

The disorder should have started in early adulthood, and five of the nine criteria are required for the diagnosis. The symptoms should not be due to schizophrenia or pervasive developmental disorder. In ICD–10, schizotypal disorder is classified together with the schizophrenias rather than with the personality disorders, although the ICD–10 text states that the course resembles that of a personality disorder and the criteria are broadly similar.

As well as the genetics, brain scan studies are also beginning to confirm the link with schizophrenia, although the observed changes in schizotypal disorder are not identical to those found in schizophrenia. Dickey *et al* (2002) reviewed 17 structured imaging studies (both computerised tomography and magnetic resonance imaging) of people with schizotypal personality disorder and on the available data suggested there were abnormalities in the superior temporal gyrus, parahippocampus, temporal horn region of the lateral ventricles, corpus callosum, thalamus and septum pellucidum as well as in total cerebrospinal fluid volume, and these changes were similar in type to those found in schizophrenia (see Chapter 8). The main differences between schizotypal personality disorder and schizophrenia were the lack of abnormalities in the medial temporal lobes and the lateral ventricles were of normal volume. Perhaps the normal functioning of the medial temporal lobes in individuals with the personality disorder in some way protects them from developing the psychosis. However, brain scanning studies suggest that schizotypal personality disorder probably represents a milder form of the disease, but that it lies among the schizophrenia spectrum disorders.

Dissocial personality disorder (psychopathy, sociopathy, antisocial personality disorder)

History

Pinel (1806) wrote of a condition called 'manie sans delire'. Among his cases he described a non-psychotic but ill-tempered French nobleman who, in a fit of rage, pushed a woman down a well. Pritchard (1835) described a condition called 'moral insanity', which comprised 'a morbid perversion of the natural feelings, tempers, moral dispositions and natural impulses without any defect in intellectual reason and functions or any insane delusions or hallucinations'. Back in France, Trelat (1861) coined the term 'folie lucide' to describe 'lucid madmen who in spite of their disturbed reason respond to all questions to the point and to the superficial observer looked quite normal', while impulsive behavioural states such as homicidal and suicidal monomanias were held to be cases of 'impulsive insanity' in the scheme of Dagonet (1870).

There are many 20th-century contributions to this subject. Henderson (1939) described three psychopathic types – aggressive, inadequate and creative – the last accounting for the high intelligence found among some deviant characters. Cleckley (1941) provided a series of detailed clinical descriptions of psychopathic individuals in his seminal book *The Mask of Sanity*, including a minister of the church, a lawyer, a physician and even a psychiatrist! Based on the traits that Cleckley suggested were core features of the psychopath; Hare (1991) developed a checklist of 20 items, the Revised Psychopathic Checklist (PCL–R), which forms the basis of much quantitative research into the subject.

Epidemiology

Antisocial personality disorder is the only category of personality disorder that has been consistently included in community surveys. Sociocultural and religious factors and changes in the social fabric of society may affect the rate, with societies that are fragmented having higher rates than those that are close-knit and homogeneous. Thus, low rates were found in Taiwan, ranging from 0.03% in rural settings to 0.14% in the capital (Hwu *et al*, 1989). The Epidemiologic Catchment Area study (Myers *et al*, 1984) found a rate of 3.7% in the 18- to 44-year age group, but only 1.4% in the 45- to 64-year age group, giving an overall prevalence of 2.7%.

Cooke & Michie (1999) drew on the 'individualistic–collectivist' construct of cross-cultural psychology to explain these large cultural differences. Individualistic cultures emphasise competitiveness, self-confidence and independence from others, and short-term relationships are common. By way of contrast, within collectivistic cultures subservience to the social group is emphasised, the acceptance of authority is paramount and long-term, stable relationships are common. An individualistic society such as the USA, with its emphasis on competitiveness and rivalry between individuals, is likely to promote the expression of features of antisocial personality disorder, whereas collectivistic societies – such as exist in Taiwan and among the Hulterites – will bear down on self-expression and promote stable and family relationships, and may have low rates.

Around 6.5% of all psychiatric patients have 'antisocial reactions', but higher rates, of around 18%, are observed among attenders at psychiatric emergency clinics (Robins, 1985).

The male:female ratio for the DSM–III definition of the disorder is 6:1, but when the older Schneiderian trait-based criteria are applied the ratio is lower.

Helgason (1964) observed that psychopathy occurred in 16% of men who emigrated from Iceland, while the rate was only 5% for those who remained behind; there was a rather smaller difference for women. Robins (1985) has made the interesting speculation that the higher crime rate observed in the USA than in Europe might be at least partially explained by repeated selective migration, because the American population is largely made up of successive generations of European immigrants. Higher rates are also found in urban rather than rural settings. An effect for lower social class is doubtful, and if present is likely to be small.

Clinical description

These individuals may be charming, brusque, or belligerent in their manner. There is generally an inner coldness, coupled with insensitivity to the feelings of others and a lack of empathy. People with severe antisocial personality disorder are obviously callous, and some will have committed serious crimes. In social or family situations there is a tendency to try to dominate, or at the very least demean, other people. Confrontation on some personal issue may provoke revenge, and among those with poor impulse control this may rapidly escalate into violence.

Dissocial individuals usually have a clear intellectual grasp of the moral values of society, and may even superficially acknowledge that they should change their behaviour. They repeatedly fail to learn from experience, or fail to respond to conventional regimes of punishment. Some may be so grossly insensitive as to be genuinely unaware of the feelings of others, but most are all too keenly aware of the foibles and weaknesses of other people and take advantage of them. A sham apology, or expression of contrition, may sometimes be made, but there is little genuine guilt or remorse.

Boredom and a low tolerance of frustration are common and they are often unable to sustain the tedium of a job, or the day-to-day responsibilities of a marriage. They may resort to thrill-seeking behaviours, such as gambling, promiscuity or substance misuse. In spite of their almost total lack of respect for the rights of others, many have a superficial charm and a mask of civility, but eventually the mask drops.

While some people with the condition (perhaps in extreme form) may become criminals, it is important to note that the majority do not. Perhaps it is only the unsuccessful psychopaths who end up in prison. One study showed that serious felonies occurred only in around a fifth of those who fulfilled criteria for antisocial personality disorder. Rather more frequent are problems with aggression, work and promiscuity. Men tend to have more illegal occupations, traffic offences, arrests and greater promiscuity. Women with antisocial personality disorder more often deserted or hit their spouses, manifested child neglect and failed to work steadily.

Two psychodynamic mechanisms are commonly employed by sociopaths – rationalisation and projection. Aggressive behaviour and unkind actions are rationalised by viewing them as 'hard but honest' (those with a more vivid imagination resort to lying). Projection and projective identification permits individuals to disown their own malevolent impulses and attribute them to others. Attacks on other people are then justified, as subjects view themselves as the persecuted victim. Millon (1981) pointed out that there are many more people with milder psychopathic traits who are neither criminal nor sufficiently dysfunctional to satisfy current diagnostic criteria. The ruthless, conniving business person, the brutalising sergeant or the vindictive head teacher all discharge their hostile impulses under the guise of their respectable occupation.

Diagnosis and differential diagnosis

Equating criminality (a behaviour) with sociopathy (a personality type) has led to much confusion. Most criminals are neither sociopathic nor mentally ill, although some people with a dissocial personality may get involved in crime and it is this group who commonly become recidivists.

In a few cases of chronic schizophrenia, personality deterioration resulting in lack of inhibition may lead to a picture resembling sociopathy. During the early phases of mania there may be increased aggression, rudeness and insensitivity, which may be indistinguishable from aggressive sociopathy. A variety of brain lesions may lead to an organic personality change where disinhibition and even minor criminal acts can occur, but the good premorbid history and history of a brain lesion/trauma usually make the diagnosis obvious.

Reid (1985) advises caution when applying the label to individuals in late adolescence or early adulthood, particularly to those from disruptive environments. Many such young delinquents lack the inner affectionless core and will later mature out of their antisocial behaviour.

The label itself is damaging, and should not be applied unless the pattern has persisted for many years.

Comorbidity

The Epidemiological Catchment Area study found no association between antisocial personality disorder and anxiety, phobic disorder, obsessive–compulsive disorder, depression, mania or schizophrenia. The only disorders associated with antisocial personality disorder were alcoholism and substance misuse, confirming many of the earlier studies. Among women there was an association with somatisation disorder and a correlation was found between the number of antisocial and somatic symptoms. These findings echo earlier observations on Briquet's syndrome (see Chapter 16) that personality disorder of the 'hysterical' type is linked to antisocial behaviour and this finding has also been confirmed in family studies. The presence of raised rates of depression and anxiety among treated samples (in contrast to their low or normal rates in epidemiological community studies, i.e. non-clinical samples) has led Robins (1985) to suggest that those with antisocial personality disorder present to the psychiatric services and seek treatment only for their axis I disorder and not for their personality problems, even though the latter may seem to be gross and obvious to others.

Among those legally detained with antisocial personality disorder in a special hospital Coid (1993) observed much higher rates of comorbidity with affective disorder, as well as with other personality disorders, in particular paranoid disorder in men and borderline disorder among women.

Classification

ICD–10 defines dissocial personality disorder as shown in Box 18.5. The DSM–IV criteria are similar to the ICD–10 ones but use the term 'antisocial personality disorder', differing only in the stipulation that there should be some evidence of conduct disorder before the age of 15.

Violent offences

The association between 'psychopathy' and violent offences has been reviewed by Hart & Hare (1997), and many of the studies in that review base their assessment on Hare's PCL, which provides a quantitative estimate of the severity of the disorder. In criminal populations, psychopaths (those with high scores on the PCL–R) are more likely to be 'high-density' offenders (5.5 versus 3.7 offences per year) than non-psychopaths. Psychopaths also have much higher rates of within-institution misbehaviour (6.7 versus 0.7 offences per year). High scores on the PCL–R are strongly associated with violent offences, especially convictions for possession of weapons, robbery, assault, kidnapping and vandalism.

Violent offences committed by dissocial subjects are distinguished from violent actions committed by non-dissocial individuals by being more callous, more aggressive and more commonly associated with a 'macho' display; the age of first arrest is somewhat younger for dissocial subjects. Victims are generally male and unknown to the subject. Episodes more often

Box 18.5 ICD–10 criteria for dissocial personality disorder

Personality disorder usually coming to attention because of a gross disparity between behaviour and the prevailing social norms, characterised by:

1 callous unconcern for the feelings of others
2 gross irresponsibility, disregard for social norms, rules and obligations
3 incapacity to maintain enduring relationships, although no difficulty in establishing them
4 low tolerance to frustration; low threshold for discharge of aggression, including violence
5 incapacity to experience guilt and profit from experience, particularly punishment
6 marked proneness to blame others, or to offer plausible rationalisations.

DSM–IV criteria are slightly different and include traits of recklessness for the safety of the self and others; and also deceitfulness and conning, as indicated by repeated lying and the use of aliases. DSM–IV does not include item 3 of ICD–10 (incapacity to maintain enduring relationships) as part of its criteria, and specifies that the individual should be at least 18 years old and have shown evidence of conduct disorder before the age of 15; also the antisocial behaviour should not occur exclusively in the course of schizophrenia or a manic episode.

occur in association with alcohol. Violent episodes caused by non-dissocial individuals generally have more understandable motives, and there is usually an affective colouring to the episode, with their victims being more commonly female (Williamson *et al*, 1987). The violence of psychopaths is often motivated by revenge or retribution, whereas non-psychopaths tend to commit acts while in a state of extreme emotional arousal.

Cornell *et al* (1996) examined instrumental (i.e. predatory) versus reactive violence and found that almost all violent offenders displayed reactive violence but the minority who also showed instrumental violence had higher PCL–R scores, indicating that they were a more severely psychopathic group.

Although the strength of the association between violence and psychopathy is not in doubt, there is remarkably little understanding of the underlying mechanisms, nor has any means or therapy been devised to reverse or at least weaken this link.

Legal aspects

Maudsley (1897) was one of the first to suggest that the legal system should not treat such offence-prone individuals in the same way as common criminals:

> 'When such individuals commit an offence, the truest justice would be the admission of a modified responsibility.'

The category of 'moral imbecility' was first included in the Mental Deficiency Act 1913, and this was changed to 'moral defective' in a 1927 Act. The Mental Health Act 1959 included four legal categories for administrative purposes: subnormality, severe subnormality, mental illness, and psychopathic disorder, the last being defined as:

> 'a persistent disorder or disability of the mind (whether or not including subnormality or low intelligence) which results in abnormally aggressive or seriously irresponsible conduct on the part of the individual and requires or is susceptible to medical treatment.'

The inclusion of the treatability clause proved unworkable, because it required psychiatrists to admit such people to hospital even when little change was possible. In the Mental Health Act 1983, although a similar definition was retained, the treatability clause was replaced with the phrase 'is likely to alleviate or prevent a deterioration of his condition'. This meant that there was less obligation to admit such patients, particularly those for whom treatment would have little or no effect. However, following a recent high-profile murder, by a man with severe personality disorder who was known to the services, there has been a reversal of government thinking on this issue. Dangerous severe personality disorder is discussed in Chapter 20 (see page 480).

Aetiology

This has been more extensively studied than in the other personality disorders. There is evidence for a contribution from heredity, from childhood disorders such as conduct disorder and attention-deficit disorder, as well as from an environmental component, and in the sections that follow the contribution of each of these elements to the aetiology of psychopathic disorder will be reviewed.

The hereditary component

A familial tendency to antisocial and criminal behaviours has long been known but family studies alone cannot provide useful information on the magnitude of the genetic and environmental influences. Only twin and adoptive studies can do this, and Rhee & Waldman (2002) report a meta-analysis of 51 twin and adoptive studies of antisocial behaviours, including studies of only antisocial behaviours ($n = 12$), aggression (11), criminality (5) and diagnosis-based studies (13). This large meta-analysis probably gives the best currently available estimate for the relative contribution of hereditary and environmental influences. The heritability for antisocial behaviours was 0.41 and the environmental contribution was 0.59. The latter component comprised shared environmental influences (i.e. family influences), which accounted for 0.16 of the variance, and non-shared environmental influences (individual attributes), which accounted for 0.43 of the variance. These heritability figures are appreciable, although slightly lower than those for the functional psychoses. The meta-analysis found slightly lower figures of the heritability as determined from the parent–offspring studies when compared with the twin and sibling adoption studies, although the reasons for this are obscure.

Antisocial personality disorder and antisocial behaviours are predominantly disorders of young men and are much less frequent among women. Could this also be genetically determined? The answer is probably not. Although a phenotypic presentation of the disorder might require a high degree of genetic loading for a particular woman, the meta-analysis showed no difference between the relative contributions of heredity and environment between the two sexes. Social factors are more likely to determine the degree of expression (or inhibition) for antisocial behaviour in women.

Age also has a powerful influence on the prevalence of antisocial behaviours; there is, for example, a 10-fold increase in such behaviours during adolescence. This increase is most likely due to an environmental influence, because the meta-analysis showed that the heritability of juvenile delinquency was only 0.07 while for adults the figure was 0.43. Moffit (1994) proposed that there are two groups of juvenile delinquents: a smaller core group with childhood difficulties and juvenile delinquency, who then mature on to adult antisocial personality disorder, and in this group the condition is probably genetically determined; and a second, much larger group of more normal adolescents, who transiently venture into delinquency only during their adolescence and who lack any significant degree of genetic loading.

Although family studies do not provide quantitative information on heritability, they have shown that certain other psychiatric disorders may occur with an increased frequency among families where the proband has antisocial personality disorder. Bohman *et al* (1982) demonstrated an association with alcoholism and there are many other studies showing this link, while Cadoret *et al* (1985) found an excess of females with hysteria of the Briquet type in families where the proband was male with antisocial personality disorder.

Neuropsychiatric aspects

The first indication of cerebral involvement in antisocial behaviours was from electroencephalography (EEG) studies, which showed widespread excessive theta activity, compatible with cerebral immaturity (Hill & Watterson, 1942), and these findings have been repeatedly confirmed. Recent neuroimaging studies have focused on the amygdala and the frontal lobes, especially the prefrontal cortex. A controlled positron emission tomography (PET) study among a group of murderers showed reductions in glucose metabolism in the prefrontal cortex but not in the posterior frontal areas (Raine *et al*, 1994) and this was subsequently confirmed in a magnetic resonance imaging (MRI) study, which showed an 11% reduction in prefrontal grey matter in a community sample with antisocial personality disorder when compared with normal controls (Raine *et al*, 2000). A functional MRI study by Khiel *et al* (2001) showed that affect processing (as measured by comparing the difference in the ability to recollect negative-affect-laden words and neutral words) resulted in significantly less activation of the amygdala and other limbic structures among subjects with high scores on Hare's PCL compared with controls, while Tiihonen *et al* (2000) have shown that these subjects may also have reduced amygdala volume. Brain scanning studies in antisocial personality disorder are still in their infancy but are likely to become increasingly important, especially as the disorder accounts for a great deal of serious crime.

Birth complications may also play a role, but they appear to interact with social factors. Thus Raine *et al* (1994) collected obstetric data on a large birth cohort and also assessed maternal rejection in an objective way (e.g. mother seeking abortion or stating the child was not wanted, or the child was brought up in an institution). They found that around 2% of children with rejecting mothers (thus defined) committed a violent crime as an adult. For those with only birth complications the rate was just under 3%, but for those infants who had the combination of both birth complications and early maternal rejection the rate for violent crimes in adulthood was very much higher, at 9%. Although only 4.5% of the sample had the combination of both birth complications and maternal rejection, this subgroup accounted for around 18% of violent crime for the whole cohort. The study provides some support for the interactive bio-social model and shows how the accumulation of risk factors is probably more important any single risk factor.

The role of neuropsychological function, particularly in the realms of verbal deficits and executive function, is also important because people with antisocial personality disorder often have difficulties in literacy as well as learning from experience. The relevant studies have been reviewed by Henry & Moffit (1997). Studies have repeatedly shown deficits in verbal IQ and a large discrepancy between performance and verbal IQ for both juvenile delinquents and adult criminals. Verbal and auditory memory tests also show more impairment than visuospatial and mental flexibility functions.

Neuropsychological deficits may even predict recidivism. For example, Moffit (1994) examined a group of juveniles who were arrested at age 13 and identified a subgroup of only 12% of the sample who had neuropsychological deficits, but by the age of 18 this small subgroup accounted for 59% of the convictions.

Tests of frontal lobe function such as the Wisconsin Card Sorting Test (see below) or the Porteus Maze Test also show deficits and may explain the disinhibited and impulsive behaviours found in antisocial personality disorder. Neuropsychological studies also suggest that there are abnormalities of executive function, involving several neural networks, particularly those located in the ventromedial and dorsolateral prefrontal cortex (Dolan & Park, 2002). However, when purely psychopathic subjects are considered (as defined in terms of behavioural traits alone, e.g. by high PCL–R scores and not by criminal or violent behaviours), most but not all studies show normal frontal lobe function and the role of frontal lobe deficits is presently unclear (Henry & Moffit, 1997).

Childhood antecedents

Childhood conduct disorder, attention-deficit disorder, oppositional defiant disorder and constitutional aggression all contribute to adult antisocial personality disorder. Oppositional defiant disorder is usually diagnosed after the age of 8 years and comprises a recurrent pattern of negativistic, defiant, hostile behaviour towards authority figures, usually having lasted for more than 6 months.

The association between conduct disorder in childhood and later antisocial personality disorder is well known and the progression from conduct disorder in adolescence has been clearly demonstrated (Myers *et al*,

1998). This is one of the most important links between child and adult psychiatry, because if any prophylactic measures are to be taken to reduce the high rates of adult antisocial personality disorder (and its associated risks of crime and recidivism) the intervention will need to be directed at the child with conduct disorder; hence the strength and nature of this link needs to be understood in some detail. The link is very much stronger looking backwards rather than forwards. This is because 4–10% of all 8-year-olds display conduct disorder but only 40% of these will later develop antisocial personality disorder (Robins, 1985). Risk factors for the development of the disorder include a younger age at onset of childhood conduct disorders and a greater variety of them, the typical sequence being school problems, fighting and lying among younger school children, followed by vandalism, stealing and drinking in early adolescence. More severe behavioural manifestations such as arrests, exclusion from school and drug misuse appear last in the sequence before antisocial personality disorder.

Follow-up studies by Robins (1985) demonstrated that all adults with the disorder had shown some antisocial behaviour during childhood. This resulted in the DSM–III and DSM–IV diagnostic criteria for antisocial personality disorder incorporating a history of antisocial behaviour before the age of 15 among the diagnostic criteria. A 26-year follow-up study (Zoccolillo *et al*, 1992) of young adults who spent time in care found that 40% of the conduct-disordered group met the criteria for antisocial personality disorder, compared with only 4.3% of those with no conduct disorder. The equivalent figures for females were 35% and 0%. However, conduct disorder has been reported as an antecedent to a number of adult psychiatric conditions, including borderline personality disorder, generalised anxiety disorder and substance misuse, and may be a non-specific effect.

Risks are decreased in the presence of protective factors such as a good family background, high intelligence and resilience (Rutter, 1985). Farrington *et al* (1990) found that children from a criminogenic environment who did not later become delinquent were, at the age of 10, less daring, more neurotic, more shy and spent less leisure time with their fathers. Conversely, risk of a poor outcome for childhood conduct disorder was increased in the presence of adverse family circumstances, which included parental mental illness, marital discord, divorce, inconsistent discipline and family chaos, foster placements, and physical or sexual abuse.

Aggressive behaviour is also a key feature of antisocial personality disorder, and studies have shown that aggression is one of the most stable character traits over time – there is only gradual attenuation with increasing age. Aggression at the age of 8 correlates highly with aggression at the age of 30, as measured by spouse abuse, self-reported physical aggression and criminality. Among men, an early history of temper tantrums predicts later divorce, ill-tempered parenting behaviours and a poor work record (Coid, 1993).

Attention-deficit disorder in childhood has been the focus of considerable interest. A follow-up study of children aged 6–12 years with attention-deficit disorder showed that 9% were later incarcerated, compared with only 1% of the control group (Mannuzza *et al*, 1989). However, it seems likely that an outcome of adult antisocial personality disorder occurs only where conduct disorder occurs with the hyperactivity disorder, especially as attention-deficit disorder attenuates with age. Attempts to resolve this have focused on longitudinal studies of 'pure' groups, that is, those with hyperactivity disorder only, those with conduct disorder only and those with mixed symptoms.

Lakey & Loeber (1997) reviewed the few available longitudinal studies of pure antisocial personality disorder and found two studies that suggested there was no link to the adult disorder in the absence of conduct disorder; for the two studies that did show a link they concluded the database was too small to draw any firm conclusions. What is clear is that conduct disorder is the main childhood predictor of adult antisocial personality disorder, but conduct disorder itself is in turn strongly linked to the two childhood conditions of attention-deficit/hyperactivity disorder (ADHD) and oppositional defiant disorder (ODD). Thus, for children between the ages of 11 and 17 years, 50% of those with conduct disorder will also have ADHD and the figures for ODD are broadly similar.

Child abuse, neglect and witnessing violence may all predispose to psychopathology in adult life, but the magnitude of the contribution they make to antisocial personality disorder is uncertain; the connection is clearer with borderline personality disorder (see below). Cleckley (1964) questioned the association and commented that he had not observed any specific problems in parent–child relationships: 'during all my years of experience with hundreds of psychopaths ... no type of parent or parental influence has been regularly demonstrable'. However, certain situations are well recognised, such as cycles of deprivation and cycles of victimisation (where the abused child later becomes an abuser), and in these cases there may be an increased risk of developing antisocial personality disorder. Luntz & Widom (1994) found that, among a group of abused and neglected children, 13.5% developed adult antisocial personality disorder, compared with 7% of a control group, but such severely adverse circumstances are probably rare and may account for only a small number of those with adult antisocial personality disorder. Coercive parenting styles have also been blamed, but many parents faced with a child with severe conduct disorder may resort to coercive, harsh or otherwise unproductive parenting styles, which may thereby be the consequence rather than the cause of the disturbed behaviour.

The bio-social model of causation

Moffit (1994) has proposed a bio-social model to explain persistent offending behaviours and antisocial personality disorder. The bio-social model may be particularly relevant to the study of personality disorders, and as it now pervades our thinking on almost all psychiatric disorders, ranging from the mildest stress reaction through to the most severe psychoses, it may be worth understanding it in a little more detail.

The model was originally proposed by George Engel (1980), who spent most of his professional life treating the psychiatric disorders of the medically ill. He proposed the bio-social model to replace the then current but rather more simplistic bio-medical model for medical conditions, as a way of incorporating the missing social dimension. His work was based on systems theory and he proposed a hierarchy of biological causes, ranging from molecules, at the lowest level, through to genes, cells, tissues, organs and the central nervous system (CNS), any one of which could contribute to a disease process in the person. A defect at a lower order of causes would affect all levels above (e.g. a genetic defect could affect the CNS, etc.). The 'person' represented the highest level of organic or biological function and all the biological causes would determine the phenomenology or particular form of the disease presentation. Beyond the person level existed the whole social dimension, and this was also arranged in a hierarchy: the key two-person relationships (e.g. marriage), the family, work and the community, culture and subculture, and above these influences were the politico-historical events, which might also affect the whole nation, and these could also contribute to disease processes.

The model presupposes that no single factor will explain the whole cause but rather that there are additive and interactive effects between a variety of identified levels of the hierarchy of causes. Doctors, by virtue of their contact with the patient, are always orientated at the 'person' level and may not take into account or be aware of many key causes that lie at many other levels in the hierarchy.

The stress–diathesis model is similar but lacks the hierarchy of causes and proposes that all the biological causes reside in the diathesis (predisposition), which determines the form of the disorder, while all the social/cultural causes contribute to the stress, and illness occurs when protective mechanisms are overwhelmed in the interaction between the stressors and the person's vulnerability.

In relation to antisocial personality disorder Moffit (1994) suggested that genetic and obstetric causes may interact at a biological level and these may result in CNS abnormalities which predispose to the characteristic neuropsychological deficits. Children with these deficits reared in unfavourable environments may go on to develop conduct disorder and the more severe disorders in adult life, such as antisocial personality disorder, while such negative tendencies may be gradually extinguished for those reared in more favourable environments.

The whole social dimension and the laws and mores of a particular subculture or society may also have a far more profound effect on the likely rates of expression of antisocial behaviours and disorders than any particular psychopathology. For example, the homicide rate in the USA is more than 10 times higher than in most European countries – but no European country has such liberal gun control laws as the USA.

Emotionally unstable personality disorder

ICD–10 describes two subtypes of this personality disorder: the impulsive and the borderline. DSM–IV does not subsume these conditions under one category but classifies borderline personality disorder in the personality disorder group and in its section on 'Habit and impulsive disorders' describes a condition similar to the impulsive subtype, termed 'intermittent explosive disorder'. This is discussed below (see page 460).

Impulsive personality disorder

ICD–10 impulsive personality disorder is characterised by a marked tendency to act impulsively, with little consideration of the consequences, and behavioural explosions may also occur. The essential components are poor impulse control, a need for immediate reward, an inability to plan ahead and unpredictability.

The borderline subtype in ICD–10

The borderline personality type is defined as having all the features of the ICD–10 impulsive type together with at least two out of five features that are similar to those in DSM–IV borderline personality disorder: identity disturbance; unstable relationships; abandonment fears; self-harm; and feelings of emptiness. ICD–10 and the previous DSM classifications (DSM–III and DSM–III–R) do not include the item 'transient stress-related paranoid ideation or severe dissociative symptoms', which is a new addition to the DSM–IV criteria.

Whewell *et al* (2000) attempted to apply ICD–10 criteria for borderline personality disorder to a sample of patients with personality disorder referred for psychotherapy but found it unsatisfactory because a large subgroup of patients who lacked the impulsive element of borderline personality disorder could not be included, even though they would have fulfilled the DSM–IV criteria for the condition. Not surprisingly, almost all research studies (even non-US ones) use the DSM–IV criteria and ICD–10 criteria are rarely used, at least in research studies.

Borderline personality disorder in DSM–IV

> 'The borderline of insanity is occupied by many persons who pass their whole life near that line, sometimes on one side, sometimes on the other.' (Hughes, 1884)

The term 'borderline' has been used to denote several different things: the area between the neuroses and the psychoses; a personality disorder genetically related to schizophrenia (Kety *et al*, 1971); a psychoanalytic formulation of a particular type of personality organisation (Kernberg, 1967); and more recently as a specific type of personality disorder in DSM–IV (Box 18.6).

The modern concept of borderline personality disorder derives mainly from writings of US analysts of the 1930s and 1940s who were puzzled by those patients who proved refractory to classical psychoanalysis yet had mainly neurotic symptoms. Stern (1938) was the first to label these patients as comprising 'a borderline group of neuroses' and his use of the word borderline has been retained. Hoch & Polatin (1949), believing that their patients were more seriously ill and nearer to psychoses, applied the term 'pseudoneurotic schizophrenia', but this terminology has been dropped. Kernberg (1967), also an analyst, developed the concept of 'borderline personality organisation', which applied to all the more serious forms of personality disorder (the less serious ones had a neurotic organisation). Borderline personality organisation entailed three intrapsychic characteristics: identity diffusion, primitive defences (splitting, idealisation, devaluation, etc.) and reality testing that was sometimes impaired but not to the same degree as in psychosis. This psychological

Box 18.6 DSM–IV criteria for borderline personality disorder

A pervasive pattern of instability of interpersonal relationships, self-image and affects, and marked impulsivity beginning by early adulthood and present in a variety of contexts, as indicated by five (or more) of the following:

1 Frantic efforts to avoid real or imagined abandonment. Note: Do not include suicidal or self-mutilating behaviour covered in criterion 5.
2 A pattern of unstable and intense interpersonal relationships characterised by alternating between extremes of idealisation and devaluation.
3 Identity disturbance: markedly and persistently unstable self-image or sense of self.
4 Impulsivity in at least two areas that are potentially self-damaging (e.g. spending, sex, substance misuse, reckless driving, binge-eating). Note: Do not include suicidal or self-mutilating behaviour covered in criterion 5.
5 Recurrent suicidal behaviour, gestures or threats, or self-mutilating behaviour.
6 Affective instability due to a marked reactivity of mood (e.g. intense episodic dysphoria, irritability, or anxiety usually lasting a few hours and only rarely more than a few days).
7 Chronic feelings of emptiness.
8 Inappropriate intense anger or difficulty controlling anger (e.g. frequent displays of temper, constant anger, recurrent physical fights).
9 Transient, stress-related paranoid ideation or severe dissociative symptoms.

For diagnosis using these criteria, with the stipulation that five out of nine criteria must be met, there are a possible 151 different combinations that will yield a borderline diagnosis, with some patients having very little in common with others.

ICD–10 differs from DSM–IV and describes 'emotionally unstable personality disorder', comprising two subtypes: impulsive and borderline (see text).

structure was later incorporated into Gunderson's concept of a borderline personality disorder (see Gunderson, 2001) – a clinical entity which subsequently gained a place in the DSM–III scheme.

Epidemiology

Mattia & Zimmerman (2001) give a median prevalence rate of 1.1% based on 12 population studies; the disorder is three times more common among women than men. An increased prevalence of major depression, alcohol and other substance misuse disorders is reported in first-degree relatives.

Clinical features

The most salient features of this disorder are unstable mood, unstable interpersonal relationships, and a disturbance of identity. Depression is common; the pattern is not one of a continuous depressed mood, but rather of rapid and reactive shifts into depression, characterised by complaints of boredom, intolerance of being alone, frustration and an unpleasant sense of emptiness. Some analysts, such as Kohut (1971), have suggested that this state of 'affective hunger' is so unpleasant that some individuals may resort to impulsive behaviour, such as binge-eating, kleptomania or thrill-seeking, and take drugs or alcohol to alleviate the dysphoria. Episodes of anxiety occur, usually lasting no more than a few hours or a day or two at most; these tend to arise in the context of separation and abandonment fears. (Some such patients break down when their therapist takes a holiday or their treatment plan is altered.)

In men outbursts of anger can result in assaultive behaviour, while among women anger, dysphoria and impulsivity are more commonly turned inward, leading to wrist-cutting, self-mutilation and impulsive taking of overdoses. Sometimes a very severe state of chaotic impulsivity occurs, where subjects respond to every passing whim, behaving like a small child and often gaining admission to hospital. Their pre-admission histories are characterised by wild living, substance misuse, promiscuity, frequent outbursts of rage, running away from home and tumultuous relationships. Lacey & Evans (1986) have used the term 'multi-impulsive personality disorder' to describe this very disturbed subgroup. From a psychobiological perspective the two key domains appear to be impulsive aggression and affective instability.

Identity disturbance is an important psychodynamic feature, but this is not the same as low self-esteem, although the two may coexist. Kernberg (1967) originally derived the concept from Erikson's (1956) maturational model. A normal adolescent should negotiate the maturational steps involved in a commitment to physical intimacy, occupational choice, energetic competition and psychosocial self-definition. Failure to negotiate this maturational phase was termed 'identity diffusion' by Erikson (1956) and 'identity disturbance' by Kernberg (1967), and the latter term has been retained in DSM–IV. DSM–IV characterises identity disturbance as a persistently unstable image or sense of the self. There may be sudden and dramatic shifts in self-image, plans about career, sexual orientation or values and friends. These individuals may suddenly shift from the role of a needy supplicant for help to someone seeking revenge for past mistreatment.

People with a borderline personality enter into ambivalent relationships, which are often intense and characterised by a tendency to over-idealise or devalue their partners. Sometimes they make dependent relationships and at the same time provoke the rejection and abandonment they fear so greatly. At other times manipulative or coercive behaviour is used to humiliate those who care for them. Over the longer term, the picture is one of instability, which ameliorates with age. These patients may have short-lived psychotic episodes (so-called 'micropsychotic' episodes) that are circumscribed and fleeting.

Reliability and validity of the concept

The DSM concept of borderline personality disorder remains rather more popular in the USA than in Europe, but studies have shown that the disorder itself is just as common in Europe. For example, Kroll *et al*

(1982) found that 8.5% of the in-patients in an admission unit fulfilled criteria for the condition but the terms 'histrionic' or 'explosive' were used, or simply 'personality disorder' without specifying the category.

The validity of the syndrome has been questioned by several researchers, including Fyer *et al* (1988), who found that, in clinical populations, borderline personality disorder rarely occurred on its own but was usually associated with some other psychiatric disorder. Of their cases, 91% had at least one other psychiatric diagnosis, 30% two other diagnoses and 12% three other diagnoses, and only 9% had a pure borderline disorder. To explain these findings they suggested that the personality disorder was either an independent diagnostic entity that commonly occurred with other disorders or it represented a rather non-specific dimension of psychiatric disorders. A further difficulty with the diagnosis is that only 0.4% of out-patients were diagnosed clinically with this disorder, although the percentage rose to 14% after a structured interview was given to the same patients (Zimmerman & Mattia, 1999). Tyrer (2002), also a trenchant critic, describes borderline personality disorder as 'a controversial diagnosis of such overwhelming co-morbidity that it embraces the whole of psychiatry'. As well as overlap with axis I diagnoses, investigators point to the finding that over 50% of patients will lose the diagnostic features over time (Links *et al*, 1998). This suggests either: that its natural history is different from that of most other personality disorders, in that there is improvement in response to treatment; or that borderline personality disorder as currently defined in not a homogeneous entity but a constellation of axis I and axis II diagnoses, in which the core features are obscured by difficult behaviour that requires intervention (Tyrer, 1999).

In spite of these criticisms the construct remains in common diagnostic usage clinically and has led to an explosion of research studies based on the DSM criteria. Furthermore, these patients form a significant part of every adult general psychiatrist's workload.

Comorbidity

Comorbidity probably occurs more commonly with borderline personality disorder than with any other psychiatric disorder. The reasons for this are unclear; some of it may be intrinsic to the definition, because criteria used to define the disorder, such as binge-eating and drinking, are also criteria for other disorders, and so, not surprisingly, alcoholism and bulimia appear as common comorbid disorders. In other cases borderline personality disorder itself may predispose to other disorders; for example, the tumultuous relationships with their frequent break-ups may predispose to much heartache and depression. Third, both the personality disorder and other disorders (particularly anxiety and affective disorders) may share some causal mechanisms.

Skodol *et al* (2002) gave the following odds ratios for associated comorbidity: substance misuse (other than alcohol or cannabis) 8.7, alcohol 4.3, panic disorder 8.2, bulimia 5.2. Among in-patients even higher rates of comorbidity are observed, particularly for affective disorders. Zanarini *et al* (1998) gave figures of 82% for major depression, 56% for post-traumatic stress disorder, 49% for panic disorders, 53% for eating disorders (of which 26% were bulimia, 21% anorexia) and 10% for somatoform disorders. Because patients are admitted to hospital as a result of their axis I disorder these figures are much higher than would be expected of a community sample. An out-patient sample found a similar pattern but the comorbid rates were somewhat lower: major depression 31%, dysthymia 16%, bipolar I disorder 9%, bipolar II disorder 4.1% (Skodol *et al*, 2002).

Borderline personality disorder bears little relationship to schizophrenia and Pope *et al* (1983) found no cases of schizophrenia among a group of 33 in-patients with the personality disorder. A 10- to 15-year follow-up of around 200 people with borderline personality disorder revealed only one who subsequently developed schizophrenia (Stone, 1990). Only long-term follow-up studies can tell whether the inclusion of the item 'transient paranoid ideation' in DSM–IV makes any difference to the likelihood of a later schizophrenic denouement, but this item was not included in the previous versions of DSM or other earlier definitions.

Borderline personality disorder is also frequently comorbid with other personality disorders, particularly schizotypal, and there is considerable overlap with antisocial, histrionic and narcissistic types. Knowledge of the comorbid pattern may be helpful in making the diagnosis of the particular subtype of personality disorder, even if the underlying reasons for the association are unclear.

Aetiology

Although the aetiology is unknown, there is now good evidence for a significant genetic contribution, as well as an important environmental contribution, namely physical and sexual abuse during childhood. A family study of probands with borderline personality disorder showed that the condition was 10 times more common among first-degree relatives than among the relatives of schizophrenic probands (Loranger *et al*, 1982). Stone (1990) observed increased rates of affective disorder, alcoholism and borderline personality disorder, but not schizophrenia, among the parents of probands.

Although the original descriptions of borderline personality disorder were made by psychoanalysts and theories of psychological causation have dominated psychiatric thinking and practice for more than half a century, the twin study by Torgersen *et al* (2000) has shown that borderline personality disorder may be strongly genetically determined. The heritability for borderline personality disorder was 0.69, but when strict criteria were used (i.e. sufficient criteria to meet the number stipulated for diagnosis) the heritability rose to 0.80, although numbers were small.

As stated above, Torgersen *et al* (2000) concluded that the heritability of personality disorders overall is high, probably higher than for most axis I disorders with the possible exception of schizophrenia and bipolar disorder. Exactly what is inherited is uncertain, but Gunderson (2001), summarising previous literature, speculated that it is the traits of aggression, impulsivity and emotional dyscontrol (which are also features of antisocial personality disorder) that form the heritable component. Zanarini (1993) proposed that there is a range of 'impulsive spectrum disorders', which include antisocial and borderline personality disorder, substance misuse and eating disorders, and that the temperament element of these disorders may have a common genetic origin.

The finding of a high heritability for borderline personality disorder is clinically useful because most psychiatrists work routinely with categorical diagnoses and the large genetic component may go some way to explaining the persistence of these disorders, as well as their resistance to most treatments; in addition, it may provide some theoretical justification for the use of biological remedies, such as the selective serotonin reuptake inhibitors, for impulsivity (see Chapter 19 on the treatment of personality disorders). It may also help to lessen attitudes of harshness and rejection directed at those burdened with this diagnosis, who are still seen in some quarters as not having a 'real' illness where only an axis I diagnosis is equated with a genuine condition. Personality disorder appears to be just as strongly genetically determined as most other psychiatric disorders.

Neuropsychiatric aspects

A biological contribution may be present in cases in which there has been some noxious early influence on the brain, such as birth injury, brain damage through infection or trauma during childhood, attention-deficit disorder and other neurological conditions. Although each of these categories, when taken individually, is uncommon, Androlunis *et al* (1981) found that 38% of a series of men with borderline personality disorder had some organic contribution.

At the time of writing there was only one small MRI study of borderline personality disorder in the literature. Six subjects with 'pure borderline personality disorder' (i.e. with no other comorbid disorders) compared with normal controls were shown to have elevated activation of the amygdala and of the inferolateral prefrontal cortex in response to a stimulus that provoked noxious emotions (Herpetz *et al*, 2001). These changes were similar in type to those found in post-traumatic stress disorder and obsessive–compulsive disorder, and suggest that the 'fear' reaction is involved. Although similar brain structures seem to be involved in antisocial personality disorder (see above), the changes are in the opposite direction; in borderline personality disorder activation of the amygdala is increased whereas in antisocial personality disorder it is reduced.

Childhood antecedents

As indicated earlier, there is strong evidence for an association between borderline personality disorder and sexual abuse during childhood. Thus there is a higher rate of sexual abuse than in depressive controls, and the parents of borderline probands also show more mental illness, personality disorder, drug misuse and marital discord (Ogata *et al*, 1990). Based on his large out-patient clinic sample, Paris (2001) estimated that around one-third of his group with borderline personality disorder had experienced severe sexual abuse, including incest, regular penetration extending over a prolonged period, or the use of force, and in these cases it appeared likely that the sexual abuse had been a major aetiological factor. In a further third of the cases there were reports of only one or two episodes of molestation and the severity was very much in line with the findings of community surveys, in which 8–15% of women report some degree of molestation; in these cases Paris suggested that the sexual abuse would have been relevant only if it was combined with other aetiological factors. In the remaining third of his sample there were no reports of childhood sexual abuse.

Zanarini *et al* (2002) reported on a much more morbid sample of in-patients with borderline personality disorder drawn from downtown Boston. Rates for childhood sexual abuse among their sample were much higher: 50% reported serious abuse on at least a weekly basis, 50% reported some violence and 78% reported penetration. Results from a quantitative scale of the severity of sexual abuse correlated with all the dimensions of borderline personality disorder but particularly with the total number of episodes of self-mutilation and suicide attempts, while results from a scale of reported childhood neglect correlated with measures of depression and hopelessness. Brown & Anderson (1991) also found a direct correlation between the severity of childhood abuse in a sample of patients admitted to a US army hospital: for those reporting no abuse the rate for borderline personality disorder was 3%, for those with either physical or sexual abuse the rate was 13%, while for those reporting both physical and sexual abuse the rate was 29%. Parental brutality is less common than sexual abuse, and was present in only 6% of Stone's (1990) series, but it may worsen outcome since 12.5% of those with borderline personality disorder who were physically abused later committed suicide. Even witnessing parental violence is thought to be of causal significance.

Childhood abuse and neglect appear to be non-specifically related to all adult personality disorders rather than specifically to borderline personality disorder. In one of the few epidemiologically sound studies in this area, Johnson *et al* (1999) prospectively followed individuals whose names had been placed on the New York Central Registry for Child Abuse and Neglect and some 12–15 years later traced and interviewed them using standardised instruments and also sought information from multiple informants before assigning them a DSM–IV diagnosis. Those who had suffered abuse or neglect in childhood had a fourfold increased risk of having an adult personality disorder, but there was no specific category that was greatly increased. Although numbers were small, physical abuse was more associated with antisocial and depressive personality disorder, sexual abuse with borderline personality disorder, and neglect with antisocial, avoidant, borderline, narcissistic and passive aggressive personality disorders. Diagnoses of obsessive–compulsive and schizoid personality disorders were not associated with histories of childhood maltreatment.

There has been much confusion concerning the magnitude of the contribution of child sexual abuse to the aetiology of borderline personality disorder, especially where only clinical reports are considered, although it is undoubtedly an important factor. At one time therapists presumed child sexual abuse had inevitably occurred in all cases, and those who failed to make such disclosures were thought to be suppressing these memories. Some therapists actively suggested such abuse and in other instances patients would 'volunteer' these memories, causing much distress to their families, since they were at times false. This has come to be known as 'false memory syndrome'.

It is important therefore to assess the overall contribution of environmental stresses in the aetiology of borderline personality disorder and to discover why some children develop personality disorders and others do not. Paris (2001) provides a thoughtful review on these issues and makes the following points:

- Most children exposed to a specific adversity do not develop any sort of adult mental disorder.
- Multiple adversities have a cumulative effect. Most children can survive a single adversity, but few can survive repeated traumas, as their resilience mechanisms will become overwhelmed. Certain situations, for example where child physical and sexual abuse occur, are usually also associated with multiple other problems that children must deal with (broken homes, parents with personality disorders or substance misuse, etc.), and the cumulative effect may be more significant than any single trauma.
- Social adversities or traumatic experiences in childhood are usually mediated through dysfunctional families and it appears that the risk factors for many different adult mental disorders may be similar.
- Timing of the adverse social experience does not seem to play a crucial role. Traditional wisdom has been that the younger the age at which a trauma occurred the more damaging it might be, but an uncomplicated parental separation occurring during a child's early infancy may be much less damaging than a bitter parental divorce occurring during adolescence.

Working out the significance of an earlier history of childhood sexual abuse in an individual case is a matter of vital importance for therapists working with patients with borderline personality disorder. Patients will show a wide degree of variation in their experience of earlier traumas and assessing the relative weight of each contribution may help influence decisions as to whether to follow a mainly psychodynamic path or a cognitive approach, or even adopt a mainly biological strategy.

Histrionic personality disorder

Histrionic personalities turn to others for protection and the rewards of life. In contrast to the dependent personality, histrionic individuals take the initiative in the quest for nurture, and this leads to seductive and overdramatic behaviour. A colourful description that also covers most of the DSM–IV features was given by Kretschmer (1926):

> 'an over-lively and over-idealistic psychic sexuality, with prudishness or rejection of its physical correlate, a rapidly vanishing élan of feelings, enthusiasm for impressive persons, a preference for what is loud and lively, a theatrical pathos, an inclination for brilliant roles, to dream themselves into big purposes in life, the playing with suicide, contrast between enthusiastic self sacrificial abandonment and a naive sultry childish egotism and especially a mixture of the droll and tragic in their way of living....'

This category has always been controversial and although described in great detail is seldom diagnosed.

Box 18.7 ICD–10 criteria for histrionic personality disorder

1 Self-dramatisation, theatricality, exaggerated expression of emotion.
2 Suggestibility.
3 Shallow and labile affectivity.
4 Continually seeking excitement, being at the centre of attention.
5 Inappropriately seductive in appearance or behaviour.
6 Overconcern with physical attractiveness.

Three out of the six items are required for the diagnosis. The DSM–IV definition requires four out of eight similar items, the additional items being style of speech (excessively impressionistic and lacking in detail) and considering relationships to be more intimate than they actually are.

One of the difficulties is that it carries overtones of sexism and it represents a caricature of femininity (Chodoff & Lyons, 1958). It is more frequently diagnosed in women than men and often without due regard to the criteria (Thompson & Goldberg, 1987). There are those who believe that this diagnosis should be relegated to the group of personality disorders that requires further study (Dowson & Grounds, 1995).

The criteria for this diagnosis are similar in ICD–10 and DSM–IV, and the core features are self-dramatisation, lability of mood, sexual provocativeness, egocentricity and excessive demand for praise and approval. Initially there is an appearance of openness and social skill. However, the histrionic person is also shallow, flirtatious and manipulative. Hyperbolic speech and melodramatic descriptions are noticeable. The superficiality manifests itself as a low capacity for self-examination or introspection. The outside world is everything and introspection is avoided. Early analysts stressed fixation at an infantile level, with childlike behaviour and confusion between fantasy and reality (Wittels, 1930).

Mattia & Zimmerman (2001) gave a median prevalence of 1.3% based on six studies and Torgersen *et al* (2000) found the disorder had a high heritability, similar to other cluster B disorders, at 0.67.

The ICD–10 features of histrionic personality disorder are shown in Box 18.7.

Comorbid disorders

Histrionic personalities are prone to anxiety, particularly at times of separation, and generalised anxiety disorder and agoraphobia may occur. It was once thought that conversion symptoms and other dissociative phenomena such as amnesia, fugues and multiple personality disorder were more common among histrionic types, but their frequency is probably no greater than in the other personality disorders (Chodoff & Lyons, 1958). Somatisation is not uncommon (the combination of multiple somatic complaints and personality disorder known as Briquet's syndrome is discussed on page 397). Other personality disorders, particularly borderline and antisocial types, may coexist. Short-lived histrionic features are sometimes observed among those with depressive episodes, but this should not be confused with more long-standing histrionic personality disorder.

Anxious (avoidant) personality disorder

In contrast to those with a schizoid personality disorder, who lack any interest in other people, those with avoidant personality disorder will actively seek contact, yet at the same time are so sensitive to rejection and feelings of humiliation that relationships rarely develop. ICD–10 uses the term 'anxious personality' and DSM–IV the term 'avoidant'.

Kretschmer (1922) identified two types of schizoid individual: the anaesthetic and hyperaesthetic type. The anaesthetic type corresponds to DSM–IV schizoid personality and the hyperaesthetic to avoidant personality. These individuals are habitually self-conscious, persistently in a state of tension and express an overwhelming need for security. There is a tendency to exaggerate the negative aspects of everyday situations. They feel their loneliness and isolated experience very deeply, but also have a strong yet unexpressed desire to be accepted. Avoidant personalities tend to be excessively introspective, unsure of their identity and self-worth. The central dynamic is the struggle between affection and mistrust. Their life is restricted and one of great psychic pain. Among the more artistically inclined, the need for affection and closeness may appear in poetry, or else become sublimated into intellectual pursuits such as music or art. Other people are actively sought out, because to be alone with one's despised self may impose an even greater torment, yet others are also avoided because of feelings of shame and humiliation. They have few friends, although they may wish for more, and because of their obsequiousness are sometimes the butt of taunts and jibes. Relationships are unlikely to be sustained unless the partner provides a degree of uncritical acceptance.

A median prevalence rate of 1.1% was given by Mattia & Zimmerman (2001) based on 11 studies, while the heritability was somewhat lower than for other personality disorders, at 0.28 (Torgersen *et al*, 2000).

The ICD–10 features of avoidant personality disorder are shown in Box 18.8.

Box 18.8 ICD–10 criteria for avoidant personality disorder

1 Persistent and pervasive feelings of tension and apprehension.
2 Belief that one is socially inept, personally unappealing, or inferior to others.
3 Excessive preoccupation with being criticised or rejected in social situations.
4 Unwillingness to become involved with people unless certain of being liked.
5 Restrictions in lifestyle because of need to have physical security.
6 Avoidance of social or occupational activities that involve significant interpersonal contact because of fear of criticism, disapproval, or rejection.

Associated features may include hypersensitivity to rejection and criticism. DSM–IV does not include items 1 or 5 above but includes 'Restraint within intimate relationships because of fear of being shamed or ridiculed' and 'Reluctance to take personal risks or to engage in any new activities because they may prove embarrassing'.

Comorbid patterns and differential diagnosis

Generalised anxiety disorder is most frequently associated, but depression resulting from the miserable lives these people lead may also occur.

Social phobias are such a pervasive part of the avoidant pattern that it is difficult to say where the personality disorder ends and the social phobia begins. There are, though, several distinguishing features. First, in the avoidant personality the pattern is much more pervasive, while in social phobia individuals are usually capable of making some normal relationships, at least within the family. Second, individuals with social phobia are intensely phobic about meeting people in specific situations, such as going to a restaurant, or meeting a large group at work, but are less likely to be troubled by relationships in general. Third, other personality traits, such as low self-esteem or the pathological desire for acceptance, are common in avoidant personality disorder, but unusual in individuals with social phobia. However, a study by Fahlen (1995) found that the overlap between the two disorders was considerable – to the extent that 60% of those diagnosed with social phobia also fulfilled criteria for avoidant personality disorder and he questioned the need for two separate categories.

Some patients present with hypochondriasis, as isolated individuals totally preoccupied with various bodily sensations and constantly seeking medical contact and reassurance. Fatigue, which enables them 'legitimately' to do little and to avoid other people, is a strategy they may use to isolate themselves from others.

Dependent personality disorder

This group is characterised by excessive emotional dependence on others, with an intense need for social approval and affection. They suppress their own needs to fit in with the wishes of others. They may be self-effacing, ever agreeable, docile or ingratiating, and this may be apparent in their manners and posture. They search for an all-powerful partner who will supply them with the necessary nurturance and affection, and then cling on to them in a dependent relationship. When it breaks down, depression and feelings of isolation may supervene. Kraepelin (1913) used the term 'shiftless', Schneider (1923) called them 'weak willed' and Freud (1901–05) described oral dependent characters.

Those with dependent personality disorder perceive themselves as thoughtful, cooperative people, but not ambitious. Beneath their affability they are constantly searching for attention and approval. Self-depreciation is often used as a ploy to obtain reassurance, or at the very least to avoid reprimand. Constantly pouring oil on troubled waters, they try to deny their own hostile impulses. Self-esteem is low and decision making is difficult. Other traits include self-doubt, excessive humility, submissiveness and a self-perception of incompetence. There are often complaints of loneliness. This is a state reflecting a person's subjective distress over limited opportunities for socialisation and difficulties in establishing close interpersonal relationships. Despite their strong reliance on others, people high in interpersonal dependency have difficulties establishing and maintaining close relationships and they become vulnerable to depression when these relationships terminate or become conflictual. A transient state of dependency resembling dependent personality disorder can occur in normal people after a major loss, and recent losses should always be taken into account before diagnosing dependent personality disorder.

Dependent personalities may make relationships with assertive partners that are ostensibly very close. Many fail to enter long-standing relationships in adult life, but rather stay at home, dependent on their parents until middle age.

Mattia & Zimmerman (2001) gave a median prevalence rate for dependent personality disorder of 1.9% (based on 10 studies) and the disorder is probably more frequent among women. Torgersen *et al* (2000) gave an estimate for its heritability of 0.57. Maternal overprotection combined with adverse temperamental factors within the child may contribute. Horney (1945) highlighted pervasive feelings of weakness and helplessness and a 'poor little me' feeling. The word 'inadequate' has since been used indiscriminately in association with personality disorders, but Sullivan (1947) described an 'inadequate type' which corresponds to dependent personality disorder.

The criteria for this diagnosis are shown in Box 18.9. There is some evidence supporting the validity of dependent personality disorder (O'Neill & Kendler 1998).

Box 18.9 ICD–10 criteria for dependent personality disorder

1 Encouraging or allowing others to make one's important life decisions.
2 Subordination of one's own needs to those of others on whom one is dependent; undue compliance to their wishes.
3 Unwillingness to make even reasonable demands on others.
4 Feeling uncomfortable or helpless when alone, because of exaggerated fears of inability to care for oneself.
5 Preoccupation with fears of being abandoned by person with whom one has a close relationship and of being left to care for oneself.
6 Limited capacity to make everyday decisions without advice from others.

Three out of six items are required for diagnosis. DSM–IV requires five out of eight items. Most of the DSM–IV items are similar, but they include two additional items: difficulty in initiating projects on his or her own; and difficulty in expressing disagreement with others because of fear of loss of support or disapproval.

Comorbidity

Dependent personality is most often comorbid with depression in in-patient samples as well as with all the anxiety disorders (generalised anxiety and the phobias, particularly agoraphobia and social phobia), although the complete picture of dependent personality disorder is rarely encountered in these anxiety disorders. Depression may also share a number of features of dependent personality disorder, such as indecisiveness or feelings of helplessness, and dependent traits may become exaggerated during a depressive episode.

More severe dependent personality disorders are found among those with the somatoform disorders, particularly somatisation disorder and hypochondriasis. Here there is a lifelong pattern of dependency, with constant seeking of reassurance in the context of a medical setting.

The most commonly associated axis II disorders are histrionic, avoidant and borderline personality disorders. Patients with long-standing psychiatric illness of any type may develop a dependent pattern, but in these cases the personality before the onset of the axis I disorder is generally normal.

Differential diagnosis

Both histrionic and dependent personalities seek reassurance and affection from their environment, but in the dependent personality this is through submissiveness rather than through dramatic attention seeking. Borderline patients may form dependent relationships, but these have a grossly unstable pattern. Individuals with avoidant personality disorder also lead restrictive lives, but they fear the good faith of others and anticipate rejection, while the dependent personality is permanently optimistic and always expects to receive nurturance from all objects.

Narcissistic personality disorder

This category is not included in ICD–10, being a diagnosis that is rarely made outside the USA. Its origins and continuing inclusion in DSM–IV in the dramatic (cluster B) group derive from the influence of Freudian psychoanalysis in the USA.

People with this disorder have a grandiose sense of self-importance. They may be preoccupied by fantasies of success, power, brilliance or ideal love. They believe it is their right to receive special treatment and self-esteem is usually based on a blind, naive assumption of personal worth. These feelings of superiority are fragile, however, and there may be an exhibitionistic need for constant attention and admiration from others. Depression sometimes arises from the deep feelings of envy of people they perceive to be more successful.

These individuals overvalue their personal worth, tend to direct affection towards themselves, and may show interpersonal exploitativeness and a lack of empathy. Friendships are one way and develop only if they feel they will profit them. In romantic relationships the partner is often treated as little more than an object to bolster self-esteem. Cognitively they tend to be expansive, with a pervasive sense of well-being. They have little or no idea that their behaviour may be objectionable, and others may describe them as arrogant.

Millon (1981) suggested that the parents of narcissists brought them up to believe they were almost perfect and invariably lovable regardless of their behaviour. Horney (1939) wrote:

> 'parents who transfer their own ambitions to the child and regard the boy as an embryonic genius, or the girl as a princess, give the child the feeling that he is loved for imaginary qualities rather than for the true self.'

Mattia & Zimmerman (2001) found a very low prevalence, of 0–0.2%, using pooled data, but the heritability was high, at 0.79 (Torgersen *et al*, 2000).

Differential diagnosis

A high degree of egocentricity occurs in most of the other personality disorders, and so this trait is not in itself diagnostic. In antisocial personality disorder it is associated with a more malevolent feeling towards others, while those with narcissistic personality disorder are well disposed, believing that other people admire them. They are less impulsive and emotional than borderline personalities, less dramatic than those with histrionic personalities, and are more cohesive and successful than people with dependent personality disorder. However, in practice, any of these disorders may coexist with narcissistic personality disorder.

Passive aggressive personality disorder

Passive aggressive personality disorder is not included in ICD–10, and in DSM–IV it appears only in the chapter entitled 'Criteria sets and axes provided for further study', indicating a degree of doubt concerning the validity of the disorder.

It is characterised by a pervasive pattern of passive resistance in both the domestic and the work situation. People with this disorder resent or oppose demands that may increase their level of functioning. As a result they may not fulfil their promise in the areas of either work or relationships. Their resistance is expressed indirectly, through manoeuvres such as procrastination, stubbornness, intentional inefficiency and forgetfulness. There is a tendency for them to become sulky, irritable or argumentative when asked to do something they do not wish to do. Sometimes they are scornful or hypercritical of people making such demands. The name of the disorder is based on the unproven assumption that such people are passively expressing covert aggression.

The clinical picture shows some resemblance to oppositional defiant disorder of childhood and adolescence, which is a much more severe condition, and this diagnosis will pre-empt a diagnosis of passive aggressive personality disorder in those under 18 years of age. Although behaviour consistent with this pattern may be commonly observed in the workplace or in general practice settings, it rarely impairs people to such an extent that any clinical intervention is required.

Depressive personality disorder

Similarly, this category is not included in ICD–10, and in DSM–IV is included only in the section entitled 'Criteria sets and axes provided for further study'. It refers to a lifelong depressive temperament. Individuals have a pervasive pattern of depressive cognitions and behaviour, pessimism and low self-esteem. As well as being critical and derogatory about themselves, they may also be judgemental and hypercritical about others. Although they claim to be realistic, others view them as unduly pessimistic, humourless and unable to enjoy themselves. They tend to be introverted, quiet individuals.

The condition should not be diagnosed in the presence of major depression because all of the above symptoms may occur in depression. The distinction from dysthymia is much more difficult to make, but in depressive personality disorder most of the changes are reflected in cognitive, interpersonal and intrapsychic personality traits rather than depressive symptoms. Those with depressive personality disorder frequently have comorbid dysthymia (estimates range from 9% to 60%) and family studies confirm the overlap also. Although it is included in DSM–IV only in an appendix, there is some support for the inclusion of depressive personality disorder in DSM–V as a full category on the basis of the stability of the depressive traits over time (Phillips *et al*, 1998).

Mixed personality disorders (ICD–10) and personality disorder not otherwise specified (DSM–IV)

Only a minority of patients can be easily placed in one of the specific diagnostic categories outlined in the preceding sections. The majority of patients with a personality disorder have traits that fulfil criteria for a mixture of two or three personality disorders and in these cases DSM–IV recommends that two or three separate personality disorders should be recorded, while ICD–10 recommends a diagnosis of 'mixed personality disorder'. The more personality disorders are recorded, the greater will be the severity of the disorder; for example, people with a combination of borderline and antisocial personality disorders have more impairments than those diagnosed with either condition alone. Other cases have insufficient traits to satisfy the criteria for any one type, or are essentially either unclassifiable or very difficult to classify, and for these DSM–IV recommends the category 'personality disorder not otherwise specified'. It is not surprising that in these circumstances most clinicians prefer to use only a diagnosis of 'personality disorder', without specifying the type.

Enduring personality changes after a catastrophic experience

Personality disorders usually have their onset in adolescence or early adulthood, which implies that once personality is formed it can no longer change, regardless of external experiences. It is now recognised that a person's character may change as a consequence of stressful events, particularly if the stress is extreme. ICD–10 describes a category in which the onset of the changed personality can be clearly traced to a particular event or illness, such as a catastrophic experience, an episode of severe psychiatric illness now resolved, chronic pain syndrome or bereavement.

Persistent personality change may follow extreme stress, such that personal vulnerability is not required to explain the effects. Severe stresses include being a concentration camp victim, experiencing torture or a disaster, or prolonged exposure to life-threatening circumstances, such as being a hostage. Personality changes that follow from short-term trauma, such as a car accident, are not included in this category since pre-existing vulnerability usually plays a role. The clinical picture is usually one of social withdrawal, coupled with a somewhat hostile or mistrustful attitude to the world. Subjects may complain of feelings of hopelessness, estrangement, and a chronic feeling of being on edge, as if constantly threatened. The diagnosis should be made only if the personality changes have lasted more than 2 years. The disorder is difficult to differentiate from chronic post-traumatic stress disorder and the latter may precede it.

There is no precise equivalent in DSM–IV, but it does include a section on 'personality change due to a medical condition'. Various subtypes are described in this category, including labile, disinhibited, aggressive, apathetic, paranoid, combined types and others. Personality changes due to organic brain disease are described on page 490.

A few individuals experience permanent personality change following an episode of psychiatric disorder, even after they have otherwise fully recovered from their original illness. The clinical picture is mainly one of dependency, a demanding attitude to others, reduced interests, and passivity, with persistent claims of being ill associated with illness behaviour, dysphoria and impaired occupational and social function. Some subjects complain of being changed or stigmatised by their psychiatric illness. The personality change should have been present for at least 2 years, and there should be no evidence of a preceding personality disorder, although previous vulnerabilities will obviously play a role. As the disorder appeared for the first time in ICD–10, little is known about its validity or frequency.

Comorbidity in the personality disorders

The diagnosis of a DSM axis I and axis II disorder signifies the presence of two independent psychiatric conditions. However, comorbidity for two axis II disorders (e.g. for borderline and histrionic types) does not signify that there are two separate personalities. It only means that the clinical picture fulfils diagnostic criteria for two personality disorders.

In view of the comorbidity between axis I and axis II and the fact that the presence of a personality disorder renders the treatment of the axis I disorder more difficult and the outcome generally less good, it is surprising that, in clinical practice, little attention is paid to the evaluation of personality. A common error in the past (and it still occurs) has been to try to diagnose *either* mental illness or personality disorder, but not both. This leads to a relative neglect of axis I disorders in these patients, because 'the personality disorder explained everything'. Indeed, it is those personality disorders that are associated with the greatest social difficulties that receive most attention clinically – hence the automatic assumption that an axis II diagnosis of personality disorder is synonymous with antisocial or borderline personality disorder when in fact the disorders that are most often comorbid with axis I are those that belong to the DSM–IV cluster C group: dependent, avoidant and obsessional personality disorder. There is a further important and unresolved question: when patients who are comorbid for both axis I and axis II disorders present for treatment, which disorder is it they are seeking to alleviate? As noted previously, Robins (1985) found the prevalence of antisocial personality disorder among treatment samples was no higher than their prevalence rate in the community and on this basis surmised that patients sought treatment only for their comorbid axis I disorder, such as anxiety or depression, and had little wish to seek any changes for their personality (which patients usually do not see as disordered), even if other people perceived this to be their primary problem.

In spite of the strong association between axis I and axis II disorders, the associations between specific axis I diagnoses and categories of personality are conflicting and confusing. The preceding sections highlighted the main axis I and axis II associations for each personality disorder subtype. A rather different picture emerges studying cohorts of patients with a particular axis I disorder.

Comorbidity with schizophrenia

Early studies found that 16–26% of patients with schizophrenia appeared to have pre-existing schizoid personality disorder, and the premorbid personality traits associated with schizophrenia are further discussed on page 225. However, Cutting *et al* (1986) failed to replicate these findings. Tyrer (1988) found that 45% of a series of 109 patients with schizophrenia were presently comorbid for personality disorder, around 18% were in the schizoid cluster (schizoid or paranoid) and a few were in the antisocial group. It is uncertain to what extent these cases represent the prodrome of a schizophrenic illness or are independent personality disorders. A premorbid personality disorder in most cases of schizophrenia is unusual; the presence of a behaviour problem suggestive of a personality disorder is usually the result of the psychosis, which resolves or diminishes with treatment of the psychosis.

Comorbidity with affective disorder

There is no evidence that premorbid personality disorder makes any contribution to bipolar disorder (Tyrer *et al*, 1988). Cyclothymia, once thought to predispose to bipolar illness, is now classified as an affective disorder and the two disorders may not be easy to distinguish. Among patients with depression, particularly in-patients, high rates of borderline personality disorder may be found (Baxter *et al*, 1984), but the two disorders are probably independent and not associated. Life events are associated with depression. McGuffin *et al* (1988) showed there is a familial tendency for life events, which suggests their occurrence may be far from random or truly independent. Seivewright (1988) went further, in suggesting that personality disorder may be one of the intervening variables that modulate the effect of a life event on the individual. In certain circumstances the disorder may even be the cause of the event, and he speculated that there may be 'event-prone personalities'.

Comorbidity with 'neurotic' disorders

The neurotic disorders may be more strongly linked with the personality disorders, particularly those in the anxious/fearful cluster. In a large study of patients attending general practice, Tyrer *et al* (1988) noted that about half of those presenting with a neurotic disorder (anxiety states, phobias, neurotic depression and hypochondriasis) were comorbid for a personality disorder, usually anankastic, dependent, passive aggressive or histrionic. No definite association between any one personality type or any specific neurotic disorder was found, but higher rates of personality disorder (particularly explosive type) were observed among those with adjustment disorders.

One of the strongest comorbid associations is between avoidant personality disorder and social phobia, as demonstrated in the Collaborative Longitudinal Personality Disorder Study (CLPDS; Skodol *et al*, 1999). However, there are many who believe that since social phobia begins in adolescence, at the same time as personality disorder, the two represent variants of the one condition rather than two separate disorders (Fahlen, 1995).

Comorbidity with eating disorders

An association between personality disorder, particularly the borderline type, and eating disorders is well established, but published figures range from 21% to 97% (Westen & Harnden-Fischer, 2001). Personality disorder is more prevalent among in-patients than among out-patients with an eating disorder and is related to hospitalisation history, functioning and sexual abuse.

Bulimia is more often associated with cluster B, the dramatic personality disorders, especially borderline personality disorder, but it should be noted that the symptom of binge-eating is one of the diagnostic criteria of the personality disorder. In particular, the bulimic subtype of anorexia nervosa is particularly associated with high rates of borderline personality disorder (55%), as compared with only 7% for the pure restricting subtype of anorexia, which tends to be more associated with avoidant personality disorder. A history of sexual abuse in childhood may be common to both the personality disorder and the eating disorder, but Waller (1993) concluded that the relationship was relatively non-specific and present only among people with borderline personality disorder who had both anorexia nervosa and bulimia. Whatever the aetiological significance of the association, patients with combined disorders seem to have a more chronic course and are more difficult to treat. The topic is also discussed on page 619.

Alcohol dependence and personality disorder

The relationship between alcohol, personality and personality disorder is complex. Premorbid abnormalities of personality (not amounting to a personality disorder) have been observed among those destined to develop alcohol dependence. From 1947 to 1961, all new students at the University of Minnesota completed the Minnesota Multiphasic Personality Inventory, and those who later developed alcohol dependence were compared with their classmates. The 'pre-alcoholic' students were more impulsive, non-conforming and gregarious, had higher scores on the psychopathic deviate and masculinity/femininity scales, but were not more maladjusted (Kammeier *et al*, 1973). Women who subsequently became problem drinkers were more often pessimistic, withdrawn, self-defeating, less dependent and less self-satisfied than those who drank moderately. These findings were echoed in later investigations into the types of personality disorders found among female in-patients with severe alcohol problems, in whom the borderline–schizotypal constellation was common (Valgum & Valgum, 1989). Tyrer *et al* (1988) found that more than half of a group of people with alcoholism in a general practice population fulfilled criteria for personality disorder (mainly explosive type). Among other substance misusers the comorbidity with personality disorder is also substantial, especially with the antisocial and borderline types (Skodol *et al*, 1999) and is associated with poor outcome.

Assessment

Because severe personality disorders are usually ego-syntonic, self-report may be unreliable, and so interviews with informants (usually relatives) may give a more accurate picture. Studies of personality disorder should therefore use a structured interview to ensure reliability, obtain data from informants and base the diagnosis on the currently accepted definitions, preferably from DSM–IV or ICD–10.

Clinical assessment

Although this is the most common method of assessing personality, it is often quite unreliable. The index of overall agreement between psychiatrists is lower for personality disorder than for any other major class of psychiatric disorder; there is usually agreement on the presence of a personality disorder, but not on the specific type. Test–retest reliability is poor and the diagnosis often changes, usually to one of the neurotic disorders. Zimmerman (1994) reported a test–retest reliability (kappa score) of 0.56 for any personality disorder (range 0.11–0.84 for specific categories) and an inter-rater reliability study (again, kappa score) of

0.75 for any personality disorder (range 0.62–0.77 for specific categories). In most studies a diagnosis of antisocial personality disorder is the most reliable.

There are a number of reasons for this unreliability, particularly when the patient's own account is used to make the diagnosis. First, certain features of the personality disorder will interfere with accurate assessment; examples are exaggeration (histrionic disorder) or dishonesty (antisocial disorder), as they are features of the disorder itself, while some otherwise socially desirable traits may also be exaggerated, such as obsessionality and reliability. Second, during an axis I illness self-assessment will be distorted by the patient's negative affect. Third, traits and symptoms are often confused. For example, a patient who, during an episode of depression, reports anxiety and displays histrionic and dependent behaviour may be wrongly diagnosed as having histrionic personality disorder. Fourth, it is often wrongly assumed that those with neurotic disorders will inevitably also have personality disorders, a notion stemming from the work of Alexander (1930), who described the neurotic character. Fifth, a contrary view is also proposed, namely that psychiatric illness and personality disorder are mutually exclusive, so that a patient can have either but not both. This was a commonly held but erroneous principle before the advent of multi-axial classifications. Finally, value judgements often cloud clinical judgements when personality is assessed, and terms such as 'inadequate', 'hysterical' or 'immature' are sometimes applied inappropriately (Thompson & Goldberg, 1987).

In spite of these plentiful sources of inaccuracy, in routine work the clinician should always make an attempt to assess the patient's premorbid personality; this should cover whether a personality disorder is present and, where possible, the assignment of a DSM–IV/ICD–10 category to it. Those referring to psychiatric services – such as general practitioners and social workers – will have some knowledge of axis I diagnoses (which are usually indicated in the referring letter) but may be less well acquainted with axis II disorders and their significance, and making this part of the assessment may form part of the psychiatrist's unique contribution. Knowledge of the comorbid patterns of axis I and axis II disorders may help offer clues even before the patient is seen (e.g. eating disorders with borderline personality disorder, substance misuse with antisocial personality disorder, social phobia with anxious or avoidant personality disorder). As the history emerges, further clues may follow, such as child sexual abuse with borderline personality disorder, forensic contacts or multiple jobs and multiple partners with antisocial personality disorder, over-close relationships with dependent types and so on, while in the mental state a relative absence of severe affective or psychotic symptoms may also suggest that a personality disorder may lie behind the psychiatric referral. Once a personality diagnosis is suspected, it is helpful to clarify its presence in a general way (e.g. the presence of impaired relationships and function over a prolonged period) as well as to attempt to assign it a particular diagnostic category by going through the relevant criteria for the disorder in question. Other members of the psychiatric team will usually find it helpful to know from an early stage that they are working with someone with a personality disorder – rather than have it belatedly confirmed after enduring months of manipulative behaviour and treatment failure.

Notwithstanding the problems associated with clinical assessment outlined above, making a personality diagnosis in a research setting is likely to remain the most clinically accurate when applied with rigour, such as to meet the Longitudinal Expert Evaluation using All Data (LEAD) standard, proposed by Spitzer (1983) as a gold standard for assessing personality. He argued that the best diagnosis was arrived at by an expert on these disorders observing the patient over time and using information from many sources, including hospital records, the family and friends, and others who can provide objective information on behaviours and traits in various contexts and independent of episodes of illness.

Several studies have shown that the level of agreement between patients and informants is low, with informants reporting more pathology (Zimmerman, 1994), probably because of their greater insight – the patient's relative lack of insight into the impairment in social functioning is the hallmark of personality disorder. Relatively little is known about the effect different types of informant have on the assessment of personality. One study (Brothwell *et al*, 1992) found that close sources (e.g. spouses and cohabitees) are better informants that more distant ones, and that women are superior to men in the validity of their evaluations.

Structured assessment

Older tools

The best-known self-rating instrument is the Eysenck Personality Inventory (EPI; Eysenck & Eysenck, 1964), which contains 108 questions relating to the dimensions of neuroticism, extroversion and psychoticism, as well as a lie scale. Although widely used in studies of physical and psychiatric disorders, it suffers from the problem that current psychiatric disorder will markedly influence the N (neuroticism) scale (Kendell & DiScipio, 1968). Also, the use of dimensions does not easily fit with clinical practice and the common clinical categories.

The MMPI (Minnesota Multiphasic Personality Inventory) was developed to differentiate between the categories of abnormal personality among in-patients (Hathaway & McKinley, 1940) (though it has been updated since) but it has also been extensively studied in the healthy population. The subject is presented with 550 statements and asked to respond to each with 'true', 'false' or 'cannot say'. Unfortunately, the scales have been labelled using the standard nosology of psychiatry (e.g. paranoia, schizophrenia, psychopathy, etc.). Its use to generate the traditional categories of personality disorder is limited, and interpretation by an experienced psychologist is required. The scale is little used now.

Cattell's l6PF (1965) is a structured interview schedule seldom used clinically but commonly used by occupational psychologists. It generates 16 dimensions, for instance 'tense–relaxed', 'controlled–uncontrolled', and the terms chosen to describe these are rather idiosyncratic, such as 'harria–parmia', 'alexia–protension'.

Newer tools – screening instruments

The Iowa Personality Disorder Screen (Langbehn *et al*, 1999) was developed specifically for the purpose of screening for personality disorder and takes 5–10 minutes to administer. It consists of 11 screening items for the DSM categories, and these show an impressively high sensitivity and specificity. However, work on this tool is ongoing.

The Standardised Assessment of Personality (SAP; Mann *et al*, 1981) is an informant scale that can be used for screening, although it is more often used as a full personality assessment tool. The Standardised Assessment of Personality – Abbreviated Scale (SAPAS; Moran *et al*, 2003) consists of eight dichotomously rated items from the SAP, which are completed by the subject. It shows good sensitivity and specificity and may prove feasible for use in everyday clinical practice.

Finally, the Personality Assessment Schedule (Tyrer & Alexander, 1979) has a screening version.

Newer tools – diagnostic instruments

These can be grouped into two major classes – questionnaires and structured interviews.

Questionnaires

Although questionnaires, such as the Personality Disorder Questionnaire (PDQ; Hyler *et al*, 1990) are convenient to use, they have the serious disadvantage of generating high false positive rates, leading to overdiagnosis.

The Millon Clinical Multiaxial Inventory (Millon, 1982) is a self-administered questionnaire of 175 items. It takes 25 minutes to complete and analysis is by computer. It provides three sets of results – an individual profile, an interpretive report and a categorical assessment of personality limited to borderline, schizotypal and paranoid types. The main limitation, inherent in all questionnaires, is the failure to distinguish current mental state from personality traits and this may confound the diagnosis. A revised version that can generate DSM–IV diagnoses is presently being developed.

Structured interviews

Structured interviews such as the PAS and the Diagnostic Interview for DSM–IV Personality Disorders (DIPD–IV) (Zanarini *et al*, 1994) achieve good reliability but are lengthy and require training in their use. Other distinctions lie in their use of informants or patients or both, an important consideration since there is evidence to suggest that reliability is higher with informants than with patients alone (Modestin & Puhan, 2000).

The PAS generates diagnoses for both ICD–10 and DSM–IV. It requires either the patient or informant or both to provide information on 24 traits of personality, and emphasis throughout is placed on premorbid traits. It takes about 30 minutes to administer.

The Structured Interview for DSM–III Personality Disorders (SIDP; Pfohl *et al*, 1983) is a comprehensive semi-structured interview with 60 items. Data are gathered from the patients and an informant to generate the diagnosis.

The Personality Disorder Examination (Loranger *et al*, 1985) is a structured interview with 359 items, some traits and some behavioural measures, which also generates both DSM–IV and ICD–10 diagnoses. It takes around 3 hours to complete and its size precludes its use except in research settings.

The Structured Clinical Interview for DSM–III–R (SCID–2) was developed by Spitzer *et al* (1987) to focus exclusively on axis II diagnosis and has been adapted to make DSM–IV diagnoses. The interview begins with administration of the PDQ and the patient is asked to make a series of dichotomous yes/no choices. The SCID–2 interview then focuses on questions to which a positive response has already been given, covering all the traits in the DSM–IV personality disorder section, but the interviewer makes the diagnosis (in contrast to the Present State Examination, where the diagnosis is computer generated).

Dimensional measures

The dimensional approach to personality was first used in the EPI (see above). More recent dimensional measures include the Dimensional Assessment of Personality Pathology – Basic Questionnaire (DAPP-BQ) (Schroeder *et al*, 1992) and the Personality Disorder Inventory (PDI; Widiger *et al*, 1995).

Disorder-specific schedules

There are now many schedules that can diagnose and rate the severity of specific categories of abnormal personality. Perhaps the best known is the Diagnostic Interview for Borderline Patients (Gunderson & Austin, 1981). Others include the Structured Interview for Schizotypy (Kendler *et al*, 1989), the Schedule for Interviewing Schizotypal Personalities (Baron *et al*, 1990) and the Diagnostic Interview for Narcissistic Patients (Gunderson *et al*, 1990).

A comprehensive overview of all the available specific rating instruments, as well as the general ones, is given by Clark & Harrison (2001).

Impulse control disorders

Both DSM–IV and ICD–10 describe a group of patients with impulsive behaviour disorders, characterised by failure to resist an impulse that is usually ego-syntonic but often harmful to the individual. The person experiences increasing tension before committing the impulsive act and a sense of pleasure or gratification once it has been completed. These conditions are not personality disorders and probably represent a residual category. They include five main disorders: kleptomania, pyromania, intermittent explosive disorder, pathological gambling and trichotillomania. Compulsive buying is sometimes also considered to be an impulse disorder but is not included as such in either DSM–IV or ICD–10.

There have been no detailed epidemiological studies of these disorders but the literature suggests that the more the aggressive impulse disorders – that is, pyromania, intermittent explosive disorder and pathological gambling – are more common in men, whereas the less obviously destructive disorders – kleptomania and trichotillomania – may be more common among women.

Population base rates for these disorders may be low, but rates may be increased among psychiatric patients. Thus, Grant *et al* (2005) applied the Minnesota Impulsive Disorders Interview (Christenson *et al*, 1994), a specially devised instrument for diagnosing impulse disorders, to patients who had been admitted to two psychiatric in-patient units, a university department and a private admission facility. Most of the patients had been admitted for a variety of affective disorders and only a few patients had psychosis in this series. Impulse disorders were common, occurring as comorbid conditions among these in-patients at the following rates: kleptomania, 8%; pathological gambling, 7%; intermittent explosive disorder, 6.4%; pyromania, 3.4%; and trichotillomania, 3.4%. Some patients had more than one impulse control disorder. A French study (Lejoyeux *et al*, 2002) that applied the same interview to a group of patients with major depression found that almost a third had an associated impulse control disorder. Those with depression who also had an impulse control disorder were more likely to be bipolar than those who did not have an impulse control problem (19% versus 1.3%).

Recognising impulse control disorders as psychiatric disorders may be important, as for example a presentation of kleptomania may signify a serious underlying depression, while the destructive effect of a bipolar disorder may be mainly through associated reckless gambling, which may require a rather different and more psychosocial approach than the treatment for the primary bipolar condition.

Kleptomania

Kleptomania (from the Greek for 'stealing madness') refers to the irresistible impulse to steal unneeded items, and the DSM–IV provides a useful description. It regards the essential feature of the condition as a recurrent failure to resist the impulse to steal items that are not needed for personal use or that have little personal value. The person concerned may experience a rising sense of tension before the theft and then experience pleasure, gratification and anxiety reduction afterwards. The objects stolen usually have little value, and the person sometimes offers to pay for them, or may give them away, or sometimes hoards them. It is usually diagnosed in pre-court evaluations for shoplifting, but even among shoplifters it is rare. In one series only 13 of 338 shoplifters (3.8%) were diagnosed as having kleptomania (Arieff & Bowie, 1947) and the DSM–IV gives an estimate of around 5% of shoplifters having the disorder.

The psychopathology of kleptomania is poorly understood but the condition is likely to have diverse causes. The account below is drawn mainly from the review by Goldman (1991), who called the condition 'nonsensical stealing'. Depression is common among people with kleptomania. Although their sample was small, Lejoyeux *et al* (2002) found that 75% of people with kleptomania and depression gave a history of a previous manic episode, indicating that a bipolar diathesis may be important. A popular psychodynamic theory proposed by Cupchik & Atcheson (1983) in their discussion on the causes of 'thieving among upstanding citizens' is that the theft represents an effort to obtain symbolic compensation for an actual or anticipated loss. Since the objects stolen usually have little monetary value, the act of theft is more for 'intra-psychic profit'.

Some earlier analysts, such as Fenichel, emphasised the sexual significance and associated secrecy and likened the behaviour to the sexual act, with the objects stolen sometimes having a fetishistic significance for the individual. Certainly there are case reports of kleptomania being associated with sexual excitement during the act of stealing, while more recent series of people with kleptomania have documented the presence of dysfunctional sexual lives.

Kleptomania may occur in severe premenstrual tension and in pregnancy, and is a rare presentation of postnatal depression. It may also occur in bulimia, where the objects stolen are sometimes, although not always, items of food.

The repetitive and compulsive nature of the condition has drawn parallels with obsessive–compulsive disorder, but in the latter the thoughts are usually unpleasant and egodystonic, and the person tries to resist them, whereas in kleptomania the thoughts are more pleasurable (even if antisocial), are egosyntonic, and the act itself is associated with tension relief.

Kleptomania may also have a biological basis. Thus, in cases of kleptomania associated with depression, successful treatment of the depression with antidepressants will usually lead to a resolution of the kleptomania as well. There are also case reports in the literature describing its first appearance in elderly people with depression, incipient dementia or in association with strokes and brain tumours (for references, see Goldman, 1991). These observations suggest the possibility of an underlying neuropsychiatric substrate and are of interest in the light of recent brain imaging studies. Thus, Grant *et al* (2006) applied diffusion tensor imaging and measured trace and fractional anisotropy (see page 217) in a study comparing 10 women with DSM–IV kleptomania and 10 control women. They found significantly lower mean frontal fractional anisotropy in their participants with kleptomania, which was interpreted as signifying decreased white matter micro-structural integrity in the inferior frontal brain regions. Kleptomania therefore has a complex bio-psychosocial aetiology, with considerable variation between individuals regarding the most relevant underlying causative factors.

Shoplifting

Shoplifting itself is not a psychiatric disorder and in English law is classed as a type of theft, but it is briefly considered here because it may be the presenting feature for a wide variety of psychiatric disorders.

In an observational study, Buckle & Farrington (1984) found that about 2% of customers who enter a store will shoplift. Because the economic losses associated with shoplifting are huge, the retail industry has invested considerable sums of money and energy in trying to detect shoplifters; as a consequence, many vulnerable people with psychiatric disorders are inevitably picked up and prosecuted. Most shoplifting is for financial gain, but in pre-court evaluations different case series report that somewhere between 5% and 15% of those detained are suffering from psychiatric disorders. Bradford & Balmaceda (1983) diagnosed 40% of their series of 50 shoplifters (most commonly middle-aged women with low self-esteem) as having depression. Gudjonsson (1990) in a review wrote that the mechanism that transmutes a depression into shoplifting is unclear but speculated that depressed people shoplift because they experience some tension relief and mood elevation during the act of theft, while at the same time do not believe they will be caught. In other cases there is a more direct wish to be caught and punished, or the theft may represent a cry for help. Distraction, absent-mindedness and impaired concentration (e.g. forgetting to pay) may play a role in severe anxiety states, as well as in organic brain disorders, particularly in the elderly. Among those with learning difficulties the person's sense of right and wrong and personal morality may not be fully developed. Although shoplifting is rare among people with schizophrenia, it can result from the disinhibition sometimes associated with acute psychosis, as well as in chronic states, which may be accompanied by genuine poverty, destitution and scavenging behaviours, where the motivation is probably for gain (and in this context may be quite understandable).

DSM–IV excludes recurrent stealing behaviours due to schizophrenia, mania or dementia from its category of kleptomania.

Although the value of the items stolen may be quite trivial, a full psychiatric evaluation is required in all the cases referred on by lawyers, the court, or the probation service, because the underlying psychiatric disorder may be severe and sometimes requires immediate attention. As noted above, kleptomania itself is an uncommon cause of shoplifting and may be difficult to treat. Being caught and prosecuted may inhibit some people, while those cases associated with depression may respond to an SSRI. A number of behavioural regimes (for review see Gudjonsson, 1990) have also been tried, but for the truly resistant cases of kleptomania a self-imposed ban on entering any store may be the only answer.

Pyromania

Pyromania is a rare disorder in adults and is characterised by multiple episodes of deliberate fire setting. These individuals have a fascination with fire and may experience tension or affective arousal before setting a fire. They may be both curious and fascinated by fire and may go to watch fires in their neighbourhood or set off false alarms. They often derive pleasure from institutions, personnel and equipment associated with fire and may spend time at their local fire department, set fires to become affiliated with the fire department, or may even become fire fighters (according to DSM–IV).

Fire setting is rather more common among juveniles. It may result in a great deal of property damage. In juveniles the condition usually presents as one feature of a more global conduct disorder, but it can occasionally also occur with attention-deficit hyperactivity disorder, adjustment disorder and learning difficulties. There are few longitudinal studies and so the relationship between adult pyromania and juvenile fire setting is unclear, but presumably many adult cases will have had their onset in childhood. Children and adolescents with fire-setting behaviours are often both curious about and fascinated by fire, in contrast to adult arsonists, who rarely show such an interest.

Pyromania needs to be distinguished from intentional fire setting (arson), where the motivation may be for revenge, profit, sabotage, to attract attention or even to make a political statement. Arson is more comprehensively reviewed elsewhere in *Seminars in Practical Forensic Psychiatry* (Chiswick & Cope, 1995). Pyromania as defined in DSM–IV and ICD–10 excludes fire setting as a consequence of mental illnesses such as depression, schizophrenia or alcoholism. After these exclusions, 'pure' pyromania in adults is extremely rare. For example, in one series of 283 convicted arsonists, although mental health problems were present in 90% (36% with a major mental disorder – either schizophrenia or bipolar disorder – and 64% with alcohol or drug problems), there were only 3 cases of pyromania (1%) (Ritchie & Huff, 1999).

Intermittent explosive disorder

DSM–IV includes this category as one of the impulse control disorders on axis I rather than as a specific personality disorder, although ICD–10 includes it as one of the personality disorders.

The degree of aggressiveness is out of proportion to any precipitating social stress and is triggered by minor conflict. The episodes occur independently of any other diagnosis. Individuals or their relatives usually describe the episodes as 'spells' or 'attacks'. Associated with the violent outbursts are feelings of tension, relief after the episode, followed by remorse. Many describe racing thoughts and an energy surge during the event, followed by lowering of mood and decreased energy. Most have a lifetime comorbidity with a mood disorder, including bipolar disorder. In general, onset is in adolescence and men predominate by a 4:1 ratio, although some women describe similar symptoms premenstrually. There is some doubt as to whether a pure category really exists, as most individuals with intermittent explosive disorder are usually comorbid for some other personality disorder, substance misuse, a psychosis or organic personality change. However, in view of the favourable response to mood stabilisers, such as lithium or sodium valproate and the selective serotonin reuptake inhibitors, there is a suggestion of a link to bipolar disorder, with the episodes representing micro-psychotic episodes of very rapid onset. There is little research on this disorder, although a detailed description is provided by McElroy (1999).

Pathological gambling

Gambling may be defined as staking something of value, generally money, on a game, or an uncertain event, or some other contingency. Professional gamblers carefully plan their gambling and attempt to decrease the element of risk, for example by having access to information not available to others. In contrast, pathological gambling is usually impulsive, and often associated with repeated and heavy losses, often to a state of financial and social ruin. The DSM–IV diagnosis has been shown to be reliable and valid, with good classification accuracy (Stinchfield, 2003).

DSM–IV defines the essential feature of the disorder as a chronic and progressive failure to resist impulses to gamble, such that the behaviour leading to much damage to personal and family life. Efforts to stop or resist gambling generally fail, and the behaviour shows some resemblance to an addiction (it is sometimes described as a non-substance addiction). Deprived of the opportunity to gamble, the person becomes restless and irritable; over time there is an increase in the size and frequency of the stake required to achieve the desired level of excitement. Repeated losses induce a strong urge to return yet again to try to win back the losses. In pathological states the gambling will persist even in the face of mounting debts, marital break-up or other legal problems. Some gamblers steal to maintain their habit and the morbid tendency may come to light only through a court case involving theft or embezzlement.

Pathological gambling is a serious problem and may be associated with other addictions, particularly to alcohol and tobacco, but may also lead to disturbances in eating, sleeping, sexual behaviour and relationships, as well as impaired function at work. Some patients present with depression or following an overdose.

The possibility that pathological gambling is not a unitary phenomenon but has several forms each with its own aetiology, natural history and so on has been suggested and should be the focus of further research. A comprehensive account of the topic is presented in a review by Raylu & Oei (2002).

Gambling itself is a common pastime and it is estimated that 39% of the British population engage in some form of regular gambling, while in the USA a figure of 61% has been given (Moran, 1983). Naturally, pathological gambling is much less common but is not rare: a recent review based on 120 studies gave a lifetime rate of 1.6% (Shaffer *et al*, 1999), although surveys of prison populations show that around 10% of prisoners are pathological gamblers (Royal College of Psychiatrists, 1977). Pathological gambling is probably more common and more obvious among men, who typically gamble on horse and dog racing, where there can be dramatic losses. Women prefer bingo and football pools, in which morbid patterns are less obvious because the losses are smaller and spread over longer periods of time.

The condition begins in adolescence for males and later in life for females. It waxes and wanes but tends to be chronic. Comorbidity is thought to include other addiction and impulse control disorders, such as substance misuse and alcoholism, as well as major depression, but there is some controversy as to whether suicide and suicide attempts are more common in gamblers.

Psychological dependence on gambling is demonstrated by the presence of withdrawal symptoms and craving following cessation of the activity.

Aetiology

The experience of risk taking is generally thrilling and pleasurable, and this is probably the main motivation. The gambling itself is a significant emotional event for those who indulge in it, and large changes in heart rate may occur. The experience of winning is said to produce a sense of euphoria resembling the effects of amphetamines or opiates. There are also suggestions that gambling will at least temporarily help people switch out of negative internal mood states, such as feelings of loneliness or other forms of dysphoria. The obvious self-destructive nature of the behaviour has provoked much analytical speculation, but there has been little scientific study of the problem. In his autobiographical novel *The Gambler,* Dostoyevsky described the rewarding sense of power obtained from gambling. Freud (1928), commenting on this book in his paper 'Dostoyevsky and parricide', suggested that gambling arose from unconscious guilt concerning patricidal urges.

Social factors are likely to play a role, such as early exposure to gambling and having a father who drank or gambled, especially among male gamblers. Female gamblers are more likely to come from families where their mothers also gambled and to have spouses who have raised rates of alcohol use and who are often absent. The likelihood of gambling appears to correlate with the number of gamblers in one's social circle, but in pathological gambling, although it is initially a social activity, in its later, morbid phase it usually becomes a lone preoccupation.

Learning theorists point out that the usual sequence of repeated gambling losses with occasional random wins provides a pattern of intermittent reinforcement, the most potent schedule for conditioning. In this respect a big win is thought to be particularly hazardous, and the financial reinforcement of winning prolongs the habit.

Recent evidence suggests that a mixture of biological and psychosocial factors are relevant to the development of this condition (Sharpe, 2002). Thus, in a recent MRI study of pathological gamblers, subjects were asked to watch videos of gambling behaviours to stimulate gambling urges. Their MRI scans showed decreased activation in the orbital prefrontal cortex, the basal ganglia and the thalamus when compared with controls. The direction of these changes in the orbitofrontal cortex is similar to the findings for antisocial personality disorder, where the decreased reaction to fear in the frontal cortex has been linked to impulsivity and disinhibition (Potenza *et al*, 2003).

Personality disorder, particularly antisocial, may also contribute, but pathological gambling can arise in the absence of any other disturbance of the personality. Childhood attention-deficit/hyperactivity disorder is also a risk factor and gambling may occur during an episode of depression as a way of obtaining symptomatic relief, similar to secondary drinking or kleptomania. Reckless gambling may sometimes accompany an episode of mania, in which gross degrees of financial irresponsibility are common.

Management

Various treatment approaches are offered, encompassing most known types of psychotherapy. Counselling and support for the family may also be helpful. During history taking it will often become apparent that help has been sought only to alleviate the consequences of gambling, such as debt, or a distressing marital situation or some other legal problem, and that there is little wish to stop gambling. Both psychodynamic psychotherapy and aversive behavioural therapy have been attempted, but neither can claim much success. Most gamblers find the notion of complete abstinence abhorrent, but a few may accept the wisdom of a moratorium for a few months, after which more controlled gambling may be permitted. Cognitive–behavioural therapy may be helpful, along with a 12-step group programme (Petry & Roll, 2001).

Among the more severe cases there is usually a disturbed appreciation of the value of money, and in these instances it is wisest for all the family income to be paid into an account over which the spouse has sole control. Gamblers Anonymous, which uses the Alcoholics Anonymous model, allows both the patient and spouse to share information about their struggles with the morbid impulses and provide mutual support; it may be more helpful than the more traditional medical and psychiatric approaches.

There is little more optimism on the pharmacological front, but if a psychiatrist is to play a role then a drug treatment is one possible option; the more recent studies are reviewed by Grant & Kim (2002). Earlier interest lay with the effects of mood stabilisers, such as lithium, valproate and carbamazepine, perhaps with an underlying assumption that affective disorder played some role, but there is little evidence for the efficacy of these drugs. Similarly, a controlled trial of olanzapine, an atypical antipsychotic, was also negative. However, six open trials of various selective serotonin reuptake inhibitors are beginning to suggest these drugs may help even in the absence of depression, with as many as 50–70% of participants responding. However, the one controlled trial revealed a high placebo response rate as well, which suggests that non-drug factors, such as being sufficiently motivated to take a drug and so enter treatment, may also be important. These trials (see Grant & Kim, 2002) suggest that high doses (higher than those used for depression, but in the same range as those used for obsessive–compulsive disorder) are required and should be tried for at least 10–12 weeks.

Naltraxone is an opiate antagonist at the mu-opioid receptor, which is the site where beta-endorphins, morphine and heroin act by modulating the neuronal input of GABA (gamma-aminobutyric acid) into dopaminergic neurones in the mesolimbic pathways. Two small trials have suggested that naltraxone is 75% effective, although only in high doses, but liver function may be disturbed with elevated transaminases.

Treatment should probably entail a combination of family support (if only to ensure that the family's money is controlled by someone other than the gambler), psychological help and, if requested, pharmacological intervention. The prevalence of pathological gambling is high, perhaps similar to that of bipolar disorder, and it can also result in a lifetime of destructive behaviour, yet very little is known about its origins or treatment.

Trichotillomania

Francois Hallopeau (1889), a French dermatologist, introduced the term trichotillomania to denote an irresistible urge to pull one's hair. This is often associated with subsequent rituals, such as mouthing the hair afterwards, or even ingesting it (trichophagy). Most sufferers report a state of tension before pulling their hair out, and this is included among the diagnostic criteria within DSM–IV (see Box 18.10). The hair pulling is not described as painful; rather, individuals report tingling and pruritis in the affected areas. Afterwards there may be a sense of gratification and release.

Box 18.10 DSM–IV criteria for trichotillomania

1 Recurrent pulling out of one's hair resulting in noticeable hair loss.
2 Increasing sense of tension prior to hair pulling.
3 Pleasure, gratification or sense of relief when pulling out the hair.
4 Not due to another mental disorder, or a general medical condition (e.g. a dermatological condition).
5 Causes significant distress or impairment in social or occupational functioning.

As well as the scalp, the eyebrows, eyelashes, beard and pubic hair may be involved. Hair pulling tends to occur during states of relaxation – while sitting down watching television, reading, studying, for example – but it usually is done in secret. Hair-pullers commonly also engage in nail biting, thumb sucking, head banging, gnawing and other types of self-mutilation. Greenberg & Sarner (1965) have described the inventiveness some patients have in devising methods to remove their hair. As well as pulling it out singly or in tufts, some would rub their scalps with their palms or their pillows until baldness supervened. Others tangled their hair in a comb or brush and then used these instruments to epilate themselves. Bizarre cases were also noted in this series: a patient with schizophrenia who, after years of hair pulling, set fire to himself, while in another case a mother was induced by her son to do the hair pulling for him. Children (usually aged 1–5 years) who swallow their hair may develop a tracheo-bezoar and present with epigastric pain, vomiting and a palpable mass, a condition sometimes leading to surgery and occasionally having a fatal outcome.

The disorder is not uncommon, occurring in around 1% of new psychiatric referrals, and usually presents to dermatological clinics before psychiatric services. However, patients often feel ashamed of their habit, which may not always be declared. The onset is typically in childhood and adolescence, and there is a marked female preponderance. A study of associated psychiatric comorbidity (Christianson *et al*, 1991) showed an increased lifetime prevalence for major depression, simple phobia, generalised anxiety disorder, and possibly also for alcohol and substance misuse. High rates of hair pulling were found in participants with obsessive–compulsive disorder, skin picking, body dysmorphic disorder and tic disorder. There was no association with personality disorder or any particular personality disorder subtype (the rates were slightly less than in the general psychiatric outpatient population). It may be more common among individuals with learning impairment, and may also occur in schizophrenia. Depression and substance misuse may lead to exacerbations, but are not thought to be causal. The course is usually chronic but with relapses and remissions. Patients may spend 1–3 hours a day in hair pulling, which leads eventually to severe baldness.

The differential diagnosis is occasionally with hypothyroidism, tinea capitis and syphilis, but is mainly with alopecia areata. Both disorders present with bald patches, but in trichotillomania the short, broken strands of hair will appear alongside normal hairs, while in alopecia all the hairs are short. In addition, when the hair regrows there is no change in pigmentation in trichotillomania, which can occur in alopecia. Among those who deny the habit of hair pulling a scalp biopsy will demonstrate the traumatic nature of the disorder with categen hairs, absence of inflammation and scarring, and dilated follicula infundibula. Hair follicle changes, known as tricomalacia, are said to be characteristic and differentiate the disorder from alopecia.

Management

The disorder often starts in childhood, has a prolonged course, and behavioural strategies appear to be the most useful. These include self-monitoring, covert desensitisation and habit reversal. The last technique involves asking the patient to practise some alternative motor response, such as grasping or clenching the hands for 3 minutes, which competes with the urge to pull hair. The behavioural regimen relies on identifying situations where the habit takes place, commonly while reading or watching television, and response prevention is attempted in these situations. Relaxation therapy is sometimes also helpful. Another component of the behavioural regime is 'overcorrection' or positive attention, which requires patients to brush or comb their hair or repair eye make-up (for eyelash pullers) after each episode of hair pulling.

Arzin *et al* (1980) reported a successful outcome for 34 hair-pullers and provided a detailed account of the behavioural methods they used.

Facial screening by covering the patient's scalp with a soft cloth is sometimes helpful. Patients will often deliberately cover affected areas out of feelings of shame, but also to protect these from further damage.

There is conflicting evidence for the efficacy of drugs. Swedo *et al* (1989) conducted a cross-over trial of desipramine and clomipramine in non-depressed women with trichotillomania. Both drugs were helpful but there was some advantage for clomipramine, which suggests a possible link with obsessive–compulsive disorder. However, a recent controlled trial showed no significant benefit from fluoxetine (60 mg daily) when compared with waiting list controls, although the same trial demonstrated significant benefits for behavioural therapy (Van Minnen *et al*, 2003).

Hypnotherapy has been reported as helpful in individual cases (Zalsman *et al*, 2001) and so may be worth trying.

While both behaviour therapy and drug treatment may offer some relief in the short term, little is known about relapse rates or long-term outcome. A recent longitudinal study found a poor prognosis even with psychiatric treatment (Keuthen *et al*, 2001).

A comprehensive review of treatment options is provided by Walsh & McDougle (2001).

References

Adler, A. (1964) *Problems of Neurosis*. New York: Harper.

Alexander, F. (1930) The neurotic character. *International Journal of Psychoanalysis*, **11**, 291–311.

American Psychiatric Association (1994) *Diagnostic and Statistical Manual of Mental Disorders* (4th edn) (DSM–IV). Washington. DC: APA.

American Psychiatric Association (2000) *Diagnostic and Statistical Manual of Mental Disorders* (4th edn, text revision) (DSM–IV–TR). Washington. DC: APA.

Androlunis, P. A., Gluech, B. C., Stroebel, C. F., *et al* (1981) Organic brain dysfunction and borderline personality disorder. *Psychiatric Clinics of North America*, **4**, 61–66.

Arieff, A. J. & Bowie, C. J. (1947) Some psychiatric aspects of shoplifting. *Journal of Clinical Psychopathology*, **8**, 565–576.

Arzin, N. H., Nunn, R. G. & Frantz, S. E. (1980) Treatment of hair pulling (tricotillomania): a comparative study of habit reversal and negative practice training. *Journal of Behaviour Therapy and Experimental Psychiatry*, **11**, 13–20,

Baron, M., Gruen, R., Asnis, L., *et al* (1983) Familial relatedness of schizophrenic and schizotypal states. *American Journal of Psychiatry*, **140**, 1437–1442.

Baron, M., Asnis, L. & Gruen, R. (1990) Schedule for Interviewing Schizotypal Personalities: a diagnostic interview for schizotypal features. *Psychiatry Research*, **4**, 213–228.

Battaglia, M., Gasperini, M., Sciuto, G., *et al* (1991) Psychiatric disorders in the families of schizotypal subjects. *Schizophrenia Bulletin*, **17**, 659–665.

Baxter, L., Edell, W., Gerner, R., *et al* (1984) Dexamethasone suppression test and axis I diagnoses of inpatients with DSM–III borderline personality disorder. *Journal of Clinical Psychiatry*, **45**, 150–153.

Bleuler, E. (1922) Die probleme der Schizoidie und der Syntonie. *Zeitschrift für die gesamte Neurologie und Psychiatrie*, **78**, 373–388.

Bohman, M., Cloinger, R., Sigvardsson, S., *et al* (1982) Predisposition to petty criminality in Swedish adoptees: genetic and environmental heterogeneity. *Archives of General Psychiatry*, **39**, 339–341.

Bradford, J. & Balmaceda, R. (1983) Shoplifting: is there a specific psychiatric syndrome. *Canadian Journal of Psychiatry*, **28**, 248–253.

Brothwell, J., Casey, P. & Tyrer, P. (1992) Perception of irrelative merits of subjects' and informants' assessment of personality status. *Irish Journal of Psychological Medicine*, **9**, 90–93.

Brown, G. R. & Anderson, B. (1991) Psychiatric morbidity in adult inpatients with childhood histories of sexual and physical abuse. *American Journal of Psychiatry*, **148**, 55–61.

Buckle, A. & Farrington, D. P. (1984) An observational study of shoplifting. *British Journal of Criminology*, **24**, 63–73.

Cadoret, R. J., O'Gorman, T. W., Troughton, E., *et al* (1985) Alcoholism and antisocial personality – interrelationships, genetics and environmental factors. *Archives of General Psychiatry*, **42**, 161–167.

Casey, P. R. (1989) Personality disorder and suicide intent. *Acta Psychiatrica Scandinavica*, **79**, 290–295.

Casey, P. & Butler, E. (1995) The effects of personality on response to ECT in major depression. *Journal of Personality Disorders*, **9**, 134–142.

Casey, P. & Tyrer, P. J. (1986) Personality, functioning and symptomatology. *Journal of Psychiatric Research*, **20**, 363–374.

Casey, P. & Tyrer, P. (1990) Personality disorder and psychiatric illness in general practice. *British Journal of Psychiatry*, **156**, 261–265.

Casey, P., Dillon, S. & Tyrer, P. J. (1984) The diagnostic status of patients with conspicuous psychiatric morbidity in primary care. *Psychological Medicine*, **14**, 673–681.

Cattell, R. B. (1965) *The Scientific Analysis of Personality*. Harmondsworth: Penguin.

Cheng, A. T. A., Mann, A. H. & Chan, K. A. (1997) Personality disorder and suicide. A case–control study. *British Journal of Psychiatry*, **170**, 441–446.

Cheng, A. T., Chen, T. H., Chen, C. C., *et al* (2000) Psychosocial and psychiatric risk factors for suicide: a case–control psychological autopsy study. *British Journal of Psychiatry*, **177**, 360–365.

Chiswick, D. & Cope, R. (1995) *Seminars in Practical Forensic Psychiatry*, pp. 44–47. London: Gaskell.

Christenson, G. A., Faber, R. J., De Zwaan, M., *et al* (1994) Compulsive buying: descriptive characteristics and psychiatric comorbidity. *Journal of Clinical Psychiatry*, **55**, 5–11.

Chodoff, P. & Lyons, H. (1958) Hysteria, the hysterical personality and 'hysterical' conversion. *American Journal of Psychiatry*, **114**, 734–740.

Christianson, G. A., McKenzie, T. B. & Mitchell, J. E. (1991) Characteristics of 60 adult chronic hair pullers. *American Journal of Psychiatry*, **148**, 365–370.

Clark, L. A. & Harrison, A. J. (2001) Assessment instruments. In *Handbook of Personality Disorders: Theory, Research and Treatment* (ed. W. J. Livesley), pp. 277–306. New York: Guilford Press.

Cleckley, H. (1941) *The Mask of Sanity* (2nd edn). St Louis, MO: Mosby.

Cleckley, H. (1964) *The Mask of Sanity* (4th edn). St Louis, MO: Mosby

Clifford, C. A., Murray, R. M. & Fulker, D. W. (1984) Genetic and environmental influences on obsessional traits and symptoms. *Psychological Medicine*, **14**, 791–800.

Cloninger, C. R. (1987) A systematic method for clinical description and classification of personality variants. *Archives of General Psychiatry*, **44**, 573–588.

Coid, J. (1993) Current concepts and classification of psychopathic disorder. In *Personality Disorders Reviewed* (eds P. Tyrer & G. S. Stein), pp. 113–164. London: Gaskell.

Cooke, D. J. & Michie, C. (1999) Psychopathy across culture: North America and Scotland compared. *Journal of Abnormal Psychology*, **108**, 58–68.

Cooney, J. M., Farren, C. K. & Clare, A. (1996) Personality disorders among first ever admissions to an Irish public and private hospital. *Irish Journal of Psychological Medicine*, **13**, 6–8.

Cornell, D. G., Warren, J., Hawk, G., *et al* (1996) Psychopathy in instrumental and reactive violent offenders. *Journal of Consulting and Clinical Psychology*, **64**, 783–790.

Costa, P. T. & McCrea, R. R. (1992) The five-factor model of personality and its relevance to personality disorders. *Journal of Personality Disorder*, **6**, 343–359.

Cupchik, W. & Atcheson, J. D.(1983) An occasional crime of the moral majority. *Bulletin of the American Academy of Psychiatry and Law*, **11**, 343–352.

Cutting, J., Cowen, P. J., Mann, A. H., *et al* (1986) Personality and psychosis: use of the Standardized Assessment of Personality. *Acta Psychiatrica Scandinavica*, **73**, 87–92.

Dagonet, H. (1870) Des impulsions dans la folie et de la folie impulsive. *Annales Medico-Psychologique*, **4**, 5–32, 215–259.

Dickey, C. C., McCarley, R. W. & Shenton, M. E. (2002) The brain in schizotypal personality disorder: a review of structural MRI and CT findings. *Harvard Review of Psychiatry*, **10**, 1–15.

Dolan, M. & Park, I. (2002) The neuropsychology of antisocial personality disorder. *Psychological Medicine*, **32**, 417–427.

Dowson, J. H. & Grounds, A. T. (1995) *Personality Disorders: Recognition and Clinical Management*. Cambridge: Cambridge University Press.

Engel, G. L. (1980) The clinical application of the biopsychosocial model. *American Journal of Psychiatry*, **137**, 535–544.

Erikson, E. H. (1956) The problem of ego identity. *Journal of the American Psychoanalytical Association*, **4**, 56–121.

Essen-Möller, E. (1956) Individual traits and morbidity in a Swedish rural population. *Acta Psychiatrica Scandinavica*, suppl. 2, 100.

Eysenck, H. & Eysenck, S. B. G. (1964) *Manual of the Eysenck Personality Inventory (EPQ)*. London: University of London Press.

Fabrega, H. J., Ulrich, R., Pilkonis, P., *et al* (1993) Personality disorders diagnosed at intake at a public psychiatric facility. *Hospital and Community Psychiatry*, **44**, 159–162.

Fahlen, T. (1995) Personality traits in social phobia I: comparisons with healthy controls. *Journal of Clinical Psychiatry*, **56**, 560–568.

Farmer, A. E., McGuffin, P. & Gottesman, I. I. (1987) Twin concordance for DSMIII schizophrenia. Scrutinising the validity of the definition. *Archives of General Psychiatry*, **44**, 634–641.

Farrington, D., Loeber, R. & Van Kammen, W. B. (1990) Long-term criminal outcomes of hyperactivity–impulsivity–attention deficit and conduct problems in childhood. In *Straight and Devious Pathways from Childhood to Adulthood* (eds L. N. Robins & M. Rutter). Cambridge: Cambridge University Press.

Fazel, S. & Danesh, J. H. (2002) Serious mental disorder in 23,000 prisoners: a systematic review of 62 surveys. *Lancet*, **359**, 545–549.

Foster, T., Gillespie, K. & McClelland, R. (1997) Mental disorders and suicide in Northern Ireland. *British Journal of Psychiatry*, **170**, 447–452.

Freud, S. (1901–05) Three essays on sexuality. In *The Complete Works of Sigmund Freud* (standard edn, 1953) (ed. J. Strachey), Vol. 7. London: Hogarth Press.

Freud, S. (1908) Character and anal eroticism. In *Collected Papers* (English translation, 1929), Vol. 2. London: Hogarth Press.

Freud, S. (1928) Dostoyevsky and parricide. In *The Complete Works of Sigmund Freud* (standard edn, 1961) (ed. J. Strachey), Vol. 21, p. 177. London: Hogarth Press.

Fyer, M. R., Frances, A., Sullivan, T., *et al* (1988) Co-morbidity of borderline personality disorder. *Archives of General Psychiatry*, **45**, 348–352.

Goldman, M. J. (1991) Kleptomania: making sense of the nonsensical. *American Journal of Psychiatry*, 148, 986–996.

Grant, J. E. & Kim, S. W. (2002) Effectiveness of pharmacotherapy for pathological gambling: a chart review. *Annals of Clinical Psychiatry*, **14**, 155–161.

Grant, J. E., Levine, M. D., Kim, D., *et al* (2005) Impulse control disorders in adult psychiatric inpatients. *American Journal of Psychiatry*, **162**, 2184–2188.

Grant, J. E., Correia, S. & Brennan-Krohn, T. (2006) White matter integrity in kleptomania: a pilot study. *Psychiatry Research*, **147**, 233–237.

Greenberg, H. R. & Sarner, C. A. (1965) Trichotillomania: symptoms and syndrome. *Archives of General Psychiatry*, **12**, 482–489.

Gudjonsson, G. H. (1990) Psychological and psychiatric aspects of shoplifting. *Medicine, Science and the Law*, **30**, 45–51.

Gunderson, J. G. (2001) *Borderline Personality Disorder: A Clinical Guide*, p. 54. Washington, DC: American Psychiatric Press.

Gunderson, J. & Austin, V. (1981) The Diagnostic Interview for Borderline Patients. *American Journal of Psychiatry*, **138**, 896–903.

Gunderson, J., Ronningstam, E. & Bodkin, A. (1990) The Diagnostic Interview for Narcissistic Patients. *Archives of General Psychiatry*, **47**, 676–680.

Gunn, J. (1988) Personality disorder: a clinical suggestion. In *Personality Disorders. Diagnosis, Management and Course* (ed. P. Tyrer), pp. 33–42. London: Wright.

Hallopeau, F. (1889) Alopecie par grattage: trichomanie on trichotillomanie. *Annales de Dermatologie et de Syphiligraphie*, **10**, 440–441.

Hare, R. D. (1991) *Manual for the Psychopathic Checklist – Revised*. Toronto: Multi-Health Systems.

Hart, S. D. & Hare, R. D. (1997) Psychopathy and association with criminal conduct. In *Handbook of Antisocial Behavior* (eds D. M. Stoff, J. Breiling & J. D. Maser). New York: John Wiley & Sons.

Hathaway, S. R. & McKinley, J. C. (1940) A Multiphasic Personality Schedule (Minnesota). Construction of the schedule. *Journal of Psychology*, **10**, 245–254.

Haw, C., Hawton, K., Houston, K., *et al* (2001) Psychiatric and personality disorders in deliberate self-harm patients. *British Journal of Psychiatry*, **178**, 48–54.

Heikkinen, M., Henriksson, M., Isometsa, E., *et al* (1997) Recent life events and suicide in personality disorders. *Journal of Nervous and Mental Disease*, **185**, 373–381.

Helgason, T. (1964) *Epidemiology of Mental Disorders in Iceland*. Copenhagen: Munksgaard.

Henderson, D. K. (1939) *Psychopathic States*. London: Chapman & Hall.

Henry, B. & Moffit, T. E. (1997) Neuropsychological and neuroimaging studies of juvenile delinquency and adult criminal behaviour. In *The Handbook of Antisocial Behavior* (eds D. M. Stoff, J. Breiling & J. D. Maser), pp. 289–304. New York: John Wiley & Sons.

Herpetz, S. C., Dietrich, T. M., Wenning, B., *et al* (2001) Evidence of abnormal amygdala functioning in borderline personality disorder: a functional MRI study. *Biological Psychiatry*, **50**, 292–298.

Hill, D. & Watterson, D. (1942) Electroencephalographic studies of psychopathic personalities. *Journal of Neurology and Psychiatry*, **5**, 47–52.

Hoch, P. H. & Polatin, P. (1949) Pseudoneurotic form of schizophrenia. *Psychiatric Quarterly*, **23**, 248–276.

Horney, K. (1939) *New Ways in Psychoanalysis*. New York: W. W. Norton.

Horney, K. (1945) *Our Inner Conflicts*. New York: Norton.

Hughes, C. H. (1884) Moral (affective) insanity: psycho-sensory insanity. *Alienist and Neurologist*, **5**, 296–315.

Hwu, H. F., Yeh, E. K. & Chang, L. Y. (1989) Prevalence of psychiatric disorders in Taiwan defined by the Chinese Diagnostic Interview Schedule. *Acta Psychiatrica Scandinavica*, **79**, 136–147.

Hyler, S. E., Skodol, A. E., Kellman, H. D., *et al* (1990) Validity of the Personality Disorder Questionnaire – revised: comparison with two structured interviews. *American Journal of Psychiatry*, **147**, 1043–1048.

Jackson, H. J. & Burgess, P. J. (2002) Personality disorders in the community: results from the Australian National Survey of Mental Health and Well-being, Part II: Relationships between personality disorder, axis I mental disorders and physical conditions with disability and health consultations. *Social Psychiatry and Psychiatric Epidemiology*, **37**, 251–260.

Jackson, H. J., Whiteside, H. L., Bates, G. W., *et al* (1991) Diagnosing personality disorders in psychiatric inpatients. *Acta Psychiatrica Scandinavica*, **83**, 206–213.

Johnson, J. J., Cohen, P., Brown, J., *et al* (1999) Childhood maltreatment increases risk for personality disorders during early adulthood. *Archives of General Psychiatry*, **56**, 600–606.

Jung, C. G. (1921) *Psychologische Typen*. Zurich: Rascher.

Kammeier, M. L., Hoffman, H. & Lopes, R. G. (1973) Personality characteristics of alcoholics as freshmen and at the time of treatment. *Quarterly Journal of Studies on Alcohol*, **34**, 390–399.

Kass, F., Skodol, A. E., Charles, E., *et al* (1985) Scaled ratings of DSM–III personality disorders. *American Journal of Psychiatry*, **142**, 627–630.

Kendell, R. E. & DiScipio, W. J. (1968) Eysenck Personality Inventory scores of patients with depressive illness. *British Journal of Psychiatry*, **114**, 767–770.

Kendler, K., Lieberman, J. A. & Walsh, D. (1989) The Structured Interview for Schizotypy (SIS): a preliminary report. *Schizophrenia Bulletin*, **15**, 559–571.

Kernberg, O. F. (1967) Borderline personality organisation. *Journal of the American Psychoanalytical Association*, **15**, 641–685.

Kety, S., Rosenthal, D., Wender, P. H., *et al* (1971) Mental illness in the biological and adoptive families of adopted schizophrenics. *American Journal of Psychiatry*, **128**, 302–306.

Keuthen, N. J., Frain, C., Deckersbach, T., *et al* (2001) Longitudinal follow-up of naturalistic outcome in patients with trichotillomania. *Journal of Clinical Practice*, **62**, 101–107.

Khiel, K. A., Smith, A. M., Hare, R. D., *et al* (2001) Limbic abnormalities in affective processing by criminal psychopaths as revealed by functional magnetic resonance imaging. *Biological Psychiatry*, **50**, 677–684.

Kohut, H. (1971) *The Analysis of the Self.* New York: International University Press.

Kraepelin, E. (1913) *Psychiatrie: Ein Lehrbuch* (8th edn), Vol. 3. Leipzig: Barth.

Kretschmer, E. (1918) *Der sensitive Beziehungswahn*. Berlin: Springer-Verlag.

Kretschmer, E. (1922) *Korperbau und Charakter*. Berlin: Springer-Verlag.

Kretschmer, E. (1926) *Hysteria* (English translation). New York: Nervous and Mental Diseases Publishing Company.

Kroll, J., Carey, K., Lloyd, S., *et al* (1982) Are there borderlines in Britain? A cross validation of US findings. *Archives of General Psychiatry*, **39**, 60–63.

Lacey, J. H. & Evans, C. D. H. (1986) The impulsivist: a multi-impulsive personality disorder. *British Journal of Addiction*, **81**, 641–649.

Lakey, B. & Loeber, R. (1997) Attention deficit hyperactivity disorder, oppositional defiant disorder, conduct disorder, and adult antisocial behaviour: a life span perspective. In *The Handbook of Antisocial Behavior* (eds D. M. Stoff, J. Breiling & J. D. Maser), pp. 51–59. New York: John Wiley & Sons.

Langbehn, D. R., Pfohl, B. M., Reynolds, S., *et al* (1999) The Iowa Personality Disorder Screen: development and preliminary validation of a brief screening interview. *Journal of Personality Disorders*, **13**, 75–89.

Lejoyeux, M., Arbarataz, M., McLoughlin, M., *et al* (2002) Impulse control disorders and depression. *Journal of Nervous and Mental Disease*, **190**, 310–314.

Lewis, G. & Appleby, L. (1988) Personality disorder: the patients psychiatrists dislike. *British Journal of Psychiatry*, **153**, 44–49.

Links, P. S., Heslegrave, R. & van Reekum, R. (1998) Prospective follow-up study of borderline personality disorder: prognosis, prediction of outcome and axis II co-morbidity. *Canadian Journal of Psychiatry*, **43**, 265–270.

Livesley, J. (2001) *Handbook of Personality Disorders: Theory, Research and Treatment*. New York: Guilford Press.

Livesley, W. J., Schroeder, M. L., Jackson, D., *et al* (1994) Categorical distinction in the study of personality disorder: implications for classification. *Journal of Abnormal Psychology*, **103**, 6–17.

Loranger, A. W. (1990) The impact of DSM–III on diagnostic practice in a university hospital. *Archives of General Psychiatry*, **47**, 672–675.

Loranger, A. W., Oldham, J. M. & Tulis, E. H. (1982) Familial transmission of DSM–III borderline personality disorder. *Archives of General Psychiatry*, **39**, 795–799.

Loranger, A. W., Susman, V. L., Oldham, J. M., *et al* (1985) *Personality Disorder Examination (PDE). A Structured Interview for DSM–III–R and ICD–9 Personality Disorders. WHOI ADAMHA Pilot Version*. White Plains, NY: New York Hospital, Cornell Medical Centre.

Luntz, B. K. & Widom, C. S. (1994) Antisocial personality disorder in abused and neglected children grown up. *American Journal of Psychiatry*, **151**, 670–674.

Macmillan, D. & Shaw, P. (1966) Senile breakdown in standards of personal and environmental cleanliness. *British Medical Journal*, **ii**, 1032–1037.

Maier, W., Uchtennann, D., Klingler, T., *et al* (1992) Prevalence of personality disorders (DSM–III–R) in the community. *Journal of Personality Disorder*, **6**, 187–196.

Mann, A. H., Jenkins, R., Cutting, J. C., *et al* (1981) The development and use of a standardised assessment of abnormal personality. *Psychological Medicine*, **11**, 839–847.

Mannuzza, S., Gittleman Klein, R., Horowitz Kongi, P., *et al* (1989) Hyperactive boys almost grown up: IV. Criminality and its relationship to psychiatric status. *Archives of General Psychiatry*, **46**, 1073–1079.

Mattia, J. L. & Zimmerman, M. (2001) Epidemiology. In *Handbook of Personality Disorders: Theory, Research and Treatment* (ed. W. J. Livesley), pp. 107–123. New York: Guilford Press.

Maudsley, H. (1897) *Responsibility in Mental Disease*. New York: Appleton.

McElroy, S. L. (1999) Recognition and treatment of DSM–IV explosive disorder. *Journal of Clinical Psychiatry*, **60**, suppl. 15, 12–16.

McGuffin, P., Katz, R., Aldrich, J., *et al* (1988) The Camberwell Collaboration Depression Study 2. Investigation of family members. *British Journal of Psychiatry*, **152**, 766–775.

Miller, P. K., Byrne, M., Hodges, A., *et al* (2002) Schizotypal components in people at high risk of developing schizophrenia: early findings from the Edinburgh High-Risk Study. *British Journal of Psychiatry*, **100**, 179–184.

Millon, T. (1981) *Disorders of Personality, DSM–III Axis II*. New York: John Wiley & Sons.

Millon, T. (1982) *Millon Clinical Multiaxial Inventory Interpretative Scoring System* (2nd edn). Minneapolis: National Computer Systems.

Modestin, J. & Puhan, A. (2000) Comparison of assessments of personality disorder by patients and informants. *Psychopathology*, **33**, 265–270.

Moffit, T. E. (1994) Neuropsychology tests predict persistent male delinquency. *Criminology*, **32**, 101–124.

Moran, E. (1983) Gambling. In *Handbook of Psychiatry, 4. The Neurosis and Personality Disorders* (eds G. F. M. Russell & L. A. Hersov), pp. 385–390. Cambridge: Cambridge University Press.

Moran, P. A., Jenkins, R., Tylee, A., *et al* (2000) The prevalence of personality disorder among UK primary care attenders. *Acta Psychiatrica Scandinavica*, **102**, 52–57.

Moran, P., Leese, M., Lee, T., *et al* (2003) Standardised Assessment of Personality – Abbreviated Scale (SAPAS): preliminary validation of a brief scale for personality disorder. *British Journal of Psychiatry*, **183**, 228–232.

Myers, J. K., Weissman, M. M., Tischler, G. L., *et al* (1984) Six-month prevalence of psychiatric disorders in three communities, 1980–1982. *Archives of General Psychiatry*, **41**, 951–967.

Myers, M. G., Stewart, D. G. & Brown, S. A. (1998) Progression from conduct disorder following treatment for adolescent substance abuse. *American Journal of Psychiatry*, **155**, 479–485.

Ogata, S. N., Silk, K. R., Goodrich, S., *et al* (1990) Childhood sexual and physical abuse in adult patients with borderline personality disorder. *American Journal of Psychiatry*, **147**, 1008–1013.

O'Neill, F. A. & Kendler, K. (1998) A longitudinal study of interpersonal dependency in twins. *British Journal of Psychiatry*, **172**, 154–158.

Paris, J. (2001) Psychosocial adversity. In *Handbook of Personality Disorders: Theory, Research and Treatment* (ed. W. J. Livesley), pp. 231–241. New York: Guilford Press.

Patience, D. A., McGuire, R. J., Scott, A. I. F., *et al* (1995) The Edinburgh Primary Care Depression Study: personality disorder and outcome. *British Journal of Psychiatry*, **167**, 324–330.

Petry, N. M. & Roll, J. M. (2001) A behavioural approach to understanding and treating pathological gambling. *Seminars in Clinical Neuropsychiatry*, **6**, 177–183.

Pfohl, B., Stangi, D. & Zimmerman, M. (1983) *Structured Interview for DSM–III Personality Disorders (SIDP)*. Iowa City: University of Iowa.

Phillips, K. A., Gunderson, J. G., Triebwasser, J., *et al* (1998) Reliability and validity of depressive personality disorder. *American Journal of Psychiatry*, **155**, 1044–1048.

Pinel, P. H. (1806) *A Treatise on Insanity* (transl. D. Davis, 1962). New York: Hafner Publishing.

Pope, H. G., Jonas, J. M., Hudson, J. I., *et al* (1983) The validity of DSM–III borderline personality disorder. *Archives of General Psychiatry*, **40**, 23–30.

Potenza, M. N., Leung, H. C., Blumberg, H. P., *et al* (2003) An FMRI Stroop task study of venteromedial prefrontal cortical function in pathological gamblers. *American Journal of Psychiatry*, **160**, 1990–1994.

Pritchard, J. C. (1835) *Treatise on Insanity*. London: Gilbert & Piper.

Rado, S. (1956) Schizotypal organization: preliminary report on a clinical study of schizophrenia. In *Changing Concepts of Psychoanalytic Medicine* (eds S. Rado & G. E. Daniels), pp. 225–236. New York: Grune & Stratton.

Raine, A., Bremian, P. A. & Mednick, S. A. (1994) Birth complications combined with early maternal rejection aged 1 year predispose to violent crime at age 18 years. *Archives of General Psychiatry*, **51**, 984–988.

Raine, A., Lencz, T., Bihrie, S., *et al* (2000) Reduced prefrontal gray matter volume and reduced antonomic activity in antisocial personality disorder. *Archives of General Psychiatry*, **57**, 119–127.

Raylu, N. & Oei, T. P. (2002) Pathological gambling. A comprehensive review. *Clinical Psychology Review*, **22**, 1009–1061.

Reid, W. H. (1985) Antisocial personality disorder. In *Psychiatry I* (eds R. Michels, J. D. Cavender, H. K. H. Brodie, *et al)*, pp. 1–11. Philadelphia: J. B. Lippincott.

Rhee, S. H. & Waldman, D. (2002) Genetic and environmental influences on antisocial behaviour: a meta analysis of twin and adoptive studies. *Psychological Bulletin*, **128**, 490–529.

Rhinehart, N. J., Bradshaw, J. L., Brereton, A. V., *et al* (2002) A clinical and behaviour review of high functioning autism and Asperger's disorder. *Australia and New Zealand Journal of Psychiatry*, **36**, 762–770.

Ritchie, E. C. & Huff, T. G. (1999) Psychiatric aspects of arsonists. *Journal of Forensic Science*, **44**, 733–740.

Robins, L. (1985) Epidemiology of anti-social personality disorder. In *Psychiatry 3* (eds R. Michels, J. O. Cavenar, H. K. Brodie, *et al*), pp. 1–14. Philadelphia: J. B. Lippincott.

Royal College of Psychiatrists (1977) *Submission of Evidence to the Royal Commission on Gambling*. London: Royal College of Psychiatrists.

Rutter, M. (1985) Resilience in the face of adversity: protective factors and resistance to psychiatric disorder. *British Journal of Psychiatry*, **147**, 598–611.

Sara, G., Raven, P. & Mann, A. (1996) A comparison of DSM–IIIR and ICD–10 personality criteria in an out-patient population. *Psychological Medicine*, **26**, 151–160.

Schafer, S. & Nowlis, D. P. (1998) Personality disorders among difficult patients. *Archives of Family Medicine*, **7**, 126–129.

Schneider, K. (1923) *Die psychopathischen Personlichkeiten*. Vienna: Deuticke.

Schroeder, M. L., Wormsworth, J. A. & Livesley, W. J. (1992) Dimensions of personality disorder and their relationship to the big five dimensions of personality. *Psychological Assessment*, **4**, 47–53.

Seivewright, N. (1988) Personality disorder, life events and onset of mental illness. In *Personality Disorders. Diagnosis, Management and Course* (ed. P. Tyrer). London: Wright.

Shaffer, H. J., Hall, M. N. & Bilt, J. (1999) Estimating the prevalence of disordered gambling behaviour in the United States and Canada: a research synthesis. *American Journal of Public Health*, **89**, 1369–1376.

Sharpe, L. (2002) A reformulated cognitive–behavioural model of problem gambling. A biopsychosocial perspective. *Clinical Psychology Review*, **22**, 1–22.

Sheldon, W. H. (1940) *The Varieties of Human Physique: An Introduction to Constitutional Psychology*. New York: Harper.

Shepherd, M., Cooper, B., Brown, A. C., *et al* (1966) *Psychiatric Illness in General Practice*. Oxford: Oxford University Press.

Singleton, N., Meltzer, H., Gatward, R., *et al* (1998) *Psychiatric Morbidity Among Prisoners in England and Wales*. London: Statistics Office.

Skodol, A. E., Oldham, J. M. & Gallaher, P. E. (1999) Axis II comorbidity of substance use disorders among patients referred for treatment of personality disorders. *American Journal of Psychiatry*, **156**, 733–738.

Skodol, A. E., Gunderson, J. G., McGlashan, T. H., *et al* (2002) Functional impairment in patients with schizotypal, borderline, avoidant or obsessive compulsive personality disorder. *American Journal of Psychiatry*, **159**, 276–283.

Spitzer, R. L. (1983) Psychiatric diagnosis: care clinicians still necessary? *Comprehensive Psychiatry*, **24**, 399–411.

Spitzer, R. L., Williams, J. & Gibbon, M. (1987) *Structured Clinical Interview for DSM–III–R (SCID–II)*. New York: Biometrics Research, New York State Psychiatric Institute.

Stern, A. (1938) Psychoanalytic investigation of and therapy in the borderline group of neuroses. *Psychoanalytic Quarterly*, **7**, 350–354.

Stinchfield, R. (2003) Reliability, validity and classification accuracy of a measure of DSM–IV diagnostic criteria for pathological gambling. *American Journal of Psychiatry*, **160**, 180–182.

Stone, M. H. (1990) Treatment of borderline patients: a pragmatic approach. *Psychiatric Clinics of North America*, **13**, 265–286.

Stone, M. H. (1993) *Abnormalities of Personality. Within and Beyond the Realm of Treatment*. New York: Norton.

Sullivan, H. S. (1947) *Conceptions of Modern Psychiatry*. New York: Norton.

Suominen, K. H., Isometsa, E. T., Henriksson, M. M., *et al* (2000) Suicide attempts and personality disorder. *Acta Psychiatrica Scandinavica*, **102**, 118–125.

Swedo, S. E., Leonard, H. L. & Rapoport, J. L. (1989) A double blind comparison of clomipramine and desipramine in the treatment of trichotillomania (hair pulling). *New England Journal of Medicine*, **321**, 497–501.

Thompson, D. J. & Goldberg, D. (1987) Hysterical personality disorder. The process of diagnosis in clinical and experimental settings. *British Journal of Psychiatry*, **150**, 241–245.

Tiihonen, J., Hodkins, S., Vaurio, O., *et al* (2000) Amygdaloid volume loss in psychopaths. *Society for Neuroscience Abstracts*, 2017.

Torgersen, S., Lygren, S., Andersien, P., *et al* (2000) A twin study of personality disorders. *Comprehensive Psychiatry*, **41**, 416–425.

Trelat, U. (1861) *La Folie Lucide*. Paris: Delahaye.

Tyrer, P. (1988) *Personality Disorders. Diagnosis, Management and Course*. London: Wright.

Tyrer, P. (1989) General neurotic syndrome and mixed anxiety–depressive disorders. In *Classification of Neurosis*, pp. 153–160. Chichester: John Wiley & Sons.

Tyrer, P. (1999) Borderline personality disorder: a motley diagnosis in need of reform. *Lancet*, **354**, 2095–2096.

Tyrer, P. (2002) Practice guidelines for the treatment of borderline personality disorder: a bridge too far. *Journal of Personality Disorders*, **16**, 113–118.

Tyrer, P. & Alexander, J. (1979) Classification of personality disorder. *British Journal of Psychiatry*, **135**, 163–167.

Tyrer, P., Casey, P. & Gall, J. (1983) The relationship between neurosis and personality disorder. *British Journal of Psychiatry*, **142**, 404–408.

Tyrer, P., Casey, P. & Ferguson, B. (1988) Personality disorder and mental illness. In *Personality Disorders: Diagnosis, Management and Course* (ed. P. Tyrer), pp. 93–104. London: Wright.

Vaillant, G. E. (1977) *Adaptation for Life*. Boston: Little, Brown.

Valgum, S. & Valgum, P. (1989) Co-morbidity for borderline and schizotypal personality disorders. A study of alcoholic women. Progress in neuropsychopharmacology and biological psychiatry. *Journal of Nervous and Mental Disease*, **177**, 279–284.

Van Minnen, A., Hoogduin, K. A., Keijsers, G. P. J., *et al* (2003) Treatment of trichotillomania with behaviour therapy or fluoxetine. A randomised waiting list controlled trial. *Archives of General Psychiatry*, **60**, 517–522.

Waller, G. (1993) Association of sexual abuse and borderline personality disorder in eating disordered women. *International Journal of Eating Disorders*, **13**, 259–263.

Walsh, K. H. & McDougle, C. J. (2001) Trichotillomania. Presentation, etiology, diagnosis and therapy. *American Journal of Clinical Dermatology*, **2**, 327–333.

Westen, D. & Harnden-Fischer, J. (2001) Personality profiles in eating disorders: rethinking the distinction of axis 1 and axis 2. *American Journal of Psychiatry*, **158**, 547–562.

Westen, D. & Shedler, J. (1999) Revising and assessing axis 11, Part 1: Developing a clinically and emperically valid assessment method. *American Journal of Psychiatry*, **156**, 258–272.

Whewell, P., Ryman, A., Bonnano, D., et al (2000) Does the ICD–10 classification accurately describe subtypes of borderline personality disorder? *British Journal of Medical Psychology*, **73**, 483–489.

Widiger, T. A., Mangine, S., Corbitt, E. M., *et al* (1995) *Personality Disorder Interview – IV: A Semi-structured Interview for the Assessment of Personality Disorders*. Odessa, FL: Psychological Assessment Resources.

Williamson, S., Hare, R. D. & Wong, S. (1987) Violence: criminal psychopaths and their victims. *Canadian Journal of Behavioural Science*, **19**, 454–462.

Wing, L. (1981) Asperger's syndrome: a clinical account. *Psychological Medicine*, **11**, 115–129.

Wittels, F. (1930) The hysterical character. *Medical Review of Reviews*, **36**, 186–190.

World Health Organization (1992) *International Classification of Diseases and Related Health Problems* (ICD–10). Geneva: WHO.

Zalsman, G., Hermesh, H. & Sever, J. (2001) Hypnotherapy in adolescents with trichotillomania: three cases. *American Journal of Clinical Hypnotherapy*, **44**, 63–68.

Zanarini, M. C. (1993) BPD as an impulse spectrum disorder. In *Borderline Personality Disorder: Etiology and Treatment* (ed. J. Paris), pp. 67–85. Washington, DC: American Psychiatric Press.

Zanarini, M. C., Frankenburg, F. R., Sickel, A. E., *et al* (1994) *Diagnostic Interview for DSM–IV Personality Disorders (DIPD-IV)*. McLean Hospital, 115 Mill Street, Belmont, Massachusetts.

Zanarini, M. C., Frankenburg, F. R., Dubo, D., *et al* (1998) Axis I co-morbidity of borderline personality disorder. *American Journal of Psychiatry*, **155**, 1733–1738.

Zanarini, M. C., Yong, L., Frankenburg, F. R., *et al* (2002) Severity of reported childhood sexual abuse and its relationship to severity of borderline psychopathology and psychosocial impairment among borderline inpatients. *Journal of Nervous and Mental Disease*, **190**, 381–387.

Zimmerman, M. (1994) Diagnosing personality disorders: a review of issues and research methods. *Archives of General Psychiatry*, **511**, 225–245.

Zimmerman, M. & Coryell, W. H. (1990) Diagnosing personality disorders in the community. *Archives of General Psychiatry*, **51**, 225–245.

Zimmerman, M. & Mattia, J. M. (1999) Differences between clinical and research practices in diagnosing borderline personality disorder. *American Journal of Psychiatry*, **156**, 1570–1574.

Zoccolillo, M., Pickles, A., Quinton, D., *et al* (1992) The outcome of childhood conduct disorder: implications for defining adult personality disorder and conduct disorder. *Psychological Medicine*, **22**, 971–986.

CHAPTER 19

Treatment and outcome of the personality disorders

Michael Stone

While it would be wrong to talk of a cure in connection with the personality disorders, they may be amenable to treatment. A generation ago a diagnosis of personality disorder was generally equated with untreatability, but advances in the fields of diagnosis, psychotherapy and psychopharmacology have now provided clinicians with a range of treatment options. These have dramatically changed our perception of the treatability of these disorders, to the extent that the American Psychiatric Association has published guidelines for the treatment of borderline personality disorder (BPD) (Oldham *et al*, 2001). None the less, many patients remain beyond the reach of any therapy, either because they are too severely affected or are too contemptuous of therapy.

The word 'enduring' is included in the ICD–10 definition of personality disorders (see Chapter 18). This implies long-lasting although not necessarily permanent features. Personality is in effect a stable mechanism. It represents the sum of a huge number of programmes, each with a high survival value, for example for getting along with parents, attracting sexual partners, rearing one's children or coping with bosses. Costa & McCrae (1986) pointed out that personality is resistant to change, whether it is normal and in harmony (and therefore in no particular need of change) or highly disagreeable to others, making it problematic (and therefore greatly in need of change).

Certain general principles are common to the management of the personality disorders. These derive mainly from the writings of a few psychoanalysts with a special interest in the area, but the same principles equally apply to treatment in general psychiatric settings. In this chapter the principles of psychotherapy will be outlined first; this is followed by a consideration of pharmacological interventions and the possible role of electroconvulsive therapy (for comorbid depression). The long-term outcomes of the personality disorders are then briefly reviewed.

Psychotherapy

Personality disorders call out for some sort of therapeutic intervention because they have the capacity to spoil patients' lives and the lives of others.

Length and phases of treatment

Maladaptive traits are difficult to change, however, and in most cases strenuous efforts and prolonged treatment are required. Therapists must content themselves with small improvements and a relatively slow advance, extending over years rather than weeks or months. Waldinger & Gunderson (1984), in their survey of psychotherapists with an interest in borderline personality disorder (BPD), found that the treatment duration was between 2 and 7 years, with an average of 4 years for most cases. These figures do not even take into consideration the discouragingly high drop-out rate in BPD patients (about 40%). A general psychiatrist using supportive measures and medication may also find the duration of the therapeutic contact extends for some 3–6 years.

In the more prolonged analytical treatments of severe personality disorders, three phases are recognised:

1. a holding or containing phase, in which the therapist serves almost as a transitional object
2. a gradual weaning phase, when previously tolerated regression is increasingly questioned and during which there is a gradual process of optimal disillusionment
3. a separation phase, when autonomy and self-worth are encouraged.

For those treating the personality disorders there is no quick fix; if the maladaptive traits disappear after a few sessions or a brief course of medication, then the original diagnosis of personality disorder, at least as the cause of the presenting behaviour rather than as a coincidental diagnosis, should be questioned.

Outline of treatment approaches

Many different methods of psychotherapy have been tried in the treatment of disorders of personality. These include supportive therapy, classical psychoanalysis, psychodynamically orientated psychotherapy, cognitive–behavioural psychotherapy (Beck & Freeman, 1990; Linehan, 1993) and a host of eclectic pragmatic approaches. With each method most authorities agree that the emphasis should be on the 'here and now' rather than the 'distant past', because the aim is to change present behaviour patterns and current modes of relating. For the analytically based therapist this means greater emphasis on interpreting the transference, while cognitive therapists will explore current distortions of reality. Other approaches include the 'rational emotive' psychotherapy of Albert Ellis (1963) – a variety of cognitive therapy – and Carl Rogers' existentialism-based psychotherapy (Rogers, 1967).

Therapists should guard against too facile formulations or simplistic interpretations that view the different personality disorders as defences against this or that conflict. Alexander (1957) suggested that the treatment of personality disorders entailed providing a 'corrective emotional experience'. Fromm-Reichmann (1950) put the case even more strongly and wrote 'what these patients need is an experience, not an explanation'. This holds true whether treatment takes the form of psychoanalysis five times weekly or an admission to a general psychiatric unit.

Syntonicity

Regardless of the theoretical orientation of the therapist, the cognitive style of the patient needs to be taken into account during treatment. Unlike most axis I disorders, many people with personality disorders do not complain of symptoms. Their problems bother other people rather than themselves. Very self-centred people may see themselves as 'tough yet reasonable', while others would perceive them as narcissists. The term 'ego-syntonic' has been used to describe this, *syntonic* signifying comfort with themselves, as opposed to *dystonic*, which suggests disharmony with themselves or their environment. Some maladaptive traits, such as being moody, shy or absent-minded, even if they are ego-syntonic, impinge only lightly on friends and intimates. However, other ego-syntonic traits, such as being wilful, impulsive or callous, have a much more damaging effect and are therefore of clinical importance. Some subjects with personality disorders are ego-dystonic and regret their maladaptive traits, and their distress provides some motivation for therapeutic change. The degree of syntonicity has important implications with regard to the initiation and ultimate success of treatment.

Treatment of traits

A second feature common to almost all personality disorders is the self-defeating nature of the maladaptive traits. These patients are adept at making matters worse for themselves. People with a paranoid personality will suspect and alienate even their closest friends; those with a histrionic personality will spare no effort to become involved with the most inappropriate person; those with an obsessional personality stifle all pleasure for themselves and their families; and for almost all there will be attempts to destroy or subvert those who seek to treat them or change their ways.

Treatment goals among those with personality disorders should be limited. A wholesale change of character is unlikely but some change may be possible. Patients with a schizoid personality will never become the life and soul of the party, but there is progress if they begin to meet a friend once a week. Someone with a borderline personality will continue to make emotionally intense relationships, but if there is only sadness rather than self-mutilation when the relationship ends, these reactions will be within the normal range. For some chronically suicidal adolescents the aim is quite modest – simply the preservation of life. Even this basic goal may require a generous allocation of psychotherapeutic time, hospital admissions, medication and nursing support.

The goals for the three DSM–IV personality disorder clusters (see Chapter 18) are quite different: for the *dramatic* cluster (borderline, histrionic, sociopathy), it is to curb impulsivity and overheated emotionality; for the *eccentric* cluster (paranoid and schizotypal), to undo the cognitive disorders; for the *anxious* cluster, to alleviate the excessive inhibitedness.

It should be noted that both psychoanalysis and psychotherapy rest on the assumption that a patient's maladaptive traits and behaviour are born out of conflicts, and that resolution of these conflicts will help the patient. The method may be of relatively little use if the main difficulty is one of temperament (e.g. extreme intensity, irritability, emotional insensitivity) because temperament is largely innate or genetic (Buss & Plomin, 1984) and less likely to change in the long term as a result of purely psychological intervention.

A key goal in treating subjects with a personality disorder is the amelioration of maladaptive traits. If rudeness and stinginess are maladaptive and to be extinguished, then their opposites (politeness and generosity) represent the ideal and should be fostered. Therapists will instinctively find themselves behaving in a manner opposite to the prevailing pathological trend in the patient's personality. For example, when treating

Table 19.1 Prevailing traits and corresponding countermeasures

Personality disorder	Prevailing trait(s)	Countermeasures
Schizoid	Aloofness	Affability
Schizotypal	Eccentricity	Conventionality
Paranoid	Mistrustfulness	Candour, honesty
Borderline	Unreasonableness, seductiveness, impulsivity	Compassionate, neutrality, strict boundaries
Histrionic	Over-emotionality	Orderliness, logical approach, modulated responses
Narcissistic	Grandiosity, condescension	Sympathy, humility, not taking offence
Antisocial	Contempt for rules	Strict adherence to rules
Obsessive–compulsive	Constriction of affect	Emotional vividness
Passive aggressive	Argumentativeness	Non-defensiveness
Avoidant	Timorousness	Encouragement
Dependent	Clinginess	Kind but distant
Depressive	Pessimistic	Optimism, enthusiasm
Irritable	Angry	Calmness

an avoidant person, therapists will find themselves being more affable and outgoing than is usual for them, thereby demonstrating that the world is not such a hostile place. For the chaotic patient, sticking to the rules, insisting on punctuality and starting and finishing sessions on time are essential. For the clingingly dependent individual, almost by instinct therapists avoid over-long stays in hospital, frequent extra individual sessions or out-of-hours telephone calls. Table 19.1 shows the therapeutic counterforces that apply to the various DSM–IV personality disorders. The use of the technique of counterforces requires some care, particularly in the presence of an axis I disorder. Thus, someone with a dependent personality and depression may try to remain in hospital because of depressive feelings rather than because of dependency needs; the clinical distinction is often fine and rarely easy to make.

Likeability

Therapy with these subjects is hard work: a successful outcome depends on the presence of a certain 'glue' which binds the patient and therapist together. What is the nature of this glue? Woolcott (1985) emphasised that the most important component is the quality of *likeableness*. It is this that motivates the therapist to work assiduously on the patient's behalf. Likeableness is difficult to define, but is probably a composite of several traits, including flexibility, forgiveness, respectfulness, consideration and perseverance. Unfortunately, the medical model, with its emphasis on disease types and negative traits, pays insufficient attention to the patient's strengths and positive traits, which may be of critical importance in determining outcome. Positive qualities, such as high intelligence, artistic sensitivity or talent and strong moral fibre may also help to motivate therapists.

It is helpful to keep in mind that, from the standpoint of evolutionary psychiatry, the personality disorders can all be understood as exaggerations of otherwise adaptive strategies for survival in the larger human community. Thus, the suspiciousness of the paranoid personality is the (now pathological) extreme of the kind of wariness and mistrustfulness that are highly adaptive in, say, detectives, spies and guards. The intense clinginess and demandingness of the borderline patient are the no longer adaptive extremes of a normal desire to preserve an attachment to a love object. Jealousy may be seen as a manoeuvre to ensure faithful attachment. Even the antisocial personality represents an unwelcome exaggeration of an otherwise socially valuable tendency to adventurousness and risk taking (McGuire & Troisi, 1998; Stevens & Price, 2000).

When both patient and therapist have some degree of mutual respect, each participant is minimally anxious and therefore best able to engage in harmonious dialogue. Therapists are unable to like everybody, and in the presence of even a mild degree of dislike anxiety and defensiveness will soon paralyse any form of self-expression, while in the presence of mutual dislike therapy will soon come to an end. The paradox is that those with the most disabling disorders, who are in the greatest need of change, are usually quite unlikeable. They alienate their relatives, employers, colleagues and, however well meaning or well trained, their therapists as well. For those at the milder end of the spectrum with more likeable characteristics, psychotherapy serves as a useful catalyst for change; for those with severe disorders who are grossly unlikeable, therapy rarely proceeds far – after starting therapy (which is usually at someone else's request) they soon quit.

To some extent, likeability is also socially determined; thus, the private therapist will soon come to dislike the patient who skips a few sessions and fails to pay bills. By contrast, therapists working in a forensic setting would hardly be troubled by such behaviour and might find they are able to 'click' quite well with certain 'likeable rogues'. Even so, there are some severely dystonic individuals – for example with sadistic or sociopathic personalities – who are so grossly contemptuous of almost all other people (including therapists) that they would not be amenable to any form of psychotherapy, especially if they show the traits of the psychopath (Hare *et al*, 1990): glibness, grandiosity, deceitfulness, manipulativeness, lack of remorse, callousness and inability to take responsibility for one's actions. Such persons lack all motivation to change, regarding themselves as superior and fine, and regarding others as fools and wimps.

A final point concerns the qualities of the therapist. Just as there are some doctors who dislike almost any psychiatric patient, there are some psychiatrists who dislike or cannot effectively cope with these most taxing and devious individuals. Gunderson (1984) suggested that psychotherapists who treat people with BPD should have qualities that include 'a comfort with aggression, sensitivity to separation experience, a sense of adventurousness and clarity of conceptual organisation'. Supervision is essential for novices and often helpful even for those with experience. Working in a unit that specialises in the treatment of the personality disorders may be helpful in familiarising trainees with the more common problems and some basic skills. However, the more intensive and longer-term therapies are perhaps best left to those who are temperamentally suited to such work.

Psychotherapy for 'eccentric' disorders

Schizoid and schizotypal personality disorders

Schizotypal personality disorder is characterised by eccentric ideas and so the area of concern for the therapist includes the cognitive distortions. Rapport is often difficult to establish, and few patients will be able to tolerate or understand a classical transference-based type of interpretation. It is best for therapy to focus on candid discussions of practical, everyday issues. This should be done in conventional, simple language, discouraging strange speech on the part of the patient, with the therapist also taking care to avoid jargon. The therapist should try to help the patient to remain in tune with others at work or at home, rather than be solely at the mercy of strange ideas. In this function the therapist will serve almost as an 'auxiliary ego' and has a psychoeducative role in teaching the patient how the world works. People with schizotypal personalities are often poor at applying what is learned in one situation to new situations; repeated gentle challenges to their cognitive distortions over a lengthy period may be required.

Schizoid patients, because of their aloofness, seldom come spontaneously for treatment and psychotherapy has little effect because motivation is so poor. They keep their distance and are content to live that way. Group therapy occasionally offers some form of contact because they learn that they are not alone in harbouring strange ideas, and may find it easier to relate to peers rather than an authority figure.

Paranoid personality disorder

Patients with paranoid personalities require extraordinarily deft handling, particularly during the early phases of therapy, when only the paranoia is manifest. Outwardly paranoid people may be sure and self-confident, although at the same time dogmatic and suspicious, but inwardly they are generally insecure, fearing a sleight at every turn. Beneath the surface there may be extreme degrees of jealousy; sometimes even classical morbid jealousy may be present. Confronting or even asking questions about distorted views of the world may be interpreted as an attack.

Rapport is often difficult to establish. A paranoid patient might say at the first meeting:

> 'I don't know if I can trust you, doctor. You are a man, and my father was a man, and he beat the living daylights out of me and put me down. I just don't trust men.'

To become defensive, or even reassuring, or to throw the question back, or to seek more information about the patient's distressing circumstance would probably only serve to heighten tension. It would be far better to accept some truth in the patient's assertion and reply:

> 'How could you possibly trust me? You have only just met me. You have no way of knowing whether all those diplomas on the wall are really mine or whether I am genuine or a charlatan. If I were in your shoes I would tread very carefully as well.'

Such a reply conveys an understanding of what it must be like to be that person and see the world through the patient's eyes. If the doctor really were a charlatan he would be unlikely to be so candid. Such a high degree of openness may go some way to mitigating the patient's suspiciousness.

Once treatment has been established and trust has developed, the paranoid patient can be seen to be struggling with intense feelings of rejection, humiliation and impotence. Therapy will soon lead into a world of earlier conflicts where there are feelings of humiliation, of being put down or subjected to withering criticism, often by the same-sex parent (Frosch, 1983). Older, Freudian notions that the paranoid feelings represent repressed homosexuality are now largely discounted, as it is recognised that most subjects have a heterosexual orientation, and the high frequency of sexual jealousy tends to confirm this. However, those with paranoid personalities are extremely touchy about the idea of homosexuality, possibly because this has become a symbol for not being able to perform adequately with a partner, and the idea is associated with a more widespread sense of failure and impotence. Empathic, rather than confrontational, interventions that accept the patient's position appear to be most helpful.

Psychotherapy for 'dramatic' disorders

Patients in the dramatic cluster present with obvious distress or attention-seeking behaviour that, by implication, almost demands therapeutic intervention. Similar psychotherapeutic principles govern the treatment of these disorders, and fundamental to them is Kernberg's (1967) concept of borderline personality organisation. An organisation, or pathological organisation, refers to the relative structures of impulses, anxieties and defences. Its purpose is to protect the individual from the chaos of earlier developmental stages. It is therefore a somewhat rigid structure that has the disadvantage of depriving the individual of more advanced modes of functioning (Higgit & Fonagy, 1993). Kernberg's borderline personality organisation consists of four elements:

1 ego weakness, which includes a poor ability to tolerate anxiety, control impulses, or develop socially acceptable ways of channelling energy

2 a tendency to shift towards irrational, dream-like thinking patterns in the context of generally intact reality testing (there is no psychosis)

3 the dominance of developmentally less mature psychological defences, such as splitting, projection and projective identification

4 identity diffusion, so that mental representations of important other people are fragmented or strongly charged as either good or bad.

This formulation has been very influential in the psychoanalytic literature on personality disorder, and is thought to be common to borderline, narcissistic, histrionic and 'as if' personalities, and to a certain extent also the antisocial disorders. It may be present in up to 10% of the population, but does not represent a clinical psychiatric disorder.

Borderline personality disorder

Acting as a container

People with borderline personality disorder lead a chaotic existence and are prey to intolerable affects. Kohut (1971) used the term 'disintegrative anxiety', while Bion (1959) wrote of a 'nameless dread'. The phrase 'holding environment' is attributed to Winnicott (1965). It is a description of the mother's primary and almost exclusive concern for her infant's welfare. During analysis, 'holding' refers to the therapist's ability to create a milieu in which many different powerful affects can be both experienced and explored in safety. Winnicott believed that the quality of reliability was at least as important as the therapist's interpretation in these cases. Bion also used the term 'container', which Gunderson (1984) specifically applied to borderline individuals and suggested that the therapist should serve as a container for all the patient's powerful affects. Sometimes patients need a bigger and stronger container than a single therapist, and in these cases admission to hospital may be invaluable.

Limit-setting

Limit-setting techniques will usually be necessary for almost every borderline patient, particularly at the beginning of treatment. Firmness will be needed concerning the timing and duration of sessions, and any conditions that warrant an extra session. The express delineation of what is, and what is not, acceptable during therapy helps to place at least some responsibility on the patient. It should be noted that therapists working in a one-to-one out-patient setting have little power to set limits, and have generally to rely on their own persuasiveness. Therapists are sometimes tempted to fashion written contracts in which their suicidal patients 'agree' to refrain from hurting or destroying themselves. This serves little purpose except to provide a false sense of security for the therapist (and an anodyne, should something go wrong). Their utility in deterring a borderline patient from suicide is negligible, and is certainly no substitute for clinical judgement.

For those with severe dyscontrol, admission is often required. It is, again, a matter of clinical judgement when hospitalisation should be urged. Ironically, the borderline patient who speaks of suicidal ideation openly may be at less risk than the patient who, while obviously depressed, remains uncommunicative, evasive and secretive – and who has a record of frequent suicide gestures and attempts.

Splitting and its management

One of the key features of patients with a borderline personality is that they view everything unrealistically in black and white, in terms of good and bad. Recognition of simultaneous ambivalent feelings towards themselves or other people is avoided. Defences such as projection, externalisation and splitting are kept in operation to enforce rigid compartmentalisation. An important aim of therapy is to help to resolve the defensive need for splitting, which is characterised by persistent division within the mind of impressions of the self and others into extreme opposites of 'good' and 'bad'. This is mainly accomplished through interpreting the transference, where the patient will begin to see the therapist now as an ideal person, moments later as a hostile, depreciating wretch. In hospital, patients with borderline personality disorder will have more than one person caring for them. They will usually make attempts to split or polarise their carers by singling out certain staff members as 'wonderful', others as 'horrible'. In so doing they tend to create disharmony.

Kernberg (1975) described the need to help patients to knit back together the various split images of the self. One way of doing this is to repeat back to the patient the many contradictory statements made in therapy concerning key interpersonal relationships. A patient may begin by describing her mother as 'perfect and saintly' but in a later session speak of some earlier memory of the mother having whipped her mercilessly for some childhood trifle. Discrepancies of this sort give the therapist a chance to suggest:

> 'Well, isn't it possible that your mother is a more complex figure than you make her out to be ... that she could shift between kindness and cruelty?'

Similarly, the self-image may be equally unintegrated. A borderline patient who has been a victim of incest may, because of the early overstimulation, later become promiscuous. At one moment she may see herself as an innocent victim and at another as a whore, and therefore alternate between self-pitying and self-loathing. An important facet of therapy is to help patients to achieve a more unified and realistic picture of their personal world. It is, after all, difficult for anyone to form a unified, integrated view of, say, an incestuous father who also lavishly doted on his daughter. She will come to see her father alternatingly as generous and kind, and as a monstrous exploiter. She cannot form a simple picture of a (generally) 'nice daddy'.

Aggression and hostile feelings

Kernberg (1967) believed that the primary problem borderline patients have is their innate aggression (which may have a constitutional basis). This results in distortions of the mental picture of the self and others. A similar view is expressed by Kleinian analysts, who also believe that the seeds of later human psychopathology arise from innate destructiveness. During treatment, hostility towards the therapist will sooner or later appear in the form of some abuse of the therapeutic situation. This may be mild, such as being late or missing sessions, or more severe, in the direct expression of criticism and hostility or by acting out. These negative transference reactions should be interpreted early on in therapy, and, if necessary, repeatedly in a neutral and non-critical atmosphere. Failure to bring the issue of aggression to the fore, or being either too supportive or overly critical, would foster the feeling in the patient that the therapist cannot cope with the patient's main problem – aggression and hostility. By withstanding the patient's repeated onslaughts, the therapist gradually enables patients to become less fearful of their destructive impulses, and a degree of integration of the personality becomes possible (Higgit & Fonagy, 1992).

Kohut (1971) provided a contrasting causal model and method for treating BPD. In his view, the disorder arises as a consequence of insufficient parental attention and lack of empathy, which results in an inadequately developed sense of the self. In essence, this is a deficiency theory that postulates 'developmental arrest'. Anger is the result of narcissistic injury and deprivation, rather than due to innate aggression. In Kohut's scheme, the therapist's role is to provide a soothing or mirroring function that gradually leads to a restoration of the self. Kohut's model has little relevance to hospitalised borderline patients: Kohut worked exclusively with ambulatory patients, few of whom would be considered 'borderline' by DSM criteria. His recommendations pertain to a less handicapped population of personality-disordered patients.

Vengeance, manipulation and self-mutilation

Many of the difficulties that BPD patients experience or impose on others stem from the poor modulation of their affects; they over-react, behave impulsively or unreasonably, and coerce by suicidal threats or other forms of blackmail. Kernberg (1975) suggested that suicidal behaviour in those with BPD often coincides with intense attacks of rage on the object.

Brobyn *et al* (1987) described a patient with severe borderline personality disorder who as a child had been beaten for many years by her father. One day she was found with a knife under her sleeve waiting for her father to come home. When asked whether she intended to kill her father, she replied: 'God, no. I was going to kill myself in front of him.' The only overt manifestation of the patient's vengeful impulses was the wish to punish her father by making him watch her death, and her own murderous impulses were at least overtly denied. Ego boundaries are broken down; he is she (she will be killed instead of him) and she is he (the perpetrator of the violence).

A common situation occurs when relationships end and borderline patients cut their wrists with the intention of coercing their partner back into the relationship, or at the very least provoking guilt feelings. The vengeful element in these situations is usually obvious. Currently we are seeing an increasing number of borderline patients who deal with rejection by 'stalking' (obsessively following) the former lover (Meloy, 1996). Sometimes during treatment, as the therapeutic relationship deepens, an episode of self-mutilation or other acting out may occur as a means of expressing guilt or fear of the growing closeness, and this signifies a negative therapeutic reaction. Following episodes of self-mutilation there is sometimes (but not always) a feeling of well-being. The patient has a sense of victory over pain and death, while family and therapists are reduced to a state of bewildered impotence.

Although innate aggression was once thought to be the main cause of such behaviour, recent studies have suggested that parental abuse of various types in childhood may be a more important factor. These aggressive and manipulative behaviours should, as Gunderson & Szabo (1993) point out, be understood in the light of adaptations made in response to past traumas and be interpreted as 'unfortunate survival techniques' that result from mistreatment. In the case mentioned above (Brobyn *et al*, 1987), the patient's mother had discovered that suicidal threats seemed to diminish the harshness of the beatings the father meted out to the children. Not surprisingly, the daughter learnt to use suicidal threats when dealing with her father and later authority figures.

Much of the aggressiveness and manipulativeness found among borderline subjects amounts to vengefulness directed at the parents or other key figures. The therapist's task is to help the patient slowly to unravel the pattern, and see the uselessness and ultimate self-destructiveness of vengefulness, for example in demolishing current relationships.

Dealing with vengeance

Among people who have experienced severe maltreatment by a parent, later relationships may be clouded by high levels of vengeance and a tendency to go to extremes. Pain-seeking behaviour becomes the norm, showing itself as some point on the spectrum of sadomasochism. At the extreme masochistic end are individuals who mutilate themselves, or who select partners who inflict physical or psychological pain. At the other extreme are individuals who are pure sadists, who rarely present themselves for treatment but who are determined to inflict as much or more suffering than they received when young. Pure types are uncommon, and most borderline patients will oscillate wildly between adoration of their partners and threats to mutilate themselves, or walk out in the face of some minor unpleasantness. In their behaviour they alternate between being kind and compassionate, and being cruel and humiliating, like the abusing parent. Appropriate in this regard are van der Kolk's (1989) comments about the victim growing up to become a victimiser. Once therapists become aware that a patient is locked into a cycle of this sort, any initial sympathy and compassion may rapidly wane. The therapist will need to alternate between compassion and firmness, with the ultimate therapeutic goal of trying to help the patient to see the futility of wreaking vengeance.

Where the partner appears normal, well meaning and not cruel, the patient needs to be taught not to overreact to minor problems in the relationship, not to react impulsively or spitefully and, above all, not to treat the partner as a 'whipping boy' or transference symbol of a cruel or sexually molesting parent. For other patients, for whom the current relationship appears to be a re-enactment of the previous childhood trauma, it may be best to try to support them in their efforts to leave the relationship. While some patients are able to use the therapists' interpretations and attempts to link the present sadomasochistic pattern to the previous traumatisation, it should be remembered that people with borderline personalities are less adaptive in handling their childhood abuse than many others who have been similarly abused.

A particular difficulty arises among those with a pronounced sadistic streak. Here almost any intervention (but most of all remarking on the patient's own unkind or cruel behaviour) is interpreted as a 'put-down'. The patient might turn vengefully on the therapist and say 'You hate me' or 'You think I'm a bad person'. An interpretation that offers some explanation might be tried, such as:

> 'Look, when you locked yourself in the bathroom and cut your wrist with the razor, after your husband said he did not want to go to the movies, your reaction may have been a bit extreme for that situation and, besides, you weren't getting back at him so much as at your father.'

This might restore some calm, but among patients who are severely vengeful, sadistic or hypersensitive, such a remark may be taken as criticism and these patients often quit therapy.

With those who experienced real parental maltreatment, therapists will often feel compassion for what the patient suffered, enabling them to empathise with the patient and then gently help to pry the patient loose from maladaptive vengeance-motivated behaviour patterns. If there was no real mistreatment, and patients misperceive the parents as bad owing to their own irritability and inordinate demands, the therapist's task will be to help them to develop a more realistic picture concerning their own irritability and the effect this may have had on the parents.

Hospitalisation

> 'This syndrome is difficult to treat and tends to create massive problems of management.' (Main, 1957)

Main (1957) treated 12 patients with borderline personality disorder in a psychoanalytically orientated in-patient unit, and some years later interviewed the nursing staff involved. They recounted how deeply distressed, almost to the point of illness, they had become while caring for these patients. People with borderline personalities are often admitted to hospital for treatment of an associated axis I disorder.

There are two areas of concern for this group: regression and splitting. A few patients seem to worsen after admission, with more frequent episodes of self-mutilation, and this apparently retrograde step is termed 'regression'. Some therapists, while not condoning the deviant behaviour, view the regressed state as providing a greater opportunity for therapy and for inducing change.

The hospital milieu may be an ideal place for mapping out the various elements in the patient's 'splitting' (see above), since the different members of staff may each be the recipient of a different attitude or behaviour from the patient. The feared therapist, the adored head nurse, the despised ward clerk, and so on, may each answer to an abusive father, a fondly loved mother, and an irritating older sister. In other cases the splitting may represent one ambivalently regarded parent, who at different times inspired all these contradictory feelings. By meeting frequently, the staff can build a more integrated picture of the patient, so that those who interact directly with the patient, especially the therapist, can now help the patient to knit together these compartmentalised patterns into a more unified and adaptive personality.

Among more severe cases, the splitting may assume a more destructive quality, and with it the tendency characteristic of borderline patients to divide hospital staff, play one off against another, extract special favours, and convert staff into friends or even lovers: in short, to *actualise* transference themes rather than to think about them. These patients try to manipulate the environment rather than conform to it. As a counterforce to these anti-therapeutic tendencies, it is best if staff maintain a united front, share a common philosophy about the optimal treatment plan, and communicate frequently in ward rounds, supervision and team meetings. Once decisions are made, staff should support one another and resist any temptation to cross professional boundaries or become over-familiar with the patient, even in the face of intense pressure or subtle seductive behaviour on the part of the patient.

Patients with borderline personality disorder will often provoke crises. The therapist and the hospital staff will have to become flexible in 'rolling with the punches', shifting seamlessly from one type of intervention to another in accordance with the needs of the moment. No matter what the therapist's major orientation, a healthy degree of pragmatism is essential.

Whether the hospital stay should be brief or prolonged has proved controversial. Because of the dangers of regression, and the requirement for most general psychiatric units to care for psychotic patients, who may be even more regressed, usually only the briefest possible stay is offered to people with a personality disorder. Brief admissions may indeed be helpful, and the American Psychiatric Association's guidelines for the treatment of borderline personality disorder (Oldham *et al*, 2001) suggest the following indications for brief admissions:

- imminent danger to others
- loss of control of suicidal impulses, or serious suicidal attempt
- transient psychotic episodes
- symptoms of sufficient severity to interfere with functioning at work or with family life.

The indications for longer-term admissions include the following:

- persistent and severe suicidality, self-destructiveness with non-adherence to out-patient or day hospital programmes
- comorbid resistant axis I disorder (e.g. eating disorder)
- comorbid and resistant substance misuse or dependence that is unresponsive to out-patient treatment
- continued risk of assaultive behaviour towards others
- symptoms of sufficient severity to interfere with work or with family life that have not responded to out-patient or day hospital treatments.

Although longer-term hospitalisation may be helpful, with the current reduction in hospital bed numbers this option is becoming less available. Once in hospital, borderline patients tend to be envious of others who function at a higher level, but often disparage or may even be cruel to other patients, such as those with schizophrenia who function at a lower level, indicating the merit in segregating borderline patients in specialised units. These have the advantage that staff become more experienced at managing acting-out behaviours, and can be sympathetic yet firm in the face of manipulative behaviour, rather than only rejecting. Specialised facilities function as therapeutic communities, with a treatment programme consisting of individual therapy, ward groups and active participation by patients in the life of the unit (Jackson & Pines, 1986; Fenton & McGlashan, 1990).

Counselling for borderline personalities who were sexually abused

Many borderline patients report sexual molestation by persons within or outside the family, and have validated histories of traumatic backgrounds, including incest as well as physical or other types of abuse. Even witnessing cruelty or physical abuse being meted out to a sibling or a parent may have a traumatising effect. Flashbacks, nightmares, episodes of panic or intense anxiety, irritability, and other manifestations of post-traumatic stress disorder are commonly found among BPD patients who are admitted to hospital (Putnam & Trickett, 1993). There is evidence that women who were traumatised, particularly before the age of 14 years, tend to resort to self-mutilation, substance misuse and suicidal gestures or acts in the context of interpersonal stress, and it is their life-threatening behaviour that results in hospitalisation. Where penile penetration takes place before a girl is 10 years old, the pathological effects of incest tend to be more serious (Paris, 1994, p. 48).

People who have experienced sexual abuse as children may display a range of abnormal sexual behaviour in adulthood. Some become prematurely eroticised and have heightened sexual cravings, in the sense that they focus on sex as an antidote for all their tensions, whether sexual or not, such as feelings of loneliness, marital conflict or anxiety. Others who become hyper-eroticised may later become promiscuous. But in some cases revulsion towards the victimising relation outweighs both the love (as towards a father or older brother) and any physical pleasure that may have accompanied the incest. In these instances there may be a total rejection of sex throughout adult life, sometimes expressed as a preference for homosexual attachments. This is because an incestuous relationship results in heightened ambivalence, at first towards the original offender and then to later sexual partners.

Ambivalent sadomasochistic relationships are characteristic during adult life (Stone, 1988) unless therapy succeeds in interrupting the pattern. There may be an endless succession of ugly scenes and fights followed by passionate reconciliations. In later life, as the passion declines, there may be rather less in the way of passion and reconciliation, with only a chronic abusive relationship remaining.

Loneliness and fears of abandonment

Earlier commentators (Masterson, 1981; Rinsley, 1982) put much weight on the theme of fears of abandonment as the central issue in patients with BPD. More recent findings have stressed the importance of sexual and physical abuse as causative factors, and simple separations in non-distressing circumstances do not appear to be causal. Still, fears of being alone or being abandoned are commonplace among these individuals, even if there were no unusual separations in childhood. Innate factors, such as predisposition to depression or anxiety, may contribute in some cases. In others, parental seductiveness or over-dependency upon a particular child may in turn produce excessive dependency on the parent, and thus rob the child of experiences such as the development of hobbies, or having a wide circle of childhood friends that would help to build self-sufficiency. The task of the psychotherapist is to work out with the patient the probable causes of the inability to be alone. Even so, knowing the relevant psychodynamics will rarely remedy the problem, because the patient is now in the habit of being unable to handle separations with ease. Up to a point, the presence of the therapist is helpful (either the physical presence during sessions or virtual presence via the telephone). However, eventually some sort of behavioural intervention is required, such as encouraging hobbies or other interests, as well as a gradual weaning from the supportive presence of the therapist.

Narcissistic personality disorder

Narcissistic traits are commonly found in other personality disorders, particularly the borderline and antisocial types. Sometimes narcissistic character traits arise from being spoiled or drowned in empty praise as a child. These individuals rarely present themselves for treatment, or if they do they remain in therapy for only a very brief period. More commonly there is a diet of parental neglect and humiliation, and here the grandiosity is no more than a compensatory mechanism for obscuring thinly veiled feelings of worthlessness, unattractiveness, low self-esteem and unloveability. These patients alienate others through their sarcasm and disdain, or sometimes even through jealousy and clingingness, but such distortions should be viewed as desperate measures of the inferior yet 'true self'.

Only the latter group are prepared to engage in therapy, which aims at the delineation of these mechanisms and the enhancement of self-esteem in a genuine way, by the achievement of success through work or through the patient's own efforts, rather than through entitlement.

In relationships, people with narcissistic personality disorder should be encouraged to make durable friendships by being more compassionate and less contemptuous of others. If they reach this more mature state, with improved relationships, the older, pathological, narcissistic defences can be dropped. Some of these patients are so hypersensitive they may be able to recognise trust only in the form of positive feedback. This does not necessarily help them, because it tends to evoke the original trauma and resultant anger at not being valued for themselves (Patrick, 1985).

As for *envy*, one of the most corrosive of human emotions, psychodynamic exploration of its childhood antecedents is often ineffective. However, greater success in life may be helpful for the person, rendering it inoperative, although it does not eradicate the tendency. Envy is a personality trait found in many persons with a personality disorder, and is not specific to any one particular disorder. Envy is, however, quite common in those with a narcissistic personality disorder.

Case example

A narcissistic young surgeon complained to his therapist that no one appreciated his brilliant operating skills, and he was contemptuous of his boss, an idiot who only promoted other, ignorant doctors. During therapy he was encouraged to distinguish himself, and in due course discovered a small modification for a thyroid operation. He wrote papers and gave lectures on the subject, and was then invited to become the senior man at another hospital – and became the envy of others.

One of the most challenging subtypes of narcissistic personality disorder is that of 'malignant narcissism', as described by Kernberg (1992, p. 77). In addition to the narcissism, this constellation is characterised by antisocial behaviour, ego-syntonic sadism and a paranoid orientation, yet with a capacity for loyalty, concern for others, and a measure of guilt. These latter qualities distinguish the malignant narcissist from a purely antisocial personality. Clinically, one sees the syndrome on occasion in men in positions of power: high executives, politicians and the like. They usually treat their subordinates shabbily. Because of the power they wield, owing to their high positions, they feel justified in their actions and attitudes. This renders them extremely difficult to treat, since they do not readily acknowledge their faults. Sometimes, they become accessible to therapy only after they fail at some endeavour and lose their position.

Histrionic personality disorder

The DSM–IV concept of histrionic personality disorders encompasses some patients at the milder end of the spectrum of what was previously known as hysterical personality disorder, as well as those who lie at the more severe end of the spectrum who also manifest narcissistic and borderline features. A short-lived exaggeration of previous histrionic traits can sometimes occur in depression, in which case standard antidepressive treatment may be helpful.

With the milder disorders, there is often intense repression that serves as a defence against hidden sexual striving, often relating to incestuous fantasies. Where there has been actual incest, especially by a relative of the older generation (father, step-father, uncle, etc.), more severe histrionic personality disorder may occur. In the latter situation, there will be a strong tendency to eroticise otherwise non-sexual relationships, including that between the doctor and patient. Patients often act out conflicts, and there is greater reliance on fantasy than on logic and reality.

The aim of psychotherapy is the lifting of an abnormal inhibition. Classical psychoanalysis or psychoanalytically orientated psychotherapy, with free association and dream analysis, was originally devised for this group. Therapy is directed at undoing the repression and exposing the hidden sexual strivings. These usually focus on incestuous choices, for example the daughter who wished for her father in the absence of any actual experiences with the taboo object. Resolution of the oedipal conflict leads to a better integration of sexuality into the fabric of the personality, with less need to seek those with an 'aura of forbiddenness' or unsuitable sexual partners, and eventually there is a more appropriate selection of partners. Therapy in these cases involves fostering a more normal sexuality.

Among the more severely affected, disinhibition rather than repression or inhibition is the main problem. These patients, who manifest repeated and strident demands for praise and attention, have overlapping narcissistic and borderline features and they function at a more infantile or borderline level (Kernberg, 1967). Among borderline in-patients with prominent histrionic traits, a history of incest or molestation is common (Stone, 1989; Zanarini & Gunderson, 1990).

Non-molested people with hysterical personalities need to realise that, while potential sexual partners may symbolise one or other parent, they are not really forbidden. Those who have suffered molestation need to learn during therapy that not all partners are as exploitative and unworthy as the individuals who once misused them.

Patients with hysterical/histrionic features should be helped to rely less on emotional appeal, and more on rational solution, thereby becoming less childlike and dependent, and more self-sufficient.

Psychotherapy for 'anxious' disorders

Patients in the 'anxious' cluster struggle with inhibitions against normal assertiveness and enjoyment to which they would be entitled. They retreat from what belongs to them, in contrast to those in the 'dramatic' cluster, who reach out for what does not belong to them. Rather than place external limits, treatment should focus on the removal of internal limits or inhibitions that impair normal interactions. These patients are dominated by fear, such as sexual fears, social fears, or fears of voicing an opinion. DSM–IV includes obsessive–compulsive, dependent and avoidant personalities in this group (see Chapter 18), but some of the 'non-official' categories, such as passive aggressive, masochistic, self-defeating, the 'as if' personality and depressive personality types show similar inhibitions and require a similar approach. The typical background features, inner scripts and coping strategies of these patients are shown in Table 19.2.

Many of these individuals are well integrated and function at much higher levels than people with BPD, for example, and will respond to out-patient treatment. Techniques differ little from those employed for individuals with neurotic disorders, and may include classical techniques such as free association and the analysis of dreams, as well as psychodynamic psychotherapy. Occasionally, a few patients in the 'anxious' cluster will respond only to psychoanalysis given three to five times weekly and focusing largely on dreams. This applies particularly to severe compulsive or passive aggressive men who are either remarkably out of touch with their emotions or grossly contemptuous of psychiatry and its treatment methods but who may, in spite of their scepticism, accept evidence from more objective sources such as dreams.

Lowered self-esteem

Lowered self-esteem is common among subjects with personality disorders of any type. Even narcissistic personalities, beneath their façade of grandiosity, may be

Table 19.2 Personality disorders dominated by anxiety

	Background	Inner script	Strategy
Obsessive–compulsive	Undue parental concern with obedience	Respect is more important than love	Conform, be neat, perfect, logical and contained
Dependent	Parent was dependent or fostered dependency	I can't manage; others can take care of me	Be compliant, submissive; cling for dear life
Avoidant	Being shamed into feeling socially unacceptable	I'm no good; others are out to hurt me	Better safe than sorry
Passive aggressive	Being intruded on and bullied by parents	I have to get even in a way I don't get hurt	Procrastinate, frustrate, sabotage, do the minimum
Depressive	Disappointment, privation, loss, abuse, shaming	My life is tragic; pessimism is justified	If I cry, others might just come to my rescue
Masochistic	Love interspersed with undeserved punishment	Martyrs can sit at the right hand of God	If I suffer enough, I can buy a little love

struggling with feelings of worthlessness, while among depressive personalities pessimism and low self-esteem are almost universal.

Low self-esteem in borderline patients may partly relate to their innate tendency to depression, but also to abuse and rejection by parents. Incest victims who become borderline often blame themselves for seducing their offending relative, who may have compounded the issue by calling the victim a 'whore' or a 'tramp' at the time of the incest. Sometimes one sees lower self-esteem stemming from more mundane reasons, such as performing less well at school than one's peers, being from a poorer family than one's peers, not being as attractive, not being accepted by the cliques that form in school, and so on.

Patients often cling to their low self-image, almost with the tenacity of a delusion, and it may be helpful to elucidate the dynamic reasons behind this. A beautiful woman who had been molested as a child may have an underlying fear of men's predatoriness, especially if she were to acknowledge her attractiveness, and because of this may feel safer maintaining she is ugly. An intelligent student who fears the envy of other children or his siblings if he were to acknowledge his intelligence, sustains, defensively, a belief that he is stupid.

Unfortunately, unearthing the real reasons or providing appropriate interpretations concerning the dynamics underlying the low self-esteem rarely brings anything more than minor relief. Psychotherapy alone is unlikely to be sufficient, and the appropriate interpretations should be understood as just preliminary steps in a process that requires real life experience. The interpretations and the presence of the therapist serve to embolden the patient to test the world more forcefully. The intelligent student needs to learn that a top mark does not provoke a backlash of murderous envy, while the beautiful woman should learn that, in encounters with men, most are trustworthy and very few are carbon copies of the truly predatory and untrustworthy figures from earlier life. To acknowledge being attractive need not come at such a high price.

The curative process for lowered self-esteem is thus interactive, and similar to overcoming a phobia by behavioural means as suggested by Marks & Marks (1990). At this point a cognitive–behavioural intervention is often useful, and the therapist may try to urge the patient to take some small steps into the forbidden zone (e.g. by calling someone for a date, or applying for a non-stressful job). Anxieties that have hitherto remained dormant now rise to the surface and can be discussed and alleviated. The strength of the therapeutic bond serves to embolden patients to test the reality of their fears. Eventually the need for the low self-image is diminished, and with that the self-esteem rises to a more realistic level.

In persons whose low self-esteem stemmed largely from withering criticism and rejection from parents, there is usually the additional problem of intense ambivalence towards them; the difficulty arises from loyalty to the cruel parent and the pain involved in gradually realising that the parent was deeply at fault, perhaps even malicious. Patients often fight against the recognition of the truth, when their parents have actually been monstrous, because the parents were the only straw to which the patients could cling when they were small and helpless. Such patients prefer to blame themselves for being 'bad', as though they deserved their maltreatment, since this may be the easier notion to entertain. Perhaps in this situation psychotherapy by itself can be effective in bringing about the necessary reversal of images: that the patient is not such a bad sort after all, and that the parents were not so good. The therapist, first hearing the accounts from the patient's childhood, and then offering a more realistic appraisal of how the offending (or rejecting) parent would be viewed by ordinary people, can in many instances overturn the patient's incorrect and self-damaging appraisals.

Countertransference

'Countertransference' refers to the reactions that therapists experience in relation to their patients (see Table 19.3). It may be divided into two main types:

1 reactions that reflect unresolved neurotic feelings that stem from the therapist's background, and are thus unique to that therapist

2 reactions that essentially *all* therapists, being human, would experience in reaction to unusually powerful stimuli coming from the patient.

An example of the former might be a therapist who always felt embarrassed at having come from a poor family and who now has a patient who is quite wealthy. If the therapist felt envious, or ingratiating, or hostile (imagining the patient must have become well-to-do

Table 19.3 Common countertransference reactions to personality types

Patient's disorder	Countertransference reaction(s)
Schizoid	Boredom; lack of sympathy
Schizotypal	Disdain at the patient's 'weirdness'
Paranoid	Fear of being menaced; impatience at the patient's misreading of social situations
Borderline	Feeling put-upon; aroused; overwhelmed; rescue fantasies
Narcissistic	Offence at patient's contempt or grandiosity
Antisocial	Contempt, fear, indignation, envy (at patient's 'freedom' to do as he pleases)
Histrionic	Charmed, aroused; swamped by patient's emotionality
Obsessive–compulsive	Boredom (at excessive, dry details)
Avoidant	Impatience, disdain (at patient's lack of courage)
Dependent	Annoyance (at the clinginess); powerful (at being needed)
Passive aggressive	Annoyance, impatience (at the covert hostility)
Depressive	Impotence, despair (at being unable to help)
Hypomanic	Charm, envy, irked (at the over-familiarity)
Irritable	Outrage
Masochistic	Impatience (at patient's continued bad choices)
Sadistic	Hatred, outrage, contempt, fear

by ripping off the poor) such feelings would represent countertransference of the neurotic sort. As an example of the second type, an openly seductive patient of a famous California psychoanalyst, Leo Rangell, once came to her session clad only in a bikini. Dr Rangell felt the inescapable twinge of erotic feelings in this provocative situation, as would almost all (male) therapists, but told her:

> 'Really, you need to come for your sessions in appropriate dress, and also share with me in *words* what was prompting you to come here with so little on – or we would have to think of suspending therapy.'

This patient had BPD and no motivation to deal with her conflicts; confronted with the admonition that talking about her problems was very acceptable, but that trying to act them out was not (inviting the therapist into a sexual relationship, in this case), she quit.

It is characteristic of patients with BPD, as Higgit & Fonagy (1993) point out, that they elicit strong feelings in their therapists, as an outgrowth of their own strong, often ungovernable, feelings. Here, the countertransference may be 'normal' but still requires great skill and tact to deal with. Patients of a particularly provocative bent may elicit *both* types of countertransference. The therapist, in coping with the neurotic, irrational aspects may need supervision or some additional therapy in order to come to grips with these more personal, as opposed to the universal, components of the countertransference reactions.

Provided the countertransference feelings can be understood, they may serve as a useful tool in therapy. Searles (1979) described how a young trainee presented a session with a woman with BPD in which the patient talked non-stop, extolling the virtues of her boyfriend, without letting the trainee get a word in. The young doctor was perplexed by the meaning of the session and Searles commented:

> 'Well, if I were in your shoes I'd feel mighty jealous – having to listen to her praise someone else while sitting there with me in the room. Maybe she wished to alert you to her own hidden struggle with the emotion of jealousy by causing you to experience that very emotion.'

In a later session and at an appropriate moment the trainee enquired whether jealousy played any role in the patient's life, and she described an unbearable jealousy of her older sister, whom she felt had always been greatly favoured by her parents.

Therapeutic neutrality is easily dislodged, and the therapist can become overly emotional or responsive to affective displays by the patient. Sometimes therapists become the vehicle for the patient's intolerable self-critical part, and so are driven into the role of confronter and accuser; they then reject the patient completely and so repeat the patient's previous pattern. In the face of sexual seductiveness, therapists may defend themselves by becoming harsh, rejecting or over-critical; but occasionally rescue fantasies may develop with romantic involvement, and these may be a serious hazard for those dealing with young borderline patients in whom the 'pathetic child victim' elicits strong parental feelings in the therapist, who may as a result try to usurp the real parents.

A more neurotic countertransference can also occur, with the patient coming to symbolise an important character for the therapist, such as a detested sibling or a former sweetheart. Unless these feelings are brought to light they may undermine psychotherapy, because the therapist may become excessively fond of or may needlessly dislike the patient.

Group therapy

Groups may sometimes have a civilising influence on individuals, but there are some patients with very severe degrees of narcissism, paranoia or disruptive behaviour who cannot fit into a group. For patients who can tolerate group therapy, other group members are able to provide a form of reality orientation therapy, and so give useful insights into a patient's maladaptive traits. Sometimes this is highly effective and can be accomplished by the other group members in a language that a therapist could not afford to use in individual therapy. Empathic interpretation by the therapist in connection with feelings of narcissistic injury has also been found to be helpful. Provided there is some degree of cohesiveness, groups appear to have a comforting and containing role for the individual with BPD without resulting in any damage to other members. Groups that specialise in dealing with patients with histories of incest and sexual molestation (common among those with BPD) may be successful, as they help to decrease the sense of isolation and shame. Among borderline patients with impulsive behaviour such as binge-eating, drinking and gambling, the appropriate 'anonymous' group may be helpful. Higgit & Fonagy (1992) and others recommend that group therapy can be a useful addition to individual therapy.

Other analytical approaches

Hospital programmes

Two hospital-based psychoanalytic programmes in the UK have recently been described.

Chiesa & Fonagy (2003) have described a 36-month follow-up study of a psychosocial treatment programme at the Cassel Hospital in London. The programme was based on the traditional therapeutic community regimen of daily unit meetings, community meetings, co-responsibility for running the therapeutic community, and structured occupational therapy. This was combined with individual and group psychodynamic psychotherapy. Two groups were compared: those who had an admission for a year, and those who were admitted for a shorter period but had a further 18 months of out-patient group and individual therapy. The latter group (with the shorter in-patient stay) had a better long-term outcome.

Bateman & Fonagy (1999) described a day hospital programme (they used the term 'partial hospitalisation') that adopted a similar psychoanalytic approach to treat BPD, and found in comparison with a control group assigned to routine general psychiatric care, that, after 6 months, the treated patients showed significant decreases in parasuicidal and self-mutilating behaviours, reduced numbers of in-patient days and better social and interpersonal function.

Cognitive programmes

Beck & Freeman (1990) described a cognitive approach to the treatment of the personality disorders. Cognitive therapy relies on the inner scripts of patients (see Table 19.2), which are thought to underlie the abnormal behaviours. Certain traits appear to be amenable to a cognitive approach, particularly anger, dependency, lack of assertiveness and low self-esteem.

Anger is a common and serious problem for patients with borderline, paranoid or antisocial personality disorder. The basis for the cognitive approach to management is identification of the triggers that provoke anger. Role-play and videotape feedback are used to assist the patient in the emotional recall of previous angry outbursts, and this is then used to help identify the most likely triggers. The significance of these triggers is explored and the therapist models a more appropriate response to such situations. These techniques form the basis of anger management programmes. These are usually based on the a verbal expression of underlying hostile feelings.

For the trait of dependency, Trukatt & Carlson (1984) recommended a graduated exposure to situations that require patients to make their own decisions. Because decision-making in dependent subjects may result in heightened anxiety, anxiety management techniques form an important component of the treatment. Patients with dependent, anxious, or passive aggressive personality disorders have difficulty in saying 'no' to others, cannot set limits on the behaviour of other people, and are therefore readily exploited. In such cases, assertiveness training and teaching patients how to say 'no' in specific situations may be helpful. This can be done using the standard techniques of role-play, modelling and videotape feedback.

Beard *et al* (1990) described a combined cognitive–analytic approach. In the first few sessions, the patient and therapist together write a description of the patient's history and this is linked to the patient's present maladaptive behaviour. Then the therapist asks the patient to monitor and record whenever he or she uses such maladaptive mechanisms. The therapist introduces diagrams to help the patient see how different frames of mind can lead to different behaviours. The patient is encouraged to recognise them and to discuss them with the therapist. In due course the maladaptive behaviours should diminish. Many people (not only those with personality disorders) have difficulty in expressing their feelings verbally, but find it rather easier to describe their interpersonal problems with diagrams, which may form a useful starting point for therapy.

Perhaps the best-known of the cognitive–behavioural approaches is that of Marsha Linehan (1993), which she terms 'dialectical behavioural therapy'. Her view is that the core characteristic of BPD is a 'dysfunction in emotion regulation', which may be physiologically based, and this results in the patient's dramatic over-reaction to events and impulsive acts. In addition, she suggests that during upbringing these individuals were exposed to parents who discounted their emotional experiences. As a result these individuals (who are already prone to disproportionate emotional responses) receive inadequate training in the regulation of their emotions and have, through their upbringing, acquired a disparaging attitude to their own emotions and self-image. Treatment is aimed at reversing these trends.

Linehan (1993, pp. 19 and 121) selected the term 'dialectic' because she felt the overriding characteristic of the therapy was a reconciliation of opposites in a continual process of synthesis. The most fundamental dialectic is the need to accept patients just as they are – but within the context of trying to teach them to change. The tension between the patients' alternating high and low aspirations and expectations in relation to their own capabilities offers the therapist a major challenge, as they require moment-to-moment changes in the use of supportive acceptance versus confrontation and change strategies.

Dialectical behaviour therapy has much in common with the dynamic therapy outlined in the earlier part of this chapter. For example, Linehan (1993, p. 121) writes:

> 'Borderline patients think in extremes and hold rigid points of view with life being black or white. Dialectical thinking requires the ability to transcend polarities, and help patients not to see the world as a series of greys but to see both black and white and to achieve a synthesis of reality that does not negate the reality of either.'

Dialectical behaviour therapy incorporates strategies derived from behavioural, cognitive and supportive therapies. It generally is given for a period of 1 year and uses both individual and group methods. The individual-therapy arm of the programme adopts a cognitive approach and uses problem-solving techniques, including behavioural skills training, contingency management, detailed exploration of every thought preceding an impulsive episode, cognitive modification and exposure to significant emotional clues. These are counterbalanced with supportive techniques such as reflective empathy and acceptance. The group therapy arm of the programme adopts a mainly psycho-educational format aimed at teaching interpersonal skills, interpersonal effectiveness, distress tolerance, reality acceptance, self-management and emotional regulation. Her book about the method she developed (called dialectical behavioural therapy, DBT) (Linehan, 1993) provides a very detailed manual of how it should be conducted, but therapist training and support are an integral part of any treatment programme. In controlled studies the programme has been shown to be successful in reducing parasuicidal acts in people with BPD (Linehan *et al*, 1991), as confirmed in a larger Dutch trial (Verheul *et al*, 2003), in which parasuicidal acts and other impulsive behaviours were significantly reduced in comparison with a control group given routine therapy.

Controlled studies are now beginning to show that, provided treatment for patients with BPD is both intensive and prolonged, it may be effective. This has been confirmed in a meta-analysis of all the controlled studies of the psychotherapy of personality disorder, which gave an effect size of 1.46 for psychodynamic therapies, and 1.0 for cognitive approaches (an effect size of 0 = no effect), and although the authors suggested caution in interpreting these figures, they were based on 21 controlled studies involving more than 600 patients (Leichsenring & Leibing, 2003).

Social and prison programmes

Certain prisons specialise in the psychotherapeutic treatment of severely antisocial people, and have developed their own psychotherapeutic programmes based on the principles of a therapeutic community. Programmes vary widely and are usually specific to particular prisons, with a mixture of group and individual methods being used (Dolan & Coid, 1993). Group methods are more helpful in enabling subjects to see how destructive some of their behaviour can be, while individual therapy serves to increase an individual's capacity to experience a more normal range of affects and fantasies, and to develop trust. In some regimens there is hierarchical progress through the prison, with the possibility of early parole serving as an incentive for some inmates.

The high security offered in prison means that these regimens are probably not applicable to ambulant patients or even those with antisocial personality disorder in the hospital setting. However, such a therapeutic approach probably cannot used for the psychopath as defined by Hare's Psychopathy Checklist (Hare *et al*, 1990). Persons with marked psychopathic traits are by definition contemptuous of authority and particularly so of psychiatry. Traits such as severe callousness or the absence of any sense of remorse or shame places the more extreme psychopathic cases beyond the realms of treatment. Hare (1993) commented on the untreatability of psychopaths:

> 'The term implies that there is something to treat ... but as far as we can determine psychopaths are perfectly happy with themselves and they see no need for treatment.'

Dangerous severe personality disorder

There was a considerable public outcry in the UK following a very high-profile murder of a mother and child by a man with an established diagnosis of severe personality disorder who was known to the psychiatric services. The UK government responded by proposing new legislation and a new service for those considered to have 'dangerous and severe personality disorder' (DSPDs). These were a small group of individuals who not only suffered from severe personality disorder but also were thought to be at high risk of causing serious harm through sexual or violent offences. The numbers in this proposed new category of DSPD are thought to be relatively small (Feeney, 2003) but the notion that such individuals should become the responsibility of an already overstretched psychiatric service drew much protest from within the profession, and as a consequence the UK government has allocated more money for research and the development of special placements for this group of individuals.

A further difficulty arises in the assessment of the risk of causing a serious offence, as such predictions are notoriously inaccurate. Buchanan & Leese (2001), in a meta-analysis of 21 studies based on a test to predict a subsequent offence, calculated that, in a 1-year period, six people would have to be detained to prevent one of these people from committing a serious offence, while the remaining five would not have committed an offence even if they had not been detained. Detention on this scale is clearly morally unacceptable as well as very expensive. The concept of DSPD as a separate legal/medical category remains under review and is more comprehensively discussed by Feeney (2003).

Drug treatments

The beneficial effects of medication in patients with a personality disorder are generally quite modest, and far less impressive than when the same drugs are given to treat affective disorder or schizophrenia. Drugs may be helpful in cases of behavioural dyscontrol, self-mutilation, suicidal behaviour and psychotic episodes, particularly during the more severe phases (i.e. those that require hospital admission). Only borderline and schizotypal personality disorders show any benefit from medication. Except when there is an associated axis I disorder, the other categories, such as the antisocial types, seldom show much improvement with medication. There are suggestions, however, that small doses of a selective serotonin reuptake inhibitor (SSRI) (such as fluoxetine) may alleviate the pessimism and moodiness of some depressive persons (including those with 'depressive' personality) and may make certain avoidant persons less socially shy. Lithium may also have a role, and this is discussed below.

For most patients, perhaps the majority, some drug or drug combinations may be found to be helpful, but some patients do not respond to any sort of medication, and a few are worsened by medication. The following types of deterioration may occur:

- physiological abnormalities (e.g. obesity with olanzapine; blood cell abnormalities with carbamazepine)
- aggression with SSRIs
- dependence with benzodiazepines
- depression with beta-blockers.

It is important to stop medications that appear to be ineffective, as patients can end up taking a mixture of antipsychotics, antidepressants, lithium, a benzodiazepine and other drugs, none of which may be helping. In the treatment of a complex disorder such as BPD, medication should be seen as providing only one arm of a comprehensive treatment programme: it cannot in itself change character, but by dampening down the swings of affective dysregulation it may permit better containment of the disorder.

Borderline and schizotypal personality disorders

Placebo-controlled trials have now established a more definite role for small doses of neuroleptic medication among subjects with BPD. In a group of in-patients and out-patients with BPD, schizotypal personality disorder or both, haloperidol (7 mg daily) resulted in significant improvements in behavioural dyscontrol, psychoticism and paranoid ideation, as well as in many neurotic symptoms, especially anxiety, hostility and depression, and was significantly superior to both placebo and amitriptyline (Soloff *et al*, 1986).

An attempt at replication by the same group questioned many of the earlier findings. Using a rather lower dose of haloperidol (4 mg daily) among a group of mainly out-patients with BPD, there were few differences between the drug and placebo for most symptoms (Soloff *et al*, 1993). Haloperidol was superior to placebo only for anger and depression, as well as for objective measures of behavioural dyscontrol. Possibly the drug was less effective among out-patients because compliance was lower.

In a community sample of subjects with BPD and schizotypal personality disorder, thiothixene was shown to be superior to placebo for a variety of psychotic symptoms as well as for hostility, phobias, and anxiety and obsessive–compulsive symptoms. There were only small differences between the drug and placebo for the symptoms of somatisation, depersonalisation, derealisation and suspiciousness. There were no differences for sensitivity to interpersonal rejection or depressive hostility, and so for these symptoms a psychotherapeutic approach may be more helpful (Goldberg *et al*, 1986).

Initial open studies of the newer, atypical drugs indicated they might be effective. Zanarini & Frankenberg (2001) reported on a placebo-controlled trial of a low dose (2.5 mg) of olanzapine in 25 patients with BPD who had been recruited through newspaper advertisements (i.e. a non-clinical sample), although following an interview the researchers selected only those who fulfilled criteria for BPD. Olanzapine was superior to placebo in the realms of affect, impulsivity and interpersonal relationships but not depression. Side-effects were minimal and movement disorders did not occur; a modest degree weight gain was the only significant side-effect, although in open studies using higher doses weight gain has been a more serious problem (it has led to discontinuation of therapy).

Some patients with BPD show signs of cognitive distortions. These may take the form of focalised delusional ideas of the sort that were called 'monomania' in the 19th century. Obsessive love, stalking, erotomanic beliefs of being loved by some stranger who is scarcely aware of the patient (de Clérambault's syndrome) and dissociative reactions ('tuning out', losing time, mumbling incoherently in the midst of otherwise depression rational speech, etc.) are some examples. In these instances, small doses of the newer, 'atypical' antipsychotics have been useful in minimising the tendency to psychotic aberrations of thought. Rocca *et al* (2002) have suggested risperidone in such cases, but the other drugs in this category (olanzapine, quetiapine and ziprasidone) may confer equal benefit. The choice will often depend upon side-effects. Olanzapine, for example, is the worst offender in relation to weight gain; so many patients will prefer ziprasidone, a drug that is available in the USA but not yet in the UK.

The use of clozapine for the treatment of BPD is rather more controversial. However, in Italy Beneditti *et al* (1998) reported on 12 subjects with BPD who had psychotic-like symptoms (but not schizophrenia), who had all failed on a variety of other drug regimens. Dosage was titrated upwards until psychotic-like symptoms disappeared (25–100 mg, mean dosage 44 mg) and this was accompanied by improvements in depression, suicidality and global assessment, and the average number of days in hospital was reduced from 40 per year to less than 1 day per year. It should be emphasised that the use of clozapine for severe BPD is only experimental and at present BPD is not a licensed indication for prescribing clozapine in the UK.

Schizotypal personality disorder is thought to be linked to schizophrenia but is very rare and so trials have been difficult to organise. However, Koenigsberg *et al* (2003) collected 20 patients over 5 years and showed significant improvements in both negative and positive symptoms for low doses of risperidone (0.25 mg titrated up to 2 mg) compared with placebo.

Suicidal behaviours and anxiety

Suicidal behaviours constitute one of the main defining features of BPD, along with impulsivity and anger. One may encounter suicidal gestures (i.e. where the lethality is low, such as taking 10 aspirin pills), suicide attempts (those with high lethality, such as breathing car exhaust or jumping from the third storey), or self-mutilation (e.g. cutting a wrist sideways so there is not much blood loss; burning an arm with a cigarette). To halt this kind of behaviour, a number of measures taken together have proven useful.

It is now common to rely on an approach that uses both psychotherapy and medications. Although clinicians specialising in one particular form of psychotherapy tend to argue for the superiority of their method over competing methods, recent research is pointing to an equipotentiality of these approaches, at least as regards the diminution of self-destructive behaviours. This improvement has been noted by those utilising dialectic behaviour therapy (see above and Linehan *et al*, 1991) and by those using an individual and group psychoanalytic therapy combined with medication (Bateman & Fonagy, 1999). Similar results have been observed by Kernberg and colleagues, using transference-focused psychotherapy combined with medication (Levy *et al*, 2006). Various medications have proved useful, depending upon the main target symptoms of the borderline patients. Where depression is paramount, an SSRI is recommended. Where impulsivity and anger predominate, a mood stabiliser such as valproic acid or lamotrigine will be useful, especially where the symptom picture is that of bipolar II disorder (Frankenberg & Zanarini, 2002). Preliminary indications from the Kernberg study (in which borderline patients were randomised into three groups: transference-focused, dialectic behavioural and supportive psychotherapies) suggest that supportive therapy can have similar positive results in lowering the tendency to self-destructive behaviours. The improvement, with all three therapy approaches, begins to show itself in about 6–8 months (Levy *et al*, 2006).

In the past, a variety of other antidepressants were prescribed routinely. These included tricyclic drugs such as imipramine and amitriptyline, but the side-effect profile of these drugs is less favourable than that of the SSRIs. The monoamine oxidase inhibitors such as phenelzine and tranylcypromine had been popular until the advent of the SSRIs, but they require avoidance of tyrosine-containing foods (mature cheese, broad beans, chocolate) lest hypertensive crises occur. Use of such medications with an ambulatory suicidal and uncooperative or untrustworthy patient with BPD is hazardous, whereas the common side-effects of the

SSRIs (diminished libido, short-term memory impairment, sleep interruption) are not life-threatening.

The role of the benzodiazepines in dealing with the anxiety in patients with BPD (or in patients with 'anxious' cluster of personality disorders – avoidant and dependent) has generated considerable controversy. This arose largely from the work of Cowdry & Gardner (1988), which showed that BPD out-patients treated with alprazolam were more suicidal and angrily impulsive than were those treated with placebo, but their study was based on a small sample. The use of a shorter-acting drug may have also prejudiced their results. Experience with longer-acting benzodiazepines such as lorazepam and clonazepam seems helpful (Oldham *et al*, 2001, p. 39), and safer in the hands of most clinicians, although the problem of habituation remains. For panic episodes, to which many of these patients are prone, the benzodiazepines continue to have an important place, the more so as they act more quickly than do other medications with anti-panic properties, such as the SSRIs and the tricyclics.

Lithium and other mood-stabilising drugs

In the USA in the 1970s, studies on chronically assaultive prisoners showed a beneficial effect with lithium. Such studies would probably fail to obtain ethical approval today and so are unlikely to be repeated.

Tupin *et al* (1973), in an uncontrolled trial, showed a beneficial effect in 15 of 27 male convicts who had a pattern of easily triggered violence, but 3 became more aggressive. Among those who benefited, lithium levels tended to be at the upper limit of the therapeutic range, and the drug appeared to induce a state of reflective delay.

Sheard *et al* (1976) conducted a much larger, placebo-controlled trial in a group of chronically assaultive prisoners with a variety of personality disorders. After 3 months the rate of serious assaults dropped to zero among the lithium-treated group, but remained unchanged in the group taking placebo. When the lithium was stopped, violent episodes escalated to their previous rate within a month.

A long-term follow-up study of patients with BPD by Stone (1990) found a few individuals (around 8%) who later developed bipolar II disorder, and these subjects did well on lithium.

The presence of anger, affective features (particularly bipolar II disorder), a family history of affective disorder, alcoholism and a family history of alcoholism are indices of possible responsiveness to either lithium or lamotrigine, especially if the mood components are primarily depressive. Some patients with 'episodic dyscontrol syndromes' may respond to lithium, and lithium may also benefit around 70% of those with self-mutilation and learning difficulties (Wickham & Read, 1987).

Impulsivity and aggressive episodes

Empirical observations and a large number of open and uncontrolled studies over many years have suggested that some anti-epileptic drugs (e.g. carbamazepine and sodium valproate), certain antidepressants (especially the SSRIs and lithium) and the antipsychotics may sometimes be helpful for impulsivity and aggressive episodes or self-mutilating behaviours. More recently, however, double-blind placebo-controlled trials have reported positive findings for fluoxetine and sodium valproate for the impulsivity associated with personality disorder. Thus, Coccaro & Kavoussi (1997) recruited 40 patients with personality disorder (borderline or psychopathic) with histories of impulsive aggression but excluded those with depression. Patients entered a randomised controlled trial of fluoxetine (20–40 mg), which was significantly better than placebo on measures of aggression and irritability, with beneficial effects first appearing after 4 weeks. Impulsivity and aggression are key features of intermittent explosive disorder as well, and an open study has demonstrated beneficial effects for SSRIs as well in this condition (McElroy, 1999).

The use of sodium valproate as a mood stabiliser in bipolar disorder has grown dramatically in the past few years, and following a series of open studies its usefulness in BPD has also been demonstrated. Frankenberg & Zanarini (2002) conducted a placebo-controlled trial of divalproex sodium (Depakote) among patients who had both BPD and bipolar disorder. They showed that overall aggression, anger/hostility and interpersonal sensitivity were all significantly reduced. An open study (Pinto & Akiskal, 1998) of one of the newer anti-epileptic drugs, lamotrigine (300 mg), in nine subjects who had previously failed on a large variety of drug treatments as well as psychotherapy led to substantial improvements in global assessment ratings, and sharp falls in suicidal and impulsive behaviours, with some patients no longer meeting criteria for BPD at the end of the trial. The lamotrigine was well tolerated, except for one patient who developed a rash, but as lamotrigine rashes may occasionally develop into the fatal Stevens–Johnson syndrome, the drug should be stopped whenever a rash appears.

Electroconvulsive therapy (ECT)

The administration of ECT and its role in the treatment of axis I disorders are discussed in Chapter 5. Therapeutic pessimism may lead to a failure to prescribe either ECT or drug treatments for people with a personality disorder, and this in itself has been shown to affect outcome (Black *et al*, 1988). Remembering the tendency of these patients to act out dangerously, it may be all the more important to pursue standard physical remedies among subjects who are depressed and who also have a comorbid personality disorder.

Patients who are comorbid for personality disorder and depression may show a good initial response to ECT, but there is often an early relapse. Kramer (1982) reported on five people with BPD and depression. One had a good response with an early relapse, two had an equivocal response with rapid relapse, and two showed no response. Zimmerman *et al* (1986) confirmed these findings and found a higher readmission rate after ECT for patients with personality disorders and depression compared with those who had only depression. In a large retrospective case note study, Black *et al* (1988) showed that 68% of patients with pure depression responded well, but only 40% of those with concomitant personality disorders did so. Against this, Casey & Butler

(1995) failed to detect any difference in either the short-term or 1-year outcome between these groups.

The prescription of ECT for patients with personality disorders raises problems. In spite of evidence that the outcome may be less successful, ECT should not be withheld. In some cases a severe depression may be concealed; thus, frequent self-mutilation may lead to intensive nursing involvement, which may itself trigger further manipulative behaviour on the part of the patient, and so confuse the diagnosis. The high doses of phenothiazines used for sedation may mask the more diagnostic biological symptoms of depression, and ECT may be helpful in such cases. In addition, there are some patients who may be suffering from a drug-responsive depression but whose behaviour is so chaotic, immature or wilful that they are unable to comply with a simple course of antidepressants, let alone discuss their difficulties with a psychotherapist. Even so, these patients are just as keen to be free of their depression, and ECT may be the only type of antidepressive remedy that they can use.

Long-term outcome

Follow-up studies provide information on how well a group with a particular diagnosis will do over time and whether the diagnosis itself has long-term stability and hence meaning. For chronic conditions such as the personality disorders, short-term follow-up may provide some indication about the effect of any intervention, but only long-term studies will give a picture of the lifetime course. However, such studies have the problem of diagnostic validity, because diagnostic criteria may change from the outset of the study to the time when outcome is examined. For example, does the old diagnosis of 'pseudoneurotic schizophrenia' identify the same group of patients as DSM–IV BPD?

There are further difficulties. First, few subjects have a pure syndrome (see Chapter 18). Patients with BPD almost invariably have one or more symptom disorders of axis I (major depression, eating disorder, panic, substance misuse, etc.) and also show enough other personality traits to trigger simultaneous diagnoses of two or three other personality disorders. Second, only those with the more extreme disorders are hospitalised and are therefore diagnosed with enough documentation to serve as a starting point for follow-up studies. Finally, some traits, such as being antisocial, may themselves lead to significant later events being expressly concealed from investigators.

Mortality and suicide

Zilber *et al* (1989) studied the 5-year standardised mortality ratio (SMR) of all the patients admitted to psychiatric hospitals in Israel in 1978 ($n = 16\,147$). The SMR for all types of personality disorder in the 20- to 39-year age group was 6.9, which was similar to that found for schizophrenia (SMR = 6.3) but slightly lower than that for affective disorders (SMR = 8.5). Around half the deaths of those with personality disorder were due to natural causes, mainly infections (SMR = 3.2). Certain complications dramatically increased mortality, such as alcohol misuse (SMR = 27) or substance misuse (SMR = 21), mainly as the result of natural causes, usually infections. The risk for suicide was higher among those with a personality disorder (SMR = 2.6), although this was considerably lower than that for affective disorder (SMR = 6.1), but in the same range as that for schizophrenia (SMR = 3.2).

The mortality of subjects with antisocial personality disorders is high, and although DSM–III–R stated 'they sometimes have a violent end', reliable mortality data relating specifically to this group are lacking. Follow-up studies by Robins (1985) indicated that excess mortality in this group was mainly due to homicide, accidents, and the complications of alcohol or substance misuse.

Among those who have been incarcerated, there is more clear-cut evidence of increased mortality. Robertson (1987) followed up a population of 1347 mentally disordered offenders (all diagnoses) in the UK, and 23 years later found that 21% had died; a quarter of the deaths were by violent or unnatural means (suicide, homicide and accidents). Offenders with non-psychotic disorders (mainly personality disorders) met a violent death in 29% of cases during the follow-up period. A similar but rather smaller study in the USA showed that 7 (5.9%) out of 118 delinquents who were incarcerated had met a violent end, giving them a 76-fold higher risk of having a violent death compared with an age- and sex-matched group in the general population (Yaeger & Lewis, 1990). Those with personality disorders who end up in prison are generally at the more severe end of the spectrum, and so these alarming figures probably do not apply to community samples.

Suicide is an appreciable risk for BPD, and rates are given of around 8% (Paris *et al*, 1987; Stone, 1990), although McGlashan's (1986) series gave a figure of only 3%. This is because the BPD patients admitted to the Chestnut Lodge Hospital of McGlashan's series were older than those of the former two studies, and thus had already passed through more of the high-risk years (ages 20–30). Factors associated with suicide in Stone's (1990) series were a personal or family history of affective disorder, alcoholism and a history of incest or parental brutality. Although numbers were small, a very high suicide rate of around 40% was found for women who had all eight of the DSM–III–R criteria, those with schizoaffective features, and those who were comorbid for alcoholism and major affective disorder as well as BPD. For the milder disorders mortality rates are unknown, but even a high neuroticism score may be associated with an SMR of 2 (Allebeck *et al*, 1988).

Outcome of specific disorders

Borderline personality disorder

Disorders that impinge more on clinicians have a greater likelihood of becoming the focus of a detailed outcome investigation. Two large series of BPD patients by Fenton & McGlashan (1989) ($n = 87$) and Stone (1990) ($n = 196$) confirmed that two-thirds of the patients had a good outcome when traced 10–15 years after the index admission. In Stone's series, a better outcome was associated with high intelligence (IQ more than 130), obsessional features, artistic talent, attractiveness (among women) and attendance at Alcoholics Anonymous (among alcoholics). A worse than average outcome was associated with parental physical cruelty, a history of transgenerational incest, schizotypal features, extreme impulsivity leading to a chaotic lifestyle, and antisocial traits. The DSM–III–R criterion 'inordinate anger' worsened outcome. Since this item is not included in the criteria for Kernberg's borderline personality organisation (see above), the latter condition has a rather more benign outcome than DSM–III–R BPD. The diagnosis of BPD tended to be stable over time, although by the fourth or fifth decade only a quarter of the subjects still had sufficient features to justify such a diagnosis. A small proportion, around 11%, switched diagnosis to affective disorder, but schizophrenia developed in only one out of the 196 cases.

A recurrence of borderline symptoms has sometimes been observed among those earlier diagnosed with BDP, but now in their mid-40s, following widowhood or divorce (sometimes the result of the patient's irascibility), when patients presented once again for treatment (McGlashan, 1986).

Although at the time of the initial index admission BPD appeared to be just as severe as a schizophrenic illness, follow-up studies indicate a better outcome. Readmission rates were lower (28% and 77%, respectively) and more borderline patients had a job (66% and 18%). However, in comparison with the general population the marriage and fertility rates were significantly lower (Stone, 1990).

Antisocial personality disorder

Robins (1985) pointed out that sociopathy is a lifelong disorder, possibly marked by three distinct phases, but it can abort at any time. In early childhood there may be arguments, tantrums and stubbornness with oppositional behaviour. In middle childhood there is aggression and conduct disorder, while in adolescence there is truancy and stealing. Around 40% of conduct-disordered boys and 20% of conduct-disordered girls go on to develop adult antisocial personality disorder, which is most prominent in young adulthood. But because conduct disorder is much more common in boys to begin with, the rate of the personality disorder in adults is almost eight times higher in men than in women.

The disorder tends to attenuate with age, and in later life there is a dramatic decline in the rates of aggression and theft, the hallmarks of antisocial personality disorder. Many explanations are offered for the high rate of termination of the criminal lifestyle that occurs in the mid-40s, including increasing maturity, the development of more satisfying relationships, commitment to legitimate employment, less self-absorption, and less rebelliousness or pleasure-seeking behaviour. The decline in physical and emotional energy may result in criminal 'burnout'; fear of further incarceration may also play a role (Coid, 1993), although there are a few individuals who fail to make any adjustment in mid-life.

It should be noted that criminal burnout does not necessarily imply maturity in a psychopathic personality. Reid *et al* (1986) suggested that many ageing psychopathic individuals are still antisocial, but just less successful, lacking the physical strength and emotional stamina needed to continue in the criminal world, so they can no longer compete with younger psychopathic personalities.

Reliable figures for the outcome of antisocial personality disorder are almost impossible to find, for, as Dilalla & Gottesman (1990) pointed out, there are many young people from abysmal environments who pass through a delinquent phase and later mature out of it, and the inclusion of such cases in any series would paint an unduly optimistic picture. On the other hand, confining a follow-up study to hardened criminals from a prison setting would give too pessimistic a picture.

The presence of antisocial personality disorder worsens the outlook for those with alcohol and substance misuse. For convicted criminals, recidivism rates rise for criminals who also have the disorder. For example, the 4-year reconviction rate for discharged rapists was higher if they were also comorbid for antisocial personality disorder (Rice *et al*, 1990).

In contrast to antisocial personality disorder, psychopathy tends not to 'burn out' past the age of 40, and the prognosis is and remains bleak. There are of course numerous persons with a few psychopathic traits (who score in the mid-range of the Hare Psychopathy Checklist), such as crooked politicians and sellers of fake Rolex watches, who never improve, are not treatable, but cause only minor trouble in society.

Schizoid and schizotypal disorders

There is considerable interest in the long-term outcome of people with schizotypal personality disorder, in particular to see whether they develop schizophrenia and to determine whether there are any predictors of such an outcome. Wolff & Chick (1980) examined 22 children with schizoid disorders between the ages of 5 and 14 years, and showed that the disorder was essentially stable over time, but by age 22 two subjects (9%) had developed schizophrenia. Fenton & McGlashan (1989) followed up 105 subjects with schizotypal personality disorder, of whom 75 were comorbid for BPD (the other 30 had mainly the 'pure' disorder). Around 15 years later, 16% had developed schizophrenia, and the items that more strongly predicted a schizophrenic outcome were those specific to schizotypal personality (i.e. magical thinking, suspiciousness, paranoid ideation and social isolation), whereas the borderline features were not associated with later schizophrenia. Additional predictive factors included transient delusional experiences, lower IQ and a poorer premorbid quality of work. These findings tend to confirm the observations of Spitzer & Gibbon (1979) that schizotypal personality disorder, but not BPD, belongs within the schizophrenia spectrum of disorders.

The presence of features of schizotypal personality disorder appears to worsen the outlook for obsessional disorder (Minichiello *et al*, 1987), the combined borderline–schizotypal personality syndrome has a poorer outlook than BPD alone (Stone, 1990), and among women it is associated with higher rates of alcoholism (Valgum & Valgum, 1989).

Milder disorders

There is little long-term follow-up information on the milder personality disorders, particularly those in the 'anxious' group, or on the outcome of individual traits. Tyrer *et al* (1993) observed a negative correlation of traits with age, suggesting a gradual improvement over time. They suggested that there were two groups of personality disorders: the *mature*, which changed little with the passage of time, and the *immature*, which attenuated with increasing age. The mature group included mainly those in the eccentric and anxious groups – the anankastic, paranoid, schizoid and anxious. The immature group included those in the dramatic cluster – the antisocial, borderline and histrionic types – as well as the dependent and narcissistic types.

This suggestion is supported by two studies that assessed the presence of personality traits with age (Reich *et al*, 1988; Tyrer & Seivewright, 1988). Both studies showed that traits associated with antisocial, borderline and explosive character disorders become less frequent with older age, while increasing age had little effect on the schizoid, compulsive, anxious or hypochondrial traits. Fogel & Westlake (1990) found that 15.8% of a large cohort of subjects with major depression also had a diagnosis of personality disorder. BPD was not diagnosed in any one aged 45 or over in their study, although a few patients with BPD are encountered who are in their 50s and even 60s. Histrionic and dependent personality disorders were less frequent with increasing age, while compulsive personality disorders increased with age (3% at 25–44 years, up to 5% for those aged over 69) (Fogel & Westlake, 1990).

Additional information can be obtained from psychogeriatric studies using older samples, adopting a retrospective view of the patient's life. Bergmann (1991) examined a group of elderly subjects in the community and tried to correlate an earlier history of interpersonal difficulties and abnormal personality traits with psychiatric symptoms in old age. He identified four main groups of subjects:

1 those who in younger life were prone to anxiety in late life manifested hypochondriasis and affective symptoms, particularly depression

2 those who in earlier life had been 'insecure or rigid', had poor relationships with their parents and sometimes psychiatric disorders in childhood in later life experienced loneliness, obsessional and affective symptoms

3 a group designated 'paranoid and hostile types' in old age when younger had had many features of antisocial personality disorder, such as poor relationships with parents, 'neurotic disorders' in childhood, marital disharmony and poor work records

4 those with dependent features and who had been apparently 'inadequate' in their younger years seemed to fit in rather better later, particularly in middle age, when they assumed submissive roles and their compliance was perceived as more of an asset than a liability, although in late life these subjects also had a tendency towards depression.

Conclusions

The high morbidity and mortality of people with personality disorders, as well as the suffering caused to others, mean that treatment issues cannot be ignored. The notion that at least some may be amenable to treatment is relatively new to psychiatry, although it remains uncertain whether treatment has any influence over the longer-term trajectory. None the less, it may be best for psychiatry to leave some individuals well alone, particularly those in the severe psychopathic group. The protection of society and forensic issues take precedence over any marginal improvement that psychotherapy may bring about in a severely dangerous individual. There are, however, many other patients, perhaps with milder or less alienating character disorders, who may experience a need to change and who have a modicum of insight and some degree of motivation. A variety of psychotherapies, ranging from the psychodynamic through to the cognitive–behavioural, may offer some hope for amelioration. For those who tend to 'act out' in various ways (gambling, promiscuity, substance misuse), group therapies and especially the 12-step programme often prove valuable (Brown *et al*, 2002).

The discovery of genetic and other associations with the functional disorders has provided some theoretical justification for psychopharmacological intervention, which, particularly if combined with psychotherapy, may be beneficial. All methods of treatment aim at the same goal: the gradual conquest of pre-existing habits by new, more adaptive habits of thought and behaviour.

References

Alexander, F. (1957) *Psychoanalysis and Psychotherapy*. London: George Allen.

Allebeck, P., Allgulander, G. & Fisher, L. D. (1988) Predictors of completed suicide in a cohort of 50,465 young men: role of personality and deviant behaviour. *BMJ*, **297**, 176–178.

Bateman, A. & Fonagy, P. (1999) Effectiveness of partial hospitalisation in the treatment of borderline personality disorder. A randomized control trial. *American Journal of Psychiatry*, **156**, 1563–1569.

Beard, H., Marlowe, M. & Ryle, A. (1990) Management and treatment of personality disordered patients. The use of sequential diagrammatic reformulation. *British Journal of Psychiatry*, **156**, 541–545.

Beck, A. T. & Freeman, A. (1990) *Cognitive Therapy of Personality Disorders*. New York: Guilford Press.

Benedetti, F., Sforzini, L., Colombo, C., *et al* (1998) Low dose clozapine in acute and continuation treatment of severe personality disorder. *Journal of Clinical Psychiatry*, **59**, 103–107.

Bergmann, K. (1991) The psychiatric aspects of personality in older patients. In *Psychiatry in the Elderly* (eds R. Jacoby & E. Oppenheimer), pp. 852–871. Oxford: Oxford University Press.

Bion, W. R. (1959) Attacks on linking. *International Journal of Psychoanalysis*, **40**, 307–315.

Black, D. W., Bell, S., Hulbert, J., *et al* (1988) The importance of axis II in patients with major depression. *Journal of Affective Disorders*, **14**, 115–122.

Brobyn, L. L., Goren, S. & Lego, S. (1987) The borderline patient: systemic versus psychoanalytic approach. *Archives of Psychiatric Nursing*, **1**, 172–182.

Brown, T. G., Seraganian, P., Tremblay, J., *et al* (2002) Process and outcome changes with relapse prevention versus 12-step aftercare programs for substance abusers. *Addiction*, **97**, 677–689.

Buchanan, A. & Leese, M. (2001) Detention of people with severe personality disorder: a systematic review. *Lancet*, **358**, 1955–1959.

Buss, A. H. & Plomin, R. (1984) *Temperament: Early Developing Personality Traits*. Hillsdale, NJ: Lawrence Erlbaum.

Casey, P. R. & Butler, E. (1995) The effects of personality in response to ECT in major depression. *Journal of Personality Disorders*, **9**, 134–142.

Chiesa, M. & Fonagy, P. (2003) Psychosocial treatment for severe personality disorder. 36 month follow up. *British Journal of Psychiatry*, **183**, 356–362.

Coccaro, E. F. & Kavoussi, R. J. (1997) Fluoxetine and impulsive-aggressive behaviour in personality disordered subjects. *Archives of General Psychiatry*, **54**, 1081–1088.

Coid, J. (1993) Current concepts and classifications of psychopathic disorder. In *Personality Disorder Reviewed* (eds P. Tyrer & G. Stein), pp. 113–164. London: Gaskell.

Costa, P. T. Jr & McCrae, R. R. (1986) Personality stability and its implications for clinical psychology. *Clinical Psychological Review*, **6**, 407–423.

Cowdry, R. & Gardner, D. L. (1988) Pharmacotherapy of borderline personality disorder. *Archives of General Psychiatry*, **45**, 111–119.

Dilalla, L. F. & Gottesman, I. I. (1990) Heterogeneity of causes of delinquency and criminality: lifespan perspectives. *Development and Psychopathology*, **1**, 339–349.

Dolan, B. & Coid, J. (1993) *Psychopathic and Antisocial Personality Disorders*. London: Gaskell.

Ellis, A. (1963) *Rational Emotive Psychotherapy*. New York: Institute for Rational Emotive Therapy.

Feeney, A. (2003) Dangerous severe personality disorder. *Advances in Psychiatric Treatment*, **9**, 349–358.

Fenton, W. S. & McGlashan, T. H. (1989) Risk of schizophrenia in character disordered patients. *American Journal of Psychiatry*, **146**, 1280–1284.

Fenton, W. S. & McGlashan, T. H. (1990) Long-term outcome of obsessive–compulsive disorder with psychotic features. *Journal of Nervous and Mental Disease*, **178**, 760–761.

Fogel, B. S. & Westlake, R. (1990) Personality disorder diagnosis and age: in patients with major depression. *Journal of Clinical Psychiatry*, **51**, 232–235.

Frankenberg, F. R. & Zanarini, M. C. (2002) Divalproex sodium treatment of women with borderline personality disorder: a double-blind placebo-controlled study. *Journal of Clinical Psychiatry*, **63**, 442–446.

Fromm-Reichmann, F. (1950) *Principles of Intensive Psychotherapy*. Chicago: University of Chicago Press.

Frosch, J. (1983) *The Psychotic Process*. New York: International Universities Press.

Goldberg, S. C., Schulz, S. C., Schulz, P. M., *et al* (1986) Borderline and schizotypal personality disorders treated with low dose thiothixene vs placebo. *Archives of General Psychiatry*, **43**, 680–686.

Gunderson, J. G. (1984) *Borderline Personality Disorder*. Washington, DC: American Psychiatric Press.

Gunderson, J. G. & Szabo, A. N. (1993) Treatment of borderline personality disorder: A critical review. In *Borderline Personality Disorder: Etiology and Treatment* (ed. J. Paris), pp. 385–406. Washington, DC: American Psychiatric Press.

Hare, R. D. (1993) *Without Conscience: The Disturbing World of Psychopaths Among Us*. New York: Pocket Books.

Hare, R. D., Harpur, T. J., Hakstian, A. R., *et al* (1990) The revised Psychopathy Checklist. *Psychological Assessment*, **2**, 338–341.

Higgit, A. & Fonagy, P. (1992) Psychotherapy in borderline and narcissistic personality disorder. *British Journal of Psychiatry*, **161**, 23–43.

Higgit, A. & Fonagy, P. (1993) Psychotherapy for personality disorder. In *Personality Disorder Reviewed* (eds P. Tyrer & G. Stein), pp. 225–261. London: Gaskell.

Jackson, M. & Pines, M. (1986) Inpatient treatment of borderline personality. *Neurologia et Psychiatrica*, **9**, 54–87.

Kernberg, O. F. (1967) Borderline personality organisation. *Journal of the American Psychoanalytic Association*, **15**, 642–685.

Kernberg, O. F. (1975) *Borderline Conditions and Pathological Narcissism*. New York: Aronson.

Kernberg, O. F. (1992) *Aggression in Personality Disorders and Perversions*. New Haven, CT: Yale University Press.

Koenigsberg, H. W., Reynolds, D., Goodman, M., *et al* (2003) Risperidone in the treatment of schizotypal personality disorder. *Journal of Clinical Psychiatry*, **64**, 628–634.

Kohut, H. (1971) *The Analysis of the Self*. New York: International Universities Press.

Kramer, B. A. (1982) Poor response to ECT in patients with a combined diagnosis of major depression and personality disorder. *Lancet*, **ii**, 1048.

Leichsenring, F. & Leibing, E. (2003) The effectiveness of psychodynamic therapy and cognitive behaviour therapy in the treatment of personality disorders: a meta analysis. *American Journal of Psychiatry*, **160**, 1223–1232.

Levy, K. N., Clarkin, J. F., Yeomans, F. E., *et al* (2006) The mechanisms of change in the treatment of borderline personality disorder with transference-focused psychotherapy. *Journal of Clinical Psychology*, **62**, 481–501.

Linehan, M. M. (1993) *Cognitive–Behavioural Treatment of Borderline Personality Disorder*. New York: Guilford.

Linehan, M. M., Armstrong, H. E., Suarez, A., *et al* (1991) Cognitive–behavioural treatment of chronically parasuicidal borderline patients. *Archives of General Psychiatry*, **48**, 1060–1064.

Main, T. (1957) The ailment. *British Journal of Medical Psychology*, **30**, 129–145.

Marks, I. & Marks. J. (1990) Exposure treatment of agoraphobia/panic. In *Handbook of Anxiety, Vol. 4. The Treatment of Anxiety* (eds R. Noyes, Jr, M. Roth & G. D. Burrows), pp. 298–310. Oxford: Elsevier.

Masterson, J. F. (1981) *The Narcissistic and Borderline Disorders*. New York: Brunner/Mazel.

McElroy, S. (1999) Recognition and treatment of DSM–IV intermittent explosive disorder. *Journal of Clinical Psychiatry*, **60**, suppl. 15, 12–15.

McGlashan, T. H. (1986) The Chestnut Lodge follow-up study: III. Long term outcome of borderline personalities. *Archives of General Psychiatry*, **43**, 20–30.

McGuire, M. & Troisi, A. (1998) *Darwinian Psychiatry*. New York: Oxford University Press.

Meloy, J. R. (1996) Stalking (obsessional following). A review of some preliminary studies. *Aggression and Violent Behaviour*, **1**, 147–162.

Minichiello, W. E., Baer, L. & Jenike, M. A. (1987) Schizotypal personality disorder: a poor prognostic indicator for behaviour therapy in the treatment of obsessive–compulsive disorder. *Journal of Anxiety Disorder*, **1**, 273–276.

Oldham, J. M., Phillips, K., Gabbard, G. O., *et al* (2001) *Practice Guidelines for the Treatment of Patients with Borderline Personality Disorder*. Supplement to the *American Journal of Psychiatry*, October.

Paris, J. (1994) *Borderline Personality Disorder: A Multidimensional Approach*. Washington, DC: American Psychiatric Press.

Paris, J., Brown, R. & Nowlis, D. (1987) Long term follow up of borderline patients in a general hospital. *Comprehensive Psychiatry*, **28**, 530–536.

Patrick, J. (1985) Therapeutic ambience in the treatment of severely disturbed narcissistic personality disorders. *American Journal of Psychoanalysis*, **45**, 258–267.

Pinto, O. C. & Akiskal, H. S. (1998) Lamotrigine as a promising approach to borderline personality disorder: an open case series without concurrent DSM–IV major mood disorder. *Journal of Affective Disorders*, **51**, 333–343.

Putnam, F. W. & Trickett, P. K. (1993) Child sexual abuse: a model of chronic trauma. *Psychiatry*, **56**, 82–95.

Reich, J., Nduaguba, M. & Yates, W. (1988) Age and sex discrimination of DSM–III personality cluster traits in a community population. *Comprehensive Psychiatry*, **29**, 298–303.

Reid, W. H., Dorr, D., Walker, J. I., *et al* (eds) (1986) *Unmasking the Psychopath*. New York: Norton.

Rice, M. E., Harris, G. T. & Quinsey, V. L. (1990) A follow up of rapists assessed in a maximum-security psychiatric facility. *Journal of Interpersonal Violence*, **5**, 435–448.

Rinsley, D. (1982) *Borderline and Other Self Disorders*. New York: Aronson.

Robertson, G. (1987) Mentally abnormal offenders: manner of death. *BMJ*, **295**, 632–634.

Robins, L. N. (1985) Epidemiology of antisocial personality disorder. In *Psychiatry 3* (eds R. O. Mithels & J. O. Cavenar). Philadelphia: J. B. Lippincott.

Rocca, P., Marchiano, L., Cocuzza, E., *et al* (2002) Treatment of borderline personality disorder with risperidone. *Journal of Clinical Psychiatry*, **63**, 241–244.

Rogers, C. (ed.) (1967) *The Therapeutic Relationship and Its Impact: A Study in Psychotherapy*. Madison, WI: University of Wisconsin Press.

Searles, H. F. (1979) *Countertransference*. Madison, WI: International Universities Press.

Sheard, M., Marini, J. L., Bridges, C. I., *et al* (1976) The effect of lithium on unipolar aggressive behaviour in man. *American Journal of Psychiatry*, **133**, 1409–1413.

Soloff, P. H., George, A., Nathan, R. S., *et al* (1986) Progress in pharmacotherapy of borderline disorders: a double-blind study of amitriptyline, haloperidol and placebo. *Archives of General Psychiatry*, **43**, 691–697.

Soloff, P. H., Cornelius, J., George, A., *et al* (1993) Efficacy of phenelzine and haloperidol in borderline personality disorder. *Archives of General Psychiatry*, **50**, 337–385.

Spitzer, R. L. & Gibbon, M. (1979) Crossing the border into borderline personality and borderline schizophrenia. *Archives of General Psychiatry*, **36**, 17–24.

Stevens, A. & Price, J. (2000) *Evolutionary Psychiatry* (2nd edn). London: Routledge.

Stone, M. H. (1988) The borderline domain: the 'inner script' and other common psychodynamics. In *Modern Perspectives in Psychiatry, Vol. II* (ed. J. Howells), pp. 200–230. New York: Brunner/Mazel.

Stone, M. H. (1989) Individual psychotherapy with victims of incest. *Psychiatric Clinics of North America*, **12**, 237–255.

Stone, M. H. (1990) *The Fate of Borderline Patients*. New York: Guilford Press.

Trukatt, I. D. & Carlson, C. R. (1984) Database versus symptomatic formulation of treatment: the case of dependent personality. *Journal of Behavioural Therapy and Experimental Psychology*, **15**, 153–160.

Tupin, J. P., Smith, D. B., Clanon, T. L., *et al* (1973) The long term use of lithium in aggressive prisoners. *Comprehensive Psychiatry*, **14**, 311–317.

Tyrer, P. & Sievewright, H. (1988) In studies of outcome. In *Personality Disorders: Diagnosis, Management and Course* (ed. P. Tyrer), pp. 119–136. London: Wright.

Tyrer, P., Casey, P. & Ferguson, B. (1993) Personality disorder in perspective. In *Personality Disorder Reviewed* (eds P. Tyrer & G. Stein), pp. 1–16. London: Gaskell.

Valgum, S. & Valgum, P. (1989) Co-morbidity for borderline and schizotypal personality disorders. A study of alcoholic women. Progress in neuropsychopharmacology and biological psychiatry. *Journal of Nervous and Mental Disease*, **177**, 279–284.

van der Kolk, B. A. (1989) Compulsion to repeat the trauma. Re-enactment, revictimisation and masochism. *Psychiatric Clinics of North America*, **12**, 389–402.

Verheul, R., Van den Bosch, L., Koeter, W. J., *et al* (2003) Dialectical behaviour therapy for women with borderline personality disorder. 12 month randomised trial in the Netherlands. *British Journal of Psychiatry*, **182**, 135–140.

Waldinger, R. J. & Gunderson, J. G. (1984) Completed psychotherapies with borderline patients. *American Journal of Psychotherapy*, **38**, 190–202.

Wickham, E. A. & Read, J. V. (1987) Lithium in the control of aggression and self-mutilating behaviour. *International Clinical Psychopharmacology*, **2**, 181–190.

Winnicott, D. W. (1965) *The Maturational Processes and the Facilitating Environment*. New York: International Universities Press.

Wolff, S. & Chick, J. (1980) Schizoid personality in childhood: a controlled follow-up study. *Psychological Medicine*, **10**, 85–100.

Woolcott, P., Jr (1985) Prognostic indicators in the psychotherapy of borderline patients. *American Journal of Psychotherapy*, **39**, 17–29.

Yaeger, C. A. & Lewis, D. O. (1990) Mortality in a group of formerly incarcerated juvenile delinquents. *American Journal of Psychiatry*, **147**, 612–614.

Zanarini, M. C. & Frankenberg, F. R. (2001) Olanzapine treatment of female borderline personality disorder patients. A double blind placebo controlled pilot study. *Journal of Clinical Psychiatry*, **62**, 849–854.

Zanarini, M. & Gunderson, J. G. (1990) Childhood experiences of borderline patients. *Comprehensive Psychiatry*, **30**, 18–25.

Zilber, N., Schufman, N. & Lerner, Y. (1989) Mortality among psychiatric patients, the groups at risk. *Acta Psychiatrica Scandinavica*, **79**, 248–256.

Zimmerman, M., Coryell, W., Pfohl, B., *et al* (1986) ECT response in depressed patients with and without a DSM–III personality disorder. *American Journal of Psychiatry*, **143**, 1030–1032.

CHAPTER 20

Organic psychiatric disorders

Robin Jacobson, Irshaad Ebrahim and Michael Kopelman

Organic psychiatry is a clinical discipline concerned with disorders of cognition, behaviour and affect arising from disorders of brain structure and function. It embraces the psychiatric problems of patients with neurological disorders and the psychological consequences of organic diseases that indirectly affect the brain. It also addresses the neurological aspects of certain general psychiatric disorders (and here organic psychiatry overlaps with biological psychiatry). Organic psychiatry focuses on the cerebral mechanisms of psychological functioning and cognitive skills and abilities, and the ways in which pathological processes disturb them. Knowledge of, and application of techniques derived from, psychiatry, neurology, neuropsychology, genetics, pharmacology and medicine are essential to clinical practice.

The developmental, psychosocial and cultural contexts and the illness beliefs of the individual are closely integrated into assessment and treatment. Hence psychological and social approaches are combined with pharmacological and cognitive efforts in the treatment and rehabilitation of the patient with an organic psychiatric disorder.

Organic psychiatry increasingly overlaps with the disciplines of neuropsychology, cognitive neuroscience and biological psychiatry:

- *Neuropsychology* investigates the cognitive organisation of mental processes and functions and their disturbances in patients with brain damage. Neuropsychologists examine the assets and deficits of patients with brain disorders using neuropsychological tests designed to characterise and quantify dysfunction and to guide rehabilitation.
- In *cognitive neuroscience*, the basic processes of the mind are investigated in animal models and computer simulations and by functional brain imaging.
- The discipline of *biological psychiatry* focuses on the structural, physiological and neurochemical abnormalities underlying primary psychiatric disorders such as depression and schizophrenia.

The work of the neuropsychiatrist or organic psychiatrist is primarily concerned with the psychiatric manifestations and complications of neurological disorders, whereas that of the neurologist is mainly with the diagnosis and treatment of specific lesions or diseases. Both deal with acute organic reactions, but each with different manifestations and referral patterns of patients with chronic organic reactions. The organic psychiatrist is primarily concerned with:

- the aetiological diagnosis and management of specific organic disorders or syndromes (e.g. delirium, memory disorders and dementia)
- the management of secondary behaviours (e.g. depression after head injury or stroke)
- psychosis in epilepsy or dementia
- neurologically unexplained symptoms
- sleep disorders
- support for relatives and carers
- the coordination of care in hospital and in the community.

Also, the neuropsychiatrist will sometimes assess an organic contribution to 'functional' disorders, and medico-legal issues.

A comprehensive approach to organic psychiatry requires the integration of biological factors with the personal, family and social context. The burden on patients, relatives and carers is often severe, requiring a multidisciplinary approach to the patient and family. A multidisciplinary team approach is essential in managing the disability patients have, and consultation with neurologists, neuropsychologists, social workers, occupational therapists and other paramedical staff, and with neuro-rehabilitation units, is often needed.

The structure of this chapter is:

1. a short section on history
2. a brief discussion of syndromes and classification
3. a description of assessment procedures
4. a more detailed account of the two principal organic psychiatric presentations, delirium and dementia.

History

The roots of organic psychiatry are embedded in both psychiatry and neurology. The history of organic psychiatry has oscillated, in the main, between *localisationist* and *holistic* phases. The former developed in the early 19th century when in 1809 the phrenologists Gull and Spurzheim speculated that the cerebral convolutions reflect the juxtaposition of many discrete cerebral organs, each subserving a particular psychological function. Early advances in aphasia by Broca in 1861 and Wernicke in 1874 led to the flowering of the localisation approach, with the advent of the 'diagram makers', who sought to explain aphasia. In this era, Meynert described the motor and sensory cortex in 1867, and in 1869 Hughlings Jackson observed contralateral focal seizures. Lissauer in 1890 and Freud in 1891 described agnosia and Liepmann described apraxia in 1900.

Opponents of this localisation approach to higher mental functions included Hughlings Jackson, whose schema of a hierarchy of functions with a 'dissolution' and a regression to lower levels of function, incorporating positive and negative symptoms, after brain damage, supplied an essentially unitary view of the patient. Globalist accounts of mental function developed further in the early 20th century, with critiques by Marie, Head and Goldstein of narrow localisationist theories of language. Later, in 1929, Lashley's theory of mass action proposed that the cortex was undifferentiated and had equipotential for cognitive abilities, their degree of impairment depending on the extent but not localisation of brain damage. More recently localisationist or modular (Shallice, 1988) approaches have predominated again.

In the 19th century, the growth of neurology and neuropathology shaped the view that mental diseases are brain diseases (a view first expounded by Griesinger in 1845), while psychological systems of explanation received an enormous boost from the debate over the nature of hypnosis and hysteria. Charcot's physical explanation of hypnosis and hysteria clashed with, and later yielded to, Bernheim's psychogenic conception, which was expanded by Janet (Micale, 1990). In this context, Freud developed psychodynamic theory.

Classical neuropsychiatric disorders were described and the syndromatic approach clarified nearer the end of the 19th century. Huntington's chorea was described in 1872, Wernicke's encephalopathy in 1881, Korsakoff's syndrome in 1887 and Pick's disease in 1892. In 1907 Alois Alzheimer described the disease that bears his name. The term 'delirium' was introduced by Celsus in the first century AD, but Hippocrates' work was rich in descriptions of delirium, which remained a stable psychiatric category until the 19th century (Berrios, 1996).

The prevailing view that individual physical diseases give rise to their own specific insanities was challenged by Chaslin in 1895 and Bonhoeffer in 1909, who redefined confusion and delirium as the stereotyped manifestations of acute brain failure (Berrios, 1996). Bonhoeffer (1909) recognised that, irrespective of the type of pathology, different forms of insult or injury led to a narrow repertoire of stereotyped responses ('exogenous reaction types'), notably delirium.

The early 20th century witnessed only modest advances in organic psychiatry, largely because of the emergence of psychoanalysis and social psychiatry, the influence of Lashley and Gestalt psychology, and the move away from localisation to descriptive approaches to psychosis.

After the Second World War, three major studies in different nations examined the relationship of cognitive dysfunction to the localisation of missile wounds (Luria, 1947; Semmes *et al*, 1960; Newcombe, 1969). Geschwind (1965) rediscovered the important descriptions of the 19th-century 'behavioural' neurologists, particularly with respect to disconnection syndromes, and relaunched the study of higher cortical functions among neurologists. Luria (1966) softened the localisation–holistic polarisation and emphasised the importance of frontal-lobe function.

The advent of new technologies in the postwar era provided neuroscientists with new tools to identify and localise brain lesions. These were initially quite crude, invasive and generally yielded poor results. It was not until the 1960s, when Sir Godfrey Hounsfield and Alan Cormack introduced computed tomographic (CT) brain scanning that the immediate localisation, nature and natural history of a lesion could be identified and monitored in an essentially non-invasive manner. In the late 1970s, Edward Purcell and Felix Bloch discovered the phenomenon of nuclear magnetic resonance. The magnetic resonance scanner provided images in much finer detail than CT and has now largely supplanted CT as a *structural* diagnostic tool.

A revolution in *functional* neuroimaging was pioneered by Seymour Kety's initial investigation of brain blood flow in mental illness during the 1940s. The advent of single photon emission tomography (SPET) and David Ingvar's seminal discovery of hypofrontality in schizophrenia has spurred the development of functional techniques in neuroimaging. Positron emission tomography (PET), functional magnetic resonance imaging (fMRI) and magnetic resonance spectroscopy (MRS) are now leading areas of research into brain function and mapping. These promise to enhance clinical practice.

Syndrome definition and classification

Organic psychiatric disorders can be subdivided on the basis of three criteria (Marsden, 1985):

1 whether the impairment of intellectual or psychological function is generalised or focal
2 whether the disorder is acute or chronic
3 whether the underlying dysfunction is functional (e.g. pseudo-dementia) or neurological.

The classification of organic psychiatric disorders turns on the central distinction between the concepts of syndrome and disease, and the further need to separate organic and functional disorders. A syndromal approach is based purely on a set of observed associations of symptoms and signs, is largely atheoretical, and does not include notions of aetiology, pathology, course and treatment response, which are intrinsic to the concept of disease. The nosology of organic disorders wavers uneasily between a syndromal and an aetiological approach. The move towards a syndrome-oriented approach and an operational approach to classification, which eschews theoretical orientation, has been adopted by both ICD–10 (World Health Organization, 1992) and DSM–IV (American Psychiatric Association, 1994).

Further details of the similarities and differences between ICD–10 and DSM–IV are easily obtainable from these classification manuals. Readers are advised to familiarise themselves with both, although neuropsychiatric topics are not well covered in either classificatory system, and it is to be hoped that ICD–11 and DSM–V will show improvements (Kopelman & Fleminger, 2002).

General terminology and principal conditions

Acute and chronic reactions

'Acute organic reaction' and 'chronic organic reaction' are the terms traditionally used for the first major division of organic psychiatric disorders (Lishman, 1998). The terms imply the type of onset and, in part, the main symptoms and the likely duration of the disorder, but not the ultimate prognosis. Acute symptoms may be due to delirium (i.e. an acute confusional state), a focal neurological deficit or psychiatric disorder, whereas chronic symptoms may be due to dementia or, again, a focal neurological deficit or psychiatric disorder.

Subacute organic reactions

These have a less sudden onset than acute disorders, a longer course and present as a mixture of acute and chronic symptoms.

Delirium

Delirium is also known as acute organic reaction or acute confusional state, toxic psychosis or acute organic psychosis. The syndrome is characterised by disorientation in time and place and by global cognitive impairment (i.e. of attention, memory and consciousness). It is of acute onset and of relatively brief duration. Impaired attention and awareness are the cardinal clinical features. Other core features include disturbances of: cognition (perception, thinking and memory), the sleep–wake cycle and psychomotor behaviour.

Delirium is usually due to a widespread disturbance of cerebral metabolism and it is a common feature of physical illness or drug toxicity, especially in the elderly. While potentially reversible, delirium may herald death. It requires urgent attention.

Clouding of consciousness

Clouding describes the mildest stage of impairment of consciousness that is detectable clinically, on the continuum from full alertness and awareness to coma (Lishman, 1998). Traditionally an essential feature of delirium, the term 'clouding of consciousness' has been dropped from current US definitions on the grounds that it is little more than a metaphor referring to the deficits that constitute the core features of delirium.

Coma

Coma represents the extreme of a graded continuum of impairment of consciousness, in which the patient is in a state of unarousable unresponsiveness (Plum & Posner, 1982). The patient is incapable of sensing or responding adequately to external stimuli or inner needs, shows little or no spontaneous movement apart from respiration, and no evidence whatever of mental activity. The Glasgow Coma Scale (Teasdale & Jennett, 1974) is used to assess grades of impairment of consciousness.

Stupor

Stupor refers to a clinical syndrome of akinesis and mutism, but with evidence of relative preservation of conscious awareness (Lishman, 1998). DSM–IV defines stupor as a state of unresponsiveness with immobility and mutism. It is one form of organic catatonic disorder (on which see below).

Mutism

Mutism is a condition in which a person does not speak or attempt spoken communication despite preservation of an adequate level of consciousness. It may sometimes be the only abnormality present.

Dementia

Dementia is defined as an acquired global impairment of intellect, memory and personality, but without impairment of consciousness (Lishman, 1998). It is persistent (unlike delirium), occurs in an alert (non-drowsy) patient, who has a global disturbance of higher mental function, and causes impairment of function (with loss of occupational, social and personality competence). Dementia may be complicated by delirium. It is caused by physical disease, although no specific physical aetiology is implied by this. Although many dementias are progressive and untreatable, for about 13% of patients under the age of 65 who are referred to specialist centres the condition is potentially reversible and treatment is successful for about 1% (Hejl *et al*, 2001).

DSM–IV requires that the patient has an impaired ability to learn new information or to recall previously learned information, associated with one or more of the following cognitive disturbances: aphasia, apraxia, agnosia and disturbance in executive functioning (planning, organising, sequencing, abstracting), sufficient to compromise social or occupational functioning, and with a disease-specific course (e.g. gradual onset and continuing cognitive decline in Alzheimer's disease). Loss of a single capacity or intellectual function, such as memory or speech, however devastating, is not sufficient.

The DSM–IV definition has several limitations. First, the requirement that all demented patients have memory loss excludes disorders such as frontotemporal dementia, in the early and middle phases of which episodic memory is preserved (Snowden *et al*, 2002). The frontotemporal dementia due to Pick's disease is, in fact, classified separately within the dementia rubric. Moreover, frontal and subcortical dysfunction is generally the most characteristic finding in vascular dementia (Bowler & Hachinski, 2003). Second, personality change, one of several non-cognitive aspects of dementia, has been relegated to an associated feature and disorder in DSM–IV 'because of its relative lack of specificity for dementia'. Yet it is the hallmark of many cases of frontotemporal dementia (see page 519). Third, social and occupational impairments are hard to define and quantify; they vary with the demands of circumstances and level of support for any given disability. Fourth, by also excluding aetiological non-organic factors, the pseudo-dementias are excluded (see page 520).

Personality and behavioural disorders due to brain disease, damage and dysfunction (ICD–10)

Brain disease, damage or dysfunction often results in persistent personality changes or behavioural disorders;

these usually represent a change or accentuation of a previous trait. (Disorders may also be lifelong if the pathology originates in childhood.) Changes in the control of emotions and impulses and in motivation and social judgement are most typical, leading to affective instability, euphoria, aggressive outbursts, social indiscretion, inability to plan or persevere with goal-directed activity, marked apathy and indifference, or suspiciousness with paranoid ideation. Cognitive deficits are mainly or exclusively of frontal lobe type. The terms 'organic personality disorder' (ICD–10) or 'personality change due to a general medical condition' (DSM–IV) are used.

This disorder usually occurs with strictly focal brain damage, as in the frontal lobe syndrome (on which see below).

The existence of a personality pattern specifically associated with epilepsy is controversial. Patients with complex partial seizures arising from a temporal lobe focus tend towards humourless sobriety, circumstantiality and religiosity (the three most discriminating traits) (Waxman & Geschwind, 1975). These interictal personality changes may occur, however, in other epileptic and psychiatric disorders.

Placidity often accompanies frontal or bilateral limbic system lesions, as in the Kluver–Bucy and Korsakoff syndromes. Irritability and apathy are the characteristic personality changes found in Huntington's disease, probably the result of disrupted caudate–frontal connections.

Reduced control over aggression may occur:

- in patients with temporal lobe epilepsy
- in patients with tumours in the medial temporal, septal or hypothalamic areas
- following birth trauma, head injury and intracerebral infections
- in habitually aggressive offenders with electroencephalographic abnormalities, including the controversial syndrome of 'episodic dyscontrol' (see Chapter 20, page 460).

ICD–10 includes the 'post-encephalitic syndrome' and the 'post-concussional syndrome' here, whereas DSM–IV relegates the latter to a category of proposed disorders requiring refinement of the criteria set. ICD–10 includes a right-hemisphere organic affective disorder in its 'other organic personality and behavioural disorder' category.

Amnesic syndrome

The amnesic syndrome is best defined as 'an abnormal mental state in which memory and learning are affected out of all proportion to other cognitive functions in an otherwise alert and responsive patient' (Victor *et al*, 1971). The Korsakoff syndrome refers, by modern convention, to those cases of an amnesic syndrome that have resulted from chronic or subacute on chronic nutritional deficiency, most commonly arising from alcohol misuse. There is no reference to either 'short-term memory' or 'confabulation' in the definitions. ICD–10 describes organic amnesic syndrome, and DSM–IV amnestic disorder due to a general medical condition and also substance-induced persisting amnestic disorder.

Organic hallucinosis

Organic hallucinosis is the ICD–10 term; in DSM–IV, psychotic disorder due to a general medical condition is used. The terms refer to a syndrome of prominent persistent or recurrent hallucinations, usually visual or auditory, occurring in a setting of clear consciousness (and full awareness of the environment), attributable to a specific organic factor. Insight is variable; any delusions that occur are secondary to the hallucinations. Common causes are use of hallucinogens, sensory deprivation, brain damage and seizures, and alcohol withdrawal (though alcohol hallucinosis is coded separately in both ICD–10 and DSM–IV).

Organic catatonic disorder

Organic catatonic disorder is the ICD–10 term; in DSM–IV catatonic disorder due to a general medical condition is used. It is a disorder of diminished (stupor) or increased (excitement) psychomotor activity associated with catatonic symptoms. The extremes of psychomotor disturbance may alternate. Common causes are brain tumours, encephalitis, hypercalcaemia, liver failure and diabetic ketoacidosis.

Organic delusional (schizophrenic-like) disorder

This ICD–10 term encompasses paranoid and schizophrenia-like disorders due to specific organic factors. Persistent or recurrent delusions are required for this diagnosis to be made, and the criteria further stipulate the assumption at least of an organic aetiology. Hallucinations, thought disorder and isolated catatonic phenomena may be present. Consciousness and memory must not be affected. Examples include amphetamine psychosis and the chronic schizophrenia-like psychosis of temporal lobe epilepsy. DSM–IV describes prominent hallucinations or delusions in the category 'psychotic disorder due to a general medical condition'.

Organic mood (affective disorders)

Organic mood (affective) disorders (ICD–10) can involve: persistent depressed mood; elevated, expansive or irritable mood; or a mixed affective state. They are directly due to a specific organic factor rather than the patient's emotional response to the knowledge of having a concurrent disorder or the symptoms of it. Common causes include drugs, thyroid disease, Cushing's syndrome, cancer and strokes in the anterior left hemisphere. DSM–IV classifies a corresponding 'mood disorder due to a general medical condition' in the 'mood disorders' section.

Organic anxiety disorder

In organic anxiety disorder (ICD–10), recurrent panic attacks or generalised anxiety, or both, develop from a specific organic factor. Examples include hypoglycaemia, thyroid disorders, phaeochromocytoma, drug intoxication and withdrawal, and seizures. DSM–IV includes obsessions and compulsions as well as prominent anxiety and panic attacks in the category 'Anxiety disorder due to an general medical condition', which falls in the 'Anxiety disorders' section.

Miscellaneous disorders

ICD–10 also describes organic dissociative disorder, organic emotionally labile (asthenic) disorder, mild cognitive disorder, and other and unspecified disorders. DSM–IV additionally includes sexual dysfunction and sleep disorder, due to a general medical condition, in other sections, and mild neurocognitive disorder and various medication-induced movement disorders in the section 'Criteria sets and axes provided for further study'.

Syndromes with regional connections

Frontal lobe syndrome

Frontal lobe lesions may cause profound personality changes, but IQ, memory and other cognitive functions are commonly preserved (Stuss & Benson, 1986). (One of the first case reports was of Phineas Gage, described by Harlow in 1868. Gage was a reliable railroad foreman who became profane, irritable and irresponsible after recovery from an accident when a tamping iron was blown through his frontal lobes.)

The outstanding personality change in the frontal lobe syndrome is disinhibition, with euphoria, overfamiliarity, tactlessness, overtalkativeness and inappropriate sexual conduct. Patients may also display impulsive behaviour, irritability and aggressive outbursts, childish excitement or silliness ('moria') with inappropriate jokes, puns or pranks ('*Witzelsucht*'). Insight, especially concern for the future and for the consequences of actions, is limited, leading to gross errors of judgement. Mood is elevated, but with a shallow and fatuous euphoria rather than a true elation. Euphoria is generally episodic, often superimposed on a background of profound apathy, indifference, lack of motivation and of spontaneity, and marked slowing of psychomotor activity.

Some patients may no longer carry out the necessary activities of daily living (dressing, washing, eating, elimination), but these can be performed on coaxing or may occur at any time or place without regard for the social consequences. Medial frontal lesions may produce akinesia, which may progress to stupor, and incontinence with or without distress. Other patients have impairments of abstract reasoning, creativity, problem-solving, and mental flexibility, jump to premature conclusions and become concrete or stimulus-bound. Patients may correctly answer questions requiring judgement yet seem unable to govern their actions by the same verbal rule. They perform normally on externally driven tasks but very poorly at self-motivated learning. Impeccable behaviour during examination may conceal impaired judgement and comportment, which emerge only in the less structured settings of everyday life.

Concentration, attention and the ability to maintain a behavioural set without perseveration (Luria, 1966) and to initiate cognitive strategies, as tested by generating lists of words, are disrupted. Loss of the ability to shift cognitive set, as revealed in the Wisconsin Card Sorting Test, occurs in many cases of frontal lesion, perhaps particularly in those involving dorsolateral lesions (Milner, 1963). Sequencing of behaviour and judgements of temporal order are impaired in patients with involvement of the dorsolateral cortical margins. Planning, problem-solving and performance on simultaneous (dual) tasks are compromised. In Lhermitte's 'environmental dependency syndrome', patients feel compelled to pick up and use objects placed before them, even without invitation and against countermand.

Other evidence of a frontal lobe lesion includes adversive focal seizures, ipsilateral optic atrophy or anosmia, grasp reflex and Broca's aphasia.

Blumer & Benson (1975) describe two distinct frontal lobe syndromes:

- a 'pseudo-depressed' type, characterised by apathy with lack of initiative and indifference, sometimes attributed to convexity lesions
- a 'pseudo-psychopathic' type, marked by disinhibition with euphoria, irritability, impulsivity and antisocial behaviour, tending to follow orbitofrontal pathology.

Memory can also be involved, resulting in either impoverished recall of past memories or in florid confabulation, depending on localisation of pathology (Kopelman, 1991).

Clinically, a mixture of frontal lobe symptoms is more common than a pure set, and occasionally large 'silent' lesions can be accommodated with little clinical disturbance. In an individual patient the localisation, size, type and course of the lesion will determine the clinical picture, which in turn will be coloured by the previous personality and age at onset. The manifestations of bilateral frontal lobe pathology are more dramatic than those of unilateral lesions, which can be subtle and elusive (Mesulam, 2000). Common causes of the frontal lobe syndrome include vascular disease, tumours, head injury, multiple sclerosis, dementia and, less often, infections.

Temporal lobe syndromes

A variety of syndromes can occur with temporal lobe lesions, depending on whether the left (language dominant) or right lobe is affected, whether one or both lobes are involved, and whether or not there is associated epilepsy. Lesions restricted to the temporal poles may also be 'silent'.

Dominant temporal lesions may produce a sensory (Wernicke) aphasia alone, which may be mistaken for dementia. More posterior lesions may impair visual aspects of language, producing alexia and agraphia. Non-dominant temporal lobe lesions may yield few symptoms or signs, or sometimes visuospatial problems.

Bilateral medial temporal lobe lesions, including those involving the hippocampus, produce a severe and selective amnesic syndrome. Unilateral lesions rarely produce spontaneous complaints, probably because the intact medial temporal lobe can compensate in part. Modality-specific memory loss, affecting verbal material on the dominant side and non-verbal material (such as places, faces, music and drawings) on the non-dominant side, is usually revealed only by special testing.

Personality disturbance may occur, similar to that following frontal lesions, but is usually associated with intellectual and neurological deficits. Emotional instability, aggression and paranoid states are common and depersonalisation and sexual disorders may occur. Schizophreniform, schizoaffective and affective psychoses are well-recognised complications of temporal lobe lesions, especially epilepsy. There is support for an association of schizophrenia-like psychoses and left-sided epileptic foci.

There is a wide variety of focal seizures and complications due to temporal lobe lesions. The single most important sign of a deep temporal lobe lesion is a contralateral upper quadrantic hemi-anopia.

Kluver–Bucy syndrome

The Kluver–Bucy syndrome follows *bilateral* ablations or lesions of the medial *and* lateral temporal lobes, including amygdalae, unci and hippocampi. Originally described in monkeys, its human analogue includes (Lilly *et al*, 1983):

- excessive oral tendencies, including bulimia
- placidity and loss of fear or anger, with apathy and pet-like compliance
- visual agnosia, and sometimes prosopagnosia
- hypermetamorphosis (i.e. an irresistible impulse to touch objects in sight)
- altered sexual activity.

Common causes are Pick's disease and herpes simplex encephalitis. Individual features, such as binge-eating, may occur in Alzheimer's disease.

The amnesic syndrome

As defined above, this refers to a pattern of memory impairment in which performance on digit, word, or block span and other tests (as examples of 'primary' or working memory) is preserved, while new learning (secondary memory) is severely impaired. The patient experiences severe difficulty in recalling or recognising material acquired in previous learning episodes or experiences ('explicit' memory). There may also be a variable degree of retrograde amnesia, that is, loss of memories initially acquired before the onset of the amnesic disorder. General knowledge of the world (so-called 'semantic memory') is affected to variable degrees: knowledge of how to use language is characteristically preserved, but the name of the present prime minister will usually be forgotten. However, skill learning (procedural memory) and the facilitation of responses to previously 'primed' material are characteristically preserved: taken together, these are known as 'implicit memory' (see Kopelman, 2002).

An amnesic syndrome can result from a variety of underlying pathologies – nutritional deficiency in association with alcohol misuse, malnutrition or malabsorption syndromes (Wernicke–Korsakoff syndrome or Korsakoff's syndrome), infection (e.g. herpes simplex encephalitis or tuberculous meningitis), head injury, anoxia, vascular lesions (e.g. thalamic infarction or subarachnoid haemorrhage), or deep midline tumours.

Consistent with the above, patients with Korsakoff's syndrome will show a severe impairment in new learning as well as a variable but often extensive retrograde loss (of two decades or more). Other cognitive functions will be relatively intact, although impairments on frontal and visuospatial tests are commonly found (Jacobson & Lishman, 1987; Kopelman, 1991). Patients may appear rather apathetic and indifferent to their environment, aside from occasional episodes of irritability, and will stick to a fairly rigid daily routine. They will learn the way around the hospital or institution, but will remember remarkably little from day to day. On the other hand, Victor *et al* (1971) remarked that 25% of Korsakoff patients show recovery through time, 50% show some degree of improvement, and 25% do not change; and clinical observation suggests that improvement can occur a considerable time after the onset of the disorder. A striking feature is that, following the Korsakoff episode, these patients often lose any interest in further alcohol intake.

Korsakoff (1889) himself noted that confusion of the temporal sequence of events is a common feature in such patients, and 'confabulation' often consists of real memories jumbled up and recalled inappropriately. More recent studies have distinguished spontaneous or 'fantastic' confabulation from 'provoked' or momentary confabulation, which consists of fleeting intrusion errors or distortions in response to a memory test (Berlyne, 1972; Kopelman, 1987). Spontaneous or fantastic confabulation appears to result from ventrofrontal lobe pathology, whereas momentary confabulation may be a normal response to a 'weak' or failing memory. Spontaneous confabulation is occasionally seen in the early (acute) stage of the Wernicke–Korsakoff syndrome, but is seldom seen in the later stages. Examples of momentary confabulation can be found in approximately 50% of Korsakoff patients in the chronic stages on memory testing, but neither spontaneous nor momentary confabulation is by any means pathognomic of the Korsakoff syndrome.

Parietal lobe syndromes

Parietal lobe lesions may produce a complex and florid variety of cognitive deficits (Critchley, 1953). Lesions of either parietal lobe may yield visuospatial difficulties, including constructional apraxia, visuospatial agnosia (see page 496) and disturbance in the perception of spatial relationships. Topographical disorientation is revealed by difficulty in learning or recalling the way about (e.g. in a ward to which the patient has recently been admitted).

Lesions of the dominant parietal lobe produce conduction aphasia or anomia (see page 494). Anterior lesions may be associated with motor dysphasia, and posterior ones with sensory dysphasia. Apraxia, finger agnosia and right–left disorientation may also occur.

Non-dominant parietal lobe lesions produce disturbances of the body image and of external space, particularly involving the contralateral side. These include denial of disability ('anosognosia'); neglect of the contralateral half of space (e.g. when drawing, walking or driving); dressing dyspraxia; visuospatial disorganisation, which may lead to difficulties with driving, using machinery or laying a table, for example; and visuospatial agnosia (see page 496).

Anterior parietal lesions encroach on the primary sensory cortex, causing contralateral cortical sensory loss, which is marked by intact perception of pain, temperature, touch or vibration but an inability to interpret these sensations. As a result, there is loss of recognition of objects by palpation ('astereognosis'), of figures written on the hand ('agraphaesthesia') and defective tactile localisation (sensory extinction) or discrimination of two stimuli. Visual inattention may also occur. Posterior lesions cause a contralateral lower quadrantic hemi-anopia.

Syndromes associated with pathology elsewhere

Occipital lobe

Occipital lobe lesions are characterised by contralateral homonymous defects. Less common are complex visual recognition disorders, such as alexia without agraphia, colour agnosia, prosopagnosia and complex visual hallucinations.

Corpus callosum

Corpus callosum lesions cause intellectual deterioration, with a pattern reflecting damage to adjacent lobes and callosal disconnection. Left-sided apraxia may occur to verbal commands, and dyslexia without agraphia in posterior lesions. The *alien hand sign* is present when the patient's (usually) non-dominant hand spontaneously and automatically acts at cross-purposes to the patient's intention with the dominant hand. A patient with a corpus callosum infarct found that after buttoning a shirt with the right hand, the left hand proceeded to unbutton it. This sign may also be found with frontal and parietal lesions.

Diencephalon and brain-stem

An amnesic syndrome and hypersomnia are the most characteristic symptoms of lesions of the deep midline structures. Amnesia occurs with lesions distributed around the third ventricle, cerebral aqueduct and posterior hypothalamus. In particular, it appears that lesions in the mammillary bodies, mammillothalamic tract and anterior thalamus are critical in disrupting memory processes. Somnolence and hypersomnia, which suggest posterior midbrain or brain-stem lesions, may progress to stupor (akinetic mutism, 'coma vigil') or coma.

Generalised intellectual decline secondary to hydrocephalus, a rapidly progressive dementia and a frontal-type syndrome are other presentations. Raised intracranial pressure with headache and papilloedema are found with most obstructive lesions, but focal neurological signs may be absent. Endocrine and other neurological signs may indicate hypothalamic and thalamic involvement, respectively.

Symptoms with regional connections

Aphasia

Aphasias are acquired disorders of language secondary to brain disease. In 1861 Broca demonstrated frontal lobe damage in a 'speechless' patient and 4 years later reported left hemisphere dominance for language, now well established as characteristic of 95–99% of right-handed people and of 60–70% of left-handed people. The classification of aphasias began in 1874, with Wernicke's clinical and pathological distinction between two types of aphasia, motor and sensory (see below).

Aphasic syndromes suggest a location or type of pathology but do not invariably result from pathology at a given site. Aphasias can be divided clinically and anatomically into syndromes involving the primary language cortex (the peri-Sylvian area) and those involving other cortical or subcortical centres. Patients with disturbed repetition have peri-Sylvian pathology, whereas repetition is spared by surrounding cortical lesions.

Most people with aphasia also fall into two clinical types based on their conversational speech: non-fluent and fluent aphasias:

- non-fluent aphasia is associated with pathology anterior to the major central sulcus (the fissure of Rolando); an example is motor (Broca's) aphasia
- fluent aphasia indicates pathology posterior to the major central sulcus; an example is sensory (Wernicke's) aphasia.

There are three peri-Sylvian aphasic syndromes – primary motor (Broca's), primary sensory (Wernicke's) and conduction aphasia.

Primary motor (Broca's, expressive) aphasia

Spontaneous speech is *non-fluent*, with decreased output (fewer than 50 words and often fewer than 10 words per minute), increased effort to produce words (with grimacing and gestures), the choice of wrong words, dysarthia leading to mispronunciation and a disturbance of rhythm (dysprosody). The phrase length is short, often with single words. Telegraphic speech, which refers to the utterance of meaningful nouns and verbs and omission of prepositions and adjectives, is none the less meaningful (e.g. 'wife come hospital tonight'). Perseveration is common. Comprehension is relatively intact but repetition seriously impaired. Naming is usually poor but aided by prompting. Reading and writing are invariably affected. Neighbouring features include right hemiplegia (in over 80% of cases), an apraxia affecting the non-paralysed left side, and sometimes sensory loss and visual field defects. Pathology involves the dominant posterior inferior frontal lobe (Broca's area).

Primary sensory (Wernicke's, receptive) aphasia

This differs dramatically from motor aphasia. The key features of sensory aphasia are impaired comprehension and fluent, paraphasic speech with defective repetition. The patient speaks fluently, sometimes even excessively (logorrhoea), effortlessly and without hesitation. Articulation, phrase length and prosody are normal. Speech content is, however, filled with empty phrases and circumlocutions, with few meaningful nouns and verbs. The major types of error are: literal or phonemic paraphasias (substitutions within language), in which a similar-sounding phoneme is substituted for the correct one (e.g. hen for pen); verbal or semantic paraphasias, in which an incorrect word is substituted (e.g. mother for wife); and the use of meaningless nonsense words – neologisms.

Rapid unintelligible speech is termed 'jargon aphasia' (e.g. 'she wants to give me the subjective vocation to maintain the vocation of perfect impregnation simbling'). Naming ability is usually poor and, in contrast to motor aphasia, prompting rarely helps. Auditory comprehension is invariably impaired, often to the point that the patient understands very little. Writing and reading (both aloud and for comprehension) are impaired. Where reading is relatively intact, the term 'pure word deafness' is used. A lack of accompanying neurological signs readily leads to misdiagnosis as psychosis or confusion. Pathology lies in the dominant temporal lobe in the posterior superior portion of the first temporal gyrus.

Conduction aphasia

The hallmark of conduction aphasia is impairment of repetition of speech out of proportion to all other deficits. Following Warrington & Shallice (1969), many neuropsychologists have interpreted this disorder as reflecting a specific deficit within short-term memory or the articulatory loop of working memory.

Aphasias involving other cortical or subcortical centres

The outstanding characteristic of the transcortical or borderzone aphasias is an intact or relatively good ability to repeat spoken language, despite serious aphasia. Pathology is located outside the peri-Sylvian region, in the vascular borderzone between the territory of the middle cerebral artery and that of the anterior or posterior cerebral arteries. The transcortical, subcortical and other language disorders are discussed by Lishman (1998) and Kirshner (2002).

Anomic aphasia (nominal aphasia)

In anomic aphasia, confrontation naming is affected more than any other language function. Low-frequency names or words are particularly affected. Anomia raises the possibility of a focal lesion of the left hemisphere, although the location may be elsewhere, and it is as an early symptom in dementia. It occurs occasionally in hysteria, and may be the only residue of recovered aphasia.

Global aphasia

Here, language loss encompasses expressive, receptive, nominal and conductive components, with lesions including and extending beyond both Wernicke's and Broca's areas.

Speech dominance and handedness

The relationship of speech dominance to handedness can be determined in different ways:

- by the carotid amytal test
- by the proportions of cerebral lesions producing dysphasia
- by studies using unilateral electroconvulsive therapy (ECT)
- by fMRI (Matthews & Jezzard, 2004).

These various techniques give broadly consistent results: 95% of right-handers are left hemisphere dominant and 5% are right hemisphere dominant; 70% of left-handers are left hemisphere dominant, 15% are right hemisphere dominant and 15% show a bilateral pattern of speech representation (for a review see Kopelman, 1982; McManus, 1985).

More left-handers than right-handers become aphasic after stroke, regardless of the side of the stroke, suggesting bilateral representation of language in sinistrals: Yet left-handers recover faster. Mixed-handedness and left-handedness are associated with prelingual deafness and psychosis. It is extremely important to be aware of the figures for speech dominance in determining the side for unilateral ECT. McManus (1985) has provided a detailed genetic model of the relationship of handedness and language dominance to dysphasia.

A commonly employed assessment procedure to determine the pattern of hand preference in an individual is the Annett Handedness Questionnaire (Annett, 1970).

Alexia

Alexia is an acquired inability to comprehend written language caused by brain damage. Developmental reading disorders are referred to as 'dyslexias'. The term is also used to denote partial as opposed to complete loss of reading. There are two forms of alexia, reflected in the presence or not of agraphia.

Alexia with agraphia (parietal–temporal alexia)

Disturbances of reading appear as letter and numerical plus word blindness, and all aspects of writing (from spontaneous to dictation) are affected.

Alexia without agraphia (occipital alexia)

Reading is impaired but writing and spelling are intact. The hallmark of this syndrome is the paradoxical inability of patients to read the words they have just written. Spelled words are recognised, in sharp contrast to parietal–temporal alexia. Associated findings include right homonymous hemi-anopia and colour anomia. Pathology involves the left inferior medial occipital region and splenium of the corpus callosum.

Dyslexia

The neuropsychological classification of acquired reading disorders includes letter-by-letter dyslexia, surface dyslexia and deep dyslexia.

Letter-by-letter dyslexia is accompanied by pronounced slowness in reading and results from 'word blindness'. The clinical diagnosis is usually 'alexia without agraphia'.

Surface dyslexia is characterised by a particular difficulty in reading irregular words (e.g. pint) but not regular words (e.g. mint). It probably results from a semantic memory deficit, is usually accompanied by a naming deficit, and results from left inferior temporal lobe lesions (e.g. in herpes encephalitis).

Deep dyslexia (Grigorenko, 2001) results from a deficit of grapheme–phoneme conversion or of the 'phonological system' itself. It is diagnosed by a particular difficulty in reading non-words (e.g. rint) and associated impairments in reading abstract words, in working memory, and in other aspects of language. There is often widespread cortical atrophy or pathology in such patients.

Other language deficits
The language impairment in Alzheimer-type dementia depends on the stage of disease and disturbances in other psychological functions, such as memory and perception. Anomia, the inability to name objects and find words, is the first obvious abnormality and rapidly worsens. Naming errors are made with objects less frequently encountered in daily life, resulting in semantic substitutions (e.g. chair for table) and circumlocutions (e.g. searching for the word 'snowman' a patient said 'It's cold, it's a ... man ... cold ... frozen'). Spontaneous speech and vocabulary are impoverished. Later symptoms include simplified syntax, reliance on stock phrases, impaired comprehension and writing, verbal perseveration, vague and meaningless content, and paraphasias. Finally, language is incoherent and, occasionally, patients are mute. Changes correspond to the more posterior types of aphasia, such as transcortical sensory or Wernicke's aphasia. The later picture resembles global aphasia.

Apraxia

Apraxia may be defined as the inability to carry out voluntary skilled movement, not attributable to weakness, akinesia, incoordination, sensory loss, intellectual deterioration, poor comprehension or uncooperativeness (Heilman & Rothi, 1985).

Two principal types of apraxia were recognised in Liepmann's original description in 1900 (see Kirshner, 2002):

- ideational apraxia, in which the patient fails correctly to carry out coordinated sequences of actions such as folding a letter, inserting it into an envelope, and stamping it (however, each separate component of the sequence can be successfully performed, which is in constrast to ideomotor apraxia)
- ideomotor apraxia, in which the patient fails to perform command actions that can usually be performed spontaneously, such as waving goodbye, or stirring a cup of tea.

Ideational apraxias occur in dementia and with lesions of the corpus callosum. Ideomotor apraxias occur with lesions of the dominant left hemisphere.

Orobuccal apraxia
In orobuccal apraxia, learned skilled movements of the face, lips, tongue, cheeks, larynx and pharynx are compromised in relation to command. Lesions of the inferior frontal region and the insula are reponsible.

Dressing difficulties
Dressing difficulties, often loosely called dyspraxia, occur in several different clinical syndromes:

- in association with profound unilateral neglect, only the non-neglected side may be bathed, toileted, and dressed
- in delirium, dementia and schizophrenia, patients may wear multiple layers of clothing inappropriate to the weather
- a syndrome of true body–garment disorientation which includes difficulty relating the spatial form of garments to the body, such as orienting an arm to a sleeve, trying to put a shirt on a leg, or putting on clothes backwards, and difficulty doing up ties, zips, buttons and laces, which are often left undone.

In the true dyspraxia syndrome, right-sided or bilateral parieto-occipital lesions are more common than left-sided lesions (Damasio *et al*, 2000).

Constructional apraxia
This is often concurrent with visuospatial agnosia. It refers to when the spatial organisation of actions is altered without any apraxia for individual movements (Lishman, 1998) (see also below). Typical difficulties occur in car driving, using machinery and laying a table. Drawing and copying abilities are especially vulnerable, and are therefore the basis of many diagnostic tests. The quality of errors depends on the laterality of the (parietal) lesion, and whether the lesion is focal or diffuse as in Alzheimer's disease.

Agnosia

Agnosia is a disorder of recognition of objects, which cannot be attributed to sensory defects, mental deterioration, attentional disturbances, aphasic misnaming or unfamiliarity with the object. An agnosic patient must be shown to have intact primary sensory perception and intact ability to name the object once it has been recognised. The failure of recognition usually afflicts a single sensory modality: vision, hearing or touch.

Since Lissauer's original description in 1889, three distinct processing stages of visual object recognition have been identified: first, objects are analysed for their visual sensory properties (either occipital lobe); then a percept (apperception) is formed (lateralised to the right parietal lobe); and third, a meaning is assigned to that percept (association) (lateralised to the left hemisphere, occipitotemporal region) (McCarthy & Warrington, 1990). In visual agnosia, an object cannot be named by sight but is identified by other means, such as touch or hearing (Bauer & Demery, 2003).

Prosopagnosia

This is an inability to recognise familiar faces and to learn new ones. Patients usually see faces as faces but cannot identify whose face they are viewing. Yet the voice easily betrays the identity of the unrecognised face. A farmer with prosopagnosia would not be able to recognise cows individually any longer. People with prosopagnosia can recognise the genus but not its individual members. In extreme form patients cannot recognise their own face in a mirror.

Prosopagnosia should be distinguished from the Capgras symptom, in which the patient believes that familiar persons have been replaced by physically identical doubles or impostors. A posterior right hemisphere lesion (occipitotemporal junction) is common to almost all cases of prosopagnosia, but most also have bilateral involvement (Damasio *et al*, 2000).

Reduplicative paramnesia

In reduplicative paramnesia, first described by Pick in 1903, patients incorrectly describe the place they are in, and further maintain that a familiar place exists simultaneously in several different locations. Bilateral frontal pathology is found in most cases (McCarthy & Warrington, 1990).

Gerstmann syndrome

The Gerstmann syndrome results from dominant parietal lobe lesions and includes finger agnosia, right–left disorientation, dyscalculia and dysgraphia. These four components can appear with other deficits, and often fail to cluster together and so do not really constitute a true 'syndrome'.

Finger agnosia

Finger agnosia is shown by the loss of ability to recognise, name, identify, indicate or select individual fingers, either on the patient's own body or on another body (Lishman, 1998). The signs are bilateral, but patients do not report symptoms.

Right–left disorientation

In right–left disorientation, the patient cannot carry out instructions that involve an appreciation of right and left.

Dyscalculia

Acquired dyscalculia has many possible causes and occurs with lesions in various sites. If a patient cannot do simple additions and subtractions in the absence of dementia or dysphasia, a left parietal lesion is likely.

Body image disturbances

The body image or 'body schema' is a subjective model of the body, acquired during development; it is subject to physiological, psychological, social and cultural influences. Organic psychiatric illness may produce bilateral or unilateral disturbances of the body image.

Bilateral body image disturbances are more common with left cerebral lesions than right and are usually restricted to finger agnosia, or right–left disorientation (see above), or, rarely, autotopagnosia. Autotopagnosia is the inability to recognise, name or point on command to various body parts on the patient's own or on other bodies (while other external objects are dealt with normally). Left parieto-occipital lesions are necessary, but bilateral lesions are more common.

Unilateral body image disturbances are more common with right hemisphere lesions than left, and therefore more often affect the left side of the body. Unilateral unawareness and neglect most often affect the left side of the body with a spectrum of disorders, ranging from mild inattention to unawareness and total neglect (Critchley, 1953), due to right parietal lobe lesions, usually acute strokes.

'Hemisomatagnosia' denotes neglect of one side of the body.

Anosognosia

Anosognosia refers to a lack of awareness of disease, and was first described for left hemiplegia by Babinski in 1914. Anosognosia ranges in degree from lack of concern to frank denial of disability, and is much more common in relation to left-sided than to right-sided cases of hemiplegia. The term is also used generically for lack of insight into other disabilities, such as sensory (Wernicke's) asphasia, amnesia in Korsakoff's syndrome and cortical blindness (Anton's syndrome) (Adair *et al*, 2003).

Other anomalous and false bodily experiences and morbid emotional attitudes towards parts of the body are discussed by Lishman (1998).

Visuospatial deficits

Cerebral lesions produce a variety of disorders of spatial perception. These are difficult to classify, as they affect various mental functions, such as perception, memory, attention, motor action, symbolisation and 'central spatial representation' (McCarthy & Warrington, 1990). They include visual disorientation, constructional apraxia or impairment, unilateral visual neglect, loss of topographical memory and selective agnosias:

- In visual disorientation, the ability to localise objects in space by vision alone is impaired. Bilateral occipito-parietal lesions are responsible.
- Constructional apraxia or impairment, which may overlap with visuospatial agnosia, involves a failure to perform tasks that demand explicit analysis of the spatial properties of a visual display. Errors include a failure to copy drawings or construct patterns with blocks, misalignment of words on a page, and spatial bias. Constructional apraxia results from lesions in the parietal lobes, and is more common and severe with lesions of the right lobe than with the left.
- Unilateral visual neglect may lead patients to fail to make left turns, or lose their way on familiar routes.
- Loss of topographical memory (topographical disorientation) involves a selective impairment of the ability to recall or recognise routes; it is associated with right occipito-parieto-temporal lesions.
- Selective agnosia for buildings and landmarks occurs with bilateral or right occipitotemporal lesions.

Other forms of visuospatial deficit are discussed by Lishman (1998) and Bauer & Demery (2003).

Organic delusions

A wide variety of neurological, toxic and metabolic disorders can have organic delusions as their presenting manifestation or as later complications. Four groups of organic delusion have been proposed: simple persecutory, complex persecutory, mood-congruent, and delusions associated with specific neurological lesions or neuropsychological deficits (Cummings, 1985; Mirea & Cummings, 2000).

Simple delusions are poorly systematised and usually transient, occurring in patients with cognitive deterioration, as in delirium and dementia, and tend to respond to treatment. Fleeting paranoid delusions, elicited and modified by current stimuli, occur in delirium (Lipowski, 1990). Delusions of theft, suspicion and infidelity occur in Alzheimer's disease, but paranoid ideation, short of delusion, is more common (Burns *et al*, 1990).

Complex delusions are more bizarre, systematised and stable than simple ones. They may occur in delirium with two main themes: belief in imminent misadventure to others, and belief in bizarre happenings in the immediate vicinity. Compared with schizophrenic delusions, organic delusions are more likely to involve others as victims of the imagined drama. Complex delusions also occur in dementia (e.g. belief that a pet had been burned, belief that a woman is changing into a man) and include primary delusions, persecutory delusions, morbid jealousy and the Capgras symptom. Other causes include epileptic psychoses, herpes encephalitis, and subcortical or limbic lesions.

The content of delusions may be associated with the laterality of the lesion:

- left hemisphere damage is associated with primary delusions and systematised persecutory delusions, which are often indistinguishable from those of schizophrenia (the distinction will usually be made on other features, from the history, mental state and investigations)
- right hemisphere damage is associated with delusional reduplication of place, time and object, and delusional misidentification of people, as in the Capgras symptom (Cutting, 1990).

The onset of delusions in middle or late life should prompt a particular search for an organic cause. Organic hallucinosis and organic mood syndrome are described in Chapter 22 and organic personality change in Chapter 21.

Assessment

General considerations

A careful history taken from close relatives or friends is essential to establish the mode of onset of the disorder, the nature and duration of symptoms and their subsequent course. The patient's own account of the symptoms will frequently be distorted by confusion, memory lapses, inconsistency, denial and loss of insight. Early changes, more obvious to others, include memory loss, disturbances of behaviour, of activities of daily living and of mood, and physical symptoms.

The clinician needs to evaluate whether there are symptoms suggestive of focal pathology, such as raised intracranial pressure (which may be indicated by headaches, nausea, vomiting and ataxia), stroke-like events, a stepwise deterioration, or seizure. Incontinence and fluctuations in symptoms and behaviour should be asked about. Nocturnal worsening or restlessness may indicate impairment (clouding) of consciousness; episodic abnormal behaviour of sudden onset and ending may suggest epilepsy; and changes in behaviour inconsistent with the setting can imply organicity.

Attention to past medical and family history, use of drugs and alcohol and toxic exposure is important. The handedness of the patient should be determined to assess cerebral dominance for speech.

The formal psychiatric history remains important, to distinguish functional from organic illness, to clarify premorbid patterns of functioning (and stress reactions) and the current social and family structure, and to detect other aetiological factors, such as abnormal illness beliefs and behaviour.

A thorough physical examination is required. Twelve per cent of those admitted to psychiatric hospital have physical signs of illness directly contributing to their mental disorders (Lishman, 1998). The elderly are especially vulnerable, with about one-third having medical disorders complicating dementia (Lipowski, 1990). Physical examination alone may detect treatable organic disorders.

Neurological examination may be surprisingly negative in patients with organic mental disorders. Subtle signs include clumsiness, motor impersistence, minor Parkinsonian or gait abnormalities, and exaggerated jaw jerk (in pseudobulbar palsy).

The mental examination

The examination begins with the patient's appearance and general behaviour. Pallor, loss of weight and disorders of facial expression, posture, movement and standards of self-care suggest organicity. Observe for slow or hesitant responses, perseveration and poor grasp. Is the patient impulsive, disinhibited, insensitive, or neglectful of dress or hygiene? Does the patient tire unduly?

Nursing observations of ward behaviour may reveal indifference to events or bewilderment, which may vary during the day; a puzzled expression, aimless wandering, restlessness, stereotypies; loss of way, memory lapses and occasional transient losses of consciousness; aggressive, suspicious or paranoid behaviour; and feeding or dressing difficulties, binge-eating and incontinence.

Talk

The interview may reveal minor incoherence, wandering off the point, or perseverative or paraphasic errors. The patient may deny having difficulties, evade questions or rationalise failures. Speech may reveal a poverty of content, restriction of theme, concrete thinking or impaired reasoning ability.

Mood

Mood abnormalities include: inappropriate placidity and lack of concern, coupled with mild disinhibition or euphoria; agitated hostile moods; or shifts between the two, as in delirium. In early dementia, a quiet perplexity or emotional lability prevails. An empty, shallow quality to emotional expression also suggests organicity. Other signs include blunting of affect and the 'catastrophic reaction', in which failure at a previously accomplished task elicits an intense emotional reaction, with loud crying, negativity, withdrawal or hostility.

Thought content

In patients with organic psychiatric disorders, the effects of cognitive impairment on the direction, detail, coherence and integration of thought noted above vary with level of intelligence. Ideas of reference and delusions of persecution are common, but often poorly elaborated, vague, shallow and transient or inconsistently related. Anxious, depressive and hypochondriacal ideas frequently occur, along with perceptual distortions, illusions and hallucinations.

Cognitive assessment

Cognitive assessment is described by Hodges (1994), Kopelman (1994), Lishman (1998) and Goldberg & Murray (2002), and the Maudsley Neuropsychiatry Module (for assessment) by Church *et al* (2000); readers should also refer to Table 20.1 on page 503.

The main aim of the assessment is to establish the level of consciousness and to determine whether one or more intellectual functions is impaired.

The patient's premorbid level of intellect must be estimated from educational and occupational attainment, or from formal tests. Cognitive assessment must be adjusted according to the previous and current intellectual state, and the examiner should have a good understanding of the limitations of the tests used and of the normal range of replies. The patient's answers to questions and behaviour should be carefully recorded to allow later evaluation of change. Aphasia and perseveration (i.e. the patient repeats a previous response to a subsequent stimulus) may cause the patient's intellectual performance to be underestimated.

The following tests should be administered to all patients, whether or not organic cerebral disease is suspected. Positive findings are more likely in patients with organic disorders.

Orientation

- What day of the week is it?
- What is the time of day?
- What is the date - day, month, year?
- Where are you now?
- What is this place, street, town, county?
- Who are you?
- What is your age and date of birth?

Attention and concentration

- Is the patient's attention easily aroused and sustained?
- Is the patient easily distracted?
- Can the patient concentrate?
- Ask the patient to give in reverse order the days of the week or months of the year.
- Ask the patient to subtract serial 7s from 100, and record and time the responses. The response has to be interpreted cautiously as attention, memory and calculating ability are required.
- Assess the forward and backward digit span (delivered evenly and at 1-second intervals).

Memory

The ability to recall information immediately and after a delay should be assessed. Compare the patient's account of his or her life (autobiographical memory) with that given by others. Assess the patient's knowledge of past public events: dates of the First and Second World Wars, and more recent news events. Assess memory for recent general information: names of present monarch, of his/her children, of the prime minister, and of the president of the USA. Examine the patient's memory for recent personal events such as admission to hospital, and in particular for the temporal sequence of recent events. Test the ability to repeat a name and address immediately (up to five learning trials) and 5 minutes later, and this may be scored as items correct out of a total.

Record any selective impairment in memory for particular incidents, periods or themes in the patient's life. Retrograde and anterograde amnesia must be distinguished in relation to the onset of an acute disorder. Note any evidence of confabulation or false memories and the patient's attitude to any memory difficulties.

Intelligence

Discrepancy between the expected level of intelligence, estimated from educational and occupational attainments, and performance during the above tests suggests deterioration. An extended cognitive examination and formal IQ assessment are then indicated.

Further examination of patients with suspected organic cerebral disorder

An extended examination is required for suspected organic disorder, to demonstrate its presence, to clarify its nature and to distinguish organic and functional psychiatric illness.

Testing must not tire the patient and may need to be conducted over several sessions. The examiner must be sensitive to the patient's reaction to failure, adapt tests to the patient's general level of intelligence and note that one disability may mask another (e.g. it is difficult to detect dyspraxia in a dysphasic patient).

A simple screening routine is helpful at the start of the examination.

1. Note the patient's level of cooperation.
2. Make a preliminary assessment of the patient's level of conscious awareness.
3. Assess language function briefly by estimating conversational speech. Ask the patient to name a series of common objects, like a pen, watch or key. Present him or her with written commands to point to objects; ask the patient to write down the names of objects to which you point.
4. Assess the patient's memory, in particular new learning ability (a sensitive indicator of cerebral disorder), and then spatial and constructional ability (often a silent deficit) by asking the patient to draw simple figures.

Level of conscious awareness

Record any evidence of drowsiness, diminished awareness of the environment, or fluctuations in level of consciousness. Minor impairment may be suspected from a vague, inert or hesitant manner, or from performance in tests of attention and memory (see above). Judgement of the passage of time is often inaccurate.

- Is the patient alert or dull, awake or drowsy?
- Assess the capacity for sustained attention (or vigilance): ask the patient to signal whenever designated letters appear in a spoken list, or to cancel specific letters in a designated script.
- If somnolent, can the patient be roused to full or only partial awareness?
- If attention cannot be sustained, does the patient drift off to sleep or does attention wander?
- Are the patient's eyes open or shut, fixed or following movement?
- The level of consciousness should be recorded by defining the nature of the stimulus required to evoke responses, such as eye opening. Record this and the best verbal and best motor responses in the Glasgow Coma Scale.
- Evidence for delirium, coma or stupor should be specified in detail.

Language

Seven separate aspects of speech function must be assessed:

- motor aspects
- comprehension
- repetition
- word finding (anomia)
- reading
- writing
- verbal fluency.

Motor aspects

- Note the quality of spontaneous speech and that in response to questions. Is there any disturbance of articulation (dysarthria)?
- Test fluency or the flow of speech: are there freely flowing phrases or sentences, or hesitant, one- or two-word groupings separated by pauses.
- Does the patient have difficulty finding words, or use circumlocutions (phrases where a single word would suffice)?
- Does the patient use wrong words or non-existent words (neologisms, such as 'I've not norter with a verker'), or words that are nearly but not exactly correct (paraphasias, such as lemon = demmun, snail = stale)?
- Is the patient's grammar incorrect (paragrammatism, for example 'the boy hit the ball on the head')?
- Are words omitted and sentences cut short (telegram style, such as 'girl give flower teacher')?
- Is speech incomprehensible (jargon aphasia, for example 'I drove him when the straightway from he guards and place, I forget to talker, what')?
- Observe for perseverative errors of speech, such as repetition of phrases just spoken (echolalia), of terminal words or phrases (palilalia, as in 'I'm not so well today, today, today...'), or of a terminal syllable (logoclonia).
- Note the content of speech, looking at the meaning conveyed, circumlocutions and errors.
- Look for discrepancies between spontaneous speech and replies to questions, and between conversational speech and automatic speech or the naming of serials (e.g. days of the week) and between formal and emotional speech.

Comprehension

Comprehension must be assessed separately, whether or not speech production is impaired.

- Can the patient point correctly on command to one of several objects in view?
- Can the patient respond to yes/no questions?
- Can the patient carry out simple commands (e.g. 'Close your eyes') or more complex instructions involving the understanding of prepositions (e.g. 'Point to the window then to the ceiling'; 'Put a key between this paper clip and coin')?

Repetition

- Can the patient precisely repeat digits, words, short phrases, or long sentences (e.g. 'No ifs, ands, or buts'; 'The orchestra played and the audience applauded').

Word finding (anomia)

Ask the patient to name both common and uncommon objects, object parts (e.g. a watch, the strap, hands, buckle), body parts and colours. Naming can be tested in people with a visual impairment by sentence completion (e.g. 'You write with a...?')

Reading

- Can the patient read aloud and perform simple written commands?
- Failing this, can the patient read aloud letters or single words?
- Does the patient comprehend what is read?

Writing

- Can the patient write spontaneously and to dictation, and copy?
- What errors are made?
- Is copying better preserved than writing to dictation?
- Is spelling out loud better than that on paper?

It is important to test more than the patient's ability to write his or her signature and address, which may be relatively well preserved.

Verbal fluency

This should be assessed even in patients with no other language disturbance, since it is sensitive to frontal lobe lesions.

- Ask the patient to name as many words as possible in 1 minute beginning with the letter F, A or S, or similarly to name as many different animals as possible.

Memory

Full examination of memory functions will always be required, as described above. Special attention should be focused on recent memory and learning ability, both verbal and visuospatial, the latter tested by asking the patient to reproduce simple figures after a 5-minute interval.

Visuospatial and constructional difficulties

- Test the patient's ability to judge the relationships between objects in space, to estimate distances, to indicate the nearer of two objects, and to point out objects in the room with eyes shut.
- Can the patient connect two dots by a straight line, bisect a straight line, draw simple geometric figures, and copy a series of line drawings of increasing complexity?
- Ask the patient to draw a house, a clock face with hands, and a rough map of Great Britain, observing for hemispatial neglect or crowding into one part.
- Test the ability to construct simple designs with sticks or matches.

Visual agnosia

- Can the patient describe what he or she sees, and identify objects and persons?
- Ask the patient to name an object in view, such as a pen or key, describe its use, or if dysphasic indicate its use. If the patient fails, can he or she identify it by touch?
- Can the patient name or match colours, grasp the meaning of a whole picture, or recognise familiar faces (by pointing out a named person in a group, or naming photographs of relatives or well-known figures)?

Dyspraxia

- Test the patient's ability to carry out purposeful movements to command, such as holding out arms, crossing legs, sticking out tongue, blowing a kiss.
- Test each hand separately for opening and closing the hand, opposition of thumb and little finger and so on.
- Ask the patient to make a gesture (e.g. salute, wave goodbye, threaten somebody); then to imitate a gesture ('Do this after me'); to mime the use of an imaginary object ('Show me how to use a comb or toothbrush'); to demonstrate the use of an actual object ('Show me how to open and close a door, use a key, use a can opener'); and finally to perform complex coordinated sequences of movement (e.g. light a match; fold paper and put it in an envelope; pour water from a sealed bottle).

Frontal executive functions

The assessment of frontal executive functions in patients who are suspected of having an organic cerebral disorder is discussed by Hodges (1994), Kopelman, (1994) and Dubois *et al* (2000):

Initiation: verbal fluency tests

Verbal fluency tests (described above) include letter fluency (F, A, S), category fluency (animals, fruit, vegetables) and the 'supermarket' test. Performance reflects both temporal and frontal lobe function.

Abstraction

There are three main tests of the patient's ability to think abstractly: proverbs, similarities and cognitive estimates.

- Observe for concrete interpretation of proverbs, but note that educational level and cultural background influence the response. Concrete responses tend to be given also by patients with schizophrenia.
- The similarities test involves asking patients in what way two conceptually linked items are alike, starting with simple pairs such as 'apple and banana', 'shirt and dress', and progressing to more abstract pairs such as 'plant and animal'. Patients with frontal deficits or dementia make concrete interpretations.
- The cognitive estimates test requires common-sense judgements to answer questions such as 'What is the height of the Telecom Tower?' The 'correct' reply is anywhere between 100 and 800 feet. Each answer is scored for unusual or extreme responses. Abnormalities on this test are found in some, but by no means all, patients with frontal lobe lesions.

Response inhibition and set-shifting

There are three key tests: alternating sequences, the 'go – no go' test, and motor sequencing.

- For alternating sequences, the examiner produces a short sequence of alternating square and triangular shapes. The patient is asked to copy the sequence and then to continue the pattern. Patients with frontal impairments repeat one of the shapes rather than alternate the pair.
- In the 'go – no go' test, the patient is asked to place a hand on the table and to raise one finger in response to a single tap, while holding still in response to two taps from the examiner's unseen finger.
- Motor sequencing tests the patient's sequencing ability in the Luria three-step (fist, edge, palm hand movements) and alternating hand movements (Lishman, 1998).

Parietal function

Number functions

- The serial 7s test can be used as well as simpler addition and subtraction, multiplication and division problems.
- Test the patient's ability to handle money properly.
- Can he or she read or write numbers of more than two digits?

Topographical disorientation

- Does the patient lose his or her way about the ward, or get into the wrong bed?
- Can the patient locate different rooms on the ward or at home, and describe familiar routes?

Right–left disorientation

- Can the patient point to objects or parts of his or her own or the examiner's body, both on the left and on the right?
- Can the patient touch his or her right ear with the left hand?

Body image disturbances

- Ask the patient to name, move on command or point to individual fingers (finger agnosia) or other body parts (autotopagnosia).
- Is the left side of the body neglected in bimanual tasks, such as washing, grooming or dressing?
- When touched symmetrically and simultaneously on both sides, does the patient fail to report the stimulus presented to the contralesional side?
- Does the patient ignore, show lack of concern or deny the disability of an injured body part (anosognosia)?

Dressing difficulties

Does the patient show undue difficulty in dressing and undressing, get muddled when inserting limbs into clothing, or try to put on garments incorrectly?

General indicators of insight and judgement

- Observe for lability of mood, euphoria or catastrophic reaction. Were emotional responses exaggerated, flat or lacking?
- Ask the patient what he or she thinks is wrong, and what his or her understanding is of the problems that have been identified (whether by the patient or by others).
- Does the patient show appropriate concern about symptoms or mistakes during tests?
- Is the patient evasive?
- Does the patient minimise, deny or excuse problems?
- Is the patient's judgement good when discussing financial or domestic matters?
- To what extent does the patient recognise any need to rely on help and advice from others?

Patients who lack insight into or show lack of concern about their disabilities, if not denial of them, tend to have organic lesions, whereas excessive concern in the absence of objective memory loss usually indicates an anxiety or depressive state.

Examination of the mute or apparently inaccessible patient

Mutism

- Is mutism elective, confined to some situations or some persons but not others?
- Does the patient appear to be disturbed by the condition?
- Distinguish mutism from severe motor dysphasia, dysarthria, aphonia, poverty of speech or psychomotor retardation.
- Is partial vocalisation preserved? For example, are emotional utterances possible, or can simple, yes/no answers be given? Can the patient articulate (whisper or make lip movements of speech), phonate, grunt or cough?
- Does the patient speak occasionally, or respond after a long delay?

Detailed neurological examination of all mute patients is also required. It should focus on the level of conscious awareness, and evidence of raised intracranial pressure and of diencephalic or upper brain-stem pathology. Thus, examine for papilloedema, equality and reactivity of the pupils, quality of respiration, and long-tract signs, and test for conjugate reflex eye movements on passive head rotation.

Stupor and the inaccessible patient

Assess separately (with the help of an informant) the following features:

- To what extent can the patient dress, feed himself or herself, or manage hygiene and elimination?
- When aroused, does the patient briefly become alert and verbally responsive?
- Assess responses to graded stimulation (as in the Glasgow Coma Scale).
- Are the eyes open or shut? If open, are they watchful and do they follow moving objects? If shut, do they resist passive opening?
- Observe the physical posture at rest. Is it constrained, or bizarre, or suggestive of possible delusions?
- What happens after passive movement?
- Observe the facial expression and its emotional reaction.
- Are there spontaneous or abnormal movements?
- Test the musculature for tone, rigidity, negativism, waxy flexibility, automatic obedience and echopraxia.
- After the patient recovers, examine for memory of events occurring during stupor.

Summary

Table 20.1 suggests in tabular form a method of assessing the cognitive state. The important point is to ensure that a *basic screening* of all the subheadings has been done. More detailed testing is the province of properly qualified neuropsychologists. Table 20.1 is extracted from a larger one on psychiatric history-taking and the assessment of the mental state (Kopelman, 1994).

Laboratory investigations

The patient's age and history and the clinical findings dictate the selection of tests for any patient with a

Table 20.1 Summary assessment of the cognitive state

Area tested	Example items	Comments
Orientation	Time, place, person Possibly also ask about age, date of birth and duration of present admission and time since last out-patient visit	The sense of personal identity is commonly lost in psychogenic amnesia, but seldom in organic disorders except for profound dementia. Age orientation is commonly impaired in amnesia, dementia and schizophrenia, underestimates being more common than overestimates.
Attention/ concentration	Days of week forwards/backwards Months of year forwards/backwards Digit span forwards/backwards Subjective assessment of concentration by the patient and the examiner Serial 7s	Attention is a complex psychological function encompassing such components as simple and choice reaction time, speed of information processing, sustained attention (vigilance), selective attention, and dual-task processing. The tests suggested measure speed of information processing; the other components are best measured by formal psychological tests. Though commonly used, the serial 7s test confounds attention, memory and mental calculation. Digit span forwards is also a measure of 'primary' or 'working' memory, which is spared in the amnesic syndrome.
Memory		
General or public information (semantic memory)	Description of three recent news events (e.g. accidents, catastrophes, political or sports events) (3 points) Queen's full name and title (1 point) Number of children she has (1 point) Names of her four children (1 point if all correct) Current prime minister (1 point) Previous prime minister (1 point) President of USA (1 point) Previous president (1 point) Years of Second World War (2 points)	These items are taken from the Gresham Questionnaire and when scored out of 12 give good differentiation between patients who have amnesia or dementia and healthy controls or patients with depression. Patients should be asked for details of recent news events (and also personal memories, as below). Mildly impaired patients may be able to give an outline of events (scoring ½ mark each), but not any detail.
Remote and recent personal (or 'autobiographical') memories (facts and incidents)		This is important to sample, but usually will already have been done in the course of obtaining the psychiatric history. Ask, for example, about recent incidents in hospital. Note that the terms 'remote' and 'recent' are far preferable to 'long-term' and 'short-term', which are used in different ways by different disciplines.
Current (or new) learning (8 items)	Name and address (see right): to evaluate *immediate recall*, repeat up to five times until the patient recalls all items completely correctly to evaluate *delayed recall*, test after 5 minutes	Use a standard procedure on each occasion of testing. An 8-item example would be: Mr John Brown, 12 Brighton Road, Edinburgh, Scotland Record the patient's score (out of 8) at each learning trial and at delayed recall.
	Paragraph recall Copy designs and recall after a 5-minute delay	Read the subject a short paragraph of several lines of fairly concrete information, e.g. a brief story, and test recall immediately and after a half-hour delay. Note any intrusion errors ('momentary confabulation'). Other tests, e.g. recall of paired associates or pictures, can also be incorporated.
Language		
Naming	Ask the patient to name readily available items of clothing, furniture, desk utensils, as well as more global names (e.g. jacket/watch) and more specific items (e.g. lapel/winder), which are generally more difficult. Doctor's name and other staff or patients in ward/department	An impairment of naming and word finding is an early feature of dementia and the most common dysphasic deficit found in psychiatric practice.
Comprehension	Ask the patient to follow a single-stage instruction (e.g. 'Use your right hand to touch the tip of your nose'), a two-staged instruction ('... left ear then right ear'), a three-staged instruction ('... left knee, left ear, tip of nose'), and a four-staged instruction ('... right ear, left knee, tip of nose, left ear')	Record how complex an instruction (i.e. how many 'stages') the patient can follow correctly. This will be impaired in early dementia.

Expression	Assess phrase length, fluency and grammar, and for paraphasias and dysarthria	
Repetition ('conduction')	Ask patient to repeat 'The cow jumped over the moon'/'The rain in Spain falls mainly on the plain'.	Impaired in dementia, and occasionally in patients with a left temporoparietal lesion
Reading and writing	Ask patient to read a short paragraph and write a brief sentence.	Specific reading deficits require formal neuropsychological assessment
Disorders of form and content	Pressure of speech, flight of ideas, 'clang' associations and poverty of speech.	Should have been noted already but, if not, should be remarked upon here
Mental calculation	Ask the patient to perform simple additions, subtractions, divisions and multiplications of varying difficulty, such as: 6 + 4; 27 + 18; 19 – 6; 51 – 13; 6 x 3; 12 x 13; 12/3; 108/9	Graduate level of difficulty to determine patient's ability. If necessary, present the patient with money and get him or her to work out appropriate change for a given price of article. These simple calculations tend to give a better impression of the subject's capacity than serial 7s
Drawing and copying	Clock face Ask the patient to draw a house Ask the patient to copy a star, cube or abstract design	Draw circle and ask the patient to fill in the numbers and place the hands to current time (tell the patient what the current time is). The results can indicate perceptual and perceptuo-motor deficits, constructional apraxia or unilateral neglect. Look for omissions, distortions, displacements, intrusions
Other agnosic or apraxic deficits	Visual agnosia, motor apraxia or dressing apraxia	These are not part of the routine cognitive assessment, as they are seen relatively seldom in psychiatric practice except as part of a global dementia. Agnosia refers to a disorder in the recognition of objects independent of any primary sensory or naming deficit. Apraxia refers to an inability to carry out a voluntary skilled movement not attributable to to a primary sensory or motor deficit. Right–left disorientation and astereognosis can also be noted here. See text
Frontal function		
Verbal fluency	Ask the patient to give as many words in 1 minute beginning with the letter F, then A, then S. Or, as many words as possible from a given category, for example, animals	For FAS verbal fluency, normal people score 30 or more; 20–30 suggests mild frontal dysfunction; scores of less than 20 suggest large frontal lesions or moderately severe dementia. Note that non-frontal lesions can sometimes produce impairment on this and other 'frontal' tests. Hence, they are sometimes called 'executive' tests
Abstracting ability	Ask the patient to interpret proverbs and/or to estimate measurements such as the height of the Telecom Tower, the size of the British population, or the height of the average English woman	Patients with frontal lesions sometimes, but by no means always, give 'concrete' interpretations of proverbs and/or grossly aberrant cognitive estimates
Luria's motor tests	Make a fist, a slicing movement, and a slapping movement with the hand, in sequence, to the words 'punch', 'cut', 'slap' and then ask the patient to mimic this. Then get the patient to carry on in sequence by himself or herself	These movements are often poorly coordinated in patients with frontal lesions
Behavioural observations	Note whether the patient appears apathetic, unkempt, irritable, disinhibited, emotionally labile, without social graces	Such things should be considered here in relation to test findings
Primitive reflexes		This is part of physical examination, but is not very specific for frontal pathology

In frankly psychotic or obviously neurotic states where an organic disorder is not suspected, it is sufficient to assess orientation in time, place and person, concentration and attention, and immediate and delayed recall of a name and address (or knowledge of three recent news events). Where an organic disorder is suspected, each aspect of cognitive function (under 'Area tested') should be sampled along the lines suggested. This table is not fully comprehensive, and the more detailed assessment of deficits more commonly seen in neurological than in psychiatric practice, such as apraxia and agnosia, is described in the text. When reporting your findings, do try to order them under subheadings. The assessment of the cognitive state should be viewed as a 'screening' procedure, and is certainly no substitute for proper neuropsychological assessment by a psychologist.

Taken from Kopelman (1994) in the *British Journal of Hospital Medicine*, **52**, 277–281, with permission.

suspected organic psychiatric disorder. Investigations essential in all patients are aimed at excluding reversible causes of symptoms.

A thorough screen would include at least some of the following: full blood count and film, erythrocyte sedimentation rate, blood sugar, thyroid function tests, urea and electrolytes, calcium, liver function tests, syphilis and Borrelia serology, vitamin B12 and folate, electrocardiography, chest and skull radiographs, CT or MRI brain scan (see below on imaging).

In selected patients, further investigations will be required: examination of the cerebrospinal fluid (CSF) for cells, protein, oligoclonal bands, and HIV antibodies; infectious diseases screen; screens for autoantibodies and immunogloblins, serum copper and ceruloplasmin, jejunal biopsy (Whipple's disease); drug and toxin screen; carotid and cardiac evaluation; electroencephalography (EEG), especially to detect Creutzfeldt–Jakob disease (CJD), metabolic encephalopathy and recurrent complex partial seizures; tonsillar biopsy (to detect variant CJD); chromosome analysis and genotyping.

Brain biopsy and metabolic screening are rarely required.

Psychological tests

Only brief mention of psychological testing can be made here. Fuller accounts of modern psychological assessments can be obtained from, for example, Lezak *et al* (2004), Warrington & MacCarthy (1990) and Spreen & Strauss (1998).

It has become customary to estimate premorbid IQ using a reading test – the National Adult Reading Test – Revised. Current intelligence is most commonly assessed using the Wechsler Adult Intelligence Scale – III – UK (Wechsler, 1998). Alternative possibilities are the Standard Progressive Matrices (Raven *et al*, 1977); Advanced Progressive Matrices and Coloured Progressive Matrices are also available. The Mill Hill Vocabulary Test is sometimes used alongside the Progressive Matrices.

The Wechsler Memory Scale – III (Wechsler, 1998) is probably the best-known, internationally available assessment of memory, although it is very lengthy. Alternatives are the 'doors and people' test, the recognition memory test, and the California Verbal Learning Test. The Rivermead Behavioural Memory Test measures aspects of 'everyday' memory as well as including more formal items (Wilson, 1987).

There are relatively few published (as opposed to research) tests of retrograde memory, but the Autobiographical Memory Interview (Kopelman *et al*, 1990) is useful and widely employed in this regard.

Tests of language include the Boston Naming Test, the graded naming test, the Snodgrass test, the token test, and the reporters test.

There are many tests of frontal function but these tend to correlate poorly with one another, once the effects of age and IQ have been partialled out (Kopelman, 1991). Tests of frontal function include measures of verbal fluency (e.g. to the letters F, A, S or to a specific category such as animals), the Wisconsin Card Sorting Test and Modified Card Sorting Test, the cognitive estimates test, the Tower of London test, and the Brixton and Hayling tests (Burgess & Shallice, 1997).

Computerised methods of assessment of cognitive function have been developed. The Cambridge Neuropsychological Test Automated Battery (CANTAB) assesses visual memory, attention and spatial working memory and planning. Based on animal tests of cognitive functions with proven neural substrates, CANTAB is sensitive to deficits in patients with Alzheimer's and Parkinson's diseases (Robbins & Sahakian, 2002). The CANTAB paired associate learning task combined with a test of semantic memory may be useful in the early detection of Alzheimer's disease (Swainson *et al*, 2001; Blackwell *et al*, 2004).

Interviews for rating behavioural abnormalities in dementia and other neuropsychiatric disorders have been developed. The Present Behavioural Examination (PBE) is a structured interview that is administered to the patient's main carer to obtain reliable measures of specific behavioural abnormalities in the following categories: mental health, walking (including wandering), eating, diurnal rhythms, aggression, sexual behaviour, incontinence and individual behavioural abnormalities (e.g. plucking, searching, mumbling, 'obsessionality') (Hope & Fairburn, 1992). MOUSEPAD is a shorter version. The Neuropsychiatric Inventory assesses ten domains of psychopathology (Cummings *et al*, 1994). Other behavioural rating scales for use with neuropsychiatric patients are reviewed by Burns *et al* (2002, 2003).

Cognitive scales

A number of scales have been developed to screen or assess cognitive function. These include the Mini Mental State Examination (MMSE; Folstein *et al*, 1975) (see Table 20.2), the Newcastle Dementia Scale (Blessed *et al*, 1968), CAMCOG–R, which is the cognitive section of the Revised Cambridge Examination for Mental Disorders of the Elderly (CAMDEX–R; Roth *et al*, 1999; and see also Huppert *et al*, 1995), and the Addenbrooke's Cognitive Examination (ACE; Mathuranath *et al*, 2000; see also Nestor & Hodges, 2001). While these scales are not strictly diagnostic tests, they are very useful in grading the severity of cognitive impairment, particularly in dementia. Scores on these scales have been shown to correlate with one another, and also with the number of post-mortem plaques and/or tangles and particularly with neuronal cell loss in Alzheimer's disease. The MMSE result can be normal in patients with lesions in the right hemisphere or frontal lobes. Here the ACE, which includes verbal fluency tests, may be useful: it yields a MMSE score. Or the MMSE may be complemented by the Frontal Assessment Battery (FAB), which includes six frontal sub-tests (Dubois *et al*, 2000). The clock drawing test (Brodaty & Moore, 1997) reflects frontal and temporoparietal functioning and is a valuable screening test for mild to moderate dementia of the Alzheimer type.

Imaging

Neuroimaging may be divided into two broad categories – structural and functional. The principal structural modalities are CT and MRI. Functional neuroimaging techniques include PET, SPET, fMRI and MRS. PET and SPET scanning are described in detail in

Table 20.2 The Mini-Mental State Examination (MMSE)[a]

Sub-scale[b]	Sample item	Instructions/notes
Orientation to time	What is the date?	
Registration	Listen carefully. I am going to say three words. You say them back after I stop. Ready? Here they are... APPLE (pause) PENNY (pause) TABLE (pause). Now repeat those words back to me.	Repeat up to 5 times, but score only the first trial.
Naming	What is this?	Point to a pencil or pen.
Reading	Please read this and do what it says.	Show examinee the words on the stimulus form. CLOSE YOUR EYES

[a]Four sample items of the scale are reproduced here, by permission.

[b]The full scale comprises 11 items set out on six sub-scales. These give a total maximum score of 30. An MMSE score of 23 or less is highly suggestive of cognitive disorder.

Chapter 10, which deals with schizophrenia and other research applications of these techniques.

Computerised tomography

Computed tomography of the brain detects most cortical lesions, large vascular infarctions, demyelination and white-matter change (leucodystrophy), and hydrocephalus. No features of the CT scan are diagnostic of Alzheimer's disease, but an increase in ventricular size over 1 year and medial temporal lobe atrophy are strongly suggestive. Automated volumetric indices of brain atrophy may, however, discriminate between normal ageing and Alzheimer's disease even in its mild stages. A frontal distribution of atrophy may suggest Pick's disease, and caudate atrophy Huntington's disease, as well as neuroacanthocytosis. Atrophy may occur in psychiatric disorders such as alcoholism, schizophrenia and affective disorder (Jacoby & Levy, 1980). For all patients, it is critical that CT scan appearances are interpreted in conjunction with the total clinical picture.

Magnetic resonance imaging

Magnetic resonance imaging is a non-invasive, volume imaging technology that was introduced as a research tool in the 1980s; it is fast becoming the dominant diagnostic tool in neurology and neuropsychiatry. MRI yields fine anatomical detail in several planes, differentiates grey and white matter, outlines major blood vessels and detects small lesions, particularly in the posterior fossa and pituitary regions, areas poorly visualised by CT. MRI sensitively detects lesions such as white-matter changes and infarcts, assists in the differential diagnosis of focal tissue pathology, and detects and allows quantitative estimations of atrophy, both generalised and focal, such as hippocampal atrophy in Alzheimer's disease and white-matter lesions in various disorders (Stevens & Fox, 2001). The predominant applications in psychiatry are for the exclusion of stroke, neurological pathology or head injury as causes for symptoms such as confusion, cognitive decline, depression, psychosis, or abnormal neurological signs. MRI is contraindicated in patients with biomedical implants that have ferromagnetic properties, pacemakers, and patients who are pregnant. A past history of operations to the head and neck area is a relative contraindication.

Functional magnetic resonance imaging

Functional magnetic resonance imaging is a relatively new and non-invasive method of functional brain mapping. Like PET scanning, it demonstrates the regions where cerebral blood flow changes during the performance of cognitive tasks. For an fMRI study, a series of images is obtained with the participant alternating between performance (activation) and resting (non-activation) (Matthews & Jezzard, 2004).

Functional MRI is increasingly being applied as a research technique to the study of neuropsychiatric disorders, including schizophrenia, Alzheimer's disease, traumatic brain injury, stroke and memory disorders. Particularly noteworthy are findings related to plasticity in the adult human brain. Despite the promise of fMRI for improving the conceptualisation, assessment, and treatment of neuropsychiatric disorders, important technical and scientific issues remain. Future research will address integrating fMRI with other emerging neuroimaging and analysis techniques (Ebmeier *et al*, 2005).

Magnetic resonance spectroscopy (MRS)

Magnetic resonance spectroscopy can be used to extract *in vivo* biochemical information from body tissue. It is a safe and non-invasive tool that is useful for the study of brain chemistry and metabolism. It has potential diagnostic applications in anxiety and affective disorders, dementia, schizophrenia and neurodevelopmental disorders.

Electroencephalography

Electroencephalography is used widely when organic disorders are suspected, as it able to confirm abnormalities of brain structure and function in about 60% of cases. The EEG reading is symmetrical and usually classified into four characteristic waveforms: delta rhythms at less than 4 Hz; theta at 4–7 Hz; alpha at 8–13 Hz; and beta at over 13 Hz.

The disturbances seen in epilepsy are summarised by Binnie & Prior (1994) and are discussed in Chapter 21.

Focal abnormalities are most consistent with localised disorders such as tumours, abscesses, subdural haematomas or cerebral infarctions; diffuse slowing occurs in toxic and metabolic disorders and in advanced degenerative diseases. EEG is a sensitive indicator of deranged cerebral metabolism.

The degree of bilateral diffuse slowing correlates positively with the degree of cognitive impairment in delirium (Engel & Romano, 1959) and so serial EEGs are useful for monitoring the progress of delirium of various types. Triphasic waves occur in the delirium associated with liver failure, high-amplitude sharp waves in herpes simplex encephalitis, low-voltage activity with posterior slowing in uraemia, acceleration of alpha activity in hyperthyroidism and low-voltage activity in myxoedema. In delirium tremens the EEG may show fast activity rather than slowing. In toxic delirium associated with drugs, the EEG may show drug-specific patterns of fast-wave activity (antidepressants, benzodiazepines) or slowing (phenothiazines). Localised spike and sharp wave complexes usually suggest an intracranial cause for delirium.

In very early Alzheimer's disease the EEG is usually normal, but as the disease advances there is progressive slowing of the tracing, with less alpha and beta activity and more delta and theta activity posteriorly. Multi-infarct dementia is characterised by an asymmetric tracing, with focal slowing in over two-thirds of patients but relative preservation of the alpha rhythm. Pronounced flattening of the EEG suggests Huntington's disease, whereas repetitive spike discharges or triphasic sharp wave complexes may indicate CJD. The latter may yield a floridly abnormal EEG in a patient with mild cognitive impairment and little change evident on structural imaging (CT or MRI). In investigating dementia, a normal EEG may be found in early degenerative dementia and pseudo-dementia, and in 20% of patients with tumours or subdural haematoma.

The use and limitations of the EEG are discussed by Lishman (1998), Binnie & Prior (1994) and Philpot (2005), who also reviews evoked potentials.

Delirium

Delirium (acute organic reaction, acute confusional state, toxic confusional state, acute organic psychosis) occurs in about 10–20% of all hospitalised patients and in 10–42% of elderly patients at admission to hospital; the incidence is 11–31% after admission (Lipowski, 1990; Lindesay *et al*, 2002). Patients with dementia are particularly vulnerable to delirium. In the Eastern Baltimore mental health survey, the point prevalence of delirium in 18- to 64-year-old adults in the community was 0.4%, rising to 1.1% in those over the age of 55, and 13.6% in those over 85 (Folstein *et al*, 1991). The ICD–10 and DSM–IV diagnostic criteria for delirium are set out in Boxes 20.1 and 20.2. Delirium is often unrecognised by physicians and nurses, partly because of its fluctuating nature, its overlap with dementia, lack of formal cognitive assessment, under-appreciation of its clinical consequences, and failure to consider the diagnosis important (Inouye, 2006).

Clinical features

Traditionally, the cardinal feature of delirium is a decreased clarity of awareness of the environment – on a continuum from the mildest impairment of consciousness, through clouding, to coma – with impairment of the ability to direct, focus, sustain and shift attention. It manifests as impaired alertness, awareness and attention in a patient who is awake. A mild impairment can advance to coma if untreated. Clouding is distinguished from natural drowsiness by observing that the patient cannot be easily aroused. While ICD–10 retains the term 'clouding of consciousness', yoking it to disordered attention (Box 20.1), DSM–IV eschews the term. In DSM–IV, the disturbance of consciousness, which is manifest by a reduced clarity of awareness of the environment, is operationalised by core attentional deficits – criterion A in Box 20.2. Reduced attentiveness can range from mild distractibility, losing the thread of conversations and failing to grasp complex details to reduced interaction, a lack of spontaneous speech and neglect of bodily needs.

In delirium, arousal may be raised, with psychomotor overactivity and restlessness, screaming and excessive reactions to noise and bright lights; or it may be reduced. In either case, patients are unable to focus attention or concentrate, and are distractible.

Onset and course

The onset of delirium may be rapid (i.e. over hours, as after concussion or intoxication) or more gradual (i.e. over a few days). In the latter case, the patient

Box 20.1 ICD–10 diagnostic criteria for delirium

For a definite diagnosis, symptoms, mild or severe, should be present in each one of the following areas:

- impairment of consciousness and attention (on a continuum from clouding to coma; reduced ability to direct, focus, sustain and shift attention)
- global disturbance of cognition (perceptual distortions; illusions and hallucinations, most often visual; impairment of abstract thinking and comprehension, with or without transient delusions, but typically with some degree of incoherence; impairment of immediate recall and of recent memory but with relatively intact remote memory; disorientation for time as well as, in more severe cases, for place and person)
- psychomotor disturbances (hypo- or hyperactivity and unpredictable shifts from one to the other; increased reaction time; increased or decreased flow of speech; enhanced startle reaction)
- disturbance of the sleep–wake cycle (insomnia or, in severe cases, total sleep loss or reversal of the sleep–wake cycle; daytime drowsiness; nocturnal worsening of symptoms; disturbing dreams or nightmares, which may continue as hallucinations after awakening)
- emotional disturbances, such as depression, anxiety or fear, irritability, euphoria, apathy, or wondering perplexity.

Box 20.2 DSM–IV diagnostic criteria for 293.0, Delirium due to ... [indicate the general medical condition]

A Disturbance of consciousness (i.e. reduced clarity of awareness of the environment) with reduced ability to focus, sustain or shift attention.

B A change in cognition (such as memory deficit, disorientation, language disturbance) or the development of a perceptual disturbance that is not better accounted for by a pre-existing, established or evolving dementia.

C The disturbance develops over a short period of time (usually hours to days) and tends to fluctuate during the course of the day.

D There is evidence from the history, physical examination, or laboratory findings that the disturbance is caused by the direct physiological consequences of a general medical condition.

cannot concentrate or think clearly, universally fails to judge the passage of time, feels anxious and restless, and may be irritable, tired, hypersensitive to light and noise, and drowsy at times, with insomnia and vivid dreams or nightmares, or even transient hallucinations. The patient may try to conceal confusion by evasion or brief answers to questions, or by complaints and anger. As delirium progresses, the patient becomes more obviously confused. 'Confusion' is a term that covers a combination of impaired attention, muddled thinking, poor grasp of one's situation, forgetfulness and some degree of disorientation for time and place. Thus the patient will have difficulty naming the correct day of the week or the date. As delirium advances, patients may think they are at home instead of in the hospital; and they may misidentify doctors and nurses for relatives and friends. This tendency to misidentify the unfamiliar for the familiar is characteristic.

As delirium worsens, patients become increasingly distractible, and either drowsy or hyper-alert and excited. They may look inert, sleepy and withdrawn, and respond slowly to questions, leave long pauses between words, and plead to be left alone. Alternatively, they may be restless, fidgety, scanning the room and striking out in terror at invisible animals, for example. In either case, attention remains impaired. Patients cannot sustain a train of thought and forget the question or the beginning of their own sentence. Thinking is laboured and slow, or rapid but incoherent. Attempts to get out of bed are common in restless frightened patients, and injuries may result. Noisy expressions of fear and screams for help may attend hallucinations, as in delirium tremens (see Chapter 22, 560).

Diurnal fluctuation in the level of arousal and awareness is a common feature of delirium. Reduced responsiveness may shift unpredictably to outbursts of excitement. Sleep–wake cycles are frequently disrupted or reversed, and confusion is often more marked at night.

At any time excited, hallucinating patients may calm down and ask coherent, pointed questions about their whereabouts, the time, their family. These lucid intervals, or brief irregular episodes of more normal thinking and behaviour, are characteristic of delirium, and occur more often during daylight hours.

Perceptual abnormalities

Perceptual abnormalities in the form of illusions and hallucinations, most commonly visual but often mixed (i.e. with auditory and other misperceptions) may appear, especially at night. Perceptual illusions include distortions of shape, size and position of the patient's body and surroundings. Depersonalisation and derealisation are common, but are often poorly expressed. Perceptual abnormalities are usually fleeting and changeable, and are readily interpreted as hostile and persecutory. A merging of dream contents, waking hallucinations and fragments of true perceptions is common in delirium, and is recalled after recovery as real experience.

Memory

Impairment of memory, with reduced digit span, impaired new learning and defective recall of remote events, is an important clinical feature. Early symptoms of memory loss include minor forgetfulness or 'absent-mindedness', with muddled time sequences, or more striking memory lapses. Loss of topographical memory is often seen, with patients losing their way when wandering from home or driving to work. An early sign is disorientation for time and, later, disorientation for place. The memory deficit is global, affecting all types of material, and involves remote as well as recent events, with failure of new learning a key feature. The memory deficit is also patchy, so that partially correct information may be incorporated into confabulatory answers or delusions. After recovery, patients will have partial or total amnesia for the period of confusion, but isolated events, especially vivid hallucinations, may be remembered in detail.

Thinking

Thought processes are either slowed or accelerated. In all cases, thinking is more or less incoherent, fragmented, illogical and undirected, with poverty of content. A sustained logical train of thought is difficult, with ready disruption from internal and external factors. The capacity to select and order thoughts to solve problems, plan action, understand a situation and communicate adequately is impaired. Content of thought may be impoverished, with intrusive images lending a dream-like quality, blurring dream from waking imagery and fact from fantasy.

Ideas of reference and paranoid delusions may develop, which tend to be poorly worked out, fleeting, changeable, and readily elicited and modified by the environment.

Speech

Speech is increased or decreased in output and often hesitant or slurred. Sentences are simple, poorly organised and often repetitious, with circumlocutions, slips of the tongue and substitutions of words (paraphasia, such as 'spool' for 'spoon', 'chain' for 'chair'). Nominal dysphasia is common and writing nearly always defective.

Emotion

Lability of emotional expression is common in delirium. Anxiety, depression, irritability, anger, perplexity and suspicion are often observed in varying combination, intensity and duration. Emotional arousal may vary from panic to apathy, or shift between the two. Autonomic arousal often occurs, with tachycardia, sweating, dilated pupils, increased blood pressure and tremor, as in delirium tremens.

Psychomotor changes

Psychomotor activity is virtually always disturbed, with two contrasting patterns, but patients may shift between the two. In most patients, spontaneous motor activity is depressed but some are hyperactive and restless.

Perseverative or repetitive stereotyped motor behaviour may occur, such as aimless plucking at bedclothes or mimicry of familiar activities (e.g. sewing or work activities). Involuntary movements such as tremor and myoclonus are usually seen in drug withdrawal or metabolic disorders. Rarely, patients are catatonic.

Variability in the levels of arousal and awareness, psychomotor activity and the presence or absence of hallucinations and delusions is characteristic of delirium, both between patients and in the same patient over time.

Lipowski (1990) distinguishes three patterns of psychomotor activity: hyperactive, hypoactive and mixed subtypes. Psychomotor overactivity and heightened alertness distinguish the hyperactive variant. The most important example is delirium tremens. In the hypoactive subtype, psychomotor activity and alertness are reduced, as in Wernicke's encephalopathy and hepatic encephalopathy, but these reductions often go unrecognised. In the most common, the mixed subtype, shifts occur between states of lethargy and marked excitement, which make it difficult to gauge the correct dose of sedative drug for the patient, with the risk of over- or under-sedation.

Differential diagnosis

Delirium needs to be differentiated from:

- chronic organic disorders, including dementia
- the focal organic disorders
- functional psychiatric disorders, in particular depression, delusional disorders and mania.

The history, physical examination and investigation of the patient are the time-honoured steps to differential diagnosis from other syndromes. The major distinguishing features of delirium are its mode of onset (rapid); duration (brief; if longer than 3 months it is unlikely to be delirium); characteristic symptoms; and EEG findings (almost always abnormal – see Lipowski, 1990). Clinical features distinguishing delirium and dementia are shown in Table 20.4 (page 512). The first essential distinction to be made is whether delirium results from a neurological cause or complicates a systemic illness. This distinction can usually be made on the history and a thorough physical examination, supported by investigation.

Aetiology

The aetiology of delirium is usually multifactorial in older people. Factors that predispose to delirium include older age, visual impairment, dementia, depression and physical disease; those that independently cause delirium are listed in Table 20.3.

The most common causes of delirium vary with patient age, but from teenage years onwards frequently include drug and alcohol intoxication and withdrawal syndromes, and in the elderly infections and multiple medications.

Neurological causes can usually be recognised by the additional presence of focal neurological signs, but diffuse neurological diseases such as encephalitis may yield no focal signs. Space-occupying lesions of the nervous system usually cause headache and focal signs, but brain abscess and midline tumours may present with gradually evolving confusion. Acute onset may indicate brain-stem compression or acute hydrocephalus.

Systemic causes are usually characterised by the absence of focal neurological signs apart from delirium. Drugs are the commonest cause of confusion, particularly in the elderly. Wernicke's encephalopathy should be considered in patients with a history of alcoholism, malnutrition and persistent vomiting, as

Table 20.3 Aetiology of delirium

Type of cause	Principal examples
Degenerative	Presenile or senile dementias complicated by infection, anoxia, etc.
Space-occupying lesions	Cerebral tumour, subdural haematoma, cerebral abscess
Trauma	Concussion, intracranial haematoma
Infection	Meningitis and encephalitis (viral, bacterial, fungal, protozoal), subacute meningovascular syphilis; septicaemia; malaria; subacute bacterial endocarditis; focal infection (e.g. pneumonia); exanthemata, HIV
Vascular	Acute cerebral thrombosis or embolism, transient ischaemic attack, subarachnoid haemorrhage, hypertensive encephalopathy, vasculitis (e.g. systemic lupus erythematosus, giant-cell arteritis), air and fat embolism
Epileptic	Psychomotor seizures, petit mal status, post-ictal states
Metabolic	Uraemia, liver disorder, electrolyte disturbances, alkalosis, acidosis, hypercapnia, remote effects of carcinoma, porphyria
Endocrine	Diabetic hypoglycaemia or pre-coma; over- or under-activity of thyroid, parathyroid, adrenal; hypopituitarism
Toxic	Drug and alcohol intoxication (including therapeutic drugs: salicylate, anticholinergic drugs, lithium, psychotropic drugs, H2-antagonists, digoxin, antihypertensives, codeine, etc., and over-the-counter drugs such as antihistamines), drug withdrawal, chemical toxins (e.g. heavy metals, organic toxins). Neuroleptic malignant syndrome
Anoxia	Pulmonary, cardiac, anaemia, carbon monoxide poisoning, post-anaesthetic
Vitamin deficiency	Thiamine (Wernicke's encephalopathy), nicotinic acid (pellagra), B12 and folic acid deficiency
Other	Pain, physical restraint, bladder catheter use, surgery, large number of hospital procedures, hypothermia, heat stroke

Derived from Lishman (1998) and Burns *et al* (2004).

in hyperemesis gravidarum. Focal infections, such as of the urinary tract, may cause confusion in the elderly. The distinction of organic from functional causes of confusion is discussed by Lishman (1998). In dementia with Lewy bodies, fluctuating cognition with pronounced variations in attention and alertness occurs (McKeith *et al*, 1996).

Investigation

Investigation is an urgent procedure. It involves obtaining urea, electrolyte and blood sugar levels, and a full biochemical profile, a blood count, erythrocyte sedimentation rate, C-reactive protein, B12 and folate, chest radiography, echocardiogram, oxygen saturation/pulse oximetry, drug and toxicological screen, blood and urine cultures, a complete infectious diseases screen if indicated, and referral to physicians for CSF examination, and consideration of EEG and imaging studies. Endocrine and other tests may be indicated.

Management

The management of delirium has two major aspects, symptomatic and aetiological (Lindesay *et al*, 2002). Treatment of the underlying cause is crucial, and presupposes accurate diagnosis, which may take time. The management of delirium is similar to that of alcoholic delirium (see Chapter 22, pages 561–563).

Outcome and prognosis

There are four distinct outcomes of delirium:

1 progression to stupor (see below), coma or death

2 recovery

3 persisting symptoms or continuing delirium

4 the development of a chronic organic syndrome, such as Wernicke's encephalopathy progressing to Korsakoff's syndrome.

As a variant of the last, occasionally a functional psychosis ensues. Some patients have a subacute organic syndrome before recovery, such as an amnesic syndrome after delirium due to Wernicke's encephalopathy or head injury.

In a meta-analysis of the outcome of delirium, 14.2% of patients had died by 1 month after admission and 46.5% were in institutional care; at 6 months 55% had improved mentally and 43% remained in institutions (Cole & Primeau, 1993).

Delirium predicts poorer outcomes for hospitalised patients, with increased disability and use of institutional care, and an increased mortality over many months, as high as 50% at 5 years after discharge (van Hemert *et al*, 1994). The mortality depends more on the underlying medical disorder than on the presence of delirium. Even after recovery, the disturbance associated with delirium may result in job losses and be socially destructive.

Stupor

Stupor refers to a clinical syndrome of akinesis and mutism, but with evidence of relative preservation of conscious awareness (Lishman, 1998). There is profound lack of responsiveness and (apparent) impairment of consciousness, with reduced or absent speech (mutism) and movement (akinesis). The eyes may be open and apparently watchful, with the patient directing gaze towards the examiner and the eyes following moving visual stimuli. When the eyes are shut they may resist passive opening.

Strong painful stimuli may produce blinking or evasive action. Although spontaneous movement is typically absent, tremors, twitching or motor stereotypies can occur. The resting posture may be awkward or meaningful in the context of psychotic experience. Reflexes are often normal. Complete mutism is the rule but patients may grunt, cough, mutter or, rarely, sing. In light stupor, feeding is possible, sphincters are intact, and commands may elicit simple responses. The features overlap with those of catatonia (Taylor & Fink, 2003).

The principal causes are psychiatric – schizophrenia and depression mainly, schizoaffective and dissociative disorders secondarily – and organic (in up to a third of cases the cause will be stroke, dementia, delirium, tumour or cyst, neurosyphilis, post-encephalitic, post-epileptic, phencyclidine). The exclusion of neurological causes is essential, particularly raised intracranial pressure and midbrain or upper brain-stem lesions. Changes from initial to final diagnosis are common, particularly from a psychiatric to a neurological diagnosis; certain clinical features aid this differential diagnosis.

In stupors due to functional psychiatric disorders, feeding ability and the sphincters may be partially preserved, the facial expression may react to events, and respiration and the pupils are normal. Schizophrenic stupor is essentially catatonic but catatonic signs are diagnostically non-specific.

In depressive stupor there is severe psychomotor retardation, sadness and hopelessness in posture or expression, and silent tears may be shed, but consciousness is retained. Manic stupor (with an affect of elation) is very rare. Dissociative (hysterical) stupor occurs under stress, usually with signs of conversion. It often fluctuates and there is complete passive dependence on others.

In organic stupors, the patient is immobile yet seemingly alert, with full eye movements, and can occasionally be aroused to move ('coma vigil'); alternatively, the patient appears apathetic and somnolent and has oculomotor abnormalities. The former pattern is seen with lesions at the base of the brain anteriorly, the latter with brain-stem lesions. Stupor may also occur in metabolic and endocrine disorders, and in states of intoxication (with alcohol, barbiturates, psychotropic drugs).

In one psychiatric hospital series (Joyston-Bechal, 1966), almost half the cases of stupor resolved within 1 week and one-fifth lasted more than 1 month, but patients with prolonged stupor all had severe brain damage.

On recovery, the recollection of the mute period is absent in those with an organic cause, poor in those with an affective disorder, and often intact in patients with schizophrenia.

Dementia

Prevalence, incidence and patterns

Dementia is common and is the major cause of long-term disability in old age. Its point prevalence ranges from 3% to 8% (on average 5%) in the UK, in those over the age of 65 years, and is 15% in those over 80. There is a relative excess of dementia of Alzheimer type (DAT) among women and of vascular dementia (VaD) among men. The prevalence rate of dementia doubles over every 5-year age band. The community prevalence of dementia in people aged 65 and over in Islington, London, was 9.9%, and 6.7% on excluding those in residential care (Livingston, 1994).

Rates for the 'treated incidence' of dementia vary between 1.9 and 2.6 per 1000 for men and between 2.1 and 4.1 for women over 60 years, but are about 10–16 per 1000 for both sexes in field surveys (Cooper, 1991).

The commonest causes/types of dementia vary with age:

- under the age of 35 years, they are Huntington's disease and variant CJD (vCJD)
- under 65 years, they are Alzheimer's disease (AD), VaD, frontal lobe dementia, alcoholic dementia, dementia with Lewy bodies (DLB) and prion disease
- over 65 years, in the Islington study, they were AD in 31.3%, VaD in 21.9%, DLB in 10.9% and frontal lobe dementia in 7.8% (Stevens *et al*, 2002).

The age-adjusted prevalence of dementia in developing countries ranges from 1.7% in Ballabgarh, India, to 5.2% in Shanghai in people over 65 years, which is below the overall European prevalence rate of 6.0%. The prevalence rates of dementia and AD are also low in Ibadan, Nigeria, in rigorous community and autopsy studies (Hendrie *et al*, 1995). The association between ApoE e4 genotype and AD was absent in Ibadan, but preserved in African-Americans (Osuntokun *et al*, 1995).

The separation of presenile (before 65 years of age) from senile (after 65) dementia was based on the assumption that the causes were different. Although the expression, genetics and course of diseases may vary with age, the major findings in patients with dementia of all ages are broadly similar, and the age-specific incidence rates are unimodally distributed, so that the distinction is arbitrary.

Two principal patterns of intellectual impairment have been described in dementia (Cummings & Benson, 1992). The first, reflecting cortical dysfunction, occurs in the majority; the second, subcortical dementia, is less common. There is, however, a considerable overlap in clinical and neuropsychological presentations (Turner *et al*, 2002). The *cortical pattern* of intellectual decline includes loss of language, learning, perception, calculation and praxis skills, and manifests as aphasia, amnesia, agnosia, acalculia and apraxia. The *subcortical pattern* results from disordered motivation, mood, attention and arousal, and is revealed as psychomotor slowing, memory loss, affective disorders and impaired problem-solving (Cummings, 1986). Cortical dementias produce neuropathological changes involving primarily, but not exclusively, the association cortex and the medial temporal lobes, as in AD and selected strokes, whereas the subcortical pattern results from lesions in the basal ganglia, thalamus and brain-stem, as in Huntington's and Parkinson's diseases. Mixed subcortical/cortical patterns occur in multiple sclerosis, stroke, severe head injury, CJD and neoplastic causes.

Differential diagnosis

Dementia must be distinguished from delirium (see Table 20.4), from focal neurological (see Chapter 21) or organic syndromes (see Chapter 22), from psychiatric disorders and age-associated memory impairment and mild cognitive impairment.

Table 20.4 Differential diagnosis of delirium and dementia

	Delirium	Dementia
Onset	Acute	Usually insidious
Duration	Transient (hours to weeks)	Persistent (months to years)
Course	Fluctuating over hours; worse at night, lucid intervals	Stable over days
Conscious level/awareness	Depressed	Normal
Alertness	Abnormally low or high	Usually normal
Attention	Impaired, causing distractibility; fluctuates	Relatively normal
Sleep–wake cycle	Disrupted: often drowsy during day, insomnia at night	Usually normal
Orientation	Impaired	Impaired in later stages
Language	Incoherent, hesitant, slow or rapid	Anomia common
Memory		
primary, working memory	Shortened	Normal in early stages
secondary, short-term memory	Impaired	Impaired
Perception	Frequent illusions and hallucinations	Normal early; agnosia, misidentifications and hallucinations later
Thinking	Disorganised, delusional	Impoverished
Autonomic changes	Common	Unusual
Psychomotor changes	Common	Uncommon
Electroencephalogram	Diffuse slow-wave activity	Mild slowing (but varies with aetiology)

Functional psychiatric disorder masquerading as dementia, or pseudo-dementia, occurs in about 9% of cases of 'dementia', most often owing to depression or, rarely, schizophrenia, hypomania, persistent delusional disorder, hypochondriasis, dissociative disorder (hysteria) and the Ganser state (Lishman, 1998). Subjective complaints of memory loss are more related to depressed mood than to objective memory performance, particularly in the elderly (Hejl *et al*, 2001; Kopelman, 2002). The differentiation between anxious preoccupation with memory and other mental functions, depression and dementia can be difficult in psychiatric settings.

In the elderly, dementia must be distinguished from mild cognitive impairment (MCI), which is a transitional state between the cognition (usually memory) of normal ageing and mild dementia (AD). Criteria for MCI include memory complaints (preferably corroborated by an informant), objective memory impairment for age and education (reduced by at least 1, usually 1.5 standard deviations), largely intact general cognitive function, preserved activities of daily living and absence of dementia (Petersen *et al*, 2001). MCI differs from normal ageing and from minor forgetfulness that accompanies ageing – termed benign senescent forgetfulness or age-associated memory impairment (AAMI) – in which the recall of names and places is variably impaired while that of experience remains intact, and the activities of daily life are not impaired.

'Age-related cognitive decline' and 'mild neurocognitive disorder' are the terms used in DSM–IV and 'mild cognitive disorder' appears in ICD–10. 'Cognitive impairment, no dementia' (CIND) is a more recent and broader term.

Mild cognitive impairment may remain stable, revert to normal, or progress to dementia. The annual conversion rate of amnestic MCI to probable AD is 10–15%, whereas only 1–2% of healthy controls will progress to AD (Petersen *et al*, 2001). MCI is associated with AD at autopsy and up-regulation of choline acetyltransferase activity in the brain. Donepezil reduced the likelihood of progression from amnestic MCI to clinically possible or probable AD in the first 12 months only in a 36-month study, with greater effect in the apolipoprotein E4 carrier subgroup (Petersen *et al*, 2005).

The concept was originally focused on memory but has broadened to include MCI with multiple cognitive domains, such as language, executive function and visuospatial skills, with or without memory impairment. This may progress to AD, vascular or mixed dementias, and MCI affecting a single non-memory domain may progress to various non-AD dementias. The concepts, their operational criteria, biological markers and outcomes are heterogeneous and in a state of flux (Petersen, 2003; Davis & Rockwood, 2004).

Aetiology

The causes of dementia may be categorised as follows: primary cerebral degeneration; tumour and hydrocephalus; cerebral infection and inflammation; vascular; alcohol-induced brain damage; trauma; anoxia; toxicity; and metabolic and storage diseases (Lishman, 1998). The so-called primary degenerative dementias include AD, DLB, frontotemporal dementia (FTD) (including Pick's disease), Huntington's disease, CJD and vCJD. The most frequent cause of dementia, AD, is diagnosed by exclusion. Alcoholic brain damage resulting in 'dementia' is suggested by multiple cognitive deficits in the context of chronic alcoholism (see Chapter 22).

Potentially reversible causes of dementia are found in approximately 15% of patients below the age of 65 and in under 5% of those over 65 presenting to specialist centres with intellectual impairment. Overall, only 0.6% of patients presenting with dementia recover (Clarfield, 2003); about half of these have pseudo-dementia and half have treatable tumours, subdural haematoma, hydrocephalus, metabolic disorders (hypothyroidism, chronic hepatic failure, hypoglycaemia, and vitamin B12 and folate deficiencies) or infective and inflammatory disorders. Potentially treatable comorbid conditions are found in up to 20–25% of people with dementia (Hejl *et al*, 2001). VaD associated with hypertension, alcoholic dementia and AIDS-related dementia may be amenable to therapy.

Alzheimer's disease

Alzheimer's disease is, strictly speaking, a pathological diagnosis, which is not usually made during life. The DSM–IV diagnostic criteria for dementia of the Alzheimer type are set out in Box 20.3. Criteria A and B are common to the general DSM–IV criteria for dementia. ICD–10 primarily requires a decline in both memory and thinking (reasoning, flow of ideas, processing of information) sufficient to impair activities of daily living, which is of insidious onset, slow deterioration and has a minimum duration of symptoms and impairments of 6 months. The accuracy of the clinical diagnosis is high if a careful history and examination as well as strict diagnostic criteria are used, such as the 'gold standard' of McKhann *et al* (1984).

Box 20.3 DSM–IV diagnostic criteria for dementia of the Alzheimer type

A The development of multiple cognitive deficits manifested by both:
1 memory impairment (impaired ability to learn new information or to recall previously learned information)
2 one (or more) of the following cognitive disturbances:
  a aphasia (language disturbance)
  b apraxia (impaired ability to carry out motor activities despite intact motor function)
  c agnosia (failure to recognise or identify objects despite intact sensory function)
  d disturbance in executive functioning (i.e. planning, organising, sequencing, abstracting)

B The cognitive deficits in Criteria A1 and A2 each cause significant impairment in social or occupational functioning and represent a significant decline from a previous level of functioning.

C The course is characterised by gradual onset and continuing cognitive decline.

D The cognitive deficits in Criteria A1 and A2 are not due to any of the following:
1 other central system conditions that cause progressive deficits in memory and cognition (eg cerebrovascular disease, Parkinson's disease, Huntington's disease, subdural haematoma, normal-present hydrocephalus, brain tumour)
2 systemic conditions that are known to cause dementia (e.g. hypothyroidism, vitamin B12 or folic acid deficiency, niacin deficiency, hypercalcaemia, neurosyphilis, HIV infection)
3 substance-induced conditions

E The deficits do not occur exclusively during the course of delirium.

F The disturbance is not better accounted for by another Axis I disorder (e.g. major depressive disorder, schizophrenia).

Three phases in AD have usually been described (Lishman, 1998; Mendez & Cummings, 2003), although a variable pattern is common.

- In the earliest stages (1–3 years) the patient complains of forgetfulness and difficulty in naming and word finding. This may be accompanied by disorders of visuospatial skills, causing problems in driving and drawing. Depression occurs in reaction to the cognitive impairment, and performance anxiety may be considerable.
- In the second stage (2–10 years), these impairments become more severe and are accompanied by other 'focal' features, such as apraxia, agnosia, comprehension difficulties and a failure in mental calculation. Disorganisation in household tasks and financial affairs is marked. Anosognosia is common.
- In the terminal stages (about 8–12 years), patients become globally demented, mute, stuporose, wasted and doubly incontinent. Loss of the sense of personal identity occurs in the later stages of the disorder.

Behavioural and psychological symptoms, which occur in about 20% of community-dwelling patients and in about 80% of those in residential care, are a particular burden to carers. Apathy and agitation are the most common of these. Depressive features, delusions (particularly of theft), hallucinations, anxiety, irritability, misidentifications, wandering, restlessness, incontinence and safety issues are frequent.

The rate of progress of the disorder is very variable. Once a patient has been admitted to residential care, the life expectancy is usually less than 2 years, but the time taken to reach this point may vary from approximately 2 years to over 10. Initial language impairment, a younger age of onset and behavioural and psychological symptoms predict more rapid decline.

Neuropsychological studies have demonstrated deficits in both working memory and secondary memory. The deficit in working memory is characterised by a 'dysexecutive syndrome' (Baddeley, 1990), involving difficulty monitoring incoming information when there are two or more tasks in hand. The deficit in secondary memory involves the characteristic impairment of explicit or episodic memory, with both retrograde and anterograde components. There is controversy concerning the extent to which implicit memory (primary, procedural memory) is spared in AD, but there is general agreement that semantic memory is more extensively affected than in the amnesic syndrome. Patients with AD, however, contrast with patients who have so-called semantic dementia, in whom there is a relatively selective deficit of semantic memory (see, for example, Hodges *et al*, 1992).

The cardinal neuropathological features of AD are the presence of extracellular neuritic plaques and intracellular neurofibrillary tangles at post-mortem or cortical biopsy. Both can occur in normal ageing, where the tangles are most commonly confined to the hippocampi. They become much more widespread and prevalent in dementia. The quantity of tangles especially has been shown to relate to ante-mortem measures of the degree of cognitive impairment, but the correlation is sometimes poor because of the aggravation of the clinical impact of AD by cerebrovascular disease

(Snowdon *et al*, 1997). In addition, there is granulovacuolar degeneration in the hippocampi, aluminium and amyloid deposition, hyaline degeneration, and loss of neurons and synaptic connections, as well as depletion of the acetylcholine, noradrenaline and serotonin neurotransmitter systems. The microtubule-associated protein tau is found in plaques and particularly tangles. The reduction in neuronal counts and synaptic connections and the degree of cholinergic depletion may be better correlated with measures of ante-mortem cognitive function than are the counts of plaques and tangles. Cholinergic deficits correlate highly not only with ante-mortem cognitive scores but also with the presence of hallucinations. A community-based neuropathological study (Fernando & Ince, 2004) found that the brains of demented and non-demented people overlapped in neocortical neuritic plaque and tangle density, with no single pathological criterion reliably distinguishing the groups. Thus, cognitive status may be less tightly correlated with pathological burden than is usually assumed.

The aetiology of the disorder remains a topic of intense research interest, particularly the role of genes as causative, risk or modifying factors in AD. While increasing age is the single greatest risk factor for AD, AD in a first-degree relative doubles the risk for an individual. In under 5% of cases, AD is inherited in an autosomal dominant manner, with almost complete penetrance, presenting between 45 and 60 years. Mutations in three genes account for these familial AD (FAD) cases: beta-amyloid precursor protein (APP) gene, presenilin 1 and presenilin 2 genes. All three result in excessive production of beta-amyloid 42, the most toxic of the three common forms of amyloid. At least 16 mutations in the beta-APP gene have been identified on chromosome 21 (e.g. isoleucine substituted for valine at codon 717 of the APP gene). This led to the amyloid cascade hypothesis, the prevailing molecular model of AD. About 50% of early-onset FAD cases are associated with presenilin 1 and under 1% with presenilin 2 mutations, found on chromosomes 14 and 1, respectively. These three genes do not explain all FAD.

No single gene is causative in late-onset or sporadic AD, in which multiple combinations of risk factors, both genetic and environmental, could result in AD. The possession of the e4 allele (on chromosome 19) of apolipoprotein E (ApoE e4) is a major risk factor in the development of late-onset AD. Caucasians carrying this allele are three (heterozygotes) to eight (homozygotes) times likelier to develop AD than those without an e4 allele. None the less, between 40% and 70% of patients with late-onset AD do not carry the e4 allele. The ApoE e4 allele determines when, but not whether, an individual develops late-onset AD (Meyer *et al*, 1998); its presence reduces the age of onset of AD by about 4–5 (one allele) or 10 years (two alleles or homozygotes) (Khachaturian *et al*, 2004). Also, in late-onset cases, there is an association between AD and an increased number of mtDNA polymorphisms or the presence of mutations in complex I mtDNA. Late-onset AD also shows strong linkage to a susceptibility locus on chromosome 10 (Grupe *et al*, 2006). Several other genetic associations have been reported (see http://www.alzforum.org/res/com/gen/alzgene/) but not confirmed. Non-cognitive factors are influenced by genetic variation.

Research into putative non-genetic aetiological factors also continues, including into the possible role of toxins (e.g. aluminium) and vascular risk factors. Female sex, history of head injury in men, western rather eastern nationality, and the lack of use of hormone replacement therapy may be modifying factors.

Community studies suggest mixed (vascular and Alzheimer) dementia comprises 10–20% of all dementias over 65 years, but autopsy studies demonstrate double the rate (20–40%) of mixed pathology. In the 'Nun study', dementia in the absence of cerebral infarction required an eight-fold greater burden of neocortical neurofibrillary tangles (Snowdon *et al*, 1997).

Hyperphosphorylation of the tau protein, a microtubule stabiliser, results in axonal breakdown and deposition of paired helical filaments (PHF). Severity of cognitive impairment correlates with the deposition of PHF-tau and inversely with the amount of normal, soluble tau in the medial temporal lobes. Cerebrospinal fluid tau protein and beta-amyloid 42 protein are altered in very mild AD.

The depletions of the various neurotransmitters have given rise to efforts at replacement therapy. In particular, cholinergic depletion is the most consistent and severe loss in AD, and it is known that cholinergic-blocking drugs impair memory in healthy subjects (Kopelman & Corn, 1988). Consequently, various attempts have been made to replace acetylcholine, most successfully with anticholinesterases, in patients with AD. The three currently licensed acetylcholinesterase inhibitors (donepezil, rivastigmine and galantamine) produce 'responses' of 2–4 points on the ADAS-Cog scale (range 0–70) over 6 months in highly selected groups with mild to moderate AD (numbers needed to treat are respectively 4, 7 and 3), compared with a decline of 5–6 points per year in placebo-treated patients. Benefit is less clear on severity of disease, with no robust effect on quality of life or disability. The cognitive changes are equivalent to a 3- to 6-month delay in disease progression. Typical improvements of 1–2 points in MMSE score over 6 months contrast with an average decline of 4–5 points per year in placebo-treated patients. Rivastigmine may benefit daily living activities, and in DLB it may reduce psychotic symptoms, especially visual hallucinations. Diarrhoea, muscle cramps, nausea, vomiting, dizziness and insomnia are the most common side-effects.

A large randomised controlled trial of donepezil in clinically representative people with AD found small but statistically significant cognitive and functional benefits maintained over 2 years, but no significant effect on progression of disability, behavioural symptoms, carer well-being or input, time to institutionalisation or costs (AD 2000 Collaborative Group, 2004). Donepezil was not cost-effective, with benefits rated as below minimally relevant thresholds.

The modest benefit of acetylcholinesterase inhibitors is not surprising in view of the complexity of breakdown in neurotransmission in AD, which includes losses of glutamate (reflecting pyramidal cell depletion); losses of serotonin and noradrenaline; gamma-aminobutyric acid (GABA), somatostatin and other neuropeptides (secondary to cortical interneuronal pathology); and cellular loss and alterations of signal transduction proteins.

The glutamatergic system is involved in neurodegeneration. Memantine is an N-methyl-D-aspartate antagonist, which blocks the excitotoxic effects of excess glutamate release, considered central to memory, behavioural dysfunction and pathology in AD and VaD. Memantine may improve function and reduce care dependence in severe dementia, including AD, VaD and mixed dementias. Other drug therapies, such as cyclo-oxygenase 2 inhibitors, hormone replacement therapy and antioxidants are unproven as yet. Lithium, which inhibits glycogen synthase kinase (GSK)-3 alpha, an enzyme regulating production of beta-amyloid peptides, may (theoretically) prevent AD (Phiel *et al*, 2003).

Dementia with Lewy bodies

Dementia with Lewy bodies is a common dementia in old age, accounting for 15–20% of cases in hospital series. It shares clinical and pathological features with both Alzheimer's and Parkinson's diseases. Lewy bodies are (eosinophilic) intraneuronal inclusions, composed of abnormally phosphorylated, neurofilament proteins aggregated with ubiquitin and alpha-synuclein (McKeith, 2002). Lewy bodies, characteristically found in the substantia nigra of patients with Parkinson's disease, are also found in the hippocampus, limbic system and neocortex of patients with DLB. Selected Alzheimer-type pathology (plaques) is also present in many patients, but neurofibrillary tangles are few and tau pathology rare. Acetylcholine and dopamine are particularly depleted.

The primary clinical criteria for DLB (McKeith *et al*, 1996, 2005) are set out in Box 20.4. The 1996 guidelines demonstrated 83% sensitivity and 92% specificity against autopsy verification of DLB.

About 12% of patients diagnosed with AD may reveal Lewy bodies at autopsy. They are more likely than Alzheimer patients to exhibit Parkinsonian features, frontal cerebral atrophy and loss of neurons in the basal nucleus of Meynert and the substantia nigra (Förstl *et al*, 1993).

The differential diagnosis includes AD and other dementias, other causes of delirium, Parkinson's disease and late-onset affective and delusional disorders. Fifty per cent of people with DLB have neuroleptic sensitivity reactions, with a two- to threefold increase in mortality. Cholinesterase inhibitors improve cognition, psychosis, apathy and agitation in most patients, and could become first-line treatment. Choline acetyltransferase activity declines earlier and more extensively in DLB than in AD, suggesting that cholinesterase inhibitors may be more effective in the former than in the latter, especially in mild disease (Tiraboschi *et al*, 2002).

Box 20.4 Consensus criteria for the clinical diagnosis of probable and possible dementia with Lewy bodies

1 Central required feature
Progressive cognitive decline of sufficient magnitude to interfere with normal social or occupational function. Prominent or persistent memory impairment may not necessarily occur in the early stage but is usually evident with progression. Executive deficits on tests of attention and visuospatial abilities may be especially prominent.

2 Core features (two required for probable DLB and one for possible DLB)
A Fluctuating cognition with pronounced variations in attention and alertness
B Recurrent visual hallucinations that are typically well formed and detailed
C Spontaneous motor features of parkinsonism

3 Features suggestive of the diagnosis
A REM sleep behaviour disorder
B Severe neuroleptic sensitivity
C Low dopamine transporter uptake in basal ganglia

4 Features supportive of the diagnosis
A Repeated falls
B Syncope
C Transient loss of consciousness
D Neuroleptic sensitivity
E Systematised delusions
F Hallucinations in other modalities

5 Diagnosis of DLB is less likely in the presence of:
A Evidence of stroke from focal neurological signs or brain imaging
B Evidence of any physical illness or other brain disorder sufficient to account for the clinical features

Source: adapted from McKeith *et al* (1996, 2005).

Vascular dementia

At the turn of the 20th century, arteriosclerosis was regarded as the major cause of senile dementia. Tomlinson *et al* (1970) demonstrated that at least 50–100 ml of brain tissue had to be infarcted before VaD occurred. In 1974, Hachinski *et al* coined the term 'multi-infarct dementia', a term that predominated until re-evaluation in the 1990s. The advent of neuroimaging revealed an increasing frequency of ischaemic abnormalities in the deep white matter of patients with dementia, and that much smaller volumes of ischaemic damage may cause dementia. This revived interest in subcortical vascular disease as an important cause of VaD.

Clinically, a third to a half of patients with pathological evidence of VaD lack a clinically recognised stroke. Recently, the concept of VaD has been broadened to include the full spectrum of cerebrovascular disease that may cause dementia. This nosological revolution continues with increasing recognition that frontosubcortical dysfunction may be the salient feature (Looi & Sachdev, 2000). The focus on memory decline influenced by AD research needs to shift because subcortical and frontal functions are most commonly affected in VaD. Moreover, the need to identify early cases has been recognised in the replacement term – vascular cognitive impairment (Bowler & Hachinski, 2000, 2003).

Vascular dementia is probably the second most common type of dementia, accounting for about 20% of cases, and affecting about 8% of people aged over 65 years. The classical emphasis on distinguishing it from AD is subtly shifting, to an approach aimed at understanding their interactions. Thus AD may underlie post-stroke dementia; vascular factors predispose to AD; and the treatment of systolic hypertension in the elderly may reduce the incidence of both dementias. Vascular pathology commonly coexists with AD pathology in community cohorts, and a synergistic interaction between these two pathologies occurs.

The principal ICD–10 categories of vascular dementia

Vascular dementia of acute onset

This usually follows a succession of strokes, or a strategically placed single large infarction, such as medial thalamic infarcts and the left angular gyrus syndrome.

Multi-infarct dementia (MID)

This is characterised by abrupt episodes of hemiparesis, sensory changes, dysphasia and focal syndromes from strokes. There is a fluctuating course and a *stepwise* deterioration in intellectual functioning that early on leaves some functions relatively intact, but culminates in dementia. Nocturnal confusion, relative preservation of personality, emotional lability, somatic complaints and depression are more common in MID than in other forms of dementia, but are not diagnostic. Focal neurological signs and symptoms are present, including pseudobulbar palsy (with dysarthria, dysphagia and emotional incontinence), ataxia and small-stepped gait, usually associated with hypertension. An acute onset with a stepwise, deteriorating course and a 'patchy' distribution of deficits distinguishes MID from other dementias. The Hachinski ischaemia index (see Table 20.5) has been widely used to separate MID and AD, which overlaps pathologically in about 35% of patients. Although the index has been much criticised, sensitivities and specificities of about 80% have been achieved for the autopsy diagnosis of 'pure' VaD. The scale is, however, far less successful in identifying mixed cases (Dening & Berrios, 1992). The most discriminating clinical variables – stepwise deterioration, evidence of cerebrovascular disease and focal neurology – are enshrined in the DSM–IV diagnostic criteria and the revised ischaemia score of Ettlin *et al* (1989) for VaD.

The major predisposing factor is hypertension, but many cases of MID result from multiple, widespread cerebral emboli from the heart or extracranial arteries.

Table 20.5 Hachinski ischaemia index

Symptom	Weighted score
Abrupt onset	2
Stepwise deterioration	1
Fluctuating course	2
Nocturnal confusion	1
Relative preservation of personality	1
Depression	1
Somatic complaints	1+
Emotional incontinence	1
History of hypertension	1*
History of strokes	2**
Atherosclerosis	2*
Focal neurological symptoms	2+**
Focal neurological signs	2+**

A total score of under 5 suggests degenerative dementia, whereas one above 6 indicates vascular dementia.

*,** Revised ischaemia score of Ettlin *et al* (1989); with features of primary** and of secondary* importance. One feature of primary or two features of secondary importance = diagnosis of MID or mixture (i.e. of MID and Alzheimer's disease).
+ = DSM–IV criteria.

Source: Hachinski *et al* (1975).

Subcortical vascular dementia

This has a complex pathogenesis, which depends on the combination and siting of lacunar infarcts with more diffuse subcortical arteriosclerotic ischaemia of deep white matter (leukoaraiosis). The cerebral cortex is usually preserved and this contrasts with the clinical picture, which may closely resemble AD. Patients with chronic hypertension often present with a more insidious cognitive deterioration, sometimes punctuated by clear-cut episodes of decline or by lacunar strokes, but rarely major thrombo-embolic events. The small-vessel disease results from the occlusion of small, deep, perforating arteries. The difference between the lacunar state, first described by Marie in 1901, and diffuse leukoaraiosis (or Binswanger's disease) is a matter of degree.

Binswanger's disease

Binswanger's disease is a slowly progressive dementia associated with subacute progression of focal neurological deficits in chronically hypertensive patients. The clinical signs include a small-stepped, wide-based gait, pseudobulbar palsy, pyramidal and Parkinsonian signs, incontinence and *fluctuating* mental changes – poor concentration and memory, abulia, bradyphrenia and emotional lability. Deep white-matter demyelination and loss occurs predominantly in periventricular and occipital regions and results from diffuse ischaemic damage, with hydrocephalus *ex vacuo*. Lacunar infarcts are frequently present.

Subcortical white-matter ischaemia may be a more frequent and important cause of VaD than multiple cortical infarcts (Rockwood *et al*, 2000). In patients thought to have MID clinically, leukoaraiosis is found in at least three-quarters. Leukoaraiosis and micro-infarction found at autopsy correlated with a history of VaD, whereas macroscopic infarction did not. Leukoaraiosis, infarcts and other vascular factors are common in AD and worsen cognitive performance in AD.

Mixed cortical and subcortical vascular dementia

This is a further ICD–10 category.

Extrapyramidal syndromes with dementia

Dementia may complicate the late stages of idiopathic Parkinson's disease in about a quarter of patients. Other causes include Huntington's disease, which is important for its genetic implications, Wilson's disease and rarer disorders. These disorders present with a subcortical dementia, with the characteristic clinical features of psychomotor retardation, forgetfulness, affective disorders, impaired insight and problem-solving, dysarthria and movement disorders.

Huntington's disease

An autosomal dominant disorder of choreiform movements and subcortical dementia, Huntington's disease (HD) has a prevalence of about 4–9 cases per 100000 in the UK. The onset is insidious, most frequently between the ages of 35 and 50; however, 4% begin under 20 years (juvenile form) and 7–11% appear after the age of 60; the interval between onset and diagnosis is typically about 8 years; the average duration is 13–16 years, with wide variation, with some patients surviving up to 30 years after diagnosis.

Two-thirds of HD patients present with chorea and one-third with mental changes. Chorea consists of muscle jerks randomly distributed in space and time, brief in duration and unpredictable in appearance. Chorea is only part of a much wider motor disturbance in HD, which frequently includes dystonia, rigidity, bradykinesia and decreased voluntary movement. It is these other movement disorders that compromise function most. Eye movements are also abnormal. Dysarthria and dysphagia worsen as the disease progresses. Less common, except in juvenile HD, are cerebellar dysfunction, upper motor neuron signs, epilepsy and myoclonus. Chorea usually involves all body parts, unlike tardive dyskinesia.

Its severity may vary from restlessness – with mild, intermittent exaggeration of gesture and expression, fidgetiness of the hands, and an unstable, dance-like gait – to a continuous flow of disabling, violent movements. Chorea increases progressively early on, later tending to plateau, in contrast to the continued progression of the other motor features. Late-onset cases (after age 60) commonly present with chorea and few other features of HD. Mental and other motor abnormalities are minor or absent.

Folstein (1989) and Watt & Seller (1993) used standardised diagnostic criteria to establish a prevalence of psychiatric disorder in HD of 66–73%. There were five main psychiatric syndromes:

1 behaviour and personality disorders in about 40% of patients (irritability, violence, suspicion, apathy), which often appear first

2 major affective disorder in 41% (32% depressive, 9% bipolar) and minor depression in 3% of US patients, but in only 26% and 28%, respectively, of patients in Watt & Seller's series

3 dementia

4 paranoid and schizophreniform psychoses in up to 12% of patients

5 conduct disorder in the offspring of affected families.

Familial association with affective disorder has been found in some HD families.

Minor depression and behaviour disorder were associated with the onset of physical signs of HD, while major affective disorder and schizophrenia were not (Watt & Seller, 1993). Paulsen & Robinson (2001) reported that neuropsychiatric symptoms in HD were relatively independent of the cognitive and motor stages of disease, but apathy may correlate with cognitive decline (Craufurd & Snowden, 2002). The suicide risk is increased four to six times in HD, occurring in about 8% of patients. Denial of the disease is largely due to anosognosia.

Initial misdiagnosis of HD is common, especially in the early stages. Psychiatric misdiagnosis is more common than neurological, especially schizophrenia or paranoid psychosis, where the chorea may be ascribed to fidgetiness, 'mannerisms' or the side-effects of drugs. Affective and personality disorders are other initial misdiagnoses. Conversely, up to 15% of patients diagnosed with HD prove to have other neurological diagnoses (including parkinsonism, tardive dyskinesia and AD) (Folstein, 1989).

The subcortical dementia has an insidious onset, marked only by apathy and inefficiency in everyday life. Cognitive problems include executive deficits – poor planning, decision-making and attention – which correlate with caudate atrophy and D_1 and D_2 receptor binding levels. Psychomotor slowing and visuospatial skills involving egocentric space, such as map reading, are also impaired (Craufurd & Snowden, 2002). Memory loss is usually mild to moderate, with encoding and retrieval deficits, relatively intact retention and recognition, and only a mild, temporally flat retrograde amnesia. Judgement is often severely impaired, but insight is commonly retained until late. Language is relatively preserved in HD but speech is dysarthric; apraxia and agnosia are notably absent, in striking contrast to AD and other cortical diseases.

Social effects

The slow progression of motor symptoms, prominent dementia and psychiatric complications culminates in total dependency, exacting an immense burden on the family.

The effects on HD patients include lower socio-economic grouping, poor educational attainment, difficulty holding down employment for more than 5 years after onset of disease, and loss of independence. Families are often disorganised, with personality disorders, alcoholism, depression, violence, marital breakdown, suicide, criminality and sexual disturbance reported both in the unaffected relatives as well as in the patients themselves.

Carers are stressed in proportion to the rate of adverse behaviour of HD patients, who often refuse external help. Furthermore, help is not often offered by the extended family, who may shun the branch with an affected member, and keep the disease 'secret'. Social support is poorly developed.

The information gained by children may be distorted and incomplete. The knowledge of being at an initial 50% risk of HD breeds variously anxiety, insecurity, symptom searching, denial and survivor guilt; there is a history of depression in 35% (Watt & Seller, 1993) but most persons at risk come to terms with their status and achieve a reasonable quality of life (Folstein, 1989).

Aetiology

The gene IT15 and the mutation responsible for HD are located on the short arm of chromosome 4 (4p16.3) (Huntington's Disease Colloborative Research Group, 1993). It contains an excessive and unstable number of trinucleotide or triplet (CAG) repeats, which are translated into a polyglutamine tract. The CAG repeat is found in all people, but normally repeats 8–37 times. The gene encodes a protein called huntingtin, of unknown function, which forms fibrillar aggregates when the tract exceeds a critical length of 37 glutamines. The length of the trinucleotide repeat and the age of onset are inversely correlated, regardless of the sex of the transmitting parent (Snell *et al*, 1993; Harper & Jones, 2002). Affected children of affected fathers have an age of onset 8–10 years earlier than their fathers, while those of affected mothers have an age of onset similar to their mothers. Patients with disease of paternal origin have more triplet repeats in the gene than those whose disease has been maternally transmitted (Snell *et al*, 1993). These observations provide a molecular substrate for genetic 'anticipation'. Paternal transmission may account for the so-called 'sporadic' cases, where fathers had a range of 29–35 repeats, which are less stable when passed through the germ line. A family history is otherwise not always found, perhaps due to the early death of a parent, illegitimacy, poor history or family secrets.

Pathology

The key lesions are progressive atrophy of the caudate nuclei (evident on CT brain scan) and putamen, with spiny cell loss and astrocytic proliferation. Ventricular dilation and cerebral atrophy occur, both maximally affecting the frontal areas. Neuronal intranuclear inclusions containing huntingtin and ubiquitin develop in patients and transgenic mouse models of HD. Other molecular mechanisms are reviewed by Ho *et al* (2001).

Reduced levels of GABA in the striatal projection pathways in the basal ganglia and substantia nigra are found in HD patients compared with controls. One theory holds that, because GABA is known to inhibit dopamine release, excessive dopamine may be released from an intact nigrostriatal system onto a reduced population of striatal neurons, resulting in motor disinhibition, which provokes chorea. Levels of met-enkephalin, substance P, choline acetyltransferase, dopamine and glutamate are also reduced. Abnormalities of basal ganglia circuitry and chemistry are reviewed by Beal *et al* (2005).

Management

The burden of knowledge of this relentlessly debilitating and uniformly fatal disease falls heavily on Huntington's families. The aims of management are: to preserve the patient's mobility and independence; to treat concurrent medical illness; and to provide long-term support for the families and primary carers, for their distress, for the experience of being at risk, for specific psychiatric complications and over genetic testing.

Currently, no treatment influences the course of the disease. Rapamycin, which reduces mutant huntingtin levels in cells by accelerating its breakdown by autophagy, slows the onset and progression of pathology and clinical signs in animal models of HD (Ravikumar *et al*, 2004). RNA interference-based therapies for gene silencing have also shown promise in transgenic mouse models of Huntington's disease. In human HD, glutamate receptor antagonists and coenzyme Q have proved disappointing. Algorithms exist for comprehensive care that account for disease stage and that include the treatment of aggression, memory loss and psychiatric complications, as well as social services input for domiciliary support, day care or residential accommodation (Nance & Westphal, 2002).

Chorea may be controlled initially with neuroleptic drugs such as risperidone (up to 6 mg/day), which may also help psychiatric symptoms and activity levels (Dallochio *et al*, 1999). Haloperidol (in doses of no more than 6–8 mg/day) or tetrabenazine may reduce chorea at the expense of functional deterioration. Benzodiazepines are useful.

Depression, anxiety and obsessive–compulsive disorder respond to the drugs used for the idiopathic disorders. Depression, which should be distinguished from apathy, responds well to selective serotonin reuptake inhibitors, and severe depression to electroconvulsive therapy. Bipolar disorder is less responsive to lithium than to anticonvulsants, and schizophreniform symptoms respond to atypical antipsychotic drugs. The use of drugs in HD is reviewed by Rosenblatt *et al* (1999).

Patients with HD have special care needs, for they are not demented in the same way as AD patients. They may have preserved insight and memory until the end, hidden behind grotesque chorea. Hospital care lasts on average 4–7 years (to death).

Genetic testing

People at risk for HD vary in their ability to deal with the burden of uncertainty. Most avoid medical help until they become ill, but a few want genetic testing. Codori *et al* (1997) found that people who have genetic testing usually cope with the results regardless of the outcome. There are difficult ethical and social problems in predictive testing, including problems of inappropriate referral, other family members and disclosure of results. Testing should always be preceded by counselling that focuses on a person's motivation and the risk that she or he may not seriously have considered a bad outcome. The genetic information has a great impact on all family members, their relationships, jobs and insurance. The direct HD test is highly sensitive and specific and is considered definitive.

Genetic testing is useful in three clinical situations: confirmatory, predictive and prenatal. The probability of HD onset by a particular age for a specific CAG repeat size can be determined (Brinkman *et al*, 1997).

Prion diseases

Prion disease or transmissible spongiform encephalopathies occur when prion protein (PrPc), a normal cellular brain protein, undergoes conformational change into an insoluble form termed PrPSc (prion protein, scrapie) (Prusiner & Hsiao, 1994). Devoid of nucleic acid, prions are resistant to proteases. PrPc is rich in alpha-helical structure, whereas PrPSc has a high beta-sheet structure. Conformational change from PrPc to PrPSc occurs in three ways: spontaneously, accounting for at least 85% of cases of CJD; genetically, comprising about 10% of CJD cases and all the inherited forms (e.g. Gerstmann–Straussler syndrome); and transmissibly, by exposure to a 'seed' of PrPSc. Unlike other infectious diseases, prion diseases are both heritable and transmissible. They have long incubation periods. Lessons from the kuru epidemic in Papua New Guinea suggest incubation periods of human prions of 10–15 years in humans after exposure, with a range from 4 to 40 years (Collinge, 2000).

A wide range of point mutations and insertions in the gene *PRNP* on chromosome 20 causes inheritable prion diseases. People homozygous for a methionine–valine polymorphism at codon 129 of PrPc are at increased risk for sporadic (methionine) and iatrogenic (valine) CJD. Collinge (2005) reviews other mutations. All prion diseases have a neuropathological triad of vacuolar (spongiform) change, astrocytosis and neuronal loss. Variant CJD has a distinct pathology, with diffuse vacuolation and PrP-containing amyloid plaques surrounded by petals of spongiosis (florid or 'daisy' plaques).

There are three types (inherited, sporadic and acquired) of prion disease in humans, and four clinical syndromes: sporadic CJD, iatrogenic CJD (exposure via pituitary-derived hormones, tissue grafts or neurosurgery); variant CJD (vCJD); and inherited (autosomal dominant) prion diseases. Only CJD and vCJD are discussed here.

Sporadic CJD classically presents with a triad of dementia, myoclonus and ataxia, usually between the ages of 45 and 75 years (mean age 60). It progresses to akinetic mutism and death within a median of 4 months. Seventy per cent of sufferers die within 6 months. Frequent additional neurological features include extrapyramidal and pyramidal signs, cerebellar ataxia and cortical blindness.

Variant CJD differs from CJD clinically. It has a median age of onset of 26 (range 12–74) years (Spencer *et al*, 2002). The median length of illness is 13 (range 6–39) months. Two-thirds of patients present with psychiatric symptoms (dysphoria, withdrawal, anxiety, irritability, insomnia and loss of interest), whereas only one-third do so in sporadic CJD. Poor memory and aggression follow, with disorientation, hallucinations and most neurological features occurring late. Dysaesthesia or pain in the limbs or face is often the first neurological feature in vCJD, but infrequent in CJD. Ataxia occurs early in sporadic and late in vCJD. The MRI scan is the most helpful non-invasive investigation, showing high signal in the posterior thalamus, the 'pulvinar sign', on T_2 and especially FLAIR sequences in about 90% of cases, whereas in sporadic CJD there is high signal in the caudate and putamen in 60%. Lumbar puncture reveals a non-specific 14-3-3 protein in CJD, and sometimes in vCJD. Tonsillar biopsy is positive for PrPSc in vCJD but not CJD, and obviates the need for diagnostic brain biopsy.

Species barriers, inherited prion diseases and possible treatment (e.g. with quinacrine) are reviewed by Collinge (2000, 2005) and Prusiner (1998). vCJD is a notifiable disease.

Frontotemporal dementia

Frontotemporal dementia (FTD) contends with DLB for the most common form of primary degenerative dementia in middle age, after AD. Onset of FTD is usually between 35 and 65 years, with a range from under 30 to old age. The sex distribution is equal. The duration of illness is 2–20 years (mean 8).

The core clinical features of the frontal variant of FTD are (Neary *et al*, 1998):

- an insidious onset and gradual progression
- an early decline in social (interpersonal) conduct (e.g. loss of manners, tactlessness and disinhibition)
- early impairment in the regulation of personal conduct (e.g. passivity, inertia, overactivity and pacing)
- early emotional blunting
- early loss of insight.

This breakdown in personality and social conduct occurs in the context of relative preservation of the instrumental functions of perception, spatial skills, praxis and memory. Overeating is common, as are perseverative and stereotyped behaviours, such as humming and foot-tapping. Speech output is reduced, with echolalia, perseveration and ultimately mutism. Cognitive changes reflect frontal lobe deficits in the absence of severe amnesia, aphasia or visuospatial disorder. Early neurological signs are absent or include primitive reflexes. Akinesia and rigidity develop later, and some patients with FTD develop signs of motor neuron disease.

The EEG is normal. MRI reveals bilateral frontotemporal atrophy, and SPET anterior abnormalities. The key distinguishing features from AD are as follows: loss of social awareness, hyperorality, stereotyped and perseverative behaviour, reduced speech output, and preserved spatial orientation.

The neuropathology reveals bilateral atrophy of the frontal and temporal lobes and degeneration of the striatum. The histology is complex, with five basic patterns. A motor neuron disease type with inclusions immunoreactive for ubiquitin but not for tau is the most frequent type, followed by corticobasal degeneration with tau-positive but ubiquitin-negative inclusions. Third is Pick's disease, with neuronal loss, widespread gliosis and inflated neurons with inclusions positive for both tau and ubiquitin (Pick bodies). Fourth, familial FTD has tau-positive inclusions in neurons and glial cells. Fifth is a pattern lacking distinctive histology.

The frontal variant of FTD is heterogeneous, with disinhibited, apathetic and stereotypic presentations. Patients with the behavioural disorder of FTD account for at least 70% of non-Alzheimer frontotemporal lobar degeneration. Semantic dementia and progressive aphasia are temporal lobe variants, accounting for approximately 15% and 10% of cases, respectively (Snowden *et al*, 1996). In semantic dementia there is progressive loss of word meaning and object or face identity, but orientation and episodic memory are spared.

About 40% of cases of FTD are familial, mainly autosomal dominant. Mutations in the tau gene were first found in FTD with parkinsonism linked to chromosome 17 (FTDP-17). Over 38 mutations in the *MAPt* (tau) gene on chromosome 17q21 account for 15–20% of familial FTD cases, with *MAPt* mutation carriers characterised by tau-positive inclusions (tauopathy), but there are 17q21-linked tau-negative patients (Mackenzie *et al*, 2006; van der Zee *et al*, 2006). Familial FTD of disinhibited form has been linked to a +16 splice site mutation in the intron to exon 10 in the tau gene (Pickering-Brown *et al*, 2002). Recent clinical and pathological data indicate that amyotrophic lateral sclerosis and FTD form part of a disease spectrum.

Treatment is limited.

Dementia in HIV disease

Dementia in HIV disease – variously termed HIV dementia, HIV-1-associated dementia complex, AIDS dementia complex (ADC) – eventually develops in 20–30% of AIDS patients, half within 2 years of an AIDS diagnosis, and dementia is the AIDS-defining illness in 3%. The clinical picture reflects subcortical dementia, typically characterised by forgetfulness, slowness and poor concentration, with motor clumsiness. Apathy, reduced spontaneity, loss of libido, blunted affect, irritability, social withdrawal and defective problem-solving are common, mimicking depression. The illness may present with depression, mania (in 5%), psychosis or seizures.

Motor symptoms are initially asymptomatic, with slowing of rapid movements of the eyes and extremities on examination, followed by early gait unsteadiness, limb incoordination, tremor and leg weakness, progressing to spastic, ataxic quadriparesis, primitive reflexes and incontinence. Dementia is correlated with very low CD4 counts and elevated CSF levels of HIV RNA. Children also develop an HIV-associated neurodevelopmental disorder. HIV-1 dementia is often complicated by opportunistic infections.

Cognitive impairments in asymptomatic HIV infection are not necessarily permament or progressive. Over 1 year about 17% of patients with a CD4 count < 200, who are initially unimpaired, develop HIV-associated minor cognitive/motor disorder and 9% HIV dementia. Highly active antiretroviral therapy (HAART) has halved the incidence of HIV dementia and may reverse neurocognitive deficits (McArthur, 2002).

The pathology, imaging and differential diagnosis (from opportunistic infections and tumours) are reviewed by Grant *et al* (2005).

Other causes of dementia

Lyme disease

Lyme disease is a multisystem illness caused by infection with tick-borne spirochaetes of the *Borrelia burgdorferi* group. Characteristic early skin rashes, such as erythema chronicum migrans, herald arthropathy, carditis and neurological symptoms. Lyme encephalopathy is a chronic mild delirium, and dementia and psychosis may occur.

Tumours and mass lesions

Brain tumours may present with dementia, particularly slowly growing deep midline tumours or tumours of the corpus callosum or frontal lobes. Frontal meningiomas are important to detect as they are benign and potentially curable. Chronic subdural haematoma is another treatable cause of dementia, in which the head injury may have been remote, mild or forgotten, particularly in the elderly.

Hydrocephalus

Hydrocephalus is usually due to tumours, particularly in the posterior fossa, obstructing the cerebral aqueduct and thereby CSF flow. Features of raised intracranial pressure (e.g. headaches and papilloedema) and non-cognitive focal signs may be absent. Colloid cysts of the third ventricle, pineal masses and parapituitary tumours may present with dementia only.

Most causes of dementia due to mass lesions or raised intracranial pressure are easily diagnosed from the MRI or CT scan. However, in the elderly it can be difficult to distinguish hydrocephalus due to abnormal CSF dynamics from hydrocephalus *ex vacuo* secondary to atrophy.

In communicating hydrocephalus, the block is not within the ventricular system but in the subarachnoid space, usually around the basal cisterns. Patients present with subacute progressive dementia, which is treatable. A history of headache, ataxia and gait disturbance is usual, but signs of raised intracranial pressure may be absent. The combination of dementia, urinary incontinence and gait disorder in the absence of routine evidence of raised intracranial pressure suggests the syndrome of normal-pressure hydrocephalus, which may respond to ventricular drainage. The condition may develop many years after meningitis, severe head injury with bleeding, or subarachnoid haemorrhage, but usually has no antecedent cause.

Chronic infections

Chronic infections are important to consider, as they may be treatable. They are usually associated with systemic manifestations, meningeal involvement, abnormal CSF and brain imaging abnormalities. Dementias may be produced by slow virus infections, including HIV-1, CJD and vCJD, bacterial encephalitis, neurosyphilis, Lyme disease, chronic meningitis (tuberculous, fungal) and other viral infections.

Diffuse brain damage

In dementia due to head injury, anoxia, hypoglycaemia, or encephalitis, the cause is usually obvious from the history. Dementia becomes evident when consciousness is regained after prolonged coma.

Endocrine disorders, vitamin deficiencies and toxic and alcohol-related disorders

These are described in Chapter 22.

Pseudo-dementia

'Pseudo-dementia' describes a syndrome of disordered intellectual function that mimics dementia; it can occur in patients with primary psychiatric illness. Caine (1981) suggests four diagnostic criteria for pseudo-dementia:

1 intellectual impairment in a patient with a primary psychiatric disorder

2 the intellectual changes resemble those caused by degenerative dementias

3 the intellectual deficits are reversible

4 the patient has no identifiable neurological disease that can account for the mental changes.

'Depressive pseudo-dementia' (DPD), 'dementia syndrome of depression' and 'depression-induced cognitive impairment' are terms reflecting various perspectives on the coexistence of depression and dementia. The early concept of pseudo-dementia was based on the assumption that depression was the unitary cause of reversible dementia. Almost 50% of patients presenting with depression and cognitive impairment are cognitively intact at follow-up, but 50% or more develop dementia after 5 years (Alexopoulos *et al*, 1993). Longitudinal studies of community-residing elders reveal that depressive symptoms often precede the development of dementia (Wilson *et al*, 2004). This suggests a preclinical or early dementia in some patients with DPD, in whom a decreased 'cognitive reserve capacity' may be unmasked by depression.

Another possibility is that depressive disorders are risk factors or even predispose patients to AD, vascular and other dementias. Depressive symptoms occurring long before the onset of dementia have been shown to increase the risk for AD, and the longer an elderly person has depression, the higher the risk is of cognitive decline or AD (Jorm, 2000).

Cognitive impairment shows marked diurnal variation in depression. While most cognitive functions normalise on recovery from depression, deficits remain in learning, memory, psychomotor speed and decision-making (Murphy *et al*, 1998; Butters *et al*, 2000), which would suggest that the term 'pseudo-dementia' is unclear and misleading. Residual cognitive deficits are found in 30% of elderly patients who have recovered from depression, in association with cerebral ventricular enlargement (Abas *et al*, 1990). Depression is common in subcortical disorder, and a subcortical dementia memory profile is found in about 30% of depressed patients. Thus, major depression refers to a heterogeneous group of patients, with regard to reversibility of cognitive impairment, presence of organic markers and prediction of later dementia, with these risks depending on age, severity and duration of depression.

Pseudo-dementia accounts for about 9% of patients under the age of 65 referred to neurologists for suspected dementia. The commonest cause is depression, particularly in the elderly, who may show poor memory and concentration, apathy, social withdrawal and self-neglect (even incontinence). Depressed mood may not be evident. The clinical picture may resemble AD. The distinction may be difficult, but the correct diagnosis of depression is often suggested by:

- a history of acute onset with the absence of memory loss or intellectual decline before the onset of depressive symptoms
- the presence of depressed mood during admission
- a history of affective disorder
- an abnormal premorbid personality.

Patients with depression often complain about their cognitive difficulties much more than seems justified by their performance on intellectual tests. In contrast, truly demented patients rarely complain appropriately; and their affect is labile and shallow. The patient with depression is often inconsistent during the history, giving detailed informative and distressed accounts of symptoms and history, but then having difficulty with specific questions, often answering 'Don't know' to questions or even failing to attempt an answer (Wells, 1979; Lishman, 1998).

Variability in performance during testing, particularly improvement with encouragement and worse performance after feedback about failure, are characteristic of depression. Memory loss for recent and remote events may be equally severe, and gaps for specific periods or events are common. In contrast, the organic patient: provides near-miss or confabulatory answers to questions; furnishes facile excuses for the memory failure; produces a consistently poor performance on tests; and usually shows relative sparing of early memories.

Physical investigations are generally unhelpful in the distinction of depression and dementia, with EEG abnormalities, cerebral atrophy on CT scan, leukoaraiosis on MRI scan, and dexamethasone non-suppression occurring in both disorders. Negative neurological investigation supports the diagnosis of pseudo-dementia but may also be found in organic dementia.

Neuropsychological tests in DPD usually reveal inattention, slow information processing, and impairments of recognition and effortful memory and of verbal fluency. Cognitive impairment was reported in 70% of elderly patients with depression, particularly in memory and latency of response, to a degree comparable with that in AD, but with a different pattern of errors (Abas *et al*, 1990). Visuospatial associative learning may distinguish AD from depression (Swainson *et al*, 2001). The executive deficits found in patients with depression are disproportionately worse over the age of 60 (Lockwood *et al*, 2002). Recent advances are reviewed by Steffens *et al* (2006). Confirmation of the diagnosis of DPD follows improvement in intellectual functioning with antidepressant therapy.

Diagnosis is more difficult when depressive illness complicates dementia. At least one depressive symptom is found in almost two-thirds of patients with AD, of whom a quarter are rated as clinically depressed (Burns *et al*, 1990). In these patients, even when depression is treated, cognitive impairment remains.

The failure to extract a dichotomy on the basis of irreversibility versus reversibility, structural versus functional, or organic versus non-organic aetiology led Emery & Oxman (1992) to view depression, cognitive impairment and degenerative dementia as intersecting continua. They proposed five prototypes:

1 pure major depression

2 depressive dementia (pseudo-dementia)

3 pure degenerative dementia

4 depression of degenerative dementia

5 independent co-occurrence of degenerative dementia and depression.

The consensus of research is that the cognitive impairment with depression in the elderly is associated with a poor outcome of the depression as well as various organic abnormalities, and may itself have a poor prognosis (Alexopoulos *et al*, 2002; Stewart, 2002).

The other main varieties of pseudo-dementia include the Ganser syndrome, hysterical pseudo-dementia, simulated dementia and rarer forms, which are discussed in Chapter 16.

Useful websites

For useful websites see:

Stone, J. & Sharpe, M. (2003) Internet resources for psychiatry and neuropsychiatry. *Journal of Neurology, Neurosurgery, and Psychiatry*, **74**, 10–12 (downloadable from http://www.jnnp.com).

See also:

http://www.alzforum.org
Research forum on AD

http://www.ninds.nih.gov
The US National Institute of Neurological Disorders and Stroke

http://www.uku.fi/neuro/linksrad.htm
Links to radiology and imaging sites around the net

http://www.med.harvard.edu/AANLIB/home.html
Harvard Whole Brain Atlas

http://www.nature.com/neurosci
Nature Neuroscience and Nature Reviews

http://www.jnnp.com
Journal of Neurology, Neurosurgery, and Psychiatry

All above sites last accessed February 2006

References

Abas, M. A., Sahakian, B. J. & Levy, R. (1990) Neuropsychological deficits and CT scan changes in elderly depressives. *Psychological Medicine*, **20**, 507–520.

AD 2000 Collaborative Group (2004) Long-term donepezil treatment in 565 patients with Alzheimer's disease (AD2000): randomised double-blind trial. *Lancet*, **363**, 2105–2115.

Adair, J. C., Schwartz, R. L. & Barrett, A. M. (2003) Anosognosia. In *Clinical Neuropsychology* (eds K. M. Heilman & E. Valenstein), pp. 185–214. Oxford: Oxford University Press.

Alexopoulos, G. S., Meyers, B. S., Young, R. C., *et al* (1993) The course of geriatric depression with 'reversible dementia': a controlled study. *American Journal of Psychiatry*, **150**, 1693–1699.

Alexopoulos, G. S., Buckwalter, K., Olin, J., *et al* (2002) Comorbidity of late-life depression: an opportunity for research in mechanisms and treatment. *Biological Psychiatry*, **52**, 543–558.

American Psychiatric Association (1994) *Diagnostic and Statistical Manual of Mental Disorders* (4th edn) (DSM–IV). Washington, DC: APA.

American Psychiatric Association (2000) *Diagnostic and Statistical Manual of Mental Disorders* (4th edn, text revision) (DSM–IV–TR). Washington, DC: APA.

Annett, M. (1970) A classification of hand-preference by association analysis. *British Journal of Psychology*, **61**, 303–321.

Baddeley, A. D. (1990) *Human Memory: Theory and Practice*. Hillsdale, NJ: Erlbaum.

Bauer, R. M. & Demery, J. A. (2003) Agnosia. In *Clinical Neuropsychology* (eds K. M. Heilman & E. Valenstein), pp. 236–295. Oxford: Oxford University Press.

Beal, M. F., Lang, A. E. & Ludolph, A. C. (2005) *Neurodegenerative Diseases*. Cambridge: Cambridge University Press.

Berlyne, N. (1972) Confabulation. *British Journal of Psychiatry*, **120**, 31–39.

Berrios, G. E. (1996) *The History of Mental Symptoms. Descriptive Psychopathology Since the 19th Century*. Cambridge: Cambridge University Press.

Binnie, C. D. & Prior, P. F. (1994) Electroencephalography. *Journal of Neurology, Neurosurgery, and Psychiatry*, **57**, 1308–1391.

Blackwell, A. D., Sahakian, B. J., Vesey, R., *et al* (2004) Detecting dementia: novel neuropsychological markers of preclinical Alzheimer's disease. *Dementia and Geriatric Cognitive Disorders*, **17**, 42–48.

Blessed, G., Tomlinson, B. E. & Roth, M. (1968) The association between quantitative measures of dementia and of senile change in the cerebral grey matter of elderly subjects. *British Journal of Psychiatry*, **114**, 797–811.

Blumer, D. & Benson, D. (1975) Personality changes with frontal and temporal lobe lesions. *Psychiatric Aspects of Neurologic Disease* (eds D. F. Benson & D. Blumer), pp. 151–170. New York: Grune & Stratton.

Bonhoeffer, K. (1909) Exogenous psychoses. In *Themes and Variations in European Psychiatry* (eds S. R. Hirsch & M. Shepherd), pp. 47–52. Bristol: John Wright (1974).

Bowler, J. V. & Hachinski, V. (2000) Criteria for vascular dementia: replacing dogma with data. *Archives of Neurology*, **57**, 170–171.

Bowler, J. V. & Hachinski, V. (2003) Vascular cognitive impairment – a new concept. In *Vascular Cognitive Impairment – Preventable Dementia* (eds J. V. Bowler & V. Hachinski), pp. 321–337. Oxford: Oxford University Press.

Brinkman, R. R., Mezei, M. M., Theilman, J., *et al* (1997) The likelihood of being affected with Huntington's disease by a particular age, for a specific CAG size. *American Journal of Human Genetics*, **60**, 1202–1210.

Brodaty, H. & Moore, C. M. (1997) The clock drawing test for dementia of the Alzheimer's type: a comparison of three scoring methods in a memory disorders clinic. *International Journal of Geriatric Psychiatry*, **12**, 619–627.

Burgess, P. W. & Shallice, T. (1997) *The Hayling and Brixton Tests*. Bury St Edmunds: Thames Valley Test Company.

Burns, A., Jacoby, R. & Levy, R. (1990) Psychiatric phenomenology in Alzheimer's disease. *British Journal of Psychiatry*, **157**, 72–94.

Burns, A., Lawlor, B. & Craig, S. (2002) Rating scales in old age psychiatry. *British Journal of Psychiatry*, **180**, 161–167.

Burns, A., Lawlor, B. & Craig, S. (2003) *Assessment Scales in Old Age Psychiatry* (2nd edn). London: Martin Dunitz.

Burns, A., Gallagley, A. & Byrne, J. (2004) Delirium. *Journal of Neurology, Neurosurgery, and Psychiatry*, **75**, 362–367.

Butters, M. A., Becker, J. T., Nebes, R. D., *et al* (2000) Changes in cognitive functioning following treatment of late-life depression. *American Journal of Psychiatry*, **157**, 1949–1954.

Caine, E. D. (1981) Pseudo-dementia: current concepts and future directions. *Archives of General Psychiatry*, **38**, 1359–1364.

Church, S., Goldberg, D., David, A., *et al* (2000) *Maudsley Neuropsychiatry Module*. London: Maudsley Publications, King's College, Institute of Psychiatry.

Clarfield, A. M. (2003) The decreasing prevalence of reversible dementias. An updated meta-analysis. *Archives of Internal Medicine*, **163**, 2219–2229.

Codori, A.-M., Slavney, P. R., Young, C., *et al* (1997) Predictors of psychological adjustment to genetic testing for Huntington's disease. *Health Psychology*, **16**, 36–50.

Cole, M. F. & Primeau, F. J. (1993) Prognosis of delirium in elderly hospital patients. *Canadian Medical Association Journal*, **149**, 41–46.

Collinge, J. (2000) Prion disease. In *New Oxford Textbook of Psychiatry* (eds M. G. Gelder, J. J. Lopez-Ibor & N. C. Andreasen), pp. 404–415. Oxford: Oxford University Press.

Collinge, J. (2005) Molecular neurology of prion disease. *Journal of Neurology, Neurosurgery, and Psychiatry*, **76**, 906–919.

Cooper, B. (1991) The epidemiology of dementia. In *Psychiatry in the Elderly* (eds R. Jacoby & C. Oppenheimer), pp. 574–585. Oxford: Oxford University Press.

Craufurd, D. & Snowden, J. (2002) Neuropsychological and neuropsychiatric aspects of Huntington's disease. In *Huntington's Disease* (3rd edn) (eds G. Bates, P. S. Harper & L. Jones), pp. 62–94. Oxford: Oxford University Press.

Critchley, M. (1953) *The Parietal Lobes*. London: Edward Arnold.

Cummings, J. L. (1985) *Clinical Neuropsychiatry*. Orlando, FL: Grune & Stratton.

Cummings, J. L. (1986) Sub-cortical dementia: neuropsychology, neuropsychiatry and pathophysiology. *British Journal of Psychiatry*, **149**, 682–697.

Cummings, J. L. & Benson, D. F. (1992) *Dementia: A Clinical Approach* (2nd edn). London: Butterworth-Heinemann.

Cummings, J. L., Mega, M. S., Gray, K., *et al* (1994) The Neuropsychiatric Inventory: comprehensive assessment of psychopathology in dementia. *Neurology*, **44**, 2308–2314.

Cutting, J. (1990) *The Right Cerebral Hemisphere and Psychiatric Disorder*. Oxford: Oxford University Press.

Dallochio, C., Buffa, C., Tinelli, C., *et al* (1999) Effectiveness of risperidone in Huntington chorea patients. *Journal of Clinical Psychopharmacology*, **19**, 101–103.

Damasio, A. R., Tranel, D. & Rizzo, M. (2000) Disorders of complex visual processing. In *Principles of Behavioural and Cognitive Neurology* (2nd edn) (ed. M. Marsel Mesulam), pp. 332–372. Oxford: Oxford University Press.

Davis, H. & Rockwood, K. (2004) Conceptualization of mild cognitive impairment: a review. *International Journal of Geriatric Psychiatry*, **19**, 313–316.

Dening, T. R. & Berrios, G. E. (1992) The Hachinski ischaemia score: a re-evaluation. *International Journal of Geriatric Psychiatry*, **7**, 585–589.

Dubois, B., Slachevsky, A., Litvan, I., *et al* (2000) The FAB: a Frontal Assessment Battery at bedside. *Neurology*, **55**, 1621–1626.

Ebmeier, K. P., Sutherland, J. K. & Dougall, N. J. (2005) Functional imaging. In *Dementia* (3rd edn) (eds A. Burns, J. O'Brien & D. Ames), pp. 94–103. London: Hodder Arnold.

Emery, V. O. & Oxman, T. E. (1992) Update on the dementia spectrum of depression. *American Journal of Psychiatry*, **149**, 305–317.

Engel, G. & Romano, J. (1959) Delirium, a syndrome of cerebral insufficiency. *Journal of Chronic Disease*, **9**, 260–277.

Ettlin, T. M., Staehelin, H. B., Kischka, U., *et al* (1989) Computed tomography, electroencephalography, and clinical features in the differential diagnosis of senile dementia: a prospective clinicopathologic study. *Archives of Neurology*, **46**, 1217–1220.

Fernando, M. S. & Ince, P. G. (2004) Vascular pathologies and cognition in a population-based cohort of elderly people. *Journal of the Neurological Sciences*, **226**, 13–17.

Folstein, S. (1989) *Huntington's Disease: A Disorder of Families*. Baltimore, MD: Johns Hopkins University Press.

Folstein, M. F., Folstein, S. E. & McHugh, P. R. (1975) 'Mini-Mental State'. A practical method for grading the cognitive state of patients for the clinician. *Journal of Psychiatric Research*, **12**, 189–198.

Folstein, M. F., Bassett, S. S., Romanowski, A. J., *et al* (1991) The epidemiology of delirium in the community: the East Baltimore Mental Health Survey. *International Psychogeriatrics*, **3**, 169–176.

Förstl, H., Burns, A., Luthert, P., *et al* (1993) The Lewy-body variant of Alzheimer's disease: clinical and pathological findings. *British Journal of Psychiatry*, **162**, 385–392.

Geschwind, N. (1965) Disconnection syndromes in animals and man. *Brain*, **88**, 273–294.

Goldberg, D. & Murray, R. (2002) *The Maudsley Handbook of Practical Psychiatry* (4th edn). Oxford: Oxford University Press.

Grant, I., Sacktor, N. & McArthur, J. (2005) HIV neurocognitive disorders. In *Neurology of AIDS* (eds H. E. Gendelman, I. Grant, I. P. Everall, *et al*), pp. 363–373. Oxford: Oxford University Press.

Grigorenko, E. L. (2001) Developmental dyslexia: an update on genes, brains, and environments. *Journal of Child Psychology and Psychiatry*, **42**, 91–125.

Grupe, A., Li, Y., Rowland, C., *et al* (2006) A scan of chromosome 10 identifies a novel locus showing strong association with late-onset Alzheimer disease. *American Journal of Human Genetics*, **78**, 78–88.

Hachinski, V. C., Lassen, N. A. & Marshall, J. (1974) Multi-infarct dementia: a cause of mental deterioration in the elderly. *Lancet*, *ii*, 207–210.

Hachinski, V. C., Iliff, L. D., Zilhka, E., *et al* (1975) Cerebral blood flow in dementia. *Archives of Neurology*, **32**, 632–637.

Harper, P. S. & Jones, L. (2002) Huntington's disease: genetic and molecular studies. In *Huntington's Disease* (3rd edn) (eds G. Bates, P. S. Harper & L. Jones), pp. 113–158. Oxford: Oxford University Press.

Heilman, K. M. & Rothi, L. J. (1985) Apraxia. In *Clinical Neuropsychology* (eds K. M. Heilman & E. Valenstein), pp. 131–150. New York: Oxford University Press.

Hejl, A., Hogh, P. & Waldemar, G. (2001) Potentially reversible conditions in memory clinic patients. In *Alzheimer's Disease: Advances in Etiology, Pathogenesis and Therapeutics* (eds K. Iqbal, S. S. Sisodia & B. Winblad), pp. 123–128. New York: John Wiley & Sons.

Hendrie, H. C., Osuntoken, B. O., Hall, K. S., *et al* (1995) Prevalence of Alzheimer's disease and dementia in two communities: Nigerian Africans and African Americans. *American Journal of Psychiatry*, **152**, 1485–1492.

Ho, L. W., Carmichael, J., Swartz, J., *et al* (2001) The molecular biology of Huntington's disease. *Psychological Medicine*, **31**, 3–14.

Hodges, J. R. (1994) *Cognitive Assessment for Clinicians*. Oxford: Oxford University Press.

Hodges, J. R., Patterson, K., Oxbury, S., *et al* (1992) Semantic dementia. Progressive fluent aphasia with temporal lobe atrophy. *Brain*, **115**, 1783–1806.

Hope, T. & Fairburn, C. (1992) The Present Behavioural Examination (PBE): the development of an interview to measure current behavioural abnormalities. *Psychological Medicine*, **22**, 223–230.

Huntington's Disease Collaborative Research Group (1993) A novel gene containing a trinucleotide repeat that is expanded and unstable on Huntington's disease chromosomes. *Cell*, **72**, 971–983.

Huppert, F. A., Brayne, C., Gill, C., *et al* (1995) CAMCOG – a concise neuropsychological test to assist dementia diagnosis: socio-demographic determinants in an elderly population sample. *British Journal of Clinical Psychology*, **34**, 529–541.

Inouye, S. (2006) Delirium in older persons. *New England Journal of Medicine*, **354**, 1157–1165.

Jacobson, R. R. & Lishman, W. A. (1987) Selective memory loss and global intellectual deficits in alcoholic Korsakoff's syndrome. *Psychological Medicine*, **17**, 649–655.

Jacoby, R. J. & Levy, R. (1980) Computed tomography in the elderly: 2. Senile dementia: diagnosis and functional impairment. *British Journal of Psychiatry*, **136**, 256–269.

Jorm, A. (2000) Is depression a risk factor for dementia or cognitive decline? A review. *Gerontology*, **46**, 219–227.

Joyston-Bechal, M. P. (1966) The clinical features and outcome of stupor. *British Journal of Psychiatry*, **117**, 967–981.

Khachaturian, A. S., Corcoran, C. D., Mayer, L. S., *et al*. Cache County Study Investigators (2004) Apolipoprotein E epsilon4 count affects age at onset of Alzheimer disease, but not lifetime susceptibility: the Cache County Study. *Archives of General Psychiatry*, **61**, 518–524.

Kirshner, H. S. (2002) *Behavioural Neurology. Practical Science of Mind and Brain*. Oxford: Butterworth-Heinemann.

Kopelman, M. D. (1982) Speech dominance, handedness and electro-convulsions. *Psychological Medicine*, **12**, 667–670.

Kopelman, M. D. (1987) Two types of confabulation. *Journal of Neurology, Neurosurgery, and Psychiatry*, **50**, 1482–1487.

Kopelman, M. D. (1991) Frontal dysfunction and memory deficits in the alcoholic Korsakoff syndrome and Alzheimer-type dementia. *Brain*, **114**, 117–137.

Kopelman, M. D. (1994) Structured psychiatric interview: assessment of the cognitive state. *British Journal of Hospital Medicine*, **52**, 277–281.

Kopelman, M. D. (2002) Disorders of memory. *Brain*, **125**, 2152–2190.

Kopelman, M. D. & Corn, T. H. (1988) Cholinergic 'blockade' as a model for cholinergic depletion: a comparison of the memory deficits with those of Alzheimer-type dementia and the alcoholic Korsakoff syndrome. *Brain*, **111**, 1079–1110.

Kopelman, M. D. & Fleminger, S. (2002) Experience and perspectives on the classification of organic mental disorders. *Psychopathology*, **35**, 76–81.

Kopelman, M. D., Wilson, B. A. & Baddeley, A. D. (1990) *The Autobiographical Memory Interview*. Bury St Edmunds: Thames Valley Test Company.

Korsakoff, S. S. (1889) Psychic disorder in conjunction with peripheral neuritis. Translated and republished by M. Victor and P. I. Yakovlev (1955). *Neurology*, **5**, 394–406.

Lezak, M. D., Howieson, D. B. & Loring, D. W. (2004) *Neuropsychological Assessment* (4th edn). Oxford: Oxford University Press.

Lilly, R., Cummings, J. L., Benson, F., *et al* (1983) The human Kluver–Bucy syndrome. *Neurology*, **33**, 1141–1145.

Lindesay, J., Rockwood, K. & Rolfson, D. (2002) The epidemiology of delirium. In *Delirium in Old Age* (eds J. Lindesay, K. Rockwood & A. McDonald), pp. 27–50. Oxford: Oxford University Press.

Lipowski, Z. J. (1990) *Delirium: Acute Brain Failure in Man*. Springfield, IL: Charles C. Thomas.

Lishman, W. A. (1998) *Organic Psychiatry. The Psychological Consequences of Cerebral Disorder* (3rd edn). Oxford: Blackwell Scientific.

Livingston, G. (1994) The scale of the problem. In *Dementia* (eds A. Burns & R. Levy), pp. 21–35. London: Chapman & Hall Medical.

Lockwood, K. A., Alexopoulos, G. S. & Van Gorp, W. G. (2002) Executive dysfunction in geriatric depression. *American Journal of Psychiatry*, **159**, 1119–1126.

Looi, J. C. L. & Sachdev, P. S. (2000) Vascular dementia as a frontal subcortical system dysfunction. *Psychological Medicine*, **30**, 997–1003.

Luria, A. R. (1947) *Traumatic Aphasia* (translated and republished 1970). The Hague: Mounton Press.

Luria, A. R. (1966) *Higher Cortical Functions in Man*. London: Tavistock.

Mackenzie, I. R., Baker, M., West, G., *et al* (2006) A family with tau-negative frontotemporal dementia and neuronal intranuclear inclusions linked to chromosome 17. *Brain*, **129**, 853–867.

Marsden, C. D. (1985) Assessment of dementia. In *Handbook of Clinical Neurology, Vol. 2: Neurobehavioural Disorders* (ed. J. A. M. Frederiks), pp. 221–232. Oxford: Elsevier Science.

Mathuranath, P. H., Nestor, P. J., Berrios, G. E., *et al* (2000) A brief cognitive test battery to differentiate Alzheimer's disease and frontotemporal dementia. *Neurology*, **55**, 1613–1620.

Matthews, P. M. & Jezzard, P. (2004) Functional magnetic resonance imaging. *Journal of Neurology, Neurosurgery, and Psychiatry*, **75**, 6–12.

McArthur, J. C. (2002) Neurological manifestations of HIV infection. In *Diseases of the Nervous System, Vol. 2: Clinical Neuroscience and Therapeutic Principles* (3rd edn) (eds A. K. Asbury, G. M. McKhann, W. I. McDonald, *et al.*), pp. 1683–1709. Cambridge: Cambridge University Press.

McCarthy, R. A. & Warrington, E. K. (1990) *Cognitive Neuropsychology: A Clinical Introduction*. London: Academic Press.

McKeith, I. G. (2002) Dementia with Lewy bodies. *British Journal of Psychiatry*, **180**, 144–147.

McKeith, I. G., Galasko, D., Kosaka, K., *et al* (1996) Clinical and pathological diagnosis of dementia with Lewy bodies (DLB): report of the Consortium on Dementia with Lewy Bodies (CDLB) International Workgroup. *Neurology*, **47**, 1113–1124.

McKeith, I. G., Dickson, D. W., Lowe, J., *et al* (2005) Diagnosis and management of dementia with Lewy bodies: third report of the DLB Consortium. *Neurology*, **65**, 1863–1872.

McKhann, G., Drachman, D., Folstein, M., *et al* (1984) Clinical diagnosis of Alzheimer's disease: report on the NINCDS–ADRDA work group under the auspices of the Dept of Health and Human Services Task Force on Alzheimer's disease. *Neurology*, **34**, 939–944.

McManus, I. C. (1985) Handedness, language dominance and aphasia: a genetic model. *Psychological Medicine*, monograph suppl. 8.

Mendez, M. F. & Cummings, J. L. (2003) *Dementia. A Clinical Approach* (3rd edn). Philadelphia: Butterworth-Heinemann Health.

Mesulam, M.-M. (2000) Behavioural neuroanatomy, large-scale networks, association cortex, frontal syndromes, the limbic system, and hemispheric specialisations. In *Principles of Behavioural and Cognitive Neurology* (2nd edn) (ed. M.-M. Mesulam), pp. 1–120. Oxford: Oxford University Press.

Meyer, M. R., Tschanz, J. T., Norton, M. C., *et al* (1998) APOE genotype predicts when – not whether – one is predisposed to develop Alzheimer disease. *Nature Genetics*, **19**, 321–322.

Micale, M. S. (1990) Hysteria and its historiography: the future perspective. *History of Psychiatry*, **1**, 33–124.

Milner, B. (1963) Effects of different brain lesions on card sorting. *Archives of Neurology*, **9**, 90–100.

Mirea, A. & Cummings, J. (2000) Neuropsychiatric aspects of dementia. In *Dementia* (2nd edn) (ed. J. O'Brien, D. Ames & A. Burns), pp. 61–79. London: Arnold.

Murphy, F. C., Sahakian, B. J. & O'Carroll, R. E. (1998) Cognitive impairment in depression: psychological models and clinical issues. In *New Models for Depression. Advances in Biological Psychiatry, Vol. 19* (eds D. Ebert & K. P. Ebmeir), pp. 1–33. Basel: Karger.

Nance, M. A. & Westphal, B. (2002) Comprehensive care in Huntington's disease. In *Huntington's Disease* (3rd edn) (eds G. Bates, P. S. Harper & L. Jones), pp. 475–500. Oxford: Oxford University Press.

Neary, D., Snowden, J. S., Gustafson, L., *et al* (1998) Frontotemporal lobar degeneration. A consensus on clinical diagnostic criteria. Neurology, 51, 1546–1554.

Nestor, P. & Hodges, J. R. (2001) The clinical approach to assessing patients with early-onset dementia. In *Early-Onset Dementia: A Multidisciplinary Approach* (ed. J. R. Hodges), pp. 23–46. Oxford. Oxford University Press.

Newcombe, F. (1969) *Missile Wounds of the Brain: A Study of Psychological Deficits*. Oxford: Oxford University Press.

Osuntokun, B. O., Sahota, A., Ogunniyi, A. O., *et al* (1995) Lack of an association between apolipoprotein E epsilon 4 and Alzheimer's disease in elderly Nigerians. *Annals of Neurology*, **38**, 463–465.

Paulsen, J. S. & Robinson, R. G. (2001) Huntington's disease. In *Early-Onset Dementia: A Multidisciplinary Approach* (ed. J. R. Hodges), pp. 338–366. Oxford: Oxford University Press.

Petersen, R. C. (2003) *Mild Cognitive Impairment. Aging to Alzheimer's Disease*. Oxford: Oxford University Press.

Petersen, R. C., Doody, R., Kurz, A., *et al* (2001) Current concepts in mild cognitive impairment. *Archives of Neurology*, **58**, 1985–1992.

Petersen, R. C., Thomas, R. G., Grundman, M., *et al.* Alzheimer's Disease Cooperative Study Group (2005) Vitamin E and donepezil for the treatment of mild cognitive impairment. *New England Journal of Medicine*, **352**, 2379–2388.

Phiel, C. J., Wilson, C. A., Lee, V. M.-Y., *et al* (2003) GSK-3 alpha regulates production of Alzheimer's disease amyloid-beta peptides. *Nature*, **423**, 435–439.

Philpot, M. (2005) The neurophysiology of dementia. In *Dementia* (3rd edn) (eds J. O'Brien, D. Ames & A. Burns), pp. 179–192. London: Hodder Arnold.

Pickering-Brown, S. M., Richardson, A. M. T., Snowden, J. S., *et al* (2002) Inherited frontotemporal dementia in nine British families associated with intronic mutations in the tau gene. *Brain*, **125**, 732–751.

Plum, F. & Posner, J. B. (1982) *Diagnosis of Stupor and Coma* (3rd edn) Philadelphia, PA: F. A. Davis.

Prusiner, S. B. (1998) Prions. *Proceedings of the National Academy of Sciences USA*, **95**, 13363–13383.

Prusiner, S. B. & Hsiao, K. K. (1994) Human prion diseases. *Annals of Neurology*, **35**, 385–395.

Raven, J. C., Court, J. H. & Raven, J. (1977) *Manual for the Standard Progressive Matrices*. London: H. K. Lewis.

Ravikumar, B., Vacher, C., Berger, Z., *et al* (2004) Inhibition of mTOR induces autophagy and reduces toxicity of polyglutamine expansions in fly and mouse models of Huntington disease. *Nature Genetics*, **36**, 585–595.

Robbins, T. W. & Sahakian, B. J. (2002) Computer methods of assessment of cognitive function. In *Principles and Practice of Geriatric Psychiatry* (2nd edn) (eds J. R. M. Copeland, M. T. Abou-Saleh & D. G. Blazer), pp. 147–151. Chichester: John Wiley & Sons.

Rockwood, K., Wentzel, C., Hachinski, V., *et al* (2000) Prevalence and outcomes of vascular cognitive impairment. Vascular cognitive impairment investigators of the Canadian Study of Health and Ageing. *Neurology*, **54**, 447–451.

Rosenblatt, A., Ranen, N. G., Nance, M. A., *et al* (1999) *A Physician's Guide to the Management of Huntington's Disease* (2nd edn). New York: Huntington's Disease Society of America.

Roth, M., Huppert, F. A., Mountjoy, C. Q., *et al* (1999) *CAMDEX-R. The Revised Cambridge Examination for Mental Disorders of the Elderly* (2nd edn). Cambridge: Cambridge University Press.

Semmes, J., Weinstein, S., Ghent, L., *et al* (1960) *Somatosensory Changes After Penetrating Brain Wounds in Man*. Cambridge, MA: Harvard University Press.

Shallice, T. (1988) *From Neuropsychology to Mental Structure*. New York: Cambridge University Press.

Snell, R. G., MacMillan, J. C. F., Cheadle, J. P., *et al* (1993) Relationship between trinucleotide repeat expansion and phenotypic variation in Huntington's disease. *Nature Genetics*, **4**, 1–6.

Snowden, J. S., Neary, D. & Mann, D. M. A. (1996) *Fronto-Temporal Lobar Degeneration: Fronto-Temporal Dementia, Progressive Aphasia, Semantic Dementia*. New York: Churchill Livingstone.

Snowden, J. S., Neary, D. & Mann, D. M. A. (2002) Frontotemporal dementia. *British Journal of Psychiatry*, **180**, 140–143.

Snowdon, D. A., Greiner, L. H., Mortimer, J. A., *et al* (1997) Brain infarction and the clinical expression of Alzheimer disease. The Nun study. *JAMA*, **277**, 813–817.

Spencer, M. D., Knight, R. S. G. & Will, R. G. (2002) First hundred cases of variant Creutzfeldt–Jakob disease: retrospective case note review of early psychiatric and neurological features. *BMJ*, **324**, 1479–1482.

Spreen, S. & Strauss, E. (1998) *A Compendium of Neuropsychological Tests*. Oxford: Oxford University Press.

Steffens, D. C., Otey, E., Alexopoulos, G. S., *et al* (2006) Perspectives on depression, mild cognitive impairment, and cognitive decline. *Archives of General Psychiatry*, **63**, 130–138.

Stevens, J. M. & Fox, N. C. (2001) Structural imaging. In *Early-Onset Dementia: A Multidisciplinary Approach* (ed. J. R. Hodges), pp. 124–141. Oxford: Oxford University Press.

Stevens, T., Livingston, G., Kitchen, G., *et al* (2002) Islington study of dementia subtypes in the community. *British Journal of Psychiatry*, **180**, 270–276.

Stewart, R. (2002) The interface between cerebrovascular disease, dementia and depression. In *Vascular Disease and Affective Disorders* (eds E. Chiu, D. Ames & C. Katona), pp. 189–202. London: Martin Dunitz.

Stuss, D. T. & Benson, D. F. (1986) *The Frontal Lobes*. New York: Raven Press.

Swainson, R., Hodges, J. R., Galton, C. J., *et al* (2001) Early detection and differential diagnosis of Alzheimer's disease and depression with neuropsychological tasks. *Dementia and Geriatric Cognitive Disorders*, **12**, 265–280.

Taylor, M. A. & Fink, M. (2003) Catatonia in psychiatric classification: a home of its own. *American Journal of Psychiatry*, **160**, 1233–1241.

Teasdale, G. & Jennett, B. (1974) Assessment of coma and impaired consciousness: a practical scale. *Lancet, ii*, 81–84.

Tiraboschi, P., Hansen, L. A., Alford, M., *et al* (2002) Early and widespread cholinergic losses differentiate dementia with Lewy bodies from Alzheimer disease. *Archives of General Psychiatry*, **59**, 946–951.

Tomlinson, B., Blessed, G. & Roth, M. (1970) Observations on the brains of demented old people. *Journal of the Neurological Sciences*, **11**, 205–242.

Turner, M. A., Moran, N. F. & Kopelman, M. D. (2002) Subcortical dementia. *British Journal of Psychiatry*, **180**, 148–151.

van der Zee, J., Rademakers, R., Engelborghs, S., *et al* (2006) A Belgian ancestral haplotype harbours a highly prevalent mutation for 17q21-linked tau-negative FTLD. *Brain*, **129**, 841–852.

van Hemert, A. M., van der Mast, R. C., Hengeveld, M. W., *et al* (1994) Excess mortality in general hospital patients with delirium: a 5-year follow-up of 519 patients seen in psychiatric consultation. *Journal of Psychosomatic Research*, **38**, 339–346.

Victor, J., Adams, R. D. & Collins, G. H. (1971) *The Wernicke–Korsakoff Syndrome*. Philadelphia, PA: F. A. Davis.

Warrington, E. K. & McCarthy, R. A. (1990) *Cognitive Neuropsychology. A Clinical Introduction*. London: Academic Press.

Warrington, E. K. & Shallice, T. (1969) The selective impairment of auditory verbal short-term memory. *Brain*, **92**, 885–896.

Watt, D. C. & Seller, A. (1993) A clinico-genetic study of psychiatric disorder in Huntington's chorea. *Psychological Medicine*, monograph suppl. 23.

Waxman, S. G. & Geschwind, N. (1975) The interictal behaviour syndrome of temporal lobe epilepsy. *Archives of General Psychiatry*, **32**, 1580–1586.

Wechsler, D. (1998) *Weschler Memory Scale – III*. New York: Psychological Corporation.

Wells, C. E. (1979) Pseudo-dementia. *American Journal of Psychiatry*, **136**, 895–900.

Wilson, B. A. (1987) *Rehabilitation of Memory*. New York: Guilford Press.

Wilson, R. S., Mendes de Leon, C. F., Bennett, D. A., *et al* (2004) Depressive symptoms and cognitive decline in a community population of older persons. *Journal of Neurology, Neurosurgery, and Psychiatry*, **75**, 126–129.

World Health Organization (1992) *Classification of Mental and Behavioural Disorders* (10th revision) (ICD–10). Geneva: WHO.

CHAPTER 21

Psychiatric aspects of neurological disorders

Jonathan Bird and Danny Rogers

Epilepsy is the quintessential neuropsychiatric disorder and one of the greatest teaching grounds in the understanding of the relationship between brain function and behaviour. This chapter therefore begins with that condition. It goes on to consider the other two major categories of neurological disorder of psychiatric significance, head injury and cerebrovascular disease. There then follows a brief review of a miscellaneous group of other neurological disorders, which includes multiple sclerosis. Carcinomas and infectious diseases may present with neurological and psychiatric signs and symptoms, and these are next reviewed. Finally, the various psychomotor disorders are discussed, including Parkinson's disease and Tourette's syndrome.

Epilepsy

Although the question 'What is epilepsy?' is complex, the basic definition has only three elements:

1 paroxysmal abnormalities of the electrical activity of the brain, seen on electroencephalography (EEG)

2 associated abnormality of brain function, at the same time as the electrical discharge

3 a tendency to recurrence.

The first and second elements together form a seizure; the third makes the condition epilepsy. The differential diagnosis of epilepsy is shown in Box 21.1.

Box 21.1 Differential diagnosis of epilepsy

- Syncope, orthostatic hypotension
- Dysrhythmias (especially Romano–Ward syndrome or prolonged QT interval)
- Aortic stenosis
- Transient ischaemic attacks
- Hypoglycaemia
- Migraine
- Narcolepsy and cataplexy
- Night-terrors and sleep-walking
- Pseudo-epileptic attacks (non-epileptic attack disorder)
- Hysterical amnesia and fugue
- Toxic and metabolic disorders (including drugs and alcohol)

Epidemiology

About 4% of the population will have one or more seizures at some time in their life, but 0.8% will have active epilepsy that requires long-term treatment. The ages of onset are in the neonatal period, the late teens and old age (Chaplin *et al*, 1992).

Prognosis

About 70% of those who have a first seizure will have a further seizure, and about 50% of those will have fewer than ten seizures in their lives. The prognosis for further seizures is much worse if the EEG is abnormal. Thirty per cent of patients who are seizure free for 5 years will have further seizures when taken off anti-epileptic drugs (Shorvon, 1990).

Classification

The Commission of the International League Against Epilepsy (1989) (ILAE) has classified epileptic syndromes and related seizure disorders into four major groups: localisation-related; generalised; undetermined; and special syndromes.

Generalised and localisation-related epilepsies are further subdivided into idiopathic, symptomatic and cryptogenic. Seizures may be either partial (focal) or generalised. Partial seizures may become secondarily generalised. Partial seizures are either simple (without impaired consciousness) or complex (with impaired consciousness). These divisions are relevant to the aetiology, management and prognosis, and so are important distinctions to make. They are set out in Box 21.2.

Generalised seizures have no aura or warning; sudden loss of consciousness (even if very brief) is invariable. An aura (warning) is evidence of partial seizures. It is therefore important to take an accurate history and to obtain witness statements.

Stages of a seizure

Prodromes may occur for some hours or days before a fit and are not necessarily evidence of partial seizures. These consist of non-specific and rather vague mood changes or a sense of unease. Their cause is unclear, but they may be due to deep-seated focal seizure activity or,

Box 21.2 International classification of epileptic seizures

I Partial seizures (seizures beginning locally)
- A Simple partial seizures (consciousness not impaired)
  - 1 With motor symptoms
  - 2 With somatosensory or special sensory symptoms
  - 3 With autonomic symptoms
  - 4 With psychic symptoms
- B Complex partial seizures (with impairment of consciousness)
  - 1 Beginning as simple partial seizures and progressing to impairment of consciousness.
    - a With no other features
    - b With features as in A1–4
    - c With automatisms
  - 2 With impairment of consciousness at onset.
    - a With no other features
    - b With features as in A1–4
    - c With automatisms
- C Partial seizures secondarily generalised.

II Generalised seizures (bilaterally symmetrical and without lead onset)
- A
  - 1 Absence seizures
  - 2 Atypical absence seizures
- B Myoclonic seizures
- C Clonic seizures
- D Tonic seizures
- E Tonic–clonic seizures
- F Atonic seizures

III Unclassified epileptic seizures (inadequate or incomplete data).

Adapted from *Epilepsia* (1981), **22**, 489–501, with permission.

conversely, some other change in brain state which sets the scene for a seizure to occur.

The aura (from the Greek for 'gentle breeze', the wind before a storm) consists of acute perceptual, mood or behavioural changes and may occur alone, without further development or generalisation. The aura is, in itself, a focal seizure. It is likely to indicate the region of brain involved. Further spread of the abnormal epileptic activity results in a form of Jacksonian march, with characteristic progression of symptoms and signs and eventually a loss of consciousness as the discharge becomes generalised and involves the deeper subcortical structures.

The study of auras and focal seizures in relation to neuropathology and surgery has added to the understanding of functional neuroanatomy (Penfield, 1967).

In adults the usual form of generalisation is to a tonic–clonic seizure – initial rigidity with respiratory arrest, followed by generalised jerking movements. In children 'absences', with flickering eyelids and mild twitching on occasion (petit mal), is the typical form of generalised seizure, but these rarely continue after the age of 20 and very rarely start after this age. The term 'petit mal' should, properly, be used only for such seizures accompanied by 3 Hz spike and wave EEG changes. 'Atypical' absence attacks may be similar but show slower spike or polyspike and wave discharges.

Post-ictal abnormalities may give a clue to the focus. Paralysis of a limb (Todd's paresis) indicates focal motor epilepsy; dysphasias and other focal impairments can occur but may be misleading as to the origin of the seizure. Confusion, headache and muscle pains are common non-specific post-ictal changes. Occasionally more prolonged amnesic episodes, and confusional, delirious and fugue states may occur.

Ictal phenomena

As mentioned above, the nature of the aura is often the most important factor indicating the site of the focus (Palmini & Gloor, 1992). About 80% of adult seizures are of focal origin and start as partial complex seizures (although the aura may be very brief). Some are clinically generalised from the beginning, even though the EEG shows a brief focal origin.

About 75% of focal seizures originate in the temporal lobes; of these, 80% are in the deep mesial temporal structures, particularly the amygdala and hippocampus (Currie *et al*, 1971). Another 15–20% of focal seizures originate in the frontal lobes, about 5% in the parietal lobes and about 3% in the occipital lobes. The typical auras of these regions are described in Table 21.1.

While close observation of the seizure, its nature and duration may allow a considerable degree of localisation of the focus, its rapid spread is likely to result in difficulty in being precise. The absolute start of the seizure is undoubtedly the most important indicator. Behavioural or experiential changes may precede EEG changes and are likely to indicate a deeper origin, for example the amygdala or cingulate gyrus.

Temporal lobe seizures are not only the most common but also the most likely to be mistaken for 'psychiatric' disorder, owing to the appearance of atypical emotion (especially fear), as well as the possible presence of auditory or visual misperceptions and hallucinations. Derealisation and depersonalisation may cause diagnostic confusion and may be difficult to distinguish from panic disorder. It appears that the mesial temporal lobes are involved in integrating sensory input, memory and emotion and in creating a sense of self. Paroxysmal disturbance of this region is therefore likely to result in disorders of particular interest to the psychiatrist (Gloor, 1990).

Frontal lobe seizures are less common than temporal lobe seizures, although probably more widespread than previously realised. Most frontal seizures involve motor activity. The patient may have experienced no aura because of the immediate loss of consciousness. They are often very brief and frequent and are more likely to be nocturnal. However, seizures arising in the cingulate region, in particular, may give rise to affective changes as well as complex automatisms akin to those seen in temporal lobe epilepsy. Frontal seizures with an unclear precise origin may cause bimanual/bipedal automatisms, such as clapping or stamping, associated with complex verbalisations like singing and at times with other semi-purposive automatisms (e.g. sexual manipulation) and may therefore earn the epithet 'functional' or 'hysterical'. The 'supplementary motor area' of the mesial/frontal lobe may be the origin of such seizures.

Table 21.1 Characteristics of typical epileptic aura, by origin

Site of origin	Percentage of partial seizures accounted for	Characteristics
Temporal lobe	75% (80% of these mesial – amygdala, hippocampus)	Mesial – rising epigastric aura, déjà vu, fear, derealisation, motionless stare, oro-alimentary and gestural automatisms Lateral – auditory and visual illusions, dreamy state, dysphasia if dominant lobe Posterior – dizziness, vomiting, complex visual hallucinations
Frontal lobe	15–20% (mostly supplementary motor area)	Non-specific 'cephalic' aura Motor automatisms – 'fencing' posture, versive eye and head movement, speech arrest or bizarre vocalisation (e.g. singing) Bilaterally coordinated limb movements (e.g. clapping) Contralateral clonic Jacksonian march if motor strip Brief, frequent, dramatic, nocturnal seizures, with immediate recovery Often misdiagnosed as 'hysterical'
Parietal lobe	5%	Sensory auras, tingling, numbness, sense of movement Visual distortions and formed hallucinations The sensation of an inability to move
Occipital lobe	3%	Fleeting visual phenomena – scotomas, flashes, simple hallucinations

Parietal and occipital seizures are still less common. They are often due to some progressive lesion and are less likely to be seen by a psychiatrist. However, the abnormal perceptions (somatic, sensory and visual) may be misdiagnosed as 'functional'. Of course, they are indeed functional disturbances, but as this term is usually taken to signify 'non-organic', perhaps the correct term should imply 'organic cause not yet discovered'.

Visual hallucinations may be seen in both posterior temporal and occipital seizures. Temporal seizures cause complex visual hallucinations (e.g. Lilliputian), while occipital seizures cause simple visual hallucinations such as flashes or spectra, and scotomas in the opposite half field.

Psychiatric aspects of epilepsy

A history of epilepsy, even for a patient with no seizures since childhood and not currently on any anti-epileptic medication, is associated with:

- increased psychopathology of almost all types
- increased cognitive deficits of all types
- increased psychosocial problems, including reduced educational achievement, reduced levels of employment, lower likelihood of marriage and fewer children.

People with epilepsy are 3.7 times as likely as the normal population to have had a history of depression before the onset of the epilepsy and people with a history of epilepsy are 17 times more likely to be depressed than the normal population. The suicide risk is increased fivefold in people with epilepsy. Of interest is the finding that people with schizophrenia appear to be less likely to develop epilepsy than the normal population, whereas people with epilepsy are between 2 and 4 times as likely to develop schizophrenia as the general population.

Psychoses associated with epilepsy

The psychoses associated with epilepsy are best divided into those related to the seizure and those seen interictally in people with epilepsy. The former are usually brief, the latter chronic. Seizure-related psychoses may be either ictal or post-ictal.

Ictal psychoses

Ictal psychosis includes automatisms and non-convulsive status and are the result of ongoing paroxysmal brain discharges.

Automatisms are part of the seizure associated with clouded or absent consciousness; patients experiencing an automatism usually show simple, repetitive movement or wandering with confusion and irritation. In 80% they last less than 5 minutes and very few last more than 1 hour.

Non-convulsive status may be due to simple partial status (usually with motor manifestations), petit mal status or complex partial status. Petit mal status (also called absence status) can start at any age and is associated with altered consciousness, myoclonic flickering of the eyelids and generalised 3 Hz spike and wave discharges on the EEG.

Complex partial status results in mental confusion and psychosis, with a fluctuating level of consciousness which may be associated with complex automatisms, episodic hallucinations and marked mood changes that may be misdiagnosed as a 'functional' psychosis. Early and energetic treatment with intravenous lorazepam is important as persistent intellectual deficit may occasionally occur after prolonged complex partial status. The EEG is diagnostic and is an early and essential investigation in confusional psychoses.

Post-ictal psychoses

Post-ictal psychoses are poorly studied and loosely defined, despite their relative frequency. Post-ictal confusion with accompanying EEG slow-wave changes is common and may, on occasion, last up to a few hours. Post-ictal confusional psychoses are traditionally divided into two forms – fugues and twilight states. The fugue is a prolonged episode of wandering, altered behaviour, amnesia and impaired consciousness, which may last for hours or even days. The EEG is often free of ictal or post-ictal changes. It appears likely that the fugue is a dissociative phenomenon provoked by the seizure. Twilight states are particularly characterised by abnormal subjective experiences (perceptual and affective) and are also associated with cognitive impairment and perseveration. Paranoid hallucinatory disturbances may also be present. Electroconvulsive therapy (ECT) may be dramatically effective treatment if this state does not resolve itself. Such twilight states may be due to sub-ictal, focal paroxysmal activity detectable with depth electrodes and this observation has been used to support of the notion of an epileptic origin for the episodic dyscontrol syndrome (see below), also commonly referred to as 'temporolimbic disorder'.

The current concept of post-ictal psychosis, especially in the presence of temporal lobe epilepsy, is that there is a preponderance of affective change at the same time as a significant admixture of paranoid delusional beliefs. Some studies (Wieser *et al*, 1985; So *et al*, 1990; Wolf, 1991; Mathern *et al*, 1995) have attempted to explore the underlying neurophysiology and neuropathology of the development of post-ictal psychosis but much controversy remains as to the underlying pathophysiological mechanism.

Chronic inter-ictal psychoses

There is no doubt that psychoses that are phenomenologically indistinguishable from schizophrenia (although usually of a paranoid–persecutory kind) have an increased prevalence in people with temporal lobe epilepsy (Logsdail & Toone, 1988; Savard *et al*, 1991; Mace 1993). The risk is about 3%. Commonly the presentation is of a chronic paranoid hallucinatory psychosis with 'first rank' symptoms. Certain features in the history, however, distinguish this condition from schizophrenia (Toone *et al*, 1982) – there is no increased family history of schizophrenia, there is usually a good premorbid personality and less personality deterioration, and these patients tend to have a warmer affect. There is also an increased incidence of neurological abnormality on examination. Typically, the psychosis emerges 10–15 years after the onset of epilepsy and there may be a reduction in the severity of the epilepsy as the psychosis develops. Risk factors include alien tissue lesions (hamartomas), an aura of fear, being left-handed, having a mesial temporal focus and onset of epilepsy in adolescence (Taylor, 1975). It is now established that a left temporal focus is particularly associated with psychosis, as was initially demonstrated by Flor-Henry (1969), with 62% of people with the condition having a left temporal focus, 15% a right temporal focus and 23% bilateral foci. The suggestion by Flor-Henry that right temporal foci are associated with affective psychosis has not been confirmed, and bipolar illness is no more frequently associated with epilepsy than would be expected in the general population.

Aetiological theories concerning the schizophrenia of epilepsy fall into two groups. The kindling hypothesis suggests that there is frequent or constant sub-ictal paroxysmal activity in the mesial temporal structures, which leads to the progressive establishment of abnormal limbic connections, eventually resulting in the symptoms of schizophrenia. It is, for instance, possible that the frequent association of ictal fear or rage with ordinary sensory input would eventually result in established paranoid delusions about the significance of everyday occurrences. The second hypothesis suggests that impairment of brain functioning causes first the epilepsy and then the psychosis.

The management of the psychoses of epilepsy is as with any other psychoses. The newer 'atypical' antipsychotic agents appear to be less epileptogenic than the typical antipsychotics. Chlorpromazine and clozapine are probably best avoided, although, on occasion, intractable schizophrenia with epilepsy can be successfully (albeit very cautiously) treated with clozapine. Reduction in anti-epileptic medication may be possible and appropriate if the epilepsy has been under good control.

Occasionally, transient psychoses with hallucinations, delusions, irritability and restlessness may occur when the epilepsy is brought under control, for example by the administration of a new anti-epileptic drug or surgery (Trimble, 1992). At this time the EEG may become normal, which is known as 'forced normalisation' (Landolt, 1958). Treatment with ECT or a reduction of anticonvulsant medication may be necessary. This form of 'alternating psychosis' is rare (although possibly more common in those with learning disability) but of interest.

Mood and epilepsy

Ictal emotion

Fear is the commonest ictal emotion (Daly, 1958); even when it is not recalled by the patient, witnesses may report that he or she appeared terrified. However, sudden severe depression of mood has often been reported in relation to temporal seizures (or even partial complex status). Rarely, elation is experienced, as described by Dostoevsky with his own seizures. Ictal emotions tend to lack clear and understandable precipitants, to start and stop suddenly, and to have a hard, primitive, unvarying 'organic' quality to them, which 'functional' mood disorders lack.

Depressed or altered mood may be seen both in prodromal and post-ictal stages. Of course, after a seizure, patients may be understandably distressed about the implication of the attack.

Inter-ictal mood disorder

Depression and anxiety are the commonest inter-ictal psychiatric disorders, occurring in 15–45% of patients, major affective disorder showing a prevalence of 11% in the population with epilepsy, compared with 4.9% in the general population. The lifetime prevalence of depression in epilepsy is 62%, compared with 17% in the general population.

It is not clear whether inter-ictal mood disorders are particularly associated with any form of focus of epilepsy (although there is an indication that a left-sided focus is more likely to be associated with an affective disorder than a right-sided focus) and conflicting results have been obtained in different surveys. Associated features include high anxiety and high hostility scores, an 'endogenous' picture in 40%, a relationship with a long history of epilepsy and currently taking phenobarbitone (Robertson *et al*, 1987, 1994). After a temporal lobe neurosurgical resection there is a 10% risk of the development of significant affective disorder.

The aetiology of depression in epilepsy is undoubtedly a mixture of biological and psychosocial factors. Increased monoamine levels result in an increased seizure threshold (supported by the fact that many antidepressants actually reduce seizure frequency) and the corollary of this is that reduced monoaminergic activity, as presumed in depression, may be epileptogenic. The psychosocial factors involved are likely to include the experience of external locus of control and epilepsy combined with learned helplessness. Secondary social and family reactions such as stigma, overprotection and poor financial status are likely to contribute. People with epilepsy suffer more negative life events than the general population. There is also the fact that sexual dysfunction is found in 14–66% of individuals with epilepsy.

The management of depression with epilepsy will include exploration of all the above issues and appropriately alternating anti-epileptic medication, as well as counselling and psychotherapy. If antidepressants are required, they must be used with an awareness that some of the older ones are potentially epileptogenic, although a number of modern antidepressants are clearly effective and safe and may actually reduce seizure frequency. Antidepressants must be started at low dosage and increase must be slow. It is probably best to avoid maprotiline, amoxapine, clomipramine and bupropion. The safest antidepressants appear to be most of the selective serotonin reuptake inhibitors (SSRIs), venlafaxine, mirtazapine and trazodone, even though a number of these contain warnings against their use in epilepsy. Nearly all antidepressants will increase seizure frequency when taken in overdose.

There are a number of important interactions between anti-epileptic drugs and antidepressants. Phenobarbitone, phenytoin and carbamazepine are all liver-enzyme inducers and are likely to reduce levels of antidepressant. The SSRIs, on the other hand, may increase levels of phenytoin and carbamazepine. Mirtazapine and carbamazepine, it has been suggested, result in an increased risk of agranulocytosis and there are rare reports of the serotonin syndrome on a combination of fluoxetine and carbamazepine. However, in the great majority of people with epilepsy requiring treatment with antidepressants, these interactions are largely irrelevant.

Interestingly, ECT may be an effective treatment, even in those still having natural seizures, although the patient's anticonvulsants may well increase the seizure threshold.

Personality and epilepsy

The individual with epilepsy was traditionally thought of as 'spiritless, stupid, unsociable, slow to learn and bewildered', as Aretaeus, a Kappadocian physician of the Roman era wrote; however, he also recognised that this might be 'either from the nature of the disease or from wounds during the attack'. The debate about whether any enduring personality characteristics are due to the brain disorder or are secondary to the social, medical and other effects of epilepsy has continued since then. During the Dark Ages epilepsy was widely thought to be due to possession by demons, even though Hippocrates had declared it to be the result of to brain malfunction in 400 BC. The witchhunters' guide *Malleus Maleficarum* (1486) instructed its readers in ways to distinguish between natural and spiritual manifestations, in a fashion rather similar to current-day lists of the distinguishing features of true and pseudo-epileptic seizures.

The enlightened neurological physician Gowers wrote in 1883 that any personality deterioration in epilepsy is a direct result of the frequency of seizures. However, at that time, the degeneracy theory of Morel held sway; this regarded epilepsy as the reflection of a hereditary stigma, part of the inevitable decline across the generations of certain families afflicted with moral insanity, mental illness, idiocy and dementia. Epilepsy was seen as a manifestation of that decline and as such showed an association with particular personality attributes. The 'epileptic personality' was regarded as pedantic, circumstantial, religiose, critical, irritable and 'viscous' (sticky) in thought. The 'epileptic' was also said to show characteristic facies – unflatteringly described by Kraepelin in 1904.

A more enlightened view developed and it then became held that such personality changes as might occur in people with epilepsy were due to stigmatisation, institutionalisation and medication, especially bromides and barbiturates, or were the result of the brain damage or inherited dysfunction that also causes the epilepsy.

However, in the 1940s and 1950s, epileptologists began to identify patients with temporal lobe seizures more reliably (from EEG) and to postulate that personality disorder could arise from persistent temporal lobe seizure discharges (Geschwind, 1965, 1979). Bear and Fedio (1977) published an influential paper detailing the results of a questionnaire study of patients with epilepsy and their relatives. The questionnaire was based on a literature search of all reports of psychiatric changes in patients with complex partial seizures. The results indicated that patients with temporal lobe epilepsy tended to show humourless sobriety, dependence, circumstantiality, obsessionality, preoccupation with religious and pseudo-philosophical concerns and irritability. A right temporal focus was said to be associated with emotionality and with hypergraphia (writing a great deal) (Okamura *et al*, 1993), while a left temporal focus was said to be associated with a ruminative intellectual tendency. When patients' questionnaires were compared with those of their relatives, patients with right temporal lobe epilepsy tended to improve on the description of their activities ('polishers'), while those with left temporal lobe epilepsy tended to over-report bad traits ('tarnishers').

It seems likely that only a subgroup of patients with temporal lobe epilepsy show this syndrome. Viscosity has been shown to be associated with left temporal foci and is seen as an inter-ictal language disturbance (Rao *et al*, 1992).

Other seizure types, apart possibly from certain of the idiopathic generalised epilepsies (Perini *et al*, 1996), do not seem to be especially related to any particular personality type, but the effects of developing epilepsy at an important stage of personality development, family attitudes, difficulty finding work and the effects of medication would all have a bearing on the individual's reaction to the diagnosis and personality. A combination of dependency, poor social skills, interrupted education, oversedation, parental overprotectiveness, low self-esteem and popular prejudice is likely to lead to social isolation, frustration and despondency.

The current evidence is that personality in epilepsy is characterised by diversity and it appears as though epilepsy accentuates extremes of behaviour. Individuals with epilepsy may show increased emotionality and yet at the same time reduced emotional life and content; they may show more irritability but at the same time more apathy. A summary of the evidence concerning personality disorders and epilepsy concludes that 'Current data do not support or refute any consistent clustering of behavioural traits in epilepsy' (Rataccio & Devinsky, 2001).

It is interesting that individuals with frontal lobe epilepsy rarely show the sort of personality difficulties seen in patients with mass lesions of the frontal regions, although some patients with long-standing epilepsy may develop impaired behavioural control (Helmstaedter *et al*, 1996).

Aggression and epilepsy

There continues to be considerable debate concerning whether aggressive behaviour is seen more commonly in people with epilepsy than in a normal control population. Compounding factors include the presence of brain damage, lower social class and stigmatisation. Pathological aggression occurs in 4–50% of patients with epilepsy, a range that indicates questionable validity. The rate of criminal offences is three times higher than in the general population and the rate of epilepsy in the prison population is 0.7% (compared with 0.5% in the general population), although prison population variables (particularly IQ and social class) may explain the difference. The crimes committed by people with epilepsy are usually non-violent. If there is any significant relationship between epilepsy and violence, it may be classified as ictal, possibly ictal and probably not ictal.

Ictal violence

Violence may be done to others in a seizure. Such episodes are usually the result of poor handling of a confused ictal or post-ictal patient, for example because someone simply got in the way of convulsing arms or because of fearful hitting out by the patient if roughly restrained. Very rarely – in 13 out of 4500 seizures in one study (Currie *et al*, 1971) and in 1 patient out of 434 in another (Rodin, 1973) – violent behaviour occurs as part of an automatism or post-ictal state. Ictal violence as a result of an automatism is usually poorly directed, purposeless, fragmentary, simple and repetitive, as well as very brief. It may consist of a continuation of a behaviour instigated before the seizure began.

Criteria for determining that a criminal act was done during a seizure are detailed in Box 21.3; this may of course be important for medico-legal purposes.

Box 21.3 Criteria for determination that a criminal act was ictal (Fenwick 1990)

- Confirmed clinical history of epilepsy – preferably with abnormal EEG and a history of automatisms.
- Lack of apparent motivation, planning or pre-meditation.
- Little attempt to conceal the crime or to escape.
- Brief duration (usually less than a few minutes).
- Inappropriate behaviour evident.
- Evidence of impaired or altered consciousness from witnesses.
- Amnesia for the behaviour.

Possibly ictal violence – the episodic dyscontrol syndrome

There has been persistent debate about whether or not deep (particularly amygdala) paroxysmal discharges that do not show on the scalp EEG could cause episodes of violent dyscontrol and thus whether impulsive outbursts of violent or potentially violent behaviour could be a form of partial epilepsy (Mark & Ervin, 1970; Bach-y-Rita *et al*, 1971; Maletzky, 1973). There have been several case reports of such disturbances seen on depth electrode recordings, although populations studied have not always been normal and have sometimes been prisoners. Also the electrophysiological activity of the normal amygdala is very poorly understood. The disorder has, however, gained diagnostic respectability in so far as it has a category in DSM–IV, as 'intermittent explosive disorder' (American Psychiatric Association, 1994).

The generally accepted features of such disorders include:

1 sudden, paroxysmal onset ('uncontrollable storms of aggression' – Maletzky, 1973)

2 behaviour (usually serious assault or destruction of property and usually related to a close family member) grossly out of proportion to any stress, precipitant or provocation

3 subsequent genuine remorse

4 hazy recollection only (or amnesia) for the episode

5 out of character, and between episodes a lack of generalised aggressiveness.

This syndrome is associated with a history of developmental delays and specific learning difficulties, previous head injury and epilepsy, and there may be non-specific EEG changes (e.g. temporal sharp wave abnormalities or posterior sharp waves). There is also sometimes a family history of violence and epilepsy. Those with episodic dyscontrol syndrome may have a chaotic personal social and work history; the condition is also briefly discussed on page 460.

Management involves the use of anti-epileptic drugs (particularly carbamazepine, although no satisfactory trial has been done) and psychological approaches to the control and the avoidance of aggression. Benzodiazepines may make the problem worse. Lithium, the SSRIs, sodium valproate, neuroleptics and propranolol have all been advocated at various times.

Probably not ictal violence

Epilepsy may be associated with criminal (violent or non-violent) behaviour for several reasons which are not directly related to the seizure. These will include:

1 organic brain disorder (e.g. in the frontal or temporal lobes), which may lead both to epilepsy and to offence behaviour

2 the social rejection and stigmatisation brought by epilepsy, and hence frustration and offence behaviour

3 the fact that both offending and epilepsy are associated with adverse social factors (low social class, non-accidental injury, violent families)

4 the fact that a tendency to antisocial behaviour (e.g. alcohol misuse, reckless driving) leads both to offence behaviour and to brain injury, which can cause epilepsy.

Non-epileptic attack disorders (pseudo-seizures, hysterical seizures)

The distinction between epileptic seizures and non-epileptic ('hysterical') seizures has taxed doctors since Roman times. Twenty per cent of patients with apparently intractable epilepsy have non-epileptic attacks, although they may have a combination of true and pseudo-epilepsy. Patients with true epilepsy are, indeed, among the most likely to have pseudo-seizures. Some 50% of episodes of 'status epilepticus' in accident and emergency departments are found to be 'pseudo-status' (*Lancet*, 1989).

The term 'non-epileptic attack disorders' describes a heterogeneous group, with a wide spectrum of morbidity. Different forms of non-epileptic seizure may present to different specialists. Pseudo-epileptic status will usually present to general physicians in an acute fashion, while neurologists are likely to see patients with pseudo-seizures of a 'generalised' form. Psychiatrists tend to see those with brief 'partial complex'-like attacks and specialist centres more often assess or manage those with an intractable combination of epilepsy and non-epilepsy. The views of these professionals differ and lead to difficulty in achieving a consensus (Betts, 1990). When distinguishing between epileptic and non-epileptic seizures, neurologists tend to list clinical findings (negative in non-epileptic seizures) and psychiatrists tend to list historical and psychodynamic features (positive patients with non-epileptic seizures). The distinction is summarised in Box 21.4. At times, however, it may seem impossible to decide whether an individual's attacks are epileptic or not, and Landouzy's term 'hystero-epilepsy' seems closest to the truth (Leis *et al*, 1992).

Box 21.4 Features more often found in non-epileptic seizures

History
- Psychiatric disorder
- Family history of psychiatric disorder
- Deliberate self-harm
- Sexual maladjustment
- Hysterical personality is present in only a few (perhaps less than 25%)

Current state
- Presence of affective disorder
- Intense current psychosocial stressors

The attack
- Emotional precipitant, with evidence of primary or secondary gain
- Gradual onset, with a prolonged warning
- Wide range of often bizarre events and behaviour (e.g. talking, screaming, struggling)
- Pelvic thrusting is particularly characteristic, as well as unresponsiveness in the absence of significant motor activity
- Varied, not stereotyped attack pattern
- Lack of true tonic and then clonic movements
- Suggestibility (regarding starting, stopping and changing nature)
- Tongue biting, incontinence and injury are rare but certainly can occur
- Nocturnal episodes may occur and the EEG will demonstrate this as an arousal phenomenon not occurring during sleep itself
- Left-sided (non-dominant) somatosensory symptoms and signs may be more frequent

Post-ictal characteristics

True confusion is rare after a pseudo-seizure; the patient may laugh or smile (it may not be an unpleasant feeling) or may recall events during the pseudo-seizure in detailed fashion.

Investigations

The EEG (e.g. ambulatory monitoring) is normal during and after an attack, although movement artefact may make interpretation difficult. Also, very localised true epileptic attacks may show no surface abnormality. The continuation of alpha rhythm during an attack in which consciousness is apparently lost almost always indicates a non-epileptic attack. However, brief frontal seizures may be very difficult to pick up on EEG. Video-telemetry, in which clinical acumen can be applied to observation of the detailed nature of the attack, even if the EEG is obscured may be invaluable here. It allows the very stereotyped (and therefore probably epileptic) or the very non-stereotyped (and probably non-epileptic) nature of the seizure to be examined.

Serum prolactin levels can also be used to distinguish true from pseudo-seizures. After generalised seizures, the level is usually over 1000 IU/ml, and even in partial attacks it may be 500 IU/ml, but in non-epileptic attacks it is usually normal, although it can be somewhat raised (Dana-Haeri *et al*, 1983). Prolactin levels taken within 20 minutes of the start of the seizure may be diagnostic in generalised attacks but less helpful in partial ones. Frontal lobe seizures may be particularly difficult to distinguish on this basis. The use of prolactin levels has not been as helpful as was initially hoped and it is vital to have a comparative baseline level.

Management of non-epileptic attack disorders

The earlier a diagnosis of non-epileptic seizures is made the better, as reinforcement of illness behaviour with drugs or medical attention can be avoided. Once it is established (preferably with EEG) that the attacks are non-epileptic, gradual withdrawal of any anti-epileptic prescribed is advised, probably as an in-patient. The attitude of ward staff should be one of 'benign neglect' so far as the attacks are concerned, and the family and other patients on the ward must also learn that this is the correct approach. Considerable psychotherapeutic discussion with patient and family will be necessary if the diagnosis of 'epilepsy' has been long established. The patient must be reassured that reducing anti-epileptics is not only safe but positively beneficial, as it returns control to the individual and reduces sedation. A family-based cognitive and behavioural approach to the change in diagnosis is usually best. This can be combined with psychotherapeutic exploration of the patient's past; it is apparently increasingly common for a history of sexual abuse to be uncovered, but the presence of non-epileptic seizures must not be taken as proof of such abuse and uncovering it is no guarantee of cure. A drug-assisted interview using diazepam or sodium amylobarbitone may help to access the patient's problems. If an 'attack' is videoed, this can be shown to the patient and discussed, using it as part of a therapeutic programme. Occasionally 'attacks' may be provoked by suggestion.

Cognitive function and epilepsy

With the increasing investigation of focal epilepsies by neuropsychologists, it has become evident that 'material-specific' focal neuropsychological deficits may occur, developing as the epilepsy develops. This is particularly relevant in individuals with left temporal lobe epilepsy, which is found in association with material-specific verbal memory deficits.

Cognitive function in people with epilepsy may be impaired by drug intoxication (Thompson & Trimble, 1982), non-convulsive status and possibly by subclinical paroxysmal discharges, such as hippocampal spike activity. It is clear that brief petit mal absence attacks may go unnoticed by the patient or those nearby and yet can significantly impair registration of memory at the time. The same may apply to brief focal discharges. Post-ictal amnesia and partial amnesias may be misdiagnosed as a dementing process, especially if frequent seizures leave the individual in an almost continuous post-ictal state.

Inter-ictal cognitive impairment and decline are much debated (Brown & Reynolds, 1981). It is clear that epilepsy need not be related to any intellectual impairment. There have been many famous people who have suffered from epilepsy, including the generals Julius Caesar, Alexander the Great and Napoleon, the writers Dostoevsky, Tennyson, Carroll, Lear and Kierkegaard, the mathematicians Newton and Pascal, artists such as Van Gogh and a number of religious leaders. Taken as a whole, patients with epilepsy will have a normal mean IQ, provided that cases of epilepsy associated as a secondary phenomenon with brain damage (congenital or otherwise) are excluded. Inter-ictal cognitive impairment may be the result of sedative anti-epileptic drugs, interrupted and poor education, parental attitudes and personal reactions to the illness.

However, specific memory and learning deficits can be associated with specific epilepsies, for example verbal memory impairment with left temporal lobe epilepsy and impaired attention with generalised epilepsy. The main determinant of cognitive impairment is the aetiology of the epilepsy. Early onset, length of illness and frequency of seizures are weakly related to cognitive impairment.

'Epileptic dementia' (a progressive decline in cognitive function) primarily related to the epilepsy may occur in a very small proportion of cases (it is debatable whether it occurs at all or is due to medication, underlying organic factors or additional pathology). It does seem, however, that there are rare cases of epilepsy – generally of early onset, long duration and high severity – that are accompanied by an inexorable but slow intellectual decline, usually associated with severe personality deterioration. This is more common in patients with a known brain lesion and may be associated with reduced reserves due to brain damage, resulting in early dementia.

In very rare cases sodium valproate has been associated with behavioural decline, with return of normal functioning on cessation of the drug. Topiramate is also associated, in about 10–15% of cases, with mental slowing and reduced verbal fluency.

Psychological induction and inhibition of seizures

A very high proportion (92%) of people with epilepsy identify psychological states as precipitants or facilitators of their seizures, especially tension, depression, tiredness and being overexcited (Antebi & Bird, 1993). More specifically, there are many single case reports of particular affective and cognitive stimuli directly provoking reflex seizures in susceptible individuals, for example mental arithmetic, playing cards or chess, reading specific lines, or even looking at a safety pin in one famous case. It seems likely that there is an interaction between the presentation of the specific stimulus and the current state of the individual.

A small proportion of patients with epilepsy (perhaps 2%, although this figure depends on the sample) are able to induce their own seizures by some conscious act of will – such as waving a hand in front of the eyes or flickering the eyelids to simulate photic flashing. Many patients (20%) are actively able to avoid situations that put them at risk and 25% of patients with an aura feel that they can abort their seizures by some act of will, such as the sudden diversion of attention or by concentration on some cognitive task.

Management of epilepsy

Inevitably, the main line of management in epilepsy is with anti-epileptic drugs (Reynolds, 1981; Chadwick, 1994). These are dealt with in detail in *Seminars in the Psychiatry of Learning Disabilities* (Frazer & Kerr, 2003) and *Seminars in Clinical Psychopharmacology* (King, 2004) and will not be covered here. The following section covers general principles of management and psychological methods.

Psychological treatment methods

Psychological treatment methods in epilepsy have been largely ignored, which is understandable in the face of the excellent success of pharmacotherapy. However, 10–20% of patients will not be adequately controlled with drugs and, apart from surgical approaches, such as selective amygdalo-hippocampectomy, psychological approaches are the only other treatment. As well as the avoidance of known psychological precipitants of seizures (see above), a number of more specific psychological and behavioural approaches may be effective in some patients (Goldstein, 1990):

- *Reward management*. Here, overt or covert (fantasised) rewards are given for reduced seizure frequency.
- *Self-control strategies*. Many patients use or can be encouraged to develop the sort of seizure inhibition strategies already described. Specific relaxation training, combined with desensitisation and various interventions during the aura period, may also be effective.
- *Conditioning procedures*. Here, the antecedents of seizures are closely studied and a behavioural approach then used.
- *Biofeedback*. Biofeedback of a variety of EEG rhythms (e.g. a sensorimotor rhythm, alpha rhythm, paroxysmal activities) can be successful. Feedback of levels of arousal may be an effective treatment (Nagai *et al*, 2004).
- *Psychotherapy*. Both individual and group psychotherapeutic approaches may well lead to improved life adjustment, reduced stress levels and thereby to reduced seizure frequency.

Head injury

Head injury has been called the 'silent epidemic', resulting as it does in 10% of all visits to accident and emergency departments and in severe permanent disability in 0.1% of the population. The incidence of head injuries is 1500 per 100 000 population each year, 130 of those being of sufficient severity to result in lasting cognitive deficit and 17 resulting in severe physical and cognitive deficit. Males are affected twice as often as females and it is the cause of 15–20% of deaths occurring between the ages of 5 and 25 years in the UK.

Head injury rehabilitation is primarily a neuropsychiatric problem, although many patients, even those with severe disabilities, do not present themselves to medical or psychiatric services – hence the relative silence of the epidemic.

Reviewing Anglo-American neuropsychiatry over the past 200 years, Ovsiew & McClelland (1995) suggested that one of the roles of contemporary neuropsychiatry is that of advocate for brain-injured members of society.

Primary injury

Primary damage to the brain occurs as a result of either rotational or horizontal acceleration or deceleration. Rotational acceleration/deceleration occurs when there is an abrupt transfer of energy to the head after rapid motion is suddenly stopped by contact with a hard object. The brain is tethered at the brain-stem and oscillates around the central axis. First, the rotational acceleration/deceleration results in diffuse shearing of long central fibres and micro-haemorrhages in the corpus callosum and rostral brain-stem. Injury is microscopic but widespread and is termed diffuse axonal injury. Wallerian degeneration of axons in the subcortical white matter and atrophic enlargement of ventricles are eventually seen after severe head injuries. Second, the rotational acceleration/deceleration causes centrifugal pressure waves to spread out so that the poles of the brain undergo repeated buffeting against the skull and tentorium, especially where there are sharp bony edges or corners. The frontal poles, orbital frontal regions, temporal poles and medial temporal structures are therefore particularly damaged. The brain-stem and midbrain may also be contused by the rim of the foramen magnum and the tentorial edge. Horizontal acceleration/deceleration injury will also cause brain contusion at the site of the injury (coup) and on the opposite side of the head (contre-coup).

Secondary injury

Secondary injury to the brain can be the result of various factors. Haemorrhage (subdural, extradural and at times intracerebral) may occur and can result, along with reactive brain swelling and acute fluid collections, in raised intracranial pressure, with a coning of the brain-stem. Later development of obstructive or communicating hydrocephalus may occur. Other, peripheral injuries can have a secondary effect on brain function, particularly hypotensive shock due to peripheral bleeding, anoxia due to respiratory or cardiovascular injury and fat emboli due to fracture of long bones.

Coma, post-traumatic amnesia and other indicators of outcome

Outcome after head injury has been extensively studied, but often without using standardised criteria or comparable measures of the severity of injury. Two main measures of injury severity have emerged: the Glasgow Coma Scale (GCS) and the length of post-traumatic amnesia (PTA).

The GCS is an accumulative 15-point scale (15 = fully alert) based on responsiveness in the three areas of eye opening, gross motor activity and verbalisation (see Table 21.2). If accurately recorded, it gives some indication of outcome. A score of 15 at 24 hours after injury is associated with a bad outcome (death, vegetative state or severe disability) in only 6%, while a score of 3 at 24 hours indicates an 80% chance of bad outcome (Jennett *et al*, 1981).

Table 21.2 The Glasgow Coma Scale

Area	Responsiveness observed	Score
Eye opening	Spontaneous	4
	To speech	3
	To pain	2
	None	1
Motor response	Obedience to commands	6
	Localisation of pain	5
	Withdrawal	4
	Flexion to pain	3
	Extension to pain	2
	None	1
Verbal response	Orientated	5
	Confused conversation	4
	Inappropriate words	3
	Incomprehensible sounds	2
	None	1

The length of post-traumatic amnesia (PTA; also termed anterograde amnesia) is probably a measure of diffuse axonal injury and is one of the best indicators of the severity of the head injury and likely later outcome, except where severe localised damage has occurred. The PTA is the time from injury to restoration of normal, continuous memory. A PTA of between 1 and 24 hours is regarded as moderate and anything over 24 hours as severe. The length of PTA correlates very roughly with eventual outcome, a PTA of more than 24 hours being likely to be associated with some permanent disability, usually of cognition or personality. Lishman (1987) suggests that a PTA of less than 1 hour predicts return to work within a month, a PTA of less than 1 week return to work within 4 months, and a PTA of more than 1 week predicts invalidism for a year, as well as a 50–70% prevalence of severe psychiatric and intellectual disability at 5-year follow-up.

Severe and disabling focal damage and slow crushing damage can occur without a coma or any PTA. Retrograde (pre-traumatic) amnesia is of little relevance and tends to shrink with time. If memory for the injury is not impaired at all, post-traumatic stress disorder may be more likely to occur. Dense and very prolonged retrograde amnesia is likely to be psychogenic.

Age at injury will significantly affect the prognosis. Older people have a relatively poor outcome in terms of mortality and intellectual impairment. Children are more resilient but are vulnerable to developmental delays as a result of specific injury, and there can be a complex and ongoing interaction between the effects of injury and the developing brain (see below on sequelae).

Stages of recovery

Recovery from traumatic brain injury (TBI) occurs in a characteristic sequence of stages. The patient passes from coma into unresponsive vigilance with a return of gross wakefulness. Mute responsiveness follows, with the patient responding to simple instructions. The next stage is a confusional state with severe attentional disturbance, confabulation, denial, perseveration, agitation, disordered sleep and considerable emotional lability at times. Acute 'hysterical' or paranoid features may be present. Subsequent improvement will progress to independence in self-care and increasingly independent intellectual and social functioning.

Neuropsychiatric sequelae

Population studies have shown that individuals with a history of TBI with loss of consciousness or confusion have a significantly higher prevalence of psychiatric disorders and suicide attempts and have a poorer quality of life (Silver *et al*, 2001). A 1-year follow-up of 196 such hospitalised adults showed a higher proportion than the general population developing psychiatric illnesses, especially depressive episodes and panic disorder (Deb *et al*, 1999). The risk of depression remains elevated for decades following head injury, especially if severe (Holsinger *et al*, 2002). Definite psychotic disorder may also emerge after TBI. Schizophreniform disorders occur more often than by chance (about 2.5%) and purely paranoid psychoses in a further 2% (Achte *et al*, 1969) (these complications are also discussed in Chapter 10, page 214). Long-term follow-studies of soldiers who received head injuries in the Second World War revealed a raised rate of the later development of chronic paranoid psychosis, often coming on 10–15 years after the original injury (Achte *et al*, 1969). Psychotic depression occurs in only 1% and very few manic–depressive disorders are apparently a result of TBI. Secondary mania may be more common and one US study gave a rate as high as 9% following TBI (Jorge *et al*, 1993).

Psychological reactions such as depression, anxiety states and irritability often occur as understandable responses to the changes wrought by the injury to lifestyle, employment and family. Premorbid personality, family support, understanding employers and appropriate psychiatric and psychological management are vital in diminishing these reactions.

It is clear that people who suffer head injuries do not constitute a 'normal' population. A study of 80 sequential admissions to one rehabilitation unit (Haas *et al*, 1987) showed that as many as 50% had evidence of premorbid specific learning disabilities. The associated attentional deficits could act as a risk factor for such injuries and premorbid cognitive difficulties should be considered in any post-injury assessments.

Frontal polar damage leads to poor judgement and insight, apathy and impaired problem solving. There is often no understanding of the impact of the disability on others. Orbitofrontal damage results in impaired social judgement, impulsivity, excitability, lack of tact and childishness. Temporal lobe damage will result in memory loss and speech difficulties; it may also lead to irritability and aggressive dyscontrol. Diffuse axonal injury characteristically leads to slowed thinking, impaired arousal and drive, poor concentration and diminished attention, as well as poor cognitive endurance due to disruption of the many subcortical connections, leading to a picture similar to that in the subcortical dementias. Attentional problems are the most common single complaint in head injury rehabilitation.

Specific neuropsychiatric and neurological sequelae include anosmia (the olfactory nerves are particularly vulnerable), other cranial nerve deficits (especially ophthalmoplegias, deafness and visual field defects) and complex movement disorders due to a combination of brain-stem, cerebellar and cortical dysfunctions (e.g. the coarse tremor of red nucleus damage, balance problems, rigidity, slowness and weakness). Communication difficulties may be profound and involve complex dysarthrias, 'pseudobulbar' disorders and impaired intonation, which can combine with impaired facial mobility and a variety of subtle perceptual difficulties to result in severely damaged social skills. A variety of more persistent 'hysterical' disorders with an organic basis may appear for the first time after diffuse brain injury, particularly when caused by anoxia (Eames, 1992).

In children especially, the sequelae can include behavioural disturbances, particularly hyperactivity and explosive outbursts, as well as specific learning difficulties. There is an increasing recognition of the potentially damaging long-term effects of TBI in children.

Aetiological factors in TBI sequelae

The sequelae of injury depend on multiple factors:

- the amount and the location of the brain injury.
- the development of post-traumatic epilepsy (see below)
- age
- premorbid personality (including constitution, psychiatric history, IQ, physical disorder and amount of alcohol ingestion)
- psychological reaction to the injury
- family, social and work factors
- compensation issues
- appropriateness of rehabilitation measures.

Post-traumatic epilepsy

Post-traumatic epilepsy (PTE) falls into two groups. Early seizures are those that occur in the first week and are seen in 2–5% of cases of TBI. These early seizures are usually focal and reflect acute brain injury. About a quarter of patients will go on to develop the second category, late PTE, which develops after 1 week. Only 3% of those without early PTE will develop later fits. Depressed fracture (15% risk) and intracranial haematoma (35% risk) are the other two main predictors for late PTE. Fifty per cent have their first fit in the first year after injury (peak at 6 months) and 80% in the first 4 years.

Development of late PTE is significantly associated with a worse psychological and social prognosis. Annegers *et al* (1998) provide some useful data indicating a 'dose–response' effect for the risks of developing epilepsy over the next 5 years, based on a large survey (of 4541 children and adults with TBI). For those with mild injury (loss of consciousness or amnesia for less than 30 minutes), the standardised incidence ratio was 1.5 (95% CI 1.0–2.2), but as the confidence interval included 1, the authors did not consider this significant. For those with moderate injury (loss of consciousness for 30 minutes up to 24 hours, or a skill fracture) the risk was increased to 2.9 (95% CI 1.9–4.1). However, for those with severe injury (loss of consciousness or amnesia for more than 24 hours, or a subdural haematoma) the risks were greatly increased, at 17.0 (95% CI 12.3–23.6). The multivariate analysis also showed that risks for later seizures were also increased for those with subdural haematoma, skull fracture and amnesia for more than 1 day, and for those aged 65 or over.

Post-concussional syndrome

After a relatively minor-seeming TBI, with brief or even no loss of consciousness, a troublesome but characteristic group of symptoms may occur, usually immediately or within the first one or two weeks after injury. This is termed post concussional syndrome (Lishman, 1988). There appear to be two groups of symptoms.

The first group appears within the first 7–14 days and becomes less prominent later on. They include headache, dizziness, fatigue, blurred vision, double vision, hypersensitivity to noise, nausea, tinnitus, and poor concentration and memory. It is thought that there may be a physical cause for these symptoms – particularly otological (labyrinthine) and cerebral circulation changes and micro-haemorrhages. Investigations such as brain-stem auditory evoked responses and magnetic resonance imaging (MRI) may show changes.

The second group of symptoms usually appears after the first 14 days and may persist for weeks or months. These include anxiety, insomnia, irritability, emotional lability, subjective memory impairment and depression. These may be more psychologically determined, as they are more related to premorbid personality, current stresses, social factors and compensation issues. Initial information processing and memory deficits are organic, and tend to improve over 3–6 months, but subjective cognitive complaints may persist.

Over 50% of people after minor head injuries have symptoms (especially headache and dizziness) for up to 2 months, but only 12% are symptomatic after 1 year. An individual's expectations of sequelae may have powerful effects.

The management of those with minor head injuries and post-concussional syndrome is symptomatic and patients should be offered early advice and reassurance about what to expect and when it is best to return to work, which should be neither too early – which would risk failure – nor too late– which would risk invalidism.

Chronic traumatic encephalopathy ('punch drunk' syndrome)

Repeated rotational TBI, particularly as seen in less successful boxers, can result in chronic traumatic encephalopathy ('punch drunk' syndrome or dementia pugilistica) (Johnson, 1969). This consists of characteristic neurological and psychiatric features with typical neuropathological findings. There is severe neurofibrillary tangle formation but with much less prominent plaque formation than in Alzheimer's dementia, although recent immunocytochemical studies have shown extensive beta-protein (plaque) deposits in severe cases. Cortical and cerebellar atrophy and cavum septum pellucidum are seen on scanning, even before any clinical symptoms appear.

The neurological symptoms result from cerebellar, pyramidal and extrapyramidal damage. Dysarthria, poverty of movement and facial immobility are seen early, followed by ataxia, tremor and spasticity. The main psychiatric features include dementia, apathy, irritability and disinhibition. Paranoid features, and in particular morbid jealousy, may also develop. Progression of neurological and psychiatric features occasionally happens even after the boxing has stopped.

Rehabilitation

The 'gold standard' review of published data on outcome and rehabilitation from traumatic brain injury (Cope, 1995) strongly supported the efficacy of rehabilitation. The process of rehabilitation after head injury must start early and continue late. It is best carried

Box 21.5 A comprehensive head injury service

A comprehensive head injury service will offer all of the following:

- acute triage and initial intensive in-patient hospital care
- a follow-up expert clinic (and team) for all TBI admissions
- intensive and comprehensive rehabilitation after initial recovery for some
- long-term sheltered or in-patient accommodation for a few
- support to patients' families.

out by a comprehensive head injury team (see Box 21.5). Such a team can reduce the need for admissions, concentrate on appropriate cases, provide training, offer consistent advice to the patient and family, and engage in research, as well as providing appropriate and comprehensive rehabilitation programmes. The team should include a neurosurgeon, a neuropsychiatrist, nurses, a neuropsychologist, social workers, physiotherapists, occupational therapists, speech therapists, cognitive therapists and teachers.

Deficits in the activities of daily living require careful *in vivo* assessment and diplomatic management by trained occupational therapists and nurses accustomed to working with patients who have had a head injury, since the combination of emotional fragility and unrealistic self-judgement with variable motivation can be very difficult to handle. Social skills may be deficient and social skills groups are sometimes useful in addition to individual behaviour programmes.

Cognitive deficits should be carefully assessed. Cognitive rehabilitation includes re-education, compensation (for permanent deficits) and substitution of new methods of functioning. Memory aids and strategies may be used, as well as computer retraining techniques. In some cases carefully graded training in problem-solving is helpful.

Severe behaviour disorders have been successfully treated using consistent token-economy behavioural-modification techniques. Some behaviour disorders are partly the result of learning poor coping mechanisms during the early period after the injury and may also result from a lack of proper rehabilitation. Specialised head injury rehabilitation units which provide retraining in a consistent and controlled fashion tend to be more often successful than those that do not.

Drug therapy is best avoided whenever possible. This is because excessive or unusual adverse effects can occur in those with TBI. There are claims that methylphenidate may improve attention and bromocriptine speed of thinking. Stimulants such as the amphetamines improve alertness. Episodic dyscontrol may be reduced by carbamazepine or sodium valproate. Sedative antidepressants, tranquillisers and anticonvulsants (particularly phenytoin) should be used only when absolutely necessary. Post-traumatic psychosis and depression must be properly treated with medication in the usual fashion. Prophylactic anticonvulsants, preferably carbamazepine or valproate, should probably be given if one or more of the poor prognostic indicators are present (namely early seizures, depressed fracture, intracranial haemorrhage).

TBI results in a huge burden of care, largely borne by the immediate relatives. Stress within the family is usually due to the behavioural, personality and cognitive changes rather than physical handicap. Only 50% of patients who have severe TBI can be left in charge of the home for any time. There are major role changes for spouses and the financial strain may be unbearable. Social isolation often results for the whole family. The rehabilitation team will need to involve the family and offer family support at every stage, and careful discharge planning will be required. Work assessment with the help of a disablement employment adviser and the vocational rehabilitation centre may be very helpful. 'Headway', the National Head Injuries Association, a self-help organisation for those with TBI and their families, can offer support and respite day care in an increasing number of centres.

After severe TBI, improvement is usually relatively rapid over the first 6 months. There is further slower physical and cognitive recovery after the next 18 months. After 2 years, further recovery is expected but usually is due to compensation, readjustment and acceptance over the following 3 years. After 5 years, little substantial improvement can be expected, although gains produced by a rehabilitation programme may actually multiply.

A genetic susceptibility to the effect of brain injury, both acutely and in its risk potential for Alzheimer's disease, is becoming increasingly recognised (Friedman *et al*, 1999; Guo *et al*, 2000).

Cerebrovascular disease

Stroke

Stroke, or cerebrovascular accident, results primarily from atherosclerosis and/or hypertension. It occurs in two forms, infarction or haemorrhage. Brief recurrent episodes are termed transient ischaemic attacks.

The nature of the sequelae of a stroke will depend on the main cerebral artery occluded or the area of haemorrhage. About 30% of people who have a stroke show permanent cerebral symptoms, often with severe cognitive impairment, 6% develop seizures and 50% die within 3 years. The focus here is on the psychiatric and cognitive symptoms.

Non-dominant middle cerebral artery occlusion may cause confusional states with few focal signs except sensory loss, inattention and anosognosia, and this may lead to diagnostic difficulties. Occlusion of the anterior cerebral artery may result in global dementia and frontal lobe personality changes. Posterior cerebral artery occlusion causes cortical blindness and denial of disability and sometimes alexia without agraphia, while transient confusion is common. Occlusion of the rostral basilar artery can result in bizarre hallucinations, disorientation and somnolence.

Multi-infarct dementia, possibly with multiple lacunar infarcts, classically presents with stepwise deterioration and progressive global dementia. Gradually progressive organic personality change may also follow, with the individual showing increasing difficulty in coping with new experiences. Anxious or irritable responses to anything unusual are common and may amount to catastrophic responses, perhaps particularly in multi-infarct dementia. Hypochrondiacal and depressive features may predominate. Eventually, emotional flattening, stereotyped reactions and irritability may be very marked.

Depression is common after stroke, occurring in around one-third of cases, and usually lasts for at least 6 months. Clinical depression must be distinguished from the reasonable resignation in an elderly person, understandable distress at the disability, underlying or exacerbated personality traits, and cognitive impairment with mental slowing. Causation is likely to be multifactorial, and a premorbid history of anxiety or depression, previous personality and a lack of family support may all contribute. Stroke lesions themselves, however, can cause depression; the correlation of severity of depression with proximity of the stroke lesion to the frontal pole is a consistent clinicopathological finding (Lyketsos *et al*, 1998). The depression responds to antidepressant medication, as does emotionalism, which affects 20–25% of survivors in the first 6 months after stroke. After a stroke, pathological crying may be attributed to partial destruction of the serotonergic raphe nuclei in the brain-stem or their ascending projections to the hemispheres, and SSRIs can be an effective and well-tolerated treatment.

Subarachnoid haemorrhage

Subarachnoid haemorrhage accounts for 5–10% of all strokes. It affects a younger population than other strokes, at a mean age of 50 years. It results in a specific pattern of deficits and has rehabilitation needs similar to those of TBI. The usual cause is a ruptured berry aneurysm, while angiomas are the cause in 5–10% (no cause is found in 15% of cases).

Persistent memory and dysphasic disability is found in 40% of cases and this may be severe in around 10%. Middle cerebral aneurysms have the most severe cognitive sequelae. Worsening cognitive sequelae after subarachnoid haemorrhage may be due to normal-pressure hydrocephalus, which can be relieved by inserting a ventriculo-peritoneal shunt (normal-pressure hydrocephalus is considered further under 'Miscellaneous neurological disorders'). A severe amnesic syndrome resembling Korsakoff's syndrome may emerge in the days or weeks following the haemorrhage but is usually short-lived.

Severe personality impairment occurs in 20% and mild changes in a further 20% of cases. Anterior communicating artery haemorrhage may result particularly in 'frontal lobe personality disorder', with disinhibition. However, rupture of the middle cerebral artery is associated with both cognitive deficit and personality change, in the form of loss of drive, withdrawal, irritability, anxiety and 'organic moodiness' (shallow, rapidly reactive depression). About 5% of patients are reported to have an improvement in personality, becoming less irritable, anxious, gloomy or obsessional.

Depression and anxiety are found in about 25% of patients, particularly in posterior communicating aneurysms which interfere with the blood supply to the hypothalamus.

Disabling anxiety and agoraphobia may present as a response to subarachnoid haemorrhage. At times symptoms rather like the post-concussional syndrome (fatigue, headache and dizziness) occur and may be psychologically determined. Psychotic disorders occasionally occur.

Subdural haematoma

Subdural haematoma presents either acutely, with stupor or coma together with some evidence of localising signs, or chronically, usually with headache, poor concentration and memory loss, although this may be fluctuating. The cause is usually a head injury, which may be trivial, but spontaneous haematomas also occur. Progression is to variable levels of consciousness down to coma, with few neurological signs, although the pupils are often unequal. Papilloedema is usually absent.

Subdural haematoma may present as a progressive generalised dementia and the true cause can be easily missed unless a computed tomography (CT) scan is performed.

In early cases, surgical evacuation of the haematoma if very successful but cognitive impairment is common if surgery is delayed.

Migraine

Migraine is thought to affect up to 20% of the adult population, although only 7% seek medical attention for it. Precise diagnosis and distinction from tension headaches may be difficult, but unilateral onset, and throbbing headache with nausea, vomiting and photophobia are characteristic; this is termed common migraine. If visual or other neurological phenomena are present, the headache is a classical migraine, or migraine with aura. A particularly severe form is cluster headache or migrainous neuralgia. This consists of marked peri-orbital pain with lacrimation, nasal blockage and sometimes Horner's syndrome. Cluster headaches are so called since attacks occur in bouts lasting several days or weeks, often at the same time each day or night. Precipitation of attacks may result from various dietary factors such as cheese, red wine, coffee or chocolate. Psychological stress has also been implicated but the headache often occurs after the stress is resolved; for example, weekend and holiday migraines are typical. Menstruation, the premenstruum and taking the contraceptive pill may provoke attacks.

Mood changes before and during an attack are common, particularly anxiety, irritability and fatigue. Depression, slowed mentation and poor concentration often occur. Elevation of mood, either before or after the attacks, has also been reported. An altered level of consciousness, mental confusion and even lapses into unconsciousness (migrainous syncope) may be experienced. Dramatic psychiatric symptoms are sometimes seen, including dreamy states, complex hallucinations, amnesia, body image disturbances, autoscopy, forced mood, automatisms and compulsive behaviour. Sacks (1992) illustrates the clinical fascination of migraine for the neuropsychiatrist.

Transient global amnesia

This acute amnesia for recent events but with preservation of alertness and memory for personal identity is thought to be due to reversible ischaemia of the inferomedial temporal lobes. It is seen in late middle age or old age and is associated with a high incidence of cerebrovascular or emotional stresses. Sometimes it is associated with epilepsy, migraine or hippocampal tumours.

The clinical hallmarks are a sudden onset of memory loss for recent events, an inability to register new impressions and retrograde amnesia. Innate abilities (e.g. musical) and personal identity are not lost, but semantic memory and frontal lobe functioning may be affected (Hodges, 1994).

Recovery occurs in less than 24 hours and persistent amnesia for the episode is usually the only deficit. Some patients may go on to develop transient ischaemic attacks or, rarely, completed stroke.

Miscellaneous neurological disorders

Multiple sclerosis

The neuropsychiatric manifestations of multiple sclerosis can be divided into the psychiatric (particularly affective) and the cognitive. The major psychiatric complication in multiple sclerosis is depression (Ron & Logsdail, 1989). Mild elation, denial of disability, optimism and laughing are classically described (Finger, 1998). Euphoria occurs in only 10% and is correlated with MRI changes. Pathological display of emotion – that is, beyond appropriate mood changes – is related to pontine, brain-stem and periventricular lesions. Transient manic, schizophreniform or confusional psychoses may relate to the disease process. It is of interest that schizophreniform psychoses are related to MRI changes in the temporal horn or occasionally may be due to high-dose steroid therapy. Multiple sclerosis rarely presents with psychiatric symptoms, but if it does then neurological signs are usually present as well, as when there is an acute encephalitic onset with confusion (Skegg, 1993).

About half the patients with multiple sclerosis attending hospital have cognitive impairment, particularly in memory, attention and abstracting ability. This may be present before any neurological signs appear. Cognitive deterioration is closely related to the course of the disease, with little evidence of deterioration when the disease is stable. The severity of the cognitive impairment correlates with the overall extent of pathology seen on MRI scans but direct correlation between particular cognitive deficits and localisation of pathology is not yet established (Ron & Logsdail, 1989).

Ron & Feinstein (1992) point out that psychiatric and cognitive abnormalities are often overlooked but add considerably to the patient's distress. Psychiatric disorders should be energetically managed in the usual fashion. Antidepressants are likely to be effective for depression. Cognitive rehabilitation, supportive psychotherapy and family support will also be needed.

Systemic lupus erythematosis (SLE)

Over 50% of patients with SLE show neuropsychiatric manifestations, usually later in the disease, but sometimes before the appearance of other symptoms (Ainiala *et al*, 2001). A wide variety of psychiatric presentations may occur, but often in episodes lasting only a few weeks. Multiple neuropsychiatric symptoms may be present sequentially or together. Thirty per cent of patients show organic reactions, usually brief acute confusional states, but occasionally progressive dementia is seen. Functional psychoses (depressive, schizophrenic or manic) occur in 16% and seizures in up to 50% of patients.

The psychiatric symptoms are almost always directly due to the pathological brain changes (inflammatory changes to small blood vessels), although the relationship is not exact. Steroid therapy is only rarely the cause of the symptoms and may be effective therapy for them.

Polyarteritis nodosa

Polyarteritis nodosa results from focal arteritis of small and medium blood vessels. Cerebral symptoms occur in 50% at the later stages of the disease. Confusional and delirious states are the most common presentation of these.

Motor neuron disease (amyotrophic lateral sclerosis)

This is a slowly progressive disorder with prominent peripheral manifestations (lower motor neuron muscular atrophy with spasticity due to cortical spinal damage). Neuropsychiatric manifestations include: pseudo-bulbar palsy, with loss of emotional control, spastic dysarthria and dysphagia; and frontal lobe dementia (Neary *et al*, 1990), which may, rarely, be of marked degree with loss of paramedial cortical cells, gliosis and spongiform changes. In many patients milder changes are seen in the cortex and subcortical nuclei.

Depression is understandably found in a proportion of patients but not as frequently as might be expected, since denial of unpleasant emotions is said to be particularly prominent in the personalities of people who develop motor neuron disease (Hogg *et al*, 1994); denial may be a useful stratagem in the face of such a debilitating condition.

Friedreich's ataxia

Friedreich's ataxia is a recessively inherited, spinocerebellar ataxia, with kyphoscolosis and pes cavus. It is due to a GAA repeat expansion of the frataxin gene on chromosome 9q13. There is dysarthria, nystagmus, cerebellar dysfunction, hypotonicity, muscle wasting and weakness. The disorder is slowly progressive. Usually there is no initial cognitive impairment but a mild cognitive decline may occur as a result of the extension of the degenerative process into the cortex and a few familial cases may have learning disability.

Personality changes have been reported, particularly immaturity and asociality. Paranoid schizophreniform disorders, with episodes of nocturnal hallucinosis and confusion, may be particularly associated with Friedreich's ataxia, although the evidence is not clear.

Myasthenia gravis

Myasthenia gravis is an autoimmune disorder of motor end-plates that results in abnormal muscle weakness after activity (Sneddon, 1980). The disorder may be significantly aggravated or even precipitated by emotional stress. The symptoms are likely to be socially embarrassing and difficult for others to understand or believe. This leads to more complex psychological reactions in the individual concerned, as well as diagnostic confusion. A diagnosis of hysteria or personality disorder is often mistakenly made initially and, even after trying standard anticholinesterase drugs, tensilon or neostigmine, the diagnosis may remain in doubt if a placebo response is suggested.

Duchenne muscular dystrophy

Duchenne muscular dystrophy is an X-linked recessive disorder in which there is a pseudo-hypertrophy of lower leg and then pelvic girdle muscles due to an abnormal dystrophin gene. There has been considerable debate about whether the associated learning difficulties are an organic or environmental part of the disorder. There is no special relationship with other psychiatric disorders.

Dystrophia myotonica

Dystrophia myotonica is an autosomal dominant myopathy, due to a CTG expansion disorder on chromosome 19q 13.3 characterised by delayed relaxation of skeletal muscles after voluntary contraction (myotonicity) – especially of the hands, forearms and facial muscles. This is accompanied by slowly progressive wasting, weakness and dysarthria. Associated features include cataract, hypogonadism, frontal balding in the male, cardiomyopathy, endocrine anomalies, respiratory arrest after barbiturate anaesthesia and a typical electromyographic (EMG) abnormality. Cerebral involvement is shown by a high rate of EEG abnormality with theta and delta waves and sometimes focal sharp wave discharges. Mental symptoms are seen in up to 80%, with mental impairment being moderate or severe in around one-third of the cases. Social and intellectual decline is seen in families affected by the disease, even in those who do not show the myotonicity. "Anticipation" refers to worsening of the disorder over successive generations. Personalities are said to be characteristic, with poor initiative "(laziness)", somnolence, fatigue and apathy, possibly due to diencephalic and perhaps frontal involvement in the disease process.

Normal-pressure hydrocephalus

This is also known as communicating hydrocephalus and results from blockage of the flow of cerbrospinal fluid (CSF) in the subarachnoid space, usually in the basal cisterns (Vanneste, 1994). Unlike obstructive, non-communicating hydrocephalus, it is not associated with high intra-ventricular pressure. It may be difficult to distinguish from hydrocephalus *ex vacuo*, which is secondary to atrophy, as seen in Alzheimer's disease. Normal-pressure hydrocephalus may be the result of subarachnoid haemorrhage, head injury or meningitis, but 40% of cases are of unknown cause, particularly in patients aged 60 or more.

The characteristic triad of clinical features comprises the gradual development of mental impairment, unsteady gait and urinary incontinence (Pujol *et al*, 1989). Memory loss, slowing of mental activity, reduced spontaneity and impoverished psychic life are the main mental features, leading eventually to a picture of severe dementia. Falling is common but seizures are rare. Initial presentation with depressive or paranoid symptoms can occur and these may be partially responsive to psychotropic medication (Pujol *et al*, 1989). Headache and papilloedema are not features. Focal neurological signs are absent. The EEG usually shows slow wave activity, and the CT scan shows ventricular enlargement, periventricular lucency and generally minimal sulcal widening. Monitoring of intracranial pressure is the most reliable method of establishing the diagnosis; it will show normal or low pressure but with characteristic pressure wave patterns.

Improvement after the insertion of a ventriculo-caval shunt may be dramatic, especially if there has been a complete block to subarachnoid CSF flow. Normal-pressure hydrocephalus is an important differential diagnosis of dementia and resistant or atypical depression, and highlights the importance of ordering a CT or MRI scan in these circumstances.

Bechet's disease

This rare syndrome, caused by a virus, primarily consists of attacks of oral ulceration, genital ulceration and uveitis/iridocyclitis. Involvement of the central nervous system (CNS) is occasionally seen and occurs as a late and ominous complication. Headache, fever, brain-stem signs and a variety of cortical dysfunctions occur in a relapsing and remitting fashion. Confusion and dementia may develop.

Sarcoidosis

Sarcoidosis, with chronic, disseminated granulomatous lesions, affects the CNS in about 5% of cases. The areas most commonly affected are the cranial nerves and the meninges. The brain substance may be involved, especially the hypothalamus and third ventricular region, resulting in somnolence, obesity, memory problems and personality change, and occasionally psychiatric reactions can occur. Fatigue may be a feature of the disease.

As with any severe debilitating condition, depression can occur, more as a result of the respiratory effects of the disease than any cerebral involvement. Thus a large multicentre survey in the USA found that 60% of sarcoid patients attending the chest clinic were depressed and that female sex, increased dyspnoea on exertion and decreased access to medical care were all associated with depression (Chang *et al*, 2001). Occasionally profound dementia or hallucinosis is reported. The diagnosis is made with chest radiography, biopsy of skin lesions and the Kveim test. Elevated levels of serum angiotension-converting enzymes and calcium are also seen, as are abnormal lung function tests. The condition is treated with prednisone; if it is severe high doses are used, and these may cause psychiatric changes, which complicate the picture.

Hallervorden–Spatz disease

This is a rare familial disorder with extrapyramidal symptoms (rigidity, dystonia, choreoathetoid movements), dysarthria, myoclonus, tremor, postural difficulties, personality change, outbursts of aggression and a gradually developing dementia. The biochemical cause of this disorder has recently been clarified and appears to be pantothenate kinase deficiency, and a mutation on the pantothenate kinase gene on band 20p13 has been described in Hallervorden–Spatz disease (Chakravarty *et al*, 2003). The MRI findings are typically of hyper-intense changes in the external segment of the globus pallidus with surrounding hypo-intensity. The hyper-intensity is related to neuronal less and axonal swelling, and the hypo-intensity to iron deposition in the substantia nigra.

An infantile form presents below the age of 6 with death typically around 8 years later; most other cases present between the ages of 7 and 15, with death some 15–20 years later.

Carcinoma

The neuropsychiatric manifestations of carcinoma fall into three categories:

- the general effect of brain tumours
- the local effects, arising from damage to the area of the brain affected by the tumour
- the non-metastatic complications of carcinoma, which include the psychological effects on sufferers and their families.

There is also the question of the role of stress in precipitating cancer, but that is not examined here.

General effects of brain tumours

The general effects of brain tumours are largely due to raised intracranial pressure; they therefore include headache, drowsiness, confusion and apathy. Raised intracranial pressure can also lead to coma if it is left untreated.

Local effects of brain tumours

Local effects will depend on the nature of the tumour (speed of growth, degree of malignancy) and its location. Rapid growth and malignancy (e.g. with gliomas) are associated with more severe mental disturbance, but slow-growing benign tumours (usually meningiomas) may present with psychiatric symptoms and personality change alone and are more easily misdiagnosed. Multiple tumours (usually metastases) are associated with a particularly high level of mental symptoms, especially confusion and cognitive impairment. Frontal and temporal lobe tumours are much more likely to present with mental symptoms than parietal, occipital or infra-tentorial tumours (Hunter *et al*, 1968). Seizures may be a presenting feature, especially with temporal and occipital tumours. In general, there are few reliable relationships between tumour site and psychiatric presentation, but the following may be significant.

Frontal lobe tumours

Often these show very few neurological signs initially but patients can present with irritability, atypical depression and apathy, memory impairment, cognitive slowing and inertia, or disinhibition, childishness and euphoria. Urinary incontinence can also occur.

Temporal lobe tumours

These may present with seizures, dysphasia, memory loss, affective disorder or, occasionally, schizophreniform disorders. Complex visual, auditory, olfactory and gustatory hallucinations characteristically result from temporal lobe tumours.

Parietal lobe tumours

These are less likely to cause psychiatric symptoms, but can result in disturbance of body image (which may suggest hysteria), depression and, rarely, personality change.

Occipital tumours

Occipital tumours are not usually associated with an increased presentation of psychiatric symptoms.

Corpus callosum tumours

These are especially associated with the development of rapid, severe cognitive deterioration. Delusional psychosis, catatonia and stupor may occur.

Tumour of the hypothalamus and third ventricle

These may present with a marked amnesic confabulatory (Korsakoff) syndrome. Removal of craniopharyngiomas from this region may result in a combination of frontal apathy, subcortical slowing, obesity and somnolence which is particularly resistant to rehabilitation. Cysts of the third ventricle may cause progressive dementia due to obstruction of CSF circulation. The combination of worsening intellectual deficit and hypersomnolence (and sometimes with apparent narcolepsy and even cataplexy) strongly suggests a diencephalic tumour.

Pituitary tumours

Pituitary tumours are said to cause mental slowing and apathy, at times with emotional lability and paranoid ideation. They may also result in multiple endocrine changes and problems due to expansion into the diencephalons and temporal regions.

Non-metastatic complications of carcinoma

Between 5% and 10% of extracranial tumours cause some form of distant neurological or myopathic disorder, with about half of these presenting with neurological manifestations. This is most frequent with lung cancer. Sensory or sensorimotor peripheral neuropathy, myopathy with bulbar palsy and sub-acute cerebellar degeneration are well-known non-metastatic effects. Of particular interest to the psychiatrist are the associated encephalopathies. Degenerative and inflammatory changes are seen and may be the result of an altered immunological state and resultant viral invasion. Limbic encephalopathy causes a Korsakoff-like disorder, but with depression, anxiety and occasionally hallucinations.

Depression and suicidal ideation are well established as occasional presenting features of carcinoma, even before a diagnosis has been made. Premonitions of illness may occur up to 6 months before any physical symptoms in up to 50% of cases. The new development of depression in middle or late life is significantly associated with a subsequent diagnosis of carcinoma.

Diagnosis

The widespread availability of CT and MRI scans has eased the fear of misdiagnosis of brain tumour as a functional disorder. The main misdiagnoses are dementia, neurotic depression and hysteria. In most studies of the psychiatric use of CT scanning, the number of tumours discovered is very small. However, the issue is of great importance. Meningiomas are particularly problematic, as early diagnosis and surgery can be curative, but they may be discovered late, when removal is difficult or permanent injury has resulted.

A number of tumours found on CT scanning may be incidental to the psychiatric disorder present. It is still necessary to have a high, but proper, index of suspicion in clinical practice since, clearly, only a small proportion of psychiatric patients can be scanned. However, in cases where there are particular indications (Box 21.6) scanning must be carried out.

Box 21.6 Clinical indications for further CT or MRI investigations for patients presenting with psychiatric disorders

- Atypical presentation, for example of depression with marked apathy
- Schizophrenia with prominent perceptual abnormalities
- Lack of response to appropriate treatment
- Progressive neurological symptoms (which should be examined for)
- Episodic dysfunctions (suggesting partial seizures)
- Headache
- Disturbance of level of consciousness
- Unexplained personality change

Infectious diseases

Infectious diseases are rarely a cause of diagnostic confusion in neuropsychiatry, except for the initial presentations of encephalitis and neurosyphilis. At one time it was feared that HIV infection would result in an avalanche of neuropsychiatric manifestations. However, psychiatric and cognitive manifestations are almost always confined to late stages of the disease, at which time other needs are usually more pressing. In developing countries, chronic parasitic infections remain prominent causes of neuropsychiatric symptoms.

Encephalitis (particularly herpes simplex)

Encephalitis is usually viral and occasionally pyogenic (meningo-encephalitis), but often the precise aetiology is unclear. The commonest single identifiable cause in the UK is herpes simplex, which may also be the most severe form.

Presentation is usually with severe, progressive headache, vomiting, papilloedema, reduced level of consciousness and coma. However, patients may present with seizures, delirium or psychotic symptoms. Focal neurological signs and psychiatric symptoms, especially those indicative of temporal lobe dysfunction (e.g. dysphasia, auditory hallucinations, bizarre behaviour), are usually suggestive of herpes simplex involvement. Early symptoms may include catatonia, thought disorder, overexcitement and delusions.

It is vital to recognise this disorder since early treatment may be life-saving and the mortality is high. Diagnosis is made with antibody titres, but early use of the EEG demonstrating periodic lateralised epileptiform discharges may give vital clues and this is one of the most important indications for an urgent EEG. Treatment is with acyclovir, an antiviral agent, and should be given even in cases of doubt. Dexamethasone may be helpful when intracerebral pressure is raised.

Encephalitides (particularly herpes simplex) carry a high risk of prolonged neuropsychiatric morbidity and also have a high mortality (Kapur *et al*, 1994). About half the survivors show a prolonged episode of disturbed behaviour, with restless distractability and poor social adjustment. This may slowly improve, but many are left with dense amnesias, mood disorders, personality change, Kluver–Bucy-type symptoms and social disinhibition. Post-encephalitic neuropsychiatric disorders form a small but significant group of people with chronic brain damage.

Other identifiable encephalitides include coxsackie B infection, Lyme disease (neuroborreliosis) as well as epidemic encephalitis (various types – transmitted by ticks or mosquitoes), equine encephalomyelitis (eastern or western – mosquito borne), infections of the echo virus and cytomegalovirus, and the various sub-acute and chronic encephalitic viral diseases (measles, mumps, rubella). The last group may cause sub-acute sclerosing panencephalitis (SSPE). This has its onset in childhood or adolescence and produces a progressive dementia and mood changes, associated with seizures and myoclonic jerks, and has a fatal course usually lasting less than 18 months. The EEG indicative of SSPE has complex repetitive generalised high-voltage slow wave discharges, which are synchronous in all leads and occur at fixed intervals of 5–10 seconds, along with involuntary jerks.

Encephalitis lethargica is largely of historic interest, but the dramatic sequelae of the 1918 epidemic is described graphically in the book *Awakenings* (Sacks, 1973). However, occasional sporadic cases are still reported, with marked features of parkinsonism, personality change, tics, stereotypies, echolalia, emotional lability, compulsive behaviour, fugues, oculogyric crises and hallucinatory states (Espir & Spalding, 1956). The putative virus was never isolated, although the timing of the onset of some of the cases coincided with influenza epidemics.

Syphilis

In developed countries, syphilis, once rare, is now on the increase. However, in the absence of routine use of venereal disease research laboratory (VDRL) testing, potentially treatable cases may be missed unless there is a high index of suspicion in unusual psychiatric presentations. Syphilis modified by the chance concurrent use of antibiotics for other disorders may be particularly difficult to diagnose.

Syphilis is classically divided into four stages – the localised primary lesion (the chancre), secondary lepto-meningitis, tertiary meningovascular syphilis and the final late stages of tabes dorsalis and general paresis (paralysis) of the insane (GPI). In addition, congenital syphilis may affect the newborn infant, although the condition may not be diagnosed until much later. The pathology of all stages relates to inflammatory responses – lepto-meningitis, obliterative endarteritis and gummas (which are granulomas).

Secondary syphilis may present with headache, lethargy, malaise and slowly progessive forgetfulness and irritability. Occasionally an acute confusional state or seizures develop. Associated cranial nerve phenomena may occur, particularly ophthalmoplegias and the legendary Argyll Robertson pupil (small, irregular pupils reacting to accommodation but not to light). Tertiary meningovascular syphilis may present with almost any focal neurological disorder, from mild headache to stupor, with cranial, particularly third-nerve palsies, aphasia, seizures, progressive dementia, hemiplegia and other manifestations of this protean disorder.

Tabes dorsalis (degeneration of the different fibres of the dorsal roots) takes the form of a slow development of 'lightning pains', which are stabbing severe pains in the legs associated with loss of proprioception and sensory ataxia. Ocular and pupillary signs are also often present.

In about 20% of untreated cases, GPI appears some 8–15 years after the primary infection. Spirochaetes are seen in cortical and subcortical tissue in at least 50% of these cases. Cerebral atrophy occurs in the anterior two-thirds of the hemispheres. The CSF VDRL test is positive in all cases, even in the absence of a serum positive VDRL, although the more sensitive and specific fluorescent treponemal antibody absorption test (FRA-ABS) is likely to be positive in serum.

Usually, GPI presents with progressive moodiness, reduced emotional control, shallow affect (apathy or mild euphoria), irritability and other frontal lobe personality changes. Forgetfulness, poor concentration and impaired insight also occur. This 'simple dementing' form comprises 50–60% of cases in the UK (Dewhurst, 1969). In developing countries a 'grandiose' form occurs in 60–70% of cases; this involves euphoria, irritability, grandiose manner and delusions and hypomanic or manic features. This is seen in only 10% of European cases. A 'depressive' form with low mood, melancholic delusions, suicidal thoughts and retardation presents in around 30% of European cases. Paranoid schizophreniform and neurasthenic presentations may also occur. Seizures develop in up to 50% of patients and may be focal. Transient cerebrovascular episodes (e.g. hemiplegia) are seen rarely.

Treatment of all forms of syphilis, including GPI, is with high-dose penicillin, which will usually arrest progress and may lead to some improvement in the mental state. Other psychotropic and supportive measures will also be necessary in most cases.

Human immunodeficiency virus (HIV)

Psychiatric patients are at an increased risk of HIV infection because of their multiple, often illness-related risk behaviour. The brain is infected very early in the disease and cerebral pathology is found in 90% of patients dying of AIDS. This pathology may be related to opportunistic infections, neoplasms or primary HIV CNS infection. Psychiatric disorders, seizures and delirious reactions of various types may occur in the later stages, possibly because of secondary pathologies such as fungal infections, toxoplasmosis or CNS lymphoma, but may also occur because of HIV alone. Finally, the early stages of HIV-associated dementia may result in a picture resembling depression. There is often multiple pathology (Table 21.3).

The current evidence is unclear, but in general there are no early neuropsychological deficits in otherwise asymptomatic HIV infections. Around 6–18 months before clinical AIDS develops, there is a marked increase in the prevalence of major depression, mania, dementia and delirium (Pajonk & Naber, 1998), but significant cognitive decline is almost entirely confined to late stages of the disorder. AIDS dementia, which may be a terminal disorder, is described in Chapter 20 (page 520), and so the account given here focuses on other psychiatric disorders and the role of the psychiatrist in the HIV team.

Psychosocial aspects of HIV

The psychosocial sequelae of HIV vary widely in different countries; for example, in Africa rejection is common, but it is much less frequent in Europe and America. Antiviral drugs were until recently widely available only in the developed world. In his editorial entitled 'One disease, two epidemics – AIDS at 25', Sepkowitz (2006) pointed out that in the richer nations the picture is one of a chronic but treatable disease, where the main problems are the side-effects of the complex drug regimens, drug resistance and the psychological problems of coping with a chronic disease, whereas in the poorer developing nations large numbers of people are still subject to severe neuropsychiatric complications, associated mood disorders, psychosis and AIDs dementia in the years before their death. This

Table 21.3 Neuropathology of HIV

Cause	Manifestations
Opportunistic infections	
Viral	Cytomegalovirus (causing encephalitis), ventriculitis, retinitis and inflammation of the choroid plexus in about 20% Herpes simplex, herpes zoster and progressive multifocal leuco-encephalopathy due to papavovirus
Fungal	Crytococcus – with meningoencephalitis, in 5% *Candida* – with multiple abscesses or meningitis
Parasites	Toxoplasmosis – causing multiple focal necrotic lesions and abscesses in 20%
Neoplasms	Lymphomas: 5%, usually highly malignant, non-Hodgkin's B-cell lymphomas. Epstein–Barr virus may be implicated in the pathogenesis Kaposi's sarcoma: may occur, usually as a secondary from elsewhere
Primary HIV CNS infection	Aseptic meningitis may be an early feature, presenting with headache, fever, neck stiffness and cranial nerve palsies. Vasculitis may also develop. Myelopathy, peripheral neuropathy and myopathy may also develop as a result of primary HIV infection HIV encephalitis with multinucleated giant cells containing viral sequences, distributed multi-focally, in 25% HIV leucoencephalopathy: diffuse with matter damage with inflammation and demyelination, in 13%

used to be picture in the UK before the introduction of effective antiviral regimens.

In the developed world, HIV is still associated with increased rates of psychiatric morbidity, but the severe, life-threatening organic pictures (AIDs dementia) are thankfully now much less frequent. Most of the more recent work emphasises a strong association with substance misuse, as it is now thought that injections are the route of infection in around a third of the cases in the USA, for example (Bing *et al*, 2001). These authors conducted a large national survey based on a representative probability sample ($n = 2864$) of people attending HIV clinics for treatment. The prevalence rates for common psychiatric disorders in the HIV population were compared with rates found in a previous national household survey and the comparative figures were: for major depression 36% (for those with HIV infection) versus 7% (in the national household survey), indicating a fivefold increase; for generalised anxiety disorder the respective figures were 15.8% versus 2.1%; panic attacks 10.5 % versus 2.5%; no drug misuse 50% versus 90%. The absolute rate for drug dependence in the HIV population was 12%. These figures are broadly similar to those reported in the UK a decade previously by King (1989), who made an ICD–9 diagnosis (neurotic depression, and neurotic anxiety and adjustment reactions) in around a third of patients, which was similar to rates reported in other medical settings. In the study by Bing *et al* (2001) factors that independently predicted psychiatric disorder in the HIV population were: drug dependence (odds ratio OR = 3.7), heavy alcohol use (1.35) but not light or moderate alcohol use, and being unemployed (1.59) or having a disability (1.86). The severity of the HIV infection in terms of the number of symptoms was also a predictor for psychiatric disorder. Affective disorders are sometimes associated with more serious disease and occasionally the presence of *Pneumocystitis carinii* infections.

Two subgroups of patients with psychiatric disorder have been shown to be especially at risk of HIV: those who are severely mentally ill and those who misuse substances. It might be expected that those who fit both these categories – the 'dual-diagnosis group' – will have even higher rates. Dausey & Desai (2003) quote studies in the mid-1990s that gave an average HIV seroprevalence rate of 7.8% (range 4–22%) among those who were seriously mentally ill, but in recent years this has fallen, and in their study the rate was 2.4% in singly diagnosed patients, although this is still much higher than the population HIV base rates, of around 0.3–0.4%. Those with dual diagnosis are indeed a high-risk group: their rate was 4.7% (about double the risk for singly diagnosed patients) and HIV was more likely if the person had had sex for money or gifts, had had sex with an intravenous drug user, had shared needles, or reported being raped (Dausey & Desai, 2003). Homelessness may be an additional risk factor (Susser *et al*, 1993). While every effort should be made to target this highly vulnerable group, it is known that both the dual-diagnosis group and the homeless are notoriously difficult to engage in any sort of treatment programme, particularly on a long-term basis,

Children may also suffer from HIV and a recent French study of HIV-positive children presenting to a psychiatric clinic (47% with depression and 29% with attention-deficit/hyperactivity disorder) found that 80% of the children had CD4 lymphocyte counts close to zero, and on this basis the authors concluded that, at least for children, a psychiatric presentation indicated severe infection and that a depressive presentation should be regarded as part of the encephalopathy (Misdrahi *et al*, 2004).

Psychiatric disorders, seizures and delirious reactions of various types may occur in the later stages, possibly because of secondary pathologies such as fungal infections, toxoplasmosis or CNS lymphoma, but may also occur because of HIV alone. Finally, the later stages of HIV-associated dementia may result in a picture resembling depression.

Price & Goyette (2003) summarise the role of the psychiatrist in the HIV treatment team, particularly in areas where there is a high risk of HIV:

- HIV/AIDs may first appear in people with pre-existing mental illness and those attending psychiatric clinics, especially in certain high-risk groups such as intravenous drug users, some patients with a deteriorated chronic psychosis or those with severe personality disorders who are engaging in high-risk behaviours (through choice, ignorance or poverty, e.g. through prostitution). Some patients presenting with purely somatic symptoms of depression such as weight loss and anorexia, which are also symptoms of HIV, may be suspected of having HIV and in these cases HIV testing should be encouraged and appropriate counselling instituted.

- Most referrals to the psychiatrist who works with the HIV team concern newly emergent psychiatric disorder in patients already diagnosed as having HIV. The onset of an episode of psychoses in these cases is particularly alarming and both referrers and sufferers demand immediate attention. Depression may have many causes apart from the HIV and it is the psychiatrist's task to clarify these. Antidepressant drugs may interact with retrovirals: thus, the non-nucleoside reverse inhibitors and protease inhibitors may elevate levels of selective serotonin reuptake inhibitor, and St John's wort can result in sub-optimal antiretroviral levels. Drug interactions are also described between reverse protease inhibitors and benzodiazepine anxiolytics and hypnotics such as aprazolam, midazolam and triazolam. New anti-retroviral drugs are constantly being introduced and the prescribing psychiatrist should always consult with the pharmacy for interactions before introducing a particular psychotropic drug.
- The prognosis of HIV in recent years has dramatically improved with the introduction of the protease inhibitors. However, patients have to follow complex drug regimens, often taking many different tablets several times a day. Non-compliance is common: for example, Gordillo *et al* (1999) gave a figure of 50%, as well as dangerous, since omitting medication for even a few days can lead to the emergence of resistant strains of this rapidly mutating virus. Psychiatric disorder can affect compliance and a study based on the General Health Questionnaire in an Australian HIV clinic found that 44% of non-complaint HIV sufferers were 'GHQ positive', which was more than four times the rate for the compliant patients (Sternhill & Corr, 2002). In a Spanish study, poorer compliance rates were also associated with younger individuals, intravenous drug use, depression and lack of perceived social support (Gordillo *et al*, 1999). Price & Goyette (2003) describe cases of non-compliance in the HIV clinic where there is comorbid depression, personality disorder, relationship difficulties, substance misuse, manipulative behaviour and attendance at multiple therapeutic agencies. These patients may split treatment teams, but psychiatrists are all too familiar with such patterns of behaviour and can help the general medical team to unravel such complex interactions before they destroy the therapeutic efforts of the team.

Tuberculosis

Epidemiological studies of tuberculosis (TB) today show that while rates are generally low in most Western countries, there are small pockets, such as in New York, where rates may be rising. TB tends to be a disease confined to the urban poor, the elderly and those with AIDS; in the UK, immigrants from Asia may be especially vulnerable. Some of the de-institutionalised patients with schizophrenia have joined the ranks of the urban poor and this group may also be at particular risk, as may those still in asylums or in nursing homes, and the disease should always be suspected among those in the high-risk groups. Tuberculosis is undoubtedly a major problem in developing countries, and Daniel (1991) estimated that half the world's population is infected with *Mycobacterium tuberculosis*, with each year seeing 30 million active cases, 10 million new cases and 3 million deaths from TB (6% of all deaths worldwide). Most of these deaths are due to pulmonary TB, and neuropsychiatric presentations are rare.

Typhoid

This acute infectious disease is caused by *Salmonella typhi* and, rarely, *paratyphi*. Diarrhoea and gastro-intestinal presentation are most frequent, but acute pyrexial confusional states occur in severe cases. In addition, post-typhoid psychosis, usually schizophreniform, has been reported and is common in Africa, as is post-typhoid amnesia. Focal cortical symptoms due to meningitis may also occur.

Typhus

This disease is caused by the parasite *Rickettsia prowazekii*, which is carried by the body louse. There is direct CNS infection, with microscopic nodules in vessel walls and thrombosis. Before the introduction of chloramphenicol and tetracycline, 60% of those infected died.

The disease presents with fever, headache, insomnia, delirium, meningism, focal cortical symptoms, cranial nerve signs and acute delirium alternating with stupor. Cerebellar and peripheral neurological symptoms may occur and survivors often show persistent cortical damage. Other rickettsia cause Q fever, trench fever and rocky mountain spotted fever.

Malaria

Malaria is a protozoan disease transmitted by the bite of the *Anopheles* mosquito. It is the most important of the human parasitic diseases, as it affects approximately 200 million people worldwide, and it is also probably the most common non-traumatic encephalopathy, causing approximately one million deaths a year. Four species of the genus *Plasmodium* (*P. vivax, P. malaria, P. ovale* and *P. falciparum*) are responsible; most cases of cerebral malaria and fatalities are due to infection by *P. falciparum* (termed malignant tertian malaria, or black water fever). The disease has been eradicated from Europe and North America, but remains common in tropical Africa, South America and parts of South-East Asia. Where malaria is endemic, the disorder should always be considered in the differential diagnoses of psychiatric disorders, and it should also be considered in travellers returning from endemic areas, especially among those who have not taken adequate prophylaxis or stopped their anti-malarials too soon.

Cerebral malaria occurs in around 2% of affected individuals. Sporules of the parasite cause thrombosis in the cerebral capillaries, with haemorrhage and oedema; this results in a diffuse symmetrical encephalopathy and so focal signs are unusual. There may be some passive resistance to head flexion but other signs of meningeal irritation are absent. The eyes may be divergent and a point reflex is common. Muscle tone may be increased or decreased, and tendon reflexes are variable, with the plantar being flexor or extensor. Abdominal and cremasteric reflexes are absent. Generalised convulsions occur in 50% of adults with cerebral malaria and in a higher proportion of children, while retinal haemorrhages are present in 15% of patients.

According to Daroff *et al* (1967), cerebral malaria can present with five different neuropsychiatric syndromes. In order of frequency these are:

1 disturbances of consciousness, stupor and coma, or acute delirium

2 acute psychosis or personality change

3 movement disorders with tremors

4 a stroke-like syndrome with focal neurological disorders

5 sub-acute or chronic cases, with depression or apathy without fever (increased slow waves may be detected on the EEG in some of these cases).

Neurological sequelae are associated with childhood cases. Thus, in one large series from Gambia, 23% had sequelae on discharge (most commonly fits, paresis and ataxia), but this rate had fallen to 8.6% at 1 month and 4.4% by 6 months. These complications were more likely if the original illness was associated with a longer period of unconsciousness, multiple convulsions and deeper levels of coma (Van Hensbrock *et al*, 1997).

Equally disconcerting are recent findings in endemic areas that cerebral malaria can result in long-standing cognitive deficits that can be detected at the population level. Thus, in one study in an endemic area of Sri Lanka, Fernando *et al* (2003) found, after controlling for parental educational level, that malarial infections were major predictors of children's performance in the key subjects of language and mathematics. In another study, subtle cognitive deficits of executive function and information processing were impaired. Reduced levels of consciousness during the original illness raised the risk by a factor of four. Thus, malaria not only kills many people but in endemic areas leaves many individuals with lasting mild to moderate cognitive deficits (Holding *et al*, 1999).

Trypanosomiasis

Sleeping sickness or African trypanosomiasis is caused by the trypanosome parasite and is transmitted by the tsetse fly of the *Glossina* genus. An initial febrile illness is followed months or years later by progressive neurological impairment and death. Around 20 000 new cases are reported each year in Africa, and in contrast to malaria the disease tends to affect only the native population in endemic areas, and rarely occurs in tourists.

Involvement of the CNS (stage II disease) is characterised by an insidious development of a variety of neurological symptoms in the form of tremors, incoordination, convulsions, paralysis and confusion, headaches, apathy and daytime somnolence with restlessness at night. A listless gaze accompanies loss of spontaneity, and speech becomes halting and indistinct. Extrapyramidal signs include choreiform movements, tremors and fasciculation and a Parkinsonian picture. In the final phase progressive neurological involvement results in coma and death. Treatment is with suramin, pentamidine and organic arsenicals. The South American variety of trypanosomiasis (Chagas disease) is caused by *T. cruzi* transmitted by the kissing bug. The acute phase generally lasts 1 month and there is an insidious progression to the secondary stage, with cardiomyopathy, myositis, facial swelling and thyroid involvement. CNS involvement is less common but meningo-encephalitis and seizures may occur. Diagnosis is made by detecting antigens to *T. cruzi*, and treatment is with nifurtimox or benznidazole (Kirchhoff, 1991).

Fungal CNS infections

The main agents are cryptococcus, actinomyces and coccidiomycoses and these may cause sub-acute or chronic meningeal symptoms with an insidious onset. A primary psychiatric presentation for these infections is rare. With the advent of HIV, these infections have become more common. Most respond to antifungal therapies, such as amphotericin B and micanazole.

Toxoplasmosis

The obligate intracellular protozoan *Toxoplasma gondii* is responsible for congenital toxoplasmosis (a cause of learning disability) as well as adult toxoplasmosis. Ingestion of poorly cooked meat is the most common form of transmission, and infection is often latent or subclinical. Ingestion of food and water contaminated with oocysts from cat excreta may also cause infection.

Infection during pregnancy is a particular hazard because the organism may be transmitted through the placenta. Congenital toxoplasmosis is severe if the infection occurs early in the first trimester, but most infected infants are asymptomatic at birth. Neonatal screening programmes using Guthrie card tests, which incorporate an IgM specific for *Toxoplasma* may help detect cases at birth, but screening tests in pregnancy are no longer routinely carried out because detection made little difference to outcome. It is estimated that there are 500–600 new cases of congenital toxoplasmosis each year in the UK.

Congenital toxoplasmosis may be evident in the first few days of life and if severe presents with seizures, microcephaly, spasticity, opisthotonos, chorio-retinitis, microphthalmus, optic atrophy and other eye lesions and there may be internal hydrocephalus. The liver and spleen may be enlarged with a raised bilirubin level and pneumonitis. Calcified nodules may be present on CT scan. Symptoms of the infantile form (non-congenital) are similar but do not show cerebral calcification. Learning disability, which may be severe, is a later manifestation.

Treatment is with pyrimethamine plus sulphadiazine and all affected infants should be treated to prevent subclinical infection and later recrudescences of infection. In cases of infection diagnosed during pregnancy, women should be offered treatment as well as the possibility of an abortion. However, a recent study has shown that treating infected women in pregnancy fails to prevent intracranial or ocular complications and the authors suggest this may be because the damage has occurred before any treatment can be instituted (Gilbert *et al*, 2001).

Cysticercosis

Cysticercosis is the result of the encystment of the larvae of *Taenia solium* (pork tapeworm) in the tissues. CNS involvement occurs in 50–70% of cases. Worldwide it may be the most common cause of neurological disease. Calcified cysts are found in the muscle, skin and various organs and CNS involvement is due to cysts in the brain. These result in seizures, raised intracranial pressure and meningitis if the cysts are in the meninges. A variety of focal neurological symptoms may also occur, depending on the site of the cysts. Psychiatric sequelae follow as a consequence of the general deterioration in more severe cases, or are due to the associated epilepsy. Dementia, affective disorders and schizophreniform states have been reported (Tavares, 1993). The diagnosis should be considered in anyone with a neurological disorder who has lived in an endemic area. The cysts may be demonstrated by CT and MRI scan. The CSF may show meningitic changes but diagnosis is by specific enzyme-linked immunoabsorbent assay (ELISA) antibody tests, and in doubtful cases a biopsy may be necessary.

Niclosamide is used to treat the intestinal infections; praziquantel appears to be the first drug to be helpful against cerebral cysts but needs to be administered together with corticosteroids to prevent inflammation; phenytoin may help control fits.

Other worm larvae – *Toxocara* (dog and cat round worms), trichiniasis (from pork), *Schistosomiasis* (bilharzias) and *Echinococcosis* (hydatid cyst) – may all rarely affect the CNS.

Whipple's disease

This is a rare multi-system disease with immunological deficits. It presents, more commonly among men over 50, with weight loss, lassitude, malabsorption, arthralgia and lymphadenopathy. A slowly progressive dementia with myoclonus, ophthalmoplegia and trigeminal neuralgia occurs in some of the reported cases (Halperin *et al*, 1982). The cause is *Tropheryma whipplei* and bound basilliform bodies are found on microscopy. Diagnosis is by PAS-positive macrophages found on jejunal biopsy. Prolonged antibiotic therapy may sometimes be helpful.

Psychomotor disorders

Parkinson's disease

Parkinson's disease (PD) is one of the most common neurological disorders of later life. Marttila & Rinne (1981), summarising the epidemiological studies, gave an estimated prevalence of 0.6–1.8% for those aged over 50 years in Caucasian populations. The classical and neurological manifestations are:

1 'pill rolling' tremor at a frequency of 4–8 Hz, present at rest but disappearing during sleep; the tremor may affect the hands (pronation/supination), jaw, tongue, head or lower limbs

2 rigidity affecting the muscles of the limbs, trunk and neck and said to have a 'lead pipe' quality; if tremor is superimposed upon the rigidity then the phenomenon of cogwheel rigidity may be observed

3 akinesia, which results in poverty of movement and slowness of initiating movement; akinesia probably explains the mask-like facies and infrequent blinking.

The numerous other symptoms include oculomotor abnormalities, postural changes, flexed posture, festination, excessive salivation, seborrhoea, constipation, subjective sensory disturbance and marked fatigue (Lishman, 1987).

Up to 70% of patients with PD exhibit psychiatric symptoms (Ring & Serra-Mestres, 2002) and these fall into four main groups: affective disorders; psychotic disorders; changes in personality or personality traits; and cognitive decline.

Affective disorders

An association between PD and depression is well established. In a review of 26 studies, Cummings (1992) reported the mean rate of depression as 40% (range 4–70%). A more recent study (Schrag *et al*, 2001) reported moderate to severe depression in 19.6% of 97 patients with PD forming part of a population-based study. Higher depression scores were associated with advancing disease severity, recent disease deterioration, higher akinesia scores, greater cognitive impairment and the occurrence of falls. They were related more to the patient's perceptions of handicap than to rated disability.

It is unclear whether this depression is best regarded as reactive to a serious disabling illness or whether it is an integral part of the disease process itself, but it is tempting to speculate on the role of brain monoamines, as both parkinsonism and depressive disorders are thought to result from a functional deficiency of central monoamines, particularly dopamine and serotonin (the topic is briefly discussed in Chapter 3, page 61). Standard antidepressive treatment such as tricyclic antidepressants and ECT appear to be effective in treating the depression (for reviews see Cummings, 1992). ECT may alleviate not only the depression but sometimes also the motor symptoms of PD (Abrams, 1989). The SSRIs are probably now the drugs of choice for treating depression. If selegiline (which is a potent monoamine oxidase inhibitor) is being used to treat PD, SSRIs are contraindicated but tricyclics may be used.

Anxiety disorders (such as generalised anxiety, panic and phobic disorders) are found in up to 40% of patients with PD, especially younger patients (Ring & Serra-Mestres, 2002). Apathy is another frequent symptom in PD, and although often related to depression it can be found in patients without mood disorder. It has been suggested that its presence is related to dysfunction of forebrain dopaminergic systems.

Psychotic disorders

The most common psychoses associated with PD are those due to the antiparkinsonian drugs, while psychoses not associated with treatment are usually indicative of the onset of dementia.

The psychoses associated with PD show some variability between individuals, but in general are characterised by affective changes, auditory, visual and olfactory hallucinations, and persecutory and paranoid delusions. Visual hallucinations are common; in cases where the psychosis is drug induced, visual hallucinations occur in up to 20% of cases.

All the antiparkinsonian drugs have been implicated. Thus, L-dopa may cause psychosis as well as a variety of other psychiatric symptoms, including delirium, depression, agitation, hypersexuality, impulsivity, lethargy, anxiety, insomnia and vivid dreaming. Treatment of these psychoses is problematic because many antipsychotics can themselves cause parkinsonian symptoms. Dosage reduction is a useful initial option but this may lead to an exacerbation of the parkinsonism itself. Small doses of quetiapine are recommended, as this atypical drug is thought to have minimal extrapyramidal side-effects.

Personality

Reviewing the literature on the personality of patients with PD, Todes & Lees (1985) concluded that introspective, over-controlled, and anhedonic personality traits together with suppressed aggressivity are frequently found, but qualified their report by questioning whether these behavioural patterns were of causal significance or were prodromal symptoms of the disease. Giovannoni *et al* (2000) described a small group of patients who became addicted to their L-dopa therapy, who would increase their dosage and soon become tolerant and develop increasingly severe dyskinesia and cyclical mood disorders, sometimes with hypomania or even mania. They termed this disorder 'hedonistic homeostatic dysregulation'. They postulated addiction to L-dopa as the cause, which supports a role for dopamine in other addiction syndromes. Personality changes may reflect early symptoms of the PD itself, since motor symptoms occur only after the striatal dopamine content has been reduced by at least 80%, with a preceding gradual fall in dopamine activity progressing over 20–30 years.

Cognitive disturbances

Cognitive disturbances in PD may be subdivided into:

1 generalised global dementia

2 focal and specific cognitive deficits

3 drug-induced confusional states

4 depression-related cognitive difficulties.

Dementia in PD is rather less common than was once thought, probably having a lifetime risk for those over the age of 65 of 10–20%, in comparison with 5–10% in the general population of similar age. Gibb & Luthert (1994) estimate a threefold increased risk over the general population. As in the general population, age is the most important single determinant for the prevalence of dementia among people with PD. Thus, dementia is very rare among those under 40 years, but the prevalence rises to 65% for those over 85 (Mayeux *et al*, 1990). A study by Stern *et al* (1993) showed that the risks of dementia were greater for: those aged over 70 years; those with more severe PD; those with facial masking as a presenting sign; and those with confusional psychosis while taking L-dopa. Typically, a patient who has been stable and well maintained for many years on L-dopa or a related drug presents with a confusional state, paranoid delusions, visual hallucinations and memory loss.

All the common antiparkinsonian medications may precipitate reversible confusional states. These are most often encountered with antimuscarinic compounds and selegiline, with elderly PD patients being at greater risk. Patients with PD and depression show a greater intellectual decline, with particular problems in frontal lobe tasks.

Neuropsychological investigations of patients with PD have shown specific impairments even in the early stages of the disease, which include deficits of behavioural regulation in sorting or planning tasks, defective use of memory stores, and impaired manipulation of internal representation of visuospatial stimuli (Dubois & Pillon, 1997). These abilities are commonly considered to be controlled by the frontal lobes. This suggests functional continuity or complementarity between the basal ganglia and association areas of the prefrontal cortex. Ascending cholinergic and catecholaminergic neuronal related symptoms may contribute to this frontal-lobe-like symptomatology which appears to be associated with PD.

Progressive supranuclear palsy

Progressive supranuclear palsy is a degenerative disorder. The features are supranuclear ophthalmoplegia (mainly of vertical gaze downwards) with normal vestibulo-occular reflexes, pseudo-bulbar palsy, prominent dysarthria, rigidity of the neck and upper trunk, and cognitive disorder (Ring & Serra-Mestres, 2002). It is a tau-opathy that affects 4–6% of those with an akinetic rigid syndrome attending a movement disorder clinic. Some 80% of sufferers have cognitive impairment characteristic of subcortical dementia, with bradyphrenia, executive deficits, forgetfulness, visuospatial problems and behavioural abnormalities of the frontal lobe type, such as inertia and stereotyped behaviour (a characteristic neuropathological picture of intracellular accumulations of filamentous tau inclusions).

Tourette's syndrome

Tourette's syndrome (TS) is a genetic disorder characterised by both multiple motor and one or more vocal (phonic) tics or noises, which occur many times a day, in bouts. A tic is a sudden, rapid, recurrent, non-rhythmic, stereotyped motor movement or vocalisation, which is experienced as irresistible, but can be suppressed for varying lengths of time. The number, frequency and complexity of the tics change over time, but for a diagnosis of TS they should be present for more than 1 year and usually begin before the age of 18 years.

Once thought to be a rarity, TS is found in all cultures, ethnic and religious groups, in whom it presents with similar clinical characteristics. Its exact prevalence is unknown but the generally accepted figure is 0.5/1000 (approximately 110 000 patients in the USA and 25 000 in the UK). The majority of studies agree that it occurs 1.5–3 more times commonly in males than in females. It is found in all social classes.

The age at onset of symptoms ranges from 2 to 15 years, with a mean of 7 years. The most frequent initial symptoms involve the eyes, for example excessive blinking. Although TS is usually referred to as a tic disorder, individuals with it often demonstrate a variety of complicated movements, including forced touching, licking, spitting, jumping, squatting and a variety of complexities of gait. The onset of the vocalisations, at a mean age of 11 years, is usually later than that of the motor tics. A variety of utterances are common, including sniffing, coughing, throat clearing, barking, grunting, snorting, low- and high-pitched noises and inarticulate sounds. Coprolalia (the inappropriate uttering of obscenities) occurs in about 30% of clinic patient populations but is uncommon in children or mildly affected cases and has a mean age of onset of 13–14.5 years, disappearing later in up to a third of patients. Overall, coprolalia occurs in less than 10% of patients with TS. Copropraxia (inappropriate obscene gestures) is reported in 1–21% of clinic samples with the palm-backed V sign being common in Europe. Echolalia and echopraxia (copying behaviours) occur in 10–44% of clinic patients. Palilalia (the repetition by the patient of the last word or phrase in a sentence or last syllable of a word uttered by the patient) occurs in 6–15% of patients. Such symptoms are noticeable as the syndrome develops into its fullest form, while other, more subjective symptoms, such as sensory tics, mental coprolalia and coprographia may be revealed only on direct questioning. Many patients will then also report associated sensory symptoms, including premonitory urges that increasingly prompt their tics, and momentary relief that can follow the performance of a tic. These may also explain repetitive urges to stretch one's shoulder or clear the throat.

Tics and vocalisations are usually aggravated by anxiety and stress, as well as a wide range of visual and auditory cues, while sleep, alcohol, relaxation, or concentrating on an enjoyable task usually lead to their temporary disappearance. Stimulants such as caffeine, methylphenidate and amphetamines can exacerbate tics. Characteristically, the course of TS over the person's lifetime is punctuated by the appearance of new tics and the disappearance of old ones. Many TS symptoms improve or may even disappear after adolescence.

Differential diagnosis

Tics are not uncommon in childhood and in the DSM-IV scheme the various tic disorders are distinguished on the basis of their duration and the variety of types present. Transient tic disorder lasts for more than 4 weeks but less than 12 months, while chronic motor or vocal tic disorders last more than 12 months. For a diagnosis of TS there should be multiple motor tics and at least one vocal tic.

Associated psychopathology

It is now recognised that TS is associated with a wide variety of behaviours and psychopathologies (Robertson, 2000). The psychopathology most commonly recognised as characteristic of TS is obsessionality. Most case series report an increased rate of obsessive–compulsive disorder (OCD) and obsessive–compulsive behaviours (OCB). Epidemiologically based studies and family studies have shown raised rates of OCB in first-degree relatives. However, the phenomenology observed shows some difference from the obsessions and compulsions found among those without TS. Thus, obsessions among people with TS are significantly more often sexual, violent and symmetrical, and touching, counting and self-damaging compulsions more frequent.

Hyperactivity, distractibility and impulsivity are relatively common in TS. There appears to be an association with attention-deficit disorder (ADD) with and without hyperactivity, and rates of 20–90% of ADD are reported among TS samples, in comparison with rates of around 10% in the general population of a similar age. The two disorders may in some cases be genetically related, but whatever the reason for the association, the combination adds greatly to the burden of the disorder and the strain on carers.

About one-third of clinic populations with TS manifest self-injurious behaviour and rage attacks. This can result in serious injury, such as retinal detachment owing to head banging, dermatological problems resulting from repetitive skin picking, or orthopaedic problems from knee banging.

Controlled studies have shown increased rates of depression. Depression is more severe among those with a longer history of TS, which suggests that it may be reactive to having a chronic, disabling and stigmatising disorder (Robertson *et al*, 1993).

Aetiology

It is now recognised that TS is probably transmitted in an autosomal dominant pattern. The vulnerability that the child inherits is for developing a tic disorder, but the precise type and severity of the tic disorder may vary in different generations. Penetrance in female gene carriers is approximately 70%, but in male carriers it is about 99%. The genetics are comprehensively reviewed by Leckman (2002) and different pedigrees show linkage to sites on several different chromosomes, but so far no single gene or site appears to predominate.

The EEG is essentially normal in TS; in particular, there is no evidence of any paroxysmal activity synchronous with the tics. The principal abnormality is the absence of the Bereitschaftspotential before the tics. CT scans do not show any consistent gross defects, but MRI studies reveal abnormalities primarily in the basal ganglia and lateral ventricles. Several abnormalities have been noted in studies using functional neuroimaging such as positron emission tomography (PET) and single-photon emission computed tomography (SPECT). Although limited owing to the small numbers involved, these findings suggest decreased metabolic activity and cerebral blood flow in the basal ganglia.

Treatment

Psychosocial measures and pharmacological interventions for the individual, as well as various manoeuvres for helping the family, are all important in managing the condition. For many patients with a mild disorder, explanation and reassurance are often sufficient. In a similar way, the parents of mildly affected children can often be reassured by the diagnosis, explanations about the nature of disorder, information about the self-help groups and booklets for teachers.

Drug therapy is the mainstay of treatment for the motor and vocal symptoms, as well as for some of the associated behaviours. The medications most commonly used are dopamine antagonists (particularly those affecting D_2 receptors) such as haloperidol, sulpiride and risperidone. Extrapyramidal side-effects, sedation and dysarthria are common with haloperidol, but less so with the others. Butyrophenones may also impair concentration and scholastic achievement and cause tardive dyskinesia. Sulpiride causes fewer extrapyramidal problems, but gynaecomastia, galactorrhoea, menstrual irregularities and possible depression have been reported. Haloperidol can be started at a dose of 0.5 mg daily and sulpiride at 100–200 mg daily.

There is now much interest in the use of the newer, atypical drugs in TS because the experience of their use in schizophrenia has shown that they are better tolerated than the older drugs.

A placebo-controlled trial (Gaffney *et al*, 2002) showed that successful tic reduction occurred in 60% of risperidone-treated cases compared with only 26% of the placebo-treated cases, but weight gain (a mean of 2.8 kg) was a significant side-effect. Risperidone liquid preparations started at low doses (e.g. 0.1–0.2 mg) can be gradually titrated up until a useful tic reduction is achieved. There are also several uncontrolled case series describing beneficial effects for quetiapine and for olanzapine.

Clonidine, which is an α_2-adrenergic agonist, is also used with some success and it may be the agent of choice if a child has TS and ADD. In general, clonidine has fewer and milder side-effects than the neuroleptics, but drowsiness, insomnia, dry mouth, headaches and postural hypertension do occur. In the trial of risperidone described above (Gaffney *et al*, 2002) clonidine was shown to be as effective as risperidone for the tics, but not for obsessional symptoms. Clonidine can also be used as a transdermal patch. The SSRIs and clomipramine can be used to treat obsessive–compulsive aspects of the syndrome; augmentation of anti-obsessional effects of SSRIs by neuroleptics has been reported.

Sydenham's chorea

Sydenham's chorea, also known as St Vitus dance, is characterised by sudden, involuntary, irregular, jerky movements of the extremities, frequently associated with emotional instability and muscle weakness. The onset may be gradual, with complaints that a child is nervous. The patient may become clumsy and stumble, fall or drop objects. There are often complaints from teachers at school of poor attention and deteriorating handwriting. Facial grimacing and a variety of speech disorders occur. Most of the choreiform movements subside during sleep and are exaggerated by emotions. Characteristically, if the patient is asked to extend the arms, hands and fingers, flexion of the wrists and hyperextension of the metacarpopharyngeal joints are observed. Other signs consist of an inability to hold the tongue still when it is protruded and spasmodic contractions of the hands when the patient intentionally grips objects or the examiner's hands (the 'milk maid grip').

Sydenham's chorea is found in 10–30% of children with rheumatic fever, most commonly in prepubertal girls. It is rare in black and adult populations, although it can reappear in adulthood as chorea gravidarum. Obsessive–compulsive symptoms have been noted in the context of Sydenham's chorea (Chapman *et al*, 1958).

Wilson's disease

Wilson's disease – hepatolenticular degeneration – is an uncommon, recessively inherited disorder of copper metabolism. It has a worldwide prevalence of around 1 per 30 000. It is caused by deficiency of a copper carrier membrane protein, a copper-transporting ATPase known as ATP7B, normally situated in the trans-golgi. There has been considerable recent interest in the gene that codes for this enzyme, which is on the long arm of chromosome 13 at the 13q14 site. Mutations within this gene, of which there are many, have been shown to be responsible for Wilson's disease, but different mutations are responsible for the disease in different ethnic groups. Thus, a study of 60 patients with Wilson's disease from Brazil sequenced all 21 exons of the ATP7B gene and identified 25 mutations, 12 of them for the first time, but the most common European mutations were not present at all, a finding the authors stated was compatible with a history of mainly Mediterranean migration (Deguti *et al*, 2004). However, a different pattern was found in Saudi Arabia, where 16 out of 30 cases of Wilson's disease were homozygous for the 4193 del C mutation, which is located on exon 21 of the ATP7B gene (Majumdar *et al*, 2003).

It was first described by Wilson (1912), who recognised both hepatic and neurological involvement as well as the familial nature of the disorder. He described the characteristic symptoms, which include generalised tremor, dysarthria, dysphasia, muscular rigidity, emaciation, spasmodic contractions, sclerosis of the liver and emotionalism, and it can present with almost any psychiatric disorder. Approximately 40% of cases of Wilson's disease present with liver disease, usually between the ages of 3 and 12 years. Around 50% have a psychiatric or neurological presentation, usually in adolescence or early adult life. Approximately half of this group will have clinically detectable liver disease. The remainder present with skeletal, renal or haemolytic disease, and these features may also be present in the other clinical categories.

There is an accumulation of copper in the liver, brain, kidney, cornea and bone. Copper deposits in the liver cause a focal necrosis that ultimately leads to a coarse nodular postnecrotic sclerosis. In the kidneys, copper is deposited in the tubular epithelial cells and results in aminoaciduria. Post-mortem studies of the brain show a striking brick red pigmentation in the basal ganglia as well as spongy degeneration of the putamen, leading to the formation of small cavities. Copper is deposited in the peri-capillary areas and within the astrocytes. In the eye, deposits in the cornea, particularly in Descemet's membrane, are responsible for the characteristic yellow to green to brown Kayser–Fleischer ring. It is almost always associated with neurological or psychiatric disorder. Most cases present in the first two decades, although it may develop later. Early onset (7–15 years) is more fulminant and later onset (19–35 years) less so. The disease presents with hepatic involvement in half the cases – acute hepatitis, fulminant hepatitis, chronic active hepatitis and sclerosis. The release of copper may also cause haemolytic anaemia.

The neurological disorder is primarily a disorder of motor function, and there are no sensory symptoms. Tremors and rigidity are common early signs. The tremor may be of the intention type (cerebellar) or it may be due to basal ganglia damage and resemble the tremor of Parkinson's disease. Most commonly it is a bizarre tremor and has been described as 'wing beating'. It is generally absent at rest and may be so violent that the patient is thrown off balance. Rigidity and spasm of the muscles are often present.

The nature of the psychiatric disorder in Wilson's disease has been examined in several retrospective series (Dening, 1985; Dening & Berrios, 1989; Akil *et al*, 1991). In one series around a fifth of the cases presented initially to the psychiatric clinic. The reported frequency for psychiatric symptoms ranges from 26% to 60%. The two most frequently observed clinical pictures are:

1 affective symptoms, with emotional lability, incongruity and a picture of neurotic depression

2 a picture of behavioural/personality change, with aggression, irritability and childish behaviour accompanied by schizoid, hysterical and psychopathic personality traits.

Anxiety, attempted suicide, organic delusional states, catatonia and psychosis have also been reported. In most series, schizophrenia-like psychoses are rare or absent. Although dementia is a recognised outcome, severe cognitive impairment is rare.

The diagnosis of Wilson's disease is easy, provided that it is suspected. The condition should be suspected in any patient under 30 who develops an unexplained CNS disorder, particularly unexplained personality change, cognitive impairment, psychosis or catatonia; and suspicion should be increased if there is any liver disease, or if the patient has a blood relative with Wilson's disease. However, a recent study found that the correct initial diagnosis was made in only around a third of cases and in the remaining two-thirds the diagnosis was reached only after a mean delay of around 2 years. For those presenting with a neuropsychiatric picture, the main initial other diagnoses were schizophrenia, neurodegenerative disorders, SSPE, metachromatic leucodystrophy and various congenital myopathies, which reflect the differential diagnosis of Wilson's disease (Prashanth *et al*, 2004). The diagnosis is confirmed by the presence of Kayser–Fleischer rings and low ceruloplasmin levels combined with low serum copper levels with increased 24-hour urinary copper excretion. While both corneas should always be inspected for Kayser–Fleischer rings, only slit-lamp examination is definitive, and their presence is usually, but not always, associated with neurological damage. CT and MRI studies show that ventricular dilatation, cortical atrophy and basal ganglia hypodensities are commonly present. If the diagnosis is confirmed, it is essential to screen the patient's siblings, because asymptomatic cases can be treated prophylactically and this can sometimes lead to a remission.

Treatment involves the copper chelating agents, such as penicillamine, a breakdown product of penicillin, or trientine, for those intolerant of penicillamine, zinc, which acts to prevent dietary copper absorption by inducing intestinal mucosal metallothionein synthesis, or tetrathiomolybdate, which forms a stable complex with dietary protein and copper in the gut, and with albumen and copper in blood. A diet restricting foods high in copper (liver, cocoa, chocolate, mushrooms, shellfish, nuts, dried fruits and vegetables) is preferred. Penicillamine (1–3 g daily) can prevent virtually every manifestation of the disease. It should be continued for life, as the mortality of those who stop treatment is high. Hepatic disorder responds less well than neurological, but there are recent reports that liver transplantation can cure both the hepatic and neurological aspects of the disease. Liver transplantation appears to convert the copper kinetics from a homozygous to a heterozygous state, thus providing a phenotypic cure (Podgaetz *et al*, 2003).

Dystonia

Dystonia is a syndrome dominated by sustained muscle contractions. These produce abnormal postures. It can be classified by the sites involved, age at onset and cause. When it starts in childhood it typically produces generalised dystonia. Toe walking is a common presentation in children, with dystonic abnormal postures of the feet. When dystonia affects more than one contiguous part of the body, it is called segmental. If it affects all the muscles in one half of the body it is called hemi-dystonia and this is associated with structural disorder in the contralateral basal ganglia or thalamus. The commonest distribution of dystonia is focal. Focal dystonias usually present in middle age and are more common in women.

Spasmodic torticollis or idiopathic cervical dystonia is the most common focal dystonia (Dauer *et al*, 1998). It is caused by involuntary contractions of the neck muscles, which result in abnormal postures or involuntary movements of the head in any of the three possible planes of rotation. At the time of diagnosis, extra-cervical dystonia is found in 20% of patients and there may be a concomitant head or hand tremor. Adult-onset cervical dystonia does not become generalised.

The aetiology is unknown but a genetic abnormality is suspected. Some 10% of cases are precipitated by neck injury and 10% by psychological trauma. While 10–20% of patients may experience remission, nearly all relapse within 5 years and are left with persistent disease. Most medications have only a 10% chance of being helpful and this is at the cost of systemic side-effects. By contrast, intramuscular botulinum toxin injections have a 90% chance of helping and have few significant side-effects, but these need to be repeated at 3-monthly intervals. Sufferers find the disorder distressing but it is generally agreed that there is no increase in formal psychiatric illness (Jahanshahi & Marsden, 1988).

If the dystonia affects eye closure, it is called essential blepharospasm. The aetiology, supported by animal models, appears to be multifactorial, representing the influence of a genetic background and an environmental trigger, such as dry eye or local ocular disease (Hallett, 2002). Unilateral blepharospasm is often due to hemifacial spasm, a peripheral disorder caused by pressure on the facial nerve by a kinked blood vessel outside the brain-stem. If dystonia affects muscles of the lower face and jaw it is called oromandibular. When dystonia affects the trunk with no other signs it is often misdiagnosed as hysteria. When the dystonic movements appear only with certain actions, the term occupational dystonia is applied and writer's cramp is a good example of this.

Writer's cramp is a focal dystonia and is characterised by postural cramps when the patient attempts to write. There may be pain, postural and action tremor and abnormalities of hand grip. Sufferers may develop an increase in muscular tension and an atypical dystonic limb posture when writing is attempted. If only writing is affected this is called 'simple writer's cramp'; if the abnormal activity also occurs with any other activity it is called 'dystonic writer's cramp'. Although distressing, there does not seem to be any association with psychiatric disorder (Grafman *et al*, 1991). 'Musician's focal dystonia' is another variant; it can lead to the end of a successful career. It is characterised by the onset of involuntary muscle contractions and movements, and may appear in musicians after years of fine and repetitive movements during performances. Patients usually present to their general practitioners and then to neurological or rheumatology clinics and so are rarely seen in psychiatric settings.

Recent PET studies of people with writer's cramp have shown significant overactivity in the primary sensory cortex during attempts at writing, with a suggestion that there is a defect in sensorimotor integration resulting in co-contractions of muscles (Lerner *et al*, 2004). Functional MRI studies have shown abnormal activations of the contralateral basal ganglion, motor cortex and ipsilateral cerebellar hemisphere, which the authors suggested implies a dysfunction of the basal ganglia and the subcortical–cortical loop (Hu *et al*, 2006).

Dystonias can be paroxysmal. They can be symptomatic of Wilson's disease, Huntington's chorea, Hallervorden–Spatz (all discussed earlier in this chapter) and the organic acidurias. The most common causes of secondary dystonia are stroke, cerebral palsy and drugs. Neuroleptic drugs can cause dystonia, often as part of a mixed movement disorder, including chorea, parkinsonian features, motor restlessness or akathisia.

Dystonia can also occur as a genetically determined neuropathic disease. L-dopa-responsive dystonia is rare but important to diagnose and is sometimes referred to as the Segawa syndrome. Some familial cases are due to a mutation of the guanosine 5'-triphosphate cyclohydrolase I gene (Van Hove *et al*, 2006). The disorder usually presents in childhood, with leg-onset dystonia. The child may fall and become wheelchair bound. A feature of two-thirds of cases is marked diurnal variation (patients are much better on getting up in the morning). Dopamine can restore almost normal movement. All children with dystonia should receive dopamine as a trial, even if they do not display diurnal variation. The condition has been recognised only relatively recently and so cases that have been missed in childhood (because during their childhoods the condition was unrecognised) can present in adulthood. Thus, Chaila *et al* (2006) described four female siblings with the disorder, who had lifelong dystonia and unsteadiness (one had scoliosis), who all showed an excellent response to L-dopa more than 40 years after the onset of their symptoms.

At one time it was common for patients with any of the dystonias to be misdiagnosed as having a psychiatric disorder. However, psychogenic dystonia is in fact relatively uncommon and should be diagnosed only if there is clear-cut evidence of a conversion reaction or malingering. When such psychogenic dystonia is present, though, it can be severe enough to lead to permanent contractures that warrant surgical procedures.

Basal ganglia calcification

About 50% of patients with basal ganglia calcification have a deficiency of parathyroid hormone; a few of these cases are related to chronic renal failure, or vascular, anoxic or infective cerebral lesions. However, many cases are idiopathic and a few may be familial.

Basal ganglia calcification seen on a CT scan is often an incidental and non-significant finding. In more severe cases the changes may be associated with dementia and extrapyramidal motor disorders presenting in people in their 50s or occasionally with a schizophreniform psychosis presenting in those in their 30s. The dementia is subcortical, with slowing of mentation, forgetfulness and lack of focal cortical deficit (Cummings *et al*, 1983). Although dementia and schizophreniform disorders are the commonest psychiatric presentations (found in 50% of published cases), depression and occasional mania are also seen (Trautner *et al*, 1988).

Fahr's disease (familial basal ganglia calcification) is inherited in an autosomal dominant fashion and begins in early adult life with progressive dementia, convulsions and rigidity. Doubt has been cast both on the familial nature of the disorder and on its relationship to psychotic disorder in particular but also to dementia. In an extensive review, Flint & Goldstein (1992) concluded that it is related to learning disability and pseudo-hypo-parathyroidism and is not a distinct disease entity.

References

Abrams, R. (1989) ECT for Parkinson's disease. *American Journal of Psychiatry*, **46**, 1391–1393.

Achte, K. A., Hillbom, E. & Aalberg, V. I. (1969) Psychoses following war brain injuries. *Acta Psychiatrica Sandinavica*, **45**, 1–18.

Ainiala, H., Loukkola, M., Peltola, J., *et al* (2001) The prevalence of neuropsychiatric syndromes in systemic lupus erythematosus. *Neurology*, **57**, 496–500.

Akil, M., Schwatz, J. A., Dutchak, D., *et al* (1991) The psychiatric presentations of Wilson's disease. *Journal of Neuropsychiatry and Clinical Neurosciences*, **3**, 377–382.

American Psychiatric Association (1994) *Diagnostic and Statistical Manual of Mental Disorders* (4th edn) (DSM–IV). Washington, DC: APA.

Annegers, J. F., Hauser, W. A., Coan, S. P., *et al* (1998) A population based study of seizures after traumatic brain injury. *New England Journal of Medicine*, **338**, 20–24.

Antebi, D. & Bird, J. M. (1993) The facilitation and evocation of seizures. *British Journal of Psychiatry*, **162**, 759–764.

Bach-y-Rita, G., Lion, J. R., Climent, C. E., *et al* (1971) Episodic dyscontrol: a study of 130 violent patients. *American Journal of Psychiatry*, **127**, 1473–1478.

Bear, D. M. & Fedio, P. (1977) Quantitative analysis of inter-ictal behaviour in temporal lobe epilepsy. *Archives of Neurology*, **34**, 454–467.

Betts, T. (1990) Pseudo-seizures that are not epilepsy. *Lancet*, **336**, 163–168.

Bing, E. G., Burnam, M. A., Longshore, D., *et al* (2001) Psychiatric disorders and drug use among human immunodeficiency virus-infected adults in the United States. *Archives of General Psychiatry*, **58**, 721–728.

Brown, S. W. & Reynolds, E. H. (1981) Cognitive impairment in epileptic patients. In *Epilepsy and Psychiatry* (eds E. H. Reynolds & M. R. Trimble). Edinburgh: Churchill Livingstone.

Chadwick, D. (1994) Epilepsy. *Journal of Neurology, Neurosurgery and Psychiatry*, **57**, 264–277.

Chaila, E. C., McCabe, D. J., Delanty, N., *et al* (2006) Broadening the phenotype of childhood-onset dopa-responsive dystonia. *Archives of Neurology*, **63**, 1185–1188.

Chakravarty, A., Mukherjee, A. & Sen, A. (2003) Familial paediatric rapidly progressive extrapyramidal syndrome: is it Hallervorden–Spatz disease? *Pediatric Neurologist*, **29**, 170–172.

Chang, B., Steimel, J., Moller, D. R., *et al* (2001) Depression in sarcoidosis. *American Journal of Respiratory Critical Care Medicine*, **163**, 329–334.

Chaplin, J. E., Lasso, R. Y., Shorvon, S. D., *et al* (1992) National general practice study of epilepsy. The social and psychological effects of a recent diagnosis of epilepsy. *BMJ*, **304**, 1416–1417.

Chapman, A. H., Pilkey, L. & Gibbons, M. J. (1958) A psychosomatic study of eight children with Sydenham's chorea. *Paediatrics*, **21**, 582–595.

Commission of the International League Against Epilepsy (1989) Proposal for revised classification of epilepsies and epileptic syndromes. *Epilepsia*, **30**, 389–399.

Cope, D. (1995) The effectiveness of traumatic brain injury rehabilitation: a review. *Brain Injury*, **9**, 649–670.

Cummings, J. L. (1992) Depression and Parkinson's disease: a review. *American Journal of Psychiatry*, **149**, 443–454.

Cummings, J. L., Gosenfeld, L. F., Houlihan, J. P., *et al* (1983) Neuropsychiatric disturbances associated with idiopathic calcification of the basal ganglia. *Biological Psychiatry*, **18**, 591–601.

Currie, S., Heathfield, K. W. G., Henson, R. A., *et al* (1971) Clinical course and prognosis of temporal lobe epilepsy – a survey of 666 patients. *Brain*, **92**, 173–190.

Daly, D. (1958) Ictal affect. *American Journal of Psychiatry*, **115**, 97–108.

Dana-Haeri, J., Trimble, M. R. & Oxley, J. (1983) Prolactin and gonadotrophin changes following generalised and partial seizures. *Journal of Neurology, Neurosurgery and Psychiatry*, **46**, 331–335.

Daniel, T. M. (1991) Mycobacterial disease. In *Harrison's Principles of Internal Medicine* (12th edn) (eds J. D. Wilson, E. Braunwald, K. J. Isseelbacher, *et al*), pp. 637–645. New York: McGraw-Hill.

Daroff, R. B., Deller, J. J., Kastl, A. J., *et al* (1967) Cerebral malaria. *Journal of the American Medical Association*, **202**, 681–682.

Dauer, W., Burke, R., Greene, P., *et al* (1998) Current concepts on the clinical features, etiology and management of idiopathic cervical dystonia. *Brain*, **121**, 547–560.

Dausey, D. J. & Desai, R. A. (2003) Psychiatric comorbidity and the prevalence of HIV infection in a sample of patients in treatment for substance abuse. *Journal of Nervous and Mental Disease*, **191**, 10–17.

Deb, S., Lyons, I., Koutzoukis, C., *et al* (1999) Rate of psychiatric illness one year after traumatic brain injury. *American Journal of Psychiatry*, 156, 374–378.

Deguti, M. M., Genschel, J., Cancado, E. L. R., *et al* (2004) Wilson's disease. Novel mutations in the ATP7B gene and clinical correlates in Brazilian patients. *Human Mutation*, **23**, 398.

Dening, T. R. (1985) Psychiatric aspects of Wilson's disease. *British Journal of Psychiatry*, **147**, 677–682.

Dening, T. R. & Berrios, G. E. (1989) Wilson's disease. Psychiatric symptoms in 195 cases. *Archives of General Psychiatry*, **46**, 1126–1134.

Dewhurst, K. (1969) The neurosyphilitic psychoses today: a survey of 91 cases. *British Journal of Psychiatry*, **115**, 31–38.

Dubois, B. & Pillon, B. (1997) Cognitive deficits in Parkinson's disease. *Journal of Neurology*, **244**, 228.

Eames, P. (1992) Hysteria following head injury. *Journal of Neurology, Neurosurgery and Psychiatry*, **55**, 1046–1053.

Espir, M. L. E. & Spalding, J. M. K. (1956) Three recent cases of encephalitis lethargica. *BMJ*, *i*, 1141–1144.

Fenwick, P. (1990) Prolonged confusion following convulsions due to generalised non-convulsive status epilepticus. *Neurology*, **40**, 1689–1694.

Fernando, S. D., Gunawardena, D. M., Bandara, M. R., *et al* (2003) The impact of repeated malaria attacks on the school performance of children. *American Journal of Tropical Medicine and Hygiene*, **69**, 582–588.

Finger, S. (1998) A happy state of mind. *Archives of Neurology*, **55**, 241–250.

Flint, J. & Goldstein, L. H. (1992) Familial calcification of the basal ganglia: a case report and review of the literature. *Psychological Medicine*, **22**, 581–595.

Flor-Henry, P. (1969) Psychosis and temporal lobe epilepsy: a controlled investigation. *Epilepsia*, **10**, 363–395.

Frazer, W & Kerr, M. (eds) (2003) *Seminars in the Psychiatry of Learning Disabilities*. London: Gaskell.

Friedman, G., Froom, P., Sazbon, L., *et al* (1999) Apolipoprotein E-E4 gina type predicts a poor outcome in survivors of traumatic brain injury. *Neurology*, **52**, 244–248.

Gaffney, G. R., Perry, P. J., Lund, B. C., *et al* (2002) Risperidone versus clonidine in the treatment of children and adolescents with Tourette's syndrome. *Journal of the American Academy of Child and Adolescent Psychiatry*, **41**, 330–336.

Geschwind, N. (1965) Disconnection syndromes in animals and man. *Brain*, **88**, 237–294, 585–644.

Geschwind, N. (1979) Behavioural changes in temporal lobe epilepsy. *Psychological Medicine*, **9**, 217–219.

Gibb, W. R. G. & Luthert, P. J. (1994) Dementia in Parkinson's disease and Lewy body disease. In *Dementia* (eds A. Burns & R. Levy), pp. 719–737. London: Chapman and Hall.

Gilbert, R. E., Gras, L. & Wallon, M. (2001) Effect of treatment on mother to child transmission of *Toxoplasma gondii*: retrospective cohort study of 554 mother child pairs in Lym, France. *International Journal of Epidemiology*, **30**, 1315–1316.

Giovannoni, G., O'Sullivan, J. D., Turner, K., *et al* (2000) Hedonistic homeostatic dysregulation in patients with Parkinson's disease on dopamine replacement therapies. *Journal of Neurology, Neurosurgery and Psychiatry*, **68**, 423–428.

Gloor, P. (1990) Experimental phenomena of temporal lobe epilepsy. Facts and hypotheses. *Brain*, **113**, 1673–1685.

Goldstein, L. H. (1990) Behavioural and cognitive behavioural treatments for epilepsy. *Bristol Journal of Clinical Psychology*, **29**, 257–269.

Gordillo, V., del Amo, J., Soriano, V., *et al* (1999) Sociodemographic and psychological variables influencing adherence to antiretroviral therapy. *AIDS*, **13**, 1763–1769.

Grafman, J., Cohen, L. J. & Hallett, M. (1991) Is focal hand dystonia associated with psychopathology? *Movement Disorders*, **6**, 29–35.

Guo, Z., Cupples, L., Kurz, A., *et al* (2000) Head injury and the risk of AD in the Mirage study. *Neurology*, **54**, 1316–1323.

Haas, J., Cope, D. & Hall, K. (1987) Premorbid prevalence of poor academic performance in severe head injury. *Journal of Neurology, Neurosurgery and Psychiatry*, **50**, 52–56.

Hallett, M. (2002) Blepharospasm, recent advances. *Neurology*, **59**, 1306–1312.

Halperin, L. L., Landis, D. M. D. & Kleinman, G. M. (1982) Whipple disease of the nervous system. *Neurology*, **32**, 612–617.

Helmstaedter, C., Kemper, B. & Elger, C. (1996) Neuropsychological aspects of frontal lobe epilepsy. *Neuropsychologia*, **34**, 399–406.

Hodges, J. R. (1994) Semantic memory and frontal executive functioning. *Journal of Neurology, Neurosurgery and Psychiatry*, **57**, 605–608.

Hogg, K. E., Goldstein, L. H. & Leigh, P. N. (1994) The psychological impact of motor neurone disease. *Psychological Medicine*, **24**, 625–632.

Holding, P. A., Stevenson, J., Peshu, N., *et al* (1999) Cognitive sequelae of severe malaria with impaired consciousness. *Transactions of the Royal Society of Tropical Medicine and Hygiene*, **93**, 519–534.

Holsinger, T., Steffens, D. C., Phillips, C., *et al* (2002) Head injury in early adulthood and the life time risk of depression. *Archives of General Psychiatry*, **59**, 17–22.

Hu, X. Y., Wang, L., Liu, H., *et al* (2006) Functional magnetic resonance imaging study of writer's cramp. *Chinese Medical Journal*, **119**, 1263–1271.

Hunter, R., Blackwood, W. & Bull, J. (1968) Three cases of frontal meningiomas presenting psychiatrically. *BMJ*, *iii*, 9–16.

Jahanshahi, M. & Marsden, C. D. (1988) Depression in torticollis: a controlled study. *Psychological Medicine*, **18**, 925–933.

Jennett, B., Snoek, J., Bond, M. R., *et al* (1981) Disability after severe head injury: observations on the use of the Glasgow Coma Scale. *Journal of Neurology, Neurosurgery and Psychiatry*, **44**, 285–293.

Johnson, J. (1969) Organic psychosyndromes due to boxing. *British Journal of Psychiatry*, **115**, 45–53.

Jorge, R. E., Robinson, R. G., Starkstein, S. E., *et al* (1993) Secondary mania following traumatic brain injury. *American Journal of Psychiatry*, **150**, 916–921.

Kapur, N., Barker, S. & Burrows, E. H. (1994) Herpes simplex encephalitis: long-time magnetic resonance imaging and neuro-psychological profile. *Journal of Neurology, Neurosurgery and Psychiatry*, **57**, 1334–1342.

King, D. J. (2004) *Seminars in Clinical Psychopharmacology* (2nd edn). London: Gaskell.

King, M. B. (1989) Psychosocial status of 192 outpatients with HIV infection and AIDS. *British Journal of Psychiatry*, **154**, 237–242.

Kirchhoff, L. V. (1991) Trypanosomiasis. In *Harrison's Principles of Internal Medicine* (12th edn) (eds J. D. Wilson, E. Braunwald, K. J. Isselbacher, *et al*), pp. 791–794. New York: McGraw Hill.

Lancet (1989) Pseudostatus epilepticus. *Lancet*, **ii**, 485.

Landolt, A. (1958) Serial EEG investigations during psychotic episode in epileptic patients and during schizophrenic attacks. In *Lectures on Epilepsy* (ed. A. M. Lorentz de Haas), pp. 21–113. Amsterdam: Elsevier.

Leckman, J. F. (2002) Tourette's syndrome. *Lancet*, **360**, 1577–1586.

Leis, A. A., Ross, M. A. & Summers, A. K. (1992) Psychogenic seizures: ictal characteristics and diagnostic pitfalls. *Neurology*, **42**, 95–99.

Lerner, A., Shill, H., Hanakawa, T., *et al* (2004) Regional cerebral blood flow correlates of the severity of writer's cramp symptoms. *Neuroimage*, **21**, 904–913.

Lishman, W. A. (1987) *Organic Psychiatry. The Psychological Consequences of Cerebral Disorders* (2nd edn). Oxford: Blackwell Scientific.

Lishman, W. A. (1988) Physiogenesis and psychogenesis in the 'post-concussional syndrome'. *British Journal of Psychiatry*, **153**, 460–469.

Logsdail, S. J. & Toone, B. K. (1988) Post-ictal psychosis – a clinical and phenomenological description. *British Journal of Psychiatry*, **152**, 246–252.

Lyketsos, C., Treisman, G. & Lipsey, J. (1998) Does stroke cause depression? *Journal of Neuropsychiatry*, **10**, 103–107.

Mace, C. (1993) Epilepsy and schizophrenia. *British Journal of Psychiatry*, **163**, 439–445.

Majumdar, R., Al Jumah, M. & Fraser, M. (2003) 4193 del C, a common mutation causing Wilson's disease in Saudi Arabia: a rapid molecular screening of patients and carriers. *Molecular Pathology*, **56**, 302–304.

Maletzky, B. M. (1973) The episodic dyscontrol syndrome. *Diseases of the Nervous System*, **34**, 178–185.

Mark, V. H. & Ervin, F. R. (1970) *Violence and the Brain*. New York: Harper and Row.

Marttila, R. J. & Rinne, U. K. (1981) Epidemiology of Parkinson's disease. *Journal of Neural Transmission*, **51**, 135–148.

Mathern, G. W., Pretorius, J. K., Babb, T. L., *et al* (1995) Unilateral hippocampal mossy fibre sprouting and bilateral asymmetric neuron loss with episodic postictal psychosis. *Neurosurgery*, **82**, 228–233.

Mayeux, R., Chen, J., Mirabello, E., *et al* (1990) An estimate of the incidence of dementia in idiopathic Parkinson's disease. *Neurology*, **40**, 1513–1517.

Misdrahi, D., Vila, G., Funk-Brentano, I., *et al* (2004) DSM-IV mental disorders and neurological complications in children and adolescents with human immuno deficiency virus type I infection (HIV I). *European Psychiatry*, **19**, 182–184.

Nagai, Y., Goldstein, L. H., Fenwick, P. B. C., *et al* (2004) Clinical efficacy of galvanic skin response bio feedback training in reducing seizures in adult epilepsy: a preliminary randomized controlled study. *Epilepsy and Behaviour*, **5**, 216–233.

Neary, D., Snowden, J. S., Mann, D. M. A., *et al* (1990) Frontal lobe dementia and motor neuron disease. *Journal of Neurology, Neurosurgery and Psychiatry*, **53**, 23–32.

Okamura, T., Fukai, M., Yamadori, A., *et al* (1993) A clinical study of hypergraphia in epilepsy. *Journal of Neurology, Neurosurgery and Psychiatry*, **56**, 556–559.

Ovsiew, F. & McClelland, J. (1995) Anglo-American neuropsychiatry in historical perspective. *Current Opinion in Psychiatry*, **8**, 45–47.

Pajonk, F.-G. & Naber, D. (1998) Human immunodeficiency virus and mental disorders. *Current Opinion in Psychiatry*, **11**, 305–310.

Palmini, A. & Gloor, P. (1992) The localising value of auras in partial seizures. *Neurology*, **42**, 801–810.

Penfield, W. (1967) Epilepsy: the great teacher. The progress of one pupil. *Acta Neurologica Scandinavica*, **43**, 1–10.

Perini, G. I., Tosin, C., Carraro, C., *et al* (1996) Inter-ictal mood and personality disorder in temporal lope epilepsy and juvenile myoclonic epilepsy. *Journal of Neurology, Neurosurgery and Psychiatry*, **61**, 601–605.

Podgaetz, E., Chan, C. & the Liver transplant team (2003) Liver transplantation for Wilson's disease: our experience with review of the literature. *Annals of Hepatology*, **2**, 131–134.

Prashanth, L. K., Taly, A. B., Sinha, S., *et al* (2004) Wilson's disease: diagnostic errors and clinical implications. *Journal of Neurology, Neurosurgery and Psychiatry*, **75**, 907–909.

Price, S. & Goyette, J. (2003) The role of the psychiatrist in the care of patients with hepatitis C and HIV/AIDs. *Psychiatric Quarterly*, **74**, 261–276.

Pujol, J., Leal, S., Fluvia, X., *et al* (1989) Psychiatric aspects of normal pressure hydrocephalus. A report of five cases. *British Journal of Psychiatry*, **54**, 77–80.

Rao, S. M., Devinsky, O., Grofman, J., *et al* (1992) Viscosity and social cohesion in temporal lobe epilepsy. *Journal of Neurology, Neurosurgery and Psychiatry*, **55**, 149–152.

Rataccio, A. L. & Devinsky, O. (2001) Personality disorders in epileps. In *Psychiatry Issues in Epilepsy* (eds A. B. Ettinger & A. M. Kanner). Philadelphia, PA: Lippincott.

Reynolds, E. H. (1981) The management of seizures associated with psychological disorders. In *Epilepsy and Psychiatry* (eds E. H. Reynolds & M. R. Trimble). Edinburgh: Churchill Livingstone.

Ring, H. A. & Serra-Mestres, J. (2002) Neuropsychiatry of the basal ganglia. *Journal of Neurology, Neurosurgery and Psychiatry*, **72**, 12–21.

Robertson, M. (2000) Tourette's syndrome, associated conditions and the complexities of treatment. *Brain*, **123**, 425–462.

Robertson, M., Trimble, M. R. & Townsend, H. R. A. (1987) Phenomenology of depression in epilepsy. *Epilepsia*, **28**, 364–372.

Robertson, M., Channon, S., Baker, J. E., *et al* (1993) The psychopathology of Gilles de la Tourette syndrome: a controlled study. *British Journal of Psychiatry*, **162**, 114–117.

Robertson, M., Channon, S. & Baker, J. (1994) Depressive symptomatology in a general hospital sample of outpatients with temporal lobe epilepsy: a controlled study. *Epilepsia*, **35**, 771–777.

Rodin, E. (1973) Psychomotor epilepsy and aggressive behaviour. *Archives of General Psychiatry*, **28**, 210–213.

Ron, M. A. & Feinstein, A. (1992) Multiple sclerosis and the mind. *Journal of Neurology, Neurosurgery and Psychiatry*, **5**, 1–3.

Ron, M. A. & Logsdail, S. J. (1989) Psychiatric morbidity in multiple sclerosis: a clinical and MRI study. *Psychological Medicine*, **19**, 887–895.

Sacks, O. (1973) *Awakenings*. London: Duckworth.

Sacks, O. (1992) *Migraine – Revised and Expanded*. London: Picador.

Savard, G., Andermann, F., Olivier, A., *et al* (1991) Postictal psychosis after complex partial seizures: a multiple case study. *Epilepsia*, **32**, 225–231.

Schrag, A., Jahanshahi, M. & Quinn, N. (2001) What contributes to depression in Parkinson's disease? *Psychological Medicine*, **31**, 65–73.

Sepkowitz, K. A. (2006) One disease, two epidemics – AIDS at 25. *New England Journal of Medicine*, **354**, 2411–2414.

Shorvon, S. D. (1990) Epidemiology, natural history and genetics of epilepsy. *BMJ*, **336**, 93–96.

Silver, J., Kramer, R., Greenwald, S., *et al* (2001) The association between head injuries and psychiatric disorders: findings from the New Haven NIMH Epidermiologic Catchment Area Study. *Brain Injury*, **15**, 935–939.

Skegg, K. (1993) Multiple sclerosis presenting as a pure psychiatric disorder. *Psychological Medicine*, **23**, 909–914.

Sneddon, J. (1980) Myasthenia gravis: a study of social, medical and emotional problems in 26 patients. *Lancet*, **i**, 526–528.

So, N. K., Savard, G., Andermann, F., *et al* (1990) Acute post-ictal pychosis. *Epilepsia*, **31**, 188–193.

Stern, Y., Richards, M., Sano, M., *et al* (1993) Comparison of cognitive changes in patients with Alzheimer's and Parkinson's disease. *Archives of Neurology*, **50**, 1040–1045.

Sternhell, P. S. & Corr, M. J. (2002) Psychiatric morbidity and adherence to anti-retroviral medication in patients with HIV/AIDs. *Australian and New Zealand Journal of Psychiatry*, **36**, 528–533.

Susser, E., Valencia, E. & Conover, S. (1993) Prevalence of HIV infection among psychiatric patients in a New York City men's shelter. *American Journal of Public Health*, **83**, 568–570.

Tavares, A. M. (1993) Psychiatric disorders in neuro-cysticerosis. *British Journal of Psychiatry*, **163**, 839.

Taylor, D. T. (1975) Factors influencing the occurrence of schizophrenia-like psychosis in patients with temporal lobe epilepsy. *Psychological Medicine*, **5**, 249–254.

Thompson, P. J. & Trimble, M. R. (1982) Anticonvulsant drugs and cognitive functions. *Epilepsia*, **23**, 531–544.

Todes, C. J. & Lees, A. J. (1985) The pre-morbid personality of patients with Parkinson's disease. *Journal of Neurology, Neurosurgery and Psychiatry*, **48**, 97–100.

Toone, B. K., Garralda, M. E. & Ron, M. A. (1982) The psychoses of epilepsy and the functional psychoses: a clinical phenomenological comparison. *British Journal of Psychiatry*, **141**, 256–261.

Trautner, R. J., Cummings, J. L., Read, S. L., *et al* (1988) Idiopathic basal ganglia calcification and organic mood disorders. *American Journal of Psychiatry*, **145**, 350–353.

Trimble, M. R. (1992) Behavioural changes following temporal lobectomy, with specific reference to psychosis. *Journal of Neurology, Neurosurgery and Psychiatry*, **55**, 89–91.

Van Hensbrock, M. B., Palmer, A., Jaffar, S., *et al* (1997) Residual neurological sequelae after cerebral malaria. *Journal of Paediatrics*, **131**, 125–129.

Van Hove, J. L., Staygaert, J., Matthijs, G., *et al* (2006) Expanded motor and psychiatric phenotype in autosomal dominant Segawa syndrome due to GTP cyclohydrolase deficiency. *Journal of Neurology, Neurosurgery and Psychiatry*, **77**, 18–23.

Vanneste, J. A. L. (1994) Three decades of normal pressure hydrocephalus – are we wiser now? *Journal of Neurology, Neurosurgery and Psychiatry*, **57**, 1021–1025.

Wieser, H. G., Hailemariam, S. & Regard, M. (1985) Unilateral limbic epileptic status activity: stereo-EEG, behavioural, and cognitive data. *Epilepsia*, **26**, 19–29.

Wilson, S. A. K. (1912) Progressive lenticular degeneration: a familial nervous disease associated with cirrhosis of the liver. *Brain*, **34**, 296–309.

Wolf, P. (1991) Acute behavioural symptomatology at disappearance of epileptiform EEG abnormality: paradoxical or forced normalisation. In *Neurobehavioural Problems in Epilepsy* (eds D. Smith, D. Treiman & M. R. Trimble), pp. 127–142. New York: Raven Press.

CHAPTER 22

Toxic, metabolic and endocrine disorders

Roger Howells

Most toxic, metabolic and endocrine disorders are rare. Collectively, however, they are numerous, and form an important but often unrecognised source of psychiatric morbidity. Presentations range from personality disorder to profound dementia. Behavioural change, mood disturbance, fatigue and apathy are common. Cognitive change is frequently absent, but when present it can be subtle and easily missed.

It could be argued that the greatest impediment to correct diagnosis is the emphasis that psychiatrists give to diagnosing functional psychiatric syndromes, without giving sufficient consideration to organic syndromes. However, there are other difficulties; for example, telltale biochemical, endocrine or toxicological derangements may fluctuate and be missed on isolated screening tests, and physical signs may unfold late or insidiously, or be hidden by the side-effects of medication.

How can routine practice be improved? In this context it is important to 'think organic', that is, it is unwise to assume a 'functional' or 'psychological' aetiology without adequately excluding an organic cause. The practice of attempting to test, or refute, functional diagnoses should be firmly encouraged.

How far should organic investigations be taken? The availability of tests should neither dictate nor limit the diagnostic enquiry. While it makes no sense to screen every patient for metachromatic leucodystrophy, the clinician should have a mental list of the possible causative conditions and be prepared to apply tests whenever the patient's presentation is suggestive.

What benefits accrue from detecting more organic diagnoses?

- There is the chance of either a cure or the partial reversal of some conditions, removing the necessity for indefinite psychiatric care.
- Rarer organic disorders are brought into sharper relief and become better managed.
- If disorders are inherited, other family members usually derive benefit from screening and genetic counselling.
- Identification of various linked multi-system conditions is of great importance for their adequate management.

This chapter is divided into two sections. The first looks at the toxins that can lead to a psychiatric presentation. The term 'psychotoxicology' embraces this aspect of neuropsychiatry. The second examines those metabolic and endocrine disorders that may present to a psychiatrist.

Psychotoxicology

The range of cerebral intoxicants is wide but has been drawn together in the form of a simple classification (Box 22.1). As alcohol is associated with the most extensive physical and psychiatric effects it is given prominence in the following account.

Alcohol

Ethyl alcohol (ethanol) is but one of many psychoactive substances in an alcoholic beverage – these other substances are called *congeners* and include higher alcohols, such as amyl alcohol and butyl alcohol, and acetaldehyde. Vodka might contain approximately 3 mg/100 ml of congeners, whereas a cognac or bourbon can contain in the region of 250 mg/100 ml. Absinthe may contain as many as five alcohol congeners. However, the precise contribution of congeners to the toxicity of alcoholic beverages is at present unclear. Dopamine, glutamate, opioid and GABA-ergic systems have a role in mediating the effects of alcohol (Lingford-Hughes & Nutt, 2003).

The neurological and psychiatric sequelae of alcohol misuse commonly coexist (Box 22.2).

Drunkenness and coma

The classification of alcohol intoxication is similar in DSM–IV (American Psychiatric Association, 1994) and ICD–10 (World Health Organization, 1992). In DSM–IV, the diagnosis of 'alcohol intoxication'

Box 22.1 Intoxicants of the brain with the potential to cause psychiatric symptoms

- Alcohol
- Medicinal drugs
- Drugs of misuse
- Plants and plant-derived substances
- Environmental elements and other chemical substances

Box 22.2 The neurological and psychiatric sequelae of alcohol misuse

Group I. Disorders related to alcohol intoxication
- Drunkenness
- Coma
- Memory blackouts
- Pathological intoxication (*manie à potu*)
- Traumatic head injury

Group II. Alcohol dependence syndrome

Group III. Alcohol withdrawal syndromes
- Simple alcohol withdrawal (with or without fits)
- Alcoholic hallucinosis (acute/sub-acute)
- Alcohol withdrawal delirium (delirium tremens)

Group IV. Alcohol-related nutritional syndromes
- Wernicke–Korsakoff syndrome (vitamin B1, thiamine)
- Nicotinic acid deficiency disorders (vitamin B6, niacin)
- Polyneuropathy
- Optic neuropathy

Group V. Alcohol-related disorders of uncertain pathogenesis
- Alcoholic hallucinosis – chronic
- Alcohol-associated cerebral atrophy and dementia
- Central pontine myelinolysis
- Marchiafava–Bignami disease
- Alcoholic personality change
- Cerebellar degeneration
- Alcohol amblyopia

Group VI. Foetal alcohol syndromes

Group VII. Hepatocerebral disorders

Group VIII. Miscellaneous alcohol-related disorders
- Alcohol-induced hypoglycaemia
- Alcohol-related electrolyte and acid–base disturbance
- Alcohol-related stroke, hypertension and dysrhythmias

Note that not all these sequelae are discussed in the text.
Source: Adapted from Adams & Victor (1989), with permission of the McGraw-Hill Companies.

requires that there has been maladaptive behavioural or psychological change following recent alcohol use, along with signs of intoxication (e.g. slurring of speech, incoordination, or impairment of attention or memory) in the absence of other physical or mental disorder. In ICD–10 'acute intoxication' carries a qualification such as uncomplicated or pathological intoxication.

It is well recognised that alcohol affects individuals differently. The degree of acquired physical tolerance is especially important, but influential factors include age, gender, weight, prior experience with alcohol, learned expectations concerning the effects of alcohol, personality and culture.

After one or two drinks a non-tolerant occasional drinker will display mild changes in mood, behaviour, cognition and motor control. If more is consumed and the blood alcohol level rises above 100 mg/100 ml, lability of mood and disinhibited behaviour, accompanied by impairment of judgement, memory and attention, slurring of speech and incoordination will be manifested. Similar symptoms may occur after head injury, post-ictally and because of hypoglycaemia. Beyond 200 mg/100 ml these changes become marked. At around 300 mg/100 ml depression of medullary function occurs, with the attendant risk of cardiorespiratory failure and coma. High blood alcohol levels inhibit gluconeogenesis and may induce severe hypoglycaemia, especially in malnourished individuals, children and adolescents; the usual signs may be missed if the individual is comatose and hypothermic. Hypovolaemia, lactic acidosis and acute renal failure are additional risks. The median lethal blood alcohol level is 400–500 mg/100 ml.

Intoxicated patients require careful appraisal and management. The margin between narcosis and dangerous respiratory depression is narrower than with other central nervous system depressants such as anaesthetic agents. There is *great* danger attached to the practice of leaving a severely intoxicated person to 'sleep it off'. Coma due to alcohol is a medical emergency, as death may occur through aspiration or respiratory depression. Careful consideration should be given to alternative explanations of coma in the patient who misuses alcohol, particularly stroke, head injury, drug overdose, subdural haematoma, hypoglycaemia, liver failure, circulatory failure and hypothermia. If a patient is comatose or close to coma, a decision will have to be taken as to whether intensive treatments such an intravenous fructose (which may increase the rate of fall of alcohol levels by approximately 25%) or dialysis are warranted. Similar risks exist in police stations: in 1994 almost 25% of the 32 deaths in custody were due to alcohol poisoning (Norfolk & Cartwright, 1996).

Memory blackouts

Loss of memory for actions and events occurring when intoxicated with alcohol is termed a memory blackout, or more correctly alcohol-induced amnesia. Normally the gap in memory is for a matter of hours, although it can be longer. Memory blackouts are widely experienced by dependent drinkers, but are also reported by occasional drinkers quite early in their drinking history.

Two distinctive types of memory loss have been delineated during a memory blackout: 'en-bloc' and 'fragmentary' memory loss. En-bloc memory loss has a discrete onset and terminates with a sense of lost time and apprehension. It is seldom followed by return of the lost memory (Goodwin *et al*, 1969*a*,*b*); large amounts of alcohol are required to induce en-bloc memory loss. Fragmentary memory loss is characterised by partial loss of memory, in which islets of recollection remain. These islets of memory loss often coalesce to produce a somewhat imperfect record of the lost events.

Memory blackouts are important because they are often referred to by drinkers and have to be distinguished from the memory impairment of thiamine deficiency and even fugue. They have considerable medico-legal significance. Alcohol-induced amnesia may account for a patient awaking in a strange place in a 'fugue state'. A range of emotional reactions may be induced by the experience, from little worry at all to anguished fear – for example fear that someone might have been injured or killed through drunken driving or other actions (Edwards *et al*, 2003).

Pathological intoxication

Unusual susceptibility to alcohol is a well-recognised sequel to brain insults, but the question as to whether there are individuals who undergo a 'pathological' reaction to alcohol (*manie à potu; pathologische alkoholreaction*) has been debated for over a century (Banay, 1944). The condition is not uncommon, particularly in medico-legal practice. Both DSM–IV and ICD–10 define it as maladaptive behavioural change, usually aggressive, owing to recent ingestion of alcohol insufficient to induce intoxication in most people, which is atypical of the person when not drinking, and not due to any other physical or mental disorder.

The four main features of the condition are as below (Coid, 1979):

1 it follows the consumption of alcohol (possibly an unexpectedly small quantity)

2 irrational violence occurs, with or without delirium or psychosis

3 there is terminal sleep

4 a degree of amnesia is present for the events that occurred.

Many authorities are sceptical about the validity of pathological intoxication as a clinical entity. May & Ebaugh (1953), for example, concluded that 'amnesia and violence are symptoms ... indications for a careful diagnostic evaluation' – a contention that they justified with illustrative case histories. The controversy has been thoroughly reviewed by Coid (1979). While alcohol is considered to have a direct effect on aggression, even before drinking is begun, beliefs about alcohol's effects, for example how a drunk person is expected to behave, and whether drunkenness is perceived as an excuse for violence, plays a part in the occurrence of disordered conduct and violence (Heather, 1994).

Traumatic head injury

Traumatic head injuries in patients who misuse alcohol are frequently an accompaniment of intoxication and not remembered. Of all the potential sequelae, bleeding into the subdural spaces presents particular diagnostic difficulties. Subdural collections, which can be bilateral, can swell and exert pressure effects – sometimes without localising signs. Furthermore, the condition may be present for months before it manifests, being suspected only when the patient's mental state deteriorates and delirium or coma supervenes. The clinical features may be subtle, with the patient merely complaining of intermittent headache, or there may be a florid presentation with fluctuating consciousness. Skull percussion may reveal lateralised tenderness, sufficient to arouse deeply stuporous patients (Robinson & Stott, 1980). Dementia may emerge insidiously in long-standing cases and be mistaken for the effects of continuing inebriation and social decline. If suspected, the absence of a clear history of trauma should not deter further investigation. Radiological procedures, particularly computed tomography (CT) or magnetic resonance imaging (MRI), will usually reveal the diagnosis, although a normal scan in a deteriorating patient should arouse suspicion that there could be bilateral haematomas with no mass effect.

Box 22.3 The main elements of the alcohol dependence syndrome

1 Narrowing of the repertoire of drinking behaviour
2 Salience of drink-seeking behaviour
3 Increased tolerance to alcohol
4 Repeated withdrawal symptoms
5 Repeated relief or avoidance of withdrawal symptoms by further drinking
6 Subjective awareness of a compulsion to drink
7 Reinstatement of the syndrome after abstinence

Alcohol dependence syndrome

Physical dependence will inevitably follow the sustained intake of alcohol, although the exact quantity required varies between individuals. The alcohol dependence syndrome has seven principal components (Box 22.3) (Edwards & Gross, 1976); these are chiefly manifestations of physical dependency, but they are also affected by personality and cultural factors (Drummond, 1991).

The severity of alcohol dependence may be measured using the Severity of Alcohol Dependence Questionnaire (SADQ), a self-rated instrument with good validity which can be completed in a few minutes (Stockwell *et al*, 1979). The criteria for alcohol dependence syndrome should be sought whenever an alcohol history is being taken. Patients, their families and their doctors are often unaware that the inability to respond to advice to 'stop drinking' is due to established dependence, which causes aversive and potentially dangerous symptoms whenever abstinence is attempted. The presence of anorexia and/or night sweats is usually indicative of alcohol dependence.

Alcohol withdrawal syndromes

When a dependent drinker withdraws from alcohol, an extensive range of physical and mental changes are triggered, collectively termed the 'alcohol withdrawal syndrome'. These changes can be grouped into three major syndromes: simple alcohol withdrawal, alcoholic hallucinosis (acute/sub-acute) and alcohol withdrawal delirium. There is usually considerable overlap between the three syndromes, and a patient experiencing alcohol withdrawal delirium will almost always have experienced the other two previously. Withdrawal features are precipitated by both complete *and* partial withdrawal, and if drinking has recommenced this will disguise the clinical presentation. The occurrence appears to be directly related to cessation of intake (Victor & Adams, 1953), the severity being linked to the quantity and duration of alcohol consumption (Isbell *et al*, 1953) and the pattern of recent drinking (Mello & Mendelson, 1970).

Box 22.4 Clinical features associated with simple alcohol withdrawal

Physical
- Generalised tremor
- Sweating
- Nausea or vomiting
- Fever
- Tachycardia
- Hypertension
- Brisk reflexes
- Epileptic seizures
- Headache
- Visual disturbance
- Disturbance of gait
- Paraesthesia

Mental
- Anxiety
- Depression
- Insomnia
- Irritability
- Anorexia[1]
- Malaise
- Possible illusions
- Possible elemental hallucinations

[1] Anorexia is also a feature of established alcohol dependency.
Sources: Victor & Adams (1953) and Salum (1972).

Simple alcohol withdrawal
This is known by a variety of broadly equivalent terms, notably the 'tremulousness syndrome', 'alcohol withdrawal' (DSM–IV) and 'withdrawal state – uncomplicated' or 'withdrawal state – with convulsions' (ICD–10).

About 3–12 hours after cessation of drinking, a dependent drinker will experience tremulousness associated with one or more of a range of physical and mental changes (Box 22.4). Many of these symptoms are reported by patients who continue to drink because they regularly enter partial withdrawal (e.g. at night or at work). Tremulousness, which can range from mild to severe, is generalised but is typically most evident in the upper limbs; patients will mention embarrassed attempts to conceal their shaking hands.

Box 22.5 Differential diagnosis of delirium in the dependent drinker

- Intoxication
- Alcohol withdrawal delirium
- Thiamine deficiency (Wernicke's disease)
- Head trauma
- Infection
- Post-ictal states
- Liver failure
- Water–sodium imbalance
- Endocrine disorders
- Hypoglycaemia
- Hyperglycaemia
- Pancreatic dysfunction
- Nicotinic acid deficiency
- Hypophosphataemia

The simple withdrawal features reach peak intensity at 24–36 hours into the withdrawal period, thereafter subsiding, although it is not uncommon for insomnia, anxiety and depression to persist for 1–2 weeks or more. Appetite tends to return after 3–5 days. Epileptic seizures ('rum fits') can complicate this otherwise benign syndrome, typically 12–18 hours into withdrawal. These seizures are usually generalised and are thought to be more common in those with a pre-existing history of epilepsy. Hypoglycaemia, hyponatraemia and hypomagnesaemia are potential causes of seizures in the drinker and should be excluded. Post-ictal delirium should be distinguished from the other causes of delirium in the dependent drinker (Box 22.5).

Alcoholic hallucinosis – acute/sub-acute
Perceptual disturbance is a common accompaniment of alcohol withdrawal in the dependent drinker, and alcohol is the commonest cause of hallucinosis in the general population. In dependent drinkers hallucinations can occur:

1 in partial withdrawal

2 where drinking has recommenced but the features of withdrawal are incompletely suppressed

3 in established withdrawal, with or without alcohol withdrawal delirium

4 as a consequence of nutritional, traumatic, ictal, toxic, metabolic or biochemical disturbances

5 due to unknown mechanisms.

In a small proportion of individuals hallucinations may become chronic, whether or not abstinence has been achieved. Careful history-taking is required to establish which type, or types, of alcohol hallucinosis a patient is describing. Withdrawal hallucinations are not usually associated with impaired cognition, but where this occurs it is more correct to use the term 'alcohol withdrawal delirium' (delirium tremens) (see below).

Hallucinations usually occur 12–48 hours into withdrawal. Characteristically, they are most pronounced during the first night – a practical point that must be borne in mind when prescribing medication for the first 24 hours of withdrawal. They are usually fleeting but may last several minutes, holding the individual in a state of perplexity or terror. Insight is variable; full insight is often impeded by the potential threat of the perceived image. One patient likened the experience to watching a horror film alone. These experiences often affect the person's mood. Legrain (1892) observed:

> 'The patient is gloomy, sad and restless. It seems as if the nocturnal tragedies at which he is present continue to impress him during the day, and that he seeks in his surroundings for their explanation.'

Patients report a range of phenomena: vivid dreams, dreams intruding into the waking periods of a broken night's sleep, illusions and misperceptions, simple elemental hallucinations (e.g. clicks and snatched glimpses of a form) and fully formed hallucinations (such as music and conversation, or insects, birds and people). In a survey of 50 consecutive cases, the distribution of affected perceptual modalities was: visual (58%), auditory (16%), and mixed auditory and visual (26%); hallucinations in other modalities were infrequent but certainly occurred (Victor & Hope, 1958). Alcohol withdrawal hallucinations, although usually acute or sub-acute, in a minority of individuals do become chronic.

Patients may be reluctant to disclose their experiences; some fear disclosing what they privately construe as madness. Such symptoms, however, are important clues to the level of a patient's consumption and should be specifically enquired about. The following case history was obtained by the author and is representative.

Case example

A 35-year-old man awoke after dozing in his chair some 16 hours after his last drink. He had earlier been out to buy new jeans and there on his jeans was a shiny spider. He brushed it away but to his horror it transformed into a teaming mass of spiders. In terror he ran downstairs, filled a bucket with a strong bleach solution and immersed his jeans. As he watched, dozens of spiders seemed to come to the surface. After his wife rebuked him he realised it must have been his 'imagination'.

It should be noted that third-person auditory hallucinosis in clear consciousness is not unique to schizophrenia but also occurs in alcoholic hallucinosis (Sabot *et al*, 1968) and that they may be difficult to distinguish (Cohen & Johnson, 1988; Galfond, 1989). This is especially so when the patient conceals or disregards a drinking history, the drinking is accompanied by other substance misuse, secondary delusions arise, or the hallucinosis is long-lasting.

The disorder can be coded in DSM–IV under the heading 'substance-induced psychotic disorder', where 'with onset during withdrawal' and 'with hallucinations' should be added. In ICD–10 the disorder is classified in the alcohol section as psychotic disorder, either as 'schizophrenia-like' or 'predominantly hallucinatory'.

Alcohol withdrawal delirium (delirium tremens)

This usually occurs within 18–36 hours of abstaining from alcohol, although it can occur later. In contrast to alcoholic hallucinosis, there is usually cognitive impairment, although a mild degree of cognitive impairment can sometimes occur with alcohol withdrawal hallucinosis. A classic triad of symptoms occurs:

1 clouding of consciousness and confusion

2 vivid hallucinations and illusions, affecting any sensory modality

3 marked tremor.

Delusions, agitation, insomnia or sleep-cycle reversal, and autonomic overactivity are often present.

In DSM–IV, alcohol withdrawal delirium is placed within the category 'substance withdrawal delirium' and alcohol is specified. In ICD–10, alcohol withdrawal delirium is qualified 'without convulsions' or 'with convulsions'.

Literature is replete with accounts. The following one is by the great French novelist and observer of psychosocial pathology, Émile Zola (1876):

'Gervaise stayed with him until the evening. When the doctor came on his six o'clock round he made him hold up his hands. There was hardly a tremor left, just a slight trembling of the finger tips. But as darkness fell Coupeau gradually got more distressed. Twice he sat up in bed and searched the floor, into the dark corners. Suddenly he lashed out as though he were squashing some creature against the wall.... "The rats! The rats!" Then after a silence, as he was drowsing off he began to struggle a bit and talk disconnectedly. "Oh Christ, they are digging holes in my skin!" ... He aimed blows at the void ... to protect himself from the bearded men he could not see.'

While certainly encountered, more severe degrees of delirium are much rarer – most probably because it is now better recognised that it is potentially dangerous to leave a dependent drinker in withdrawal without some form of medication.

Severe alcohol withdrawal delirium presents abruptly and dramatically, but typically after prodromal simple withdrawal symptoms have occurred. Prodromal symptoms are easily overlooked, particularly when a dependent drinker is unexpectedly cut off from alcohol, as happens following admission to a medical or surgical unit a day or two earlier.

The individual is profoundly disorientated and experiences vivid, often terrifying hallucinations with secondary delusions. Visual hallucinations are most common, but are usually accompanied by auditory and tactile hallucinations (Salum, 1972). Tremulousness is common and pronounced agitation almost always occurs. The patient's mood is typically elevated but may become low in intervals of lucidity. Autonomic changes are usually striking – pupil dilation, fever, tachycardia and profuse sweating are seen. The blood pressure may be high, but in an important minority hypotension is evident. Hypotension is an ominous development usually indicating dehydration and impending circulatory collapse. Thomas Sutton's account in 1813 was remarkable in that it pointed to the dangers of hypovolaemia (blood-letting) (Sutton, 1813). Subcutaneous haematomas are relatively common, and it is reported that in the severest cases pseudo-opisthotonos, which comprises retraction of the head and hyperextension of the back, occurs (Salum, 1972). Epileptic seizures occur in approximately a third of cases, and these often precede the onset of delirium. The delirium fluctuates in intensity and is usually worse at night or under conditions of minimal sensory stimulation. The delirious episode usually ends abruptly as the exhausted individual falls into a long terminal sleep. Memory for the preceding events is usually incomplete and can be absent altogether. Most episodes (80%) end within 72 hours or less. Ward staff should be warned that relapses can occur after apparent recovery, and that the condition may persist for a week or more with periods of lucidity between episodes.

Mortality from severe alcohol withdrawal delirium still occurs; figures of 5–15% are often quoted. Hyperthermia in combination with dehydration will precipitate circulatory collapse. Self-injury and infections also contribute to mortality. Dependent drinkers undoubtedly do die from delirium tremens when alone at home.

Two points deserve to be stressed. First, in clinical practice patients commonly present with symptoms from more than one type of withdrawal syndrome. Thus, symptoms such as drenching nocturnal sweats suggest the autonomic overactivity of nocturnal delirium, yet may not be accompanied by impairment of consciousness. Second, patients may or may not progress from a milder state to a more severe one. Detoxification regimens started early, and of sufficient dosage, will stem the progression to withdrawal delirium.

Management of alcohol withdrawal states

Alcohol withdrawal presents in very many guises and clinicians should have a high index of suspicion in all newly referred psychiatric patients (Howells & Patrick, 1989). Ideally, an informant should be spoken to, indicators of dependency should be sought, and specific enquiry should be made about withdrawal symptoms – such as nocturnal sweats, morning shakes, nausea, anorexia and perceptual disturbance. Enquiry about the type of beverage being consumed is important; strong lagers are typically used by dependent drinkers as an inexpensive source of alcohol.

In order to plan treatment, the severity of withdrawal needs to be gauged. The amount and duration of recent drinking appear to be linked to severity of withdrawal; knowledge of the nature of past withdrawal symptoms, particularly the presence of fits, may also be helpful. The time of the last drinking episode should be recorded and, where possible, a breath alcohol measurement should be made.

A minimum physical examination should assess the following:

- autonomic arousal (temperature, pulse, blood pressure, sweating)
- the severity of tremor and agitation
- signs of liver disease and/or failure (cognitive impairment associated with restlessness, drowsiness, slurred speech, yawning, hiccups, liver flap, foetor hepaticus, various cutaneous signs and ascites)
- physical features of Wernicke's disease (ophthalmoplegia, nystagmus, ataxia, or neuropathy)
- dehydration (buccal dryness, reduced skin turgor, low jugular vein pulse, postural drop in blood pressure and a fast, low-amplitude pulse)
- whether infection is present.

Table 22.1 The components of supportive care required for the nursing management of a patient in alcohol withdrawal

Requirements	Intervention
Control of environmental stimuli	Provide a quiet private room Control the lighting Only one staff member to be in contact Use a uniform, laboratory coat or name badge
Foods and fluids	Offer fluids every 60 minutes Normal, familiar diet at meal times Record the intake
Physical comfort	Support the patient's position with pillows Raise the bed-head if necessary
Body temperature	Apply or remove blankets
Rest and sleep	Allow rest and sleep between assessments Talk to the patient only if an exchange is initiated by the patient
Elimination	Assist to the bathroom or commode Record the output
Reality orientation	Orientate with respect to time, place and person
Reassurance	Use positive encouragement Ensure hourly contact
Rehabilitation	Discuss only if it is raised by the patient Agree if the patient says he/she wants to stop drinking
Visitors	No visitors when intensive supportive care is under way
Smoking	Only if patient asks, and limit it because of the fire risk

Source: Based on Naranjo & Sellers (1986).

Mental state examination should assess mood, anxiety, the presence or absence of abnormal perceptions and thoughts, cognition (especially orientation and memory) and the degree of insight.

In-patient management will be necessary if the patient has features of incipient delirium (particularly cognitive impairment, with autonomic overactivity or severe agitation), physical complications, a strong history of withdrawal seizures, or a history of poor compliance with out-patient detoxification regimens, or poor home support.

Practical rating instruments are used to monitor autonomic and psychological indices, such as the Selected Severity of Alcohol withdrawal (SSA) or its revised derivative, the Clinical Institute Withdrawal Assessment for Alcohol (CIWA-Ar) scale (Sullivan *et al*, 1989).

Simple withdrawal features of a mild degree may respond to structured in-patient nursing procedures (Table 22.1).

Patients in simple withdrawal or with uncomplicated alcohol withdrawal hallucinosis can undergo alcohol withdrawal as out-patients, attending daily to pick up a prescription and for clinical review. The medication of choice is a benzodiazepine drug such as chlordiazepoxide. Benzodiazepines have cross-tolerance with alcohol, better efficacy and less toxicity than most other candidate drugs, and have excellent anticonvulsive properties. Chlordiazepoxide is used in the dose range 20–40 mg four times a day. Under-medicating patients receiving out-patient detoxification is dangerous. The prescription of one or two extra p.r.n. doses of medication for the first two nights is often helpful as symptoms are severest to begin with, at a time when the ideal dosage for symptom control is unknown. Decrements are made each day to enable the drug to be withdrawn after 7–14 days or sooner. Each day when the patient returns, breath alcohol analysis should be performed and the adequacy of the medication in achieving symptom control in the preceding 24 hours should be assessed, treatment adjustments being made accordingly. Loss of night sweats, reduction in tremor and return of appetite herald recovery.

Since anorexia, poor diet and impaired absorption of vitamins occur in dependent drinkers, a poly-vitamin supplement is indicated in all in-patient detoxifications (Taylor *et al*, 2003). Parenteral administration (with Pabrinex) overcomes the impairment of gut absorption that is thought to occur in patients who misuse alcohol, but it is important if there is a suspicion of Wernicke's encephalopathy (see below), malnutrition or peripheral neuropathy. It carries a risk of causing an anaphylactic reaction. Precautionary arrangements should always be made.

Patients with a history of recurring withdrawal seizures may warrant prophylactic treatment with an anticonvulsant, although the risks of prescribing anticonvulsants in this group are considerable. As alcohol withdrawal seizures are usually generalised, partial seizures always warrant investigation.

Alcohol withdrawal delirium (delirium tremens) requires intensive nursing care as an in-patient. Minimum investigation comprises a full blood count and erythrocyte sedimentation rate, serum electrolytes and liver function tests, blood glucose analysis, chest and skull radiographs, and close observation of fluid balance.

Benzodiazepines are the drugs of choice. Chlordiazepoxide is usually used (diazepam in some centres or where sensitivity to chlordiazepoxide is known). Taylor *et al* (2003) set out the management. An initial or 'stat' dose is determined, followed by a regimen for the first 24 hours. Thereafter a standardised reducing regimen can be implemented. The dosage is estimated according to the clinical signs and symptoms of withdrawal, and the breath alcohol concentration on admission and after 1 hour. Should there continue to be significant further symptoms after the initial regimen has been implemented, medical review of the patient is required – 'as required' (p.r.n.) prescribing of chlordiazepoxide should not be routinely used.

In extremis, more rapid control can be achieved with slow intravenous injection of diazepam (with which there is a risk of overdosage). Alternative regimens in the past used drugs such as chlormethiazole, propranolol, phenothiazines (which risk precipitating hypotension and fits), chloral hydrate, and even the reintroduction of alcohol. While they are generally effective, they are not recommended – their associated complications have made benzodiazepines the first-line agents. Fluid and electrolyte problems are discussed separately below; details of the accompanying physical complications are available elsewhere.

Box 22.6 The principal clinical features of the Wernicke–Korsakoff syndrome

Wernicke's disease

1 Disorders of cognition and consciousness. Three presentations are recognised:
'quiet' delirium (disorientation, apathy, drowsiness, impaired attention and memory)
stupor
coma

2 Ocular abnormalities:
nystagmus (horizontal and/or vertical)
lateral rectus palsy (bilaterally)
conjugate gaze palsy

3 Ataxia (mild to severe gait ataxia)

4 Polyneuropathy (the legs alone are affected in most cases)

Korsakoff syndrome

1 Memory impairments:
preserved primary memory
impaired recent memory
extensive retrograde amnesia

2 Other criteria include relatively poor insight into the deficit, absence of impairment of consciousness, and the absence of global cognitive impairment

3 Other reported cognitive impairments include frontal lobe dysfunction, visuoperceptive deficits and impairment on abstracting tasks

Note: confabulation, usually of the spontaneous type, occurs early as the Korsakoff state emerges, but does not persist. (Confabulation should not be regarded as a prerequisite for the diagnosis.)

Source: Adapted from Victor *et al* (1989).

Wernicke–Korsakoff syndrome

Ophthalmoplegia, nystagmus, gait ataxia and mental confusion (delirium) constitute the cardinal features of Wernicke's disease (also known as Wernicke's encephalopathy), a disorder of abrupt onset first described in 1881 by Carl Wernicke in Germany. In 1887 Sergei Korsakoff, a prominent Russian psychiatrist, described an illness characterised by pronounced impairment of recent and retrograde memory – cerebropathia psychica toxaemica. Korsakoff's 'psychosis' was subsequently linked to Wernicke's disease: that is, a proportion of cases of acute Wernicke's disease proceed to Korsakoff syndrome, and Wernicke–Korsakoff syndrome is the unitary disorder comprising the two. In patients with either clinical presentation, post-mortem neuropathological examination (further confirming their unitary nature) reveals lesions in the following nuclei: medial dorsal, medial mamillary, dorsal hypothalamic, central grey, oculomotor, and medial vestibular. The nucleus basalis of Meynert is also affected.

The cause of the Wernicke–Korsakoff syndrome was discovered to be thiamine deficiency. This appears to be due to poor appetite and malnutrition, as well as malabsorption and other factors.

The manifestations of Wernicke's disease and Korsakoff syndrome (Box 22.6) rarely present in their entirety, but the classical clinical triad indicative of Wernicke's disease (ophthalmoplegia/nystagmus, delirium and ataxia) should always be actively sought. More than 70% of these patients may not have eye signs, and the point has been made that the delirium and ataxia may be impossible to distinguish from simple intoxication or drunkenness in the accident and emergency department (Thomson *et al*, 2002). Coincidental disorders such as alcohol withdrawal delirium can obscure the picture. While Korsakoff syndrome is usually the sequel, it can present without an explicit history of Wernicke's disease. In these cases, it seems likely that the preceding episode of Wernicke's disease may have occurred unnoticed, outside hospital.

Wernicke's disease is mostly encountered in dependent drinkers, although psychiatrists must be well acquainted with the range of settings in which it can occur (Box 22.7).

Box 22.7 Circumstances in which thiamine deficiency may cause Wernicke's disease

Dietary deficiency
- Alcoholism, anorexia nervosa, inadequately formulated total parenteral nutrition, starvation
- Refeeding syndrome
- Persistent vomiting
- Hyperemesis gravidarum, alcoholism, bulimia nervosa

States of impaired absorption
- Alcoholism, pernicious anaemia, gastrointestinal carcinoma, chronic diarrhoea, gastroduodenal surgery
- Increased metabolic demand in the context of deficiency
- Through giving a glucose load to a thiamine-deficient person who misuses alcohol
- Hyperthyroidism

Others
- Dialysis (haemodialysis or peritoneal)
- Cancer
- HIV syndromes

It should be emphasised that a diagnosis of Wernicke's disease is made clinically. Serum thiamine levels can be inferred from red cell transketolase and other enzymes but the results will not be ready soon enough to influence management and, moreover, serum levels do not necessarily mirror levels within the central nervous system (CNS). If the disease is suspected, treatment with parenteral thiamine should not be delayed. Wernicke's disease is a medical emergency, because without rapid intervention permanent brain damage (i.e. Korsakoff syndrome) is a likely, although not invariable, consequence. In one series it was the sequel in 84% of cases (Victor *et al*, 1989). Without treatment patients face a significant risk of mortality; severely deficient patients can become stuporous, enter coma and die in 1–2 weeks or develop beriberi heart disease.

The Royal College of Physicians' guidelines on managing patients at risk of Wernicke's disease propose one pair of Pabrinex intravenous injection ampoules by slow injection (over 30 minutes) in 100 ml normal saline, and for established Wernicke's disease two pairs of Pabrinex ampoules 3 times daily for 3 days. The same authority gives guidelines on magnesium, phosphate and potassium supplements (Thomson *et al*, 2002). They note that there is a small risk of inducing anaphylaxis with these injections; therefore resuscitation facilities must be available. It is essential to correct thiamine deficiency *before* giving a carbohydrate load.

The ocular palsies that occur in Wernicke's disease are remarkably responsive to treatment, a helpful diagnostic point to note. Initially patients should have bed rest because of the small but significant risk of cardiovascular collapse from 'beriberi' heart disease induced by thiamine deficiency, a disorder in which there is peripheral vasodilation and associated oedema, cardiac dilation and ultimately high-output cardiac failure. Supportive nursing measures are required (see Table 22.1). Nicotinic acid (niacin, nicotinamide) deficiency can coexist with thiamine deficiency and must be suspected if patients fail to respond to thiamine.

While the ophthalmoplegia, ataxia and delirium resolve rapidly with treatment, nystagmus can persist as a permanent marker of the episode. If significant brain damage has been incurred, the disorders of memory characteristic of Korsakoff syndrome come into sharper relief (Kopelman, 1987*a*), often heralded by spontaneous confabulation (Kopelman, 1987*b*). However, confabulation generally recedes and is not a feature of patients with established Korsakoff syndrome. Partial recovery of memory is usual, but the onset of this is delayed for several weeks or months, thereafter proceeding slowly over many months (Victor *et al*, 1989). Serial psychometric measurements are an objective way of monitoring recovery. Less than a quarter of patients recover their memory completely. The deficit may be so great as to necessitate indefinite nursing.

Nicotinic acid deficiency disorders

Deficiency of nicotinic acid (niacin, nicotinamide) is most commonly found among people who misuse alcohol and may have a significant mortality. It may coexist with other vitamin deficiency disorders. It is due to poor dietary intake, decreased uptake, decreased conversion to the active coenzyme form, decreased storage and an increased requirement. It presents with the well-known triad of skin lesions, gastrointestinal disorders and mental changes. Some members of the triad may not be present or may go unrecognised. The skin lesions (erythema, pigmentation and hyperkeratosis) occur on parts of the body exposed to sunlight and are easily missed. The gastrointestinal disorders, such as diarrhoea, constipation and nausea, may be attributed to 'gastritis' and dismissed. Furthermore, the mental changes of delirium, hallucinations, insomnia, anxiety and depression are indistinguishable from those of alcoholism. In less severe deficiency states, the clinical presentation is similar to neurasthenia (fatigue, loss of appetite, headache, disturbed sleep, anxiety, irritability and depression). Left untreated, a delirious state may arise (acute nicotinic acid encephalopathy) or dementia may develop insidiously.

The acute delirious state contrasts with that of Wernicke's disease in that it is usually accompanied by agitation and excitement. Stupor, coma and death may supervene before the diagnosis is made. While the presentation may be clinically indistinguishable from alcohol withdrawal delirium, the development of extrapyramidal rigidity is an important pointer to the presence of nicotinic acid deficiency, as is treatment resistance in alcohol withdrawal delirium or Wernicke's disease. Administration of the deficient vitamin has a strikingly beneficial effect on the clinical course.

Post-mortem findings are of central chromatolysis in the Betz cells of the motor cortex, thalamic neurons, pontine neurons and anterior horn cells.

Alcohol-related disorders of uncertain pathogenesis

Alcoholic hallucinosis – chronic

Hallucinations in cases of acute withdrawal hallucinosis, alcohol withdrawal delirium and in other conditions in people who misuse alcohol are commonly and erroneously grouped together under the term 'alcoholic hallucinosis'. The recorded drinking histories in such cases are often meagre, and it is not made clear whether other causes have been adequately excluded. Before making the diagnosis of chronic alcoholic hallucinosis, other cerebral disorders and substance misuse should be rigorously sought and excluded. Chronic hallucinosis presents a particular diagnostic problem when accompanied by changes in mental state, personality and behaviour resembling those seen in schizophrenia (such as downward social drift).

Management is straightforward: absolute abstinence should be enforced, and the misuse of other substances excluded by regular screening. A low starting dose of neuroleptics should be titrated against the symptoms. Periodically, attempts should be made to reduce or withdraw the medication.

Alcohol-associated cerebral atrophy and dementia

The issue as to whether or not alcohol toxicity itself causes a *primary* dementia remains unresolved. There are many complicating factors. First, any directly toxic effects are difficult to dissociate from other potential influences (i.e. nutritional deficiencies, hepatocerebral disorder, misuse of other substances, head injury, Alzheimer's disease, arteriosclerotic disease and other dementing processes). Second, even the most elegant neuropsychometric protocols are affected by such problems as uncooperativeness, apathy and mood disturbance in the patient who is alcohol dependent. Third, studies of the relationship between alcohol and cognitive function are influenced by the timing of cognitive testing in relation to periods of abstinence. Finally, gaining reliable drinking histories from patients who misuse alcohol has proved to be notoriously difficult.

There is compelling evidence that cortical atrophy, especially frontal atrophy, occurs in Wernicke–Korsakoff syndrome. This evidence comes from CT and MRI studies, morphological studies and cerebral blood flow studies, but whether this is due to thiamine deficiency or the action of alcohol *directly* is unresolved.

Whether alcohol is the direct cause of some of the structural and functional deficits detectable in the brains of many chronic drinkers is far less certain. Ron (1983) reported cerebral shrinkage in half to two-thirds of individuals who were chronic misusers of alcohol, often from quite early in their drinking careers. There are also reports of widespread cognitive deficits, in memory, psychomotor speed, visuospatial and abstracting abilities and complex reasoning, which can persist after 'drying out'. Some dispute the existence of a primary alcoholic dementia and instead relate the changes to the effects of thiamine deficiency. There is evidence that favours a direct and more diffuse neurotoxic effect of alcohol as well; the issues are discussed by Lishman (1998).

Central pontine myelinolysis

Central pontine myelinolysis is an acute, usually fatal disorder first described in people who are dependent on alcohol and undernourished individuals. The aetiology is uncertain, but the direct cause does not appear to be alcohol toxicity or vitamin deficiency. The disorder typically occurs in conjunction with life-threatening illnesses, which are often unrelated to alcohol use. Rapid correction of hyponatraemia may lead to central pontine myelinolysis, and disturbances of serum potassium levels have also been incriminated. The presence of clinical features such as pseudo-bulbar palsy, quadriplegia, delirium and coma may lead to the diagnosis being made before death, but more usually it is made at post-mortem. The lesions are visible on MRI. Histological examination of the brain will show circumscribed areas of demyelination both in the pons and less commonly in certain extrapontine sites.

Marchiafava–Bignami disease

This disorder is characterised by demyelination of parts of the corpus callosum, the anterior commissure, and other areas of the brain, such as the third layer of the frontal and temporal cortices. While the majority of cases described have been patients with chronic alcoholism, it is not exclusive to them. Nutritional factors are thought to be implicated.

The presentation can be very varied. Affected patients may exhibit neurological signs such as dysarthria, dysphasia, dyspraxia, ataxia and hemiparesis, typically accompanied by physical deterioration that leads to stupor and coma. Marchiafava–Bignami disease may present as a frontal lobe syndrome, or as a progressive dementia evolving over 3–6 years. The diagnosis is notoriously difficult to make in life because of the variability of the clinical picture; other complications of alcoholism can further obscure the presentation. A frontal lobe syndrome in someone who misuses alcohol should alert the clinician to the possibility of Marchiafava–Bignami disease, as should symptoms suggestive of a corpus callosal tumour. MRI is capable of detecting corpus callosal lesions early in the course of the disease.

Hepatocerebral disorders

The term 'hepatic encephalopathy' has been used to describe the organic reactions of the brain to liver disease. Acute severe hepatic dysfunction, such as that caused by viruses and drugs, is relatively uncommon in people who misuse alcohol. Patients with acute severe hepatic dysfunction exhibit euphoria, depression, hypersomnia, posturing and behavioural change of a bizarre and socially inappropriate nature (Collis & Lloyd, 1992). The presence of psychiatric symptoms is almost always a grave prognostic indicator, as chemical and histological changes are severe and extensive by then. Coma usually supervenes within a few days unless there is effective management of the many complications. Cerebral oedema is found at post-mortem, and histological changes are usually non-specific.

However, hepatocerebral disturbance in people who misuse alcohol is more usually sub-acute, chronic, or acute on chronic, occurring as a consequence of the development of a shunt between the portal and systemic circulation (toxins from the portal system enter the cerebral circulation unchanged by the liver). Quite which toxic substance is responsible is unclear; two possibilities involve impaired hepatic removal of ammonia from the gut with an increase in false transmitter precursors, and increased endogenous benzodiazepine activities.

Days to weeks before the onset of delirium, stupor or coma, there may be an array of symptoms that are essentially reversible. These include changes in personality, such as irritability, jocularity, neurotic symptoms, depressed or elated mood, restlessness and schizophreniform psychosis. Daytime hypersomnia with nocturnal wakefulness is usually present early on. It is often cautioned that hypersomnia, coupled with a fixed, staring appearance and a reduction in spontaneous movement, is early evidence of clinical deterioration. Recent memory is often impaired and confabulation can be striking. Attention and orientation may be affected. Delirium is typically of the 'quiet' type, but there may be episodes of irritability and overactivity. Hallucinations are usually simple or elemental, although complex visual hallucinations may occur. Catatonia and stupor are well-recognised developments, and deterioration into coma is a real risk. Hypoglycaemia, electrolyte imbalance, renal failure, infection and cerebral oedema may all contribute to the altered mental state in hepatic failure. However, delirium in someone who misuses alcohol and who has liver disease should not be assumed to be hepatocerebral, as it is not always so.

As the patient deteriorates, extrapyramidal, cerebellar and pyramidal signs unfold. Initially there may be incoordination, impaired handwriting and constructional apraxia. Foetor hepaticus ('liver breath') is typically present. In the course of time a flapping tremor (asterixis), dysarthria and muscle rigidity may develop. Pyramidal signs become increasingly pronounced, fits may occur and the patient becomes comatose, with flaccid tone, absent reflexes and extensor plantars (Lishman, 1998).

At post-mortem, protoplasmic astrocytes are typically increased in size and number in the cortex and many other brain regions. There is usually patchy necrosis and neuronal loss in the deep cerebral cortex.

Some patients develop persistent global cognitive impairment, particularly where the acute episodes have been prolonged or frequent. This has been termed 'acquired hepatocerebral degeneration'. Attention is impaired but orientation in time and place is often intact. Memory is affected, particularly in the acquisition and retention of new material, but not disproportionately as in Korsakoff syndrome. Insight is generally lacking. A variety of neurological signs are usually present, particularly choreoathetosis, dysarthria, ataxia and pyramidal signs. These patients may periodically deteriorate as acute organic episodes are superimposed.

The assessment of the degree of cerebral disorder in a patient with liver failure is reviewed by Pappas & Jones (1983); they recommend that the mental state is staged and provide a scheme. It is important to note that verbal skills may be relatively well preserved, and thus mild degrees of cerebral disorder may go unnoticed unless psychometry is performed.

A normal electroencephalogram (EEG) will usually exclude the diagnosis of hepatocerebral disorder. EEG changes may antedate changes in mental state and persist after apparent clinical improvement.

The patient with hepatocerebral disorder should not drink alcohol. Dietary protein restriction and other measures are required. If sedation is required a very low starting dose must be used; the risk is proportionate to the degree of liver disorder and this may not be a function of liver enzymes alone. A benzodiazepine can be used cautiously; Taylor *et al* (2003) provide guidance on the use of drugs in hepatic impairment. The patient should be made aware of the potential dangers of medications, particularly sedatives, whose absorption, protein-binding, metabolism and distribution will be altered (Collis & Lloyd, 1992).

Renewed drinking, dietary indiscretion, a gastrointestinal bleed, inappropriate medication and infection are but a few of the potential causes of a resurgence of psychiatric disturbance in a previously well-managed patient.

Miscellaneous alcohol-related disorders

Alcohol-induced hypoglycaemia

Hypoglycaemia is an often overlooked cause of morbidity in those who misuse alcohol and should always be excluded. It is predominantly a disorder of more chronic, dependent drinkers who are malnourished. It has also been described in young people after first exposure to alcohol and in children after self-poisoning with alcohol-containing mouthwash. The origin is thought to be a reduced hepatic output of glucose, due to reduced hepatic stores of glycogen and suppression of gluconeogenesis during metabolism of alcohol. This is a situation potentiated when there is anorexia, for then gluconeogenesis is the main source of glucose.

Hypoglycaemia typically occurs 2–16 hours after a large intake of alcohol. At a blood glucose level just under 2.0 mmol/l, autonomic symptoms appear and gradually intensify, heralding the onset of delirium. Hypoglycaemia may induce generalised seizures, which should not be mistaken for withdrawal seizures. Stupor may also occur. At a blood glucose level of around 0.6 mmol/l, life-threatening hypoglycaemic coma is usually evident and recovery will often be incomplete. The treatment is immediate administration of glucose intravenously, and thiamine should be given concurrently to avoid precipitating Wernicke's disease.

Alcohol-related electrolyte and acid–base disturbance

Fluid loss may be substantial in severe delirium, requiring close monitoring and prompt correction. As much as 6 litres of fluid a day may need to be given, of which no more than 1 litre should be in the form of normal saline. Conversely, hyponatraemia may complicate the consumption of large quantities of relatively dilute alcoholic drinks. It is a potential cause of convulsions and is managed by fluid restriction. Hyponatraemia, hypokalaemia, hypophosphataemia and hypomagnesaemia may all occur in people who misuse alcohol and have been associated with withdrawal delirium.

Psychiatrists should also be aware of the dangers (including heart failure and sudden death) of the 'refeeding syndrome' – hypophosphataemia, hypomagnesaemia, and hypokalaemia with or without critical thiamine deficiency occur as a consequence of the resumption of oral nutrition after prolonged calorie deprivation. Alcohol-dependent individuals, vagrants, and individuals with self-neglect in the context of severe mental illnesses are all at risk (Crook *et al*, 2001).

Medicinal drugs

Cerebral intoxication with medicines is a frequent cause of psychiatric morbidity. This can go unrecognised if there is ignorance of the adverse effects of a medication, or when patients overlook, deny or understate their usage. The young and elderly are especially vulnerable, as are those individuals with physical illness, alcohol dependency or a requirement for more than one drug at a time. Drugs produce mental changes either by direct intoxication or, once physical tolerance has developed, as a consequence of withdrawal. Intoxication can occur at normal dosage, as an idiosyncratic reaction, or through interaction with other substances, but more usually it is due to excessive dosage, by accident or deliberately.

Delirium is a characteristic manifestation of drug intoxication, often with hallucinations. Other manifestations are dementia, psychosis in clear consciousness, mood change, lethargy and anxiety. Predominantly physical adverse reactions, such as neuroleptic malignant syndrome, tardive dyskinesia and lithium intoxication, usually have accompanying mental changes.

Many drugs have the ability to cause delirium. Information on adverse psychiatric reactions to drugs can be obtained most efficiently by a search on the internet-based version of the *British National Formulary* (http://bnf.org/bnf/), while *Martindale* (Sweetman, 2006) remains the most authoritative paper-based resource (and now also available online from http://www.pharmpress.com).

Three types of drug intoxication have been selected for more detailed discussion here: intoxication as a result of drugs with anticholinergic activity; intoxication from drugs with central stimulant properties; and intoxication from over-the-counter medications.

Box 22.8 Classes of drugs with anticholinergic activity

- Antispasmodic drugs
- Antimotility (gastrointestinal) drugs
- Antihistamines
- Compound nasal decongestants
- Antipsychotics
- Antidepressants
- Antiparkinsonian drugs
- Antiemetics
- Premedication agents
- Drugs for urinary incontinence
- Topical antipruritic drugs
- Mydriatic and cycloplegic drugs

Anticholinergic (antimuscarinic) intoxication

Anticholinergic poisoning from plants and medicines has been recognised since ancient times. In 38 AD the retreating troops of Mark Antony are said to have consumed *Datura stramonium* as they left Partia, and developed confusion with many deaths. The same mistake was made by British troops in Jamestown, Virginia, in 1676.

Drugs with antimuscarinic activity inhibit the actions of acetylcholine on autonomic effectors innervated by postganglionic cholinergic nerves, as well as having a direct effect on smooth muscles that lack cholinergic innervation. Atropine is the best known of this class of drug, although there are very many others (see Box 22.8 and Table 22.2, below). It should be noted that anticholinergic poisoning can occur as a result of ingestion of a number of plants, notably *Atropa belladonna* (deadly nightshade), *Datura stramonium* and *Hyoscyamus niger* (henbane).

The clinical picture has been described as 'hot as a hare, blind as a bat, dry as a bone, red as beet and mad as a hatter'. However, it should not be forgotten that intoxication commonly unfolds in an insidious fashion (Johnson *et al*, 1981). The symptoms of anticholinergic intoxication are essentially those of atropine intoxication. Small doses of atropine cause a dry mouth and reduce bronchial secretions. Inhibition of sweating is followed by fever. Larger doses impair pupillary accommodation, and cause pupil dilation and thus blurred vision. Tachycardia is common. Still larger doses inhibit parasympathetic control of the bowel and bladder, resulting in difficulty passing urine and reduced bowel sounds. Doses as great as 5 mg of atropine produce difficulty in swallowing, restlessness, fatigue and headache, together with dry, hot skin. Beyond this, the skin is hot, dry and scarlet in colour. Ataxia, restlessness and excitement occur. Delirium and hallucinations ensue and can be followed by coma. Impairment of recent memory is a prominent feature. The hallucinations may be auditory or visual. Without effective intervention there is a significant chance that the patient will die through brain-stem depression, hyperpyrexia or injury (while delirious).

Anticholinergic intoxication should not be confused with the neuroleptic malignant syndrome, which has certain features in common (notably tachycardia, labile blood pressure, hyperpyrexia and fluctuating levels of consciousness; Howells, 1994). The vital distinguishing features of anticholinergic intoxication are dilated pupils, with dry skin and mucous membranes.

Anticholinergic drug intoxication is managed with physostigmine, an anticholinesterase, in accordance with a management plan such as that of Heiser & Gillin (1971).

Anticholinergic intoxication has become more uncommon within psychiatric drug prescribing, as the use of tricyclic antidepressants and thioridazine has lessened. Clozapine is the atypical antipsychotic drug with especially prominent anticholinergic properties.

Central nervous system stimulants and anoretics

In 1924 ephedrine, extracted from the ancient Chinese herb Ma Huang, was introduced into Western medicine as a bronchodilator. Shortly afterwards it was synthesised chemically, and amphetamine was synthesised as a substitute for ephedrine. The structures of the two compounds are remarkably similar, as are their actions and those of the further synthetic derivatives that constitute this group of drugs.

Ephedrine, pseudo-ephedrine, phenylephrine and phenylpropanololamine are ingredients of cold remedies and constitute some of the most widely used over-the-counter drugs. Analysis of the non-proprietary drugs used in the UK (as listed in edition 47 of the *British National Formulary*) reveals some 55 compounds with these ingredients. In the UK the use of centrally acting stimulants (dexamphetamine sulphate or methylphenidate) is restricted principally to the treatment of narcolepsy, and hyperactivity and/or attention-deficit disorder in adults and children. Drugs with amphetamine-like properties are scarcely available for use as anoretic pills; however, these are widely available on the internet – such compounds number more than 20 and include drugs such as benzphetamine, cloforex, diethylproprion, fenproporex, pemoline and phenmetrazine.

The toxic effect of amphetamine is to induce a paranoid psychosis, with ideas of reference, delusions of persecution, and auditory and visual hallucinations, almost always in a setting of clear consciousness (Connell, 1958). Depression and somnolence are common in withdrawal. Intoxication with ephedrine produces a virtually identical clinical picture. First-rank symptoms of schizophrenia are reported to be present in approximately 35% of cases, delusions in 100% and auditory hallucinations in 90% (Whitehouse & Duncan, 1987).

While children and the elderly are especially vulnerable, misuse and dependence also occur in other age groups. Similar effects are reported with anoretic agents and other centrally acting stimulants. Related compounds have been sold for indications such as 'lack of drive', as in the following example.

Case example

A middle-aged Jamaican man with unstable paranoid schizophrenia and aggression was brought to England for clinical review. It transpired that he had been buying large quantities of fenethylline (Captagon) which he had been able to purchase legally over the counter. A clear temporal relationship was demonstrated between the use of the drug and the occurrence of his symptoms. The patient understood and accepted the link but confessed an inability to change his habit.

These drugs achieve special significance when considering the differential diagnosis of schizophrenia – a diagnosis that, arguably, should be made only if symptoms are present when a person has been shown to be completely free of such substances. In the author's experience the clinical situation can be complicated by patients who conceal their drug use, volunteer symptoms that were present when they *were* taking the drug, and by misleading results from drug screening tests. Commonly used immunoassay techniques may fail to detect the presence of diethylpropion, phentermine and other drugs, while the more reliable (but less widely available) gas chromatographic assays can fail to detect pemoline.

Over-the-counter drugs

The misuse of over-the-counter drugs has long been recognised. In the late 1980s it was estimated that some five billion doses of phenylpropanolamine were taken annually in the USA (Forman *et al*, 1989), revealing the extent of the problem.

Chronic affective disturbance, psychosis, delirium and personality change are the consequences of intoxication, dependence or withdrawal from these drugs (Jacobs, 1987). There are at least 80 over-the-counter products whose constituents have the potential to cause significant psychiatric symptoms (Table 22.2 shows some of the more common ones). Intoxication has been reported from topical nasal compounds, eye drops, inhalations and even substances administered topically.

The hidden morbidity from these compounds is likely to be high, particularly in children, who are commonly given cold remedies containing drugs with the potential to cause intoxication. Evidence for this can be adduced from Sweden, where in 1979 the Swedish adverse drug reaction committee received 61 reports of psychic disturbance from phenylpropanolamine – restlessness, irritability, aggression and sleep disturbance. The majority were in children, including three of the five individuals who had psychotic symptoms (Norvenius *et al*, 1979).

Case example

A physician gave his 2-year-old son 5 ml of a preparation of triprolidine and pseudo-ephedrine at bedtime because of an irritating cough and runny nose. The child awoke saying there were 'ants crawling in his bed'. This was assumed to be due to pyrexia. The next night the medicine was overlooked and the child had no sleep disturbance. On the third night the medicine was given again and the hallucinations recurred. On reflection it was thought that these could have been induced a number of times over the preceding 9 months, but the link had not been made. (Drennan, 1984)

Dependence in adults is often concealed and is difficult to detect from drug screening. It may become extreme. Dependence does not always begin accidentally; some compounds, particularly phenylpropanolamine and ephedrine, have long been regarded as convenient amphetamine substitutes.

Drugs of misuse

A detailed exposition of this group of drugs is beyond the remit of this chapter; however, many of these drugs represent important sources of brain intoxication. It should be noted that certain substances have prolonged effects that persist beyond the period during which an effect may reasonably be assumed to be operating. Flashbacks are a well-known example of this, but other effects include personality disorder, affective disorder,

Table 22.2 Constituents of over-the-counter products available in the UK with the potential to cause cerebral intoxication and/or dependence

Group	Constituents
CNS stimulants with amphetamine-like effects	Ephedrine, methylephedrine, pseudo-ephedrine, phenylephrine, phenylpropanolamine, oxymetazoline (eye drops)
Drugs with anticholinergic side-effects	Atropine, belladonna alkaloids, homatropine, hyoscine, chlorphenhydramine, diphenhydramine, promethazine, doxylamine
Alcohol	
Drugs with caffeine-like effects (xanthines)	Caffeine, theophylline
Opioids	Morphine, codeine, pholcodine, dextromethorphan
Miscellaneous drugs	Bismuth carbonate, menthol, chloroform

cognitive impairment and late-onset psychotic disorder. Interested readers are referred to *Seminars in Alcohol and Drug Misuse* (Chick & Cantwell, 1994).

Plants and plant-derived substances

Here, the broad notion of intoxication from material derived from plants is introduced. The interested reader is encouraged to consult further sources such as Emboden (1972), Efron *et al* (1979) and Jacobs (1987).

Intoxication from various plants occurs in at least four ways.

1 Accidental exposure may occur through contamination, as in the instance of ergot-contaminated grain (*Claviceps purpurea*) or through accidental ingestion, as with nutmeg (*Myristica fragrans*) and deadly nightshade (*Atropa belladonna*).

2 Intoxication may occur as a result of traditional rites, rituals and practices. Examples range from the excessive use of caffeine-containing beverages, and the drinking and chewing of khat (*Catha edulis*) in Arabia and Somalia, to chewing a quid of pituri (*Duboisia hopwoodii*) (Australia) or drinking sinicuichi (*Heimia salicifolia*) (Central America).

3 Intoxication may be due to deliberate misuse of plant substances, either those available within one's culture, or by seeking out substances from other cultures or lands. The author had one patient who obtained peyote (*Lophophora williamsii*) from a south London herbalist shop and had regularly misused magic mushrooms (*Psilocybe*).

4 Intoxication may occur as a result of poisoning by another person.

The range of potential plant intoxicants is much wider than is often appreciated (Table 22.3 shows some of them). The chief relevance to the clinician is in differential diagnosis, particularly but not exclusively in transcultural practice; it should always be recalled that major psychiatric symptoms such as hallucinations can be caused by plant intoxicants.

Caffeine intoxication

Of the plant-derived substances with the potential to cause intoxication, caffeine (a xanthine) is surely the most popular and widely consumed. It is present in tea, coffee, soft drinks such as cola, and chocolate, and also in some 27 or more over-the-counter compounds. Other xanthines are found in tea, coffee and chocolate, particularly theobromine and theophylline, the latter having a potent stimulant effect on the CNS.

Caffeine has a stimulant effect on the CNS, as well as wide-ranging systemic effects. The clinical features of intoxication include restlessness, nervousness, excitement, insomnia, flushed face, diuresis, gastrointestinal disturbance, muscle twitching, rambling flow of thought and speech, tachycardia or cardiac dysrhythmia, periods of inexhaustibility, and psychomotor agitation. After prolonged use, physical tolerance

Table 22.3 Plants with hallucinogenic potential

Latin name	Local name	Location
Amanita muscaria	Fly agaric	Temperate
Conocybe, Psilocybe	Magic mushrooms	Ubiquitous
Pancratium trianthum	Kwashi	West Africa
Catharanthus roseus	Madagascar periwinkle	Ubiquitous
Acorus calamus	Sweet flag	North America
Sarcostemma acidum	Soma	India
Lophophora williamsii	Peyote	Central America
Cannabis sativa	Pot, ganja, etc.	Ubiquitous
Catha edulis	Khat, qat	Arabia, north-east Africa
Argyreia nervosa	Silver morning glory	Tropics
Erythroxylon coca	Coca, coke	South America
Alcohornea floribunda	Niando	West Africa
Cytisus canariensis	Canary Island broom	Ubiquitous
Sophora secundiflora	Mescal bean	Central America
Claviceps purpura	Ergot	Temperate
Coleus blumei	El macho, el nene	Mexico, Asia
Lobelia inflata	Indian tobacco	North America
Heimia salicifolia	Sinicuichi	Central America
Mimosa hostilis	Vino de Jurema	Brazil
Myristica fragrans	Nutmeg	Tropics
Olmedioperebea sclerophylla	Rape dos indios	Brazil
Psychotria viridis	–	Equador
Atropa belladonna	Deadly nightshade	Ubiquitous
Datura innoxia	Thorn apple	Central America
Datura stramonium	Jimson weed	Ubiquitous
Duboisia hopwoodii	Pituri	Australia
Hyoscyamus niger	Henbane	Europe
Mandragora officinarum	Mandrake, Satan's apple	Southern Europe
Methysticodendrom amnesianum	Culebra-Borrachera	Columbia
Foeniculum vulgare	Fennel	Europe

Sources: Emboden (1972), Efron *et al* (1979), Jacobs (1987).

Table 22.4 Approximate caffeine content of beverages

Beverage	Caffeine content
Boiled coffee	100–500 mg/225 ml vessel
Roasted ground coffee	125 mg/225 ml vessel
Instant coffee	60–100 mg/225 ml vessel
Decaffeinated coffee	2–4 mg/225 ml vessel
Tea	30–100 mg/225 ml vessel
Cola drinks	23–50 mg/330 ml can
Chocolate drink	5–50 mg/225 ml vessel
Chocolate bar	(Approximately 30 mg/bar)

Sources: Wells (1984), Ashton (1987), Greden & Walters (1992).

and dependence ensues (Greden & Walters, 1992). Withdrawal symptoms include headache, hypersomnia, irritability, lethargy, poor concentration and anxiety, all of which are countered by the inclusion of caffeine in many cold cures and over-the-counter compound analgesics. It is usual for the symptoms of intoxication and withdrawal, if recognised at all, to be attributed to other circumstances. The complications of caffeine use are not trivial and this is recognised by their inclusion in ICD–10 under 'Mental and behavioural problems due to caffeine use' and prominent coverage in DSM–IV, where they are listed under 'Caffeine-related disorders'.

To gauge the contribution of tea or coffee consumption to a patient's symptoms, consideration must be given to the individual's age and size, whether there is consumption of other caffeine-containing substances such as soft drinks, and whether other drugs that increase (oral contraceptive, cimetidine) or reduce (rifampicin, smoking) the half-life are being used. The nature of the beverage, size of the vessel, frequency of consumption and mode of preparation should be noted; boiling and percolating coffee dramatically increases the dosage, as does a long period of brewing tea. Merely asking about the number of cups of tea or coffee taken in a day is insufficient, although it does serve as a useful starting point (Table 22.4).

Caffeine consumption (and thus toxicity) has been shown to be increased in psychiatric patients with a dry mouth due to anticholinergic drug treatment. Furthermore, individual susceptibility to intoxication is variable; some individuals develop intoxication from as little as 250 mg of caffeine a day.

Caffeine may mimic or augment a range of neurotic disorders, such as panic disorder, generalised anxiety disorder, minor mood disturbance and neurasthenia. It may also aggravate stress reactions and affective disorder, impair personal effectiveness, and in exceptional circumstances, following a sudden increase in consumption, even induce delirium (Bruce & Lader, 1986). The psychiatrist in family practice should be aware that caffeine enters breast milk and can cause babies to become restless, sleepless and 'difficult'.

Environmental elements and other chemical substances

One large group of brain intoxicants may be categorised together as the environmental intoxicants – metallic and non-metallic. The latter include solvents and vapours, herbicides and pesticides.

Metals and metal compounds

Aluminium

Aluminium accumulation can occur as a result of dialysis, from industrial exposure, from parenteral nutrition, from certain foodstuffs, from the ingestion of aluminium-containing antacids and phosphate-binding agents, and in other ways. Occupational exposure to aluminium has been associated with memory impairment and actual dementia, as well as a range of neurological disturbances. While aluminium is present in senile plaques and neurofibrillary tangles in the brains of people with Alzheimer's disease, the relationship between aluminium exposure and that disease has yet to be clarified. It should be pointed out that anomalies in the levels of other metals, such as iron and zinc, are also found in Alzheimer's disease. Impairment in performance on the symbol digit test was found in people exposed to drinking water contaminated with aluminium sulphate in the Camelford area of Cornwall (Altmann *et al*, 1999). Methodological issues preclude firm conclusions as to whether organic brain damage was induced by this exposure.

Arsenic

Natural geological contamination of ground water can induce chronic arsenic poisoning – notably in parts of Bangladesh, but also elsewhere around the world. Arsenical compounds are widely employed as herbicides, insecticides and rodenticides, as well as within the metal, paint and dye industries. Acute poisoning can cause headache, nausea, vomiting, diarrhoea, burning of the mouth and throat, abdominal pain, delirium, coma, fits, peripheral neuropathy with profound paraesthesia, and heart failure. The actual clinical presentation reflects the dose received.

Sub-acute intoxication is most likely to present to psychiatrists; this is characterised by fatigue, weakness, muscle aches and anorexia. Schizophrenia-like psychoses occur, as also do cognitive impairments, particularly deficits in recent memory and new learning. Arsenic intoxication should be suspected if a significant number of these features are present in the context of possible poisoning or occupational exposure. Pronounced paraesthesia in the extremities along with scaly dermatitis and/or hyperpigmentation of the trunk and limbs provide additional evidence of exposure. Mees' lines are transverse white lines on the fingernails that suggest an earlier episode of exposure to arsenic. Arsenic can be identified in urine, hair and nails.

Bismuth

Intoxication with bismuth is commonly caused by the treatment of gastrointestinal complaints with bismuth compounds, particularly bismuth subgallate, bismuth subnitrate and tripotassium dicitratobismuthate. Bismuth subcitrate and bismuth subsalicylate appear to be safer. Intoxication is characterised by depression, anxiety, irritability, phobias, insomnia and delusions. It may be associated with myoclonus, tremor, ataxia and other motor problems. The clinical resemblance to Creutzfeldt–Jakob disease has been remarked upon. Many of these clinical problems are reversible. Patients can develop hallucinations in the visual, auditory and/or gustatory modalities and delirium can occur. Memory impairment and progressive dementia are reported.

Hyperdensities in the basal ganglia, cortex and cerebellum are sometimes evident on brain imaging. Blood bismuth levels can be measured, as can the 24-hour urine bismuth level.

Gold
While gold has been used medicinally for centuries, it is mainly used now in the treatment of rheumatoid arthritis. Toxic symptoms include depression, hallucinations, delirium, ataxia, blurred vision, tremor and peripheral neuropathy.

Lead (including tetraethyl lead)
Despite efforts to remove lead from our environment, intoxication by accumulation is still an occupational hazard, particularly for printers, painters and workers manufacturing batteries. The main systemic features are gastrointestinal upset, mild anaemia, occasionally a 'lead line' on the gingival margins, fatigue and muscle weakness. Acute brain intoxication results in irritability, auditory and visual hallucinations, memory difficulties, delirium and coma. It can manifest more insidiously with insomnia, headache, irritability and cognitive decline. Generalised seizures and raised intracranial pressure are reported complications. The diagnosis can be confirmed by the presence of high blood and urine lead levels in association with a hypochromic anaemia with basophil stippling. Antidotes for lead intoxication include sodium calcium edetate, penicillamine and dimercaprol. Recovery after severe poisoning is often incomplete; sequelae include mental handicap, seizures and neurological dysfunction.

Organic lead poisoning from tetraethyl (or tetramethyl) lead occurs as a result of industrial exposure or, more usually, of sniffing petrol. Typically it causes excitement, which progresses to delirium. Accidental exposure can lead to insidious accumulation of organic lead, in which case ataxia, peripheral nerve damage, anorexia, fatigue, nervousness, insomnia and memory loss occur. Chronic organic lead intoxication has been reported to simulate both schizophrenia and hypomania.

The effects of lead on children and the developing brain may be more serious. A meta-analysis of eight studies suggested that a 2.6-point decrease in IQ score is associated with an increase in blood levels from 10 to 20 mg/dl (Schwartz, 1994).

Tetraethyl lead has been removed from petrol (and most cars now use lead-free petrol) and as a consequence there has been an 80% reduction in mean blood levels in children in the USA, a major triumph of a public health measure (Needleman, 1998).

Manganese
Manganese intoxication is a particular hazard for manganese miners, battery and steel plant workers, welders, and glass workers. Three presentations of intoxication are identifiable. In the first few months after exposure, ataxia and speech problems occur in conjunction with fatigue, anorexia, insomnia, memory difficulties, hallucinations and mania. This state of 'manganese madness' can closely resemble mania and schizophrenia. In the next phase, neurological symptoms such as incoordination, sleepiness and speech problems become more prominent. Finally, progressive parkinsonism, personality change and even dementia appear, a state referred to as 'manganism' (Hartman, 1988).

Mercury
Mercury intoxication results from exposure to the elemental liquid or vapour, a mercury salt, or an organic mercury compound, the latter causing the most significant pathological changes in the brain (Vroom & Greer, 1972). Systemic features of chronic poisoning include gingivitis, loosening of the teeth, excessive salivation, a metallic taste, anorexia, renal damage, anaemia, hypertension, tremor, peripheral neuropathy and ataxia (Jefferson & Marshall, 1981). Psychiatric features include fatigue, lassitude, depression or irritability and insomnia. Certain individuals develop a curious behavioural syndrome termed 'erythism'. The remarkable feature is an inability to function in front of observers, coupled with timidity, nervousness and social anxiety. While memory difficulties and dementia are reported sequelae, delirium and psychosis are rare.

During the 19th century, hat makers used mercury to help make the wool more pliable but there was no knowledge of the toxic effects of inhaled mercury vapour, which could send people psychotic, and the phrase 'mad as a hatter' originates from this situation, later to be immortalised in Lewis Carroll's *Alice's Adventures in Wonderland* as 'the Mad Hatter'.

Acute organic mercurial poisoning can produce a severe disorder characterised by paraesthesia, incoordination, blindness, parkinsonism and/or a clinical picture resembling amyotrophic lateral sclerosis. Intoxication in children can present with a combination of pruritic skin rashes and neurobehavioural disabilities, a syndrome that has been termed acrodynia. To date there is no firm evidence of mercury intoxication resulting from dental fillings of amalgam containing mercury (Herrström & Högstedt, 1993), although dental staff may be exposed to unsafe levels of mercurial compounds in their daily work.

Nickel
Nickel carbonyl is a gas given off during the refining of nickel. It is said to have a toxicity five times that of carbon monoxide, and inhalation is reported to induce pulmonary oedema, delirium, fits and death.

Thallium
Thallium salts are used in the manufacture of optical lenses, semiconductors, fireworks and jewellery, and also as catalysts in a range of chemical processes. There are regular reports of their use with murderous intent, which probably reflects the fact that thallium salts are odourless, colourless and tasteless (Moore *et al*, 1993). Acute thallium poisoning typically presents with prominent gastrointestinal and neuromuscular symptoms. Neurological and psychiatric features may be delayed for a few days; these include paraesthesia, hyperaesthesia, headaches, ptosis, optic atrophy, prominent myalgia, myopathy, fits, psychosis, delirium, and dementia. Sudden death may result from cardiac arrhythmias. The episode of poisoning is marked 2–3 weeks later by hair loss, parotid enlargement, skin lesions and sometimes Mees' lines on the nails.

The impact of thallium poisoning can be alleviated with regular oral doses of Berlin blue and other measures. The differential diagnosis includes intoxication with lead, gold, carbon monoxide, organophosphates and such conditions as Guillain–Barré syndrome, diabetic polyneuritis and porphyria.

Other metals

The organic tin compounds trimethyl tin and triethyl tin are toxic to the nervous system. Inhalation and transcutaneous exposure to trimethyl tin has been associated with headache, fits, delirium and impairment of recent memory, as well as anorexia, fatigue and personality change. Triethyl tin causes oedema of myelin and symptoms suggestive of raised intracranial pressure.

Poisoning with vanadium compounds has been shown to cause a range of respiratory complaints, depressed mood, anorexia, visual disturbance and tremor.

Zinc intoxication can cause fatigue, lethargy and delirium.

Reports of the neuropsychiatric effects of intoxication with barium, boron, selenium, cadmium, platinum, silicon and tellurium are few.

The laboratory investigation of *past* metal exposure is difficult since blood and urine levels of many metals have returned to normal by the time patients present to the psychiatrist.

Organic solvents, gases and vapours

Intoxication with this class of chemical is now chiefly encountered as a result of deliberate misuse. The condition is probably increasing in frequency. Thus, McGarvey *et al* (1999) in their review suggested that the rate of experimentation with solvents in US high schools was around 20%. They examined a high-risk population of incarcerated juvenile offenders and indeed found that 20% had experimented with solvents but that 8.5% had used them more than 40 times a year.

There is often an association with other illicit drug use, school problems, truanting, child abuse, comorbid psychiatric disorders and CNS impairment, and serious medical problems among chronic users, which clearly elevates the risk of death.

A large range of products containing organic solvents are misused, notably lighter fuels, adhesives, typewriter correction fluid, dry cleaning fluids, aerosols and nail-polish remover. Pure solvents, antifreeze, petroleum, fire-extinguishers, whipped-cream aerosols and even asthma inhalers (fluorinated hydrocarbons) have also been similarly misused. In the UK, the majority of solvent misusers now employ butane; previously, adhesives containing toluene and acetone were most widely used.

Fluorinated hydrocarbons (freons) and butane appear to be disproportionately associated with fatalities, possibly due to their cardiotoxicity. Intoxicated individuals can become sensitised to the effects of endogenous and exogenous catecholamines. Deaths also occur through asphyxiation, accidents and liver failure. A study of deaths associated with solvent misuse in Virginia showed that 95% of those who died were male, and most (70%) were under 22 years of age. Deaths from the misuse of volatile substances accounted for 0.3% of all deaths of males aged 13–22 years, and around a quarter of these deaths were of children aged 13–16. The chief volatile substances that caused deaths were gas fuels (i.e. butane and propane) (46%), chlorofluorocarbons (26%) and then a variety of other hydrocarbons.

The problem of inhalant misuse in young people is serious but has not attracted as much interest or therapeutic concern as other types of addiction (Bowen *et al*, 1999).

Organic solvents have toxic effects on the central nervous system, liver, lungs, haemopoietic system, kidneys and heart. Teratogenic changes and a neonatal syndrome have been long suspected. Products often contain more than one solvent whose effects can be additive or synergistic with one another. The diagnosis and treatment of acute poisoning with volatile substances has been outlined by Meredith *et al* (1989).

Toluene usefully illustrates the general effects of solvent intoxication. As with other CNS depressants, toluene inhalation causes an initial excitatory effect, followed by a depressive phase that may result in narcosis and even loss of consciousness. The excitatory phase is characterised by euphoria, disinhibition, excitement, tinnitus, dizziness and diplopia. Sneezing and coughing, gastrointestinal disturbance, fits and paraesthesia, illusions, hallucinations (visual or auditory), delirium and coma are also reported (Ron, 1986). Regular use can cause physical tolerance and withdrawal phenomena (headache and lethargy), constituting a state of dependency (Westermeyer, 1987). While the evidence that toluene misuse routinely causes severe or lasting neuropsychological or psychiatric disorder is meagre, there are data suggesting that dose-dependent MRI changes may occur, particularly to the periventricular white matter. UK epidemiological data for deaths from the misuse of volatile substances identify deprivation as the factor associated with regional variation.

Solvent misuse should be suspected in the presence of an odour on the breath, freeze marks on the face, a peri-oral rash, glue on the hands or garments, and possession of solvent containers. Behavioural changes include social withdrawal and anorexia, as well as those of intoxication. Laboratory detection is difficult; blood levels of solvents are detectable for 12 hours to 5 days, depending on the type of solvent. Toluene is detected in urine as increased hippuric acid levels, although if testing is delayed for more than 2 days it can be missed.

Straight-chain aliphatic hydrocarbons

Small straight-chain aliphatic hydrocarbons such as methane and ethane are thought to have a toxic effect by inducing hypoxia. Aliphatic hydrocarbons of higher molecular weight, such as propane to octane, act as CNS depressants, thus producing intoxication in a manner generally similar to toluene. N-hexane deserves special mention. It is a widely used solvent that not only produces a peripheral nerve distal axonopathy, but also, with high-level exposure, acute intoxication and CNS axonal degeneration. Like methyl butyl ketone (MBK), n-hexane is metabolised to 2,5,-hexanedione (2,5,-HD), which is reponsible for most of its neurotoxic effects. Butane misuse now exceeds toluene misuse, possibly reflecting the fact that it is conveniently packaged as lighter fuel.

Benzene

Acute intoxication with the aromatic hydrocarbon benzene produces features generally similar to those with toluene, although dyspnoea and impaired gait may persist for several weeks. Chronic exposure is linked to the subsequent development of aplastic anaemia and leukaemia.

Carbon tetrachloride
Carbon tetrachloride is a particularly toxic halogenated hydrocarbon solvent, but is now less commonly encountered. Transient exposure can cause irritation to the eyes, nose and throat, nausea and vomiting, dizziness, drowsiness, diplopia and headache. Continued higher-level exposure leads to delirium, stupor, fits, coma and sudden death. Severe delayed systemic effects occur in the hepatic, renal and gastrointestinal systems.

Methyl bromide
Intoxication from methyl bromide, an insecticide, has been reported to induce persistent sequelae such as hallucinations, memory difficulties, aphasia and incoordination. In children it can be mistaken for Reye's syndrome.

Methylene chloride
Methylene chloride is a ubiquitous solvent and refrigerant. It is metabolised to carbon monoxide, which exerts narcotic and hypoxic effects on the brain.

Trichloroethylene
Trichloroethylene exposure can cause cranial neuropathies, particularly trigeminal neuropathy. At higher levels of exposure the features are those of acute solvent intoxication. Alcohol potentiates the effects of trichloroethylene.

Trichloroethane
Trichloroethane was once a common aerosol propellant, but is now mainly used as an industrial degreasing solvent, in garment cleaners and in correction fluids. Acute low-level exposure (500 p.p.m.) is thought to have only slight behavioural effects. However, permanent neurological sequelae have been associated with acute, massive exposure, probably as a result of cerebral hypoxia.

Methanol
Methanol poisoning is often due to the adulteration of alcoholic beverages. Initially a state of intoxication occurs which resembles that with ethanol. In the body it is oxidised to formaldehyde and formic acid, which can give rise to severe metabolic acidosis and retinal ganglion cell damage, resulting in scotomata and blindness. Symptom onset can be delayed for up to 3 days; these symptoms include visual changes, tiredness, delirium, stupor and coma. The three main components of treatment are intravenous sodium bicarbonate, ethanol and early haemodialysis.

Isopropanol
Intoxication with the alcohol isopropanol can result from either ingestion or exposure to the vapour. Features of intoxication are similar to those with ethanol, but more delayed and prolonged. Gastric symptoms can be severe; vomiting with aspiration is a recognised danger. Muscle spasms arise as a result of the chelation of calcium by the oxalate produced from the metabolism of isopropanol; this is a useful pointer to the diagnosis.

Ethylene glycol and other glycols
Ethylene glycol is widely employed as a solvent and in antifreeze, and may be taken as an alcohol substitute. Inebriation can be rapidly followed by CNS depression, narcosis, coma and death. A severe metabolic acidosis usually arises and acute renal failure is a further complication. The treatment is similar to that for methanol intoxication.

The effects of diethylene glycol and propylene glycol resemble those of ethylene glycol, although propylene glycol is considerably less toxic.

Petroleum ethers
Petrol sniffing results in acute exposure not only to a wide range of organic solvents (benzene, toluene, olefins, naphthenes and paraffin) but also to tetraethyl lead (see above).

Other esters
Dimethyl sulphate, glyceryl trinitrate, amyl nitrate, butyl nitrite and isobutyl nitrite are esters that have all been known to cause delirium after intense exposure.

Chlorinated pesticide compounds
These chemicals cause CNS stimulation. Dichlorodiphenyl-trichloroethane (DDT) now has major restrictions on its use because, being highly fat-soluble, it is biomagnified in the food chain of animals (Klaassen, 1990). Poisoning causes facial paralysis, dizziness, tremor, delirium and fits.

Chlorinated cyclodienes such as aldrin, dieldrin, heptachlor and chlordane produce the signs and symptoms of DDT poisoning but, being more potent CNS stimulants, often induce epileptic-type seizures before other symptoms. Compared with DDT, poisoning with these chemicals is more lethal.

Lindane, a commonly used topical treatment for head lice, is the gamma isomer of benzene hexachloride. Acute poisoning results in tremors, ataxia, delirium and fits.

Organophosphate pesticides
Organophosphate compounds have replaced many chlorinated hydrocarbons as agricultural pesticides; exposure to these chemicals is a major cause of death and morbidity worldwide. Their use is not restricted to agriculture, as they are also found in a range of occupational and domestic contexts – and are constituents of chemical weapons, too. For example, O-isopropyl methylphosphonofluoridate (Sarin) is a colourless, odourless gas that acts by inhibiting acetylcholinesterase.

Malathion, diazinon and parathion are but three examples of many thousands of these chemicals. They act as irreversible acetylcholinesterase inhibitors, first stimulating and then blocking synaptic transmission in cholinergic neurons throughout the nervous system. Intoxication has three phases. Acute features include headache, vomiting, abdominal pains, sweating, excess salivation and lacrimation, wheezing, miosis and blurred vision, muscle weakness, cramps and fasciculations. Delirium and impaired memory are additional features. Hyperglycaemia, hypertension or hypotension may develop. Affected individuals' breath may smell of garlic. In the second phase, after 1–4 days, weakness and/or paralysis can develop in the proximal limb, neck and respiratory muscles. Cranial neuropathies, fatigue, irritability and memory difficulties are other features of this second phase, but tend to recede after 2 weeks. A third phase, of delayed effects, may occur, particularly the development of a distal sensorimotor neuropathy. Some organophospate compounds can also induce corticospinal damage in this phase. Lasting emotional and affective symptoms occur in individuals exposed to these chemicals, although it is not certain that discrete, persistent neuropsychological deficits occur (Minton & Murray, 1988).

The treatment of organophosphate poisoning involves taking measures to stop further absorption and the administration of atropine, with or without pralidoxime mesylate, a cholinesterase reactivator. It is only the initial effects that respond to these measures, and so treatment must be rapidly instigated.

Carbamate insecticides such as carbyl are also cholinesterase inhibitors.

Miscellaneous chemicals

Carbon monoxide

Carbon monoxide is a colourless, odourless, non-irritative gas formed by the incomplete combustion of organic material. Inadequately maintained gas appliances have become a notorious cause of carbon monoxide poisoning, and such poisoning in exhaust-filled cars is sometimes used as a means of suicide. Carbon monoxide reduces the oxygen-carrying capacity of blood and causes hypoxia. Klaassen (1990) points out that a higher metabolic rate predisposes to carbon monoxide toxicity, hence children succumb earlier than adults.

Exposure results in transient weakness, headache, nausea and vomiting, dimness of vision and syncope. However, there may be no prodromal warning before consciousness is lost. Delirium can be a presenting feature or occur as consciousness is regained, and can last as long as 4 weeks. Individuals who have experienced high levels of exposure can develop a syndrome of delayed neurotoxicity. Permanent sequelae include extrapyramidal and pyramidal motor disturbance, affective and personality disturbance, amnesic syndrome and other cognitive deficits, even dementia. The diagnosis is confirmed by high blood carboxyhaemoglobin levels. The initial management is to remove the person to fresh air, to administer 100% oxygen and to give cardiopulmonary support.

Carbon disulphide

Carbon disulphide, an organic solvent, is a constituent of lacquers and varnishes and is used in the manufacture of rubber and plastics, notably rayon. It causes both axon destruction and indirect damage by inducing arteriosclerosis. Acute psychiatric features of exposed chemical workers include fatigue, depression, irritability, insomnia, acute mania and delirium. More chronic behavioural, motor and cognitive changes can develop.

Hydrogen disulphide

Hydrogen disulphide is a product of decaying organic matter that contains sulphur; it is typically encountered in sewage works. Higher concentrations induce a rapid loss of consciousness, sometimes preceded by delirium.

Nitrous oxide

Nitrous oxide has been misused as a euphoriant for over a century. While acute exposure can cause delirium, prolonged exposure leads to the development of combined degeneration of the posterior and lateral columns of the spinal cord, akin to that found in vitamin B12 deficiency.

Ketamine

Ketamine causes excitability, depersonalisation, hallucinations and delirium in a minority of patients in whom it is used for anaesthesia. It is a substance of misuse.

Metabolic and endocrine disorders

This section includes rarities that require listing along with more common conditions (Box 22.9), to prevent underdiagnosis. Illustrative of this is the condition neuroacanthocytosis (discussed below), a hitherto overlooked entity that is now recognised as an important differential diagnosis of Huntington's chorea.

Multi-system disorder is a topic that requires mention. Certain of the conditions discussed here have a significant chance of being associated with other disorders, which will either precede their onset, coincide, or occur after the presenting condition has been treated. The multiple endocrine neoplasia (MEN) disorders and the polyglandular autoimmune syndrome type II are examples of such linked conditions and are of considerable relevance to psychiatric practice. The MEN I disorders include adenomas and hyperplasias of the pituitary, parathyroid and pancreas, as well as thymomas, schwannomas and skin lipomas. The MEN IIa disorders include phaeochromocytoma, medullary thyroid carcinoma, and various brain tumours; and the final group, MEN IIb, includes a variety of mucocutaneous lesions, such as neuromas in various sites and Marfan's syndrome. The polyglandular autoimmune disorders include Addison's disease, thyroiditis, hypoparathyroidism, diabetes mellitus, pernicious anaemia, vitiligo, myasthenia gravis and other conditions. Patients with one of these disorders require investigations for associated conditions, sometimes indefinitely, and where conditions are inherited, family members will require screening (Schimke, 1991).

Endocrinopathies

Hyperthyroidism

Hyperthyroidism is a hypermetabolic state, typically of insidious onset. The three commonest causes account for 99% of cases: diffuse toxic hyperplasia (Grave's disease); toxic solitary goitre (toxic adenoma); and toxic multinodular goitre. The commonest of these is Grave's disease, and it is in this type of hyperthyroidism that the distinctive eye signs are particularly identified. It should be noted that hyperthyroidism can also be due to exogenous thyroxine or iodide administration/exposure, thyroid carcinoma or tumours outside the thyroid gland.

Sustained hyperthyroidism is uncommon in psychiatric practice, occurring in 0.2–2.6% of psychiatric in-patients (White & Barraclough, 1988), approximately the same as in the general population (McLarty *et al*,

Box 22.9 Disorders of metabolism with psychiatric manifestations

Organ failure or dysfunction

- Endocrinopathies
  - Hyperthyroidism
  - Hypothyroidism
  - Cushing's syndrome
  - Adrenocortical deficiency
  - Hyperparathyroidism
  - Hypoparathyroidism
  - Acromegaly
  - Hypopituitarism
  - Diabetes mellitus
  - Diabetes insipidus (Riggs *et al*, 1991)
  - Hypoglycaemia and insulinoma
  - Phaeochromocytoma
- Hepatic dysfunction (see under alcohol)
- Pancreatic dysfunction (Estrada *et al*, 1979)
- Renal dysfunction (Lishman, 1998)
- Respiratory dysfunction (see acidosis and alkalosis, below)

Deficiency of substrates of cerebral metabolism

- Hypoxia
- Hypoglycaemia (see under endocrinopathies and section on alcohol, above)

Disorders of electrolyte, acid–base and fluid balance

- Hypernatraemia
- Hyponatraemia (see also under water intoxication)
- Hyperkalaemia
- Hypokalaemia
- Hypercalcaemia (see under endocrinopathies)
- Hypocalcaemia (see under endocrinopathies)
- Hyper- and hypomagnesaemia
- Hyper- and hypophosphataemia
- Zinc deficiency
- Acidosis
- Alkalosis
- Water intoxication
- Water depletion (see under hyper- and hyponatraemia, above)
- Uraemia

Vitamin disorders

- Vitamin deficiency (Carney, 1990)
- Vitamin excess (Lipowski, 1990)

Disorders of temperature regulation

- Hypothermia
- Hyperthermia

Miscellaneous disorders

- Wilson's disease (see Chapter 21, page 550)
- Porphyria
- Mitochondrial myopathy
- Neuroacanthocytosis
- Metachromatic leucodystrophy
- Paraneoplastic syndromes (Cornelius *et al*, 1986)
- Carcinoid syndrome (Major *et al*, 1973)
- Kufs' disease (Greenwood & Nelson, 1978)
- Adrenoleucodystrophy (Eldridge *et al*, 1984)
- Leigh disease (Kalimo *et al*, 1979)
- Familial idiopathic calcification of the basal ganglia (Flint & Goldstein, 1992)
- Cerebrotendinous xanthomatosis (Adams & Victor, 1989)
- Hallervorden–Spatz syndrome (Dooling *et al*, 1974)
- Gaucher disease (Winkelman *et al*, 1983)
- Niemann–Pick disease (Adams & Victor, 1989)
- GM2 gangliosidosis (Adams & Victor, 1989)
- Whipple's disease (Weeks *et al*, 1996) (now considered to be infective – *Tropheryma whippelii*)

Source: Adapted from Lipowski (1990).
Note: Certain disorders not discussed in the text are referenced.

1978). Psychiatric symptoms, however, are virtually universal when hyperthyroidism occurs, particularly overactivity, nervousness, anxiety, irritability and emotional lability (Lishman, 1998). A shortened sleep period and increased appetite are usually present. Depression can occur, but is not usually either sustained or severe, in contrast to hypothyroidism (Whybrow *et al*, 1969). Checkley (1978) was unable to demonstrate a clear temporal relationship between hyperthyroid illness and manic episodes, which suggests that hyperthyroidism does not predispose to manic illness. Psychosis is well recognised but uncommon (about 1%). Close examination of the mental state will often reveal a mixture of affective and psychotic disturbance in the context of mild global impairment of cognition. Chorea, periodic paralysis, myopathy and myasthenia are recognised neurological accompaniments.

Fulminant episodes of delirium occur in some 3–4% of hyperthyroid patients (Lipowski, 1990). Such a state is usually accompanied by high fever, tachycardia, hypotension, vomiting and diarrhoea, and is termed a 'thyroid crisis' or 'thyroid storm'. It can be precipitated by inadequate preparation for thyroidectomy, non-thyroidal surgery or infection, but often a precipitant is not found. Occasionally, the presentation is more subtle, with apathy, prostration, stupor and coma without a high temperature. Thyroid crisis constitutes a medical emergency. Supportive measures include the administration of fluids, dexamethasone or hydrocortisone, glucose and B vitamins. The patient may require cooling and digitalisation. Thyroid hormone synthesis should be blocked with propylthiouracil or carbimazole (by nasogastric tube) and release of thyroid hormone inhibited with iodine. Adrenergic antagonists have an important role in the absence of heart failure. Control is usually regained within 24 hours.

A small minority of hyperthyroid patients, more usually older ones, present with apathetic detachment without restless overactivity, a state termed 'apathetic' hyperthyroidism by Lahey (1931), who contrasted it with the more normal presentation of 'activated' hyperthyroidism. These patients usually have a masked hyperthyroid state without striking clinical signs. A goitre, if present, is usually small. Appetite is usually poor and weight loss considerable. These patients are at risk of developing cardiac complications, becoming stuporous, and sinking into terminal coma.

The differentiation of anxiety and hyperthyroidism can be difficult. While physical signs of Grave's disease, particularly the eye signs, are strong evidence of hyperthyroidism, these may well be absent. Hyperthyroid patients are sensitive to higher temperatures, have increased appetite, and yet lose weight (Lishman, 1998). The onset of anxiety is often at an earlier age than is the case with hyperthyroidism. A 24-hour heart-rate chart is often helpful, as hyperthyroid patients tend to have a sleeping pulse rate above 90 beats per minute. Serum levels of free triiodothyronine (T3), free thyroxine (T4) and thyroid stimulating hormone (TSH) should be determined.

It has been pointed out that in acute psychiatric admissions there is a high incidence of hyperthyroxinaemia. In these cases, serum TSH is generally high or normal, not low; it tends to normalise within 2 weeks and treatment is not indicated (Hein & Jackson, 1990). Elevation of the serum T3 level without a raised T4 level (T3 toxicosis) can occur, although this is usually an early phenomenon. T4 toxicosis is occasionally seen in particularly ill or elderly patients.

The prognosis of psychiatric symptoms in hyperthyroidism is good, although it should be cautioned that psychotic symptoms and delirium can appear for the first time when treatment begins.

Hypothyroidism

Hypothyroidism is a hypometabolic state caused almost exclusively by inadequate thyroidal secretion of T3 and T4. Endemic or sporadic hypothyroidism present from birth is termed 'cretinism', and is usually accompanied by mental retardation. It is noteworthy that milder cases may be missed at birth and, while usually recognised in childhood, they may present in adulthood. Myxoedema is the term applied to hypothyroidism in the child or adult. It is very much more common in women, and is most frequently a disorder of middle life. On account of its insidious onset it is often overlooked. The commonest causes are over-treatment of hyperthyroidism, end-stage chronic thyroiditis or multinodular goitre. Inhibition of hormone synthesis or release by antithyroid drugs is another significant cause, lithium being the main culprit in psychiatric practice. Carbamazepine and phenytoin can also affect thyroid function.

As physical features accrue, the diagnosis becomes more obvious. Fatigue, poor appetite, slowed activity, aches and pains, constipation and cold intolerance are core features. Mucopolysaccharides infiltrate the dermis of the skin, causing it to become characteristically thickened and doughy. The patient may develop a hoarse voice and an expressionless face, and suffer hair loss. Marked slowing of the recovery phase of the ankle jerk is a useful clinical sign. Patients may present with angina, impotence and hearing difficulties.

Psychiatric features occur early in virtually every case and were noted by both Sir William Gull in his original description of hypothyroidism, and by W. M. Ord, who coined the term myxoedema (Tonks, 1964). Fatigue accompanied by mental and physical slowing is a central psychiatric feature. Memory for recent events may be impaired (Hadden, 1882). Apathy and tranquillity are not always present – oppositional, explosive personality attributes are well described, as is paranoia. When depressed mood develops it can be severe and respond poorly to treatment. Insight is present to begin with, but fades as the disorder intensifies. Cognitive impairments range from quite subtle degrees of mental slowing, impaired concentration and impaired memory for recent events to states of frank dementia (de Fine Olivarus & Röder, 1970).

Delusions (usually paranoid) and auditory or visual hallucinations, if present, are usually accompanied by impaired cognition and clouded consciousness. Such a presentation is well illustrated by the following case (Asher, 1949).

Case example

A housewife aged 60 was admitted with delusions of persecution and hallucinations. For 16 months she had noticed that her voice was croaking and she felt cold weather badly, but she had noted no other myxoedematous symptoms – no gain in weight, falling out of hair or deafness. During the week before admission she had an idea that her landlord was trying to poison her 'because she knew all about the shootings in the garden'. She heard voices talking to her continuously, and locked herself in her room to protect herself from imaginary enemies. On examination she was completely confused and disorientated.

Hypothyroidism may be mistaken for depression, dementia, personality disorder and hypochondriacal neurosis. Serum TSH or free T4 are the initial investigations; a normal TSH will exclude primary hypothyroidism, but not hypothyroidism due to pituitary or hypothalamic disease. Tests for thyroid antibodies should be requested and repeated in patients in whom clinical suspicions linger. In approximately a third of patients with hypothyroidism the EEG is abnormal, with a slowing of the dominant rhythm and a reduction of the background activity, which corrects after treatment (Hooshmand & Sarhaddi, 1975).

Thyroid replacement treatment must be started cautiously, as angina and heart failure can arise. Most of the psychiatric symptoms in hypothyroid patients can be expected to respond to treatment. Women positive for thyroid antibodies may be more prone to post-partum depression.

Lithium and the thyroid gland

Lithium treatment affects the thyroid gland directly by inhibiting release of iodine, T3 and T4, and indirectly by inducing thyroid auto-antibodies. It is said to occur in 2–5% of patients, although reports from studies in different geographical areas vary. In one study in Scotland it was found to have a rate of about 10%, to occur more in women, particularly women of early middle age, and more in the first 2 years of treatment (Johnston & Eagles, 1999), but it can occur at any time during the course of lithium treatment and, therefore, thyroid status must be checked before the patient starts lithium and every 6 months thereafter. Weight gain and lethargy are useful clinical indices to monitor. Lithium-induced goitre is rarely of noticeable proportions. If lithium is stopped, the effects it has exerted on the thyroid reverse in 1–2 months. If it is necessary to continue treatment when there is evidence of hypothyroidism, treatment with thyroxine will restore euthyroid status. Lithium given in pregnancy can cause neonatal hypothyroidism, and early in pregnancy (up to 6 months after conception) Ebstein's anomaly in the foetal heart.

T3 and T4 supplementation for affective disorders

The role of the hypothalamic–pituitary–thyroid axis in the genesis and management of affective disorder is discussed in Chapter 5. Presently lithium augmentation seems to be a more effective strategy than thyroid supplements (Anderson, 2003). Some authorities favour the use of thyroid supplements in the treatment of patients with 'rapid cycling' manic–depression.

Cushing's syndrome

Cushing's syndrome is due to excessive pituitary secretion of adrenocorticotrophic hormone (ACTH) in about 75% of cases. Other causes include adrenal tumours, and ACTH-secreting tumours such as oat cell carcinoma of the lung. It may be confused with simple obesity, hirsutism, and functional ovarian tumours. It is four times more common in women. It usually presents in the third or fourth decade but can occur at any age.

Surveys report psychiatric symptoms in 50–80% of cases of Cushing's syndrome. Affective disorder is the most frequent psychiatric disturbance; it is predominantly depressive, although mania has been described (Haskett, 1985). The depression may range from mild to severe in intensity; suicide has been reported in 3–10% of cases and therefore represents a significant risk (Jefferson & Marshall, 1981). Severe retardation, delusions, hallucinations, agitation and behavioural disturbance are recognised accompaniments of the depression. Patients are also prone to emotional lability, anxiety, apathy and fatigue. Schizophreniform illness is described but relatively infrequent. Frank delirium is rare, but when present is likely to be associated with high cortisol levels, physical complications secondary to the disorder, advanced disease and older age. Cognitive impairments, for example amnesia and attentional deficits, are not uncommon (Starkman *et al*, 1986).

The cause of the psychiatric manifestations of Cushing's syndrome is at present uncertain. A higher incidence of depression is reported if the origin is pituitary and not adrenal (Cohen, 1980). The severity of depression is not directly related to steroid levels, although both delirium and psychosis tend to be commoner when steroid levels are very high (Kelly *et al*, 1983). Neurodegeneration of the hippocampus and frontal lobes has been linked to raised cortisol levels. Furthermore, steroid synthesis inhibitors, such as ketoconazole and other cortisol-lowering drugs, have been shown to be effective in the treatment of depression associated with hypercortisolaemia (McQuade & Young, 2000). Psychiatric disorder responds well to the correction of the underlying physical disorder. The two usually resolve in parallel, sometimes in days, although affective disturbance may persist for as long as a year.

Steroid-induced mental disturbances

In contrast to Cushing's syndrome, steroid treatment is most commonly associated with mild elation of mood, although depression certainly occurs (Ling *et al*, 1981). The presentation of steroid-induced mental disturbances are typically very variable. Symptoms can include emotional lability, euphoria, anxiety, distractibility, pressured speech, insomnia, depression, perplexity, agitation, auditory and visual hallucinations, intermittent memory impairment, mutism, disturbances of body image, delusions, apathy and hypomania. These symptoms tend to occur in the first 3 weeks of treatment, although they can start for the first time after years of steroid treatment.

Dosage is correlated with the risk of developing mental disturbance, but neither dosage nor duration of treatment appears to influence the time of onset, duration, severity or type of mental disturbance. Hall *et al* (1979) reported that patients receiving more than 40 mg of prednisone a day (or equivalent) tend to get psychiatric reactions. Females appear to be more prone to mental disturbance. Past mental illness does not necessarily predispose to steroid-induced mental disturbances.

Milder reactions respond well to a gradual reduction in dosage. There is a tendency for patients to relapse, so observation should continue for a reasonable period. More severe reactions will require symptomatic psychiatric treatment, especially if the patient's physical condition leaves little room for dose reduction. The use of tricyclic drugs for steroid-related depression can cause a dramatic deterioration in mental state, namely the development of florid hallucinations and delusions (Hall *et al*, 1978). Alternate-day steroid regimens have been associated with less severe mental changes in some patients.

A steroid withdrawal syndrome is described, the trigger for which appears to be abrupt withdrawal. Such patients may experience lethargy and weakness, myalgias, depression or delirium. What first appears to be a withdrawal 'reaction' may in fact be a complication of the illness for which treatment is being prescribed. In patients with a steroid withdrawal syndrome evidence of suppression of the hypothalamic–pituitary–adrenocortical axis can be obtained using the short Synacthen (tetracosactide) test.

Adrenocortical deficiency

Adrenocortical insufficiency is mostly due to disease of the adrenal cortex (primary type), but may have a secondary cause, notably pituitary, hypothalamic or iatrogenic. Three-quarters of cases of acquired primary adrenocortical insufficiency (Addison's disease) are due to autoimmune disease and the prevalence is twice as great in women. Easy fatigability, progressive weakness, anorexia, cold intolerance, hypotension, syncope, pain and skin changes are often prominent physical complaints. Anorexia and weight loss usually appear early, in some patients months or years before other symptoms (Drake, 1957).

Psychiatric symptoms invariably occur, and the earliest features are slowly progressive fatigue, weakness and apathy. When present, depression, irritability, anxiety and paranoia tend to have a fluctuating course (Cleghorn, 1951). Affective and schizophreniform psychoses are rare, but may herald an acute adrenal crisis. Memory impairment is commonly present. If suggestive electrolyte abnormalities are present, adrenocortical insufficiency should be excluded in patients presenting with dementia, an amnesic syndrome, neurosis, depression, anorexia nervosa or a chronic fatigue syndrome (Roberts *et al*, 2004).

All patients with adrenocortical insufficiency require specialist medical management. The psychiatric manifestations respond well to steroid replacement – the glucocorticoid component is reported to have the most decisive effect.

Hyperparathyroidism

Hypercalcaemia, due to primary hyperparathyroidism, is an important cause of psychiatric morbidity. If overlooked, a patient may suffer years of remediable psychiatric illness. Hypercalcaemia occurs for many reasons, including renal failure, carcinoma, immobilisation, bone disease, vitamin D excess, sarcoidosis and thyrotoxicosis. Fatigue, weakness, anorexia, constipation, thirst and polyuria are symptoms frequently associated with hypercalcaemia, and thus necessitate a serum calcium estimation when encountered.

Primary hyperparathyroidism may develop at any age, but mostly in middle life. Petersen (1968) reported that up to two-thirds of patients have mental changes, a third of these being severe. Psychiatric features can be divided into two main types: the more common is disturbed mood and drive, which may be the sole manifestation; delirium is associated with higher calcium levels (Christie-Brown, 1968), and has been termed parathyroid crisis.

The earliest changes are subtle – personality change, depressed mood and insidiously progressive fatigue, listlessness and apathy. Impaired attention, mental slowing and impaired memory can develop, but actual dementia is a rare presentation. Schizophreniform psychosis is also rare, although persecutory delusions and hallucinations are not uncommon as calcium levels rise. Elevated calcium is a significant cause of stupor and catatonia. Depression can become very severe, profound psychotic features being accompanied by a significant risk of suicide. Antidepressants have a temporary role, but the depression is often resistant, and so the definitive treatment is to reverse the hypercalcaemia.

Case example

A 58-year-old woman was referred for an urgent psychiatric opinion, as she had stated that she felt she could no longer carry on and wished to die. At interview the patient sat in a languid, drooping fashion in an armchair. During the previous 2 months she had lost 7 kg in weight. Her mood was unaffected by external events. There was a considerable degree of psychomotor retardation, but no evidence of thought disorder, delusional thinking or hallucinations, or memory defect. Orientation was correct in all respects. The patient's level of consciousness was diminished, resembling that seen in pre-stuporous states. The most striking abnormality was an elevated serum calcium level of 3.12 mmol/l and a lowered serum phosphate level of 0.48 mmol/l. The disorder was revealed to be an extreme case of intoxication as a result of 15 years of therapy with vitamin D tablets and calcium tablets after thyroid surgery. (Keddie, 1987)

Where origin of the symptoms described above is in doubt, the EEG is a useful investigation. Slowing of the background rhythm and the appearance of bilateral high-voltage delta episodes are suggestive of a metabolic cause (Cooper & Schapira, 1973).

Correction of serum calcium usually results in reversal of psychiatric symptoms, although exceptions have been reported (Öztunç *et al*, 1986). Hypomagnesaemia may also make a significant contribution to the mental state in some patients.

Hypoparathyroidism and hypocalcaemia

Hypoparathyroidism is most commonly secondary to damage or removal of the parathyroid glands, usually as a consequence of thyroid surgery. More rarely, there may be primary parathyroid disease, or end-organ unresponsiveness to circulating parathyroid hormone – pseudohypoparathyroidism. Patients with hypoparathyroidism are often female, have a history of surgery to the neck, and may present with tetany, cramps, cataracts or generalised seizures. A skull radiograph may show symmetrical calcification within the basal ganglia in primary hypoparathyroidism, but extrapyramidal features such as chorea are relatively rare.

Cases of secondary hypoparathyroidism tend to present with more acute psychiatric disorders, such as delirium characterised by florid psychotic manifestations and irritability. Depression, manic–depression, schizophreniform psychosis, nervousness and irritability are all reported. Primary hypoparathyroidism, on the other hand, unfolds insidiously with symptoms such as emotional lability, impaired concentration and intellectual impairment (Denko & Kaelbling, 1962). The cause can be easily missed and slow progression over months or years may leave the patient demented.

Pseudo-hypoparathyroidism tends to be congenital and causes intellectual retardation which is poorly responsive to medical intervention. The nature of familial calcification of the basal ganglia, its psychiatric presentations, and its relationship to pseudohypoparathyroidism have been reviewed by Flint & Goldstein (1992).

Patients who have low (though still normal) serum calcium levels are prone to develop intermittent psychiatric symptoms if their levels dip further. This can be alleviated with calcium supplements. (Similarly, the induction of intermittent psychiatric symptoms by irregularly dipping hormone levels may well operate in other borderline metabolic derangements.)

The prognosis of psychiatric symptoms associated with secondary hypoparathyroidism is good, although some symptoms may take a few months to resolve once calcium levels are normal. The prognosis of dementia due to primary hypoparathyroidism is less certain, but cases that have reversed well are certainly described.

Acromegaly

This condition, also called Marie's disease, results from hypersecretion of growth hormone after puberty and is usually caused by a pituitary adenoma. Characteristic overgrowth of the head and extremities occurs (with a consequent rapid increase in shoe size), often accompanied by headache, hypertension and glucose intolerance.

The psychiatric manifestations were extensively studied by Manfred Bleuler and colleagues at the

Zurich Psychiatric Clinic (Bleuler, 1951). An 'endocrine psychosyndrome' was proposed which was claimed to be common to many endocrine conditions. Apathy and lack of spontaneity were frequently present. Altered emotions were also common, including cheerfulness, self-satisfaction, elation, resentfulness coupled with anxiousness, tenseness and unpleasantness. Mood swings were noted, and libido was generally reduced. Psychosis was uncommon, except as a complication of the disease process. In the absence of raised intracranial pressure there were no striking cognitive deficits, other than those attributable to apathy and indifference. Patients were often regarded by others as egocentric, inconsiderate and touchy. It is likely that psychiatric changes reflect an amalgam of influences, consisting of metabolic changes, raised intracranial pressure, and the psychological reaction to illness and altered appearance (Avery, 1973; Margo, 1981).

Hypopituitarism

This disorder is most commonly due to a pituitary adenoma with a prolonged onset, rather than the result of infarction caused by postpartum haemorrhage (Sheehan's syndrome), as was once the case. Other causes include basal skull fracture or infection, sarcoidosis and craniopharyngioma in children. Much of the information about the psychiatric effects of hypopituitarism is based on the studies of Hans Kind (1958), who worked with Manfred Bleuler in Zurich. The psychiatric effects reflect underfunctioning of the adrenal cortex, thyroid and other metabolic disturbances.

Most patients with hypopituitarism have psychiatric disturbance, usually an involutional state characterised by varying degrees of apathy, inertia and insouciance. Impotence and impaired libido are early symptoms. The patient's mood is depressed, and when this is combined with apathy and memory impairment the patient may appear to be demented (Kind, 1958). Delirium usually reflects actual or impending metabolic upset. Patients with hypopituitarism are peculiarly prone to coma, which is often lethal. Schizophreniform psychosis is rare.

The weight loss, impaired appetite, scanty axillary and pubic hair, and amenorrhoea of hypopituitarism should not be mistaken for anorexia nervosa. In hypopituitarism, the patient's attitude to food is less intense, drive is much less, the facial lanugo hair to be found in anorexia nervosa is absent, and the degree of weight loss is usually less.

Psychiatric symptoms typically respond well to hormone replacement, although long-standing apathy may not reverse completely. If vasopressin production and release have been disturbed, it may come to light only after steroid replacement has begun, resulting in the polydipsia and polyuria characteristic of diabetes insipidus.

Diabetes mellitus

Diabetes mellitus is characterised by hyperglycaemia due to absolute or relative insulin deficiency. Estimates of the UK prevalence range between 1% and 3%. The lifetime risk of developing it is 10%. Type 2 diabetes accounts for 90% of all cases; causes include insulin resistance linked to obesity, excess growth hormone, thyroxine, cortisol or adrenalin (as in phaeochromocytoma), pregnancy, certain medications (conventional and atypical antipsychotics, beta-blockers, and diuretics) and liver disease (Holt, 2004).

Five types of coma may occur: hypoglycaemic, ketoacidotic, hyperosmolar non-ketotic, alcoholic ketoacidotic and that due to lactic acidosis. In diabetic ketoacidosis the level of consciousness correlates best with plasma osmolality. Hyperosmolar coma is especially common in elderly people. The key signs and laboratory findings comprise lethargy, changes in cognition, profound dehydration, polydipsia and polyuria, shallow respiration, hypotension and tachycardia, hyperthermia, extreme hyperglycaemia and minimal ketoacidosis. Salicylate poisoning and stroke are two important differential diagnoses of diabetic coma.

Emotional upset is associated with poor diabetic control, and many mechanisms can be postulated, including altered diet, alcohol use, changes in routine and activity levels, carelessness and so forth. Occasionally, obvious manipulation occurs, which may respond well to an individual or family psychotherapeutic approach. The study of the role of life circumstances in diabetic control is complex because of the many confounding variables (Rubin & Peyrot, 1992).

Insulin and oral hypoglycaemic drugs are potentiated by alcohol and monoamine oxidase inhibitors. Selective serotonin reuptake inhibitors (SSRIs) may reduce serum glucose by as much as 30% and cause appetite suppression, resulting in weight loss. Tricyclic drugs have even greater potential to disrupt glucose control – they can increase serum glucose levels by up to 150%, increase appetite, and reduce the metabolic rate. However, they are considered safe unless the disease is advanced or the control is poor. Amitryptyline, imipramine and citalopram are used to treat painful diabetic neuropathy. The newer atypical antipsychotics appear to be associated with the precipitation of hyperglycaemia and diabetes even among those who did not previously have diabetes, and sometimes there is a worsening of pre-existing diabetes, which may relate to drug-induced weight gain. These changes are most likely with clozapine and olanzapine but have been observed for all the atypicals, although the extent to which newer drugs are more diabetogenic than the older, typical drugs is unclear (the topic is also discussed on page 259). Sodium valproate may give false-positive urine tests for glucose in patients with diabetes (MacHale, 2002). The oral hypoglycaemic drug chlorpropamide can cause facial flushing if taken after the ingestion of alcohol, and metformin may cause anorexia as a side-effect.

Hypoglycaemia and insulinoma

Hypoglycaemia may induce permanent damage as the CNS (but for conditions of extreme starvation) has a single source of energy, glucose, and the reserves of glycogen and glucose are small. The damage is not uniform, but occurs in a rostrocaudal fashion – the middle layers of the cerebral cortex (but for the striate area) and the hippocampus are most affected, followed in turn by the basal ganglia and anterior thalamus. The brain-stem and spinal cord are most resistant (*Lancet*, 1985).

Hypoglycaemia may be extremely subtle in its presentation, considerably more subtle than acute diabetic hypoglycaemia. The causes can be obscure (e.g. insulinoma, ingestion of the Caribbean ackee fruit, and deliberate poisoning with, or misuse of, hypoglycaemic medicines). It is helpful to subdivide hypoglycaemia into acute, sub-acute and chronic forms (Marks & Rose, 1987).

In its acute form, hypoglycaemia unfolds with a characteristic progression of symptoms – a feeling of emptiness, weakness, hunger, sweating, palpitations, tremor, faintness, headache and blurred vision, delirium, and coma. Seizures occur in 10–20% of adults (*Lancet*, 1985). The person's behaviour may be out of character, inappropriate and even violent. In children, mental symptoms are more those of lassitude, somnolence and coma accompanied by generalised seizures. When hypoglycaemia is nocturnal, only sweats will be recalled, but in the daytime fatigue and underperformance occur (Gale & Tattersall, 1979). The triad of hypoglycaemia, CNS symptoms and prompt relief after intravenous glucose (Whipple's triad) forms the basis of diagnosis.

Malouf & Brust (1985) studied prospectively 125 cases of hypoglycaemia presenting acutely at hospital accident and emergency departments during a 12-month period. Sixty-five of these patients were obtunded, stuporous or in coma; 38 had acute focal or generalised cognitive impairments and/or psychiatric symptoms; 10 were dizzy or tremulous; 9 had seizures, and 3 had suffered sudden hemiparesis. Diabetes, alcohol (see alcohol-induced hypoglycaemia, above) and/or sepsis accounted for 90% of the predisposing conditions. Despite the series including several patients with coma of a substantial degree, only one patient died from hypoglycaemia, although four had residual neurological signs (indices of persisting psychological impairment were not sought). There is evidence that several severe episodes of hypoglycaemia can cause permanent memory impairment (Sachon *et al*, 1992).

In sub-acute hypoglycaemia the symptoms of excess sympathetic activity are usually absent; the picture is more that of languor, apathy and withdrawal, which is often discontinuous. Sometimes there is behavioural disinhibition. Cognitive impairment is often present and delirium can occur (Lishman, 1998).

Chronic hypoglycaemia may be punctuated by episodes of either of the two aforementioned presentations and is the rarest of the three. Personality change occurs, mirroring ongoing brain damage. Memory is often affected but left untreated, and this can result in dementia.

Insulinoma is a notable cause. Insulin-secreting tumours (insulinomas) of the beta-cells in the islets of Langerhans of the pancreas are a rare but important source of psychiatric morbidity – they are one of the 'great mimics', along with syphilis and Wilson's disease. Approximately 10% are malignant. They affect all age groups but are commonest after childhood and before 60. Insulinomas are MEN type I disorders. Two-thirds of patients have adenomas of two or more endocrine systems and one-fifth have tumours of three or more systems; there can be many years between the presentations of each disorder.

The effects of an insulinoma usually unfold insidiously and comprise sub-acute and/or chronic hypoglycaemic symptoms, punctuated by acute hypoglycaemic episodes which progressively increase in frequency (Lishman, 1998). Diagnosis is made difficult by the changeability of the presenting phenomena in a given individual. They can present with the clinical picture of neurosis, personality disorder, mania, depression, schizophrenia, epilepsy, 'funny turns', sleep disorder, delirium and dementia (Service *et al*, 1976). Patients may experience memory blackouts during and after acute episodes, although these frequently go unnoticed. The diagnosis is suggested where the illness is episodic and recurrent. Careful questioning may elicit physical symptoms suggestive of hypoglycaemia, but only a minority of patients notice a link with meals or exercise.

Investigation is best undertaken in a metabolic unit. While the ratio of plasma insulin to serum glucose is usually maintained at 0.3, in the presence of an insulinoma the ratio is usually >0.4 and rises with fasting; the diagnosis is made by demonstrating fasting hypoglycaemia in conjunction with normal or raised plasma insulin levels (Kaplan, 1991). Rising cortisol levels during fasting excludes hypothalamic–pituitary disorder as the cause of the hypoglycaemia.

The C-peptide of proinsulin normally varies in parallel with plasma insulin. If insulin has been administered surreptitiously, the level will be found to be suppressed, thus allowing misuse of insulin to be detected.

Surgery is the definitive treatment for insulinoma, although medical treatments also have a place. First-degree relatives should be screened.

Phaeochromocytoma

Phaeochromocytomas are tumours derived from chromaffin cells, which secrete catecholamines and other substances. About 10% of these tumours are malignant. In the USA there are about 36 000 affected individuals (Melicow, 1977). Roughly 90% of the tumours are located in the adrenal medulla, 10% being bilateral (Robbins & Cotran, 1979). They occur at any age, but mostly in the fourth and fifth decades. They present in many clinical guises: as 'turns'; as diabetes in which there is severe hypertension; as angina with normal coronary arteries; as pre-eclampsia in pregnancy; and in many more ways. The variability of the presentation is partly due to the variation in the nature and quantity of catecholamines released. In one study the majority of cases had presented with paroxysmal attacks of less than an hour, in which the four most prominent symptoms were headache, perspiration, palpitations and pallor (Thomas *et al*, 1966). Attacks usually progress in frequency and severity, although the form is fairly uniform for each individual. During attacks the blood pressure is usually high and accompanied by tachycardia. Glucose intolerance, elevated packed cell volume, polycythaemia, orthostatic hypotension, cardiac ischaemia and cardiomyopathy can all occur.

Psychological accompaniments include intense anxiety, fear, overarousal, delirium, depression, psychosis and dementia. Epileptic fits can occur. Reported precipitants of attacks include bending, turning in bed, sexual intercourse, straining, excitement and physical exertion, but a precipitant may not be identified (Melicow, 1977). Tricyclic antidepressants enhance the effects of circulating catecholamines, and indeed all drugs must be carefully considered before being used in a patient suspected of having a phaeochromocytoma.

A high index of suspicion is required in psychiatric patients with anxiety disorders or depression, and in those who present with 'turns'. Work-up should include thorough blood pressure monitoring, retinoscopy, a blood glucose and three 24-hour urinary vanillylmandelic acid (VMA) estimations using acidified containers, which should be kept cold. Further investigations involve pharmacological tests, intravascular sampling and imaging techniques.

Suspected phaeochromocytoma is one of the few *absolute* contraindications for electroconvulsive therapy (Drake & Ebaugh, 1956).

Hypoxia

Hypoxia of the brain causes psychological symptoms whose severity are related to the rate at which hypoxia occurs, its duration, the cause and the context (Gibson, 1985; Lishman, 1998). Four brain areas are thought to be especially vulnerable: the arterial boundary zones, the thalamus, Ammon's horns and the cerebellum. It can present with lethargy, mental slowing, impaired judgement, hallucinations and delirium. Permanent psychological sequelae include regional psychological deficits, amnesic syndrome and dementia. When evaluating a patient with chronic cognitive impairment, it should always be established whether the patient could have been hypoxic at any time. General anaesthesia, cardiovascular events, lung disease, carbon monoxide poisoning, hypoglycaemia, epilepsy, anaemia, cerebral malaria or activities such as climbing or diving are potential causes. Cyanide and carbon disulphide poisoning are but two examples of toxic causes. Acute mental changes – disturbance of mood, memory, judgement and orientation – at altitude tend to become apparent at 4000–5000 m (Nelson, 1982). Coma from hypoxia has a worse outcome than coma of equivalent severity from hypoglycaemia (Malouf & Brust, 1985).

Disorders of electrolyte, acid–base and fluid balance

Hypernatraemia

Hypernatraemia, defined as a serum sodium level above 150 mmol/l, is present in the following four circumstances: excessive water loss (e.g. pyrexia, extensive burns, ventilator loss, hypercatabolism and diabetes insipidus); water loss exceeding sodium loss (e.g. sweating, vomiting, diarrhoea, and conditions in which there is osmotic diuresis); inadequate fluid intake (e.g. with impairment of consciousness); and after the excessive administration of sodium (e.g. salt poisoning, sodium in dialysate) (Jefferson & Marshall, 1981). Hypernatraemia causes brain shrinkage, and in extreme cases subdural, subarachnoid or intracerebral haemorrhages occur. The main symptoms are relatively non-specific irritability, lethargy, weakness, illusions and visual hallucinations, delirium, stupor and coma. The more rapid the development of hypernatraemia, the more pronounced the symptoms are; when the onset is insidious the diagnosis can be easily overlooked. Physical signs of dehydration are less marked than with salt depletion and may be delayed. These include tachycardia, low-amplitude pulse, depressed jugular venous pressure, reduced skin turgor, sunken eyes and postural hypotension. Too rapid correction of the electrolyte imbalance may induce cerebral oedema and fits.

Hyponatraemia

Hyponatraemia commonly accompanies numerous systemic diseases and is due to depletion or dilution of sodium reserves (Arieff & Guisado, 1976). It is often iatrogenic, being due to incorrect intravenous infusion regimens or diuretic treatment, and can be induced by many drugs (e.g. carbamazepine, lithium, amitriptyline and phenothiazines). Hyponatraemia can be induced deliberately, but also accidentally through excessive beer drinking ('beer potomania'). Other causes include renal disorder, the syndrome of inappropriate of anti-diuretic hormone secretion (SIADH), hepatic cirrhosis, congestive heart failure and Addison's disease.

The neurobehavioural symptoms of acute hyponatraemia are due to brain swelling, and are described below in the section on water intoxication. Chronic hyponatraemia may present with lethargy, muscle weakness and somnolence. Serum urea, electrolytes, creatinine and liver function tests should be assayed, serum and urinary osmolality measured, and the patient examined for the presence of oedema. The treatment of hyponatraemia is complex; it has been outlined by Sterns (1987). Rapid correction of hyponatraemia is hazardous as it can cause acute brain shrinkage and is implicated in the development of central pontine myelinolysis.

Hyperkalaemia

Hyperkalaemia is due to reduced renal excretion or transcellular potassium shifts. Diminished renal excretion is due to reduced glomerular filtration rate (acute oliguric renal failure or chronic renal failure) or reduced tubular secretion (potassium-sparing diuretics or Addison's disease). Transcellular shifts occur with acidosis, cell destruction (trauma, burns, rhabdomyolysis and haemolysis), hyperkalaemic periodic paralysis and diabetic hyperglycaemia. Overzealous fist-clenching during venepuncture or an overnight delay in sending a sample to the laboratory can also cause hyperkalaemia, but this is artefactual.

Hyperkalaemia causes an organic brain syndrome characterised by weakness, dysarthria and a range of neuromuscular symptoms (Webb & Gehi, 1981), which can be mistaken for neurotic illness. In more severe disturbances, delirium and an ascending flaccid paralysis can occur.

Hyperkalaemic periodic paralysis is an autosomal dominant condition which may be mistaken for hysteria. Episodes of paralysis can occur spontaneously, after exercise or following excessive dietary potassium. The occurrence of myotonia suggests the diagnosis, and an electrocardiogram can confirm it.

There are three particular aspects to the treatment of hyperkalaemia – reduction of cardiac excitability (calcium gluconate therapy), the transfer of potassium into intracellular fluid (sodium bicarbonate or glucose and insulin therapy), and the elimination of potassium from the body (diuretic administration and renal dialysis).

Hypokalaemia

Hypokalaemia is due to inadequate intake of potassium, excessive renal loss (e.g. diuretics, mineralocorticoid excess, antibiotics and chronic renal failure), vomiting and diarrhoea, and shifts into the intracellular compartment (as a result of alkalosis, periodic hypokalaemic paralysis or insulin therapy). Hypokalaemia produces neuromuscular symptoms (weakness and/or paralysis), lassitude and, more rarely, delirium.

Periodic hypokalaemic paralysis is a rare condition characterised by episodic weakness and/or paralysis following the ingestion of a high load of carbohydrate. The lack of an obvious precipitant may result in it being taken for a hysterical conversion disorder (Mitchell & Feldman, 1968).

Hypermagnesaemia and hypomagnesaemia

The effects of magnesium and calcium disturbances can be difficult to dissociate. Hypermagnesaemia may result from the use of magnesium-containing antacids and from renal failure. Among the symptoms reported are nausea, vomiting, malaise, drowsiness, dysarthria, gait ataxia, difficulty in voiding urine and defaecating, hyporeflexia and coma. Hypermagnesaemia from habitual use of an antacid is a cause of reversible dementia in the elderly.

Isolated hypomagnesaemia is rare. Hypomagnesaemia has a large range of causes, of which alcoholism is one of the most common. Psychiatric manifestations include personality change, apathy, depression, agitation, anxiety, disorientation, hallucinations and delirium. Magnesium deficiency may aggravate Wernicke–Korsakoff syndrome (Flink, 1986), may induce seizures and may be accompanied by myoclonus, chorea and athetosis. Serum levels may be normal in the presence of whole-body depletion, as 99% of magnesium is in intracellular stores or bone. In order to make the diagnosis a 24-hour urine collection is required.

Hyperphosphataemia and hypophosphataemia

Discrete psychiatric symptoms have not been linked to hyperphosphataemia.

Hypophosphataemia has been associated with a range of neurobehavioural features, from irritability to delirium or coma (Knochel, 1977), but it is not clear whether these features are due to associated metabolic disturbances.

Hypophosphataemia is encountered in a hitherto often unrecognised but important presentation to the psychiatrist – the 'refeeding syndrome'. Malnourished patients' intracellular phosphate stores can be depleted despite normal serum phosphate concentrations. As they start to feed, a shift from fat to carbohydrate metabolism occurs and secretion of insulin occurs. This stimulates cellular uptake of phosphate and can precipitate profound hypophosphataemia. Hypokalaemia, hypomagnesaemia and low thiamine are among other associated metabolic derangements that can coexist. It is usually seen within 4 days of starting to feed. Malnourished homeless individuals admitted for assessment of psychosis, chronic alcohol misusers undergoing detoxification, patients with eating disorders and others with extreme self-neglect are all liable to develop the refeeding syndrome (Catani & Howells, 2007). The consequences can be life-threatening – a potential cause of an in-patient death. Phosphate concentrations of less than 0.50 mmol/l produce the clinical features, which include rhabdomyolysis, leucocyte dysfunction, respiratory failure, cardiac failure, hypotension, arrhythmias, seizures, coma and sudden death. The early clinical features of refeeding syndrome are non-specific and may go unrecognised. The management is discussed by Hearing (2004).

Zinc deficiency

Zinc deficiency causes anorexia and weight loss, impaired taste and olfaction, and altered mood and behaviour. It is especially prevalent worldwide in communities where mainly cereals are consumed because phytate inhibits zinc absorption; the deficiency then presents with growth retardation and hypogonadism (Prasad, 2003). It can cause a paranoid state, memory impairment and cerebellar symptoms (Henkin *et al*, 1975). Zinc deficiency may present to the psychiatrist as fatigue states, depression, anorexia and progressive dementia. As patients with anorexia nervosa and low serum zinc levels have been reported to respond to zinc supplementation, it is reasonable to consider zinc supplementation in anorexia nervosa as an adjunct to psychological and other measures (Yamaguchi *et al*, 1992).

Serum zinc levels are subject to various factors. There is a pronounced diurnal variation, with peak levels at 10.00 h, and large fluctuations occur following meals. Levels increase after prolonged fasting, and are low in hypoalbuminaemia, pregnancy, oestrogen therapy and in the presence of certain malignancies. Low activity of serum alkaline phosphatase, which is a zinc-dependent enzyme, may indicate zinc deficiency.

Acidosis

Metabolic acidosis is caused by hyperglycaemia, salicylate overdosage, renal disease and any condition causing alkali loss. Deep, fast breathing (Kussmaul breathing) is often a prominent clinical feature. Fatigue, progressive depression of consciousness and seizures occur. Salicylate poisoning constitutes a medical emergency. Restlessness, facial flushing, sweating, hyperventilation, tinnitus and an impaired sensorium are all features. Blood levels should always be measured and the patient is best managed in a medical unit.

Respiratory acidosis is associated with carbon dioxide retention and was studied in end-stage chronic obstructive airways disease by Westlake *et al* (1955). Delirium with hallucinations (auditory and visual) may occur, but some patients exhibit progressive impairment of consciousness alone. The nursing staff may report that an affected patient is becoming increasingly oversensitive, obstreperous and 'difficult'. Both acidosis and hypercapnia can independently cause coma. Hypercapnia is associated with headache, sweating, muscle twitching (particularly facial) and raised intracranial pressure.

Alkalosis

The causes of metabolic alkalosis include chloride depletion, hyperadrenocorticism, severe potassium depletion and excessive alkali intake. As the arterial pH exceeds 7.55, irritability, muscle weakness, apathy, delirium and stupor occur.

Respiratory alkalosis as a result of hyperventilation is relatively common in psychiatric practice; typically it is a result of anxiety or habit. Hyperventilation, however, has many causes – salicylate poisoning, metabolic acidosis, hypercapnia, pregnancy and many others should always be ruled out. In the anxious person, hyperventilation produces a range of symptoms that can reinforce any original anxiety, so creating a vicious circle of events. These include fatigue, general weakness, atypical chest pain, tachycardia, palpitations, dyspnoea, light-headedness, faintness, impaired concentration and memory, derealisation, blurred vision, paraesthesia, tetany and mild delirium. Hallucinations have been described as a result of hyperventilation, and it may precipitate epilepsy.

Hyperventilation is best managed by teaching the patient about how it arises, ideally in the company of a friend or relative. Voluntary hyperventilation is performed, and the patient is taught how to respond, emphasising diaphragmatic breathing. The classic remedy of breathing into a paper bag may be of value in acute situations, but understanding, rehearsal and prevention are more effective (Missri & Alexander, 1978).

Water intoxication

The excessive drinking of water is a relatively common practice among psychiatric patients, particularly those with schizophrenia. A survey by de Leon *et al* (2002) of a group of chronic patients mainly with schizophrenia gave rates for a significant degree of polydipsia (i.e. with a risk of water intoxication) of around 5%. The criteria used to detect those at risk was a greater than 4% change in diurnal body weight (7.00–15.00 h), since changes in diurnal body weight of this magnitude are known to be associated with a lowering of serum sodium of around 10 mmol/l. Although mainly occurring among patients with schizophrenia, it also occurred among other groups and the odd ratios (ORs) were increased for those who smoked heavily (OR = 4.3), those taking antimuscarinic drugs (OR = 1.9) and those who had been hospitalised for longer (OR = 1.9).

It is an important source of morbidity and mortality. It may be seen as a reaction to the consumption of MDMA ('ecstasy'). The early features of water intoxication include headache, blurred vision, polyuria, vomiting, tremor and exacerbation of psychosis. It can go unnoticed until delirium, a generalised epileptic fit or even coma occur. Muscle cramps, ataxia and stupor can also occur (Ferrier, 1985). Copying the conduct of others may be part of the explanation for the activity. Surveys suggest that there is rarely a compulsion – the majority want to do it.

The diagnosis of water intoxication is made when a symptomatic patient has a plasma sodium of less than 120 mmol/l. To confirm that overdrinking of water has occurred, staff and other informants should be questioned about the patient's behaviour, and observations undertaken. Such observation tends to reveal a common pattern: drinking begins around breakfast time and continues through the day until the evening. Fluid retention is maximal late in the afternoon or in the early evening and then tends to reverse to normal, or near normal, overnight. It follows that the serum sodium level should be estimated in the late afternoon, and *not* in the morning, as is more customary.

Other causes of polydipsia and polyuria should be excluded: these comprise diabetes mellitus, chronic renal failure, hypercalcaemia and diabetes insipidus (Illowsky & Kirch, 1988). The possibility of hypothalamic lesions and pituitary tumours should be borne in mind. The effects of drugs such as lithium, alcohol and diuretics must also be excluded. The syndrome of inappropriate antidiuretic hormone secretion (SIADH) is identified by the presence of a low serum sodium concentration in the presence of relatively concentrated urine, and confirmed by further tests. It should be noted that amitriptyline, desipramine, tranylcypromine, thioridazine, fluphenazine, trifluoperazine, haloperidol and other psychotropic drugs can induce hyponatraemia.

Management approaches include monitoring the patient's weight, trying to distract the patient, optimising medication, and stopping all fluid intake and awaiting the urinary excretion of excess water (Crammer, 1991). There have been reports that tetracycline, demeclocycline and naloxone may help in the management. Among patients with schizophrenia the older, typical drugs do not appear to be helpful and there are reports showing that risperidone may also be ineffective; there are, however, now several reports in the literature indicating the clozapine may restore water balance in this dangerous syndrome (Canuso & Goldman, 1999).

Uraemia

Mental changes are a feature of both acute and chronic renal failure. The relationship between the level of urea and the nature and degree of mental changes is not necessarily causal, since patients with renal failure can have mental disturbances for a host of reasons. There is a wide range of symptoms; apathy, detachment and fatigue are prominent early on, and may be misconstrued as a depressive episode. Other patients become expansive and irritable. Impaired concentration is complained of at an early stage, and more global cognitive problems develop subsequently. Activities become slowed and speech becomes slurred. Delirium is a feature of both acute and chronic renal failure, foreshadowed by higher urea levels and rapid fluctuations. Auditory and visual hallucinations occur and are accompanied by delusions, often persecutory in type. Epileptic seizures are an additional complication. Patients ultimately become stuporous and enter coma. Myoclonus, muscular twitches, asterixis, choreoathetosis and catatonia are all reported. EEG changes occur and these comprise background slowing, bouts of paroxysmal slow waves and reduced rapid eye movement (REM) and slow wave sleep. As renal function is being corrected, underlying medical complications should be actively sought.

If dialysis is too rapid, patients may develop any of the following constellation of symptoms – headache, cramps, lethargy or agitation, hallucinations, delusions and behavioural changes. This is sometimes referred to as the 'dialysis disequilibrium syndrome'. 'Dialysis dementia' is the term given to a potentially more lethal condition that can develop abruptly or insidiously after months or years of dialysis with aluminium-containing dialysis fluids. Intoxication with aluminium in renal failure also occurs through the use of aluminium-containing phosphate buffers. It may be heralded by speech disorder, ranging from hesitancy to frank dysphasia, delirium, progressive dementia and personality change. The dementia of chronic low-level aluminium overload in renal failure appears to resemble a slow-onset version of dialysis delirium, rather than Alzheimer's disease (Kerr *et al*, 1992).

Hypothermia and hyperthermia

Hypothermia is defined as a drop in the core temperature to 35°C or less. At less than 30°C consciousness is impaired, and coma is the rule at 26.7°C or less. Hypothermia causes delirium and other mental changes. It is most likely to be encountered among elderly patients with psychiatric illness, as a consequence of drug overdose or self-neglect.

Hyperthermia ('heat stroke') is defined as occurring at a core temperature of 40.6°C or more. It is classified as exertional or non-exertional in nature. In psychiatric patients, it is especially common in those taking medication with anticholinergic effects during hot weather. Hyperthermia is a feature of neuroleptic malignant syndrome and complicates overdosage with lithium, monoamine oxidase inhibitor (MAOI) antidepressants and amphetamines.

Hyperthermia causes agitation, delirium and/or coma. Lethargy, hallucinations, stupor and seizures are other well-recognised features. Delirium appears to be the predominant presenting symptom. Affected individuals have hot, dry skin, tachycardia and flaccid muscles with reduced or absent reflexes (Petersdorf, 1991). Hypotension and hypoventilation are usually present.

Hyperthermia is a medical emergency; patients can die within a few hours if left untreated. Hyperthermia must be anticipated during hot weather, particularly with in-patients receiving medication with strong anticholinergic properties.

Miscellaneous disorders

Porphyria

The porphyrias are a set of metabolic disorders caused by a partial deficiency of enzymes responsible for haem synthesis. The word 'porphyria' derives from the Greek *porphuros*, which means red or purple. Excessive production of haem precursors results, and these precursors are readily oxidised to porphyrins. Characteristic clinical presentations include episodes of acute porphyria and/or photosensitive skin reactions. The porphyrias are of importance in psychiatry because of their ability to present with a range of major psychiatric manifestations, sometimes in the absence of physical symptoms. Furthermore, they may be precipitated or exacerbated by drugs used in psychiatry. The details of the biochemistry of porphyria were reviewed by Elder *et al* (1990).

Four types of porphyria are virtually indistinguishable clinically – as the liver is the main site of excess porphyrin production, these are called acute hepatic porphyrias. These are rare before puberty, more common in women, and are associated with fatality in about 5% of hospitalised cases. They present with three core features: abdominal pain, psychiatric disturbances and peripheral neuropathy. Skin lesions are found in most types of porphyria.

Fifty cases of acute intermittent porphyria (AIP) were evaluated by Goldberg (1959), who found that neurological or psychiatric symptoms were the predominant feature at presentation in about 25%. Abdominal pain is even more common, occurring in as many as 90% of cases. Approximately 50–75% of cases exhibit psychiatric symptoms (Ackner *et al*, 1962), including personality change, neurotic disorders, depression, schizophreniform psychosis, hallucinations, delirium and dementia. Epilepsy and coma may occur. Between episodes, few residual cognitive deficits were found in a sample of 25 cases of AIP (Wetterberg & Österberg, 1969). The initial neurological manifestation is usually a rapidly spreading, symmetrical, predominantly motor polyneuropathy. Cranial nerve lesions and a Guillian–Barré-type syndrome can occur in more severe cases, ending with fatal cardiac or respiratory failure.

The most famous case of alleged prophyria and its psychiatric complications, which even featured in a play and a film, is that of King George III, who suffered from episodes of insanity. His personal physician, Dr Willis, kept a daily diary of his prolonged illness and all 47 volumes of this are in the British Museum. Within this diary there are four references to discoloured urine: 'bluish urine', 'bilious urine', 'deep colour' and 'blood water'. Macalpine & Hunter (1966) documented a strong family history of psychiatric disorder among the European royal relatives of George III, as well as other relatives and proposed a familial genetic disorder; they suggested porphyria on the grounds that there was documentary evidence of urine discoloration. They also found mildly elevated porphyria levels in two descendants. However, the hypothesis is unlikely because George III suffered from very severe episodes of mania which went on for months on end, which are quite typical of bipolar I disorder, whereas mania of similar duration and severity has nowhere else been described in association with porphyria. The biochemical evidence has also been questioned; thus, Arnold (1996) suggested the bluish urine was probably due to urinary indican, and indicanuria is the result of constipation and bowel stasis and the activity of intestinal flora, with severe constipation being a common feature of severe, prolonged psychotic illness.

Drugs are probably the most important precipitants of porphyria, including tricyclic and MAOI antidepressants, barbiturates, most older anticonvulsants, sulpiride, zuclopenthixol, thioridazine, ketoconazole and amphetamines. Unfortunately, because of the infrequency of the condition there is little systematic information available on associations with the newer, more commonly prescribed psychotropics such as the SSRIs and the atypical antipsychotics. Other precipitants include fever, alcohol, menstrual change, starvation and pregnancy.

Porphyria has been mistaken for hysteria, affective disorder, schizophrenia and dementia. Physical examination may reveal neuropathy, hypertension or a laparotomy scar. Leucocytosis and fever can occur during acute attacks. In AIP, urine left to stand may turn to a purple red colour.

Each enzyme deficiency has a characteristic pattern of plasma, erythrocyte and excretory (urinary and faecal) abnormalities that forms the basis of biochemical diagnostic procedures. It should be noted that lead intoxication, gastrointestinal bleeding, liver disease and certain other conditions also cause the excretion of porphyrins to be increased. Biochemical diagnosis is best made during symptomatic illness, as afterwards biochemical parameters may return to normal. Most laboratories will be able to identify porphyria with urinary and faecal tests, which must include measurement of urinary porphobilinogen if acute porphyria is suspected. Urine, faecal and blood porphyrias should be determined to avoid errors in the identification of individual porphyrias. Screening of relatives for latent forms is best conducted by reference laboratories.

Much of the initial treatment is supportive. Exposure to sunlight and trauma to the skin should be avoided. Suspected drug precipitants should be removed, but chlorpromazine has been widely used to control mental disturbance, and diazepam can be used to control seizures. Paraldehyde is a safe and effective reserve agent. Intravenous infusion of haem arginate may alleviate acute attacks – out-of-hours sources are listed in the *British National Formulary*. Glucose infusions may also have a role. The prognosis for psychological symptoms is said to be good.

Mitochondrial myopathy

The mitochondrial myopathies are a rare group of metabolic disorders that are clinically and biochemically heterogeneous, but share the common feature of structural mitochondrial abnormalities on skeletal muscle biopsy (Morgan-Hughes, 1986). The majority of cases present before the age of 20. Three overlapping clinical groups are reported (Petty *et al*, 1986). The first is characterised by external ophthalmoplegia and limb weakness, the second by limb weakness alone, and the third by predominantly CNS manifestations – ataxia, dementia, deafness, involuntary movements, pigmented retinopathy and seizures. Mitochondrial myopathy may present as a chronic fatigue syndrome, hysteria or progressive dementia at a young age. The family history should be explored carefully. Presently there is no definitive treatment.

Neuroacanthocytosis

Neuroacanthocytosis refers to a constellation of metabolic disorders, often familial, characterised by neurological disorder in conjunction with acanthocytic red blood cells (red cells with spiky projections). Various other terms have been applied to these disorders, particularly choreoacanthocytosis, which signals the frequent association of chorea with acanthocytosis. The clinical, haematological and pathological features include orofacial dyskinesia, biting of the tongue and lips, dysarthria, chorea, tics, dystonia, parkinsonism and muscle disorder. Cases presenting with solely psychiatric features are not uncommon (Wyszynski *et al*, 1989). Personality change (of the frontal lobe type), depression, anxiety, paranoid delusions and obsessive–compulsive disorder are all described. Seizures occur and can be the presenting feature. While mild cognitive impairments occur, progressive dementia is also well recognised.

The diagnosis should be entertained in any patient presenting with movement disorder, personality change and progressive intellectual deterioration. It should be excluded in all suspected cases of Huntington's chorea and in atypical cases of tic disorder. It has been suggested that more than 3% of true acanthocytes in a blood film is significant – echinocytes and other artefacts must be excluded. One negative film does not exclude the disorder. It should be noted that caudate head shrinkage on brain imaging, a feature commonly seen on the scans of patients with Huntington's chorea, also occurs in patients with neuroacanthocytosis. However, in both conditions cortical atrophy may be the only feature on the scans, especially in younger patients. Screening and counselling are an important aspect of management.

Metachromatic leucodystrophy

Metachromatic leucodystrophy is a lysosomal storage disease. While rare, it warrants inclusion here as it exemplifies a recurring rule within this chapter, namely that a psychiatric disorder may have an unusual cause, one that may be readily overlooked or not even known about. Other lysosomal storage diseases with psychiatric manifestations include Gaucher disease, Niemann–Pick disease, GM2 gangliodiosis and neuronal ceroid lipofuscinosis (Kufs' disease).

In metachromatic leucodystrophy, the enzyme aryl sulphatase is deficient and levels of lysosomal galactosyl sulphatide are high throughout the nervous system. The inheritance is autosomal recessive. Progressive impairment of motor function occurs, which in the adult form may be preceded by a range of mental changes, including personality change, affective disorder and schizophrenia-like psychosis (this is further discussed on page 214). The prognosis is poor – progressive dementia accompanies a relentless deterioration in neurological function.

The diagnosis is strongly suggested by low or absent urinary aryl sulphatase A; in addition, metachromatic material may be seen in Schwann cells obtained by sural nerve or rectal biopsy. Protein levels in the cerebrospinal fluid are usually raised and in established cases brain imaging will reveal cerebral atrophy and periventricular white-matter changes.

References

Ackner, B., Cooper, J. E., Gray, C. H., *et al* (1962) Acute porphyria: a neuropsychiatric and biochemical study. *Journal of Psychosomatic Research*, **6**, 1–24.

Adams, R. D. & Victor, M. (1989) *Principles of Neurology* (4th edn). New York: McGraw-Hill.

Altmann, P., Cunningham, J., Dhanesha, U., *et al* (1999) Disturbance of cerebral function in people exposed to drinking water contaminated with aluminium sulphate: retrospective study of the Camelford water incident. *BMJ*, **319**, 807–811.

American Psychiatric Association (1994) *Diagnostic and Statistical Manual of Mental Disorders* (4th edn) (DSM–IV). Washington, DC: APA.

Anderson, I. (2003) Drug treatment of depression: reflections on the evidence. *Advances in Psychiatric Treatment*, **9**, 11–20.

Arieff, A. I. & Guisado, R. (1976) Effects on the central nervous system of hypernatremic and hyponatremic states. *Kidney International*, **10**, 104–116.

Arnold, W. N. (1996) King George III's urine and indigo blue. *Lancet*, **347**, 1811–1813.

Asher, R. (1949) Myxoedematous madness. *BMJ*, *ii*, 555–556.

Ashton, C. H. (1987) Caffeine and health. *BMJ*, **295**, 1293–1294.

Avery, T. L. (1973) A case of acromegaly and gigantism with depression. *British Journal of Psychiatry*, **122**, 599–600.

Banay, R. S. (1944) Pathological reaction to alcohol. I. Review of the literature and original case reports. *Quarterly Journal of Studies on Alcohol*, **4**, 580–605.

Bleuler, M. (1951) The psychopathology of acromegaly. *Journal of Nervous and Mental Disease*, **113**, 497–511.

Bowen, S. E., Daniel, J. & Balster, R. L. (1999) Deaths associated with inhalant abuse in Virginia from 1987–1996. *Drug and Alcohol Dependency*, **53**, 239–245.

British National Formulary (2004) *British National Formulary* (47th edn). London: British Medical Association/Royal Pharmaceutical Society of Great Britain.

Bruce, M. S. & Lader, M. (1986) Caffeine: clinical and experimental effects in humans. *Human Psychopharmacology*, **1**, 63–82.

Canuso, C. M. & Goldman, M. B. (1999) Clozapine restores water balance in schizophrenic patients with polydipsia–hyponatremia syndrome. *Journal of Neuropsychiatry and Clinical Neuroscience*, **11**, 86–90.

Carney, M. W. P. (1990) Vitamin deficiency and mental symptoms. *British Journal of Psychiatry*, **156**, 878–882.

Catani, M. & Howells, R. (2007) Risks and pitfalls for the management of refeeding syndrome in psychiatric patients. *Psychiatric Bulletin* (in press).

Checkley, S. A. (1978) Thyrotoxicosis and the course of manic–depressive illness. *British Journal of Psychiatry*, **133**, 418–424.

Chick, J. & Cantwell, R. (eds) (1994) *Seminars in Alcohol and Drug Misuse*. London: Gaskell.

Christie-Brown, J. R. W. (1968) Mood changes following parathyroidectomy. *Proceedings of the Royal Society of Medicine*, **61**, 1121–1123.

Cleghorn, R. A. (1951) Adrenocortical insufficency: psychological and neurological observations. *Canadian Medical Association Journal*, **65**, 449–454.

Cohen, S. I. (1980) Cushing's syndrome: a psychiatric study of 29 patients. *British Journal of Psychiatry*, **136**, 120–124.

Cohen, S. I. & Johnson, K. (1988) Psychosis from alcohol or drug abuse. *BMJ*, **297**, 1270–1271.

Coid, J. (1979) Mania à potu: a critical review of pathological intoxication. *British Journal of Psychiatry*, **9**, 709–719.

Collis, I. & Lloyd, G. (1992) Psychiatric aspects of liver disease. *British Journal of Psychiatry*, **161**, 12–22.

Connell, P. H. (1958) *Amphetamine Psychosis*. Maudsley Monograph No. 5. London: Chapman & Hall.

Cooper, A. F. & Schapira, K. (1973) Case report: depression, catatonic stupor, and EEG changes in hyperparathyroidism. *Psychological Medicine*, **3**, 509–515.

Cornelius, J. R., Soloff, P. H. & Miewald, B. K. (1986) Behavioral manifestations of paraneoplastic encephalopathy. *Biological Psychiatry*, **21**, 686–690.

Crammer, J. L. (1991) Drinking, thirst and water intoxication. *British Journal of Psychiatry*, **159**, 83–89.

Crook, M., Hally, V. & Pantelli, S. (2001) The importance of the refeeding syndrome. *Nutrition*, **17**, 632–637.

de Fine Olivarus, B. & Röder, E. (1970) Reversible psychosis and dementia in myxedema. *Acta Psychiatrica Scandinavica*, **46**, 1–13.

de Leon, J., Tracey, J., McCann, E., *et al* (2002) Polydipsia in a psychiatric hospital: a replication study. *Schizophrenia Research*, **57**, 293–301.

Denko, J. & Kaelbling, T. (1962) The psychiatric aspects of hypoparathyroidism. *Acta Psychiatrica Scandinavica*, **38**, 7–70.

Dooling, E. C., Schoene, W. C. & Richardson, E. P. (1974) Hallervorden–Spatz syndrome. *Archives of Neurology*, **30**, 70–83.

Drake, F. R. (1957) Neuropsychiatric-like symptomatology of Addison's disease: a review. *American Journal of Medical Sciences*, **234**, 106–113.

Drake, F. R. & Ebaugh, F. G. (1956) Phaeochromocytoma and electroconvulsive therapy. *American Journal of Psychiatry*, **113**, 295–301.

Drennan, P. C. (1984) Visual hallucinations in children receiving decongestants. *BMJ*, **288**, 1688.

Drummond, D. C. (1991) Dependence on psychoactive drugs: finding a common language. In: *International Handbook of Addiction Behaviour* (ed. I. B. Glass), pp. 1–14. London: Routledge.

Edwards, G. & Gross, M. M. (1976) Alcohol dependence: provisional description of a clinical syndrome. *BMJ*, *i*, 1058–1061.

Edwards, G., Marshall, E. J. & Cook, C. H. (2003) *The Treatment of Drinking Problems* (4th edn). Cambridge: Cambridge University Press.

Efron, D. H., Holmstedt, B. & Kline, N. S. (1979) *Ethnopharmacological Search for Psychoactive Drugs*. New York: Raven.

Elder, G. H., Shith, S. G. & Smyth, S. J. (1990) Laboratory investigation of the porphyrias. *Annals of Clinical Biochemistry*, **27**, 395–412.

Eldridge, R., Anayiotos, C. P., Schelsinger, S., *et al* (1984) Hereditary adult-onset leukodystrophy simulating chronic progressive multiple sclerosis. *New England Journal of Medicine*, **311**, 948–953.

Emboden, W. (1972) *Narcotic Plants*. London: Studio Vista.

Estrada, R. V., Moreno, J., Martinez, E., *et al* (1979) Pancreatic encephalopathy. *Acta Neurologica Scandinavica*, **59**, 135–139.

Ferrier, I. N. (1985) Water intoxication in patients with psychiatric illness. *BMJ*, **291**, 1594–1596.

Flink, E. B. (1986) Magnesium deficiency in alcoholics. *Alcoholism: Clinical and Experimental Research*, **10**, 590–594.

Flint, J. & Goldstein, L. H. (1992) Familial calcification of the basal ganglia: a case report and review of the literature. *Psychological Medicine*, **22**, 581–595.

Forman, H. P., Levin, S., Stewart, B., *et al* (1989) Cerebral vasculitis and hemorrhage in an adolescent taking diet pills containing phenylpropanolamine: case report and review of literature. *Pediatrics*, **83**, 737–741.

Gale, E. A. M. & Tattersall, R. B. (1979) Unrecognized nocturnal hypoglycaemia in insulin-treated diabetics. *Lancet*, *i*, 1049–1052.

Galfond, D. (1989) Psychosis from alcohol or drug abuse. *BMJ*, **298**, 524.

Gibson, G. E. (1985) Hypoxia. In *Cerebral Energy Metabolism and Metabolic Encephalopathy* (ed. D. W. McCandless), pp. 43–78. New York: Plenum.

Goldberg, A. (1959) Acute intermittent porphyria. A study of fifty cases. *Quarterly Journal of Medicine*, **28**, 183–209.

Goodwin, D. W., Crane, B. & Guze, S. B. (1969*a*) Alcoholic 'blackouts': a review and clinical study of 100 alcoholics. *American Journal of Psychiatry*, **126**, 191–198.

Goodwin, D. W., Crane, B. & Guze, S. B. (1969*b*) Phenomenological aspects of the alcoholic blackout. *British Journal of Psychiatry*, **115**, 1033–1038.

Greden, J. F. & Walters, M. D. (1992) Caffeine. In *Substance Abuse: A Comprehensive Textbook* (eds J. C. Lowinson, P. Ruiz, R. B. Millman & J. G. Langrod), pp. 357–370. Baltimore, MD: Williams and Wilkins.

Greenwood, R. S. & Nelson, J. S. (1978) Atypical neuronal ceroid-lipofuscinosis. *Neurology*, **28**, 710–717.

Hadden, W. B. (1882) The nervous symptoms of myxoedema. *Brain*, **5**, 188–196.

Hall, R. C. W., Popkin, M. K. & Kirkpatrick, B. (1978) Tricyclic exacerbation of steroid psychosis. *Journal of Nervous and Mental Disease*, **166**, 738–742.

Hall, R. C. W., Popkin, M. K., Stickney, R. N., *et al* (1979) Presentation of the steroid psychoses. *Journal of Nervous and Mental Disease*, **167**, 229–236.

Hartman, D. E. (1988) *Neuropsychological Toxicology*. New York: Pergamon.

Haskett, R. F. (1985) Diagnostic categorization of psychiatric disturbance in Cushing's syndrome. *American Journal of Psychiatry*, **142**, 911–916.

Hearing, S. D. (2004) Refeeding syndrome. *BMJ*, **328**, 908–909.

Heather, N. (1994) Alcohol, accidents, and aggression. *BMJ*, **308**, 1254.

Hein, M. D. & Jackson, I. M. (1990) Review: thyroid function in psychiatric illness. *General Hospital Psychiatry*, **12**, 232–244.

Heiser, J. F. & Gillin, J. C. (1971) The reversal of anticholinergic drug-induced delirium and coma with physostigmine. *American Journal of Psychiatry*, **127**, 1050–1054.

Henkin, R. I., Patten, B. M., Re, P. K., *et al* (1975) A syndrome of acute zinc loss. Cerebellar dysfunction, mental changes, anorexia, and taste and smell dysfunction. *Archives of Neurology*, **32**, 745–751.

Herrström, P. & Högstedt, B. (1993) Clinical studies of oral galvanism: no evidence of toxic mercury exposure but anxiety disorder an important background factor. *Scandinavian Journal of Dental Research*, **101**, 232–237.

Holt, R. I. G. (2004) Diagnosis, epidemiology and pathogenesis of diabetes mellitus: an update for psychiatrists. *British Journal of Psychiatry*, **184**, s55–63.

Hooshmand, H. & Sarhaddi, S. (1975) Hypothyroidism in adults and children. EEG findings. *Clinical Electoencephalography*, **6**, 61–67.

Howells, R. B. (1994) Neuroleptic malignant syndrome. Don't confuse with anticholinergic intoxication. *BMJ*, **308**, 200–201.

Howells, R. B. & Patrick, M. (1989) Delirium tremens. *BMJ*, **298**, 457.

Illowsky, B. P. & Kirch, D. G. (1988) Polydipsia and hyponatraemia in psychiatric patients. *American Journal of Psychiatry*, **145**, 675–683.

Isbell, H., Fraser, H. F., Wickler, A., *et al* (1953) An experimental study of the aetiology of 'rum fits' and delirium tremens. *Quarterly Journal of Studies on Alcohol*, **16**, 1–33.

Jacobs, M. R. (1987) *Addiction Research Foundation's Drugs and Drug Abuse*. Toronto: Alcoholism and Drug Addiction Research Foundation.

Jefferson, J. W. & Marshall, J. R. (1981) *Neuropsychiatric Features of Medical Disorders*. New York: Plenum.

Johnson, A. L., Hollister, L. E. & Berger, P. A. (1981) The anticholinergic intoxication syndrome: diagnosis and treatment. *Journal of Clinical Psychiatry*, **42**, 313–317.

Johnston, A. M. & Eagles, J. M. (1999) Lithium-associated clinical hypothyroidism. Prevalence and risk factors. *British Journal of Psychiatry*, **175**, 336–339.

Kalimo, H., Lundberg, P. O. & Olsson, Y. (1979) Familial subacute necrotizing encephalomyelopathy of the adult form (adult Leigh syndrome). *Annals of Neurology*, **6**, 200–206.

Kaplan, L. M. (1991) Endocrine tumors of the gastrointestinal tract and pancreas. In *Harrison's Principles of Internal Medicine* (12th edn) (eds J. D. Wilson, *et al*), pp. 1386–1393. New York: McGraw-Hill.

Keddie, K. M. G. (1987) Case report: severe depressive illness in the context of hypervitaminosis D. *British Journal of Psychiatry*, **150**, 394–396.

Kelly, W. F., Checkley, S. A., Bender, D. A., *et al* (1983) Cushing's syndrome and depression – a prospective study of 26 patients. *British Journal of Psychiatry*, **142**, 16–19.

Kerr, D. N., Ward, M. K., Ellis, H. A., *et al* (1992) Aluminium intoxication in renal disease. *Ciba Foundation Symposium*, **169**, 123–135.

Kind, H. (1958) Die Psychiatrie der hypophyseninsuffizienz Speziell der simmondsschen Krankeit. *Fortschritte der Neurologie und Psychiatrie*, **26**, 501–563.

Klaassen, C. D. (1990) Nonmetallic environmental toxicants: air pollutants, solvents and vapors, and pesticides. In *Goodman and Gilman's The Pharmacological Basis of Therapeutics* (8th edn) (eds A. G. Gilman, T. W. Rall, A. S. Nies, *et al*), pp. 1615–1639. New York: Pergamon Press.

Knochel, J. P. (1977) The pathophysiology and clinical characteristics of severe hypophosphatemia. *Archives of Internal Medicine*, **137**, 203–219.

Kopelman, M. D. (1987*a*) Amnesia: organic and psychogenic. *British Journal of Psychiatry*, **150**, 428–442.

Kopelman, M. D. (1987*b*) Two types of confabulation. *Journal of Neurology, Neurosurgery & Psychiatry*, **50**, 1482–1487.

Lahey, F. H. (1931) Non-activated (apathetic) type of hyperthyroidism. *New England Journal of Medicine*, **204**, 747–748.

Lancet (1985) Editorial. Hypoglycaemia and the nervous system. *Lancet*, *ii*, 759–760.

Legrain, M. (1892) Alcoholism. In: *A Dictionary of Psychological Medicine* (ed. D. H. Tuke), p. 69. London: Churchill.

Ling, M. H., Perry, P. J. & Tsuang, M. T. (1981) Side effects of corticosteroid therapy. *Archives of General Psychiatry*, **38**, 471–477.

Lingford-Hughes, A. & Nutt, D. (2003) Neurobiology of addiction and implications for treatment. *British Journal of Psychiatry*, **182**, 97–100.

Lipowski, Z. J. (1990) *Delirium: Acute Confusional States* (2nd edn). New York: Oxford University Press.

Lishman, W. A. (1998) *Organic Psychiatry* (3rd edn). Oxford: Blackwell Scientific.

Macalpine, I. & Hunter, R. (1966) The 'insanity' of King George III: a classic case of porphyria. *BMJ*, *i*, 65 – 71

MacHale, S. (2002) Managing depression in physical illness. *Advances in Psychiatric Treatment*, **8**, 297–305.

Major, L. F., Brown, L. & Wilson, W. P. (1973) Carcinoid syndrome and psychiatric symptoms. *Southern Medical Journal*, **66**, 787–789.

Malouf, R. & Brust, J. C. M. (1985) Hypoglycaemia: causes, neurological manifestations, and outcome. *Annals of Neurology*, **17**, 421–430.

Margo, A. (1981) Acromegaly and depression. *British Journal of Psychiatry*, **139**, 467–468.

Marks, V. & Rose, C. F. (1987) *Hypoglycaemia*. New York: Raven Press.

May, P. R. A. & Ebaugh, F. G. (1953) Pathological intoxication, alcoholic hallucinosis, and other reactions to alcohol: a clinical study. *Quarterly Journal of Studies on Alcohol*, **14**, 200–227.

McGarvey, E. L., Clavet, G. J., Mason, W., *et al* (1999) Adolescent inhalant abuse: environments of use. *American Journal of Drug and Alcohol Abuse*, **25**, 731–741.

McLarty, D. G., Ratcliffe, W. A., Ratcliffe, J. G., *et al* (1978) A study of thyroid function in psychiatric in-patients. *British Journal of Psychiatry*, **133**, 211–218.

McQuade, R. & Young, A. H. Y. (2000) Future therapeutic targets in mood disorders: the glucocorticoid receptor. *British Journal of Psychiatry*, **177**, 390–395.

Melicow, M. M. (1977) One hundred cases of pheochromocytoma (107 tumors) at the Columbia–Presbyterian Medical Center, 1926–1976. A clinicopathological analysis. *Cancer*, **40**, 1987–2004.

Mello, N. K. & Mendelson, J. H. (1970) Experimentally induced intoxication in alcoholics: a comparison between programed and spontaneous drinking. *Journal of Pharmacology and Experimental Therapeutics*, **173**, 101–116.

Meredith, T. J., Ruprah, M., Liddle, A., *et al* (1989) Diagnosis and treatment of acute poisoning with volatile substances. *Human Toxicology*, **8**, 277–286.

Minton, N. A. & Murray, V. S. G. (1988) A review of organophosphate poisoning. *Medical Toxicology*, **3**, 350–375.

Missri, J. C. & Alexander, S. (1978) Hyperventilation syndrome, a brief review. *JAMA*, **240**, 2093–2096.

Mitchell, W. & Feldman, F. (1968) Neuropsychiatric aspects of hypokalemia. *Canadian Medical Association Journal*, **98**, 49–51.

Moore, D., House, I. & Dixon, A. (1993) Thallium poisoning. *BMJ*, **306**, 1527–1529.

Morgan-Hughes, J. A. (1986) Mitochondrial diseases. *Trends in Neuroscience*, **9**, 15–19.

Naranjo, C. A. & Sellers, E. M. (1986) Clinical assessment and pharmacotherapy of the alcohol withdrawal syndrome. In *Recent Developments in Alcoholism* (ed. M. Galanter), vol. 4, pp. 265–280. New York: Plenum.

Needleman, H. L. (1998) Childhood lead poisoning. *American Journal of Public Health*, **88**, 1871–1877.

Nelson, M. (1982) Psychological testing at high altitude. *Aviation Space and Environmental Medicine*, **53**, 122–126.

Norfolk, G. & Cartwright, J. (1996) Deaths in police custody are being analysed retrospectively. *BMJ*, **312**, 911.

Norvenius, G., Widerlöv, E. & Lönnerholm, G. (1979) Phenylpropanolamine and mental disturbances. *Lancet*, *ii*, 1367–1368.

Öztunç, S., Guscott, R. G., Soni, J., *et al* (1986) Psychosis resulting in suicide in a patient with primary hyperparathyroidism. *Canadian Journal of Psychiatry*, **31**, 342–343.

Pappas, S. C. & Jones, E. A. (1983) Methods for assessing hepatic encephalopathy. *Seminars in Liver Disease*, **3**, 298–307.

Petersdorf, R. G. (1991) Hypothermia and hyperthermia. In *Harrison's Principles of Internal Medicine* (12th edn) (eds J. D. Wilson, *et al*). New York: McGraw-Hill.

Petersen, P. (1968) Psychiatric disorders in primary hyperparathyroidism. *Journal of Clinical Endocrinology and Metabolism*, **28**, 1491–1495.

Petty, R. K. H., Harding, A. E. & Morgan-Hughes, J. A. (1986) The clinical features of mitochondrial myopathy. *Brain*, **109**, 915–938.

Prasad, A. S. (2003) Zinc deficiency. *BMJ*, **326**, 409–410.

Riggs, A. T., Dysken, M. W., Kim, S. W., *et al* (1991) A review of disorders of water homeostasis in psychiatric patients. *Psychosomatics*, **32**, 133–148.

Robbins, S. L. & Cotran, R. S. (1979) *The Pathologic Basis of Disease* (2nd edn). Philadelphia, PA: W. B. Saunders.

Roberts, A. D. L., Wessely, S., Chalder, T., *et al* (2004) Salivary cortisol response to awakening in chronic fatigue syndrome. *British Journal of Psychiatry*, **184**, 136–141.

Robinson, R. & Stott, R. (1980) *Medical Emergencies, Diagnosis and Management*. London: Heinemann.

Ron, M. A. (1983) The alcoholic brain: CT scan and psychological findings. *Psychological Medicine*, monograph supplement 3.

Ron, M. A. (1986) Volatile substance abuse: a review of possible long-term neurological, intellectual and psychiatric sequelae. *British Journal of Psychiatry*, **148**, 235–246.

Rubin, R. R. & Peyrot, M. (1992) Psychosocial problems and interventions in diabetes. A review of the literature. *Diabetes Care*, **15**, 1640–1657.

Sabot, L. M., Gross, M. M. & Halpert, E. (1968) A study of acute alcoholic psychoses in women. *British Journal of Addiction*, **63**, 29–49.

Sachon, C., Grimaldi, A., Digy, J. P., *et al* (1992) Cognitive function, insulin-dependent diabetes and hypoglycaemia. *Journal of Internal Medicine*, **231**, 471–475.

Salum, I. (1972) Delirium tremens and certain other acute sequels of alcohol abuse. *Acta Psychiatrica Scandinavica*, suppl. 234, 1–145.

Schimke, R. N. (1991) Disorders affecting multiple endocrine systems. In *Harrison's Principles of Internal Medicine* (12th edn) (eds J. D. Wilson, *et al*). New York: McGraw Hill.

Schwartz, J. (1994) Low level lead exposure and children's IQ: a meta analysis and search for a threshold. *Environment Research*, **65**, 42–55.

Service, J. F., Dale, A. J. D., Eleveback, L. R., *et al* (1976) Insulinoma. Clinical and diagnostic features of 60 consecutive cases. *Mayo Clinic Proceedings*, **51**, 417–429.

Starkman, M. N., Schteingart, D. E. & Schork, M. A. (1986) Correlation of bedside cognitive and neuropsychological tests in patients with Cushing's syndrome. *Psychosomatics*, **27**, 508–511.

Sterns, R. H. (1987) Severe symptomatic hyponatremia: treatment and outcome. *Annals of Internal Medicine*, **107**, 656–664.

Stockwell, T., Murphy, D. & Hodgson, R. (1979) The severity of alcohol dependence questionnaire: its use, reliability and validity. *British Journal of Addiction*, **78**, 145–155.

Sullivan, J. T., Sykora, K., Schneiderman, J., *et al* (1989) Assessment of alcohol withdrawal: the revised Clinical Institute Withdrawal Instrument for Alcohol Scale (CIWA-Ar). *British Journal of Addiction*, **84**, 1353–1357.

Sutton, T. (1813) *Tracts on Delirium Tremens, on Peritonitis and on some other Inflammatory Affections*. London: Underwood.

Sweetman, S. C. (2006) *Martindale: The Complete Drug Reference* (34th edn). London: Pharmaceutical Press.

Taylor, D., Paton, C. & Kerwin, R. (2003) In *2003 Prescribing Guidelines*. London: Martin Dunitz.

Thomas, J. E., Rooke, E. D. & Kvale, W. F. (1966) The neurologist's experience with phaeochromocytoma. A review of 100 cases. *JAMA*, **197**, 100–104.

Thomson, A. D., Cook, C. C. H., Touquet, R., *et al* (2002) The Royal College of Physicians report on alcohol: guidelines for managing Wernicke's encephalopathy in the accident and emergency department. *Alcohol and Alcoholism*, **37**, 513–521.

Tonks, C. M. (1964) Mental illness in hypothyroid patients. *British Journal of Psychiatry*, **110**, 706–710.

Victor, M. & Adams, R. D. (1953) The effect of alcohol on the nervous system. In *Metabolic and Toxic Disease of the Nervous System* (eds H. H. Merritt & C. C. Hare). Research Publications of the Association for Research in Metabolic and Nervous Disease, Vol. 32. Baltimore, MD: Williams & Wilkins.

Victor, M. & Hope, J. M. (1958) The phenomenon of auditory hallucinations in chronic alcoholism. A critical evaluation of the status of alcoholic hallucinosis. *Journal of Nervous and Mental Diseases*, **126**, 451–481.

Victor, M., Adams, R. D. & Collins, G. H. (1989) *The Wernicke–Korsakoff syndrome and related neurological disorders due to alcoholism and malnutrition* (2nd edn). Philadelphia: F. A. Davis Company.

Vroom, F. Q. & Greer, M. (1972) Mercury vapour intoxication. *Brain*, **95**, 305–318.

Webb, W. L. & Gehi, M. (1981) Electrolyte and fluid imbalance: neuropsychiatric manifestations. *Psychosomatics*, **22**, 199–203.

Weeks, R. A., Scott, J., Brooks, D. J., *et al* (1996) Grand rounds – Hammersmith Hospital: cerebral Whipple's disease. *BMJ*, **312**, 371–373.

Wells, S. J. (1984) Caffeine: implications of recent research for clinical practice. *American Journal of Orthopsychiatry*, **54**, 375–389.

Westermeyer, J. (1987) The psychiatrist and solvent-inhaler abuse: recognition, assessment, and treatment. *American Journal of Psychiatry*, **144**, 903–907.

Westlake, E. K., Simpson, T. & Kaye, M. (1955) Carbon dioxide narcosis in emphysema. *Quarterly Journal of Medicine*, **24**, 155–173.

Wetterberg, L. & Österberg, E. (1969) Acute intermittent porphyria: a psychometric study of twenty-five patients. *Journal of Psychosomatic Research*, **13**, 91–93.

White, A. J. & Barraclough, B. (1988) Thyroid disease and mental illness: a study of thyroid disease in psychiatric admissions. *Journal of Psychosomatic Research*, **32**, 99–106.

Whitehouse, A. M. & Duncan, J. M. (1987) Ephedrine psychosis revisited. *British Journal of Psychiatry*, **150**, 258–261.

Whybrow, P. C., Prange, A. J. & Treadway, C. R. (1969) Mental changes accompanying thyroid gland dysfunction: a reappraisal using objective measurement. *Archives of General Psychiatry*, **20**, 48–63.

Winkelman, M. D., Banker, B. Q., Victor, M., *et al* (1983) Non-infantile neuronopathic Gaucher's disease: a clinico-pathologic study. *Neurology*, **33**, 994–1008.

World Health Organization (1992) *International Classification of Diseases and Related Health Problems* (ICD-10). Geneva: WHO.

Wyszynski, B., Merriam, A., Medalia, A., *et al* (1989) Choreoacanthocytosis. Report of a case with psychiatric features. *Neuropsychiatry, Neuropathology and Behavioral Neurology*, **2**, 137–144.

Yamaguchi, H., Arita, Y., Hara, Y., *et al* (1992) Anorexia nervosa responding to zinc supplementation: a case report. *Gastroenterology Japan*, **27**, 554–558.

Zola, E. (1876) *L'Assommoir* (trans. L.Tancock, 1970). Harmondsworth: Penguin.

CHAPTER 23

Sleep disorders

Gregory Stores and Irshaad Ebrahim

Throughout history, sleep and its processes have been viewed with some fascination. The scientific investigation of sleep can be traced to a small series of experiments in the 1920s performed by Nathaniel Kleitman, who proved that sleep-deprived individuals were less sleepy and impaired the next morning than in the middle of their sleepless night. The discovery of the electroencephalogram (EEG) by the German psychiatrist Hans Berger and the subsequent delineation of the sleep and wake EEG set the scene for Kleitman's discovery of rapid eye movement (REM) sleep in 1953. Another pioneering psychiatrist, William Dement, working with Kleitman, successfully staged sleep into REM and non-REM (NREM) periods and characterised the hypnogram. In 1972, Christian Guilleminault, a French psychiatrist, helped set up the first sleep disorders centre, at Stanford University, and by 1974 the Stanford team had developed the diagnostic technique called polysomnography (PSG).

Although it is not obvious from the usual content of higher training courses in psychiatry or from psychiatric textbooks, sleep disorders are a central issue in psychiatry.

This chapter is mainly concerned with sleep disorders from the psychiatric perspective. More general and detailed accounts are provided by Kryger *et al* (2005) concerning adults and Stores (2001*a*) regarding children and adolescents. An overview for the general public and patients is given by Stores (2007).

Normal sleep and its stages

The nature of sleep

Sleep may be defined in a variety of ways. Behaviourally, sleep is a reversible state of reduced awareness of and responsiveness to the environment. Usually (but not necessarily) sleep occurs when the person is lying down, quietly, with little movement. Physiologically, sleep has characteristic features that distinguish it from other states of relative inactivity, such as coma.

Within sleep, two physiologically distinct states have been defined: NREM sleep and REM sleep. Both are active processes and not merely a cessation of daytime activity.

Wakefulness is maintained by cortical noradrenaline (norepinephrine), dopamine and acetylcholine from terminals of brain-stem neurons. For sleep to occur, activity in the ascending reticular activating system must diminish. In addition, however, NREM sleep depends on activity especially in the basal forebrain systems, while the pons is primarily responsible for the control of REM sleep. Serotonin and gamma-aminobutyric acid (GABA) neurons, as well as various peptides, are involved in NREM sleep; REM sleep may be described as a cholinergic state, since it is dominated by acetylcholine activity.

The functions of sleep

No one theory accounts for all the complexities of sleep and it seems likely that sleep serves multiple purposes. Whatever else, we may deduce that sleep is restorative, as both physical and psychological impairment follows persistent sleep disturbance. Animals totally deprived of sleep for long periods die, with loss of temperature regulation and multiple system failure. The adverse effects of chronic partial sleep deprivation on mood, behaviour and cognitive function can be substantial.

The emerging discipline of proteomics – the study of the structure and functions of newly identified peptides and proteins – is beginning to shed some light on the basic control of sleep. The discovery of the neuropeptide hypocretin (orexin) and the role it has in sleep and wakefulness provides an exciting avenue for future research in sleep and neuropsychiatric disorders (Ebrahim *et al*, 2002).

Sleep stages

Conventionally, standardised criteria are used to identify different sleep stages according to their characteristic physiological features, especially in the EEG, electro-oculogram (EOG), and electromyogram (EMG); the integrated diagnostic test is called the polysomnogram (PSG).

Sleep is entered through NREM sleep. NREM sleep itself is divided into four stages of increasing depth of sleep:

- *Stage I* occurs at sleep onset or following arousal from another stage of sleep. The EEG is low voltage with mixed frequencies and reduced alpha activity compared with the waking state. Vertex sharp waves are seen in the EEG and slow, rolling eye movements occur. This stage represents 4–5% of the main sleep period.

- *Stage II* contains more slow activity, and sleep spindles and K complexes are seen. It accounts for 45–55% of overnight sleep.
- *Stage III* contains yet more slow EEG activity. It accounts for 4–6% of total sleep time.
- *Stage IV* is characterised by the slowest activity and constitutes 12–15% of sleep.

The combination of stages III and IV is called slow wave sleep (SWS), or delta sleep. This is the deepest form of sleep, from which awakening is particularly difficult. The arousal disorders described later (confusional arousals, sleepwalking and sleep terrors) arise from SWS.

REM sleep is physiologically very different. Brain metabolism is highest during this stage of sleep, which is characterised by a low-voltage, mixed-frequency, non-alpha EEG, and spontaneous rapid eye movements are seen. EMG activity is virtually absent in skeletal musculature; that is, all skeletal muscles lack tone during REM sleep – this is called REM atonia and is an important feature of the symptom of cataplexy in narcolepsy (see below). Heart rate, blood pressure and respiration are all variable, body temperature regulation ceases temporarily and penile or clitoral tumescence occurs. REM sleep usually takes up 20–25 per cent of total sleep time and is most abundant in the last third of the night. As most dreaming occurs in REM sleep, this form of sleep is sometimes called 'dreaming sleep'.

Following sleep deprivation, recovery sleep is initially mainly in the form of NREM sleep, suggesting its importance. On the other hand, the prominence of REM sleep in early development implies its value in cognitive processing and dreaming is viewed in psychodynamic theory as emotionally important. However, loss or reduction of REM sleep in adults does not necessarily have either cognitive or emotional consequences. It is likely that both deep NREM and REM sleep in the first few cycles of overnight sleep ('core sleep') have the greatest restorative value.

Sleep architecture

NREM and REM sleep alternate cyclically throughout the night. The cycle starts with a phase of NREM sleep that lasts about 80 minutes and is followed by about 10 minutes of REM sleep. This 90-minute *sleep cycle* is repeated three to six times each night. Each REM period typically ends with a brief arousal or transition into light NREM sleep. In successive cycles the amount of NREM sleep decreases and the amount of REM sleep increases. SWS is usually confined to the first two sleep cycles. The diagrammatic representation of overnight sleep structure is known as a hypnogram and a simplified version is shown in Fig. 23.1.

This conventional sleep staging is concerned with the macrostructure of sleep, but there is increasing interest in the microstructural 'fragmentation' of sleep by frequent, brief arousals (seen mainly in the EEG) that last a matter of seconds without obvious clinical accompaniments. This subtle type of sleep disruption, overlooked

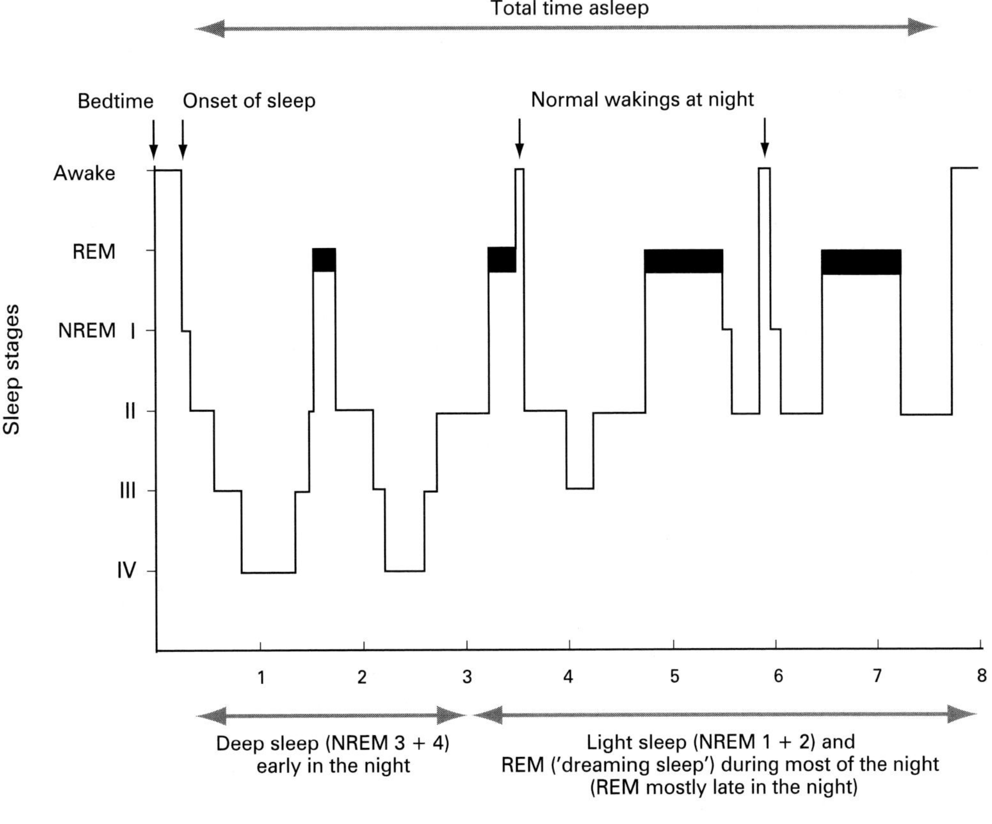

Fig. 23.1 The overnight sleep of a healthy young adult. Adapted with the publisher's permission from Stores (2001*a*) *A Clinical Guide to Sleep Disorders in Children and Adolescents*, Cambridge University Press.

by conventional sleep staging, is increasingly associated with impairment of daytime performance, mood and behaviour, more so than any one stage of sleep.

Circadian sleep–wake rhythms

The timing of sleep (but not its amount) is regulated by a circadian 'clock' in the suprachiasmatic nucleus (SCN) of the hypothalamus. Without an environmental cue to give the time of day (or *zeitgeber*), the duration of the endogenous 'free running' sleep–wake cycle in humans has generally been considered to be about 25 hours, although some doubt has been cast on this recently with the suggestion that the intrinsic circadian pacemaker is close to 24 hour in human adults, consistent with other species. From an early age the individual's sleep–wake rhythm has to synchronise with the 24-hour day–night rhythm. The main *zeitgeber* by which this is achieved ('entrainment') is sunlight, but social cues, such as mealtimes and social activities, are also important.

The SCN also controls other biological rhythms, including body temperature and cortisol production, with which the sleep–wake rhythm is normally synchronised. In contrast, growth hormone in adults is locked to the sleep–wake cycle and is released with the onset of SWS, whatever its timing.

Within each 24-hour period, the level of alertness and tendency to sleep varies. Sleep tendency is greatest is the early hours of the morning and, to a lesser extent, in the early afternoon (the 'post-lunch dip'). Alertness is generally highest in the evening (the 'forbidden zone') before the onset of sleepiness. However, individual differences are seen: some people are very alert early in the day ('larks') and others in the evening perhaps until late ('owls').

Melatonin is related to the light–dark cycle rather than the sleep–wake cycle. It is secreted by the pineal gland during darkness and suppressed by exposure to bright light. It influences circadian rhythms via the SCN pacemaker, which, in turn, regulates melatonin secretion by relaying light information to the pineal gland.

Changes with age

Changes in basic aspects of sleep are prominent from birth to old age, although individual differences are seen at all ages. As with other biological variables, any one sleep measure at a given age will show a relatively normal (bell-shaped) distribution. Changes of clinical significance include the following.

- *Total sleep time* decreases with age. Average daily values are as follows: newborns, 16–18 hours; young children, 10 hours; adolescents, 8 hours or more; adults, 7.5 hours and possibly not less than this in elderly people.
- *NREM sleep* shows an overall decrease across the life span. SWS is particularly prominent in young children who sleep very soundly. Its decline begins in early adolescence and continues throughout adulthood. Deep sleep decreases in the elderly.
- The *proportion of REM sleep* declines from 50% or more of total sleep time in the newborn (more than this in premature babies) to 20–25% by 2 years. This figure remains fairly constant thereafter.
- *NREM–REM sleep cycles* occur at intervals of 50–60 minutes in infants, who often enter REM at the onset of their sleep period. This interval between sleep cycles remains until adolescence, when the periodicity changes to 90–100 minutes, and this interval persists into adult life. The proportions of NREM and REM in each sleep cycle is about equal in early infancy, but gradually NREM sleep (especially SWS) predominates in the earlier cycles and REM sleep in the later cycles.
- *Continuity of sleep* is greatest in early childhood and least at the extremes of age. Although repeated brief waking at night is more common in infancy and early childhood than later, it remains a normal occurrence throughout life and increases in frequency again in old age. The clinical problem arises when there is difficulty returning to sleep after such awakenings.
- *Circadian sleep–wake rhythms* change considerably during the first year. Full-term neonates show 3- to 4-hour sleep–wake cycles. Sleep periods have largely shifted to the night and wakefulness to daytime by 12 months.
- *Napping* is normal very early in life, then gradually diminishes and usually stops by about 3 years of age. However, a physiological tendency to nap early in the afternoon remains throughout life and is made use of in some societies in the form of a siesta. A brief early afternoon nap can be restorative if overnight sleep is restricted but inadvisable when there is difficulty getting to sleep at night.

Classification of sleep disorders

The second edition of the *International Classification of Sleep Disorders* (ICSD-2) (American Academy of Sleep Medicine, 2005) is the standard tool for the diagnosis of sleep disorders in clinical practice. This classification of sleep disorders outlines diagnostic categories, each with specific criteria that can be used for both clinical and research purposes. It describes more than 90 sleep disorders in eight categories and includes, for the first time, sections for paediatric sleep disorders. Box 23.1 shows a summary of the classification.

Box 23.1 Structure of the ICSD-2 classification of sleep disorders

- Insomnia
- Sleep-related breathing disorders
- Hypersomnias of central origin
- Circadian rhythm disorders
- Parasomnias
- Sleep-related movement disorders
- Isolated symptoms, apparently normal variants and unresolved issues
- Other sleep disorders

Source: American Academy of Sleep Medicine (2005).

ICSD-2 contains useful summaries of each of the sleep disorders, including clinical features, possible complications, course, predisposing factors, prevalence, age at onset, sex ratio, familial pattern, polysomnographic and other laboratory features, and differential diagnosis. A glossary of basic terms and concepts is also provided. Overall, ICSD-2 is more comprehensive and informative than the current ICD and DSM systems.

Assessment and diagnosis of sleep disorders

Sleep complaints are divisible into three broad categories:

1. inadequate amount of sleep or not sleeping enough (insomnia or sleeplessness)
2. sleeping too much (excessive daytime sleepiness or hypersomnia)
3. episodes of disturbed behaviour related to sleep (parasomnias).

It is essential to try to identify the exact sleep disorder underlying a sleep problem. Treatments based on symptoms alone may well be ineffective or even make the problem worse. Some sleep disorders may cause more than one type of complaint and a patient may have more than one sleep disorder.

Screening questions

The following basic screening questions should be asked of any person complaining of sleep symptoms and, indeed, of anyone with a physical or psychological disorder:

- Do you have any difficulty getting off to sleep or staying asleep?
- Are you very sleepy during the day?
- Do you have any disturbed episodes at night?

Positive answers call for a detailed sleep history; additionally, the patient's bed partner and/or cohabitee(s) should be interviewed.

Sleep history

Essential elements of a sleep history include:

- the precise nature of the sleep complaint, its onset, development and current patterns
- medical or psychological factors that occurred at the onset of the sleep problem or that might be maintaining it
- the patterns of occurrence of the symptoms – that is, factors making them better or worse, weekdays compared with weekends, or work compared with holiday periods
- effects on mood, work, social life and family members
- past and present treatments for sleep problems and their effects
- past and present medication or other treatments for other illnesses or disorders.

In addition, detailed information is required concerning the following:

- the patient's typical 24-hour sleep–wake schedule
- sleep hygiene (see below).

When enquiring about the patient's typical 24-hour sleep–wake schedule, it is often useful to start with the evening meal, followed by preparation for and timing of bedtime, time and process of getting to sleep, events during the night, time and ease of waking up and getting up, level of alertness, and mental state and behaviour during the day. An attempt should be made to establish the duration, continuity and timing of the patient's overnight sleep, as these are the most important aspects of sleep for daytime functioning. It is also important to identify events of particular diagnostic significance (e.g. loud snoring).

Compilation of a sleep history can be aided by the use of a sleep questionnaire, such as the Pittsburgh Sleep Quality Index for adults (Buysse *et al*, 1989) or the Children's Sleep Habits Questionnaire (Owens *et al*, 2000). Some are general in their scope, while others are directed to particular aspects of sleep, including the effect of excessive sleepiness on daytime function in a number of important real-life situations, such as the Epworth Sleepiness Scale (Johns, 1992).

Other relevant histories

These include the following:

- Medical and psychiatric history should include past and current treatment details, as sleep disturbance is associated with a wide range of illnesses or disorders and their treatments.
- Social history should include occupational, marital and recreational factors (drinking, smoking, drug use) that may affect sleep
- Family history is often positive, for example in sleepwalking and related disorders.

Breathing difficulties and nocturia as well as painful or uncomfortable conditions, may result in sleep disturbance. Severe obstructive sleep apnoea can cause cardiopulmonary and cardiovascular complications.

Physical and mental state examination

Particular attention should be paid to the following:

- evidence of any systemic illness, including cardiorespiratory disease or neurological disorder, such as Parkinson's disease or stroke, that may disturb sleep
- obesity, oral and pharyngeal abnormalities, retrognathia (underdeveloped lower jaw), or mid-face deformity, which may all predispose to obstructive sleep apnoea

- depression or other psychiatric disorder
- intellectual impairment, especially features of dementia or learning disability (including specific syndromes) in view of their associations with sleep disturbance.

Sleep diary

Systematic recording of a sleep diary each day over 2 weeks or more, using a standardised format, avoids the bias or distortion of retrospective generalisations. The diary should record the times of:

- going to bed
- getting to sleep
- awake periods during the night
- final awakening
- getting up.

This will allow estimates to be made of total sleep time, sleep efficiency (proportion of time in bed the patient is actually asleep) and the number of awakenings. The occurrence and nature of night-time episodes of disturbed behaviour can also be determined, and daytime events including sleepiness can be assessed. Previously unrecognised patterns of occurrence of these sleep phenomena may become apparent, including temporal patterns, any shift in the timing of the sleep period, or the relationship to stressful events or other factors.

Investigations

Actigraphy

If the details of sleep physiology are not needed, monitoring of body movements by means of wristwatch like devices ('actigraphs' or 'actometers') may be used at home. These can provide an objective record of sleep–wake patterns and quantify basic sleep variables (Sadeh & Acebo, 2002) (see Fig. 23.2). The most robust indication for the use of actigraphy is in the investigation of sleep–wake rhythm disorders, such as delayed sleep phase disorder (see later).

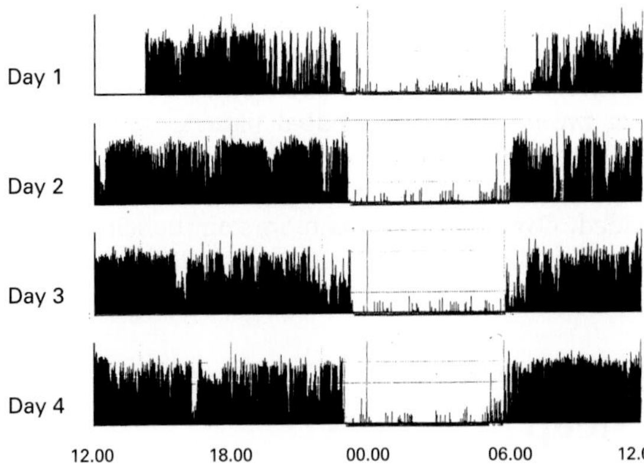

Fig. 23.2 Printout of an actometry recording over 4 days and nights. Awake periods consistently show a high rate of body movements, in contrast to few movements when asleep.

Polysomnography (PSG)

Physiological sleep studies are indicated if preliminary assessment and screening tests, such as actigraphy or oximetry, prove inconclusive. Traditionally this has entailed admission to a sleep laboratory; however, advances in mobile technology now allow for accurate home studies. Home studies are cheaper and also decrease the 'first night effects' (sleep disturbances attributable to the unfamiliar sleeping environment) which are prominent in laboratory recordings and mean that more than one night of PSG is required to allow adaptation to take place.

Basic PSG entails the recording of EEG, EOG and EMG only. This allows sleep to be staged and a 'hypnogram' showing sleep architecture to be compiled (see Fig. 23.2). Usually the recording is made overnight but it may be extended during the day if appropriate. Where indicated, basic recording can be extended to include additional physiological measures, especially the following:

- respiratory variables (and audio-video recordings) for sleep-related breathing problems such as sleep apnoea
- additional EEG channels (combined with video) if nocturnal epilepsy is suspected
- anterior tibialis EMG for the detection of periodic limb movements in sleep (PLMS).

Main indications for PSG are:

- the investigation of excessive daytime sleepiness, including the diagnosis of sleep apnoea or narcolepsy
- the diagnosis of parasomnias where their nature is unclear from the clinical details
- where an objective check is needed on the accuracy of the sleep complaint, or response to treatment.

Other uses of PSG include the distinction between penile erectile dysfunction caused by organic factors (in which the normal erection during REM sleep is impaired) and that caused by psychological factors (in which erection during REM sleep is maintained). However, this distinction is not absolute.

Other investigations

Further special investigations may be appropriate, depending on the nature of the sleep problem and the purpose of the assessment. Examples are:

- human leucocyte antigen (HLA) typing for the investigation of narcolepsy
- toxicology screening where drug problems are suspected
- psychometric assessment or developmental assessment
- the measurement of hypocretin (orexin) in the cerebrospinal fluid (CSF) of patients with suspected narcolepsy, which is an established diagnostic test in certain specialist centres (Mignot, 2002)
- the multiple sleep latency test (MSLT).

The last involves the recording of basic PSG variables and quantification of the degree of daytime sleepiness by measuring the time a person takes to fall asleep during five opportunities to do so during the day. The stage of sleep entered may also be informative, for example the early onset of REM sleep in narcolepsy (which, however, can also occur in several other conditions, as mentioned later). Generally, MSLT is feasible only for patients from about the age of 8 years.

Therapeutic approaches

In clinical practice, a combined biological and psychosocial approach and in-depth knowledge of available therapies are essential to provide benefit to patients. Box 23.2 outlines the range of available treatments, as well as general principles of management.

Sleep hygiene refers to ways of promoting satisfactory sleep in anyone whose sleep is persistently disturbed. Basic principles of good sleep hygiene are considered in more detail later in relation to insomnia.

Explanation and, if appropriate, reassurance form an essential part of any treatment and may be effective in their own right, without the need for more specific measures. An optimistic view should be taken of most sleep disorders. The patient's confidence in the recommended measures, and a willingness to comply fully with treatment, are important determinants of success or failure.

Box 23.2 Examples of treatment approaches for sleep disorders in adults

General principles
- Explain the problem, reassure where appropriate and provide support
- Encourage good sleep hygiene
- Where possible treat any underlying cause of sleep disturbance, whether medical or psychiatric
- Take safety or protective measures (for hazardous parasomnias)

Specific measures
- Psychological (mainly for insomnia)
- Bedtime routine
- Positive associations with bedtime
- Specific behavioural treatments

Chronotherapy (for circadian rhythm sleep disorders)
- Sleep phase retiming
- Light therapy

Medication
- Hypnotics (very selectively and short term)
- Stimulants (for excessive sleepiness)
- Melatonin (for some circadian rhythm disorders)

Physical measures
- Continuous positive airway pressure for obstructive sleep apnoea
- Surgery, especially adenotonsillectomy for obstructive sleep apnoea in children

Sleep and psychiatry

Sleep disorders and clinical psychiatry are intimately related in a number of important respects.

- Sleep disturbance is a common feature of almost all psychiatric conditions.
- Persistently disturbed sleep gives rise to a range of psychological problems in the domains of abilities and performance, mood and general behaviour, and these may compound the difficulties of someone who is already psychiatrically disturbed.
- In some cases a primary sleep disturbance may be the partial cause of a psychiatric disorder.
- Certain psychotropic medications are capable of causing significant sleep disturbance.
- Some primary sleep disorders may be mistaken for primary psychiatric conditions.

Certain implications for psychiatric practice follow from these connections.

- Psychiatrists should be well versed in sleep disorders medicine, whatever the age group of their patients or their psychiatric sub-specialty.
- Liaison psychiatrists need to be familiar with the effects on sleep of physical illness and its treatment.
- Detailed enquiries about sleep should be a basic part of the assessment of any psychiatric patient, to avoid a significant sleep disturbance being missed.
- Conversely, the possibility of a primary psychiatric disorder should always be considered in any patient complaining of sleep problems, and ascertaining the temporal sequence of the sleep and psychiatric disturbance may help make this distinction.

Greater attention to sleep disorders in the population in general, as well as among those with a psychiatric disorder, should be expected to improve quality of life and the ability to cope with other difficulties. Fewer demands would be made on general medical and mental health services (Weissman *et al*, 1997) and the considerable overall economic cost of sleep problems would be reduced (Hossain & Shapiro, 2002).

Effects of sleep disturbance on psychological function

Bonnet (2005), Dinges *et al* (2005) and Ferrara & De Gennaro (2001) have comprehensively reviewed the clinical and experimental evidence that sustained sleep disturbance can have serious adverse psychological effects.

Experimental studies of *total sleep loss* demonstrate a progressive deterioration in cognitive function, mood and behaviour, and this is related to length of sleep loss. However, inter- and also intra-individual differences in susceptibility are seen and task characteristics are also important.

Variations for similar reasons are reported in *partial sleep deprivation* experiments, which are much closer to real-life sleep disturbance, for example as caused by late-night social activities, job demands and other aspects of modern lifestyle. These studies raise the question of how much sleep is needed for optimal daytime functioning and whether this requirement is being met. It has been argued that there is a 'national sleep debt' in the USA and other Western countries and that if people slept longer than they do habitually, their well-being during the day, and performance, might improve.

Experimental evidence suggests that a consistent reduction of the total sleep time by at least an hour compared with the individual's unrestricted sleep period is likely to affect daytime performance and behaviour. Disruption of overnight sleep by repeated interruptions and disturbance of natural sleep–wake rhythms (e.g. in shift-work or jet lag) are also harmful. The effect of chronic sleep restriction to 6 hours per night over a 4-week period has been shown to be equivalent to total sleep deprivation of two night's duration (van Dongen *et al*, 2003).

The usual subjective effects of sleep disturbance are mood changes, especially irritability, depression or even aggression, and complaints of fatigue and poor concentration. More dramatic effects are described with prolonged and severe sleep disturbance, such as disorientation, illusions, hallucinations, persecutory ideas and inappropriate behaviour, with impaired awareness (automatic behaviour) caused by frequent microsleeps.

Psychometric studies have shown that sleep disturbance can produce a range of cognitive impairments, again depending on its duration and individual susceptibility. Sustained attention (vigilance) is particularly vulnerable and creativity (divergent intelligence) may be altered. A meta-analysis of research findings in adults indicated that the mean level of functioning of sleep-deprived individuals is equivalent to that of only the ninth percentile of non-sleep-deprived individuals. From a psychiatric viewpoint, mood was more affected by sleep deprivation than cognitive performance and much more than psychomotor function, which was still significantly worse than in the non-sleep-deprived groups (Pilcher & Huffcutt, 1996).

Although these observations concerning the psychological effects of sleep disturbance have been made on normal adults and patients, it is likely that they will also apply to children and the elderly. Indeed, as reviewed by Fallone *et al* (2002), evidence is accumulating concerning the harmful effects of unsatisfactory sleep on performance by children and adolescents at school. Similarly, among the elderly limited research on the topic suggests that disturbed sleep has adverse effects on mood, behaviour and cognitive function. For this reason, every attempt should be made to improve sleep in the expectation that quality of life will be significantly improved.

Fortunately, it seems that in both adults and children the effects of sleep loss are reversed after much less sleep than that originally lost.

The importance of detection and treatment of sleep disturbance, particularly insomnia, at an early stage was emphasised by Ford & Kamerow (1989), who considered that this could have significant value in the prevention of psychiatric disorder. The early detection of insomnia forms a critical part of schizophrenia relapse prevention programmes (this is further described in Chapter 12). Insomnia was also reported by Breslau *et al* (1996) to be a significant predictor of major depression in young adults. Gillin (1998) suggested that, regardless of whether there was a previous psychiatric history, insomnia and hypersomnia are independent risk factors for the later development or recurrence of depression, anxiety states and substance misuse.

The possible significance of various forms of sleep disturbance in psychiatric disorders is illustrated by a report of a close association between nightmares and suicide in the general population (Tanskanen *et al*, 2001).

The following possibilities suggest that sleep disturbance may be a cause of psychiatric illness, or at least a contributory factor in its development.

- From childhood to old age, people with a history of insomnia are described as having a significantly increased risk of severe depression. A causal link is contained in the suggestion that sleep deprivation late in pregnancy and in labour and childbirth at night may trigger postnatal depression. Abnormal circadian sleep–wake rhythms have been implicated in various depressive disorders, including seasonal affective disorder. Treatment by light therapy is said to correct the abnormality and relieve the depression.
- Changes in REM sleep, especially reduced REM latency, and also a reduction in deep NREM sleep have been closely linked with certain types of severe depression and are thought to be of aetiological significance. However, the meaning of reduced REM latency remains obscure. It is not specific to depressive illness, and also occurs in schizophrenia, borderline personality disorder, eating disorders, post-traumatic stress disorder (PTSD), narcolepsy and the Kleine–Levin syndrome, as well as during recovery from sleep loss. Explanations for this widespread occurrence remain conjectural (Le Bon *et al*, 1997).
- The therapeutic effect of sleep deprivation in some forms of depression is another tantalising hint about the possible causal link between sleep disturbances and depression. Total sleep deprivation can have a mood-elevating effect in major depressive illness but the effect is readily reversible with recovery sleep, including brief naps. It may even trigger manic episodes in patients with bipolar illness. Partial sleep deprivation (i.e. being deprived of sleep, especially in the early morning hours) also has an antidepressant effect. This may be because REM sleep is more affected in the early morning hours, as REM sleep deprivation achieved in other ways can improve depression. Advancing the timing of the overnight sleep phase can enhance the beneficial effect of both total sleep deprivation and also antidepressant medication.
- Disordered REM sleep mechanisms have been said to be fundamental in the development of the symptoms of PTSD, although this view has been contested (Reynolds, 1989). It has even been suggested that some forms of psychosis are a manifestation of brainstem pathology, as indicated by the REM sleep abnormalities (Howland, 1997). Interest has been growing in the possibility that a primary sleep disturbance is responsible for some cases of attention-deficit hyperactivity disorder (ADHD). This claim has been made for both children (Walters *et al*, 2000) and adults (Naseem *et al*, 2001). Various causes of

the sleep disturbance have been held responsible, such as sleep–wake cycle disorders and obstructive sleep apnoea.

- The fatigue element of chronic fatigue syndrome, and possibly other features of the condition, may be exacerbated by the various types of sleep disturbance that are described in these patients. Similarly, the sleep disturbance commonly seen in dementia may worsen the degree of intellectual impairment. Better sleep may improve the patient's general well-being and lessen the burden on carers.

Associations between sleep disorders and psychiatric disorders

It is difficult to identify any psychiatric disorder, acute or chronic, in which sleep is unlikely to be disturbed. Benca (2000) provides a comprehensive coverage regarding adults. Sleep disturbance in children and adolescents with disorders of development (including those with psychiatric disorders) is reviewed by Stores & Wiggs (2001).

Depression

Sleep disturbance (mainly insomnia, but also hypersomnia in many patients) is a recognised clinical feature of depression. Benca (2000) and Brunello *et al* (2000) have reviewed the aetiological, therapeutic and prognostic significance of the fundamental sleep changes in depression, and have highlighted the various areas of uncertainty, in need of research.

People with depression commonly report insomnia, with difficulty in falling asleep, prolonged or frequent awakenings in the night, and early-morning waking, often accompanied by profound depression and sometimes accompanied by vivid and disturbing dreams. A minority report hypersomnia, especially those with bipolar disorders or seasonal affective disorder.

Polysomnography of people with depression shows a wide variety of changes but not all patients show all of them. Sleep disruption is common, with prolonged latency to sleep onset, and there may be increased amounts of wakefulness in the night, with classical early-morning waking. There is reduced total sleep time and reduced sleep efficiency (see page 604). There is also loss of SWS and a decrease in SWS as a percentage of total sleep. Probably the most consistently reported change is the reduced latency to REM sleep onset. An increased proportion of REM in the first third of the night and an increase in the percentage of REM sleep compared with total sleep may occur. Sometimes there is an increase in the total number of REM episodes and REM density (frequency of eye movements during a period of REM) across the night. None of these changes is consistent enough to serve as a diagnostic marker.

Treatment is for the underlying condition, with remedies ranging from cognitive–behavioural therapy (CBT) to medication and electroconvulsive therapy (ECT), although the presence of severe sleep disorder is usually taken as an indication for the use of antidepressant medication. Sedative antidepressants are preferred, such as the tricyclics, as well as trazodone and mirtazapine, while the minority with hypersomnia may benefit from the more stimulating selective serotonin reuptake inhibitors (SSRIs).

Mania

Sleep disorder, usually severe restless insomnia but occasionally hypersomnia, is a key feature of mania. Because of their great distractibility, patients with mania are difficult to study, but Hudson *et al* (1992) compared the sleep architecture in groups of participants with mania or depression and normal control subjects. Although mania and depression present with opposite clinical pictures, their sleep patterns in PSG studies are almost identical. Thus, those with mania in comparison with controls showed disturbed sleep continuity, shortened REM latency, increased REM density and an increase in the proportion of stage I sleep. The only difference between mania and depression in this study was that participants with mania had less total sleep time; otherwise, their sleep architecture was similar.

Schizophrenia

Sleep is commonly impaired in schizophrenia and people with acute psychoses have significant sleep disruption, although not so consistently as in depression and PSG findings are also more variable. PSG findings that have been reported include decreased REM latency and a decreased proportion of SWS. Total sleep time and sleep continuity may also be reduced. A study of neuroleptic-naive patients showed significant reductions in delta wave sleep, particularly in the 1–2 Hz frequency range (Keshavan *et al*, 1998). Deficits in slow-wave sleep (SWS, or delta sleep) have been found to be associated with the more enduring aspects of schizophrenia, such as negative symptoms, ventriculomegaly and impaired frontal lobe metabolism, and because of this Keshavan *et al* (1998) argued the sleep disorder is a primary and integral feature of the illness rather than an epiphenomenon.

At a clinical level, routine enquiry into sleep is very important in the management of schizophrenia because worsening sleep is commonly a predictor of a relapse. Dencker *et al* (1986) followed 23 patients in remission who had ceased their antipsychotic medication, and 81% of these relapsed. One month before their relapse – and before any psychotic symptoms had appeared – there was a statistically significant increase in wake episodes after sleep onset (WASO) (also called middle insomnia). Based on these findings, the onset of disrupted sleep continuity may be a predictor of relapse in schizophrenia. Enquiring about sleep in patients with schizophrenia may therefore enable the clinician to intervene early to prevent or reduce the severity of relapse.

Anxiety and tic disorders

Sleep problems associated with various anxiety disorders have been well documented, although not all of them are widely known, for example sleep-related panic attacks (Shapiro & Sloan, 1998). Obsessive–compulsive disorders are associated with poor sleep quality, and tic disorders, including Tourette's syndrome, with sleeplessness and parasomnias.

Post-traumatic stress disorder

Difficulty in falling asleep and remaining asleep and recurrent distressing nightmares of the traumatic event are all core features of PTSD as defined in DSM–IV (American Psychiatric Association, 1994). There is, in fact, a wide range of sleep disorders that can accompany PTSD, although the emphasis has traditionally been placed only on the nightmares. In the latter, patients are often woken in the night by terrifying re-enactments of the trauma, and as a consequence suffer from broken sleep, which may in turn result in daytime exhaustion, malaise and sleepiness; sometimes the content of the nightmares is unrelated to the traumatic event.

Numerous PSG studies have revealed a much more complex and variable picture, which has been reviewed by Harvey *et al* (2003). Sleep-onset insomnia and sleep-maintenance insomnia both occur in PTSD and it is thought that hyperarousal underlies this. However, studies of waking threshold reveal that this is raised compared with controls, and thus those with PTSD are more difficult to awaken. Some PSG studies have demonstrated that objective records of sleep show better sleep than subjective reports have indicated; thus, it would seem that sleep state misperception is not uncommon in PTSD. Some studies have found an increase in REM sleep but others have not; there are more consistent findings with regard to REM density, which is increased.

Other primary sleep disorders have also been reported in PTSD. For example, among women who have experienced sexual or criminal assault there may be a raised rate of breathing-related sleep disorder, which in some cases PSG studies have shown to be due to obstructive sleep apnoea, and treating this will alleviate the PTSD. The symptoms of PTSD often attenuate with time but specific psychological treatments for the PTSD usually help the sleep disorder (Harvey *et al*, 2003).

Dementia

The consequences for patient care, and for carers themselves, of the severe sleep disruption associated with dementing disorders are very serious and the cost implications high (see later).

Alcohol and substance use disorders

Insomnia and other forms of sleep disturbance are also common in those who misuse alcohol or other substances, or on stopping the misused substance (Roehrs & Roth, 2001). The PSG findings in people who misuse alcohol show that in the first half of the night alcohol decreases the latency to sleep onset, increases SWS and mildly suppresses REM. As alcohol levels diminish in the second half of the night there is a rebound increase in REM sleep. Chronic alcoholics frequently complain of disrupted sleep and show loss of SWS.

During acute alcohol withdrawal there is prolongation of sleep latency, reduction of total sleep time, loss of SWS and an increase in REM and REM sleep density. The first few months of abstinence after alcohol withdrawal are often a critical period and sleep disorder at this time can predict relapse: 60% of those with sleep disorder relapse – usually resorting to self-medication with alcohol – compared with only 30% of those who had good sleep. Treatment of sleep disorder at this juncture is important but not always easy, since benzodiazepine hypnotics are best avoided because of risks of further dependence. Attendance to sleep hygiene principles, continued psychotherapeutic support and the use of a sedative antidepressant may help, but there are no controlled trials in this important area (Benca, 2000).

Child psychiatry and sleep

Many childhood psychiatric disorders, including such diverse disorders as autism, learning disability and ADHD may also be accompanied by sleep disorders (Stores & Wiggs, 2001).

Psychotropic medication as a possible cause of sleep disturbance

In general, sleep can be expected to improve with successful treatment of a psychiatric disorder but sometimes psychotropic medication has unwelcome effects on sleep and wakefulness; the topic is reviewed by Schweitzer (2005).

Antidepressants and antipsychotics

In general, tricyclic antidepressants may be sedating during the day, at least initially. This sedative effect is more pronounced with amitriptyline, trimipramine, imipramine and doxepin. Monoamine oxidase inhibitors may also cause daytime sleepiness but are not usually sedating. Insomnia is consistently reported as a problem in a significant proportion of patients taking SSRIs, and daytime sedation in a similar proportion. Other antidepressants associated with complaints of daytime sedation are trazodone, mirtazapine, maprotiline, amoxapine, venlafaxine and bupropion. Insomnia is also reported in a minority of patients taking the last two of these drugs.

The SSRIs are associated with increased sleep disturbances in some patients. PSG has shown that fluoxetine decreases sleep efficiency. Dorsey *et al* (1996) showed that fluoxetine is associated with significantly more eye movements and arousals during NREM sleep and also an increased frequency of periodic limb movement disorder. Rush *et al* (1998) observed a prolonged latency to REM sleep (i.e. the time from sleep onset to the onset of the first REM period). Their study also demonstrated increased suppression of REM sleep (i.e. a decrease in the total amount of REM sleep), which was greatest with fluoxetine. These changes may therefore explain the sleep disorder associated with the SSRIs.

Sedation is a common side-effect of the traditional antipsychotic drugs, especially chlorpromazine (less so with haloperidol). Clozapine is frequently linked with a high incidence of daytime sedation, much more than is risperidone or olanzapine. Psychotropic medications, especially some antidepressants, have been identified as a reversible cause of REM sleep behaviour disorder (Schenck & Mahowald, 2002). Sleepwalking may be associated with the use of lithium or other psychotropic drugs (e.g. Landry *et al*, 1999), and there are claims that haloperidol and fluvoxamine can cause circadian sleep–wake rhythm disorders (Dagan, 2002).

Box 23.3 Primary sleep disorders at risk of misdiagnosis as primary psychiatric disorders

- Delayed sleep phase syndrome
- Other circadian-rhythm sleep disorders
  - advanced sleep phase syndrome
  - jet lag
  - nightshift work
  - irregular sleep–wake schedule
  - non-24-hour sleep–wake syndrome
- Obstructive sleep apnoea syndrome
- Narcolepsy
- Other causes of pathological sleepiness:
  - idiopathic hypersomnia
  - Kleine–Levin syndrome
- Isolated sleep paralysis
  - REM sleep behaviour disorder
- Other sleep disorders associated with abnormal behaviour
  - hypnagogic/hypnopompic hallucinations
  - hypnic jerks
  - sensory sleep starts
  - restless legs syndrome
  - sleepwalking/sleep terrors
  - overlap parasomnia disorder
  - sleep-related eating disorders
  - nocturnal frontal lobe epilepsy

From Stores (2003*a*).

Benzodiazepines

Benzodiazepines, particularly those with a long half-life (e.g. diazepam, nitrazepam and flurazepam), cause daytime somnolence. A brief period of insomnia is a feature of withdrawal, especially from short-acting benzodiazepines and if withdrawal is abrupt. Vivid and frightening dreams occur because of a REM rebound effect as a result of the pronounced REM-suppressant properties of the benzodiazepines in general.

Because of their potential respiratory depressant effects, benzodiazepines are best avoided in patients with obstructive sleep apnoea (see later) or severe respiratory disorders. The anxiolytic agent buspirone appears to have no adverse effects on sleep and wakefulness. The same seems true of non-benzodiazepine hypnotics such as zopiclone.

Stimulants

Stimulant medication for ADHD is generally considered to cause difficulty getting off to sleep and staying asleep, especially if the last dose is taken later in the day, although in some children bedtime problems are lessened by the improvement in their behaviour produced by a late dose.

Misdiagnosis of sleep disorders as primary psychiatric conditions

Many sleep disorders have been misconstrued as psychological or psychiatric disorders, especially when familiarity with the clinical manifestations of sleep disorders is limited. Box 23.3 gives examples of such sleep disorders, which are described later in this chapter, and below are a few examples:

- The unsatisfactory sleep patterns in circadian rhythm sleep disorders have variously been misinterpreted as awkward 'adolescent' behaviour or some other type of psychological shortcoming. The common pattern in adolescence is one of a delayed sleep–wake phase.
- The psychological problems of people with severely disrupted sleep caused by obstructive sleep apnoea are frequently misconstrued as a primary depressive disorder or dementia.
- Narcolepsy/cataplexy is commonly not recognised for years as a neurological disorder, instead being seen as laziness, attention-seeking behaviour, conversion symptoms or depression. Kleine–Levin syndrome, where periods of excessive sleepiness and various behavioural abnormalities alternate with periods of normality, is often thought to be psychological in nature. Similarly, the complex behaviour enacted during sleepwalking episodes can be misinterpreted as malingering or a dissociative state.

More detailed discussion of these and other examples of concern in psychiatric practice is available in Stores (2003*a*).

Insomnia

Insomnia is the most common sleep-related problem. At any one time it affects about a third of adults, and perhaps as many as 10–15% will have the problem for some months or years. However, only a minority seek medical advice. Insomnia is more common in women and the elderly, as well as in certain occupational groups, notably shift-workers. Sleeplessness is also a problem in a significant proportion of children, especially adolescents. It is also common in people with medical or psychiatric disorders, the majority of whom sleep badly, although this aspect of their difficulties is often overlooked.

Insomnia should not be considered as a condition or diagnosis in itself but rather as a symptom, and its cause needs to be clarified for each individual. The cause is likely to be reflected in the duration of the insomnia. Insomnia can be classified as *transient* (lasting several days to perhaps a week or two), *short-term* (lasting up to several weeks) and *chronic* (lasting more than a few weeks and possibly months or even years).

The term insomnia covers various complaints, occurring singly or in combination, which need to be specified, as their cause (and treatment) may well differ. The complaint may be:

- difficulty falling asleep (defined as taking 30 minutes or more (sleep onset insomnia)
- recurrent waking during the night
- waking early in the morning and not being able to return to sleep.
- feeling unrefreshed after a night's sleep of an apparently adequate duration.

In each case the complaint may well be associated with distress or impaired functioning during the day.

Sometimes an attempt to identify the nature of a person's 'insomnia' reveals that the sleep pattern is within normal limits but that the person is worried because of mistaken expectations of sleep or as part of a generally pessimistic or worried attitude. In some cases sleep studies provide no objective support for the complaint and these patients are said to have 'sleep state misperception'. Causes of this include over-concern about health and well-being. A few people are constitutionally 'short sleepers', needing only 4–5 hours sleep a night to function well.

Transient insomnia

This is the most common type of insomnia and is something many people will experience sooner or later. Common causes include: worrying about a coming interview, a family dispute or some other stressful or upsetting experience, being excited (e.g. about going on holiday), sleeping somewhere new or in a noisy or otherwise unsatisfactory place, being ill for a few days, menstruation-related insomnia, withdrawing from hypnotic drugs, and jet lag (see below).

Because the causes of transient sleep disorder are themselves often temporary, the sleep would be expected to return to normal without any special measures. However, in certain circumstances a more active approach may be justified because even a few nights of poor sleep can cause daytime problems such as feeling unwell and making mistakes; it can even predispose to driving accidents.

If the circumstances causing the sleep disturbance cannot be altered and sleep disorder is almost inevitable, hypnotic medication for (at most) several nights may be justified, partly to help prevent the daytime problems mentioned above but also to avoid a brief sleep problem developing into a long-term difficulty. The prescribed hypnotic should be short-acting to avoid hangover effects during the day (*Drug and Therapeutics Bulletin*, 2004).

As in other types of sleep disturbance, good sleep hygiene is important in minimising the effects of influences that disturb sleep (see Box 23.5 on page 603).

Jet lag

The effects of jet lag are usually short-lived but travellers who frequently cross several time zones on each flight can develop sleep disturbances that have serious effects on mood and performance; these are made worse if alcohol, sedatives or stimulants are used to alleviate symptoms.

The symptoms of jet lag fall into two groups. The first is due to the flying itself and sitting in the confines of a pressurised, often cramped aircraft cabin. These include dry eyes, irritated nasal passages, headache, and sometimes oedema and muscle cramps in the legs. The second group of symptoms is due to the altered timing or the 'lag' component. These include daytime sleepiness, difficulties in falling asleep, disturbed night-time sleep for a few days, gastrointestinal disturbance, poor psychomotor coordination, mood disturbance, decrements in cognitive function and general malaise. The problems arise from the sleep–wake rhythm and other bodily circadian rhythms (e.g. temperature) getting out of step with the 24-hour light–dark cycle because the rapid travel across time zones does not allow the body to adapt. The effect is greater when travelling eastwards.

Various measures can help, especially for long-haul trips, including avoiding becoming sleep deprived before, during and after the journey, and shifting the timing of the sleep period in the appropriate direction before the journey. It is also best to avoid working in the first 24 hours after arrival or making key decisions when the body clock expects you to be asleep.

Short-term insomnia

Difficulty sleeping may last several weeks for such reasons as drawn-out illness, worries about being ill, and bereavement (the effects of which may last months or longer if the grieving process is impeded). Stress reduction and attention to the principles of sleep hygiene are important but there is also a limited place for the short-term use of hypnotics in these circumstances.

In certain psychiatric disorders, but particularly bipolar affective disorder, short-term insomnia may show a fluctuating course as the symptoms of the disorder change. Treatment of the underlying condition (whether mania or depression) is required but the sleep disorder may require special attention, and the affected person should be helped to understand the underlying cause of the sleep problem.

Chronic insomnia

Some 10–15% of adults suffer from insomnia that lasts many months or years. Short-term insomnia can readily become more persistent in the absence of effective treatment. The longer the sleep problem has lasted, the more difficult it is to see how it started, partly because the picture may have become confused by the psychological effects of not sleeping well. The patient's attention may become focused on daytime fatigue or depression, without realising that these are the result of persistently not sleeping well. Sometimes the original cause no longer exists but bad sleep habits may have become established and maintain the problem. In other circumstances, there may be a definite cause that is not easily identified and therefore will continue to be overlooked until specific enquiries are made. Especially (although not only) in the elderly there may be more than one cause of the sleep problem.

Chronic insomnia is associated with:

- psychological and occupational difficulties
- educational problems in young people
- reduced quality of life
- increased risk of depression
- chronic dependence on hypnotic medication and sometimes alcohol as an (ineffective) means of sleeping better
- more frequent use of health services.

The causes of chronic insomnia (listed in Box 23.4) may operate in combination. All of them may result in excessive sleepiness, fatigue or underperformance during the day because of lack of sleep. PSG may demonstrate poor sleep continuity (e.g. increased sleep latency, increased intermittent wakefulness), decreased sleep efficiency, increased stage I sleep, decreased stage

Box 23.4 Causes of chronic insomnia

- Psychological factors
  - Psycho-physiological insomnia
  - Conditioned or learned insomnia
  - Sleep state misperception
- Poor sleep hygiene (see Box 23.5 for advice on sleep hygiene)
- Circadian rhythm sleep disorders
  - Shift work sleep disorder
  - Delayed sleep phase syndrome
  - Advanced sleep phase syndrome
  - Irregular sleep–wake pattern
  - Non-24-hour sleep–wake disorder
- Restless legs syndrome
- Medical conditions and treatments
- Psychiatric disorder
- Other causes
  - Idiopathic insomnia
  - Primary insomnia

II and III sleep, increased muscle tension and increased amounts of activity during sleep.

Psychological factors

Probably the most common reason for persistently not sleeping well is some form of psychological difficulty not severe enough to amount to a psychiatric illness. This includes states of hyperarousal (e.g. from being excessively stressed about everyday problems). Especially in people of an obsessional disposition, things may prey on the mind during the night (the 'racing mind'). Lying in bed worrying or thinking about the day's events at work or at home, or other issues, makes it difficult to relax sufficiently to sleep. Realising that it is difficult to get to sleep, and then worrying about the effect that this will have on next day, raises the level of arousal still further, making the problem worse. Insomnia caused by this state of sleep-preventing tension and arousal and preoccupation with not being able to sleep is called *psychophysiological insomnia*.

Insomnia due originally to a particular cause may persist even after the cause has ceased to operate, because being in bed has become associated with being awake, agitated and distressed rather than being content and relaxed. This is a form of *conditioned* or *learned insomnia*.

Some people have a mistaken idea of how much sleep they need or misinterpret how much sleep they are actually getting. In such cases the complaint of persistent insomnia is unaccompanied by PSG evidence of a sleep disturbance (*sleep state misperception* or *pseudo-insomnia*).

Poor sleep hygiene

This refers to circumstances that can prevent people sleeping well. The psychological factors just described are examples of this but there are other causes (see Box 23.5, page 603).

Mistiming of sleep phase (circadian rhythm sleep disorders)

The period of sleep can sometimes occur at the wrong time and this can cause difficulty getting to sleep and other problems, such as excessive daytime sleepiness. Common causes of mistimed sleep include jet lag and shift-work, which can produce long-standing difficulties.

Many people have to work at night and a relatively large proportion of them will suffer from some degree of *shift-work sleep disorder*. Psychological problems and physical complaints can arise as a result of having to be active at night, when their biological clock dictates that they should be asleep. Mistakes and accidents are common and can be very serious (Akerstedt, 1995).

In their account of accidents attributed to sleep disorders, Walsh *et al* (2005) give an account of two nuclear power disasters, at Chernoby (occurring at 12.30 a.m.) in the Ukraine and Three Mile Island (occurring at 4 a.m.) in the USA, in both of which much of the human error was blamed on the sluggish thinking of the shift-workers (both occurred at the circadian nadir of human alertness and performance).

The daytime sleep to which shift-workers must resort is often impaired in both duration and quality. Family and marital problems can develop from the chronic sleep disturbance itself, plus the restrictions on normal family and social life imposed by the shift-work patterns. Self-treatment with alcohol or other substances worsens the situation. There are various measures that can help minimise these adverse effects of shift-work, including the organisation by employers of shift-work patterns that are least disruptive of circadian sleep–wake patterns.

As a result, for example, of persistently working late, socialising or watching television until the early hours, not going to sleep until late can become a habit. However, this habit might then give way to not being able to go to sleep earlier no matter how much the person may want to do so, because the biological clock controlling sleep and wakefulness becomes reset. This condition is called the *delayed sleep phase syndrome* (DSPS) (Dagan, 2002) and is described below.

The sleep phase can also become displaced in the opposite direction, that is, advanced in time (*advanced sleep phase syndrome*). Sleep begins early and ends early in the morning, by which time sleep needs have been met. This tendency can occur naturally in the elderly and possibly to a mild extent in depression, although it is important not to mistake the early-morning wakening in the advanced sleep phase syndrome with the early-morning wakening of depression.

Exposure to bright light in the evening can help to re-time the sleep period; otherwise, gradually delaying bedtime sometimes helps.

The hormone melatonin has also been used to treat DSPS and other circadian rhythm disorders (Arendt, 2000). As discussed later, in relation to its use as a treatment for insomnia in general, there are uncertainties about its use. In the UK melatonin is available only on a named-patient basis. Exposure to bright light in the morning has some value in promoting overnight sleep and improving its timing.

In the *irregular sleep–wake pattern*, sleep is disorganised: there are variable periods of sleep and wakefulness, and difficulty in sleeping at the right time or for long enough. This can sometimes occur in dementia and other neurological disorders, as well as with drug and alcohol misuse, including the period of recovery.

The sleep–wake cycle of blind people may last longer than the normal period of 24 hours (*non-24-hour sleep–wake disorder*).

Restless legs syndrome

This condition affects 10–15% of adults and also occurs in children, accounting for some cases of 'growing pains'. It consists of creeping, crawling, prickling or otherwise uncomfortable feelings in the legs, especially in the evening or at night, which are relieved by moving them, for example by walking around the bedroom. It can cause severe difficulty in getting to sleep and much distress. It may occur during pregnancy or in people with a physical condition, such as iron deficiency anaemia or rheumatoid arthritis. Usually it is accompanied by *periodic limb movements in sleep*, which, if frequent, are thought by some to impair the restorative value of sleep (see the section below on excessive daytime sleepiness). Drug treatments are available for both these conditions, and include dopaminergic agents and clonazepam (*Drug and Therapeutics Bulletin*, 2003).

Medical conditions and treatments

Brief illnesses can easily disturb sleep as part of feeling generally unwell or being uncomfortable or distressed. Sleep usually returns to normal on recovery. Chronic medical conditions are very likely to disturb sleep for much longer. Even where the duration of sleep seems satisfactory its quality may be impaired by frequent interruptions or subclinical arousals. Dramatic awakenings or apparent parasomnias due to a physical disorder should not be confused with the primary parasomnias (see below) or psychiatric disorder. Those working in the field of liaison psychiatry will need to be familiar with the particular types of sleep disorder associated with specific physical illnesses.

Some medical conditions, such as eczema and certain types of arthritis and malignancy, cause discomfort and pain at night. Cardiac and respiratory disorders (e.g. asthma or emphysema) and duodenal ulcers or other gastrointestinal disorders also often disturb sleep, including the associated problem of being worried about being ill. Nocturia (e.g. from prostatic enlargement or diabetes) is another cause. Further examples are seen in virtually all chronic physical illness.

Culebras (2000) describes the sleep disorders associated with neurological disease, such as neurodegenerative disorders, including Parkinson's disease (in which various sleep disorders are common), cerebrovascular disease, brain injury and neuromuscular disorders. Patients who undergo surgical procedures or spend time on intensive care units are also prone to sleep disruption, which can be severe.

Every effort should be made to treat the sleep disturbance of medically ill patients. Sometimes relieving the underlying medical condition or adjusting the medication may help, but if no improvement in the basic condition is possible, specific treatment for the sleep disturbance should be tried. However, the common practice of routinely prescribing hypnotic drugs to hospital in-patients should be avoided, as this can lead to long-term use and dependence following discharge, as well as other adverse consequences.

Certain drugs used to treat medical conditions are thought to disturb sleep (Schweitzer, 2005). Examples include some treatments for cardiac and respiratory disorders, some antihypertensive medications, corticosteroids and antiparkinsonian drugs. It is worth considering if there was any change in sleep when medication was started or the dose increased. The problem usually takes the form of difficulty sleeping, but other changes are possible, including nightmares or other disturbed behaviour at night (discussed below).

Psychiatric conditions

A basic distinction needs to be made between a psychiatric disorder causing a sleep disturbance and the reverse, that is, where a sleep disturbance precedes and therefore probably partially causes the psychiatric condition.

Other causes of not being able to sleep

The quality and restorative value of sleep is severely disrupted by fragmentation in obstructive sleep apnoea (discussed later), in which repeated awakenings are sometimes associated with a fear of not being able to breathe.

Idiopathic insomnia or *childhood-onset insomnia* refers to a constitutional condition in which there is a lifelong difficulty sleeping that is not attributable to environmental, psychological or medical factors. However, before this diagnosis is made it is important not to assume a constitutional cause for any sleeping difficulty but to enquire about other, more likely – and usually treatable – causes.

The term *primary insomnia* indicates that the insomnia is not caused by medical or psychiatric conditions or other sleep disorders. Psychophysiological insomnia, learned insomnia and sleep-state misperception are subtypes of primary insomnia.

Groups at high risk of insomnia

The predisposition to disturbed sleep of long-distance air travellers and shift-workers has been described above. Higher rates of insomnia are also reported in lower socio-economic groups, including the unemployed, and people who are separated or divorced. Other groups at particular risk for sleep disruption and its psychological and other consequences are described below.

Young children and adolescents

About a third of children between the ages of 1 and 3 years have sleep problems, including waking at night demanding their parents' attention, whose sleep therefore also suffers. Many adolescents have sleep problems of a different type, partly because of their lifestyle and late-night social activities, but also because of biological changes in sleep patterns occurring at puberty which contribute to the DSPS. Misunderstanding the teenager's sleep problems can lead to disputes and upset affecting the sleep of other family members.

See Stores (2001*a*) for a clinical guide to sleep disorders in children and adolescents.

Women

A need for more sleep is common in the first few weeks of pregnancy, after which the problem usually disappears. Difficulty in getting off to sleep or staying asleep becomes more frequent during later stages of the pregnancy as a result of leg cramps, backache or other physical discomfort caused by the enlarging foetus. Anxieties about being pregnant and impending motherhood may also disturb sleep and sometimes produce frightening dreams.

It is important to know whether the sleep problems are new and attributable to being pregnant or whether there was a pre-existing sleep disorder that may have been made worse by the pregnancy. In general, explanation and reassurance that sleep will improve, as well as good sleep hygiene (with the involvement of the partner), are preferable to using medication.

Mothers of newborn babies commonly suffer seriously disrupted sleep through having to feed their baby repeatedly during the night. By the age of about 6 months babies are usually capable of confining feeding to daytime and it is important to avoid prolonging demands for night-time feeds by gradually eliminating this as soon as possible. Establishing a regular sleep pattern aids this process. Mothers often continue to bear the brunt of disturbed nights beyond infancy, into the toddler years. Such disturbance is avoidable, much more than is usually thought, by training the child into good sleep habits from an early stage or using behavioural means to correct undesirable habits if they begin to develop.

Insomnia (as well as hypersomnia) can occur premenstrually and insomnia is often a feature of the menopause, usually in the form of reported nocturnal awakenings caused by the 'hot sweats', and may be accompanied by other menopausal symptoms.

Many women cannot sleep because their bed partner snores or has jerking legs (periodic limb movements). However, especially with increasing rates of obesity, snoring is not confined to males.

The elderly

Changes in sleep patterns associated with later life include less deep sleep, increased night-time waking and fragmentation, less time asleep while in bed, and a shift forward in time of the sleep phase. These changes combine to make complaints about unsatisfactory sleep, daytime sleepiness and fatigue particularly common, especially if there are also medical illnesses or psychological problems. Bereavement, loneliness or financial difficulties may also lead to interrupted sleep. Certain sleep disorders that can impair the quality of sleep, such as obstructive sleep apnoea and periodic limb movements in sleep, appear to occur more often in the elderly. Waking at night to urinate is also a common cause of disrupted sleep at this age.

It should not be assumed that poor sleep is an inevitable part of getting older. As with younger people, an optimistic view should be taken that sleep can be improved with accurate diagnosis of its cause (Shochat *et al*, 2001).

In general, behavioural measures are preferable to medication, which has particular hazards in the elderly. Successful treatment can reduce considerably the demands on carers and may even lessen the need for nursing home placement (Chenier, 1997).

People with a learning disability

Particularly high rates of sleep disturbance (especially sleeplessness but also sleep apnoea, for example) are described in people with a learning disability, somewhat in relation to the cause of the disability and its severity (see Stores & Wiggs, 2001). Improvement in the duration or the quality of their sleep may be one of the few ways of improving psychological well-being when the basic underlying condition cannot be altered. Contrary to the common supposition by both professionals and relatives, success can usually be achieved (even with severe and long-standing sleep problems) if an accurate diagnosis is made of the type of sleep disorder, which may be predominantly behavioural or physical, or a combination of the two, depending on the cause of the learning disability (Wiggs & France, 2000).

People with dementia

Sleep disturbance is acknowledged to be a very serious problem in patients with dementia and a particularly significant additional problem for carers (Bliwise, 2000). Apart from the changes to be expected as part of the ageing process, much more severe disruption of sleep often occurs, including restlessness, wandering, confusion and agitation at night ('sundowning') with very irregular sleep patterns throughout the 24-hour period. Hypersomnia and sleep-related hallucinations can be additional problems.

REM sleep behaviour disorder (see later) is associated with neurodegenerative diseases, including various forms of dementia but especially dementia with Lewy bodies. Additional causes of sleep disturbance include depression and possibly acetylcholinesterase inhibitors.

Treating the sleep problems of people with dementia can be very difficult and depends on the cause. Boeve *et al* (2002) have provided some guidance.

The treatment of insomnia

As with all sleep disorders, a thorough diagnostic assessment and a multi-modal treatment approach emphasising the biological and psychosocial aspects will usually provide relief from symptoms.

Medication

Kupfer & Reynolds (1997) suggest five basic principles for the use of hypnotic medication for chronic insomnia:

- use the lowest effective dose
- use intermittent dosing (2–4 times/week)
- prescribe medication for short-term use only (no more than 3–4 weeks)
- discontinue medication gradually
- be alert for rebound insomnia after discontinuation.

Table 23.1 Speed of onset and elimination half-lives of commonly used hypnotic drugs

Drug name	Speed of onset (min)	Elimination half-life (h)
Benzodiazepene hypnotics		
Loprazolam	30–60	6–12
Lormetazepam	30–60	10–20
Lorazepam	30–60	10–20
Nitrazepam	20–50	15–38
Metabolites of nitrazepam	–	20–200
Z-drugs		
Zopiclone	15–30	3.5–6
Zolpidem	10–30	2.5
Zaleplon	30	1

Data from the *Maudsley Guidelines* (Taylor *et al*, 2003) and *Drug and Therapeutics Bulletin* (2004).

In the UK, the National Institute for Health and Clinical Excellence (NICE) and the Committee on Safety of Medicines have compiled detailed reports on hypnotic prescribing. They recommend short-term use (less than 4 weeks) and emphasise the use of behavioural or other non-pharmacological measures in the treatment of insomnia. Nevertheless, each year there are around 10 million prescriptions for hypnotics in the UK, mostly for benzodiazepine hypnotics (6 million prescriptions) and the remainder for other drugs with similar actions, the so-called 'Z-drugs' – zaleplon, zolpidem and zopiclone – with 80% of the prescriptions being for patients aged over 65 (*Drug and Therapeutics Bulletin*, 2004).

Although the Z-drugs are chemically distinct from the benzodiazepines, the two classes of drug act in a similar way, by binding to specific $GABA_A$ benzodiazepine receptors in the brain and in this way enhance neuronal inhibition by the neurotransmitter GABA. As zaleplon has a particularly rapid action and short half-life, it can be used to promote sleep both at bedtime and on waking during the night.

Different benzodiazepine receptor subtypes are thought to mediate different functional effects. Thus, the α_1 receptor has been linked to sedative, hypnotic and amnesic effects, and the α_2 and α_3 receptors to anxiolytic effects. Benzodiazepines and zoplicone are non-selective agonists at the latter sites, while zolpidem and zaleplon are more selective for the α_1 sub-units, which theoretically should minimise their non-hypnotic effects, but whether this selectivity has any clinical relevance is unclear at present.

The pharmacodynamic characteristics of the various hypnotics (Table 23.1) may have important implications for drug selection. Thus, for patients who have difficulty falling asleep, a drug with a rapid onset of action may be helpful, whereas for those troubled by nocturnal awakenings a drug with a longer elimination half-life may be preferred. Any hypnotic may be associated with daytime hangover effects, although these are less likely with the Z-drugs, which have much shorter elimination half-lives.

Adverse effects of benzodiazepine hypnotics

The main adverse effects of the benzodiazepine hypnotics are as follows:

- *Hangover effects*. These include changes of mood, reduced alertness, poor memory, impaired performance and skills (e.g. those required for driving a vehicle or operating machinery). They occur mainly with compounds of long half-life (e.g. flurazepam) and are worsened by taking alcohol and some psychotropic drugs with a sedative action.
- *Tolerance (i.e. increasing use to produce the same effect) and dependency.*
- *Transient (1 or 2 nights) 'rebound' insomnia* following discontinuation of compounds of shorter half-life (e.g. temazepam), even after brief administration. If possible, temazepam should not be prescribed because it is a controlled drug and was misused in the past.
- *Withdrawal effects* following the development of dependency after long-term use. Withdrawal symptoms include various physical complaints (e.g. tremor, involuntary movements, tinnitus, nausea and vomiting) and psychological disorder, as well as insomnia and disturbing dreams. There is a risk that the insomnia will be confused with the original sleep problem and that medication should therefore be continued. The potential problems on withdrawal (including anxiety and depression) and the careful procedure required for successful withdrawal are discussed by Lader (1994).
- *Paradoxical disinhibition.*

Benzodiazepines also have respiratory depressant effects and are therefore contraindicated in patients with sleep-related breathing problems, including obstructive sleep apnoea. There is also a particular risk of oversedation in older patients, who are then at risk of becoming unsteady and injury from falls. Other groups at particular risk for adverse effects include pregnant women, patients with renal or hepatic insufficiency and people in occupations such as nursing or fire-fighting, who are likely to be required to wake up suddenly, to be alert and do their job.

Adverse effects of non-benzodiazepine hypnotics

Non-benzodiazepine hypnotics (zolpidem, zopiclone and zaleplon) are considered to carry significantly less risk of adverse effects than the benzodiazepines (Wagner & Wagner, 2000). Like the benzodiazepines, Z-drugs occasionally produce paradoxical stimulant effects and adverse psychiatric reactions. Other side-effects include gastrointestinal disturbance (nausea, dyspepsia) and, with zopiclone, a bitter or metallic taste.

When the Z-drugs were introduced, claims were made that they had a lesser tendency for misuse and dependency, but it is now clear that dependency is common with the Z-drugs and there is no information as to whether the tendency differs from the rate with the benzodiazepine hypnotics. For both groups a history of other substance or alcohol misuse is a strong predictor of dependency.

Melatonin

The demonstrated value of melatonin lies mainly in its use for circadian rhythm sleep disorders (Zhdanova, 2000). Although it has a sleep-inducing effect, its use for insomnia in other circumstances is not well supported at present, and there is little information concerning appropriate dosage, time of administration or long-term side-effects and safety, whether in adults (Sack *et al*, 1997) or in children (Stores, 2003*b*). Often the dose used is well above physiological amounts and there are also concerns about the purity and content of commercially available forms.

Role of antidepressants and other classes of drug
Antidepressant drugs with a sedative effect (including amitriptyline, mirtazepene and trazodone) are probably best reserved for those whose insomnia is associated with depression: there is no evidence that these drugs can help insomnia in patients who are not depressed and they have associated risks, such as cardiac side-effects with amitriptyline.

Sedative antihistamines such as promethazine and diphenhydramine, are widely used as over-the-counter remedies, but there is little trial evidence suggesting efficacy, and hangover effects and rebound insomnia are common.

A number of other substances, including valerian, a herbal preparation which may be bought over the counter, have been said to help in some cases of insomnia but there is insufficient information to assess such claims adequately, and it has also (though rarely) been associated with cardiotoxicity and hepatotoxicity.

Self-medication
The use of self-medication with products bought over the counter, usually antihistamines, should be discouraged because there is little evidence that such products are helpful. Even if they do seem to be effective, increasing dosage may be needed to maintain the same effect and they may cause daytime drowsiness and poor concentration.

Alcohol should not be used for difficulty getting to sleep because of the rebound effect, which causes disturbed sleep later in the night.

Similarly, stimulant drugs should not be used to combat sleepiness during the day without medical advice. The cause of the sleepiness should always be sought and treated in its own right.

Sleep hygiene

This refers to ways in which a good sleep pattern can be promoted. The principles of good sleep hygiene apply to anyone but, combined with the appropriate specific treatment, they are particularly useful for those with a sleep disorder. Observing these principles is the best form of self-help, and good sleep hygiene is sometimes sufficient in itself to treat a disorder.

Advice about sleep hygiene is set out in Box 23.5. Each point will not apply to everyone equally.

Behavioural treatments for insomnia

These involve treatment programmes for people with established insomnia, based on the observation that psychological and behavioural factors are often responsible for insomnia becoming long-lasting. Some incorporate the principles of sleep hygiene described in Box 23.5. The effectiveness of these methods is being subjected increasingly to evidence-based review (e.g. Morin *et al*, 1999).

Box 23.5 Principles of sleep hygiene

- People sleep best when they are comfortable, that is, with a suitable mattress and pillows.
- The bedroom should not be too hot or too cold. It should be darkened and also peaceful.
- Disturbance by a sleeping partner should not be overlooked (e.g. snoring, restless sleep or the partner's own inability to sleep soundly for other reasons).
- In general, bed should be a place only for sleeping or sexual activity; the bedroom should not be a place to work or somewhere to be entertained or excited by television.
- Sleeping habits, including bedtime and getting-up time, should be consistent.
- Going to bed when sleepy will maintain the link between being in bed and going to sleep rather than lying there awake and worrying about not being able to sleep.
- It is advisable not have a clock nearby the bed, otherwise the temptation is to keep checking for how long it has not been possible to get to sleep.
- Lying awake thinking through problems or making plans should be avoided by making time to deal with such matters before going to bed.
- If not asleep after about half an hour, it is advisable to get out of bed, move to another room, engage in a quiet or non-stimulating activity and then go back to bed when sleepy.
- Being in bed should not be associated with disputes or difficulties with a sleeping partner or other negative experiences.
- Caffeine (contained in tea, cola drinks and chocolate drinks) and nicotine are stimulants. Many people will have difficulty getting to sleep or will wake during the night if they drink coffee late in the day or close to bedtime. Tobacco has an alerting effect and should be avoided for this and many other reasons.
- Excessive alcohol in the evening can cause rebound insomnia later in the night and hence should be avoided.
- Milky or malt-containing drinks appear to help some people to sleep.
- Napping during the day is best avoided, except for anything more than 20 minutes or so in the early afternoon (corresponding to the physiological 'post-lunch dip' in levels of alertness). Napping longer than this leads to deep sleep, awakening from which can cause prolonged grogginess ('sleep inertia'). Repeated naps and napping late in the day carries the risk of not being able to get off to sleep easily at bedtime, and possibly waking in the night, because of a reduction in the 'sleep drive'.
- It is advisable to maintain a healthy lifestyle – having a good diet, being generally fit and not being overweight.
- Daily exercise is recommended, but not too close to bedtime because of its stimulant effect.
- Regular, consistent exposure to sunlight can help to maintain an appropriate sleep–wake rhythm.
- Another person's hypnotic drugs or other medication should never be used.

A programme of behavioural treatment, including cognitive–behavioural treatment, needs to be designed for each individual, often with the help of a psychologist or someone else with special knowledge of the behavioural approach to insomnia. Like other treatments, it is important to persist with the treatment, especially as the sleep problem can sometimes worsen before improvement occurs. A detailed account, with references to evaluation studies, is provided by Morin *et al* (2001), from which the account below is drawn.

Cognitive therapy

This involves correcting mistaken ideas and negative thoughts about sleep, which can make insomnia worse. Sometimes basic education about sleep requirements can be very therapeutic. For example, many people worry unnecessarily that they are not sleeping long enough because they have unrealistic ideas about how long they should sleep for. Alternatively, they may mistakenly think that their daytime problems are caused entirely by not sleeping as well as they would like to. Anxiety levels, and further difficulty sleeping, are likely to increase if they feel they have no control over their sleep. These unhelpful cognitions can be challenged using a cognitive approach and changed by providing more accurate information about sleep and by replacing negative cognitions with more positive attitudes and beliefs.

Certain concerns are commonly encountered when trying to treat someone with insomnia. For example, if postponing bedtime is advocated as part of a sleep-restriction programme (see below), some patients say that:

- they will miss the most refreshing portion of the night's sleep
- they will be unable to stay awake until the prescribed time
- they will be unable to get out of bed when they are unable to fall asleep.

Other patients worry excessively that their insomnia will lead to a deterioration in their mental and physical health. Such cognitions are often intertwined with a degree of emotional distress and other maladaptive behaviour patterns, each of which may need tackling.

The cognitive therapist needs to elicit all the distorted cognitions concerning sleep and slowly engage in a socratic debate with the patient, assess the evidence and strength of belief, and present alternative information so the patient's irrational beliefs can gradually be changed. Where simple exchange of factual data is not be sufficient to lead to useful changes, full cognitive–behavioural therapy may still be effective.

Stimulus control

Stimulus control is another way in which people's anxieties about sleep when they go to bed can be reduced. Application of the general principles of sleep hygiene is important, but where insomnia has already become a serious problem, it may be necessary to emphasise these aspects of treatment and work on them in a systematic way.

The aim is to re-establish the link between bed and the bedroom and sleep, rather than with feeling frustrated and distressed by not being able to sleep. Bad habits, such as falling asleep while watching television, should be discouraged to strengthen the link between bedroom and sleep.

Sleep restriction

This involves restricting the time spent in bed to the time actually spent sleeping: time spent lying awake in bed should be kept to an absolute minimum. The aim is to increase so-called 'sleep efficiency', that is, the ratio of time asleep to time in bed. If, for example, a person lies in bed for 8 hours but spends the first 2 hours awake, he or she will need to avoid going to bed until 6 hours before he or she has to get up. To begin with, this may be difficult because of the need to be strict about not going to bed until late. This restriction usually means even less sleep is obtained initially than before treatment, because at first there will still be some difficulty getting off to sleep. However, it is important to persist and still to get up at the usual time, and also not to nap during the day, in order to maintain the physiological 'drive' to sleep at night. Soon it should be possible to fall asleep quicker and to sleep soundly, after which point the time in bed can be gradually lengthened until a satisfactory period of overnight sleep is achieved. Morin *et al* (2001) advise patients to go to bed only when they feel sleepy, and to get out of bed if they are unable to sleep within 10–15 minutes and to return to bed only when sleepy. The time of rising in the morning should be regular and relatively fixed.

Relaxation

People who sleep badly are often anxious and tense at night, and possibly also during the day, and so ways of helping them relax may be useful. Muscle relaxation exercises at bedtime, breathing exercises and ways of avoiding a racing mind, or stopping unwelcome thoughts interfering with sleep, may all play a role (Harvey, 2001). Other measures that might be helpful include 'paradoxical intention', where the patient is encouraged to attempt to stay awake. Psychotherapy for anxiety, perhaps with cognitive–behavioural therapy, may also be helpful.

Excessive daytime sleepiness

Excessive daytime sleepiness (EDS) or 'problem' sleepiness implies a tendency to sleep that is greater than that seen in most other people, with the additional connotation that this increased tendency interferes with everyday function, to the person's disadvantage. The condition is thought to affect at least 5% of adults (and possibly many more) and increasing concern is being expressed about its personal, medical, educational, occupational, social and economic consequences (Walsh *et al*, 2005). The corresponding figure for young people is unknown, but as sleepiness is associated with many conditions in children and adolescents the problem cannot be rare at this age. Recognition and help are hampered by sleepiness not being viewed as a medical problem by sufferers or their relatives, and by the symptoms being readily misconstrued as laziness, awkwardness, or lack of interest or motivation; the problem may also be mistaken for depression.

The EDS may take a variety of forms:

- almost continuous sleepiness throughout the day
- the need for frequent (voluntary) daytime naps
- discrete involuntary 'sleep attacks', usually described as an overwhelming urge to sleep and found most frequently in narcolepsy
- periodic episodes of excessive sleepiness followed by periods of normal alertness, as occur in the periodic hypersomnias such as the Kleine–Levin syndrome.

The severity of EDS is judged as:

- *mild* – general slowing up of activities and complaint of tiredness without actually falling asleep
- *moderate* – inability to stay awake in circumstances conducive to sleep, such as watching television
- *severe* – falling asleep when active, for example when eating or talking.

Experimental findings and clinical reports illustrate a range of adverse effects of EDS:

- impaired cognitive function, perhaps especially sustained attention and creativity
- poor school or occupational progress
- increased number of accidents, including road traffic accidents
- associated behaviour disturbance, including irritability, aggression, depression and, in children (in contrast to adults), overactivity
- impaired social relationships, activities and opportunities
- personal and family problems arising from misinterpretation of pathological sleepiness.

The Epworth Sleepiness Scale (Johns, 1992) is often used to measure the degree of sleepiness. It provides a score from 0 to a maximum of 24; a score above 10 indicates excessive sleepiness. The MSLT (described above) provides an objective measure of sleepiness. On MSLT, sleep-onset REM periods are a characteristic finding in narcolepsy.

Sleepiness should be distinguished from a complaint of tiredness in the sense of fatigue, exhaustion or lack of energy, in which there is no prominent increased tendency to sleep; this usually has other causes, such as physical illness or depression.

Occasionally, excessive sleepiness is simulated as a way of avoiding difficult situations. For example, 'pseudo-narcolepsy' has been described (Hicks & Shapiro, 1999).

ICSD-2 describes the various sleep disorders that might underlie EDS. For present purposes, these causes are grouped according to whether sleep is curtailed, impaired in quality or pathologically increased. The conditions that are considered in this approach are listed in Box 23.6. Each requires its own specific treatment approach.

As there are many causes of EDS, a thorough clinical assessment of all aspects of a patient's sleep–wake cycle is necessary when searching for the cause. The following are important pointers:

Box 23.6 Possible causes of excessive sleepiness

Insufficient sleep

- Chronic lack of sleep
- Circadian rhythm sleep disorders
- Irregular sleep–wake pattern
- Delayed sleep phase syndrome
- Non-24-hour sleep–wake syndrome

Disrupted (poor quality) sleep

- Caffeine, alcohol, nicotine excess
- Medical and psychiatric conditions
- Medications
- Illicit drugs (including withdrawal)
- Obstructive sleep apnoea
- Periodic limb movement disorder

Increased tendency to sleep

- Narcolepsy
- Idiopathic central nervous system hypersomnia
- Other neurological disorders
- Kleine–Levin syndrome (intermittent EDS)
- Other causes of intermittent EDS

- Is there evidence of insufficient nocturnal sleep (i.e. reduced sleep quantity)?
- Is the timing of nocturnal sleep time normal and is this consistent every night?
- Is there any evidence of nocturnal sleep disruption (i.e. poor sleep quality)? For example, are there symptoms of sleep apnoea (snoring, interrupted breathing) or of other medical conditions that may disrupt sleep continuity?
- Is there any evidence of a neurological disorder, such as periodic limb movements or epilepsy?
- Is the patient on medication that may disrupt sleep?
- Has the presence of a substance misuse disorder (alcohol, recreational drugs) been excluded (including a urine drug screen)?
- Are there any reports or evidence of behaviours in sleep, such as sleepwalking or sleep terrors?
- Is there a history of daytime sleep attacks, loss of muscle tone associated with emotional arousal, sleep paralysis or hypnagogic hallucinations?
- Are there episodes of periodic (lasting days to weeks) EDS associated with disturbed behaviour, hyperphagia and personality changes?

Driving and excessive daytime sleepiness

Being sleepy while driving can be as dangerous as drinking and driving. Car accidents are likely to be severe because a sleeping driver does not swerve or apply the brakes. Typically in such accidents the sleeping driver runs into the vehicle in front or weaves about the carriageway or drifts off it. Such accidents by drivers of private cars, lorries and goods vehicles (and also those in charge of trains, boats or planes) are more likely to occur in the following circumstances:

- where the driver is short of sleep or prone to disrupted sleep patterns (e.g. shift-workers)
- during the early hours of the morning when the tendency to sleep is greatest (and also to a lesser extent in the early afternoon, at the time of the post-lunch dip)
- after long periods of continuous driving
- where the driving conditions are monotonous (as in motorway driving)
- where the inside of the vehicle is comfortable and warm
- following alcohol consumption or the use of sedative medication or other drugs
- if the driver has a sleep disorder that itself causes excessive sleepiness (e.g. obstructive sleep apnoea).

The most important warning sign is the driver's own awareness of feeling sleepy. It is essential to realise that, especially if the driver feels the need to fight off sleep, falling asleep can occur very rapidly, without further warning. In these circumstances it is essential to stop driving as soon as possible and take a break for at least 30 minutes, during which time at least two cups of caffeinated coffee should be drunk, followed by a nap for about 20 minutes.

Circadian rhythm sleep disorders

Circadian rhythm sleep disorders may cause a combination of insomnia and EDS (Dagan, 2002).

Delayed sleep phase syndrome

In DSPS, the sleep phase becomes delayed, with the result that it is physiologically impossible to go to sleep earlier by choice, in spite of feeling tired and having been awake for a long time. Likewise, getting up and staying awake during the day are difficult because sleep requirements have not been met. Rarely there is a family tendency for the sleep phase to be delayed.

The extent of the delay can be considerable – until the middle of the night or even later. The person's sleep is then sound but obviously not long enough by the time it is necessary to get up for work or other daytime activities. This lack of sleep causes both great difficulty in getting up and daytime sleepiness (feeling groggy or exhausted), especially during the first part of the day, after which the tiredness may wear off.

The characteristic clinical features of DSPS about which specific enquiries should be made are:

- persistently severe difficulty getting to sleep
- uninterrupted sound sleep once asleep
- if awakened before the time dictated by the circadian time-keeping system, the patient may show 'sleep drunkenness' (see below)
- considerable difficulty getting up for school or work
- sleepiness and underfunctioning especially in the morning and afternoon, giving way to alertness in the evening and early hours
- sleeping in very late when able to do so at weekends and holidays (which maintains the sleep phase delay).

Information on these points may be obtained by means of a sleep diary kept over 2–3 weeks. Questions directed at these specific aspects of the sleep–wake pattern should be asked. Actometry over a similar period is a valuable way of describing the sleep schedule objectively, especially if there is doubt about the accuracy of the clinical information or difficulty obtaining it. Polysomnography conducted at the preferred sleep times is essentially normal for age. Other measures of the phase of the endogenous circadian pacemaker in these cases, such as core body temperature, show the same expected delay in the timing of the acrophase (peak time) and the nadir.

Because of physiological changes in sleep timing and requirements, plus altered lifestyle, DSPS is common in adolescence (the prevalance is at least 7%) and can be difficult to correct, but it is important to do so because of its serious effects on everyday living. Methods of treatment include strict sleep hygiene; attention to sleep habits; consistent bedtime and getting up times; exposure to bright light, preferably daylight soon after waking; and, depending on the magnitude of the sleep phase delay, either gradually advancing the timing of the sleep period or gradually moving the sleep phase round the clock, which will need much organisation and commitment on the part of the patient and the family. Melatonin at bedtime at the start of the treatment programme can be helpful. The person must be motivated to make the lifestyle changes involved. Sometimes this is not the case, for example where a young person prefers to sleep late in order to avoid school. The latter is an example of 'motivated sleep phase delay' and here other help may be needed to improve attitudes or emotional state.

Irregular sleep–wake schedule

This can occur at any age as a result of lack of consistency and routine in the way a person lives. This may result from a habitually disorganised way of life, with irregular mealtimes, inconsistent late-night social activities and variable times of going to bed and waking up. In addition, stress and use of recreational and illicit drugs may combine to disrupt basic circadian rhythms. The result may be loss of a clear sleep–wake rhythm, with difficulty in getting off to sleep, staying asleep or confining sleep to night-time. Sleep is likely to be broken into a number of blocks, possibly of different duration, within each 24-hour period. Correction of such a situation can be difficult. Education about the importance of regular sleep, and consistency and moderation in other activities, is important, combined with attention to specific causes such as interpersonal problems, substance misuse or psychiatric disorder.

Non-24-hour sleep–wake syndrome

The non-24-hour sleep–wake syndrome ('entrainment failure') is much less common than the regular type of circadian disorder or DSPS. It is essentially the result of failure to entrain to a 24-hour period, and as a result the sleep phase advances each night. This can result from damage to the brain pacemaker mechanisms controlling sleep and wakefulness, as in children with widespread cerebral damage or maldevelopment (usually associated with severe learning disability), or from localised hypothalamic dysfunction. Alternatively, blindness can be a cause because of the absence of light perception as the main *zeitgeber* for the entrainment of endogenous sleep–wake rhythms.

In these conditions there is a tendency to fall asleep around one hour later each night, and so the main complaint is increasing sleeplessness. There is also a need to sleep progressively later each morning. This causes increasing daytime sleepiness if the affected person has to get up at a set time. The sleep period gradually works its way around the clock, so there is a temporary phase when the person's sleep pattern is normal before the cycle repeats itself. Often the sleep–wake pattern is complicated by the disruptive effects of the psychological consequences of the patient's highly abnormal sleep. Treatment can be difficult. The main aim is to boost environmental cues to entrainment, combined with very regular bedtimes and wake times, as well as firmly fixing the timing of other daily events, including mealtimes and social activities.

Disrupted (poor-quality) sleep

General factors

If a person complains of excessive sleepiness but the total duration is satisfactory, the patient may be experiencing disrupted sleep which has poor restorative quality. In these cases an exogenous cause is most likely and the following disruptive influences should be considered:

- large quantities of caffeine-containing drinks, notably coffee, cola drinks and 'stimulant' drinks
- alcohol or nicotine excess
- medical conditions such as nocturnal asthma, nocturia or epilepsy
- psychiatric states
- medications, including hypnotic and sedative drugs, and particularly their rebound effects, and (possibly) stimulants for ADHD
- illicit drug use, including withdrawal effects.

However, the following common sleep disorders also may be responsible.

Obstructive sleep apnoea (OSA)

Many people snore occasionally without it being of particular significance, apart from being a nuisance to the sleeping partner or others nearby. However, in cases where there is loud and persistent snoring and where breathing is repeatedly interrupted by apnoeic episodes and the person is sleepy or affected in other ways, further investigation is essential. Partners, other family members or friends should encourage the sufferer to seek advice, as the person is often unaware of the condition.

OSA is a common condition affecting people of all ages, including children, and can cause serious problems (Strollo & Davé, 2005). At least 3 in every 100 adults are affected, especially the overweight and women after the menopause. Unfortunately only around 10% of those affected seek medical advice, partly because it is not realised that OSA is the reason for their fatigue, depression or intellectual difficulties during the day. Sometimes they are treated for the physical or psychiatric complications of OSA without the basic condition being recognised (Smith *et al*, 2002).

Muscle hypotonia, neck pressure as a result of obesity or a narrower than normal pharynx cause the upper airway to be obstructed repeatedly during sleep in OSA. The consequent repeated interruptions of breathing each last for up to 10 seconds or more. Each apnoeic episode produces oxygen desaturation and hypercapnia. This stimulates arousal – sometimes with actual awakening – the airway opens and respiration resumes with a large intake of breath, causing a loud snore produced by vibration of the soft palate and adjacent structures. The sufferer may also make gasping or choking sounds, moan or mumble or move about, perhaps violently. Some people wake up at the end of an apnoeic episode in a frightened or confused state perhaps feeling that they are suffocating.

The apnoeic episodes may happen hundreds of times a night, interrupting sleep each time, so that sound, refreshing sleep is impossible. Great difficulty waking up and headache may be experienced. During the day the sufferer is likely to be very sleepy, unable to concentrate or remember things properly, irritable, constantly exhausted, anxious or depressed. Performance at work declines and even dementia may be suspected. Relationships with other members of the family may suffer, and there may be loss of interest in sex; men sometimes become impotent. Overall, the person's quality of life can be seriously impaired. Rates of hypertension, myocardial infarction, heart failure and stroke are raised in patients with OSA.

Sufferers also have increased rates of driving accidents after falling asleep at the wheel. They have more accidents at work because of difficulty sustaining attention.

Investigations for OSA include careful assessment of the sleep problem and the person's general condition as well as extended polysomnography, including respiratory measures. The degree of sleepiness during the day (and other daytime problems) also need to be assessed (often by means of sleepiness scales), partly to evaluate treatment.

Treatment is usually possible and can produce dramatic improvements. Maintaining a patient's upper airway during sleep by means of continuous positive airway pressure (CPAP) is the main treatment for adults. Mandibular advancement appliances can also be helpful. Other important aspects of treatment include: weight reduction in the high proportion of OSA sufferers who are overweight; avoidance of alcohol near bedtime because alcohol depresses breathing and makes apnoeas worse; avoidance of benzodiazepines, which have the same effect; and careful use of any other medication that can impair breathing during sleep. Some people suffer from OSA only when lying on their back and they can be helped by encouraging them to sleep on their side, for example by placing pillows behind their back. Sometimes physical abnormalities that interfere with breathing can be removed surgically; these include nasal polyps and, in children, enlarged tonsils and adenoids. More complicated causes are more difficult to treat; these include the various congenital upper-airway abnormalities in Down syndrome and other causes of obstruction in various neurodevelopmental disorders in which OSA is particularly common (Stores, 2001*c*).

Periodic limb movement disorder

Periodic limb movements in sleep are brief and stereotyped contractions, mainly affecting the legs, detected by anterior tibialis monitoring during polysomnography (Stiasny *et al*, 2002). If frequent and associated with arousals, they have been considered a possible cause of EDS, via disruption of nocturnal sleep. They are also thought to cause ADHD symptoms in some children because the daytime tiredness resulting from sleep disruption can take this form, in contrast to the reduced activity of adults with disturbed sleep. The condition may occur in its own right but often coexists with restless legs syndrome, REM sleep behaviour disorder, OSA and narcolepsy. It is also associated with various metabolic disorders, antidepressant drugs and withdrawal of various other medications. Treatments include dopaminergic medications and clonazepam.

Conditions in which sleep tendency is increased

There are some conditions in which prolonged or otherwise excessive sleep is an intrinsic part of the disorder, rather than a consequence of it. It is important to establish the pattern of occurrence because in some conditions such as narcolepsy the excessive daytime sleepiness is persistent; in others it is intermittent.

Narcolepsy

Narcolepsy is a debilitating lifelong disorder of the central nervous system (CNS) which may follow a variable clinical course (Thorpy, 2001). It was first described by Gelineau in 1880 and is sometimes known as Gelineau's syndrome. Its prevalence has been estimated as 2–5/10 000, with onset in at least a third of cases occurring during childhood or adolescence. It usually begins with excessive daytime sleepiness and sleep attacks during the second and third decades of life. Other symptoms, including cataplexy, sleep paralysis and hypnagogic hallucinations, may follow. These added symptoms reflect the intrusion of REM sleep and its atonic motor component into normally wakeful periods. In time, sleep fragments and variable periods of non-REM and REM sleep may drift around the clock, alternating with periods of wakefulness.

The precise cause is unknown; however, recent human and animal data have provided strong evidence that the pathophysiology of narcolepsy involves the neuropeptide hypocretin (orexin) (Siegel, 1999). Hypocretin-containing neurons are found in the lateral hypothalamus, where they project to various parts of the brain, including nuclei believed to regulate sleep. Disrupting hypocretin neurotransmission, at the level of either the neurotransmitter or the receptor, results in animals exhibiting many of the classic symptoms of narcolepsy. This is supported by the fact that hypocretin is undetectable in cerebrospinal fluid in a large percentage of patients with narcolepsy (Mignot *et al*, 2002). In addition, post-mortem examination of the brains of people who had narcolepsy has revealed an 85–95% decrease in the number of hypocretin-containing cells.

Patients with narcolepsy usually present with complaints that they fall asleep too readily, both in circumstances where drowsiness is expected but also in unusual circumstances. They may occur at work, or even while eating a meal or holding a conversation. Sleep attacks may occur several times a day.

Cataplexy consists of sudden loss of motor tone, commonly following a transient emotional or physical event such as crying, laughing, a surprise or a sudden effort. The patient may even fall to the ground, the jaw may sag and there may be some muscle jerking. In contrast to epileptic attacks the patient is fully conscious throughout and fully aware of the attacks.

Two other common features of the narcoleptic syndrome are hypnagogic hallucinations and sleep paralysis, both of which may also occur in normal people. Hypnagogic hallucinations are frightening, complex, visual hallucinations or dream imagery occurring at the onset of sleep, while hypnopompic hallucinations occur on waking. Sleep paralysis occurs at the onset or offset of sleep; there is a sudden paralysis of all the body muscles, but sparing of the muscles involved in breathing. Patients are fully aware of their paralysed state, which is short-lived, but often they cannot get themselves out of it, although they may do so immediately if touched by another person.

Hypnagogic hallucinations (produced by the dreaming element of REM sleep) and cataplexy and sleep paralysis represent the skeletal muscular paralysis of REM sleep. In addition, overnight sleep is disrupted by frequent awakenings, producing a background of daytime sleepiness (sometimes with automatic behaviour) against which the narcoleptic sleep attacks occur.

The diagnosis of narcolepsy is dependent on maintaining a high index of suspicion, as there is considerable scope for misdiagnosis. Diagnostic errors include symptoms being misinterpreted over long periods as psychiatric symptoms of neurosis, depression or personality disorder (Kryger *et al*, 2002). In addition, cataplexy has been misinterpreted as conversion disorder and a few narcoleptic patients with complex hypnagogic hallucinatory experiences have been diagnosed as having schizophrenia (Douglass *et al*, 1991). Denial, aggression and depression may well result from the frightening experiences and limitations imposed by the condition. It is possible that some cases do not come to medical attention at all (Stores, 2006). The possibility of narcolepsy should be considered, alongside various medical, psychiatric or other primary sleep disorders, in any person (whatever the age) with EDS and psychiatric problems.

There is limited diagnostic value of human leucocyte antigen (HLA) testing (principally for the DQB1*0602 antigen), as it occurs in more than 30% of the normal population. However, a negative result makes the diagnosis of narcolepsy unlikely, since this trait is present in more than 96% of patients with narcolepsy. Physiological sleep studies (overnight PSG) may be helpful to exclude other causes of sleepiness and to demonstrate the classical features of narcolepsy, such as increased stage I sleep, short sleep latencies and often sleep-onset REM period and an increased number of awakenings. The MSLT typically shows a mean REM sleep latency of less than 10 minutes over the five sessions of the test and the occurrence of REM sleep at sleep onset (SOREM) in two or more of the tests is diagnostic of the syndrome. In young patients serial investigations may be required before a diagnosis can be made confidently.

The cornerstone of treatment is medication and advice on optimising alertness and daytime functioning. The drug of choice for treatment of the daytime sleepiness associated with narcolepsy is the wake-promoting agent modafinil, which does not produce dependence. Failure to control the daytime sleepiness may require the use of other stimulant drugs. Choices include methylphenidate, methamphetamine and pemoline. Pemoline has been associated with hepatic failure and as such must be used with caution and regular monitoring of liver function. Antidepressants (tricyclics, SSRIs and venlafaxine) are useful for the treatment, if necessary, of the other manifestations of the syndrome, that is, the sleep paralysis, cataplexy and hypnagogic phenomena. A new drug, gamma-hydroxybutyrate (GHB), is increasingly being used for the management of cataplexy. Regular sleep, adequate sleep routines, planned naps during the day and timing of activities in relation to likely symptoms are important. Explanation of the disorder to all concerned is required, as well as support for what can be a very distressing and limiting condition, often associated with psychological problems.

Idiopathic CNS hypersomnia

Other conditions to consider in the differential diagnosis of narcolepsy include certain other neurological disorders such as postviral and head injury states, and a rare disorder called idiopathic CNS hypersomnia, in which there is chronic, excessive daytime sleepiness unexplained by medical or psychiatric factors and without the characteristic abnormal REM sleep features of narcolepsy.

Sleep drunkenness

Sleep drunkenness refers to a state of considerable difficulty in attaining full alertness for a prolonged period after waking, despite sound overnight sleep. Confused, automatic and inappropriate behaviour and also unsteadiness (simulating drug intoxication) may be evident in this state. Sleep drunkenness is a feature of idiopathic CNS hypersomnia, although it can also be seen in severely sleep-deprived states or other circumstances or conditions that deepen sleep, including those caused by CNS depressant medication.

Intermittent excessive sleepiness

The classic example of this pattern, and one of particular psychiatric interest, is the Kleine–Levin syndrome (Arnulf *et al*, 2005). This apparently rare condition typically begins in adolescent males, often following an infection or some other type of stressful experience or injury. Periods of excessive sleepiness lasting hours to weeks occur at intervals of weeks to months, with return to normality in between. In each episode the patient sleeps for excessively long periods. Overeating (sometimes leading to obesity) and various forms of hypersexual behaviour characterise the waking state during an attack in classical cases, together with various other disturbances (including disorientation and hallucinations) suggestive of a mild organic confusional state. At the end of each episode a short period of depression or elation with sleeplessness may occur. Incomplete forms with only excessive sleepiness have been described. There is a tendency towards spontaneous resolution of the condition, but this may take many years. The condition is easily misconstrued as something other than an illness (Pike & Stores, 1994). Preventive measures seem inconsistent in their effect, but good results with lithium have been reported in some cases.

Other possible causes of intermittent excessive sleepiness are major depressive disorder (25% of sufferers complain of EDS), intermittent substance misuse, some neurological disorders, including status epilepticus, seasonal affective disorder (SAD) and menstruation-related sleep disorders. Excessive daytime sleepiness and other sleep complaints are described occasionally in the Munchhausen syndrome. Occasionally prolonged sleep may be simulated in order to escape from a difficult situation.

Idiopathic recurring stupor (Tinuper *et al*, 1994) may be confused with intermittent excessive sleepiness. In this condition patients have high plasma and CSF levels of an endogenous benzodiazepine-like substance (endozepine-4) and regular episodes of stupor (possibly confused with hypersomnia) with widespread fast activity in their EEG. Episodes are promptly resolved by treatment with flumazenil, a benzodiazepine antagonist.

Parasomnias

'Parasomnia' is the term used for recurrent episodes of disturbed behaviour, experiences or physiological change that occur exclusively or predominantly during sleep. Some involve subtle change, but many are dramatic (Stores, 2001*b*). Many parasomnias can be considered primary sleep disorders (over 20 of which are described in ICSD-2); others are secondary manifestations of various physical and psychiatric disorders. Parasomnias seem to be a particular source of diagnostic imprecision, and their confusion with each other often leads to inappropriate management. Commonly there is uncertainty and undue concern about the possible psychological significance of a parasomnia.

Some of the more common primary parasomnias are listed in Table 23.2 in relation to the stage of sleep with which they are usually associated. This link with the stage of sleep gives the timing of their occurrence some diagnostic value. However, as in any episodic disorder, it is also necessary to obtain, as far as possible, all the subjective and objective details of the onset of the episode and the precise sequence of events until the episode is concluded. A patient may have more than one type of parasomnia, or an associated sleep disorder of a different type.

When relatives have been alarmed by witnessing the patient's night-time episodes, their descriptions may be distorted by an understandable emphasis on the

Table 23.2 Primary parasomnias related to stage of sleep

Stage of sleep	Parasomnias
Presleep period or sleep onset	Sleep 'starts' Hypnagogic imagery Sleep paralysis Rhythmic movement disorder
Light NREM sleep	Bruxism Periodic limb movements
Deep NREM sleep	Arousal disorders (confusional arousals, sleep walking, sleep terrors)
REM sleep	Nightmares REM sleep behaviour disorder
Awakening	Hypnopompic imagery Sleep paralysis
Various stages of sleep	Nocturnal enuresis Sleep-talking Parasomnia overlap disorder Sleep-related eating disorders

more dramatic features. A diary record completed at the time, or the making of a home video, may provide helpful diagnostic information. If the diagnosis remains unclear, home-based or in-patient monitoring, combining audio-video and either EEG or sleep recording, will be required.

Primary parasomnias occurring in the presleep period or at the onset of sleep

Sleep 'starts'

Sleep starts (usually an occasional sudden jerk) are essentially benign but can be alarming, especially if they take a sensory form such as a sudden flash of light or loud bang, crack or snapping noise (for which the term 'exploding head syndrome' has been used).

Hypnagogic hallucinations

Hypnagogic hallucinations (or imagery) may accompany sleep starts but are also common experiences in their own right. The more usual form (unassociated with narcolepsy) can be frightening; it consists of a combination of a dream-like state and altered awareness of the environment in which things may be seen, heard, felt, smelled, tasted or distorted. These experiences, and their counterparts on waking (hypnopompic imagery), very rarely signify physical or psychological disorder.

Rhythmic movement disorder

Rhythmic movement disorder (RMD) refers to recurrent stereotyped movements, mainly of the upper part of the body (Hoban, 2003). These usually occur at sleep onset but can also occur in relation to nocturnal waking and sometimes at the end of the sleep period. Head banging is the best-known form; head rolling and rolling or rocking movements of the body are in the same category. These movements may be accompanied by rhythmic vocalisations. Most children exhibit some form of sleep-related rhythmic movements in their first year, but usually the behaviour stops spontaneously by 3–4 years of age and it only occasionally continues into adult life, when it can be a cause of great embarrassment.

Treatment is not usually needed except perhaps for protective measures such as padding on the cot sides in the case of young children. In this respect, sleep-related RMD contrasts with that occurring repeatedly during the day, which is often a feature of severe developmental delay or other forms of serious psychiatric condition. Various treatments, including behavioural approaches, have been described where intervention is really necessary.

Primary parasomnias occurring mainly in light NREM sleep (stages I and II)

Forceful grinding and clenching of the teeth in a paroxysmal fashion (*bruxism*) usually occurs in light sleep in bursts that last 4–5 seconds but may occur at any stage of sleep. It is thought to be common and to be caused by a number of physical or psychological factors. It may be aggravated by alcohol, although the cause is not always clear. Stress may precipitate or exacerbate the condition. Complications include headache and dental damage in severe cases. Treatment is directed to the cause as far as possible, but in cases where dental damage is occurring a rubber guard should be worn.

Primary parasomnias occurring in deep NREM sleep (stages III and IV) (mainly in the first part of the overnight sleep)

The so-called 'disorders of arousal' (i.e. confusional arousals, sleepwalking and sleep terrors) are common parasomnias in childhood, but in a minority they persist into adult life. The arousal is, in fact, a partial arousal from deep NREM sleep (SWS) to a lighter stage of NREM sleep or REM sleep. A range of behaviours can occur (from simple to complicated) while the patient remains asleep. Some people predisposed to arousal disorders also have such arousals arising from light NREM and REM sleep. Typically, there is only one episode on the night in question, but there can be multiple episodes throughout the night, usually less dramatic each time. Partial arousals can occur during daytime naps.

Predisposing factors are:

- genetic, as there is often a family history
- young age, because this is when SWS is more marked
- sleep loss or irregular sleep–wake patterns, which make full arousal from SWS difficult
- the sleep disrupting effects of stress or trauma.

Precipitating factors include fever, systemic illness, CNS depressant medication, internal or external sleep-interrupting stimuli, and other disorders in which sleep is interrupted, such as OSA. Psychological factors may precipitate and maintain the occurrence of these episodes, and also influence their severity.

Because of the degree of disturbance and the obvious distress, episodes of confusional arousals, agitated sleep-walking and sleep terrors are often the cause of much concern to parents.

However, in most children, no matter how dramatic the behaviour, partial arousals and most other primary parasomnias do not seem to signify a psychological disturbance. Their occurrence can be considered as a temporary, 'developmental' phase, although spontaneous resolution may take several years. Therefore, appropriate management usually consists of explanation, reassurance and perhaps protective measures where a child's safety is at risk.

Psychological or physical problems should be suspected if the parasomnias:

- are frequent
- persist into late childhood, adolescence or adult life
- recur after a period of remission
- start late in development
- follow a traumatic experience
- in the case of nightmares, contain a recurrent, suggestive theme.

Covert trauma such as sexual abuse should be carefully considered if partial arousals (or other sleep disorders with an intense fear element) appear without apparent reason.

Three main forms of arousal disorder have been described. Sleepwalking and sleep terrors are well known; confusional arousals are often less well recognised. All have in common a strange combination of behaviour suggesting the individual is simultaneously awake and asleep, with confusion, disorientation, unresponsiveness to the environment, automatic behaviour and little or no recall of events. In later childhood and subsequent ages (unlike earlier) there is a tendency to wake up at the end of an episode. Adults in particular may recall fragments of events that have occurred during the episode.

- *Confusional arousals* occur mainly in infants and toddlers, and present as agitated and confused behaviour, intense crying, calling out, or thrashing about. The child does not respond when spoken to and more forceful attempts to intervene may be met with resistance and increased agitation. Parents are often alarmed and, feeling the need to console their child, may make vigorous attempts to waken him or her, mostly without success. Episodes usually last 5–15 minutes, but it can be much longer before the child calms down and returns to restful sleep.

- *Sleepwalking episodes*, which last up to 10 minutes or so, are usually less dramatic. Young children may crawl or walk about in the cot; at a later age they may walk around the room or go to other parts of the house, such as the toilet or the parents' bedroom. Urinating in inappropriate places is common. In later childhood, adolescence or adulthood, wandering may extend further within or outside the house, which has an increased risk of accidental injury. Sleepwalking may take an agitated form with a risk of injury from crashing through windows or glass doors, for example.

- *Sleep (night) terrors* tend to occur in older children and adolescents, as well as adults. Classically, parents are awoken by their child's piercing scream, which marks the very sudden onset of the partial arousal. The patient appears to be terrified, with staring eyes, intense sweating and rapid pulse, and may jump out of bed and rush about frantically, as if pursued, in which case injury from running into furniture or windows is a serious risk. The event usually lasts no more than a few minutes at most and ends abruptly. At that point the patient (especially an adult) may wake up and describe a feeling of primitive threat or danger but not the elaborate narrative of a nightmare.

PSG is appropriate only if, in spite of careful clinical evaluation, the distinction cannot be made between partial arousals and other parasomnias, including nocturnal epilepsy and sleep apnoea awakenings.

Explanation with reassurance often reduces parents' anxiety. However, the environment should be made as safe as possible, to minimise the risk of injury. Relatives should refrain from trying to waken or restrain the person during the episode, as this is likely to cause confusion and distress. It is much better to wait until the episode subsides and then calmly to encourage the affected person back to restful sleep. If there is no recall of the episodes, there may be little point in recounting them, especially as this may become a source of anxiety.

General principles of regular and adequate sleep routines are an important part of treatment, with avoidance of sleep loss or disruption. Medication is rarely appropriate and, if used at all (e.g. a benzodiazepine), should be only short term, to cover particularly difficult situations. If the episodes are frequent and consistent in their time of occurrence, 'anticipatory waking' (involving waking the person for a while before the episode is due) can be helpful. If there is evidence of an underlying psychological problem, the usual enquiries and help will be needed.

Primary parasomnias occurring in REM sleep (mainly later in night)

Nightmares

Nightmares (frightening dreams) are the obvious example of a REM-related parasomnia. Unfortunately, the term 'nightmare' is sometimes mistakenly used for any type of recurrent dramatic night-time episode. Occasional true nightmares, occurring later in the night, are common from early childhood and are characterised by awakening with vivid recall of a sequence of events, often with personal involvement. The sufferer may remain frightened after waking and be unable to return to sleep for some time, but reassurance and comforting are usually possible. The dreams may be spontaneous or precipitated by illness and stress. Especially in children, nightmares may coexist with bedtime fears. Abrupt withdrawal from REM-suppressing substances (including most antidepressants, benzodiazepines, methylphenidate and alcohol) can precipitate nightmares. Preventive measures include avoidance of disturbing experiences or DVDs/videos before going to bed. Treatment is that of any identifiable underlying cause, including the use of psychotherapy if appropriate.

REM sleep behaviour disorder

REM sleep behaviour disorder (Schenck & Mahowald, 2002) is of particular psychiatric and medico-legal interest. It is characterised by a pathological preservation of muscle tone in REM sleep which allows dreams to be acted out. If the dreams are violent, the patient punches, kicks, leaps or runs about or displays apparently purposeful behaviour in line with the content of the dream. This often causes self-injury or injury to anyone nearby, especially bed partners, who may be at serious risk of harm.

It was initially thought to be the preserve of elderly males but is now known to occur in both genders and in patients of all ages, including children. However, women come to medical attention less often than men because their attacks are less aggressive. There is a strong association with neurodegenerative disorders, especially Parkinson's disease and Lewy-body dementia, and with narcolepsy. Often, a prodromal period is described, sometimes extending back over many years, with persistent sleep-talking, loud vocalisations, limb twitching or gross limb and body jerking.

An acute form of REM sleep behaviour disorder has been reported in association with the use of or withdrawal from alcohol or antidepressant drugs, and misuse of cocaine, amphetamines and other substances.

Because of its links with organic factors, REM sleep behaviour disorder is increasingly viewed as a secondary parasomnia rather than as a primary sleep disorder. Diagnosis rests on eliciting the typical history and demonstrating on PSG the REM sleep abnormalities associated with the disturbed behaviour. Clonazepam is a very effective treatment, even in the presence of neurological disease.

Primary parasomnias occurring on awakening

Hypnopompic imagery has been described above, under 'Hypnagogic hallucinations'.

Sleep paralysis is another condition mainly associated with waking either in the morning or during the night. In ICSD-2 it is classified as being associated with REM sleep. The brief period of paralysis (which spares eye and respiratory movements) with preservation of consciousness can be very frightening, especially if associated with a feeling of difficulty breathing or inability to speak. Complex hallucinatory phenomena may accompany the paralysis, mimicking a psychotic illness (Stores, 1998). Although sometimes part of the narcolepsy syndrome (when it mainly occurs at sleep onset), sleep paralysis is common as an occasional, isolated experience, even in childhood and adolescence.

Parasomnias inconsistently associated with stage of sleep

Nocturnal enuresis

The common condition of nocturnal enuresis used to be considered an arousal disorder and is still often regarded as the result of particularly deep sleep. Although there is a tendency for bedwetting to occur in the first half of the night, it can occur in any stage of sleep. Voiding of urine at night can also be linked with partial arousals, OSA or nocturnal epilepsy.

Sleep-talking

Sleep-talking occurs in all sleep stages (mainly REM) and, although often spontaneous, it may occur in association with a number of other parasomnias. Usually it has no particular clinical significance.

Parasomnia overlap disorder

Parasomnia overlap disorder has the clinical and PSG features of sleepwalking, sleep terrors and REM sleep behaviour disorder. Some of these patients have a physical or psychiatric disorder, but in others the condition seems to be idiopathic. It is an example of a number of clinical conditions (often involving strange behaviour) which are the result of a mixture of different sleep stages and wakefulness (Mahowald & Schenck, 1992).

Sleep-related eating disorders

Sleep-related eating disorders (Winkelman *et al*, 1999) can be a feature of various underlying sleep disorders such as sleepwalking, OSA and narcolepsy. There may or may not be an association with abnormal eating patterns during the day.

Parasomnias secondary to physical disorder

The parasomnias secondary to physical and psychiatric disorders (Box 23.7) are classified within the ICSD-2 system (see Box 23.1). The main physical disorder to give rise to parasomnias is epilepsy.

There are various types of epilepsy, both generalised and localised, in which the seizures are closely related to the sleep–wake cycle:

- *Nocturnal frontal lobe seizures* (Provini et al, 2000) illustrate this problem well. This not uncommon form of epilepsy is often misdiagnosed because of the complicated motor manifestations (e.g. kicking, hitting, rocking, thrashing and cycling or scissor movements of the legs) and vocalisations (from grunting, coughing,

Box 23.7 Examples of secondary parasomnias

Physical
- Nocturnal epileptic seizures
- REM sleep behaviour disorder secondary to neurological or other physical disease or medication
- Other physical disorders, e.g. respiratory, cardiac, gastrointestinal, neurological

Psychiatric
- PTSD parasomnias
- Nocturnal panic attacks
- Other psychiatric disorders
- Pseudoparasomnias

muttering or moaning to shouting, screaming or roaring) that often characterise the seizures. These dramatic manifestations are often mistakenly interpreted as a non-epileptic basis for the attacks. Diagnosis rests on awareness of this form of epilepsy and recognition of its clinical features. EEG recordings (even during episodes) are of limited diagnostic value.

- *Other forms of sleep-related epilepsy* at risk of misdiagnosis include seizures of temporal lobe origin with prominent affective symptoms, benign partial epilepsy of childhood with centrotemporal (Rolandic) spikes and benign occipital epilepsy (Autret *et al*, 1999).

The distinction between epilepsy and the primary parasomnias should be possible in most cases. This is achieved by careful clinical evaluation combined with the appropriate special investigations, for example sleep studies and long-term EEG monitoring by various means, such as combined video/EEG monitoring or home EEG monitoring. The occurrence of attacks both at night and during the day favours epilepsy. However, the diagnosis may remain difficult because of the variable clinical manifestations and EEG accompaniments of some seizures.

Other parasomnias of (non-epileptic) physical origin include those associated with respiratory disorders such as asthma or OSA, cardiac arrhythmias, gastrointestinal conditions (e.g. gastro-oesophageal reflux), headaches of a migrainous type, nocturnal muscle cramps, restless legs syndrome and periodic limb movements when symptomatic of underlying physical illness.

Parasomnias secondary to psychiatric disorders

The clinical manifestations of some primary psychiatric disorders include episodic disturbances of behaviour or experience related to sleep. These call for psychiatric help rather than attention to the parasomnia alone.

In the first part of this chapter examples were given of the many primary psychiatric disorders (or their treatment) for which sleep disturbance, including parasomnias, is a common feature. Sometimes, as in anxiety states, nightmares are an understandable occurrence. Sleep disturbance is acknowledged to be a prominent feature of PTSD. Emphasis has been placed mainly on nightmares, but other dramatic parasomnias are described in adults, some of which do not seem to fit into conventional categories. In Tourette's syndrome, by contrast, the origin of the reported parasomnias (including sleepwalking) is less obvious.

Nocturnal panic attacks, mentioned previously, may not be recognised as such because of the features they share with other causes of apparently fearful behaviour at night, such as nightmares, night terrors, OSA awakenings and partial seizures. It is diagnostically helpful if panic attacks also occur during the day with other phobic symptoms, but this is not always the case. Data from the few sleep panic attacks that have been recorded suggest they occur more commonly during NREM sleep at the transition to SWS (Benca, 2000).

In what might be termed 'pseudo-parasomnias', dramatic behaviour, sometimes bizarre or violent, is enacted at night but actually while the person is awake, as shown by PSG (Thacker *et al*, 1993; Molaie & Deutsch, 1997). Much care is obviously required to distinguish between a conscious attempt to simulate a sleep disorder and supposed limited awareness of the occurrence of such events and the reasons for them.

Legal aspects of sleep disorders

Sleep disorders medicine may be relevant to legal issues in a number of ways, as antisocial acts may be committed while asleep or in a sleep-related state.

Driving accidents may be caused by falling asleep at the wheel as a result of sleep loss, sleep apnoea or other causes of excessive daytime sleepiness. In such cases the person causing the accident may be considered culpable if he or she is deemed responsible for the circumstances leading to sleepiness, including any failure to take appropriate precautions.

Workplace accidents may also occur as a result of sleepiness during work, and sleepiness is known to have made a contribution to some well-known disasters; Chernobyl and Three Mile Island were alluded to above, to which may be added the *Exxon Valdez*, Bopal and the *Challenger* space shuttle disasters.

The sleep-related act may, though, consist of direct violence to others, or even homicide. The most common sleep disorders associated with such behaviours are those of arousal, including sleepwalking, sleep terrors, sleep drunkenness and REM sleep behaviour disorder. There are also reports of various other primary and secondary parasomnias, and other types of sleep disorder (including OSA and some other causes of hypersomnia), in relation to which violence can occur (Broughton & Shimizu, 1997).

Various sexual offences have been reported to occur during episodes of sleepwalking or other states related to sleep (Fenwick, 1996). Examples of sexual acts performed while the person was asleep but without actual sleepwalking behaviour (for which the term 'sleep sex' has been coined), and sometimes involving sexual abuse of children, have been published (Rosenfeld & Elhajjar, 1998).

Both types of case raise the issue of the complexity of behaviour that is possible during sleep. Courts have varied in their awareness of this and, therefore, their willingness to accept sleep automatism as a defence. The main legal issue in cases of sleep-related violence or sexual misconduct is whether the offence was committed in a state of automatism, that is, without the offender being conscious of his or her actions and therefore not being responsible for them. Fenwick (1996) provides a useful medical definition of an automatism:

> 'An automatism is an involuntary piece of behaviour over which an individual has no control. The behaviour is usually inappropriate to the circumstances, and may be out of character for the individual. It can be complex, co-ordinated and apparently purposeful and directed though lacking in judgment. Afterwards the individual may have no recollection or only a partial and confused memory for his actions. In organic automatisms there must be some disturbance of brain function sufficient to give rise to the above features.'

For a person to be convicted of a crime, the law requires that a criminal act has occurred (*actus rea*) and this must be paired with a culpable mental state (*mens rea*), which means a knowing intent to commit a crime. It is the latter element that must be shown to be lacking when a defence of automatism is used. However, the medical and legal concepts of automatism differ. The medical concept refers to absence of conscious awareness or volitional intent. Legally, two forms of automatism are distinguished:

1 *Sane automatism*. This is considered to result from an external cause and generally leads to acquittal. The external factor could be a blow on the head, for example. The person does not have an illness and without the external trigger nothing would have occurred.

2 Insane automatism. This is due to an intrinsic or endogenous cause (e.g. a disease of the mind) and generally leads to commitment to a psychiatric hospital.

The sleep disorder automatisms generally fall into the second category.

Until recently, the verdict of guilty due to insane automatism meant a committal to a psychiatric hospital, but the Criminal Procedure (Insanity and Unfitness to Plead) Act 1991 permitted a much wider set of disposals, ranging from hospital orders to a supervision disorder or even an absolute discharge.

The medico-legal aspects of sleep disorders medicine have been discussed by Mahowald & Schenck (1999). The same authors have suggested guidelines, including the following, to help determine the likelihood that an illegal act is attributable to a sleep disorder (especially sleepwalking):

- There is convincing evidence of a history of sleepwalking or a related sleep disorder, and similar episodes with a benign outcome have occurred in the past.
- The act was without premeditation, was motiveless and was out of character.
- The duration of the act was only a few minutes.
- The victim merely happened to be present.
- There is lack of awareness during the event and at least some degree of amnesia for it afterwards.
- The offender feels remorse after return to consciousness and makes no attempt to conceal the action.
- There is potentiation of the sleep-related act, for example by alcohol, medication or sleep deprivation.

References

Akerstedt, T. (1995) Work hours, sleepiness and accidents. *Journal of Sleep Research*, **4**, suppl. 2, 1–3.

American Academy of Sleep Medicine (2005) *International Classification of Sleep Disorders: Diagnostic and Coding Manual* (2nd edn) (ICSD-2). Rochester, MN: American Sleep Disorders Association.

American Psychiatric Association (1994) *Diagnostic and Statistical Manual of Mental Disorders* (4th edn) (DSM–IV). Washington, DC: APA.

Arendt, J. (2000) In what circumstances is melatonin a useful sleep therapy? Consensus Statement, WFSRS Focus Group, Dresden November 1999. *Journal of Sleep Research*, **9**, 397–398.

Arnulf, I., Zeitzer, J. M., File, J., *et al* (2005) Kleine–Levin syndrome: a systematic review of 186 cases in the literature. *Brain*, **128**, 2763–2776.

Autret, A., de Toffo, I. B., Corcia, Ph., *et al* (1999) Sleep and epilepsy. *Sleep Medicine Reviews*, **3**, 201–217.

Benca, R. M. (2000) Psychiatric sleep–wake disorders. In *New Oxford Textbook of Psychiatry* (eds M. G. Gelder, J. J. López-Ibor & N. C. Andreasen), vol. 1, pp. 1021–1026. Oxford: Oxford University Press.

Bliwise, D. L. (2000) Sleep and nocturnal delirium in the dementias. In *Sleep Disorders and Neurological Disease* (ed. A. Culebras), pp. 257–274. New York: Marcel Dekker.

Boeve, B. F., Silber, M. H. & Ferman, T. J. (2002) Current management of sleep disturbances in dementia. *Current Neurology and Neuroscience Reports*, **2**, 169–177.

Bonnet, M. H. (2005) Acute sleep deprivation. In *Principles and Practice of Sleep Medicine* (4th edn) (eds M. H. Kryger, T. Roth & W. C. Dement), pp. 51–66. Philadelphia, PA: Elsevier Saunders.

Breslau, N., Roth, T., Rosenthal, L., *et al* (1996) Sleep disturbance and psychiatric disorders: a longitudinal and epidemiological study of young adults. *Biological Psychiatry*, **39**, 411–418.

Broughton, R. J. & Shimizu, T. (1997) Dangerous behaviour at night. In *Forensic Aspects of Sleep* (eds C. Shapiro & A. McColl Smith), pp. 65–83. Chichester: Wiley.

Brunello, N., Armitage, R., Feinberg, I., *et al* (2000) Depression and sleep disorders: clinical relevance, economic burden and pharmacological treatment. *Biological Psychiatry*, **42**, 107–119.

Buysse, D. J., Reynolds, C. F., Monk, T. H., *et al* (1989) The Pittsburgh Sleep Quality Index: a new instrument for psychiatric practice and research. *Psychiatry Research*, **28**, 193–213.

Chenier, M. C. (1997) Review and analysis of caregiver burden and nursing home placement. *Geriatric Nursing*, **18**, 121–126.

Culebras, A. (ed.) (2000) *Sleep Disorders and Neurological Disease*. New York: Marcel Dekker.

Dagan, Y. (2002) Circadian rhythm sleep disorder (CRSD). *Sleep Medicine Reviews*, **6**, 45–55.

Dencker, S. J., Malm, U. & Lepp M. (1986) Schizophrenia relapse after drug withdrawal is predictable. *Acta Psychiatrica Scandinavica*, **73**, 181–185.

Dinges, D. F., Rogers, N. L. & Baynard, M. D. (2005) Chronic sleep deprivation. In *Principles and Practice of Sleep Medicine* (4th edn) (eds M. H. Kryger, T. Roth & W. C. Dement), pp. 67–76. Philadelphia, PA: Elsevier Saunders.

Dorsey, C. M., Lukas, S. & Cunningham, S. L. (1996) Fluoxetine induced sleep disturbance in depressed patients. *Neuropsychopharmacology*, **14**, 437–442.

Douglass, A. B., Hays, P., Pazderka, F., *et al* (1991) Florid refractory schizophrenias that turn out to be treatable variants of HLA-associated narcolepsy. *Journal of Nervous and Mental Disease*, **179**, 12–17.

Drug and Therapeutics Bulletin (2003) Managing patients with restless legs. *Drug and Therapeutics Bulletin*, **41** (11), 81–83.

Drug and Therapeutics Bulletin (2004) What's wrong with prescribing hypnotics? *Drug and Therapeutics Bulletin*, **42** (12), 89–93.

Ebrahim, I. O., Howard, R. S., Kopelman, M. D., *et al* (2002) The hypocretin/orexin system. *Journal of the Royal Society of Medicine*, **95**, 227–230.

Fallone, G., Owens, J. A. & Deane, J. (2002) Sleepiness in children and adolescents: clinical implications. *Sleep Medicine Reviews*, **6**, 287–306.

Fenwick, P. (1996) Sleep and sexual offending. *Medicine, Science and the Law*, **36**, 122–134.

Ferrara, M. & De Gennaro, L. (2001) How much sleep do we need? *Sleep Medicine Reviews*, **5**, 155–170.

Ford, D. E. & Kamerow, D. B. (1989) Epidemiologic study of sleep disturbances and psychiatric disorders. An opportunity for prevention? *JAMA*, **262**, 1479–1484.

Gillin, J. C. (1998) Are sleep disturbances risk factors for anxiety, depression and addictive disorders. *Acta Psychiatrica Scandinavica Supplementum*, **393**, 39–43.

Harvey, A. G. (2001) I can't sleep, my mind is racing! An investigation of strategies of thought control in insomnia. *Behavioural and Cognitive Psychotherapy*, **29**, 3–11.

Harvey, A. G., Jones, C. & Schmidt, D. A. (2003) Sleep and post-traumatic stress disorder: a review. *Clinical Psychology Review*, **23**, 377–407.

Hicks, J. A. & Shapiro, C. M. (1999) Pseudo-narcolepsy: a case report. *Journal of Psychiatry and Neuroscience*, **24**, 348–350.

Hoban, T. F. (2003) Rhythmic movement disorder in children. *CNS Spectrums*, **8**, 135–138.

Hossain, J. L. & Shapiro, C. M. (2002) The prevalence, cost implications, and management of sleep disorders: an overview. *Sleep and Breathing*, **6**, 85–102.

Howland, R. H. (1997) Sleep-onset rapid eye movement periods in neuropsychiatric disorders: implications for the pathophysiology of psychosis. *Journal of Nervous and Mental Disease*, **185**, 730–738.

Hudson, J. I., Kipinski, J. F., Keck, P. E., *et al* (1992) Polysomnographic characteristics of young manic patients. *Archives of General Psychiatry*, **49**, 378–380.

Johns, M. W. (1992) Reliability and factor analysis of the Epworth Sleepiness Scale. *Sleep*, **15**, 376–381.

Keshavan, M. S., Reynolds, III, C. F., Miewald, J. M., *et al* (1998) Delta sleep deficits in schizophrenia: evidence from automated analyses of sleep data. *Archives of General Psychiatry*, **55**, 443–448.

Kryger, M. H., Walld, R. & Manfreda, J. (2002) Diagnoses received by narcolepsy patients in the year prior to diagnosis by a sleep specialist. *Sleep*, **25**, 36–41.

Kryger, M. H., Roth, T. & Dement, W. C. (eds) (2005) *Principles and Practice of Sleep Medicine* (4th edn). Philadelphia, PA: Elsevier Saunders.

Kupfer, D. J. & Reynolds, C. F. (1997) Management of insomnia. *New England Journal of Medicine*, **336**, 341–346.

Lader, M. (1994) Anxiety or depression during withdrawal of hypnotic treatments. *Journal of Psychosomatic Research*, **38**, suppl. 1, 113–123.

Landry, P., Warnes, H., Nielsen, T., *et al* (1999) Somnambulistic-like behaviour in patients attending a lithium clinic. *International Clinical Psychopharmacology*, **14**, 173–175,

Le Bon, O., Staner, L., Murphy, J. R., *et al* (1997) Critical analysis of the theories advanced to explain short REM latencies and other sleep anomalies in several psychiatric conditions. *Journal of Psychiatric Research*, **31**, 433–450.

Mahowald, M. W. & Schenck, C. H. (1992) Dissociated states of wakefulness and sleep. *Neurology*, **42**, suppl. 6, 44–52.

Mahowald, M. W. & Schenck, C. H. (1999) Medico-legal aspects of sleep medicine. *Neurologic Clinics*, **17**, 215–234.

Mignot, E., Lammers, G. J., Ripley, B., *et al.* (2002) The role of cerebrospinal fluid hypocretin measurement in the diagnosis of narcolepsy and other hypersomnias. *Archives of Neurology*, **59**, 1553–1562.

Molaie, M. & Deutsch, G. K. (1997) Dangerous events presenting as parasomnia. *Sleep*, **20**, 402–405.

Morin, C. M., Hauri, P. J., Espie, C. A., *et al* (1999) Non pharmacologic treatment of chronic insomnia. An American Academy of Sleep Medicine review. *Sleep*, **22**, 1134–1156.

Morin, C. M., Daley, M. & Ouellet, M.-C. (2001) Insomnia in adults. *Current Treatment Options in Neurology*, **3**, 9–18.

Naseem, S., Chaudhary, B. & Collop, N. (2001) Attention deficit hyperactivity disorder in adults and obstructive sleep apnea. *Chest*, **119**, 294–296.

Owens, J. A., Spirito, A. & McQuinn, M. (2000) The Children's Sleep Habits Questionnaire (CSHQ). Psychometric properties of a survey instrument for school-aged children. *Sleep*, **23**, 1043–1051.

Pike, M. & Stores, G. (1994) Kleine–Levin syndrome: a cause of diagnostic confusion. *Archives of Disease in Childhood*, **71**, 355–357.

Pilcher, J. J. & Huffcutt, A. I. (1996) Effects of sleep deprivation on performance: a meta-analysis. *Sleep*, **19**, 318–326.

Provini, F., Plazzi, G., Montagna, P., *et al* (2000) The wide clinical spectrum of nocturnal frontal lobe epilepsy. *Sleep Medicine Reviews*, **4**, 375–386.

Reynolds, C. F. (1989) Sleep disturbance in posttraumatic stress disorder: pathogenetic or epiphenomenal? *American Journal of Psychiatry*, **146**, 695–696.

Roehrs, T. & Roth, T. (2001) Sleep, sleepiness, sleep disorders and alcohol use and abuse. *Sleep Medicine Reviews*, **5**, 287–297.

Rosenfeld, D. S. & Elhajjar, A. J. (1998) Sleep sex: a variant of sleepwalking. *Archives of Sexual Behaviour*, **27**, 269–278.

Rush, A. J., Armitage, R., Gillin, J. C., *et al* (1998) Comparative effects of nefazodone and fluoxetine on sleep in outpatients with major depressive disorders. *Biological Psychiatry*, **44**, 3–14.

Sack, R. L., Hughes, R. J., Edgar, D. M., *et al* (1997) Sleep-promoting effects of melatonin: at what dose, in whom, under what conditions and by what mechanisms? *Sleep*, **20**, 908–915.

Sadeh, A. & Acebo, C. (2002) The role of actigraphy in sleep medicine. *Sleep Medicine Reviews*, **6**, 113–124.

Schenck, C. H. & Mahowald, M. W. (2002) REM sleep behavior disorder: clinical, developmental, and neuroscience perspectives 16 years after its formal identification. *Sleep*, **25**, 120–138.

Schweitzer, P. K. (2005) Drugs that disturb sleep and wakefulness. In *Principles and Practice of Sleep Medicine* (4th edn) (eds M. H. Kryger, T. Roth & W. C. Dement), pp. 499–518. Philadelphia, PA: Elsevier Saunders.

Shapiro, C. M. & Sloan, E. P. (1998) Nocturnal panic – an under-recognized entity (editorial). *Journal of Psychosomatic Research*, **44**, 21–23.

Shochat, T., Loredo, J. & Ancoli-Israel, S. (2001) Sleep disorders in the elderly. *Current Treatment Options in Neurology*, **3**, 19–36.

Siegel, J. M. (1999) Narcolepsy: a key role for hypocretins (orexins). *Cell*, **98**(4), 1–20.

Smith, R., Ronald, J., Delaive, K., *et al* (2002) What are obstructive sleep apnea patients being treated for prior to this diagnosis? *Chest*, **121**, 164–172.

Stiasny, K., Oertel, W. H. & Trenkwalder, C. (2002) Clinical symptomatology and treatment of restless legs syndrome and periodic limb movement disorder. *Sleep Medicine Reviews*, **6**, 253–265.

Stores, G. (1998) Sleep paralysis and hallucinosis. *Behavioural Neurology*, **11**, 109–112.

Stores, G. (2001*a*) *A Clinical Guide to Sleep Disorders in Children and Adolescents*. Cambridge: Cambridge University Press.

Stores, G. (2001*b*) Dramatic parasomnias. *Journal of the Royal Society of Medicine*, **94**, 173–176.

Stores, G. (2001*c*) Sleep–wake function in children with neurodevelopmental and psychiatric disorders. *Seminars in Pediatric Neurology*, **8**, 188–197.

Stores, G. (2003*a*) Misdiagnosing sleep disorders as primary psychiatric conditions. *Advances in Psychiatric Treatment*, **9**, 69–77.

Stores, G. (2003*b*) Medication for sleep–wake disorders. *Archives of Disease in Childhood*, **88**, 899–903.

Stores, G. (2006) The protean manifestations of childhood narcolepsy and their misinterpretation. *Developmental Medicine and Child Neurology*, **48**, 307–310.

Stores, G. (2007) *Understanding Adult Sleep Disorders*. Poole: Family Doctor Publications/British Medical Association.

Stores, G. & Wiggs, L. (2001) *Sleep Disturbance in Children and Adolescents with Disorders of Development: Its Significance and Management*. London: MacKeith Press.

Strollo, P. J. & Davé, N. B. (2005) Sleep apnoea. In *Sleep Disorders and Psychiatry* (ed. D. J. Buysse), pp. 77–105. Washington, DC: American Psychiatric Publishing.

Tanskanen, A., Tuomilehto, J., Viinamäki, H., *et al* (2001) Nightmares as predictors of suicide. *Sleep*, **24**, 844–847.

Taylor, D. Patron, C. & Kerwin, R. (2003) *The Maudsley (2003) Prescribing Guidelines* (7th edn). London: Martin Dunitz.

Thacker, K., Devinsky, O., Perrine, K., *et al* (1993) Nonepileptic seizures during apparent sleep. *Annals of Neurology*, **33**, 414–418.

Thorpy, M. (2001) Current concepts in the etiology, diagnosis and treatment of narcolepsy. *Sleep Medicine*, **2**, 5–17.

Tinuper, P., Montagna, P., Plazzi, G., *et al* (1994) Idiopathic recurring stupor. *Neurology*, **4**, 621–625.

Van Dongen, H. P. A., Maislin, G., Mullington, J. M., *et al* (2003) The cumulative cost of additional wakefulness: dose–response effects on neurobehavioral functions and sleep physiology from chronic sleep restriction and total sleep deprivation. *Sleep*, **26**, 117–126.

Wagner, J. & Wagner, M. L. (2000) Non-benzodiazepines for the treatment of insomnia. *Sleep Medicine Reviews*, **4**, 551–581.

Walsh, J. K., Dement, W. C. & Dinges, D. F. (2005) Sleep medicine, public policy and public health. In *Principles and Practice of Sleep Medicine* (4th edn) (eds M. H. Kryger, T. Roth & W. C. Dement), pp. 648–656. Philadelphia, PA: Elsevier Saunders.

Walters, A. S., Mandelbaum, D. E., Lewin, D. S., *et al* (2000) Dopaminergic therapy in children with restless legs/periodic limb movements in sleep and ADHD. Dopaminergic Therapy Study Group. *Pediatric Neurology*, **22**, 182–186.

Weissman, M. M., Greenwald, S., Niño-Murcia, G., *et al* (1997) The morbidity of insomnia uncomplicated by psychiatric disorders. *General Hospital Psychiatry*, **19**, 245–250.

Wiggs, L. & France, K. (2000) Behavioural treatments for sleep problems in children with physical illness, psychological problems or intellectual disabilities. *Sleep Medicine Reviews*, **4**, 299–314.

Winkelman, J. W., Herzog, D. B. & Fava, M. (1999) The prevalence of sleep-related eating disorder in psychiatric and non-psychiatric populations. *Psychological Medicine*, **29**, 1461–1466.

Zhdanova, I. V. (2000) The role of melatonin in sleep and its disorders. In *Sleep Disorders and Neurological Disease* (ed. A. Culebras), pp. 137–157. New York: Marcel Dekker.

CHAPTER 24

Anorexia nervosa and bulimia nervosa

Janet Treasure

Anorexia nervosa

Historical background

Historical accounts of young women who eat very little are plentiful, but the causes and meaning ascribed to such behaviour have varied. The religious interpretation was that extreme piety led to this asceticism. Bell (1985) in his book *Holy Anorexia* described the practices of Italian holy women from the 13th century, and questioned whether there are similarities with anorexia nervosa. Once scientific thinking began to hold sway, 'miraculous maids' such as the tragic Welsh fasting girl Sarah Jacob became a curiosity, as they appeared to defy the laws of nature. In 1869 doctors and nurses from Guy's Hospital set up a watch committee to provide rigorous proof as to whether Sarah Jacob could indeed survive without food or drink (Fowler, 1871). She died after six days.

Richard Morton (1694) is usually credited with the first medical descriptions of patients with anorexia nervosa. In his book on wasting illnesses, *Phthisiologia, Or, a Treatise of Consumptions*, he described two patients whose illness appeared to be due to voluntary food restriction. One was an 18-year-old girl who:

> 'fell into a total suppression of her Monthly Courses from a multitude of Cares and passions.... From which time her appetite began to abate ... she was wont by her studying and continuing pouring upon Books to expose herself both day and night ... she was like a Skeleton only clad with skin.'

This girl unfortunately died from the condition, but the second patient, a 16-year-old schoolboy, who 'fell gradually into a total want of appetite, occasioned by studying too hard and the Passions of the Mind', was cured by advice, which was to 'abandon his studies, to go into the country Air, and to use Riding and a milk diet'.

Unequivocal descriptions of anorexia nervosa appeared in the 19th century. Marcé (1860), a young French psychiatrist, wrote of:

> 'young girls who at the period of puberty become subject to inappetancy carried to the utmost limits ... these patients arrive at the delirious conviction that they cannot or ought not to eat.... All attempts made to constrain them to adopt a sufficient regimen are opposed with infinite strategies and unconquerable resistance.'

Sir William Gull (a physician at Guy's Hospital) and Charles Lasegue (a French psychiatrist) brought the illness to the attention of the medical community between 1868 and 1888 with articles and case presentations. Lasegue's (1873) account is particularly vivid and well observed:

> 'gradually she reduces her food further and further, and furnishes pretexts for so doing ... the abstinence tends to increase the aptitude for movement.'

He describes the lack of insight into the dangerousness of the weight loss and gives a typical patient riposte when confronted: 'I do not suffer and therefore must be well.'

Attempts to classify the illness reflect some of the uncertainties that remain today:

> 'the want of appetite is, I believe, due to a morbid mental state.' (Gull, 1873)

> 'the cases were not strictly insane; there was however something wrong in the nervous equilibrium, and usually something queer in the family history.' (Ryle, 1936)

The name given to the disorder has changed over time, as beliefs about both the aetiology and the psychopathology have shifted. Marcé used the expression 'hypochondriacal delirium', probably because many of his patients explained their reluctance to eat in terms of abdominal discomfort, and he considered that the lack of appetite and abdominal complaints were hysterical. Lasegue did not refer to Marcé and used the term 'anorexia hysteric'. The current French term is *anorexie mentale*. Although Gull (1868) initially called the syndrome 'apepsia hysterica', 5 years later he replaced 'apepsia' with 'anorexia', as he observed that food, if taken, was digested, indicating that the stomach was not at fault. He later argued that, because men could be afflicted and the deficit was central rather than peripheral, 'nervosa' was a better term than 'hysterica'. In recent years many have questioned whether 'anorexia' is appropriate (the root is *orexis*, meaning appetite). There are physiological, psychological and behavioural features characteristic of starvation that lead to the premise that appetite should still be present in patients with anorexia, but that there must be a block at some level between the perception of hunger and the motivation to eat.

In the West, explanations of the reluctance to eat now focus on dissatisfaction with weight and shape rather than on abdominal discomfort. It is interesting that the German name for the condition, *Magersucht*, describes more accurately the current content of the psychopathology, as it means 'thinness addiction'.

Treatment recommendations were remarkably similar from all sources, and centred upon removal of the patient from her family and home surroundings:

> 'The hypochondriacal delirium, then, cannot be advantageously encountered so long as the subjects remain in the midst of their own family and their habitual circle: the obstinate resistance that they offer, the sufferings of the stomach, which they enumerate with incessant lamentation, produce too vivid an emotion to admit of the physician acting with full liberty and obtaining the necessary moral ascendancy. It is therefore indispensable to change the habitation and the surrounding circumstances and to entrust the patients to the care of strangers.' (Marcé, 1860)

> 'the patient should be fed at regular intervals and surrounded by persons who would have most control over them ... the inclination of the patient must be in no way consulted.' (Lasegue, 1873)

Clinical description

The historical clinical descriptions are still relevant to current clinical practice. The onset of the illness commonly occurs within a few years of the menarche, at a median age of 17, but patients as young as 8 and as old as 60 have been described. The female:male ratio is 10:1. (For this reason, for the sake of simplicity, in much of the discussion below, the patient is referred to as 'she'.) The onset is insidious, and the gradual weight loss is frequently unnoticed by the family or is even commended as an adoption of a healthy lifestyle. Parents often do not react until the weight loss has been considerable. The family may even protest that their daughter eats large amounts, if her plate is piled with large quantities of vegetables or salads or other low-calorie foods.

As observed by Morton (1694), the contrast between the degree of emaciation and the level of mental and physical activity is striking. Often the first indication that something is amiss is that menstruation ceases. Parents may describe a change in temperament, where their previously 'good girl' has become 'difficult', emotional and excessively conscientious.

It is usually held that anorexia nervosa is more common within the upper social classes. However, this may reflect a referral bias since case registers do not confirm the association, but instead suggest a relationship with educational achievement.

In the majority of cases it is easy to make the diagnosis of anorexia nervosa. The following is a vignette of a typical case.

Case example

Susan was a 21-year-old undergraduate at Oxford University, reading philosophy. Her eating became erratic after difficulties in a relationship in her first year. Her weight fell from 63 kg to 42 kg, when her body mass index (weight/height^2) was 14 kg/m^2 and she developed amenorrhoea. She was sent home from college as she could not cope with her studies; her tutors noted that her academic performance had deteriorated and her friends were concerned about her misery. She refused to accept that she had anorexia nervosa, and stated that she was a fraud, wasting medical time. Her parents insisted that she eat, but she described feeling 'gross' and contemplated suicide: 'Nothing could be worse than having to eat'. Even low-calorie foods were threatening. She could not finish anything she ate, not even a tomato or a slice of cucumber or a pot of yogurt; it was 'too excessive and greedy to do so'. She weighed herself five or six times a day and would feel her thighs for excess flesh with disgust. The only time she felt happy was when she lost weight, and conversely she became despondent and despairing when she failed to do so, or if she lost control in any way.

She became obsessed with food and would go for frequent long walks that included visits to supermarkets, where she handled many items but bought nothing. She became preoccupied by a new interest in preparing food for others and even dreamed about force-feeding and woke up terrified. Her interest turned from philosophy to diet magazines, recipe books and cooking. She was driven to be always on the go, and even in bed she would furtively clench and stretch her muscles.

Mental state

The clinical features of anorexia nervosa are entwined with those of starvation. It is useful to digress slightly to highlight which features are secondary to weight loss and which will therefore be ameliorated by nutritional rehabilitation.

Keys *et al* (1950) outlined the profound effects that starvation has on physiology and psychology. They reported the Minnesota experiment, in which a series of 32 male conscientious objectors were semi-starved for 6 months to 76% of their previous weight, and followed-up during 12 weeks of rehabilitation. The men started to toy with the food and increase the use of spices and salt, and to dawdle for 2 hours over a meal. Food became the principal topic of conversations and dreams, and their attention to food-related items increased. The men became emotionally unstable, irritable and aggressive. Social activity decreased; it was 'too much trouble' and 'too tiring'. Sexual interest also dwindled, one man ruefully observing: 'I have no more sexual feeling than a sick oyster'. We can conclude from this study that much of the food-related behaviour, psychological distress and social isolation seen in anorexia nervosa is weight-related.

It is often difficult to pinpoint the core primary features of anorexia nervosa, that is, the characteristic psychopathology. The explanations given for the refusal to eat vary over time and place. Currently, the control of weight or shape is central. Fatness epitomises moral degradation and is equated with sloth, gluttony and selfishness. These strongly held views and overvalued ideas constitute what has been described as a morbid fear of fatness, which is present in both the ICD–10 and the DSM–IV descriptions (World Health Organization, 1992; American Psychiatric Association, 1994) (see Box 24.1). However, Crisp (1980) believed that the key component is a phobia of normal weight.

In addition to the global attitudes about fatness or weight, there may be sensitivity to a particular part of the body. This feature has been termed a disturbance of body image. It is not always present and it has been difficult to measure experimentally, as it may be a metaphor for more abstract discontent.

The sufferer may acknowledge that she is thin, but will explain that she needs a margin of safety to ensure that her body does not become too fat. To elicit this feature, the patient should be asked to give her 'ideal weight', which will be well below her premorbid weight.

Box 24.1 Diagnostic criteria for anorexia nervosa given in ICD–10 and DSM–IV

ICD–10 anorexia nervosa

1 Significant weight loss (BMI < 17.5 kg/m^2) or failure of weight gain or growth
2 Self-induced weight loss
   (a) avoidance of fattening foods
   (b) vomiting
   (c) purging
   (d) excessive exercise
   (e) use of appetite suppressants
   (f) use of diuretics
3 Psychopathology
   (a) fear of fatness
   (b) low weight threshold
4 Widespread endocrine disorder
   (a) amenorrhoea
   (b) raised levels of growth hormone
   (c) raised levels of cortisol
   (d) reduced levels of thyroid hormone T_3

DSM–IV anorexia nervosa

1 Refusal to maintain normal minimum weight (15% below expected)
2 Fear of weight gain or fatness even though underweight
3 Abnormal perception of weight, size or shape
4 Amenorrhoea (minimum three cycles)

This preoccupation with weight and shape is a contemporary phenomenon and was not present in the classical descriptions of the illness, and is frequently absent in males. In non-Western cultures, for example in Hong Kong, the explanations are in terms of internal physical discomfort. Some patients explain that eating impairs their academic performance (though others may pursue their academic work with excessive zeal). Changes in the content of the psychopathology (termed pathoplasticity) over time and across cultures resemble those seen in other psychiatric illnesses, such as hysteria, and an example of how eating disorders can appear in a non-Western society (in Fiji) is given in Chapter 31 (page 789).

In contrast to externally imposed starvation, which produces mental and physical inertia, anorexia nervosa is associated with heightened activity until over 30% of initial body weight is lost. Excessive exercise to 'burn off' calories occurs. In others the activity is driven by a compulsion for tidiness or cleanliness.

Physical state

A typical patient with anorexia nervosa will have gaunt facial features, with the rest of the body hidden under layers of bulky clothes. The hands, feet and nose are pinched, blue and cold. Skin and hair are dry and downy, and lanugo hair may be present on the cheeks, nape of the neck, forearms and legs. In severe cases a proximal myopathy will be present, as may a petechial rash. The pulse rate is slow (60/minute) and blood pressure low (90/60 mmHg).

Additional psychiatric disorders

Over 80% of people with anorexia nervosa have additional psychiatric morbidity during the course of their lives. Depression (70%) and obsessive–compulsive disorder (30%) are the most frequent. These syndromes are also common among first-degree relatives (Halmi *et al*, 1991). Indeed, it has been suggested that obsessive–compulsive personality disorder represents the broader phenotype, as it is often present in childhood, after recovery and at a higher level in first-degree relatives.

Low mood, anhedonia, lack of concentration, pessimism and sleep disturbance often occur in anorexia. However, these symptoms also developed in the participants in the starvation study by Keys *et al* (1950), mentioned above. Therefore they are not specific to anorexia nervosa but are a more general consequence of starvation, and these symptoms usually disappear with weight gain. It is difficult, if not impossible, to distinguish these depressive features from those of an affective disorder. Specific characteristics of anorexia nervosa, such as a preoccupation with food, may help, although when the weight loss is severe, hunger itself will diminish. Active suicidal ideation is rare. Patients with anorexia nervosa usually state that they do not want to die, vigorously deny that their behaviour is putting their life in danger, and reject the idea that they are undertaking a slow, passive form of suicide. Once the illness becomes chronic and the quality of life diminishes, more active suicidal ideation occurs and accounts for over half of the mortality in this group.

Although it has been argued, because of the frequent history of affective disorders within the families, that anorexia nervosa is a variant of an affective disorder (Cantwell *et al*, 1977), the clinical features, epidemiology and course of the two conditions suggest they are distinct (Halmi, 1985; Strober & Katz, 1987). In addition, there is no reciprocal increased risk of an eating disorder among families with affective disorder (Strober *et al*, 1990).

Obsessional symptoms, particularly centred around food and eating, are present in the majority of cases. For example, there are often rituals about which plate a patient can use and who can wash it. Any disturbance to the routine, such as an unexpected visitor, leads to refusal to eat. Often the rituals are associated with calorie counting; for example, one patient noted with despair how she would drive 10 miles out of her way to buy a wheat cereal product from a large supermarket, as this brand had 10 fewer calories per serving than other brands. Other rituals relate to body shape or size. More general cleaning or checking rituals can also arise. In most cases the obsessional behaviour diminishes with weight restoration. Again, starvation in its own right produces rituals and obsessive behaviour around food, as documented in Aleksandr Solzhenitsyn's *One Day in the Life of Ivan Denisovich* (1963):

> 'picking up Shuhov's bread ration he handed it to him ... though he was in a hurry he sucked the sugar from his bread with his lips, licked it under his tongue ... he broke his ration in two, one half he stuck into his bosom into a little pocket he had specially sewn into his jacket ... he considered eating the other half but food gulped down is no food at all; it's wasted; it gives you no feeling of fullness ... so he crawled barefoot up to his bunk, widened a little hole in his mattress and there amid the

sawdust, concealed his half ration.... Meanwhile the sugar in his mouth had melted....'

The ritualised meal is regarded as a reward to be earned and is associated with great pleasure, which compensates for the hassles and discomforts of everyday life. Again this is clearly described by Solzhenitsyn:

> 'Shukov with his two bowls.... And now they had nothing more to say to one another – the sacred moment had come.... He set to. First he only drank the liquid, drank and drank. As it went down filling his whole body with warmth, all his guts began to flutter inside him at that meeting with that skilly. Gooo-ood! There it comes, that brief moment for which a zek lives. And now Shukov complained about nothing.... This was all he thought about now....'

Approximately a third of women who present with obsessive–compulsive disorder later in life have a history of anorexia nervosa (Kasvikis *et al*, 1986). Anxiety and panic disorder are less common. Personality disorders, particularly in the avoidant, anankastic and emotionally unstable domains, are present in approximately half those referred for psychiatric treatment of anorexia (see also page 456). Patients with a mixed pattern of anorexia nervosa and bulimia may show borderline features and impulsively harm themselves, steal or misuse alcohol. Personality traits such as poor self-esteem and a lack of confidence in their academic abilities or their physical looks are common. Perfectionist traits are usual; flawed work may be destroyed and repeated, or personal belongings strictly ordered.

Measurement

A structured interview, the Eating Disorder Examination, is regarded as the gold standard method to measure symptoms (Cooper & Fairburn, 1987). Several self-report questionnaires are also in common use. The Eating Attitudes Test (EAT) is a self-report questionnaire that has been validated in clinical samples, but it has poor sensitivity and specificity when used in the community (Garner & Garfinkel, 1979). The same group (Garner *et al*, 1983) later produced another self-report questionnaire, the Eating Disorders Inventory, which incorporates factors from the EAT as well as personality dimensions.

Epidemiology

Anorexia nervosa can present to a variety of medical specialties, under several different diagnostic guises. Therefore it is not sufficient to calculate the incidence solely from psychiatric case registers, because some cases will be missed. The ascertainment of missed or misdiagnosed cases was meticulously undertaken in a study at the Mayo Clinic, in Rochester, Minnesota (Lucas *et al*, 1991). These workers examined the medical records of all the Mayo Clinic epidemiological archives, which extended back over 50 years, for any mention of terms relating to an eating disorder. Most of the patients had not been hospitalised. The authors found a considerable variation in incidence over time. Thus, for girls in the 10- to 19-year age group, the incidence of the disorder for the years 1935–39 was 16.6 per 100 000 per year; this then fell to an all-time low of 7.0 for the years 1950–54 but then rose once more, to 26.3 for the period 1980–84. For the whole 50-year period, the overall age-adjusted incidence rate per 100 000 person-years was 14.6 for females and 1.8 for males. The authors speculated that the changes over time could be cyclical and might relate to changing fashions concerning idealised body image. The incidence of anorexia nervosa within primary care in the UK has remained constant over the past two decades, at 20 per 100 000 for females aged 10–39, which corresponds to the main at-risk age period (Turnbull *et al*, 1996).

Establishing the prevalence of anorexia nervosa is fraught with even more difficulties, as large populations need to be screened and all studies so far have found that 'cases' actively avoid participation. A Swedish study sought to avoid these difficulties by carrying out a survey of a group at high risk for the condition: 15-year-old schoolchildren. Among this group the prevalence was found to be 700 per 100 000 per year for girls and 90 per 100 000 for boys (Rastam *et al*, 1989). The prevalence figures found in the large Mayo Clinic study were a little lower, at 270 per 100 000 per year for females and 22.5 for males (Lucas *et al*, 1991), but it should be noted that case ascertainment in that study was derived from medical records, whereas the Swedish school survey was based on a whole-population survey.

Certain groups in whom weight and appearance are at a premium are at high risk. Ballet dancers and models have a prevalence rate of 4–6%. Dieticians also may have increased rates.

There have been case reports of anorexia nervosa from Asia and Africa. However, the incidence of anorexia nervosa in Curacao in the Caribbean was similar to that in the Netherlands (Hoek *et al*, 1998). It has been argued that cases of anorexia nervosa can be seen in non-Western societies if the 'fear of fatness' criterion (a culture-bound symptom) is removed (Lee, 1991).

Aetiology

Theorists have produced a variety of explanations for anorexia nervosa. For example, Orbach (1986) argues that anorexia nervosa is a hunger strike undertaken to resolve the conflict between the expectations of a traditional female role and those of the modern woman. Nutritional knowledge and dietary fashion have changed eating behaviour over time. The carbohydrate avoidance of the 1960s and 1970s has been replaced by the exclusion of fat. Others blame fashion or the media.

Families have also been implicated (Selvini-Palazzoli & Viaro, 1988). Rigidity (resistance to change), enmeshment (over-close involvement between a child and a parent so that each is poorly differentiated), conflict avoidance and overprotection have all been described as characteristic features of the family of a child with anorexia nervosa (Minuchin *et al*, 1978), but more recent work has either failed to find this constellation or has found that it may be a non-specific response to a severe illness (Blair *et al*, 1995). Bruch (1974) suggested that early parenting experiences contribute to later difficulties, leading to a poor sense of identity, uncertainty about the relevance and meaning of internal states, and an overwhelming sense of ineffectiveness. Crisp (1980) suggested that a conflict relating to sexual maturity is often a causal factor, and the significance of puberty was discussed further in a review that took a developmental perspective (Gowers & Shore, 2001).

No prospective study has been large enough to put any of these hypotheses to the test. There have been two recent systematic reviews of aetiological studies of eating disorders, by Stice (2002) and by Jacobi *et al* (2004). The latter obtained risk factors from both longitudinal and cross-sectional studies. The risk factors identified include gender, ethnicity, early childhood eating and gastrointestinal problems, elevated weight and shape concerns, negative self-evaluation, sexual abuse, other adverse experiences and general psychiatric morbidity.

A recent study included a quantitative meta-analysis of changes in incidence rates over time and place, as well as a qualitative examination and summary of historical evidence; it concluded that anorexia nervosa is not a culture-bound syndrome, in contrast to bulimia nervosa, which is considered to be closely tied to culture (see below) (Keel & Klump, 2003).

Genetic factors

Findings from the largest and most systematic studies suggest a 7–12-fold increase in the prevalence of anorexia nervosa and bulimia nervosa among the relatives of probands with eating disorders (Strober *et al*, 2000). The clustering of eating disorders within the families of patients provides strong support for familial transmission of both disorders (Lilenfeld *et al*, 1998). Estimates from twin studies indicate that roughly 58–76% of the variance in the liability to anorexia nervosa is due to heritable factors. For both anorexia nervosa and bulimia nervosa, the remaining variance in liability appears to be due to non-shared environmental factors (i.e., factors that are unique to siblings in the same family) rather than shared or common environmental factors (i.e., factors that are common to siblings in the same family). There is preliminary evidence from affected relative pairs for linkage to chromosome 1 (Grice *et al*, 2002). However, this study awaits replication, as do many of the association studies.

Developmental trauma

There are parallels between some of the risk factors found in schizophrenia and those found in anorexia nervosa and it is possible that neurodevelopmental mechanisms may play a role. Thus, a case linkage study based on an in-patient psychiatric register ($n = 781$) from Sweden found an increased risk of anorexia nervosa in girls born with a cephalo-haematoma (odds ratio = 2.4) and those born prematurely (odds ratio = 3.2), especially if the baby was small for gestational age (odds ratio = 5.7) (Cnattingius *et al*, 1999). In common with most psychiatric disorders, there is a higher level of premorbid sexual and physical abuse (Fairburn *et al*, 1999; Karwautz *et al*, 2001).

The biology of eating

Anorexia nervosa is characterised by a severe energy deficit. However, the peripheral systems signalling energy deficits appear to be functioning normally, in that leptin and insulin are decreased and ghrelin levels are increased. This implicates the *central* control of appetite as a causal mechanism. People with anorexia nervosa have abnormal activation in the orbitofrontal cortex and anterior cingulate cortex in response to food cues. This persists even after recovery (Uher *et al*, 2003). Also, people with anorexia nervosa have an abnormal distribution of serotonin receptors, both in the acute state and after recovery.

Box 24.2 Questions for the assessment of the medical sequelae of eating disorders

- When was your last period?
- Do you feel the cold badly? How does the cold affect your peripheral circulation?
- Have you noticed any changes in your body hair, head hair, skin or nails?
- Have you noticed any weakness in your muscles? What about climbing stairs or brushing your hair?
- Are you troubled by aches in your bones or have you had fractures?
- What is your sleep like? Do you have to wake to go to the toilet?
- Have you fainted or had dizzy spells?
- Have you noticed palpitations?
- Have you had any pain or trouble with your teeth? What about temperature sensitivity? Do you attend to mouth hygiene after you have vomited?
- Have you vomited blood or lost blood from your back passage?
- Do you suffer from bloating or abdominal pain?
- Have you noticed if the glands on your face have become swollen?

Medical consequences

Medical problems often arise. (For a more complete review see Treasure & Szmukler, 1995.) Box 24.2 displays the questions that are useful to ask. Boxes 24.3 and 24.4 outline common problems related to weight loss and weight control measures, and Box 24.5 outlines the investigations that are of value.

Metabolism

Fatal hypoglycaemia can supervene rapidly and without warning, especially in the context of exercise or, in severe cases, even simply a change in routine. Asymptomatic hypoglycaemia is often found on routine testing of in-patients, and does not require active management other than the usual refeeding regimen. High results on tests of liver function reduce with refeeding of the patient. Ironically, in view of the low-fat diet of these patients, a high cholesterol level is often present.

Salt and electrolyte balance

Electrolyte abnormalities are frequent in the underweight subgroup who vomit and misuse laxatives. Plasma potassium levels occasionally fall below 3 mmol/l. As a consequence of low potassium, the electrocardiogram may show prolonged QT intervals

Box 24.3 Medical consequences of starvation

- *Reproductive function:* loss of menstruation, fertility and difficulties during pregnancy
- *Musculoskeletal:* myopathy, particularly of the limb girdle muscles; pathological fractures; tooth decay
- *Cardiovascular:* palpitations and syncope
- *Renal:* nocturia; renal stones
- *Skin and hair:* loss of head hair, increase in body hair, dry skin, Raynaud's sign (acrocyanosis), chilblains
- *Metabolic:* hypoglycaemia, liver dysfunction, high cholesterol, hypothermia
- *Gastrointestinal:* delayed gastric emptying, constipation
- *Central nervous system:* poor concentration, difficulty in undertaking complex thought
- *Psychological symptoms:* depression, obsessive–compulsive behaviour

Box 24.4 Medical consequences of weight control methods used by patients with eating disorders

- *Gastrointestinal tract:* tooth decay, salivary gland hypertrophy, bleeding in the upper and lower gastrointestinal tract, abdominal distension, constipation
- *Renal:* oedema, dehydration, stones, failure
- *Cardiovascular:* dysrhythmias, postural hypotension
- *Central nervous system:* tetany, fits
- *Metabolic:* dehydration, hypokalaemia, hyponatraemia
- *Drug effects:* caffeine, slimming tablets such as diethyl proprion, amphetamine and ecstasy can be misused; toxicity leads to nervousness and overt psychotic features

and U-waves. Fatal arrhythmias can occur without warning. Sodium, magnesium and phosphate levels are also sometimes reduced. Too rapid correction of these abnormalities can tip the patient into an acute confusional state, while too rapid correction of a low potassium level can trigger dangerous arrhythmias.

Although the electrolyte abnormalities are profound, they develop slowly and there is a degree of metabolic adaptation. Supervision to prevent vomiting and oral potassium supplements are the first line of management for hypokalaemia. Oedema may result from the rehydration after laxative misuse and vomiting have ceased, and this oedema may be a component of the 'refeeding syndrome' (see page 581). Patients may gain as much as 5 kg in a week on a refeeding regimen.

Box 24.5 Useful investigations for anorexia

1 Physical examination
- Skin for petechial rash, lanugo hair, Raynaud's sign (acrocyanosis), chilblains, callus on hand, self-mutilation
- Mouth and teeth for caps, loss of enamel, abrasions
- Lying and standing blood pressure for dehydration
- Abdomen for constipation
- Ability to rise from a squat for proximal myopathy

2 Blood count
- Anaemia (Hb 9–12 g/l) (the anaemia is usually normocytic and normochromic)
- White-cell count between 2000 and 4000 per ml
- Platelet deficiency (rare)
- Erythrocyte sedimentation rate (normal)

3 Blood chemistry

Urea and electrolyte levels are usually in the normal range unless there are other complications:
- Urea levels are usually low in restricting anorexia but may be increased with vomiting and laxative misuse
- Potassium < 3.5 mmol/l where there is vomiting or laxative misuse
- Bicarbonate > 30 mmol/l where there is vomiting or < 18 mmol/l where there is laxative misuse

Other tests:
- Aspartate transaminase, alkaline phosphatase and gamma-glutamyl transaminase levels may all be increased
- Cholesterol level > 6.5 mmol/l
- Amylase (salivary isoenzyme) increased (after persistent vomiting)
- Phosphate levels decreased
- Carotene levels increased
- Protein levels usually normal

4 Blood hormones

These are of no use diagnostically and do not need to be determined routinely. However, the following trends have been reported:
- Levels of luteinising and follicle stimulating hormones decreased
- Oestrogen levels decreased
- Thyroid hormone T_4 decreased
- Levels of growth hormone increased
- Cortisol levels increased
- Prolactin levels normal
- Basal thyroid stimulating hormone normal (a delayed response to thyrotropin-releasing hormone may occur)
- Basal adrenocorticotrophic hormone normal (decrease in response to corticotrophin-releasing hormone)
- Basal insulin levels reduced (increased sensitivity to insulin)

Haematology

Marrow suppression is common, leading to haemoglobin levels reduced to 9 g/100 ml and white-cell counts of less than 4000 per ml. Platelet suppression is rare, but is a sign of dangerous weight loss. The erythrocyte sedimentation rate (ESR) is low and usefully distinguishes the anaemia and weight loss of anorexia nervosa from that of inflammatory bowel disease. Surprisingly, people with an eating disorder are often free of the common viral infections, but tuberculosis and other chronic infections occur sporadically.

Endocrine system

The endocrine dysfunction reflects both the acute and the chronic nutritional disturbance. Amenorrhoea is one of the diagnostic criteria for anorexia nervosa, but it may be masked by withdrawal bleeds from the oral contraceptive pill. The hypothalamic–pituitary–gonadal axis regresses to a prepubertal state. Luteinising hormone (LH) and follicle stimulating hormone (FSH) are reduced, oestrogen and progesterone levels are undetectable, and pelvic ultrasonography reveals ovaries diminished in size, but with a multifollicular appearance, and a small uterus.

All of the hormonal components of the hypothalamic–pituitary–adrenal axis are increased; this is thought to reflect increased hypothalamic secretion of corticotrophin-releasing hormone (CRH), and there is an impaired response to the dexamethasone suppression test.

A Polish study found low levels of T_4 but T_3 was only occasionally reduced, while reverse T_3 levels were normal. The levels of thyroid stimulating hormone (TSH) also tended to be low. The altered thyroid function may explain the lipid disorder of a raised cholesterol level and decreased high-density lipoprotein levels sometimes found in anorexia nervosa (Smorawinska *et al*, 2001).

The endocrine abnormalities disappear with weight recovery.

Gastrointestinal system

Gastric emptying is delayed and leads to distension and discomfort once refeeding is instituted. In the most extreme cases, acute gastric distension may occur, which can be fatal. It is therefore common to start refeeding gradually, with 'half portions' (approximately 1000–1500 kcal). Constipation is common and may become intractable in cases of laxative misuse.

Central nervous system

Concentration is impaired and the capacity for complex thought diminished. Cerebral atrophy (ventricular dilatation and widened sulci) may be related to vomiting or raised cortisol levels, and resolves in most cases following weight gain.

Long-term health problems

The detrimental medical consequences in both the short and the long term can be used in the context of a motivational approach to facilitate change. It is usual to find one item on the health checklist that is of personal concern to the individual. For example, some patients are extremely concerned about the loss of their periods and the implications this will have for their future fertility. The showing and explanation of their own pelvic ultrasonography scans of their ovaries and uterus may be particularly motivating for such women. Others may be concerned about the risk of osteoporosis, which becomes more severe with the length and severity of the illness and weight loss. Pathological fractures may appear after 10 years of amenorrhoea.

Assessment

The diagnosis of anorexia nervosa in adolescents or adults rarely poses difficulties. However, engaging the patient in treatment is much more tricky. Ambivalence about treatment is usual, and patients are often unforthcoming and angry at being coerced into seeing a doctor by concerned relatives and friends.

Even if the family has brought the patient for assessment, it is important to establish an individual relationship with the sufferer from the outset. The skills of motivational interviewing can often help to engage the patient. This involves gentle probing for the benefits of anorexia nervosa (these may be idiosyncratic but often include emotional avoidance, a signal of distress, etc.) in addition to the costs in terms of physical health, education and career, social and romantic life, and psychological and spiritual well-being. Arguments are best avoided, as are any comments that may be interpreted as critical or hostile, as patients are usually acutely sensitive to these (Treasure & Ward, 1997).

Later in the interview it is appropriate to narrow the focus to the development of symptoms, by taking a weight and eating history. Both the rate of change of weight as well as the absolute weight are good indicators of acute medical risk (see Table 24.1). Two types of anorexia are sometimes described: a pure 'restricting type', where the patient only has anorexia nervosa symptoms without any bulimic symptoms; and a 'bulimic type', where the patient shows features of both anorexia and bulimia. Patients with the restricting form of the illness usually maintain a regular meal pattern, while those who are in the prodrome of the bulimic form will have prolonged periods of abstinence.

It is important to establish whether symptoms associated with bulimia nervosa are present, because these may terrify the patient and reinforce her need to have rigid control over her diet. Direct questioning may lead to denial. It is better to normalise these reversing behaviours with probes such as:

- 'It is a common occurrence when people are as underweight as you that they have episodes when their eating seems excessive or out of control. Has this ever happened to you?'
- 'At times like this people experience discomfort and may even vomit. Has this happened to you? Have you ever had to make yourself sick to give you some relief?'
- 'Often people who are underweight suffer badly from constipation. Has this ever happened to you? Have you had to take something to help?'
- 'Sometimes people with this illness are driven to be very active. Does this apply to you?'
- 'Many people with this problem use other methods to control their weight, such as health-shop preparations or street drugs. Perhaps you have had to do this?'

The weight history establishes the relationship between eating and life circumstances and context. Weight, physical and psychiatric histories of all the other family members are also required, and may provide material that can be used in later psychotherapeutic sessions.

Table 24.1 Features associated with medical risk

	Examination	Moderate risk	High risk
Nutrition	Body mass index (BMI) (kg/m^2)	< 15	< 13
	BMI centiles *	< 3	< 2
	Weight loss per week	> 0.5 kg	> 1.0 kg
			Purpuric rash or ulcers
Circulation	Systolic blood pressure	< 80 mmHg	< 70 mmHg
	Diastolic blood pressure	< 60 mmHg	< 50 mmHg
	Postural drop	> 10 mmHg	> 20 mmHg
	Pulse rate	< 50 beats/min	<40 beats/min
	Oxygen saturation	< 90%	< 85%
	Extremities		Dark blue or cold
Musculoskeletal	Squat test[a]	Unable to get up without using arms for balance	Unable to get up without using arms as leverage
Core temperature		< 35°C	< 34.5°C
Investigations	Full blood count, urea , electrolytes (including PO_4), liver function tests, albumin, creatinine kinase, glucose	Concern if outside normal limits	K < 2.5 mmol/l Na < 130 mmol/l PO_4 < 0.5 mmol/l Glucose < 2.5 mmol/l
	Electrocardiography		Prolonged QT interval

[a]The squat test gives a clinical indication of muscle power and may be used to monitor progress. The patient squats on her haunches and has to stand up without, if possible, using her hands to get additional support.
*Body mass index centiles are appropriate for people under 18 years.

The formulation should detail constitutional risk factors, patterns of interaction and behaviour, precipitating events, and factors that perpetuate the illness (the last often lie within the family).

Acute medical risk

It is essential that all psychiatrists are able to assess medical risk in anorexia nervosa and Table 24.1 gives a rough guide to the relevant factors. However, if there is doubt concerning the gravity of the medical risk, priority should be given to the overall physical examination of the patient.

Treatment

The classical treatment, advocated by Gull, was to remove the patient from her home environment to a nursing home, where 'moral management' would be applied. There has been a distinct move away from this approach over the past 20 years, and novel specific psychotherapeutic treatments have recently been developed.

In-patient treatment was regarded as standard, as reflected in the American Psychiatric Association's (2000) guidelines, and in-patient therapy is highly effective in correcting malnutrition in the short term, although the long-term outcome is less certain. However, a wider range of management strategies may be more cost-effective and acceptable. For example, the plan of management may include day and out-patient care, with complex mixes of types of therapy and numbers of hours, over a variety of durations, sometimes on an individual basis and at other times with various members of the family. Indeed, in the 2004 guidelines from the National Institute for Health and Clinical Excellence (NICE, 2004) the first-line approach recommended for anorexia nervosa was out-patient therapy.

Planning treatment for someone with anorexia nervosa is not a simple affair that can be solved by entering a few key words and searching the literature for systematic reviews of evidence-based treatments, as these usually focus only on the well-known generalities of treatment, tend to be guarded in their conclusions and may offer little useful guidance for a particular patient. In addition, the process of negotiating a joint treatment plan is difficult, as people with anorexia nervosa often have mixed feelings about treatment. In formulating the treatment plan, the clinician will need to take into account:

1 the acute medical risk (Table 24.1), which in turn determines the speed and efficiency of the refeeding that needs to be instituted

2 the symptomatic presentation – whether it is the restricting or bulimic type of anorexia

3 the factors that determine the long-term prognosis.

Matching treatment to risk

There needs to be a careful evaluation of the risks and resources and hence prognosis for the individual case. Matching the intensity and type of treatment to need involves a careful risk assessment of medical, clinical and psychosocial factors. The first question is whether starvation requires acute management, that is, whether are there signs of high medical risk (see Table 24.1). If so, it is essential to manage this in a safe environment. This can be at home if there is shared care of some form (family or community psychiatric nurse) or there are high levels of motivation. However, the skills of teams on paediatric, medical or specialised eating disorder units may also be needed, and criteria for admission are shown in Box 24.6. Nurses on general psychiatric units rarely have the time or skill to manage life-threatening starvation.

Box 24.6 Clinical and psychiatric grounds for admission

A Medical indications
1 Body mass index below 13.5 kg/m^2 (or a rapid rate of fall)
2 Syncope
3 Proximal myopathy
4 Hypoglycaemia
5 Electrolyte imbalance
6 Petechial rash and platelet suppression

B Psychiatric indications
1 Risk of suicide
2 Chronicity (duration > 5 years)
3 Comorbidity with impulsive behaviour
4 Intolerable family situation
5 Extreme social isolation
6 Failure of out-patient treatment

Admission and involuntary admission

In-patient treatment in a specialised unit skilled in refeeding should be considered if the person falls into the high-risk category (see Table 24.1). If, despite maximal support (including meeting with the family) in an out-patient department, the individual remains at risk yet declines admission, then the psychiatrist should consider whether to use the Mental Health Act.

Stabilisation of 'at risk' patients

Nutritional risk

The deficits in anorexia nervosa develop slowly and are general rather than specific. Therefore, it is preferable to rectify them slowly, orally and with ordinary food supplemented with multi-vitamin/multi-mineral preparations (e.g. Sanatogen Gold, Forceval 1–2 or Seravit capsules). In the first phase (3–7 days) a 'soft diet' of approximately 30–40 kcal/kg/day spaced in small portions throughout the day is recommended.

Fluid and electrolyte balance

Some weight change strategies such as vomiting, diuretic and laxative misuse can result in severe dehydration (or over-hydration), acute renal failure and electrolyte imbalance. Oral replacement is preferable (e.g. using Diorylate). Serum potassium levels may remain low even with potassium supplements if vomiting persists.

Medication

The risk of harm, for example from the consequences of QT prolongation, needs to weighed against the negligible evidence of benefit from antidepressants, antipsychotics and antihistamines in patients with low weight. Small doses of promethazine or some of the newer antipsychotic agents can help the severe anxiety and overactivity associated with refeeding.

Complications of refeeding

Severe medical complications collectively known as 'the refeeding syndrome' can occur, especially in those with a BMI less than 12 kg/m^2, or in those who binge and purge as well as those with concurrent physical conditions. Close monitoring is necessary, as a range of electrolyte disturbances, including hypokalaemia, hypocalcaemia and hypomagnesaemia and physical complications can occur during refeeding. Fatal consequences such as acute gastric dilatation and hypophosphataemia can occur quickly. Acute gastric dilatation can occur with rapid nasogastric feeding or if the patient binges. Hypophosphataemia can develop if a high carbohydrate load has been given; if severe, this can cause cardiac and respiratory failure, delirium and fits.

What is effective therapy in anorexia nervosa?

Adolescents: short-duration cases

A systematic review (Treasure & Schmidt, 2004) concluded that the majority of adolescent cases (in particular those with a short duration of illness) could be managed within out-patient services. However, even in this group, which has a good prognosis, approximately 20% may need a higher intensity of care, such as in-patient treatment. Involvement of the family is beneficial for younger, early cases. Indeed, this was the only recommendation in the NICE (2004) guidelines on anorexia nervosa that reached the level of evidence warranting a B grading (i.e. some data from a randomised controlled trial). However, traditional family therapy is not necessary. Indeed, parental counselling may be more effective, especially in families with high expressed emotion (on which see Chapter 10, page 228).

Adults: long-duration cases

In the adult group, which has a poorer prognosis, there is less certainty about what works. Thus, the NICE (2004) guidelines were unable to recommend any specific treatment. Similarly, a Cochrane review of out-patient therapy concluded that there was no evidence on which to choose between different treatments (Hay *et al*, 2003). The placebo response is minimal in anorexia nervosa. Specialised therapy (family, focal or cognitive analytical) improves the outcome. Some treatments are less acceptable than others and have high drop-out rates. There have been several randomised controlled trials of various types of medication as adjuncts to in-patient care but there is no clinically significant benefit in terms of weight gain in this context.

The general principles of treatment

In this section we use the word 'therapist' for the person treating the person with anorexia nervosa. In specialist teams it is usual for treatment to be given by nurses or psychologists, but no matter what the professional background, the approach needs to address areas of both physical and psychological health.

A key aspect of treatment is weight monitoring. This is important as an outcome measure and also is a key indicator of medical risk. The therapist needs to have a set procedure for monitoring weight and medical risk at the beginning of each session. If the patient is at medium to moderate risk, then the examination should include further aspects of medical monitoring, such as cardiovascular function (blood pressure, heart rate and peripheral circulation) and an examination of limb

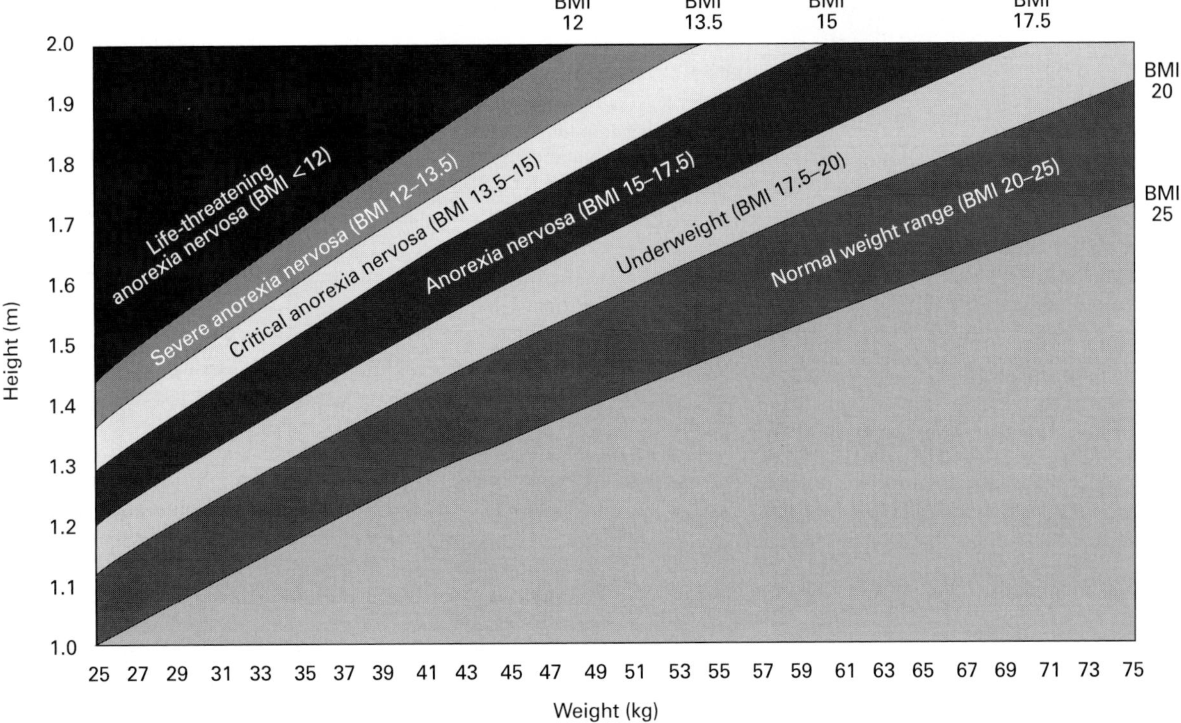

Fig. 24.1 The Maudsley body mass index (BMI) chart.

girdle muscle function. If the patient is at high risk, then this needs to be shared with other key members of the care network (general practitioner, parent, community general psychiatrist). (A specific underweight risk chart is presented in Fig. 24.1.) The therapist should then have a conversation about weight, starting with questions like the following:

> 'Is this what you expected your weight to be? Are you surprised at what it is?'

For patients who are in the zone of moderate to high risk, there needs to be a longer conversation discussing whether they intend to instigate any plans to decrease the nutritional risk. Is this something they can do themselves or do they need help? What level of help should this be – family, day patient or in-patient care? What changes in eating can be implemented? Go through this in a step-by-step approach in which patients visualise increasing their food intake during the day, and then describe how this could be done, whether on their own or by asking for the support of others. It is important to warn patients that weight gain in the short term can be distressing; for example, there can be an uncomfortable perception of gastric bloating and sometimes the appetite can vigorously re-emerge. This leads some patients to fear they will never be able to stop eating. In addition to the physical rebound of appetite there can be a rebound of emotions that had been suppressed during the acute phase, resulting in heightened anxiety, irritability and impulsiveness. This may be a distressing period in which there is a battle between that part of the patient that wants to get a bigger life, get well and accept weight gain, and the persisting anorexic attitudes, where suppression of eating and loss of weight are still perceived to have positive consequences. Weight gain, however, disrupts the factors that maintain the illness.

We have developed a conceptual model of the maintaining factors that are important in anorexia nervosa, as shown in Fig. 24.2. This includes the positive aspects of anorexia, such as the ability to connect with others through communicating distress or the ability to avoid emotions (often the person with anorexia nervosa is fearful of expressing negative emotions, and possibly also this is something that the family would find difficult to tolerate). The response of other people, particularly the family, is often a key factor that perpetuates the illness.

These positive benefits are often grounded in some of the extreme personality traits that predispose to the disorder. The need for perfection, order, exactness and fear of making mistakes can make the certainty and control of a world centred upon food and weight seem to be highly beneficial. Similarly, those predisposed to anorexia because of their high levels of anxiety discover that the limited horizons of the anorexic world enables them to avoid the challenges of maturation and individuation.

The therapeutic alliance

At all stages the therapeutic relationship needs to be collaborative, with a kind, consistent and persistent approach. It is helpful to hold in mind the trans-theoretical model of change. Many people with anorexia nervosa are not ready to change and are in pre-contemplation or contemplation rather than action. Indeed, they may have been brought or pressurised into coming to the clinic by concerned others. Their stance is that they do not see anything wrong. This means that the initial task is to develop a relationship in which the person with anorexia nervosa is willing to work with professionals, initially to reflect on her position

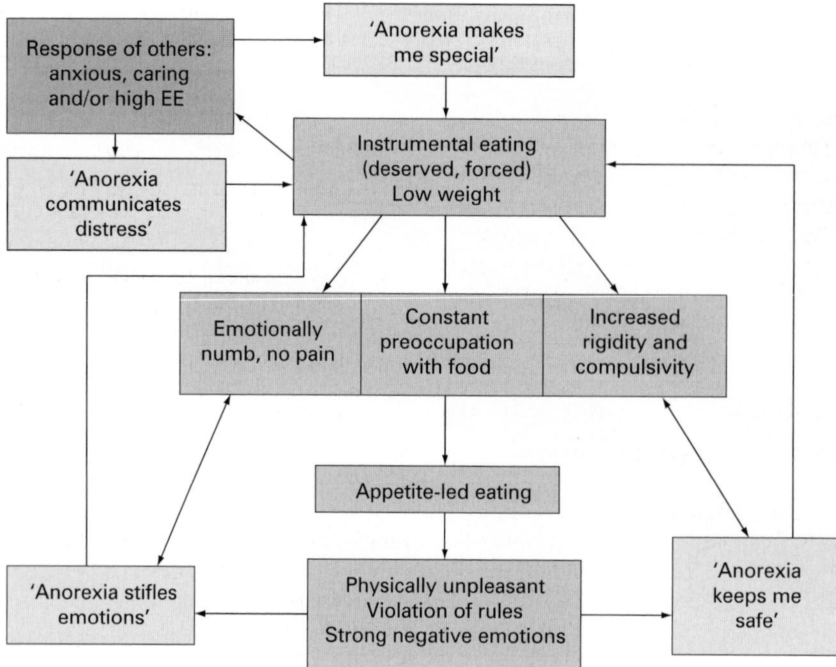

Fig. 24.2 Factors maintaining anorexia nervosa. EE, expressed emotion.

and that of others close to her rather than actively to go for change. High levels of therapist anxiety arising from concerns about malnutrition can lead to the wish to force change, but coercive strategies merely lead to resistance by deception or drop-out. This can be intensely frustrating for the therapist, who may respond with higher levels of coercion or by withdrawal from the problem. It is all too easy to get caught up in unhelpful struggles for control in the relationship. An astute therapist will gauge exactly where the person with anorexia nervosa is and adjust reactions accordingly. For example, there is no point in trying to institute change strategies before the person is ready to implement them. The therapist needs to be able to uncover the positive benefits of anorexia nervosa and replace them with more adaptive strategies and at the same time to make the negative aspects more salient. This requires working to shift the balance between the pros and cons of the illness. Only at the point within therapy when the person has reached the stage of active change can work on goal setting, problem solving and making change plans become a meaningful activity.

The initial phase of treatment

The first task within therapy is to gauge the degree of medical risk and establish whether the patient has the resources to attain minimal levels of nutritional safety.

The second task of the initial phase of treatment is to explore the mixed feelings about change (described above). The decisional balance can be explored by making lists of benefits and disbenefits and also employing cognitive techniques such as asking the patient to write letters to 'anorexia the friend' and 'anorexia the enemy'.

In order to make the negative aspects of anorexia nervosa more salient, the therapist needs gently to explore all domains of life. It helps if the therapist is knowledgeable about the wide range of consequences of an eating disorder and is able to cue responses from each of these domains (see Box 24.7). Over several sessions the therapist encourages the individual to expand upon these negative areas in as much detail as possible. Strategies such as reflective listening are important, where the therapist explores and empathises and subtly highlights negative aspects of anorexia nervosa.

Other strategies used to highlight negative aspects of the current behaviours are to ask the patient to project herself into the future and to consider the consequences of life still with the anorexia nervosa and contrast this with a life in which her future health is good. A complementary approach is to ask the person with anorexia to reflect on the hopes and ambitions of the past. These approaches are used to draw out discrepancies between the current state of health and an idealised state.

The second phase of treatment: working on change

The next phase of treatment centres upon the maintaining factors, within the patient and also within the family. Traits such as perfectionism, compulsiveness and anxiety may all serve as powerful maintaining factors. Their treatment follows the same approach as with the anorexia nervosa symptoms. For example, these traits are examined in terms of how they are helpful or less helpful, both for the person's own function as well as within her social network. Another common maintaining factor is extremely low self-esteem and feelings of worthlessness, with their compensatory patterns of thought and avoidance or submission. The challenge is to shift these fixed patterns of behaviour.

Box 24.7 The domains commonly affected by anorexia nervosa

Physical
- Worry about periods
- Sensitivity to the cold
- Loss of head hair
- Growth of body hair
- Loss of stamina

Psychological
- Anhedonia and low mood
- Irritability
- Rituals and preoccupations relating to body shape and food, merging into more general obsessive–compulsive phenomenology

Family
- Respond with high distress and anger
- Become intrusive or rejecting in relationship to the symptoms

Romantic life
- Loss of interest
- Loss of libido

Social life
- Loss of interest in relationships
- Isolation and withdrawal
- Difficulty engaging with peers

Career
- Recognition of problem by others
- Poor concentration

Forensic
- Stealing of food and other items
- Drugs and smoking used to lose weight and to control appetite

Spirituality
- Feelings of alienation
- Feelings of being morally wrong

These negative aspects of the illness are made more salient by including them in the written formulation that is given to the patient.

Work with the family

The amount of work with the family depends on the developmental age of the person: the younger she is, the more appropriate intensive involvement becomes; in addition, people with a severe form of illness often benefit from having the family involved.

In all cases it is important to include the family for part of the first assessment. The family should be offered general information about the illness as well as specific help. They should also be taught skills for managing particular symptoms and how to side-step unhelpful modes of responding. In cases where there is moderate to high medical risk, it is regarded as good practice to discuss this with the family members and ensure that they are clear about the management of this risk, and how they can help modify this risk as well as monitor it. The exact approach needs to be a process of negotiation, experimentation and review. Similarly, it can be helpful to involve the parents or other family members if patients remain 'stuck' and have poor progress despite a long period of out-patient therapy, or have an ominous long-term risk because of poor physical health and psychosocial stunting.

If there is a large amount of face-to-face contact between the person with the eating disorder and her family, it is possible that their patterns of interaction are unwittingly maintaining the problem. One of the strongest predictors of outcome and dropping out of treatment for anorexia nervosa is high expressed emotion among family members and this may need to be addressed.

Anorexia nervosa is a clear signal of distress and strikes at the core of family life – that is, meals. Family members become anxious, depressed, angry, over-solicitous or withdraw, and may blame themselves and experience stigma. These extreme reactions merely increase the anorexic behaviours. It is useful to teach family skills to help avoid these unhelpful modes of interaction.

We teach parents reflective listening skills so that they can listen to their daughters' distress and empathise with it. The skills of clear communication and assertiveness are useful when managing anorexia nervosa. The focus needs to be on restoring nutritional health, with a clear plan of implementation, such as how much is eaten, and when and how this will be achieved. This will involve a process of gradual goal setting and negotiation. A functional analysis of the patterns of interaction is sometimes helpful, as this may reveal how the anorexic behaviours are being reinforced by the time and attention given to them. The therapist needs to work with the family to try to reduce this pattern and encourage non-anorexic behaviours and interactions, and ensure that these are also given high priority. It is usually possible for a parent to work with the person with anorexia nervosa to help her overcome her symptoms but it is less easy or appropriate for partners to be so closely involved in this task.

Medication

There is no evidence that any medication gives additional benefit to the skilled nursing available in a specialised in-patient unit. However, minor tranquillisers such as promethazine are often given for the extreme distress about food. There is interest, derived from open studies, in some of the newer antipsychotic drugs but so far there is no high-quality evidence for their effectiveness. Medication for symptomatic treatment such as drugs to increase gastric emptying or oestrogens for osteoporosis have been tried but there is no evidence for their effectiveness. Any potential benefit has to be balanced against negative effects such as prolongation of the QT interval and the risks of abnormal cardiac conductivity.

Overall, for restricting anorexia nervosa the benefits of drug treatment are small, and need to be balanced against side-effects. In practice, compliance with medication is usually poor, perhaps because this represents sacrificing control. Alternatively, the patient may discover from her own research that weight gain can be a side-effect of medication, especially of the newer atypical antipsychotics.

In-patient treatment

In-patient treatment is required for those who are at high risk and who do not respond to out-patient management and care. The treatment team needs to be skilled in implementing feeding in conjunction with psychological care. Refeeding severely malnourished patients can be problematic and requires specialist expertise (see above). A subgroup of patients with very severe anorexia nervosa often require repeated and lengthy admissions with prolonged rehabilitation in order to attain a degree of nutritional stability.

There are two main aims of in-patient treatment:

1 to ensure nutritional safety, which can usually be attained at specialist units

2 to ensure that the person with anorexia nervosa can optimise her nutritional, psychological and social health within the community.

Prognostic factors and outcome

Most published studies on prognosis and outcome represent the experience of relatively small clinical groups from tertiary referral centres and hence are biased towards the more severe cases. This has arisen because there may be variable filters or selection processes, which can skew the case mix. Nevertheless, there is some consistency among studies in that markers of the severity of the illness (duration, BMI) are related to outcome, whether this is defined as mortality or degree of recovery (Nielsen *et al*, 1998).

Case example

Clarissa rapidly lost weight after starting a diet for fun. Her parents were divorced and she lived with her father. It was several months before her mother became so worried about her weight that she arranged to have the family doctor call when she was visiting her daughter at home. Clarissa was admitted to a local psychiatric unit, where she was offered the freedom to eat as she wished. She later recounted, 'They didn't make me eat, so I didn't'. She collapsed on the third day with a cardiac arrest. She was successfully resuscitated but required ventilation on an intensive-care unit for several days. Her parents were warned about the nature and danger of her illness and agreed to put their daughter on a treatment order of the Mental Health Act. She was transferred to a specialised unit, where she refused to eat and drink for 2 days, despite the nurses sitting with her for several hours after meals and encouragement from fellow sufferers. The nurses told her that they were not going to let her die, but they understood how difficult it was for her to eat and they would help by assisting her more actively. Two nurses gently but firmly ensured that several spoons of porridge were eaten. This did not need to be repeated. She gained weight and left the hospital after 14 weeks. She was seen intensively as an out-patient and managed to maintain her weight.

Follow-up studies have found that, on average, up to half of patients recover fully (i.e. a return to normal weight and menstruation): weight is restored in 60%, menstrual functioning resumes in 55%, and normal eating behaviour in 40%. On average, the duration of the illness is 6 years. Psychosocial adaptation is often impaired: typically, only two-thirds of participants in follow-up studies are in employment or in a normal educational career, very few are married, and approximately a third have a negative attitude to sexuality (there is wide variation between studies).

Factors that are associated with poor outcome are:

- severe weight loss
- long duration of illness
- high level of reversing behaviours (vomiting, over-exercise)
- failure to attain normal weight
- additional comorbidity (e.g. obsessive–compulsive disorder)
- poor premorbid psychological adjustment.

Normal-weight bulimia nervosa (see below) develops in approximately a quarter of cases of anorexia nervosa. Affective disorders and obsessional disorders are less common and are more usually present in those who have failed to recover.

Bulimia nervosa

History

The word 'bulimia' is derived from the Greek *bous*, meaning ox, and *limos*, meaning hunger. A state of pathological voracity has been recognised for centuries. However, in many accounts the bulimia was considered to be a symptom of a physical disorder. Four of the 14 historical examples described by Parry Jones & Parry Jones (1990) were of people infested with parasitic worms, while the symptoms in the remaining cases resembled those seen in pyloric stenosis. Other historical accounts describe a fluctuating course rather similar to the Kleine–Levin syndrome. Binge eating in association with obesity was described by Stunkard (1959) and Bruch (1974) used the term 'thin fat people' to describe ex-obese individuals who regurgitated food after indulging in large meals.

Russell (1979) described a similar pattern of behaviour developing after an episode of anorexia nervosa. He used the term 'bulimia nervosa' to describe the syndrome in which bulimia was associated with purging and a morbid fear of fatness. It took Russell 6 years to collect 30 cases, but today the condition is common, indicating that the prevalence has increased rapidly over the past three decades.

Definition

Several systems for classifying binge-eating disorders have evolved. Broad criteria were used for 'bulimia' in DSM–III (American Psychiatric Association, 1980). They differed from Russell's criteria for bulimia nervosa in that purging, a morbid fear of fatness and a history of anorexia nervosa were not considered necessary. In DSM–III–R (American Psychiatric Association, 1987) the criteria were tightened, the preoccupation with weight and shape was included, and frequency cut-off points were introduced (a minimum of 2 binges a week over 3 months). The ICD–10 criteria for bulimia nervosa (World Health Organization, 1992) differ from

Box 24.8 Criteria for a diagnosis of bulimia nervosa

DSM–IV
1 Recurrent episodes of binge-eating
2 Feeling of lack of control of eating during binge
3 Regular use of methods of weight control
  (a) vomiting
  (b) laxatives
  (c) diuretics
  (d) fasting/strict diet
  (e) vigorous exercise
4 Minimum average of 2 binges a week over 3 months
5 Persistent over-concern with shape or weight

ICD–10
1 Episodes of overeating
2 Methods to counteract weight gain
  (a) vomiting
  (b) laxatives
  (c) fasting
  (d) appetite suppressants
  (e) metabolic stimulants
  (f) diuretics
3 Morbid fear of fatness with a sharply defined weight threshold
4 Often a history of anorexia nervosa

those of DSM–IV (see Box 24.8) in that frequency criteria are not present. The link with anorexia nervosa is mentioned but is not essential.

Clinical description

The median age of onset of bulimia nervosa is 18, which is slightly later than that of anorexia nervosa; again, females predominate at a ratio of 10:1. All social classes are affected. Patients usually have normal body weight. It is more common in groups where weight and shape issues are important, such as ballet dancers, models and actresses. Approximately a third of patients have a history of anorexia nervosa and another third a history of obesity.

A characteristic set of attitudes to shape and weight is a key feature; it resembles the overvalued ideas that are common in anorexia nervosa and has been termed ‘a morbid fear of fatness’. Preoccupation with weight and shape concerns is the driving force behind the abnormal eating behaviours and can interfere with concentration and social life.

A history of weight loss preceding onset is typical and there is usually an attempt to follow a strict diet, with protracted periods of fasting. Bingeing has not been clearly defined but there is a move to use operational criteria such as objective overeating (1000 kcal or more) accompanied by a sense of loss of control, followed by feelings of shame and disgust.

The content of binges varies, from an array of ‘forbidden’ palatable foods to foodstuffs that would normally be regarded with disgust (leftovers, or food from the dustbin). The usual precipitants for binges are transgressions of self-imposed dietary rules, or feelings of depression, anxiety, loneliness and boredom. Swollen parotid glands can give the face a rounded appearance; the teeth may be capped or smooth and shiny, and a callus may be present on the dorsum of the hand (Russell’s sign).

Extreme attempts to control weight and shape are used and are notable for both their ingenuity and for the tenacity with which patients pursue them in the face of dangers to their health. The most common method is self-induced vomiting. Dehydration and severe electrolyte abnormalities can develop. Women with coexistent medical problems use some of the most dangerous methods of weight loss. Patients with diabetes mellitus will omit their insulin and run their blood glucose at high levels, which can lead to coma and severe complications such as retinopathy and neuropathy and a multiplication of the risk (Nielsen *et al*, 1998). Patients with Crohn’s disease may fail to comply with steroid treatment, and those with thyroid disease may take thyroxine to excess.

Case example

Charlotte grew up in a rural community. Her father used physical and sexual violence to control the family. She left home at the age of 16, and with little money for food she lost weight. She began to binge eat, and self-induced vomiting and laxative misuse rapidly ensued. She binged several times a day on a gruel that she made from flour and water. Her laxative consumption gradually increased so that, in the mornings, after taking a full bottle of laxatives, she vomited and was unable to walk without feeling faint. She described her body with loathing and spent over an hour each morning finding suitable clothes from her wardrobe (size range 10–16). She lost many friends because she often phoned to cancel an arrangement at the last minute if she felt too fat to go out. Her first job was in a bakers, which she quickly lost as she was caught stealing food. She was unable to maintain any job for longer than a few months as her concentration was poor and she had many days off sick. Her debt gradually increased and was a source of grave concern. She had a series of short relationships, usually with men who abused her in a variety of ways. She tried a variety of medications to control her weight. Initially she obtained diet pills from private slimming clinics, but then bought amphetamines or ecstasy. Over the years, excessive alcohol consumption became a regular part of her life, and she described being less concerned about her weight when drunk. She was regularly admitted to hospital after episodes of self-harm, which usually involved cutting herself or overdoses.

Measurement

The interviews and schedules described for anorexia nervosa also apply for bulimia nervosa. The Bulimia Investigatory Test, Edinburgh (BITE) (Henderson & Freeman, 1987) and the Eating Disorders Examination Questionnaire (EDE-Q) (Fairburn & Begley, 1994) are widely used self-report questionnaires.

Differential diagnosis

Binge eating can accompany a variety of medical conditions. A tendency to gluttony may occur in frontal lobe dementia. Prader–Willi syndrome is also associated with gross episodes of overeating, as is the Kleine–Levine syndrome.

Comorbidity

Additional psychiatric features are common; depressive and anxiety symptoms predominate. These patients often have disorders of impulse control: self-mutilation (10%), suicide attempts (30%), promiscuity (10%) and shoplifting (20%). Alcohol misuse occurs in 10–15%. Patients often fulfil the criteria for borderline personality disorder; the association between eating disorders and personality disorders is also discussed in Chapter 18 (page 456).

Epidemiology

The incidence of cases of bulimia nervosa presenting to primary care in the UK is similar to that found elsewhere in the world. It increased during the 1980s and reached a plateau in the 1990s. There is an associated age cohort effect, with a marked increase in the risk for women born after the 1950s; this has been shown in studies that have used the most sophisticated methods, that is, with an initial screening instrument followed by a later interview. The prevalence rate of bulimia nervosa in young women has consistently been found to be about 1%. However, the prevalence of a range of clinically relevant eating problems that do not necessarily meet the full criteria – including eating disorder not otherwise specified and atypical eating disorders – could be as high as 7% of young women. Bulimia nervosa is therefore 5–10 times more common than anorexia nervosa.

Aetiology

Two systematic reviews of risk factors are useful sources of information (Stice, 2002; Jacobi *et al*, 2004). Sociocultural risk factors (Western influences) appear to be of more relevance for bulimia nervosa than for anorexia (Klump *et al*, 2003). Evidence from case–control and cohort studies converges in suggesting that bulimia nervosa seems to arise as the result of exposure to:

1 premorbid dieting and related risk factors (premorbid and parental obesity, an innate tendency to overeat and enjoy food, critical comments by the family about weight, shape or eating)

2 general risk factors for psychiatric disorders (including exposure to parental psychiatric disorders such as depression, alcohol and substance misuse during childhood, low parental contact and yet high parental expectations, abuse and neglect).

The two classes of risk factor contribute independently to the risk.

There is a familial disposition to bulimia nervosa; the risk for first-degree relatives is increased fourfold. The variance in liability due to common genetic factors for bulimia nervosa is between 54% and 83%. Eating disorder symptoms (binge eating, self-induced vomiting and dietary restraint) are also moderately heritable, as are pathological attitudes such as body dissatisfaction, eating and weight concerns, and weight preoccupation. Klump *et al* (2001) suggested that the heritability estimates for bulimia nervosa may be more variable across cultures than those for anorexia nervosa. For example, in a culture where there is a large variability in exposure to the thin ideal or in access to food, genetic estimates may be much lower. The inherited risk may be part of a tendency to obesity secondary to heightened appetite. A preliminary but unconfirmed study (Bulik *et al*, 2003) suggested that there is linkage to chromosome 10. Affective lability and impulsivity, which are common features, may also result from inherited factors or may arise in the context of developmental adversity.

Assessment

People with bulimia nervosa are less ambivalent about treatment than people with anorexia nervosa. They generally wish to stop bingeing. However, they may still be quite reluctant to change their weight control strategies. Eating pathology and the methods of weight control they have adopted need to be fully assessed. It is important to ascertain during history taking whether there are any significant medical consequences. The enquiry should cover teeth, salivary glands, gastrointestinal function (bleeding, regurgitation), and kidney and endocrine function. A physical examination and a screen for electrolyte abnormalities are also required. The presence of any other psychiatric comorbidity should be established, as this may lead to treatment difficulties. Social difficulties and current life stresses should be also sought, as they may play a role in maintaining the illness. The initial assessment should also focus on the patient's reasons for 'giving up bulimia' because, during treatment, the therapist can also utilise these reasons to encourage perseverance.

Treatment

Treatment research in bulimia nervosa has been summarised in several systematic reviews, which are in the Cochrane library (Hay & Bacaltchuk, 2000, 2001; Hay *et al*, 2003); drug treatments have been reviewed by Bacaltchuk *et al* (2000). The NICE (2004) guidelines gave a grade A recommendation for cognitive–behavioural treatment (CBT) for bulimia nervosa. CBT is the form of psychological treatment that has been best researched to date. A manual that describes the standard CBT treatment adopted in treatment studies for bulimia nervosa is available (Fairburn *et al*, 1993).

The CBT model of the maintenance of bulimia nervosa is shown in Fig. 24.3. CBT delivered in a self-help or guided self-help format seems to be almost as efficacious as a full course of CBT (usually 20 sessions). There is also evidence supporting the use of interpersonal treatment, although this is less strong. Medication is less effective than psychological treatments, and the combination of medication and psychological treatment seems to be more effective than either treatment on its own, but has higher drop-out rates.

Many centres adopt a stepped-care approach, starting with the least intensive, least costly and least invasive intervention. As the first step, a CBT self-help book

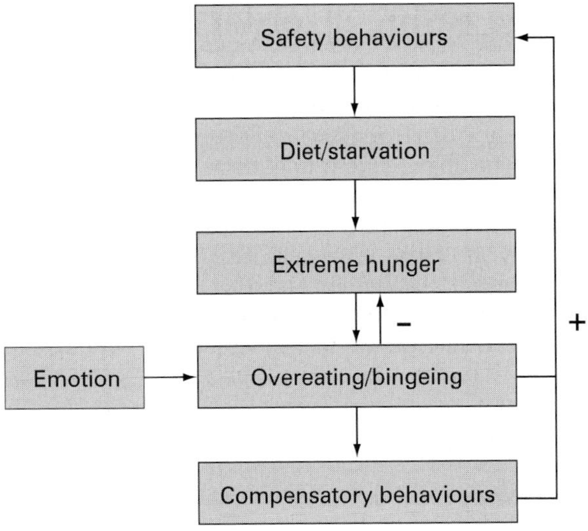

Fig. 24.3 Cognitive model for bulimia nervosa.

may be valuable (Cooper & Fairburn, 1993; Fairburn, 1995; Schmidt & Treasure, 1997) or a CD-ROM can be helpful.

Cognitive–behavioural treatment

The cognitive model for bulimia nervosa is illustrated in Fig. 24.3. The first phase of treatment includes an explanation about the cognitive model of bulimia nervosa and the vicious circle of bingeing. One of the basic maintaining cycles is that the over-consumption of food leads to regret and anxiety about having broken strict dietary rules. This then leads to reversing behaviours (fasting, vomiting, laxatives, etc.). However, these in turn exacerbate feelings of starvation, which leads to more craving and a predisposition to overeat, and the so cycle starts again.

Phase 1: building motivation

As indicated above, people with bulimia nervosa are generally less ambivalent about change than are those with anorexia nervosa, but even so it is still worth spending time discussing their mixed feelings about change. The positive aspects of bulimia nervosa will centre on the regulation of weight and emotions. Often patients may have been trying to control their weight for many years and will report feelings of prolonged victimisation about their weight, shape and eating, and may have experimented with numerous diets that have had little effect. They may have discovered that vomiting is an effective method of losing large amounts of weight. Bulimic behaviours can dampen down intense emotional reactions and hence may be reinforcing for those who have a degree of emotional dysregulation.

In parallel to the approach with anorexia nervosa (see Box 24.7), it is helpful to probe for the negative consequences of bulimia nervosa in all domains of life. The impact on physical health includes temperature sensitivity of the teeth, loss of dental enamel and toothache. Cramps, fatigue and gastrointestinal pain and disturbance are common. Rebound oedema occurs following the use of diuretics, vomiting or laxatives, which commonly features in reversing behaviours.

The common associated psychological features include depression, guilt, irritability and poor concentration. A subgroup share the same compulsive behaviours as seen in anorexia nervosa. A disruption in the social network is also common, as people with bulimia nervosa become unpredictable; for example, they let people down and arrive late because of their tendency to spend long periods of time checking their body. The profound change in mood can result in neglect and disinterest in friendships or avoidance because of the fear of eating with others, while in the work situation mood changes can result in impaired concentration and increased sick leave. People with bulimia nervosa are more likely to get involved in romantic relationships than those with anorexia nervosa, but these relationships may be impaired by the disorder. Because the illness has a later onset, often when people have left home, there is less family involvement. Otherwise, problems may arise over the use of the bathroom, or eccentric behaviours around food, including stealing from others. There may also be additional problems with drug and alcohol misuse.

In this initial phase of treatment, the therapist examines the decisional balance and the motivation to change. The therapist builds up feelings of dissonance by encouraging people to project themselves, still ill, into the future. Any positive aspects of the bulimia need to be replaced with other strategies; for example, someone who has always had a weight problem may need to think about introducing more exercise. People who use bulimia as an emotional regulator should be encouraged to find other self-soothing and comforting strategies, such as relaxation.

Phase 2: a functional analysis

The therapist works with patients to help them to construct and investigate their own functional analysis. This includes tracking the vicious circle of unhelpful behaviours and looking at the events and the feelings that trigger a binge, as well as the thoughts and emotions that accompany the reversing activities.

A key therapeutic tool is the food diary. This is used to monitor eating patterns throughout the day and is used to look for links between eating, emotions and behaviours. Patients are encouraged to record what and how much they eat, the time they eat it and also to record what they were thinking and feeling at the time.

Phase 3: challenging cognitions

The next phase of treatment involves identifying the thoughts that trigger the emotions and behaviours of bulimia nervosa. Often there are a large number of negative automatic thoughts, linked to low self-esteem. People with bulimia nervosa display many of the common errors of thinking found in depression, such as focusing on negative aspects and discounting any positive ones. This is often accompanied by an extreme black-and-white way of thinking, in which something is either all bad or all good. Another common thinking trap is the use of conditional statements ('should', 'must' and 'ought'). There may also be a tendency to jump to conclusions and assume that bad things will happen. One of the tasks of cognitive therapy is to teach the person to catch and monitor these extreme and unhelpful thinking errors.

The next step is to challenge these appraisals. Sometimes it is helpful to ask patients with bulimia to consider what other people would say if they could hear these thoughts. Other challenges to these thinking biases include exploring the consequences of the thought and whether it is helpful to have such a thought.

Phase 4: implementing change
In the later stages of treatment the therapist and patient work together to set detailed goals and targets, which should include a clear plan to implement change and how to overcome blocks. Teaching skills such as assertiveness and problem solving may help the patient overcome the common hassles and difficulties that often seem to overwhelm someone with bulimia nervosa. Associated depression or anxiety may lead to avoidance or decreased activity.

The main aim is for the patient to be able to eat normal meals, regularly, throughout the day, and these should be shared with others whenever possible. It is sometimes helpful to list foods in terms of how frightening they are and to plan a gradual programme of exposure. Thoughts about body shape and weight can be tackled with techniques such as cognitive restructuring and behavioural experiments. Extreme behavioural reactions sometimes occur, and these include excessive focusing on bodily appearance, with mirror gazing or body checking, or the opposite phenomenon of avoidance and failing to attend at all to appearance. Some people focus excessively on thin models in magazines rather than considering the generality of women's size and shape.

At the very end of treatment, plans should be developed to cope with a brief lapse as well as strategies to help prevent a proper relapse.

Outcome

Since bulimia nervosa has been recognised only since 1979, there are few long-term outcome follow-up studies, but one of the largest is that of Keel *et al* (1999). These workers followed 173 people who met DSM–III criteria for bulimia nervosa (the study covered patients presenting during the 1980s, when DSM–III was the diagnostic standard), who were followed for an average of 11 years. At follow-up, only 10% continued to meet full diagnostic criteria for bulimia but a further 20% continued to engage in some bingeing or purging behaviours. The remaining 70% were either in full or partial remission and, taking into account other follow-up studies, these authors suggested that around 50% could attain full remission. At follow-up, only 0.6% had developed anorexia nervosa which met full diagnostic criteria, indicating that the illness type probably remained true to form and there was no switching from bulimia to anorexia during the follow-up period. Mortality was low (0.5%) as there was only one death due to suicide, which the authors contrasted with the very much higher crude mortality rate associated with anorexia nervosa, of 5.9% (Sullivan, 1995). There were very few predictors of a good outcome, but a poorer outcome was associated with a longer duration of illness, as well as substance misuse at the initial presentation (Keel *et al*, 1999).

Binge eating disorder

As the criteria for the condition now known as bulimia nervosa have evolved and become more specific, there has been a corresponding increase in the size of the group who do not exactly fulfil these diagnostic criteria, that is, who have 'eating disorder not otherwise specified'. Spitzer *et al* (1991) suggested that an additional category of 'binge eating disorder' could be defined from within this group and this condition appears in DSM–IV as a proposed category pending further research (American Psychiatric Association, 1994).

Epidemiology

The incidence may be highest in individuals with type II diabetes and obesity. In weight control clinics the prevalence rate is around 30%, with a female preponderence (a 3:2 sex ratio), and in non-patient community samples a prevalence rate of 0.7–4% is reported in DSM–IV.

Clinical features

People with binge eating disorders have a bimodal age at onset. Some develop their symptoms early, that is, at the mean age of 11 years, and a second group develop the disorder in their mid-20s. People with binge eating disorder have episodes of bingeing as defined for bulimia nervosa but they do not compensate for this with extreme behaviours such as vomiting or taking laxatives, fasting or the use of excessive exercise, which occurs in bulimia, and their absence is the main diagnostic distinction from bulimia. Thus, these people are often obese. Indicators of impaired control include eating very rapidly, eating until feeling uncomfortably full, eating large amounts of food when not hungry, eating alone because of embarrassment over how much one is eating, and feelings of disgust, guilt or depression after overeating. There is some distress both during and after the binge episodes and there may also be long-term concerns over body weight and shape. The levels of psychopathology observed in individuals with binge eating disorder fall between the high levels seen in bulimia nervosa and the low levels seen in simple obesity. Emotional and personality difficulties are common and there may be impaired work and social functioning.

Aetiology

Many of the risk factors for bulimia nervosa are shared by people with binge eating disorder. A history of sexual or physical abuse is common, as is a history of bullying by peers.

Treatment and outcome

Most of the treatments applied in bulimia nervosa, such as self-help approaches using CBT manuals or the CD-ROM for bulimia, have been applied to people with binge eating disorder. Efficacy in terms of reduction in binge eating is good, although there is usually little success in terms of weight loss for those who are obese.

Antidepressants or anti-obesity drugs are being evaluated and do appear to be effective in reducing weight. The outcome of community-ascertained binge eating disorder is better than that reported in bulimia nervosa. Thus, in one study, by 5 years only 18% had any form of clinical eating disorder, although 39% fulfilled the criteria for obesity (Fairburn *et al*, 2000).

References

American Psychiatric Association (1980) *Diagnostic and Statistical Manual of Mental Disorders* (3rd edn) (DSM–III). Washington, DC: APA.

American Psychiatric Association (1987) *Diagnostic and Statistical Manual of Mental Disorders* (3rd edn, revised) (DSM–III–R). Washington, DC: APA.

American Psychiatric Association (1994) *Diagnostic and Statistical Manual of Mental Disorders* (4th edn) (DSM–IV). Washington, DC: APA.

American Psychiatric Association (2000) Practice guideline for the treatment of patients with eating disorders (revision). American Psychiatric Association Work Group on Eating Disorders. *American Journal of Psychiatry*, **157**, 1–39.

Bacaltchuk, J., Hay, P. & Mari, J. J. (2000) Antidepressants versus placebo for the treatment of bulimia nervosa: a systematic reveviw. *Australian and New Zealand Journal of Psychiatry*, **34**, 310–317.

Bell, R. M. (1985) *Holy Anorexia*. Chicago, IL: University of Chicago Press.

Blair, C., Freeman, C. & Cull, A. (1995) The families of anorexia nervosa and cystic fibrosis patients. *Psychological Medicine*, **25**, 985–993.

Bruch, H. (1974) *Eating Disorders: Obesity, Anorexia Nervosa and the Person Within*. London: Routledge & Kegan Paul.

Bulik, C. M., Devlin, B., Bacanu, S. A., *et al* (2003) Significant linkage on chromosome 10p in families with bulimia nervosa. *American Journal of Human Genetics*, **72**, 200–207.

Cantwell, D. P., Sturzenburger, S., Burroughs, J., *et al* (1977) Anorexia nervosa: an affective disorder? *Archives of General Psychiatry*, **34**, 1087–1090.

Cnattingius, S., Hultman, C. M., Dahl, M., *et al* (1999) Very preterm birth, birth trauma and the risk of anorexia nervosa among girls. *Archives of General Psychiatry*, **56**, 634–638.

Cooper, Z. & Fairburn, C. G. (1987) The Eating Disorder Examination. A semi-structured interview for the assessment of the specific psychopathology of eating disorders. *International Journal of Eating Disorders*, **6**, 1–8.

Cooper, P. & Fairburn, C. G. (1993) *Bulimia Nervosa and Binge Eating. A Guide to Recovery*. London: Constable and Robinson.

Crisp, A. H. (1980) *Anorexia Nervosa: Let Me Be*. London: Plenum.

Fairburn, C. G. (1995) *Overcoming Binge Eating*. New York: Guilford Press.

Fairburn, C. G. & Begley, S. (1994) Assessment of eating disorders: interview or self-report questionnaire? *International Journal of Eating Disorders*, **16**, 363–370.

Fairburn, C. G., Marcus, M. D. & Wilson, G. T. (1993) Cognitive behaviour therapy for binge eating and bulimia nervosa: a comprehensive treatment manual. In *Binge Eating: Nature, Assessment and Treatment* (eds C. G. Fairburn & G. T. Wilson), pp. 361–404. New York: Guilford Press.

Fairburn, C. G., Cooper, Z., Doll, H. A., *et al* (1999) Risk factors for anorexia nervosa: three integrated case–control comparisons. *Archives of General Psychiatry*, **56**, 468–476.

Fairburn, C. G., Cooper, Z., Doll, H. A., *et al* (2000) The natural course of bulimia nervosa and binge eating disorder in young women. *Archives of General Psychiatry*, **57**, 659–665.

Fowler, R. (1871) *A Complete History of the Case of the Welsh Fasting Girl (Sarah Jacob)*. London: Henry Renshaw.

Garner, D. M. & Garfinkel, P. E. (1979) The Eating Attitudes Test: an index of the symptoms of anorexia nervosa. *Psychological Medicine*, **9**, 273–279.

Garner, D. M., Olmsed, M. P. & Polivy, J. (1983) Development and validation of a multidimensional eating disorder inventory for anorexia and bulimia. *International Journal of Eating Disorders*, **2**, 15–34.

Gowers, S. G. & Shore, A. (2001) Development of weight and shape concerns in the aetiology of eating disorders. *British Journal of Psychiatry*, **179**, 236–242.

Grice, D. E., Halmi, K. A., Fichter, M. M., *et al* (2002) Evidence for a susceptibility gene for anorexia nervosa on chromosome 1. *American Journal of Human Genetics*, **70**, 787–792.

Gull, W. W. (1868) The address in medicine to the annual meeting of the British Medical Association at Oxford. *Lancet*, 8 August, 171–176.

Gull, W. W. (1873) Proceedings of the Clinical Society of London. *BMJ*, *i*, 527–529.

Halmi, K. A. (1985) Relationship of the eating disorders to depression: biological similarities and differences. *International Journal of Eating Disorders*, **4**, 667–680.

Halmi, K. A., Eckert, E., Cohen, J., *et al* (1991) Comorbidity of psychiatric diagnosis in anorexia nervosa. *Archives of General Psychiatry*, **48**, 718.

Hay, P. J. & Bacaltchuk, J. (2000) Psychotherapy for bulimia nervosa and binging (Cochrane review). *Cochrane Database Systematic Reviews*, **(4)**, CD000562.

Hay, P. J. & Bacaltchuk, J. (2001) Bulimia nervosa. *Clinical Evidence*, **6**, 642–651.

Hay, P., Bacaltchuk, J., Claudino, A., *et al* (2003) Individual psychotherapy in the outpatient treatment of adults with anorexia nervosa. *Cochrane Database of Systematic Reviews*, **(4)**, CD003909.

Henderson, M. & Freeman, C. L. (1987) A self-rating scale for bulimia. The BITE. *British Journal of Psychiatry*, **150**, 18–24.

Hoek, H. W., van Harten, P. N., van Hoeken, D., *et al* (1998) Lack of relation between culture and anorexia nervosa – results of an incidence study on Curacao. *New England Journal of Medicine*, **338**, 1231–1232.

Jacobi, C., Hayward, C., de Zwaan, M., *et al* (2004) Coming to terms with risk factors for eating disorders: application of risk terminology and suggestions for a general taxonomy. *Psychological Bulletin*, **130**, 19–65.

Karwautz, A., Rabe-Hesketh, S., Hu, X., *et al* (2001) Individual-specific risk factors for anorexia nervosa: a pilot study using a discordant sister-pair design. *Psychological Medicine*, **31**, 317–329.

Kasvikis, Y. G., Tsakiris, F., Marks, I. M., *et al* (1986) Past history of anorexia nervosa in women with obsessive–compulsive disorder. *International Journal of Eating Disorders*, **5**, 1069–1075.

Keel, P. K. & Klump, K. L. (2003) Are eating disorders culture-bound syndromes? Implications for conceptualizing their etiology. *Psychological Bulletin*, **129**, 747–769.

Keel, P. K., Mitchell, J. E., Miller, K. B., *et al* (1999) Long term outcome of bulimia nervosa. *Archives of General Psychiatry*, **56**, 63–69.

Keys, A., Brozak, J., Henshall, A., *et al* (1950) *The Biology of Human Starvation*, Vol. II, pp. 850–857. Minneapolis, MN: University of Minnesota Press.

Klump, K. L., Miller, K. B., Keel, P. K., *et al* (2001) Genetic and environmental influences on anorexia nervosa syndromes in a population based twin sample. *Psychological Medicine*, **31**, 737–740.

Klump, K. L., McGue, M. & Iacono, W. G. (2003) Differential heritability of eating attitudes and behaviors in prepubertal versus pubertal twins. *International Journal of Eating Disorders*, **33**, 287–292.

Lasegue, E. C. (1873) On hysterical anorexia. *Medical Times Gazette*, **2**, 265–269.

Lee, S. (1991) Anorexia nervosa in Hong Kong: a Chinese perspective. *Psychological Medicine*, **21**, 703–712.

Lilenfeld, L. R., Kaye, W. H., Greeno, C. G., *et al* (1998) A controlled family study of anorexia nervosa and bulimia nervosa: psychiatric disorders in first degree relatives and effects of proband co-morbidity. *Archives of General Psychiatry*, **55**, 603–610.

Lucas, A. R., Beard, M. C., O'Fallon, M. W., *et al* (1991) 50-year trends in the incidence of anorexia nervosa in Rochester, MN: a population-based study. *American Journal of Psychiatry*, **148**, 917–922.

Marcé, L. A. (1860) On a form of hypochondriacal delirium occurring consecutive to dyspepsia and characterized by refusal of food. *Journal of Psychological Medicine and Mental Pathology*, **13**, 204–206.

Minuchin, S., Rosman, B. L., Liebman, R., *et al* (1978) *Psychosomatic Families: Anorexia Nervosa in Context*. Cambridge, MA: Harvard University Press.

Morton, R. (1694) *Phthisiologia: Or, a Treatise of Consumptions*. London: Smith & Walford.

NICE (2004) *Clinical Guideline for Eating Disorders: Core Interventions in the Treatment and Management of Anorexia Nervosa,*

Bulimia Nervosa and Related Eating Disorders. Guideline No. CG009. London: National Institute for Health and Clinical Excellence.

Nielsen, S., Moller-Madsen, S., Isager, T., *et al* (1998) Standardised mortality in eating disorders – a quantitative summary of previously published and new evidence. *Journal of Psychosomatic Research*, **44**, 413–434.

Orbach, S. (1986) *Hunger Strike*. Harmondsworth: Penguin.

Parry Jones, B. & Parry Jones, W. L. (1990) Bulimia: an archival review of its history. *Psychosomatic Medicine*, **10**, 129–143.

Rastam, M., Gillberg, C. & Garton, M. (1989) Anorexia nervosa in a Swedish urban region: a population-based study. *British Journal of Psychiatry*, **155**, 642–646.

Russell, G. F. M. (1979) Bulimia nervosa: an ominous variant of anorexia nervosa. *Psychological Medicine*, **9**, 429–488.

Ryle, J. A. (1936) Anorexia nervosa. *Lancet*, *ii*, 893–899.

Schmidt, U. & Treasure, J. (1997) *A Clinician's Guide to Management of Bulimia Nervosa (Motivational Enhancement Therapy for Bulimia Nervosa)*. Hove: Psychology Press.

Selvini-Palazzoli, M. & Viaro, M. (1988) The anorectic process in the family: a six-stage model as a guide for individual therapy. *Family Process*, **27**, 129–148.

Smorawinska, A., Korman, E. & Rajewski, A. (2001) Disturbances of the thyroid function in patients with anorexia nervosa. [In Polish.] *Endokrynologia, Diabetologia i Choroby Przemiany Materii Wieku Rozwojowego*, **7**, 81–84.

Solzhenitsyn, A. (1963) *One Day in the Life of Ivan Denisovich*. Harmondsworth: Penguin.

Spitzer, R. L., Devlin, B., Walsh, A., *et al* (1991) Binge eating disorder: to be or not to be in DSM-IV. *International Journal of Eating Disorders*, **10**, 627–629.

Stice, E. (2002) Risk and maintenance factors for eating pathology: a meta-analytic review. *Psychological Bulletin*, **128**, 825–848.

Strober, M. & Katz, J. L. (1987) Do eating disorders and affective disorders share a common etiology? A dissenting opinion. *International Journal of Eating Disorders*, **6**, 171–180.

Strober, M., Lampert, C., Morrell, W., *et al* (1990) A controlled family study of anorexia nervosa: evidence of familial aggregation and lack of shared transmission with affective disorders. *International Journal of Eating Disorders*, **9**, 239–254.

Strober, M., Freeman, R., Lampert, C., *et al* (2000) Controlled family study of anorexia nervosa and bulimia nervosa: evidence of shard liability and transmission of partial syndromes. *American Journal of Psychiatry*, **157**, 393–401.

Stunkard, A. J. (1959) Eating patterns and obesity. *Psychiatric Quality*, **33**, 284–292.

Sullivan, P. F. (1995) Mortality in anorexia nervosa. *American Journal of Psychiatry*, **152**, 1073–1074.

Treasure, J. L. & Schmidt, U. (2004) Anorexia nervosa. *Clinical Evidence*, **11**, 1192–1203.

Treasure, J. & Szmukler, G. (1995) Medical and surgical complications of chronic anorexia nervosa. In *Handbook of Eating Disorders: Treatment and Research* (eds G. Szmukler, C. Dare & J. L. Treasure), pp. 197–220. Chichester: Wiley.

Treasure, J. L. & Ward, A. (1997) A practical guide to the use of motivational interviewing in anorexia nervosa. *European Eating Disorders Review*, **5**, 102–114.

Turnbull, S., Ward, A., Treasure, J., *et al* (1996) The demand for eating disorder care. An epidemiological study using the general practice research database. *British Journal of Psychiatry*, **169**, 705–712.

Uher, R., Brammer, M. J., Murphy, T., *et al* (2003) Recovery and chronicity in anorexia nervosa: brain activity associated with differential outcomes. *Biological Psychiatry*, **54**, 934–942.

World Health Organization (1992) *The Tenth Revision of the International Classification of Diseases* (ICD–10). Geneva: WHO.

CHAPTER 25

Perinatal psychiatric disorders

George Stein

History

Among the very earliest descriptions of serious mental illness is Hippocrates' account of puerperal insanity. Hippocrates, who lived in the 5th century BC in ancient Greece, cited the case of the wife of Epicrates, in the town of Cyzicus, who gave birth to twins, then developed severe insomnia, became restless on the 6th day, delirious on the 11th day, speechless on the 16th day and died on the 17th day. Hippocrates offered two explanations: first, that the lochia had been suppressed and redirected to the brain, which had caused mania; and second, that the mania was the result of an influx of blood into the breast (Brockington, 1996).

Many more clinical descriptive accounts followed over the next 2000 years (see Brockington, 1996, for details) but the modern era probably starts with Esquirol's account, based on his work at the Salpêtriére during the Napoleonic era. He described 92 cases, of which 37 started within 2 weeks of childbirth. Of the 92 cases, 49 were of mania, 35 melancholy and monomania, whereas 'dementia' (probably schizophrenia) occurred in only 8 – a pattern not dissimilar to the diagnostic profile of present-day admissions. Gooch (1829), a lecturer in midwifery at St Bartholomew's Hospital in London, made the important distinction between fatal and non-fatal delirium, the fatal type being due to sepsis, the non-fatal variety being caused by insanity.

Esquirol had a brilliant pupil, Marcé (1858), who wrote the first substantive textbook on the subject, *Traité de la folie des femmes encientes, des nouvelles accoucheés et des nourrices*. He described 310 cases, of which 79 were his own; 9% started in pregnancy, 58% had an early puerperal onset and 33% had a later onset and were termed 'lactational psychosis'. He considered ways in which these illnesses both resembled and differed from non-puerperal mental disorder, which was to be a recurring conundrum of the 20th-century literature.

Patients with a puerperal psychosis were admitted to the new asylums of the 19th century often for 1 or 2 years, until their illnesses remitted spontaneously. This comprised around 7% of all admissions (Brockington, 1996). They suffered from a high mortality, of around 10%, usually the result of debility, infection or suicide, but the introduction of electroconvulsive therapy (ECT) in the 1940s led to a dramatic fall in the mortality of the illness. Today, the prognosis is generally held to be good, although there are still occasional suicides (the biggest single cause of maternal mortality in the first post-partum year).

An important innovation in the management of puerperal mental disorder was made by Thomas Main (1958), a psychoanalyst, when he arranged for the first joint admission of a mother and baby to the Cassel Hospital in London, and so ushered in the modern era of joint admissions for mothers with their babies, which is now common practice in the UK, Australia and some European countries but is rather uncommon elsewhere and is not practised in the USA.

The most recent developments have focused less on the puerperal psychoses and more on the early detection and treatment of milder cases of postnatal depression found in the community. Post-partum disorders comprise a significant portion of the case load of any catchment area team, and are usually classified into three groups:

1 the severe and life-threatening post-partum psychoses, which follow around 2/1000 deliveries

2 the postnatal depressions and other related disorders, such as panic disorder, anxiety and obsessional states, all starting in the postnatal period, and which (as a spectrum of neurotic disorders) occur in around 10% of women

3 the 'maternity blues', which occur in around 50% of women and which is a normal reaction and not a clinical disorder.

A fourth group of disorders – bonding difficulties which may result in child abuse – have a complex multi-factorial aetiology, but a perinatal psychiatrist may be required to assess such cases and this topic is covered later in this chapter. The chapter also briefly covers premenstrual syndrome and the menopause.

Puerperal psychoses

The onset of puerperal psychoses may be abrupt and frightening both for the patient and for those around. Sometimes, but not always, the first 2 days are relatively symptom free, and then the illness sometimes gradually, but often abruptly, declares itself between days 3 and 7, with the peak time onset being around days 5 and 6. Thus, most cases will have started in the first 2 weeks, although a small number may start at any time in the first 6 months, occasionally during the first premenstrual phase, or with the onset of weaning. Early signs include restless activity, disinhibition, fleeting anger and negativistic behaviour, profound insomnia, anxiety and a state of fear. Because many women are experiencing the maternity blues at this time, the initial diagnosis is often confused with severe blues, but the appearance of bizarre psychotic material will alarm relatives or nurses on the post-partum wards and a psychiatric referral is usually made as an emergency. The initial state is usually one of delirium with an undifferentiated, rapidly changing psychotic state. This early undifferentiated picture sometimes shows some resemblance to delirium tremens, except there is no alcohol misuse.

Karnosh & Hope (1937) described puerperal delirium as:

> 'panic, sudden aversion and mistrust of relatives, misidentification, hallucinosis, sing song chat, and disintegration of poor affect, together with a rapid pulse and fever ranging from 99°–102°F. This delirium usually abates but mania, depression, schizophrenia, occasionally normality and rarely even death may ensue.'

The presence of an elevated temperature ('milk fever') is only an occasional feature appearing at the onset of a psychosis (in the developed world such infections are rare) but may be a source of diagnostic confusion: it still requires that blood cultures and other tests for infection are instituted. The initial undifferentiated picture of delirium usually passes fairly rapidly into a more classical psychotic picture.

Affective disorders

Puerperal mania

Puerperal mania is among the most florid conditions encountered in psychiatric practice, and the motor symptoms of mania, hyperactivity and distractibility are marked. The onset may be abrupt, but more often there is increasing irritability or elation, with severe blues around the 4th or 5th day post-partum. Sleep is invariably severely disturbed, with patients waking in the early hours and then displaying manic behaviour. Some women have a pleasant or humorous grandiosity, but many are paranoid or querulous, believing themselves to be totally competent mothers and fiercely resenting any suggestion otherwise. A degree of sexual disinhibition is common. One patient, after trying to throw herself through a closed window pane, arrived in hospital wearing pink high-heeled shoes, sprayed herself heavily with perfume, and told the ward staff she had come to a party. Savage (1875) wrote:

> 'patients are often seized with an erotic tendency. I have several times judged a case of insanity to be puerperal from the mincing gait and lascivious looks of the patient.'

Patients with puerperal mania tend to have more confusion and more disorganised communications, are less competent and require more in the way of task supervision than patients with non-puerperal mania (Brockington *et al*, 1982). Some episodes of puerperal mania switch into depression, which may persist for few months, but others may settle into euthymia without passing through a depressive phase. Mixed affective states are also commonly encountered post-partum, and these are particularly dangerous because they combine the boundless energy of mania with the suicidal urges of depression.

Post-partum psychotic depression

Severe depression usually presents sub-acutely, in the first 10 days. It is often confused with severe blues, but the mood fails to lighten and depressive delusions appear, such as delusions of unworthiness, delusions concerning the baby (e.g. that the baby would be better off dead), infanticidal urges or declarations that the baby should be adopted. These may be accompanied by severe psychomotor retardation, depressive stupor or suicidal acts. Although the diagnosis is obvious, the condition is extremely dangerous – much more so than the rather more florid manic conditions.

Hospitalisation for depression usually occurs as an emergency at the request of relatives, staff on post-natal wards or social workers who are fearful for the life and safety of both mother and baby. These severe depressions follow around 1 per 1000 births. A small number of single women with severe personality disorder and multiple social problems may also gain admission to mother and baby units, with also initially apparently life-threatening situations, although their depressions are generally less severe, and the relative absence of the biological symptoms of depression makes the diagnosis of a non-psychotic disorder more obvious.

Puerperal schizophrenia and schizoaffective disorder

Puerperal schizophrenia is rare, and rates of 4–16% in series of women with puerperal psychoses are given in most UK studies (Kendell *et al*, 1987). Higher rates are reported from some non-Western countries, such as 22–34% in India (Agrawal *et al*, 1990), even when modern diagnostic criteria are used. Most cases of puerperal schizophrenia are the result of pregnancies occurring in women with previous schizophrenia, although in some instances the schizophrenia may start after childbirth. Although rare, the prognosis is much worse than for puerperal affective disorder, and the ability to care for the new-born infant is often severely impaired.

As with the other puerperal psychoses, schizophrenia may have a delirious onset and this may progress through both manic and melancholic phases before the full picture of 'dementia' emerges (Savage, 1875); the disorder is then indistinguishable from non-puerperal schizophrenia. Delusions and hallucinations often focus around the baby. Thus, one woman with previous paranoid delusions believed her baby to be a cat. Another, with catatonic features and marked echolalia, began to scream loudly every time her baby cried.

Most authorities do not believe that puerperal schizophrenia comprises a separate schizophrenic subgroup, but at least in the early phases there often is an affective colouring to the clinical picture. Although pure pictures of mania, depression or schizophrenia may occur in the postnatal period, many cases present with a mixed picture of both schizophreniform and affective features. Sometimes it is possible to discern a classic schizo-manic or schizo-depressive picture, in which case a diagnosis of schizoaffective disorder should be made.

Case example

Jane became confused immediately after delivery. She gradually became more depressed and was admitted 5 days after delivery. She expressed a delusional belief that her husband was an imposter and also feared that her baby would be sexually abused by a child molester, and asked her doctor to teach her baby not to talk to strangers. She was unable to cope with the day-to-day management of her baby because she said opposing forces were inserting clicks into her mind. After a 4-month admission with little improvement, the addition of lithium to her antipsychotic drugs led to a rapid resolution of her illness and her diagnosis was changed from schizophrenia to schizoaffective disorder.

Distinguishing schizoaffective disorder and other puerperal psychoses from schizophrenia is a matter of the greatest importance because the long-term prognosis with regard to infant and child care is sometimes very poor with regard to schizophrenia, but generally good in schizoaffective disorder and other non-specific psychoses. Some cases may present with a picture of confusion, perplexity and retardation, and are diagnosed as cycloid psychoses (see Chapter 9, page 193). Mixed manic and depressive pictures or mixed affective states are also quite common, with some women showing rapid switches in and out of mania and depression in a single day, while a more common pattern is for some women to present initially with mania and then switch into a state of depression after a few weeks.

In most of the published series, these mixed pictures are usually classed as 'psychotic disorder not otherwise specified'. Kendell *et al* (1987) found 10% fitted this picture, a Dutch study gave a figure of 30% (Klompenhouwer & Van Hulst, 1991) and an Indian series gave a figure of 47% for these mixed pictures (Agrawal *et al*, 1990). The presence of a large number of patients with these mixed pictures was one of the arguments used to support the notion that puerperal psychosis was a unique and different category of psychosis and should be listed separately in the ICD and DSM schemes, although such a view has little support today. A small number of patients are admitted during the puerperium in a psychotic state that resolves rapidly after a few days and these patients are said to have a brief psychosis.

Epidemiology

Puerperal psychosis is not a common disorder and Marcé's (1858) original estimate of 2.2 per 1000 deliveries has stood the test of time. However, a large obstetric unit, with say some 3000–5000 deliveries a year, will usually have several cases each year and so midwives working in these units will be familiar with the disorder. There is some variation in the reported rates: for example, in the Edinburgh series Kendell *et al* (1987) reported a rate of 1 per 1000 births, while Janssen (1964) in Sweden found an admission rate of 4.8 per 1000 deliveries admitted to a university hospital. Presumably, the increased availability of hospital beds and lower threshold of severity required for admission may explain some of this variation. Although in the literature there are many reports of uncontrolled case series, there are very few proper epidemiological studies (i.e. which examine cases only from a defined catchment area).

Paffenbarger (1964) examined all the case notes of women aged between 15 and 47 who were admitted to either public or private hospitals in Hamilton County, Ohio, during the years 1940–58 and identified 314 cases. There was a relatively lower rate (lower than among non-childbearing women) of admission during pregnancy, at 7–9 per month, but this rose dramatically in the first month after delivery to 164 cases, giving an 18-fold increased risk for the first month, and there was a total of 242 admissions during the first 6 months.

Kendell *et al* (1987) matched information from the Edinburgh psychiatric case register with data from the Scottish maternity discharge computer for all women who had delivered in Edinburgh during 1970–78. As in Paffenbarger's study, the relative risk of admission was decreased in pregnancy (0.65) but rose dramatically in the first month after delivery to 22, and when primigravid women alone were considered this relative risk rose to 35. Risk factors of this magnitude are unusual in medicine and almost unheard of in psychiatry and are presumably due to some unknown, possibly biological factor associated with childbirth.

A series of 381 women from Baragwanath Hospital in Johannesburg, South Africa (Allwood *et al*, 2000), had an overall incidence of 2–3 cases per 1000 births and the pattern of diagnosis was similar to that in the developed world. Risk factors in this study were being a primiparous patient, a family history of psychiatric disorder, a medical illness, season of the year and psychosocial stresses (including the need for a special care baby unit or the death of the baby).

There is an obvious interest in whether obstetric factors are associated. All the more recent controlled studies (e.g. those of Paffenbarger and Kendell) have found links with primigravidity, with Paffenbarger estimating the risk for primigravid women as about double. However, 19th-century authors such as Marcé, writing when multiparous birth was much more common, suggested a multigravid predominance (see Brockington, 1996, p. 243, for review). Paffenbarger (1964) found links with maternal hypertension, increasing maternal age, cervical dystocia and a slightly shorter pregnancy. Kendell *et al* (1987) did not replicate these findings but instead found an association with Caesarean section. The Danish series of Videbech & Gouliaev (1995) found no increased rate of obstetric complication of any type.

In most European studies, the sex of the child was unrelated, but in one African study (Allwood *et al*, 2000) there was an association with having a male child, whereas in a study from India having a female infant was associated (Agrawal *et al*, 1990), as appears to be the case with postnatal depression as well (see page 646). The most likely explanation is sociocultural and may relate to the place of women in Indian society and the rejection of female infants.

The search for environmental triggers for the puerperal psychoses has yielded few clues and, apart from primigravidity, none of the associations reported appears to be very strong or, if an association has been found in a series, this has not been replicated. At a clinical level, it is striking how few women even with very difficult labours develop psychiatric sequelae and how often the deliveries of patients who have even severe psychosis have been completely normal.

Aetiology

Genetics

'It is a fact', wrote Savage (1875), 'that the neuroses of pregnancy and childbirth are often associated with a hereditary tendency.' Thuwe (1974), pooling the data of ten series published between 1911 and 1973, found that in 40% of 614 cases there was a family history of mental illnesses. Illnesses in the relatives were not confined to the psychoses, but rather there was a mixture of depression, manic–depression, psychopathy, alcoholism and suicide. Thuwe also found that around 10% of the children of patients with puerperal psychosis developed an acute psychotic illness later in life, and this was a six-fold increase over the rate in the control groups.

In a large family study, Protheroe (1969) reported that for female probands with a puerperal affective disorder, the risk for any affective disorder for siblings was 10% and for parents 14.7%, and these figures were similar to those reported for probands with non-puerperal affective disorder.

Family studies of probands with puerperal mania have yielded two interesting findings:

1 The overall level of genetic loading may be less for puerperal mania than for non-puerperal mania. Kadramas *et al* (1979), for example, found that probands with puerperal mania had fewer affected first-degree relatives than the relatives of probands with non-puerperal mania.

2 Within the whole class of women with bipolar disorder, there may a small but highly specific familial subgroup who are especially liable to puerperal mania. A family study has shown that within the bipolar spectrum some families have a predisposition to the development of puerperal psychosis. Thus, Jones & Craddock (2001) compared the post-partum course of bipolar women with a family history of a puerperal psychosis with that of women without such a history. A puerperal episode occurred in 20 out of 27 women (74%) who had a family history of puerperal psychosis, but in only 38 out of 125 (30%) where such a family history was absent. When only first episodes were considered the odd ratio rose to 6, indicating that childbirth acts as an extremely potent trigger for psychosis in a subgroup of patients with a bipolar affective disorder who carry a familial (probably genetic) tendency to develop a puerperal psychosis.

Social factors

Although social factors are important in the aetiology of the less severe pregnancy and post-partum depressions, there is little evidence that they play much of a role in the more severe psychotic illnesses. Savage (1875) remarked on how few cases 'could be traced back to fright, grief or losses' and more systematic studies of life events in the UK have failed to establish any links between recent life events and severe post-partum depression (Dowlatshahi & Paykel, 1990).

Post-partum psychoses affect all social classes, but increased rates of admission are associated with single women and, in one African study, with stresses associated with the baby dying or being in intensive care (Allwood *et al*, 2000).

Classification

The illness itself has altered little over the past 150 years, but the way it has been classified has changed frequently, in line with changing views concerning its aetiology. In the first part of the 19th century there were good descriptions of two separate illnesses, puerperal (early-onset) and lactational (late-onset) insanity, but these illnesses were not connected with schizophrenia or manic depression, which had not yet been described. Towards the end of the 19th century, the newly discovered bacteria came into prominence in medicine and an infective cause of puerperal psychosis was thought possible, particularly as the onset was delirious, and there was a high death rate, and so these illnesses were considered to be organic psychoses. The advent of antibiotics and of ECT in the 1940s lowered the death rate, but the florid psychotic picture remained and led many, especially in America, to believe that these disorders were mainly the result of schizophrenia.

The advent of the antidepressant drugs, lithium (to which these disorders are often extremely sensitive) and modern classificatory schemes, starting with the Research Diagnostic Criteria (RDC) (Spitzer *et al*, 1978), led to a further about-turn in diagnosis, with most of these disorders now being considered affective and closely related to bipolar disorder. From time to time there have been suggestions that they comprise a separate and independent group of psychoses, but such a position has never been widely held.

The present position as described in DSM–IV (American Psychiatric Association, 1994) and ICD–10 (World Health Organization, 1992) is that childbirth acts as a trigger for a variety of mainly affective disorders and that they should be diagnosed and classified under their respective categories – depression, mania, schizoaffective disorder and so on.

The relevant post-partum period has also been poorly and variably defined. The DSM–IV onset specifier is within the first 4 weeks. ICD–10 suggests 6 weeks, while the Royal College of Obstetricians and Gynaecologists takes the whole of the first post-partum year after delivery to define the puerperium in *The Confidential Enquiries into Maternal Deaths in the United Kingdom* (National Institute for Clinical Excellence, 2001).

To code an episode in according to ICD–10, the relevant code from the affective disorders section is taken and to show an onset associated with childbirth a code of the obstetric section (099.3) of ICD–10 is added on. ICD–10 does not have a section describing the main post-partum syndromes but only a short section describing a few puerperal syndromes and these include postnatal depression and puerperal psychoses not classified elsewhere. It also specifies that episodes should have started within 6 weeks of delivery.

Classification in DSM–IV represents an advance on ICD–10 because it recognises a post-partum onset and it is possible to add a post-partum onset specifier to any affective episode that starts within 4 weeks of childbirth. This means that the vast majority of puerperal illnesses (which are affective) can be separately coded, which is not possible with ICD–10 or with the previous DSM systems. The post-partum onset specifier is applied to the current or most recent episode of major depression, mania or mixed episodes in major depressive, bipolar I, bipolar II or brief psychotic disorder.

Treatment

'Tonics and a change of scenery are useful' wrote Savage (1875) and the same principles apply today, although the tonics of today are modern psychotropics and treatment depends on a combination of hospital admission, drug therapy and community nursing support for the patient and her family. In severe cases hospital admission is always advisable and will often require the immediate implementation of a section of the Mental Health Act. If possible and where facilities are available the baby, should be admitted with the mother, and an early initial assessment should be made to see whether continued joint nursing is possible or whether a brief separation is advisable.

The pharmacological treatment of the psychoses that occur after childbirth is similar to their treatment at other times, although there may be one or two minor differences in strategy. For a majority of women their post-partum admission will be their first psychiatric contact and they will be a drug-naive population. Thus, even normal doses of psychotropic drugs may result in quite severe side-effects, such as excessive sedation and dyskinesias, while cholinergic side-effects may result in bladder problems or an excessive dry mouth, leading to episodes of oral thrush. Manic symptoms need sedation with some of the new atypicals, such as olanzapine, while very severe hyperactivity may respond to lorazepam. Classical manic and schizoaffective pictures may require lithium therapy as well. As puerperal mania is often associated with a profound disorder of sleep, the restoration of normal sleep is essential and a sedative antipsychotic combined with a hypnotic may be helpful, while the night nursing staff should take care of the baby at night to ensure the mother has a period of unbroken sleep.

A few women with very severe mania or depression may not eat or drink because they are either delirious or stuporous; they may also neglect their personal hygiene and may then be prone to infection. Nursing staff may need to wash these patients regularly and monitor their pulse and temperature. ECT should be considered for such unresponsive and dangerous states (though they are rare), because the response is usually excellent. Martin (1958) gave ECT to 28 patients (27 with depression, 1 with mania), all of whom had an excellent initial response, although 10 women (36%) relapsed within 3 weeks and required a second course of ECT, which was usually successful. An antidepressant, lithium or both should be given for a few months following a successful course of ECT, to prevent relapse.

In spite of its proven efficacy, ECT is unpopular with patients and their families and most patients prefer treatment with medication. The response rate to a single antidepressant, such as a tricyclic, in the severe puerperal depressions is low and probably worse than in non-puerperal cases of depression (Dean & Kendell, 1981), but many patients do well with lithium augmentation. There is only one uncontrolled study on the use of lithium in puerperal women and this suggested that lithium may be effective for confusional, depressive and schizoaffective syndromes, as well as for its more usual indication of mania (Silberman *et al*, 1975). Patients presenting with complex mixed affective and schizophreniform pictures often require an antipsychotic, an antidepressant and lithium, while ECT is best held as a reserve option for the small minority of women who fail to respond to pharmacotherapy.

Schizophrenic illnesses should be managed as described in Chapter 11, but during the first 3 or 4 months affective syndromes often appear to be superimposed and may require separate treatment. Although affective disorders often resolve quickly, usually in a period of weeks, a schizophrenic illness may take several months to resolve, and so decisions concerning the longer-term care of infants should, if possible, be delayed. Once the initial episode has resolved, it is essential to ensure compliance with medication, by using drugs with fewer side-effects, such as the atypicals, or occasionally with the use of depot medications. Monitoring by community psychiatric nurses for a prolonged period is essential, because relapses in the second or third post-partum year may have a catastrophic effect on child care.

Most women with a severe post-partum illness who have been admitted to hospital are either unable or unwilling to breast-feed and so the issue of psychotropic drugs being ingested by the baby rarely arises for the more severe cases. However, many of those with milder illness or those being treated in the community wish to continue to breast-feed while taking medication and this topic is reviewed below (see also Table 25.1).

Hormones have little place in the management of acute psychotic illnesses, except in a few instances where there is a premenstrual exacerbation of a puerperal disorder, particularly depression. These exacerbations are usually a sign that the illness is resolving, because the symptoms are appearing only intermittently, and they may sometimes be abolished by increasing the dose of antidepressant or the use of progesterone suppositories for 2 weeks before menstruation, although there are no systematic trials on how to manage these premenstrual exacerbations, which commonly occur in post-partum illnesses. These exacerbations tend to subside over the next 6–12 months and they do not usually signify the onset of a more prolonged premenstrual syndrome.

Mother and baby units

As mentioned above, the tradition of joint admission of mother and baby into psychiatric units is largely confined to the UK and some Commonwealth countries, such as Australia. The underlying aim of such admissions is to sustain and facilitate the mother–infant relationship while working towards the mother's recovery from illness and her rehabilitation. Before the introduction of joint admissions, infants were cared for separately, either by other family members or, where these were lacking (e.g. for single mothers), by social services, who would place the baby in foster care. In a small minority of cases, infants were not reunited with their mother even when her illness had resolved – these mothers lost their babies. A joint admission serves as a powerful statement of the need to preserve the bond, even in the face of a severe mental disturbance, which is presumed to be temporary. Moreover, any difficulties in later being reunited with their babies no longer occur. Mother and baby units used to be placed in acute psychiatric units in district general hospitals, and a few still remain there. These had the advantage of easy access to paediatric and obstetric liaison facilities, and earlier fears that babies might come to harm as a result of infections or from other psychiatric patients proved unfounded. However, a report from the Royal College of Psychiatrists (2000) recommended that women should no longer be nursed in general psychiatric wards but in specialised mother and baby units, with each unit serving a population of 1.3 million. Such an ideal has yet to be achieved, but there are now a few large units in specialised teaching hospitals. However, as large numbers of in-patient beds have closed, the levels of acute disturbance have risen on ordinary in-patient units, to the extent that they are no longer deemed to be a safe environment in which to care for mothers and babies. This loss of dedicated mother and baby beds has meant that many women are now being admitted to ordinary psychiatric units without their babies and so do not obtain the advantages of a joint mother and baby admission. Some trusts purchase an admission to private mother and baby facilities, where the in-patient units have fewer seriously ill patients and the environment may be more congenial.

Effects of psychiatric disorder on mothering abilities

Mothers with severe depression, that is, with psychomotor retardation, difficulties in concentration and feelings of exhaustion, may have insufficient energy to complete the practical tasks required for infant care. Depressed, irritable women, or those with hostile, infanticidal or suicidal thoughts, may require especially close observation. Occasionally, women with psychotic depression try to smother their babies with a pillow or drown them in the bath. This can occur even after admission to hospital, and those with severe psychotic depression may require a nurse to be present with them at all times.

Patients with mania are also unsafe, particularly during their overactive phase. Their distraction can make them forget to complete a feed or to change their baby, or walk away during changing and leave the baby unattended on a nappy-changing table. Others may wake their babies up from sleep to cuddle them in a sentimental fashion, or give unnecessary feeds or feed inappropriately, for example with solids. Their irrational anger is usually directed at their husband or the nurses, but may occasionally be directed towards the baby. Grandiosity, disinhibition and general lack of sensitivity may all diminish the quality of infant care, and sometimes the mother hands the baby round the ward for anyone, however unsuitable, to look after. Infant care is generally poor until the mother's distractibility has resolved and she has a reasonable degree of concentration. During phases of severe mania or catatonic excitement, mothers must be separated from their infants, and nurseries where babies sleep should be locked to prevent access. In a few cases it may be advisable to remove the baby from the ward while a severe psychotic phase is being treated.

In women with schizophrenia, thought disorder may result in major defects in practical competence, while negative symptoms such as apathy and emotional blunting can grossly impair the sensitivity required for good infant care. The presence of negative symptoms, which may be long lasting, is a poor prognostic sign. Delusions may preoccupy a woman's mind to such an extent that the infant is excluded or neglected. Delusions and hallucinations that focus around the baby may be particularly dangerous, as patients with schizophrenia sometimes act on the basis of their delusions. Dangerous mistakes such as bathing the baby in cold water, giving the baby feeds that are boiling hot, substituting sterilising fluid for milk or other bizarre practical errors may occur. One patient, in a distracted state, repeatedly let her baby's face slip under water while she was bathing the infant, so that nursing staff always had to be present at bathing time to rescue the baby from drowning. Some cases of puerperal schizophrenia may respond well to medication after some months; in other cases the child is brought up by relatives (usually the father or the infant's grandparents). Where social support is poor and the illness fails to respond to medication, the social services may have to remove the baby for fostering or adoption.

The nurses on mother and baby units serve several functions. Perhaps most importantly, when the mother is obviously failing or the situation is dangerous, they need to intervene and either take over the care or speedily remove the infant from the mother. They also need to nurse and observe the mother for her primary psychiatric disorder, as well as provide instruction on basic mothering skills. Primigravid women suffer from the dual handicap of both having a psychosis and being inexperienced in mothering, and new learning is difficult during a psychotic episode, with psychotropic medication being an additional impeding factor. It is sometimes better to wait until more florid psychotic symptoms have subsided before attempting to teach basic mothering skills. Nursery nurses are commonly employed solely to look after the babies when mothers are unable to do so, while some of the older nurses who themselves have had children may offer advice based on their own experiences of child care, as well as provide a more 'maternal' type of support.

In a few of the more severe cases where the illness fails to resolve, or other factors (see page 657) militate against successful infant care, the mother–infant relationship may be seriously impaired. Margison (1982) recommends that mother–infant interactions should be assessed over four separate areas over a 2-week period, to clarify this:

1 the practical competence of the mother in feeding, bathing and changing the baby

2 untoward incidents, such as handling the baby roughly or leaving the baby unattended, or verbal or physical attacks on the baby

3 what mothers say about the babies, particularly the content of any delusions or hallucinations

4 a mother's overall affective response to the baby – whether it is normal and loving, detached or in some way bizarre.

A scale to measure the quality of mother–infant attachments, the Bethlem Mother–Infant Interaction Scale, has been developed in a specialised mother and baby unit. It can be used to quantify the interaction (Kumar & Hipwell, 1996). The scale covers seven dimensions of infant care: eye contact, vocal contact, physical contact, maternal mood and its degree of synchrony with the infant's needs, the ability to have a general routine of care, and an assessment of risk. Experienced nursing staff are usually able to tell, without the use of scales, fairly quickly whether a mother will be able to care capably and safely for her infant, although a rating scale may help in systematising observational data, and is useful for research.

Outcome and risks of recurrence

Information is available for several different types of outcome:

1 the natural history of the disease and the interval before spontaneous resolution occurs, as described in the pre-treatment era

2 the outcome of treated cases

3 the risk of relapse following subsequent pregnancies

4 the risk of further affective episodes over the long term.

Knowledge of the natural history of the disease in untreated cases is helpful in estimating when a spontaneous resolution may occur, especially for those patients who show little response to treatment. The 19th-century authors described a rather lengthy illness which nevertheless usually did eventually remit. Savage (1875) found among 84 women with puerperal psychosis that only a third were better after 6 months. Among the 54 women with melancholia, 50% were better by 6 months and 85% by 1 year – but 8% had died.

In the post-treatment era these figures had improved dramatically. Janssen (1964) found that 75% of patients with puerperal psychosis had admissions of less than 6 weeks, 15% were ill for 6–12 weeks and only 3% for more than 6 months, and there were no deaths.

Two long-term studies have provided data concerning the much longer-term risk of further puerperal and non-puerperal relapse. Schopf & Rust (1994) followed 119 women who had an admission for a post-partum disorder and found that 66 (55%) had a non-puerperal episode over the next 20 years. In a 23-year follow-up study, Robling *et al* (2000) found that 75% had a further episode, most of which were non-puerperal, and around one-third of this sample experienced at least three further episodes, indicating that a puerperal episode frequently represented the opening of a recurrent affective disorder.

There is an increased risk of further psychotic breakdown following a subsequent pregnancy; relapses typically have an almost identical clinical picture and time of onset to the index episode. Summarising information from several different sources, Brockington (1996) estimated a 20–25% risk for each subsequent pregnancy. Among those women who have an index puerperal episode and who continue to have children, one in three will experience a further puerperal episode at some time. In a study by Dean *et al* (1989), women with a bipolar disorder who had both previous puerperal and non-puerperal episodes were at greater risk (50%) of a subsequent puerperal breakdown than those with only a previous puerperal episode, for whom the rate was 36%. If, however, the previous history is of a non-puerperal depression alone, the literature suggests that these women are less likely to experience a puerperal recurrence than those with a previous puerperal episode. That is, most women with a history of depression, provided this has been non-puerperal, can be reassured that postnatal depression is unlikely. What is uncertain is whether these women will have rates of postnatal illness that are above baseline rates, which are quite high anyway. Bratfos & Haug (1968) found that 62% of women with a history of depression (puerperal or non-puerperal) and who had had at least one child did not have subsequent puerperal episodes. However, for those who had had a previous puerperal depressive episode, risks of recurrence were high. In the series reported by Garvey *et al* (1983), out of 54 women with previous puerperal episodes, 37 (67%) did not experience puerperal depression following their later childbirths, but the other 17 women (33%) did and 75% of their subsequent pregnancies were also followed by depression. Of these, 8 women (15%) experienced puerperal depression after every single pregnancy, replicating an observation made in the 19th century, when grand multiparity was more common, that there were a few women who developed a depression after every single pregnancy.

Patients often ask about their risks of developing postnatal depression following a subsequent delivery and the studies described above provide some factual data on which to base a response:

- if the previous episode was non-puerperal, the risk is low and may be only marginally increased above baseline rates
- if the previous episode was puerperal, the risk is definitely raised, at probably around 25%
- if the previous episodes were both puerperal and non-puerperal, the risk may be even higher, at about 50%
- if there were two or more previous puerperal episodes, the risk may be very greatly raised (although there are no available published figures), because there is a chance that such a woman will be among those who inevitably develop a postnatal illness after every pregnancy.

These figures were derived from studies on both unipolar and bipolar disorder, and so probably apply to both conditions. A recurrence of bipolar disorder may entail a very severe illness.

Puerperal schizophrenia is a far less common condition and there are therefore very few reports on its recurrence rate. Yarden *et al* (1966) gave a figure of 45% and Protheroe (1969) 47%. Yarden *et al* (1966) also investigated whether pregnancy had any longer-term deleterious effect on the course of schizophrenia and in a controlled study showed there was no difference in subsequent hospitalisation rates among women with schizophrenia who became pregnant and a matched control group with schizophrenia who had not been pregnant.

Suicide

Suicide is presently very rare in pregnancy in the UK, but this has not always been the case. In the years 1900–47, 12.6% of all women of childbearing age who died by suicide were pregnant; this figure then fell to 1.3% for the years 1943–80 (Kleiner & Greston, 1984).

Presumably the advent of contraception, more liberal abortion laws, and a change in the attitude of society towards single mothers and unwanted pregnancy explain much of this fall. The UK suicide statistics for 1973–84 also suggest a very low standardised mortality ratio (SMR) for suicide (i.e. in comparison with an age- and sex-matched general population group) of 0.05 for pregnancy and 0.17 for the postnatal period, but there were certain high-risk groups – pregnant teenagers, single mothers, those with stillbirths and mothers with a mental illness – among whom the methods of suicide used were commonly violent (Appleby, 1991).

In a detailed study of the Danish national psychiatric case register (Appleby *et al*, 1998) for the two decades of 1973–93, the SMR for suicide for women who had a hospital admission for a post-partum psychiatric disorder was raised 70-fold. When only the first 2 post-partum years were considered, the SMR for this group was raised 19-fold, but this high risk persisted over a 15-year period, at 17-fold. These observations suggest that although post-partum illness is rare, it carries a substantial risk of both early and late suicide, and these risks will be present with each recurrence (whether puerperal or non-puerperal). The increased rate of late suicide in this group suggests that these women (i.e. women with a history of hospital admission for depression after childbirth) may have a rather more severe and dangerous form of depression, and so later episodes – even long after the child-bearing years – should be viewed with seriousness and treated vigorously.

The rate for episodes of parasuicide may be reduced after childbirth – Appleby (1991) gave a figure for the relative risk of around 0.43 for the first post-partum year; for these episodes, personality disorder and social crises rather than serious mental illness were the main causes.

Prophylaxis

After an episode of puerperal psychosis or severe depression, many women will none the less wish to have more children and will seek advice on the risks of recurrence (detailed above) and the possibility of prevention. The scientific literature on this important practical matter is surprisingly sparse, comprising only a few uncontrolled reports.

Hamilton (1962) gave a mixture of oestrogen and testosterone in oil to 40 women and noted that none had a recurrence. Dalton (1985), an advocate of progesterone therapy, suggested that progesterone might prevent further episodes of non-psychotic depression, but her claims were never substantiated. As most puerperal illnesses are thought to be affective, Stewart *et al* (1991) administered lithium to 25 women with previous manic or schizo-manic illnesses, and only two women (8%) relapsed, which was lower than the expected rate of around 25% (see above), although a few women developed mild or attenuated illnesses, indicating that a relapse had occurred that had been partially treated rather than prevented. Stewart *et al* (1991) administered the lithium during pregnancy, but current practice, if lithium is to be used, is to start the drug only after delivery, and then usually to wait until all transfusions, intravenous drips and other serious obstetric complications have resolved.

Following a small open trial using nortriptyline to prevent postnatal depression, Wisner *et al* (2001) went on to conduct a randomised, double-blind, placebo-controlled trial of 50 mg nortriptyline started immediately after birth and then continued for 20 weeks. Relapse rates of 25% were found in both the placebo and the nortriptyline-treated women, and so the drug appeared to offer no protection. A later open study of selective serotonin reuptake inhibitors (SSRIs) suggested that these may be beneficial in prophylaxis, but this has yet to be proved in a randomised controlled trial. Despite this negative finding, there may be rather more to preventing a puerperal relapse than the simple prescription of one antidepressant. The strategy for relapse prevention used in the author's clinic is described below.

A strategy for relapse prevention

When women seek prophylactic advice, a careful history of the previous episode or episodes should be obtained, because puerperal relapses are usually remarkably similar to the original index illness. Critical information includes:

- the time of onset – so that a prophylactic regimen can be instituted before this
- the diagnostic category, as indicated in the case notes – so that drugs known to ameliorate this particular disorder can be selected
- whether any particular treatments appeared to work well in the previous episode
- the overall duration of the illness.

Armed with this information, it is usually possible to give an estimate of the likely risks of a recurrence as previously described, and also relatively easy to select which medications may be beneficial, and decide when they should be started and how long they should be taken for.

It is also essential to assess the severity, duration, dangerousness and the amount of harm incurred by the previous illness to establish how necessary prophylaxis is. Some illnesses involve lengthy hospitalisations, treatment with ECT, or have resulted in severe marital conflict, with marital violence, or contributed to an impaired relationship with the baby, which may extend well into childhood and have caused much damage. In these cases the need for a prophylactic regimen will be pressing and most women in this situation will be very keen to take anything that may prevent such a disastrous illness repeating. In other cases the illness may have been relatively brief, perhaps lasting for a few months only, and may have lifted quickly following a few sessions of counselling or a short course of an antidepressant, and caused little damage to ongoing family relationships; in these cases prophylaxis is perceived to be more optional, with many women being happy to 'take a chance' that a recurrence will not occur.

During the assessment interview, which takes place in pregnancy, the risks of a recurrence and possible treatment regimens should be outlined to the patient. No decision needs to be taken following the first interview, but a comprehensive care plan will have to be agreed before the end of the pregnancy, and if possible the patient's partner should also be involved. The following regimens are offered and they should all start on the first day after delivery. Because most of the more serious illnesses are bipolar in origin (both mania and depression) lithium may have a role to play in the prophylaxis of the more serious illnesses.

For previous mania, schizo-mania, cycloid psychosis

A small dose of an atypical antipsychotic (e.g. 5 mg olanzapine) can be prescribed but over-sedation can occur. Halperidol (5–15 mg) is also effective but dyskinesias may occur. Lithium is also usually helpful and an open study by Stewart *et al* (1991) supports its use, but breast-feeding is contraindicated because lithium is expressed in breast milk and can result in neonatal lithium toxicity, which presents with hypotonia or diarrhoea and vomiting. If lithium is used, a lithium level should be taken after a few days.

Whatever regimen is implemented, the patient should be monitored very closely (e.g. every 3 or 4 days in the first 2–3 weeks after delivery) because this is the peak time when a relapse may occur. Some patients taking these drug regimens will develop mild, attenuated illnesses with broken sleep and this should be quickly dealt with by altering the medication, or adding a hypnotic. These minor mood swings and insomnia indicate that a recurrence has probably occurred but it is being suppressed with the medication, and so the early detection and swift treatment of these premonitory symptoms are essential to prevent more serious developments.

For previous depression

If the previous illness responded well and without significant side-effects to a particular SSRI or tricyclic and the patient has confidence in that particular drug, then the same drug should be used to prevent the next episode and this should be started on day 1. If tricyclics are selected they should be started in doses of 20–30 mg at night, because higher doses may be poorly tolerated and can lead to over-sedation. Fortnightly monitoring is usually sufficient but this should continue for at least 3 months because many illnesses have a later onset, and as soon as any symptoms appear the dosage should be raised to the more usual therapeutic range. The use of these low doses of tricyclics as prophylactic treatment for the 25% who do relapse is also useful, as this will make the subsequent dosage escalation into the therapeutic range much easier than if treatment had had to commence for the first time once a full-blown depression had appeared. If an SSRI is used, the drug is started in full dosage (e.g. 50 mg sertraline or 20 mg fluoxetine) from the first day and dosage titration is not used. Breast-feeding is safe with both tricyclics and SSRIs.

For more severe depression (i.e. that has resulted in previous hospital admission or dangerous episodes)

Lithium may be given in combination with either a tricyclic or an SSRI and this appears to be highly effective, although there are no supporting trial data. There should be close monitoring. It should be noted that breast-feeding is not possible with a regimen that includes lithium (see above) but is thought to be safe with either a tricyclic antidepressant or an SSRI on its own. Women who have had a previous severe and damaging episode are highly motivated to do everything possible to prevent a recurrence and are usually willing to forego breast-feeding. The motivation of those with previous milder episodes is rather more variable.

Other aspects of care

Hormonal therapy in the form of progesterone was once popular and its use was much publicised by Dalton (1985), although there never were any scientific studies to support its use and it is little used today. Oestrogen preparations probably should not be used at all because there are no data to support their prophylactic effectiveness and they are associated with an increased risk of deep-vein thrombosis, a known hazard of the puerperium.

As well as instituting pharmacotherapy, the psychiatrist needs to remain in close contact with the patient throughout the early puerperium, so that he or she can intervene quickly to treat any minor mood changes or sleep disorder. Appointments with the patient should continue until the risk period (as defined by the previous episode) has clearly passed, when the medication can be gradually tapered off.

Non-psychotic postnatal depression

There has been increasing recognition and interest in the milder, non-psychotic depressions found in routine community surveys and in psychiatric out-patient clinics. Community surveys in the UK and many other countries reveal that around 10% of women are depressed postnatally and around 1.6% will be referred to psychiatric out-patient clinics; the account below focuses more on the clinic cases that lie at the more severe end of the spectrum because it is this group that the psychiatrist will be working with.

Presentation and symptoms

The illness presents as an ordinary depression (see Chapter 1) and does not differ markedly from depression occurring at other times. Out-patients will usually lack the severe and life-threatening features of the rare cases of psychotic depression that result in hospitalisation. The illness may start straight after delivery or on the 4th or 5th day (maternity blues which have apparently failed to resolve) or insidiously, around 8–12 weeks after delivery. A few cases have an onset with the first premenstrual phase or with weaning.

In many cases, particularly when there are ongoing social or relationship difficulties, the illness may represent a continuation of a pregnancy depression. Low mood, depressive thoughts and feelings of inadequacy are common. Weeping is ubiquitous, and the frequency and intensity of crying spells provide some indication of the severity of the illness. Daily weeping episodes occur at the onset but these gradually diminish in frequency as the illness resolves. Anhedonia is an almost universal complaint and usually presents as a failure to gain any pleasure from caring for the newborn baby. A normal mother may have increased emotional lability during her first few weeks, but unless she is also suffering from a depression she will usually derive immense pleasure from caring for her baby. As well as emotional lability some women have increased irritability, aggression and hostility – usually directed at the husband or partner but occasionally at older children or, rarely, at the newborn baby.

Feelings of exhaustion, poor concentration, psychomotor retardation and confusion are also common; these result in difficulties achieving tasks that need some effort, such as the practical aspects of mothering like feeding or changing the baby. Some mothers will vacillate in a state of indecisiveness. Others are perplexed and complain of feeling confused about the different advice they receive from different health professionals or their own families. Housework becomes an impossible chore and in cases where there is severe hypersomnia mothers may take to their beds, neglecting essential domestic work and child care, which are often taken over by relatives.

Depressive sleep disorder, with difficulty getting off to sleep, early morning wakening and occasional nightmares, should be distinguished from the broken sleep resulting from the demands of the infant. Diurnal mood variation is common; depression may be worse in the morning but some patients report being worse in the afternoon or evening. Weight loss may be an unreliable sign, because most women will be losing weight during the puerperium, shedding the weight gained during pregnancy. A small minority will be dieting to try to restore their figure and a small number of women may have comorbid eating disorders.

Suicide is rare, but suicidal thoughts are common and frighten the patient, the family and other carers, and may act as a trigger for referral. Infanticidal thoughts are less common, but usually accompany suicidal thoughts, and some patients make half-hearted gestures where they imagine placing a cushion briefly over the baby's face or consider drowning the baby in the bath. Some women who have not otherwise abused their babies may describe brief attacks where infanticidal urges have been half-heartedly acted on but not been carried through, and they may report such episodes only years later, usually with remorse. Infanticide today is extremely rare and a declaration of such thoughts should alert the clinician to a risk of suicide, which is far more likely. A decrease in sexual feelings is common after childbirth but during a postnatal depression is almost universal. The return of sexual feelings is usually delayed until well after the resolution of any underlying depression and may be further delayed by the use of antidepressant drugs such as the SSRIs.

Comorbidity

A wide spectrum of anxiety disorders may also present postnatally but usually they appear with the depression and remit as the depression resolves. Generalised anxiety disorder is the commonest and presents with a picture of mixed anxiety and depression, with the content of the anxiety usually revolving about issues of infant care and infant health. Panic disorder and panic attacks may be particularly frightening and some women may not permit their husband or partner to leave for work in an attempt to avoid separation anxiety, which might trigger a panic attack. In most cases the panic occurs in women with a history of panic attacks. The high rate of anxiety disorders and mixed anxious–depressive pictures led Pitt (1968) to apply the term 'atypical depression' to postnatal depression, but today these illnesses are not regarded as atypical or significantly different from major depressive disorder, which is sometimes accompanied by anxiety.

Obsessional symptoms are common and worrying, and occasionally merit a separate diagnosis of an episode of obsessive–compulsive disorder, but more frequently the obsessional symptoms are associated with the depression and tend both to appear and to resolve with the depression. Obsessional phenomena among postnatal women are often both weird and frightening and may include intrusive thoughts of harming the baby; for example, one woman had recurrent thoughts of putting her baby in the oven, another had recurrent visual obsessions of knifing her baby, while a third had obsessions of throwing her baby downstairs every time she reached the top of the stairs. Themes of sexual abuse are also quite common. Although it is extremely rare for a patient to act on an obsessive thought, they are not always harmless: one women had a curious obsession about wasting water and as a consequence refused to cool the baby's feed down with running cold water and instead gave the baby over-heated feeds.

Agoraphobia may sometimes start for the first time after childbirth, but this generally resolves as the depression improves. A few women develop kleptomania and these cases may present through the courts. Acute depersonalisation starting with the depression can sometimes turn into a chronic depersonalisation syndrome, which may take years to remit; a few of these women console themselves by shoplifting and end up in court.

During a postnatal illness, once menstruation has resumed, a premenstrual exacerbation of almost any premenstrual symptom is common, particularly towards the end of the first post-partum year. Any acting out episode such as an overdose, a marital dispute or a violent episode will usually coincide with a premenstrual phase. As the postnatal depression resolves, the premenstrual tension becomes more distressing because the abrupt deterioration in mood is less well tolerated than a more continuous depression.

More problematic cases

Most published studies are based on community samples and they paint a picture of a mild, self-limiting disorder that responds readily to a few sessions of counselling or a short course of an antidepressant. While such a benign picture may apply to women detected in a community screening programme, many of those attending the psychiatric clinic present with a more complex and challenging picture, and below some of the more problematic types of case are outlined.

- Some women are troubled with severe morbid thoughts, distressing nightmares or strange obsessions or near delusional thoughts, even though they are not psychotic. Small doses of an atypical antipsychotic such as risperidone (2 mg) or olanzapine (2.5–5 mg) at night or an older (typical) drug such as trifluoperazine (2 mg) may be helpful in these cases.

- A small minority of new mothers have severe depressions, which may be complicated by suicidal or infanticidal thoughts, but for a variety of social reasons (e.g. other small children at home) they cannot be admitted to hospital, or hospital admission has itself proved to be unhelpful. In these cases the input from the team should be high, with frequent visits. The support of other family members who can stay with the patient should be enlisted. Drug therapy should be more vigorous, perhaps using higher doses, with an earlier consideration of lithium augmentation; if a day hospital or other day facilities are available they should be used.
- In some cases, there appear to be risks to the baby or more commonly other children in the family and in these cases social services should be involved. More often than not these risks are transient and with good collaborative work the family can resolve them and remain together. The crisis will pass but the use of family aides, short-term fostering and intensive visiting may be required. Regular case conferences provide a structure to coordinate the efforts of all the professionals involved (these cases are further discussed on page 656). The risks to the infant usually fall far short of those described for child abuse.
- Patients with borderline personality disorder, or those with pre-existing borderline traits that are exacerbated by a postnatal depression, may present with difficult and unpredictable behaviour. These women often have a poor response to antidepressants, show impulsive behaviour in the form of overdoses, may occasionally be involved in child abuse, show poor compliance with therapy and often have abusive relationships with both spouses and therapists. They enter into repeated emotional and social crises, particularly during the pre-menstrum, which the team should anticipate in their care plan.
- A few women, often those with a strong family history of alcoholism, either continue their pregnancy drinking behaviours or turn to drink in the postnatal period, usually in association with depression. Drunken mothers were a major social problem during the 19th century and the Licensing Act 1902 (section 21) permits the police to arrest and charge a woman for 'being drunk in charge of a child under the age of seven'. Intoxicated women become too sleepy, irritable or insensitive to care properly for their infants, while those addicted to drugs may be subjected to bizarre or irritable mental states. Some women are sufficiently motivated by the fear of losing their child to enter treatment programmes to curb their drinking, but many are unable to do so and so for safety's sake it may be best to remove the child.
- In contrast to the above severe illnesses, which may be relatively brief, some women have prolonged milder yet unresponsive puerperal illnesses (to both pharmacological and psychotherapeutic approaches); these disorders sometimes persist for 3 or 4 years. Occasionally there is an associated medical disorder such as a hypothyroidism, hypopituitarism, hypertension or the prolonged use of an antihypertensive drug, but in most cases nothing is found. Supportive monthly interviews may be helpful until the illness itself resolves spontaneously, which it usually does.
- Reactions to the baby are not always joyful. A few women became very anxious or almost phobic or dislike dealing with their baby but seem to function quite well otherwise, and in these cases an early return to work may be helpful, with infant care being delegated to relatives or child-minders. Often these women relate better to their offspring when they are a bit older but cannot cope with the infant phase.
- Women with medically ill or very premature babies are naturally highly anxious but do not have a raised rate of depression. However, if they do develop a depression, the content of the depression revolves around their infant's health and there may be wide mood swings which follow all the ups and downs of the child's medical progress. Antidepressants can help dampen the severity of the mood swings and these women usually welcome any psychological support as well.
- In contrast, women with babies with a handicap often have overpowering feelings of hurt and anger ('Why me?', 'Why my baby?'), but despite their distress rarely seek psychiatric help, which they may perceive as yet another humiliation or punishment.

Epidemiology and aetiology

Most epidemiological research into postnatal depression is based on the use of the Edinburgh Postnatal Depression Scale (EPDS). Cox *et al* (1987) devised this scale by adapting questions from the Hospital Anxiety and Depression Scale (Zigmund & Snaith, 1983) but excluded physical symptoms because after childbirth these are common and are of physical rather than psychogenic origin. The scale has ten questions, each with four levels of severity, and the score ranges from 0 to 30, with a score of 12 or above usually indicating a depressive disorder.

The scale has been widely applied in many countries and among many different ethnic groups. These studies have shown that postnatal depression is a universal phenomenon, with rates of around 10%, although in some countries (e.g. Japan) rates may be a little lower, while in deprived inner-city areas rates may be a little higher; for example, in down-town Dallas, Texas, USA, Yonkers *et al* (2001) reported a rate of 16%. Only a few studies have examined the period prevalence or given a duration for the episodes. Beeghly *et al* (2002) found that around one-third of mothers who were depressed at 2 months were also depressed at 6 and 12 months, a finding that replicates Pitt's (1968) much earlier observation that 50% of women he found to be depressed at 3 months were still depressed at 1 year, indicating that the duration, although variable, was usually of several months, but in some cases can extend to 1 or even 2 years.

Although EPDS-based studies have repeatedly demonstrated a high prevalence of depression in the first post-partum year, the critical issue of whether postnatal depression is itself a separate entity from ordinary depression depends on whether its prevalence is raised above comparative population base rates, and also whether there is an increased inception rate in the first few months after delivery. The evidence for both these tests seems equivocal and certainly far less strong than for the severe puerperal psychoses.

Evans *et al* (2001) followed a large cohort of women (12 000) through pregnancy and the post-partum period, using a threshold of 12/13 on the EPDS to diagnose depression. They reported rates for depression of: 8.4% at 18 weeks of pregnancy, 13.5% at 32 weeks of pregnancy; 9.1% at 8 weeks post-partum; and 8.1% at 8 months post-partum. They concluded there was no evidence to support the existence of a subgroup of women with a specific disorder of postnatal depression. A similar large study from Norway (Eberhard-Gran *et al*, 2002) found the rate of depression, again as diagnosed by the EPDS, in a group of women 6 weeks after delivery to be 8.9%, while the rates among women drawn from the same district who were 'non-post-partum' was 13.6%. However, once a correction was made for confounding variables known to predispose to depression, namely life events, relationship difficulties and a history of depression, a modest increase in the liability for depression (odds ratio 1.6) was demonstrated for the postnatal period.

Yonkers *et al* (2001) screened a large cohort of deprived Hispanic and Afro-American women in Dallas and, using a cut-off score of 12 on the EPDS, found a rate of 16% for postnatal depression. Women who screened positive for postnatal depression were then interviewed, but only half (8%) qualified for a DSM–IV diagnosis of major depression, and of these, 2% had a pre-pregnancy onset, 2% had a pregnancy onset, and only 4% had a true postnatal onset. These observations suggest that while screening can detect large numbers of women with some depression during the postnatal period, once stricter diagnostic criteria are applied and only cases with a postnatal onset are included the rates are much lower. There probably still is a 'postnatal effect' in terms of onset, and postnatal illnesses appear to have a typical form and usually respond well to treatment, but these studies show that the evidence base underlying the validity of postnatal depression as a specific entity is not so strong as was once thought.

Patients attending psychiatric clinics are at the more severe end of the spectrum and more often have a true postnatal onset, but they represent only a small proportion of the cases. The aetiological role of the puerperium as a risk factor in clinic cases probably lies somewhere in the intermediate range between the very high rates associated with post-partum psychotic disorders, where the increased risk is raised by a factor of 18- to 35-fold (see above), and the much lower risks of the community cases, which are only marginally above base rates.

A wide variety of other factors have been found to be associated with depression in the postnatal period and these are similar to the causal social factors associated with depression (as outlined in Chapter 3). They include life events, a poor marriage, relationship problems with the partner, the absence of a confiding relationship and other young children at home. Most studies also identify a history of depression – especially postnatal depression, severe maternity blues or depression in pregnancy – but also feelings of elation in pregnancy as factors associated with postnatal depression. Obstetric factors do not appear to be prominent in most series, and where a particular obstetric item is identified in one series it has usually failed to be replicated in other studies.

Cultural factors are also undoubtedly important. Thus, in Western society, where equality of the sexes prevails, the sex of the infant has little bearing on the rates of postnatal depression. However, in India, where the social status of women is low, the birth of a female infant is often a source of disappointment, especially to a woman's in-laws. Chandran *et al* (2002) interviewed a large cohort of women from rural southern India and found an overall rate of 11% for ICD–10 postnatal depression, which was similar to the European rates, and also identified the usual known risk factors such as adverse life events, no help post-partum, and low income. However, they also found rates were more than doubled for women who had a daughter where a son was wanted, as well as for women who were having difficulties with their in-laws, factors that have never been reported in any Western series. Patel *et al* (2002) also describe how disappointment in having a female infant interacts and exacerbates marital disharmony in cases of postnatal depression (see page 787).

Treatment

The account below is largely based on the personal experiences of the author, as there are not many treatment studies.

The initial diagnostic consultation is often the most important and offers many useful opportunities for psychotherapy and support. Patients usually present with a diffuse set of complaints, such as depressive symptoms, disappointment in motherhood, sleep disorder or shame associated with their morbid thoughts, which seem to be out of character for the person concerned. The act of sharing such thoughts with a professional may provide immediate cathartic relief. For other symptoms, which may be experienced by the woman for the first time, such as panic attacks, depersonalisation, or failure to develop warm feelings for the baby, an explanation in itself may be reassuring.

During the initial interview, the strengths and weaknesses of a patient's present family set-up and family of origin should be explored, to give some idea of the direction of future management. Towards the end of the initial consultation, if there is evidence of a clear-cut depressive episode, the patient should be told she has a definite illness, which should be named as 'postnatal depression'. The simple act of naming the illness by someone in authority, such as the doctor, appears to have a beneficial effect for many women, as it provides an explanation for the feelings of depression and failure, and husbands or partners are usually also reassured that the cause is a treatable medical disorder that usually has a benign outcome.

Psychotherapy

There are now several reports showing that psychotherapy in the form of cognitive–behavioural therapy (CBT) or interpersonal psychotherapy are effective in postnatal depression. Thus, O'Hara *et al* (2000) selected women with DSM–IV major depression and conducted a trial of 12 sessions of interpersonal therapy (see Chapter 6): the patient's depression was placed in an interpersonal context and sessions were utilised to review the patient's current and past interpersonal relationships. Around a third (37%) of those who received therapy recovered (as judged by scores on the Hamilton Rating Scale for Depression), compared with only 13% of the waiting-list controls. In this trial, although the effects of psychotherapy were demonstrable, there were many women (63%) with major depression who did not improve, and so other (somatic) remedies should also be considered.

Appleby *et al* (1997) conducted a rather more complex randomised controlled trial which compared fluoxetine (20 mg) with placebo, and six sessions of CBT to one session of simple counselling. The CBT was conducted by health visitors in the community who were trained to offer reassurance and practical advice in four areas: feelings of not coping, lack of enjoyable activities, lack of practical support, and other difficulties. The CBT group improved by 39%, while in the pharmacotherapy section of the study there was a 40% difference between fluoxetine and placebo. There was thus little difference in the degree of improvement obtained from either CBT or fluoxetine. The study also showed quite a marked improvement in the placebo groups; for example, the placebo patients who received only one session of counselling showed an almost 50% reduction from baseline scores on the Hamilton scale over the 12 weeks of the study. These observations indicate that many cases of depression detected in the community are at the more benign end of the spectrum and may resolve spontaneously, but this optimistic benign picture may not hold for the more severe cases referred to psychiatric departments.

Cooper *et al* (2003) have shown that many different types of psychotherapy – such as counselling, CBT and psychodynamic therapy – are equally effective for postnatal depression. As in other fields, what probably matters more than the specifics of a particular psychotherapeutic technique is the empathic quality of the therapeutic relationship. In conducting psychotherapy with postnatal women, due allowance should be made for real practical difficulties, such as illnesses in babies and the needs of other children in the family. During the early stages of psychotherapy, and particularly with the more severe illnesses, women prefer to talk about their symptoms, and sympathetic listening, permission to talk expansively on symptomatic distress and a cognitive approach are beneficial. Feelings of rejection or hostility directed at the spouse or other children are commonplace and some new mothers also complain of an inability to experience warmth towards the baby. As the depression lightens, the more traditional psychotherapeutic themes of relationships with parents and other family members begin to emerge. Motivation to remain in psychotherapy usually lasts for the duration of the depression, but once the depression lifts most women cease contact and long-term, dependent relationships with therapists or treatment teams are unusual.

Group therapy, often led by a community psychiatric nurse or psychologist, where all the participants suffer from postnatal depression, is often helpful and may provide a highly supportive environment. Previously well-integrated individuals derive most benefit from groups, and patients will often strike up close friendships with each other. However, as many women cannot tolerate group therapy, individual therapy should always be offered as well.

Drug therapy

Many women, particularly those with brief or mild episodes of postnatal depression, will neither wish for nor require pharmacotherapy. O'Hara *et al* (2000) found that 40% of women with postnatal depression in the community would reject drug treatment. However, those referred to specialist services appear to have more severe illnesses and are more willing to take medication; they may even have started it before their referral. Antidepressant therapy at this time is similar to antidepressant therapy at other times and is described in Chapter 4, but a few points deserve mention.

Both SSRIs and tricyclics are effective in postnatal depression and safe in mothers who are breast-feeding (see below). The more benign side-effect profile of the SSRIs has led to their becoming the first choice of drug in the treatment of depression in most instances. In postnatal depression reducing side-effects is especially important and will also facilitate compliance. Appleby *et al* (1997) confirmed the effectiveness of fluoxetine (see above). Tricyclics may be useful in certain cases where sleep disturbance is prominent because of their sedative effects, and they also have an advantage in that dosage can be gradually titrated upwards, starting from very low doses, where side-effects are minimal, and many patients will respond to relatively low doses (e.g. for amitriptyline in the 30–75 mg range). However, certain tricyclic side-effects are disliked by postnatal women, for example daytime drowsiness and dizziness, for fear of dropping the baby.

Failure to respond to the initial prescription is quite common; increasing the dose or a switching to a drug of a different group may be helpful. Lithium augmentation (with either a tricyclic or an SSRI antidepressant) is often a useful strategy in resistant cases, possibly because the more severe puerperal cases may have an underlying bipolar diathesis. If lithium is used, breast-feeding should cease, but most of those with a severe depression will have given up breast-feeding by this stage. A less common but more dangerous risk is the potential teratogenicity of lithium, and before giving lithium women should *always* be actively forewarned about the teratogenic risks, because a few women may be planning further pregnancies, while others may be unreliable in their use of contraception.

Once the condition has resolved, drug therapy should continue for a further 6–12 months, because case register studies (e.g. Kendell *et al*, 1981) have shown that morbidity remains high in the second post-partum year. Drug tapering should be gradual and supervised closely, as relapses are common and not always easy to treat. Relapses after further pregnancies are common, although precise figures for non-psychotic depression are not available. Antidepressants can be used prophylactically and started immediately after delivery to minimise the risk of recurrence, as described above for puerperal psychosis.

Breast-feeding and psychotropic drugs

Women with very severe mental illness are usually unable to breast-feed. Women with illness of moderate severity who wish to breast-feed but need to take a psychotropic drug can usually do so, but will need psychiatric support and advice on the optimum choice of drug. Those with milder disorders often successfully breast-feed while taking medication, or make a choice either to breast-feed or to take medication but not both together. A few women select to breast-feed for 2–3 months without medication to ensure that their infants

Table 25.1 Database on breast-feeding and psychotropic drugs

Drug	Summary of reported findings
Tricyclics	Generally well tolerated by mothers and infants
Amitriptyline	Milk:serum ratio 0.7–1.6, mean around 1. Infant plasma levels low or undetected. One woman on 100 mg daily had maternal plasma level of 128 ng/ml and the infant level was 7.5 ng/ml, but there is variability. The use of 10 mg tablets allows for dosage titration to ensure minimum effective dosage. Widely used in the pre-SSRI era
Doxepin	One case report of infant respiratory depression, drowsiness, hypotonia and poor infant feeding
SSRIs	
Fluoxetine	Hendrick *et al* (2001*a*) found infant fluoxetine levels low or undetectable, but norfluoxetine was detected ($n = 20$). Maternal dosage was critical: thus, at 20 mg/day, mean fluoxetine and norfluoxetine level was 8.9 ng/ml; at 30 mg the mean level was 62.5 ng/ml. Breast milk: maternal plasma ratio usually around 1, but in one woman breast milk showed a six-fold increase but infant levels were low at 25 ng/ml. Another infant had a high plasma level, at 265 ng/ml, but was asymptomatic. Variability and occasional high values probably relate to slow metaboliser status. There have been two adverse clinical reports: one of excessive crying, decreased sleep diarrhoea and vomiting; one of somnolence, decreased feeding, hypotonia
Sertraline	Small amounts only in breast milk. Undetected in infant plasma, but desmethyl sertraline present in 24%. Significantly higher levels in women on 100 mg daily or above. One report of a withdrawal syndrome in the infant of a mother who abruptly stopped sertraline, which consisted of restlessness, insomnia and poor feeding. Otherwise no adverse reports
Paroxetine	Levels of paroxetine and its metabolite were undetectable in infant blood (Hendrick *et al*, 2001*b*). No adverse reports
Citalopram	Levels undetected in infant blood. No adverse reports
Typical neuroleptics	
Chlorpromazine	Maternal plasma:breast milk ratio 0.5. One report of lethargy
Haloperidol	Present in breast milk. One report of delayed development in a woman breast-feeding on chlorpromazine and haloperidol, but infants exposed to haloperidol alone did not show this
Thioxanthenes	May improve breast-feeding (possibly by increasing prolactin). No adverse reports
Sulpiride	Limited data
Atypicals	
Olanzapine	Limited data. One report of jaundice and drowsiness
Clozapine	Maternal plasma:breast milk ratio approximately 1. Theoretical risk of fits and agranulocytosis in the infant, hence probably contraindicated. No reports on its use or adverse reports
Amisulpride, risperidone, quetiapine, aripiprazole	No information; but because of this and theoretical risks, manufacturers advise avoiding them
Mood stabilisers	
Lithium	Maternal plasma:milk ratio 0.3 – 0.7. Infant lithium levels highly variable. Lithium toxicity in infants a known hazard, presenting as cyanosis, lethargy, hypothermia and hypotonia. Close infant lithium monitoring may not be sufficient to prevent toxicity as any current illness (e.g. infant diarrhoea) can rapidly cause electrolyte imbalance and toxicity. Avoid
Valproate	Breast milk levels 1–10% of maternal plasma levels. Infant blood levels low at 4–12% of maternal blood levels. One report of thrombocytopenia and anaemia, which reversed on stopping the valproate
Carbamazepine	Breast milk levels 7–95% of maternal blood levels. Infant levels 6–65% of maternal levels. Adverse reports: two cases of hepatic dysfunction, one report of drowsiness and irritability. Seizures reported in one case of an infant whose mother was on fluoxetine, carbamazepine and buspirone, indicating the increased risks to infants of mothers on polypharmacy
Benzodiazepines	
Diazepam	Maternal milk:plasma ratios are low, at 16–30%, but there are reports of 'floppy infant syndrome', with hypotonia and lethargy. Hence avoid

Data based on Yoshida *et al* (1999) and Taylor *et al* (2003).

have received what they believe to be a good supply of maternal antibodies and immunity and then wean the infant and start an antidepressant.

All psychotropic drugs are small molecules and are highly fat soluble; they enter the breast milk to a variable degree and also cross the infant's blood–brain barrier. Most of the commonly used psychotropic drugs appear to be 'relatively safe', but no drug is completely safe, although, by the same token, none is absolutely contraindicated. This means that the psychiatrist will need to be acquainted with the existing database on the various psychotropic drugs, to offer some advice to the mother who wishes to breast-feed. This database is in fact at present remarkably thin and derived from only a few case reports and a few studies of maternal and infant plasma levels as well as breast milk levels (Table 25.1).

Breast-feeding while taking a psychotropic drug should be avoided where the infant has a hepatic, renal or neurological disorder, or is premature, or has some other particular problem. Maternal drug dosages should be kept to a minimum, as there is uncertainty regarding how newborn infants can handle the higher plasma levels of psychotropic drugs. It should be noted there will always be a small proportion of mothers (and presumably infants as well) who may be slow metabolisers (see Chapter 11), and because metaboliser status will be unknown to the prescriber, the level of psychotropic drugs in the maternal breast milk may be highly variable.

Advice is often given that breast-feeding should be done before psychotropics are taken, but as most infants feed on demand this may not be possible.

The Maudsley guidelines (Taylor *et al*, 2003) suggest that if a woman has done well in pregnancy on a particular drug, then the same drug should be continued during the puerperium. For postnatal illness, these guidelines recommend: paroxetine or sertaline as antidepressants; sulpiride as an antipsychotic; lorezapam for sedation; and zolpidem for sleep. These guidelines state that mood stabilisers should be avoided if at all possible.

The main risk to the infant is of drug toxicity, and although full-blown syndromes are rare, women often report their babies are lethargic, sleepy or irritable and the psychiatrist should make specific enquiry about these symptoms and the infant's general welfare at each visit. If the infant's symptoms appear to be clinically significant, maternal drug dosage should be reduced or alternatives to breast-feeding should be considered.

Maternity blues

Transient mild depression and crying spells after childbirth are frequent and have been called the baby blues, third-day blues, the maternity blues and the transitory syndrome, the last capturing the evanescent nature of the mood swing. The syndrome is reviewed in detail by Stein (1982). Crying spells are the hallmark of the maternity blues and are reported in 50–70% of new mothers. Often, there is a very brief cry due to emotion in the first few hours after delivery, and this may be accompanied by feelings of happiness or tears of joy, but around 10% of women describe feeling acutely depressed, strange or depersonalised immediately after delivery.

A rather more severe, prolonged spell of weeping sometimes occurs between the third and fifth day, and this weepiness sometimes occurs with an altered mood, although the mood is not necessarily depressed. Anxiety, elation, irritability or a state of emotional lability may accompany these weeping spells. Common reasons given for the weeping include feelings of rejection by the husband or nursing staff, or minor ailments in the baby or themselves. Illness in a newborn baby usually takes precedence over all other causes of maternal anxiety, while among multigravid women the reason given for the weeping usually revolves around the other children at home.

More severe depressive feelings, sometimes with a violent or bizarre content and reminiscent of the thought pattern observed in depressive illness, occur in around 10% of women and are more common among those with previous depression (Stein, 1980). This more intense depression usually lasts only for a few hours and rarely for the whole day, but may recur in bouts on two or three successive days. Irritability or angry feelings directed at the husband or partner or hospital staff are common, while transient negative feelings towards the baby and an early lack of maternal affection can be elicited in up to 40% of women; these usually resolve without any adverse consequences. Although forgetfulness, confusion and poor concentration are common complaints, psychometric testing has failed to detect any objective measure of cognitive impairment. Elation is present in over 80% of women on day 1, but this falls to 40% by day 4, although a few women are elated every day. This elation falls far short of hypomania. Emotional lability, particularly on the blues day, is also common.

Insomnia, dreaming and nightmares are common, while transient hallucinations on wakening (hypnopompic hallucinations) occur in around 10% of women. Rapid eye movement and stage IV sleep are decreased in pregnancy, but may show a rebound increase on nights 2 and 3 post-partum, approximately coinciding with the blues (Karacan *et al*, 1969). A mild headache, generally bilateral and frontal, occurs in around a third of women, usually between days 3 and 6, and this appears to be more common among those women with a personal or family history of migraine (Stein, 1984). For most women, the maternity blues is a brief acute episode lasting no more than a few hours and for 1 or 2 days only, but a few women may have a rather more continuous pattern of disturbance. Just occasionally, a very severe, brief, almost psychotic episode occurs for 2–3 days as a part of the maternity blues, and this was the original 'milk fever'.

The only established clinical associations with the maternity blues are anxiety and depression during late pregnancy, previous premenstrual tension, and subsequent postnatal depression. Parity, social factors and obstetric complications do not appear to be related.

Aetiology – a hormonal and biochemical hypothesis

The clinical picture

A single cause for all the diverse post-partum syndromes is unlikely, but there is some evidence pointing to a biological basis for the puerperal psychosis and the maternity blues. The clinical picture of the maternity blues, with its fixed time interval of onset 3–4 days after delivery, combined with the organic affective picture and the lack of significant psychosocial correlates, suggests the possibility of an underlying biological cause. For puerperal psychoses the onset is also at a relatively fixed interval after childbirth, and occurs at the same time as the blues, and the initial clinical picture also has elements of an organic affective state such as delirium.

The puerperium acts as a trigger for these organic affective changes. Mood changes and affective disorder are also known to follow menstruation and weaning, and occasional exacerbations follow premenstrual phases during the first post-partum year. However, they have by far the greatest risk in the first month after childbirth. Kendell *et al* (1987) reported a 35-fold increased risk for mania for this period, while the maternity blues occur in 50% of women at this time. This suggests that there must be some quite potent biological change during the puerperium that acts as a trigger for severe affective psychoses in predisposed women, but results in only a minor mood swing among women who lack such a predisposition.

A specific trait in some women but not others

The hormonal changes following childbirth are probably similar in all women, but why do some women succumb and others not? There is good evidence, at least for the puerperal psychoses, that possessing an inherited manic–depressive diathesis is of critical importance, and even within cohorts of women with manic depression there appears to be a familial (possibly genetic) subset who are more liable to puerperal disorders, as identified by Jones & Craddock (2001). There is also evidence that there is a subset of women with depression who are peculiarly sensitive to the mood effects of sex hormone withdrawal. Bloch *et al* (2000) recruited two groups of eight women, one with a history of puerperal depression and a control group who had also had children but who had never had puerperal depression. All the women were asymptomatic at the start of the experiment and were given a gonadotrophin-releasing hormone agonist, leuprolide. This blocks the release of both follicle-stimulating hormone (FSH) and luteinising hormone (LH) and so drastically lowers oestrogen and progesterone levels and induces a state of hypogonadism. To cover this, micro-ionised oestrogen and progesterone were administered for 8 weeks and then withdrawn under placebo-controlled double-blind conditions so the women did not know they were experiencing hormone withdrawal. Five out the eight women (62%) with a history of puerperal depression became depressed during this experiment, compared with none of the women who lacked such a history. These findings strongly suggest that the presence of a 'hormone-withdrawal sensitive affective trait', which is probably quite widely distributed in the population, may be a prerequisite for puerperal depression. This trait is distinct from the bipolar trait, but individuals who possess both traits may be especially liable to develop the more severe puerperal illnesses.

The individual hormones

The puerperium is a time of massive hormonal change. Not only do the levels of oestrogen and progesterone fall dramatically, but there are also fluctuations in cortisol and thyroid hormones, and changes in many other biochemical systems as well.

Oestrogens

Oestrogen levels rise from 2 ng/ml in early pregnancy to around 15 ng/ml at term, and then fall abruptly with delivery. The placenta and to a lesser extent the foetal adrenal gland are the main sources and both of these are lost after delivery. Oestrogen may be aetiologically important because oestrogen receptors are widely distributed in the brain, and oestrogen itself has some effects on mood, has neurological effects and interacts with a variety of amine systems. Thus, there are a few case reports that suggest that oestrogens can induce dyskinesias and that chorea gravidarum (chorea in pregnancy) is due to an oestrogenic effect mediated via striatal dopamine.

Cookson (1982) suggested that the fall in oestrogen levels after delivery exposes dopamine receptors which have been rendered supersensitive by high levels of oestrogen during pregnancy. In support of an oestrogen–dopamine hypothesis, Wieck *et al* (1991) administered the apomorphine challenge test, a measure of dopamine receptor function, on the fourth post-partum day to a group of high-risk women and found evidence of increased dopamine receptor sensitivity among those who became psychotic. Oestrogen also interacts with adrenergic receptors, particularly β-adrenergic receptors, as well as with several different serotonergic receptors. Nott *et al* (1976) found that the change in oestrogen levels failed to correlate with measures of mood but that there was an association with sleep. It is unknown which of the many hormone–neurotransmitter interactions are relevant.

Progesterone

Progesterone also shows a massive (10-fold) rise in pregnancy, with peak luteal phase levels of about 10–20 ng/ml, rising to 65–233 ng/ml in late pregnancy. The placenta manufactures about 250 mg of progesterone daily and there is a 100-fold fall after delivery. Progesterone has fewer interactions with amine neurotransmitter systems than oestrogen, but systemic administration of progesterone and its metabolites (e.g. allopregnanolone) produces anxiolytic, hypnotic and anti-epileptic effects by enhancing $GABA_A$ receptors, which are thought to be the benzodiazepine receptors. An abrupt fall in progesterone and its metabolites may therefore simulate an acute benzodiazepine withdrawal syndrome and this may help explain why anxiety, depression and occasionally psychosis occur after parturition.

Harris *et al* (1994) found that greater decreases in progesterone between late pregnancy and the early puerperium were correlated with mood. Allopregnanolone levels also correlated negatively with mood. Nappi *et al* (2001) measured levels of serum allopregnanolone and progesterone in 40 post-partum women and found that those who experienced the maternity blues had significantly lower levels of allopregnanolone but not progesterone. Dalton (1985) also claimed that progesterone administered by suppository or injection (it is degraded in the stomach when ingested orally) has both therapeutic effects in postnatal depression and when administered immediately after delivery could prevent further relapses, although such claims were never subjected to scientific scrutiny. Evidence that either hormone has useful therapeutic effects is thin, but if hormones are to be used in the puerperium, progesterone (unlike oestrogen) is not associated with any increased risk of thrombo-embolism and may therefore be a safer option, although of unknown efficacy.

Cortisol

Cortisol levels rise slowly during pregnancy, sharply during labour and fall after delivery. Elevated plasma cortisol levels and changes in the hypothalamic–pituitary–adrenal (HPA) axis are the only consistent endocrine change found in association with depression and the clinical picture of labile mood found in the maternity blues resembles the dysphoria found in Cushing's disease, while severe psychotic depressions can also occur in Cushing's disease.

Levy (1987) conducted an interesting study of the dysphoria that follows major surgery and demonstrated the presence of a syndrome that had a similar frequency, symptomatic pattern and severity to the maternity blues. After surgery, although there are no changes in sex hormone levels, there are changes in cortisol levels. During the early puerperium over 80% of women are dexamethone suppressors, indicating an abnormality in the HPA axis, a pattern that resembles that found in depression, and one study has reported an association between post-partum mood and ante-partum cortisol levels (Handley *et al*, 1980).

Thyroid changes

A transient biochemical hypothyroidism has been described between the fifth and tenth month post-partum. A Japanese study reported significantly lower levels of FT_3 (free tri-iodothyromine) among women who had the blues 5 days post-partum, and among these women FT_3 levels were also lower at 37 weeks of pregnancy (Ijuin *et al*, 1998).

Both hypo- and hyperthyroidism may occur in the puerperium, but it is unclear if the rates are significantly increased above base rates, and it is unlikely that thyroid hormones play a major role in the aetiology of the puerperal disorders. Hatotani (1983) reported beneficial effects for thyroxine in some cases of repeatedly relapsing puerperal psychoses and this may provide a theoretical basis for trying thyroid augmentation of antidepressants in resistant cases of postnatal depression.

Physiological changes

Almost every bodily system shows some change in the early puerperium as the body switches back to the non-pregnant state. Mood changes are maximal around the third to fifth day, and at this time colostrum changes to milk, which may be related to oxytocin. Body weight generally rises for the first 3 days and is then lost at a rate of 0.5 kg/day between days 4 and 6, but the severity of the mood disturbance shows no correlation with the magnitude of the weight loss (Stein, 1980). Similar abrupt weight loss associated with increased water and electrolyte excretion have also been described in some patients with bipolar disorder, in whom the weight loss occurs synchronously with the switch in mood (Crammer, 1959).

Brain amines are probably involved in the pathogenesis of depression. These cannot be measured directly, so attempts have been made to measure precursors or platelet amines in the hope that they reflect central changes. The levels of free and total plasma tryptophan, the precursors of brain serotonin, do correlate with mood disturbance (Stein *et al*, 1976; Gard *et al*, 1986), but these changes are unlikely to be causal because administering tryptophan to women with the maternity blues has no beneficial effects (Harris, 1980). Changes have also been reported in platelet monoamine oxidase, platelet β-adrenoreceptor levels and plasma endorphin levels during the puerperium, but these are of uncertain significance.

The puerperium is a time of both rapid hormonal change and the onset of affective disorder – but which of the myriad changes occurring at this time are the most relevant ones remains a mystery.

Psychiatric disorders in pregnancy

Pregnancy is generally held to be a time of maternal well-being, but individual reactions vary so widely that generalisations are probably meaningless. The prevalence of psychiatric disorders during pregnancy probably resembles that of non-pregnant women of a similar age. Thus, Kelly *et al* (2001) used a self-rating scale to detect DSM–IV psychiatric disorders in a cohort of pregnant women in Seattle, and found that 21% had 'depression' but only 4% qualified for a current diagnosis of DSM–IV major depression, and most women had either minor depression or anxiety–depression. Around 5% had an anxiety state, with 1% suffering from panic disorder, and eating disorders were also fairly common (5%, with 2% having anorexia nervosa and 3% suffering from bulimia). As previously noted, in the study by Evans *et al* (2001), depression was more prevalent during pregnancy (13.5%) than at 8 weeks post-partum (9.1%). Depression may be more common in the first and third trimesters, with some sparing of the mid-pregnancy period.

The causes of depression in pregnancy are similar to those found among non-pregnant women and appear to be mainly social, including adverse life events, relationship difficulties, the absence of a confiding relationship, a history of depression, and in some clinic population studies a history of abuse when a child (Spinelli & Endicott, 2003).

Anxiety in pregnancy is almost ubiquitous and generally centres on fears of abnormality in the foetus or personal problems. Among women who have had previous difficulties, such as a stillbirth, foetal abnormality, a difficult labour, or previous postnatal depression, the worry revolves around the risk of the same problem recurring.

There has been some interest in the effect that maternal stress and anxiety have on the developing foetus and the more recent studies have been reviewed by Glover & O'Connor (2002). The adverse outcome most consistently associated with maternal anxiety is pre-term labour or low birth weight for gestational age. The mechanisms are unclear, but Teixeira *et al* (1999) showed that high state and trait anxiety as measured by questionnaire was associated with increased uterine artery resistance as measured by Doppler ultrasound, and increased uterine artery resistance itself is known to be associated with intrauterine growth restriction and pre-eclampsia. A longitudinal study (O'Connor *et al*, 2002) measuring anxiety in late pregnancy and infant outcome at 4 years found a significant correlation between maternal anxiety in the third trimester and the presence of behaviour disorder or emotional problems in both boys and girls at 4 years. Although the authors postulated that the maternal anxiety in some way affected the mother's pregnancy (e.g. by leading to an elevated maternal cortisol level) and developing foetus, the more usual explanation for two family members having the same or similar conditions is a genetic one.

The more severe depressions – those requiring hospital admission – are much less common during pregnancy than they are postnatally, but the recent literature is very sparse on these cases. Clouston (1896) managed to collect only 15 cases over 15 years and estimated they comprised around 1% of all admissions, having an onset in either the first or third trimester. New cases of psychoses are also rare in pregnancy, usually starting in the eighth or ninth month, but there are a few women who regularly become depressed during each pregnancy but then get better after delivery (see Brockington, 1996).

Pregnancy usually has a beneficial effect on the course of anorexia nervosa, possibly because women are highly motivated to ensure adequate nourishment for their foetus if not for themselves. However, weight gain for anorexic mothers is less than for normal mothers and their babies may weigh a little less. One small series suggested has suggested there may be an excess of premature births and a raised perinatal mortality rate (Brinch *et al*, 1988).

The vomiting of bulimia nervosa should be distinguished from the rather more common condition of hyperemisis gravidarum. This usually has an onset between the third and sixth week of pregnancy and generally resolves spontaneously between the 12th and 16th week, although in some cases it may persist for the duration of the pregnancy. Bulimia will usually predate the pregnancy and appetite is generally preserved, but it is lost in hyperemesis (although it returns once the vomiting ceases). In severe cases of hyperemesis there is rapid weight loss, dehydration and, if the condition is prolonged, Wernicke's encephalopathy may occasionally supervene. The cause is unknown, and although at one time hyperemesis was suspected of having a psychogenic origin, this is no longer believed to be the case. Women experiencing such profuse vomiting are naturally anxious about their condition.

Patients with schizophrenia tend to default on antenatal care, may not eat properly or neglect themselves in other ways and so may require an increased input from the team during pregnancy, which may include hospital admission, if indicated.

Management of depression in pregnancy

The treatment of depression during pregnancy is similar to its treatment at other times, but differences exist in the social context, degree of motivation and the ubiquitous fear that any psychotropic drug might cause foetal damage, which needs to be taken into account in the treatment plan.

Psychotherapy may be helpful, particularly for some cases of depression. A randomised controlled trial of a group of women with major depression compared 16 weeks of interpersonal therapy against an education programme (Spinelli & Endicott, 2003). Scores on the Hamilton Rating Scale for Depression fell equally (by around a third) for the two groups during the first 4 weeks, but by the end of the trial there was a significant difference between the two groups, with 50% of those receiving interpersonal therapy improved compared with only 30% of those who had the education programme. Put another way, these figures suggest that 30% of pregnant women who become depressed may experience spontaneous remission (i.e. the women in the control group), a further 20% will benefit from the specific effects of psychotherapy, while the other 50% will show little change after 16 weeks. Thus, there is still a need for other remedies, such as antidepressants. Although this trial demonstrated specific benefits for interpersonal therapy, it is likely that other types of psychotherapy with skilled therapists are equally effective.

The use of antidepressant drugs in pregnancy

Pregnant women with depression respond well to antidepressant drugs, which appear to be reasonably safe in pregnancy, although they should be used sparingly. The topic has been reviewed in an editorial by Hampton (2006) aptly entitled 'Antidepressants and pregnancy: weighing the risks and benefits, no easy task'. It is now beginning to emerge that there are small risks with the use of antidepressants, and one of the SSRIs (paroxetine) has recently been identified as being associated with cardiac abnormalities, while there is also increasing evidence of a risk for a variety of neonatal syndromes. Against these risks, there are also significant risks in leaving a serious depression untreated; these include weight loss in pregnancy, an increased need to smoke and drink during pregnancy (both of which may be harmful to the foetus), poor attendance at the antenatal clinic, and the effects of a large overdose taken in a suicide attempt; a completed maternal suicide will usually kill the baby as well.

Drug therapy in pregnancy is further complicated by powerful fears among most women that any drug taken during pregnancy may harm the baby. These fears became very much more severe and widespread following the thalidomide disaster in 1968, when thalidomide was prescribed for vomiting in pregnancy and resulted in an epidemic of infants who were born missing one or more limbs (phocomelia). Before this the tricyclic antidepressants had been prescribed to large numbers of pregnant women without any particular difficulty or any observed increased rate of malformation. One harmful effect of these fears is that some women will immediately cease taking their antidepressant when they discover they are pregnant and will thereby trigger a depressive withdrawal syndrome. Thus, Cohen *et al* (2006), in a study of 201 women with previous recurrent major depression, a group for whom there is good evidence in favour of long-term maintenance therapy, found that for women who were followed up, 44 out of the 65 (68%) who discontinued their antidepressants suffered a depressive relapse, whereas only 21 out of the 82 (26%) women who continued with their medication relapsed. It is therefore generally recommended that patients with recurrent or previous severe depression who are currently taking antidepressants and then discover they are pregnant should either continue their medication or gradually withdraw it, but only under supervision.

Major birth defects occur at a rate of around 2% in the USA, so a small number of birth defects are to be expected, and the key question is whether a particular drug is associated with a raised rate or a particular type of malformation. First-trimester exposure is particularly important as foetal development is most rapid in this phase, with the central nervous system being at its most vulnerable between 14 and 35 days after conception – the phase of neural tube closure – although the risk is not confined to this critical period.

While prospective clinical trials in this area are clearly not possible, considerable effort has gone into following up women who have taken antidepressants during pregnancy and ascertaining the outcome in relation to their infants. In a meta-analysis of 414 cases of documented first-trimester exposure to tricyclic antidepressants (as a group), no excess of congenital malformations were identified (Altshuler *et al*, 1996).

There is a database of 2750 infants whose mothers had taken SSRIs during pregnancy (2000 with fluoxetine, 300 with citalopram, 200 with sertraline, 200 with paroxetine and 50 with fluvoxamine), among whom no increase in teratogenicity has been observed when compared with the offspring of women who did not have such exposure (Altshuler, 2002). However, the manufacturers of paroxetine in a post-marketing survey have identified a raised rate of congenital cardiac abnormalities (mainly ventricular septal defects) and the US Food and Drug Administration (2006) has issued guidance that paroxetine should not be used in pregnancy or among women who are planning to become pregnant. One study (Chambers *et al*, 1996) found no difference between the rates of major abnormalities between women who took fluoxetine in pregnancy and controls, but did report a significant difference in the frequency of minor abnormalities (15% versus 6.5%), although it is important to note these minor abnormalities were all surface abnormalities of no cosmetic or functional significance and were diagnosed by a paediatrician specially trained in their detection.

Four studies have compared pregnant women taking antidepressants and pregnant women exposed to known non-teratogenic agents (such as penicillin or dental radiography) and found no differences in terms of pregnancy outcome, rates of intrauterine death, methods of delivery, or offspring characteristics such as gestational age and birth weight (Wisner *et al*, 1999).

There is accumulating evidence for neonatal disturbances occurring immediately after delivery. The most serious of these disorders is persistent pulmonary hypertension, a fairly rare condition but one that carries substantial morbidity and a mortality rate of around 10%. In the study by Chambers *et al* (2006) the pattern of antidepressant consumption in the mothers of 337 infants with persistent pulmonary hypertension was compared with the pattern in the mothers of 836 controls. Women who had taken an SSRI in the second half of pregnancy had a greatly increased risk (odds ratio 6.1; 95% CI 2.2–16.8), but no increased risk was found for other antidepressants.

For both the tricyclics and the SSRIs a neonatal withdrawal syndrome has been identified for infants whose mothers have taken antidepressants in late pregnancy. For tricyclics, the syndrome consists of neonatal jitteriness, irritability, tachypnoea, tachycardia, feeding difficulties, sweating and occasional cholinergic symptoms such as functional bowel disturbance and urinary retention. Withdrawal fits have also been described in association with maternal clomipramine use. A similar syndrome of transient poor neonatal adaptation has been described in association with maternal fluoxetine use. This comprised jitteriness, hypoglycaemia, hypothermia, poor muscle tone, respiratory distress, weak or absent crying and desaturation (a fall in blood oxygen levels) on feeding. This picture was present in 31% of the infants of mothers who had taken fluoxetine in late pregnancy and represented an eight-fold increased rate over controls, while only 9% who had only early exposure (first trimester) to fluoxetine developed such a syndrome.

A large ($n = 119\,547$) Canadian study extending over 3 years (1998–2001) found that 14% of women had depression in pregnancy; at the start of the study 2.3% of the women were on an SSRI, but by the end of it this had risen to 5%. The infants of SSRI-exposed mothers were more likely to have lower birth weight (but not very low birth weight – below the 10th percentile), neonatal respiratory distress (14% versus 8%), feeding problems (3.9% versus 2.4%) and jaundice (9% versus 7%) (Oberlander *et al*, 2006).

The later prognosis for children appears to be unaffected by prenatal exposure to antidepressants. Thus, Nulman *et al* (1997) applied a battery of psychometric tests to a group of children (aged between 16 and 86 months) exposed to tricyclics ($n = 129$) or fluoxetine ($n = 55$) and non-exposed controls ($n = 84$) and found no differences on any of the neurobehavioural tests they applied. More recently Misri *et al* (2006) reported on the 'internalising behaviours' of 4- and 5-year-old infants of mothers who had been exposed to SSRIs in pregnancy, and although there were some differences from control children, these could be wholly accounted for by the raised levels of maternal anxiety. These studies, although preliminary, suggest that there are no long-term effects of maternal antidepressants on infant development and behaviour, but in the light of epidemiological evidence now emerging that very large numbers of pregnant women are currently taking SSRIs, further work is clearly warranted.

The decision on whether to prescribe or not is essentially a clinical one. There are no firm guidelines that take into account some of the more recent revelations concerning the risks of the SSRIs. The clinical decision will rest largely on the severity of the depression. In severe depression the risks of leaving the patient untreated may be high and the decision to proceed with medication may be clear cut. In contrast, with mild dysthymic states it may be best to adopt a 'wait and see' policy. For women with depression of moderate severity the decision may be more difficult and in these cases, once all the potential risks and benefits of treatment and non-treatment have been discussed, the patient's own wishes may be a determining factor. Even where the patient initially declines somatic therapy, the psychiatrist should maintain contact and offer continued psychotherapeutic support, which may help in itself. In addition, the course of the depression itself can fluctuate and may abruptly become severe; this will often lead some women to change their mind about medication.

If a decision is made to prescribe an antidepressant, one will need to be selected. At the time of writing there are no guidelines that incorporate some of the more recent findings directing the selection of any particular drug or drug group in pregnancy and the views expressed here are those of the author. Until the more recent discovery of adverse effects of the SSRIs in pregnancy, most authorities published guidelines favouring the use of the SSRIs, and even with the observations on persistent pulmonary hypertension the SSRIs (but not paroxetine) can still be used. The older tricyclics may still have certain advantages. First, pregnancy depressions are often remarkably sensitive to relatively small doses of tricyclics (e.g. 30 mg daily), but if this does not work, doses can be quickly titrated up to 75 mg (e.g. for amitriptyline), which will generally be sufficient for a therapeutic response. Second, sleep disturbance is common in normal pregnancy and may be exacerbated by depressive sleep disorder, which usually responds very well to sedative tricylics such as amitriptyline administered at night, whereas SSRIs may sometimes worsen sleep disorder. Thirdly, as pregnancy nears term, antidepressants should be reduced or even stopped to avoid any neonatal withdrawal syndrome. This is easily done for the tricyclics because they can be tapered down to an extremely low dosage (e.g. 10 mg) before the expected date of delivery and then maintained until delivery and afterwards, which will help prevent any withdrawal syndrome occurring in either the mother or baby.

For women who have been previously well stabilised on a particular antidepressant, whether an SSRI (other than paroxetine – see above) or a tricyclic, there does not appear to be sufficient evidence to justify changing to another drug. It may be wise to try to reduce the dose or even stop an SSRI when the mother is near term, to reduce the risk of neonatal complications. Fluoxetine will have to be stopped at least 2 weeks before the expected date of delivery because the drug has a very long half-life. Stopping paroxetine at this time may be undesirable since a paroxetine withdrawal syndrome may be precipitated, which may not be helpful immediately before delivery. The database for the other antidepressants is too small to make any meaningful recommendations.

ECT may occasionally be required in resistant or severe suicidal depression in pregnancy, and is a safe procedure, the only hazard being the risk of the anaesthesia. Pregnancy is associated with slower gastric emptying, which increases the anaesthetic risk for gastric reflux, and anaesthesia may result in aorto-caval compression in late pregnancy, which can theoretically reduce foetal circulation. Close collaboration between the maternity services, the anaesthetist and the psychiatrist are required on the rare occasions when ECT is used.

Antipsychotic drugs, teratogenicity and other neonatal complications

Although antidepressants are the most frequently prescribed psychotropic drugs in pregnancy, there will be occasions when other drugs are required, particularly for those with serious mental illness. As with antidepressants, there are three areas of concern:

1 Are there direct teratogenic effects?

2 Will neonates experience a neonatal withdrawal syndrome?

3 Are there long-term neurobehavioural changes in the infant as a consequence of taking psychotropics in pregnancy?

Although some data are available for the antidepressants, information on other drugs is much more sparse. In the UK, a national teratology information service is based at the University of Newcastle (see http://www.nyrdtc.nhs.uk/Services/teratology/teratology.html). This service will carry out individual risk assessments for pregnant women exposed to drugs.

Teratogenic effects are at greatest risk in the first trimester, from weeks 3 to 11, when the neural tube and other major organs are developing. In the second and third trimesters drugs may affect foetal development or have a direct toxic effect on foetal tissues, while drugs given in the third trimester may have adverse effects on labour or on the neonate after delivery.

Antipsychotics may have to be continued in some patients with established and severe psychoses, because the risks of a psychotic breakdown in pregnancy as a result of drug discontinuation far outweigh the risks of continuing therapy. Considerable experience with the older, conventional ('typical') antipsychotic drugs led to a general consensus that there was little or no significant elevation for the rates of major foetal abnormality. One report (Rumeau-Roquette *et al*, 1977) suggested that chlorpromazine (now little used) raised the rates by 0.4% (base rates of abnormalities are 1–2%). There have been no reports of adverse effects with trifluoperazine. There were no teratogenic effects in an older trial in which haloperidol was used to treat a large series of cases of hyperemesis gravidarum in the first trimester (van Waes & van de Velde, 1969). A more recent multicentre controlled trial of haloperidol and penfluridol (a long-acting butyrophenone, but little used in the UK) conducted within the European Network of Teratology Information Services found there was no overall increase in the rates of congenital anomalies in comparison with the control group. However, there were two cases of limb defects (one with haloperidol, one with penfluridol) and this, combined with two previous isolated case reports of limb defects, led the authors of this study to suggest that the possibility of an association between butyrophenone exposure and limb defects could not be ruled out. They therefore recommended a level II ultrasound scan with an emphasis on limbs in any women who had a first-trimester exposure to a butyrophenone (Diav-Citrin *et al*, 2005).

For the atypicals, McKenna *et al* (2005) have reported on data derived from three separate teratology services in Canada, Israel and the UK. Data were obtained on 151 pregnancy outcomes where there had been exposure to olanzapine ($n = 60$), risperidone ($n = 49$), quetiapine ($n = 36$) and clozapine ($n = 6$). Among women exposed to an atypical antipsychotic, there were 110 live births (72.8%), 22 spontaneous abortions (14.5%), 15 therapeutic abortions (9.9%) and 4 stillbirths (2.6%). Among babies of women in this group, there was one major malformation (0.9%) and the mean birth weight was 3341 g (s.d. = 685 g). There were no statistically significant differences in any of the pregnancy outcomes of interest between the exposed and comparison groups, with the exceptions of the rate of low birth weight, which was 10% in exposed babies compared with 2% in the comparison group ($P = 0.05$) and the rate of therapeutic abortions ($P = 0.003$). The authors concluded that these results suggest that atypical antipsychotics do not appear to be associated with an increased risk of major malformations. This appears to be the best currently available information on the atypicals.

In general, if a patient has done well on a particular antipsychotic drug and a clinical decision has been made that antipsychotics are essential, it may be best to stick with the medication that the patient is familiar with rather than take the risk of switching drugs, especially as no particular antipsychotic drug has been identified as being either 'safe' or 'unsafe'. An increasing number of pregnant women are being exposed to atypical drugs each year and so far there have not been any adverse reports indicating teratogenicity, although there are a few reports of maternal hyperglycaemia.

Neonatal syndromes of two types have been described with antipsychotic drugs:

1 occasional extrapyramidal syndromes
2 withdrawal syndromes associated with discontinuation, which present as crying, agitation and increased suckling, similar to neonatal antidepressant withdrawal syndromes.

In general, high-potency antipsychotics are preferred in pregnancy, as they have fewer anticholinergic and hypotensive side-effects; as all the newer atypicals are high-potency drugs, probably any of them may be used.

Mood stabilisers and benzodiazepines

Lithium is probably the safest of the mood stabilisers in pregnancy, but as it has known risks of teratogenicity it should not be used unless absolutely necessary – a few women who have been well stabilised on lithium are liable to severe, frequently relapsing bipolar disorder and in these cases the risks of discontinuation and relapse outweigh the teratogenic risk, which is rather lower than initially thought (1 in 1000–2000). Lithium is associated with an increased risk of cardiac abnormality, particularly Ebstein's anomaly (tricuspid valve displacement into the right ventricle, resulting in an enlarged right atrium and small right ventricle, and usually an associated atrial septal defect). This can be detected with a foetal ultrasound scan, which should be offered to all pregnant women who are on lithium. Neonatal goitre and arrhythmias are also described.

The other mood stabilisers are anti-epileptic and while they may be required to be used as anti-epileptics in pregnancy, they should probably be discontinued if they are solely being used as mood stabilisers, because they are associated with raised rates of serious neural tube defects (spina bifida) (carbamazepine at a rate of 0.5–1.5% and sodium valproate at a rate of 1–5%). If they are used, a folic acid supplement should be co-administered during pregnancy and vitamin K after delivery.

Benzodiazepines have been associated with a possible increased risk of cleft palate if taken in the first trimester, and may result in the 'floppy baby syndrome' if taken near term; they should therefore be avoided.

In general, psychotropic prescribing in pregnancy should be kept to a minimum, with the lowest possible doses, but if the severity of the disorder requires psychotropic medication, then the patient should remain under the care of the psychiatric team throughout the pregnancy as well as afterwards, to ensure that all other aspects of psychiatric care are optimised during this period.

Maternal alcoholism

Drinking behaviours are common in pregnancy. Kelly *et al* (2001) found 17.5% of their sample of pregnant women scored at least 1 on the CAGE questionnaire (see page 419), which indicates at least a degree of alcohol misuse (7.5% scored 2 and 2.2% scored 3, although none scored 4). Other types of substance misuse were present in 5% of the women and 8% had both substance misuse and a psychiatric disorder. These women probably represent a very vulnerable subgroup who should, whenever possible, be identified during the antenatal period.

Maternal alcoholism must be quite severe to cause the full-blown foetal alcohol syndrome. Neonates with this syndrome have an odd facial appearance: a short nose and a broad flat nasal bridge, short palpebral fissures, abnormal ears and palmar creases, dental malocclusion, maxillary hypoplasia (small chin), psychomotor disturbance and sometimes microcephaly. It is not known for certain whether lesser degrees of drinking may cause lesser degrees of foetal damage but this is possible, so women found to be drinking in pregnancy should be appropriately counselled and, if they agree, be referred to an alcohol treatment programme. The infants of mothers who are addicted to drugs or alcohol may require admission to a special-care baby unit for treatment of a drug withdrawal syndrome, with an appropriate drug-tapering regimen.

In the postnatal period a few women, often with a strong family history of alcoholism, either continue their pregnancy drinking behaviours or turn to drink, sometimes in association with depression. Some women are sufficiently motivated by the fear of losing their child to enter treatment programmes to curb their drinking, but many are not.

Intoxicated women become too sleepy, irritable or insensitive to care properly for their infants, who should never be exposed to carers prone to abnormal alcohol- or drug-induced mental states. Mothers who misuse alcohol or drugs are able to keep their children only if other family members (usually partners or grandmothers) assume a leading role in child care. Unfortunately, many of these women are unable to sustain longer-term relationships with their partners and, as a result of their addictive and other maladaptive behaviours, will have broken off from their families of origin, leaving the social services little option but to remove the child for long-term fostering or adoption.

Effects of post-partum psychiatric disorder on others

Puerperal mental disorder never occurs in a vacuum and derives at least some of its importance from the dramatic effect it may have on others, particularly the baby but also partners and other family members. Reactions to the baby may vary from positive feelings of love and warmth through to disinterest, neglect and abuse, and, rarely, even to infanticide. Even when abuse has not occurred, maternal mental illness may have demonstrable effects on infant development.

Infant development

There has been some recent interest in whether a postpartum illness may have a longer-term effect on infant and child development. Cohorts of infants of mothers who have had a particular psychiatric disorder have been examined, both using psychometric tests and by direct observation of mother–infant interactions with videos, and then followed up. Murray (1992) showed that infants aged 18 months of mothers who had postnatal depression were less likely to form secure attachments than infants of non-depressed control mothers, performed worse on an object concept task, and also showed mild behavioural difficulties. Male infants appeared to be more affected than females and the IQ of the 4-year-old sons of women with postnatal depression was around 1.5 standard deviations lower than that of boys of non-depressed control mothers. These changes persisted when the same children were followed up aged 11 (Hay *et al*, 2001). There is also a suggestion of increased rates of hyperactive and distractible behaviours among the male but not among the female offspring of women who have had postnatal depression.

By contrast, the children of mothers who have experienced a puerperal affective psychosis that resulted in hospital admission do not seem to be impaired. Hipwell *et al* (2000) suggested that this might be because these infants are usually separated from their mothers during the most intense symptomatic phase, but as recovery is often complete there is negligible exposure to the disturbed mother.

Maternal eating disorder may also have subtle effects on infant development. Stein *et al* (1994) took videos of mothers with eating disorders and control mothers while they were feeding their 1-year-old infants. Mothers with an eating disorder were more intrusive and expressed more negative emotion during meal times. Not surprisingly, their infants gained less weight than the infants of control mothers and infant weight appeared to relate to the degree of mother–infant conflict as shown on the video, as well as to the mother's concern over her own body shape.

Although the studies described above have found demonstrable effects on child development, none of the infants or families included in them became involved in serious child abuse cases. The implication is that a maternal axis I condition alone (with the possible exception of some cases of schizophrenia) is not of itself a major cause of child abuse or neglect. It is probable that the additional effect of other difficulties – such as personality disorder, a criminal history, low IQ or substance misuse – is what results in a devastating effect on child care, particularly when superimposed on a maternal depression.

Child abuse and neglect

Adult psychiatrists, particularly those specialising in perinatal psychiatry, are becoming increasingly involved in the assessment of cases of child abuse and neglect, although child protection issues are traditionally more the work of social service departments and child psychiatrists. The account here highlights the areas where adult psychiatrists may become involved.

The causes of child abuse and neglect are multifactorial. Serious mental disorder is much more commonly associated with child neglect than with child abuse.

Paediatricians were first alerted to parental child abuse by a paper by Caffey (1946), a paediatric radiologist who saw puzzling radiographs of six infants who presented with the unusual combination of multiple fractures of long bones and subdural haematomas. The fractures were all at different stages of healing, which suggested the infant had received multiple episodes of trauma over a prolonged period, and this was combined with bilateral subdural haematoma, which was presumed to be due to a shaking injury. In all cases the parents denied any history of injury. Kempe *et al* (1962) drew further attention to the problem in a famous paper entitled 'The battered child syndrome' and suggested the phenomenon was quite widespread.

Over the next two decades several case series were published and identified the characteristic features. Thus, in one large Australian series (Ryan *et al*, 1977) bruises were present in 31% of the cases, fractures in 20% and subdural haematoma in 11%. Injuries around the mouth were common, with split lips, lacerations of mucus membranes, torn frenulum or injuries to the palate, presumably related to attempts to stop the infant screaming. Blows on the head may rupture the eardrum and cause deafness or damage the external ear. A series of non-accidental injuries tends to cause multiple complex fractures at different stages of healing, whereas genuine accidents are more likely to cause single, linear fractures. Blows to the abdomen may cause visceral injuries such as ruptured spleen, kidney, stomach or bowel and may have a high mortality. Subperiosteal haematomas may result from limb wrenching, while shaking can cause both retinal haemorrhages and bilateral subdural haematomas. Bite marks are always suspicious but may be misleading; they are sometimes inflicted by an older sibling. Burns, scalds and chemical burns may all occur, while simple trauma may cause widespread bruising and petechial haemorrhages.

Attempts at asphyxiation sometimes present with complaints of cyanotic attacks. Some mothers smother their infants with a pillow in a desperate attempt to suppress crying, while others hold their face under water during a bath. Video surveillance methods have shown that some women who report cyanotic episodes have deliberately smothered their babies.

Poisoning occurred in 5% of the cases reported by Ryan *et al* (1977). Sodium chloride was the most common poison used and caused hypernatraemia. Water intoxication from forced feeding of drinks results in hyponatraemia. Laxatives and emetics, CNS depressants, insulin, oral anti-diabetics, anticoagulants and almost all other drugs have been reported to have been used as a poison in isolated cases.

Serious non-accidental injury usually presents initially to either the accident and emergency department or the paediatric department; the initial diagnosis is usually the province of the paediatrician, but at a later stage many of the women involved will require psychiatric

Table 25.2 Relative importance of different screening characteristics in parents and infants for child abuse as determined by discriminant function analysis

Checklist characteristics	Abusing families (%) (*n* = 106)	Non-abusing families (%) (*n* = 14146)	Conditional probability (%)[a]
Parents with a child under 5 (baseline)	–	–	0.7
History of family violence	30.2	1.6	12.4
Parent indifferent, intolerant or overanxious towards child	31.1	3.1	7.0
Single or separated parent	48.1	6.9	5.0
Socio-economic problems, such as unemployment	70.8	12.9	3.9
History of mental illness, drug or alcohol addiction	34.9	4.8	5.2
Parent abused or neglected as a child	19.8	1.8	7.6
Infant premature, low birth weight	21.7	6.9	2.3
Infant separated from mother for more than 24 h after delivery	12.3	3.2	2.8
Mother < 21 years old at time of birth	29.2	7.7	2.8
Step-parent or co-habitee present	27.4	6.2	3.2
Less than 18 months between birth of children	16.0	7.5	1.6
Infant mentally or physically handicapped	2.8	1.1	1.9

[a] Conditional probability refers to the percentage of families with a characteristic that go on to abuse or neglect their newborn in the first 5 years of life.
From Browne & Herbert (1997), p. 120.

care, particularly as they break down at various points during the ensuing legal process.

Neglect is rather more common among the infants of mothers with psychiatric disorder than it is in the general population. It may involve a failure to protect the child from exposure to any kind of danger or a failure to carry out important aspects of the child's care, such as protection from common hazards, providing adequate food and clothing, or seeking appropriate medical care. There may be evidence of poor hygiene, sometimes severe nappy rashes, after babies have been left in wet nappies for too long, or even being left alone unsupervised. Infections and other illnesses may be more frequent because the house may be unclean and minimum standards of hygiene are not maintained, while the accompanying emotional neglect may cause developmental delays.

Failure to gain weight that is not due to some medical disorder, or 'non-organic failure to thrive', is one of the most common presentations of physical neglect, and in around a third of such cases no medical condition is found. These infants seem mute and lifeless at home, but thrive, gain weight and become happy and playful in hospital. Such cases are less dramatic than those of physical abuse, but neglect can also result in considerable long-term damage. Neglect is usually detected initially by health visitors, social workers or general practitioners, but the psychiatrist will become involved where mental illness is thought to be a contributing cause.

Background factors

Child abuse is a social phenomenon and not a medical disorder. It has a multiplicity of causes. Browne & Herbert (1997) screened the parents of a very large cohort of children born in Surrey with a 12-item checklist of factors thought to predispose to child abuse. Five years later 0.7% of the children had become the focus of a social service enquiry into suspected or actual maltreatment or neglect. The results of this large study are summarised in Table 25.2. They are important, as they quantify the probability that a parent or child with a particular risk factor will become involved in later child abuse.

One important risk factor not included in Table 25.2 is the presence of a low IQ, which is commonly found in cases of both neglect and abuse. Sheridan (1956) found that of 100 mothers charged with neglect, the mean IQ was 80, with a mode of 75, and only 14 mothers had an IQ above the norm. Some women with lowish intelligence, particularly if well supported by other relatives, are able to cope with the demands of their children, but the addition of any other adverse factor, such as a personality problem, poor support or failure to comply with a treatment programme, makes child removal far more likely (Tymchuk & Andron, 1990). Smith *et al* (1973) reported a similar low average IQ (of 80) for women who were responsible for cases of non-accidental injury that had led to a hospital admission. In addition, these workers found that 62% of these mothers had a personality disorder, 11% had a criminal record and 7% were 'aggressive psychopaths', but only 3% were psychotic (two with paranoid schizophrenia and two with psychotic depression). Of the fathers, 37% were 'aggressive psychopaths' and 29% had a criminal record. Other background social factors included lower social class, relative youth, an unwanted pregnancy, being from a large family and social isolation.

Abusive parents more often see negative intentions in their children's behaviour than do normal parents, and have more unrealistic expectations of what is developmentally appropriate. They tend to find even normal infant or child behaviour more stressful.

Oliver (1985) demonstrated that cycles of familial violence and abuse of children could be established: that is, the abused children became abusive parents. This pattern might extend over several generations. Personality disorder, mental illness, suicide attempts, drug and alcohol dependence in both mothers and fathers, epilepsy, learning disability and criminality were all conspicuous features in these families. More comprehensive accounts of child abuse are given elsewhere (e.g. Browne, 2002).

Functional mental disorder, which is the main area of concern of adult psychiatrists, is only weakly associated with child abuse and child removal. Browne & Herbert (1997) found that only 5% of mothers with mental illness later became involved in social services child-care proceedings. However, where mental disorder is severe and chronic it may be an important cause and the presentation is almost always one of neglect rather than abuse. Howard *et al* (2001) examined a group of mothers who had a psychosis (mostly schizophrenia but also a few affective disorders) and found that 90% kept their children, although they often lived under grossly impoverished and unsatisfactory conditions; long-term fostering arrangements or child removal were required only for the other 10%. This was associated with the mothers being of younger age, being involuntarily admitted, having a criminal record and, in the particular district studied (Southwark, in London), being of black African origin.

'Nuclear schizophrenia', as defined by the Present State Examination (PSE), appears to have a very poor prognosis with regard to child care. Da Silva & Johnston (1981) found that only one of 17 mothers who had an admission for PSE-defined nuclear schizophrenia during the puerperium was able to keep her children.

In bipolar disorder, mothers can keep their children provided that there are long intervals free of illness, that episodes of mania are brief and patients are well supported by their partners, and that their families can take over child care during the episodes of mania. However, if these conditions are not met and no other family members are available to help out, small children cannot be exposed to mothers with mania, particularly if the underlying affect is one of paranoid aggression and in cases where episodes are frequent or prolonged, or admission is difficult to facilitate. Fostering arrangements may be needed during episodes, which, if repeated, may eventually culminate in a more permanent separation.

Assessment and management – the role of the adult psychiatrist

Under the Children Act 1989, the statutory responsibility for the provision of child care lies with the local-authority social services department. Social services may call on any number of different professionals, such as lawyers, the police, paediatricians, psychologists and child and adult psychiatrists to assist them in this daunting task. The initial task of the case conference is to work together with the parents and other relevant professionals to reach a consensus on the level and type of risks involved and to make a decision about whether the child's name should be placed on the Child Protection Register.

In the year 1999–2000, a total of 29 300 children were registered under the following categories: neglect (35%), physical abuse (23%), sexual abuse (12%), emotional abuse (17%) and combinations of categories (13%). Around 14% of the registrations were re-registrations, indicating the need for continued surveillance even after the case has apparently improved and been closed. The overall rate of new registrations was 27 per 10 000 (0.27%) children under the age of 18, but was highest for infants under 1 year of age, at 71 per 10 000 (0.7%), suggesting that postnatal depression may also play a role, in conjunction with other factors.

The case conference will also discuss other issues of child care, such as attendance at parent craft training, or day centres, or specific tasks the parents should accomplish in the home, or whether additional help in the form of family aides is required, and a whole variety of other measures. An adult psychiatrist may become involved in these proceedings and may be required to submit a psychiatric report in some cases of postnatal depression where child care appears to have been affected. In many of these cases the difficulties are transitory; social workers may have adopted an unduly pessimistic view, because postnatal depression is usually a self-limiting disorder. With more vigorous therapy and extra support for the family, the child-care issues usually resolve as the depression lightens. However, in a minority of cases the risks are more severe and long term. Other factors, such as low IQ and personality disorder, are more prominent in these cases and the likely outcome will be removal of the child. In these instances it is essential for the psychiatrist *not* to be *both* the treating doctor (usually a sector psychiatrist) *and* the person who writes a medico-legal report for social services and the court – a task that can be undertaken by an independent expert psychiatrist. This is because the patient may later quite understandably have difficulty in trusting anyone who has contributed to her losing her children, yet will continue to need treatment and support from the sector psychiatric team.

Reder & Duncan (1997) suggest that adult psychiatrists (whether independent experts or the local sector psychiatrist) should confine their reports to issues of mental state, diagnosis and prognosis, while critical assessments parental skills should be dealt with by child psychologists or child psychiatrists, who are more familiar with this perspective. In preparing such reports, as well as providing a comprehensive account of the mental disorder, it may also be helpful to assess the risk factors identified in Table 25.2, and also obtain the patients' IQ from a formal assessment by a psychologist.

In the face of a deteriorating situation, the social worker can apply to a magistrate for an emergency protection order (under section 44 of the Children Act 1989) and remove the child. This order can last for 7 days and can then be extended for a further 7 days, but if more prolonged intervention is required an interim care order (section 37), which lasts for 8 weeks, may be instituted, which can be renewed for a further four weekly periods, but eventually social services are required to draw up a long-term plan for the child, which may involve permanent removal. To do this they must apply to the court for a full care order (section 31) and the only criterion that can justify this is that significant harm to the child might otherwise arise.

Once the court is considering the grave step of child removal, some women break down, especially before important meetings or court cases, and may need admission or support from the team. The picture is rarely one of a classical depression, but more often of an angry depression in an immature patient with personality disorder and lowish IQ, and there may be demanding or more frequent acting out behaviours.

Finally, once a child has been removed from a mother, most women are quite bereft and suicidal, and many will require long-term psychiatric care, occasional admissions and support extending over many years, a task that usually falls to the catchment area psychiatrist. As noted above, it is therefore important that those who care for the patient's depression or other psychiatric difficulties are not a part of the social service team involved in child removal (Reder & Duncan, 1997).

On occasions, women who are undergoing this arduous legal process confide that they have developed homicidal impulses directed towards their social worker, and although actual homicides are rare, assaults are a well recognised hazard of child protection work. There is a duty for the treating psychiatrist to assess this risk and pass the information on to the relevant person, even though this may occasionally entail breaking a patient's confidence.

Filicide, neonaticide and infanticide

Filicide refers to the homicide of children aged under 16, neonaticide to the killing of infants very soon after delivery (usually on the first day) and infanticide to the killing of infants under 1 year of age. The last category is the most strongly associated with psychiatric disorder. In England and Wales, the Infanticide Act 1938 provides for a verdict of infanticide:

> 'for the killing of a child under the age of 12 months by its mother under circumstances that would otherwise amount to murder, if the balance of the mother's mind is thought to have been disturbed at the time.'

It is usually dealt with leniently by the court, by either a probation or hospital order. The Infanticide Act does not apply in Scotland, nor is there any similar legislation in the USA. In these countries, when mental illness is thought to have contributed, a plea of diminished responsibility is submitted and a verdict of manslaughter rather than murder is applied. For the 5 years 1995–99, in England and Wales 172 infants under 1 year were officially registered as the victims of homicide. It is possible this figure is an underestimate because a small and as yet undefined proportion of the large number of cot deaths are also now thought to be due to homicide. Of the homicide cases, 23% (around 40, or approximately eight cases per year) received a verdict of infanticide and a further 15% received a verdict of some other type of manslaughter (Brookman & Maguire, 2003). The frequency of the infanticide verdict appears to be unchanged because, in the decade 1976–85, the rate was also around seven cases per year (Home Office, 1985).

Psychiatric interest is greatest for infanticide in the context of a psychotic illness, but because of the rarity of this event in recent times only the older literature is able to provide some insights. Hopwood (1927) examined 166 women admitted to Broadmoor following infanticide between 1900 and 1927; indeed, this was the commonest reason for a female admission to Broadmoor at that time, comprising 42% of all female admissions. Around 70% of the cases occurred during lactation rather than in the very early puerperium, and these women had what Hopwood termed an 'exhaustional psychosis'. The clinical picture comprised symptoms of restlessness, insomnia, delusions, hallucinations, confusion, depression, disorientation and occasionally stupor – a picture consistent with an untreated puerperal psychosis. In addition to exhaustion psychoses, 13% had manic depression, 10% 'dementia' (i.e. schizophrenia) and 5% epilepsy – these women killed their child during an epileptic automatism (one mother placed her child in the fire and the kettle in the cradle). Most cases (60%) of 'exhaustion psychoses' resolved spontaneously fairly quickly, but 30% of these women attempted suicide and 6% died.

Hopwood's study confirms that in the pre-ECT and pre-drug era, a puerperal psychosis was a very dangerous condition. These early observations remain relevant to present-day practice and indicate that an untreated or a partially treated or a relapsing puerperal psychoses is a dangerous condition for the mother, where the risk is of suicide, and also for the baby, where the risk is infanticide. Every effort should be made to get symptoms under control as quickly as possible.

Neonaticide is rather more of a social and historical phenomenon than the result of specific psychopathology. In ancient Sparta, weak or sickly newborn infants were left to die at the foot of Mount Taygetus. In 18th-century Japan, peasants would kill some newborn infants by suffocating them with wet paper, a procedure known as *makibi* ('thinning out') and this was used as a means of population control. In 19th-century Europe, young mothers would often conceal illegitimate pregnancies and then either smother or drown their newborn infant. Selective female infanticide probably still continues today in some parts of rural China (Brockington, 1996). Neonaticide is rare today in the UK but does still occur: between 1995 and 1999 there were 27 infant homicides on the first post-partum day, which comprised around 16% of the total number of infant homicides.

Infanticide and filicide are rare and tragic outcomes of a chain of events and circumstances. Psychotic illness is responsible for only a small minority of cases; the majority result from repeated child abuse. Resnick (1969) found five possible motives in his series:

1 altruistic filicide, where the parent, who may be suicidal or otherwise psychotic, feels unable to abandon the child and so kills the child to relieve real or imagined suffering (it is thought that psychotic depression in the parent most commonly underlies this type of behaviour)

2 acute psychotic filicide, where a parent kills the child as a result of delusions or hallucinations focusing on the baby

3 accidental filicide (the commonest 'motive'), particularly for older children, relates to the child being killed as a result of child battering, when there is irritation with the child but no homicidal intent

4 the killing of an unwanted child

5 spousal revenge, where the offspring is killed in order to get back at the spouse.

D'Orban (1979) conducted a similar study, of 89 women admitted to Holloway Prison who had either killed or attempted to kill their child. Only 27% suffered from a psychotic illness or were seriously mentally ill at the time. Rather more frequent were battering mothers (40%). Most of these women suffered from a personality disorder. One-third had a reactive depression at the time of the offence. Low IQ was prominent in this group, with over a third having an IQ below 90, and three women had a formal diagnosis of learning difficulties. Battering mothers often came from large families, where there had been a history of maltreatment at the parents' hands, and parental discord and separation were also significant background features. A few killed in the context of a Medea complex, where the baby reminded them of a hated partner; a few of the infants were unwanted and there was also one case of a mercy killing.

Infants under 1 year of age appear to be at greatest risk of being victims, with the risk being four times that of the general population; those between 1 and 5 years of age have the same risk and those between 5 and 15 years have a lower risk. Within the first year, the first 6 months may be a particularly vulnerable period (Marks, 2001).

Falkov (1996) reported on the psychopathology of 100 cases of the perpetrators of filicide, and around half had either a definite or a probable psychiatric diagnosis. Of those with a definite psychiatric disorder (32 cases), there were 10 cases of psychosis but only one had a puerperal psychosis. The other illnesses were: postnatal depression (3), other depression (8), personality disorder (6), alcoholism (5), drug dependency (4) and Munchausen by proxy (2) (some women had more than one diagnosis). Eight perpetrators attempted suicide at the same time as killing the child, indicating their mental state was abnormal. In contrast to the pattern found in child abuse, 'all available' children tended to be killed rather than just the most vulnerable one. In this series, two-thirds of the victims were already subject to child protection proceedings and as many as one-third of the perpetrators had been in contact with the adult psychiatric services in the month before the killing.

Reder & Duncan (1997) in their commentary on their study entitled 'Adult psychiatry – a missing link in the child protection network', advocated far greater awareness and involvement by adult psychiatrists in child protection issues. Most healthcare trusts now try to ensure that all clinical staff are aware of local child protection protocols.

Male reactions and marriages

During a wife's pregnancy some men become disturbed; this has been termed the 'couvade syndrome' (from French *couver*, meaning to brood or hatch). Trethowan & Conlon (1965) found a raised incidence of nausea, vomiting, early-morning sickness, abdominal pains, anxiety, insomnia, weakness and headaches among men whose wives were pregnant, compared with married men whose wives were not pregnant. About one in nine men developed such symptoms, which usually started in the third month and abated after parturition.

Anthropologists have been interested in couvade rituals, some of which are designed magically to transfer the pangs of labour to the husband. For example, the Dyaks of Sarawak perform a pantomime of obstructed labour on the husband when the wife is in difficulties during labour. Some couvade rituals take place after delivery, such as special diets for men, and these are seen as a way of protecting the newborn child from disease.

Psychoanalysts have speculated on the role in these male reactions of envy of women's creativity, and repressed hostility related to the sexual taboos imposed by pregnancy and the implied rejection. The clinician should note that some men may become temporarily disturbed, or even ill, or act out by having affairs, or may even leave the relationship during their wife's pregnancy. The last in particular may have a devastating effect on a woman's mental state, especially if she has depression. An explanation provided to the woman that some men may have a strange reaction to their wife's pregnancy is sometimes helpful because often these reactions are transitory and resolve after parturition, but in the present era of high divorce rates some women are abandoned at this time.

After delivery, a postnatal depression in a woman may be associated with a psychiatric disorder in her partner. Zelkowitz & Milet (2001) studied 50 women with postnatal depression and found that their partners were three times more likely to have a psychiatric diagnosis at 2 months, usually anxiety, depression or adjustment disorder, than the partners of women who were free of postnatal depression (23% versus 8%). In half the cases the partner's depression was still present at 6 months These findings suggest that a woman's postnatal depression may somehow light up psychiatric disorder in her partner.

Most studies have shown that a poor marriage and the absence of a close confiding relationship have a major causal role in both puerperal and non-puerperal depression (see page 56). However, postnatal depression itself may have a major impact on the spouse and consequently the marriage as well. Loss of libido is almost universal in postnatal depression and this may result in a weakening of the affectionate bond. Psychoanalysts point to the change from a two-person to a three-person situation, with its potential for destructive envy. Certain symptoms of depression – irritability, hostility, self-preoccupation and a loss of sensitivity to the needs of others – may also have a subtly corrosive effect on a relationship, particularly if the illness becomes prolonged.

The clinician should note any marital deterioration and in all cases try to see the spouse, preferably with the patient. This may give the partner an opportunity to unburden himself of the stress of trying to cope with a wife with depression or may have a cathartic effect if he has become independently psychiatrically ill.

Stillbirth

A stillbirth is a devastating event and even with modern obstetric care around 0.5% of women will experience the loss of a foetus between 24 weeks and term. In most published series almost all the women had typical grief reactions. The pattern is usually one of initial shock followed by numbness, disbelief and denial. Guilt may be prominent as women desperately search for an explanation. Some women harshly criticise themselves for minor peccadillos during pregnancy, such as drinking small amounts of alcohol, eating the wrong foods or failing to heed the doctor's advice. Sometimes their anger is directed at the obstetric team, particularly if an intervention has failed. Women may experience depression or a post-traumatic syndrome, or both, with intrusive nightmares featuring their experiences of labour. Only a minority succumb to a prolonged postnatal depression, but even among those who have recovered, anniversary reactions of a depressive type are common.

Clarke & Williams (1979) found that although rates of depression among women who had had a stillbirth were increased at 3 months post-partum, by 6 months the rate was no higher than among non-pregnant women. Turton *et al* (2001) studied mothers who had conceived again and found that rates of depression during the second pregnancy were lower if women had not conceived for at least a year after the stillbirth. It seemed as if those women who had given themselves adequate time to recover from the tragedy did better. In a second paper (Hughes *et al*, 2002), this group found that during the next pregnancy around 20% of women developed post-traumatic stress disorder (PTSD) and this was strongly comorbid with depression. However, 1 year after the birth of the next live child this figure had fallen to 4%, indicating that the trauma associated with a stillbirth tended to ameliorate with the passage of time.

Women who have experienced a stillbirth need to see their obstetrician to clarify whether there was any reason for their loss and whether such an event can be prevented in the future. There has also been interest in a programme of active management, where women are encouraged to see and hold their dead baby or take a lock of hair and have photos taken of the baby. While such a programme may suit some women, many will be much too distraught to permit such close contact with their dead infant. Turton *et al* (2001) found that, overall, active management of seeing and holding the baby was associated with later higher levels of anxiety and also tended to worsen the symptoms of PTSD; further, it was associated with a greater degree of disorganised attachment behaviour in their next infant.

Counselling with a professional after a stillbirth may help diminish the severity of the grief reaction, but few women present for psychiatric help, preferring instead to seek support from fellow sufferers through organisations such as the Stillbirth and Neonatal Death Society (SANDS). The work of Turton *et al* (2001) suggests the long-term psychiatric prognosis may be better if women wait at least a year after the loss before embarking on a further pregnancy, by which time they have more fully recovered, and that so-called 'active management' is probably not helpful.

Premenstrual syndrome

Around 20–40% of women experience some premenstrual symptoms but these are severe in only 3–5%. The hormonal basis of the condition was first recognised by R. T. Frank (1931), who described 15 women with severe symptoms, although Hippocrates had described women with mood changes before menstruation in ancient Greece. The observation that the premenstrual syndrome (PMS) does not occur before puberty or after the menopause, and the cyclical nature of the symptoms, have led to the suggestion that the hormones involved in ovulation are in some way responsible for the disorder. However, repeated studies have shown that these hormone levels are within the normal range; the cause instead appears to lie in a differential reactivity between women to normal hormone levels. The aetiology is in fact unknown, but there appears to be a definite genetic contribution, as demonstrated by twin studies (van den Akker *et al*, 1987; Kendler *et al*, 1998). There is an association with affective disorder, since around two-thirds of those presenting to PMS clinics also give a lifetime history of affective disorder (Halbreich *et al*, 1985) and there is commonly a psychosocial contribution, such as a history of childhood sexual abuse (Golding *et al*, 2000). Most women presenting for treatment are over 30 years of age and the condition is most severe in the 5–10 years before the menopause, but it may be severe from the menarche onwards.

The main psychological symptoms of PMS are depression, irritability and lethargy, but a wide variety of other, mainly neurotic symptoms may also occur. The depression is usually labile, often associated with weeping, in contrast to the fixed continuous low mood encountered in a depressive illness. A picture of atypical depression with hypersomnia, food craving and a reactive mood occurs in some cases, while in others there are agitation and hostility. Irritability is characteristic (partners often report increased anger or temper premenstrually). There are premenstrual phase effects for school marks, the frequency of minor misdemeanours, suicide attempts and hospital admission rates for affective disorder but not schizophrenia.

The somatic symptoms include painful swelling of the breasts (mastalgia), swelling of the abdomen, fingers or ankles, while cognitive symptoms include impaired efficiency in work tasks and sometimes clumsiness. Among those with a predisposition to migraine, premenstrual headache may be troublesome. Premenstrual alcohol craving, heightened sexual urges and brief hypomanic episodes are all described. Although rare, recurrent menstrual and premenstrual psychoses are described, and there may be premenstrual exacerbations of a post-partum psychosis as well.

Diagnostic criteria

To make the diagnosis, ICD–10 requires only a history of a single physical or mood symptom occurring on a cyclical basis without functional impairment. DSM–IV recognises a rather more severe variant, premenstrual dysphoric disorder (PMDD) (see Box 25.1). DSM–IV includes PMDD in an appendix entitled 'Criteria sets and axes for further study' and this condition is not in the main text of the book, indicating that PMDD is not fully accepted as an officially recognised psychiatric disorder; rather, its nosological status is still under consideration.

To make the diagnosis of PMDD there should be a clear history of a premenstrual exacerbation and a resolution of the symptoms with onset of menstruation or shortly after, and the criteria should be confirmed by prospective daily ratings for at least two cycles. A small number of women report an ovulatory exacerbation. There should also be a clear account that the symptom complex interferes with school, work, relationships or some of other aspect of daily living to qualify for a diagnosis of PMDD, according to DSM–IV. However, such a severe degree of functional impairment is not necessary to diagnose PMS in the ICD–10 scheme or even in routine clinical practice.

Box 25.1 DSM–IV diagnostic criteria for PMDD

1 Clinically significant emotional and behavioural symptoms during the last week of the luteal phase, which remit with the onset of the follicular phase.
2 At least 5 of the following 11 symptoms, of which one symptom must be (i), (ii), (iii) or (iv). The 11 symptoms are: (i) marked depressed mood; (ii) anxiety tension; (iii) anger, irritability, increased interpersonal conflict; (iv) affective lability; (v) decreased interest; (vi) difficulty in concentrating; (vii) lethargy, lack of energy; (viii) overeating, specific food cravings; (ix) hypersomnia or insomnia; (x) feeling overwhelmed or out of control; (xi) other physical symptoms – breast tenderness, headaches, muscle pain, feeling bloated.
3 The condition should be of sufficient severity to cause marked impairment of social and occupational function.
4 The condition should have occurred in the majority of the menstrual cycles during the previous year.
5 The symptoms cannot be explained as an exacerbation of another disorder such as depression, panic disorder or personality disorder.

Treatment

Non-pharmacological approaches

Placebo-controlled trials, even for the more severe version of premenstrual tension, namely DSM–IV PMDD, show that 30% of patients improve, indicating that the condition has a fairly high rate of spontaneous remission, and this should always be borne in mind when assessing the claims for any particular remedy.

The most commonly used non-pharmacological approaches include special diets, exercise, cognitive therapy and relaxation. Dietary recommendations are to increase complex carbohydrates and dietary fibre to 20–40 g daily, reduce intake of refined sugar, reduce salt intake and taking frequent small meals to lessen the tendency for blood sugar levels to fluctuate, even though frank hypoglycaemia has never been demonstrated in PMS. Some authors recommend a reduction in caffeine intake (by drinking less tea and coffee), which is a generally helpful measure for any anxiety disorder. Exercise is recommended. Although there are no controlled studies, exercise is known to increase brain endorphin levels and in many people leads to a feeling of well-being. Twelve sessions of CBT proved to be significantly superior to a programme of group awareness and a waiting-list control condition, and cognitive therapy seems a promising approach, particularly in the light of its success in other psychiatric disorders (Kirkby, 1994). Relaxation therapy is also superior to simply charting the symptoms and leisure reading (Goodale *et al*, 1990). Psycho-educational programmes have also proved helpful and a simple explanation of the origin of the symptoms should form a part of any treatment programme.

Antidepressants

Reduction in brain 5-HT transmission is believed to be associated with poor impulse control, irritability and dysphoria, as well as increased carbohydrate craving, all of which are features of PMDD. A special drink that results in acute tryptophan depletion lowers central serotonin by removing its precursor, L-tryptophan, and this has been shown to aggravate the symptoms of premenstrual tension (Menkes *et al*, 1994). In addition, a placebo-controlled trial has shown that large doses of L-tryptophan (6 g daily) have a beneficial effect on the mood symptoms of PMDD, which again suggests a role for serotonin (Steinberg *et al*, 1999).

The first trial of an SSRI (fluoxetine) in PMS was described by Menkes *et al* (1992), who conducted a placebo cross-over trial in 16 women with PMS; 15 of the 16 improved while taking fluoxetine, but only 3 of the 16 improved while taking placebo. All the women who improved on fluoxetine relapsed when the fluoxetine was withdrawn. There are now over 30 reported studies, including 20 randomised trials, involving more than 1100 patients, showing that the SSRIs are effective and mostly well tolerated in up to 70% of women with PMDD (Steiner & Pearlstein, 2000). Patients appear to respond fairly quickly to low doses of SSRIs and increasing the dosage only leads to more side-effects. Curiously, the somatic symptoms of PMS, such as breast pain, swelling and clumsiness, also improve with SSRI therapy, but this may be due to an altered perception associated with the improvement in mood. An interesting finding has been the demonstration that these drugs are just as effective if given during the luteal phase only (i.e. half cycle treatment) and in one trial with citalopram intermittent dosing proved to be more effective than continuous dosing (Wikander *et al*, 1998). Open-label studies have shown these drugs can be used for 12–18 months, but it is important to note that not all patients can tolerate SSRIs.

Hormones and hormonal therapies

The facts that PMS is manifest only between the menarche and the menopause and is suppressed during pregnancy strongly suggest an association with ovulation. Strategies to suppress ovulation have therefore been used in its management, and these include the use of gonadotrophin-releasing hormone (GnRH) agonists, oestrogen, progesterone and danazol.

The use of GnRH agonists is of theoretical interest only. GnRH is responsible for the release of the pituitary hormones, follicle-stimulating hormone (FSH), which primes the ovarian follicle, and luteinising hormone (LH), which causes the release of the ovum into the fallopian tube. GnRH agonists cause anovulation by chronic down-regulation of GnRH receptors in the hypothalamus, and this leads to decreased secretion of FSH and LH, resulting in greatly lowered oestrogen and progesterone levels, absence of cyclical hormonal changes and anovulation; the symptoms of PMS are also abolished.

These preparations cannot be used long term in clinical practice because they cause such a profound fall in oestrogen levels as to result in osteoporosis. To counteract this fall, oestrogen and progesterone can be added back to the regimen, but when this is done mood and anxiety symptoms may recur. In a small controlled study, Schmidt *et al* (1998) rendered women with and without PMS anovulatory for 3 months through the use of monthly injections of the GnRH analogue leuprolide. The women with previous PMS experienced a resurgence of their mood and anxiety symptoms when either oestrogen or progesterone was reintroduced, but this did not occur among the women with no previous PMS. The authors suggest that women with PMDD appear to have a special sensitivity to the mood effects of oestrogen and progesterone.

Gynaecologists have used oestrogen implants to manage PMS because they suppress ovulation, but the main use of oestrogen is as hormone replacement therapy (HRT) for the management of the menopause (see below). Several studies also show its efficacy in the prevention of premenstrual migraine. By suppressing ovulation, oestrogen implants also appear to help reduce the symptoms of PMS (Magos *et al*, 1986). Implants of oestradiol (100 mg) are inserted into the subcutaneous fat of the lower abdominal wall and women are also given an oral progestin (5 mg norethisterone) to counteract the risk of unopposed oestrogen causing endometrial cancer. Implants tend to lose effectiveness after 4–8 months and sometimes rebound depression or anxiety can occur when they wear off, and they may need to be replaced.

Progesterone, once fashionable for the treatment of PMS, is no longer recommended, as several placebo-controlled double-blind trials have failed to demonstrate any efficacy for progesterone-based products, even including a trial of a preparation of oral micronised progesterone (Freeman *et al*, 1995). However, the continuous administration of high-dose progestins can cause anovulation, which is required to suppress the symptoms of PMS. Thus, medroxyprogesterone acetate (MPA) (Provera, or the injectable version, Depot Provera) has had some success in the management of PMS. In a one trial, women who received 15 mg MPA daily had a significant reduction in their symptoms compared with those taking either placebo or norethisterone. Ovulation was usually suppressed on this low dosage but breakthrough bleeding was a problem.

Danazol acts by inhibiting pituitary gonadotrophins. It is mainly anti-oestrogenic and anti-progestogenic and may suppress ovulation, but androgenic side-effects have limited its use. Oral contraceptives have also been investigated and although a few women report improvements, others report worsening of symptoms; placebo-controlled trials show no efficacy. Androgens have also been used for premenopausal (and also perimenopausal) symptoms, and it is suggested that they benefit women with decreased libido and fatigue. Dosage is restricted to a narrow therapeutic window because there is a risk of virilising side-effects with the higher doses.

Other remedies

A variety of other medications have been used to treat PMS or particular symptoms in the PMS complex, and these are reviewed by Pearlstein & Steiner (2000). Mineral supplements have been used for some time and a large multicentre trial of calcium supplements (1200 mg daily in two doses) showed that calcium was effective in 48% of cases, compared with 30% on placebo, in reducing all the emotional and physical symptoms of PMDD except for fatigue and insomnia (Thys-Jacobs *et al*, 1998). The administration of magnesium (200 mg daily) was helpful only for reducing fluid retention and had little effect on emotional symptoms (Walker *et al*, 1998). Vitamin B6 has been in vogue for many years and comprises a group of compounds, including pyridoxal and pyridoxamine. It is converted to pyridoxal phosphate, a coenzyme that is essential in the metabolism of most transmitters, including serotonin. Earlier reviews cast doubt on its efficacy, but a meta-analysis of nine controlled studies suggested weak beneficial effects for vitamin B6 in doses of 50–100 mg daily (Wyatt *et al*, 1999). True deficiency of vitamin B6 is not described in PMS, so it is uncertain what, if anything, the supplements are doing.

Diuretics were fashionable for many years to treat 'fluid retention', although direct weighing of people who claim to retain fluid reveals only small fluctuations in weight. Because thiazides can cause potassium loss, if a diuretic is prescribed a potassium-sparing diuretic such as spironolactone may be preferable. Ammonium chloride is an old remedy and is combined with caffeine in the over-the-counter remedy Aquaban. Bromocriptine is useful for breast pain but is associated with vomiting and side-effects; more recent dopamine agonists such as cabergoline have fewer side-effects and are much better tolerated.

Prostaglandin-related treatments, such as the non-steroidal anti-inflammatory drugs (NSAIDs) naproxen and mefenamic acid, have shown some benefits, but the risk of more serious side-effects such as gastrointestinal haemorrhage or agranulocytosis with mefenamic acid probably preclude their use in a relatively benign condition such as PMS.

Lithium is not effective in PMS but occasional patients with premenstrual hypomania or other exacerbations of bipolar affective disorder may benefit, and in one reported case there was a rise in plasma lithium levels premenstrually despite a constant lithium intake (Kukopoulos *et al*, 1985).

Other treatments that have been used include evening primrose oil, beta-blockers, calcium channel blockers, thyroxine, light therapy and sleep deprivation.

In the more severe cases, hysterectomy and oophorectomy may be curative because they abolish the menstrual cycle. Usually women will have some other indication for such surgery, such as fibroids or endometriosis. Surgery will need to be followed with oestrogen replacement therapy. Cyclical mood changes can occasionally persist after hysterectomy.

The menopause

The menopause is defined as the cessation of a woman's menstrual periods for 12 months. It represents a normal physiological development and is not a physical or mental disorder. These changes usually take place between the ages of 45 and 55 years but may occur many years earlier. The decline in ovarian function leads to a fall in oestrogen production and the lowered oestrogen levels in association with a raised FSH level may be helpful in diagnosis. Hot flushes are experienced by 75–85% of women as they approach the menopause; when they occur at night they may significantly impair sleep and this may contribute to daytime fatigue and irritability. The mechanism of the hot flush is thought to be via the lowered oestrogen level, which decreases endogenous opioid peptide activity, and this in turn results in less opioid inhibition of central noradrenergic activity – particularly in the thermo-regulatory centres. Quite large fluctuations in skin temperature (up to 5°C) may occur during a hot flush (Stuenkel, 1989).

Urogenital atrophy is the second most common manifestation of oestrogen deficiency and epithelial changes in the vagina result in a more alkaline pH and frequent episodes of vaginitis. Thinning of the vaginal epithelium and atrophic vaginitis can result in painful intercourse, with consequent effects on libido and feelings of self-worth. Because the lower third of the urethra is also oestrogen sensitive, complaints of urinary frequency, dysuria and urgency are also common. Later and more serious effects of decreased oestrogen levels include osteoporosis and increased rates of atherosclerosis.

Ever since Kraepelin (1896) first suggested that the menopause might cause a condition called 'involutional melancholia' there has been controversy surrounding the question of whether the menopause is associated with increased rates of affective disorder or depressive symptoms, as detected in community surveys. Burt *et al* (1998) reviewed epidemiological surveys and found that five out of six cross-sectional surveys but only one out of four longitudinal surveys reported an increased rate of depressive symptoms around the menopause. However, one study found a doubling of the rate of depressive symptoms following an artificial or surgically induced menopause, while in another study there was an association between physical and depressive symptoms at this time. Burt *et al* (1998) concluded that there probably is an association but that it may not be particularly strong, as it did not show in all the studies; nor is the link necessarily hormonal, as cultural and social factors may independently contribute to depressive symptoms at this time of life; in this connection it is of interest that in countries where older age is venerated and associated with a higher social status, such as in India and Japan, the only menopausal symptoms reported regularly are the menstrual changes (Prados, 1967).

Although Kraepelin subsequently retracted his original proposal that ovarian involution could cause melancholia, Eagles & Whalley (1985) found that the greatest difference between rates of admission for female and male admissions for affective disorder was between the ages of 45 and 55 years, which correspond to the perimenopausal and menopausal years, although such a temporal link does not prove hormonal causation – socio-cultural explanations may be equally plausible.

There are definite medical indications for HRT, particularly following oophorectomy, when HRT may help prevent osteoporosis, premature heart disease and stroke, and it is also helpful for those with troublesome hot flushes or atrophic vaginitis. HRT is not without risk, however; for example, increased rates of breast cancer are reported and it is now thought that a substantial number of the cases of breast cancer in the community are related to HRT, Endometrial cancer may also occur.

The effect of HRT on mood is much more controversial. Hormonal therapies for affective disorders have been suggested for over 50 years and have always attracted a few enthusiasts, but even at times of obvious hormonal change, such as the puerperium and the menopause, the majority of practitioners have not used these remedies, nor are the published data on their efficacy very convincing.

In cases of depression presenting around the menopause, the doctor's task is to clarify the diagnosis and ascertain the patient's main source of distress, which may be socially determined, due to a general medical condition, or due to a major depressive disorder, in which case standard psychiatric remedies should be applied. A few women may present with depression and severe premenstrual tension in their perimenopausal years and they may benefit from hormone implant therapy, which may also be combined with antidepressant therapy, but the widespread prescribing of HRT has no psychiatric justification and therefore should probably be avoided.

References

Agrawal, P., Bhatia, M. S. & Malaik, S. C. (1990) Post-partum psychosis: a study of indoor cases in a general hospital psychiatric clinic. *Acta Psychiatrica Scandinavica*, **81**, 571–575.

Allwood, C. W., Berk, M. & Bodemer, W. (2000) An investigation into puerperal psychoses in black women admitted to Baragwaneth Hospital. *South Africa Medical Journal*, **90**, 518–520

Altshuler, L. (2002) The use of SSRIs in depressive disorders specific to women. *Journal of Clinical Psychiatry*, **63**, suppl. 7, 3–7.

Altshuler, L., Cohen, L., Szuba, M. P., *et al* (1996) Pharmacological management of psychiatric illness during pregnancy: dilemmas and guidelines. *American Journal of Psychiatry*, **153**, 592–606.

American Psychiatric Association (1994) *Diagnostic and Statistical Manual of Mental Disorders* (4th edn) (DSM–IV). Washington, DC: APA.

American Psychiatric Association (2000) *Diagnostic and Statistical Manual of Mental Disorders* (4th edn, text revision) (DSM–IV–TR). Washington, DC: APA.

Appleby, L. (1991) Suicide during pregnancy and in the first postpartum year. *BMJ*, **302**, 137–140.

Appleby, L., Warner, R., Whitton, A., *et al* (1997) A controlled study of fluoxetine and cognitive behavioural counselling in the treatment of post-natal depression. *BMJ*, **314**, 932–936.

Appleby, L., Mortensen, P. B. & Faragher, E. B. (1998) Suicide and other causes of mortality after postpartum psychiatric admission. *British Journal of Psychiatry*, **173**, 209–211.

Beeghly, M., Weinberg, M. K., Olsen, K. L., *et al* (2002) Stability and change: level of material depressive symptomatology during the first postpartum year. *Journal of Affective Disorders*, **71**, 169–180.

Bloch, M., Schmidt, P. J., Danaceau, M., *et al* (2000) Effects of gonadal steroids in women with a history of postpartum depression. *American Journal of Psychiatry*, **157**, 924–930.

Bratfos, O. & Haug, J. O. (1968) The course of manic depressive psychosis: a follow up of 215 patients. *Acta Psychiatrica Scandinavica*, **44**, 89–112.

Brinch, M., Isager, T. & Tolstrup, K. (1988) Anorexia nervosa and motherhood: reproduction pattern and mothering behaviour of 50 women. *Acta Psychiatrica Scandinavica*, **77**, 611–617.

Brockington, I. (1996) *Motherhood and Mental Health*. Oxford: Oxford University Press.

Brockington, I. F., Winokur, G. & Dean, C. (1982) Puerperal psychosis. In *Motherhood and Mental Illness* (eds I. F. Brockington & R. Kumar), pp. 37–69. London: Academic Press.

Brookman, F. & Maguire, M. (2003) *Reducing Homicides: A Review of the Possibilities*. Home Office Online Report 01/03. London: Home Office.

Browne, K. (2002) Child protection. In *Child and Adolescent Psychiatry* (4th edn) (eds M. Rutter & E. Taylor), pp. 1158–1174. Oxford: Blackwell Science.

Browne, K. & Herbert, M. (1997) *Preventing Family Violence*. Chichester: Wiley.

Burt, V. K., Altshuler, L. L. & Rasgon, N. (1998) Depressive symptoms in the peri-menopause: prevalence, assessment and guidelines for treatment. *Harvard Review of Psychiatry*, **6**, 121–132.

Caffey, J. (1946) Multiple fractures in long bones of infants suffering from subdural haematoma. *American Journal of Radiology*, **56**, 163–173.

Chambers, C. D., Johnson, K. A., Dick, L. N., *et al* (1996) Birth outcomes in pregnant women taking fluoxetine. *New England Journal of Medicine*, **335**, 1010–1015.

Chambers, C. D., Hernandez-Diaz, S., Van Marter, L. J., *et al* (2006) Selective serotonin-reuptake inhibitors and risk of persistent pulmonary hypertension of the newborn. *New England Journal of Medicine*, **354**, 579–587.

Chandran, M., Tharyan, P., Muliyil, J., *et al* (2002) Postpartum depression in a cohort of women from a rural area of Tamil Nadu, India. Incidence and risk factors. *British Journal of Psychiatry*, **181**, 499–504.

Clarke, M. & Williams, A. J. (1979) Depression in women after perinatal death. *Lancet*, *i*, 916–917.

Clouston, T. S. (1896) *Clinical Lectures on Mental Diseases* (4th edn). London: Churchill.

Cohen, L. S., Altshuler, L. L., Harlow, B. L., *et al* (2006) Relapse of major depression during pregnancy in women who maintain or discontinue antidepressant treatment. *JAMA*, **295**, 499–507.

Cookson, J. C. (1982) Postpartum mania: dopamine and oestrogens. *Lancet*, *ii*, 672.

Cooper, P. J., Murray, L., Wilson, A., *et al* (2003) Controlled trial of short- and long-term treatment of post-partum depression: 1. Impact on maternal mood. *British Journal of Psychiatry*, **182**, 412–419.

Cox, J., Holden, J. M. & Sagovsky, R. (1987) Detection of post-natal depression: development of the 10-item Edinburgh Postnatal Depression Scale. *British Journal of Psychiatry*, **150**, 782–786.

Crammer, J. L. (1959) Water and sodium in two psychotics. *Lancet*, *i*, 1122–1126.

Da Silva, L. & Johnston, E. C. (1981) A follow-up study of severe puerperal psychiatric illness. *British Journal of Psychiatry*, **139**, 346–354.

Dalton, K. (1985) Progesterone prophylaxis used successfully in postnatal depression. *The Practitioner*, **229**, 507–508.

Dean, C. & Kendell, R. E. (1981) The symptomatology of puerperal illnesses. *British Journal of Psychiatry*, **139**, 128–133.

Dean, C., Williams, R. J. & Brockington, I. F. (1989) Is puerperal psychosis the same as bipolar manic depression? A family study. *Psychological Medicine*, **18**, 637–647.

Diav-Citrin, O., Shechtman, S., Ornoy, S., *et al* (2005) Safety of haloperidol and penfluridol in pregnancy: a multicenter, prospective, controlled study. *Journal of Clinical Psychiatry*, **66**, 317–322.

D'Orban, P. T. (1979) Women who kill their children. *British Journal of Psychiatry*, **134**, 560–571.

Dowlatshahi, D. & Paykel, E. S. (1990) Life events and social stress in puerperal psychosis: absence of effect. *Psychological Medicine*, **20**, 655–662.

Eagles, J. M. & Whalley, L. J. (1985) Ageing and affective disorders. The age at first onset of affective disorders in Scotland 1969–1978. *British Journal of Psychiatry*, **147**, 180–187.

Eberhard-Gran, M., Eskild, A., Tambs, K., *et al* (2002) Depression in postpartum and non-postpartum women: prevalence and risk factors. *Acta Psychiatrica Scandinavica*, **106**, 426–433.

Evans, J., Hero, J., Francomb, H., *et al* (2001) Cohort study of depressed mood during pregnancy and after childbirth. *BMJ*, **323**, 257–260.

Falkov, A. (1996) *Study of Working Together. 'Part 8' Reports. Fatal Child Abuse and Parental Psychiatric Disorder.* London: Department of Health.

Food and Drug Administration (2006) Paxil and the risk of birth defects. *FDA Consumer*, **40**(2), 4.

Frank, R. T. (1931) The hormonal basis of premenstrual tension. *Archives of Neurology and Psychiatry*, **26**, 1053–1057.

Freeman, E. W., Rickels, K. & Sondheimer, S. J. (1995) A double blind trial of oral progesterone, alprazolam, and placebo in the treatment of severe premenstrual syndrome. *JAMA*, **274**, 51–57.

Gard, P. R., Handley, S. L., Parsons, A. D., *et al* (1986) A multivariate investigation of post-partum mood disturbance. *British Journal of Psychiatry*, **148**, 567–575.

Garvey, M. J., Tuason, V. B., Luming, A. E., *et al* (1983) Occurrence of depression in the post-partum state. *Journal of Affective Disorders*, **5**, 97–101.

Glover, V. & O'Connor, T. G. (2002) Effects of ante-natal stress and anxiety. *British Journal of Psychiatry*, **180**, 389–391.

Golding, J. M., Taylor, D. L., Menard, L., *et al* (2000) Prevalence of sexual abuse history in a sample of women seeking treatment for premenstrual syndrome. *Journal of Psychosomatic Obstetrics and Gynaecology*, **21**, 69–80.

Gooch, R. (1829) Puerperal psychosis. In *Three Hundred Years of Psychiatry* (eds R. Hunter & I. Macalpine, 1963), pp. 768–800. Oxford: Oxford University Press.

Goodale, I. L., Domar, A. D. & Benson, H. (1990) Alleviation of premenstrual syndrome symptoms with the relaxation response. *Obstetrics and Gynaecology*, **75**, 649–655.

Halbreich, U., Endicott, J. & Schacht, S. (1985) Relationship of premenstrual dysphoric changes to depressive disorders. *Acta Psychiatrica Scandinavica*, **77**, 331.

Hamilton, J. A. (1962) *Postpartum Psychiatric Problems.* St Louis, MO: Mosby.

Hampton, T. (2006) Antidepressants and pregnancy: weighing risks and benefits, no easy task. *JAMA*, **295**, 1631–1633.

Handley, S. L., Dunn, T. L. & Waldron, G., *et al* (1980) Tryptophan, cortisol and puerperal mood. *British Journal of Psychiatry*, **136**, 498–508.

Harris, B. (1980) Prospective trial of L-tryptophan in the maternity blues. *British Journal of Psychiatry*, **137**, 233–235.

Harris, B., Lovett, L., Newcombe, R. G., *et al* (1994) Maternity blues and major endocrine changes: Cardiff puerperal mood and hormone study II. *BMJ*, **308**, 949–953.

Hatotani, N., Nomura, J., Yamaguchi, T., *et al* (1983) Clinical endocrine studies of postpartum psychoses. In *Neurobiology of Periodic Psychoses* (eds N. Hatotani & J. Nomura), pp. 93–104. Tokyo: Igateu-Shoin.

Hay, D., Pawlby, S., Sharp, D., *et al* (2001) Intellectual problems shown by 11-year-old children whose mothers had post-natal depression. *Journal of Child Psychology and Psychiatry*, **42**, 871–890.

Hendrick, V., Stowe, Z. N., Altshuler, L. L., *et al* (2001*a*) Fluoxetine and norfluoxetine levels in nursing infants and breast milk. *Biological Psychiatry*, **50**, 775–782.

Hendrick, V., Fukuchi, A., Altshuler, L., *et al* (2001*b*) Use of sertraline, paroxetine and fluvoxamine in nursing women. *British Journal of Psychiatry*, **179**, 163–166.

Hipwell, A., Goosseus, F., Melhuish, E., *et al* (2000) Severe maternal psychopathology and infant mother attachment. *Development and Psychopathology*, **12**, 157–175.

Home Office (1985) *Criminal Statistics, England and Wales, for 1984.* London: HMSO.

Hopwood, J. S. (1927) Child murder and insanity. *Journal of Mental Science*, **73**, 95–107.

Howard, L. M., Kumar, R. & Thornicroft, G. (2001) Psychosocial characteristics and needs of mothers with psychotic disorders. *British Journal of Psychiatry*, **178**, 427–432.

Hughes, P., Turton, P., Hopper, E., *et al* (2002) Assessment of guidelines for good practice in psychosocial care of mothers after stillbirth: a cohort study. *Lancet*, **360**, 114–118.

Ijuin, T., Douchi, T., Yamamoto, S., *et al* (1998) The relationship between maternity blues and thyroid dysfunction. *Journal of Obstetrics and Gynaecological Research*, **24**, 49–55.

Janssen, B. (1964) Psychic insufficiencies associated with childbearing. *Acta Psychiatrica Scandinavica*, **39**, suppl. 172, 41–56.

Jones, I. & Craddock, N. (2001) Familiality of the puerperal trigger in bipolar disorder: results of a family study. *American Journal of Psychiatry*, **158**, 913–917.

Kadramas, A., Winokur, G. & Crowe, R. (1979) Postpartum mania. *British Journal of Psychiatry*, **135**, 551–554.

Karacan, I., Williams, R. L., Hursch, C., *et al* (1969) Some implications for the sleep pattern for post-partum emotional disorder. *British Journal of Psychiatry*, **115**, 929–932.

Karnosh, L. J. & Hope, J. M. (1937) Puerperal psychoses and their sequelae. *American Journal of Psychiatry*, **94**, 537–550.

Kelly, R. H., Zatzik, D. F. & Anders, T. F. (2001) The detection and treatment of psychiatric disorders and substance abuse among pregnant women cared for in obstetrics. *American Journal of Psychiatry*, **158**, 213–219.

Kempe, C. H., Silverman, F. N., Steele, B. F., *et al* (1962) The battered child syndrome. *JAMA*, **181**, 17–24.

Kendell, R., Rennie, D., Clarke, J. A., *et al* (1981) The social and obstetric correlates of psychiatric admission in the puerperium. *Psychological Medicine*, **11**, 341–350.

Kendell, R. E., Chalmers, J. C. & Platz, C. (1987) Epidemiology of the puerperal psychoses. *British Journal of Psychiatry*, **150**, 662–673.

Kendler, K. S., Karkowski, L. M., Corey, L. A., *et al* (1998) Longitudinal population-based twin study of retrospectively reported premenstrual symptoms and lifetime major depressive disorder. *American Journal of Psychiatry*, **155**, 1234–1240.

Kirkby, R. J. (1994) Changes in premenstrual symptoms and irrational thinking following cognitive–behavioral coping skills training. *Journal of Consulting Clinical Psychology*, **62**, 1026–1032.

Kleiner, G. J. & Greston, W. M. (1984) Overview of demographic and statistical factors. In *Suicide in Pregnancy* (eds G. J. Kleiner & W. M. Greston), pp. 23–40. Littleton, MA: John Wright.

Klompenhouwer, J. C. & Van Hulst, A. M. (1991) Classification of post-partum psychoses. *Acta Psychiatrica Scandinavica*, **84**, 255–281.

Kraepeline, E. (1896) *Psychiatria: Ein Lehrbuck für Studierende und Ärzte* (5th edn). Leipzig: Abel.

Kukopoulos, A., Minnai, G. & Muller-Oerlinghausen, B. (1985) The influence of mania and depression on the pharmacokinetics of lithium: a longitudinal single-case study. *Journal of Affective Disorders*, **8**, 159–166.

Kumar, R. & Hipwell, A. E. (1996) Development of a clinical rating scale to assess mother–infant interaction in a psychiatric mother and baby unit. *British Journal of Psychiatry*, **169**, 18–26.

Levy, V. (1987) The maternity blues in post-partum and post-operative women. *British Journal of Psychiatry*, **151**, 368–372.

Magos, A. L., Brincat, M. & Studd, J. W. W. (1986) Treatment of the premenstrual syndrome by subcutaneous oestradiol implants and cyclical norethisterone: placebo controlled studies. *BMJ*, **292**, 1629–1633.

Main, T. F. (1958) Mothers with children in psychiatric hospital. *Lancet*, *ii*, 845–847.

Marcé, L. V. (1858) *Traité de la folie des femmes encientes, des nouvelles accouchées et des nourrices*. Paris: Baillière.

Margison, F. (1982) The pathology of the mother–child relationship. In *Motherhood and Mental Illness* (eds I. F. Brockington & R. Kumar), pp. 223–238. London: Academic Press.

Marks, M. (2001) Parents at risk of filicide. In *Clinical Assessment of Dangerousness* (eds G. F. Pinard & L. Pagani), pp. 159–180. Cambridge: Cambridge University Press.

Martin, M. E. (1958) Puerperal mental illness. A follow-up study of 75 cases. *BMJ*, *ii*, 773–777.

McKenna, K., Koren, G., Tetelbaum, M., *et al* (2005) Pregnancy outcome of women using atypical antipsychotic drugs: a prospective comparative study. *Journal of Clinical Psychiatry*, **66**, 444–449.

Menkes, D. B., Taghavi, E., Mason, P. A., *et al* (1992) Fluoxetine treatment of severe premenstrual syndrome. *BMJ*, **305**, 346–347.

Menkes, D. B., Coates, D. C. & Fawcett, J. P. (1994) Acute tryptophan depletion aggravates premenstrual syndrome. *Journal of Affective Disorders*, **32**, 37–44.

Misri, S., Reebye, P., Kendrick, K., *et al* (2006) Internalizing behaviors in 4-year-old children exposed in utero to psychotropic medications. *American Journal of Psychiatry*, **163**, 1026–1032.

Murray, L. (1992) The impact of post natal depression on infant development. *Journal of Child Psychology and Psychiatry*, **33**, 543–561.

Nappi, R. E., Petralgia, F., Luisin, S., *et al* (2001) Serum allopregrianolone in women with postpartum blues. *Obstetrics and Gynaecology*, **97**, 77–80.

National Institute for Clinical Excellence (2001) *Why Mothers Die, 1997–1999. The Fifth Report of the Confidential Enquiries into Maternal Deaths in the United Kingdom.* London: Royal College of Obstetricians and Gynaecologists.

Nott, P. H., Franklin, M., Armitage, C., *et al* (1976) Hormonal changes and mood in the puerperium. *British Journal of Psychiatry*, **128**, 379–383.

Nulman, I., Rovet, J., Stewart, D. E., *et al* (1997) Neurodevelopment of children exposed in utero to antidepressant drugs. *New England Journal of Medicine*, **336**, 258–262.

Oberlander, T. F., Warburton, W., Misri, S., *et al* (2006) Neonatal outcomes after prenatal exposure to selective serotonin reuptake inhibitor antidepressants and maternal depression using population-based linked health data. *Archives of General Psychiatry*, **63**, 898–906.

O'Connor, T. G., Heron, J., Golding, J., *et al* (2002) Maternal anxiety and children's behavioural/emotional problems at 4 years. *British Journal of Psychiatry*, **180**, 502–508.

O'Hara, M., Stuart, S. & Gorman, L. (2000) Efficacy of interpersonal therapy for postpartum depression. *Archives of General Psychiatry*, **57**, 1039–1045.

Oliver, J. E. (1985) Successive generations of child maltreatment in social and medical disorders in the parents. *British Journal of Psychiatry*, **147**, 484–490.

Paffenbarger, R. S., Jr (1964) Epidemiological aspects of postpartum mental illness. *British Journal of Preventive and Social Medicine*, **18**, 189–195.

Patel, V., Rodriguez, M. & De Souza, N. (2002) Gender, poverty, and postnatal depression: a study of mothers in Goa, India. *American Journal of Psychiatry*, **159**, 43–47.

Pearlstein, T. & Steiner, M. (2000) Non-antidepressant treatment of premenstrual syndrome. *Journal of Clinical Psychiatry*, **61**, suppl. 12, 22–27.

Pitt, B. (1968) Atypical depression following childbirth. *British Journal of Psychiatry*, **114**, 1325–1335.

Prados, M. (1967) Emotional factors in the climecterium of women. *Psychotherapy and Psychosomatics*, **15**, 231–244.

Protheroe, C. (1969) Puerperal psychoses: a long term study, 1927–1961. *British Journal of Psychiatry*, **115**, 9–30.

Reder, P. & Duncan, S. (1997) Adult Psychiatry – a missing link in the child protection network. *Child Abuse Review*, **6**, 35–40.

Resnick, P. J. (1969) Child murder by parents. A psychiatric review of filicide. *American Journal of Psychiatry*, **126**, 325–334.

Robling, S. A., Paykel, E. S., Dunn, V. J., *et al* (2000) Long-term follow-up of severe puerperal psychiatric illness. A 23-year follow-up study. *Psychological Medicine*, **30**, 1263–1271.

Royal College of Psychiatrists (2000) *Perinatal Mental Health Services. Recommendations for Provision of Services for Child Bearing Women*. Council Report 88. London. Royal College of Psychiatrists.

Rumeau-Roquette, C., Goujard, J. & Huel, G. (1977) Possible teratogenic effect of phenothiazines in human beings. *Teratology*, **15**, 57–64.

Ryan, M. G., Davis, A. A. & Oates, R. K. (1977) One hundred and eighty-seven cases of child abuse and neglect. *Medical Journal of Australia*, *ii*, 623–628.

Savage, G. H. (1875) Observations on the insanity of pregnancy and childbirth. *Guy's Hospital Reports*, **20**, 83–117.

Schmidt, P. J., Nieman, L. K., Danaceau, M. A., *et al* (1998) Differential behavioral effects of gonadal steroids in women with and in those without premenstrual syndrome. *New England Journal of Medicine*, **338**, 209–216.

Schopf, J. & Rust, B. (1994) Follow-up and family study of postpartum psychosis. Part I: Overview. *European Archives of Psychiatry and Clinical Neuroscience*, **244**, 101–111.

Sheridan, M. D. (1956) The intelligence of 100 neglectful mothers. *BMJ*, (4958), 91–93.

Silberman, R. N., Beenen, F. & De Jong, H. (1975) Clinical treatment of postpartum delirium with perphenazine and lithium carbonate. *Psychiatrica Clinica*, **8**, 314–326.

Smith, S. M., Hanson, R. & Noble, S. (1973) Parents of battered babies: a controlled study. *BMJ*, *iv*, 388–391.

Spinelli, M. & Endicott, J. (2003) Controlled trial of interpersonal therapy versus a parenting education programme for depressed pregnant women. *American Journal of Psychiatry*, **160**, 555–562.

Spitzer, R. L., Endicott, J. R. & Robins, E. (1978) Research Diagnostic Criteria: rationale and reliability. *Archives of General Psychiatry*, **35**, 773–782.

Stein, A., Woolley, H., Cooper, S. D., *et al* (1994) An observational study of mothers with eating disorders and their infants. *Journal of Child Psychology and Psychiatry*, **35**, 733–748.

Stein, G. S. (1980) The pattern of mental change and body weight change in the first post-partum week. *Journal of Psychosomatic Research*, **24**, 165–171.

Stein, G. S. (1982) The maternity blues. In *Motherhood and Mental Illness* (eds I. F. Brockington & R. Kumar), pp. 119–154. London: Academic Press.

Stein, G. S. (1984) Headaches in the first post-partum week and their relationship to migraine. *Headache*, **21**, 201–205.

Stein, G. S., Milton, F., Bebbington, P., *et al* (1976) Relationship between mood disturbance and free plasma tryptophan in post-partum women. *BMJ*, *ii*, 451.

Steinberg, S., Annable, L., Young, S. N., *et al* (1999) A placebo controlled trial of L-tryptophan in premenstrual dysphoria. *Advances in Experimental Medicine and Biology*, **467**, 85–88.

Steiner, M. & Pearlstein, T. (2000) Premenstrual dysphoria and the serotonin system: pathophysiology and treatment. *Journal of Clinical Psychiatry*, **61**, suppl. 12, 17–21.

Stewart, D. E., Klompenhouwer, J. L., Kendell, R. E., *et al* (1991) Prophylactic lithium in puerperal psychosis: the experience of three centres. *British Journal of Psychiatry*, **158**, 393–397.

Stuenkel, C. A. (1989) Menopause and oestrogen replacement therapy. *Psychiatric Clinics of North America*, **12**, 133–152.

Taylor, D., Paton, C. & Kerwin, R. (2003) *The South London and Maudsley NHS Trust 2003 Prescribing Guidelines* (7th edn). London: Taylor & Francis.

Teixeira, J. M., Fisk, N. M. & Glover, V. (1999) Association between maternal anxiety in pregnancy and increased uterine artery resistance index: cohort based study. *BMJ*, **318**, 1288–1289.

Thuwe, I. (1974) Genetic factors in puerperal psychosis. *British Journal of Psychiatry*, **125**, 378–385.

Thys-Jacobs, S., Starkey, P., Bernstein, D., *et al* (1998) Calcium carbonate and the premenstrual syndrome: effects on premenstrual and menstrual symptoms. *American Journal of Obstetrics and Gynecology*, **179**, 444–452.

Trethowan, W. H. & Conlon, M. F. (1965) Couvade syndrome. *British Journal of Psychiatry*, **111**, 57–60.

Turton, P., Hughes, P., Evans, C. D. H., *et al* (2001) Incidence, correlates and predictors of post-traumatic stress disorder in the pregnancy after stillbirth. *British Journal of Psychiatry*, **178**, 556–560.

Tymchuk, A. J. & Andron, L. (1990) Mothers with mental retardation who do or do not abuse or neglect their children. *Child Abuse and Neglect*, **14**, 313–323.

van den Akker, O. B., Stein, G. S., Neale, M. C., *et al* (1987) Genetic and environmental variation in the menstrual cycle: histories of two British samples. *Acta Genetica Medica Gemollogica (Rome)*, **36**, 541–548.

Van Waes, A. & van de Velde, E. (1969) Safety of haloperidol in the treatment of hyperemesis gravidarum. *Journal of Clinical Pharmacology*, **9**, 62–64.

Videbech, P. & Gouliaev, G. (1995) First admission with puerperal psychosis: 7–14 years of follow-up. *Acta Psychiatrica Scandinavica*, **91**, 167–173.

Walker, A. F., de Souza, M. C., Vickers, M. F., *et al* (1998) Magnesium supplements alleviate premenstrual symptoms of fluid retention. *Journal of Women's Health*, **7**, 1157–1165.

Wieck, A., Kumar, R., Hirst, A. D., *et al* (1991) Increased sensitivity of dopamine receptors and recurrence of affective psychoses after childbirth. *BMJ*, **303**, 613–616.

Wikander, I., Sundblad, C., Andersch, B., *et al* (1998) Citalopram in premenstrual dysphoria: is intermittent treatment during luteal phases more effective than continuous medication throughout the menstrual cycle? *Journal of Clinical Psychopharmacology*, **18**, 390–398.

Wisner, K. L., Gelenberg, A. J., Leonard, H., *et al* (1999) Pharmacologic treatment of depression during pregnancy. *JAMA*, **282**, 1264–1269.

Wisner, K. L., Perel, J. M. & Perindl, K. S. (2001) Prevention of recurrent postnatal depression: a randomized clinical trial. *Journal of Clinical Psychiatry*, **62**, 82–86.

World Health Organization (1992) *The Tenth Revision of the International Classification of Diseases and Related Health Problems* (ICD–10). Geneva: WHO.

Wyatt, K. M., Dimmock, P. D., Jones, P. W., *et al* (1999) Efficacy of vitamin B-6 in the treatment of premenstrual syndrome: systematic review. *BMJ*, **318**, 1375–1381.

Yarden, P. E., Max, M. D. & Eisenbach, Z. (1966) The effect of childbirth on the prognosis of married schizophrenic women. *British Journal of Psychiatry*, **112**, 491–499.

Yonkers, K. A., Ramin, S. M., Rush A. J., *et al* (2001) Onset and persistence of postpartum depression in an inner-city maternal health clinic system. *American Journal of Psychiatry*, **158**, 1856–1863.

Yoshida, K., Smith, B. & Kumar, R. (1999) Psychotropic drugs in mothers' milk: a comprehensive review of assay methods, pharmacokinetics and of safety of breast feeding. *Journal of Psychopharmacology*, **13**, 64–80.

Zelkowitz, P. & Milet, T. H. (2001) The course of post-partum psychiatric disorders in women and their partners. *Journal of Nervous and Mental Disease*, **189**, 575–582.

Zigmund, A. S. & Snaith, R. P. (1983) The Hospital Anxiety and Depression Scale. *Acta Psychiatrica Scandinavica*, **67**, 361–370.

CHAPTER 26

Psychosexual medicine for psychiatrists

Peter Trigwell and Gill Kirk

Sexual problems are common and important. Psychiatrists need to be able to assess, understand and offer effective help for such problems. Indeed, the current curriculum for basic specialist training and the MRCPsych examination includes a section on 'gender issues and psychosexual disorders' (Royal College of Psychiatrists, 2001). The curriculum states that the trainee should be able to demonstrate a working knowledge of following:

- the classification of sexual problems and dysfunction
- the organic–psychological interface of sexual dysfunction
- the management and treatment options available for psychosexual disorders
- sexual identity disorders and paraphilias.

In addition, they should be able to assess and formulate a management plan for people with psychosexual problems.

Sexual problems carry with them a certain stigma, as do many other conditions seen in psychiatric services, and they are not easy problems to talk about, either for patients or for professionals. Patients may not mention them until they have already developed a therapeutic relationship with their psychiatrist, or other member of the multidisciplinary team. Even then, they are not likely to disclose a problem without being prompted by appropriate questions. A clinician who asks such questions as a usual part of taking a history will detect twice as many sexual problems as one who waits for the patient to raise the subject (Burnap & Golden, 1967). Despite this, most psychiatrists rarely take a detailed sexual history, and if problems are detected many psychiatrists are unsure what to do to help.

Members of the general public tend to believe that psychiatrists are interested in, and able to help with, sexual difficulties (at least of psychogenic aetiology), but the reality is that many psychiatrists feel far from confident in this area. This chapter aims to provide readers with a basic understanding of sexual problems and a framework within which they are confidently able to assess, formulate and treat (or decide to refer on for treatment) their patients' sexual problems.

In both of the main psychiatric classification systems – ICD–10 (World Health Organization, 1992) and DSM–IV (American Psychiatric Association, 1994) – sexual problems are subdivided into three areas:

- sexual dysfunction
- gender identity disorders
- paraphilias.

This chapter concentrates on sexual dysfunction. This is partly for reasons of space but is also in recognition of the prevalence and importance of problems with sexual functioning, and because they may present to psychiatrists quite frequently. Paraphilias and gender identity disorders are also covered, but *briefly* and towards the end of this chapter.

The clinical importance of sexual dysfunction

Prevalence and incidence

Difficulties with sex are rather more common than most people would suspect. Many men who present with erectile dysfunction are surprised (and sometimes relieved) to learn that over 10% of men in the general population (across the whole age range) suffer with erectile problems at any one time. Kinsey's surveys of sexual function in the mid-20th century found there to be an exponential rise in prevalence of 'more or less permanent erectile impotence' with increasing age. The figures he reported were 0.1% at age 20, 0.8% at age 30, 1.9% at 40, 6.7% at 50, 27% by the age of 70, and over 50% for men aged 75 years or more (Kinsey *et al*, 1948). Another large but more recent study has reported a rate of 52% for 'minimal, moderate or complete' erectile dysfunction in the general population across the age range. That study also found that the prevalence of complete erectile dysfunction rises from 5% for men at 40 to 15% for men at 70 years of age (Feldman *et al*, 1994). Other figures available from large-scale surveys of sexual dysfunction include prevalence figures of 6% for premature ejaculation, 16% for anorgasmia and 2.6% for female dyspareunia (Gebhard & Johnson, 1979).

Although such figures on classifiable sexual dysfunctions are available, perhaps what is really of clinical importance is sexual dissatisfaction. Just as with other areas of physical dysfunction, patients with sexual dysfunction (and their partners) vary with regard to the level of dissatisfaction reported. The relationship between these two areas is unclear. In a questionnaire study of 100 married couples, Frank *et al* (1978) looked

Table 26.1 Rates of sexual dysfunction in clinic populations and medical conditions

Clinic population/medical condition	Reported types and rates of dysfunction	References
Diabetes mellitus	Erectile dysfunction in 50% of men overall (25% in their 30s, 75% in their 60s)	McCulloch *et al* (1980), Rubin & Babbott (1958)
Family planning clinic (women)	Sexual problems in 12.5%. Of these, over 75% wanted help	Begg *et al* (1976)
Genitourinary medicine clinic (sexually transmitted infections)	Sexual dysfunction in 25% of men and 29% of women	Catalan *et al* (1981)
General practice, urology, obstetrics and gynaecology	Sexual problems in an average of 15%	Burnap & Golden (1967)
Gynaecology	17% with sexual dysfunction (anorgasmia)	Levine & Yost (1976)
Mastectomy	No sexual activity in 33% after one year	Maguire *et al* (1978)
Multiple sclerosis	Erectile dysfunction in 43–62%	Vas (1978), Lilius *et al* (1976)
Peripheral vascular disease	Erectile dysfunction in 40–50%	Wagner & Metz (1981)
Psychiatric clinic	**Sexual/marital problems in 12%**	Swan & Wilson (1979)
Stroke	50% do not resume sexual activity after stroke	Hawton (1984)

at the three areas of sexual dysfunction, sexual difficulties and sexual dissatisfaction. A higher proportion of women than men reported sexual difficulties (such as problems relaxing and a lack of interest). Around 60% of the women and 40% of the men had some degree of sexual dysfunction, and yet the figures for sexual dissatisfaction were 20% for the women and around 30% for the men. Apart from suggesting that sexual dysfunction is common, these figures give an indication that other aspects of the relationship may be more important in causing dissatisfaction, which may, in turn, be more likely to lead to people consulting healthcare professionals about their sexual problems (Frank *et al*, 1978; Bancroft, 1989).

Considering how common sexual dysfunction is in the general population, and its association with both psychiatric and medical conditions, it is unsurprising that a high incidence of such problems has been found in studies carried out in a broad range of clinic populations and medical conditions, as shown in Table 26.1. Despite the size of the problem, little exists in the way of specialist services to help these people. With regard to psychogenic sexual dysfunction, psychiatrists sometimes find themselves in receipt of referrals from medical colleagues trying to find psychosexual help for their patients. Where it has been possible to provide such services, it has been found that, in addition to general practice, the majority of referrals come from urology, genitourinary medicine, gynaecology and diabetology (as shown in Table 26.2).

Table 26.2 The first 1000 referrals to a psychosexual service, by referral source

Referral source	Number (*n* = 100)	Percentage (%)
General practice	529	52.9
Urology	209	20.9
Genitourinary medicine	58	5.8
Gynaecology	56	5.6
Diabetology	30	3.0
Other (various medical/surgical)	73	7.3
Unknown from database	45	4.5

Source: Database of the Leeds Psychosexual Medicine Service.

The effects of sexual dysfunction

In addition to the emotional distress caused, sexual dysfunctions have a range of clinically important effects, on the relationship, the children and the individual.

Effects on the relationship

When sex is going well it is often just a small part of what is perceived as a good relationship. When sex becomes a problem, however, it can soon develop into a preoccupying issue for the person or couple involved. If left unresolved, this can lead to a deterioration in the more global (non-sexual) aspects of the relationship because repeated 'failures' of sexual functioning may provoke a whole range of negative emotions in both partners. These include embarrassment, humiliation, guilt, anger, hopelessness and low self-esteem. Along with a lack of positive reinforcement as a result of the sexual dysfunction, these negative emotions may lead to an avoidance of sex. If not addressed, major relationship problems may arise.

Problems with sex are often cited by people presenting in psychosexual clinics as the primary reason for the failure of previous relationships. By way of an example, a UK survey found that 21% of men with erectile dysfunction reported that their relationship had broken down, and a further 9% that their relationship was in difficulty, as a result of their sexual problem (Impotence Association, 1997).

On occasion, couples may adjust and 'normalise' with regard to the sexual problem, or even choose to enter into the relationship in the first place knowing that there is a serious sexual difficulty (even one that may prevent sexual intercourse). In such cases it must be remembered that, for them, 'improving' sexual function may not necessarily be a welcome change and may even upset the current dynamics of their relationship. This illustrates the importance of considering each case individually and not seeing patients in isolation from their partner.

Effects on children

Sexual problems can have a negative effect on the couple's children. This occurs as a result of their deleterious effects on the relationship and their tendency to cause discord. Divorce is a common outcome of couple relationship problems. In the early 1960s, almost 90% of children lived with two biological, married parents throughout their childhood and adolescence. By the late 1980s this figure had dropped to around 50% (Wadsworth, 1986). Recent research has shown that divorce has long-term risks for the children involved. These include more social, emotional, behavioural and academic problems. Hetherington & Stanley-Hagan (1999) warned that the stresses on children during and following divorce should not be underestimated, and that when adverse outcomes do occur 'they may be difficult to modify through educational or short-term therapeutic interventions'. The damaging element appears to be the parental discord rather than the divorce or separation *per se* (Hetherington & Stanley-Hagan, 1999). Furthermore, O'Connor *et al* (1999) found a long-term correlation between parental divorce and depression, which was explained by the 'quality of parent–child and parental marital relations (in childhood), concurrent levels of stressful life events and social support'. To add to this concern, they also found a long-term association between parental divorce and the children's later experience of a divorce in adulthood, highlighting the risk of a repeating cycle of this problem (O'Connor *et al*, 1999).

Effects on the individual

Clinically significant anxiety states can be precipitated by sexual and relationship problems. Perhaps more commonly, depression may be caused in susceptible individuals. Sexual and relationship problems cause depression, but people who are depressed often also suffer with secondary sexual dysfunction, although the absence of longitudinal studies has made it difficult to determine the precise incidence of depressive disorders that can be attributed to sexual dysfunction. Sexual dysfunction may be an integral part of the depressive symptomatology, as in the case of loss of libido (Beck, 1967; Mathew & Weinman, 1982), or may be a consequence of antidepressant medication, causing impaired sexual arousal in the form of erectile dysfunction or retarded ejaculation, as well as a loss of interest in some people (Segraves, 1988, 1989; Balon *et al*, 1993; Bazire, 2001).

Normal sexual functioning

For sex to work well, at least from a physiological perspective, four basic elements are necessary:

1 *Intact endocrine functioning (i.e. normal levels of sex hormones)*. Several substances are important. Testosterone is the main sexual driver in both men and women, although with much lower levels in the latter. Sex hormone binding globulin (SHBG) is also important, however, as much of the testosterone detectable in the bloodstream is bound to it. As a result of this, a high SHBG level can mean a low free (active) testosterone level. High prolactin levels can impair sexual drive in either sex, as can a raised oestradiol level in women (the level of oestradiol obviously varies with the stage of the menstrual cycle).

2 *Intact vascular supply to the genital areas*. The external genitalia in both sexes are supplied by the internal pudendal artery, which is one of the terminal branches of the anterior trunk of the internal iliac artery (Snell, 1981).

3 *Intact neural supply to the genital areas*. Although this is an oversimplification, in essence genital arousal (erection in the male, and vaginal and vulval engorgement and lubrication in the female) is mediated via parasympathetic fibres, and ejaculation or orgasm mainly via the sympathetic system. The parasympathetic supply runs from sacral outflow S2, 3 and 4, via the pelvic splanchnic nerves and the nervi erigentes to the genitalia. Sympathetic supply to the same area is via fibres from the thoracic and upper lumbar rami. The latter pass to the pelvic plexus (usually situated in front of the bifurcation of the abdominal aorta) and then on to the genitalia, either via discrete bundles or as a scattered network of fibres, sometimes within the pudendal nerve, although this distribution is quite variable (Bancroft, 1989).

4 *Appropriate cognitions (i.e. sexually stimulating thoughts and images)*. Although often not recognised by patients, or some healthcare professionals, this is of fundamental importance to normal sexual functioning. Problems with cognitions assume aetiological significance in cases of psychogenic sexual dysfunction (as in the classic examples of performance anxiety and 'spectatoring', as described below). Sexual functioning suffers when thoughts are not sexually stimulating, or in the presence of anxious or unpleasant thoughts, because arousal via the autonomic nervous system is impaired.

'Normal' sexual response

In normal sexual functioning the sexual response is generally considered to comprise the following stages:

1 drive/desire

2 arousal

3 plateau

4 orgasm

5 resolution.

Schematic representations of the male and female sexual responses are shown in Figs 26.1 and 26.2, respectively. Both the male and female response curves may be divided into these five stages, as described below, with the addition in the case of the male curve of the 'refractory period'.

A large variety of female responses have been observed. Those shown in Fig. 26.2 represent three common patterns (A, B and C). 'A' is the cycle of a woman who, on that particular occasion, passes through all four stages, including orgasm. 'B' is that of a woman who becomes highly aroused but does not reach orgasm. 'C' represents the rapid response to orgasm that might occur during masturbation.

The general assumption is that, with regard to any one particular episode of sexual activity, these physiological stages occur in sequence, that is, from 1 to 5. In fact, each stage is rather more independent than

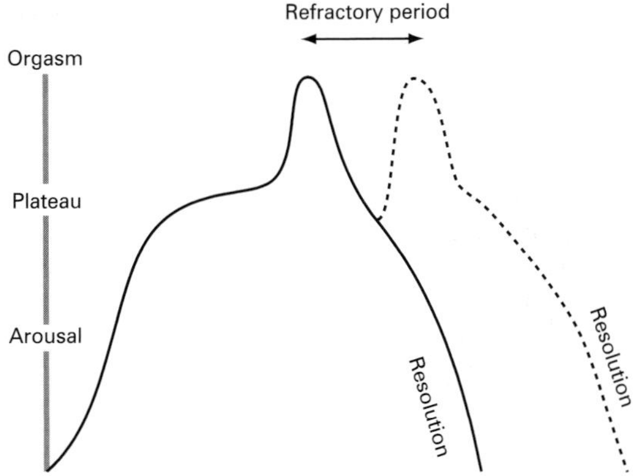

Fig. 26.1 The male sexual response curve. Adapted from *Sex Therapy: A Practical Guide*, Hawton, K. (1985), by permission of Oxford University Press. (© K. Hawton 1985.)

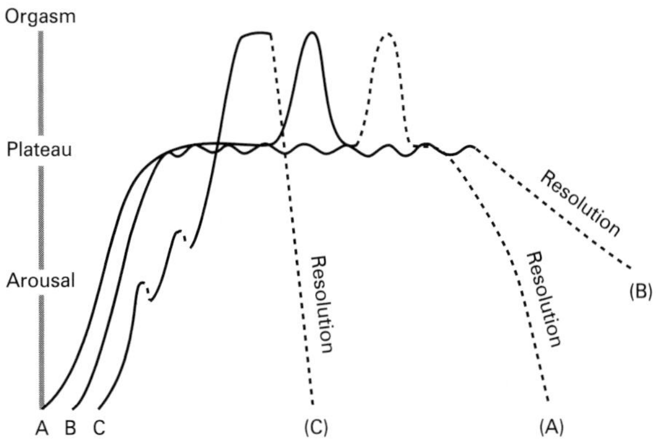

Fig. 26.2 The female sexual response curve: three common patterns (A–C). Adapted from *Sex Therapy: A Practical Guide*, Hawton, K. (1985), by permission of Oxford University Press. (© K. Hawton 1985.)

that. For example, ejaculation may occur without any sign of erection in a man with an erectile disorder, this being possible in view of the differences in neurological control of each of these stages.

Drive/desire

The initial stage of 'drive/desire' may be considered to represent an individual's current level of interest in sex, but these are not identical concepts. Sexual drive is the perception of a need for sexual activity. It is a basic human need that is largely biologically (hormonally) driven and not necessarily specific to an object or person. By contrast, sexual desire is the object- or person-specific correlate of that drive. In other words, one may have thoughts about sex in general and an urge towards sexual activity as a result of intact drive, but this tends to be experienced as an interest in and longing for sexual contact with a particular person, that is, desire.

Arousal

Arousal is the stage during which more focused sexual thoughts and activity begin to occur. Perhaps the most noticeable correlate of the arousal stage is genital vascular engorgement, leading to penile erection in males and vulval and clitoral engorgement and vaginal lubrication in females. Research has confirmed the anatomical and physiological similarities between male and female genitalia. In basic terms, the glans penis is homologous with the clitoris, the shaft of the penis with the labia minora and the scrotum with the labia majora. There is no anatomical difference to suggest that the process of sexual arousal would vary to any great extent between the genitalia of men and women. In addition, the spinal centres of reflex control of the sex organs are similar and the involved afferent and efferent nerves entirely correspond (as described above). The response to tactile stimulation is also identical in both sexes, and from the physiological perspective erection in the male is identical with turgidity of the erectile tissue of the clitoris (Ellenberg, 1977). In both men and women, arousal builds via a complex mechanism of feedback loops, as illustrated in Fig. 26.3.

Plateau

During the plateau stage the individual remains in a state of high sexual arousal. The duration of this stage is obviously very variable between individuals, and within one individual on different occasions, and dependent on circumstances. It may or may not lead to orgasm.

Orgasm

Orgasm is difficult to define, which is probably why most texts avoid even attempting to do so. In his

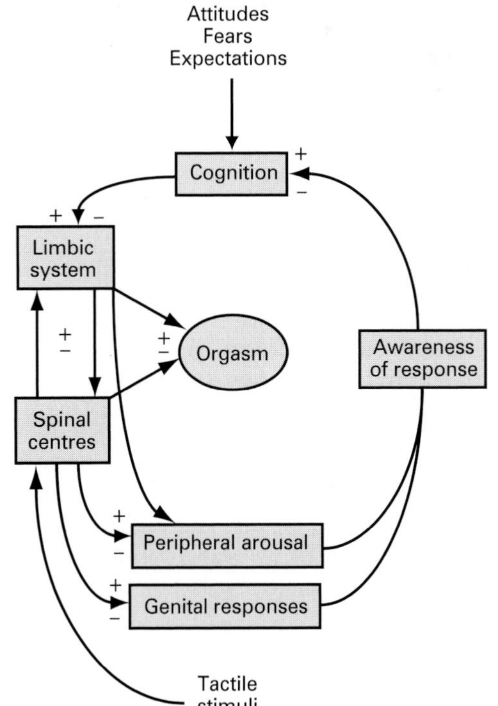

Fig. 26.3 The psychosomatic circle of sex. Redrawn from *Human Sexuality and Its Problems* (2nd edn), John Bancroft (1989), by permission of the publisher, Churchill Livingstone.

seminal and still outstanding textbook, Bancroft (1989, p. 12) describes orgasm as:

> 'still largely a neurophysiological mystery, [which] involves both central processes in the brain and widespread peripheral effects experienced as acute increases in the intensity of erotic sensation and muscle contractions which are largely involuntary.'

It is the muscle contractions that produce ejaculation (i.e. emission of seminal fluid) in men. The experience of ejaculation tends to occur at the same time as a more central sensation of orgasm, but the two are not identical and occur as different components of the overall experience of orgasm in the male. The process of ejaculation itself involves three main stages (Bancroft, 1989):

1 the pooling of seminal fluid in the bulbar urethra (which may be perceived by the man as the 'moment of ejaculatory inevitability' or point of no return)

2 tight closure of the bladder neck sphincter

3 the rhythmic contraction of the muscles of the penile base, causing expulsion of seminal fluid in three to seven ejaculatory spurts at intervals of 0.8 seconds.

In women, the muscular contractions at orgasm are of the circum-vaginal/perineal muscles, also at 0.8-second intervals. Older texts tend to discriminate between two types of female orgasm. 'Vaginal orgasm' (i.e. due to vaginal penetration and penile thrusting only) was felt to be more powerful and in some way more 'mature' than 'clitoral orgasm' (due to direct clitoral stimulation of some sort), which was viewed as inferior and immature in comparison. This notion is not now considered valid.

There is still a degree of controversy surrounding the idea of female ejaculation at the point of orgasm. This is connected with the concept of the Grafenberg or 'G' spot (Ladas *et al*, 1982). In essence, it does seem that some women have vestigial prostatic tissue around the urethra, corresponding to a small area of increased sensitivity along the anterior vaginal wall. These women may emit a small amount of what is basically prostatic fluid from the urethra at orgasm, and it is this that constitutes female ejaculation (Goldberg *et al*, 1983).

Resolution

The final stage of the normal sexual response is resolution, when the body returns to its normal 'resting' state in terms of heart rate, respiration rate, skin flushing, and genital engorgement and lubrication. This is obviously an important time for physical and emotional closeness in a loving relationship; however, for some, especially if making love at the end of a long and busy day, sleep may follow rapidly. This can sometimes be a source of discontent for the sexual partner.

Refractory period

An addition to the five stages noted above is the refractory period in men. This is the period after orgasm during which it is not possible to experience further physiological genital arousal. It increases in duration with increasing age, so that in a teenager it may be only a few minutes, whereas it could extend to hours or even days in an elderly man (Hawton, 1985).

Classification of sexual problems

The fact that sexual response tends to occur in the sequential stages mentioned above is reflected in the way sexual dysfunction is classified. Currently, the most useful classificatory system is DSM–IV, which most specialists tend to use in preference to ICD–10 because it is much more detailed (see Table 26.3). In DSM–IV, 'sexual and gender identity disorders' are classified under three main headings:

- sexual dysfunctions (the main focus of this chapter)
- gender identity disorders (briefly covered below, pages 691–692)
- paraphilias (briefly covered below, pages 692–694).

Management of sexual dysfunction

A brief history of sex therapy: schools of thought

The history of Western approaches to understanding and dealing with sexual problems is briefly summarised in Box 26.1.

Anthropological studies across the world have shown that there is no universal social or psychological value in any form of sexual behaviour or attitude: the meaning or value is determined by the social context. The Western concept of sexuality has been highly influenced by Christianity, a religion with a very ambivalent attitude to sex. This has included early asceticism, which declared the virtue of celibacy and viewed sexuality as sinful. During the Reformation there was a renewed emphasis on the role of marriage as the only sanctified arena for sexual fulfilment, as well as the context for creating a new awareness of human community through the family.

It is important to grasp that before the Enlightenment and the advent of scientific (physiological and anatomical) explanations for bodily phenomena, common understanding was often in magical or supernatural terms. Corresponding remedies would also be in this vein (spells and charms), or involve seeking to redress the sin that was believed to have caused the dysfunction in the first place.

In the late 19th century, Havelock Ellis and Richard von Krafft-Ebing (author of *Psychopathia Sexualis*) were among the leading early exponents of sexology, together with Sigmund Freud. From the early 20th century onwards, Freud's work emphasised the importance of sex and sexuality in the development and understanding of both sexual dysfunction and other psychopathology. His ideas originated in his collaboration with Josef Breuer and led to his theories of childhood sexual development. These include progressive development through oral, anal, phallic, latency and genital phases. Psychoanalytic theory proposes that failure to negotiate any of these stages may lead to later problems; thus, fixation due to trauma or blocking of a libidinal urge may emerge as a perversion if the fixation is later expressed, or as a neurosis if it is repressed. Although most of these earlier psychoanalytic formulations have

Table 26.3 The classification of sexual dysfunctions

DSM–IV	ICD–10
Sexual dysfunctions Specifiers: Lifelong-acquired type Generalised/situational type Due to psychological/combined factors	*Sexual dysfunction, not caused by organic disorder or disease*
Sexual desire disorders	
Hypoactive sexual desire disorder	Lack or loss of sexual desire
Sexual aversion disorder	Sexual aversion and lack of sexual enjoyment
	Excessive sexual drive
Sexual arousal disorder	
Female sexual arousal disorder	Failure of genital response
Male erectile disorder	
Orgasmic disorder	
Female orgasmic disorder	Orgasmic dysfunction
Male orgasmic disorder	
Premature ejaculation	Premature ejaculation
Sexual pain disorder	
Dyspareunia (not due to a general medical condition)	Non-organic dyspareunia
Vaginismus (not due to a general medical condition)	Non-organic vaginismus
Sexual dysfunction due to a general medical condition (GMC)	
Female hypoactive sexual disorder due to ... [insert GMC]	
Male hypoactive sexual disorder due to ... [insert GMC]	
Male erectile disorder due to ... [insert GMC]	
Female dyspareunia due to ... [insert GMC]	
Male dyspareunia due to ... [insert GMC]	
Other female sexual dysfunction due to ... [insert GMC]	
Other male sexual dysfunction due to ... [insert GMC]	
Substance-induced sexual dysfunction	
Sexual dysfunction not otherwise specified	Unspecified sexual dysfunction, not caused by organic disorder or disease Other sexual dysfunction, not caused by organic disorder or disease

Sources: World Health Organization (1992); American Psychiatric Association (1994).

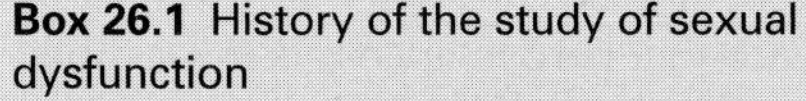

Box 26.1 History of the study of sexual dysfunction

Pre-Freud (medieval/magical)

↓

Psychoanalytic (sexual problems viewed as arising from deep intrapsychic conflicts)

↓

Behavioural (learning theory/deconditioning – Wolpe)

↓

Masters & Johnson added to psychodynamic/Balint tradition

↓

Integrated behavioural and cognitive approaches ('modified Masters & Johnson')

↓

Modern technology/biomedical advances

↓

Pragmatic (integrating biological and psychological approaches as necessary)

been superseded, modern psychiatry remains indebted to the psychoanalytic movement for the reappraisal of the importance of sex and sexuality in the aetiology of later mental illness and personality development, and for ideas regarding the psychological context in which sexual dysfunctions develop.

In the field of sex therapy, the psychoanalytic approach has largely been succeeded by other psychological schools of thought, particularly the cognitive–behavioural. Behaviourism is based on Pavlovian and Skinnerian learning theory, so that behavioural treatments have developed using the principles of learning, established by experiment, to change maladaptive behaviours by weakening or eliminating habits while initiating and strengthening adaptive alternatives. More recently, the cognitive model put forward by Beck and others has taken further forward the development of organised cognitive–behavioural forms of therapy. In addition, some influential practitioners have moved from a psychoanalytic to a more cognitive–behavioural approach to treating sexual problems, perhaps the most notable of these being the American therapist Helen Singer Kaplan (Kaplan, 1989). Modern psychosexual therapy has developed out of these streams of thought into an integrated approach that may combine psychodynamic, systemic and cognitive–behavioural approaches.

The development of various therapeutic approaches, as outlined above, has been closely related to parallel changes in social and cultural attitudes over time. These have included changes relating to fertility and birth control, diversity in sexuality and the role of women. Noteworthy modern milestones have included reform of the English law regarding homosexuality with the Sexual Offences Act 1967, work of the pioneers of birth control, including Marie Stopes and Margaret Sanger, and the social and sexual revolution of the 1960s onwards. Despite increasingly liberal views, controversy still remains in some quarters over the ethics of sexual behaviour and the practice of birth control; Freud apparently once suggested that the greatest invention would be a form of contraception that did not induce neurosis.

As mentioned above, a medical and psychiatric interest in sex and its disorders first developed in the late 19th century, followed in the 20th century by a more systematic study of sex and sexual dysfunction. This has grown into a discipline of both popular and scientific interest; the Institute for Sex Research founded by Alfred Kinsey is a well-known embodiment of the latter. More recently, the work of Alex Comfort has reached millions through his publicly acclaimed *Joy of Sex* books (Comfort, 1972). In addition, he worked to expand the horizons of the field by looking at how people who are elderly or who have a disability fare, paralleling social and cultural shifts towards the increased inclusion of these groups within society. The work of William Masters and Virginia Johnson since the 1960s has also had a particularly strong influence in the field of sex research and therapy, mainly through their description and use of a 'sensate focus' approach as the basis for treating sexual problems (Masters & Johnson, 1966, 1970).

Over recent years there have been major advances in biomedical techniques and treatments for sexual dysfunction, such as the development of agents for the treatment of erectile dysfunction (e.g. sildenafil citrate). The psychosexual practitioner employs a combined, bio-psychosocial approach to help patients overcome their sexual problems.

Modern sex therapy

The modern approach to sex therapy, as outlined in the following sections of this chapter, may broadly be described as a 'modified Masters & Johnson', cognitive–behavioural approach.

Assessment

The essential first stage in dealing with sexual dysfunction is a thorough assessment. The history should be taken in a chronological fashion; it is often most helpful to take background details first and only later in the interview to come on to the 'history of the presenting complaint' (i.e. the sexual problem), although it is important to be flexible with regard to the order. In essence, what is required is a thorough psychiatric-style history, but with a separate and detailed section on sexual history and functioning, which should also be essentially chronological.

In eliciting the patient's sexual history, it is best to begin by finding out about the sources that may have contributed to the individual's attitudes towards sex and sexuality. These might include religious beliefs, attitudes within the family towards sex, sex education, discussion with others about sex when growing up, masturbatory behaviour, and so forth. The history of sexual activity with other people should follow, beginning with the first sexual experience that the patient had with another person, including detail as to the basic level of interest and functioning in the areas of arousal, plateau (sustained arousal) and orgasm. Each sexual experience and relationship should be covered in turn, concentrating on these same areas of functioning. In other words, it is important to take a history that will facilitate an understanding of the development of the current problem and its nature, in accordance with the stages of sexual response as detailed earlier.

It is often necessary in this field to tolerate a degree of uncertainty with regard to the relative importance of physical and psychological factors. None the less, the therapist should attempt to decide whether the problem is primarily *organic* or *psychogenic*. Table 26.4 lists the type information that may be relevant, using erectile dysfunction as the example.

When making a diagnosis, it is also important to consider whether the dysfunction is 'primary' (having been present for the whole of the individual's sexual life) or 'secondary' (having emerged after a period of normal sexual functioning).

It is best, whenever practicable, to interview the patient alone, their partner alone, and the couple together. This helps to ensure that as much relevant and meaningful information as possible is gathered. In taking a history in this way, it is essential to clarify with each individual whether there is any information that he or she does not wish to be disclosed when the partner is present, and to respect this request. On occasion this may cause a particular difficulty, notably where there is ongoing infidelity about which the partner is unaware. This would generally be considered to make successful sex therapy with that particular couple impossible.

Physical examination and investigations are required, as with all psychiatric assessments. As a minimum, blood pressure measurement and blood glucose and urine testing should be performed, along with appropriate physical examination (checking whether the external genitalia are normal and whether there are any signs of hormonal disturbance, or of excessive alcohol or drug use, etc.). Where indicated by the history and examination, testosterone and SHBG (see page 670), luteinising hormone, prolactin, urea and electrolytes, liver function tests, thyroid function tests and full blood count should be performed.

Formulation and diagnosis

The aim of assessment is to generate a formulation of the patient's or couple's problems. This means a description of the problem (i.e. diagnosis) plus an explanation in terms of the apparent aetiological

Table 26.4 Indicators of the aetiology of erectile dysfunction

Area of enquiry in taking history	Organic	Psychogenic
Onset	Gradual	Sudden (may have a clear psychosocial precipitant
Extent	Generalised (i.e. in any setting, alone or with a partner)	Situational (e.g. erectile dysfunction when with a partner but not when alone)
Early-morning tumescence	Lack/loss of erections on waking	Erections still occur on waking
Ejaculation	May be normal (i.e. still occur despite no erection)	May be premature, normal or delayed
Life events	Often nil of note	Possibly relationship changes/life events or difficulties
Medical history	Cardiovascular, neurological, endocrine, surgical or traumatic risk factors	Possibly no identified physical risk factors
Drugs and medications	Possible use of drugs/medications associated with sexual dysfunction	No use of drugs/medications associated with sexual dysfunction
Lifestyle	Possibly smoking, alcohol use (especially excessive or harmful use)	May be no lifestyle risk factors identified

This table is merely an *aide memoire*. It is important to remember that organic and psychological factors often coexist.

factors (predisposing, precipitating and perpetuating). The formulation thus includes as clear an explanation as possible as to why this problem has arisen at this time for this individual or couple. Sometimes, when dealing with sexual dysfunction, the aetiology may not be immediately clear. This may particularly be the case in relation to the relative importance of physical and psychological factors. It is therefore important to set up treatment in a way that will allow ongoing assessment. (See the description of sensate focus approach on pages 675 to 678.)

Sharing the formulation

This is a crucial stage in helping the patient or couple. The formulation is discussed and, hopefully, agreed. This is done so that both parties understand the nature of the problem, what is being proposed as the underlying cause, and what is being suggested as the plan for therapy. It is also an opportunity to give the couple hope and encourage a positive approach towards dealing with their problems.

Agreeing goals of therapy and treatment strategy

A treatment plan is generated. This is done by considering which of the various treatment options is likely to be appropriate and acceptable, discussing this with the patient (and partner, if part of the treatment strategy) and then implementing the treatment plan over a number of sessions. It is essential to agree goals with the patient or couple that reflect their needs and wishes, rather than basing the aims of therapy on the therapist's own view of what would be a desirable outcome. Supervision is a key feature, as for any other psychological therapy.

Treatment

Where necessary, physical treatments can be offered in conjunction with psychological work. This may mean co-working with other specialties such as urology and gynaecology, although prescribing oral agents should be within the capabilities of the general adult psychiatrist. Specific physical treatments are discussed below, where relevant to specific conditions.

General approach to sex therapy

Broadly speaking, sex therapy has three main components:

- homework assignments (sensate focus approach)
- dealing with blocks (cognitive 'troubleshooting')
- education (an important element, to a variable extent, in every case)

This general approach is the core of sex therapy (Hawton, 1985). Specific techniques for particular conditions are also used, as described later, but on the background of this general approach to the therapy.

Homework assignments (sensate focus approach)

The sensate focus approach is used to provide a structure that allows couples to rebuild their sexual relationship over time. It consists of pre-planned stages, with clearly described homework assignments to carry out between sessions with the therapist. Although it is an effective basis for the treatment of most cases of sexual dysfunction, it must be remembered that sometimes it will not be suitable or effective, perhaps necessitating referral to a more specialised service.

Sensate focus is both a treatment and an ongoing assessment. As well as helping the couple rebuild their sexual relationship, the technique will permit identification and clarification of the specific blocks that are maintaining the sexual dysfunction. There are four stages of sensate focus:

- non-genital sensate focus
- genital sensate focus
- vaginal containment
- vaginal containment with movement.

Non-genital sensate focus

Following discussion of the formulation and an agreement to pursue sex therapy, the couple are asked to agree to abstain from penetrative sexual intercourse and to not touch each other's genital areas (or the woman's breasts) until this becomes appropriate in later stages of the approach. These elements of sexual activity are temporarily 'banned', in order to remove the sense of a need to 'perform' sexually. However, it is obviously essential for the couple still to have sessions of time together in order to give and receive physical (sensual, but not yet sexual) pleasure. It is suggested that they should have sessions lasting around 30 minutes two or three times during the week when they will engage in touching and caressing. One partner will first explore and caress the other's body (apart from the 'banned areas'), perhaps using massage, stroking, kissing, and so on. The partner who is receiving this physical contact will give feedback to the 'active' partner. In doing so he or she should begin each sentence with the word 'I', in order to try to minimise the possibility of criticism. For example, he or she may say 'I really like what you were just doing' or 'I would prefer it if you did that more firmly', rather than 'You're not very good at that'. After a period of time which suits the couple, preferably around half of the session, they should swap roles. They should stop the session if they become bored or if serious anxiety is provoked in either partner, but otherwise the actual duration of the session would be determined by what feels right for that particular couple.

These sessions should improve trust and closeness, increase the awareness of what each partner likes and dislikes, and may assist the therapist in clarifying difficulties. The couple should not proceed to the next stage of the programme until they have been able to enjoy several sessions of successful non-genital sensate focus. These sessions should always be carried out in a private, warm and comfortable environment, with subdued lighting and precautions being taken to avoid being disturbed.

Genital sensate focus

In this next stage of the programme the couple will be allowed to touch the genital and breast areas, which were previously 'out of bounds'. It is important to avoid any suggestion to the couple, however, that they should go straight to these areas; this stage should be added to the previous activity carried out during non-genital sensate focus. Penetrative sexual intercourse remains banned during this stage. Each partner should continue to focus on the sensations being experienced, proceeding on to the more overtly sexual areas if that feels acceptable. They should not strive to become aroused or put any pressure on each other to do so. In fact, a truly adult-to-adult agreement by the couple *not* yet to proceed to penetration should make physiological genital arousal much less relevant.

Specific details regarding gentle touching and switching attention from one part of the body to another should be given by the therapist. It may be helpful to describe the genital touching, at least initially, as 'genital exploration', to distinguish it from behaviour specifically aimed at producing arousal. The couple should continue to feel relaxed and concentrate on the giving and receiving of pleasure, and feedback should continue, as in the previous stage.

Vaginal containment

The title of this stage sounds very clinical to some couples, and so the therapist may choose to use different words to describe it. In essence, however, this stage involves the gradual introduction of penetrative sexual intercourse while trying to minimise the anxiety that may be induced in some couples with regard to penetrative sex. This may be the case in men suffering premature ejaculation or erectile dysfunction, or women with the problem of vaginismus (described in more detail below). The couple should move on to this stage during a session of mutual pleasuring when they both feel relaxed and sexually aroused. Female superior is the most suitable position; the male superior ('missionary') position is not usually recommended at this stage, as it increases the likelihood of ejaculation and is not a position in which a woman with sexual anxieties would feel in control.

Once penetration has occurred the couple should remain still, concentrating on pleasant genital sensations, although the man may move a little to stimulate himself if his erection begins to wane. Containment should last however long the partners feel comfortable with, following which they should withdraw and continue pleasuring each other as previously described. Hawton (1985) suggests that vaginal containment is repeated two or three times in any one session.

Vaginal containment with movement

This is the final stage of sensate focus. It is generally most appropriate for the woman to move first, slowly initially but perhaps more vigorously with time to establish or re-establish full sexual intercourse. Thereafter, the therapist may suggest to the couple that they experiment with different positions, while remaining cognisant of their particular anxieties and any specific sexual activity that is unacceptable to either of them.

Dealing with blocks (cognitive 'trouble-shooting')

Most couples encounter difficulties at some stage of the sensate focus approach. It is important to view these as a source of additional information regarding the aetiology of the couple's problems. When initiating sex therapy it is, therefore, helpful to discuss with the couple the need for them to return to the clinic even if their homework assignments do not seem to go well. Difficulties can be positively reframed as providing useful information and therefore increasing the likelihood of eventual success through therapy. Minor blocks to therapy are common and include partners not initiating sessions owing to feelings of embarrassment, tiredness or an initial lack of motivation. This can be addressed by discussing the need for them to prioritise their sessions together in order to ensure that they take place. They should be informed that many couples find things a little difficult initially. Major blocks are less common but important.

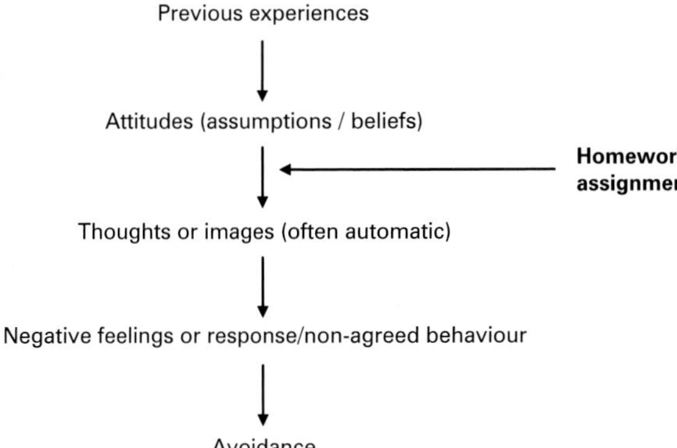

Fig. 26.4 The cognitive model applied to problems with homework assignments in sex therapy.

The successful management of these is crucial within sex therapy and perhaps is the core skill of an effective sex therapist. They should be addressed using the cognitive model shown in Fig. 26.4.

The automatic negative thoughts or images that block sexual activity may concern the nature of the assignment or the possible consequences as perceived by the patient(s). The therapist should help the couple to identify automatic thoughts and images, then to identify underlying attitudes or beliefs and to encourage the partners to review evidence for them while considering alternative and more helpful interpretations of the situation. Myths and misunderstandings regarding sex are often exposed at this point, so it is very important to have sessions in clinic with both partners present if at all possible. Sometimes it may become necessary to alter the focus of therapy temporarily, in order to address the problems encountered, and then to return to the sensate focus approach at an appropriate later time.

Box 26.2 sets out various strategies to facilitate progress in sex therapy.

Education

Education will occur informally throughout clinic sessions with the couple. Sexual anatomy, physiology and response should be discussed and clarified. It may also be helpful to suggest reading for the couple, using a general text (e.g. *The Book of Love*, Delvin, 1974), or specific texts (e.g. *Men and Sex*, Zilbergeld, 1978; *Becoming Orgasmic*, Heiman & LoPiccolo, 1999), depending on the specific problems occurring.

A specific education session is also helpful in most cases; it should be tailored to the educational level, age and cultural background of the individuals concerned. This may be a few sessions into treatment, perhaps around the time of commencing genital sensate focus. The aim of this session is to provide information, to dispel sexual myths (such as those listed on page 680), to alleviate anxieties, to enhance understanding and confidence, and to identify any important blind spots or fallacies that might perpetuate the couple's problems. Diagrams and photographs may be a helpful adjunct.

It is important throughout therapy to be flexible regarding the approach and to adjust the pace of

Box 26.2 Strategies to overcome blocks to therapy

Strategies for minor difficulties

- Acknowledge difficulty and offer encouragement
- Suggest easier or alternative homework assignments

Strategies for major difficulties

- Identify negative thoughts and attitudes
- Offer interpretation
- Explore a series of explanations

Other useful strategies

- Identify the positive benefits of homework assignments
- Attribute positive intentions to actions
- Suggest positive relabelling or reframing of events
- Give reassurance about the normality of the experience
- Give permission
- Use paradoxical intention (see Box 26.3)
- See the partners individually
- Use confrontation (see Box 26.3)

Box 26.3 Paradoxical intention and confrontation

The use of *paradox* is a technique first developed in systems and family therapy work (Selvini Palazzoli *et al*, 1978). It should be used with care, in selected cases when other approaches have failed, and possibly only by a specialist in this area. In essence, it involves giving a suggestion to the couple that may appear contrary to the goal of therapy but which the therapist feels may work. One simple example would be to suggest that a couple who have been striving to arouse each other should avoid arousal. Another would be to describe or summarise a particular and apparently intractable problem in the couple's relationship, but then say that it should stay as it is rather than that the couple should try to change it. This can focus the couple's efforts on what remains, to them, a problem worth tackling.

On occasion it may also be necessary to *confront* a lack of progress in a very direct way, for example if sessions are simply not taking place. The reasons behind this may be elucidated but it is also important to be clear with the couple that, analogous to taking antibiotics for a chest infection, progress will be possible only if the treatment is actually applied.

Although the sex therapy approach described in this chapter will enable a general psychiatrist to help many patients with sexual problems, there will be some cases that require more specialised techniques, and so referral to a specialist psychosexual medicine service.

progress through the stages to suit each couple and their particular difficulties. As with any psychotherapy, it is also important to prepare for termination from the start of therapy. This can be assisted by extending the intervals between later sessions, attempting to prepare the couple for any future problems that could arise and which they might now be able to deal with more effectively, and perhaps setting a follow-up assessment for some 3 months after the final treatment session.

Specific techniques for specific conditions

Many of the possible sexual dysfunctions can be dealt with by applying specific techniques in parallel with or on the background of the general sex therapy approach described above. More specific techniques under the headings of the sexual dysfunctions to which they apply are described below.

Lack or loss of sexual interest

The techniques used to increase sexual interest apply equally to women and men.

Drive versus desire

Despite the fact that the terms 'drive' and 'desire' are often used interchangeably by patients and professionals when discussing sexual feelings, they are not the same. *Drive* is a fundamental biological urge that is not subject specific, whose total absence is suggestive of an organic pathology. *Desire* is subject specific (i.e. usually a specific person) and can be variable in intensity or even absent without this reflecting the presence of pathology, whether physical or psychological. Thus, it is possible to experience loss of or absence of desire without loss of drive, so that a person may lose interest in sex with a partner while continuing to have sexual thoughts and feelings from time to time.

It is always important to elicit in the history and mental state examination which of these is present or altered, in order to consider physical versus psychological problems in the aetiology of a loss or lack of sexual interest. It is also important to remain alert to the tendency to categorise the partner with a lower sexual interest as having a problem, although this may be neither helpful nor accurate.

Treating loss of drive

Treatment for a total loss of drive may be the identification and treatment of an organic disorder, such as testosterone deficiency. This treatment, or hormonal augmentation in peri- or postmenopausal women, should be undertaken only by suitably medically qualified professionals, such as endocrinologists or gynaecologists.

Treating loss of desire

Treatment for a loss of desire, in both men and women, is based on addressing the specific areas of difficulty identified in the assessment and formulation. It is important to be as clear as possible about the aetiology of the loss of desire. This is often secondary to general relationship problems, or because the couple's lives have changed, becoming much busier over the years and as a result they spend far too little time together. *Timetabling* is a useful technique to clarify whether this process of 'growing apart' is the problem, and to demonstrate it to the couple. Each of them is asked to complete a timetable covering every hour of all seven days of a typical week, and to classify the time according to the following categories:

- work at work (employment)
- work at home (including housework, etc.)
- family time
- extended-family time
- social time (with friends)
- couple time (just the two of them)
- personal time (for the individual).

They are then (perhaps between the next two sessions) asked to do the same for a typical week at a time in the past, before their problem(s) arose. The results are often striking and quite powerful with regard to increasing understanding of the problem and motivating the couple to address it (Butcher, 1999). In fact, it should be recommended to all busy and active couples who have been together for several years, as a way of showing the importance of setting time aside to be together as a couple. A relationship in which couple time is virtually nil is not conducive to a healthy and satisfying sex life.

If the loss of desire is a consequence of more specific relationship problems, these must be addressed in order to allow the later rebuilding of a satisfactory sexual relationship through sensate focus. Such relationship problems are approached through couple work, aimed at facilitating an equal discussion in which both parties can put across their point of view and be heard. Various techniques may be employed in this regard, including making lists of the aspects of the partner's behaviour or personality that are cherished or disliked, considering priorities and whether these coincide, and timetabling (as above).

Apart from identifying a basic lack of time together, the couple may discuss the fact that when they are together they are very tired. This can be a good basis on which to discuss what sort of life together they actually want, and can realistically achieve. This may change as their lives progress: people with small children, or couples in jobs that do not synchronise free time, or who are caring for elderly relatives, may begin to understand more clearly why their partnership is suffering.

The roles people adopt throughout their lives may also influence how they see themselves and how their partners see them. Taking women as the example, the range of interpersonal roles through which they pass might be as follows:

- daughter
- sister
- friend
- work colleague

- girlfriend
- lover
- wife
- mother
- grandmother.

Any one individual may occupy several roles at any one time. The problem is that, for some people, certain roles are more immediately powerful than others, in terms of how the individual sees her- or himself (self-identity) and the effect this has on behaviour. In particular, the mother role may virtually eclipse all others, and particularly may be viewed as much more important than the lover role. Behaviour in and around the sexual relationship that seems acceptable as a young lover lacking many responsibilities may just not be seen as appropriate for a mother of young children. This tends, of course, to be an unconscious problem, manifesting in a loss of interest in sex and leading to wider relationship problems. It may be particularly striking in a woman who perceived her own mother (perhaps her only model for that role) to be serious, judgemental and sexless. Such issues will need to be addressed if they are thought to make a contribution to the loss of interest in sex.

Often, in the case of general relationship problems, simply improving communication and allowing the two partners to express themselves freely in a non-threatening environment, with facilitation by a third party, is enough to begin a process that, if fostered, strengthens honesty, trust and respect on both sides. As communication improves, the therapist may 'withdraw' more and more from the conversation (perhaps in part physically by rearranging the three chairs), to allow the couple to communicate directly with each other more effectively than has been possible for some time.

In their popular textbook *Therapy with Couples*, Crowe & Ridley (2000) describe the overall goals of such therapy:

- improved couple adjustment (communication, negotiation and satisfaction)
- increased flexibility of interaction in the relationship
- reduction of any symptoms or individual problems
- decrease in labelling one partner as the 'problem'
- if the relationship or the individual problems cannot be improved, a reduction of expectations ('live with it')
- any improvement should be able to last without further therapeutic help.

The same authors stress the fundamental importance of clear and agreed goals of therapy, and describe the 'alternative levels of intervention hierarchy'. This is a sequence of interventions of increasing therapist action and ingenuity; the more problems the couple has, the further along this sequence the therapist may need to go in attempting to help them (Box 26.4).

There is insufficient space to expand on these elements of couple therapy in this chapter, but for those interested in reading more, Crowe & Ridley (2000) provide an excellent and detailed guide.

Box 26.4 Interventions used in couple therapy

- Reciprocity negotiation (agreeing each to alter a specific element or elements of his/her behaviour as requested by the partner, in a reciprocal fashion)
- Communication training
- Induce arguments
- Timetables and tasks
- Paradox
- Adjust to the symptom
- Cease treatment or use other therapies

After Crowe & Ridley (2000).

Another problem sometimes encountered is that of one or other partner complaining that he or she no longer finds the partner attractive. If this is the case, the person will have to consider what the options are, and whether or not the relationship should continue. Before this decision is reached, and to help the person to think through this problem, it may be helpful to ask him or her to consider what brought the couple together originally, under the following three headings:

1 attraction

2 goals (what they want out of life, what they want to do or to achieve)

3 beliefs (what life is about, what is important, how one should live and behave).

By reviewing these areas some individuals find they still wish to remain with their partner, and seek ways of addressing their relationship difficulties and improving its physical aspects. Such a favourable outcome tends to occur if the individual still sees a high level of 'closeness of fit' between themselves and their partner, despite a perception that immediate physical attraction has waned. However, in other cases, the declared loss of attraction and interest may remain, and may ultimately lead to the end of the relationship.

Depression affecting sexual interest

If a psychiatric contributory factor such as loss of libido as a component of a depressive illness is identified, this should be treated. Ideally, approaches that minimise the use of medication should be tried because of the risk of further suppressing sexual interest. There is some evidence to suggest that trazodone may increase libido in both men and women who are depressed: one study reporting an improvement in libido and erections in two-thirds of patients studied (Kurt *et al*, 1994). This is in contrast to many other antidepressants and lithium, which decrease sexual desire. It should also be remembered that if sexual desire is of great importance to the patient, an antidepressant-induced impairment of libido may mask the degree of recovery from the depressive illness.

Drugs affecting sexual interest

Many drugs, both prescribed and illicit, can affect sexual interest (Box 26.5).

Box 26.5 Psychotropic drugs that may affect sexual interest

- Antidepressants (clomipramine and other tricyclic antidepressants; selective serotonin reuptake inhibitors; venlafaxine; monoamine oxidase inhibitors, etc.)
- Lithium
- Anxiolytics and hypnotics (e.g. benzodiazepines)
- Anticonvulsants
- Acamprosate
- Antipsychotics (may help to restore libido impaired by untreated schizophrenia but have a deleterious effect on erectile and orgasmic performance and satisfaction)

Sources: Bazire (2001); Taylor *et al* (1997); Clayton & Shen (1998).

If sexual interest is being suppressed by a drug, then there should be a careful discussion between the patient, the sex therapist and the prescribing doctor, in order to weigh up the advantages and disadvantages of continuing with the drug, trying an alternative, or stopping the treatment. Restoring sexual interest may be important but interfering with the prescribing relationship between the patient and another doctor – and possibly unleashing a whole new set of problems – would not be desirable. This is also an area in which informed consent is very important.

Prognosis of impaired sexual interest

Of all the types of sexual dysfunction, low sexual desire has the least favourable prognosis (Hawton *et al*, 1986). For women this condition has a particularly poor long-term outcome. Although initial resolution of the problem (at the end of therapy) has been reported for approximately 30% of patients, at follow-up 1–6 years later only some 3% remain free of the problem (Hawton *et al*, 1986). This may in part be due to some affected women having psychological issues relating to low self-esteem, or perhaps because the loss of sexual interest is a consequence of ongoing problems in the general (non-sexual) aspects of the relationship. It is important, as with all psychological management, to remember to see the patient as a whole, and not to view the psychosexual problem in isolation.

Impaired arousal

In women

In premenopausal women, in the absence of impaired sexual interest, impaired physiological arousal (vaginal engorgement and lubrication) appears to be relatively uncommon. Alternatively, it may be more common as a problem than realised but not complained of, possibly in part because it is less obvious than impaired sexual arousal in men (erectile dysfunction). When assessing the problem it is important to establish at what point during sex the impaired arousal occurs.

Box 26.6 Common myths of sexuality

- Sex should be natural and spontaneous – asking for it spoils it
- All physical contact must lead to sex
- Men always want and are ready for sex
- Sex is for male pleasure – a woman's duty is to fulfil his need, not her own
- Men must take charge of and orchestrate sex
- If women aren't orgasmic they should fake it
- Women expect men to know all about sex
- Men should not have or at least not express certain feelings
- Anything other than the missionary position is dirty
- Women must wait for the man to initiate sex
- For men, in sex, as elsewhere, it is performance that counts
- Women must maintain a 'good' reputation
- Women must be attractive, obedient and passive, because men expect it
- Having sex means having intercourse
- For the couple to have sex, the man must have an erection
- Good sex always ends in orgasm
- Good sex means both partners having an orgasm, preferably at the same time
- There is something wrong with a man who has a lower sex drive than a woman
- In general, women receive more stimulation from a large penis than a small one
- Nice girls don't get turned on – and they certainly never move during lovemaking
- Don't show affection to men because they will want sex
- If a woman shows interest in making love, she must be promiscuous
- Most homosexuals exclusively adopt the passive or active role in their sexual relationship
- In this enlightened age, none of the previous myths has had any effect on any of *us*

Source: Drawn from Zilbergeld (1978) and others.

The partner's sexual technique may inhibit arousal, or expectations on the part of either partner may be unrealistic. Discussion and challenging of the 'myths of sexuality' may be helpful in the latter circumstance, for both men and women (Box 26.6).

It can be useful for the woman to share with her partner her own experience of successful arousal techniques. In general and in the absence of an organic cause for the arousal impairment (e.g. diabetes, multiple sclerosis, severe vascular disease or any of the list of medications that are known to impair arousal, as listed in Box 26.5), the approach to this area of difficulty follows the usual sensate focus pattern, with promotion of communication about sexual matters. The sharing of responsibility for sexual arousal between the couple will also be important.

Where there are ongoing difficulties stemming from previous sexual trauma or abuse, individual psychotherapeutic work to help the woman deal with the trauma may be indicated, and sensate focus work should be postponed. In such circumstances, and as far as allowed by the woman concerned, explanation to the partner as to what the problem is and why most physical activity is being postponed is helpful.

There are various ways in which the woman or couple may attempt to maximise arousal. Sexual fantasies can be used to increase arousal but need a tactful and considered approach if they are to be suggested at all. Some couples may react with horror or see using fantasies as a betrayal of their partner and threatening to the relationship. It can be helpful to explain that sexual arousal achieved through the use of fantasy eventually becomes linked with the partner, and as this association strengthens, the need for the use of fantasy decreases. Sensitivity to the couple and good judgement are needed to avoid causing distress, but in suitable cases the therapist may recommend the use of erotic literature, videos or vibrators as further ways to enhance sexual arousal.

Postmenopausal women may benefit from gynaecological assessment for atrophic vaginitis, which usually responds to local application of oestrogen cream. This treatment should be supervised by a doctor (general practitioner or gynaecologist) experienced in its use, as should other types of hormone replacement therapy (HRT).

In men

Erectile dysfunction with a clear organic cause is usually dealt with by the patient's general practitioner, or in secondary care by a urologist or andrologist. Ageing, vascular (arterial) disease, neurological disease, trauma, post-surgical complications and diabetes are some of the physical causes of erectile dysfunction. In addition, a large number of drugs can induce sexual dysfunction, and most commonly erectile dysfunction, as a side-effect. These include antidepressants, anticholinergics, antihypertensives, antipsychotics, corticosteroids, diuretics, hypnotics, lithium carbonate, oestrogens and opiates, among others. Table 26.5 lists some of the common agents implicated in erectile dysfunction; this is not an exhaustive list and more detailed information may be available in the relevant datasheets and with the local drug information service. For prevalence figures of erectile dysfunction in various clinical settings see Table 26.1 on page 669.

Table 26.5 Medication associated with erectile dysfunction

Type of drug	Examples	Alternative drugs with lower risk of erectile dysfunction
Antihypertensives	Beta-blockers (e.g. propranolol, atenolol) Thiazide diuretics Hydralazine	Alpha-adrenergic blockers ACE inhibitors Calcium channel blockers
Diuretics	Thiazide diuretics Potassium-sparing diuretics Carbonic anhydrase inhibitor	Loop diuretics
Antidepressants	Selective serotonin reuptake inhibitors Tricyclic antidepressants Monoamine oxidase inhibitors	Newer agents may have lower risk (e.g. nefazodone, mirtazepine), but a specialist opinion may be required before treatment is changed
Antipsychotics	Phenothiazines Risperidone	Newer agents may have lower risk (e.g. quetiapine), but specialist opinion may be required before treatment is changed
Mood stabilisers	Carbamazepine Lithium	
Hormonal agents	Cyproterone acetate Luteinising hormone-releasing hormone analogues Oestrogens	Dependent on diagnosis and options available
Lipid regulators	Gemfibrozil Clofibrate	Statins
Anticonvulsants	Phenytoin Carbamazepine	Need specialist neurological advice
Antiparkinsonian drugs	L-dopa	Needs specialist neurological advice
Dyspepsia and ulcer-healing drugs	H2 antagonists	Proton pump inhibitors
Miscellaneous	Allopurinol Indomethacin Disulfiram Phenothiazine Antihistamines Phenothiazine antiemetics	Cyclizine

Adapted from Ralph & McNicholas (2000).
Note that this table aims to suggest alternative medication that may be less likely to cause erectile dysfunction, but all the suggested alternatives are also liable to cause erectile dysfunction to some extent, and may themselves be the primary cause in a patient presenting with organic erectile dysfunction.

Impact of psychotropic medication

In the day-to-day practice of adult general psychiatry it is important to bear in mind the effect that prescribed medication may have on the desire, arousal and orgasm of patients. All too often patients are too embarrassed to raise these issues themselves, so psychiatrists (and other healthcare professionals) should seek out information about them in an appropriate manner, regardless of whether the patient currently has a partner or not.

Compliance with treatment can be markedly affected if patients experience adverse sexual side-effects. Hyperprolactinaemia and other disturbance of the hypothalamic–pituitary–adrenal (HPA) axis caused by neuroleptics (and sometimes other drugs or causes) may also occur. These difficulties may not be only sexual, and effects can be long term. In particular, reproductive capability should be discussed with patients when obtaining informed consent for the use of such drugs.

Some agents are more likely than others to cause erectile dysfunction. Buproprion, desipramine, fluvoxamine and reboxetine are all thought less likely to cause sexual dysfunction, while lithium, fluphenazine, thioridazine, tricyclic antidepressants and selective serotonin reuptake inhibitors (SSRIs) are all commonly associated with erectile dysfunction. Smoking and alcohol consumption are common contributory factors in the aetiology of erectile dysfunction; nicotine in cigarettes may cause spasm of the penile arteries (Virag *et al*, 1985).

A particular problem for general adult psychiatrists is young men with psychosis who, once they discover that their sexual dysfunction is related to their antipsychotic medication, choose to discontinue it and may even disengage from services or conceal their illness to avoid further exposure to antipsychotics. There may also be pressure from the patient's sexual partner. It is obviously important to discuss this issue with this group of patients in order to try to avoid difficulties arising through non-adherence to treatment.

Physical treatments

Commonly used physical treatments for erectile dysfunction include vacuum devices with constriction bands, intracavernosal injections or intraurethral pellets of prostaglandin, and oral therapy such as sildenafil citrate (Viagra) and, more recently, sublingual apomorphine (Uprima). New and more acceptable oral treatments for erectile dysfunction were becoming available at the time of writing.

The physiological mechanism of erection involves the relaxation of vascular smooth muscle in the walls of the trabecular spaces in the corpora cavernosa. Noradrenergic transmission controls the tonic contraction of this muscle in the non-erect penis, so that blockade of this control mechanism with alpha-blocking drugs will result in an erection. Alternatively, intracavernosal injection of an alpha-agonist, such as metaraminol, will cause the erect penis to detumesce. This is used in the treatment of drug-induced priapism (Stein, 1995). Largely based around this system, various drugs have been developed for use in the treatment of erectile dysfunction (Box 26.7). At the time of writing, the oral therapies have a somewhat lower efficacy rate but a better side-effect profile than more locally administered medication, such as injections.

Box 26.7 Drugs used in the treatment of erectile dysfunction

Yohimbine is a presynaptic alpha$_2$-adrenergic receptor blocker which decreases sympathetic (adrenergic) and increases parasympathetic (cholinergic) activity, and is thought to have a boosting effect on noradrenergic activity in the corpora cavernosal tissues. In the UK yohimbine is not licensed for the treatment of erectile dysfunction but is still sometimes prescribed on a named-patient basis.

Alprostadil is prostaglandin E1, and is the main intracavernosal injection agent used in the UK at present (although papaverine and phentolamine are still used occasionally).

Alprostadil is also available in a transurethral form (as a pellet passed into the penile urethra, known as MUSE – medicated urethral system for erection).

Sildenafil citrate (Viagra) is a phosphodiesterase type-5 (PDE-5) inhibitor. During sexual stimulation, nitric oxide, which is released from blood vessels, activates chemical messengers, including cyclic guanosine monophosphate (GMP). These act as vasodilators and increase penile blood flow, filling the corpora cavernosa. Cyclic GMP in penile tissue is denatured by phosphodiesterase type-5. Sildenafil works by inhibiting this enzyme, so that vasodilation continues and the erectile response is 'boosted'. In contrast to injections or pellets of prostaglandin E1, this means that sildenafil is an 'erection enhancer' rather than an 'erection inducer'. It has to be taken about 1 hour before sex is expected to occur, and is then at peak level of effectiveness for approximately 4 hours. Sildenafil, in common with all PDE-5 inhibitors, is contraindicated in patients taking nitrates or in patients in whom vasodilation or sexual activity are inadvisable. In addition, in the absence of information, manufacturers of the PDE-5 inhibitors contraindicate these drugs for people with hypotension, recent stroke, unstable angina and myocardial infarction (British Medical Association, 2004).

Tadalafil (Cialis) is also a PDE-5 inhibitor, but with a longer duration of action than sildenafil. It has a half-life of around 17 hours and is thought to be at peak level of effectiveness from approximately 30 minutes after being taken until up to 36 hours later. (This newer preparation has the same contraindications as sildenafil, as listed above.)

Vardenafil (Levitra) is the third generally available PDE-5 inhibitor. It is recommended to be taken 25–60 minutes before sexual activity (British Medical Association, 2004). Its half-life and absorption characteristics are similar to those of sildenafil, and it has the same contraindications (as listed above).

Sublingual **apomorphine** (Uprima) is a centrally acting dopaminergic agonist that has been introduced very recently for the treatment of erectile dysfunction in men. Nitric oxide (as mentioned above) is known to play an essential role in the production of erections evoked by central neurotransmitters and mediators. The latter include dopamine as well as oxytocin, excitatory amino acids and serotonergic (5-HT$_{2c}$) agonists; hence the erectogenic effect of apomorphine.

Before prescribing a drug it is essential that the doctor does the following:

- informs the patient about the potential side-effects of any suggested treatment, particularly where failure to respond to a problem could have severe consequences
- advises against dosage manipulation without medical guidance
- records in the notes that this discussion has occurred.

One particularly important warning to give patients is of the urgent need to detumesce an erection lasting over 2 hours. Priapism of this duration is a surgical emergency due to the risk of cavernosal necrosis. Trazodone can, rarely, cause priapism as an unwanted side-effect and is sometimes used in cases of depression with erectile dysfunction.

Where appropriate, surgical intervention may be considered, either vascular or to correct a deformity or insert an implant. It must be understood, however, that insertion of rods, whether silastic or with hydraulics, requires virtual ablation of the cavernosal tissue. This is an absolute last resort, because if the procedure fails (e.g. due to infection) and the rods have to be removed there will be no erectile tissue remaining with which to do further work.

Some patients self-medicate with a variety of 'alternative' medications, such as ginseng. The potential for interactions with other medications must be remembered and enquiry should always be made about what non-prescribed substances patients are using (Medicines Control Agency, 2002).

Prescribing regulations for drug treatments for erectile dysfunction

In response to financial concerns for the National Health Service (NHS) on the introduction of Viagra (sildenafil citrate), the Department of Health decided that a patient can be prescribed drug treatment for erectile dysfunction on the NHS only if he also has one of the following conditions:

- diabetes
- multiple sclerosis
- Parkinson's disease
- poliomyelitis
- prostate cancer or prostatectomy
- radical pelvic surgery
- renal failure treated by dialysis or transplant
- severe pelvic injury
- single-gene neurological disease
- spinal cord injury or spina bifida.

Patients who do not fall into any of these categories can be treated in one of two ways: they can receive NHS treatment from 'specialist services' if they are felt to be suffering from 'severe distress' in relation to their erectile dysfunction; or they can receive private prescriptions from their general practitioner. In the current guidelines, 'severe distress' is not clearly defined. The Department of Health has given guidance, however, on the frequency of dosing, recommending that one treatment per week should be adequate for most patients. This can be problematic for more sexually active patients or perhaps those going on holiday, so that some flexibility would seem reasonable.

Combination therapy

A patient with erectile dysfunction with a likely psychological cause (possibly coexisting with an organic cause) may be referred to a psychosexual service, where one exists. Alternatively, a general psychiatrist may be approached for an opinion and advice. Lack of an identifiable organic cause, sudden onset and a situational pattern all suggest that the problem is psychogenic (see Table 26.4, page 675). Depending on the 'psychological mindedness' of the patient, it may be possible to identify and address the causes of the erectile dysfunction through therapy without using adjunctive therapy such as drugs (see below). This is not always possible, however, and an important part of the assessment is checking whether patients share the same aims and philosophy of treatment as the psychosexual service they are engaging with. This may not be the case, for a variety of possible reasons, such as cultural factors, educational level, intellectual capacity and the patient's conceptual framework. There should be no bar to combination therapy – where drugs, or even other physical treatments, are used alongside psychological therapy if necessary.

When setting up a psychosexual service it is important to consider how this will be achieved when needed. It may mean establishing good working relationships with allied services such as urology and diabetology, especially where local trust prescribing practices dictate that only certain specialties can prescribe drugs for erectile dysfunction.

Psychological approaches to the treatment of erectile dysfunction

Psychological approaches involve the identification and resolution of marital or couple conflict, and the sensate focus approach for couples, as described above. It is also important to assess whether the problem (as is often the case in psychogenic erectile dysfunction) is one of performance anxiety (Fig. 26.5).

'Spectatoring' refers to the process of psychologically or emotionally 'standing back' from what is happening during sex, to 'observe' (and worry about) one's own sexual 'performance' (e.g. the strength of erection). In other words, the person is having anxious rather than sexually stimulating cognitions. The result is an inhibition of the usual feedback loop of sexual arousal, via interference with stimulation of the genital vasculature by autonomic nerves. The initial 'failure' of erectile functioning may have had various causes, such as anxiety, excessive alcohol, environmental factors (cold) and so on, but the resultant 'spectatoring' sets up a cycle of repeating failure, as shown in Fig. 26.5.

If performance anxiety is the problem, a description of it using the diagram shown in Fig. 26.5 will lead to its recognition and confirmation by the man concerned. Sensate focus, as described above, can then be applied to help the couple rebuild their sexual relationship without performance anxiety causing problems.

Men who do not have a sexual partner but have a problem with erectile dysfunction may find themselves

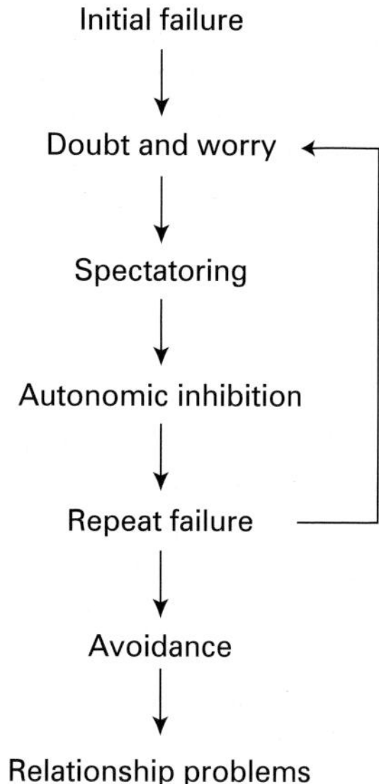

Fig. 26.5 Performance anxiety.

in something of a 'catch 22' situation. They may avoid or fail to secure relationships as a result of their sexual dysfunction, but have no setting within which to use sensate focus techniques to overcome their difficulty. In the past, this situation was often made worse by the fact that sex therapy was not offered to single people, only to couples, but today help is offered for sexual problems to whoever presents to services, whether they are in a relationship or not. Even so, in the case of erectile dysfunction in a single man, a psychological (behavioural) approach has definite limitations. What can be offered are explanation and education (the formulation) as a means of reducing anxiety, combined with a simple technique called 'waxing and waning', which serves to increase the man's confidence in his erectile functioning, but it can be used only where the erectile dysfunction is situational. This technique involves pausing during masturbation and allowing the erection to reduce before continuing masturbation, with a return of the erection. If this is done several times during each masturbation session, confidence may improve and also demonstrate to the person that the normal lessening of the strength of an erection which sometimes occurs during love making does not necessarily signify the impending loss of the erection altogether.

In addition, of course, medication may help by improving the patient's confidence in his ability to have an erection if the need arises, and so reduce the likelihood of avoidance of future relationships.

Prognosis with psychological treatments

Follow-up studies suggest that with psychological treatment alone, successful resolution of the problem will occur in around 75% of those treated, with 60% remaining in remission at follow-up between 1 and 6 years later (Hawton & Catalan, 1986).

Prognosis with physical treatments

Intracavernosal injections may achieve beyond 90% technical success but are often unacceptable to patients (and partners), with priapism, penile pain and fibrosis as recognised complications (Ralph & McNicholas, 2000). Vacuum devices may be more acceptable, though they require some dexterity and practice to master and can be expensive. The introduction of the newer oral agents for the treatment of erectile dysfunction has widened the range of treatment options and boosted success rates for the treatment of erectile dysfunction. In patients treated with sildenafil, 50–88% of patients report improvement in erectile response and, provided the appropriate prescribing precautions are in place, the drug appears to be safe (Ralph & McNicholas, 2000). At the time of writing the only newer oral agent was sublingual apomorphine, for which a 67% success rate was reported from early trial work (Morales, 2001).

Surgical interventions, including implantation of silastic rods or rods with hydraulic systems, are outside the scope of this chapter but it is worth noting that both technical success and patient and partner satisfaction rates are high with penile implants (Ralph & McNicholas, 2000). As mentioned above, however, it is essential to appreciate that such intervention involves the total ablation of cavernosal tissue, so that failure has serious implications.

Difficulties with orgasm

In women

Range of orgasmic response in women

It is important to understand that there is a range of orgasmic response in women. Most surveys suggest that some 7–10% of women have never had an orgasm (Kinsey *et al*, 1953; Hunt, 1975; Tavris & Sadd, 1977; Masters *et al*, 1995). For some this is a problem, while for others there is no significant distress or concern. For example, one study described (in a non-random sample of couples) that 63% of women reported arousal or orgasm disorders – although 'happily married' – and 85% were satisfied with their sexual relationship (Frank *et al*, 1978). Thus, orgasmic problems do not necessarily mean that sexual dissatisfaction or relationship distress will follow.

Cultural factors play a large part in forming the individual woman's expectations in this area, as do her own religious and personal beliefs, values and experiences. There has been a significant and continuing increase in the level of interest displayed in this area by the media, and sometimes the resulting proliferation of articles, tapes and books about female orgasm may be helpful – but for others it causes further problems. This is particularly the case when a woman feels that she is expected to 'perform', and when partners believe that every woman should be orgasmic and judge their own sexual performance by the response of the woman concerned.

Box 26.8 Kegel's (pelvic floor) exercises

Kegel's exercises are a helpful adjunct. They improve tone, power and control of the pelvic floor muscles. The first step is their identification. This is followed by sessions of repeated contraction and relaxation of these muscles, gradually building up the frequency and duration of these exercises over several weeks.

For those who are orgasmic but find their orgasmic capacity impaired, Kegel's exercises (Box 26.8) to strengthen the pubococcygeus muscle may help by improving sexual sensation and response. Where a woman is not orgasmic, thorough assessment should indicate which areas need to be addressed. For example, some women 'switch off' when highly aroused. This loss of arousal may indicate that exploration is needed to address any fear associated with orgasm, such as anxiety regarding 'losing control', which may suggest a need for individual psychological therapy. In other cases, improvements in sexual technique achieved through sensate focus exercises may be sufficient.

Sexual growth programme for women

Some women who present with either anorgasmia or a perceived lack of sexual interest will actually give a history of very little sexual experience or none at all. There may be a sense of anxiety, fear or revulsion with regard to even the idea of engaging in sexual intercourse. This may have prevented them having any experiences with a partner, but presentation to a doctor usually means that they have now have decided to try to resolve this problem. In such cases a 'sexual growth programme' is often essential if any progress is to be made.

In essence, a sexual growth programme seeks to address an individual's anxieties and psychological discomfort about sex in a graded and organised way. It has similarities to systematic desensitisation and should be taken forward at a pace that is acceptable to, and largely set by, the patient herself. It starts with education about sexual anatomy and functioning, particularly the very wide variation in the appearance of female external genitalia. This should be accompanied by discussion of fears and concerns with regard to sex, using a calm, 'permission giving' approach. There will then follow a series of homework tasks, at an appropriate pace, with continuing discussion and cognitive troubleshooting of blocks in subsequent sessions with the therapist.

The tasks follow a sequence:

1 *General self-examination*. The patient is likely to need to start by spending some time looking at herself in a mirror, initially clothed but later moving on to viewing herself naked. This may be difficult for the patient, in which case encouragement and working through of issues highlighted will be necessary. Later, examination of the body in general by touching will occur.

2 *Genital self-examination*. This is also initially by looking (e.g. with a hand mirror) and later by touching and digital exploration. Many women find the stages of this approach easier if they take place after relaxation, whether by specific techniques or simply a long bath.

The two examination stages are a way to help the woman become comfortable with her own body, with her genitals and with herself as a sexual being. Most women will acknowledge the need to achieve this before they can be comfortable with another person in a sexual situation, and so permit the closeness and intimacy that they seek.

3 *Touching for pleasure*, with discussion of issues or problems encountered in therapy sessions.

4 *Enhancing sexual arousal*, particularly for women wishing to achieve orgasm for the first time. Here, care and tactful awareness of the patient's views as to what is acceptable should be considered before discussing the use of erotic literature or, possibly, the use of a vibrator.

5 *Sharing discoveries* with the partner (if there is one), and dealing again with concerns or difficulties that might arise.

Helpful reading (which is also recommended by both Relate and the Family Planning Association) is the book *Becoming Orgasmic* by Heiman & LoPiccolo (1999), as it includes a readily understood account of all the stages of a sexual growth programme.

Prognosis of female anorgasmia

The outcome of therapy of women with anorgasmia is uncertain, as few figures are available. One study reported a good level of response in the 'problem resolved although difficulties still experienced' category, but with very small numbers (Hawton *et al*, 1986).

In men

Broadly speaking, men may have five types of problem with the orgasm stage of sexual response:

1 premature ejaculation

2 retarded ejaculation (but able to ejaculate sometimes)

3 retrograde ejaculation (into the urinary bladder)

4 absent ejaculation (never ejaculates)

5 ejaculation but with reduced or lack of central sense of orgasm.

Premature ejaculation

What constitutes premature ejaculation? This is a complex question, especially because what is felt to be fine for one couple may be seen as premature by another. Perhaps the best definition might be 'ejaculation that occurs too soon in the subjective view of the couple concerned'. Most people would agree that ejaculation before penetration or within 1 or 2 minutes thereafter would be premature. However, if a man or couple present complaining that ejaculation is too soon because it occurs 10–15 minutes after thrusting commences, the first action to take would be to educate and facilitate discussion of realistic expectations. Those writing in the US literature are beginning to use the term 'rapid ejaculation' as an alternative.

Premature ejaculation is usually best treated with a behavioural approach, such as that used in the excellent self-help manual *PE: How to Overcome Premature Ejaculation* by Helen Singer Kaplan (Kaplan, 1989). This incorporates 'masturbation training' and the 'stop–start technique' (otherwise eponymously described as Seman's technique). The theoretical basis for this approach is that the fundamental problem in premature ejaculation is an inability to control the ejaculatory reflex. The key to success in treatment is for the man to become proficient in identifying the 'moment of ejaculatory inevitability' (MOEI), which is the point at which the man can sense that ejaculation is imminent and when even a cessation of all sexual activity would fail to prevent it. The patient is likely to understand this as 'the point of no return'.

Many patients suffering with premature ejaculation will already have tried distraction techniques during sex as a way to try to delay ejaculation. Typically these include such things as thinking non-sexual thoughts (e.g. about cricket or a problem at work), or inflicting pain on oneself by pinching. Other common techniques include masturbating before sex or taking a cold shower. Such attempts do not work (quite apart from the fact that they obviously reduce the man's enjoyment of sex). What is actually required is for the man to learn or train himself to control the ejaculatory reflex. This necessitates proficiency at identifying the MOEI, which in turn requires the man to focus on physical genital sensations during sex. Thus, the therapist will ask him to carry out sessions of masturbation, alone and when not expecting to be disturbed. During these he will concentrate on the pleasurable sensations in his genital area and will try to identify the MOEI. He will attempt to *stop* just before he reaches that point, and will then wait for several seconds to allow the feeling of being close to ejaculation to subside. He should not wait so long as to allow the erection to subside, and should *start* masturbation again when he no longer feels that ejaculation is very close. In this way, he should practise 'stop–start' three times, allowing himself to continue on to ejaculation the fourth time it approaches.

Going too far (failing to stop before ejaculation) should not be seen as a failure, but as a way for him to learn to identify the MOEI accurately and to improve his ability to stop just before it on the next occasion. Sessions should occur two or three times each week, with an attempt as time goes on to increase the duration of each session (from commencement to ejaculation), and so to begin to experience improved control. Meanwhile, if he is in a sexual relationship, the couple should continue to have physical pleasurable time together, but along non-genital sensate focus lines as described above.

When the patient has achieved improved control so that masturbation sessions can last for several (e.g. 7–10) minutes, he should be instructed to continue but with a lotion on his hand during masturbation (e.g. 'baby oil' or an artificial vaginal lubricant). Ejaculation may be a little quicker with a lubricant, but he should continue stop–start sessions until a reasonable degree of control is achieved once more.

Stop–start can next be brought into sessions with his partner, in the setting of genital sensate focus with manual stimulation by the partner (whom he can tell or signal to in some way when a stop or pause is necessary). Later stop–start stages are stimulation by the partner with a lotion, vaginal containment without movement (initially using the female superior position because ejaculation is generally quicker in the traditional 'missionary' position, due to the pulling down of skin at the base of the penis). Finally penetrative intercourse takes place, but still with appropriate stop–start elements. The ultimate aim is for the man to be able to have some control over his ejaculatory reflex, even simply by 'slowing down' when necessary rather than actually stopping as such.

Some patients cannot follow this approach, but as it is the best available, every effort should be made to facilitate it, by additional explanation and exploration of concerns or, if there is a language difficulty, by providing translated written material.

Some men come to the clinic with relatively fixed ideas of a medical intervention to slow things down and refuse to try the behavioural approach; in these cases there is little point arguing and it is best to go along with the patient. Physical treatments can be provided, preferably as an adjunct to the behavioural approach outlined, but sometimes as the sole treatment. Topical anaesthetic or 'freeze' sprays and gels have been suggested as useful and can be bought over the counter, but are not to be recommended as they have anaesthetic effects on the partner's vulval and vaginal tissue or other areas of her body. A better and often effective alternative is treatment with an SSRI. Of these, paroxetine would seem to have most research evidence to support its use in premature ejaculation (Waldinger *et al*, 1994; Ludovico *et al*, 1996). This medication should be initially taken daily for 3 months and then, if effective, on an 'as required basis' on the day of sex, but may be only a temporary solution as the problem is likely to return when medication is stopped.

An addition to stop–start is the 'squeeze technique', as pioneered by Masters & Johnson (1970). Despite what many people may think, this is not a simple technique to apply correctly. It is very anatomically specific and if incorrectly used (which is easy to do) it can cause discomfort and can therefore be ineffective. Thus, given that stop–start is very often successful without it, it may be best in general to avoid using the squeeze technique.

Prognosis The prognosis of premature ejaculation is the best of any condition treated with sex therapy. With the behavioural treatments, a 96% success rate is reported by Hawton *et al* (1986), while Kaplan (1989) claims that 'over 90% of premature ejaculators can be cured within an average of 14 weeks of treatment'. This 'cure rate' refers to initial remission, however, so that the patient's newly learnt skills may be needed again in the future if there is a relapse.

Retarded ejaculation

Conventionally, retarded ejaculation has been considered to be a consequence of the man 'holding back' or at least being unable, for psychological reasons, to ejaculate in the presence of a woman or intravaginally. This may be due to a specific problem between the couple concerned, or because of a more general problem on the part of the man. Some men may develop a strikingly dichotomised view of women. In other words, they may view all women as belonging to one of two 'groups' or 'types':

- easy, dirty, bad, sexually available women (akin to a very traditional view of a 'whore')
- good, clean, virtuous, mother-like women.

They may see it as reasonable to have sex with, and ejaculate in the presence of, the former but certainly not the latter. They then tend to choose a woman of the second type as their wife and mother for their children, and so it is not surprising that a problem with ejaculation and sex arises in their relationship.

Other psychological formulations have been advanced for failure to ejaculate. Psychoanalysts explain it as an expression of the patient's unconscious fears of the dangers associated with ejaculation, while systems theory suggests that the key lies in understanding the meaning of the symptom in terms of the effect on the relationship between the sexual partners.

More recently these traditional views of psychogenic retarded ejaculation have been challenged, mainly because such concepts have led to little success in the realms of treatment. Apfelbaum (2000) has suggested that the problem should be reformulated based on the concept of 'autosexuality'. He proposed that men with retarded ejaculation can achieve an erection that is satisfactory for intercourse automatically in response to a certain situation, but do so without experiencing any actual subjective sexual arousal. Because many of the men who experience retarded ejaculation with their partner are able to achieve orgasm alone, the problem of retarded ejaculation can be viewed as 'partner anorgasmia' or situational anorgasmia with a partner (Apfelbaum, 2000). The suggestion is that retarded ejaculation has been inappropriately treated in the past by viewing it as almost analogous to vaginismus in women (see below), and by using a behavioural approach that produces a tremendous pressure to perform to orgasm, amounting almost to 'sexual coercion'. It may be preferable to view it like female anorgasmia, where the focus during therapy is on the negative emotions of the woman towards her partner, her fears and underlying feelings. Apfelbaum proposes that the way forward is to help the man openly to face his negative feelings rather than go on denying them (i.e. hostility towards or distance from the partner and consequent lack of arousal), along with the introduction and maximisation of sexual arousal itself.

Retarded ejaculation presenting as an infertility problem is sometimes treated with superstimulation as described by Masters & Johnson (1970) or a high-speed vibrator applied to the glans penis (Crowe, 1998). Desipramine, neostigmine and yohimbine have all been suggested to be of benefit. When none of the above has worked, digital prostate massage may be tried. If unacceptable or unsuccessful this may sometimes lead to a urologist undertaking electro-ejaculatory stimulation. Rectal vibratory excitation (with great caution to avoid damage) might also be considered.

Prognosis Retarded ejaculation is often difficult to treat, either for psychological reasons as outlined above or because it is a side-effect of medication (i.e. those medications that reduce sexual interest or arousal, as listed in Box 26.5 on page 680). Its prognosis when treated with sex therapy is also somewhat unclear, owing to a lack of published data. What figures are available suggest a possible resolution rate of around 50%, but these are based on very small numbers (Hawton & Catalan, 1986). Prognosis also appears to be related to severity, to whether the condition is primary or secondary, and to the existence of concomitant relationship discord.

Retrograde ejaculation

Retrograde ejaculation occurs when there is a failure of the bladder neck sphincter to close at the start of ejaculation. Seminal fluid will thus pass up into the bladder instead of being emitted from the external urethral meatus, so that the patient may complain of a 'dry run'. If suspected, this problem can be confirmed by the presence of sperm in the urine. It may be helpful to ask the patient whether his urine is cloudy after sex, or to arrange for a sample to be examined under a microscope.

Retrograde ejaculation may be caused by surgery to the bladder neck, prostatectomy, division or impairment of the sympathetic nerve supply, or blockade of the $alpha_1$ drive to the bladder neck (by medication). Diabetic neuropathy and the side-effects of some antipsychotic medication are particularly important causes to consider. Retrograde ejaculation has been reported with chlordiazepoxide, various neuroleptics (including chlorpromazine, fluphenazine, perphenazine, pimozide, thioridazine, clozapine and trifuoperazine), monoamine oxidase inhibitors, tricyclic antidepressants, trazodone and narcotics (Hutchison *et al*, 2002).

It is possible to retrieve sperm from the bladder and wash it, using a specialised process, if fertility is an issue.

Absent ejaculation

Absent ejaculation (i.e. ejaculation never occurs, despite high arousal) should lead to physical examination and investigation, as it may indicate a physical, possibly neurological, disorder.

Lack of orgasmic experience with ejaculation

Some men, albeit rarely, present complaining that although ejaculation (emission) does occur they do not, or no longer, experience a subjective 'central' sense of orgasm or climax. In these cases, an organic or neurological cause should be ruled out before assessing issues of submaximal arousal, relationship problems or depression.

Sexual pain or 'dyspareunia'

In women

This symptom always indicates the need for full gynaecological assessment to exclude an organic cause. Possible causes include insufficient vaginal lubrication owing to a general medical condition; pelvic pathology such as vaginal or urinary tract infections, vaginal scar tissue, endometriosis or adhesions; postmenopausal vaginal atrophy; urinary tract irritation or infection; or gastrointestinal conditions (American Psychiatric Association, 1994).

Superficial pain, including general soreness in the outer part of the vagina, suggests a remediable physical cause, such as infection, the presence of pathology in local structures or allergy to semen, which may be helped by use of a condom.

If psychological causes are likely, and this is usually after all other causes have been excluded, impaired sexual arousal may result in painful penetration – although this usually improves as lubrication increases during intercourse. Sometimes deep pain from repeated buffeting of the cervix (which would normally lift somewhat during arousal but which has not altered in position owing to the lack of physiological response in the absence of arousal) adds to this difficulty. By far the most common psychological cause of superficial dyspareunia in women is 'vaginismus', as outlined in the next section.

Deep dyspareunia that cannot be fully resolved by gynaecological intervention, whether medical or surgical, may sometimes be helped by changing to those sexual positions that allow the woman greater control over the depth of penetration, such as entry from behind while lying on the side, or the female superior position.

In men

Ejaculatory pain and dyspareunia are uncommon and require urological assessment to exclude an organic cause, such as infection of the glans, urethra, seminal vesicles, prostate or bladder. Hyperaesthesia or over-sensitivity of the glans after ejaculation is not uncommon in normal men. Actual pain during intercourse in men usually has a physical cause.

Vaginismus

The term 'vaginismus' refers to the problem of difficulty with penetrative sex as a result of involuntary contraction or possibly spasm of the pubococcygeus muscles (surrounding the entrance to the vagina) when penetration is attempted. This occurs as a reflex reaction, due to the 'expectation' that penetration will be painful. The original aetiology may be around aversive sexual experiences, such as rape or abuse, but is often rather simpler than that. Any cause of superficial vaginal or vulval pain during intercourse may result in an expectation that future penetration will hurt. Such causes include sex in the presence of a vaginal thrush (*Candida*) infection, a first or early sexual experience that was painful owing to clumsiness, or a poorly performed clinical vaginal examination. The involuntary muscle spasm that follows (when penetration is expected and generally with a phobic element) can be painful in itself, but will be much exacerbated by continued attempts at penetration when the introitus is, in effect, 'closed'.

Some women presenting to the clinic may be frustrated or irritated by having seen a series of physical medical specialists for multiple investigations without being given a diagnosis in physical terms.

There are several components to the effective treatment of vaginismus:

- explanation
- addressing couple factors
- relaxation
- reassurance
- desensitisation
- psychotherapy for unresolved traumatic experiences, when necessary.

The essential first step is an early and clear explanation in the form of a formulation discussed with the patient and, whenever possible, her partner. Treatment follows a systematic desensitisation approach, ensuring that the therapist is flexible in setting up the programme and that its pace is set at all times by the female patient. This sense of control and safety within the treatment programme gives rise to confidence and is essential for a successful outcome.

Desensitisation may need to begin in the form of a sexual growth programme (as described above – see page 685). Thereafter, using learning theory as part of the explanation of the treatment, the female patient will be given homework tasks to carry out, while the couple agree to refrain from attempts at penetrative sex and are invited to engage in non-genital sensate focus sessions together, if acceptable to them.

The homework tasks will take the patient through stages designed to help her discover that insertion of an appropriate object into the vagina can occur without continued discomfort or any adverse consequences. It is important to start small and gradually build up. The patient should never move on to a later stage until the current stage has become comfortable and problem free. She may begin by attempting, when alone and in a non-sexual way, to insert one finger. She should use lubrication (e.g. Sensilube, Liquid Silk or another proprietary substance) and proceed slowly, if possible keeping her finger inserted for a few minutes, allowing enough time for the anxiety experienced to subside, or at least begin to do so, in order that the next session will be easier, and so on.

Kegel's exercises (Box 26.8) are a helpful adjunct, as they help to improve the condition and awareness of activity of the muscles around the introitus, while also enabling the patient to recognise the difference between the sensations of vaginal muscle contraction and relaxation. Another helpful manoeuvre if the woman is having difficulty inserting her finger is to contract the pelvic floor muscles tightly while her finger is at or on the introitus, as it may slip in more easily when she then relaxes.

The next stage may be to insert two fingers, or possibly a tampon. Most therapists find graded 'vaginal trainers' very useful. These are plastic torpedo-shaped objects in four sizes (from finger sized to a size approximating an erect penis) so that the patient can work slowly up through the series. They are *not* vaginal dilators. It is crucial for the patient to understand that the model is one of learning, not dilating or stretching, as the size of the vagina is generally not the problem. The aim is, in effect, eventually to use the partner's erect penis as the final stage, but in a way that keeps the woman in control (i.e. female superior and at her pace).

It is important for therapists to identify and address blocks that may arise during treatment. Sometimes these can occur at an early stage, as many women find initiating the introduction of their own fingers or vaginal trainers difficult. Extra encouragement, explanation and advice may suffice. Some therapists, however, may use more direct intervention, namely performing a therapeutic vaginal examination – during which important issues are sometimes disclosed by the patient. Alternatively, this may simply allow progress with insertion of a finger by the patient, with help and reassurance by the therapist. The involvement of a chaperone should always be considered, and this approach should be carried out only by suitably (medically) qualified therapists.

When treating women for vaginismus, it is also important to remember that the couple's relationship may be built around the impossibility of sex and the expectation of non-consummation, which may continue to suit one or both partners. Progress with treatment of the vaginismus may, as a result, lead on to secondary sexual dysfunction in the male partner (e.g. erectile dysfunction or premature ejaculation), which may also require treatment.

Prognosis

Vaginismus generally has a good outcome with treatment but the course of therapy is often far from straightforward. Masters & Johnson (1970) and some of their successors reported close to 100% success, but these excellent figures were probably due to case selection and the intensive nature of the treatment they were able to carry out. However, even in the more 'real life' setting of an NHS psychosexual clinic, the outcome of sex therapy for vaginismus continues to be reported as very good, one study reporting that it is resolved or largely resolved in 79% of cases (Hawton, 1982).

Sexual aversion and phobias

Sexual aversion and phobias *per se*, in men or women, rarely present to clinics, but may be components of other sexual dysfunctions, and any phobic element should be identified in the initial assessment. Sometimes the phobia relates to earlier traumatic sexual experiences, and this indicates the need for specific work to deal with issues such as incest or rape. However, if the phobia is relatively straightforward, simple behavioural or cognitive–behavioural techniques using imaginal and *in vivo* exposure may be helpful.

The key to success with sexual aversion or phobia is a thorough assessment to identify exactly which element(s) of sex have caused this response, and then to focus on these. Unless sexual aversion is absolute, sensate focus, if well set up and proceeded with gradually, may be the best approach, as it will also allow clarification of the precise problem.

Substance-induced sexual dysfunction

Substance-induced sexual dysfunction may involve prescribed or non-prescribed (legal or illicit) drugs. Treatment involves identifying this problem and then reconsidering with the patient, and any prescribing doctor also involved, the indications or reasons for using the drug, the relationship (if any) between dose and effects, the acceptability to the patient of this, and consideration of any alternatives to the present treatment.

Alcohol, tobacco and recreational drug use are frequently implicated in sexual dysfunction, but often neglected both by patients and professionals when considering aetiology.

Sexual dysfunction due to a general medical condition

Where sexual dysfunction is due to a general medical condition, treatment involves education and explanation to help the patient and partner come to terms with the diagnosis. Efforts should be made to minimise the impact of the disease on sexual functioning. Treatment for the disease may involve the use of agents that themselves contribute to sexual dysfunction, so the patient needs to be as fully informed as possible in making decisions.

Adjunctive biological therapies may be used to try to improve any sexual dysfunction. For example, many urologists have subsidiary erectile dysfunction services to which patients with conditions such as prostate cancer can be referred to access appropriate biological therapies.

The potential impact on sexual functioning of any medical procedure or intervention should also be borne in mind. Even simple procedures such as having a cervical smear or colposcopy can produce effects in patients that healthcare professionals, whose perception of the procedure may be very different to that of the patient and partner, may overlook or fail to recognise.

Overall prognosis in sex therapy

In general, the prognosis for sex therapy is variable between problems and between patients with the same problem, as well as between follow-up studies. Approximately 50–70% of couples report substantial benefits (Bancroft, 1998). Hawton's group completed a prospective study of prognostic factors in sex therapy and found that the motivation for treatment (especially in the male partner), the quality of the non-sexual relationship, and progress by the third therapy session all had prognostic significance (Hawton *et al*, 1986). These authors assessed long-term outcome for sex therapy and concluded that it was excellent for vaginismus and good for erectile dysfunction, but often poor for premature ejaculation, although for this condition a repeated course of behavioural treatment is often helpful. The prognosis for female impaired sexual interest was poor and this was often secondary to general relationship problems (Hawton *et al*, 1986). Perhaps the prognosis in such cases is, therefore, actually dependent on identifying and effectively addressing the general relationship problems themselves (as described on page 679).

Rating scales used in psychosexual medicine

In the UK, there is a general lack of use of assessment and outcome scales in this field, as revealed in a recent national survey (Holland, 2002). Regarding the use of rating scales in research, however, the following are examples of scales that are useful and frequently used.

- *Golombok Rust Inventory of Marital Satisfaction (GRIMS)* (Rust *et al*, 1988). This is a 28-item self-report measure of satisfaction with and functioning of the general (non-sexual) part of the relationship. Despite its name, it can be used with unmarried people who are in a current relationship. It is often used when considering possible aetiological factors in cases of sexual dysfunction, as it can indicate whether the dysfunction might be secondary to a generalised relationship problem.

- *International Index of Erectile Function (IIEF)* (Rosen *et al*, 1997). This is a 15-item self-report measure of erectile functioning (frequency, quality, duration, etc.), ejaculatory functioning, satisfaction and enjoyment, desire and sexual confidence. It was produced by an international consensus group and has been used very widely, particularly in research into the effects of biological treatments for erectile dysfunction, as it is able to detect treatment-related changes in patients with erectile dysfunction. It is psychometrically sound and has been linguistically validated in 10 languages and is also cross-culturally valid.
- Female Sexual Functioning Questionnaire (SFQ) (Pfizer Global Research and Development, 1997; Heiman *et al*, 2000). This is a 34-item self-report measure of sexual functioning and sexual satisfaction in women. It addresses all aspects of the sexual response cycle as well as pain, in keeping with DSM–IV diagnostic criteria. Importantly, and somewhat unusually, the arousal questions generate two separate domains of 'arousal: sensation' and 'arousal: lubrication'. Both the physical and the cognitive aspects of sexual response are evaluated within the questionnaire. Use of the SFQ in clinical trials in a large sample of women (some 900 in total) has demonstrated its excellent psychometric properties, including discriminative and construct validity, test–retest reliability, internal consistency and sensitivity to change (Heiman *et al*, 2000). The seven domains identified through factor analysis are 'desire', 'arousal: sensation', 'arousal: lubrication', 'orgasm', 'pain', 'enjoyment' and 'partner'. It is possible to analyse results at item, domain and total score level (Basson *et al*, 2000; Heiman *et al*, 2000).

Ethical considerations

Sexuality is a fundamentally important area of most people's lives. This includes you, your partner, your patients and their partners, your colleagues and so on. Increasing awareness of sexual issues (and particularly the associated human rights) means that this area is also important to your organisation, at many levels, from the individual care of patients in hospital to the prescription of medications that may alter fertility or sexual functioning, as well as to your individual practice and conduct as a clinician.

Sexuality can be a difficult area to approach, for many reasons. Some relate to the clinician's personal attitudes and experiences, and some relate to the patient. Personal sensibilities can be affected by religious, moral and cultural values and beliefs. Often these are virtually universal, such as the taboo on intercourse with prepubescent children, but there is considerable diversity on other issues, such as the acceptability of premarital sex, contraceptive practices, termination of pregnancy, and whether sex should actually be enjoyed for any purpose other than procreation. All psychiatrists should consider and acknowledge their own personal and professional attitudes, responsibilities and prejudices, in order to try to cultivate a sensitive approach to sexual issues. Practising asking patients about these important areas not only immediately improves overall management of patients and their partners and families, but also reduces the embarrassment felt by the enquiring practitioner.

Potential areas of difficulty for therapists

It is important that psychiatrists or anyone else working with people with sexual problems should be non-judgemental, accepting of the lifestyle choices made by their patients and their partners, and respectful of the importance of sexuality to these people. Therapists must not impose their own principles or preferences on patients, nor should they assume that their patient's view of what is right, wrong, good or bad in sex is necessarily similar to their own. Having said that, it is important to acknowledge that any individual therapist may find it difficult to work with clients whose sexual preferences or practices are found to be too alien or even disturbing.

One useful way to think about these concerns is to consider the difference between 'benign variation' and 'malignant variation' (Gordon, 1994). Although an individual may enjoy a type of sexual activity that some others would not wish to engage in, it may be viewed as an example of benign variation if many people in society would see it as acceptable. Possible examples are oral sex and anal intercourse, or perhaps 'virtually any sexual activity that occurs in private and between consenting adults'. There are other examples that would, however, be seen by the vast majority of society as wholly unacceptable under any circumstances. These would include paedophilia, and can be considered examples of malignant variation.

It is important for any individual working with people with sexual problems to consider for him- or herself what behaviours or preferences would fall into each of these categories. Discussion in supervision or with another colleague working in the same field can facilitate thorough consideration of the issues and the ethical dilemmas faced when there is some such aspect to the case that the therapist finds troubling. A particularly important example might be how to proceed when asked for help with an erectile dysfunction by a man with a previous conviction for sexual assault or rape.

Appropriate behaviour for therapists

The general behaviour of any professional working in this field is very important. He or she must behave in an appropriate way at all times, using language appropriate to the sensibilities of the patient, using a chaperone where necessary, and responding as far as possible to a patient's request for therapy by a person of a particular gender. Appropriate dress, conduct and the maintenance of clear boundaries are all essential elements of good professional conduct.

Supervision and good-quality record keeping are also essential, particularly when dealing with potentially sensitive subjects such as sexual dysfunction. Keeping the patient's records separate from general psychiatric or medical notes is important as it facilitates openness on the part of the patient. In the service run by the main author, patients are reassured that their notes are kept separately in the department and that only a brief entry is made in the main hospital notes to indicate that the patient has been seen in the psychosexual medicine service.

The importance of consulting the partner whenever possible

An important word of warning is to remember that your patients are not usually isolated and alone, so changing their sexual function is likely to have an impact on their partners. It is vital to try to engage the couple wherever possible to address problems, not just for the obvious reasons of increasing the likelihood of accurate formulation and successful treatment, but to ensure that any improvement in sexual functioning will be welcomed, and understood, and will not compromise the overall relationship.

Services for sexual dysfunction

Demand for services

Attitudes towards sexuality are changing throughout society. In particular, we are seeing an increasing proportion of older adults presenting with sexual dysfunction. The recent advent of effective oral therapies for erectile dysfunction that are relatively free of side-effects, as highlighted in the media, may be partly responsible for this. In addition, there is an increasing acceptance that older people need not give up the pleasures of life just because they are ageing. This is also the case for people with disabilities and those from cultural groups who may have previously found it particularly difficult to present for help with sexual problems (such as Muslim Asian women, whose only apparent route towards help may be via a white male general practitioner). It is also notable that different cultural groups may present in different ways with the same condition. For example, white couples in the UK with the problem of non-consummation due to primary vaginismus may present in their late 30s, when they wish to have children, whereas Asian couples describe more family pressure and concern leading to a much earlier referral via infertility services.

Provision of services

Psychosexual medicine is a developing sub-specialty area within psychiatry. Its boundaries overlap with several other medical and surgical specialties and many of the cases seen have mixed physical and psychological aetiology. These features are shared with the sub-specialty of liaison psychiatry, as is the likelihood that demand for services will continue to grow. Some established services do exist in the public, private and voluntary sectors. A range of staff, skill mixes and specialties may be involved, including nurses, psychologists and medically qualified practitioners from psychiatry, urology, genitourinary medicine, gynaecology, and so on. Any service will be shaped by what staff are available, their degree of training for such work and their need for further training (with attendant cost implications). It is important to give some thought to facilities, including consideration of clinic hours and accessibility, privacy and soundproofing, access to good supervision for all staff, clerical support and all the other usual features of providing a psychological therapy service to patients.

If there is no dedicated service, the task of treating psychosexual disorders will fall to the local adult general psychiatrist and it is hoped that the outline given in this chapter may be helpful. Every general adult psychiatrist should be alert to the sexual aspects of their patients' lives, and should incorporate enquiry about this into routine assessment. For patients presenting with a psychosexual disorder they should be able to make an assessment and attempt a formulation, paying due attention to both the organic and the psychological aspects of aetiology. In what appear to be relatively straightforward cases, sensate focus and other techniques or relevant physical treatments should be used, with referral on to specialised services for difficult or complex cases, or those requiring highly skilled therapy.

This chapter has concentrated on sexual dysfunction, as these will present to psychiatrists quite frequently. Gender identity disorders and paraphilias are less likely to do so but brief overviews are included below.

Gender identity disorders

The types of gender identity disorder in the main psychiatric classificatory systems are shown in Table 26.6. Much of this account is drawn from DSM–IV (American Psychiatric Association, 1994).

As outlined by Bancroft (1989), gender can be manifested in at least seven different ways:

1 chromosomes

2 gonads

3 hormones

4 internal sexual organs

5 external genitalia and secondary sexual characteristics

6 the gender assigned at birth ('It's a boy')

7 self-concept of gender identity ('I'm a girl').

Problems of gender identity are largely subsumed within the concept of 'transsexualism'. Transsexual individuals persistently feel an incongruity between their anatomical sex and gender identity. They will tend to complain of a sense that they are 'trapped inside the wrong body'. Their own gender identity does not match the appearance of their genitals and secondary sexual characteristics (Masters *et al*, 1995). The biologically male transsexual wishes to live as a woman and may wish to change to female anatomy, and vice versa. The male-to-female type is much more common than the female-to-male type. One estimated prevalence for the former is 1 in 100 000 men (Pauly, 1974).

DSM–IV requires two key elements to make the diagnosis: first, there must be a strong and persistent

Table 26.6 Classification of gender identity disorders

DSM–IV	ICD–10
	Psychological and behavioural disorders associated with sexual development and maturation *Specifier:* heterosexuality, homosexuality, bisexuality, prepubertal
Gender identity disorder in children *Specifier:* sexually attracted to males, females, both, neither	Gender identity disorder in childhood
Gender identity disorder in adolescents or adults *Specifier:* sexually attracted to males, females, both, neither	Transsexualism Dual-role transvestism Sexual maturation disorder Ego-dystonic sexual orientation Other psychosexual development disorders Psychosexual development disorder, unspecified
Gender identity disorder not otherwise specified	Gender identity disorder, unspecified
Sexual disorder not otherwise specified	Other gender identity disorders

cross-gender identification and a desire – almost an insistence – that one is of the opposite sex; and second, there should also be evidence of persistent discomfort about one's own assigned sex.

The onset is usually in childhood. In boys there tends to be a preoccupation with female toys, dress, and maternal or female heroes and roles, while in girls there may be tomboyish behaviour, and a wish to be called by a male name. However, as many children transiently pass through such phases, diagnosis should not be made too early. That said, parents are often aware that their child has a problem with regard to their sexual identity. During adolescence the condition becomes more obvious, and there may be very frequent cross-dressing accompanied by a wish or insistence that one is of the opposite sex. Referral to services may result because of parental concern at the behaviour as well as increasing isolation, teasing and rejection by peers. In adults there are obviously serious difficulties in the realms of sexual relationships, with individuals making relationships with same-sex partners, which may be constrained by the preference that their partners neither see nor touch their genitals.

The differential diagnosis of a gender identity disorder includes a simple non-conformity to the stereotypical or expected sex role behaviours (in these cases a primary wish to be of the opposite sex is lacking). In addition, certain rare congenital intersex conditions such as the androgen insensitivity syndrome and congenital adrenal hyperplasia should be considered. Finally, in some cases of schizophrenia there may be delusions of being of the opposite sex and, rarely, when these are accompanied by transsexual urges serious genital self-mutilation can occur (American Psychiatric Association, 1994).

Treatment for gender identity disorders

Psychotherapy alone has generally been unsuccessful in resolving the distress felt by these people as a result of their predicament (Tollinson & Adams, 1979). As a result, services to help such people, possibly with what is often their ultimate and stated goal of gender reassignment (or 'sex change'), require a multi-specialty team approach, including psychiatric/psychological, endocrinological and surgical elements. In view of the irreversible nature of surgical gender reassignment, a cautious approach is taken to offering it. This includes up to a 2-year trial period, during which time patients are required to live openly as a person of the opposite sex. They will be expected to adopt hairstyles, clothing and mannerisms of that sex, and to assume a name that fits with their new gender. If they are able to do all of this, they will move on to hormonal and possibly surgical treatment, as required.

Prognosis with treatment

Varying success rates have been reported. Green & Fleming (1990) reviewed 11 different follow-up studies and concluded that 87% of male-to-female transsexuals have a 'satisfactory outcome', with this number rising to 97% for female-to-male transsexuals, although the latter do not necessarily opt for any attempt at surgical construction of a penis.

Paraphilias

The essential features of a paraphilia are recurrent, intense, sexually arousing fantasies, sexual urges or behaviours generally involving:

- non-human objects, as in fetishism
- suffering or some sort of humiliation in oneself or one's partner, as in sexual sadism or masochism
- children or other non-consenting persons.

In some cases the paraphilic preference occurs only episodically, such as at time of stress, but for other individuals the unusual behaviour may become the major sexual activity throughout life. Social and other sexual relationships may suffer if others find the unusual sexual behaviour repugnant and many individuals with these disorders are unable to enter into an affectionate relationship that shows some reciprocity. Individuals with exhibitionism, paedophilia and voyeurism make up the majority of apprehended sex offenders. The range of paraphilias in the main psychiatric classificatory systems is shown in Table 26.7. The account below is derived mainly from DSM–IV.

The preferred stimulus, even within a particular paraphilia, is often highly specific. Individuals with a particular paraphilia may seek out a hobby or occupation that brings them in contact with the desired stimulus (e.g. selling women's shoes or lingerie to satisfy a fetish) and paedophiles may seek out work with children. Most do not report that the behaviour causes them any

Table 26.7 Classification of the paraphilias

DSM–IV: Paraphilias	ICD–10: Disorders of sexual preference
Fetishism	Fetishism
Exhibitionism	Exhibitionism
Paedophilia *Specifiers:* Sexually attracted to males, females, both, limited to incest Exclusive type/ non-exclusive type	Paedophilia
Sexual masochism	Sadomasochism
Sexual sadism	
Transvestic fetishism	Fetishistic transvestism
Voyeurism	Voyeurism
Paraphilia not otherwise specified	Disorder of sexual preference, unspecified
Frotteurism	Other disorders of sexual preference
	Multiple disorders of sexual preference

distress, their only problem being social dysfunction as a result of the reaction of others. A minority do report guilt, shame and depression at feeling a need to engage in sexual behaviour that they know is socially unacceptable and which they themselves may also regard as immoral. The overwhelming majority of people with paraphilias are male, although sexual masochism is (rarely) reported in females.

'Polymorphously perverse' is a phrase used to describe individuals who find sexual excitement and gratification through many different paraphilic behaviours, such as those listed above.

Space permits here only an outline of some of the more prevalent paraphilias. A comprehensive review is given in the book *Sexual Deviation* by Rosen (1996).

Paedophilia

According to DSM–IV, the paraphilic focus involves sexual activity with prepubescent children (13 years or under). Individuals report an attraction to children of a specific age range, some to male children, and some to female children. Some are attracted only to children (exclusive type), others to both children and adults (non-exclusive type). They may rationalise their activities in terms of it having 'educational value' for the child or the child also deriving 'sexual pleasure' or the child being 'sexually provocative'. Because of the ego-syntonic nature of paedophilia, most individuals with paedophilic fantasies and behaviours do not experience significant distress. Some limit their activities to their own families but others are highly predatory and go to great lengths to search out suitable victims. The disorder usually begins in adolescence, although some individuals report that they did not become aroused by abnormal fantasies until middle age. The course is chronic, and recidivism rates are high, with rates for those attracted to males being twice as high as for those attracted to females (American Psychiatric Association, 1994).

Paedophilia is a problem of major concern for most societies because, in the absence of any cure, long-term incarceration, with its associated huge expense, is the only solution for the more severe and resistant cases. The aetiology is unknown but Bradford (2001) has drawn parallels with obsessive–compulsive disorder (OCD) by suggesting that the repetitive fantasies of the paedophile resemble the repetitive phenomena of OCD. This provides some sort of a rationale for the use of the SSRIs, which have proved to be helpful in some cases of paedophilia, as they generally reduce interest.

Paedophilic behaviours have also been associated with organic brain disorders such as temporal lobe epilepsy, Tourette's syndrome, frontal and temporal lobe lesions, post-encephalitic syndromes and multiple sclerosis (Bradford, 2001). There may also be an association with a history of childhood attention-deficit hyperactivity disorder (ADHD). Kafka & Prentky (1998) found that around half of a group of paedophiles (both offenders and non-offenders) had a history of ADHD, and there was also a high prevalence of other psychiatric comorbidity – dysthymia (69%), major depression (48%), anxiety disorder (43%) and panic disorder (12%) – with the psychiatric disorders being strongly associated with the subgroup who had had ADHD. On this basis the authors suggested that the type of dysregulation found in ADHD may have made some contribution to the paedophilia. However, the majority of individuals with paedophilia lack any associated psychiatric comorbidity.

Individuals with paedophilia do not usually volunteer for treatment, but many will eventually become involved through their contact with the criminal justice system. Some of the less severe cases may respond to a cognitive approach combined with a relapse prevention programme (Bradford, 2001). The SSRIs seem to be effective in some cases (see above); open studies have shown beneficial effects, and these drugs are well tolerated, although there are no randomised controlled trials and so the place of these drugs in management is still uncertain (Greenberg *et al*, 1996).

Collaboration between the forensic psychiatrist and endocrinologist is required for the use of anti-androgen regimens. These have generated rather more interest in North America and mainland Europe than in the UK, and have been reviewed by Bradford (2001). Anti-androgen drugs act by reducing or blocking the action of testosterone. Cyproterone acetate is a competitive antagonist for testosterone and therefore blocks its action at the receptor level. Medoxyprogesterone acetate (Provera), which can also be administered as a long-term injection (Depot Provera), is a progestogen that acts by blocking the synthesis of the gonadotrophin follicle-stimulating hormone (FSH) and reduces testosterone output. It also induces the enzyme testosterone reductase, thereby increasing the rate of metabolic breakdown, so that both mechanisms combine to reduce circulating testosterone levels. One placebo-controlled study has shown that regimens based on the use of anti-androgen drugs may reduce recidivism rates (Bradford & Pawlak, 1993), but these regimens have side-effects such as weight gain, a tendency to precipitate type-2 diabetes, deep-vein thrombosis, headaches, nausea and feminisation, which limits their use.

An even more powerful way of reducing FSH and testosterone levels is through the use of analogues of gonadotrophin-releasing hormone (GnRH). These drugs cause a very profound fall in testosterone levels, shrinking of the testicles and effectively a reversible 'chemical castration'. In a remarkable study by Rosler & Witzum (1998), a group of 30 highly recidivistic paedophiles, all of who had been in prison many times, were treated with triptorelin, a GnRH analogue. The drug took 3 months to take full effect. While taking the drug none of the patients reported any deviant sexual fantasies or urges, and nor did they commit any offence against a child. However, the drug abolished all sexual activity, both normal and paraphilic, and also caused a marked degree of osteoporosis, which had to be treated with calcium supplements and vitamin D.

Transvestism

This is defined as persistent wearing of clothes of the opposite sex (cross-dressing). There is a broad range of such behaviour, from the occasional wearing by a man of one female garment to regularly dressing entirely in female clothing. It is usually done by a heterosexual man for the purpose of sexual excitement or sometimes for coping with stress. Cross-dressing in order to fulfil a social role without sexual excitement is part of transsexualism (Sims, 1988).

Exhibitionism

In exhibitionism, the main sexual expression and gratification is derived from exposure of the genitals to a person of the opposite sex (Snaith, 1983). This leads to the most common sexual offence in the UK ('indecent exposure'). There are two types (Rooth, 1971):

- Type I accounts for some 80% of cases. Inhibited young men, emotionally immature, who struggle against the impulse, usually expose a flaccid penis, feel guilty afterwards and have a good prognosis.
- Type 2 accounts for the other 20% of cases. Men with a sociopathic personality expose the erect penis, often masturbate while exposing and show little guilt. They may take sadistic pleasure in what they are doing and have a much worse prognosis.

Fetishism

Fetishism means 'the worship of inanimate objects', but in a modern sense refers to a repeated sexual preoccupation and excitement with non-living objects, which have a central importance in achieving sexual arousal and orgasm (Sims, 1988). The object of the fetish may be an article of clothing (e.g. shoes of the opposite sex), a substance (e.g. rubber) or a texture (e.g. fur). The fetishistic object may be used in sexual behaviour either alone or with the involvement of another person.

Voyeurism

Voyeurism is the viewing, to achieve sexual excitement, of unsuspecting people who are naked, undressing or engaged in sexual activity. Masturbation may take place during or after viewing.

Frotteurism

Frotteurism involves touching and rubbing against a non-consenting person. This usually occurs in a crowded place (e.g. an underground train), as it gives the perpetrator a better chance of avoiding arrest. While rubbing his genitals against the victim's thighs or buttocks, or touching her genitalia or breasts with his hands, the perpetrator may fantasise an exclusive, caring relationship with the victim (American Psychiatric Association, 1994).

Sadomasochism

Sadomasochism means sexual arousal in response to the infliction of pain, psychological humiliation or ritualised dominance or submission. Sadism is the infliction of pain or suffering on another for sexual excitement and masochism is sexual excitement gained from the passive experience of being made to suffer (Sims, 1988). Masochistic acts include physical restraint (bondage), blindfolding (sensory deprivation), beatings and piercing, and any other painful procedures; these may occasionally result in serious injury or even death. One particularly dangerous form of sexual masochism, called auto-eroticism or hypoxyphilia in DSM–IV, involves heightening sexual arousal by means of oxygen deprivation. This can be achieved by means of chest compression, ligatures, the use of a noose or a plastic bag, or via a vasodilating agent such as amyl nitrate, which temporarily decreases oxygen supply to the brain. It is estimated that hypoxyphilia is responsible for one or two deaths per million each year in the USA (American Psychiatric Association, 1994).

Necrophilia

Necrophilia involves achieving sexual excitement through contact with a dead body. It is very rare and may be associated with murder (Hucker & Stermac, 1992).

References

American Psychiatric Association (1994) Sexual disorders. In *Diagnostic and Statistical Manual of Mental Disorders* (4th edn) (DSM–IV), pp. 493–538. Washington, DC: APA.

Apfelbaum, B. (2000) Retarded ejaculation: a much misunderstood syndrome. In *Principles and Practice of Sex Therapy* (3rd edn) (eds S. R. Leiblum & R. C. Rosen), pp. 205–241. London: Guilford Press.

Balon, R., Yeragani, V. K., Pohl, R., *et al* (1993) Sexual dysfunction during antidepressant treatment. *Journal of Clinical Psychiatry*, **54**, 209–212.

Bancroft, J. (1989) *Human Sexuality and its Problems* (2nd edn). Edinburgh: Churchill Livingstone.

Bancroft, J. (1998) Sexual disorders. In *Companion to Psychiatric Studies* (6th edn) (eds E. C. Johnstone, C. Freeman & A. Zealley), pp. 529–550. Edinburgh: Churchill Livingstone.

Basson, R., Berman, J., Burnett, A., *et al* (2000) Report of the international consensus development conference on female sexual dysfunction: definitions and classifications. *Journal of Urology*, **163**, 888–893.

Bazire, S. (2001) Selecting drugs, doses and preparations – sexual dysfunction. In *Psychotropic Drug Directory 2001/2002*, pp. 165–171. Salisbury: Mark Allen Publishing Ltd.

Beck, A. T. (1967) *Depression. Clinical, Experimental and Theoretical Aspects*. London: Staples Press.

Begg, A., Dickerson, M. & Loudon, N. B. (1976) Frequency of self-reported sexual problems in a family planning clinic. *Journal of Family Planning Doctors*, **2**, 41–48.

Bradford, J. W. M. (2001) The neurobiology, neuropharmacology and pharmacological treatment of the paraphilias and compulsive sexual behaviour. *Canadian Journal of Psychiatry*, **46**, 26–33.

Bradford, J. & Pawlak, A. (1993) Double-blind placebo cross-over study of cyproterone acetate in the treatment of the paraphilias. *Archives of Sexual Behavior*, **22**, 383–402.

British Medical Association (2004) Drugs for erectile dysfunction. In *British National Formulary*, Vol. 48, pp. 417–420. London: BMA.

Burnap, D. W. & Golden, G. S. (1967) Sexual problems in medical practice. *Journal of Medical Education*, **42**, 673–680.

Butcher, J. (1999) Female sexual problems: loss of desire – what about the fun? *BMJ*, **318**, 41–43.

Catalan, J., Bradley, M., Gallwey, J., *et al* (1981) Sexual dysfunction and psychiatric morbidity in patients attending a clinic for sexually transmitted diseases. *British Journal of Psychiatry*, **138**, 292–296.

Clayton, D. O. & Shen, W. W. (1998) Psychotropic drug-induced sexual function disorders. *Drug Safety*, **19**, 299–312.

Comfort, A. (1972) *The Joy of Sex*. London: Mitchell Beazley.

Crowe, M. (1998) Sexual therapy and the couple. In *Seminars in Psychosexual Disorders* (eds H. Freeman *et al*), pp. 59–83. London: Gaskell.

Crowe, M. & Ridley, J. (2000) *Therapy with Couples*. Oxford: Blackwell Science.

Delvin, D. (1974) *The Book of Love*. London: New English Library.

Ellenberg, M. (1977) Sexual aspects of the female diabetic. *Mount Sinai Journal of Medicine*, **44**, 495–500.

Feldman, H., Goldstein, I., Hatzichristou, D. G., *et al* (1994) Impotence and its medical and psychosocial correlates: results of the Massachusetts male ageing study. *Journal of Urology*, **151**, 54–61.

Frank, E., Anderson, C. & Rubenstein, D. (1978) Frequency of sexual dysfunction in 'normal' couples. *New England Journal of Medicine*, **299**, 111–115.

Gebhard, P. H. & Johnson, A. B. (1979) *The Kinsey Data: Marginal Tabulations of the 1938–1963 Interviews Conducted by the Institute for Sex Research*. Philadelphia, PA: Saunders.

Goldberg, D. C., Whipple, B., Fishkin, R. E., *et al* (1983) The Grafenberg spot and female ejaculation: a review of initial hypotheses. *Journal of Sex and Marital Therapy*, **9**, 27–37.

Gordon, P. (1994) The contribution of sexology to contemporary sexuality education. *Sexual and Marital Therapy*, **9**, 171–180.

Green, R. & Fleming, D. T. (1990) Transsexual surgery follow-up: status in the 1990s. *Annual Review of Sex Research*, **1**, 163–174.

Greenberg, D. M., Bradford, J. W. M., Curry, S., *et al* (1996) A comparison of treatment of paraphilias with three serotonin reuptake inhibitors. A retrospective study. *Bulletin of the Academy of Psychiatry and Law*, **24**, 525–532.

Hawton, K. (1982) The behavioural treatment of sexual dysfunction. *British Journal of Psychiatry*, **140**, 94–101.

Hawton, K. (1984) Sexual adjustment of men who have had strokes. *Journal of Psychosomatic Research*, **28**, 243–249.

Hawton, K. (1985) *Sex Therapy: A Practical Guide*. Oxford: Oxford University Press.

Hawton, K. & Catalan, J. (1986) Prognostic factors in sex therapy. *Behaviour Research and Therapy*, **24**, 377–385.

Hawton, K., Catalan, J., Martin, M., *et al* (1986) Long-term outcome of sex therapy. *Behaviour Research and Therapy*, **24**, 665–675.

Heiman, J. R. & LoPiccolo, J. (1999) *Becoming Orgasmic* (2nd edn). London: Piatkus.

Heiman, J., *et al* (2000) Development of a sexual function questionnaire for clinical trials of female sexual dysfunction. *International Journal of Fertility and Women's Medicine*, **45**, 200.

Hetherington, E. M. & Stanley-Hagan, M. (1999) The adjustment of children with divorced parents: a risk and resiliency perspective. *Journal of Child Psychology and Psychiatry*, **40**, 129–140.

Holland, A. R. (2002) An evaluation of assessment and outcome tools used by psychosexual therapists across the UK. MSc dissertation, University of Central Lancashire.

Hucker, S. J. & Stermac, L. (1992) The evaluation and treatment of sexual violence, necrophilia, and asphyxiophilia. *Psychiatric Clinics of North America*, **15**, 703–719.

Hunt, M. (1975) *Sexual Behaviour in the 1970s*. New York: Dell.

Hutchison, T. A., Shahan, D. R. & Anderson, M. L. (eds) (2002) Drugdex System, Internet Version. Micromedex, Inc., Colorado. See http://www.micromedex.com/products/updates

Impotence Association (1997) *Key Findings of the Impotence Association Patient and Partner Erectile Dysfunction Survey 1997*. London: Impotence Association.

Kafka, M. P. & Prentky, R. A. (1998) Attention deficit hyperactivity disorder in males with paraphilia and paraphilia related disorders: a comorbidity study. *Journal of Clinical Psychiatry*, **59**, 388–396.

Kaplan, H. S. (1989) *PE: How to Overcome Premature Ejaculation*. New York: Brunner/Mazel.

Kinsey, A. C., Pomeroy, W. B. & Martin, C. E. (1948) *Sexual Behaviour in the Human Male*. Philadelphia, PA: Saunders.

Kinsey, A. C., Pomeroy, W. B., Martin, C. E., *et al* (1953) *Sexual Behaviour in the Human Female*. Philadelphia, PA: Saunders.

Kurt, U., Ozkardes, H., Altug, U., *et al* (1994) The efficacy of anti-serotonergic agents in the treatment of erectile dysfunction. *Journal of Urology*, **152**, 407–409.

Ladas, A. K., Whipple, B. & Perry, J. D. (1982) *The G Spot and Other Recent Discoveries About Human Sexuality*. New York: Holt, Rinehart and Winston.

Levine, S. B. & Yost, M. A. (1976) Frequency of sexual dysfunction in a general gynaecological clinic: an epidemiological approach. *Archives of Sexual Behaviour*, **5**, 229–238.

Lilius, H. G., Valtonen, E. J. & Wilkstrom, J. (1976) Sexual problems in patients suffering from multiple sclerosis. *Journal of Chronic Diseases*, **29**, 643–647.

Ludovico, G. M., Corvasce, A., Pagliarulo, G., *et al* (1996) Paroxetine in the treatment of premature ejaculation. *British Journal of Urology*, **77**, 881–882.

Maguire, G. P., Lee, E. G., Bevington, D. J., *et al* (1978) Psychiatric problems in the first year after mastectomy. *BMJ*, *i*, 963–965.

Masters, W. H. & Johnson, V. E. (1966) *Human Sexual Response*. London: Churchill.

Masters, W. H. & Johnson, V. E. (1970) *Human Sexual Inadequacy*. London: Churchill.

Masters, W. H., Johnson, V. E. & Kolodny, R. C. (1995) *Human Sexuality* (5th edn). New York: HarperCollins.

Mathew, R. J. & Weinman, M. L. (1982) Sexual dysfunction in depression. *Archives of Sexual Behavior*, **11**, 323–328.

McCulloch, D. K., Campbell, I. W., Wu, F. C., *et al* (1980) The prevalence of diabetic impotence. *Diabetologia*, **18**, 279–283.

Medicines Control Agency (2002) Reminder: use of traditional Chinese medicines and herbal remedies. *Current Problems in Pharmacovigilance*, **28**, 6.

Morales, A. (2001) Apomorphine to Uprima: the development of a practical erectogenic drug: a personal perspective. *International Journal of Impotence Research*, **13**, suppl. 3, 29–34.

O'Connor, T. G., Thorpe, K., Dunn, J., *et al* (1999) Parental divorce and adjustment in adulthood: findings from a community sample. *Journal of Child Psychology and Psychiatry*, **40**, 777–789.

Pauly, I. B. (1974) Female transsexualism: part I. *Archives of Sexual Behavior*, **3**, 487–507.

Pfizer Global Research and Development (1997) *The Female Sexual Functioning Questionnaire (SFQ)*. Manchester: Pfizer.

Ralph, D. & McNicholas, T. (2000) UK management guidelines for erectile dysfunction. *BMJ*, **321**, 499–503.

Rooth, F. G. (1971) Indecent exposure and exhibitionism. *British Journal of Hospital Medicine*, **5**, 521–533.

Rosen, I. (1996) *Sexual Deviation* (3rd edn). Oxford: Oxford University Press.

Rosen, R. C., Riley, A., Wagner, G., *et al* (1997) The International Index of Erectile Function (IIEF): a multidimensional scale for assessment of erectile dysfunction. *Urology*, **49**, 822–830.

Rosler, A. & Witzum, E. (1998) Treatment of men with paraphilia with a long-acting analogue of gonadotrophic releasing hormone. *New England Journal of Medicine*, **338**, 416–465.

Royal College of Psychiatrists (2001) *Curriculum for Basic Specialist Training and the MRCPsych Examination* (CR95). London: Gaskell.

Rubin, A. & Babbott, D. (1958) Impotence and diabetes mellitus. *JAMA*, **168**, 498–500.

Rust, J., Bennun, I., Crowe, M., *et al* (1988) *The Golombok Rust Inventory of Marital State (GRIMS)*. Windsor: NFER-NELSON.

Segraves, R. T. (1988) Sexual side-effects of psychiatric drugs. *International Journal of Psychiatric Medicine*, **18**, 243–252.

Segraves, R. T. (1989) Effects of psychotropic drugs on human erection and ejaculation. *Archives of General Psychiatry*, **46**, 275–284.

Selvini Palazolli, M., Boscolo, L., Cecchin, G., *et al* (1978) *Paradox and Counter-paradox*. New York: Jason Aronson.

Sims, A. C. P. (1988) *Symptoms in the Mind: An Introduction to Descriptive Psychopathology*. London: Ballière Tindall.

Snaith, R. P. (1983) Exhibitionism: a clinical conundrum. *British Journal of Psychiatry*, **143**, 231–235.

Snell, R. S. (1981) *Clinical Anatomy for Medical Students*. Boston, MA: Little, Brown.

Stein, G. (1995) Drug treatment of the personality disorders, premenstrual tension, impotence, and male sexual suppressants. In *Seminars in Clinical Psychopharmacology* (ed. D. King), pp. 446–479. London: Gaskell.

Swan, M. & Wilson, L. J. (1979) Sexual and marital problems in a psychiatric out-patient population. *British Journal of Psychiatry*, **135**, 310–314.

Tavris, C. & Sadd, S. (1977) *The Redbook Report on Female Sexuality*. New York: Delacorte Press.

Taylor, D., Duncan, D., Mir, S., *et al* (1997) Antidepressant-induced sexual dysfunction: new antidepressants. *Drug Information Quarterly*, **4**, 6–9.

Tollinson, C. D. & Adams, H. E. (1979) *Sexual Disorders: Treatment, Theory, Research*. New York: Gardner Press.

Vas, C. J. (1978) Sexual impotence and some autonomic disturbances in men with multiple sclerosis. In *Sexual Consequences of Disability* (ed. A. Comfort), pp. 45–60. Philadelphia, PA: Stickley.

Virag, R., Bouilly, P. & Frydman, D. (1985) Is impotence an arterial disorder? *Lancet*, *i*, 181–184.

Wadsworth, M. E. J. (1986) Grounds for divorce in England and Wales: a social and demographic analysis. *Journal of Biosocial Science*, **18**, 127–153.

Wagner, G. & Metz, P. (1981) Arteriosclerosis and erectile failure. In *Impotence: Physiological, Surgical Diagnosis and Treatment* (eds G. Wagner & R. Green), pp. 63–72. New York: Plenum.

Waldinger, M. D., Hengeveld, M. W. & Zwinderman, A. H. (1994) Paroxetine treatment of premature ejaculation: a double-blind, randomized, placebo-controlled study. *American Journal of Psychiatry*, **151**, 1377–1379.

World Health Organization (1992) *International Classification of Mental and Behavioural Disorders* (ICD–10). Geneva: WHO.

Zilbergeld, B. (1978) *Men and Sex*. London: HarperCollins.

CHAPTER 27

Clinical epidemiology

Matthew Hotopf

Introduction

Epidemiology is usually defined as the study of diseases in populations. The word itself is derived from three separate Greek roots: *epi*, which means 'on, upon, befall' (as in epidermis), *demo*, which means 'man, people' (as in democracy) and *ology*, which means study, and so the word literally means 'the study of that which befalls man' (Timmreck, 1994). In the 17th and 18th centuries the word 'epidemic' was applied to almost any harm that appeared to be common and seemed to spread as if by contagion, such as epidemic madness, epidemic stealing and diseases such as the plague (*Oxford English Dictionary*, 1989). It was only in the 19th century, with the identification of bacteria, that epidemics (and their study, epidemiology) became strongly associated with infectious diseases, but it soon became clear that many of the methods used for tracking infectious diseases, such as accurate case identification and determining precisely when and where cases had occurred, as well is their frequency in different settings, had a far wider application across medicine.

Morgan & Cooper (1975) provide a brief overview of the history of psychiatric epidemiology and they credit Durkheim, the French sociologist, as among the first to apply epidemiological methods, in his studies of suicide. Durkheim examined successive 5-year average suicide rates in different European countries and showed these were remarkably constant for each country, but differed widely between countries, with the Protestant north European countries having rates that were three to four times higher than the Mediterranean and presumably Catholic countries such as Italy. To test his hypothesis further Durkheim looked at how suicide rates varied within just one country and he selected Germany because some provinces of Germany were strongly Catholic, while others had a predominantly Protestant population. He showed that the Protestant provinces (less than 50% Catholic) had a relatively high mean suicide rate, of 192/100 000, while the rate for provinces with 90% or more Catholics, had rates that were less than half this, at 75/100 000. Those provinces that were 50–90% Catholic assumed an intermediate position with regard to suicide rates, at 135/100 000. Durkheim conducted similar analyses comparing suicides rates between married and divorced people, among those who were fertile against those who were childless, and even without the help of modern statistical tests found large differences between these different social groups. He concluded that suicide, as a phenomenon, was a collective act, in that it was related to societal forces, and that the Catholic religion in some way appeared to offer a degree of protection. His findings with regard to religion have been replicated to some extent in a more recent study by Neeleman *et al* (1997), who showed that people with stronger religious beliefs tended to have lower suicide rates, although the size of the effect was much smaller than that found by Durkheim in the 19th century.

In the early 20th century, in the southern United States, there was an alarming rise in the prevalence of pellagra, a debilitating neuropsychiatric disease presenting with neurasthenic symptoms, occasionally psychoses and dementia, as well as skin rashes. It was thought the cause was a specific communicable disease, possibly because of its known association with unsanitary conditions. In 1914, the US public health authority appointed Joseph Goldberger to investigate the cause of pellagra. Goldberger first observed that in institutions where pellagra was rife, all the cases seemed to occur only among the inmates and none of the staff were affected. He wrote 'that this pattern seemed to be no more comprehensible on the basis of an infection than is the absolute immunity of the asylum employees' (Goldberger, 1914). Furthermore, fresh cases seemed to occur among inmates who had been there for a long time and who had little contact with the outside world rather than the new entrants, who had recent contact with the outside world. In a more detailed survey of an orphanage in Jackson, Mississippi, he found that the pellagra cases seemed to be confined to those aged 6–12 years; he was personally involved in the survey and he noted that the younger children (below the age of 6) received a daily ration of fresh milk, while most of those aged 12 or over were sent out to work on the farms, where they received supplementary food. However, those in the 6–12 age group subsisted only on the orphanage diet. To confirm his hypothesis that a dietary deficiency was responsible, Golderger then conducted a dietary survey of households in seven villages in South Carolina, where the prevalence of pellagra was known to be very high. There were no cases of pellagra in households consuming more than 19 quarts of fresh milk per fortnight, but a 22.5% rate among households consuming less than one quart per fortnight, and a similar pattern was found for the consumption of fresh meat.

This simple but well-designed survey based only on good case identification, and the ascertainment of the age and occupational distribution of cases and non-cases, followed by a basic dietary survey, led to the identification of the probable cause of pellagra as a specific dietary deficiency. The disease was then easily prevented by ensuring an adequate supply of fresh milk and meat protein, and all this was clarified long before laboratory scientists had isolated vitamin B6 and identified its deficiency as the definitive biochemical cause of pellagra.

There are two main strands of epidemiology. First, it provides a framework in which to *describe* diseases (or, more correctly for psychiatry, disorders or illnesses). Such descriptive statistics include the frequencies of disorders, such as of schizophrenia or depression, or suicide rates, as were used in Durkheim's studies. It is important to know whether disorders are on the increase or in decline, and whether they vary dramatically between countries or regions. Having this knowledge allows services to be planned, but also helps develop hypotheses about possible causes. Further, it is especially important for patients and their families that their doctors are able to describe the prognosis of disorders. How many people with first-onset psychosis make a full recovery and never require psychiatric treatment again? How many develop severe symptoms and require psychiatric care for the rest of their lives?

The second main strand of epidemiology is to make links between a cause and an effect, and the studies of Goldberger on pellagra described above are a good example of this approach. Such *analytic* studies test hypotheses that exposures (or risk factors) cause disorders or, once the disorder is established, whether the exposure is associated with a good or bad outcome. Included among analytic studies are treatment trials. In this regard reviews, particularly those that include meta-analyses of all the currently available studies, provide comprehensive evidence about current knowledge of a disorder or its treatment.

Exposures and outcomes

In most studies, investigators measure three main things:

- exposures
- outcomes
- potential confounders, which are other exposures that may influence the outcome.

The term 'exposure' encompasses a wide range of different factors that might be important in the aetiology of a disorder. These include simple demographic variables such as age and gender; biological entities such as genotype, intrauterine infection or brain abnormalities; psychological variables such as experiences of parenting; or social factors such as life events, deprivation and income inequality. Clearly, these exposures may be measured in many different ways, but the methodological principles behind linking exposure to outcome are essentially similar.

The term 'outcome' is also used broadly – to psychiatrists the most obvious outcomes are diagnostic categories such as schizophrenia. While some researchers may choose to 'split' psychiatric categories into diagnostic groups as defined in ICD–10 (World Health Organization, 1992) or DSM–IV (American Psychiatric Association, 1994), others may 'lump' together broad categories (e.g. 'mental disorder'). Both approaches are valid, and the approach chosen will depend on the question under study. Other outcomes may be dimensions, such as neuroticism, depression score or disablement.

Potential confounders are described in more depth below, but are essentially any variable that may confuse the observed relationship between exposure and outcome.

Development of measures: reliability and validity

All quantitative research involves measurement of variables, which may be outcomes or exposures. In physical science there are often objective criteria on which to base measurement (weight, length, electrical resistance etc.). In psychiatry (and much of medicine besides) such objective, external measures are lacking, and our measurement is therefore particularly prone to error. In developing questionnaires, rating scales or diagnostic interviews it is necessary to assess their reliability and validity.

Reliability

There are two main types of reliability: inter-rater reliability and test–retest reliability. The term is also used, though, to describe the 'internal' integrity of an instrument, that is, inter-item reliability.

Inter-rater reliability

Inter-rater reliability indicates whether two or more researchers using the same measure on the same subject will gain similar answers. The measurement of inter-rater reliability depends on the type of variable generated by the questionnaire. If it generates a binary outcome, such as the presence or absence of a specific diagnosis, reliability could be described as the *percentage agreement* between the two researchers. However, this would not take account of agreements that happened just by chance. Instead, *Cohen's kappa* takes into account that some of the observed agreements would be expected by chance. Kappa can a value anywhere between –1 and +1, where positive values indicate above chance agreement (1 indicates perfect agreement) and negative values indicate below chance agreement.

If the measure generates an ordered categorical outcome, for example levels of certainty about the presence of a diagnosis (definite, probable, possible, absent), a *weighted kappa* can be used. This gives more emphasis to serious levels of disagreement between raters than to trivial ones.

If the measure is a continuous variable, such as a symptom score, the *intraclass correlation coefficient* may be used, which will take a value between 0 and 1, with 1 again indicating perfect agreement.

Test–retest reliability

Test–retest reliability involves the same rater using the same measure to assess the same subject twice over an interval of time. The same parameters can be used as for inter-rater reliability. Test–retest reliability is important for measures that assess stable psychological traits, such as personality or intelligence, but is less useful for gauging the reliability of psychological symptoms, as these fluctuate over time.

Inter-item reliability

Split-half reliability describes the integrity or coherence of a questionnaire and assesses whether the questions assess the same underlying construct. It can be measured by calculating a correlation between the scores of the first and second half of the questionnaire, or odd-numbered versus even-numbered questions. Alternatively, Cronbach's α can be used, which provides the average correlation between all possible ways of splitting the items.

Validity

Validity refers to the extent to which an instrument (which in this context usually means a questionnaire or interview) *actually* measures what it sets out to measure. There are three main types of validity:

- *Content validity* (which includes 'face validity') refers to the degree to which the measure covers what it is meant to cover – for example, one would expect a measure of depression to include items on low mood, anhedonia and fatigue.
- *Construct validity* is a more abstract term meaning the degree to which results from a measure fit with underlying theoretical constructs pertaining to that measure. For example, if the phenomenon under study changes with age, one would expect the results of the test to reflect this.
- *Criterion-related* validity (*concurrent* or *predictive*) is the degree to which the measure compares with an alternative criterion. In concurrent validity the measure is compared with a 'gold standard' – and the results are summarised as the sensitivity and specificity of the measure (these are discussed further below). Predictive validity is assessed by how well the measure is able to *predict* a subsequent outcome that fits into the construct being examined – for example, an IQ test used in children should go some way to predict future academic performance, or a measure of suicidal ideas should be able to predict future suicide attempts to some extent.

Concurrent validity – sensitivity and specificity

It will be easiest to define and discuss sensitivity and specificity in relation to an example and some actual numbers. Say a general practitioner (GP) decided to screen all attenders with the 12-item General Health Questionnaire (GHQ-12), to improve his or her detection of common mental disorders. It would be important to know the concurrent validity of the questionnaire – in other words, how it performs against a 'gold standard' psychiatric interview. The GP might therefore compare the results of the GHQ-12 with those on the Revised Clinical Interview Schedule

Table 27.1 Definitions of sensitivity and specificity

GHQ-12 results (test)	CIS-R results (gold standard)		
	Positive	**Negative**	**Total**
Positive	a	b	$a+b$
Negative	c	d	$c+d$
Total	$a+c$	$b+d$	$a+b+c+d$

Sensitivity $= a / (a+c)$

Specificity $= d / (b+d)$

Positive predictive value $= a / (a+b)$

Negative predictive value $= d / (c+d)$

Likelihood ratio (LR) of positive result $= \dfrac{\text{sensitivity}}{(1-\text{specificity})}$

Pre-test odds of having disorder $= (a+c) / (b+d)$

Post-test odds of having disorder $= (a+c) / (b+d) \times \text{LR}$

Post-test probability of having disorder $= \dfrac{\text{post-test odds}}{(1 + \text{post-test odds})}$

Table 27.2 Example calculations of sensitivity and specificity for a sample of 49 patients

GHQ-12 results (test)	CIS-R results (gold standard)		
	Positive	**Negative**	**Total**
Positive	23	9	32
Negative	1	16	17
Total	24	25	49

Sensitivity $= 23/24 = 0.96$

Specificity $= 16/25 = 0.64$

Positive predictive value $= 23/32 = 0.72$

Negative predictive value $= 16/17 = 0.94$

Likelihood ratio (LR) of positive result $= 0.96/0.36 = 2.67$

Pre-test odds of having disorder $= 0.96$

Post-test odds of having disorder $= 2.56$

Post-test probability of having disorder $= 2.56/3.56 = 0.72$

(CIS-R), which is a structured diagnostic interview. It is then possible to give the sensitivity and specificity of the GHQ-12 (in relation to the CIS-R) (Table 27.1). Say the doctor uses both measures on 49 patients, and the results are as shown in Table 27.2.

Note, first, that the frequency of psychiatric disorders rated on the CIS-R is high (nearly half the patients score positive). Note also that the frequency of patients who are positive on the GHQ-12 is higher still – this is usually the case when a questionnaire is being used to detect possible cases, and indicates that at least some of the 'positives' on the questionnaire are false positives. The *sensitivity* is a measure of the ability of a measure to pick up genuine cases – in this instance the sensitivity is close to one, indicating that the GHQ-12 identifies nearly all those who are true cases. The *specificity* is a measure of the ability of the measure to identify correctly those who are free from the disorder. Here the specificity is much lower, indicating that the GHQ-12 was performing less well. There is a play-off between sensitivity and specificity: the more sensitive a measure is, the more likely it is also to pick up false positives, and vice versa. The positive predictive value describes the chances that an individual scoring positive on the test will actually have the disorder when the gold standard is applied. Similarly, the negative predictive value is the chance that an individual who tests negative will be free from the disorder. Note that the positive and negative predictive values are sensitive to the frequency of the disorders under study. If the disorder is very rare, it is likely that a higher proportion of those who test positive will not have the disorder compared with when it is very common.

The odds, the likelihood ratio and proportion

The GP knows from past experience that a high proportion (in fact 49%) of his patients have psychiatric disorder. How much of a difference does the test make? The likelihood ratio of a positive value gives us an idea of the 'added value' that the test makes, but to use it we have first to calculate the *odds* of a patient having a disorder. Note that the odds is different from the probability and is calculated as the proportion with the disorder divided by the proportion without a disorder (here, 24/25 = 0.96). The *likelihood ratio* of a positive test is defined as the amount by which a positive test result increases the odds of a patient having the disorder, in this case 2.67. If a patient scores positive on the GHQ-12, the odds that he or she has a disorder now increases by 2.67-fold, to 2.56. What does this mean in terms of proportions? We now use the following formula:

$$\text{probability} = \text{odds}/(1 + \text{odds})$$

which now equals 72%. Hence the positive test result has changed the probability that the patient has a disorder from 49% to 72%.

Measures of disorder frequency: prevalence and incidence

One of the basic functions of epidemiology is to describe the frequency of disorders in the population. There are two main measures of frequency – prevalence and incidence.

The prevalence is the total number of individuals with the disorder, divided by the population from which they are drawn.

$$\text{Prevalence} = \text{total cases}/\text{total population}$$

Prevalence estimates will include some patients who have had the disorder for many years and others who have only just developed it. Prevalence is therefore a function of the number of new cases developing over a given time period (i.e. the incidence – see below) and the chronicity of the disorder (i.e. its average duration).

Prevalence may be subdivided into *point prevalence*, which is the proportion of the population who have the disease at the point in time when it is measured, and *period prevalence*, which is the proportion of the population who have experienced the disorder over a defined interval. In psychiatry there are advantages to using period prevalence, as many disorders relapse and remit and a point prevalence may not reflect the true proportion of the population who have been affected by the condition under study. Lifetime estimates of prevalence are also commonly reported. There has been considerable controversy over the accuracy of lifetime prevalence estimates when obtained from psychiatric interviews. The problem with such estimates is that they depend on recall of clusters of symptoms (e.g. for depression: low mood, anhedonia, sleep disturbance, etc.) many years before. Recall of such complex information is likely to be very inaccurate.

Note also that in order to calculate the prevalence (and incidence) it is important to have accurate information about the denominator. *Denominator error* occurs if the investigator attempts to define a population using some routinely available data (e.g. census or electoral register) but these are inaccurate because not everyone provided information in the census or signed up to the electoral register. This may lead to an overestimate of prevalence (or incidence) if the numerator is being accurately recorded.

Incidence is the proportion of individuals in a given population who develop a disorder within a specific time period. Note that the population at risk includes *only* individuals who have never had the disorder. The numerator is therefore the number of individuals who develop the disorder, and the denominator is the population at risk divided by the time period.

There are two main approaches to measuring incidence – risk and rate – and these are illustrated here with the data shown in Fig. 27.1. Consider a population of 10 individuals who are followed for 1 year to determine who develops a disorder. Three possible outcomes are possible for each individual: remain well; develop the condition under study; or be *censored* – in other words, stop contributing to the study because of death, migration or withdrawal of consent. When calculating the *risk*, the problem of censoring is ignored. The numerator is all new cases of the disorder and the denominator is the population at risk. In the study illustrated in Fig. 27.1 we would state that two cases (4 and 7) developed the disorder, so the risk is 2/10 or 0.2.

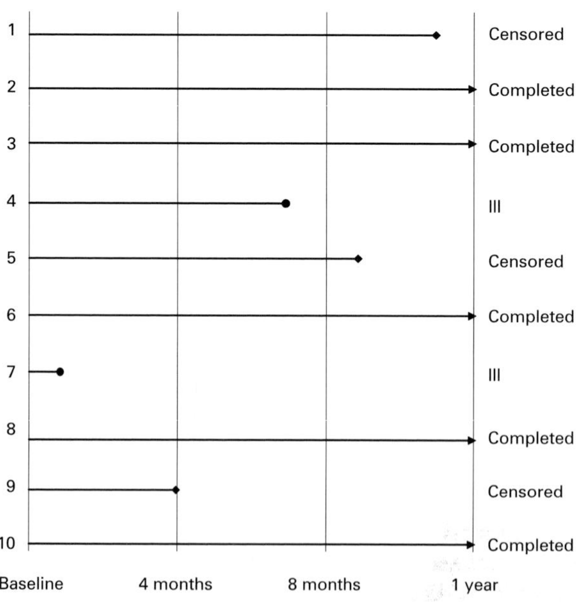

Fig. 27.1 Calculation of risk and rate ratios (see text for explanation).

When calculating the *rate*, a more precise estimate is made, to take into account the differing amounts to time at risk each individual contributes. Individuals who become ill can no longer contribute to 'time at risk', nor can individuals who die or who are censored. The denominator for the rate is the total *person time at risk* in the study. From Fig. 27.1, only five individuals (2, 3, 6, 8 and 10) contribute an entire year of time at risk. Case 7 hardly contributes any time, becoming ill after 1 month. Case 4 becomes ill at 7 months, and cases 1, 5 and 9 are all censored, at 11, 9 and 4 months, respectively. The total person time at risk here is 7.7 years, and the rate is 2 per 7.7 person years at risk. Because it is a more accurate measure, the rate is the preferred expression of incidence.

Measures of the strength of associations: risk difference, risk ratios, rate ratios and odds ratios

In analytical studies, an attempt is usually made to describe the *strength* of an association between and *exposure* (or risk factor) and an *outcome* (or disorder). In cohort studies the incidence of a disorder is compared in two groups – one exposed to a risk factor, the other not exposed. The study estimates incidence risks or rates for each group.

The risk difference is the difference in risk between the exposed and unexposed group. Risk (rate) ratios are ratios of the risk (rate) in the exposed population divided by the risk (rate) in the unexposed population. A risk ratio of 3, for example, indicates that individuals with the exposure are three times as likely to develop the outcome as those unexposed.

$$\text{risk difference} = \text{risk}_{\text{exposed}} - \text{risk}_{\text{unexposed}}$$

$$\text{risk ratio} = \text{risk}_{\text{exposed}} / \text{risk}_{\text{unexposed}}$$

$$\text{rate ratio} = \text{rate}_{\text{exposed}} / \text{rate}_{\text{unexposed}}$$

Another widely used measure of impact is the odds ratio, which is used especially in case–control studies. The relationship between the odds ratio and risk or rate ratio is described in detail by Hotopf (2003) but can be illustrated in the following example.

Imagine that we are interested in determining the effect of unemployment on suicide rates in men of working age. We might identify a population of 1 million men for whom we know the employment status. Assume that 5% of the population are unemployed and we follow the population for 1 year assessing suicide rates, to obtain the figures shown in Table 27.3. From these figures it is possible to calculate the rate ratio:

$$\text{odds ratio} = 36/12 = 3$$

Now let us assume that it was impossible to identify the employment status of the entire population at the start of the study, and instead a case–control design was used. In the case–control study, the exposure status for cases (i.e. people who die by suicide) and controls (i.e. people who do not die by suicide) are compared. Assuming that it was possible identify all 132 suicides in the population and compare them with a randomly selected sample of individuals who did not commit suicide, and assuming that the rate of unemployment in this randomly selected group was similar to that of the general population, we could compare the odds of exposure in the cases with that in the controls. This might generate a table like Table 27.4. From this it is possible to calculate the odds ratio:

$$\text{odds ratio} = 0.158/0.052 = 3.04$$

The odds ratio in this example is a close approximation to the rate ratio; however, the two are not identical. The odds ratio approximates to the rate or risk ratios where the outcome under study is rare. When it is not rare, the odds ratio is higher than the risk ratio.

A key question for preventive medicine is determining how much impact a risk factor has on the overall rate of a disorder. Returning to the unemployment and suicide example, we might want to know how much unemployment contributes to the total suicide rate, and whether removing the exposure (i.e. providing conditions of full employment) would have a sizeable impact on suicide rates. The population attributable risk (PAR) gives an estimate of this:

$$\text{PAR\%} = \left[\frac{P_e(I_e - I_u)}{P_t \times I_t}\right] \times 100$$

where:

P_e = number of persons exposed = 50 000
P_t = total population = 1 000 000
I_e = incidence in exposed = 36/100 000/year
I_u = incidence in unexposed = 12/100 000/year
I_t = incidence in total population = 13.2/100 000/year

PAR = 9%

In other words, this shows us that, of the 132 suicides that occurred in the year, 9% were attributable to unemployment. This implies that if unemployment was removed as a risk factor, the suicide rate would fall by this amount. Thus the population attributable risk can be defined as the proportion of a population's experience of a disorder which can be explained by the presence of a risk factor.

Population attributable risk has major practical limitations. First, it may be impossible to remove a risk factor completely from a population. For example, certain occupational groups are at high risk of suicide, but it is not feasible to remove the exposure (e.g. being a farmer or a doctor) from the population! Second, the risk factor may not be directly causal; it may be, for example, that the unemployed group are at higher risk

Table 27.3 Illustration of rate of suicide by employment status

	Employed	Unemployed
Denominator	950 000	50 000
Number of suicides	114	18
Suicide rate	12/100 000/year	36/100 000/year

Table 27.4 Illustration of rate of unemployment by suicide status in a case–control study

	Cases of suicide	Controls
Total	132	264
Employed	114	251
Unemployed	18	13
Odds of exposure	0.158	0.052

of suicide because other problems – perhaps chronic mental disorders – lead to their becoming unemployed, and these would remain important risk factors even if they were returned to work.

Study designs

Ecological studies

The ecological study plots the average exposure of a population against the rate of some outcome in the same population. This approach requires routinely available estimates of prevalence or incidence, as well as the data on exposure. The problem in psychiatry, and the reason that ecological studies are not a common design, is that there are relatively few reliable estimates of prevalence or incidence that apply between many populations. One exception is suicide rates. An example of an ecological study assessing suicide is that by Neeleman *et al* (1997), who assessed the relationship between suicide rates in 19 Western countries and the strength of religious belief and participation in the same countries. This 'exposure' had been measured in a major survey on religious belief which had previously been performed. The authors found that countries where less strong religious conviction was the rule were likely to have higher suicide rates.

Ecological studies may give important clues on the aetiology of a disorder relatively cheaply. However, because they do not measure the exposure or the outcome at the level of the individual, it is not possible to use them to link exposures and outcome at the level of the individual. This is referred to as the *ecological fallacy*. Another problem with ecological studies is *ecological bias*, which is essentially a form of confounding – because important information on potential confounders is often lacking, it is often possible to explain associations described in ecological studies by factors that might link the exposure and outcome. If, for example, it was found that suicide rates were highest in areas with the most developed mental health services, a naive interpretation would be that mental health services are bad for mental health, and have caused this excess. An alternative explanation is that there are unmeasured confounders, such as social deprivation or urban environments, which are associated with both suicide and the extent of local mental health services.

Despite these concerns, there is growing recognition that the ecological study may have important applications. Many exposures cannot be measured within individuals in a meaningful way – this particularly applies to variables that are more correctly measured at a societal level, such as income distribution, ethnic density, and religiosity of the society. Perhaps the most important advantage of ecological studies is that they can give clues about differences in rates of disorders between populations, and thus can provide important clues as to why (for example) there might be such dramatic international differences in suicide rates.

Cross-sectional study

Cross-sectional studies involve the identification of a population and measurement of a disorder within that population. They therefore provide prevalence estimates, but also have an important function in describing risk factors and associations. There are several important examples of large cross-sectional studies in psychiatry, such as the US Epidemiologic Catchment Area (ECA) study (Regier *et al*, 2002) and National Comorbidity Study (Blazer *et al*, 1994), and the UK National Psychiatric Morbidity Survey (Meltzer *et al*, 1995).

The first step in the design of a cross-sectional study is the identification of a population. For the purposes of most studies, population means individuals living within a defined geographical area. However, it can be any group of individuals of interest to the researchers, as long as that group can be defined in a reproducible way. Thus, cross-sectional studies may be carried out within specific settings, such as primary care, general hospital out-patient departments, or among employees of a firm or pupils within a school. In some circumstances the researcher may be interested in defining a population of individuals with a disorder – such as patients with schizophrenia – and measuring the prevalence of another disorder – such as tardive dyskinesia – within this group.

The key to providing a valid prevalence estimate within a cross-sectional study is to ensure complete ascertainment of the population defined. Thus, if a cross-sectional study of school refusal was carried out, it would clearly be important not to limit the interviews to those children attending school, as the group of most interest are those least likely to be there! Another example might be a cross-sectional study that interviewed individuals within their own home. If the survey was performed during working hours, it is likely that the healthiest members of the community would be at work, and the survey would exaggerate rates of illness as a consequence.

Because psychiatric diagnostic interviews can take a long time to administer and are therefore expensive, two-stage surveys are a common design in psychiatric epidemiology. Such surveys screen a population with a brief measure (usually a questionnaire) and then perform the psychiatric interview in a subset of responders. Usually the researchers attempt to interview all those who scored positive on the questionnaire and a sample of those who scored negative. The rationale for this goes back to the concurrent validity of the questionnaire. No questionnaire performs its task perfectly, so a proportion of those who score positive on the questionnaire will not have the disorder under study (i.e. false positives) and a proportion of those who score negative will in fact have the disorder (i.e. false negatives). The prevalence for the whole population can be calculated, provided the sampling procedure is taken into account.

Table 27.5 provides an illustration of this calculation. Suppose 10 000 individuals have been administered the screening questionnaire. All 1000 respondents who scored positive are interviewed, and half of them (500) are diagnosed with the disorder. Of all those who who screen negative, 10% (900) are interviewed and 5% of these are diagnosed with the disorder. From this it can be shown that 500 + 450 cases would have been detected in the entire population of 10 000, making the overall prevalence 9.5%.

Apart from generating a prevalence estimate and 95% confidence intervals (see below), cross-sectional studies

Table 27.5 Illustration of the calculation of prevalence in cross-sectional surveys

	Screen positive	Screen negative
Total surveyed	1000	9000
Sample interviewed	1000 (i.e. 100%)	900 (i.e. 10%)
Prevalent cases	500	45
Expected cases in total sample	500	450

can also provide important information on the cause and impact of a disorder. They can give information on the demographic characteristics of sufferers – for example age, gender, social class and race. Often more specific risk factors for the disorder are measured (such as recent life events, or drug use). Because cross-sectional studies (like case–control studies) measure exposures after the onset of the disorder, the direction of causation may not be clear. Furthermore, they are subject to both recall and prevalence bias (see below).

Cross-sectional studies provide an ideal sampling frame for case–control studies (see below). There are also a number of important examples where cross-sectional studies have been repeated with the same participants over time (e.g. the Health and Lifestyle Survey, British Household Panel Study). These are termed *panel studies*, and are in essence a hybrid form of cross-sectional and cohort study.

Cohort studies

In a cohort study the sample is defined according to its *exposure status* and followed up over time to determine who develops the disorder(s) of interest. The key strength of the cohort study is its longitudinal design, which means that participants are assessed before the onset of the disorder. Thus, cohort studies can usually give an insight into the direction of causation (see below) and are not susceptible to recall bias. Cohort studies allow rare exposures to be studied, and can assess the effect of such exposures on multiple outcomes. The classic cohort studies identify groups of people exposed to toxins (in general epidemiology, tobacco smoke and asbestos are good examples) and compare the incidence of diseases with that among a non-exposed group.

The cohort study is best suited to situations where the outcome is common. For rare outcomes (such as suicide and schizophrenia) cohort studies, unless very large, have limited utility. To illustrate this, suppose that a research team designs a cohort study to determine the effect of birth asphyxia on schizophrenia. They may identify babies with birth asphyxia (the 'exposed' group) and babies without such a history (the 'unexposed' group). They then have to follow the babies until adulthood in order to see whether any of them have developed schizophrenia. Assuming that by 25 years of age the risk of schizophrenia is 0.5% in those without birth asphyxia, the team would have had to follow (on average) 200 babies for each individual with schizophrenia in the unexposed cohort. In order to have a reasonable chance of detecting a twofold increase in the risk of schizophrenia over the course of the study, they would have had to follow over 10 000 individuals for 25 years. This example illustrates that cohort studies can be very expensive and time-consuming, especially if the outcome is rare.

Cohort studies need to follow up as many of the original sample as possible. For psychiatric disorders this is particularly important, as the individuals who cannot be traced may be the ones of most interest. For example, individuals with schizophrenia frequently become homeless, or may not be cooperative with requests to participate in research. *Non-response bias* is therefore a major concern in cohort studies. In the reporting of these studies, the investigators should describe the characteristics of those who could not be traced and how they differ from those who were traced. The analysis of a cohort study then involves the calculation of a risk ratio or rate ratio (see above).

Because of the problem of rare outcomes, and also the fact that most psychiatric disorders are multifactorial in aetiology, the classic cohort study is relatively rare in psychiatric epidemiology. Two approaches can be used to overcome some of these difficulties yet still retain the advantages of cohort design. First, there are a number of large population-based cohort studies in the UK – for example, the three birth cohort studies that have followed individuals born in a certain year over the course of their lives, and looked at many exposures and outcomes at different ages. These cohort studies have looked at many different aspects of health, and because of their size and inclusion of relevant exposures they have provided important data for psychiatric epidemiologists (e.g. Jones *et al*, 1994; Hotopf *et al*, 1999*a*). The second common approach is the retrospective or historical cohort study. To return to the example of birth asphyxia and schizophrenia, instead of following babies born now, the investigators could examine the hospital records of babies born 25 years ago, and – provided sufficient information on asphyxia was available – could then trace the babies to identify individuals who had developed schizophrenia. This is a cheaper approach, because the long follow-up time is not required, but the problem of tracing the sample may be even greater.

Prognostic studies

Studies on prognosis essentially use a cohort design in which the participants are patients with a disorder, who are followed over time. There is usually no comparison group, as such studies are essentially descriptive – giving insights into the natural history of the disorder, rather than its cause. The main methodological consideration is ensuring that an *inception cohort* is defined, meaning that to be included patients must be as close as possible to the start of their first episode of illness. Most psychiatric disorders have a fluctuating course, with relapses and remissions. If a study assessing the prognosis of psychotic illness gathered a sample of individuals at different stages of their illness, it would tend to give an overly pessimistic view of prognosis, because it would preferentially include individuals whose illness had an established chronic course. Determining that the cohort of individuals are all in their first episode ensures that those who get better quickly and never suffer further symptoms are included.

Another consideration with such studies is that the sample should be truly representative of the general population. If patients are recruited from specialist centres, there may be important *referral biases*, where more unusual cases are included, perhaps with a poorer outcome. Thus, many of the earlier prognostic studies in the UK, for example of depression, were conducted from the Maudsley Hospital, which is not only a tertiary referral centre but also has an inner-city catchment area, both factors that may skew the outcome in a negative direction.

Case–control study

In a case–control study, individuals with a disorder are compared with individuals who are free from the disorder. In psychiatric epidemiology the exposure is usually some event in the past (e.g. obstetric complications; childhood abuse or neglect; life events). In biological psychiatry the 'exposure' may be assessed by neuroimaging or neuroendocrine tests, as some of the methodological issues are identical. Unlike cohort studies, case–control studies are useful for rare disorders, and it is possible to determine the relationship between many different exposures and the disorder under study. Case–control studies are usually quicker and cheaper to perform than cohort studies, because the disorder has already occurred and it is not necessary to follow individuals over many years. Unless very large, case–control studies are not useful for rare exposures because insufficient cases and controls will have experienced them to make useful comparisons. Like cross-sectional studies, case–control studies are unable to determine direction of causality, and are susceptible to recall bias.

The most important issue in case–control studies is the selection of both cases and controls. The key problem is *selection bias*, which occurs when the risk factor under study has an effect on the likelihood that the individual will be recruited to the study. This can work for both cases and controls. For example, some neuroimaging studies in psychiatry involve selecting patients with severe chronic psychotic illness recruited from 'centres of excellence' and comparing them with controls who may be PhD students from the same centres. For both cases and controls, equal and opposite selection factors may generate misleading results. Cases may be unlikely to give a true representation of psychotic illness, because those most readily available tend to be those with chronic symptoms (an instance of *prevalence bias*, on which see below). The controls are unlikely to represent the typical 'normal' brain because they have been drawn from a highly educated sample. For this reason, much emphasis is placed on attempting to select as representative a sample of cases as possible, and investigators may go to great pains to identify all cases of a disorder within a population. The key to the selection of controls is that they should be drawn from a similar population and be similar to the cases in all respects apart from the disorder under study.

The analysis of the case–control study involves a comparison of the odds of exposure in the cases compared with the controls – and is expressed as the odds ratio (see above).

The randomised controlled trial

In the randomised controlled trial (RCT) two or more interventions to treat (or sometimes prevent) a disorder are compared. Unlike studies of risk factors, where it would be unethical for the investigator to assign individuals to receive a potentially harmful exposure, RCTs are ethical because the intervention is expected to do good. The key ethical principle behind the RCT is equipoise: to perform an RCT the investigator should demonstrate that there is no evidence to suggest that a treatment is better than placebo, or that one active treatment is no better than another. (In other words, if one treatment was already known to be far superior to another, it would not be ethical to randomise.)

The key methodological feature of the RCT is randomisation with concealed allocation. The rationale behind randomisation is that each participant has an identical chance of receiving each treatment. Then, if the trial is sufficiently large, potential confounders will be evenly distributed between the groups, and selection bias can be avoided. This allows trials to be able to measure accurately quite small effect sizes. Randomisation may be performed using random number tables (available in most statistics books) or computer generated random numbers. In *simple randomisation* the participants are assigned to groups according to each random number in the sequence. The problem with this method is that the random groups may not be balanced: it is possible that, simply by chance, the two groups are of different size, and this is statistically inefficient. *Balanced randomisation* overcomes this by allocating participants in blocks. A typical block size would be eight, and the investigator would arrange that within this block four participants would receive the intervention and four the control condition (see Fig. 27.2).

Randomisation usually ensures even distribution of important confounders between groups, but in smaller trials this cannot be guaranteed – by chance there may be big differences in the distribution of confounders. To get around this, the investigator can perform a *stratified randomisation*, where the sample is divided according to the presence of the variable. For instance, in a trial of fluoxetine for chronic fatigue syndrome, the presence of depression was thought to be a key variable, and the investigators stratified the randomisation on this (Vercoulen *et al*, 1996).

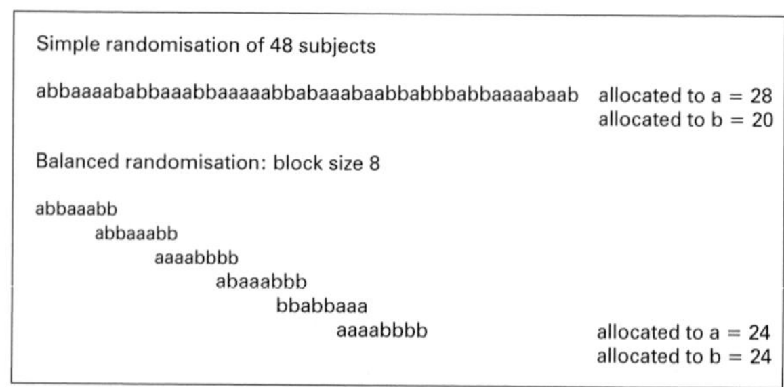
Simple randomisation of 48 subjects

abbaaaababbaaabbaaaaabbabaaabaabbabbbabbaaaabaab allocated to a = 28
allocated to b = 20

Balanced randomisation: block size 8

abbaaabb
abbaaabb
aaaabbbb
abaaabbb
bbabbaaa
aaaabbbb

allocated to a = 24
allocated to b = 24

Fig. 27.2 Distinction between simple randomisation and balanced randomisation. In the simple randomisation the total in each group is unlikely to be balanced. In balanced randomisation the investigator has decided to randomise within blocks of eight. In each block of eight, there must be four participants on each treatment.

In *minimisation* this process is taken a step further, and a wide range of key variables are identified; participants are then effectively matched on each of these to ensure that they are as similar as possible.

The practical process of randomisation has received considerable attention since it was reported that studies that reported 'positive' results were more likely to have methods where it was easy to cheat on the randomisation process. If the investigator had considerable faith in a new treatment, he or she might consciously or unconsciously manipulate the randomisation process in order to ensure that patients with a good prognosis were assigned to the experimental treatment. *Concealment of allocation* refers to the degree to which it is predictable to the researcher which treatment the patient will receive. The best method is to have randomisation performed by an independent third party who is not aware of the study questions.

RCTs usually have a list of inclusion and exclusion criteria to ensure that patients entered are similar. The rationale for exclusion criteria may be:

- to prevent patients with contraindications for the treatments being entered
- to ensure that certain clinical subtypes with particular profiles that might confuse the results are excluded
- to prevent certain groups who are considered 'high risk' (e.g. patients with suicidal ideas) from participating (a practice that may prevent embarrassment of the investigators and sponsors, but which is not useful to clinicians, who see such patients all the time).

It is good practice for trials to report the number of individuals approached, the number who refused to participate or were excluded, and the number randomised. Altman (1996) recommended summarising this information with a 'CONSORT statement'.

An RCT usually involves a clinical assessment before randomisation and then a series of subsequent assessments. Depending on the condition or treatment under study, these may take place soon after randomisation, or involve long follow-up.

As with cohort studies, drop-outs from RCTs are a major problem. The trialist should attempt to follow everyone up, including patients who drop out of treatment. Many trials simply compare those in the two groups who have completed the trial according to protocol. This may mean that a sizeable proportion of those randomised (one-third in average antidepressant trials) are left out. This is misleading and can be a source of potential bias. A better approach is to use *intention to treat* analysis, where all randomised participants, no matter how long they were on treatment, are included in the analysis.

The analysis of RCTs depends on the nature of the outcome. For categorical outcomes (e.g. recovery or admission to hospital) the approach will be similar to cohort studies and a relative risk or rate ratio may be calculated. The number needed to treat, which expresses the number of individuals whose recovery can be attributed to the intervention, can also be calculated. This is a clinically useful measure which describes the number of individuals who would have to be placed on a treatment in order to produce one good outcome. For example, most RCTs of antidepressants versus placebo indicate that, at 6 weeks, two-thirds of those treated with antidepressants are better, compared with one-third of those treated with placebo. In other words, a doctor would have to prescribe antidepressants to three patients in order to help one get better. Put formally, the number needed to treat is the inverse of the risk difference (see Box 27.1).

Box 27.1 Calculation of number needed to treat

Risk of recovery on antidepressant	2/3
Risk of recovery on placebo	1/3
Risk difference	1/3
Number needed to treat (NNT)	3

Many RCTs describe results in terms of change of scores on symptom rating scales. In these cases it is preferable to present results as differences in the change scores from baseline.

Systematic reviews and meta-analysis

Reviews are an important source of information for clinicians and researchers. Most reviews (such as most textbook chapters) are written by an expert with a special interest who has, over time, collected a body of knowledge which he or she distils into a summary of available evidence. This approach (referred to as *narrative* reviews) has been criticised because the methods are not reproducible: important articles may be missed, and the reviewer may overemphasise results that confirm his or her point of view. *Systematic reviews* involve a systematic effort to identify all relevant literature; inclusion and exclusion criteria are then applied to that literature and results are extracted in a systematic way. Systematic reviews include a 'methods' section that describes the search strategy. *Meta-analysis* is a statistical synthesis of the main findings of the reviews.

Just as with primary research, systematic reviews should aim to answer a specific question, and state aims and objectives explicitly. The reviewer performs a literature search, which will usually involve a combination of electronic searches (e.g. MEDLINE), tracing other articles in the reference lists of identified studies, contacting experts in the field to determine whether they know of other relevant literature (published or unpublished), contact with the pharmaceutical industry for unpublished results, and so on. The reviewer should state the inclusion and exclusion criteria. For reviews of treatment, the exclusion criteria will commonly include non-randomisation or inadequate concealment of allocation (see above).

One of the most useful products of systematic reviews is a description of common problems in researching a particular field. Systematic reviews should involve a critique of previous literature (e.g. Hotopf *et al*, 1997). The results section should include information on the number of studies identified from the literature search, the numbers excluded and included, and the characteristics of the studies included.

Meta-analysis involves pooling together the results of a number of (usually) RCTs. The rationale for this approach is to improve statistical power. Because the majority of randomised trials in psychiatry are too small to give useful information, pooling the results of many similar studies will improve the precision of the effect size.

Meta-analyses have been criticised for lumping 'apples and oranges' together. For example, different trials of the same intervention may take place in different settings (out-patient, in-patient, primary care), with disorders of differing severity or chronicity. For pharmacological treatments, the drug prescribed in different trials may have been identical but the dosage may have been different. For non-pharmacological treatments, such as psychotherapy or trials of the way in which community care is delivered, the treatment may differ radically between trials. This *heterogeneity* between trials should be explored in meta-analyses (Thompson, 1994). It is possible to use a statistical test of heterogeneity to assess whether all the trials included in a meta-analysis are 'pulling the same way'. If this test indicates that significant heterogeneity between trials exists, the researchers should investigate why this might be. This would involve testing whether the effect size differs according to the type of study included.

Publication bias

An important problem with meta-analysis is *publication bias*. It is a fact of life that researchers and journal editors like to have 'positive' results. There is considerable evidence that papers that show that one treatment has a clear advantage over another are more likely to be published than those that do not. Publication bias is the result: papers that are 'negative' end up in the desk-drawer of the researcher. Meta-analysis assumes that no publication bias has occurred. It is not difficult to see how substantial publication bias could radically alter the conclusions of a meta-analysis. Publication bias is best avoided by a comprehensive search strategy. There has been an 'amnesty' on unpublished RCTs by major medical journals to encourage investigators with unpublished results to place these in the public domain.

The funnel plot is a method to assess the potential role of publication bias (Egger & Davey Smith, 1998). It relies on the fact that small studies are more likely to be susceptible to publication bias than large ones. If researchers complete a large RCT they are likely to want to see it published even if the result is negative because of the effort involved. If publication bias does exist, it is most likely to be due to small negative trials not being published. The funnel plot is a graphical representation of the size of trials plotted against the effect size they report. As the size of trials increases, they are likely to converge around the true, underlying effect size. For the large trials one would expect to see an even scattering of trials either side of this true, underlying effect. When publication bias occurs one expects an *asymmetry* in the scatter of small studies, with more studies showing a positive result than those showing a negative result.

Choosing a study design

The choice of a study design depends on the type of question being asked, the nature of the disorder and the exposure, and the time and resources available. The first question a researcher should ask is whether the question has been answered already, and the step before any serious research project should be to identify systematic reviews on the topic, or to perform one.

For some types of question the study design may be obvious. Studies on treatment efficacy are usually best answered by a RCT or a systematic review and meta-analysis of RCTs. When the researcher wants to describe the prevalence of a disorder, cross-sectional studies provide the obvious solution. However, it is more difficult to settle a question about the aetiology of a disorder, or the potential harmful effect of an exposure, and study design will often be a trade-off between methodological considerations and resources.

The question next to ask it whether there are existing sources of data. Previous research studies may have collected the data necessary to answer the question. Weich *et al* (1998) were able to use data from the British Household Panel Study to determine whether the gender difference in rates of depression was accounted for by differences in social roles, which the study showed not to be the case. This was an extremely economical way of answering a well-focused question, which would otherwise have required major resources. Sometimes data exist that are not part of a research study but which still allow the question to be answered. For example, Andreasson *et al* (1987) used data routinely collected by the Swedish military on conscription to demonstrate a strong association between cannabis use and subsequent psychotic illness. For rare side-effects of drugs, large databases such as the UK General Practice Research Database, are an ideal resource.

If existing data do not exist, the choice of whether to use a case–control, cohort or cross-sectional study will depend on the relative frequency of the outcome and exposure, and how easy they are to measure. Case–control studies manipulate the frequency of the outcome (by sampling according to participants' disorder status) and cohort studies manipulate the frequency of the exposure (by sampling according to the participants' exposure status). Thus, case–control studies are best for rare disorders, and cohort studies for rare exposures. When both are common, cross-sectional designs may be the best option, as they will provide an estimate of prevalence, and be less prone to selection biases.

Causation

In analytical studies, researchers attempt to make a link between two variables. In aetiological studies these are a risk factor and a disorder; in treatment studies they are a treatment and its effect. Some measure of the size of the effect (e.g. an odds ratio) is then given. In this section we explore some of the factors that may interfere with the accurate estimation of the 'effect size', in respect of causation.

Confounding

Confounders are variables associated with both the exposure and the outcome, and can lead to a spurious association or eliminate a real one. To be a confounder, a variable has to be an independent risk factor for the outcome *and* to vary systematically with the exposure under study. However, confounders are not on a causal pathway between exposure and outcome. For example, depression is more common in patients with rheumatoid arthritis than in those with osteoarthritis; however, because rheumatoid arthritis is three times more common in women, the association could be confounded by gender. Note that confounding is a reflection of the relationship between variables in real life – unlike bias (see below), it is not a result of error in the design of studies.

There are five main methods of dealing with confounding:

1 *Restriction* is a method by which individuals with the confounding variable are removed from the study altogether. In the previous example, one could restrict the study to females (or males) and determine whether depression is still more common in rheumatoid arthritis.

2 *Matching* involves artificially making the two groups similar in terms of the confounding variable, so the investigator might ensure that each female patient with rheumatoid arthritis was matched with a female patient with osteoarthritis. Matching is intuitively easy to understand, but makes the analysis somewhat more complicated as specific statistical methods that take account of the matching have to be used.

3 *Stratification* is a method used in the analysis where instead of lumping all subjects together, the sample is split according to the presence of the confounder – thus males and females would be analysed separately. It is possible using stratification to calculate a combined estimate of the size of the effect (e.g. odds ratio) using specific statistical techniques.

4 *Modelling* is a general term for multivariate statistical techniques where a regression equation is generated that takes account of the effect of the exposure and confounder together. There are many different types of modelling, but these include multiple regression (for a continuous outcome variable such as symptom score) and logistic regression (for a binary outcome variable such as presence of a disorder).

5 The final approach to confounding is *randomisation*, which is dealt with in the section on RCTs. Because it is not ethical to assign participants in studies on risk factors to receive a potentially hazardous exposure, randomisation is limited to treatment or preventive studies. However, it is the best method for managing confounders because it will theoretically deal with unknown confounders, which cannot be taken into account by any of the other methods.

Bias

Bias refers to errors in the design of a study which may generate misleading results. Unlike confounding, bias comes about as a result of the study design or execution. Bias is classified into selection bias and information bias.

Selection bias

Selection bias refers to the way in which participants in a study are selected and the impact this may have on the study's results. It is a particular problem in case–control studies, but not exclusive to them. An example was given under case–control studies. Selection bias tends to be a particular problem when studies identify cases from clinical populations, especially in specialist settings.

Non-response bias

Non-response bias is a form of selection bias of particular importance in cohort studies (but relevant to all study designs), where the individuals of greatest interest may be those who are least likely to participate. This can cause misleading results if the exposure under study also influences participation.

Prevalence bias

Prevalence bias is a subtype of selection bias that is a problem in case–control and cross-sectional studies where investigators identify prevalent cases, some of whom may have had the disorder for many years. With disorders such as depression, where relapse and remission are the rule, prevalent samples will be biased because they will over-represent those with chronic depression. It is then difficult to determine whether exposures act to cause or maintain the disorder.

Information bias

Information bias refers to errors made in the gathering of information from participants. There are two main types of information bias – recall bias and observer bias.

Recall bias

Recall bias particularly occurs when a disorder has an impact on the participant's recall. For example, patients with depression, when asked about recent life events, may be more inclined to dwell on negative events, and overlook positive ones, as this is a feature of depressive thinking. In schizophrenia research it is notoriously difficult to gain good information on early experiences, such as obstetric complications, and mothers of people with schizophrenia may be inclined to put a good deal more effort into remembering remote events than mothers of healthy controls. Recall bias is best prevented by using documentary evidence. Other strategies are to use a control group of individuals with another disorder not thought to be associated with the risk factor under study, where similar recall effects would be expected to act.

Observer bias

Observer bias relates to the way in which researchers ask questions of participants in studies. If the researcher is aware of the hypothesis under study, and also knows which group the participant is from, he or she may ask questions in subtly different ways. For example, if the study was assessing the efficacy of cognitive therapy versus standard care for depression, the researcher may probe depressive symptoms in a less persistent way to the group who have had cognitive therapy. 'Blinding' is an important approach to prevent observer bias, but it is not always possible to blind the researcher – in case–control studies it may be very obvious which participants have a psychiatric disorder and which do not. Observer bias may be overcome by using highly structured interviews or pen-and-paper questionnaires so that every participant is asked the same question in the same way.

Reverse causation

In reverse causation, the association between the risk factor and the disorder is a valid one, but the interpretation is turned around. For example, a study might find that there is a strong association between job loss and depression, and this might be interpreted as indicating that those who lose their jobs are at greater risk of becoming depressed. However, an alternative hypothesis is that depression is an important cause of job loss – individuals who become depressed perform less well at work and are therefore more at risk of losing their jobs. A classic problem of reverse causation is the issue of whether the higher rates of schizophrenia seen in city dwellers is due to features of urban life or whether those suffering from schizophrenia are more likely to migrate to the cities ('urban drift'). Issues of reverse causation can be addressed using longitudinal study designs, such as cohort studies, where the risk factor is measured *before* the onset of the disorder.

Chance

Type 1 and type 2 error

Most studies aim to describe reality by taking a *sample* of the total population. However, the sample will not exactly describe the true underlying population distribution: there is always a degree of *sampling error.* Tossing a coin 10 times will yield different combinations of heads and tails. Statistically the *most likely* result would be five heads and five tails, but any combination of heads and tails is possible. More extreme results (e.g. all tails or all heads) become less probable with increasing numbers of tosses of the coin. In other words, increasing the number of tosses increases the *precision* with which the underlying 'true' situation can be estimated.

In any analytic study, we hope that the results of our study reflect reality. Nevertheless, if 10 identical studies were performed they would all come up with slightly different results. The size of the difference would depend on the size of the sample in each study. Studies that report an association between two variables may either be describing the true underlying situation, or by chance have committed a *type 1 error* (see Table 27.6). Type 1 error occurs where an association is detected by chance, and the probability that this has occurred is assessed by statistical testing. By convention, the type 1 error rate is often set at the arbitrary level of $P < 0.05$.

Studies that report a 'negative finding' (i.e. do not show an association between two variables) may either be describing the true underlying situation, or may by chance have committed a type 2 error. Type 2 error occurs when a genuine association is missed by chance. In designing a study, the power calculation takes into account an acceptable type 2 error rate, usually set at 10–20%, meaning that most studies accept that there is a 10–20% chance that they will fail to detect a true effect. Statistical power is the converse of the type 2 error rate (and is therefore usually set at 80–90%). More powerful studies require bigger sample sizes.

Table 27.6 The relationship between the results of a study and 'true life'

Study	'True life'	
	Association exists	**No association exists**
Association demonstrated	✓	Type 1 error
No association demonstrated	Type 2 error	✓

✓ indicates the study results represent 'true life'.
Most studies set the type 1 error rate (α) at 0.05 or less, and the type 2 error rate (β) at 0.1–0.2. The power of a study is $1-\beta$ (ie 80–90%).

Points to consider if a study reports one or more positive associations

If a statistically significant association is reported, it is of course still possible that the finding could be due to chance. There is no *P* value that can 'prove' an association. By convention we often take 'statistical significance' to mean $P < 0.05$. This means that 1 time in 20 we expect to detect the difference by chance, and there is no way of knowing whether the study we are reporting or reading about is that one time. This is why researchers seek to replicate one another's results.

'Significant' *P* values come about for several reasons. First, it may be that the study is very big, and even differences that are in clinical terms trivial show up as statistically significant. The important thing to look for is the effect size (e.g. how big the odds ratio is) rather than the *P* value.

Second, the more hypotheses tested, the greater the likelihood is that a 'significant' association will be found by chance. If researchers collected data on 40 possible risk factors for schizophrenia, they could expect two to be associated at $P < 0.05$ *just by chance*.

There is a balance to be reached between wasting data and 'data trawling'. The best way to overcome this dilemma is to set out with one or two main hypotheses that form the centre of the research protocol, and on which the power calculation is based. All additional findings can be labelled 'secondary analyses', and be seen as a useful by-product of the main research. An alternative approach to multiple statistical testing is to use a *Bonferroni correction*. This works on the principle that the level of statistical significance set should be adjusted to take account of the number of tests performed. Thus, if we set $P < 0.05$ for a single significance test, this should be reduce to $P < 0.005$ if we perform 10 comparisons. This approach is generally considered too conservative and may lead one to miss significant positive findings. A better approach is to express results in terms of their *precision* (see section below on confidence intervals).

Another way of getting spurious *P* values is by using subgroup analyses. Here the researcher breaks down

Table 27.7 Power calculations for different effect sizes: sample size required to detect differing levels of recovery rates for a new treatment at 95% confidence and 80% power

Recovery rate on new antidepressant (compared with 66% improvement on imipramine)	Number required to be randomised
33%	82
40%	128
50%	320
55%	654
60%	2096

the statistical analysis according to certain characteristics of the participants. For example, a researcher may have performed a randomised trial comparing a new atypical antipsychotic with haloperidol in patients with treatment-resistant psychosis. The main results show no overall difference, but the researcher may investigate whether there are any particular subgroups of patients in whom there was a difference. For example, he might hypothesise that patients with pronounced positive symptoms will respond better to the atypical antipsychotic. Such analyses are often reported as showing positive evidence for the new intervention, but are best avoided as it is notoriously easy to generate a type 1 error in this way.

Points to consider if the study reports a 'negative finding'

The key question to consider when a negative finding is presented is whether the sample size was sufficient to pick up a true difference – that is, are the results due to type 2 error? In evaluations of new antidepressants, the new treatment is often pitted against a reference compound. Studies often report no difference in treatment effect between the two drugs, suggesting perhaps that the new treatment is as good as the old one. However, comparisons between two active treatments require large samples. If one assumes that two-thirds of patients treated with imipramine respond within 6 weeks, Table 27.7 indicates the sample size required to detect differing levels of recovery rates for a new treatment at 95% confidence and 80% power. It indicates that a sample size of 82 would be able to detect only a very big difference between the treatments, and that to detect a difference of 10 percentage points in recovery rates (which would be a clinically meaningful difference) would require over 650 participants. Thus, an underpowered study that demonstrates no difference between two treatments *does not* indicate that the treatments have similar efficacy!

Assessment of chance – *P* values and confidence intervals

There is a long tradition of using *P* values to determine the chance that a study has committed a type 1 error. A wide range of statistical tests can be used to determine the *P* value. The choice of the test depends on the nature of the data and a discussion of individual tests is beyond the scope of this chapter. In any case, this approach has limitations – the *P* value is somewhat uninformative, and increasing emphasis has been placed on describing the confidence interval for a parameter. Just as the traditional type 1 error rate of 0.05 has been used as a cut-off for *P* values, the 95% confidence interval has been most widely used, but it is perfectly valid to present 90% or 99% confidence intervals. The confidence interval of a parameter describes the range of results that might be expected after doing the same study on different samples. Put formally, the 95% confidence interval indicates that if the same study were repeated, there would be a 95% chance that the parameter would be estimated within the range described.

Table 27.8 Parameters and their null values

Parameter	Null value
Differences in means, risk difference	0
Odds ratio, rate ratio, risk ratio, hazard ratio	1
Number needed to treat	∞

Confidence intervals may be calculated for most parameters we estimate. For example, it is possible to calculate a confidence interval around purely descriptive statistics like a mean or a proportion. It is also possible to show a confidence interval around a comparative parameter such as a difference between two means, a relative risk or a number needed to treat. When the 95% confidence interval crosses the null value of a parameter, this indicates that there is no difference at the $P = 0.05$ level between the groups compared. It is important here to know the null value (see Table 27.8).

Internal versus external validity

Most of the previous discussion has concentrated on threats to the *internal validity* of research studies. However, a common complaint about research is that participants may be so dissimilar from patients seen in normal clinical practice that it is impossible to generalise from the research findings. This complaint particularly applies to RCTs, which are indeed performed in different settings and with different patient groups to those seen in standard practice. In general, complaints about lack of generalisability of RCTs have been misplaced. There are very few examples of treatments working on one group of patients with a disorder but not on others. In some circumstances the practicalities of recruiting patients makes it difficult to ensure that those entered into the study are similar to those seen in clinical practice; this particularly applies to patients with psychotic or manic illness, where the most severely affected are least likely to give their consent to participate. In other circumstances, RCTs impose unnecessarily long lists of exclusion criteria. Elsewhere it has been argued that there is a need for pragmatic RCTs which apply standard trial methodology on representative samples of patients (Hotopf *et al*, 1999*b*).

Critical appraisal

This chapter has discussed a number of aspects of clinical epidemiology, with particular emphasis on developing understanding of the principal study designs and their associated flaws. Critical appraisal is the approach of putting this knowledge into practice when assessing research findings. While some knowledge of study designs and common flaws helps, critical appraisal is a skill that requires practice. This is best gained by:

- reading new research with a sceptical frame of mind
- following correspondence about published studies
- discussing studies with colleagues
- presenting and attending journal clubs
- when given a 'fact' (even in this book!), being prepared to ask 'what's your evidence?'

Acknowledgement

I am grateful to Dr William Lee for his comments on an earlier draft.

References

Altman, D. G. (1996) Better reporting of randomised controlled trials: the CONSORT statement. *BMJ*, **313**, 570–571.

American Psychiatric Association (1994) *Diagnostic and Statistical Manual of Mental Disorders* (4th edn) (DSM–IV). Washington, DC: APA.

Andreasson, S., Allebeck, P., Engstrom, A., *et al* (1987) Cannabis and schizophrenia: a longitudinal study of Swedish conscripts. *Lancet*, *ii*, 1483.

Blazer, D. G., Kessler, R. C., McGonagle, K. A., *et al* (1994) The prevalence and distribution of major depression in a national community sample: the National Comorbidity Survey. *American Journal of Psychiatry*, **151**, 979–986.

Egger, M. & Davey Smith, G. (1998) Bias in location and selection of studies. *BMJ*, **316**, 61–66.

Goldberger, J. (1914) The cause and prevention of pellagra. *Public Health Report*, **29** (no. 37), 2354.

Hotopf, M. (2003) The case–control study. In *Practical Psychiatric Epidemiology* (eds M. Prince, T. Ford, R. Stewart, *et al*). Oxford: Oxford University Press.

Hotopf, M., Lewis, G. & Normand, C. (1997) Putting trials on trial: the costs and consequences of small trials in depression. A systematic review of methodology. *Journal of Epidemiology and Community Health*, **51**, 354–358.

Hotopf, M., Mayou, R., Wadsworth, M., *et al* (1999*a*) Childhood risk factors for adult medically unexplained symptoms: results of a national birth cohort study. *American Journal of Psychiatry*, **156**, 1796–1800.

Hotopf, M., Churchill, R. & Lewis, G. (1999*b*) The pragmatic randomised controlled trial in psychiatry. *British Journal of Psychiatry*, **175**, 217–223.

Jones, P., Rodgers, B., Murray, R., *et al* (1994) Child development risk factors for adult schizophrenia in the British 1946 birth cohort. *Lancet*, **344**, 1398–1402.

Meltzer, H., Gill, B., Petticrew, M., *et al* (1995) *OPCS Surveys of Psychiatric Morbidity in Great Britain, Report 1: The Prevalence of Psychiatric Morbidity Among Adults Living in Private Households*. London: HMSO.

Morgan, H. G. & Cooper, B. (1975) Historical background. In *Epidemiological Psychiatry*, pp. 3–23. Springfield, IL: Charles C. Thomas.

Neeleman, J., Halpern, D., Leon, D., *et al* (1997) Tolerance of suicide, religion and suicide rates: an ecological and individual study of 19 Western countries. *Psychological Medicine*, **27**, 1165–1171.

Oxford English Dictionary (1989) 2nd edn. Prepared by J. Simpson & E. Weiner. Volume 5, p. 328. Oxford: Clarendon Press.

Regier, D. A., Myers, J. K., Kramer, M., *et al* (2002) The NIMH Epidemiologic Catchment Area program. Historical context, major objectives and study population characteristics. *Archives of General Psychiatry*, **41**, 934–941.

Thompson, S. G. (1994) Why sources of heterogeneity in meta-analysis should be investigated. *BMJ*, **309**, 1351–1355.

Timmreck, T. C. (1994) *An Introduction to Epidemiology*, p. 2. Boston, MA: Jones and Bartlett.

Vercoulen, J., Swanink, C. & Zitman, F. (1996) Fluoxetine in chronic fatigue syndrome: a randomized, double-blind, placebo-controlled trial. *Lancet*, **347**, 858–861.

Weich, S., Sloggett, A. & Lewis, G. (1998) Social roles and gender difference in the prevalence of common mental disorders. *British Journal of Psychiatry*, **173**, 489–493.

World Health Organization (1992) *International Classification of Mental and Behavioural Disorders* (ICD–10). Geneva: WHO.

CHAPTER 28

Principles of nosology

Anne Farmer and Muna Adwa

Classification in psychiatry has had a long and rather chequered history, and it was only in the last decades of the 20th century that some degree of consensus was achieved, as reflected in the acceptance of two main international classifications: the 10th revision of the *International Classification of Diseases* (ICD–10) (World Health Organization, 1992) and the fourth edition of the *Diagnostic and Statistical Manual of Mental Disorders* (DSM–IV) (American Psychiatric Association, 1994). In this chapter we first consider the diagnostic process in relation to mental experiences. We then examine why a scientific approach to the measurement of psychopathology is important. Next, the development of ICD–10 and DSM–IV and their broad structure are reviewed. Finally, we consider the strengths and weaknesses of these nosological approaches and what the future may hold in terms of the classification of mental disorder.

Eliciting psychopathology

Teasing apart what is pathological from what is part of normal experience

When a psychiatrist takes a history and undertakes a mental state examination, he or she is trying to discover whether the mental experiences described by the patient are pathological or merely part of everyday or 'normal' experience. For example, someone who reports 'feeling depressed' may mean that he or she is experiencing transient low spirits that are mild and self-limiting. Alternatively, the description of low mood may be an indicator of a mental disorder. Establishing whether depression is a symptom of a psychiatric disorder, or merely a part of everyday life, requires answers to a number of supplementary questions related to:

- the intensity of the experience (how bad is it?)
- how long it has lasted (how much has there been of it?)
- how much the experience has interfered with daily activities (how disabling has it been?).

We also recognise that clinically significant depression is also associated with a number of co-occurring symptoms such as poor sleep, reduced appetite, lack of self-esteem and slowed thoughts. Knowing what supplementary questions to ask and their significance allows us to determine whether the low mood is pathological or not.

By careful cross-examination undertaken in a systematic way, the clinician builds up a picture of the mental experience of the respondent (Wing *et al*, 1974). This process also incorporates an attempt to arrive at an objective (clinical) judgement about the nature and severity of each symptom. For example, although patients can complete self-report questionnaires about their mood, these can only indicate the patient's subjective view of the symptoms. This is somewhat different to the psychiatric history and mental state examination, where the clinician is making an objective assessment about the nature and severity of individual symptoms.

Having determined what pathological features are present, it is then possible to assign the individual to a diagnostic category. In a clinical setting, a diagnosis is assigned by matching the symptom profile of the patient to a 'mental template' acquired through clinical experience. This mental template is derived from groups of individuals who share particular psychopathological features.

In order to complete the diagnostic process, it is also important that those having such symptoms are able to articulate and communicate their experiences and that the clinician is sufficiently empathic to understand and interpret their significance. This interaction between sufferer and observer depends on what is considered pathological in the culture(s) to which they both belong, which, in turn, may be influenced by language, education, religious beliefs or politics.

Different schools of psychopathology

The use of systematic enquiry to establish the presence or absence of psychopathology, as outlined above using depression as an example, is termed *phenomenological psychopathology*, which relates to objective descriptions of morbid mental experiences, or *phenomena*, and does not rely on any theories about what may have caused them. Phenomenological psychopathology was described by Jaspers (1959) as 'representing, defining and classifying psychic phenomena as an independent activity'.

There are two other main approaches to assessment of psychopathology, namely *psychodynamic* and *experimental* psychopathology. Psychodynamic psychopathology is derived from psychoanalytical theory, which proposes that unconscious mental processes generate mental events. While the phenomenological approach examines the details of the abnormal phenomena, the psychodynamic approach concentrates on the unconscious mechanisms assumed to have caused them. In contrast, the approach used in experimental psychopathology consists of testing hypotheses that compare normal and abnormal experiences. The approach utilises a number of different scientific methods, including animal models of human behaviour.

Diagnosis

Syndromes not diseases

Mental disorders are defined according to the clustering together of subjective complaints (symptoms) and observable abnormalities in behaviour, cognition or speech (signs) that are considered pathological. Consequently, what are described in the various categories of diagnosis are *syndromes* rather than 'true' disease entities. This is because the definition of disease requires the presence of demonstrable pathology, which is not yet possible for most psychiatric conditions. Because of this the term 'disorder' is preferred, rather than disease, and DSM–IV and ICD–10 are classifications of psychiatric disorders that are essentially syndromes. Although these two classifications have international acceptance, they are only a 'best guess'; that is, they represent our current state of knowledge about mental disorder. As such, they need to be continually reassessed and modified in the light of new understanding about the aetiology of mental states. Hence, at the time of writing, plans are being made for the development of ICD–11 and DSM–V. We discuss both the strengths and the limitations of the current system below. However, first we consider why making a diagnosis is important.

Why assign a diagnostic category?

It may seem odd to some readers that this question is even being posed. Most doctors take the need to apply a diagnosis as self-evident and, indeed, in most of the rest of medicine the making of a diagnosis has such a central role that its importance is rarely questioned.

The word 'diagnosis' is derived from two Greek roots: *dia,* meaning the way through, and *gnosis,* meaning knowledge. Scadding (1967) viewed diagnosis as a medical *process* rather than a single act, and his definition of diagnosis holds right across medicine, including psychiatry:

> 'Diagnosis is the process by which a patient's symptoms and signs are assessed and investigated with a view to the categorisation of his or her case with other cases of a similar sort which have been studied in the past so that the patient may benefit from the application of established knowledge to the problem.' (Scadding, quoted by Mindham *et al,* 1992, p. 688)

However, in psychiatry the diagnostic process is less clear cut than it generally is in other fields of medicine and its usefulness has sometimes been challenged. Psychiatric diagnoses, at least until the latter part of the 20th century, were often unreliable and a source of frequent differences between clinicians; nor has it always been the case that the two main classifications have had broad international agreement (as it is now). In particular, in the middle of the 20th century a strong case was made for diagnosis to be abandoned in relation to psychiatry. Much of the early criticism came from psychoanalysts, mainly on the grounds that psychiatric diagnoses were far too reductionist and failed to convey the essence of what may be a very complex situation (Menninger, 1963). Criticisms were also made on the basis of what we have described above, namely that most diagnoses are syndromal, and for most disorders attempts have failed to discover coherent links between clinical features and specific aetiological factors or to find biological tests related to pathogenesis. Also, psychiatrists' reliance on clinical descriptions of signs and symptoms is a process of low epistemological (theory and methods of knowledge) ranking.

The case against making a diagnosis

Since the majority of psychological symptoms and signs that are considered pathological cannot be verified by any biological tests, it is clear that their presence can be considered merely a matter of opinion. Indeed, psychiatrists may (and some would say frequently do) disagree with one another about what is or is not pathological. This calls into question both the reliability and the validity of the diagnostic process. Szasz (1960), a critic of modern psychiatry, though a psychiatrist himself, argued that the mental events that are defined as abnormal are produced by the mind and, since it is not an organ of the body, the mind cannot be diseased in the same way as it is possible for the body to be diseased. That is, the mind cannot show demonstrable pathology or lesions.

The obvious answer to this criticism is that the mind must be 'located' in the brain. Although it remains true that few pathological abnormalities can be shown in those experiencing mental disorder, it is argued that this is because the brain abnormalities are subtle and the technologies that can identify them are only now being developed.

Szasz disliked the concept of diagnosis because he did not believe there was any such thing as mental illness. He wrote:

> 'labelling individuals displaying or disabled by problems in living as mentally ill has only impeded and retarded the essentially moral and political nature of the phenomena to which psychiatrists address themselves.' (Quoted in Mindham *et al,* 1992)

In his clinical examples, hysteria, which was a common diagnosis in the 1950s, is extensively discussed, but little attention is given to the major sources of psychiatric morbidity, such as schizophrenia, affective disorders or dementia. Szasz concluded with a scathing dismissal of psychiatry itself:

> 'It is customary to define psychiatry as a medical speciality concerned with the study, diagnosis and treatment of mental illnesses. This is a worthless and misleading definition. Mental illness is a myth. Psychiatrists are not concerned with mental illnesses and their treatments. In actual practice they deal with personal, social and ethical problems of living.' (Quoted in Mindham *et al,* 1992, p. 686)

Psychiatry, he argued, is nothing more than the institutional denial of the tragic nature of life:

> 'Individuals who want to reject the reality of free will and responsibility can medicalise life and thereby entrust its management to the health professionals.'

He believed that many psychiatric diagnoses are primarily driven by non-medical forces, such as social, personal, economic, legal and political factors rather than being solely derived from clinical considerations.

In the 1960s, when Szasz wrote his book, his views were rejected by the bulk of the profession and he was regarded as an 'anti-psychiatrist'. However, more recently, especially with advances in the field of social psychiatry, it is clear that much of what he said about the factors underlying psychiatric diagnoses had some truth in it, as evidenced by the inclusion of a social dimension in the DSM–IV multi-axial classification scheme (Axis IV, psychosocial stressors), although the language he used was perhaps a little extreme.

An additional criticism of the medical model of psychiatric disorder is that the current categories are merely hypothetical constructs, and it is inappropriate to talk about 'illness' or 'disease' but better to discuss maladaptive behaviour, communication difficulties or problems with living (Erikson, 1964; Scheff, 1966). Furthermore, it has been suggested that assigning a psychiatric diagnosis is stigmatising and the process detracts from the individual's dignity. Such 'labelling' also leads society to react against the individual (Scheff, 1966). Indeed, it has been shown that the presence of a psychiatric 'label' remains a strong influence on general practitioners' decisions to refer depressed and anxious patients to psychiatrists (Farmer & Griffiths, 1992).

Although there have been vigorous proponents of a 'disease free' approach to psychopathology over several decades, there has not been one consistent and testable alternative hypothesis proposed regarding the nature of mental disorders that can be used as a viable alternative. It is as if de-medicalising the measurement of psychopathology leads to a loss of the scientific rigour that is required for its evaluation.

The case in favour of making a diagnosis

Arguably, the most important reason for retaining a medical model when describing and categorising psychopathology is that abnormal mental states cause considerable suffering and impairment. Disability is associated with increased morbidity and, as is well recognised, abnormal mental states are also associated with increased mortality, which is partly, but not solely, due to the high rates of suicide among those who experience them. In the past, little could be done to treat such distress, but this is no longer true. Both drug and psychotherapeutic treatments have been shown to reduce or even eliminate many symptoms.

The individual's unique personal experience is certainly important in modifying both the presenting features and the response to treatment. Failure to distinguish different types of mental disorder or between mental illness and health will lead to failure to differentiate the needs of someone with schizophrenia from another who has panic disorder. The diagnosis is therefore central to the individual's treatment plan and management. Thus, certain diagnostic groups respond preferentially to certain types of treatment but not to others. A simple example is that lithium carbonate is an effective mood stabiliser for individuals with bipolar disorder but is of little benefit in the treatment of schizophrenia. In addition, assigning an individual to a group with others who share similar psychopathological features allows predictions to be made about the course and prognosis of the illness.

At an administrative level, another reason for categorising mental disorders is to address the needs of sufferers and their carers, and to plan services. Cases need to be accurately identified and diagnosed in epidemiological surveys to estimate the magnitude of the problem in the community, so that services can be planned and costed with reasonable accuracy.

Problems of terminology

Mental experiences require the ability to communicate intimate thoughts and feelings, which may be open to varied interpretation. Many everyday words have been used to describe psychopathology such as 'guilt', 'worry' and 'tension', but their precise definition may become confused with their 'lay' meaning. On the other hand, some terms with a precise medical meaning, such as 'schizophrenia', have been given an alternative meaning by the media and taken up by the lay public. In the case of 'schizophrenia' it is sometimes used to mean a 'split personality' or sometimes an individual's dilemma in having two choices, neither of which is remotely similar to the medical meaning of the term. Further, some descriptive terms have lost their meaning in translation from other languages, for example the English translation of the writings of French and German phenomenologists and psychiatrists (e.g. Esquirol, 1833; Jaspers, 1959).

The concept of disease and definitions of mental disorders

As alluded to above, because, as psychiatrists, we have trained as doctors, our response to the presence of psychopathology is to talk about 'illness' and 'disease'. Various attempts have been to made to define disease, starting with Cohen's (1960) definition that disease is present when there is 'statistical deviation from the average'. However, there are considerable problems with the definition of disease or illness when applied to psychopathology. Most medical conditions have certain key pathognomonic symptoms or signs which make diagnosis and the definition of disease a relatively straightforward process.

By contrast, psychiatric conditions tend to be poorly delineated and much of our thinking concerning disease definition for these vaguer conditions derives from the writings of Scadding (1967), a chest physician. Chest medicine, like psychiatry, has many non-specific symptoms, such as cough, sputum or shortness of breath, which are not pathognomonic of any one disease and which may occur in many different conditions. Scadding introduced the concept of harm or 'biological disadvantage' into his definition of disease, since significant disease processes usually result in harm to the individual. Thus, he viewed a disease essentially as a syndrome that both is statistically abnormal and results in significant biological disadvantage.

Kendell (1975) tried to retain the objective and observable component of biological disadvantage, which he interpreted for psychiatry to mean lowered fertility or decreased life span. While this may be true for certain severe organic and functional psychoses, most psychiatric disorders have little or no impact on either fertility or life span.

Another important contribution to the debate came from Kraupl-Taylor (1971), a psychotherapist working at the Maudsley Hospital in London, who specialised in the treatment of severe personality disorders. Patients with these disorders frequently defy conventional diagnostic approaches yet are severely dysfunctional and of great concern to others; they also often present with complaints of suffering. Kraupl-Taylor introduced the concepts of 'therapeutic concern' and 'subjective distress' to the concept of 'disease'. His definition of a disease was as follows:

> 'Then there are three kinds of people who are members of the class of patients: (1) people who feel therapeutic concern for themselves, but do not arouse it in the social environment, (2) people who do not feel therapeutic concern for themselves but do arouse it in their environment, and (3) people who feel therapeutic concern for themselves and also arouse it in their environment.' (Kraupl-Taylor, 1971, p. 359)

This definition was criticised by Kendell (1975) for its lack of objectivity; Kendell went on to add that it was no more than a tautology: 'doctors treat diseases, therefore diseases are what doctors treat'. It was also criticised on the grounds that the definition was far too flexible, especially as it permitted the definition of disease to vary with changes in the social environment. Despite these criticisms, subjective distress and concern on the part of others are now central to the modern concept of psychiatric disorder.

Modern definitions of disorder appear to comprise three elements:

1 a statistically abnormal syndrome

2 some suggestion of harm, in the form of biological or social disadvantage or social dysfunction

3 subjective distress.

Thus, the definition of a psychiatric disorder in the DSM–IV (American Psychiatric Association, 1994) is:

> 'A clinically significant behavioural or psychological syndrome associated with present disorders (painful symptoms) or disability (impairment in one or more areas of functioning) or with significant increased risk of suffering, pain, disability or important loss of freedom.'

The judgement as to whether the symptom is 'painful' is made by the patient and corresponds to Kraupl-Taylor's notion of therapeutic concern. The World Health Organization's (1992) definition, given in ICD–10, is similar:

> 'Disorder is not an exact term but is used here to imply the existence of a clinically recognisable set of symptoms or behaviours associated in most cases with distress and interference with personal functions. Social deviance or conflict alone without personal dysfunction should not be included in mental disorder as defined here.'

This definition causes some difficulties with socially deviant individuals who are said to have psychopathic personality disorder, since such individuals would not be included in the ICD–10 definition of mental disorder. None the less, the definition does include the need for a 'clinically recognisable set of symptoms or behaviours', that is, the syndrome itself. This is practical, applicable and generally acceptable. However, it underscores the importance of carefully eliciting and quantifying the symptoms and signs of mental disorder when taking the history and performing the mental state examination.

Are dimensions better than categories?

So far we have talked exclusively about identifying disorder and distinguishing this from health, that is, defining categories of case/non-case. However, some researchers and clinicians have argued the use of dimensional approaches to psychopathology has greater validity (Persons, 1986; Bentall *et al*, 1990; Costello, 1992).

Most psychopathological symptoms can be quantified; indeed, symptoms like low mood or anxiety can be readily conceptualised as dimensions, running from mild and within the normal range to severe and pathological. It can be argued that measuring psychopathology is similar to measuring blood pressure. We all have a recordable blood pressure but when this is high we are at risk of developing stroke, myocardial infarction or other diseases. Although blood pressure is a continuous measure, it is none the less possible to impose a cut-off or threshold to decide at what point medical intervention is required. Similarly, it is highly likely that we have all had some experience of mental symptoms such as feeling anxious or depressed. Like defining the cut-off for hypertension, the important question is 'how much' or 'how severe' it is. A severity or duration criterion can be applied to form the threshold between health and disorder for most mental symptoms. Even symptoms that appear to be clear dichotomies (present or absent), such as delusional beliefs, can be quantified (e.g. how much of the time they dominate thought or behaviour). It has even been argued that conceptualising mental disorder as a series of points on a number of continuous measures is a more valid approach than our continued reliance on categories (Costello, 1992).

Dimensions have the theoretical advantage that there is no loss of information and so maximum flexibility is preserved. There are no typical or atypical forms: most cases will fall near the centre position and a few 'outliers' will occupy positions at the extremes of the axis. Dimensions are favoured by psychologists because attributes such as intelligence, memory and personality traits are distributed on a continuum.

The alternative to a dimensional approach is a categorical one, and most psychiatrists work within the categorical frameworks given in ICD–10 and DSM–IV. A categorical approach assumes that all members of a class are relatively homogeneous in some chosen respect and that different categories are mutually exclusive. A nosological system should therefore have sufficient categories to cover all possible disorders. In the dimensional approach it is assumed (and probably correctly) that clinical phenomena are distributed on a continuum, whereas in a categorical system the assumption is that these phenomena are distributed in a binary, or all-or-none fashion.

Despite the obvious theoretical advantages of a dimensional approach, most clinicians think, work and diagnose in a categorical way. This is because most clinical work involves making binary decisions, for example whether to admit to hospital or not, to prescribe a drug or not, or to support a medico-legal or insurance claim or not. The presence or absence of a particular diagnostic category can be used to justify such decisions.

Prototypal classification

So far we have talked about the symptoms and signs of mental disorder and some of the issues regarding their measurement. These are the basic building blocks from which the familiar diagnostic categories are constructed. A third, and rather less commonly used, type of description of the main symptoms and signs of a disorder is termed a prototypal classification. This classifies patients according to the way they resemble a prototypal description that includes the core features of the disorder. Descriptions of conditions found in textbooks adopt a prototypal approach and the earlier chapters of this textbook contain prototypal descriptions of most of the common conditions encountered in psychiatry. Prototypal descriptions are especially helpful in the training situation, as they facilitate a rapid grasp of the essence of a disorder, but are less useful in a research setting, as they may be too vague, and boundaries between conditions are poorly defined. Most research projects therefore utilise diagnostic criteria, such as DSM–IV or ICD–10.

Early attempts to classify mental disorders and the origins of psychiatry

Before the 18th century most people lived in small villages and worked on the land, and so it was possible to care for those with mental disorders at home. During the 18th century, the Industrial Revolution swept through England, and large numbers of people with mental illnesses were found concentrated in a relatively hostile urban environment. This led to a growth in the number of private 'madhouses' as well as the opening of new 'asylums', placed some distance outside the rapidly expanding new towns. The Asylums Act of 1808 recognised for the first time the role of the state in providing care for the insane and each county was required to build its own asylum. More significantly, that Act stipulated that each new asylum should have a physician superintendent, who then often appointed deputies and other medically qualified assistants.

Similar changes took place elsewhere in Europe. For example, in Paris people with mental illnesses were admitted to hospitals such as the Salpetrière and the Bicêtre, and so they became segregated and alienated from society; they were said to suffer from 'mental alienation' and the doctors who cared for them became known as 'alienists'. The asylum physician superintendents and the alienists became the first medical specialists to work full time and exclusively with mental illness and in this sense were the first true psychiatrists. Thus, it was around this time that psychiatry began to develop as a specialty separate from medicine.

From a historical perspective it can be seen how the asylums and the new profession of psychiatry evolved almost as a by-product of the social chaos engendered by the Industrial Revolution. Some of the asylums developed affiliations with local medical schools and this facilitated a more systematic study of psychopathology. This trend occurred particularly in Germany, perhaps more so than in England or France. Thus, J. C. A. Heinroth was appointed the first professor of psychiatry (the title was actually professor of psychotherapy) at the University of Leipzig in 1827 (Marx, 1990). The word *psychiatrie* also originated in Germany: it was first used by J. C. Reil (1759–1853), in 1808 in an article and referred to the healing of the mind by the doctor (from the Greek: *psyche,* mind; *iatros,* doctor). Reil believed that all physicians should have the ability to treat the patient's mind (Marx, 1990).

From the 19th century until the middle of the 20th, psychiatrists from different countries developed their own nosologies of mental disorders. These were influenced by the philosophies and practices relating to the insane prevailing in each country. Some of the eminent men who shaped ideas about psychopathology at the time included: Pinel, Esquirol, Falret, Magnan, Morel and Charcot in France; Bucknill, Tuke, Maudsley and Pritchard in the UK; and Reil, Heinroth, Griesinger, Kahlbaum, Hecker, Kraepelin and Schneider in Germany. In the next section we focus on the work of Kraepelin, the most important of the 19th-century nosologists.

Kraepelin's contribution to classification

The German psychiatrist Emil Kraepelin (1856–1926) meticulously examined patients over many years. In the 1890s he devised a card system for collecting, sorting and comparing information on groups of patients. His approach to classification, published in the fifth edition of his textbook in 1896, has had, and continues to have, considerable influence on classifications of mental disorders. He observed not only the pattern of his patients' symptoms, but also their course over time, in order to try to discover common features that would help to distinguish between patient groups and be of value in assessing prognosis. On the basis of both cross-sectional and longitudinal observations, he was able to classify mental disorders into three main classes:

1 organic psychosis

2 endogenous psychosis

3 deviations of personality and reactive states.

This classification he hoped would lead to the discovery of the underlying aetiology of mental disorders. He also hoped that prevention and treatment of mental disorders could be based on this aetiological knowledge. Kraepelin's three main classes of disorder remain relevant today. His definition of 'organic psychosis' can be applied to current definitions of the dementias and confusional states. His definition of 'endogenous psychosis' includes present-day concepts of schizophrenia and psychotic affective disorders, while that of 'reactive states' could apply to non-psychotic unipolar depression, and anxiety and personality disorders (Jablensky, 1997).

Kraepelin further divided the endogenous (or functional) psychoses into dementia praecox and manic–depressive insanity. 'Dementia praecox' was an umbrella term, introduced by Kraepelin to bring together three rather different presentations of the illness: *hebephrenia*, described first by Hecker (1871); *catatonia*, described by Kahlbaum (1874); and *dementia paranoides*, which Kraepelin himself added as a subtype of his syndrome in 1913. Kraepelin separated these conditions from manic–depressive insanity (bipolar disorder), where full recovery occurred between episodes of illness. The term 'dementia praecox' was gradually dropped in favour of the term 'schizophrenia', largely as a result of Eugene Bleuler's influential work, originally published in 1911, entitled *Dementia Praecox or the Group of Schizophrenias* (Bleuler, 1911).

Different diagnostic practices in the USA and the UK

The change of name, along with an apparent subtle shift in emphasis, had a marked and lasting effect on diagnostic practice, which ultimately led to large diagnostic differences between the USA and northern Europe. The USA, where Bleuler's influence was the greater, had substantially higher first-admission rates of schizophrenia than in Kraepelin-influenced northern Europe, where there were much higher rates of manic–depressive psychosis.

These transatlantic differences were examined in a series of studies undertaken in the 1950s and 1960s, called the US/UK Diagnostic Series (Bellak, 1958; Kramer, 1961). Research teams in the USA and UK were trained to use a structured interview with all patients newly admitted to hospital with psychosis, to establish current psychopathology. The data obtained from the interviews were scored by a computer and a 'study' diagnosis was then compared with the admitting doctor's diagnosis. While the standardised study diagnoses showed good agreement for the rates of different psychotic disorders in the USA and the UK, the hospital diagnoses reflected the national differences noted above. These studies therefore indicated that the national differences in rates of schizophrenia and manic–depressive illness were due to diagnostic practices and did not reflect true differences in the incidence or prevalence of the disorders.

The studies also showed that training doctors to use a standardised interview could greatly improve the reliability between them (inter-rater reliability). Subsequently, the degree to which diagnostic practice differed on a more global scale was investigated in the International Pilot Study of Schizophrenia (IPSS) (World Health Organization, 1973) (see also Chapter 31, page 794). As well as examining the incidence and prevalence of schizophrenia in nine countries, this study also compared local diagnostic practices. As in the US/UK Diagnostic Series, a structured interview, the Present State Examination, was employed by the project team to elicit current psychopathology and cases were assigned to a single category according to the eighth edition of the *International Classification of Diseases* (World Health Organization, 1974) using a computerised diagnostic system called CATEGO (Wing *et al*, 1974). Over 1000 patients were interviewed in nine different countries. The results showed that for seven of the nine countries clinical diagnoses were consistent and largely in agreement with the project diagnosis. However, in two sites, Washington, DC, and Moscow, the local psychiatrists diagnosed schizophrenia more frequently than the project team. The study confirmed that inter-rater reliability could be dramatically improved if a structured interviewing approach was used and if a standardised diagnostic procedure such as a computerised scoring program was adopted.

In order to produce a computerised scoring program it was necessary to formulate diagnoses as a series of coding algorithms – a somewhat different approach to the methods for eliciting psychopathology being used clinically at the time. This requirement, along with proposals from other sources about how to overcome the unreliability of diagnosis in psychiatry, led to the introduction of operational definitions of psychiatric disorders.

Operational definitions

The operational approach to defining scientific concepts was originally proposed by Bridgman, a physicist, in 1927, and the idea was taken up and modified in 1961 by Hempel (a philosopher) for use in psychiatry. Hempel (1961) suggested that instead of stating that the typical features of a disease are features A, B, C, D and E, an unambiguous statement is presented defining precisely how much of A, B, C, D and E must be present to fulfil the definition. For example, to define the 'A' criterion of low mood in diagnosing unipolar depression operationally, it is necessary to specify that the mood must have been persistently low, and interfering with daily activity, for at least two weeks. Similar precisely quantified definitions (B, C, D and E) are also required to specify the number and type as well as the severity of additional symptoms that must be present to fulfil the diagnostic criteria for unipolar depression. Although such methods for defining psychiatric disorder are very familiar now, when first introduced they were heralded as revolutionary.

The first definition of a psychiatric disorder that lent itself to being cast in an operational format was that originally proposed for schizophrenia by Schneider. First published in German in 1939, the English translation appeared in 1959. A list of what he termed 'first rank' symptoms was diagnostic of schizophrenia provided they occurred in the absence of 'coarse brain disease'. Subsequent studies did show that these symptoms allow very high inter-rater agreement. Indeed, the first-rank symptoms have had considerable impact on the diagnosis of schizophrenia throughout Europe and subsequently in the United States and are included in the criteria for schizophrenia in both DSM–IV and ICD–10.

At the time he was writing, Schneider was not intending to produce an operational definition of schizophrenia. Consequently, the first operational definitions to be published *de novo* were the St Louis criteria (Feighner *et al*, 1972) and these were soon followed by a number of others, some for a broad range of disorders and some just for schizophrenia (Carpenter *et al*, 1973) or its subtypes (Tsuang & Winokur, 1974). However, of these, it was the Research Diagnostic Criteria (RDC) published in 1978 (Spitzer *et al*, 1978) together with the St Louis criteria of Feighner that were highly influential in the development of DSM–III (American Psychiatric Association, 1980), which was the first 'official' classificatory scheme to appear in an operationalised format.

Operational definitions: their structure

At this stage it may be worth examining the operational definition of one particular psychiatric disorder to see how the principles outlined in the previous sections of this chapter have been incorporated into modern diagnostic criteria. The three elements that underlie the concept of disorder in general – namely a syndrome, biological disadvantage or social dysfunction, and subjective distress – are all included in separate clauses. In addition, for the definition of a particular disorder, a fourth element – the boundaries between the disorder and its near neighbours – is also specified. The example selected is the DSM–IV criteria for hypochondriasis (Table 28.1), but there is no particular reason for selecting this condition and most of the definitions given in the DSM and ICD systems follow a very similar format, although, as noted in Table 28.1, DSM–IV has more 'specifier' subtypes than ICD–10.'

Monothetic and polythetic diagnoses

The diagnosis of hypochondriasis is made only when *all* the criteria (A–F) in the definition (Table 28.1) are present. A diagnosis of this type is called monothetic. Monothetic criteria are easy to memorise and understand but are not very reliable because this will be determined by the reliability of the weakest item. A more serious disadvantage of monothetic criteria is that they fail to cope adequately with the very varied presentation of many common psychiatric disorders, for example personality disorders. To avoid this difficulty, polythetic definitions may be used.

According to Sokal (1974), a polythetic classification is one in which members of a class share a large proportion of their properties but do not necessarily agree on the presence of any one property; that is, there is no single pathognomonic feature. A typical polythetic definition comprises a list of all possible symptoms that a patient with a given disorder may have, with the stipulation that a certain number of these items are required to make the diagnosis. For example, the DSM–IV definition of borderline personality disorder (see page 448) has nine items, of which five are required to make the diagnosis. Polythetic criteria are more robust and reliable than monothetic criteria but,

Table 28.1 An example of an operational definition of a psychiatric disorder: DSM–IV hypochondriasis (adapted with permission from DSM–IV–TR. Copyright 2000 American Psychiatric Association)

Criterion	Comment
A. Preoccupation with a fear of having a serious disease, or the belief that one has such a disease, based on a misinterpretation of bodily symptoms	This clause describes the core features of the disorder or the syndrome itself
B. The preoccupation persists despite appropriate medical evaluation and reassurance	This clause describes two specific operational tests, medical evaluation and reassurance. For the diagnosis, an examination has to be performed and negative results obtained, and reassurance must be given, without benefit
C. Belief in criterion A is not of delusional intensity (as in delusional disorder, somatic type) and is not restricted to a circumscribed concern about appearance (as in body dysmorphic disorder)	This is an exclusion clause and describes the borders of the syndrome and what conditions should be considered to be outside the specified syndrome. The two most important differential diagnoses, delusional disorder and body dysmorphic disorder, are highlighted
D. The preoccupation causes clinically significant distress or impairment in social, occupational or other important areas of functioning	Subjective clinical distress and functional impairment are key features for the definition of most DSM–IV psychiatric disorders and are gradually assuming greater prominence in disorder definition as there are so few objective criteria
E. The duration of the disturbances is at least 6 months	Transient hypochondriacal feelings, e.g. after an episode of flu or some other physical illness, are relatively common, but the condition must be severe and not trivial to qualify for a DSM–IV diagnosis of psychiatric disorder because such a designation will imply medical or other interventions. These milder conditions are effectively excluded by stipulating a 6-month period, which is the duration criteria for many DSM–IV disorders
F. The preoccupation is not better accounted for by generalised anxiety disorder, obsessive–compulsive disorder, panic disorder, major depressive disorder, separation anxiety or another somatoform disorder	This clause specifies the other similar or related conditions that should be excluded, i.e. the differential diagnoses. DSM–IV has excellent sections covering the differential diagnosis of most of the conditions it includes
Specifier: 'with poor insight'. Used if, for most of the time during the present episode, the person does not recognise that the concern about having a serious illness is excessive or unreasonable	DSM–IV, more than ICD–10, has subtypes, which are called specifiers. Here, the specifier subtypes are 'with insight' and 'with poor insight'

to return to the example of borderline personality disorder, theoretically there are 93 different combinations of items that can satisfy the criteria for the diagnosis (Frances *et al*, 1990).

Strengths and weaknesses of operational definitions

Having a set of precise operational rules for defining psychiatric disorders has certainly improved inter-rater agreement for diagnosis (reliability). Also, both ICD–10 and DSM–IV have received widespread international acceptance, both for clinical use and in research. Indeed, it is now quite difficult to get research studies of mental disorder published if participants are not defined using either or both classifications.

Balanced against these advantages are a number of disadvantages. First, there are many different operational definitions, especially for schizophrenia and affective disorders, none of which has proven validity. Second, although highly reliable, operational definitions such as those incorporated into DSM–IV and ICD–10 leave out much clinically relevant information about the person's condition. For example, information related to psychiatric history, family history and previous response to medication is usually omitted from operational definitions. Similarly, items that are difficult to rate, such as negative symptoms of schizophrenia, are often not included. Third, it is frequently the case that improved reliability has been largely brought about by employing a highly restrictive and prescriptive format for operational definitions. Also, assigning a diagnosis is a 'top down' procedure, with the rater attempting to fit the person's experience to a predetermined set of criteria. Individuals who fail to fulfil one or more item fall outside the diagnosis and end up in a 'not elsewhere specified' or 'atypical' category. It has been noted with some definitions that the majority of patients end up in such a category, which can then be larger than the main diagnostic groups (Farmer *et al*, 1992).

The US system – the Diagnostic and Statistical Manual (DSM)

In 1917 the American Psychiatric Association (APA) adopted a simple classificatory system to obtain statistics from US mental hospitals. By 1934 the APA switched to using the American Medical Association's 'standard classified nomenclature of disease', which was largely based on the sixth edition of Kraepelin's textbook of psychiatry. The first edition of the *Diagnostic and Statistical Manual of Mental Disorders* (DSM–I) was published in 1952. Psychoanalytic influence was dominant at the time and the term 'reaction' was used throughout the classification, reflecting the influence of Adolf Meyer's psychobiological view that mental disorders represented reactions of the personality to social, biological and psychological factors. DSM–II appeared in 1968 but showed little advance on DSM–I, as the psychoanalytic influence was still strong, except the aim was to base the classification as closely as possible on the then current ICD, ICD–8, but, as this schedule continued to include aetiological criteria within its definitions of psychiatric disorder, neither classification proved to be satisfactory..

The introduction of operational definitions for mental disorders in DSM–III represented a real paradigm shift in trying to employ *scientific evidence* as the main guiding principle in classification. The APA decided, in the face of many competing schools of psychiatric nosology, that DSM–III should be atheoretical and as free as possible of any assumptions regarding causation and pathogenesis. It also decided to abolish the psychotic–neurotic dichotomy, which had dominated psychiatric nosology for the previous half century (the word 'neurosis' no longer appears in DSM).

The national and international bodies charged with producing the ICD and DSM classifications convene committees of experts, who employ various criteria to make decisions about the constituent elements of the diagnostic categories, such as current diagnostic practice, historical perspective, and personal and clinical opinion, as well as the research evidence available at the time. In addition, starting with the DSM–III criteria, field trials of draft versions of the proposed criteria have been done to test their applicability and clinical utility.

The revised version of DSM–III, DSM–III–R, was published in 1987, DSM–IV in 1994 and DSM–IV–TR ('text revision') in 2000. The impact of these three subsequent versions of the classification was very much less than that of DSM–III, as they are all essentially refinements that have taken into account the most recent scientific developments, and all three manuals have the same basic structure and an atheoretical clinical approach. As well as operational definitions for all major psychiatric disorders, personality disorders are also operationally defined. In addition to these main categories, the DSM criteria are multi-axial: each patient can be rated on five different axes. Axis I consists of the main psychiatric syndromes, while axis II lists any co-occurring personality disorders. Axis III refers to any concurrent physical health problems, while axis IV lists important psychosocial stressors that have occurred in the previous year. Finally, axis V evaluates the highest level of functioning in the previous year. In practice, axes IV and V are seldom used, even in research, and most clinicians use only axes I and II.

The World Health Organization system – ICD

The *International Classification of Diseases* (ICD), published by the World Health Organization, covers all diseases, not just psychiatric conditions. ICD finds its origins in the International Statistical Congress held in Paris in 1853. Two medical statisticians, William Farr from London and Jacques Bertillon from Paris, presented a list of causes of death which became known as 'Bertillon's classification of the cause of death'. This was revised every five years by the International Statistical Institute and was later taken over by the French government, which published the 'International list of the causes of death'. After the Second World War the World Health Organization took over this task and included diseases as well as causes of death. This new list was renamed *The International Statistical Classification of Diseases, Injuries and Causes of Death* and was published in 1948, and this became ICD–6, which included a separate psychiatric section. As noted above, there was an attempt to align DSM–II more closely with ICD–8, but there continued to be clear differences of interpretation on the boundaries between schizophrenia, affective disorder and personality disorder. The paradigm shift that took place in the US with the publication of DSM–III has now led to a high degree of convergence of between ICD–10 and DSM–IV, the two major classification schemes now in current use.

In the present (10th) edition of ICD, psychiatric disorders are included in chapter 6, or 'F', which is why all the ICD codes for mental disorder have this prefix. The main ICD–10 has been produced in several different formats, each tailored to specific circumstances. These include the following:

1 A version for use in general clinical psychiatry. The main volume of ICD–10 includes 'the clinical descriptions and diagnostic guidelines' for use mainly by psychiatrists and clinical psychologists in everyday practice, and contains 'traditional' descriptive definitions of disorders. This version is also known as 'the blue book'.

2 A version for researchers. The version for use by researchers, the Diagnostic Criteria for Research (DCR–10; World Health Organization, 1993), contains explicit or operational definitions of disorder (this is sometimes known as 'the green book').

3 A version suitable for primary care. There is also a shortened version for primary care (ICD–10–PHC; World Health Organization, 1996) and this was added because the presentation of psychopathology in primary care and general hospital settings may be quite different to that seen in psychiatric practice (Ustun *et al*, 1995).

ICD–10 also introduced the 'Family of documents', covering neurological disorders and disorders of the elderly, which are not primarily related to psychopathology. Although ICD–10 is a primarily descriptive classification, in some areas aetiology does form part of the organisation of classification, particularly regarding organic brain syndromes and substance-related disorders.

Disorders are arranged into ten groups of categories:

F0 the dementias and other organic brain syndromes

F1 mental disorders due to substance misuse

F2 schizophrenia and other non-affective psychoses

F3 affective disorders

F4 neurotic, stress-related and somatoform disorders

F5 disorders of eating, sleep and sexual functioning

F6 personality disorders

F7 mental retardation

F8 disorders of psychological development

F9 behavioural and emotional disorders with onset in childhood or adolescence.

Features of ICD–10

ICD–9, the previous edition of the World Health Organization's nosology, was published in 1965, and consequently it was quite out of date by the time 10th edition was finally published, in 1992. ICD–9 included a neurotic–psychotic conceptual dichotomy for disorders which was abolished in DSM–III and subsequent versions of DSM and was largely avoided in ICD–10, although the terms 'neurotic' and 'psychotic' are still retained as descriptive terms, for example in 'neurotic, stress-related and somatoform disorders' (F40–F48).

The arrangement of disorders in ICD–10 is according to major common themes and this means that, for example, cyclothymia (F34.0) is included in affective disorders (F3) rather than in F6 (disorders of adult personality and behaviour). Similarly, schizotypal disorder, previously regarded as a personality disorder, is included in F2 (schizophrenic illness). Mood disorders in F3 employ the term 'bipolar' rather than 'manic–depressive', which had been used in ICD–9, since there is now much research evidence to suggest that a bipolar–unipolar dichotomy is a more appropriate way to classify mood disorders (Farmer & McGuffin, 1989). Both depression and mania are also subdivided according to severity in ICD–10, unlike in previous classifications.

Anxiety disorders such as phobic disorders, panic and generalised anxiety, and obsessive–compulsive disorder, as well as reactions to stress, adjustment and dissociative disorders are grouped together in F4. The increasing evidence for somatoform disorders and chronic fatigue syndrome has ensured that these disorders also have their own categories in ICD–10.

In general, the rules of taxonomy require that each patient be restricted to the membership of a single diagnostic category. Unlike DSM–IV, ICD–10 is not multiaxial. While in theory this seems to be desirable, in practice clinicians frequently encounter patients who they consider cannot be adequately described without using two or more categories. Although ICD–10 does allow more than one diagnosis to be recorded, the authors recommend that there is one main diagnosis and subsidiary or secondary ones. It is also recommended that precedence is given to that diagnosis most relevant to the purpose for which the diagnoses are being collected. In clinical work this is often the disorder that gave rise to the consultation or contact with health services. On other occasions it may well be the main 'lifetime' diagnosis. The classification also has an in-built hierarchy, with lower numbers taking precedence; thus, an F0 (organic disorders) category has greater 'significance' than an F6 diagnosis (personality disorder).

Multiple diagnosis, hierarchies and comorbidity

As noted above, it is a common clinical observation that some patients may have two or more psychiatric diagnoses. A patient with dementia may become depressed. Are these two conditions independent or has one led to the other? Jaspers (1959) was the first to describe an explicit diagnostic hierarchy and in his scheme the more severe and pervasive disorder was regarded as primary and causal, and the less severe disorder as secondary. Organic disorder took precedence over all other disorders, followed by schizophrenia; manic–depression was at the third level, and at the fourth and lowest level were the neuroses and personality disorders.

Comorbidity

Diagnostic hierarchies have the drawback that they make the unproven assumption that one disorder is more fundamental or more pervasive than another. Comorbidity makes no assumption as to cause and effect but merely documents that two or more disorders have been simultaneously diagnosed in the same individual. In contrast to hierarchies, comorbidity offers an atheoretical approach and this has found increasing utility in research settings.

Caron & Rutter (1991) make a distinction between *false comorbidity* and *true comorbidity*. False comorbidity can arise because the definition of a disorder may be so fundamentally flawed that only a few patients fulfil the diagnostic criteria of just one disorder. This occurs with the current official descriptions of personality disorder (see Chapter 18): many individuals fulfil criteria for several different types of personality disorder yet clearly only have one personality.

False comorbidity can also be the result of an artificial subdivision of disorders. For example, in the DSM–IV scheme generalised anxiety disorder is separated from panic disorder, but many individuals can be diagnosed with both conditions, indicating that there may not be a significant boundary between the two in clinical populations.

True comorbidity can be established in an epidemiological survey and it may have a variety of differing causes. Schizophrenia is often comorbid with substance misuse, which may occur through a variety of different mechanisms. For example, some people will become psychotic through taking stimulants such as amphetamines, while others with schizophrenia will drift into inner-city areas where substance misuse is endemic; a third group may report that cannabis soothes their psychotic symptoms. A hierarchical explanation would assume the schizophrenia had 'caused' the drug misuse, but such an oversimplification is not tenable in complex clinical situations.

Comorbidity merely documents that the two conditions have occurred together. It makes no assumptions about cause and effect, and is therefore scientifically more accurate. However, while it is, for these reasons, more useful in a research setting, in the clinical world doctors still prefer one primary diagnosis and tend to prefer hierarchical explanations for any other diagnoses the patient may have.

Diagnostic interview instruments and rating scales

Structured and semi-structured diagnostic interviews

The introduction of operationalised formats to define mental disorders meant that it was very easy to construct diagnostic interviews and rating scales to assess the presence, severity and duration of psychopathology. Although the first 'modern era' diagnostic interviews and rating scales were produced in the 1960s, their numbers proliferated following the introduction of operationally defined classifications in the 1970s. Initially constructed as 'pencil and paper' tests, both interviews and rating scales were readily adapted to computerised application, either self-administered or administered by an interviewer. In addition, the scoring algorithms could be included in a computerised 'package', so the results were available at the click of a mouse.

As discussed above, the first diagnostic interviews scored by computerised algorithms were those introduced in the US/UK Diagnostic Series in the 1960s. The Present State Examination scored by the CATEGO program has passed through several editions over 30 years. The tenth edition of the Present State Examination was incorporated in the Schedules for Clinical Assessment in Neuropsychiatry (SCAN) (Wing *et al*, 1990), which has the approval of the World Health Organization and is still widely used today. The latest version of the CATEGO scoring program (CATEGO5) is used to assign ICD–10 and DSM–IV codes to SCAN data.

Also developed for the US/UK studies was the Mental Status Examination, which was a prototype for the Schedules for Affective Disorders and Schizophrenia (SADS), which had been designed to cover the items included in the Research Diagnostic Criteria following their publication in the late 1970s (Spitzer & Endicott, 1978). Following the introduction of DSM–III, the lead author of the SADS, Professor Robert Spitzer, published the Structured Clinical Interview for DSM–III (SCID) (Spitzer *et al*, 1992), an interview designed to cover the new classification. Later, a second interview, the SCID-II, was added in, specifically to deal with diagnosing people with a personality disorder. Both the SADS and the SCID have been updated to incorporate DSM–III–R and DSM–IV classifications and continue to enjoy wide international use.

These three interviews, SCAN, SADS and SCID, have been designed to evaluate psychopathology in clinical samples, and so they concentrate on psychopathology at the severe (and psychosis) end of the spectrum. Those using the interviews require some clinical experience as well as training in the use of the interview itself. Around the same time, diagnostic interviews for epidemiological use were also developed, which focused on more common and milder disorders.

In 1980, the National Institute of Mental Health in the USA commissioned the development of a structured diagnostic interview for a large epidemiological study of the mental health of 15,000 respondents from the general population living in five US cities (Regier *et al*, 1984). This was known as the Epidemiologic Catchment Area study and led to the development of the Diagnostic Interview Schedule (DIS) (Robins *et al*, 1981), which in turn led to the creation of the Composite International Diagnostic Interview (CIDI) by the same team. In contrast to the SCAN, SADS and SCID, these interviews do not require any clinical experience to administer and can be reliably used by lay interviewers who have been trained in their use.

All the above interviews have since received the approval of the World Health Organization for use in international research and have been translated and back-translated into several languages. Despite their ease of application, it is still imperative that investigators do not use these interviews without undergoing training to a sufficient level to ensure that all raters score the interview in the same way and achieve acceptable inter-rater agreement (Farmer *et al*,

2002). All published studies in which such diagnostic interviews have been used should report a measure of the inter-rater agreement.

Scales for screening and for measuring change

Rating scales, which again can be self-administered or administered by an interviewer, have a rather different function to diagnostic interviews.

Self-report scales

Self-report scales are of limited usefulness and have numerous systematic sources of error. Perhaps the most common bias found in almost all self-rating scales is the *response set*, which refers to the tendency either to agree with all the statements made in the questionnaire or, for a few patients, to disagree with every item, without seriously considering their meaning. Related to this is the issue of *social desirability*, as most people tend to favour giving a positive answer to symptoms they regard as socially desirable, but become more defensive or may even deny the presence of socially undesirable symptoms (and most psychiatric symptoms have an element of social undesirability). Errors of *central tendency* reflect the reluctance of some respondents to use either of the extreme points of the scale, instead preferring the more central points. This tendency makes a four-point scale preferable to either a three- or a five-point scale. *The halo effect* refers to the tendency to make a judgement early on in the process of rating and then to apply this to all subsequent items. *Proximity errors* refer to the tendency to rate all adjacent items similarly.

Self-rating scales have two main general uses:

1 to rate change in psychopathology over time, for example in drug trials

2 to screen for the presence of psychopathology, for example psychiatric 'case finding' in epidemiological or primary care settings.

Some self-rated questionnaires have been used for both purposes, but they are rarely used in routine clinical work as, for example, people with a severe mental illness are likely to lack insight or to have impaired concentration, and therefore be unable to fill in even a simple form.

There are now a large number of self-rated scales covering all the different categories of disorder, many of which are described elsewhere in this book.

Observer-rated scales

It was the revolution in psychopharmacology of the late 1950s, and the need to measure the effects of the newly introduced antidepressants, that led to the development of the first interviewer-administered questionnaire, the Hamilton Rating Scale for Depression (HRSD) (Hamilton, 1960). The Hamilton 'family' of self-report and interviewer-administered interviews are still widely used in drug trials. Other interviewer-rated questionnaires used in measuring change in depression and anxiety symptoms are the Comprehensive Psychopathological Rating Scale (CPRS) (Asberg & Shalling, 1979) and a shorter version of the full 65-item CPRS covering depression items, the Montgomery–Asberg Depression Rating Scale (MADRAS) (Montgomery & Asberg, 1979).

Observer scales are more trouble to use than self-rated instruments, since interviewer training and attention to inter-rater reliability are required, whereas self-report questionnaires can be readily sent by post for completion. In addition, interviews that are used for diagnostic purposes are subject to observer bias. Although the general assumption is that observer-rated scales give more accurate and conservative results than data derived from self-reporting scales, a study in a clinic sample of people with depression that compared two self-report scales with two observer-rated scales of depression found high levels of agreement between all four scales, with little advantage for one method of rating over another (Feinberg *et al*, 1981).

Screening questionnaires

Among the first screening instruments for general psychiatric morbidity in primary care populations was the General Health Questionnaire (GHQ), first published in 1978. Devised to screen for common, less severe forms of (mainly) depression and anxiety, the GHQ was compared against a 'gold standard', namely the Present State Examination, undertaken by a clinician, to calculate the sensitivity, specificity and other psychometric properties of the screening process (see Goldberg & Williams, 1988).

Screening questionnaires such as the GHQ are usually sent by post for completion at the start of a study. Only a proportion of those responding are then contacted for further examination, by either telephone or face-to-face interview. The screening provides an opportunity to select a specific subset of the total population for further enquiry (this is described in Chapter 27, page 702).

Research procedures

Poly-diagnostic approaches

The fact that several different sets of operational definitions have been published since the 1970s (and more for schizophrenia) does not affect the clinician, who is usually expected to use the most recently published ICD or DSM definition, but for the researcher the constant revisions of the definitions of psychiatric disorder can be problematic. The issue is not whether operational definitions should be used in research but which set to choose, since there are now a number of equally reliable sets of criteria and no evidence that one definition is more valid than another. If the most recent criteria are selected for practical and pragmatic reasons, it may be difficult to compare results with earlier studies that employed different operational definitions. This can cause problems with the interpretation of epidemiological changes over time (Regier *et al*, 1984). It has been shown that for some of the earlier definitions there may be little overlap between participants defined according to different operational criteria (Brockington *et al*, 1978). Also, different methods used to collect participants can influence the numbers assigned to different diagnostic categories by different sets of operational definitions (Farmer *et al*, 1992).

One solution to such problems is to use a polydiagnostic approach and to collect sufficient information on each participant to be able to apply multiple sets of criteria. Although the statistical analyses need to take account of the multiple testing that this produces, the advantage of such an approach is that, in addition to defining participants according to the most recently published criteria, a comparison becomes possible with older criteria used in earlier studies. The computerised OPCRIT checklist (McGuffin *et al*, 1991) was produced so that multiple definitions of various psychoses and affective disorders could be applied to interview and case-note information using a simple 90-item checklist. OPCRIT has been used in a number of epidemiological and genetic studies (Williams *et al*, 1996) and can be applied with good inter-rater agreement (McGuffin *et al*, 1991).

A similar system but relating to attention-deficit hyperactivity disorder in children (Hypescheme) allows the rater to obtain sufficient information to apply the two main operational definitions of the disorder (currently ICD–10 and DSM–IV) not only to that disorder but also to various other comorbid disorders (Curran *et al*, 2000).

Consensus and best-estimate diagnostic procedures

In research, a number of sources of information may be used to assign a diagnostic category. As well as structured or semi-structured interviews with a relative or other informant, case notes may also be available. In order to collate the information from all these sources a best-estimate or consensus diagnosis can be applied if a group of researchers collectively review all information sources (Leckman *et al*, 1982). Although costly and time-consuming, this approach has practical and common-sense appeal, and has been shown to compare well with computer-generated diagnoses (Craddock *et al*, 1996).

The future of psychiatric nosology

Some readers of this chapter will be frustrated that this discussion of diagnostic issues and attempts to achieve a resolution of these complex issues has quoted widely from studies dating from several decades past. This is mainly because this topic has attracted little or no research in recent years. It is as if the whole diagnostic issue has been 'put on hold'.

Until the precise aetiology and hence the pathology of mental disorders can be established, we can only define syndromes, which, at best, can only achieve good reliability. Valid definitions of the disease processes associated with psychopathology remain elusive. Future generations may be able to apply new technologies as they become available, especially in the fields of genetics and neuroimaging, and these may provide insights into brain structure and function and their role in psychiatric disorder, which in turn may inform the diagnostic criteria. The committees that are currently considering criteria for DSM–V and ICD–11 have already begun to employ some of the new evidence in reshaping diagnostic categories. However, until pathological processes are properly delineated, each set of operational definitions will remain no more than a 'working hypothesis', requiring continued re-evaluation, and so the process of revision and repeated fine-tuning of diagnostic criteria that started in the 1980s with DSM–III is likely to continue long into the future.

Developments in the clinical world may also affect psychiatric nosology. For example, recent changes in the way health services are organised have led to the suggestion that new ways of defining disorder should also take much greater account of clinical realities, such as service utilisation, the need for care, quality of life, treatment response and outcome (Ustun *et al*, 1995; Jenkins *et al*, 1997). The multi-axial approach of DSM–IV has been little used, yet covers far more than a solely phenomenological diagnosis. Perhaps it is time for clinicians to adopt a more multi-axial approach, since this gives a much more holistic and complete account of an individual than merely assigning a diagnosis.

References

American Psychiatric Association (1980) *Diagnostic and Statistical Manual of Mental Disorders* (3rd edn) (DSM–III). Washington, DC: APA.

American Psychiatric Association (1987) *Diagnostic and Statistical Manual of Mental Disorders* (3rd edn, revised) (DSM–III–R). Washington, DC: APA.

American Psychiatric Association (1994) *Diagnostic and Statistical Manual of Mental Disorders* (4th edn) (DSM–IV). Washington, DC: APA.

American Psychiatric Association (2000) *Diagnostic and Statistical Manual* (text revision) (DSM–IV–TR). Washington, DC: APA.

Asberg, M. & Shalling, D. (1979) Construction of a new psychiatric rating instrument, the Comprehensive Psychopathological Rating Scale (CPRS). *Progress in Neuro-Psychopharmacology*, **3**, 405–412.

Bellak, L. (1958) *Schizophrenia: A Review of the Syndrome*. New York: Logos Press.

Bentall, R. P., Claridge, G. S. & Slade, P. D. (1990) The multi-dimensional nature of schizotypal traits: a factor analytic study with normal subjects. *British Journal of Clinical Psychology*, **28**, 363–367.

Bleuler, E. (1911) *Dementia Praecox or the Group of Schizophrenias* (trans. S. M. Clemens, 1950). New Haven, CT: Yale University Press.

Bridgman, P. W. (1927) *The Logic of Modern Physics*. New York: Macmillan.

Brockington, J. F., Kendell, R. E. & Leff, J. P. (1978) Definitions of schizophrenia: concordance and prediction of outcome. *Psychological Medicine*, **8**, 387–398.

Caron, C. & Rutter, M. (1991) Co-morbidity in child psychopathology, concepts, issues and research strategies. *Journal of Child Psychology and Psychiatry*, **32**, 1063–1080.

Carpenter, W. T., Strauss, J. S. & Bartko, J. J. (1973) Flexible system for the diagnosis of schizophrenia. *Science*, **182**, 1275–1278.

Cohen, J. A. (1960) A coefficient of agreement for normal scales. *Educational and Psychological Measurements*, **20**, 37.

Costello, C. G. (1992) Research on symptoms versus research on syndromes. Argument in favour of allocating more time to the study of symptoms. *British Journal of Psychiatry*, **160**, 304–309.

Craddock, N., Asherson, P., Owen, M. J., *et al* (1996) Concurrent validity of the OPCRIT diagnostic system: comparison of OPCRIT diagnoses with consensus best estimate lifetime diagnoses. *British Journal of Psychiatry*, **169**, 1–6.

Curran, S., Newman, S., Taylor, E., *et al* (2000) Hypescheme: an operational criteria checklist and minimum dataset for molecular genetic studies of attention deficit and hyperactivity disorders. *American Journal of Medical Genetics (Neuropsychiatric Genetics)*, **96**, 244–250.

Erikson, K. (1964) Notes on the sociology of deviance. In *The Other Side* (ed. H. Becker). New York: Free Press.

Esquirol, J. E. D. (1833) *Observations of the Illusions of the Insane*. London: Renshaw & Rush.

Farmer, A. E. & Griffiths, H. (1992) Labelling and illness in primary care: comparing factors influencing general practitioners' and psychiatrists' decisions regarding patient referral to mental illness services. *Psychological Medicine*, **22**, 717–726.

Farmer, A. E. & McGuffin, P. (1989) The classification of the depressions. Contemporary confusion revisited. *British Journal of Psychiatry*, **155**, 437–443.

Farmer, A. E., Wessely, S., Castle, D., *et al* (1992) Methodological issues in using a polydiagnostic approach to define psychotic illness. *British Journal of Psychiatry*, **161**, 824–830.

Farmer, A. E., McGuffin, P. & Williams, J. (2002) *Measuring Psychopathology*. Oxford: Oxford University Press.

Feighner, J. P., Robins, E., Guze, S. B., *et al* (1972) Diagnostic criteria for use in psychiatric research. *Archives of General Psychiatry*, **26**, 57–67.

Feinberg, M., Carroll, B. J., Smouse, P. E., *et al* (1981) The Carroll rating scale for depression. III. Comparison with other rating scales. *British Journal of Psychiatry*, **138**, 205–209.

Frances, A., Pincus, H. A., Widiger, T. A., *et al* (1990) DSM–IV: work in progress. *American Journal of Psychiatry*, **147**, 1439–1448.

Goldberg, D. P. & Williams, P (1988) *User's Guide to the General Health Questionnaire*. London: NFER-Nelson.

Hamilton, M. (1960) A rating scale for depression. *Journal of Neurology, Neurosurgery and Psychiatry*, **23**, 56–62.

Hecker, E. (1871) Die Hebephrenie. *Virchows Archiv für Patholgische Anatomie*, **52**, 392–449.

Hempel, C. G. (1961) Introduction to problems of taxonomy. In *Field Studies in the Mental Disorders* (ed. J. Zubin), pp. 3–22. New York: Grune & Stratton.

Jablensky, A. (1997) The 100-year epidemiology of schizophrenia. *Schizophrenia Research*, **28**, 111–125.

Jaspers, M. K. (1959) *Allgemeine Pscyhopathologie* (7th edn) (trans. J. Hoenig & M. W. Hamilton, 1962). Manchester: Manchester University Press.

Jenkins, R., Lewis, G., Bebbington, P., *et al* (1997) The National Psychiatric Morbidity Survey of Great Britain: initial findings from the household survey. *Psychological Medicine*, **27**, 775–789.

Kahlbaum, K. L. (1874) *Catatonia* (trans. Y. Levi & T. Pridon, 1973). Baltimore, MD: Johns Hopkins University Press.

Kendell, R. E. (1975) *The Role of Diagnosis in Psychiatry*. Oxford: Blackwell Science.

Kraepelin, E. (1896) *Psychiatrie. Ein Lehrbuch für studirende und Artze* (5th edn). Leipzig: J. A. Barth. Translated in part in Cutting, J. C. & Shepherd, M. (eds) (1986) *Schizophrenia: The Origin and Development of Its Study in Europe*. Cambridge: Cambridge University Press.

Kraepelin, E. (1913) *Psychiatrie*, Vol. 3, Part 2 (trans. as *Dementia Praecox and Paraphenia*). Edinburgh: Livingstone.

Kramer, M. (1961) Some problems for international research suggested by observations as differences in first admission rates to mental hospitals of England & Wales, and of the United States. In *Proceedings of the Third World Congress of Psychiatry*, Vol. 3, pp. 153–160.

Kraupl-Taylor, F. (1971) A logical analysis of the medico-psychological concept of disease. *Psychological Medicine*, **1**, 356–364; **2**, 7–16.

Leckman, J. F., Sholomskas, D., Thompson, W. D., *et al* (1982) Best estimate of lifetime psychiatric diagnosis: a methodological study. *Archives of General Psychiatry*, **39**, 879–883.

Marx, O. M. (1990) German Romantic psychiatry. *History of Psychiatry*, **1**, 351–381.

McGuffin, P., Farmer, A. E. & Harvey, I. (1991) A polydiagnostic application of operational criteria in studies in psychotic illness: development and reliability of OPCRIT system. *Archives of General Psychiatry*, **48**, 764–770.

Menninger, K. (1963) *The Vital Balance: The Life Processes in Mental Health and Disease*. New York: Viking Press.

Mindham, R. H. S., Scadding, J. G. & Cawley, R. H. (1992) Diagnoses are not diseases. *British Journal of Psychiatry*, **161**, 686–690.

Montgomery, S. & Asberg, M. (1979) A new depression scale designed to be sensitive to change. *British Journal of Psychiatry*, **134**, 382–389.

Persons, J. B. (1986) The advantages of studying psychological phenomena rather than psychiatric diagnoses. *American Psychologist*, **41**, 1252–1260.

Regier, D. A., Myers, J. K., Krammer, M., *et al* (1984) The NIMH Epidemiologic Catchment Area program. Historical context major objectives and study population and characteristics. *Archives of General Psychiatry*, **41**, 934–941.

Regier, D. A., Kaelber, C. T., Rae, D. S., *et al* (1998) Instruments for mental disorders. Implications for research and policy. *Archives of General Psychiatry*, **55**, 109–115.

Robins, L. N., Helzer, J. E., Croughan, J., *et al* (1981) National Institute of Mental Health, Diagnostic Interview Schedule: its history, characteristics and validity. *Archives of General Psychiatry*, **38**, 381–389.

Scadding, J. G. (1967) Diagnosis, the clinician and the computer. *Lancet*, *ii*, 877–882.

Scheff, T. (1966) *Being Mentally Ill*. Chicago, IL: Aldine.

Schneider, K. (1939) *Clinical Psychopathology* (trans. M. Hamilton, 1959). New York: Grune & Stratton.

Sokal, R. R. (1974) Classification: purposes, principles, progress, prospects. *Science*, **185**, 115–123.

Spitzer, R. L. & Endicott, J. R. (1978) *Schedule for Affective Disorders and Schizophrenia*. New York: New York State Psychiatric Institute.

Spitzer, R. L., Endicott, J. R. & Robins, E. (1978) Research Diagnostic Criteria: rationale and reliability. *Archives of General Psychiatry*, **35**, 773–782.

Spitzer, R. L., Williams, J. B. W., Gibbon, M., *et al* (1992) The Structured Clinical Interview for DSM–III–R (SCID): history, rationale and description. *Archives of General Psychiatry*, **49**, 624–629.

Szasz, T. S. (1960) *The Myth of Mental Illness*. New York: Harper.

Tsuang. M. T. & Winokur, G. (1974) Criteria for subtyping schizophrenia. *Archives of General Psychiatry*, **31**, 43–47.

Ustun, T. B., Goldberg, D., Cooper, J., *et al* (1995) A new classification of mental disorders based upon management for use in primary care. *British Journal of General Practice*, **45**, 211–215.

Williams, J., Farmer, A. E., Ackenheil, M., *et al* (1996) A multicentre inter-rater reliability study using the OPCRIT computerized diagnostic system. *Psychological Medicine*, **26**, 775–783.

Wing, J. K., Cooper, J. E. & Sartorius, N. (1974) *The Measurement and Psychiatric Symptoms*. Cambridge: Cambridge University Press.

Wing, J. K., Babor, T., Brugha, T., *et al* (1990) SCAN: Schedules for the Clinical Assessment in Neuropsychiatry. *Archives of General Psychiatry*, **47**, 589–593.

World Health Organization (1973) *Report on International Pilot Study of Schizophrenia. Vol. 1*. Geneva: WHO.

World Health Organization (1974) *The Eighth Revision of the International Classification of Diseases* (ICD–8). Geneva: WHO.

World Health Organization (1992) *The Tenth Revision of the International Classification of Diseases and Related Health Problems* (ICD–10). Geneva: WHO.

World Health Organization (1993) *Diagnostic Criteria for Research – Geneva. International Classification of Diseases 10th Edition*. Geneva: WHO.

World Health Organization (1996) *Diagnostic and Management Guidelines for Mental Health Disorders in Primary Care ICD–10*. Chapter V, Primary care version. Bern: Hogrefe & Huber.

CHAPTER 29

Mental health services

Rosalind Ramsay and Frank Holloway

This chapter provides an account of contemporary policy and practice in the organisation and provision of mental health services for adults of working age in England. (Healthcare has been devolved to the constituent countries of the UK.) It begins with a brief discussion of the evolution of psychiatric services both in England and in a number of other countries. The components of a comprehensive mental health service are then presented and discussed in turn. Throughout there is an attempt to relate policy and practice to the expanding evidence base that has been provided by mental health services research.

The focus of this chapter is on the practical service response to people with a severe mental illness, such as schizophrenia, rather than people with much more prevalent less severe mental health problems, which are described in Chapter 30. It is important to be aware of the salience of cultural, ideological, economic and political factors in the evolution and current state of mental health services. This is reflected most starkly in changes in mental health law over time, as legislation has addressed the particular public concerns about mental illness then current.

Our evidence base is, of course, provisional, qualified and subject to change as knowledge advances. Some distinction should be made between the role of mental health services as a means to deliver effective *treatments* for mental illness and the provision of *care* that minimises the effect of mental illness on the individual, the family and society. Service structures are, in themselves, not treatments but a vehicle for the delivery of treatment and care.

The evolution of mental healthcare

Beginnings

Before the 18th century, there was very little organised care in England for people with a mental illness. Mental healthcare depended almost exclusively on family members, alms-giving and generic provision for the indigent within the evolving framework of the Poor Law. Those who were behaviourally disturbed were kept in workhouses, Bridewells and gaols. The Bethlem Hospital in the City of London, which was for several hundred years the sole specialist facility in the kingdom for those who were mentally ill, was recorded in 1403 as containing six insane inmates (Scull, 1979).

People with financial resources might be looked after at home, taken into the paid care of a family or be treated in a private 'mad-house' run by a 'mad-doctor'. (This term was used to describe those members of the medical profession who claimed expertise in the treatment of mental illness and had no overtly pejorative connotation.) The 'mad-house' or asylum came to dominate practice and thought about mental healthcare during the 18th century. A handful of public asylums, initially funded through private benefactions, opened in this period, of which St Luke's was the first, in London in 1751.

The 18th-century 'mad-doctors' deployed both physical and mental or 'moral' approaches to the treatment of their patients. Physical treatments included blood-letting, purges, blistering and cold-water immersion, and aimed to alter the hypothesised organic basis of madness (Porter, 1987). However, influential practitioners were sceptical of the efficacy of physical treatments. William Battie, one of the founders of St Luke's Hospital, wrote in his 1758 *Treatise on Madness* that 'management did much more than medicines' (quoted in Porter, 1987, p. 207). Moral management owed much to the associationistic psychology of John Locke, and was based on the belief that some forms of madness were acquired as a result of life experiences and could be cured by psychological means, while others were inherent in the individual. This physical–psychological dualism persists to this day.

The 19th century and the rise of the asylum

Increasing concern about conditions of care and the potential for inappropriate detention in the 'mad-houses' and asylums resulted in a series of Acts of Parliament, culminating in the Lunatics Act 1845. This set up the Lunacy Commission, which built on the role of the commissioners who had overseen London's asylums since 1774. A reform movement at the turn of the 19th century, drawing from the example of Pinel at the Bicêtre in revolutionary Paris and emanating in England from the York Retreat, promoted 'moral treatment' within an asylum.

Moral treatment consisted of a range of approaches that emphasised kindness and the minimisation of coercion, the importance of activity and the development of self-control by those who were mentally ill, living together within a community (Porter, 1987). Its proponents drew an optimistic distinction between incurable organic brain disease and functional disorders that might be amenable to moral treatment (Scull, 1979). The aim was for patients to be discharged when their condition had recovered or improved.

The County Asylums Act 1845 compelled every county and borough to provide asylum treatment for its pauper lunatics, reflecting best practice as presented to a select committee of Parliament. The tradition of service responsibility for a defined geographical area has persisted in the UK. In both the USA and the UK, a comprehensive system of public asylums evolved during the 19th century. Success rates were initially high: Bockhoven (1954) reported that, over a 20-year period (1833–52), 71% of inmates at Worcester State Hospital admitted after less than 1 year of illness were successfully discharged. However, as the asylums expanded, conditions for patients deteriorated and medico-cultural perspectives on mental illness changed, discharge rates declined and the system entered its 'long sleep'.

During the subsequent era of custodial care, cost containment became a priority (Scull, 1979). The 'long sleep' was conceptually closely linked with 19th-century degeneracy models of lunacy, which eclipsed associationism. Reflecting popular concerns over inappropriate detention, the Lunacy Act 1890 provided for tight legal restrictions on admission to the asylum, but showed rather little concern for the fate of the inmate once admitted. However, even during this period there was some interest in community care, as evidenced by the founding in 1879 by a hospital chaplain of the Mental After Care Association.

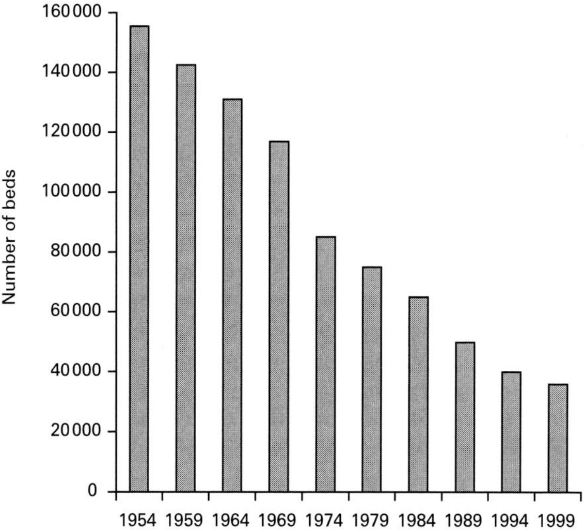

Fig. 29.1 Psychiatric bed numbers in England and Wales, 1954–99.

Deinstitutionalisation

Informal admission to an asylum became possible only with the passage of the Mental Treatment Act 1930, which also encouraged local authorities to develop out-patient clinics and after-care services. This Act marks the formal beginning of community-care policies in England, although implementation was disrupted by the Great Depression of the 1930s and the Second World War. By the 1930s Freud's ideas had begun to have an impact on educated public opinion, and psychological explanations for and responses to mental illness had again gained credibility.

The expansion of institutional care for people with a mental illness, a worldwide phenomenon, was first halted in Britain and the USA in the mid-1950s (see Fig. 29.1). The reasons for the subsequent sustained decline in mental hospital bed numbers are complex and not fully understood. Major factors were the introduction of effective antipsychotic medication, a shift in professional attitudes back towards the active physical and social treatment of mental illness, and increasing public acceptance of those who are mentally ill.

Many traditional mental hospitals were transformed in the years after 1945, as both the concept of the 'therapeutic community' (developed by military psychiatrists during the Second World War) and the 'open door' movement influenced psychiatric practice. In the prewar mental hospital all the doors were locked and there was little interchange between hospital and community. Postwar hospitals developed schemes for the rehabilitation and resettlement of long-stay patients, while an increasing proportion of patients were managed by relatively brief and often repeated in-patient stays on acute wards, with out-patient follow-up on discharge.

The introduction of effective antipsychotic and antidepressant medications in the 1950s and the rise of the psychiatric unit within the district general hospital reinforced a medical model of psychiatric treatment within local services. The Mental Health Act 1959 gave sanction to the medical approach to mental illness by taking hospital admission out of the legal arena. Informal admission became the norm, while compulsory detention in hospital was permitted on the recommendation of registered medical practitioners.

During the 1950s and 1960s the potentially damaging effect of institutions on their inmates was increasingly recognised (Barton, 1959; Goffman, 1961; Wing & Brown, 1970). The white paper *Better Services for the Mentally Ill* (Her Majesty's Stationery Office, 1975) identified the components of a comprehensive psychiatric service, which was to be organised around the psychiatric unit at the local general hospital. This would include day hospitals, out-patient clinics and community psychiatric nursing services, which could offer follow-up in the patient's home. Subsequently, the major thrust of professional practice and government policy has been to provide care for those who have a mental illness (and indeed other client groups, including the elderly, people with a physical disability and people with a mental handicap) in non-institutional settings.

A series of scandals in mental illness and mental handicap hospitals further undermined confidence in institutional provision, at a time when the thinking of 'anti-psychiatrists' such as R. D. Laing (1960) and Thomas Szasz (1961) was fashionable. The Mental Health Act 1983 was introduced after a debate focused on the rights of the decreasing minority of patients detained in hospital against their will. It marked a return to the legalistic constraint of psychiatric practice and the revival of a Mental Health Act Commission charged with the oversight of the welfare of detained patients (Jones, 1991). The user movement and the concept of patient advocacy, which originated in the USA, began to have an impact on services in the UK during the 1980s.

Community care

The decline in bed numbers after 1954 was not matched by the development of effective community mental health services. There was persistent evidence of family burden, poor-quality discharge planning, lack of organised follow-up and little help with the practical aspects of daily life for patients discharged from psychiatric hospital (Brown *et al*, 1966; Melzer *et al*, 1991).

The white paper *Caring for People* (Department of Health, 1989*a*) set out reforms to the system of community care and introduced parallel systems to be run by health and social services: the Care Programme Approach (CPA) and Care Management, the latter a mechanism for purchasing social care. The CPA has since been the framework under which mental health services have been operating. When introduced in 1990, it was little more than a requirement on services to maintain a register of patients discharged into the community. It has become increasingly elaborate. Flexibilities introduced in the most recent round of National Health Service (NHS) and social care reform, the NHS Plan (Department of Health, 2000*a*), have encouraged mental health and social care providers to form integrated services and to overcome a harmful and artificial dichotomy introduced in *Caring for People*.

During the 1990s a mental hospital closure programme that had begun in the 1980s gathered momentum. Reprovision programmes were strongly influenced by 'normalisation', a concept introduced from mental handicap services that emphasised the social nature of disability and the development for 'handicapped' people of socially valued roles (Wolfensberger, 1983). The Team for the Assessment of Psychiatric Services (TAPS) project studied the well-conducted closure programmes of two mental hospitals in north London, Friern Barnet and Claybury. The project carefully followed up the cohorts discharged. The conclusions were optimistic. A 5-year follow-up of 670 discharged long-stay patients found that the survivors did well in their new community-based settings, exhibiting improved social functioning and showing no evidence of symptomatic deterioration. Their quality of life was much enhanced in the new services (Leff & Trieman, 2000).

The majority of the large mental hospitals that had served the country were replaced by smaller, more local psychiatric units that were either free standing or attached to a district general hospital. The 1990s were also characterised by the general adoption of the model of the community mental health team (CMHT): a multidisciplinary team responsible for the provision of comprehensive care to adults within a defined subcatchment area of the local service, preferably working out of a non-stigmatised local team base.

Another influence on policy in the 1990s was the growing public concern about the risks presented by people with a mental illness to the community, stoked up by dramatic reporting in tabloid newspapers. The murder of Jonathan Zito by Christopher Clunis in December 1992 was a particularly seminal event and resulted in the publication of an inquiry report that graphically portrayed the deficiencies in the mental health and social care system in London up to the early 1990s (Ritchie, 1994). Risk assessment and risk reduction became central tasks of mental health services. The Mental Health (Patients in the Community) Act 1995 introduced supervised discharge, a form of compulsory after-care that fell short of compulsory community treatment.

Mental health services in the 'new' NHS

The white paper *Modernising Mental Health Services* (Department of Health, 1998*a*) sketched a broad strategy for the future, on the principles of 'safe, sound and supportive'. Based on the premise that 'community care has failed', this included a commitment to reform the Mental Health Act 1983 along lines that would reinforce public safety. The *National Service Framework for Mental Health* (Department of Health, 1999*b*) set seven standards for a modernised mental health service. These covered mental health promotion, primary care and access to services, the care of people with a severe mental illness, the needs of carers and the prevention of suicide. Under the aegis of *The Mental Health Policy Implementation Guide* (Department of Health, 2001*b*) and subsequent documents set out a model for the modernised mental health service. This model differed from the prevailing orthodoxy of the 1990s, based on the generic CMHT. It recommended a number of 'functionally differentiated' teams to work with patients and carers at different times during an individual's illness career, with 'seamless' care being glued together by the CPA and supported by strengthened information systems. (A compendium of recent policy documents, including the *Policy Implementation Guide* and its supplements, as well as all publications from the National Institute for Mental Health in England, can be accessed via the NIMHE website, http://www.nimhe.org.uk, and on the Department of Health website, http://www.dh.gov.uk.)

The *National Service Framework* and *Policy Implementation Guide* drew on and made copious reference to the evidence base for service organisation. All health professionals can access the Cochrane Collaboration collection of meta-analytic reviews, which bring together good-quality trial data on specific treatments and, where it exists, patterns of service organisation. (The Cochrane Collaboration reviews are available through the National electronic Library for Health website, http://www.nelh.nhs.uk.) The National Institute for Health and Clinical Excellence (NICE) also produces evidence-based appraisals of treatment technologies and clinical guidelines – of which the first was on schizophrenia (NICE, 2002). (NICE appraisals and guidelines can be found on the NICE website, http://www.nice.org.uk.) The roll-out of emerging policy is supported by the NIMHE (which has been incorporated within the Care Standards Improvement Partnership).

Mental health services worldwide

The USA

There are close parallels in the evolution of mental healthcare between the UK and the USA, where a pattern of 'cycles of reform' has been identified (see Table 29.1). Both countries experienced a vast expansion in mental hospitals throughout the 19th century, similar therapeutic pessimism in the second half of the

Table 29.1 Cycles of reform in the USA

Paradigm	Date	Location
Moral treatment	1800–1850	Asylum
Mental hygiene	1890–1920	Mental hospital or clinic
Community mental health	1955–1970	Community mental health centres
Community support	1975	Community settings
Recovery	1990	Self-help

19th century and a deinstitutionalisation movement starting in the 1950s. In the USA a 'mental hygiene' movement during the early years of the 20th century offered promise of change that was not fulfilled and a thriving private sector developed, offering mainly psychodynamic treatment. Deinstitutionalisation was more extreme in the USA than in the UK. Rapid downsizing of the state mental hospitals produced a very visible problem on urban streets of homeless people who are mentally ill that persists to this day.

The Community Mental Health Centers Act 1963 initiated a federal policy of public mental health services based on such centres. This bold experiment was later judged to have failed people with a severe mental illness (Mollica, 1983), a failure that held back the adoption of CMHTs in the UK. A further reform movement sought to provide more effective community support for people with a severe mental illness. Ground-breaking research in Madison, Wisconsin, by Stein & Test (1980), introduced 'assertive community treatment' (ACT) (which is considered further below). ACT has gone on to become the dominant paradigm for community services for those who are severely mentally ill in the USA and has greatly influenced UK policy.

More recently, the concept of 'recovery' has become influential in the USA. This emphasises the importance of empowerment and acknowledges the personal struggle of those who experience mental illness and their capacity to regain control of their lives and sense of self. It offers the optimistic prospect for people with a mental illness to transcend its effects on their life (Davidson & Strauss, 1992; Jacobson & Greenley, 2001).

Two European models

The psychiatric reforms introduced in Italy in 1978 by Law 180 led to a bold and largely successful attempt to provide psychiatric care without access to a mental hospital. Italian services function with a remarkably low number of hospital beds, in a mixture of general hospital, private and university settings (some 17 beds per 100 000 population) (Piccinelli *et al*, 2002). The 'Italian experience' was highly influential in the UK in the 1980s as the hospital closure programme was set in motion.

Less influential, but striking in its parallels with the UK, was the introduction in France from 1960 of a model of 'sectorised psychiatry', with a sector of some 70 000 population being served by a multidisciplinary team required to provide preventive, rehabilitative and curative care (Kovess *et al*, 1995).

Australia

More recently, a thoroughgoing reform of the Australian mental health system, which had previously been reliant on traditional large mental hospitals, has seen the introduction of community treatment teams along lines reminiscent of the *Policy Implementation Guide* and the down-sizing and closures of mental hospitals. In addition, the Australian states have introduced forms of compulsory community treatment. Success in team development and in reducing bed numbers has been reported, although 74% of the health and social care costs associated with schizophrenia are still taken up by in-patient care (Carr *et al*, 2003).

The uniqueness of the UK

There are a number of important and unique features of the UK mental health system. The first is the gatekeeping role of primary care. This results in a smaller proportion of mental healthcare being provided within specialist mental health services than in other advanced industrial countries, which, in general, allow direct access to secondary care. (Direct access is possible in the UK, but usually only after some very visible crisis has occurred, involving, for example, the police or presentation to an accident and emergency department.)

The second is the current relative insignificance of the private sector in the UK (important exceptions being the role of private providers of long-stay medium-security and low-security hospital beds and private-sector psychotherapy). Current plans to increase use of the private sector are controversial and it is unclear how these changes will affect mental health services.

A third feature is the funding of mental healthcare, which is not insurance based and is free at the point of delivery.

Finally, the UK system is comprehensive, covering all residents, in stark contrast to the USA, where public mental health services cater only for those without health insurance.

These unique features, and sociocultural differences in attitudes towards mental illness and the availability of family support, make the direct extrapolation of the results of mental health services research from one country to another problematic.

Components of a comprehensive mental health service

There are three potential approaches towards describing the components of a mental health service. First, one can look at the *needs* of individual patients (and their carers) and then describe the service arrangements that might be put in place to meet those needs. There is a very extensive and sophisticated literature on the assessment of need in psychiatry (see Andrews & Henderson, 2000). One widely used measurement tool, the Camberwell Assessment of Need (Phelan *et al*, 1995), assesses 20 domains of need from both the user perspective (reflecting 'wants') and the professional perspective (expert-defined 'needs'). People with a severe mental illness tend to have needs that are unusual in the general population (e.g. treatment for

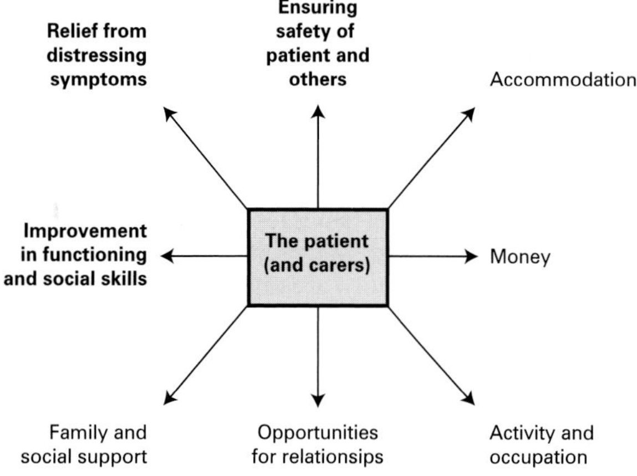

Fig. 29.2 The needs of people with mental illnesses. Needs in bold are specific to people with mental illnesses and will be met by mental health services. Other needs are common to everyone but people with severe mental illnesses may require additional support to meet them.

psychotic symptoms, management of the side-effects of psychotropic medication, help to address deficiencies in personal and social skills, and management of risks of harm to self and others). However, these specific needs go hand in hand with a wide range of ordinary human needs (e.g. accommodation, occupation, food, money, company of others, and access to physical healthcare), which, because of disability caused by mental illness, may require a service response. Services may also have to make specific tailored responses to meet quite common needs (e.g. for help with substance misuse problems, treatment of neurotic symptoms or help with literacy) among special populations, such as people with psychotic illnesses. Fig. 29.2 shows, in a simplified fashion, the general and specific needs of people with severe mental illness. Competent services must combine the provision of social care and support with the delivery of effective treatments. Throughout the focus should be on the social recovery of the individual.

Box 29.1 Core elements of a comprehensive mental health service

- Systems for the identification of people in need
- Systems for consultation and liaison with primary care, general medical care, the criminal justice system and community agencies
- Mechanisms for care planning and care coordination
- Systems of case management and assertive outreach
- Systems for practical support with tasks of daily living
- Crisis response systems
- Systems to support and educate carers
- Hospital beds
- Day care, rehabilitation, work and leisure opportunities
- Residential care and access to housing
- Access to effective physical, social and psychological treatments

Second, the *core elements* of a service system can be described (see Box 29.1). These include both arrangements for undertaking key tasks (assessment, crisis response, management of risky behaviours, provision of treatments, etc.) and specific kinds of services within which these key tasks can be undertaken (e.g. community teams, hospital beds and day care provision).

Finally, and conceptually least satisfactory, is a catalogue of *services*.

For ease of explanation, the rest of this chapter is organised around service elements rather than the key tasks of services or patient (and carer) needs. It is important to recognise that most tasks of treatment and care can, in principle, be carried out in a variety of settings and that needs may be met in a variety of different ways. No one, for example, 'needs' a day hospital or day centre, but important needs for treatment, care and social support can be met through a day facility.

Mental health services in England – an outline

The defining features of the English mental health system are familiar to all practitioners but deserve emphasis. Care is funded out of general taxation (although some people have to contribute to aspects of social care). The Department of Health sets both overall priorities and an increasingly prescriptive policy and practice framework, which is aggressively performance managed. Responsibility for commissioning is devolved locally to primary care trusts (PCTs), which work in partnership with the local authority, with oversight from Strategic Health Authorities. Services are provided largely by mental health trusts, which tend to cover a wide geographical area and serve a large population. Local PCTs will also purchase services from the private and voluntary sector, particularly for social care, and may have arrangements with other trusts for some specialist services, such as eating disorders, mother and baby care, neuropsychiatry and forensic provision. Increasingly the norm is for operational and budgetary integration between health and social services. Trusts are likely to operate from more than one hospital site and many community sites, to work with more than one local authority and to be commissioned by more than one PCT. Trusts have statutory duties to balance their books financially and a duty, under clinical governance, to provide quality services. Social care is monitored by the Commission for Social Care Inspection (CSCI), while the quality of healthcare is monitored by the Healthcare Commission (HC) (the two bodies are due to merge by 2008).

Within a local mental health economy (commissioned by a PCT) the catchment area will be broken down into sub-units or sectors, with a population of between 25000 and 100000. The sector service will consist of community services and an allied in-patient unit. Depending on the level of development, perceived local need and fidelity to the *Policy Implementation Guide*, there may be catchment-area or sector specialist teams subsuming various functions (crisis intervention/home treatment, early onset, assertive outreach, etc.). Sectors

Box 29.2 Key principles of the Care Programme Approach

- All services to have a Care Programme Approach policy
- Applies to all patients accepted by mental health services
- Assessment of health and social care needs (including financial, occupational and accommodation needs)
- Assessment of risks
- Nominated care coordinator
- Production of an agreed care plan (including contingency and crisis plans with relapse indicators)
- Information sharing and collaboration between agencies and with carers
- Regular reviews convened by care coordinator
- Data to be held on an electronic patient record

Based on Department of Health (1999*c*).

may be geographically defined but are now more usually based on practice lists (with special arrangements required for people who are not registered with a general practitioner).

Arrangements for other functions, such as psychology, vary. The norm is a balance between psychology provision within the various teams and a separate psychological treatment service.

The bulk of community service referrals come from primary care, with varying arrangements for direct patient access. Systems for supporting primary care mental health vary, although there is an expectation that secondary care will provide 'link workers' who visit practices, discuss shared cases and facilitate access to secondary care.

All people under treatment by secondary mental health services are expected to be under the CPA (Department of Health, 1999*c*). This demands a structured assessment of patient need (including risk assessment), the development of a care plan (including relapse plans) and regular review of the care plan (see Box 29.2). Increasingly, CPA reviews are captured on an electronic database that is available within the local mental healthcare economy. Meeting the requirements of the CPA will draw on a wide range of health and social care services, as well as the resources of the individual and any carers. The rest of this chapter describes this range of services (Box 29.3).

Box 29.3 The types of mental health services

- Community services
- Emergency services and crisis response
- Hospital beds
- Accommodation and residential care
- Day care and occupation
- Services for special needs groups
- User-led services
- Services for carers

Community mental health services

Community services

Over the past 40 years different models of service delivery have evolved in the UK. Even in one city, there may be a range of service models in place. For example, in London, Johnson *et al* (1997) reported that 'There are very large variations in service availability, both between Trusts and within Trust catchment areas'. At that time, most London trusts had made substantial progress in setting up multidisciplinary teams, but among those in the more deprived areas only 21% had community mental health centres (CMHCs), while 57% had CMHCs only in some areas, and much out-patient work continued to take place on hospital premises rather than on a community site. In 57% of the trusts in the more deprived areas, intensive home-based treatment in working hours was not available, while in 36% it was usually available in some but not all of the catchment area.

Community mental health teams

These teams (also known as primary care liaison teams) are the mainstay of the system (Department of Health, 2001*b*):

> 'CMHTs have an important, indeed integral, role to play in supporting service users and families in community settings. They should provide the core around which newer service elements are developed.'

The *Policy Implementation Guide* devoted to the CMHT (Department of Health, 2002*a*) identifies its functions rather than specifying the precise structure:

> 'local flexibility and close working relationships between all key stakeholders will enable the best arrangements to be developed in each locality.'

The CMHTs provide a service for adults of working age with a range of mental health problems. The functions of a CMHT include:

- offering opinions and advice on the management of mental health problems by other professionals, in particular, advice to primary care, and a triage function
- providing treatment and care for people with a time-limited disorder who will benefit from a specialist intervention
- providing treatment and care for people with more complex and enduring needs.

In some areas some of these functions may be provided by separate teams, for example if there is a rehabilitation team.

The *Policy Implementation Guide* advises that, by using an integrated multidisciplinary approach with adequate outreach, the CMHT can:

- increase capacity within primary care through collaboration
- reduce the stigma associated with mental health problems

Box 29.4 Key aspects and tasks of a CMHT

- Working with primary care and providing a single point of entry to specialist mental health services
- Assessment (including social services assessments)
- Team approach (with each user assigned a care coordinator from the team)
- Regular reviews of care plans
- Interventions (including psychological therapies, physical healthcare, medication management, basics of daily living, help in accessing work and education, carer support and help, and treatment of substance misuse)
- Liaison with other health services (including in-patient care and discharge from in-patient care, primary healthcare and other agencies)
- Discharge and transfer arrangements (including discharge from the CMHT, routine transfers and emergency transfers)

Based on Department of Health (2002*a*).

- ensure that care is delivered in the least restrictive and disruptive manner possible
- stabilise social functioning and help patients stay in the community.

The CMHT should be able to improve the care provided by primary care services by giving advice and support, establishing effective liaison with local general practitioners and other referrers, carrying out prompt expert assessments, and offering treatment. The CMHT also needs to gather detailed information about local resources that may be useful to its patients, and assist patients and carers in accessing these resources. The key aspects and tasks of the CMHT are listed in Box 29.4.

Healthcare and social care staff now usually work under single management. The team should have a mix of nursing, social work, psychology and medical skills but use a single integrated set of notes.

Each CMHT should have clear responsibility for a local population, which may be partly defined by local authority boundaries, and links to specific general practices. The recommended maximum case-load is 300–350 patients per team, or 35 for a full-time care coordinator or key worker, but these figures require modification if patients have more complex needs and will also depend on the local demography and stage of development of other community teams. The population served by a CMHT will vary between 10000 and 60000, according to the levels of morbidity and size of the patch.

Case management and assertive outreach

Community care has led to a fragmentation of mental health services, and there is a need for some form of coordinating mechanism. Case management systems are intended to provide this coordination, offering vulnerable patients long-term, flexible support (Holloway *et al*, 1991).

The core case management activities are:

- the assessment of need
- the development of a comprehensive care plan
- the arrangement of service delivery
- the monitoring and assessment of what is being provided.

Case management developed during the 1980s to become a major element of the mental healthcare system in the USA. Two contrasting models of case management can be distinguished:

1 *The brokerage model*. The case manager acts as a service broker, responsible for, but not necessarily providing, the assessment and implementation of a package of care. This is similar to the role of a care manager in a UK local authority social services department, where the care manager is responsible for purchasing the social component of community care.

2 *The clinical model*. A skilled mental health professional is directly concerned with all aspects of the patient's physical and social environment. The case manager works directly with the patient to offer a range of interventions as well as arranging access to appropriate services. Clinical case management activities therefore include engaging patients in treatment, delivering and monitoring a package of care, practical help, training, support and counselling, advocacy, and brokerage of other services (Burns & Firn, 2002).

Stein & Test (1980) developed a particular model of clinical case management, the ACT programme in Madison, Wisconsin. This team-based approach involves a multiprofessional group of staff caring for a defined group of patients. Team members generally share responsibility for their clients, and attempt to provide all the psychiatric and social care required by the individual, rather than obtaining care from other agencies. Teams have low staff:client ratios (10–15 clients per member) and will continue to contact and offer services to reluctant or uncooperative patients. Like other forms of clinical case management, ACT aims to keep people in contact with services, to reduce the frequency and duration of hospital admissions, and to improve outcome, especially social functioning and quality of life.

What distinguishes ACT from other forms of clinical case management is its emphasis on team working and team responsibility, while the other forms tend to emphasise professional autonomy and individual responsibility, the link being between the single case manager and his or her clients. Also, ACT has a more clearly defined model of practice, while case management is defined by more theoretical concepts. In practice there may be considerable overlap between these approaches.

Stein & Test (1980) reported reduced hospitalisation, improved social functioning, reduced symptoms and enhanced employment from their service in Madison, Wisconsin. Their work was replicated by Hoult *et al* (1983) in Sydney and subsequently a large research literature emerged. Marshall & Lockwood (1998) concluded that ACT, correctly targeted on high users of in-patient care, could improve outcome, give higher patient satisfaction and lower costs. Few studies in Europe have found that ACT makes a significant difference to hospitalisation (Killaspy *et al*, 2006). There is

Box 29.5 Key aspects and tasks of assertive outreach

- Multidisciplinary assessment and care plan
- Individual care coordinator for each service user (and some sharing of care across the team, allowing for continuity of care)
- Services that are sensitive to clients' age, gender and culture
- Daily team review meetings and weekly team reviews
- Review meetings for individual service users at least every 6 months
- Range of psychosocial and medical interventions, including:
  - assertive engagement, with frequent contact
  - practical support over the basics of daily living
  - support for carers
  - medication management
  - cognitive–behavioural therapy
  - treatment of comorbid substance misuse
  - help for clients to build social networks and address their training and employment needs
  - relapse prevention work
  - crisis support
  - liaison with in-patient and respite services
- Discharge and transfer as needed

Based on Department of Health (2001*b*).

debate over the reason for this – whether it is due to a failure to apply the method properly (a failure in 'programme fidelity') or because control (i.e. comparison) services in Europe contain many of the key features (Burns & Guest, 1999).

In spite of this lack of evidence, within health services in England there has been a requirement to develop assertive outreach services. The *Policy Implementation Guide* (Department of Health, 2001*b*) states that these services can improve engagement, reduce both the number and length of hospital admissions, increase stability in the lives of service users and their carers, improve social functioning and be cost-effective. The key aspects and tasks of assertive outreach are listed in Box 29.5. It is aimed at adults with a severe and persisting mental illness who have a high level of disability and previous difficulty in maintaining contact with services, as well as a high use of in-patient or intensive home-based care. The clients of assertive outreach services have multiple complex needs, including, for example, a history of violence or persistent offending, persistent self-harm or neglect, poor treatment response, a dual diagnosis, admission under the Mental Health Act in the past and unstable accommodation or homelessness.

Each team is likely to cover a population of about 250 000 and to have a case-load of around 90 service users, aiming for a ratio of service users to care coordinators of 12:1 (ideally 10:1). Care coordinators – who can be a community psychiatric nurses (CPN), an 'approved' social worker (ASW), an occupational therapist (OT), a psychologist or a team leader – need to be able to understand the needs of service users and coordinate care and provide a broad range of interventions. Medical staff should be active members of the team but not care coordinators. There may also be support workers who have themselves personal experience of mental health problems or treatment or may have other appropriate life experiences.

Each team will have a finite number of places, and the team needs to discharge patients in order to accept new referrals. Although there is no time limit on the availability of ACT services, studies of the natural history of psychotic illness predict a stabilisation over time (Burns & Guest, 1999). Reasons to consider discharge include clinical and social stability (e.g. no serious deterioration over the past 2 years), persistent refusal by an individual to engage with this approach, or transfer to a different service. Individuals may move to the care of either the CMHT or the general practitioner.

Burns & Guest (1999) discuss some of the questions raised by work in an ACT. These include concerns over the boundaries between care coordinators and their clients, whom they may be seeing very frequently and in their own homes, and over the dilemma of the difference between engagement and harassment for individuals who do not wish to have contact with the team.

Early intervention in psychosis

The new early intervention services are for people generally between 14 and 35 years with a first presentation of psychotic symptoms or within the first 2 or 3 years of their illness. At present there is often a delay between the onset of symptoms and the individual and his or her carers engaging in treatment. This delay may be due to a lack of awareness, ambiguous early symptoms and stigma. Key therefore is early detection, to reduce the pre-treatment delay, as there is a possible critical period during which useful secondary prevention work may take place. There is better recognition now of the social and emotional problems of early psychosis and of the importance of cognitive therapy for this group, who need a multi-component approach to treatment (Garety & Jolley, 2000). Services aim to maximise work and social functioning, and also to prevent relapse and treatment resistance. A controlled trial of the Lambeth Early Onset (LEO) service showed improved outcomes for the experimental group (Craig *et al*, 2004).

The Department of Health (2001*b*) *Mental Health Policy Implementation Guide* sets out a number of components of early intervention services. They should raise awareness of psychotic illness and focus on the individual's symptoms, aiming for early detection and sustained engagement using an assertive outreach approach. One of the principles of early-intervention services is the maintenance or re-establishment of users with appropriate mainstream provision, so teams need to foster a range of close links with other agencies across the voluntary and statutory services.

Crisis resolution and home treatment services

People with a severe mental illness who are in crisis should be treated in the least restrictive environment (consistent with the need to protect them and the public) as close to home as possible. An individual's care plan should specify the action to be taken in a crisis (as stipulated by standard 5 of the National Service Framework). The National Service Framework discusses the need for a range of services to prevent or anticipate crises if possible, to ensure prompt and effective help if a crisis does occur, and to ensure timely access to an appropriate hospital bed or alternative bed or place in the least restrictive environment and as close to home as possible. There should also be access to services 24 hours a day, 365 days a year (according to standard 4).

The development of crisis intervention teams owes much to Caplan's theory that, in a crisis, individuals' traditional patterns of coping break down. Caplan (1964) hypothesised that in their response to an adverse event there is a critical period during which individuals are more responsive to therapeutic intervention, when the disequilibrium of the crisis provides an opportunity for more adaptive coping skills to emerge.

The Department of Health (2001*b*) has provided detailed guidance on crisis resolution/home treatment teams. This states that such teams can offer an alternative to in-patient care. The *Policy Implementation Guide* (Department of Health, 2001*b*) states that the majority of service users and carers prefer community-based treatment and that the clinical and social outcomes achieved by such treatment are as good as those achieved in hospital.

Four stages to the work of a crisis intervention team with an individual can be identified: assessment, planning, intervention and resolution. Different aspects of the intervention may include:

- intensive support with frequent contact (up to several times a day in the early phases) and ongoing risk and needs assessment
- delivery and administration of medication, involving the service user in decisions about its use, and monitoring of side-effects
- practical help with the basics of daily living, such as help with benefits, housing and child care
- support and involvement of the family or carer
- interventions aimed at increasing resilience, for example problem solving, stress management and brief supportive counselling
- relapse prevention, looking at early warning signs, and identifying and reducing any conditions that leave a service user vulnerable to relapse
- crisis planning, with 24-hour contact details for the service user and the family or carer
- respite care, with access to facilities, preferably in a non-hospital setting, and to day care
- links to in-patient services, with involvement in the discharge planning.

Box 29.6 sets out the principles of a crisis resolution/home treatment service, and Box 29.7 its functions.

Each service is likely to cover a population of about 150 000 and to have a case-load of 20–30 service users at any one time. This number will depend on factors such as the geography and demography of the area, the epidemiology and health and social services boundaries.

Box 29.6 Principles of a crisis resolution/home treatment service

- Available 24 hours a day, 7 days a week
- Rapid response
- Intensive support during the early stages
- Active involvement of users and carers
- Assertive approach to engagement
- Time-limited contact
- Learn from the crisis

Based on Department of Health (2001*b*).

Box 29.7 Functions of a crisis resolution/home treatment service

- To act as a gatekeeper to mental health services, rapidly assessing individuals with acute mental health problems, and referring them to the most appropriate service
- For individuals with acute severe mental health problems, if home treatment is appropriate, to provide immediate multidisciplinary community-based treatment, 24 hours a day, 7 days a week
- to remain involved with the patient until the crisis has resolved and the individual is linked into ongoing care
- If admission to hospital is necessary, to be involved in discharge planning and provide intensive care at home to enable early discharge

There should be a multidisciplinary team with a range of skills to provide the different interventions. Referrals will come from different sources, including the in-patient unit as a facilitator of early discharge, and clear pathways of care are needed. There is now evidence that a home treatment team can result in a substantial saving in in-patient bed-days (Johnson *et al*, 2005).

Other services as an alternative to admission

In addition to specific crisis resolution and home treatment services, a range of alternatives to hospital admission has evolved. These include clinic-based crisis intervention, acute care fostering (supplemented by home care) and non-hospital alternative residential care (e.g. community in-patient units or women-only residential crisis facilities), as well as acute day care facilities (see below) (Holloway, 2000).

Particularly for individuals who lack family support or who have housing problems, admission to a residential unit may be necessary in a crisis. However, we know little about the various options for providing non-hospital alternative residential units for patients in need of respite in a therapeutic environment away from acutely ill patients with a psychosis. The provision of such units may allow patients more choice about the help they receive. Boardman & Hodgson (2000) recommend that these units be integrated with other community services, although each one also needs to have its own identity, with its own separate space and activities, and ideally situated within the local community, not on an acute hospital site.

Some non-hospital residential units have been developed for women only. The longest-running example of this type in the UK, Drayton Park, is able to manage women in acute mental health crisis within a relatively short length of stay (Killaspy *et al*, 2000).

Acute day care

Acute day care, although evidence based, is not fashionable, having been overtaken by the emphasis on home treatment teams. However, no study has directly compared acute day care and a home treatment team. Home treatment has several disadvantages: first, as Marshall (2003) has pointed out, it often requires two members of staff to visit a patient if there are any concerns about staff safety; and second, there is the time lost in travelling to patients' homes. There would appear to be some advantages to acute day care: for example, it may allow staff to manage patients in a safer environment, while providing one-to-one treatment, and it also gives the option of group therapies. The addition of outreach work and respite facilities would add to the flexibility of acute day care to manage a range of patients. (There is further information about day care in the 'Day care and occupation' section below.)

Another service involved in crisis care for psychiatric patients is the accident and emergency department in a general hospital. In some departments there are specialist psychiatric liaison teams who can take a lead in assessing and managing patients presenting with a range of mental health problems, including deliberate self-harm, substance misuse and somatoform disorders. These teams need to work closely both with the general hospital staff and with local community teams. A particular problem liaison services face at the moment is the need to ensure that, within the accident and emergency department, patients complete their attendance episode within 4 hours (Henderson *et al*, 2003).

NHS Direct

This is a nurse-led telephone helpline for England and Wales, which gives 24-hour advice and information. There is a similar service in Scotland, NHS 24. The staff of NHS Direct use a computerised decision-support system when giving advice. In an emergency, NHS Direct will access emergency services immediately or refer the caller to a crisis helpline. It also has an internet site (http://www.nhsdirect.nhs.uk) and has published a home-care advice manual for callers. The need for such a service came from two sources: consumerism and the growth of the 24-hour society; and from the growing demand for primary care and emergency services. It is not a substitute for existing services but functions as an additional service.

The NHS Direct mental health project established a mental health lead in each call centre. The project's aims included: establishing a list of local statutory first-line and crisis services; developing links with local services, including referral protocols; and providing support, training and supervision for the helpline advisors (Boardman & Steele, 2002).

In-patient services

The traditional psychiatric hospital performed an array of functions, including meeting patients' basic needs for food, shelter, clothing and a minimal income, and offered opportunities for occupation, leisure and social interaction. With experience gained through reprovision programmes for long-stay patients and the development of community services, it has become clear that the vast majority of patients can be managed outside hospital (Thornicroft & Bebbington, 1989). However, there will continue to be a need for in-patient care, to manage patients who are a serious risk to themselves or to others or who fail to comply with treatment (Stein & Test, 1980), and for patients whose assessment or treatment cannot be provided in a community setting.

Reports on acute in-patient services from the Sainsbury Centre for Mental Health (1998), the mental health charity MIND (Rose, 2000) and the Department of Health (2002*b*), as well as individual reports from the Commission for Health Improvement (CHI, which has now been taken over by the Healthcare Commission), have all highlighted similar problems with in-patient psychiatric care over recent years. These include high bed occupancy rates, poor hygiene, a lack of space, boredom, a lack of privacy, scarcity of therapeutic interventions, violence, substance misuse and bed-blocking. There are also staff recruitment and retention difficulties for in-patient services, as staff move to more attractive posts in the new community teams. With the development of alternatives such as home treatment teams and crisis homes, the threshold for admission to acute care has risen, as indicated by the higher proportion of involuntary admissions (Fitzpatrick *et al*, 2003). No studies have demonstrated the therapeutic effectiveness of hospital care compared with other services, and they have come to be seen as a place of last resort (Muijen, 2002).

Until recently, mental health policy concentrated on the development of community services as a way of reducing the demand for in-patient care. The *National Service Framework for Mental Health* (Department of Health, 1999*b*) refers to the failings of hospital care and how to reduce its use further, while the NHS Plan (Department of Health, 2000*a*) makes no mention of hospital care (Muijen, 2002).

The first steps to address the problems of in-patient services came with what was called 'the refurbishment offer', whereby money was made available to improve the physical environment of wards (Appleby, 2001). There have also been requirements to remove fixed curtain rails (the means of hanging in many in-patient suicides) and, in line with the Patients' Charter target, to establish single-sex accommodation for all in-patients (NHS Executive, 2000).

In 2002 the Department of Health published its *Mental Health Policy Implementation Guide* on adult acute in-patient care (Department of Health, 2002*b*). This acknowledged the poor standards of care on many in-patient units and the fact that, in government initiatives to date, 'inpatient practice and service delivery arrangements have not received the same focussed attention or policy guidance' as community services. The *Policy Implementation Guide* looked to put in-patient services within a whole system of care. Each trust should set up a local acute care forum, to identify strengths and weaknesses and to bring about change. Acute care forums need to work together to carry out a service mapping exercise to identify benchmarks and good practice standards. The report also called for each ward to have a lead consultant, to ensure expert input into matters of service delivery, and for the support and supervision of staff and overall coordination of acute services. Staff should welcome patients on arrival on a ward and have available a range of therapeutic and recreational resources. Specific attention is needed for the physical and psychological safety of women.

The importance of this document is more as a sign of a sensible readjustment of priorities than as an attempt to impose centralised solutions. The fundamental issue that hospital care still struggles with is how to create an optimally therapeutic environment while maintaining safety (Muijen, 2002). Although there is mention of the current 'inadequate arrangements for safety, privacy, dignity and comfort' and of the 'lack of activity that is meaningful to recovery', there is little attention given to the overarching importance of the ward's atmosphere. Haigh (2002) regretted the lost opportunity to prioritise a more therapeutic environment, and argued that more importance should have been given to relationships than to administrative and technical requirements. There are also questions regarding the case-mix on acute wards and whether basing wards around geographical sectors allows for specialist expertise in the management of particular problems or in meeting specific cultural needs (Muijen, 2002).

One particular challenge facing in-patient services is how to manage substance misuse in dual diagnosis patients (Department of Health, 2002*c*). Illicit drug use is a widespread problem within acute in-patient units, including psychiatric intensive care units (PICUs). Local practice varies, for example, in the use of searches of patients or their property, and in random drug and alcohol screening (Williams & Cohen, 2000). Some units have used treatment contracts, but strategies such as withdrawing leave can make a patient feel more frustrated and bored, and substance misuse more attractive, while having discharge from the ward as a sanction can lead to the withdrawal of services from needy individuals, or may be an empty threat if statutory frameworks prevent it taking place. There are no easy answers. The dual diagnosis *Policy Implementation Guide* (Department of Health, 2002*c*) refers to the need for: improved training; organisational support for in-patient units; the building of collaborative relationships with other agencies such as the police, housing and substance misuse services; and good clinical supervision. (For further information about dual diagnosis services see 'Special patient groups', below.)

Psychiatric intensive care units and low-security environments

Psychiatric intensive care is for patients who are compulsorily detained and in an acutely disturbed phase of their illness, needing more secure conditions (Department of Health, 2002*b*). These patients have a lower capacity for self-control, with a corresponding increase in risk, which does not allow their safe and therapeutic management on an acute unit. Care and treatment should be patient centred, multidisciplinary, intensive, comprehensive and collaborative, and have an immediacy of response to critical situations. Length of stay will depend on a patient's clinical need and the assessment of risk, but should generally not exceed 8 weeks.

Low-security units deliver intensive, comprehensive, multidisciplinary treatment and care for patients who have disturbed behaviour in the context of a serious mental illness and who require the provision of security. They work on the principles of rehabilitation and risk management, and provide a homely but secure environment that has occupational and recreational opportunities and links with community facilities. Patients are compulsorily detained and usually need to stay for up to 2 years.

Detention in a PICU or low-security unit constitutes a loss of freedom for the individual, and staff will liaise with referring services to ensure that admission is appropriate to the individual's needs. Admission criteria are likely to include a significant risk of aggression, absconding with associated serious risk, suicide risk or vulnerability (e.g. due to sexual disinhibition or overactivity) in the context of a serious mental illness. PICUs and low-security units need to agree with the referrer the benefits to be gained from the admission, and this agreement should include a clear rational for assessment and treatment. Links should also be made with a range of agencies, under the categories of social support, user agencies, legal and judicial, community and in-patient mental health and medical services in primary and secondary care.

Long-stay patients

This term refers to patients who have been in hospital for more than a certain length of time, typically between 6 months and 2 years. Over the past 40 years, with the push to reprovide care for patients not in a hospital but in smaller residential settings in the community, the number of long-stay patients has fallen. However, there are still patients with complex needs who prove difficult to place. It has become clear that some patients will continue to accumulate in hospital wards and have protracted stays. These 'new long-stay' patients (with a stay of between 1 and 5 years) form a mixed group with complex needs.

Accommodation, supported housing and residential care

Most people with a mental illness live independently or with their families. Some patients need intensive domiciliary care in order to live in community settings, while others are supported by their families in the face of very severe disabilities. A minority, because of their symptoms, behavioural disturbance and disability associated with their illness, require temporary or permanent supported accommodation. There is a wide range of potential accommodation options (see Table 29.2).

Table 29.2 A classification of residential services (costs of care generally increase down the list)

Facility	Description
Community care	
Independent living	Own house, flat, bedsit
Independent living with support	Domiciliary support (from home care team, etc.) or sheltered housing project with *in situ* support
Living with family; supported lodgings (for people living alone)	May involve considerable support from informal carers
Group home; shared housing; supported housing (for groups)	Shared accommodation with varying levels of support
Staffed housing (low staffing)	Daily contact with staff team
Staffed housing (high staffing)	24-hour staff cover (sleep-in)
Staffed housing (very high staffing)	24-hour staff cover (night waking); may offer rehabilitation or long-term care
Very highly staffed housing	
Residential home	
Nursing home	
Registered mental nursing home	
Hospital care	
Acute ward	Short stay
Hospital; hostel	Long-stay in domestic environment
Rehabilitation unit	Medium stay – may be open or locked
Continuing care unit	Long stay
Intensive care unit	Locked short stay
Low-security unit	Locked long stay
Medium-security unit	Locked with significant perimeter security
Special hospital	Locked with high security

Specialist accommodation for people who are mentally ill is provided by the statutory sector (health and social services and housing departments) and the non-statutory sector (housing associations, voluntary organisations and the private sector). There has been a strong policy emphasis during the past two decades on the use of the non-statutory sector and a mixed economy of care. The funding of supported accommodation for people with a mental illness is complex and subject to frequent change.

Access to ordinary housing for people with a mental illness who have become homeless is also a major issue, particularly in areas of the country where there is a severe shortage of social housing. Housing legislation places responsibility on local housing authorities to provide for people who are deemed vulnerable because of mental illness. Unfortunately, in practice, this generally means that patients who have become homeless, often as a consequence of a relapse in their illness, are placed in unsatisfactory and stressful bed-and-breakfast accommodation. There is a shortage of all forms of housing for people who are mentally ill, and this is particularly acute in the case of high-support and specialised provision, for which choice is limited and out-of-area placement common.

Principles underlying residential care

There are a number of key principles for residential services:

- As far as possible, people should be catered for locally.
- The degree of support offered should match the level of disability.
- Provision should be non-stigmatising, offer a homely environment and promote choice and independence for residents.
- Institutional practices – such as 'block treatment' (where everyone is managed in the same way), lack of personal possessions for residents and social distance between care staff and residents – should be avoided.
- There should be flexibility to cater for changing needs, either by altering the level of support offered within a setting or by offering a more appropriate setting.
- Services should be competent to deal with the particular problems that residents experience or present; these may include, in addition to the symptoms and behaviours associated with severe mental illness, comorbid substance misuse, organic mental disorders and primary or comorbid developmental disorders, notably in the autistic spectrum.

One constant dilemma facing staff in residential care settings is balancing respect for the rights of the individual and the promotion of independence with the duty to provide a safe and structured environment, especially where an individual has severe disabilities or presents significant risks. There is no easy resolution to this dilemma, and services must negotiate a tightrope between allowing people to 'rot with their rights on', on the one hand, and being unduly controlling and coercive on the other.

Accommodation options

The traditional forms of residential care available for people with a mental illness were:

- the group home (a minimally staffed shared house)
- the more highly staffed hostel, which could either offer 'rehabilitation' with an expectation that the resident would move on into less supported accommodation or provide a permanent home
- a long-stay hospital bed, for those with the most severe disabilities.

Good-quality mental health services now offer a much wider range of accommodation options (see Table 29.2), although many services will not be able to cater locally for uncommon conditions, such as people with acquired brain damage and those with primary or comorbid autistic spectrum disorders.

Most people want to live independently and a popular alternative to traditional forms of care is an extension into the mental illness sector of the sheltered housing model seen in the provision of services for other vulnerable groups, such as elderly people. Some residents require only occasional visits from a housing worker or social work aide to ensure that minimum standards are being met and the rent is paid.

For those who need more intensive supervision and support, a 'core and cluster' model may be employed. In this model a central highly staffed unit (residential, but also possibly offering day care) supports other residents who live in a cluster of surrounding independent properties; some of these cluster residents will have moved on from the core unit. Adult fostering and boarding-out schemes are unfashionable but highly cost-effective. For a relatively modest cost, landlords or landladies offer patients considerable practical assistance with daily living and monitoring of their mental state within their own home, mimicking the devoted care that some family members are able to provide. Foster care for people who are mentally ill has been practised in the Belgian town of Gheel for at least 700 years. There is evidence that the outcome for foster care is best for patients discharged into small family homes with few other residents (Linn *et al*, 1980).

Recent experience with hospital closure programmes, notably the TAPS study, indicates that even highly disabled long-stay patients can live successfully in ordinary housing with the support of non-professional care staff (Trieman *et al*, 1998). However, a small but significant proportion of long-stay patients are identified as 'difficult to place' and require specialised facilities that are highly staffed (Trieman & Leff, 2002). Older chronically disabled patients may readily be discharged into residential care and nursing homes, but in practice these are often far from their local area. Although the physical environment of such homes is often excellent, levels of activity among residents are often very low. For patients discharged into the private sector, close follow-up is essential.

The most thoroughly evaluated form of residential provision is the hospital hostel, a specialised professionally staffed residence for 'new long-stay' patients (Garety & Morris, 1984). Hospital hostels can offer individually planned (often behaviourally orientated) interventions in an intensively staffed setting that is also a homely environment. Improved functioning and quality of life have been demonstrated for patients who would otherwise have been resident on hospital back wards or inappropriately placed in acute wards; despite the high staffing levels, hospital hostels can be cost-effective compared with these unsatisfactory alternatives.

Challenging behaviours

Some patients cannot be cared for even within the highly supported environment of a hospital hostel or an open rehabilitation unit. This small residual group of patients who exhibit 'challenging behaviours' went almost un noticed in the large mental hospitals, but are very apparent as the 'new long-stay' within modern, community-orientated services. No generally agreed service model has yet emerged in the era of deinstitutionalisation for this patient group, which is diagnostically heterogeneous but characterised by non-compliance with treatment, absconding, violence, disturbance at night and bizarre behaviour (Holloway *et al*, 1999). Some of these patients will improve – over a period of years – with intensive rehabilitation and aggressive pharmacological management (Trieman & Leff, 2002), although others appear to have intractable problems. When behavioural disturbance, risk or offending behaviour is extreme, patients may be treated in a special hospital or medium-secure unit, although the latter were not designed or resourced to provide long-term care. More recently, long-term low-security units have opened to provide continuing, institutionally based care in a development that suggests a return to the asylum concept.

Day care and occupation

Day care (referred to in the American literature as partial hospitalisation) for people with a mental illness dates back to the 1930s, when a day hospital was opened in Moscow, apparently owing to a lack of mental hospital beds. Subsequently day care has attracted passionate advocates, not least the many service users who have perceived their day hospital or day centre as a vital aspect of their lives, but it has always been outside the mainstream of mental health services.

A day care service may function as:

- an alternative to admission
- an aid to early discharge of in-patients
- a site for intensive treatment for people with severe personality disorders or specific psychological problems, such as anxiety disorders
- a site for short-term rehabilitation
- a source of long-term structure, support and social contact for patients.

The specific types of day care are listed in Box 29.8.

Acute day hospitals

The extensive literature on day care as an alternative to in-patient admission has been summarised in a meta-analytic review (Marshall *et al*, 2003). Consistent findings are that acute day care is feasible, cost-effective and reduces the number of in-patient bed-days. Time to recovery may be quicker for day patients. There is

Box 29.8 Types of day care

- Acute day care: an alternative to admission on an acute ward
- Transitional day care: for patients discharged after a brief in-patient stay
- Therapeutic day care: offering specific packages of treatment that cannot be provided on an out-patient basis
- Long-term supportive day care: including structured and unstructured settings; drop-ins; sheltered work; sheltered leisure
- Generic day care: use of mainstream facilities open to the general public (e.g. adult education, training schemes)

no evidence of a long-term difference in clinical or social outcome between acute day care and in-patient treatment. However, approximately 40% of patients presenting for admission cannot be managed within an acute day hospital, because of the presence of behavioural, physical or social problems or the need for compulsory treatment (Creed *et al*, 1997). (For further information about acute day care see 'Crisis resolution and home treatment services', above.)

Acute day care can also be offered at the transition from in-patient to out-patient status, and a policy of doing this can result in significant bed savings (Endicott *et al*, 1979). Transitional day care can be offered in a stand-alone facility or by allowing patients to return during the day to the in-patient ward: it occurs in a *de facto*, unplanned fashion when ward occupancy levels go over 100%.

Therapeutic day hospitals

Day hospitals can be a setting for more intensive therapeutic interventions than can be delivered on an out-patient basis. An important controlled trial carried out at the Halliwick Day Hospital in London compared psychoanalytically oriented day hospital care with standard care for patients with borderline personality disorder. Sustained clinical gains were identified in terms of episodes of self-harm and self-reported depression, anxiety, distress and functioning (Bateman & Fonagy, 2001). However, a meta-analysis of randomised controlled trials of therapeutic day care compared with out-patient care found limited evidence of its value, and the authors noted the methodological limitations of the Halliwick trial (Marshall *et al*, 2001).

Long-term day care

Day centres can act as a source of long-term structure and support for patients with chronic disabilities. Surprisingly, despite their very clear importance in many people's lives, evidence from randomised controlled trials is lacking for the efficacy of non-medical day centres (Catty *et al*, 2001). A multicentre controlled trial of day treatment centres run by the Veterans Administration in the USA found that, overall, there was no evidence of efficacy in reducing admissions. Centres with low readmission rates were characterised by an accepting, low-key atmosphere, slower patient flows and an emphasis on recreation and occupation rather than 'therapy' (Linn *et al*, 1979).

From the users' perspective, long-term day care plays a psychological role akin to the 'latent' functions of work. Work, in addition to its obvious role in providing people with money (its 'manifest' function), provides a structure to one's time, enforces activity, offers social relationships outside the home and produces external goals for achievement (Jahoda, 1981). Day care users stress the importance of having somewhere to go, the support of staff and fellow attenders and the availability of activities of any therapeutic function (Holloway, 1989).

There is little empirical evidence surrounding day care activities. Although individual assessments, particularly of daily living skills, may be carried out within a day unit, most activities involve groups of attenders. Groups should vary in the demands they make on members, and foster the use of a range of social and functional skills. Practical activities, work assessment, social skills training, family therapy and other specific therapeutic interventions may all form part of a day care programme.

The influential Fountain House model of psychosocial rehabilitation, which originated in New York in the 1950s, emphasises the empowerment of service users (who become 'members'), the importance of productive activity (with members contributing to the running of the service) and the opportunity for gainful employment (Beard *et al*, 1982).

Drop-ins and social clubs

Patients often find evenings and weekends particularly difficult, and some services are now available out of working hours. Voluntary organisations can be particularly successful at providing informal 'drop-ins', which can complement the more formal statutory day care. Access to leisure activities is a major problem for some patients, who may be restricted by lack of money, social anxiety, impaired social skills or simply lack of motivation.

One important aspect of day care is that it provides users with a ready-made social network. It is important that this artificial social network encourages appropriate, socially skilled behaviour. Ideally, services should be encouraging patients to maintain or develop social networks that have nothing to do with the mental health system. Professional support systems should therefore also be making use of 'generic' resources – those that are open to members of the public. Adult education courses and local leisure centres are particularly valuable forms of generic provision.

Work and vocational rehabilitation

People with severe mental illness have very high rates of unemployment (in the region of 75%). Until recently, interest in providing work opportunities for people who are mentally ill was waning, being seen as a reminder of the asylum era, when the more capable patients were put to productive work in ways that now appear exploitative. However, it is clear that work in itself is potentially highly therapeutic, as well as bringing potential financial benefits and access to the wider social world. Most people with a mental illness want to be employed. A range of provision is required to encourage them to retain or to return to employment. This will include rapid access to effective treatment (so that job loss is prevented), educational opportunities, work assessment and training, careers counselling, sheltered work, 'social firms', sheltered placements in ordinary firms and access to open employment.

Within community mental health services, occupational therapists often take the lead in supporting people to return to meaningful occupation, in whatever form, including open employment. Psychiatrists will need to liaise with occupational health departments to encourage the managed return of their patients to work. They should also be aware of the Disability Discrimination Act 1995, which requires employers to make 'a reasonable adjustment' if an applicant or employee has a disability: adjustments could include the availability of part-time work, work in less pressurised environments and increased supervision.

Two specific models for helping those people with a severe mental illness who have the potential (and the desire) to return to open employment can be identified:

1 pre-vocational training ('train and place')

2 supported employment ('place and train').

Within supported employment programmes, which were first developed to aid people with learning disabilities to obtain work, people are found entry-level jobs and supported in these by project workers; this is known as the individual placement and support model (Drake *et al*, 2001). There is very strong evidence, from a literature that emanates almost entirely from the USA, that supported employment programmes are more effective than pre-vocational training, which is no more effective than standard care (Crowther *et al*, 2001).

However, supported employment is not a panacea for the occupational needs of people with a mental illness. The evidence from controlled trials shows that only a minority of patients will be in employment at follow-up, and job loss is frequent. The contemporary economy in the UK lacks the sort of unskilled jobs that could be taken on by individuals with the cognitive and social disabilities common among people with a severe mental illness.

One major additional problem for people with a disability in the UK who return to work is the benefits system, which provides very strong disincentives for people to seek to return to low-paid employment (the 'benefits trap'). A valuable option is voluntary work, which can be both a stepping stone and an alternative to open employment. There is also a potential role for mental health service providers, who will often be relatively large local employers, in offering employment opportunities to people with mental health problems.

Special patient groups

There is evidence that women and people from Black and minority ethnic groups often have negative experiences of mental health services (National Institute for Mental Health in England, 2002*a*). Women consistently report sexual harassment on mixed-sex wards and women patients may have very specific problems relating to men, such as child sexual abuse and recent domestic violence. Black people are over-represented in specialist mental health services, are more likely to be detained under the Mental Health Act 1983 and are more commonly treated in conditions of security. Both women and people from ethnic minorities are under-represented within senior management and senior professional roles in the health services. There is now a strong policy emphasis on the provision of health and social services in a manner that is sensitive to cultural and gender issues. Policy has also identified the need for a specialised service response for people with a comorbid mental illness and substance misuse (dual diagnosis) and for those with a personality disorder.

Black and minority ethnic groups

England is now a multicultural society, with about one in eight people belonging to minority ethnic communities, for whom disadvantage and discrimination remain common (National Institute for Mental Health in England, 2003*a*). There is a complex epidemiology surrounding ethnicity and mental illness (National Institute for Mental Health in England, 2002*a*). The Race Relations (Amendment) Act 2000 placed all public authorities under a duty to promote race equality, by eliminating unlawful discrimination and by promoting equality of opportunity and good race relations. All health organisations must have a race equality scheme that addresses cultural diversity and equality in terms of service planning, delivery and training, and that tackles institutional racism, where it exists (see Box 29.9).

There are a number of important practical steps that services need to undertake to provide appropriate treatment for people from ethnic minorities.

1 Ethnic monitoring of both service users and staff is required. Without this, obvious questions about which minorities present locally for treatment and the potential disadvantages experienced by minority ethnic users and staff cannot be addressed.

2 Interpreting services must be made available.

3 The cultural competence of staff needs to be developed, so that they are aware of both the general importance of culture on the presentation and

Box 29.9 Institutional racism

'Institutional racism is the collective failure of an organisation to provide an appropriate and professional service to people because of their colour, culture or ethnic origin. It can be seen or detected in processes, attitudes and behaviour which amount to discrimination through unwitting prejudice, ignorance or thoughtlessness and racist stereotyping which disadvantages minority ethnic people.'

Sir William Macpherson, chair of the Stephen Lawrence Inquiry (1999)

management of mental illness and the specific cultural and religious issues relevant to the patients they will regularly encounter.

4 Mental health services should work with local community leaders and voluntary sector providers. Local voluntary organisations have a vital role to play in linking statutory mental health services with minority ethnic groups and in meeting specific care needs.

5 The National Institute for Mental Health in England (2003*a*) has also recommended the introduction of community development workers, although there is as yet no evidence of their efficacy.

Women's services

Women's Mental Health (National Institute for Mental Health in England, 2002*b*) sets out very clear recommendations for gender sensitivity in generic mental health provision and the development of specific services for women. It contains numerous descriptions of good practice, although few of these have been subjected to rigorous evaluation.

The best established women-specific services are for eating disorders, which cater for an overwhelmingly female patient group, and perinatal psychiatry. A comprehensive perinatal service might consist of liaison with obstetric services prenatally and postnatally; mother and baby beds targeted at mothers with post-partum psychosis; and community services providing specialist care in the puerperium for mothers with both major and minor mental illness and support for health visitors. The National Service Framework (Department of Health, 1999*b*) required health economies to develop local protocols for the management of postnatal depression, which uncommonly requires referral to secondary services. A specific commitment within the NHS Plan (Department of Health, 2000*a*) was for women-only day services, designed to address therapeutic issues that are specific to women. There are recommendations surrounding women-only residential services, including hostels, crisis units and women-only areas within in-patient units. Finally, there are suggestions for the development of dedicated services for specific groups of women, including victims of domestic and sexual violence, child sexual abuse and women who repeatedly harm themselves. Women from certain minority ethnic groups, notably from the Indian subcontinent, may be particularly difficult for services to reach and special initiatives may be required.

Dual diagnosis

Comorbid substance misuse (misuse of alcohol, drugs or both) and mental illness is common, with a prevalence that varies markedly between inner urban, suburban and rural catchment areas (Farrell *et al*, 1998; Wright *et al*, 2000; Weaver *et al*, 2001). The relationship between mental illness and substance misuse is complex, since substance misuse can be both a cause (e.g. drug-induced psychosis, depressive symptoms secondary to alcohol dependence) and a consequence (e.g. self-medication for psychosis or social anxiety) of mental illness, or occur quite independently. There is a strong association between some personality disorders and substance misuse.

Because of its association with acquisitive crime, contemporary social policy has focused on the misuse of illicit drugs. Every local health economy has a multi-agency drug action team, tasked and funded to purchase treatment for drug misusers. Alcohol misuse is, in fact, both a greater societal problem and commoner among people with a severe mental illness (and missed alcohol misuse is an important cause of treatment refractoriness).

The drugs misused by people who have a severe mental illness reflect those used by the general population. Cannabis and stimulants are commonly misused. Opiate misuse is rare among people with a severe mental illness and clinically relatively non-problematical since opiate misusers are easily engaged with services in which substitute prescribing with methadone is available and opiates do not exacerbate psychosis. However, opiate misuse has a high profile because of the severe physical consequences associated with the use of needles and the high death rate among opiate misusers, who, because of their chaotic lifestyle and dysphoria, may have contact with adult mental health services.

The prison population and homeless people have high levels of substance misuse, combined with much psychiatric morbidity. General psychiatrists experience particular problems with people who misuse stimulants, which are toxic to people with a diathesis for psychosis, are addictive and expensive (resulting in acquisitive offending behaviour) and lack a clear-cut treatment technology.

Four models for managing comorbid substance misuse have been identified:

1 the sequential model, in which the comorbid individual has to be effectively treated for one or other problem first

2 the parallel model, in which the organisationally separate mental health and substance misuse services provide care at the same time

3 the integrated model, in which a specialist co-morbidity team or specialist substance misuse workers embedded within a mental health team provide care for those with comorbidity conditions

4 the mainstreaming model, in which mental health staff, with training and supervision, are expected to provide basic substance misuse interventions, with an option for referral to specialist substance misuse services if necessary.

There is a lack of data from the UK on the efficacy of these models of care for people with a dual diagnosis. There is, though, a general consensus that the sequential model is ineffective. The US literature offers qualified support for the integrated model (Drake *et al*, 1999; Tyrer, 1999), and the presence of a substance misuse worker within an ACT team (see above) is one of the criteria for fidelity to the ACT model. Reflecting the ambiguous evidence base, current policy in England is not prescriptive, although it does advocate the availability of basic substance misuse skills within mainstream services (Department of Health, 2002*c*). These include the ability to identify and assess substance misuse, the rudiments of a motivational approach to encouraging change in behaviour, and the ability to link with local specialist substance misuse services. Policy also encourages experimentation in the development of specialist dual diagnosis teams to work with mainstream services.

Personality disorder

Historically, psychiatrists have been reluctant to care for people with a personality disorder, a diagnosis that has often been used to exclude people from the care system. Primary personality disorder is common in the general population (in the region of 10–13% of the adult population) and very common among the prison population (National Institute for Mental Health in England, 2003*b*). By contrast, primary personality disorder is uncommon among the case-loads of CMHTs, but comorbidity of mental illness and personality disorder is frequent (Keown *et al*, 2002). CMHTs experience particular difficulty in working with people with antisocial and borderline personality disorders, who tend to present with affective disturbance and self-harming behaviours, often with a triple comorbidity of substance misuse.

A range of potentially effective psychological treatments for personality disorder have been described: dynamic psychotherapy, cognitive analytical therapy, cognitive therapy, dialectic behavioural therapy and treatment within a therapeutic community (Bateman & Tyrer, 2002). These treatments are complemented by psychopharmacological approaches aimed at treating comorbidity and reducing the impulsivity that is such a feature of DSM–IV 'cluster B' personality disorders (Bateman & Tyrer, 2002). For the offender population there is a further range of treatments: 'thinking skills', anger/violence management, sex offender programmes and forensic psychoanalytic psychotherapy (Craissati *et al*, 2002).

Currently, potential demand for these treatments (other than medication, which has limited efficacy) far outstrips supply. There is a very limited evidence base surrounding service arrangements for people with a personality disorder. Policy requires local mental health economies to consider developing a range of services (National Institute for Mental Health in England, 2003*b*) and as a minimum should establish a specialist personality disorder team. This team should be located within the local psychological therapy service but adopt a more assertive approach and work to the rubric of the CPA, which might offer one or more of the modalities of evidence-based psychological treatment. In areas with a high level of morbidity this team might be complemented by a specialist day unit for the treatment of personality disorder, an approach supported by a single highly influential controlled trial (Bateman & Fonagy, 2001).

Brief crisis admission of people with a personality disorder is both necessary and common, although it can be minimised by the development of agreed crisis plans for those who frequently present for admission. Very disturbed individuals will require treatment within specialist in-patient units, although such units will serve a wide catchment area. There is a separate service development stream for offenders with personality disorders that lies within the remit of forensic psychiatry (National Institute for Mental Health in England, 2003*b*).

Service users and carers

In *Shifting the Balance of Power*, the Department of Health (2002*d*) sets out the tasks required to achieve a patient-centred NHS, in which services will be built around the needs of patients rather than on the established workings of the organisations delivering care. This reflects a trend towards increased democracy within society and in the decision-making processes of public bodies, which need to be open and accountable to the people they serve. It also builds on existing work on service users and carers.

Under the Carers (Services and Recognition) Act 1995 carers must have an assessment of their own caring, physical and mental health needs, and a written care plan, while the Carers and Disabled Children's Act 2000 enables a local authority to provide services directly to carers. The National Service Framework for Mental Health (Department of Health, 1999*b*) includes a standard for carers. This states that all individuals who provide regular and substantial care for a person on the CPA should have an assessment of their own caring, physical and mental health needs, repeated at least annually, with a written care plan. Provided the service user consents, carers should receive information about their relative's medication, other treatment and care, and what to do in a crisis. Similar provision should be available for the carers of older adult patients. The NHS Plan (Department of Health, 2000*a*) proposed the recruitment of extra staff to work with carers, the strengthening of carer support networks and the provision of more respite care.

The National Service Framework also states that service users need to be involved in developing services. Users and carers, including those from Black and minority ethnic groups, should help assess service performance and they should take part in the training of healthcare professionals. Chapter 10 of the NHS Plan aims to change the existing culture and embed patient and public views at the centre of service delivery. According to the Department of Health (2001*a*):

> 'Improved patient and public representation and support is at the heart of the NHS Plan's drive to build a modern service around the needs of the individual patient. The enhancement of the basic level of scrutiny provided by the Community Health Councils of the 1970s is long overdue. The new organisations and services knit together to form a radical and powerful system which will ensure that patient and public pressure will build a more responsive and accountable NHS.'

These new organisations are patient advice and liaison services (PALS) and patients' forums. Both will operate locally at trust level.

In-house PALS are available to both service users and their carers. They may provide advice and information about the services in the local trust, as well as on-the-spot problem solving, and help with accessing systems of consultation and involvement for service users and their carers. PALS should be able to identify themes for service improvement and feed these into the trust board.

Patients' forums have been established in trusts 'to provide direct input from patients, their representatives and carers into how local NHS services are run' (Department of Health, 2000*a*, p. 94). Patients' forums have the rights to monitor and review every NHS service that is used by the patients they represent. Forums make reports and recommendations to trust boards and they monitor the performance of their local PALS. Patients' forums comprise patients who have recently used trust services and members of local patients' groups and voluntary organisations, and they are independent of the trusts.

The Health and Social Care Act 2001 has made it a legal duty for trusts to consult service users, carers and the general public (directly or through representatives) about and involve them in the planning and provision of services, and on any proposals to change service provision. It also sets out requirements for trusts to have independent complaints advocacy services (ICAS) available. Patients' forums should commission these at a local level, and NHS Direct and PALS will help direct service users and carers to this service. The Commission for Patient and Public Involvement in Health, established in 2003, sets standards and issues guidance to patient forums and ICAS.

Developments in practice – working with service users

There are different ways of viewing users (Pilgrim & Rogers, 2001):

- as patients
- as providers
- as consumers
- as survivors.

In their role as providers we can consider the place of user-led services. These are generally in the voluntary sector, although they are sometimes supported by statutory organisations. The voluntary sector has traditionally offered services that are not otherwise available, and professional boundaries, which might hinder such developments, are less evident. An example of a user-led service is the Hearing Voices Network, which works positively with people's psychotic experiences. There are also examples of community services employing people with a history of mental illness as members of community teams who can help in service delivery, particularly in engaging and organising the care of other users.

Service users who want to be more involved in their own care may value the option of keeping their own records. To foster working in partnership with patients as consumers, there have been pilot studies looking at patient-held records (Warner *et al*, 2000). Another step in this direction has been the requirement (since April 2004) for mental health professionals to send copies of letters to the service user concerned.

As a survivor, a service user may train to become a patient advocate. Advocates are trained to help people with mental health problems in making their own informed choices, and to help protect their rights and interests. Peer advocacy involves support from advocates who have experienced mental health problems themselves, while self-advocacy – the ultimate aim of peer advocacy – occurs when people are able to speak out for themselves. Crisis cards are a simple form of self-advocacy. The cards carry details of whom to contact in an emergency. Advanced directives contain more detailed instructions about the help and support that an individual prefers, including where help should be provided and the type of medication to be given (Thomas & Bracken, 1999).

Carer organisations

Carer groups for the families of people with a mental illness have been formed in many countries. Notable UK examples are listed in Table 29.3. The emphasis is usually on voluntary activity, largely supported by carers, but some groups have engaged with mental health professionals and may have a small number of paid staff. These organisations aim to provide mutual support and sometimes other functions, such as information sharing. A family carer may start a group or in some cases an empathic mental health professional initiates the development. Group members can become educators of mental health professionals, advisors in policy developments, advocates for community acceptance of mental illness, and educators and trainers of other families (Leggatt, 2001).

Conflicts of interest between carers, users and professionals may occur when consumers blame their families for their problems, the symptoms of mental illness are directed at family members, or users and carers do not have common goals. Western cultures place high value on the enforcement of confidentiality, but Leggatt (2001) argues that confidentiality is not absolute and that there are situations in which it is legal and ethical to breach it. If professionals develop a commitment to ongoing involvement with family carers as a partnership, this will help to overcome any problems with maintaining confidentiality.

Clinical governance and outcome research

The white paper *Working for Patients* (Department of Health, 1989*b*) introduced medical audit into the NHS. Medical audit was seen as the process of setting explicit standards, measuring areas of medical practice against these standards and implementing any changes needed to improve patient care. It subsequently evolved into clinical audit. By 1997, attempts were additionally being made to improve organisational quality, for example by monitoring waiting lists (following on from standards in the 1991 Patient's Charter) and to explore patient views, for example through patient surveys and complaints systems (Palmer, 2002).

Since the Labour government came to power in 1997, there have been further moves to make quality central to national health policy:

> 'Every part of the NHS, and everyone who works in it, must take responsibility for improving quality ... and it must be the quality of the patient experience as well as the clinical result.' (Department of Health, 1997)

Table 29.3 UK care organisations

Organisation		Role/services provided
MIND	Mind The Mental Health Charity	The leading mental health charity in England and Wales; it works for a better life for everyone with experience of mental distress
SANE	SANE	Campaigns for greater awareness and understanding of serious mental illness; it supports care (including through its helpline, SANELINE) and promotes research into the causes and treatment of serious mental illness
Rethink (previously known as NSF, the National Schizophrenia Fellowship)	rethink severe mental illness	Dedicated to improving the lives of everyone affected by severe mental illness, whether they have a condition themselves, care for others who do or are professionals or volunteers in the mental health field
Manic Depression Fellowship	MD FELLOWSHIP	Works to enable people affected by manic depression to take control of their lives; it provides information on bipolar disorders and support groups
Turning Point	TURNING POINT turning lives around	Works at the cutting edge of the struggle to help people with problems related to drink, drugs, mental health and learning disabilities to build a better and more independent life
YoungMinds	YoungMinds for children's mental health	Committed to improving the mental health of all children and young people
Mencap	MENCAP Understanding learning disability	Works with people with a learning disability to fight discrimination and campaigns to ensure that their rights are recognised and that they are respected as individuals

Adapted from the SANE website, http://www.sane.org.uk.

Lelliott (2000) identified two key drivers for the quality agenda: professional interest and concern about variations in practice; and public concern about the quality of medical practice. There have also been concerns about perceived failures of self-regulation and questions about doctors' accountability, as well as about a growing culture of blame. There is now a culture of inspection or accreditation and regulation. Patients as customers have become more vocal, and there is a greater demand for 'value for money'.

There was further discussion of clinical governance in the consultation paper *A First Class Service – Quality in the New NHS* (Department of Health, 1998*b*). Clinical governance is about bringing together local activity for improving clinical quality into a single coherent programme, and assuring both trust boards and the public that systems exist and are effective. It can be defined as follows:

> 'a framework through which NHS organisations are accountable for continuously improving the quality of their services and safeguarding high standards of clinical care by creating an environment in which excellence in clinical care will flourish.' (Department of Health, 1998*b*)

A First Class Service lists the main components of clinical governance as:

- clear lines of responsibility and accountability for the overall quality of clinical care
- a comprehensive programme of quality improvement activities
- clear policies aimed at managing risk
- procedures for all professional groups to identify and remedy poor performance.

Alongside clinical governance come strengthened professional self-regulation and the development of values and structures to support lifelong learning.

The roots of clinical governance lie in the commercial sector. High-profile misdemeanours had led the government to recommend standards for financial management to companies in the private sector, and later in the NHS (Palmer, 2002). Corporate governance works as both an assurance mechanism and as a control mechanism. The explicit duties, responsibilities and accountability structures serve to assure the public by indicating who are the individuals overseeing the financial integrity of an institution, while the rules of conduct are the control measures dictating the practices and procedures that ensure financial probity (Oyebode *et al*, 1999).

Further support for the development of robust clinical governance followed with the report from the Bristol Royal Infirmary Inquiry (2001) into unexpected deaths on the paediatric cardiac surgery unit. One theme that emerged through the inquiry was about providing care of an appropriate standard. The report included recommendations on standards of care in NHS organisations and on monitoring standards and performance both locally and nationally, serving to sharpen the debate on clinical governance (Oyebode *et al*, 1999).

Clinical governance must be seen in the context of other structures (Fig. 29.3), first outlined by the Department of Health (1997). These include the National Service Frameworks and the National Institute for Health and Clinical Excellence (NICE, previously the National Institute for Clinical Excellence), both of which set clear standards of service, and the Healthcare Commission (HC, previously the Commission for Health Improvement), the National Performance Framework and the National Survey of Patient and User Experience, which monitor standards.

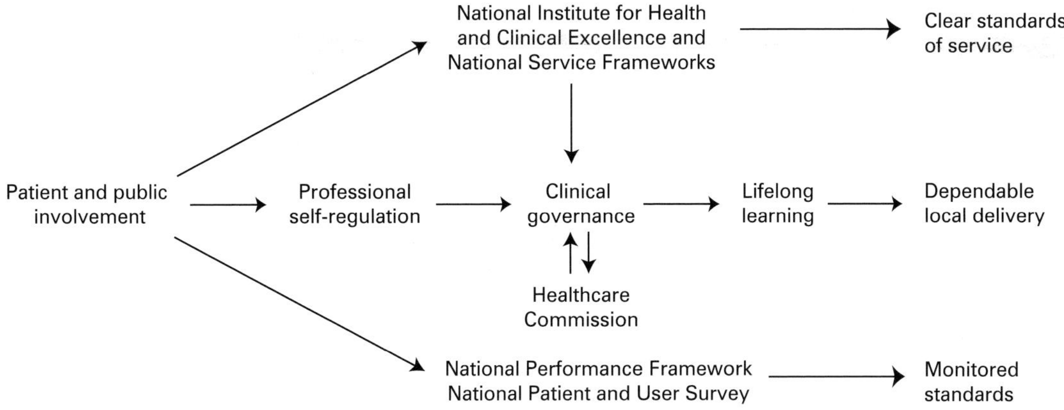

Fig. 29.3 Setting, delivering and monitoring standards. Adapted from *A First Class Service* (Department of Health, 1998*b*) and Wattis & McGinnis (1999).

A series of National Service Frameworks covering different topics offer guidance on the shape and structure of services. The first one to be published was the *National Service Framework for Mental Health* (Department of Health, 1999*b*), which focused on adult services. Since then there have been further NSFs with relevance to mental health: the *NSF for Older Adults* and the *NSF for Children*.

NICE is an independent organisation responsible for providing national guidance on the promotion of good health and the prevention and treatment of ill health. It was established in 1999. It covers England and Wales; the Health Technology Board for Scotland and Scottish Intercollegiate Guidelines Network develop guidance for the NHS in Scotland.

The HC was established in 2004 with the overall function of encouraging improvement in healthcare and public health in England and Wales. It replaced the Commission for Health Improvement (CHI). The HC focuses on service users and the public, and looks at a number of issues, including the availability of and access to healthcare, its quality and effectiveness, and the economy and efficiency of healthcare. It has developed criteria and an assessment process based on 'Standards for Better Health' (Department of Health, 2004). Trusts need to complete an annual health check against these standards and there are also due to be improvement reviews focusing on particular aspects of the standards and for specific populations and conditions.

Alongside the HC there are other mechanisms for monitoring the quality of care, such the National Performance Framework and the National Patient and User Survey. The National Performance Framework aims to address a number of different areas of care, and measures the quality of care using a set of performance indicators. Early indicators for mental health included emergency psychiatric readmission rates and suicide rates. The annual National Patient and User Survey requires service users to give information on their perception of local services.

The Commission for Social Care Inspection (CSCI) is the single independent inspectorate for all social care services in England. It inspects, regulates and reviews them.

The National Patient Safety Agency (NPSA) is a Special Health Authority set up in England and Wales in 2001 to help healthcare staff learn from patient safety incidents occurring in the NHS. It follows recommendations from *An Organisation with a Memory* (Department of Health, 2000*b*), which examined key factors at work in organisational failure and learning, and which proposed solutions based on developing a culture of openness, reporting and safety consciousness within NHS organisations. It recommended the introduction of a national system for identifying patient safety incidents in healthcare, to gather information on causes, and to learn and act to reduce the risk of similar events. It aims to promote an open and fair culture in the health service, encouraging staff to report incidents and 'near misses'. This should be without fear of personal reprimand, so that staff can feel that by sharing their experiences they will be able to learn lessons and improve patient safety. One of its specific targets has been the reduction to zero of the number of suicides by mental health patients as a result of hanging from non-collapsible bed and shower curtain rails on in-patient units.

Supporting clinical governance have been professional self-regulation and lifelong learning. The principle of self-regulation is that the individual professions are best able to determine and enforce standards of practice, and that this is in the public interest. However, successive failures of this system are leading to a tightening of the regulatory framework.

The NPSA is responsible for the National Clinical Assessment Service (NCAS), which was developed following recommendations in the Chief Medical Officer's report *Supporting Doctors, Protecting Patients* (Department of Health, 1999*d*). The Scottish Executive coordinates a system of external clinical advisory teams (ECATs), which provide a similar role. The NCAS aims to provide a support service to trusts when they have concerns over the performance of an individual doctor, 'helping local organisations to manage performance problems swiftly, effectively and sensitively'.

Lifelong learning is a concept that comes from industry. With the accelerating rate of change in technology, skills and society, only by retaining, developing and replacing skills can staff continue to function at a high level. A key issue in modernising the NHS is the balance between basic training and continuing professional development to meet retraining needs.

One of the needs for clinicians is to develop clinically effective practice – self-evidently a 'good thing' but not easy to achieve. The term 'clinical effectiveness' covers

Box 29.10 National Confidential Inquiry into Suicide and Homicide by People with Mental Illness

Aims

- To provide a national clinical survey of suicides and homicides by people who use mental health services
- To recommend changes to clinical practice
- To identify training needs
- To become a national research resource

The inquiry is particularly interested in the circumstances of suicide and homicide in 'priority groups', for whom recommendations are most needed. Current priority groups are patients who:

- were in-patients at the time of the incident
- were discharged from in-patient care less than 3 months earlier
- were subject to enhanced CPA
- were not compliant with medication
- had missed their final appointment with services
- were from an ethnic minority
- were homeless.

a range of activities (Lelliott, 2000). These include identifying the evidence and making evidence-based messages available. The UK Cochrane Centre and the NHS Centre for Reviews and Dissemination at the University of York both produce reviews on mental health topics, and the latter produces two periodicals, *Effective Health Care* and *Effectiveness Matters*. Clinical practice guidelines are another way to package evidence-based messages. The dissemination of information on clinical effectiveness can be facilitated by NICE and also through the developing National electronic Library for Health. The National Confidential Inquiry into Suicide and Homicide by People with a Mental Illness (see Box 29.10) now comes under the umbrella of NICE. Lelliott (2000) states that the implementation of evidence-based messages is a local issue, and the mechanism must be through clinical governance.

Higgitt & Fonagy (2002) discuss the difficulties of translating information on clinical effectiveness into an individual's clinical practice. Publication in a journal is a relatively uncontrolled and untargeted process. 'Dissemination' refers to the development of practice guidelines and overviews of a topic targeted at a particular audience. 'Implementation' is a more active process, with sanctions and incentives, and monitoring and adjustment to local needs. Summarising the evidence on changing clinical practice, Higgitt & Fonagy (2002) suggest it is unlikely that clinicians will change their behaviour unless they see a direct benefit for their patients, and unless they are convinced of the appropriateness of the evidence-based advice to do so. Palmer & Lelliott (2000) argue that there are a number of steps in implementing clinical standards in practice. These involve communication and marketing, leadership, training and peer support or social influence, as well as adequate resource allocation and management, and practical support through, for example, reminder systems and audit.

Outcome research

Performance indicators to date have tended to focus on what services do, giving information about admissions, readmissions, prescriptions and so on, but this leaves open the question of what services achieve. Outcomes work from the NIMHE has been looking at introducing routine outcome measures into clinical practice. These fall into three categories:

1 symptom change, including any change in substance misuse

2 quality of life

3 user and carer satisfaction with services.

Outcome measures that have been developed include the Health of the Nation Outcome Scale (HoNOS). It consists of 12 scales covering behaviour, impairment, psychiatric symptoms and social functioning. The scale rates the clinician's view of the patient's state in these areas to give an indicator of clinical outcome. Repeat measures allow professionals to see how the outcome changes as the result of an intervention, such as admission to acute care. For maximum usefulness, routine assessments should be carried out every 2 weeks. Any member of a multidisciplinary team may do the HoNOS rating, but it is best performed by the clinician who is most knowledgeable about the patient's state during the rating period, for example the care coordinator under the CPA. To improve reliability, it is best if the same rater does all the ratings for a particular patient. Raters require some training in how to carry out the assessment. Other methods of assessing clinical outcome and getting the views of stakeholders such as patients and carers require different approaches.

Data from the HoNOS form part of the mental health minimum dataset (MHMD). Work on the MHMD comes under the Mental Health Information Strategy (see http://www.icservices.nhs.uk/mentalhealth/dataset), which describes the way in which *Information for Health* (NHS Executive, 1998) will be implemented to support mental health services. Problems in information management in health and social care led to the development of the Information Strategy in England. Some of the problems that mental health services have in this area are common to all NHS units. However, there are additional difficulties in mental health services, which generally work across multiple sites and liaise with many different agencies, and these make for greater complexity in data structures, software applications and electronic communications than in other specialties (Elphick, 2000). The Mental Health Information Strategy aims to guide local organisations towards specific informatics developments in mental health.

The National Clinical Audit Support Programme (NCASP), managed by the NHS Information Authority, aims to support the production of national comparative data on the quality and effectiveness of care in mental health. It will use information from the MHMD when this is available.

Conclusions

Mental health services are complex and evolving systems. Recent years have seen an accelerating pace of change, with the relentless production of directives from the Department of Health on how mental health services should look and how we should be working. However, we still lack evidence on what works best and, to complicate the situation further, there are different opinions to consider: not only those of clinicians, but also the views of service users and the wider community.

References

Andrews, G. & Henderson, S. (2000) *Unmet Need in Psychiatry*. Cambridge: Cambridge University Press.

Appleby, L. (2001) A brighter future for in-patient wards. *Psychiatric Bulletin*, **25**, 391.

Barton, R. (1959) *Institutional Neurosis*. Bristol: Wright.

Bateman, A. & Fonagy, P. (2001) Treatment of borderline personality disorder with psychoanalytically oriented partial hospitalisation: an 18 month follow-up. *American Journal of Psychiatry*, **156**, 1563–1569.

Bateman, A. & Tyrer, P. (2002) *Effective Management of Personality Disorder*. Leeds: NIMHE.

Beard, J. H., Propst, R. & Malamud, T. J. (1982) The Fountain House model of psychiatric rehabilitation. *Psychosocial Rehabilitation Journal*, **5**, 47–53.

Boardman, A. & Hodgson, R. (2000) Community in-patient units and halfway hospitals. *Advances in Psychiatric Treatment*, **6**, 120–127.

Boardman, J. & Steele, C. (2002) NHS Direct – a telephone helpline for England and Wales. *Psychiatric Bulletin*, **26**, 42–44.

Bockhoven, J. S. (1954) Moral treatment in American psychiatry. *Journal of Nervous and Mental Disease*, **124**, 167–194.

Bristol Royal Infirmary Inquiry (2001) *Learning from Bristol. Report of the Public Inquiry into Children's Heart Surgery at the Bristol Royal Infirmary 1984–1995*. London: HMSO.

Brown, G. W., Bone, M., Dalison, B., *et al* (1966) *Schizophrenia and Social Care*. Oxford: Oxford University Press.

Burns, T. & Firn, M. (2002) *Assertive Outreach in Mental Health – A Manual for Practitioners*. Oxford: Oxford University Press.

Burns, T. & Guest, L. (1999) Assertive community treatment. *Advances in Psychiatric Treatment*, **5**, 348–356.

Caplan, G. (1964) *Principles of Preventive Psychiatry*. New York: Basic Books.

Carr, V. J., Neil, A. L., Halpin, S. A., *et al* (2003) Costs of schizophrenia and other psychoses in urban Australia: findings from the low prevalence (psychotic) disorders study. *Australian and New Zealand Journal of Psychiatry*, **37**, 31–40.

Catty, J., Burns, T. & Comas, A. (2001) Day centres for severe mental illness. *Cochrane Database of Systematic Reviews*, **(2)**, CD001710.

Craig, T. K. J., Garety, P., Power, P., *et al* (2004) The Lambeth Early Onset (LEO) Team: randomised controlled trial of the effectiveness of specialised care for early psychosis. *BMJ*, **319**, 1067–1071.

Craissati, J., Horne, L. & Taylor, R. (2002) *Effective Treatment Models for Personality Disordered Offenders*. Leeds: NIMHE.

Creed, F., Mbaya, P., Lancashire, S., *et al* (1997) Cost-effectiveness of day and in-patient psychiatric treatment. *BMJ*, **314**, 1381–1385.

Crowther, R. E., Marshall, M., Bond, G. R., *et al* (2001) Helping people with severe mental illness to obtain work: systematic review. *BMJ*, **322**, 204–208.

Davidson, L. & Strauss, J. S. (1992) Sense of self in recovery from severe mental illness. *British Journal of Medical Psychology*, **65**, 131–145.

Department of Health (1989*a*) *Caring for People. Community Care in the Next Decade and Beyond*. London: HMSO.

Department of Health (1989*b*) *Working for Patients*. London: HMSO.

Department of Health (1997) *The New NHS, Modern, Dependable*. London: HMSO.

Department of Health (1998*a*) *Modernising Mental Health Services. Safe. Sound. Supportive*. London: Department of Health.

Department of Health (1998*b*) *A First Class Service – Quality in the New NHS*. London: HMSO.

Department of Health (1999*a*) *Clinical Governance: Quality in the New NHS*. HSC 1999/065. Leeds: Department of Health.

Department of Health (1999*b*) *The National Service Framework for Mental Health. Modern Standards and Service Models*. London: Department of Health.

Department of Health (1999*c*) *Effective Care Co-ordination in Mental Health. Modernising the Care Programme Approach*. London: Department of Health.

Department of Health (1999*d*) *Supporting Doctors, Protecting Patients*. London: Department of Health.

Department of Health (2000*a*) *The NHS Plan. A Plan for Investment. A Plan for Reform*. London: Department of Health

Department of Health (2000*b*) *An Organisation with a Memory*. London: Department of Health.

Department of Health (2001*a*) *Patient Representation in the New NHS*. London: Department of Health.

Department of Health (2001*b*) *The Mental Health Policy Implementation Guide*. London: Department of Health.

Department of Health (2002*a*) *Mental Health Policy Implementation Guide. Community Mental Health Teams*. London: Department of Health.

Department of Health (2002*b*) *Mental Health Policy Implementation Guide. Adult Acute Inpatient Provision*. London: Department of Health.

Department of Health (2002*c*) *Mental Health Policy Implementation Guide. Dual Diagnosis Good Practice Guide*. London: Department of Health.

Department of Health (2002*d*) *Shifting the Balance of Power: The Next Steps*. London: Department of Health.

Department of Health (2004) *National Standards, Local Action. Health and Social Care Standards and Planning Framework 2005/06–2007/08*. Annex I. Leeds: Department of Health.

Drake, R. E., McHugo, G. J., Bebout, D. R., *et al* (1999) A randomised controlled trial of supported employment for inner city patients with severe mental illness. *Archives of General Psychiatry*, **56**, 627–633.

Drake, R., Essock, S., Shaner, A., *et al* (2001) Implementing dual diagnosis services for clients with severe mental illness. *Psychiatric Services*, **52**, 469–476.

Elphick, M. (2000) Mental Health Information Strategy. *Psychiatric Bulletin*, **24**, 426–428.

Endicott, J., Cohen, J., Nee, J., *et al* (1979) Brief vs standard hospitalisation: for whom? *Archives of General Psychiatry*, **36**, 706–712.

Farrell, M., Howes, S., Taylor, C., *et al* (1998) Substance misuse and psychiatric comorbidity: an overview of the OPCS national psychiatric morbidity survey. *Addictive Behaviours*, **23**, 909–918.

Fitzpatrick, N. K., Thompson, C. J., Hemingway, H., *et al* (2003) Acute mental health admissions in inner London: changes in patient characteristics and clinical admission thresholds between 1988 and 1998. *Psychiatric Bulletin*, **27**, 7–11.

Garety, P. & Jolley, S. (2000) Early intervention in psychosis. *Psychiatric Bulletin*, **24**, 321–323.

Garety, P. & Morris, I. (1984) A new unit for long-stay patients: organisation, attitude and quality of care. *Psychological Medicine*, **14**, 183–192.

Goffman, E. (1961) *Asylums: Essays on the Social Conditions of Mental Patients and Other Inmates*. New York: Doubleday.

Haigh, R. (2002) Acute wards: problems and solutions. Modern milieux: therapeutic community solutions to acute ward problems. *Psychiatric Bulletin*, **26**, 380–382.

Henderson, M., Hicks, A. E. & Hotopf, M. H. (2003) Reforming emergency care: implications for psychiatry. *Psychiatric Bulletin*, **27**, 81–82.

Her Majesty's Stationery Office (1975) *Better Services for the Mentally Ill*. London: HMSO.

Higgitt, A. & Fonagy, P. (2002) Reading about clinical effectiveness. *British Journal of Psychiatry*, **181**, 170–174.

Holloway, F. (1989) Psychiatric day care: the users' perspective. *International Journal of Social Psychiatry*, **35**, 252–264.

Holloway, F. (2000) Mental health policy, fashion and evidence-based practice. *Psychiatric Bulletin*, **24**, 161–162.

Holloway, F., McLean, E. K. & Robertson, J. A. (1991) Case management. *British Journal of Psychiatry*, **159**, 142–148.

Holloway, F., Wykes, T., Petch, E., *et al* (1999) The new long stay in an inner city service: a tale of two cohorts. *International Journal of Social Psychiatry*, **45**, 93–102.

Hoult, J., Reynolds, I., Charbonneau-Powis, M., *et al* (1983) Psychiatric hospital versus community treatment: the results of a randomised trial. *Australian and New Zealand Journal of Psychiatry*, **17**, 160–167.

Jacobson, N. & Greenley, D. (2001) What is recovery? A conceptual model and explication. *Psychiatric Services*, **52**, 482–485.

Jahoda, M. (1981) Work, employment and unemployment: values, theories and approaches in social research. *American Psychologist*, **36**, 184–191.

Johnson, S., Ramsay, R., Thornicroft, G., *et al* (1997) *London's Mental Health. The Report for the King's Fund London Commission.* London: King's Fund.

Johnson, S., Nolan, F., Pilling, S., *et al* (2005) Randomised controlled trial of acute mental health care by a crisis resolution team: the north Islington crisis study. *BMJ*, **331**, 599.

Jones, K. (1991) Law and mental health: sticks and carrots? In *150 Years of British Psychiatry. 1841–1991, Vol. 1* (eds G. E. Berrios & H. Freeman), pp. 89–102. London: Gaskell.

Keown, P., Holloway, F. & Kuipers, E. (2002) The prevalence of personality disorders, psychotic disorders and affective disorders amongst the patients seen by a community mental health team in London. *Social Psychiatry and Psychiatric Epidemiology*, **37**, 225–229.

Killaspy, H., Dalton, J., McNicholas, S., *et al* (2000) Drayton Park, an alternative to hospital admission for women in acute mental health crisis. *Psychiatric Bulletin*, **24**, 101–104.

Killaspy, H., Bebbington, P., Blizard, R., *et al* (2006) The REACT study: randomized evaluation of assertive community treatment in north London. *BMJ*, **332**, 815–820.

Kovess, V., Biosguerin, B., Antoine, D., *et al* (1995) Has sectorization of psychiatric services in France really been effective? *Social Psychiatry and Psychiatric Epidemiology*, **30**, 132–138.

Laing, R. D. (1960) *The Divided Self.* London: Tavistock.

Leff, J. & Trieman, N. (2000) Long-stay patients discharged from psychiatric hospitals: social and clinical outcomes after five years in the community. The TAPS project. *British Journal of Psychiatry*, **176**, 217–223.

Leggatt, M. (2001) Carer and carer organisations. In *Textbook of Community Psychiatry* (eds G. Thornicroft & G. Szmukler), pp. 475–486. Oxford: Oxford University Press.

Lelliott, P. (2000) Clinical standards and the wider quality agenda. *Psychiatric Bulletin*, **24**, 85–89.

Linn, M. W., Caffey, E. M., Klett, J., *et al* (1979) Day treatment and psychotropic drugs in the aftercare of schizophrenic patients. *Archives of General Psychiatry*, **36**, 1055–1066.

Linn, M. W., Klett, J. & Caffey, E. M. (1980) Foster home characteristics and psychiatric patient outcome. The wisdom of Gheel confirmed. *Archives of General Psychiatry*, **37**, 129–132.

Marshall, M. (2003) Acute psychiatric day hospitals. *BMJ*, **327**, 116–117.

Marshall, M. & Lockwood, A. (1998) *Assertive Community Treatment for People with Severe Mental Disorders*. Oxford: Cochrane Library.

Marshall, M., Crowther, R., Almaraz-Serrano, A., *et al* (2001) Day hospital versus out-patient care for acute psychiatric disorders. *Cochrane Database of Systematic Reviews*, **(3)**, CD003240.

Marshall, M., Crowther, R., Almaraz-Serrano, A., *et al* (2003) Day hospital versus admission for acute psychiatric disorders. *Cochrane Database of Systematic Reviews*, **(1)**, CD004026.

Melzer, D., Hale, A. S., Malik, S. J., *et al* (1991) Community care for patients with schizophrenia one year after hospital discharge. *BMJ*, **303**, 1023–1026.

Mollica, R. F. (1983) From asylum to community. The threatened disintegration of public psychiatry. *New England Journal of Medicine*, **308**, 367–373.

Muijen, M. (2002) Acute wards: problems and solutions. Acute hospital care. *Psychiatric Bulletin*, **26**, 342–343.

NHS Executive (1998) *Information for Health.* HSC(98)168. London: HMSO.

NHS Executive (2000) *Safety, Privacy and Dignity in Mental Health Units. Guidance on Mixed Sex Accommodation for Mental Health Units.* London: Department of Health.

National Institute for Clinical Excellence (2002) *Schizophrenia. Core Interventions in the Treatment and Management of Schizophrenia in Primary and Secondary Care. Clinical Guideline 1.* London: NICE.

National Institute for Mental Health in England (2002*a*) *Cases for Change. Anti-discriminatory Practice.* Leeds: NIMHE.

National Institute for Mental Health in England (2002*b*) *Women's Mental Health.* Leeds: NIMHE.

National Institute for Mental Health in England (2003*a*) *Inside Outside. Improving Mental Health Services for Black and Minority Ethnic Communities in England.* Leeds: NIMHE.

National Institute for Mental Health in England (2003*b*) *Personality Disorder: No Longer a Diagnosis of Exclusion.* Leeds: NIMHE.

Oyebode, F., Brown, N. & Parry, E. (1999) Clinical governance: application to psychiatry. *Psychiatric Bulletin*, **23**, 7–10.

Palmer, C. (2002) Clinical governance: breathing new life into clinical audit. *Advances in Psychiatric Treatment*, **8**, 470–476.

Palmer, C. & Lelliott, P. (2000) Encouraging the implementation of clinical standards into practice. *Psychiatric Bulletin*, **24**, 90–93.

Phelan, M., Slade, M., Thornicroft, G., *et al* (1995) The Camberwell Assessment of Need (CAN): the validity and reliability of an instrument to assess the needs of people with a severe mental illness. *British Journal of Psychiatry*, **167**, 589–595.

Piccinelli, M., Politi, P. & Barale, F. (2002) Focus on psychiatry in Italy. *British Journal of Psychiatry*, **181**, 538–544.

Pilgrim, D. & Rogers, A. (2001) Users and their advocates. In *Textbook of Community Psychiatry* (eds G. Thornicroft & G. Szmukler), pp. 465–474. Oxford: Oxford University Press.

Porter, R. (1987) *Mind-Forg'd Manacles*. London: Athlone Press.

Ritchie, J. H. (1994) *The Report of the Inquiry into the Care and Treatment of Christopher Clunis*. London: HMSO.

Rose, D. (2000) *Users' Voices* (MIND report). London: Sainsbury Centre for Mental Health.

Sainsbury Centre for Mental Health (1998) *Acute Problems. A Survey of the Quality of Care in Acute Psychiatric Wards.* London: Sainsbury Centre for Mental Health.

Scull, A. T. (1979) *Museums of Madness*. Harmondsworth: Penguin.

Stein, L. I. & Test, M. A. (1980) Alternative to mental hospital treatment. I. Conceptual model, treatment program, and clinical evaluation. *Archives of General Psychiatry*, **37**, 392–397.

Stephen Lawrence Inquiry (1999) *Report of an Inquiry by Sir William Macpherson of Cluny.* London: The Stationery Office.

Szasz, T. S. (1961) *The Myth of Mental Illness: Foundations of Theory of Personal Conduct*. New York: Deel.

Thomas, P. F. & Bracken, P. (1999) The value of advocacy: putting ethics into practice. *Psychiatric Bulletin*, **23**, 327–329.

Thornicroft, G. & Bebbington, P. (1989) Deinstitutionalisation – from hospital closure to service development. *British Journal of Psychiatry*, **155**, 739–753.

Trieman, N. & Leff, J. (2002) Long-term outcome of long-stay psychiatric inpatients considered unsuitable to live in the community. TAPS Project 44. *British Journal of Psychiatry*, **181**, 428–432.

Trieman, N., Smith, H. E., Kendal, B., *et al* (1998) The TAPS Project 41: Homes for life? Residential stability five years after hospital discharge. *Community Mental Health Journal*, **34**, 407–417.

Tyrer, P. (1999) Severe mental illness and substance misuse. *BMJ*, **318**, 137–138.

Warner, J. P., King, M., Blizard, R., *et al* (2000) Patient-held shared care records for individuals with mental illness. *British Journal of Psychiatry*, **177**, 319–324.

Wattis, J. & McGinnis, P. (1999) Clinical governance and continuing professional development. *Advances in Psychiatric Treatment*, **5**, 236.

Weaver, T., Rutter, D., Maden, P., *et al* (2001) Results of a screening survey for co-morbid substance misuse amongst patients in treatment for psychotic disorders: prevalence and service needs in an inner London borough. *Social Psychiatry and Psychiatric Epidemiology*, **36**, 399–406.

Williams, R. & Cohen, J. (2000) Substance use and misuse in psychiatric wards. *Psychiatric Bulletin*, **24**, 43–46.

Wing, J. K. & Brown, G. W. (1970) *Institutionalism and Schizophrenia.* London: Cambridge University Press.

Wolfensberger, W. (1983) Social role valorization: a proposed new term for the principle of normalization. *Mental Retardation*, **21**, 234–239.

Wright, S., Gournay, K., Glorney, E., *et al* (2000) Dual diagnosis in the suburbs: prevalence, need and in-patient service use. *Social Psychiatry and Psychiatric Epidemiology*, **35**, 297–304.

CHAPTER 30

Psychiatry in general practice

Greg Wilkinson

> 'We are convinced that for the good of general medicine, this particular study of psychological medicine, dealing as it does with so many complex problems should be merged in the general routine of medical practice.' (Andrew Wynter, 1875)

The historical origins of general practice

The practice notes of the astrological physician Richard Napier (1559–1637) provide a description of the mental illnesses recognised in an era long before psychiatry and general practice existed as separate specialties (MacDonald, 1989). Napier considered about 5% of his patients to be suffering from symptoms that he regarded as due to a mental disorder. Within this group the most common conditions were: 'troubled in mind' (33%), 'melancholy' (20%), 'mopish' (15%), 'mad and lunatic' (5.5%) and 'distracted' (5.4%). If 'troubled in mind' can be equated with 'anxiety', 'melancholy' with 'depression', and 'mad' and 'lunatic' with 'psychoses', these figures show some similarity to the prevalence of these disorders in general practice today, even when modern diagnostic criteria are applied. For example, Casey *et al* (1984), applying ICD–9 criteria, found that 7% of all general practice consultations were 'psychiatric'; the main groups were anxiety (20%), depression (30%) and schizophrenia (5%).

Loudon (1983) provides a description of the origins of general practice as a profession in Great Britain. Until 1800, medical care was provided by three groups of doctors:

1 the physicians, who were a learned profession trained at the universities and who dealt with internal disorders

2 the surgeons, who were craftsmen whose sphere was external disorders requiring surgery or other manual interference

3 the tradesmen apothecaries, whose only legal role was to dispense prescriptions written by the physicians.

After the Rose case in 1704, apothecaries won the right to 'practise physic' (to visit, advise and prescribe), but even so they could charge only for the medicine they supplied (Clark, 1966). The surgeons had insufficient work and as there was more work and money to be made in dispensing, many surgeons became 'surgeon apothecaries'. These apothecaries were the first general practitioners (GPs). There was also stiff competition from untrained chemists and midwives, while an additional financial pressure came in 1812 with the imposition of the glass tax to help finance the Napoleonic Wars (medicine was always dispensed in glass containers). To defend their position, the apothecaries and the surgeon apothecaries formed a trade association in 1812, the Association of Apothecaries and Surgeon Apothecaries, and then pressed for protective legislation. The Apothecaries Acts of 1812 and 1815 stipulated that apothecaries should have a period of training (an attachment of 5 years to an established apothecary) and if they passed a professional examination they were qualified to become a Member of the Royal College of Surgeons and a Licentiate of the Society of Apothecaries (MRCS–LSA). The licence permitted the apothecaries to practise surgery, midwifery and physic, and was an accepted medical qualification until the 1960s, while the Medical Act of 1858 led to a unification of all medical education, so that surgeons, physicians and GPs all started with the same basic medical training, which is the present-day system.

General practice flourished during the 19th century, mainly as a result of the increasing wealth of the middle classes, and by 1840 GPs comprised over 80% of the medical profession, with one GP per 1000 population. Marinker (1988) described the competition between the hospital-based physicians and surgeons and the GPs during the 19th century. This eventually led to the exclusion of the GPs from the hospitals, so a patient could be admitted to hospital only if the GP first referred the patient to a physician or a surgeon. The referral system, which originally started as a restrictive trade practice for the benefit of physicians and surgeons, has survived, as it is cost-effective, and with medical logic has helped in the development of a rational hospital service. The referral system permits the GP to act as a gatekeeper to expensive, high-technology specialist medical care. The gatekeeper has two functions:

1 to contain the majority of care within general practice

2 to select the most appropriate specialist advice.

There are some 30 000 GPs in the UK. Almost all (95%) of the UK population is registered with a GP, and 60–70% of these registered patients consult at least once each year; only about 10% will not consult at all in any 3-year period. Thus, the GP can be regarded as a personal physician who has access to the medical history and social background of patients. By virtue of the continuity of care GPs provide, not only for the patient but often for the whole family, they are in a unique position to manage psychiatric illness.

The scientific study of psychiatric disorders in general practice began with Shepherd's classic study *Psychiatric Illness in General Practice*, which describes a large-scale survey carried out in 12 general practices in Greater London between 1961 and 1962 (Shepherd *et al*, 1966). The authors demonstrated for the first time that the vast bulk of psychiatric disorders were identified and treated by GPs and not by mental health specialists. The main conclusions were as follows.

- Psychiatric morbidity was one of the more common reasons for consulting a GP. About 14% of the population at risk consulted their family doctor at least once over a 12-month period for a complaint diagnosed as entirely or largely psychiatric.
- Conditions given a psychiatric diagnosis made up about two-thirds of all psychiatric morbidity and these were mainly neurotic conditions – only 5% of patients with a psychiatric diagnosis suffered from psychoses – while the remainder were not recognised or given a diagnosis. Although labelled 'minor', these neurotic conditions were often of long duration and disabling.
- GP treatment consisted largely of drugs or discussion, but almost a third of patients with psychiatric disorders received no treatment.
- GPs dealt with the bulk of identified psychiatric morbidity themselves, referring only 5% to specialist psychiatric services.

Much of the subsequent research in this area, which forms the main body of this chapter, has elaborated and amplified Shepherd's observations on the epidemiology of common mental disorders; the social and medical factors that contribute to them; and how GPs deal with them. The term 'common mental disorders' (abbreviated to CMDs) will appear frequently in this chapter; it refers to the totality of neurotic disorders in the community or in the surgery. The CMDs do not include alcohol and substance misuse or psychotic disorders, but it is important to note that these conditions also make a substantial contribution to GPs' workload.

What is general practice psychiatry?

The topic of general practice psychiatry is poorly defined, yet it covers a vast area of medical activity, with perhaps more than half a million psychiatric consultations taking place in any one week in the UK, which is far more than occurs in the specialist psychiatric services. The topic can be viewed from a variety of perspectives. Thus, this chapter could have adopted a mainly clinical approach and focused on how a GP might deal with individual patients, and the common psychiatric syndromes, as described in the earlier chapters of this book, although in rather less detail. An epidemiological approach could also be justified, because such large numbers of patients with CMDs are involved: this would focus more on issues of prevalence, outcome and associated socio-demographic features, in order to provide information for funding and administrative bodies as well as finding ways of optimising treatments for the community as a whole. Much of this chapter takes the latter approach, and because these studies are mainly statistical this chapter contains many tables and a considerable amount of numerical data, perhaps more than any other chapter in this book.

This chapter also looks at how GPs treat the CMDs and issues such as psychiatric diagnosis in general practice and unrecognised psychiatric disorder, as well as other topics, such as the way GPs use psychotropic drugs and further education in psychiatry for GPs. GPs also deal with alcohol and substance-related psychiatric disorder, children and adolescents, and other branches of psychiatry, but these topics are dealt with in other volumes of the College Seminar Series. The chapter starts with a description of the prevalence and social correlates of the common mental disorders in the UK today, as found in the large survey by the Office for Population and Census Statistics (OPCS), as this forms the essential backcloth for understanding the nature of the work of primary care psychiatry.

The prevalence of psychiatric disorder in the community

The World Health Organization's study *The Global Burden of Disease* (Murray & Lopez, 1996) estimated that mental disorder was responsible for 38% of all years lost through disability for women and 25% for men, in the established market economies. Not surprisingly, governments in these countries have commissioned large-scale surveys to try to understand what lies behind this vast amount of disability. In their comprehensive review, Melzer *et al* (2003) identified nine such large-scale surveys from America and various European countries, which all had broadly similar findings; of these, the OPCS survey was the largest and most recent in the UK.

The OPCS has been conducting household surveys since 1971. Fully analysed data are available for the 1993 survey, which was the largest ($n = 10018$) cross-sectional psychiatric survey carried out in the UK. Psychiatric status was assessed by lay interviewers, who used the Clinical Interview Schedule, Revised (CIS-R) (Goldberg *et al*, 1970), which covers 14 key symptoms over the previous week or month. A cut-off of 12 or more symptoms was used to define 'caseness' and algorithms were used to assign an ICD–10 diagnosis. As the respondents were also part of the National Household Survey, a huge amount of additional socio-demographic data were also at hand. A novel feature of this particular survey was the inclusion of information on disability, with respondents being asked to rate the effect their mental symptoms had on limiting their 'activities of daily living' (ADLs). ADLs are commonly impaired in physical disease and are also routinely assessed by occupational therapists in certain subgroups of psychiatric patients, for example those with cognitive impairment or chronic schizophrenia,

Table 30.1 Prevalence of individual neurotic disorders (CMDs) by ICD–10 diagnoses in the OPCS community survey

ICD–10 type	Rate per 1000	% of group with neurotic disorders (i.e. CMDs)
Mixed anxiety and depression	77	48
Generalised anxiety disorder	31	19
Depressive episode	21	13
All phobias	11	7
Obsessive–compulsive disorder	12	8
Panic disorder	8	5
All neurotic disorders (CMDs)	160	100

where the issue of competence at living alone may be in question, and they are also routinely assessed in Care Programme Approach assessments. The OPCS survey recorded difficulties with: ablutions, transport, medical care, household activities, practical activities, paperwork and managing money.

Diagnostic subtypes of the common mental disorders

A breakdown of the diagnostic subtypes of CMDs and their prevalence as found in the OPCS survey is shown in Table 30.1. The most frequent diagnosis is 'anxiety depression', an ICD–10 category used only when symptoms of both anxiety and depression are present, but are not severe enough to qualify for a single diagnosis of either generalised anxiety disorder or major depressive disorder. Note also that the prevalence of depression itself constitutes only a relatively small proportion (13%) of the cases said to be CMDs.

Overall prevalence of neurotic disorder and relation to disability

The overall prevalence of neurotic disorder (all types) in the community for those in the 15- to 64-year age range was found to be 15.5%, a figure that is broadly in agreement with the findings of similar surveys. To assess the presence of impairment, respondents were also asked whether their 'mental symptoms stopped them from doing things'. Half of those with a neurotic disorder (8.3% of the total) replied positively and this group were said to have 'limiting disorder', but the other half (7.2%) reported no functional impairment.

Severity criteria that are sufficient to qualify for a DSM–IV diagnosis usually include the clause 'and should result in a significant degree of functional impairment', indicating that around half the respondents identified as 'cases' in the OPCS survey would therefore not have qualified for a DSM–IV diagnosis. At the more severe end of the spectrum, 3.4% of the respondents reported a limitation on at least one ADL and this was termed 'disabling disorder'; it is this smaller group who are likely to be clinically more relevant (see Table 30.8, page 756).

The main socio-demographic factors contributing to neurotic disorder

The main socio-demographic factors contributing to neurotic disorder and 'disabling disorder' are given in Table 30.2, which shows the results of the multivariate analysis. It confirms many of the already known associations between the CMDs and socio-demographic factors: being a lone parent, being unemployed or economically inactive, recent life events, absence of social support, and having left school before the age of 16. A few items emerge as being protective and these include older age, absence of life events and a good support network.

Sex ratio

Most studies show higher rates of anxiety and affective disorder for women than for men. The OPCS confirmed this for the CMDs, but one important finding was that for 'disabling disorder' the sex ratio was equal. The authors suggested that at the milder levels of severity, women more readily report symptoms than men, but for disorders causing severe disability there is less inhibition about consulting and so the prevalence is equal.

The overall prevalence of depressive disorders is 8.56%, although some variation is reported across study sites in Europe (Ayuso-Mateos *et al*, 2001); there is a notable a female predominance, with rates of 10.05% for women and 6.61% for men. It is possible that some men with anxiety and affective disorders resort to self-medication with alcohol and drugs, resulting in lower rates for males. The presence of comorbid physical disease may increase the rate of psychiatric disorder, particularly in women. When physical disorder is excluded, Vazquez-Barquero *et al* (1992) found the sex ratio was equal.

Sex differences in the prevalence of CMDs are not explained by differences in the socio-economic status or the number or type of social roles occupied by men and women. Weich *et al* (2001) found that the presence of a CMD at baseline was associated with a subsequent reduction in social role occupancy, but this did not vary between men and women. Neither the number nor the type of social roles occupied, nor socio-economic status, explained the gender difference for the CMDs. The sex ratio in depressive disorders is also discussed in Chapter 3 (page 50, on the aetiology of depression) and Chapter 31 (page 792, on its wide cross-cultural variation).

Age

Age plays an important role in the prevalence of most mental disorders and the OPCS survey found that older age was significantly protective against CMDs. Major illnesses such as the functional psychotic disorders, personality disorders and substance misuse, which figure prominently in secondary care, are also more common in those under 45 years of age. Affective disorders are common and peak in middle age, while cognitive impairment is most frequent in old age.

Educational level

Leaving school before 16 was a consistent predictor of CMDs in the OPCS study, with 19% of such respondents

Table 30.2 Odds ratios for a comprehensive set of factors associated with neurotic disorder: results of a multivariate analysis

Variable	Reference category	Category	Disorder (odds ratio)	Disabling disorder (odds ratio)
Age group (years)	16–24	55–64	0.62*	0.71
		45–54	1.02	1.15
		35–44	1.06	1.05
		25–34	1.07	0.92
Gender	Male	Female	1.68*	0.92
Age left education	16 years or more	Up to 15 (including no education)	1.26*	1.60*
Work status	Working full time	Economically inactive	1.42*	3.32*
		Unemployed	1.30	1.63*
		Working part time	1.13	1.03
Ethnicity	White/European	Other	1.17	2.97*
		Asian/Oriental	1.15	1.46
		West Indian/African	0.79	0.66
Urban residence	Urban	Semi-urban or rural	1.14	1.19
Family type	Couple, no children	Child of lone parent	0.97	0.74
		Child of couple	0.89	1.45
		One person	1.17	1.55
		Lone parent	1.43*	1.97*
		Couple with children	1.14	1.79
Number of life events	None	Two or more	3.16*	3.25**
		One	1.75*	1.80*
Social support	No lack	Unknown	1.46	2.03
		Severe lack	2.14**	2.23**
		Moderate lack	1.25	1.12
Number of physical illnesses	None	Two or more	3.46**	6.42**
		One	1.86*	2.69*

*Significant at $P < 0.05$ level; **odds ratio greater than 2. Confidence limits have been omitted.

having a CMD. However, when 'disabling disorders' are considered, the effect is much larger (see Table 30.8, page 756): around half (52%) of those with a disabling disorder had left school before 16, which indicates that poor education was a major contributor to disabling CMDs. Children leave school before 16 for many non-educational reasons, such as childhood physical or psychiatric disorder, truancy and low IQ, each of which may independently contribute to CMDs, so this may partly explain the association. However, this association has been repeatedly found in other national surveys; for example, in the USA there was a raised rate (odds ratio, OR) of mood disorders among those who had completed only 11 years of education relative to those who completed 17 years (OR = 1.3) in the Netherlands (OR = 1.55), while in Australia secondary school non-completers, relative to those with a post-school qualification, had raised rates of affective disorders (OR = 1.55). Better education confers a higher level of personal competence and this appears to have a protective effect on the subsequent development of CMDs, but the strong association of poorer education with disabling CMDs emphasises the need to ensure people are educated to the highest possible level they are able to attain (for references see Melzer *et al*, 2003).

Physical illness

Physical illness emerged as a significant factor causing CMDs; the presence of one illness gave an OR of 1.86, but if two diseases were present the OR rose to 3.46. Physical disease itself may cause disability, but the survey specifically tried to isolate disability caused by mental problems from the impairment caused by some physical diseases. The complex relationship between physical and mental disease is further elaborated in Chapter 17.

Life events

Life events are known to be associated with CMDs, although the bulk of the scientific literature concerns their association with depression. The OPCS survey found that one recent life event elevated the risk for CMDs by a factor 1.75 and two life events by 3.16. The survey also was able to give a quantitative estimate for the frequency of each life event in the community, as well as the potential for a particular event to result in a CMD (Table 30.3); in addition, the survey looked at the influence of protective factors, such as social support. Types of event that registered high rates (greater than 30% of respondents) were: separations, problems with relatives, financial crises and problems with the police. A more detailed discussion of the association of life events and depression is given in Chapter 3 on page 54, but the OPCS survey shows that this association also holds for the CMDs in general, even though depression itself formed only a small minority (around 13%) of cases constituting the CMDs.

Table 30.3 Six-month prevalence of particular life events in the community and proportion of those with the life event who have a CMD

Item	Frequency of item over a 6-month period (%)	% with item who develop a CMD
Baseline rate of the CMDs	–	15
Number of events		
0 life events	49	10
1 life event	30	17
2 life events	18	29
Degree of support		
Adequate support	62	14
Moderate lack of support	26	17
Severe lack of support	9	29
Individual events		
Relative seriously ill	13	23
Close relative died	15	23
Separation	5	30
Problems with relatives	9	37
Seeking work for 1 month or more	11	22
Financial crises	5	36
Problem with police	1.6	39
Something lost or stolen	7	25

Rates of CMDs for individual life events should be compared with the baseline rate for CMDs of 15%.

Lone parents

Lone parents constituted 12.3% of the head of households in the OPCS sample and lone parents had raised rates of CMDs (OR = 1.43). Around 10% of all the children of the survey respondents were living with lone parents and a third of these children (n = 200) were living with a lone parent who also had a CMD. Although these only comprised of 3% of the total number of children of the respondents, the authors made a point of highlighting the special needs of these children, as their lone parent was suffering from a mental disorder. Thus some of these children may have been at risk. The authors also suggested that these lone parents might usefully be targeted for help as their number is relatively small and the psychological distress associated with being a lone parent may be far more amenable to change through some social or psychological intervention, than some of the other major causes of CMDs, such as unemployment or physical illness, where a change may be far more difficult to achieve.

Urban–rural differences

Urban–rural differences have been found in many older studies, with anxiety being more prevalent in the rural areas and depression in the urban areas (Prudo *et al*, 1984; Vazquez-Barquero *et al*, 1992). Is this because city life is more stressful than living in the countryside? The more recent pan-European ODIN study (Dowrick *et al*, 2000*b*) showed that these urban–rural differences existed only in some, not all European countries. Thus, in both the UK and Ireland rates for depression were two to three times higher in urban than in rural areas, but in Norway and Finland urban and rural rates for psychiatric disorder were approximately equal, indicating that urban–rural differences are not universal. To try to understand what lay behind these differences, Paykel *et al* (2000) analysed in greater depth the UK data, as elicited from the OPCS survey, and confirmed higher rates of CMDs, alcoholism and drug misuse in urban environments. They also found that once the factors known to cause CMDs – poverty, deprivation, life events, poorer education, unemployment and so on – are taken into account, urban–rural differences tended to disappear. They concluded that the large differences found in the UK were largely attributable to higher rates of adverse social factors in UK cities. Presumably, in the more equitable societies of Scandinavia, the city environments are less socially adverse, while the study of Paykel *et al* (2000) suggests that it is the more benign social environment of the countryside rather than simply its scenic beauty that is protective.

Inequality and psychiatric disorder, social class and social deprivation

Much of the earlier literature on social disadvantage reported an association between psychiatric disorder and lower social class (as defined by occupation). Thus, for example, in a survey of women in Edinburgh conducted by Surtees *et al* (1983), which defined social class by occupation according to the classification of Goldthorpe & Hope (1974), the rate of psychiatric disorder for unemployed working-class women was more than double (29% versus 14%) that for unemployed middle-class women and similarly for employed women (14% versus 7%). However, the more recent OPCS survey failed to detect any significant effect for social class on the prevalence of the CMDs. Possible reasons for this may be that recent socio-economic changes have resulted in greater numbers of 'working-class wealthy' and 'middle-class poor', and so there has been an eroding of wealth differentials between the various occupational groups. What did emerge from the OPCS survey was a link between indicators of poverty and wealth and the prevalence of the CMDs (Table 30.4). This suggests that the relevant factor in the development of CMDs is probably *financial deprivation* rather than occupationally defined social class. The importance of financial deprivation is also evident in studies of unemployed people, which show that once the financial impact of unemployment is controlled for, unemployed people are no more psychologically distressed than those in work (Kessler *et al*, 1987).

What is social deprivation?

Even though occupationally defined social class no longer shows much correlation with psychiatric disorder, widespread inequalities in the community persist. It is to these inequalities that the term 'social deprivation' refers, and it is this parameter that shows the strongest link with a wide variety of both physical and mental disorders, making it all the more important to understand exactly what the term means and how 'social deprivation' is measured.

Table 30.4 Multivariate analysis of markers of wealth, education and occupation, adjusted for age group and gender

Variable	Reference category	Category	Disorder (odds ratio)	Disabling disorder (odds ratio)
Type of accommodation	Detached house	Flat, bedsit or other	1.31	1.42
		Terraced	1.19	1.40
		Semi-detached	0.95	1.25
Housing tenure	Owned	Rent, other	1.31*	1.22
		Rent from local authority or housing association	1.46*	1.60*
		Mortgage	1.17	1.23
Car or van ownership	2+	None	1.46*	1.80*
		One	1.20	1.27
Age left school	16 years plus	Up to 15 (including no education)	1.32*	1.72*
Work status	Working full time	Economically inactive	1.68*	4.26*
		Unemployed	2.16*	2.97*
		Working part time	1.20	1.13
Social class	I+II	IV+V	0.93	1.07
		III M	0.97	0.91
		III NM	1.17	1.13

*Identified odds ratios that are significant at the 5% level. Note the absence of significant associations between social class and disorder, even including disabling disorder.

Social deprivation is a rather more complex concept than occupationally defined social class, and also entails far more than simple poverty. Our understanding of social deprivation derives from two quite separate strands: first, the writings of sociologists such as Townsend, who were trying to understand the causes and consequences of poverty; and second, the work of Brian Jarman, a GP.

Townsend (1987) wrote that deprivation has two key qualities. The first is *unacceptability*, which he illustrated with a definition given by Berthoud, also a sociologist:

> 'deprivation involves conditions and experiences which have become more unacceptable to society as a whole ... the word deprivation as it is commonly used, appears to imply a situation that is unacceptably below some minimum standard, even though more general inequality may be accepted as at least inevitable if not desirable. If inequality can be seen as a hill, then deprivation is a ravine into which people should not be allowed to fall.' (Berthoud, 1976, pp. 175, 180)

The second quality Townsend considered central to deprivation is that it is a multifaceted phenomenon and *covers a wide range of categories*, both in the material field and in the more social realms. Deprivation relates more to the conditions people find themselves living in than the resources that are available to them, although the two are obviously linked.

Townsend devised an index and an interview to measure deprivation, based on 13 separate categories and a total of 77 individual items. In the 1980s this index was used to study deprivation in different districts of London. Although this index is now little used and has been replaced by much simpler, census-based measures, it provides an insight into the sociologist's understanding of the term 'social deprivation' (Box 30.1 gives examples of items in the index).

The second strand to our understanding of deprivation derives from a rather different source, the work of Brian Jarman, a GP who worked in an inner-London practice. In common with other GP colleagues he had observed that his own personal workload was heavy

Box 30.1 Categories included in Townsend's index of deprivation

Material deprivation

- Dietary deprivation: e.g. at least 1 day in past 2 weeks with insufficient to eat; no fresh meat or fish most days.
- Clothing deprivation: inadequate footwear for all weathers, inadequate protection against heavy rain.
- Housing deprivation: no exclusive indoor toilet or bath, no electricity.
- Deprivation of home function: no car, no central heating, no carpets.
- Deprivation of environment: nowhere for children to play safely, no garden; air pollution, noise
- Deprivation of location: no nearby park, no shops, litter problems.
- Deprivation of work: poor working environment, polluted air, dust, noise, unsocial hours, standing for much of the day.

Social deprivation

- Lack of employment rights: unemployed, no paid holiday, no sick pay, work more than 50 hours per week.
- Deprivation of family activities: difficulties for children to play indoors, health problems in a relative, relative with a disability at home.
- Lack of integration into the community: alone or isolated, unsafe environment, racial harassment.
- Lack of formal community participation: did not vote, not a member of any union or work-related association.
- Lack of recreational activities: no holidays, less than 3 hours per week of recreational activity.
- Education deprivation: fewer than 10 years' education, no formal qualifications.

Note that only a few representative items are included in the above list. Townsend's index is little used today but illustrates the breadth of categories which lie behind in the concept of 'social deprivation'.

Box 30.2 Items comprising the Jarman-8 under-privileged area (UPA) index

Proportion of:

- older people living alone
- single-parent households
- unemployed people
- people who have moved house
- children under 5 years
- unskilled people
- overcrowded households
- ethnic minority households

and much more influenced by social than by strictly medical factors. He conducted a large-scale survey of his fellow GPs, sending them a list of 21 items, each of which they were asked to rate on a scale of 0–9 according to its contribution to GP workload. Some items were socio-demographic factors related to patients and others related to the general practice itself, such as its size, the accessibility of other local health service provision, the availability of district nurses, or ease of making out-patient appointments in the local hospital and so forth. The factor that came out highest (i.e. as contributing most to GP workload) was 'elderly person living alone'.

Jarman (1983) distilled the results of his survey and eventually selected eight socio-demographic variables according to two criteria:

1 the GPs had identified them as making a major contribution to their workload

2 they were routinely identified in the national census (and therefore the data were readily available).

These items are given individual weightings and produce the Jarman-8 index 'under-privileged area' (UPA) score. The items (but not weightings) are listed in Box 30.2. With the use of local census data it is possible to give a Jarman deprivation score for a post-code area, a council ward, or the catchment area of a particular general practice or hospital. Jarman-8 UPA scores correlate highly with the prevalence of both psychosocial and medical disorder. For example, surveys have shown increased rates of depression, anxiety, schizophrenia, heart disease and non-insulin-dependent diabetes in areas of higher deprivation.

Moser (2001) calculated that if all of England and Wales experienced the same rates as the least deprived fifth of the population, the overall rates of depression would fall by 10% and coronary heart disease by 11%. The effect was greater for people in the age range 25–44 years. Thus, for men in this age range the rate for treated depression in the most deprived areas was 50% higher than it was in the least deprived areas. Similarly, the Hampshire Depression Project found a large effect for deprivation on rates of depression, with the Jarman UPA scores accounting for 48% of the variance of depressive symptoms between the different general practices in Hampshire (Ostler *et al*, 2001). Some childhood psychiatric disorders may also correlate with deprivation; thus, Foreman *et al* (2003) found a strong correlation between the prevalence of conduct disorder and Jarman-8 UPA scores for individual post-code areas.

Deprivation and government funding for healthcare

Because deprivation is associated with a wide range of both medical and psychiatric conditions, there has been interest in refining the way it is measured. Thus, central government has always needed a method of distributing National Health Service (NHS) funds to ensure that the poorer, more populous regions of the country, which have higher morbidity and a higher mortality rates, receive more money than the less densely populated rural shires. The government's Resource Allocation Working Party (RAWP) in the mid-1970s used a very crude formula based on the numerical size, age and sex distribution of the population and the square root of the standardised mortality ratio (SMR) of a district to estimate its financial allocation. More recently, health economists at the University of York (Smith *et al*, 1996) have combined elements of the older RAWP formula with items from the Jarman-8 UPA index to provide two separate indices of deprivation, the first to predict the service needs for acute physical care and the second to predict needs for the psychiatric services. Items that comprise this York index for psychiatric care are shown in Box 30.3. As with the Jarman index, each item is given a numerical weighting ('old alone' has the highest rating, 'new Commonwealth' the lowest) and the resulting formula is used to calculate the York Psychiatric Index, which is used to calculate the amount allocated for the psychiatric services of each district.

The amount of money spent on mental health services is probably the most important single determinant of both their quantity and quality. The old district health authorities, which served approximately the same areas as their local authorities, used to be the recipients of government money, but these have been replaced by primary care trusts (PCTs), with the presumed intention of ensuring that primary care (i.e. the GPs) have a greater say in how the money should be spent. The actual calculation of how money is allocated to each PCT is very complex and the methods used to calculate this are published on government websites, but Glover (2003) provides a simplified overview. Essentially, it entails taking into account:

- the weighted population of each district (the age structure is critical because older people have greater health needs)

Box 30.3 Items comprising the York Psychiatric Index

Proportions of households with:

- a lone parent
- old alone (i.e. elderly person living alone)
- dependants with no carer
- ethnic minorities (new Commonwealth)
- standardised mortality ratio (square root)
- chronically sick and disabled

- the estimated health need of some districts (e.g. some inner cities they have more sick people)
- local cost-of-living indices (as some districts are more expensive than others)
- indices of deprivation (as indicated above, the York index is used for psychiatric services, and the Jarman index for general medical services)
- any other local factors that may be relevant.

The previous year's allocation is taken as the base and adjustments either up or down are made to this figure.

Separate calculations are made for mental health and the acute services (GP and acute hospital services). Mental health services received on average 11.85% of the total health budget, but districts showed a wide range (9–15%) in the proportion of the budget allocated to mental health.

Table 30.5 Mental illness in community, general practice and specialist settings: Goldberg & Huxley's (1980) concept of levels and filters

Level/filter	Rate/1000/year
Level 1: Mental illness in the community	260–315
Filter 1: The decision to consult	
Level 2: Total general practice morbidity	239
Filter 2: GP recognition	
Level 3: Conspicuous general practice morbidity	101.5
Filter 3: The decision to refer	
Level 4: All psychiatric patients	23.5
Filter 4: The decision to admit	
Level 5: Psychiatric in-patients	5.71

Pathways to care: levels and filters

Psychiatric morbidity varies in severity from the few extremely ill patients who are in hospital through to the many people in the community who may experience a few psychiatric symptoms but are not sufficiently distressed to seek help. Goldberg & Huxley (1980, 1992) employed the concepts of *levels* and *filters* (Table 30.5) to describe this wide range of severity of disorder and the pathways that patients take to reach specialist care. This model not only has been influential in research into general practice psychiatry but has also provided a convenient way of organising the large and diffuse literature on morbidity in primary care. The model comprises *five levels*; and, to move from one level to the next, it is necessary to pass through one of *four filters*.

Level 1 refers to psychiatric and emotional disorder in the community as measured by community surveys. Investigations using this approach suggest that the probable prevalence of psychiatric disorder in the community is about 20%. For example, Goldberg & Huxley (1992) reported an annual period prevalence of 260–315 per 1000 per year. Only a proportion of people with such a disorder in the community will consult a GP, and they pass through *filter 1* to reach *level 2*.

Filter 1 is the decision made by the patient to seek help and the act of consulting. The major determinant of contacting a GP is the severity of the disorder, which will mainly be the level of psychiatric symptoms but with an independent contribution from social dysfunction; even so, some people with high levels of psychiatric symptoms do not have any contact with professionals who might be able to help them (Bebbington *et al*, 2000).

Level 2 comprises the total of all psychiatric morbidity that presents to GPs. Goldberg & Huxley (1992) gave an estimate of 239/1000 cases per year in Manchester. Some of these cases are diagnosed by the GP and have 'conspicuous morbidity', while a substantial number are unrecognised and are said to have 'hidden psychiatric morbidity'. This group of patients do not pass through *filter 2* and so fail to reach *level 3*.

Level 3 consists of conspicuous psychiatric morbidity, that is, morbidity identified and recognised by the GP (annual period prevalence around 101.5/1000/year).

Levels 4 and 5 consist, respectively, of all patients who are referred to psychiatric services (both in-patient and out-patient) (annual period prevalence around 23.5/1000/year); or are admitted to hospital, and therefore represent the severe end of the spectrum (annual period prevalence around 5.71/1000/year).

There is a change in the sex ratio among patients at the various levels: in general practice (level 3) the female:male ratio of cases is 2.38:1, whereas in secondary care (levels 4 and 5) it is 1.37:1. Thus, with increasing severity, sex differences in psychiatric disorder tend to equalise. In primary care the CMDs are the main diagnostic group, whereas in secondary care the psychoses are predominant, but personality disorder and alcohol and substance misuse are problems commonly encountered in both primary and secondary care.

Psychiatric morbidity in the community (level 1) has been described above in the context of the OPCS survey and so in the following sections only psychiatric morbidity at the levels 2 and 3 is further discussed; this is followed by a description of the first three filters in the Goldberg & Huxley (1980) model (see Table 30.5). Morbididity at levels 4 (all psychiatric patients) and 5 (psychiatric in-patients) and filter 4 (admission to hospital) are all topics more related to secondary care and so are not considered further here, as they are covered in the previous chapters of this book.

Level 2 – psychiatric morbidity in general practice

This is defined as the total psychiatric morbidity that presents to GPs and it comprises two groups: those who are recognised and are said to have conspicuous psychiatric morbidity and those whose condition is not recognised by the GP and are said to have 'hidden' psychiatric morbidity. An early study by Goldberg & Blackwell (1970), which has since been replicated many times, illustrates the nature of the problem. Using the General Health Questionnaire (GHQ) to screen for probable 'caseness', 31% of GP attendees were identified as probable cases but the GPs picked up only 20%: the remaining 11%, or roughly one-third of the cases,

Table 30.6 Diagnostic profile of psychiatric cases presenting to the GP

Diagnosis	Weekly prevalence per 1000 adults aged 16–64 years	No. of patients on GP list of 1650	No. of patients on GP list of 2000
Psychotic illness*	4	4	5
Mixed anxiety and depression	92	96	116
Generalised anxiety	47	49	59
Depressive episode	28	29	35
All phobias	19	20	24
Obsessive–compulsive disorder	12	12	15
Panic disorder	7	8	9
All neuroses	173	180	218
Drug dependence	42	44	53
Alcohol dependence	81	84	102

Table shows the expected numbers of patients on the average GP's lists, assuming 63% of the list are aged 16–64 years. A list of 1650 is an optimal size; 2000 is a common size in areas where there is a shortage of GPs.
*Note how uncommon psychosis is in general practice, with only one new presentation of schizophrenia every 5 years.

were missed and they continued to have 'hidden morbidity'. Ormel & Giel (1990) found that GPs missed around half the cases and tended to give non-specific diagnoses to the recognised cases, but the recognised cases had a better outcome in terms of decreases in psychopathology and improved social functioning. Better recognition and outcome were associated with purely psychological presentations, recency of onset, diagnostic category and a lower rate of psychiatric comorbidity.

Hidden psychiatric morbidity is a cause for concern because it indicates a substantial amount of unrecognised and therefore unmet need. This may be a particular worry in health service systems, as in the UK, where the GP serves as the gatekeeper to a wide array of other medical, social and voluntary services, and hence GP recognition is essential if patients are not to miss out.

Level 3 – conspicuous psychiatric morbidity

Level 3 refers to patients with psychiatric morbidity that is recognised by the GP. Psychiatric illness defined by modern research criteria occurs in around a quarter to a third of all new episodes of illness seen in general practice. Anxiety and depression and associated problems comprise the bulk of this morbidity. In addition to these CMDs, a GP will be confronted sooner or later by the full range of psychiatric disorders. This is illustrated in Table 30.6, derived from data from the Office of National Statistics (Cohen *et al*, 2004). Although depression and anxiety have the highest overall rates of occurrence in general practice, psychoses, substance-related disorder and personality disorder also make an impact, and because these conditions are more difficult to treat, they may also make a greater demand on the GP's time.

The vast bulk of the psychiatric morbidity presenting to the GP is contained within primary care. Thus, an earlier large study of Manchester GPs by Whitehouse (1987) found that when all CMDs were considered only 5% were referred to a psychiatrist, 0.6% to social services and 0.5% to community psychiatric nurses (CPNs). Out of 1729 patient consulting for anxiety, 75% received a prescription and only 2.8% were referred to a paramedical person. Today, with the more widespread availability of counselling in the surgery, a rather higher proportion will be referred for counselling, but these figures none the less indicate that GPs will personally treat large numbers of people with psychiatric disorder and in this sense for much of their time will function as 'psychiatrists', a role for which they merit far better training as well as greater support.

Most psychiatric disorders in the community have a benign outcome

Tennant *et al* (1981) found that 1 month after the initial diagnosis around half the cases had resolved; where the disorder had been triggered by a threatening event, 80% had resolved. Remission had little to do with medical intervention, such as consultation or taking a psychotropic drug, but seemed to be related to neutralising or 'fresh start' events that appeared to give hope. Brodaty (1983) also found that, of those with a positive GHQ screen at consultation, only 50% were still positive at 4 months, and 40% at 6 months.

Some disorders may become chronic

Although most illnesses are transient (have a natural tendency to remit), the OPCS survey found that 63% of cases had lasted for 6 months. Mann *et al* (1981) found that 25% of consultees in an inner-London practice who were 'GHQ positive' at consultation were still positive at 1 year. In that study the more chronic outcome was associated with greater illness severity, increasing age, physical illness and receiving a prescription for a psychotropic drug. The reasons underlying a delay in resolution of CMDs have been much less studied than the causes of an onset, but similar factors appear to operate. Separation or divorce, becoming and remaining unemployed, health limiting daily activities, and caring for a sick relative all decreased the chances of recovery. Severity of disorder was associated with both less likelihood of recovery and longer time to recovery. Low social support increased the chances of a fresh onset and decreased the chances of recovery (Pevalin & Goldberg, 2003). Seivewright *et al* (1991) showed that people with personality disorder also made a contribution to chronic morbidity in general practice by having significantly more contacts over a 3-year period as well as by taking more psychotropics (benzodiazepines).

Table 30.7 Diagnostic composition of the group of patients with enduring and disabling mental illness

Diagnosis	Percentage of group
Psychosis	
Schizophrenia	23.6
Bipolar affective disorder	8.7
Other	3.8
Total (psychosis)	36.1
Non-psychosis	
Severe anxiety/depression	45.4
Alcohol/drug misuse	7.5
Personality disorder	3.0
Other	6.9
Total (non psychosis)	63.9

From Kai *et al* (2000).

Some disorders are both chronic and disabling

The most problematic patients are those with both chronic and severely disabling mental disorders. The OPCS survey reported a 6-month period prevalence of 3.4% for 'severe disabling disorder', but Kai *et al* (2000), using a duration criterion of 2 years or more, found a rather smaller proportion were disabled. In that study, disability was defined as failure to fulfil any one of four roles as a result of their mental symptoms: hold down a job; maintain personal hygiene and self-care; perform necessary domestic chores; or participate in recreational activities. By applying a case-finding methodology in primary care they found a point prevalence of 1.29% of patients with both enduring psychotic and non-psychotic illness (36.1% and 63.9%, respectively). The different psychiatric diagnostic groups that contributed to this severe chronic morbidity are shown in Table 30.7. These patients with a chronic disability contribute considerably to GP workload and include a significant proportion of older people (24.6% aged over 65 years). Only half of these patients were in contact with mental health services and 25% of those with psychosis were not in contact with mental health services at all. However, almost all patients were being seen frequently in primary care, which would have considerable workload and resource implications.

The underlying causes of this longer-term severe morbidity are poorly understood. For the psychotic group, who comprise around a third of the cases, the main determinant is likely to be the severity of the underlying mental illness. However, for the non-psychotic group, who comprise around two-thirds of the cases, social and other causes are important, with the severity of the underlying mental disorder itself having a less important role. Thus, the OPCS survey found important effects for social factors such as being unemployed or economically inactive and poorer education, as well as for serious medical disorders. These items were particularly important for 'disabling neurotic disorder', as shown in Table 30.8. Lowering unemployment rates and improving education levels in the community are obviously desirable goals, but they are beyond the reach of psychiatry and call for changes in the wider socio-economic or political arena.

The combination of high frequency of contact, sometimes extending over several years, and severity of disorder may make considerable demands on a GP's time and emotional resources – a few patients who were particularly demanding at one time acquired the description of 'heart-sink patients', although the term is little used now. The present-day shift of focus and funding of mental health policy towards those with chronic psychosis rather than supporting those with chronic neurotic disorders remains a source of tension, especially as many of those with chronic neurotic disorders appear to be just as severely disabled.

The magnitude of the economic burden of mental illness to the community is well known, but in terms of days of work lost, minor psychiatric disorder clearly takes largest share. Shiels *et al* (2004) studied the diagnoses most commonly given on medical certificates. The results are summarised in Table 30.9. Mild mental disorder accounted for nearly 40% of total certified sickness and was responsible for ten times more 'sickness days' than severe mental illness.

Filter 1 – the decision to consult

The recognition of any medical disorder hinges critically on two decisions. The first, made by the patient, is that there is sufficient 'illness' or 'discomfort' to consult a doctor. The second, made by the doctor, is that 'something is wrong'; it is this decision that initiates the diagnostic process. Eisenberg (1986) points out that patients are driven to consult a doctor more because of ill-defined states of dysphoria and social dysfunction in daily living than for specific symptoms or any pathology.

Not surprisingly, physical illness and illness severity are the main determinants of consultation. However, but minor psychiatric morbidity in the form of CMDs may also play a significant role, and this was investigated by Williams *et al* (1986). In the 1970s, in response to public anxiety concerning the effect of noise on residents who lived near Heathrow Airport,

Table 30.8 Relative contribution (%) of each high-risk group to total morbidity

Total number in sample (n = 10018)	Neurotic disorder (n = 1562)	Disabling disorder (n = 341)
Lone parents	10	12
Two or more physical illnesses	16	30
Unemployed	14	16
Economically inactive	31	52
Left school at age 15 or earlier	36	52

High-risk groups overlap and so totals are greater than 100%.

Table 30.9 Proportion of total days certified on all sickness certificates, by diagnostic group

Diagnostic category	Percentage of total days certified
Mild mental disorder	39.7
Musculoskeletal	15.4
Injury	7.1
Post-operative recovery	5.5
Respiratory	5.2
Symptoms not otherwise specified	4.9
Circulatory	4.7
Severe mental disorder	3.0
Nervous system/sense organ	2.8
All the rest	< 2.0

From Shiels *et al* (2004).

the government commissioned a large survey that recorded noise levels in different London districts at varying distances from the airport, together with the GHQ scores of residents. Noise in fact had little effect on GHQ score, but Williams *et al* (1986) used the information gathered in this survey to try to work out whether minor psychiatric morbidity (i.e. a high GHQ score) had any influence on consulting behaviour. They obtained GP records of all the respondents in this survey and noted which had consulted their GP in the 2 weeks before the survey. Minor psychiatric morbidity (a high GHQ score) doubled consultation rates (26% for men, 33% for women) and around 20% of all consultations could be solely attributed to it. A similar study in Cantabria (Vazquez-Barquero *et al*, 1992), in northern Spain, also confirmed that minor psychiatric morbidity doubled consultation rates, and that lower educational levels increased rates for men, but the highest consultation rates (of around 90%) were observed for those who had both physical and psychiatric disorder. The diagnostic profile of cases found in community surveys is broadly similar to that found in the surgery, with the possible exception that somatisation, and neurasthenic presentations are more frequent in the surgery than in the community (Goldberg & Huxley, 1992).

Filter 2 – GP recognition and non-recognition of psychiatric disorders

Studies of the ability of GPs to recognise cases correctly have identified both illness factors and GP factors, especially GP time, as being important, and these are reviewed below.

Patient/illness factors contributing to non-recognition

Freeling (1993) identified illness factors that influenced the ability of GPs to recognise depression. More frequent recognition of depression was associated with patients specifically stating they were depressed, and also if the GP developed a feeling that they were depressed, derived mainly from non-verbal cues during the interview. In contrast, depressions that had lasted for more than 1 year or those showing greater mood reactivity were less likely to be recognised. The presence of comorbid serious physical disease raised the non-recognition rate of depression by a factor of five. Presumably, in these instances, the GP is more preoccupied with issues of organic pathology and so will either neglect any associated psychiatric disorder or will assume the level of distress can be adequately explained solely by the physical disorder.

Although most of the earlier studies on GP recognition of depression focused on the dichotomous distinction between 'recognition versus non-recognition', more recent work has shown that GP diagnosis is a more quantitative affair, with a curvilinear relationship between GP rates for recognition and increasing severity of depression. Thus, in the Hampshire Depression Project (Thompson *et al*, 2001) the Hospital Anxiety and Depression – Depression subscale (HAD-D) was administered to a large number of patients in general practice. Using the recommended cut-off score for the HAD-D of 7, GPs had made a formal diagnosis of depression in only 33% of cases, but 75% of those who scored below the threshold score were diagnosed as having 'an emotional disorder', giving an overall diagnosis rate of 84%. With increasing severity of the depression, the recognition rate rose: for patients with an HAD-D score of 12, GPs recognised 59% of the cases; for those with an HAD-D score of 16, they identified 75% of cases.

In the Hampshire Depression Project the only factor independently to increase GP recognition of psychiatric disorder was unemployment (OR = 1.7), possibly because GPs may already have been sensitised to the association between depression and unemployment, and so looked out for it. This may also be because GPs are responsible for the certification of this depressed unemployed group, which may be numerically quite large. A recent government intervention has been to place personal employment advisers in GP surgeries in the hope that these patients can achieve a more rapid resolution of their employment difficulties, and that this will translate into an improvement in their depression and potential savings of state benefits, but the scheme has yet to be evaluated.

Thompson *et al* (2001) concluded that 'GP recognition of depression was not as poor as had been claimed in the past', and cautioned against burdening GPs with extra tuition on depression because increasing the general sensitivity of GPs to depression may increase the false positive rates of diagnosis, which in turn will increase the false positive rates of treatment, and this would be unlikely to improve the care of depression as a whole. The recent very high rates of prescribing of the selective serotonin reuptake inhibitors (SSRIs) bears some witness to this; for example, 3% of the population of Sweden are taking an SSRI (Isacsson *et al*, 1999) and so the extent of GP under-recognition and under-treatment of depression is now very much less than it used to be.

Does recognising depression in general practice matter, and are patients with unrecognised depression worse off than those who receive a diagnosis? Sireling *et al* (1985) found that 12 weeks after consultation, patients with unrecognised depression had significantly higher scores for depressed mood, loss of energy and irritability compared with those with recognised depression. However, unrecognised depressions tend to become recognised with the passage of time. By 6 months, of those cases that were previously unrecognised, 20% had been recognised and a further 20% had remitted, but 20% remained unrecognised (Freeling, 1993). Kessler *et al* (2002) also found that although many patients with depression do not receive a diagnosis at a single consultation, most are given a diagnosis at subsequent consultations.

Many GPs feel that the whole area of research into GP diagnosis – with the conclusion that GPs miss many cases of significant psychiatric disorder – has done a disservice to GPs, in that much of the so-called 'non-recognition' is actually deliberate. Thus, when confronted with a patient with symptoms, but where the situation is known to be intractable or where no change can realistically be effected, GPs often choose not to make a diagnosis of a CMD, preferring instead to direct their diagnostic and therapeutic endeavours to cases where some change may be possible.

In support of this, Dowrick & Buchan (1995) found that recognition made little difference to outcome when all cases of depression (both new and chronic cases) were considered; further, feedback to the GP that a patient was depressed made no difference to the outcome. These authors concluded that a GP diagnosis of depression was only a marker of severity and that most of the depression seen in the community was beyond the reach of medical intervention, and mainly owing to intractable medical and social problems – a hypothesis that receives some support from the OPCS survey (see Table 30.8, page 756).

GP variation in recognition rates

GPs vary widely in their rates of recognition of psychiatric disorder but the reasons for this are obscure. Whitehouse (1987) examined recognition rates for CMDs in five urban practices. CMDs were recorded at mean rate of 8% for all GP attendees, a figure consistent with known inner-city rates. Around two-thirds of the GPs in the study had recording rates for CMDs of between 5% and 10%, indicating they were probably setting their diagnostic thresholds at conventional levels. However, the range of recording a CMD diagnosis was very wide, at 1–24%, indicating that there must be a few GPs who either virtually deny the existence of the CMDs, or at the other extreme are over-diagnosing (by a factor of 3), with attendant risks of over-treatment and over-medication. The possibility that this may be an artefact due to greater patient choice should also be considered, since patients are now free to choose which doctor within a practice they see, and those with psychological problems will tend to gravitate to GPs whom they perceive to be sympathetic to such difficulties. Probably the majority of GPs (those who set their diagnostic thresholds at conventional levels) will miss an occasional case of depression, but for those patients who attend the small minority of GPs who set their diagnostic thresholds at very high or otherwise unconventional levels there may be a risk that their depressions will be completely ignored.

Attempts have been made to see whether the GP's attitude to depression influences diagnostic ability. Dowrick *et al* (2004) devised a GP 'attitude to depression scale' but found no correlation between the GPs' attitude to depression and their diagnostic acumen. Diagnostic accuracy was, however, associated with:

1 a preference for psychotherapy over antidepressants

2 a sense of ease in managing depression

3 a belief in the possibility of successful treatment within the general practice setting.

A study of Turkish GPs identified 'interest in psychiatry' as an important factor in their ability to recognise and treat depression, even after controlling for age, gender and attendance at courses on depression (Soykan & Oncu, 2003). Therefore, those devising courses of continuing medical education (CME) for GPs should always aim to stimulate an interest in psychiatry as well as convey factual material.

Millar & Goldberg (1991) found that those GPs who are skilled in the detection of psychiatric problems elicit more cues from their emotionally distressed patients than those GPS who are poor at recognition. These workers also showed that doctors with fewer skills tend to prevent their patients from giving them verbal and non-verbal cues, by conducting a more hurried, theory-led interview, while a patient-led interview that clarifies the patient's problem and facilitates discussion was used more often by the more skilled doctors. While such observations are in all the expected direction, changing the ways GPs interview or manage their patients with depression is likely to prove difficult.

General practitioner time

A psychiatrist expects to be able to spend around 1 hour with a patient to reach a diagnosis, and even with the advantage of specialised knowledge few psychiatrists would claim to be able to reach an accurate diagnosis on the basis of a single interview lasting 10 minutes or less, yet this is precisely what is expected of GPs. It should therefore come as no surprise that increased consultation time is associated with better recognition rates for psychiatric disorder. Thus, in a large Scottish study of GP attendees, Stirling *et al* (2001) found a caseness (high GHQ score) rate of 44% and the average consultation time was 8.71 minutes. A 50% increase in consultation time was associated with a 32% increase in the recognition rate for psychiatric disorder. However, the study also showed that GP time was in itself a complex phenomenon and that increasing levels of distress (higher GHQ scores) were associated with longer consultation time. Social deprivation (which is associated with more psychiatric disorder) was associated with shorter consultation times. Thus, practices in the poorest districts had 20% shorter consultation times than practices in wealthy areas. A Welsh GP, J. Tudor Hart, described what he called 'the inverse care law' (Hart, 1971) – namely, the availability of good medical care is inversely proportional to its need – and this study, which demonstrated that the poor received less GP time than the wealthy, provides some support for this rule (Stirling *et al*, 2001).

In a study of the way GP consultations for depression are perceived by patients, Pollock & Grime (2002) noted that many patients had detected a sense of time pressure and as a result would self-impose a rationing of their own time to relieve the pressure they thought the doctor was working under. Gask *et al* (2003) confirmed this, and added that patients often felt guilty about taking up the doctor's time, to the extent that some would even question whether depression was a legitimate reason for seeing the doctor, while among others poor self-worth appeared to be associated with a generally low expectation of what the NHS could provide. These more subtle interview studies have shown how the illness itself can undermine consultations for depression in general practice, so it is important to try to counter the influence of depressive guilt and low self-esteem on the consultation and treatment process.

GP time is one of the most precious commodities the NHS has to offer, and is highly valued by most patients. It therefore seems bizarre that it has become so strictly rationed (less than 10 minutes per consultation in the UK), while equally prosperous nations with state-funded health-care, such as Canada (where the average GP consultation time is 15 minutes) and Sweden (21 minutes) are able to be much less harsh in their allocation of GP time (Stirling *et al*, 2001).

GP diagnosis and attempts to improve GP diagnosis by teaching modern classification

The use of ICD–10 (World Health Organization, 1992) or DSM–IV (American Psychiatric Association, 1994) is central to modern secondary care psychiatry and has led to considerable improvements in the quality of diagnosis. All in-patients are now routinely assigned an ICD–10 diagnosis and many clinics use these schemes for their out-patient work. Can similar benefits from better diagnosis be found in primary care as well? Attempts have been made to devise similar classification schemes that are appropriate for primary care, the first of these being the International Classification for Primary Care based on ICD–9, which has now been supplanted by the ICD–10 PHC (primary health care) (World Health Organization, 1996) derived from ICD–10.

Croudace *et al* (2003) sought to test whether better knowledge and the routine application of the ICD–10 PHC scheme might help improve diagnostic accuracy and so lead to a better patient outcome in general practice. A group of GPs in the Bristol area were trained in a series of workshops in the use of ICD–10 PHC, while a control group of GPs received no training. The study showed that guideline practice had no effect on GPs' diagnostic behaviour in terms of detection rates, nor did it influence patient outcome in terms of GHQ score, disability or measures of quality of life. This indicates that these official guidelines failed to add to the GPs' diagnostic ability or quality of care for their patients, with the underlying implication that psychiatric diagnosis may be a rather different endeavour in primary care than in secondary care.

An earlier and thoughtful editorial in the *British Journal of General Practice* highlighted some of the differences between making a psychiatric diagnosis in primary care as opposed to secondary care:

> 'psychiatric disorder like most illness behaves as a continuously distributed variable and the more valid question from the general practitioner perspective might therefore be "how much of it is present". In psychiatry the question is different – deciding what the disorder actually is. General practitioners are less preoccupied than psychiatrists by questions of phenomenology and psychiatric classification but are more concerned with the distinction between psychiatric disorder and physical disorder, as well as psychiatric disorder that merits intervention versus that which is best left alone. In General Practice, the question is often compounded because of the high incidence of transient morbidity and also an illness will often be seen in its early stages, before the full clinical picture has developed. For these reasons, the classifications in current use are quite inappropriate for primary care.' (After Sharp & King, 1989)

Very few GPs use the ICD–10 PHC routinely in their diagnostic work, probably because they find that such phenomenologically driven diagnoses add little in the general practice setting.

Filter 3 – referral to specialist psychiatric services

A generation ago, only a GP could refer a patient to a consultant psychiatrist and only the psychiatrist could determine hospital admission. The diagnostic acumen of GPs was then held in high esteem, and they were the main gatekeepers to secondary care. Such exclusive 'doctor to doctor' referrals still occur but are rather less common; however, primary care teams still continue to refer patients to secondary care, which is now provided by the community mental health team (CMHT).

Two UK studies have attempted to clarify referral patterns between modern primary care teams and their local CMHTs, but these have presented conflicting results. The smaller study, by Ashworth *et al* (2002), of 29 practices, found no significant demographic or practice correlates to explain inter-practice variations in referral rates. However, a rather larger study (of 161 practices), by Hull *et al* (2002), is more informative and reported an average annual referral rate from primary care to secondary care of 1% of the population per year, with a sixfold variation in referral rates between practices. The main sources of referral to CMHTs found in that study are shown in Table 30.10; it can be seen that only 21% of the referrals to the CMHT came from general practice.

An effect for ethnicity was found in the study of Hull *et al* (2002), which found that practices in areas with large Asian populations had lower referral rates, which may relate to the strong stigma concerning mental illness in this community.

Table 30.10 Sources of 7812 referrals to community mental health teams in East London

Source of referral	% of all referrals
General practice	21
Mental health service (other services)	35
Local authority service (mainly social services)	14
Self-referral	8
General hospital	3
Other (courts, day services, voluntary, etc.)	19
Annual average rate for the population	1

Source: Hull *et al* (2002).

Neither study found any effect for deprivation, possibly because all the practices in both studies were deprived inner-London surgeries. Larger practices had more people on antipsychotic medication and also referred more people for long-term CMHT input. Also, because large practices could afford more on-site psychology and counselling services, they tended to refer fewer patients to out-patient and in-patient services.

Referrals to the CMHTs had three possible outcomes:

1 The CMHT acted as a 'brokerage' and immediately referred the patient on, for example to a specialised service such as eating disorders, a voluntary organisation, or some other service (31% of referrals).

2 CMHT workers undertook short-term work, of 8–10 weeks (33% of referrals).

3 The patient was taken on for long-term work and a CPN was assigned to the patient (32% of referrals).

The GPs expressed a variety of opinions on their local CMHTs, at one extreme describing them as being responsive and accepting but in other instances as being 'obstructive' or 'mysterious' because of their tightly defined referral criteria. The authors also suggest that the 'consultation liaison' model (see page 777) was probably the most useful in helping GPs make more appropriate referrals. CMHTs should be receptive to their local GPs but at the same time need to limit referrals, as even a small increase in GP referral rates could rapidly overwhelm secondary care; for example, if the present average of 1% of patients being referred were to increase to 1.5%, this would lead to a 50% increase in numbers presenting to their CMHTs.

A recent development in the psychiatric services in the UK has been the development of 'crisis teams' (see page 731), with the primary aim of minimising the number of admissions to expensive hospital beds. GPs now contact crisis teams directly for any psychiatric emergency and use the CMHTs for help only with the management of the more long-term, less acute, less seriously ill patients. In addition, GPs refer to the local NHS psychology services as well as to psychotherapists in the private and voluntary services. The older concept of the GP acting as a 'filter' for secondary care services is probably now outdated, and it fails to convey the complexity and wide variety of arrangements that now exist between primary and secondary care.

Ethnicity

The UK is now a multi-ethnic society and it may be helpful to review some basic socio-demographic data (as provided by the 2001 census). Around 7% of the population described themselves in the census as belonging to an ethnic minority. Of these, 50% were born in the UK, compared with 95% of those describing themselves as White. The numerical sizes of the larger ethnic minorities are shown in Table 30.11. People in ethnic minority groups tend to be younger, with a greater proportion of children under 16.

This trend was highest for Bangladeshi/Pakistani groups, at 38%, compared with 30% of the Black population, 27% of the Indian population and 20% of the White population. The pattern was reversed for the elderly; thus, 16% of the White population was over 65, but only 5% of the Black population and 3% of the Bangladeshi population.

Table 30.11 Age and size of ethnic groups in the UK: 2001 census data (1000s)

Ethnic group	Under 25	Over 25	Total	%
White	17 788	40 140	57 928	93
Indian	403	584	928	1.6
Pakistani/Bangladeshi	458	343	802	1.3
Black (Caribbean and African)	476	629	1 105	1.9
Remaining groups	553	504	1 057	1.8
All ethnic minority groups	1 890	2 060	3 951	6.8

The census found that people from the ethnic minorities tended to live in large cities; 45% of the total 'non-White' population live in London. For 'Blacks', the number living in London was even higher, at 69%, whereas people from the Indian subcontinent were more widely distributed across cities in the UK. For obvious reasons, the census gives only a very broad guide to the numbers in the major ethnic groups and provides little detailed information on the large subgroups of people who now live in the UK, although most people in these smaller minority groups tend to live in London. There was also a tendency for ethnic minorities to be living in the most deprived districts.

Average household size was highest for Pakistani or Bangladeshi households, at 4.2 persons, followed by Indian households at 3.3 persons, Black households at 2.5 persons and White household at 2.3 persons.

The most obvious implication of the census data is that multi-ethnicity is mainly a feature of inner-city general practices, particularly for London. The greater number of children in ethnic minority groups has significance for child health and child psychiatric services as well as for education.

Ethnicity and the prevalence of CMDs

By far the most important survey of CMDs among people of ethnic minorities in the UK is the 4th National Survey of Ethnic Minorities (Nazroo, 1997), which complemented the OPCS survey. The survey was large (5196 individuals from ethnic minorities, who were compared with 2867 White people); the methodology was rigorous and similar to the OPCS survey. However, instead of the usual English version of the CIS-R being used, the interview was translated into six Asian languages, then independently back-translated into English to check the accuracy of the translation. ICD–9 diagnoses were generated from the interview data.

The prevalences of the main CMDs in different ethnic groups are shown in the Table 30.12. The same predominance of anxiety over depression as was found in the main OPCS survey (Table 30.2) is evident, and this applied to both Whites and those in ethnic minorities. Overall, there were no dramatic differences in the rates for CMDs between ethnic groups, but for anxiety disorders the differences between Whites and

Table 30.12 Age- and gender-standardised prevalence rates of anxiety and depression among different ethnic groups

Ethnic group	Depression (%)	Anxiety (%)
White	3.8	18
Irish or other White	6.3	28
Caribbean	6.0	13
Indian/African Asian	2.8	9
Pakistani	3.4	11
Bangladeshi	1.9	5
Chinese	1.6	7

From Shah (2003).

all other ethnic groups were significant. Thus, rates for anxiety disorders were higher among the 'Irish and other White groups' and phobic disorders may be more common among Asians, but otherwise rates for ethnic minorities were not lower than for Whites, and for a few groups may have been higher. The lower rates of depression for South Asians were not significant. As may be expected, the main socio-demographic correlates for the CMDs among those in ethnic minorities were similar to those found in the main OPCS survey: female sex, lone parenting, unemployment and life events. There were, however, a few findings that suggest ethnicity may have had some influence.

- Lone parenting was, overall, associated with a raised rate of CMDs (OR = 2.5). For South Asians, where lone parenting is uncommon, rates for CMDs were considerably elevated (OR = 3.7), possibly related to the shame associated with divorce and birth out of wedlock in these cultures. On the other hand, for African–Caribbeans, where lone parenting is common and almost half the children are raised in one-parent households (Rutter & Tienda, 2005), the association with CMDs was low (OR = 0.4) and significantly below the average rate, indicating that lone parenting is widely accepted in this community. Thus, being a lone parent may have a very different social significance between Asian and African–Caribbean cultures.

- Although there is considerable concern about whether people in ethnic minorities consult sufficiently with their GPs (perhaps because they are deterred by language and cultural problems), this survey found that consultation rates for all ethnic minority groups was higher than for Whites, and this applied at all levels of illness severity.

- There is some interest in whether living closely together with people of one's own ethnic grouping offers greater support and so confers a degree of protection against CMDs. This has been called an 'ethnic density effect'. Analysis showed only a very small (1%) protective effect for higher ethnic density, indicating that the degree of protection is small and ethnic density is probably less important than once thought.

- A younger age of immigration (below 11) increased the later risk of CMDs for South Asians and this was not explained by linguistic difficulties. Age of immigration was not relevant for African–Caribbeans.

Smaller studies have identified some additional factors appertaining to ethnicity, such as: victimisation; personal attacks; racial discrimination, for example in housing and employment; absence of a confidant; absent parents; small primary family groups; and perceived lack of social support. Most of these items were reported in single studies only and so their significance is unclear. In addition, Rutter & Tienda (2005) point out that even when an ethnic difference in some psychiatric disorder or social parameter is identified, ethnicity is unlikely to be the sole explanation; rather, there may be some other mediating variable that accounts for the difference, such as language difficulty, poor education, unemployment and so forth.

It would be impossible to describe the psychiatric difficulties of the myriad different cultures encountered in the UK today, but a comprehensive review of all the published psychiatric studies concerning CMDs in ethnic minorities is given by Shah (2003). For reasons of space, the South Asian cultures (Indian, Pakistani and Bangladeshi) and the African–Caribbean and Black African communities have been selected for further description.

South Asian cultures

Bhugra (2004) and others, using a typology set out by Hofstede (1980), suggest these cultures fit the criteria of 'collective societies' as opposed to the 'individualistic' societies that characterise the Western European or American pattern. Collective societies stress the 'we' consciousness, collective identity, group solidarity, sharing of duties and obligations, and group decision making; they are characterised by high degrees of family integrity and interdependence, as for example in the extended family. In contrast, individualistic societies emphasise the 'I' consciousness, autonomy, emotional independence, individual initiative, the right to privacy, pleasure seeking, assertiveness and self-fulfilment.

Traditionalism is also a feature of collective societies and is prominent in South Asian cultures. Traditional societies place far greater emphasis on filial piety, the use of shame to enforce behaviours, self-control and fatalism, as well as an expectation that individuals will subordinate their personal feelings in the interests of social solidarity. These generalisations probably apply to only a limited degree to the South Asian cultures as found in the UK today, which in themselves are diverse (with more than 20 languages and several different religions, even in the UK), and cultural influences will be considerably less strong among second-generation immigrants.

Suicide and attempted suicide among South Asian women

In his book *Culture and Self Harm*, Bhugra (2004) reviews the evidence that attempted suicide among South Asians may be a culture-bound disorder. Although suicide is generally frowned upon within these cultures, certain types of suicidal behaviour are tolerated or even encouraged. These include women who burn themselves in the practice of *sati* or self-immolation either when their husbands are cremated (*sahamaranam*) or after this (*anumaranam*). Suicide by drowning is not only permitted but enjoined as a religious ritual at the confluence of the River Ganges and River Yamuna, as is death by self-cremation at one of the holy places. Suicide is recommended for ascetics, while one Indian sect, the Purana, allow persons with incurable diseases to end their lives, by *mahaprasthena* (the great exit).

How do these cultural attitudes to suicide translate into the lives of Asian people in the UK? Numerous studies have shown high rates of attempted suicide and suicide among young Asian women (but not older women or Asian men). Merrill & Owens (1986) contrasted the pattern of self-poisoning among Asian and White self-poisoners and found the Asian group were 'less psychiatric', with lower rates of current psychiatric disorder, previous psychiatric treatment or personality disorder, but instead were more likely to be young, married and female, and culture conflict was more common. Bhugra (2004) found the overall rate for attempted suicide among young Asian women was raised (OR = 1.5) when compared with White and African–Caribbean women (who had approximately the same rate). He also found some evidence in favour of culture conflict among the Asian women who attempted suicide, as they were less likely to believe in arranged marriages than were a control group of Asian women (30% versus 88%), and more likely to be involved in a relationship with a non-Asian partner (22% versus 0%).

Soni Raleigh *et al* (1990), in the largest study of Asian suicide in the UK, conducted between 1970 and 1979, found high rates of completed suicide as compared with the native population, especially for females (2.7% versus 0.8%; for males the rates were 1.8% versus 0.6%). Age-specific rates for women showed a peak in the 15- to 24-year group and most (83%) were married. For males, one subgroup, Indian doctors and dentists, accounted for 20% of male suicides, compared with only 0.9% of all male UK suicides, indicating that this high-achieving group may be under considerable stress. Around 30% of Indian female suicides were by self-immolation, a method commonly used for female suicide in India and perhaps favoured because of its similarity to the culturally sanctioned practice of *sati*, but hanging was also common in this series.

The epidemiological pattern for suicide among South Asians living in the UK is therefore very different from the more usual Western pattern, where suicide is more common among the elderly, particularly males, and where among younger people single males are at high risk, whereas young married women are generally held to be a low-risk group. Bhugra (2004) cites other authors who suggest that young Indian women, given their tightly defined roles in Indian society, may be subject to very powerful social pressures. These include submission and deference to males and elders, arranged marriages, the financial pressures implied by dowries and associated marital and family conflicts, which all contribute to suicide and attempted suicide among young Asian women.

CMDs among South Asian communities in the UK

Studies of the symptom profiles of CMDs among South Asians have suggested that there is a greater tendency for somatic presentations (Bhui *et al*, 2001). This has been confirmed for the UK Pakistani community in the study by Tabassum *et al* (2000), who also found aggression was often regarded as a mental symptom in this community.

An obvious concern is whether CMDs among Asians are less often recognised by GPs than they are among Whites. The literature is equivocal, with only some studies (Wilson & Macarthy, 1994; Bhui *et al*, 2001) suggesting this occurs, although, given the already high rates of non-recognition for the White population, it is uncertain whether ethnicity further compounds the problem. One surprising finding to emerge from the study by Bhui *et al* (2001) was that Punjabi GPs, who might be expected to be well acquainted with the cultural issues, were no better at detecting CMDs among their Punjabi patients than were White GPs.

African–Caribbean and Black African communities and the CMDs

There are now two major Black communities in the UK, the African–Caribbean and the Black African (mainly West African) and they have very different cultures, but patterns of CMDs in both these communities have been rather less studied than CMDs among Asians. Modood (2005) considers the African–Caribbean culture to be closer to British culture than the Black African culture, and in this context it is of interest that a large study of African–Caribbeans attending practices in inner-Manchester found similar rates of CMDs for African–Caribbeans (13%) and Whites (14%). However, there were differences in symptom profile, with anxiety disorders being less common among the African–Caribbeans than among Whites (3% versus 9%), whereas depression was more frequent (13% versus 9%). For women the differences in rates of depression were marked (19% versus 11%) and the author commented that the depression that afflicts a high proportion of African–Caribbean women may be just as important a problem as the psychosis of young African–Caribbeans, but these women and their needs have been relatively neglected in recent years (Shaw *et al*, 1999).

The West African Black population is a relatively recent immigrant group and so has a high proportion of first-generation members; they are mainly located in London. However, as the census groups the African–Caribbeans together with Africans as 'Blacks', they have been little studied as a separate group. The only available study is that by Maginn *et al* (2004), who examined consecutive GP attendees in a south-east London general practice (in Lewisham) and found an overall caseness rate (as defined by a high GHQ score) of 37%, and 73% of these cases were recognised by the GPs. In this study, Whites had the highest caseness rates, followed by African–Caribbeans (OR = 0.73 relative to Whites), but Black Africans had substantially lower rates (OR = 0.36 relative to Whites). The reasons for this are unclear, but Peltzer (1995) suggests that African societies are more collectivist and traditional in type and many individuals have strong religious affiliations (mainly evangelical Christian). Possibly both these factors offer some protection against family breakdown, which predisposes to CMDs, whereas family breakdown is known to be frequent among both the White and African–Caribbean populations in inner cities.

Conclusion

The majority of ethnicity studies in psychiatry have been epidemiological and tended to focus on differences in prevalence, symptom profile and GP recognition rates between particular ethnic groups and the local White community, but Rait (1999), in an editorial entitled 'Counting heads may mask cultural and social factors', offers a critique of such a statistical approach as a way of gaining insight into cultural differences. She suggests that such an 'etic' approach may be unproductive, whereas an approach based on in-depth individual interviews (emic methods) may yield much richer information on the cultural aspects of mental health (see page 785 for an explanation of 'etic' and 'emic'). A deeper level of cultural knowledge may also be needed for counselling and psychotherapy among people in ethnic minorities, and this is reviewed by Pedersen (1997).

Perhaps for most GP consultations cultural issues are not relevant. For example, depression associated with unemployment or bereavement may be no different for people from ethnic minorities. However, in a few instances, say of a young Indian woman presenting with cut wrists, cultural issues may assume clinical importance.

Asylum seekers and refugees in the UK

Background and definitions

While the vast majority of those from ethnic minorities are reasonably well integrated into UK society, a rather smaller group of those who have recently arrived, namely asylum seekers, present a major challenge to medical and social services, particularly while their asylum status is being assessed. Legal immigration status, as determined by the Home Office, may be of critical importance in determining the nature of the stress a person is under, as well as benefit and NHS entitlements, and Tribe (2002) provides definitions for each category.

- An *asylum seeker* is someone requesting asylum or refuge, that is, who has asked to be given formal refugee status, but for whom the outcome of the application has not yet been determined.
- A *refugee* is a person whose residential status in the host country has been accepted and he or she is usually entitled to the full range of services available to a native resident. The UK government recognises an asylum seeker as a refugee when he or she meets the terms set out under the 1951 UN Convention relating to the Status of Refugees. This states that a refugee must have a well-founded fear of persecution because of his or her race, religion or nationality, membership of a social group or political opinion.
- An *immigrant* is a person who makes a positive choice to move to another country in a planned way without feeling forced to leave the country of origin (whereas a refugee is generally forced to flee, often in an unplanned and hurried way).

The psychiatric difficulties of immigrants and refugees are also discussed in Chapter 31 (see pages 796 and 799). Asylum seekers are likely to be anxious that their case may be rejected. Asylum seekers who have had an initial refusal have the right to appeal, and they may continue to reside in the UK while their appeals are being heard. At such times they are obviously a highly anxious group and may be worried about being deported. The Home Office also grants a small number of people 'discretionary leave' and 'humanitarian protection', when they are permitted to stay in the UK for a further defined period of time. Those asylum seekers who have had their appeals rejected and those granted discretionary leave to remain are under considerable stress and generally have fewer rights in terms of benefits, social service entitlements and NHS provision than those who have been granted full refugee status. A few asylum seekers are detained while their case is being considered, usually not because of any criminal activity, and this almost certainly is a source of considerable stress and despair. The Home Office legal category will have a strong bearing on a person's anxiety and mental symptoms and should always be ascertained in cases presenting to the GP or psychiatric services.

Between 1990 and 2005 the UK received over half a million applications for asylum. In London, the proportion of asylum seekers and refugees within the population has been estimated to be as high as 1 in 20. Their origin reflects the international situation at any one time; three-quarters of current UK asylum applications are made by people from countries in conflict. A Home Office report (Heath *et al*, 2006) showed that in the preceding year the top applying nationalities were Iranian, Eritrean, Chinese, Somalian and Afghan. Most people seeking asylum in the UK are single men under 40 years of age. Families are frequently with single parents. There are also a significant number of unaccompanied children, who have usually been sent to the UK because their parents consider conditions in their own country to be adverse.

Clinical data

Asylum seekers and refugees present a growing challenge to mental health services. The few available studies suggest that one in six refugees in the UK has a severe physical health problem. Common examples are: malnutrition; communicable diseases such as tuberculosis, hepatitis or HIV/AIDS; and physical injuries from war and torture. These medical conditions are reviewed by Burnett & Peel (2001).

The same studies show that two-thirds of refugees experience significant anxiety or depression. There are very few studies of psychiatric disorders specifically appertaining to asylum seekers, as this is a relatively new legal category, but there is an older and more extensive literature on the mental health of refugees. This has been usefully summarised in a meta-analysis (Porter & Haslam 2005) that included all 59 studies from the past 50 years that had compared the mental health of refugees with that of control groups taken from their new host country. Refugee status conferred an overall increase in psychopathology with an effect size of 0.41 ± 0.02, and as this figure was based on a large number of studies it is likely to be the most accurate presently available. Although the rate of psychopathology in this group is significantly raised, the overall figure suggests that the vast majority of refugees, like the native population they were compared with, do not have significant psychiatric disorder. Indeed, many of those who have made such painful journeys into exile are likely to be courageous and resourceful individuals who may later go on to enjoy successful lives in their new host countries.

Asylum seekers are a diverse group and do not share any specific psychopathology; the whole range of psychiatric disorders may be encountered. However, as many individuals are fleeing from war-torn areas or from despotic regimes where torture is in common use, an increased rate of post-traumatic stress disorder (PTSD) has been observed in some studies. Nevertheless there are claims that use of this diagnosis is reductive and may mask many other causes of distress or the actual needs of asylum seekers. A study of male Iraqi refugees in the UK illustrates some of the complexity of the problem. In this sample, 65% of the Iraqi men gave a history of definite and often severe torture, but only 11% qualified for a diagnosis of PTSD, whereas depression was much more common (44%). This was related to low levels of emotional support, mainly as a result of separation from wives and families, racial attacks in the UK, financial problems and the history of torture. Many of the participants in that study showed considerable despair and the authors concluded that the simple manoeuvre of permitting the men to be reunited with their wives and families would lead to much better levels of emotional support and have a far more beneficial effect than years of specialised psychotherapy for PTSD (Gorst-Unsworth & Goldenberg, 1998).

Asylum seekers are often from the same countries as refugees, but for the latter group the issue of residence has been settled. Thus, a Norwegian study that compared the rates of acute admission between immigrants, asylum seekers and native Norwegians found that immigrants and native Norwegians had the same relative risk of admission (1.07), but the relative risk for asylum seekers compared with Norwegians was greatly raised (8.84), indicating that the issue of residence may hugely increase anxiety levels (Iversen & Morken, 2003).

In a second study the same workers compared the admission diagnoses of refugees with those of asylum seekers and found that asylum seekers had much higher rates of PTSD than refugees (45% versus 11%), whereas the refugees had higher rates of compulsory admission, especially for schizophrenia (Iversen & Morken, 2004). The authors interpreted the greatly increased overall admission rates for the asylum seekers and their high rates of PTSD as reflecting the high levels of stress associated with the asylum process. By contrast, the pattern for refugees resembled that of the local population, where schizophrenia was the most frequent reason for admission in both groups, with most admissions being compulsory. Somatic presentations are also frequently high, and can reflect physical pain, which may be more acceptable than psychological pain; this aspect is more comprehensively discussed in Chapter 31 (page 790).

Pre- and post-migration adversity

Many refugees experience adversities both before and after migration that are likely to affect their health, physical and mental. Before migration, the experience of conflict is common. Some refugees will have experienced detainment and torture, or other violence. During this period, access to healthcare may be minimal. Journeys to the UK can be long and hazardous, and frequently lead to separation from families and communities. Numerical data for the magnitude of the increased contribution these parameters make to psychopathology is given in the meta-analysis by Porter & Haslam (2005), where the effect size is placed in parenthesis. Thus, age had an important bearing, with children and adolescents generally having lower rates of psychopathology (0.28) and adults intermediate rates (0.53), but for the elderly rates were markedly increased (1.21). The more middle class and better educated (0.91) fared worse those who were primarily working class (0.34), which the reviewers interpreted as being the result of a greater fall in social status for the middle classes when they were forced to leave their homeland.

Once in the UK, post-migration adversities include social isolation, poverty and cultural alienation. Current government policies, including detention, dispersal and lack of legitimate work opportunities, can compound problems. The meta-analysis showed that lack of permanent accommodation had an effect size (0.67) similar to institutional accommodation (0.65), whereas permanent residence had a beneficial effect (0.37). The ability to work in an unrestricted way also lowered rates of psychopathology (0.27), whereas restricting work and economic opportunities led to much increased rates (1.06). Not surprisingly repatriation doubled the risks for psychiatric disorder, as did ongoing conflict.

Increasingly, the deleterious effect of the asylum process has been recognised. A Dutch study showed that an asylum process that lasted for more than 2 years more than doubled the risks of psychiatric disorder (Laban *et al*, 2004) and there is also evidence that a prolonged process increases the risk in the UK. Detention almost certainly has a negative effect and the meta-analysis showed that institutional residence doubled the risks of psychiatric disorder. For many years, all asylum seekers in Australia were placed in detention centres, often in remote areas. In her account in the *Lancet*, Lawrence (2004), who was the President of the Australian Labour Party, wrote of her personal reaction of shock during a visit to a detention centre in a remote area of Western Australia, where all the inmates seemed to her to be in a state of despair. She wrote:

> 'Australia's decade of mandatory detention should be an object lesson to other governments who may be thinking of imitating Australian policy. Such a policy has a profound human cost, damaging those who are held and brutalising those who hold them. The consequences of detention will endure long after the camps are closed especially as most of the people incarcerated eventually prove to be genuine refugees.'

In September 2005 there were 1695 asylum seekers being detained in the UK.

Administrative aspects

The area of health and social benefits for asylum seekers is one of considerable political sensitivity and governments seem to oscillate rapidly in their generosity between degrees of grudging acceptance of their obligations to becoming overly harsh, according to the political mood of the day. This may explain the ever-changing regulations, which often fail to make good medical sense.

Asylum seekers are not eligible for mainstream welfare benefits. The National Asylum Support Service (NASS) is a department established by the Home Office to be responsible for support arrangements for destitute asylum seekers. However, the package of support can involve enforced dispersal across the country, often to locations with few resources for refugees, preventing continuity of healthcare. Since July 2002, asylum seekers have not been allowed to work or undertake vocational training until they are given a positive decision on their asylum case, regardless of how long they have to wait. Regulations concerning benefits and housing entitlements are constantly changing but the patient advice and liaison service (PALS) within the primary care trusts is a good source of information.

All asylum seekers and refugees are entitled to free primary healthcare services. However, as of 1 April 2004, individuals who have exhausted the appeal process and been refused political asylum have been no longer eligible for free secondary healthcare (except where deemed immediately necessary or for conditions that are life threatening). These regulations border on being unethical. For example, asylum seekers are entitled to free HIV testing but not to free HIV treatment, and this applies even to pregnant women. For mental illness, only compulsory treatment is free, whereas informal treatment is meant to be paid for, although in practice this is rarely enforced. Not only does this have far-reaching negative implications, but proposals are also under discussion to exclude 'failed' asylum seekers from access to free primary healthcare services.

Doctors are asked to see asylum seekers to assess their need for treatment. Psychiatrists may be asked to write medico-legal reports for those asylum seekers alleging torture, a report that can be significant in determining the asylum case, as well as providing information on their mental health. Diagnosing and appropriately treating mental health problems are more problematic when there are conceptual or linguistic difficulties in describing the symptoms, and cultural differences in the perception of mental health. The services of an interpreter may be required.

In summary, refugees and asylum seekers presenting to healthcare services have complex and multiple needs, which require a range of interventions. Building local networks of services for refugees is vital. This needs to include the active involvement of non-statutory services, from the larger charities, such as the Medical Foundation for Care of Victims of Torture, to local Refugee Community Groups. There are many useful refugee resources, including the Refugee Council, the HARP website (http://www.harpweb.org.uk), which provides a gateway to refugee resources, and Asylum Aid, a charity that provides advice and legal representation.

Management of depression in general practice

The vast majority of the cases of depression in the community are now treated by GPs, with the secondary care team being involved only with those at the more severe end of the spectrum. GPs will also treat many people with major depressive disorder, but they will probably also see and treat a much larger group with sub-threshold forms of disorder. ICD–10 uses the term 'mild depressive episode' to cover this group, and the ICD–10 criteria include depressed mood, loss of interest and enjoyment, fatigue and at least two of the symptoms of major depression (see Box 1.2 on page 12). The condition should have lasted for more than 2 weeks and even though patients may report some difficulty in continuing with their work or academic programme, they are usually able to carry on. DSM–IV–TR uses the term 'minor depressive disorder' to describe sub-threshold disorder, which it defines as the patient having two to four symptoms for at least a month (whereas major depression requires five or more symptoms).

There are very few studies of the outcome of these sub-threshold conditions. Wagner *et al* (2000) showed that DSM–IV minor depression in a general practice

Box 30.4 NICE guidelines (2004) for the treatment of depression

Consider patient preference and the patient's experience of previous treatment(s) when deciding on treatment.

- *Screening in primary care and general hospital settings*. Screening should be undertaken for depression in high-risk groups, for example those with a history of depression, significant physical illnesses causing disability, or other mental health problems, such as dementia.
- *Watchful waiting*. For patients with mild depression who do not want an intervention or who, in the opinion of the healthcare professional, may recover with no intervention, a further assessment should be arranged, normally within 2 weeks ('watchful waiting').
- *Antidepressants in mild depression*. Antidepressants are not recommended for the initial treatment of mild depression, because the risk–benefit ratio is poor.
- *Guided self-help*. For patients with mild depression, healthcare professionals should consider recommending a guided self-help programme based on cognitive–behavioural therapy (CBT).
- *Short-term psychological treatment.* In both mild and moderate depression, psychological treatment specifically focused on depression (such as problem-solving therapy, brief CBT and counselling) of 6–8 sessions over 10–12 weeks should be considered.
- *Prescription of an SSRI*. When an antidepressant is to be prescribed in routine care, it should be a selective serotonin reuptake inhibitor (SSRI), because SSRIs are as effective as tricyclic antidepressants and are less likely to be discontinued because of side-effects.

setting basically followed a similar trajectory to major depression, often lasting for a year or more. It frequently resulted in psychosocial impairment and an impoverishment in the quality of life in a similar way to major depression, although to a rather lesser degree.

The guidelines from the National Institute for Health and Clinical Excellence (NICE) (2004) for depression, which are summarised in Box 3.4, come down against the use of antidepressants for 'mild depression'. However, the observations of Wagner *et al* (2000) indicating that these sub-threshold conditions can sometimes last a long time and be accompanied by psychosocial impairment provide a sufficient rationale for prescribing an antidepressant and trying to curtail the illness in some cases.

GPs will also be involved, sometimes on a shared-care basis, in the long-term management of patients with recurrent major depression, chronic depression and dysthymia. The pharmacological management of depression (see Chapter 4) in primary care is the same as in secondary care, and will not be further described here. Instead, the focus is more on the types of psychotherapy and counselling GPs are able to offer, as well as the role of other paramedical personnel in the primary care team in the management of depression in general practice, as well as attempts to improve GP management of depression through training courses.

Counselling in general practice

GPs do informal counselling for much of the time, mainly for adjustment to physical illness, but also for relationship difficulties and a wide variety of other problems. However, the rather more prolonged counselling sessions traditionally used in treating anxiety or depression may be difficult for busy GPs to deliver, as they have more pressing demands on their time. In addition, because of their unique role as the family doctor in the management of physical illness, patients may have recollections of their GP being prescriptive and authoritative, and so the more informal and equal relationship needed for counselling may be difficult to achieve.

The NHS now pays for all general practices to have counsellors, although in recent years the money for counsellors has been included in the general allocation for the practice, with the expectation (not obligation) that the money will be spent on counselling services. Randomised controlled trials (RCTs) of counselling for depression in general practice have generally been positive. Thus, in one recent trial with four separate arms, patients were randomised to receive either counselling or 'treatment as usual' in two of the arms, while in the remaining two arms patient preference was used for selection to either counselling or treatment as usual. Overall, patients in all four groups did well: 83% had recovered by 12 months, although 15% had relapsed, indicating the need for continued vigilance after recovery. However, the most interesting finding to emerge from this study was that patients in the arm that had expressed a preference for counselling did significantly better than those randomised to counselling, a finding highlighting the merits of respecting 'patient choice' (Chilvers *et al*, 2001).

Cognitive–behavioural therapy (CBT) is now the accepted gold standard for the psychological treatment of depression. However, a study by Ward *et al* (2000) showed that patients who received 12 sessions of counselling did just as well as those who received 12 sessions of CBT delivered by a psychologist. Both groups did significantly better than patients allocated to treatment as usual, suggesting that at least in the general practice situation ordinary non-directive counselling by counsellors may be sufficient. A Cochrane review (Rowland *et al*, 2001) on the efficacy of counselling in general practice concluded that it was beneficial, with a mean effect size of 0.3 when compared with treatment as usual, and an effect size of this magnitude is similar to that reported for RCTs of antidepressants. There was also a trend for women to prefer counselling to antidepressants, which they commonly believed to be addictive (Churchill *et al*, 2000). One study in the review examined costs and found no overall difference in costs between counselling and treatment as usual (Bower *et al*, 2000). As might be expected, the more resistant forms of depression do not do so well with counselling. Thus, in an RCT of counselling in chronic depression, which by definition is a more resistant category, Simpson *et al* (2003) found that, apart from a small initial benefit, no difference was observed at 6 and 12 months between counselling and treatment as usual.

Problem solving may also be helpful for managing depression in general practice. This behaviourally orientated technique assumes an almost diametrically opposed stance to the more traditional non-directive counselling. After the counsellor has listened to the patient's reports of the symptoms, as well as of relationship or other difficulties, the patient is asked to describe all the problems as concretely as possible, and those identified as 'insurmountable' are discussed and broken down into smaller, more manageable problems. Patients are then invited to offer practical solutions, which they feel are within their grasp. Subsequent visits are used to monitor progress, or lack of it. The pan-European Outcomes of Depression International Network (ODIN) study of depression showed that problem solving conferred a 17% (number needed to treat, NNT = 6) advantage over 'treatment as usual' for depression presenting in general practice. The ODIN study also examined the effect of a psycho-educational group approach to prevent relapses and here there was a 14% advantage (NNT = 7) over GP treatment as usual, but these differences had disappeared by 12 months (Dowrick *et al*, 2000*b*).

A psycho-educational approach using written material was shown by Jacob *et al* (2002) to be helpful (i.e. to improve GHQ scores) in the management of depression among Asian women. Those who had been provided with the psycho-educational material in their native language recovered significantly faster than those who had not been given the material. In general, written material alone usually has little impact on the management of CMDs, but it may be rather more useful for those from ethnic minorities, especially where there are language difficulties.

Patient self-help

The NICE guideline on depression also recommends a number of other techniques which do not involve any other person, that is, no doctor or any other therapist.

These include guided self-help manuals ('bibliotherapy'), exercise and CBT-based computer programs. Thus, Proudfoot *et al* (2004), in an RCT, found that computerised CBT improved depression, negative attributional style, work and social adjustment, and these effects were independent of drug treatment or illness severity. Similarly for patients with anxiety disorders, computerised CBT helped attributional style and was also helpful for those who were more disturbed; moreover, patients felt satisfied with their treatment.

While computers do not suit many patients, these programs are becoming more popular, as evidenced by their increasing sales. However, for anything other than mild depression these methods should be used only as an adjunctive treatment, and a person such as a doctor, psychologist or counsellor should always be involved. People who are divorced, unemployed or bereaved may need more than an exercise bike or a computer screen to console them or help adjust to a new and sometimes painful reality.

Other psychiatric professionals in the GP surgery

Although counsellors form by far the largest group of mental health workers attached to general practices, there is a long history of other professionals also working in the surgery, including social workers (Corney, 1984), psychologists (Deys *et al*, 1989) and practice nurses (Wilkinson *et al*, 1993). In recent years practice nurses have played an increasing role in the follow-up of psychiatric problems and their work needs to be evaluated. Health visitors (Holden *et al*, 1989) have for many years been involved in both screening for and managing postnatal depression, while district nurses are well placed to detect depression in the elderly. In most instances, the additional input has been helpful, but in terms of numbers only the addition of counsellors has made any impact on a national basis.

During the health service reorganisations of the early 1990s, for a brief period CPNs were attached to general practices in many parts of the country. Their skills were much appreciated, both in the form of advice to the GPs, as occurs in the consultation–liaison model, where the CPN acts as the practice psychiatric adviser, and with the referral of large numbers of clients with anxiety and depression to the CPNs, to the extent that their traditional role of working with psychotic patients became undermined. Eventually, the CPNs had to be redirected back to rejoin their sector psychiatrists and continue working in secondary care with people with chronic psychosis. However, this episode inadvertently revealed the huge demand for psychiatrically skilled personnel (with more than just counselling skills) to be placed in the surgery, although this has never been easy to 'prove' scientifically. Thus, Bower & Sibbald (2000) reviewed the few available studies and concluded that the presence of an on-site mental health worker may provide the GP with an alternative to prescribing medication, and some studies also showed it provided an alternative to off-site referral. Paradoxically, other studies found an increase in the rate of off-site referral, with the most likely explanation being that the presence of the psychiatric worker sensitised the GP to psychological issues.

Mental health primary care workers

There is an obvious need for additional mental health input in primary care and Kingdon (2002) noted that the impetus and underlying logic for the development of this new category of mental health professional derives from three sources.

1 There is a huge shortage of skilled therapists such as CPNs and clinical psychologists, and this is likely to continue because training places for clinical psychologists are so few that NHS needs will never be met.

- It is now apparent that much NHS work in mental health, in both primary and secondary care, is generic in type, so that any skilled professional, regardless of their category, should be able to deal with it.
- The idea originates from the USA, where for some time graduates have been recruited directly to the psychiatric services, and after 1–2 years of training are able to join case management teams and work with patients in the community.

Kingdon (2002) also described the training programme used in Wessex for the new generic mental health practitioner (government documents use the term 'mental health primary care worker'). In essence, this consists of a 1-year placement in a CMHT, with release for 1–2 days a week for more formal training. Cost savings are said to arise because this bypasses the lengthy, more traditional hospital-based training programmes that most professionals undergo, although some might argue that taking such a short cut in training may carry risks of its own and that an apprenticeship in the hospital service may be of considerable value. The government is keen to develop this new type of generic professional and the NHS Plan (Department of Health, 2000) stated:

> 'One thousand new graduate mental health primary care workers trained in brief therapies of proven effectiveness will be employed to help general practitioners manage and treat common mental problems in all ages and groups, including children.'

It is probably far too early to judge whether this new professional grouping will take off, although one study showed that a generic mental health facilitator had no effect on GP diagnosis or management (Bashir *et al*, 2000). Also it is questionable whether there will be any real cost savings, as these workers will also need to receive a salary comparable to that of the existing professionals.

Training for general practitioners

Attempts by psychiatrists to improve the outcome of depression through GP training

Because the vast majority of patients with depression and other CMDs are treated by GPs, there has been some interest in whether short, focused training courses given to GPs may help improve their skills and translate into better patient outcome. There have been many studies of this type and the work of Rutz *et al* (1989) on the isolated Baltic island of Bornholm is a good example. This island was selected because it had a natural catchment population of 56000, which was relatively stable and so could be readily studied, and also the GP population was small ($n = 18$) and could be easily trained. The programme consisted of a series of lectures on depression, psychotherapy, suicide and antidepressants, and to ensure the GPs had understood everything the course was repeated twice. The initial findings showed a beneficial effect. Thus, referrals for depression to the clinic fell from 25% to 5%, admission days to the hospital fell by more than 60%, sick leave for depression halved and there was also a small fall in suicide rates. Unfortunately, when Rutz returned to Bornholm some 3 years later, the beneficial effects had disappeared. Even though the population had not changed, the GPs had seen a steady turnover and the message was gradually forgotten. Rutz *et al* (1992) argued that the course would need to be regularly repeated if benefits were to be maintained.

Tiemens *et al* (1999) conducted a similar training course in the Netherlands and also found that the patients of GPs who had undergone special training had better outcomes (i.e. less psychopathology, shorter illnesses) than patients of the same GPs but before their training. However, as with the Bornholm GPs, the training effects soon faded and by 1 year they were undetectable. Similarly, King *et al* (2002) reported a negative outcome to an RCT that aimed to teach GPs CBT.

The message is fairly clear: even though brief training courses on depression directed at GPs sometimes result in short-term benefits for GPs and their patients, these effects are not sustained, and hence their overall value is questionable.

Attempts to improve patient outcome through training GPs in the use of guidelines

Thompson *et al* (2000) examined the effect of teaching GPs a clinical practice guideline on depression in the primary care setting. The training was well received by the GPs, 80% of whom thought it would change their management of patients with depression, but the outcome of depressed patients at 6 weeks and 6 months was not significantly different to the outcome of patients of 'untrained' control GPs.

Baker *et al* (2001), noting the well-documented history of the relative lack of success of guideline implementation, argued that the main problem was in the way guidelines were taught; that is, they were merely distributed as a handout and such passive dissemination was ineffective. Instead, they devised an active teaching programme, where the guidelines were tailored in such a way as to try to overcome obstacles known to affect the ability of GPs to change their treatment practices. The RCT of their training programme demonstrated some impact, as those doctors who had been on their course conducted significantly more suicide assessments, and their patients with depression had lower scores on the Beck Depression Inventory at the 16-week follow-up appointment than the patients of control doctors, who had not been on the course. Unfortunately, there was no follow-up study of either the doctors or their patients, and so it is unclear whether these GPs retained their gains over the longer term.

Attempts to improve outcome through screening

The NICE (2004) guidelines recommend that screening should be undertaken in primary care and general hospital settings for depression in high-risk groups such as: those with a history of depression, people with significant physical illnesses causing disability, and those with other mental health problems, such as dementia. However, the literature suggests that routine screening in the community is costly and there is little evidence that it leads to improved psychosocial outcomes. Thus, Gilbody *et al* (2001) undertook a systematic review of all the RCTs ($n = 9$) that had examined the effects of routinely administered psychiatric questionnaires such as the GHQ, on the recognition, management and outcome of psychiatric disorders in non-psychiatric settings. Increased recognition through screening did not translate into an increased rate of intervention and had no effect on patient outcome. Routine screening is therefore rarely used in clinical practice, but there is one notable exception: health visitors often use the Edinburgh Post Natal Depression Scale to screen for postnatal depression among the women they must routinely visit during the first postpartum year.

Attempts to improve outcome at the practice level

There have been many studies of attempts to improve the outcome of depression at the practice level, but for reasons of space only one is considered here, as it illustrates certain useful points. Simon *et al* (2000) conducted a study on the effect of monitoring depressed patients in treatment and then providing their GPs with feedback on the patient's status and the adequacy of the drug treatment; a second group of patients were provided with support over the telephone from a practice care manager as well as feedback to the GP. The results showed that feedback to the GP alone was no better than 'treatment as usual', but that the combination of feedback to the GP and additional support to the patient from the practice care manager proved to be beneficial. Thus, it led to more patients being prescribed antidepressants in the therapeutic range, and also patients in the feedback plus support group had significantly lower depression scores and lower rates of major depression at follow-up than the feedback-only group or the treatment-as-usual group. This study suggests not only that intervention only with the GP may be ineffective, but that additional intervention with the patient by the care manager was useful as well as being feasible because the cost of this particular intervention, which comprised telephone contact only, was low ($80).

Summary of attempts to improve GP management of the CMDs

The quest for ways to strengthen the GP's hand at treating depression and the other CMDs is among the most daunting challenges facing primary care psychiatry today. The brief overview presented above is far from complete, representing only a very small minority of studies in this key area, but two broad themes stand out. Thus studies that have sought to achieve improved patient outcomes solely by focusing on the GP – for example by providing educational programmes on depression, training courses on guidelines, or the giving of feedback – have usually had negative outcomes; where there were any benefits, effect sizes have been small, with benefits usually fading with the passage of time. In contrast, those studies that have examined the effect of giving 'more' directly to patients, whether this means more GP time, more counselling sessions, more paramedical input, or even more computer programs have in most instances yielded quite strongly positive results, with reasonable effect sizes, sometimes even comparable to those found for antidepressants. However, taken on a national basis, giving 'more' to the huge numbers of patients with CMDs in the community would be likely to prove to be a very much more costly exercise than paying for a few education courses for GPs or issuing them with a new set of guidelines.

Somatisation disorder in general practice

Somatic presentations are undoubtedly very common in general practice. Fink *et al* (1999) found 22% of consecutive GP attendees fulfilled diagnostic criteria for an ICD–10 somatoform disorder, with the ICD–10 disorder autonomic dysfunction (see page 400 for a description) being the most frequent category, comprising 14% of the total. Most of the GPs in that study were reasonably good at recognising somatic presentations, correctly identifying 50–71% of the cases, and they also detected a psychosocial component in around two-thirds of the cases.

Patients presenting with purely somatic symptoms usually insist they have a physical illness and, at least in their earlier consultations, will seek help only for what they perceive to be a physical disorder; they are not usually receptive to the idea that their problem may be psychologically based. However, research studies have repeatedly demonstrated that there is often another comorbid psychiatric disorder, such as anxiety or depression.

Those who present to the GP with purely psychological presentations are sometimes called 'psychologisers' and are a smaller group, comprising only 5% of attendees, whereas patients with a mixture of somatic and psychological complaints are more common. Patients with exclusive somatic presentations are sometimes known as 'somatisers'. Comparisons between 'psychologisers' and 'somatisers' show that somatisers have less depression, lower levels of social dissatisfaction, are less dependent on relatives, and, as may be expected, have fewer and less severe psychological symptoms. However, they are more likely to have received medical in-patient care as an adult, and tend to have an unsympathetic attitude to mental illness (Wright, 1990; Bridges *et al*, 1991).

Among the more severe and protracted cases, the patients' insistence they have a physical disorder combined with the GPs' ever-present fear of missing a serious physical condition drives on the process of repeated and pointless medical referrals and physical investigations. Balint (1957), a psychoanalyst, described how patients in this group might be passed from one organic specialist to another without any consideration being given to a psychological contribution, in what he termed 'a collusion of anonymity'. Goldberg & Huxley (1992) also commented on the development of this type of relationship, where the GP attempts to satisfy the patient's demands by ordering more and more physical investigations while at the same time prescribing some physical remedy. The doctor colludes with the patient's denial of psychological disorder and 'it ill behoves an outsider to declare that anything is wrong'. Once the pattern has set in, it is difficult to reverse the endless requests for fruitless investigations.

Attempts to improve the management of somatisation in general practice

The management of somatisation disorder in secondary care, which is very difficult, is considered in Chapter 16 (page 398) and so here just a few recent studies aimed at improving its treatment in the general practice setting are reviewed.

First, attempts have been made to devise training programmes to improve GP recognition. Rosendal *et al* (2003) randomly allocated a group of Danish GPs into two groups. One group received a training programme comprising of 23 hours of lectures and workshops covering such topics as bio-psychosocial history-taking, somatisation disorder and reattribution theory, while a second, control group received no training. In both groups there was a very wide range in recognition rates: for the control group 2–22%, and for the intervention group 3–33%, indicating that, even with training, there are a few GPs who just cannot detect somatisation or at least do not record a diagnosis for it. Training did lead to a modest, non-significant improvement for the detection of somatoform disorders, but there was a significant improvement in the recognition rates for 'medically non-explained symptoms' (7.7% for trained GPs versus 3.9% untrained GPs). Even if improved rates of recognition fail to translate into more cures, it may still be useful, as this may lead to a reduction in the number of non-useful medical investigations and referrals.

Changing the agenda from discussing exclusively physical symptoms to exploring psychosocial issues is an accepted strategy for modifying somatising disorders, but there is a difficulty in identifying suitable opportunities for intervening during the consultation, as well as doing it in such a way that patients do not feel their symptoms have been ignored or misunderstood, or otherwise alienating them. Salmon *et al* (2004) audiotaped the consultations 36 somatisation patients had with their GPs and found that all but two interviews provided opportunities for a more psychologically focused discussion. These occurred at points during the interview where patients began to reveal their social and emotional difficulties, or changes in their mood. The implication is that, with careful listening, it may be possible to 'change the agenda' for most somatisers, but almost certainly the brief consultation times of general practice will militate against the success of such an approach.

Disclosure of emotionally significant events is also a useful psychotherapeutic technique but a randomised trial of disclosure showed no benefits to the health of somatising patients (Schilte *et al*, 2001). Dowrick *et al*

(2004) described how GPs tended to manage somatisation by 'normalisation', which usually meant giving a rudimentary reassurance that everything was normal, often accompanied by the authority of a negative test result. Normalisation of this type was usually ineffective and in a few patients might even exacerbate symptoms. More success was observed when normalisation was accompanied by a more comprehensive explanation, linking physical and psychological factors, which also led to further psychosocial intervention.

Schizophrenia in general practice

GPs play a crucial role in the clinical management of all chronic illnesses and this includes schizophrenia. They may help with:

- the early detection of prodromal symptoms
- monitoring patients and preventing relapses
- providing treatment
- the treatment and prevention of physical ill-health.

Effective GP care requires:

- liaison with the CMHT
- appropriate and tolerant attitudes
- knowledge and skills in prescribing psychotropic medication
- an awareness of how to access effective psychosocial interventions.

Patients with schizophrenia are in more frequent contact with their GPs than their psychiatrist. Melzer *et al* (1991) found that, by 1 year after discharge, 57% of patients had been in contact with their GP, 52% had visited an out-patient clinic but only 20% had seen the CPN. Personnel in the psychiatric services often have a high turnover, whereas GPs tend to stay in post for long periods and such continuity of care and contact may be greatly valued by people with a long-term condition such as schizophrenia. Patients with schizophrenia consult their GPs at around the same rate as patients with chronic physical disorders and usually present with a physical complaint rather than for their schizophrenic symptoms (Nazareth *et al*, 1993).

The carers of patients with schizophrenia are usually their parents and they need considerable support over the longer term. GPs are well placed to fulfil this role. Recent legislation has recognised the importance of carers and the considerable distress they may suffer, and so treating teams are required to assess the needs of carers and draw up appropriate plans for helping them. Distressed relatives will usually first turn to their GP when the patient is beginning to relapse.

Cohen *et al* (2004) have summarised the role of the GP in the care of patients with schizophrenia in the community in the UK today (Box 30.5).

Box 30.5 The role of the general practitioner in the management of schizophrenia

- Assessment and treatment of physical morbidity. Monitoring physical health over the longer term, for example for diabetes and cardiovascular disorder.
- Prescription of medication (especially repeats, and over the long term).
- Development of shared-care protocols with other agencies for monitoring lithium or antipsychotic drugs.
- Education of patients and carers. Support for carers.
- Monitoring of the mental state. In some services this is a CMHT responsibility, but in others this may fall to the GP, particularly for those patients the CMHT has discharged back to the GP or in inaccessible rural areas, where the GP may be the only professional visiting.
- Identification of patterns of relapse. Being proactive in relapse prevention, for example by informing the CMHT if a patient fails to collect a repeat prescription, or if new symptoms appear.
- Crisis intervention (prepare a crisis plan, and know which CMHT worker should be involved).
- Identification of risk factors for suicide: depressed mood, voicing suicidal ideation, hopelessness, recurrent relapses with inadequate symptom control. Groups thought to be at a higher risk of suicide include single young men, those recently discharged from hospital, and those with comorbid drug or alcohol misuse, poor social support or a family history of suicide.
- Identification of local networks and support groups, for example for ethnic minority groups and for those with particular religious affiliations.
- Coordinating care with social services, including housing and education, and the local mental health trust. Usually this means liaising with the CPN. Help generally with 'the system'.
- Ensuring that any female patient with a history of a serious psychiatric disorder (postpartum or non-postpartum) is assessed by a psychiatrist in the antenatal period.

Suicide and homicide prevention in general practice

Estimates suggest that patient suicide is a relatively rare event for GPs, occurring only once every 4–7 years, with pre-suicide contact occurring once every decade on average (Diekstra & Egmond, 1989). An event with such a low frequency will therefore be almost impossible to predict and has been little studied.

Stanistreet *et al* (2004) found that although there was a significant difference in the proportion of patients who had seen their GP during the 3 months before death among those who died by suicide (56%) and those who died of accidental causes (41%), this was not significant at 1 month, which is the critical period when preventive action may be taken (38% versus 30%, respectively). Those who died by suicide were more likely to have seen a mental health professional at some time (27% versus 13%). Stanistreet *et al* also showed that relatively few young men consult their GP during the period shortly before death from suicide or accidents.

Rutz (2001) has argued that prevention must extend beyond suicide risk assessment, and consider ways to reach out to young men experiencing emotional distress, mental health problems or substance misuse, and this should be accompanied by improved education on suicide for all mental health professionals. However, the rarity of the event in general practice, combined with the fact that many distressed people often contact other voluntary services, such as the Samaritans, means that GPs are not particularly well placed to implement suicide prevention strategies.

The suicide of doctors is considered separately on page 775.

Homicide is an even less frequent event, but with increasing numbers of people who are severely mentally ill now living in the community, and homicides still occurring, it may be timely to consider whether GPs have a role in trying to prevent such tragedies, for example by better training in risk assessment.

Drug prescribing by general practitioners

Trethowan (1975), in a paper entitled 'Pills for personal problems', was among the first to raise the alarm for what he called 'the relentless psychotropic drug juggernaut'. Data from surveys based in general practice suggest that somewhere between 9% and 15% of attendees are presently taking psychotropic medication, the three main drug groups being antidepressants, anxiolytics and hypnotics, although GPs also prescribe antipsychotic drugs. In part, drug prescriptions are determined by the clinical psychiatric disorders, but repeated studies have shown that other socio-demographic factors have an important and independent influence on prescribing.

A recent pan-European study found that older age, female sex, 'separated' marital status and the presence of depression or other psychiatric disorder were all independently predictive of receiving a prescription for a psychotropic drug (Kisely *et al*, 2000). A Finnish study found a fivefold difference between prescribing rates for psychotropics: for the youngest age group (18–34 years) the rate was 10%, and for the oldest age group it was 50%. That study also found that being widowed, retired, living alone or being unemployed increased rates of psychotropic drug prescribing, while being unmarried, employed and in the upper social classes (1–3) decreased the rate (Joukamaa *et al*, 1995).

A study of GP attendees in West London, an area with a high immigrant population, identified White ethnic groups, not owning a property and previous symptoms as the main predictors of a mental health intervention that included a psychotropic drug prescription (Raine *et al*, 2000).

These observations suggest that the current high consumption of prescribed psychotropic medication, in many ways like the consumption of illicit psychotropic drugs, has important social determinants, even though the psychosocial correlates of prescribed drug use are very different to those of illicit drug taking. The use of prescribed drugs is certainly far from being solely a medical endeavour.

Antidepressant prescribing

Antidepressant prescribing by GPs has increased vastly since the early 1990s, with the greatest increases being among the elderly. In 1998, a total of 23.4 million antidepressant prescriptions were issued by GPs in the UK. Middleton *et al* (2001) speculated on the causes of this increase, which could be changes in recognition rates, or the use of different management strategies, but the most likely explanation is the relatively greater tolerability of the most recent generation of antidepressants, namely the SSRIs. In support of this, Lawrenson *et al* (2000) observed a 9.8% increase in the overall rate of antidepressant prescribing between 1991 and 1996, with a 40% increase in the prescribing rates of tricyclic antidepressants, but over the same period there was a 460% increase in SSRI prescribing rates. This suggests that in previous decades many people with depression probably missed out on potentially beneficial drug treatments. Under-treatment was still observed in the late 1990s in the Hampshire Depression Project, where overall antidepressant prescribing rates were still relatively low, as only 28% of those with probable major depression, and 15% with possible depression, received antidepressants (Kendrick *et al*, 2001).

There is wide variation in antidepressant prescribing rates between practices. Thus, in the USA, Ornstein *et al* (2000) reported a tenfold range of 0.4–4% for the overall proportion of all attendees receiving an antidepressant between different practices, while in the UK, Hull *et al* (2001) reported a 25-fold difference in rate, indicating that both under-treatment and over-treatment probably still occur for depression. The study of Hull *et al* (2001) took place in the East End of London, an area with a large Asian (mainly Bangladeshi) community, who had lower rates of antidepressant prescribing, with ethnicity accounting for 28% of the variance in prescribing rates. Reasons for this are uncertain, but there is a suggestion of low rates of depression among Bangladeshis (see page 761), as well as a strong stigma against mental illness or any sort of psychotropic drug use.

Anxiolytic prescribing

This has been less studied than antidepressant prescribing, but Kisely *et al* (2000) found that prescriptions for anxiolytics were more common among females, those who were less educated (had left school earlier) and those who were unemployed. Severity of disorder was not associated with an anxiolytic prescription. The most commonly used anxiolytics were the benzodiazepines, but GPs also use small doses of various antipsychotics to manage anxiety. As expected hypnotics were more commonly prescribed for the elderly, but their prescription was not associated with any particular diagnosis (Kisely *et al*, 2000).

The benzodiazepine epidemic peaked in 1979, with a total of 18 million prescriptions in the UK. This fell to 8 million in 1988 and the number has been falling ever since, although benzodiazepine addiction still remains a problem in the community. Numerous attempts have been made to try to treat benzodiazepine dependence within the general practice setting. For example, Cormack *et al* (1989) found that an appropriate letter outlining the risks of dependency combined with a small self-help group could reduce the prescribing rate. More recent studies based in general practice have shown that transfer to diazepam, with a gradual taper, may be effective but the addition of either an SSRI or

CBT failed to confer any further advantage (Zitman & Couvee, 2001; Voshaar *et al*, 2003).

Antipsychotic drug use in general practice

Kaye *et al* (2003), using the UK's GP research database covering the period 1991–2000, found that GPs often used antipsychotic drugs. The most common diagnosis for an antipsychotic prescription was anxiety or depression; less than 10% of antipsychotic prescriptions were for schizophrenia and only 1% were for bipolar disorder. Antipsychotic prescribing was more frequent for the elderly (usually for dementia) and accounted for 15% of the total, and around 1% of the population were taking antipsychotics. Paradoxically, the most frequently prescribed drug for this period was thioridazine (38%), a drug now considered to be so hazardous that it is almost impossible to obtain. Other typical drugs, chlorpromazine, flupentixol, trifluoperazine and haloperidol, each accounted for around 10% of prescriptions. The atypicals were introduced during the study period, risperidone in 1993 and olanzapine in 1996, and their use increased progressively, both reaching around 20% of total antipsychotic prescribing by the year 2000.

In the USA, Hermann *et al* (2002) found a 20% penetration rate for the atypicals had been reached somewhat earlier, by 1997, but during the late 1990s in the UK there was considerable pressure from government for reasons of cost not to prescribe atypicals. Hermann *et al* (2002) also noted that 'office' prescriptions by psychiatrists were more often for an atypical (37%) than those given by the GP (14%).

A study of atypical antipsychotic prescribing by Italian GPs between 1999 and 2002 confirmed the increasing penetration of the atypicals, and the study also found that women and people with non-schizophrenic psychoses were the most likely to take an antipsychotic drug (Rifiro *et al*, 2005). Compliance, as measured by the 'medicine possession ratio' (derived from the patients' records), was greater with the atypical drugs than with the typical drugs (medical possession ratios for the atypicals was 2.21 versus 1.69 for typicals). The most common 'off label' reason for prescribing an atypical drug was senile dementia. It is likely that this gradual and unintended increase in the use of atypical drugs for people with senile dementia provided the background circumstance that preceded the discovery that the atypicals were associated with an increased mortality risk for patients with senile dementia, so that now the use of atypicals (olanzapine and risperidone, but not quetiapine) for these patients has been very severely curtailed.

Psychotropic drug prescribing and physical illness

The strong association between depression and physical illness is well documented and is discussed in Chapter 17. Community surveys and surveys of GP attendees confirm high rates of CMDs among those with physical illness. For example, Vazquez-Barquero *et al* (1992) found that the combination of physical and psychiatric disorder led to very high consultation rates – 89% for men and 97% for women – and so not surprisingly physical illness is associated with high rates of psychotropic drug prescribing. Also, because GPs work mainly with people who are physically ill, chronic physical illness accounts for a high proportion of psychotropic drug prescribing. However, this association does not seem to extend to patients with acute physical disorders, for whom the prescribing rate is actually lower than the average (Irwin & Cupples, 1986). Possibly, with acute disorders, GPs feel better able to resist the pressure to prescribe psychotropics because an end is sight, whereas with chronic physical illness the need to relieve the distress and 'do something' is always present.

It should be noted that some GP antidepressant prescribing may be for physical pain, as some of these drugs have analgesic effects. For example, because the non-steroidal anti-inflammatory drugs are associated with gastrointestinal haemorrhages and the newer COX-2 inhibitors were found to raise the rate of cardiac events, GPs are now increasingly using amitriptyline in low doses as an adjunct in pain relief. Lawrenson *et al* (2000) found that around one-third of all amitriptyline prescriptions in general practice were for pain. Amitriptyline in low doses (10–20 mg) is also being increasingly used as a hypnotic in general practice, as it lacks the addictive potential of the benzodiazepines.

Duration of psychotropic drug prescribing and repeat prescribing

Most psychotropic prescribing is short term. An early study by Parish (1971) found that 50% of patients took their drugs for less than 1 month, 15% for 1 year and only 5% for more than 5 years. Even before the SSRI era, Williams (1979) reported that antidepressants were taken for longer periods than tranquillisers, but it is likely today that there are very many more patients taking antidepressants, especially SSRIs, over the long term. Thus, Ornstein *et al* (2000) found that around half of patients with depression were given an antidepressant (6% of all GP attendees) and in 81% of cases this was an SSRI, but repeat SSRI prescriptions comprised 60% of the total whereas new SSRI prescription accounted for only 40%. GPs cannot see patients for every prescription renewal, and so a great deal of repeat psychotropic drug prescribing is done without consultation. Balint (1957) suggested that this tended to create a special type of doctor–patient relationship, one based on anonymity, which some patients and some GPs may actually prefer. However, such anonymity can lead to unnecessarily long psychotropic drug use. Varnam (1981) found that patients who were being seen while obtaining repeat prescriptions continued their medication for 2.7 years, whereas those who obtained repeat prescriptions without being seen continued with their medication for a mean of 4.3 years.

High and low GP prescribers, and attempts to understand GP variation

Several studies have demonstrated considerable variability in GP prescribing rates. For example, Fleming & Cross (1984) found that the top 'quintile' of GPs (ranked by prescribing rates) issued twice as many psychotropic drug prescriptions as the lowest quintile, and these GPs showed a tenfold difference for repeat prescriptions. Since more than half the prescriptions issued are repeats, these differences between GPs are quite substantial. Differences between practices did not appear to relate to either workload or patient factors, but more to GP education and experience.

Kisely *et al* (2000), in their pan-European prescribing survey, found that doctors with lower rates of psychotropic drug prescribing took a positive view of their psychiatric training and also tended to use more antidepressants. Around half the practices in that study were client-centred clinics (i.e. large group practices) and the remainder had an old-style 'personal physician model'. Antidepressants and anxiolytics were prescribed twice as frequently in the client-centred clinics as in the personal physician model.

A qualitative study of prescribing behaviour, based on in-depth interviewing of GPs in New Zealand, identified three groups of GPs ($n = 10$ for each), those who were low-cost, medium-cost and high-cost prescribers. Low-cost prescribers had been in practice for longer, took a more relaxed attitude to medicine, were more comfortable saying 'no' to patients, had longer consultation times, emphasised the listening aspect of general practice and did more formal counselling. In contrast, the high-cost prescribers viewed medical practice as a contractual matter, were more highly motivated, viewed their obligation to the patient in terms of service provision and issues of medical competence, and were acutely aware of pressure arising from patient expectation; they explained much of their prescribing practice as arising in response to this pressure (Jaye & Tilyard, 2002).

It can be seen that GP prescribing of psychotropics is a complex sociocultural phenomenon associated with a variety of socio-demographic factors, the ability to resist patient pressure, medico-legal fears on the part of the doctor and differences in medical training. It therefore encompasses far more than purely clinical indications. A huge amount of research and money go into trying to discover new drugs and this is generally accompanied by very expensive clinical trials, which seek to refine clinical indications for drug use. In contrast, the social and non-clinical factors associated with psychotropic drug use over the longer term are not well understood and have been neglected as a research topic. Yet they may be of importance, not only because of the vast amount of medication prescribed and its associated expense, but also because of the large populations involved.

Government targets and incentives for general practice psychiatry

The NHS is a highly centralised system of healthcare and the government has laid down targets and incentives for all specialties. For general practice, the majority of these targets relate to immunisation or cancer screening programmes, but there are four targets and incentives that relate to psychiatry in general practice settings. While they do not represent an overall coherent strategy, and although they are all in the right direction, they are relatively small and probably have only marginal effects. These are:

1 standards 2 and 3 of the National Service Framework

2 incentives for looking after the physical care of people who have a chronic mental illness, under the terms of the General Medical Services (nGMS) contract for GPs

3 additional payments for looking after patients in deprived catchment areas

4 the development of 'general practice specialists in psychiatry', that is, GPs who specialise in psychiatry and receive extra remuneration for doing this.

National Service Framework for Mental Health

The National Service Framework for Mental Health was published by the Department of Health in 1999. It set out a strategic blueprint for the psychiatric services for the next 10 years and defined seven 'standards' that trusts should aim to achieve. Overall, the aim is to deliver better primary healthcare, and to ensure consistent advice and help for people with mental health needs, including primary care services for individuals with severe mental illness. Standards 2 and 3 relate to primary care and access to services:

- Standard 2 states that any service user who contacts the primary healthcare team with a common mental health problem should have their mental health needs identified and assessed, and be offered effective treatments, including referral to specialist services for further assessment, treatment and care if they require it.
- Standard 3 states that any individual with a common mental health problem should be able to make contact around the clock with the local services necessary to meet their needs and receive adequate care. They should also be able to use NHS Direct, as it develops, for first-level advice and referral on to specialist help-lines or to local services.

There are no additional payments for implementing these standards in general practice.

Although round-the-clock contact with the GP is desirable, the loss of the 'personal physician' model in most parts of the country means that outside working hours only deputising services are available and so only psychiatric assessments of a very basic sort (e.g. to admit or not to admit) are made. Although the doctors making these assessments are often GPs, they usually have no knowledge of the patient or access to their records and must squeeze the assessment in with numerous other acute medical emergencies as well. An assessment of this type is a long way from the original intention of the authors for standard 3.

The new GP contract

The 2003 General Medical Services contract for GPs, on which GP salary is partly based, contains five mental health quality indicators, which relate to record keeping, the physical health of people who are chronically mentally ill, and monitoring serum lithium. On the basis of these, GPs will be able to receive extra remuneration. Other targets are added in from time to time and these schemes vary from one locality to another (because of the existence of 'local enhanced schemes', the uptake of which is highly variable).

Government payments for GPs working in deprived areas

Since 1990, GPs in England and Wales have received additional capitation payments for patients living in deprived areas. These payments are made on the assumption that workload and pressure on GP services increase directly in proportion to the number of patients registered with the practice who live in deprived council wards. The underlying aim has been to ensure retention of GPs in deprived areas, so that they could have smaller lists, and not feel the need to move to less deprived areas to retain their salary. Deprivation is measured using the Jarman UPA-8 score (which ranges from +30 to –50) and a ten-point decrease in this score has been shown to be associated with a 17% increase in consultation frequency. It should be remembered that Jarman originally devised his rating scale as a way of trying to understand and measure GP workload. To receive these payments, GPs are expected to reach their targets over a wide range of other conditions, such as immunisation or cervical cancer screening targets and so forth. A more recent modification of the system has been to calculate payments to particular practices based on enumeration districts (post-code areas), rather than council wards, and this system is more accurate and fairer, as many GPs in apparently prosperous council wards had a few council estates that were pockets of deprivation, and so were probably working just as hard as inner-city GPs. The use of deprivation payments may have helped psychiatry more than most specialties because the geographical distribution of psychiatric disorder closely follows the pattern of deprivation (Bajekal *et al*, 2001).

General practitioners with a special interest

Many GPs have an interest in a medical sub-specialty and until recently they could work in their area of special interest only by attaching themselves to the local consultant and doing clinics in their local hospital. A recent trend has been to offer contracts to GPs who are enthusiastic about their specialty and remunerate them for their special-interest work, but it is uncertain how many actually receive payment for their specialist work. Primary care organisations may wish to employ 'GPs with a special interest in psychiatry' to take on the responsibility for achieving national objectives. The grade is new and so there is no systematic data, but Pogue (2003) provides a personal account of her experience. Pogue found that her tasks were more in the administrative realm of advising PCTs on services and commissioning secondary care, as well as visiting practices in her locality, rather than in direct clinical care. She wrote that to do the job required enthusiasm for the subject, a strong psyche and a good sense of humour – the last being essential for coping with the various bureaucracies encountered.

So far, there is no consistent training programme or job description, but there is interest on the part of both the Royal College of Psychiatrists and the Royal College of General Practitioners in developing a diploma in 'Primary care mental health and education'.

Written communication between GPs and psychiatrists and patients

Good communication is essential for the practice of good medicine and the communication between GPs and psychiatrists depends almost exclusively on the quality of the letters they write to each other. How useful are these letters, and what items of information should they include? Williams & Wallace (1974) in their survey asked a group of GPs and psychiatrists in Cardiff to rank 12 items in order of relevance for inclusion in a GP referral to a psychiatrist and for the psychiatrist's response to the GP. The five most relevant items of information for each type of letter are shown in Table 30.13, along with the frequency with which these items were present in a survey by Pullen & Yellowlees (1985).

Psychiatric summaries used in the case notes are often quite lengthy documents. Craddock & Craddock (1989) found that GPs preferred to have a letter of around one A4 page, while psychiatrists preferred to have a two- to four-page summary. However, these summaries serve primarily as a long-term record of the patient's condition. These studies suggest that GPs do not wish to read a lengthy reiteration of a patient's social history, with which they are probably familiar, but are interested in the psychiatrist's diagnosis, suggested management plan and the recommended drug prescription, and also want to receive some explanation of their patient's disorder. Even though most psychiatrists will spend many hours a week dictating letters to their GP colleagues, the topic has been little researched in recent years.

Table 30.13 Key items required in letters from GPs and psychiatrists

Items required	% of letters with item
Items required by psychiatrist (n = 120) in referral letters	
Medication	62
Family history	37
Main symptom/problem	100
Reason for referral	99
Psychiatric history	72
Items required by GPs (n = 120) in letters from psychiatrists	
Diagnosis	88
Treatment	92
Follow-up	95
Prognosis	23
Concise explanation	60

After Pullen & Yellowlees (1985).

Letters to patients and patient-held records

The NHS Plan (Department of Health, 2000) requires letters between clinicians about an individual patient's care to be copied to the patient as of right, with full implementation from April 2004. The underlying rationale for this is that patients have the right to know what is being written about them, but at the same time also have the right to refuse to see such information if that is their wish. An early study, conducted long before this government directive, showed that although most patients were not perturbed by reading their notes, people with a diagnosis of psychosis or personality disorder were sometimes upset, and so any written comments about a patient's personality or personality traits should be made with caution or even completely omitted (Bernadt *et al*, 1991).

Two more recent studies on the effect of the NHS Plan directive produced conflicting results. Nandhra *et al* (2004) found that 83% of patients in the 16- to 65-year age group expressed a positive view about receiving copies of letters sent to their GPs, but 18% experienced some upset and 5% were distressed. The psychiatrists writing these letters also reported that in 25% of cases they altered the letter from their usual form because they were aware the patient might read it. One letter went astray and this raised important issues of confidentiality. A study among older patients found that only 20% wanted to receive a copy of the letter sent to their GP but rather more would have liked a simpler letter (36%) directed to themselves in addition to a letter for their carer (Dale *et al*, 2004).

Of relevance to secondary care, where many people suffer from schizophrenia, is the issue of whether written confirmation of this diagnosis will upset patients. Lester *et al* (2003) found that a patient-held record for people with schizophrenia was quite acceptable to patients and acted as a useful tool in communicating between patients, GPs and key workers, although it made no difference to outcome. Some patients obviously benefit from reading copies of their GP letters and this may lead to improved rapport and better cooperation, while a rather smaller proportion seem to get distressed, and so further evaluation of the risk:benefit ratio of this directive may be needed.

Mental health and suicide among doctors

The mental health and raised suicide rates of doctors are matters of concern for the whole profession. Around 60% of the referrals to the National Counselling Service for Sick Doctors are for GPs, 50% of which are for alcoholism and 25% for depression. A study by Murray (1976) found that the admission rate for doctors was 2.7 times greater than that for a control group of the same social class. Anxiety levels, as measured by the Middlesex Hospital Questionnaire, were raised among male GPs, but female GPs were found to have lower levels of anxiety and depression than the general population (Cooper *et al*, 1989). The SMRs for stress-related conditions may also be raised for doctors: the SMR for suicide was 335, accidental poisoning 818, and cirrhosis 311 (HMSO, 1986). GPs are at increased risk of alcoholism and one survey found rates of 5.4% for heavy drinking (6–12 units a day), which was similar to the rate of heavy drinking for patients who were on the GP lists in this survey (Anderson, 1985).

In spite of increased knowledge and greater awareness of mental health issues, doctors may not be an easy group to reach out to and help. Allibone *et al* (1981), in a study of the physical and mental health of a group of older GPs, found a high incidence of self-treatment, delay in seeking medical care and anxiety in confiding to a colleague (which was associated with underlying fears that they might be perceived as weak and unstable, to the extent that their professional credibility might be questioned, and even place their livelihood in jeopardy).

There is now good evidence that the suicide rate of doctors is raised. Sternhammer & Colditz (2004) conducted a meta-analysis of all 25 published studies on physician suicide over the previous 30 years and found a significantly elevated suicide rate ratio of 1.41 for male doctors in comparison with the general population rate, but for female doctors the risk was more than double, at 2.27. A UK study conducted around the same time found a rate of 18.8/100 000 per year for female doctors, which was significantly above the female general population suicide rate, but the male rate of 19.2/100 000 was not significantly elevated (Hawton *et al*, 2001).

Suicide rates in certain specialties may be higher. Thus, anaesthetists (possibly because of ease of access to toxic chemicals), community health doctors, GPs and psychiatrists all had significantly increased suicide rates compared with doctors working in general hospitals. Seniority had no effect. To try to understand why doctors take their own lives, Hawton *et al* (2004) conducted a psychological autopsy of 38 currently working doctors who had died by suicide. In the year before their death, 71% had occupational problems, which included working long hours, and feeling overloaded by work or unable to cope with the responsibility of work. Around 17% were facing an enquiry and for 5 out of the 38 cases (13%) the researchers thought the complaints or enquiry were the major cause of the suicide. Mental illness was present in 63% (mainly depression), alcohol misuse in 17%, relationship problems in 40%, financial difficulties in 29% and family problems in 23%, but the most common picture was of several difficulties occurring together. The most common method of suicide was self-poisoning, often with drugs taken from work. The authors suggested that the profession should learn to deal with professional and personal difficulties among colleagues with greater compassion if suicide rates among doctors are to be reduced. Such changes in attitudes could help improve the quality of care given to the wider population as well.

GP further training in psychiatry

Most psychiatrists will train over a 5- to 8-year post-graduate period, to gain sufficient skill and competence to treat psychiatric patients. Most GPs will have to draw on knowledge gained during their 5- to 8-week attachment to the psychiatric department as a medical student, and their 1 year as a supervised GP trainee, so not surprisingly many GPs will initially feel overwhelmed when they begin to encounter the large numbers of psychiatric patients in primary care. Surveys have shown that there is a strong demand among GPs for CME in psychiatry, while there is also evidence that knowledge tends to decline with the passage of years in practice. Thus, in a study where medical students, postgraduate trainees and established GPs all took the same written examination, in which all the questions pertained to patient care, postgraduate trainees came out best, and their marks increased as the number of postgraduate years increased. However, declines in knowledge were observed for those who had been in practice for 5–10 years, and worryingly persistent declines were observed for all those who had been practice for more than 10 years (Van Leeuwen *et al*, 1995).

While the need for CME for GPs in psychiatry is widely acknowledged, there is no consensus on what should be taught or how. However, the literature of the past 50 years on the topic has been usefully reviewed by Hodges *et al* (2001), from which the account below is taken.

Perhaps the first psychiatrist to venture into the field of providing GPs with an education in psychiatry, as well as stimulating their interest and improving their psychotherapeutic skills, was the Hungarian psychoanalyst Michael Balint, who immigrated to England before the Second World War. His seminal book *The Doctor, His Patient, and the Illness* (Balint, 1957) was based on weekly meetings with a group of GPs, where the discussion would focus on the doctors' reactions to their patient, the doctor–patient relationship and the way this impinged on day-to-day interactions with patients. The group setting was also used to convey some important psychotherapeutic principles, such as the importance of listening, rather than simply asking questions, as might occur in a traditional GP or psychiatric consultation, as well as the use of empathy, although formulations expressed in terms of the transference and countertransference were avoided. Balint believed that the GP, far from being a faceless diagnostician, was by far the most important therapeutic agent to interact with the patient and, using the metaphor of a drug to convey this to a medical audience, he wrote:

> 'By far the most frequently used drug in general practice is the doctor himself. No guidance is contained in any textbook as to the dosage in which the drug doctors should prescribe themselves, in what form, how frequently and what is curative and what the maintenance dose should be, and so on.' (Balint, 1957)

The methods Balint first developed in the 1950s have evolved into 'Balint groups'. A small number of these exist in the UK but the method is very much more popular in Europe. For example, a recent survey of GPs in Aarhus, Denmark, found that more than half of them were either currently attending or had attended such a psychotherapy supervision group (Nielsen *et al*, 2002).

Box 30.6 Psychiatry attribute guide for trainee GPs

- Understand the doctor–patient relationship and its therapeutic vale
- Factors leading to mental illness
- Emotional, intellectual and social development
- Recognise deviations from the expected norms of development – mental handicap, dyslexia, behavioural and personality disorders
- The roles of other health professionals in mental illness
- Liaison with social services
- Impact on family of mental illness
- Mental Health Act, Children's Act and Misuse of Drugs Regulations

Clinical skills

- Taking a psychiatric history
- Consultation skills – listening, recognising clues and providing explanation
- Mental state examination
- Prescribing drug treatment
- Formulating the psychodynamics of a case, including a Care Programme Approach
- Advising relatives
- Planning interviews to modify behaviour
- Referral for specialist advice

Knowledge and understanding of mental and emotional disorders

- Acute, life-threatening disorders and appropriate management
- Schizophrenia
- Early depression
- Postnatal depression
- Manic–depressive illness
- Substance misuse
- Mental handicap
- Dementia
- Phobias
- Bereavement/grief reactions
- Enuresis
- School refusal
- Knowledge of psychological aspects of physical illnesses and of medical and surgical treatments

Treatment

- Pharmacology of drugs used in psychiatry
- Non-pharmacological treatments available for psychiatric disorders
- Understand the placebo affect

Based on the training objectives for the psychiatric component of GP vocational training, from Page & Valentine (2003). Note that although all the topics listed above are important in secondary care, the syllabus is very different to that used for training psychiatrists.

Need for and objectives of CME in psychiatry for GPs

A coherent syllabus has been worked out for the postgraduate training of psychiatrists and for the training of undergraduate medical students in psychiatry. Recent years have also seen the development of an accepted guideline for the training of GPs on vocational training schemes and this has been published by the Joint Committee on Postgraduate Training for General Practice (Page & Valentine, 2003). A brief summary of this is shown in Box 30.6. It can be seen that the syllabus for GP psychiatry is very different from that for psychiatric trainees, and this reflects the very different case-mix and workload found in primary care as compared with secondary care. The Royal College of General Practitioners has also published a very much more detailed 27-page syllabus entitled

'Care of People with Mental Health Problems', which is due to be implemented in 2007 (see http://www.rcgp.org.uk/education/education_home/curriculum/gp_curriculum_documents.aspx).

However, the area of postgraduate education that remains of concern is the nature of the CME offered to GPs who are already established in practice, and there is still no consensus on what aspects of psychiatry can most usefully be offered to this group. In their review, Hodges *et al* (2001) were struck by the large number of articles on CME for GPs that based the selection of topics for their programme on what they termed the 'service deficit model'. Thus, the article would start by citing literature that showed some gap in mental health delivery, such as non-recognition of depression, diagnostic difficulties in general practice, or inadequate drug treatment, and so forth, and on this basis the educators would then plan their courses to remedy the presumed deficit – almost as if the underlying reason for the service deficit was the direct result of the GP's lack of knowledge. Such an approach is probably philosophically unsound, because a service deficit is rarely the result of simple lack of knowledge. However, a preoccupation in academic circles with topics like GP non-recognition of depression and GP diagnosis, combined with readily available financial support from the pharmaceutical industry and their need to sell antidepressants, has, over the last 30 years, resulted in huge numbers of CME courses on depression, and the use of antidepressant drugs, often held in hotels. This may have been a terrible waste of very valuable GP education time, which for psychiatry is severely limited in any case. Thus, when GPs and GP trainees are asked about topics they wish to learn more about, they tend not to place depression or antidepressants highly. On the basis of their survey, Hodges *et al* (2001) reported that the more highly rated topics were somatisation, psychosexual disorders, working with difficult patients and stress management. A survey of established GPs in Australia found that they wished to acquire counselling skills for both individual and family and marital problems, as well as to learn strategies to prevent their own burnout.

Around 40% of GP trainees in the UK now do a 6-month placement in a psychiatric post, and such exposure is certainly helpful in preparing doctors for general practice. Radcliffe *et al* (1999) surveyed trainees in these posts and found the psychiatric topics these GP trainees wished to learn more about were: communication skills, how to access resources, detection of psychiatric disorder, drug treatment and the management of aggression.

Box 30.7 Features of the consultation–liaison model

- There is regular, face-to-face contact between the visiting psychiatrist and other members of the primary care team. The CPN or other members of the CMHT may also be present.
- The meetings should not be less than monthly.
- Referral of individual patients takes place only after discussion at the face-to-face meeting.
- Many episodes of illness (perhaps the majority) are managed by the primary care team after discussion at the face-to-face meeting, without referral to the psychiatrist.
- Where referral takes place, there is feedback to the primary care team and the management is by them.

After Gask *et al* (1997).

Box 30.8 Summary of recommendations for CME in psychiatry for GPs

- Psychiatric educators should meet with the GPs who wish for further training and conduct a needs assessment on what topics or skills should form the focus of the course. The needs of one group of GPs may not be the same as those of another group; for example, GPs at different phases of their career may have different needs.
- Skills acquisition is a lengthier and more expensive process than didactic teaching of a topic, but may prove to be of more long-term benefit to GPs.
- Psychiatrists engaged in GP education should familiarise themselves with the context of primary care, for example by working in a GP practice or observing a GP at work to appreciate some of the constraints, such as the 15-minute as opposed to the 50-minute interview.
- Learning should be tied to real clinical practice, with GPs presenting their own clinical material whenever possible.
- Interactive methods, if available, should be used.
- Evaluation should be based on more than simple satisfaction and should test newly acquired knowledge and skills. Although evaluating altered patient outcome is of interest, this is expensive and can realistically be done only as part of a funded research programme.
- Programmes should be ongoing, rather than brief targeted courses, as the benefits of brief targeted courses fade rapidly. Doctors should be able to attend refresher courses.

After Hodges *et al* (2001).

Educational methods

A wide variety of educational methods have been used in CME for all specialties. Davis *et al* (1999) conducted a meta-analysis of the better designed studies. The educational methods used in these were classified as: 'didactic'; 'interactive', which meant the learner took some active part such as role play, video with feedback and so forth; or 'mixed', where both interactive and didactic teaching methods were used. Only the 'interactive' and 'mixed' educational methods were found to have any significant effect on physician behaviour and the effects of didactic teaching alone were non-significant. Much of the CME today, perhaps the bulk, for both GPs and psychiatrists, is didactic and so its longer-term value is uncertain.

A second variable of importance is the duration of the intervention. There is good evidence that any beneficial effects of the shorter courses that characterise most CME have faded by 1 year and only longer courses are associated with more long-lasting changes. The reviewers found the most optimistic reports came from programmes that adopted the traditional school or university teaching model, where the teacher (the psychiatrist) met the learner (the GP) on a regular, one-to-one basis, permitting an ongoing dialogue. This was even more relevant if the meeting took place in the general practice itself. In the UK this method has been called the 'consultation–liaison model', the main features of which have been outlined by Gask *et al* (1997) (Box 30.7).

Only a minority of GPs have a regular link of this kind, but many probably would welcome such arrangements, the type of link most commonly desired by GPs being one in which the GP shares actively in the assessment and treatment of the patient (Brown & Tower, 1990). Although this model is probably the most effective, it is expensive in terms of consultant psychiatrist time and may not be feasible on a national basis, especially bearing in mind the large number of GPs in the UK and the very much smaller number of psychiatrists who work in the fields of adult general or liaison psychiatry. An Australian survey found that only 1 in 11 GPs had links with a psychiatrist in a primary care setting, 1 in 6 with a psychologist and 1 in 17 with a CPN or social worker (Barber & Williams, 1996). UK figures are unlikely to be higher and so although this educational method is known to be moderately effective, it is unlikely to be widely adopted.

Box 30.8 summarises the recommendations made by Hodges *et al* (2001) based on their literature survey.

Conclusion

A vast ocean of psychiatric morbidity exists in primary care, yet only a trickle of the overall psychiatric budget is spent in primary care. Research has fairly consistently demonstrated that 'more' – more GP time, counselling sessions and paramedical and other skilled input – leads to better patient outcomes and so further improvements will largely depend on the amount government and society choose to invest in primary care psychiatry. Some of the more severe and chronic forms of neurotic disability may be beyond the reach of psychiatry, having deeper and more intractable social causes, but even so a large portion of the morbidity in primary care may benefit from standard psychiatric interventions. There is less certainty that better GP education by itself can alter patient outcome. The most obvious change in GP psychiatry since the early 1990s has been the huge increase in antidepressant prescribing, and it is time to ensure that psychological interventions also become widely available in primary care.

Acknowledgements

I would like to thank Dr Frank Holloway and Dr G. Stein for providing helpful contributions to earlier drafts of this chapter, as well as the thoughtful suggestions of Dr Anthony Furness, who works as a GP, and Dr Helen McColl, for her contributions to the section on asylum seekers.

References

Allibone, A., Oakes, D. & Shannon, H. S. (1981) The health and health care of doctors. *Journal of the Royal College of General Practitioners*, **31**, 728–734.

American Psychiatric Association (1994) *Diagnostic and Statistical Manual of Mental Disorders* (4th edn) (DSM–IV). Washington, DC: APA.

Anderson, P. (1985) Managing alcohol problems in general practice. *BMJ*, **290**, 1873–1875.

Ashworth, M., Clement, S., Sandhu, J., *et al* (2002) Psychiatric referral rates and the influence of onsite mental health workers in general practice. *British Journal of General Practice*, **52**, 39–41.

Ayuso-Mateos, J. L., Vazquez-Barquero, J. L., Dowrick, C., *et al* (2001) Depressive disorders in Europe: prevalence figures from the ODIN study. *British Journal of Psychiatry*, **179**, 308–316.

Bajekal, M., Alves, B., Jarman, B., *et al* (2001) Rationale for the new GP deprivation payment scheme in England: effects of moving from electoral ward to enumeration district underprivileged area scores. *British Journal of General Practice*, **51**, 451–455.

Baker, R., Reddish, S., Robertson, N., *et al* (2001) Randomised controlled trial of tailored strategies to implement guidelines for the management of patients with depression in general practice. *British Journal of General Practice*, **51**, 737–741.

Balint, M. (1957) *The Doctor, His Patient and the Illness*. London: Pitman.

Barber, R. & Williams, A. S. (1996) Psychiatrists working in primary care: a survey of general practitioners' attitudes. *Australia and New Zealand Journal of Psychiatry*, **30**, 278–286.

Bashir, K., Blizard, B., Bosanquet, A., *et al* (2000) The evaluation of a mental health facilitator in general practice: effects on recognition, management, and outcome of mental illness. *British Journal of General Practice*, **50**, 626–629.

Bebbington, P. E., Meltzer, H., Brugha, T. S., *et al* (2000) Unequal access and unmet need: neurotic disorders and the use of primary care services. *Psychological Medicine*, **30**, 1359–1367.

Bernadt, M., Gunning, L. & Quenstedt, M. (1991) Patients' access to their own psychiatric records. *BMJ*, **303**, 967.

Berthoud, R. (1976) *The Disadvantages of Inequality: A Study of Social Deprivation. A PEP Report*. London: Macdonald and James.

Bhugra, D. (2004) *Culture and Self-harm: Attempted Suicide in South Asians in London*. Maudsley Monograph No. 46. Hove: Psychology Press.

Bhui, K., Bhugra, D., Goldberg, D., *et al* (2001) Cultural influences on the prevalence of common mental disorder, general practitioners' assessments and help-seeking among Punjabi and English people visiting their general practitioner. *Psychological Medicine*, **31**, 815–825.

Bower, P. & Sibbald, B. (2000) Systematic review of the effect of on-site mental health professionals on the clinical behaviour of general practitioners. *BMJ*, **320**, 614–617.

Bower, P., Byford, S., Sibbald, B., *et al* (2000) Randomised controlled trial of non-directive counselling, cognitive–behaviour therapy, and usual general practitioner care for patients with depression. II: Cost effectiveness. *BMJ*, **321**, 1389–1392.

Bridges, K., Goldberg, D., Evans, B., *et al* (1991) Determinants of somatisation in primary care. *Psychological Medicine*, **21**, 473–483.

Brodaty, H. (1983) *Brief Psychotherapy in General Practice: A Controlled Prospective Intervention Study*. Unpublished MD thesis. University of New South Wales, Australia.

Brown, L. M. & Tower, J. E. C. (1990) Psychiatrists in primary care: would general practitioners welcome them? *British Journal of General Practice*, **40**, 369–371.

Burnett, A. & Peel, M. (2001) Health needs of asylum seekers and refugees. *BMJ*, **322**, 544–546.

Casey, P. R., Dillon, S. & Tyrer, P. J. (1984) The diagnostic status of patients with conspicuous psychiatric morbidity in primary care. *Psychological Medicine*, **14**, 673–81.

Chilvers, C., Dewey, M., Fielding, K., *et al* (2001) Counselling Versus Antidepressants in Primary Care Study Group. Antidepressant drugs and generic counselling for treatment of major depression in primary care: randomised trial with patient preference arms. *BMJ*, **322**, 772–775.

Churchill, R., Khaira, M. & Gretton, V. (2000) Nottingham Counselling and Antidepressants in Primary Care (CAPC) Study Group. Treating depression in general practice: factors affecting patients' treatment preferences. *British Journal of General Practice*, **50**, 905–906.

Clark, G. (1966) *A History of the Royal College of Physicians*, vol. II, pp. 476–479. Oxford: Oxford University Press.

Cohen, A., Singh, S. P. & Hagne, J. (2004) *The Primary Care Guide to Managing Severe Mental Illness*. London: Sainsbury Centre for Mental Health.

Cooper, C. L., Rout, U. & Faragher, B. (1989) Mental health, job satisfaction and job stress among general practitioners. *BMJ*, **298**, 366–370.

Cormack, M. A., Owens, R. G. & Dewey, M. E. (1989) The effect of minimal intervention by general practitioners on long term benzodiazepine use. *Journal of the Royal College of General Practitioners*, **39**, 408–411.

Corney, R. (1984) The effectiveness of attached social workers in the management of depressed female patients in general practice. *Psychological Medicine Monograph Supplements*, **6**.

Craddock, N. & Craddock, B. (1989) Psychiatric discharge summaries: differing requirements of psychiatrists and GPs. *BMJ*, **299**, 1382.

Croudace, T., Evans, J., Harrison, G., *et al* (2003) Impact of the ICD–10 primary health care (PHC) diagnostic and management guidelines for mental disorders on detection and outcome in primary care. Cluster randomised controlled trial. *British Journal of Psychiatry*, **182**, 20–30.

Dale, J., Tadros, G. & Adams, S. (2004) Do patients really want copies of their GP letters? A questionnaire survey of older adults and their carers. *Psychiatric Bulletin*, **21**, 199–200.

Davis, D., Thomson, M. A., Freemantle, N., *et al* (1999) Impact of formal continuing medical education: do conferences, workshops, rounds and other traditional continuing educational activities change physician behavior or health care outcomes? *JAMA*, **282**, 867–874.

Department of Health (1999*b*) *The National Service Framework for Mental Health. Modern Standards and Service Models*. London: Department of Health.

Department of Health (2000) *The NHS Plan. A Plan for Investment. A Plan for Reform*. London: Department of Health.

Deys, C., Dowling, E. & Golding, V. (1989) Clinical psychology: a consultation approach in general practice. *Journal of the Royal College of General Practitioners*, **39**, 342–344.

Diekstra, R. F. W. & Egmond, M. V. (1989) Suicide and attempted suicide in general practice, 1979–1986. *Acta Psychiatrica Scandinavica*, **79**, 268–275.

Dowrick, C. & Buchan, I. (1995) Twelve month outcome of depression in general practice: does detection or disclosure make any difference. *BMJ*, **311**, 1274–1276.

Dowrick, C., Gask, L., Perry, R., *et al* (2000*a*) Do general practitioners' attitudes towards depression predict their clinical behaviour? *Psychological Medicine*, **30**, 413–419.

Dowrick, C., Dunn, G., Ayuso-Mateos, J. L., *et al* (2000*b*) Problem solving treatment and group psychoeducation for depression: multicentre randomised controlled trial. Outcomes of Depression International Network (ODIN) Group. *BMJ*, **321**, 1450–1454.

Dowrick, C. F., Ring, A., Humphris, G. M., *et al* (2004) Normalisation of unexplained symptoms by general practitioners: a functional typology. *British Journal of General Practice*, **54**, 165–170.

Eisenberg, L. (1986) Mindlessness and brainlessness in psychiatry. *British Journal of Psychiatry*, **148**, 497–508.

Fink, P., Sorensen, L., Engberg, M., *et al* (1999) Somatisation in primary care. Prevalence, health care utilization, and general practitioner recognition. *Psychosomatics*, **40**, 330–338.

Fleming, D. M. & Cross, K. W. (1984) Psychotropic drug prescribing. *Journal of the Royal College of General Practitioners*, **34**, 216–220.

Foreman, D. M., Foreman, D. & Minty, E. B. (2003) How should we measure social disadvantage in clinic settings. *European Child and Adolescent Psychiatry*, **12**, 308–312.

Freeling, P. (1993) Diagnosis and treatment of depression in general practice. *British Journal of Psychiatry*, **163**, suppl. 20, 14–19.

Gask, L., Sibbald, B. & Creed, F. (1997) Evaluating models of working to the interface between mental health services and primary care. *British Journal of Psychiatry*, **170**, 6–11.

Gask, L., Rogers, A., Oliver, D., *et al* (2003) Qualitative study of patients' perceptions of the quality of care for depression in general practice. *British Journal of General Practice*, **53**, 278–283.

Gilbody, S. M., House, A. O. & Sheldon, T. A. (2001) Routinely administered questionnaires for depression and anxiety: systematic review. *BMJ*, **322**, 406–409.

Glover, G. R. (2003) Money for mental health care 2003/4. *Psychiatric Bulletin*, **27**, 126–130.

Goldberg, D. & Blackwell, B. (1970) Psychiatric illness in general practice. A detailed study using a new method of case identification. *BMJ*, *ii*, 439–443.

Goldberg, D. & Huxley, P. (1980) *Mental Illness in the Community. The Pathway to Psychiatric Care*. London: Tavistock.

Goldberg, D. & Huxley, P. (1992) *Common Mental Disorders – A Biosocial Model*. London: Routledge.

Goldberg, D., Cooper, B., Eastwood, M. R., *et al* (1970) A standardised interview useful for use in community surveys. *British Journal of Preventative Social Medicine*, **24**, 18–20.

Goldthorpe, J. & Hope, K. (1974) *The Social Grading of Occupations: A New Approach and Scale*. London: Oxford University Press.

Gorst-Unsworth, C. & Goldenberg, E. (1998) Psychological sequelae of torture and organised violence suffered by refugees from Iraq. Trauma related factors compared with social factors in exile. *British Journal of Psychiatry*, **172**, 90–94.

Hart, J. T. (1971) The inverse care law. *Lancet*, *i*, 405–412.

Hawton, K., Clements, A., Sakarovitch, C., *et al* (2001) Suicide in doctors: a study of risk according to gender, seniority and specialty in medical practitioners in England and Wales, 1979–1995. *Journal of Epidemiology and Community Health*, **55**, 296–300.

Hawton, K., Malmberg, A. & Simkin, S. (2004) Suicide in doctors. A psychological autopsy study. *Journal of Psychosomatic Research*, **57**, 1–4.

Heath, T., Jefferies, R. & Pearce, S. (2006) *Asylum Statistics United Kingdom 2005*. London: Home Office.

Hermann, R. C., Yang, D., Eltner, S. L., *et al* (2002) Prescription of antipsychotic drugs by office based physicians in the USA 1989–97. *Psychiatric Services*, **53**, 425–430.

HMSO (1986) *Morbidity Statistics from General Practice*. London: Her Majesty's Stationery Office.

Hodges, B., Inch, C. & Silver, I. (2001) Improving the psychiatric knowledge, skills and attitudes of primary care physicians 1950–2000: a review. *American Journal of Psychiatry*, **158**, 1579–1586.

Hofstede, G. (1980) *Cultural Consequences*. Beverly Hills, CA: Sage.

Holden, J. M., Sagovsky, R. & Cox, J. L. (1989) Counselling in a general practice setting, controlled study of health visitor intervention in treatment of postnatal depression. *BMJ*, **298**, 223–226.

Hull, S. A., Cornwell, J., Harvey, C., *et al* (2001) Prescribing rates for psychotropic medication amongst east London general practices: low rates where Asian populations are greatest. *Family Practice*, **18**, 167–173.

Hull, S. A., Jones, C. L, Tissier, J. M., *et al* (2002) Relationship style between GPs and community mental health teams affects referral rates. *British Journal of General Practice*, **52**, 101–107.

Irwin, W. G. & Cupples, M. E. (1986) A survey of psychotropic drug prescribing. *Journal of the Royal College of General Practitioners*, **36**, 366–368.

Isacsson, G., Boethims, G., Hendrikson, S., *et al* (1999) Selective serotonin reuptake inhibitors have broadened the utilisation of antidepressant treatment in accordance with recommendations. *Journal of Affective Disorders*, **53**, 15–22.

Iversen, V. C. & Morken, G. (2003) Acute admissions among immigrants and asylum seekers to a psychiatric hospital in Norway. *Social Psychiatry and Psychiatric Epidemiology*, **38**, 515–519.

Iversen, V. C. & Morken, G. (2004) Differences in acute psychiatric admissions between asylum seekers and refugees. *Nordic Journal of Psychiatry*, **58**, 465–470.

Jacob, K. S., Bhugra, D. & Mann, A. H. (2002) A randomised controlled trial of an educational intervention for depression among Asian women in primary care in the United Kingdom. *International Journal of Social Psychiatry*, **48**, 139–148.

Jarman, B. (1983) Identification of underprivileged areas. *BMJ*, **286**, 1705–1709.

Jaye, C. & Tilyard, M. (2002) A qualitative comparative investigation of variation in general practitioners prescribing patterns. *British Journal of General Practice*, **52**, 381–386.

Joukamaa, M., Sohlman, B. & Lehtinen, V. (1995) The prescription of psychotropic drugs in primary health care. *Acta Psychiatrica Scandinavica*, **92**, 359–364.

Kai, J., Crosland, A. & Drinkwater, C. (2000) Prevalence of enduring and disabling mental illness in the inner city. *British Journal of General Practice*, **50**, 988–994.

Kaye, J. A., Bradbury, B. D. & Jick, H. (2003) Changes in antipsychotic drug prescribing by general practitioners in the United Kingdom from 1991 to 2000: a population-based observational study. *British Journal of Clinical Pharmacology*, **56**, 569–575.

Kendrick, T., Stevens, L., Bryant, A., *et al* (2001) Hampshire Depression Project: changes in the process of care and cost consequences. *British Journal of General Practice*, **51**, 911–913.

Kessler, R., House, J. & Turner, J. (1987) Unemployment and health in a community sample. *Journal of Family Practice*, **16**, 319–324.

Kessler, D., Bennewith, O., Lewis, G., *et al* (2002) Detection of depression and anxiety in primary care: follow up study. *BMJ*, **325**, 1016–1017.

King, M., Davidson, O., Taylor, F., *et al* (2002) Effectiveness of teaching general practitioners skills in brief cognitive behaviour therapy to treat patients with depression: randomised controlled trial. *BMJ*, **324**, 947–950.

Kingdon, D. (2002) The mental health practitioner – bypassing the recruitment bottleneck. *Psychiatric Bulletin*, **26**, 328–331.

Kisely, S., Linden, M., Bellantuono, C., *et al* (2000) Why are patients prescribed psychotropic drugs by general practitioners? Results of an international study. *Psychological Medicine*, **30**, 1217–1225.

Laban, C. J., Gernaat, H. B., Komproe, I. H., *et al* (2004) Impact of a long term asylum procedure on the prevalence of psychiatric disorders in Iraqi asylum seekers in the Netherlands. *Journal of Nervous and Mental Diseases*, **192**, 843–851.

Lawrence, C. (2004) Mental illness in detained asylum seekers. *Lancet*, **364**, 1283–1284.

Lawrenson, R. A., Tyrer, F., Newson, R. B., *et al* (2000) The treatment of depression in UK general practice: selective serotonin reuptake inhibitors and tricyclic antidepressants compared. *Journal of Affective Disorders*, **59**, 149–157.

Lester, H., Allan, T., Wilson, S., *et al* (2003) A cluster randomised controlled trial of patient-held medical records for people with schizophrenia receiving shared care. *British Journal of General Practice*, **53**, 197–203.

Loudon, I. S. L. (1983) James McKenzie lecture. The origin of the general practitioner. *Journal of the Royal College of General Practitioners*, **33**, 13–18.

MacDonald, M. (1989) Psychiatric disorders in early modern England. In *The Scope of Epidemiological Psychiatry* (eds P. Williams, G. Wilkinson & K. Rawnsley), pp. 145–147. London: Routledge.

Maginn, S., Boardman, A. P., Craig, T. K., *et al* (2004) The detection of psychological problems by general practitioners: influence of ethnicity and other demographic variables. *Social Psychiatry and Psychiatric Epidemiology*, **39**, 464–471.

Mann, A., Jenkins, R. & Belsey, E. (1981) The 12-month outcome of patients with neurotic illness in general practice. *Psychological Medicine*, **11**, 535–550.

Marinker, M. (1988) The referral system. *Journal of the Royal College of General Practitioners*, **38**, 487–491.

Melzer, D., Hale, A. S., Malik, S. J., *et al* (1991) Community care for patients with schizophrenia one year after hospital discharge. *BMJ*, **303**, 1023–1026.

Melzer, D., Fryers, T. & Jenkins, R. (2003) *Social Inequalities and the Distribution of the Common Mental Disorders*. Maudsley Monograph No. 44. Hove: Psychology Press.

Merrill, J. & Owens, J. (1986) Ethnic differences in self-poisoning: a comparison of Asian and white groups. *British Journal of Psychiatry*, **148**, 708–712.

Middleton, N., Gunnell, D., Whitley, E., *et al* (2001) Secular trends in antidepressant prescribing in the UK, 1975–1998. *Journal of Public Health Medicine*, **23**, 262–267.

Millar, T. & Goldberg, D. P. (1991) Link between the ability to detect and manage emotional disorders: a study of general practitioner trainees. *British Journal of General Practice*, **41**, 357–359.

Modood, T. (2005) Ethnicity and intergenerational identities and adaption in Britain. The sociopolitical context. In *Ethnicity and Causal Mechanisms* (eds M. Rutter & M. Tieda), pp. 281–300. Cambridge: Cambridge University Press.

Moser, K. (2001) Inequalities in treated heart disease and mental illness in England and Wales, 1994–1998. *British Journal of General Practice*, **51**, 438–444.

Murray, C. & Lopez, A. D. (1996) *The Global Burden of Disease*. Boston, MA: Harvard School of Public Health.

Murray, R. M. (1976) Alcoholism amongst male doctors in Scotland. *Lancet*, *ii*, 729–733.

Nandhra, H., Murray, G., Hymas, N., *et al* (2004) Medical records: doctors and patients' experiences of copying letters to patients. *Psychiatric Bulletin*, **28**, 40–42.

National Institute for Health and Clinical Excellence (2004) *Management of Depression in Primary and Secondary Care*. Clinical Guideline 23. London: NICE.

Nazareth, I., King, M., Haines, A., *et al* (1993) Care of schizophrenia in general practice. *BMJ*, **307**, 910–911.

Nazroo, J. Y. (1997) *Ethnicity and Mental Health Findings from a National Community Survey*. PSI report no. 842. London: Policy Studies Institute.

Nielsen, J. M., Vedstel, P. & Olesen, F. (2002) The postgraduate training of general practitioners in communication and counselling. A questionnaire survey in the County of Aarhus. *Ugeskr Laeger*, **164**, 895–899.

Ormel, J. & Giel, R. (1990) Medical effects of non-recognition of affective disorders in primary care. In *Psychological Disorders in General Medical Settings* (eds N. Sartorius, D. Goldberg, G. de Girolamo, *et al*). Bern: Huber, Hogrefe.

Ornstein, S., Stuart, G. & Jenkins, R. (2000) Depression diagnoses and antidepressant use in primary care practices: a study from the Practice Partner Research Network (PPRNet). *Journal of Family Practice*, **49**, 68–72.

Ostler, K., Thompson, C., Kinmonth, A. L., *et al* (2001) Influence of socio-economic deprivation on the prevalence and outcome of depression in primary care: the Hampshire Depression Project. *British Journal of Psychiatry*, **178**, 12–17.

Page, J. & Valentine, M. (2003) Psychiatry attribute guide. In *SHO Report for General Practice*, p. 25. Joint Committee on Postgraduate Training for General Practice. See http://www.pgmd.man.ac.uk/genprac/Docs/Attribute%20Guide.doc. Last accessed 10 October 2006.

Parish, P. A. (1971) The prescribing of psychotropic drugs in general practice. *Journal of the Royal College of General Practitioners*, **21**, suppl. 4, 1–77.

Paykel, E. S., Abbott, R., Jenkins, R., *et al* (2000) Urban–rural mental health differences in Great Britain: findings from the national morbidity survey. *Psychological Medicine*, **30**, 269–280.

Pedersen, P. B. (1997) *Culture Centred Counselling Intervention*. London: Sage.

Peltzer, K. (1995) *Psychology and Health in African Cultures*. Frankfurt: IKO – Verlag fur InterKuthrelle Komunication.

Pevalin, D. J. & Goldberg, D. P. (2003) Social precursors to onset and recovery from episodes of common mental illness. *Psychological Medicine*, **33**, 299–306.

Pogue, L. (2003) Working as a GP with a special interest in mental health. *BMJ*, **327**, 33–35.

Pollock, K. & Grime, J. (2002) Patients' perceptions of entitlement to time in general practice consultations for depression: qualitative study. *BMJ*, **325**, 687.

Porter, M. & Haslam, N. (2005) Pre-displacement and post-displacement factors associated with the mental health of refugees and internally displaced persons: a meta-analysis. *JAMA*, **294**, 602–612.

Proudfoot, J., Ryden, C., Everitt, B., *et al* (2004) Clinical efficacy of computerised cognitive–behavioural therapy for anxiety and depression in primary care: randomised controlled trial. *British Journal of Psychiatry*, **185**, 46–54.

Prudo, R., Harris, T. & Brown, G. W. (1984) Psychiatric disorders in a rural and in an urban population: 3. Social integration and the morphology of affective disorder. *Psychological Medicine*, **14**, 327–364.

Pullen, I. & Yellowlees, A. (1985) Is communication improving between general practitioners and psychiatrists? *BMJ*, **290**, 31–33.

Radcliffe, J., Gask, L., Creed, F., *et al* (1999) Psychiatric training for family doctors: what do GP registrars want and can a brief course provide this? *Medical Education*, **33**, 434–438.

Raine, R., Lewis, L., Sensky, T., *et al* (2000) Patient determinants of mental health interventions in primary care. *British Journal of General Practice*, **50**, 620–625.

Rait, G. (1999) Counting heads may mask cultural and social factors. *BMJ*, **318**, 305–306.

Rifiro, G., Spine, E., Brignoli, O., *et al* (2005) Antipsychotic prescribing patterns among Italian general practitioners. *European Journal of Psychopharmacology*, **61**, 47–53.

Rosendal, M., Bro, F., Fink, P., *et al* (2003) Diagnosis of somatisation: effect of an educational intervention in a cluster randomised controlled trial. *British Journal of General Practice*, **53**, 917–922.

Rowland, N., Bower, P., Mellor, C., *et al* (2001) Counselling for depression in primary care. *Cochrane Database of Systematic Reviews*, **(1)**, CD001025.

Rutter, M. & Tienda, M. (2005) *Ethnicity and Causal Mechanisms*. Cambridge: Cambridge University Press.

Rutz, W. (2001) Preventing suicide and premature death by education and treatment. *Journal of Affective Disorders*, **62**, 123–129.

Rutz, W., Walinder, J., Eberhard, G., *et al* (1989) An educational programme on depressive disorders for general practitioners. *Acta Psychiatrica Scandinavica*, **79**, 19–26.

Rutz, W., Knorring, V. L., Walinder, J., *et al* (1992) Long term effects of an educational program for general practitioners given by the Swedish Committee for the Prevention and Treatment of Depression. *Acta Psychiatrica Scandinavica*, **85**, 83–88.

Salmon, P., Dowrick, C. F., Ring, A., *et al* (2004) Voiced but unheard agendas: qualitative analysis of the psychosocial cues that patients with unexplained symptoms present to general practitioners. *British Journal of General Practice*, **54**, 171–176.

Schilte, A. F., Portegijs, P. J., Blankenstein, A. H., *et al* (2001) Randomised controlled trial of disclosure of emotionally important events in somatisation in primary care. *BMJ*, **323**, 86.

Seivewright, H., Tyrer, P., Casey, P., *et al* (1991) A three year follow up of psychiatric morbidity in urban and rural primary care. *Psychological Medicine*, **21**, 495–504.

Shah, A. (2003) Ethnicity and the common mental disorders. In *Social Inequalities and the Distribution of the Common Mental Disorders*, Maudsley Monograph No. 44 (eds D. Melzer, T. Fryers & R. Jenkins), pp. 171–224. Hove: Psychology Press.

Sharp, D. J. & King, M. B. (1989) Classification of psychosocial disturbance in general practice. *Journal of the Royal College of General Practitioners*, **39**, 356–358.

Shaw, C. M., Creed, F., Tominson, B., *et al* (1999) Prevalence of anxiety and depressive illness and help-seeking behaviour in African Caribbeans and white Europeans: two-phase general population survey. *BMJ*, **318**, 302–306.

Shepherd, M., Cooper, A. B., Brown, A. C., *et al* (1966) *Psychiatric Illness in General Practice*. Oxford: Oxford University Press.

Shiels, C., Gabbay, M. B., Ford, F. M. (2004) Patient factors associated with duration of certified sickness absence and transition to long-term incapacity. *British Journal of General Practice*, **54**, 86–91.

Simon, G. E., VonKorff, M., Rutter, C., *et al* (2000) Randomised trial of monitoring, feedback, and management of care by telephone to improve treatment of depression in primary care. *BMJ*, **320**, 550–554.

Simpson, S., Corney, R., Fitzgerald, P., *et al* (2003) A randomized controlled trial to evaluate the effectiveness and cost-effectiveness of psychodynamic counselling for general practice patients with chronic depression. *Psychological Medicine*, **33**, 229–239.

Sireling, L. I., Paykel, E. S., Freeling, P., *et al* (1985) Depression in general practice: case thresholds and diagnoses. *British Journal of Psychiatry*, **147**, 113–119.

Smith, P., Sheldon, T. A. & Martin, S. (1996) An index of needs for psychiatric services based on inpatient utilisation. *British Journal of Psychiatry*, **169**, 308–316.

Soni Raleigh, V., Bulusul, L. & Balarajan, R. (1990) Suicides among immigrants from the Indian sub-continent. *British Journal of Psychiatry*, **156**, 46–50.

Soykan, A. & Oncu, B. (2003) Which GP deals better with depressed patients in primary care in Kapstamonu, Turkey: the impacts of 'interest in psychiatry' and continuing medical education. *Family Practitioner*, **20**, 558–562.

Stanistreet, D., Gabbay, M. B., Jeffrey, V., *et al* (2004) The role of primary care in the prevention of suicide and accidental deaths among young men: an epidemiological study. *British Journal of General Practice*, **54**, 254–258.

Sternhammer, E. S. & Colditz, G. A. (2004) Suicide rates among physicians. A quantitative and gender assessment (meta-analysis). *American Journal of Psychiatry*, **161**, 2295–2302.

Stirling, A. M., Wilson, P. & McConnachie, A. (2001) Deprivation, psychological distress, and consultation length in general practice. *British Journal of General Practice*, **51**, 456–460.

Surtees, P. G., Dean, E., Ingham, J. G., *et al* (1983) Psychiatric disorders in women from an Edinburgh community association with demographic factors. *British Journal of Psychiatry*, **142**, 238–246.

Tabassum, R., Macaskill, A. & Ahmad, I. (2000) Attitudes towards mental health in an urban Pakistani community in the United Kingdom. *International Journal of Social Psychiatry*, **46**, 170–181.

Tennant, C., Bebbington, P. & Hurry, J. (1981) The short term outcome of neurotic disorders in the community. The relation of remission to clinical factors and to neutralising events. *British Journal of Psychiatry*, **139**, 213–220.

Thompson, C., Kinmonth, A. L., Stevens, L., *et al* (2000) Effects of a clinical-practice guideline and practice-based education on detection and outcome of depression in primary care: Hampshire Depression Project randomised controlled trial. *Lancet*, 355, 185–191.

Thompson, C., Ostler, K., Peveler, R. C., *et al* (2001) Dimensional perspective on the recognition of depressive symptoms in primary care: the Hampshire Depression Project 3. *British Journal of Psychiatry*, **179**, 317–323.

Tiemens, B. G., Ormel, J., Jenner, J. A., *et al* (1999) Training primary care physicians to recognize, diagnose and manage depression: does it improve patient outcomes? *Psychological Medicine*, **29**, 833–845.

Townsend, P. (1987) *The Intentional Analysis of Poverty*. New York: Harvester Wheatsheaf.

Trethowan, W. H. (1975) Pills for personal problems. *BMJ*, *iii*, 749–751.

Tribe, R. (2002) Mental health of refugees and asylum seekers. *Advances in Psychiatric Treatment*, **8**, 240–248.

Van Leeuwen, Y. D., Mol, S. S., Pollemans, M. C., *et al* (1995) Change in knowledge of general practitioners during their professional careers. *Family Practitioner*, **12**, 313–317.

Varnam, M. (1981) Psychotropic prescribing. What am I doing? *Journal of the Royal College of General Practitioners*, **31**, 480–483.

Vazquez-Barquero, J. L., Diez-Manrique, J. F., Saite, L., *et al* (1992) Why people with probable minor psychiatric morbidity consult a doctor. *Psychological Medicine*, **22**, 495–502.

Voshaar, R. C., Gorgels, W. J., Mol, A. J., *et al* (2003) Tapering off long-term benzodiazepine use with or without group cognitive–behavioural therapy: three-condition, randomised controlled trial. *British Journal of Psychiatry*, **182**, 498–504.

Wagner, H. R., Burns, B. J., Broadhead, W. E., *et al* (2000) Minor depression in family practice: functional morbidity, co-morbidity, service utilization and outcomes. *Psychological Medicine*, **30**, 1377–1390.

Ward, E., King, M., Lloyd, M., *et al* (2000) Randomised controlled trial of non-directive counselling, cognitive–behaviour therapy, and usual general practitioner care for patients with depression. I: Clinical effectiveness. *BMJ*, **321**, 1383–1388.

Weich, S., Sloggett, A. & Lewis, G. (2001) Social roles and the gender difference in rates of the common mental disorders in Britain: a 7-year, population-based cohort study. *Psychological Medicine*, **31**, 1055–1064.

Whitehouse, C. R. (1987) A survey of the management of psychosocial illness in general practice in Manchester. *Journal of the Royal College of General Practitioners*, **37**, 112–115.

Wilkinson, G., Allen, P., Marshall, E., *et al* (1993) The role of the practice nurse in the management of depression in general practice: treatment adherence to antidepressant medication. *Psychological Medicine*, **23**, 229–237.

Williams, P. (1979) The extent of psychotropic drug prescribing. In *Psychosocial Disorders in General Practice* (eds P. Williams & A. Clare), pp. 151–160. London: Academic Press.

Williams, P. & Wallace, B. B. (1974) General practitioners and psychiatrists – do they communicate? *BMJ*, *i*, 505–507.

Williams, P., Tarnopolsky, A., Hand, D., *et al* (1986) Minor psychiatric morbidity and general practice consultations: the West London Survey. *Psychological Medicine Monograph Supplements*, **9**.

Wilson, M. & Macarthy, B. (1994) GP consultation as a factor in the lower rate of mental health service use by Asians. *Psychological Medicine*, **24**, 113–119.

World Health Organization (1992) *The Tenth Revision of the International Classification of Diseases and Related Health Problems* (ICD–10). Geneva: WHO.

World Health Organization (1996) *Diagnostic and Management Guidelines for Mental Health Disorders in Primary Care*. Bern: Hogrefe & Huber.

Wright, A. F. (1990) A study of the presentation of somatic symptoms in general practice by patients with psychiatric disturbance. *British Journal of General Practice*, **40**, 459–463.

Wynter, A. (1875) The role of the general practitioner. In *The Borderlands of Insanity*. London: Robert Hardwicke.

Zitman, F. G. & Couvee, J. E. (2001) Chronic benzodiazepine use in general practice patients with depression: an evaluation of controlled treatment and taper-off: report on behalf of the Dutch Chronic Benzodiazepine Working Group. *British Journal of Psychiatry*, **178**, 317–324.

CHAPTER 31

Cultural and international psychiatry

Vikram Patel and George Stein

Emil Kraepelin in his memoirs, describing his combined holiday and working trip to Java, in 1904 wrote:

> 'I was impressed by the coral banks of Point de Galle, the rain forest of the Pangerango and the landscape of the Serangoon. I also learned important new facts for my own field of interest. For example it was true that in spite of the high frequency of syphilis in the native patients at the asylum at Buitenzorg, paralysis was extraordinary seldom; I was not able to identify a single case amongst several hundred syphilitic patients.... A hasty examination also showed that most of the patients had dementia praecox to a greater extent than in Germany and that therefore race, climate and living conditions had no decisive influence on the origin of this disease. Furthermore I was able to make a number of observations on the special symptoms of well-known European diseases in the Javanese patients and this seemed to be very important for an understanding of the type of connection between the type of race and the mental disorder. There were no distinct melancholic states among the natives, nor suicides, so facilities similar to those in our clinics to supervise the patients were completely superfluous here. The auditory hallucinations in cases of dementia praecox are considered unimportant, probably because language and speech only have a lesser influence on the thinking process in Java. Delusions were also remarkably scarce. From these and other experiences, I became convinced that my attempt to prepare the way for a comparative psychiatry could be successful and intended to follow up these ideas as soon as possible.' (See Hippius *et al*, 1987, pp. 115–116)

If we assume that culture plays any role in psychiatric disorders, then, by definition, virtually the entire body of psychiatric knowledge *is* cultural psychiatry, with cultural factors assuming a variable degree of importance for all psychiatric disorders. The study of cultural influences on psychiatry has to a large extent been conducted from the platform of Western biomedicine, mainly because psychiatry as a discipline developed entirely in Western Europe and North America and cross-cultural psychiatry in its early years tended to focus on how people from cultures other than the Anglo-American experienced mental illnesses. At the root of this academic discipline, therefore, is the assumption that psychiatric syndromes and disorders as described in Western literature, especially in the postwar years, form the basis of a universal categorisation of mental illness. These formulations have been helpful in the comparative study of the major psychoses but have had rather less meaning in the study of the common mental disorders (CMDs) or neurotic disorders, where cultural influences may be paramount.

Psychiatry has its roots in Western medicine and this is a largely biological and scientific discipline, reflecting Western culture and values. Psychiatry was then exported to the rest of the world, largely as a result of colonisation. Thus, the early study of the influence of culture on psychiatry was based on the belief that any variations in clinical presentation found in other cultures were to be interpreted in the light of cultural differences, the 'gold standard' being the universal disease category invented in the West. However, in reality, even today, for most diagnostic categories (particularly those in the neurotic realm), which have been almost reified in various classification systems, the syndromal description does not go beyond the subjective experiences of individual patients, and these almost by definition will largely be influenced by culture.

Definitions and terms

Classifications of people

Cultural psychiatry simply signifies the study of psychiatric disorders in different 'cultures'. One major problem with this discipline has been coming to terms with exactly what 'culture' itself means. Several definitions are available. The ninth edition of the *Concise Oxford Dictionary*, for example, defines culture as 'the customs, civilization and achievements of a particular time or people', but such a definition is too brief to be helpful in the study of cross-cultural psychiatry. A more comprehensive definition is provided by Prince *et al* (1998):

> 'Culture is the totality of habits, ideas, beliefs, attitudes and values, as well as the behaviors that spring from them (language, art, marriage patterns, eating habits and so forth). Ashanti's, Germans, Koreans, and Crees feel, think, and act differently: culture accounts for a good deal of the variance.'

The same concept expressed more briefly, again by Prince *et al* (1998), is that:

> 'culture is the blueprint-for-living that is non-genetically transmitted from one generation to another.'

Murphy (1982) also highlights this aspect and states that culture for the social scientist comprises values, habits and other patterns of behaviour that a human

Table 31.1 Race, culture and ethnicity

Term	Characterised by	Determined by	Perceived as
Race	Physical appearance	Genetic ancestry	Permanent (genetic/biological)
Culture	Behaviour, attitudes	Upbringing, choice	Changeable (assimilation, acculturation)
Ethnicity	Sense of belonging, group identity	Social pressures, psychological need	Partially changeable

Source: Fernando (1991).

group consciously or unconsciously transmits from one generation to another and hence regards as traditional and worthy of reproduction.

As may be evident even without a clear definition, culture is a dynamic construct, particularly in a globalising world where all cultures are being shaped by powerful influences from other cultures. Furthermore, with the advent of major migrations of peoples from one nation to another, the cultures of both host and migrant communities are undergoing rapid and irrevocable change (take, for example, the recent acceptance of Indian food as part of British culture, or the adoption of English dress styles by Indian migrants to the UK).

In the face of the ever-changing nature of culture, alternative terms such as 'race' and 'ethnicity' have been used to define subgroups of human beings (Table 31.1). Race is, essentially, a descriptive term by which people are grouped according to how they look to the observer, based on predefined physical characteristics of presumed genetic or biological origin. Studies of the racial distribution of mental disorder should be interpreted with caution, since huge social and economic differences may explain much more of the differences in prevalence than minor genetic or cultural effects. For example, high rates of alcohol misuse are more commonly reported among 'Black' people in North America, but the bulk of the variance of these findings can be attributed to socio-economic differences between Blacks and Whites in America.

The concept of ethnicity is held to be politically more correct. This term is used to describe a group of people who share a common identity (i.e. how they describe their origins), a common ancestry (both historically and geographically) and, to some extent, shared beliefs and history. This term, however, does not describe either a single type of people or a single nation. Thus, people from the Indian subcontinent living in the UK may be defined as 'ethnic Asians', but this does not capture the fact that this apparently homogeneous ethnic grouping is at least as internally diverse as an ethnic grouping of 'European'. The term 'ethnicity' is none the less arguably the most useful term to describe subgroups of people and is routinely ascertained in the collection of national statistics such as the census and is also used in the study of the epidemiology of diseases.

Terms for the academic discipline

A number of different terms have been used to describe the study and practice of psychiatry in different cultures. The word 'trans' means 'across' but the term 'transcultural psychiatry' is possibly the least appropriate because of other connotations of the prefix 'trans', which occurs in words like transcendental, with its connotations of magic, or 'transcend', which gives the impression of going over a limit (Prince *et al*, 1998). 'Ethnopsychiatry' has limited appeal, too, because it originates from the curious anthropological interest emanating from Western universities for studying exotic cultures elsewhere.

Cultural psychiatry is, perhaps, the most appropriate term of all, originating from Wittkower's definition:

> 'that [which concerns] itself with the mentally ill in relation to their cultural environment within the context of a given cultural unit.' (Quoted by Prince *et al*, 1998)

The strength of this definition lies in its implication that all psychiatry becomes cultural psychiatry. Murphy (1982) proposed the term 'comparative psychiatry', by which he meant:

> 'the study of the relations between mental disorder and the psychological characteristics which differentiate people, nations, or cultures. Its main goals are to identify, verify, and explain the links between mental disorder and these broad psychosocial characteristics.' (Murphy, 1982)

This term seems to have gradually disappeared from contemporary psychiatry but remains a useful concept because it does not seek to define the comparative groups only along the lines of a preset criterion such as culture. In this sense, this term comes closest to the concept of an international psychiatry, as described later in this chapter.

The value of cultural psychiatry

Okpaku (1998, p. 12) lists four reasons why the study of psychiatric disorders across cultures is of value:

1. Such study can help inform clinical practice in different cultures, for example by providing guidelines on diagnosis and management that are valid for a particular local culture.
2. It can help the growth of academic psychiatry, by providing information on the validity of classification systems, so that these evolve into truly international systems.
3. There may be particular therapeutic factors that operate in one culture but that may be applicable in a much wider context.
4. Because all psychiatric disorders are multi-factorial in aetiology, the study of disorders in different settings can help elucidate their precise cause.

Studies in cultural psychiatry may compare the prevalence of disorders between several countries, as was done in the International Pilot Study of Schizophrenia (which is discussed below). High rates of immigration in recent years have meant that most countries have substantial ethnic minorities and enjoy a variety of different cultures; this has led to studies of the varied pattern of psychiatric morbidity found between the different ethnic groups within one country. Cross-cultural studies on the variation of mental disorders among ethnic groups in the UK are dealt with in Chapter 30, on pages 760–765. These studies form the basis of our knowledge of cultural psychiatry, a topic that has generated much armchair speculative theorising but rather less in the way of a core of factual knowledge and agreed general principles. Therefore, to acquaint the reader with some of the basic building blocks that comprise this topic, a few selected studies, from different parts of the world, some classical, some modern, have been described in a little more detail in this chapter.

The evolution of the discipline

The chequered history of this discipline has been well described by other authors, notably Murphy's (1982) classic text on comparative psychiatry and more recently Okpaku (1998), from which the account below is drawn.

The view that psychiatric phenomena can vary from one culture to another has existed for more than 200 years, having first appeared at around the same time as the general acceptance that abnormal behaviour can be caused by an illness (as opposed to, for example, evil spirits). In keeping with this change in belief systems in the Western world, the doctors who treated mental disorders considered one of the causes to be the higher level of intellectual attainment of civilisation in Western societies. Thus, Sir Andrew Halliday, writing in a 1820s survey of British mental hospitals, referred to 'the rarity of insanity among savage tribes of men, the contented peasantry of the Welsh mountains and those dwelling in the wilds of Ireland', and in another report wrote 'not one of our African travelers remark their having seen a single madman' (see Prince *et al*, 1998, p. 3). White psychiatrists thought that certain mental disorders were rare in Africans because their brains were considered too primitive to experience sophisticated emotional states (e.g. Le Roux, 1973). Much of the literature of the colonial era is replete with the use of words such as 'primitive' and 'savages', as well as being tainted by more insidious racism.

Political ideals sometimes also influenced the debate on causation. Thus, Benjamin Rush, an American psychiatrist who was also a fervent republican at the time of the American War of Independence, claimed that participation in the American revolution cured women of hysteria, whereas supporting the British crown encouraged hypochondriasis and the development of an illness known as 'protection fever'.

A more clinical approach starts with the study of T. D. Greenlees (1895), who observed a very high rate of mania over melancholia in the Grahamstown asylum in South Africa (there were 221 cases of mania but only 31 cases of melancholia). He wrote:

> 'Melancholia is rare among the natives and I have never found it as acute as among the white patients, while general paralysis among the pure uncontaminated native is not known.'

The introduction of a scientific quality to the investigations of comparative psychiatry can be attributed to Kraepelin. Kraepelin made an important contribution to the evolution of the discipline during his study of patients in the Buitenzorg asylum (presently the State Hospital of Bogor, outside Jakarta) in Java in 1903. In a work-filled holiday of no more than 3 weeks he examined 225 cases: 100 European patients, 100 native Javanese and 25 ethnic Chinese. Among the local Javanese patients he found prevalence rates of 67% for schizophrenia, 7% for epilepsy and 4% for mania. Alcohol-related disorders and general paralysis of the insane (GPI) were rare among the native group, but in the European patients as many as 16% of the males had GPI. Manic depression was equally common among the Europeans and Javanese. Although dementia praecox (schizophrenia) appeared to be just as common among the Javanese and Europeans, Kraepelin wrote that it was less colourful among the native population, with less frequent catatonia and auditory hallucinations, while coherent delusional ideas were absent. Later in his life, in 1925, he embarked on a study comparing the Black American and native Indian populations in America, but unfortunately died before he could analyse the data that he had so assiduously collected.

Other psychiatrists in the Far East, such as Gillmore Ellis, the director of the Singapore asylum, wrote about amok, which he believed to be an epileptic type of condition, and he also described latah (see page 805). Kraepelin took the view that neither condition represented any new or special cultural type of disorder and that both could be accommodated within existing categories.

Psychoanalytic theories have contributed to the evolution of cultural psychiatry, with early analysts such as Geza Roheim looking to anthropology and its descriptions of the myths, rituals and behaviours of non-Western peoples for support for many of their psychoanalytic theories. However, with the more recent decline in the influence of psychoanalysis on psychiatry, these theories have more relevance in trying to understand how an individual perceives an illness within the cultural context rather than a broader understanding of the influence of culture on mental illness.

One psychoanalyst, E. D. Wittkower, who was a refugee from the Nazi persecution in Europe, made one of the most important contributions to the scientific study of cultural psychiatry. He fled to Canada in the 1930s and set up the first academic unit devoted to this field, at McGill University, in 1955. A year later he launched the first journal in the field, the *Transcultural Psychiatric Research Review*, which is still one of the leading journals in the field (now called *Transcultural Psychiatry*).

Important contributions from the psychoanalytic school have also come from a handful of non-European writers, notably S. Kakar, who has written extensively on the cultural applicability of psychoanalysis in the Indian context (Kakar, 1982).

A major historical step in the thinking and philosophy associated with cultural psychiatry was the work of the Leightons with the Navajo peoples of North America. The non-judgemental way in which they described and interpreted Navajo models of illness causation was a first step in the cleansing of the old colonial and racist influences on this field. Important contributions were also made by a growing band of psychiatrists from non-European cultures who were working in their own countries, such as T. A. Lambo from Nigeria, S. Morita in Japan (who described Morita therapy) and P. M. Yap in Hong Kong (who coined the phrase 'culture-bound syndrome').

Cross-national collaborations were best exemplified by the work by Leighton, Lambo and colleagues in their pioneering comparative studies of mental illness in the United States and Nigeria. With a multidisciplinary team of psychiatrists and social scientists, the researchers descended on villages in the study area in Nigeria, spending about a week in each village, collecting a variety of social, cultural and psychiatric data. Altogether 262 villagers, 64 urban residents and an assortment of others were interviewed. Symptoms and diagnoses were based on the 1952 version of the DSM and they used the same questionnaire they had used in the Stirling County study in the USA, with a few modifications to adapt it to the local culture. The study provided extensive information on symptoms, indigenous models and the prevalence of mental disorders (Leighton *et al*, 1963). They described the indigenous systems of classification of medicine, which they considered as an important taxonomy in its own right and not simply a 'primitive' precursor of a modern classification, a viewpoint that has found increasing favour in more recent cross-cultural studies.

A collection of essays describing various indigenous classification systems, *Magic, Faith, and Healing* (Kiev, 1964) was among the earlier classic texts of cultural psychiatry.

The 'etic' and 'emic' approaches to cross-cultural psychiatry

The 'etic' approach

Before the 1960s, cultural psychiatric studies generated much narrative and anecdotal data, but this was of limited usefulness. For example, diagnostic criteria were so poorly defined that what constituted a 'case' of a particular disorder varied from site to site. There were even wide variations in the diagnostic profiles of hospitalised patients between the apparently similar cultures of the UK and the USA (Cooper *et al*, 1972). These inconsistencies led to a movement to standardise the process of psychiatric measurement and diagnosis (as discussed in Chapter 28). After standardising the interview schedules in Euro-American cultures, they were used in cross-cultural psychiatric investigations in the 1960s and 1970s. These studies relied on a number of implicit, largely untested assumptions (Beiser *et al*, 1994):

1 the universality of mental illnesses, with the implication that, regardless of cultural variations, disorders as described in Euro-American classifications occur everywhere

2 invariance, that is, the assumption that the core features of psychiatric syndromes are invariant across cultures

3 validity, with the implication that although refinement is possible, the diagnostic categories of current classifications are valid clinical constructs.

This approach, termed the 'etic' or universalist approach, became the most popular method for investigations of mental illness across cultures.

The word 'etic' was originally derived from the word *phonetic*, with the underlying assumption that the basic patterns of causation are similar across cultures, and the role of culture is limited to facilitating or inhibiting the expression of the different types of psychiatric disorder.

The main criticism of the purely etic approach is that it risks confounding culturally distinctive behaviour, which may be quite normal, with psychopathology, because of superficial similarities. A further argument against the etic approach is that, because they largely reflected American and European concepts of psychopathology, the classifications of psychiatric disorders would inevitably be culturally biased towards European concepts of normality and deviance. Some have even gone so far as to suggest that cross-cultural psychiatry should examine the influence of culture on mental illness in Euro-American societies themselves, rather than assume that these illnesses are 'natural' and free of any cultural bias and that 'the study of cultural psychiatry should start at home' (Murphy, 1977). The etic approach also tends to 'privilege biology over culture' (Eisenbruch, 1991), in that it gives little weight to the cultural and social contexts of psychiatric disorders.

An example of an 'etic' study is that by Ormel *et al* (1994), of the impact of CMDs on functional disability in 14 different countries. This is described in Box 31.1.

Box 31.1 An example of a study using the etic approach to cultural psychiatric research

Ormel *et al* (1994) carried out a study of the effect of common mental disorders on functional disability in 14 countries. The study involved a two-stage case identification procedure using the General Health Questionnaire (GHQ) in the first stage and the Composite International Diagnostic Interview (CIDI) in the second. The study was a large multinational enterprise, involving more than 25 000 patients attending general healthcare settings. The article did little justice to the key issues of the translation of instruments, the validity of various cut-off scores of the GHQ, or the diagnostic validity of the categories generated by the CIDI. Also, although the authors stated that the study covered most 'major cultures and languages', more than half the study centres were in Europe or North America. Similarly, although there was considerable variation in the effect of psychiatric disorder on disability between centres (ranging from a mean of 2.5 disability-days in Verona, Italy, to 11.9 days in Bangalore, India, and Ibadan, Nigeria), the authors highlighted the consistency between centres in the univariate associations; thus, the study was unable to explain why being a psychiatric 'case' caused so much more disability in the Indian centre than in the Italian centre. However, the study is important in its demonstration of a strong association, even after adjustment for physical disorders, between common mental disorders and functional disability in all the study centres and indicates the huge economic and social burden that common mental disorders impose across the globe.

The 'emic' approach

The field of medical anthropology, a largely descriptive specialty, places its greatest emphasis on the individual's social and cultural environment. It has been one of the key factors fuelling the development of the 'emic' approach in cross-cultural psychiatry, particularly in low-income countries. The term 'emic' is derived from the word 'phonemic'. The emic approach is used to evaluate phenomena from within a culture and their context, aiming to understand their significance and relationship with other intra-cultural elements, with little or no referral to external criteria. At a general level, this approach argued that the culture-bound aspects of biomedicine, with its emphasis on medical disease entities, were just not universally applicable and it was wrong to presume *a priori* that Euro-American psychiatric categories were appropriate throughout the world (Helman, 1991).

Purely emic studies have also drawn their share of criticism, the most fundamental one being that they are unable to provide data that can be compared

Box 31.2 An example of a study using the emic approach to cultural psychiatric research

Skultans (1991), herself an anthropologist, examined the way patients with a mental illness were treated in the province of Maharashtra in India. For many centuries the temples in this region were run by the Mahanubhav sect, which was founded in the 13th century by Cakradhara, in opposition to the ritual authority of the Brahmins. There was a long tradition of welcoming the deprived members of society such as the untouchables, or women who had lost their role in society, as well as people who were mentally afflicted, with only the Brahmins being specifically excluded from the temple. Skultans conducted her study at the Mahanubhav temple at Phaltan, which had a particularly good reputation for treating those with a mental affliction. The temple functioned both as a religious sanctuary and an asylum. Most of the supplicants came for healing on a daily basis but a few (around 30) became residents and they were often accompanied by a relative who moved in with them.

Most of the supplicants were thought to be suffering from one of four conditions:

- *karani* (witchcraft), which was the result of human malevolence, almost always instigated by another family member and usually an in-law, and which was thought to be very difficult to cure
- *bhut bhada*, a type of spirit possession that usually came out of the blue, which was not thought to be due to human malevolence, and which had a better outcome than *karani* (usually taking about 5 weeks to resolve)
- *pida*, which was the result of undeserved and unsolicited victimisation by malevolent spiritual forces
- *ved*, which denotes 'obvious madness'.

There was no medical input and no biomedical diagnoses were made, but from the case material Skultans presents it seems that some of the residents had fairly severe chronic schizophrenia, while others had more short-lived psychiatric disorders or family problems and one or two had physical illness such as asthma or cancer. In some cases she did not make any medical or psychiatric diagnosis, implying they may not have been ill in the sense understood in biomedicine. However, all women received a temple diagnosis of 'madness'.

There is no symptom-based description of madness in Maharashtrian society but only a stereotyped picture of madness, consisting of three key behavioural elements which relate to family life:

- the tearing off of clothes,
- violence towards other family members
- a lack of attention and an irreverence towards the preparation and consumption of food.

These three elements are more severely condemned in women, who are supposed to be modest at all times, and such behaviour is seen as inviting sexual exploitation, and so causes maximal distress, particularly for the families of younger women.

Much of the women's social role concerns the presentation of food, and mental affliction in women in Maharashtrian society manifests itself as withdrawal of support and services to the family. Notably, the author found that the inferior position of a woman in Indian society and her precarious situation in her husband's family were exaggerated when she became mentally ill. Thus, one reason for a woman to seek help alone was the shame attached to her mental illness. Among men, the beating of wives and mothers, absconding, and physical destruction of the home were the main types of behaviours resulting in families bringing their ill members to the temple. Since all the supplicants were essentially being brought to the temple to heal a mental disorder, it was implicit that they were considered mentally ill by their families (the emic case criterion).

The temple kept a register for each supplicant, noting the date of arrival and the home village, the nature of the trouble, and diagnosis in terms of *karani, bhut bhada* or *pida* was made. Record keeping, even if very basic, appears to be a universal component of any mental health system.

Therapy took the form of prayer and the induction of trance states or *hajeri*. The monks of the temple usually organised the trance by setting the scene with ceremonial worship, and trancing rarely took place outside this religious setting. Sometimes the carers would try to induce trances in themselves to try to drive out the malevolent spirits from the supplicant towards themselves in the hope of obtaining a cure. Trancing was more common and more often successful among the women than the men, who were usually much more severely afflicted.

Skultans (1991) did not categorise the residents in terms of psychiatric diagnoses but more in sociological terms, for example as to whether they were accompanied or not. Those accompanying the supplicants were of great importance because they became the primary carers, involved in food purchase and preparation as well as the general care of the supplicant. Some of the women were unaccompanied and had to look after themselves; they were not so severely afflicted and were usually suffering from some 'personal problem'. Some stayed for a long time, probably those with schizophrenia, and one individual and his mother stayed for more than 10 years.

This 'emic' study is highly informative, yet contains no formal psychiatric diagnoses, no control group, no rating scales, small numbers and no statistical tests, yet it describes a centuries old civilised and humane way of caring for people who are mentally ill and which appears to owe almost nothing to modern Western psychiatry.

across cultures (Mari *et al*, 1989). Thus, some authors have adopted the attitude that each culture is unique and incomparable to any other ('cultural relativism'), which, in effect, undermines the very basis of any cross-cultural study. Emic studies are usually small in scale, and may not have any numerical data, as they are often being purely descriptive, and so are unable to resolve questions of the long-term course and treatment outcome of illness episodes. The reliability of emic studies is in doubt owing to the lack of standardisation of research methods and rigorous methodology. There is scope therefore for the interpretations of individual researchers to be biased. Advocates of the emic approach have also been criticised for not suggesting plausible alternatives, such as a set of principles that would help ensure cultural sensitivity, or models on which to fashion culturally sensitive nosologies (Beiser *et al*, 1994).

A good example of an emic study (Box 31.2) is that by Skultans (1991), who examined the relationship between mental illness and family structures in Maharashtra, India, while at the same time describing the traditional system of care offered by the temple authorities for people who are mentally ill.

The new cross-cultural psychiatry

The 'etic' versus 'emic' debate started with Arthur Kleinman's (1987) accusation that 'old' transcultural psychiatrists were intent on forcing Western psychiatric categories on to non-Western societies. Skultans (1991) doubted that it was possible for a psychiatrist to enter an alien culture without carrying his or her preconceived psychiatric formulations. In essence, the central aim of the 'new' cross-cultural psychiatry would be to describe mental illness in different cultures using methods that are sensitive and valid for the local culture but which result in data that are comparable across cultures. There are strengths and weaknesses to both the etic and emic approaches in cross-cultural psychiatry and it is increasingly accepted that there must be an integration of the two approaches for the development of the 'new cross-cultural psychiatry', that is, a culturally sensitive psychiatry. Value must be given to both folk beliefs about mental illness as well as to the biomedical system of psychiatry. Kleinman (1987) described the importance of assessing the patient's own 'explanatory models', that is, how patients understand their problems – their nature, origins, consequences and remedies – since these can greatly help patient–doctor negotiations in treatment.

Health service research

One of the key problems with most cross-cultural psychiatric research is that it is essentially an academic pursuit, whose primary goals, up till now, have been either to establish the burden of mental illnesses (the epidemiological approach) or to demonstrate the influence of some narrowly defined cultural variables, most often the individual's subjective beliefs, on mental illness (the ethnographic approach), neither of which has much relevance to the problems of running a health service in a developing country. A good example of this mismatch is the consistent finding that persons with schizophrenia have a better outcome in developing countries (see below), which is of academic interest in the theoretical study of the environmental influences on the outcome of schizophrenia, but which is of no practical benefit to the large number of patients in these developing countries who either receive no treatment or whose rights are regularly abused.

It is now increasingly apparent that neither culture nor biology is the only, or even the main, variable that distinguishes the pattern and outcome of psychiatric disorders between different regions of the world. War, ignorance, abject poverty, health resources, physical illness and epidemics probably play a far larger role than cultural belief systems in explaining the differences in psychiatric morbidity between the developed and developing world.

Health systems research (HSR) offers a pragmatic model for investigating mental health problems across the world, because of its recognition that mental illness and mental healthcare are profoundly influenced not only by culture or biology but also by the complex interaction of numerous factors – social, political, economic, historical and health service.

Two key features of HSR are:

1 its multidisciplinary nature, in that it incorporates epidemiology, clinical medicine of different specialties, social sciences, health policy and so on

2 its use of a problem-oriented approach, as opposed to complex classification systems heavily biased towards European and American nosologies.

Furthermore, the focus of the research is on locally generated priorities as opposed to the expensive multinational projects, which are generally funded by the more wealthy Western nations and tend to focus on issues of concern to them.

Another advantage of the HSR approach is that there are likely to be far fewer types of health systems worldwide than different cultures. For example, even though urban Asian and African settings are different 'culturally', their systems of healthcare may be similar, so that research in one setting may inform health services in the other. In contrast, urban and rural Indian settings, even though 'culturally' related, may differ so greatly in their health systems that research in one setting may have little practical relevance to health services in other settings.

Patel (2000) discusses HSR. Some case studies are presented below.

Case studies in health systems psychiatric research

Depression and motherhood in India

A cohort study of mothers was conducted in a district general hospital in Goa, India, to investigate the predictors, prevalence and impact of postnatal depression (Patel *et al*, 2002). Goa is one of India's smallest states and has a high literacy rate (67%) and a lowish infant mortality rate (20/1000, which is more than double the rate for most European countries but much better than that of most developing nations). The average monthly income for the fathers was around US$47. A total of 270 participants were recruited and the Edinburgh Postnatal Depression Scale (see Chapter 25) was administered twice, at 6 weeks and 6 months after delivery. Around 14% of participants had scores above the cut-off of 11 points on both occasions, indicating that they had a prolonged depression. As might be expected, the rates were highest for those women whose infants had died. Gender discrimination, in the form of boy preference, is common in India, but the overall rate for postnatal depression among the mothers of female infants was only marginally and not significantly raised (female infant to male infant ratio 1.3:1, $P < 0.20$). Domestic violence and poverty are both major public health concerns in India; this study explicitly examined the aetiological role of these factors in the onset of depression, and the influence of these factors is shown in Table 31.2.

The study showed that even though the overall rates of postnatal depression were not greatly increased among mothers of female infants, these risks rose dramatically in the presence of associated poverty or a history of marital violence, and they were also increased if the mother had not yet had a male infant. It appears that the preference for male infants acts as a precipitating factor for postnatal depression, which becomes manifest only in the presence of other social stressors, such as severe poverty or marital disharmony. Effects of this magnitude for the sex of the infant on the rates of postnatal depression have not been documented in any European studies on postnatal depression.

The study is an example of HSR since it took place at the local hospital and has obvious service implications. The findings of high rates of depression in this population and the influence of the sex of the infant on these rates has been disseminated through local workshops with doctors, with information material for parents and the publication of scientific articles (Patel *et al*, 2002).

Setting up mental health services in Cambodia

A relatively stable civilian government has been in place in Cambodia since the mid-1990s, after decades of a brutal civil conflict which culminated in the genocide of a large proportion of the population. The health system has been gradually rebuilt and in 1995 the first 'Western'-style mental health services were introduced.

Somasundaram *et al* (1999) describe their attempt to introduce mental health services in Cambodia, focusing on the opening of four mental health clinics in two provinces. At the time of the research the country was still extremely poor, with poverty being defined in calorie terms, whereby an intake of less than 2100 calories per day corresponds to a monthly income of US$15 a month. A doctor's salary at the time was only $20 a month. Diagnostic criteria were the clinical diagnoses made by Cambodian medical staff who had been trained in the use of the primary healthcare version of ICD–10 (ICD–10 PHC).

The records of the first 5000 patients were analysed and these showed that 18% had psychoses, 15% epilepsy, 18% depression, 15% anxiety and 2% mania. Surprisingly, despite the war, only 3% had post-traumatic stress disorder (PTSD). Interventions included psychotropic medication, counselling, education and group and family therapy, and around 50% of the patients showed improvement. Although the clinics were originally opened up to ensure that clients with a psychosis in the community could receive antipsychotic medication, the clinics soon became overwhelmed by demands for the treatment of a large variety of psychosocial problems.

The study is an example of HSR because it used local clinicians' diagnoses rather than those of a 'research team'. The article demonstrates the efficacy and problems in implementing a low-cost, basic mental health service and relates its findings to the prevailing socio-economic circumstances in the region. The work was a continuation of ethnographic research carried out by some of the authors on traditional healing and indigenous beliefs about mental illness in Cambodia.

Culture change and mental disorder

One important limitation of cross-cultural psychiatry is that it fails to recognise that cultures are dynamic, indeed ever-changing constructs. Globalisation has had an enormous effect on culture. No longer do cultures exist in relative isolation from one another. Whereas, previously, attitudes, practices and beliefs used to evolve separately in different cultures, now cultures are integrating, with values and beliefs from one culture finding new homes in other cultures. While the process of globalisation may work in diverse ways, in reality the dominant cultures are those of industrialised societies, because of their far greater wealth and their domination of the media. This has resulted in a relatively homogeneous culture in the developed world and a process of homogenisation of cultures across the developing world; this is beginning to make redundant one of the original and key rationales behind cross-cultural psychiatry. The study below demonstrates the power of the media in bringing new disorders to previously unaffected

Table 31.2 Risk factors for postnatal depression in Goa: the influence of the sex of the infant

Risk factor in the mother	Male infant		Female infant	
	Relative risk	P	Relative risk	P
Unhappy about the infant's gender	2.6	0.27	2.4	0.01
Already had a female child	0.9	0.79	2.4	0.002
Hungry in the past month	1.9	0.09	3.0	0.001
Ever experienced marital violence	1.0	0.97	3.3	0.001

Source: Patel *et al* (2002).

populations through the impact of the introduction of Western television programmes on eating disorders in a previously media-naive population in Fiji.

Case study of culture change and mental disorders

Becker *et al* (2002) describe an innovative community-based study that assessed the effect of novel, prolonged exposure to television on disordered eating attitudes and behaviours among ethnic Fijian adolescent girls. Fiji was selected because the prevalence of eating disorders was known to be extremely low, with only one reported case of anorexia in the 1990s. The traditional Fijian attitude to eating has in general supported 'robust appetites' and correspondingly 'robust bodily shapes', and in this society the Western prevailing pressure for women to be thin was notable by its absence. Before 1995 the population of the Nadroga province of Fiji had not been exposed to television.

A prospective, multi-wave, cross-sectional design was used to compare two samples of Fijian schoolgirls (mean age 17 years) before (the 1995 group) and then after prolonged regional television exposure (the 1998 group). Participants completed a modified, 26-item version of the Eating Attitudes Test (EAT-26) supplemented with a semi-structured interview to confirm self-reported symptoms. Narrative data from a subset of 30 respondents with a range of disordered eating attitudes and behaviours, and data on television viewing habits from the exposed 1998 sample, were analysed for content relating television exposure to concerns about body image.

The researchers found that 12% of the 1995 group had EAT-26 scores greater than the cut-off of 20, but this was more than double in the 1998 group, where 29% were above the cut-off score. The rate of self-induced vomiting was 0% in 1995 but had reached 11.5% in 1998. Information on dieting was not collected in 1995 because it was presumed to be rare, but in 1998 69% of the respondents reported dieting behaviours. Key indicators of disordered eating were significantly more prevalent following exposure to television. Narrative data showed that weight loss was one way in which the girls modelled themselves after television characters, and as many as 40% of respondents believed that their career prospects would be enhanced if they were thinner, a notion that was quite novel to this society.

This naturalistic experiment describes the negative impact of television on disordered eating attitudes and behaviours in a previously media-naive population and highlights the possible role that the media may have in the continuing epidemic of eating disorders that is occurring in the West.

The influence of culture on mental disorders

The influence of culture on mental disorders is considered in four contexts:

1 symptoms of mental disorders

2 diagnosis and classification

3 epidemiology and risk factors

4 treatment.

Since this textbook concerns only general adult psychiatry, cross-cultural issues in the psychiatric subspecialities such as substance misuse, child and old age psychiatry are not covered here. The focus in this review is on the CMDs and severe mental disorders, for which, in any case, the research evidence is most comprehensive. A substantial segment of the research literature is not in the English language, or is not published in indexed journals. Thus, the review presented here cannot be considered to be fully comprehensive.

Symptoms

The prominent finding of studies in different cultures is that core symptoms of CMD can be detected in a similar presentation in most cultures (Box 31.3 briefly describes one example). For instance, the commonest complaints associated with depression and anxiety are usually somatic, in particular tiredness, weakness, multiple aches and pains, dizziness, palpitations and sleep disturbances. Typical psychological symptoms, such as loss of interest in daily or social activities, suicidal thoughts, poor concentration and anxiety or worry, can also readily be elicited from most patients. These symptom complexes all figure prominently as well in the various culture-bound syndromes (see below).

Earlier theories had suggested that, in developing countries, somatic symptoms were the 'cultural' equivalent of depression and that somatisation, the process by which psychological distress was 'converted' into somatic symptoms, was a typical formulation. This hypothesis has now been shown to be wrong in two respects: first, somatic symptoms are also the commonest presenting features of depression in developed societies (Bhatt *et al*, 1989; Katon & Walker, 1998); and second, the classic psychological symptoms of depression can also usually be elicited in developing countries (Araya *et al*, 1994; Patel *et al*, 1995). Some authors draw a distinction between somatisation and alexithymia. Somatisation is seen as a positive and adaptive way of letting the body speak when in distress and is the typical presentation of the common mental disorders in most cultures. Katon *et al* (1982) write: 'Somatization has become a metaphor for personal feelings and thoughts which are expressed to an external reference system'. Alexithymia is seen as a deficiency or inability to express personal feelings, emotions and fantasy using verbal channels, as may occur in some 'psychosomatic patients'. Alexithymia is strongly related to sensations of pain and dysphoria, which tend to occupy consciousness and thereby occlude awareness, thus making it difficult to discriminate nuances of feeling and elaborate symbolism and fantasy (Van Moffaert, 1998).

Acute presentations of depression are more likely to be somatic; as the illness becomes chronic the patient re-evaluates the illness and becomes more likely to present with psychological symptoms (Weich *et al*, 1995). Recently, attention has been drawn to the fact that 'psychologisation' may be the less common presentation of CMD and may itself be heavily influenced

Box 31.3 The Primary Mental Health Care Project, Harare, Zimbabwe

The Primary Mental Health Care Project (PMHC), Harare (Patel, 1998) was a 3-year project in primary care in Harare, Zimbabwe, aimed at describing the epidemiology of CMDs, in a general practice setting and also among the attenders of a traditional healer. Before the research began, extensive networking was undertaken by the author, and many consultations were held with key health providers, policy makers, academics and non-government organisations, to try to understand the local concepts of the CMDs. The most common condition was *kufungisisa*, which literally means 'thinking too much', or worrying excessively; most people with this complaint appear to have anxiety or depression. The next step in the research was to try to elicit the more common symptoms, explanatory models and disease idioms of primary care attenders with conspicuous CMDs.

These idioms were collated into a preliminary 14-item questionnaire, the Shona Symptom Questionnaire, which was developed and evaluated as a locally valid measure of CMD. For example, the first question on this scale incorporates the notion of *kufungisisa*, with the question 'Did you have times (in the past week) in which you were thinking deep or thinking too much?' This questionnaire was then used in a case–control investigation of the risk factors for CMD among those seeing their general practitioners and in another group who were attending traditional medical healers (a mixed group of spirit mediums, diviners, herbalists and apostolic Christian leaders). The cohorts of cases and controls were reviewed after 12 months to provide information on the outcome and incidence of CMD in an African setting.

The project found a higher rate of common mental disorders among patients attending traditional healers than among those attending primary healthcare (39% versus 27%, $P < 0.001$). The project led to the eliciting of models of illness among the Shona people of Zimbabwe (supernatural illness and thinking too much, which resemble CMD).

The most discriminatory symptoms of CMD were psychological symptoms, although some of the perceptual symptoms may be unique to the cultural setting. Female gender, older age, low education, impoverishment and infertility were identified as key risk factors for a CMD. Persistence of CMD was found in 40% of cases at 12-month follow-up. CMDs were strongly associated with disability. Similarly, economic problems (e.g. no money to buy food, loss of a job by a partner) were associated with the onset of a CMD and economic improvement with recovery from a CMD.

The two most common explanatory models of illness offered by the patients were the notion of *kufungisisa* and 'a heavy painful heart'. Supernatural causation was frequently seen as the underlying aetiology, most commonly *chivanhu*, which means being bewitched, or *mamhepo*, which means suffering from bad airs. Beliefs in witchcraft are widely held in this community.

The study's findings were disseminated through workshops, local media and journals. They had an immediate bearing on the medical curriculum; for example, material relating to spiritual distress and other local idioms, the importance of traditional healers and medical pluralism were used in teaching medical students about CMD. New programmes for debt relief and infertility were also recommended as administrative measures.

by cultural factors (as opposed to being the 'real' clinical presentation of CMD). These 'psychologised' symptoms are more likely to be identified as depression by the physician.

Somatic symptoms as idioms of distress

Somatic symptoms may have a variety of different meanings, depending on the contexts in which they occur. They may be indications of major psychopathology, such as somatoform disorder or hypochondriasis. In a psychotherapeutic or psychoanalytic situation somatic symptoms are sometimes interpreted as 'condensations' of some underlying intra-psychic conflict. In a group setting, for example during an epidemic of hysteria, the symptoms have psychic meaning for the individual. They may also be a reflection of severe social stress. These separate meanings are discussed in Chapter 16 (page 383). However, in the cross-cultural context somatic complaints may have an additional function, as 'idioms of distress'. These idioms are a well-structured and codified way of expressing distress. The use of such idioms does not imply an illness; nor is an idiom the same as a symptom – it is more of a language (Kirmayer *et al*, 1998, p. 244). There is a huge diversity of somatic idioms across the different cultures of the world, with different sensations in the various bodily organs having quite diverse meanings in different cultures (see Box 31.4).

Diagnosis and classification

The classification of depression remains a contentious issue. Diagnostic labels such as 'depression' and 'phobia' have no conceptually equivalent term in many non-European languages. These terms, derived from European cultures, have made the leap from common language to medical disorders and, in the process, have acquired biomedical significance. The inclusion of the item 'sadness' in the description of depression has led to a significant degree of under-reporting of depression in many developing nations because sadness may not feature in the clinical presentation of the mood disorder (Bebbington, 1993). Terms such as 'common mental disorders', though offering some advantages over 'depression' because they do not imply a specific mood state, can be criticised because their vagueness. Even in psychiatric settings, only a quarter of patients in one study attributed their symptoms to a mental illness, while a state of 'nerves' was cited by half (Channabasavanna *et al*, 1993).

Kirmayer *et al* (1998) suggest that many patients in developing countries present with a confluence of somatic, affective and anxiety disorders, which in the milder cases should be distinguished from a culture-specific idiom of distress and in the more severe cases from a genuine depressive illness. Another difficulty in the classification of depression lies in the clinical validity of the distinction between depression

Box 31.4 Some examples of idioms of distress

- In Iran the idiom of 'heart distress' (*narahatiye qualb*) is common (Good *et al*, 1985) and is conceptually related to feelings of loss and grief. A second meaning found in this population derives from the notion that the heart is the source of emotions and its discomfort may relate to issues surrounding female sexuality.
- Among Turkish immigrant women in Denmark the sensation of chest tightness or *sikinti* (the Turkish word *siki* means tight) denotes anguish and has a social meaning relating to social isolation, poverty, being uneducated and lacking control over one's destiny (because of immigrant status).
- In some Mediterranean countries (e.g. Morocco), pain in the head may symbolise authority problems, and often represents conflicts between a son and his father, while gastrointestinal symptoms in these countries, particularly in men, are symbols of sexual problems, such as impotence. In females, feelings of anxiety are somatised through the heart, in the form of palpitations or complaints of a deficit of 'clean blood' (Van Moffaert, 1998).
- Some African–Caribbean communities also consider blood as central to health and they complain of *sangue dormido*, or 'low blood'.

There are many more such cultural idioms of distress which are used to communicate specific anxieties or social difficulties, but the degree of distress used in an idiom falls far short of the severity expected for a state of illness. However, it is essential for psychiatrists to be familiar with the idioms used by the ethnic groups whom they are likely to be treating.

An example of a somatic syndrome that probably does reach 'illness' severity is the Korean syndrome of *hwa-byung*. This is characterised by a number of somatic complaints, such as a feeling of heaviness in the chest, burning, or a mass in the epigastric region, muscular aches and pains, dry mouth and indigestion and palpitations. Emotional symptoms include anxiety, depression and irritability. The condition is thought by sufferers to be due to the suppression of feelings of anger and resentment, which form a sort of physical mass in the chest (Kirmayer *et al*, 1998). The condition occurs among Korean migrants to the USA. Korean psychiatrists relate *hwa-byung* to the cultural socio-moral sentiment of *haan*, which in Korean society denotes the accumulation of anger, resentment and despair associated with collective and individual victimisation.

and anxiety. A World Health Organization (WHO) multinational study in general healthcare found that 'comorbidity' of depression and anxiety exceeded 50% (Goldberg & Lecrubier, 1995), confirming previous similar observations made in primary care (Sen & Williams, 1987). The lack of distinction between these syndromes across many cultures has prompted some Western psychiatrists to suggest a return to the older concept of neuroses, albeit with new names such as 'cothymia' (Tyrer, 2001), which shows some resemblance to the concept of 'common mental disorders' as applied to culturally diverse populations.

Neither DSM–III (American Psychiatric Association, 1980) nor DSM–III–R (American Psychiatric Association, 1987) included any concession to the different cultural presentations of depression, but the present DSM–IV (American Psychiatric Association, 1994) includes a very lucid descriptive paragraph that acknowledges the importance of cultural influences in the presentation of depression:

> 'Culture can influence the experience of and communication of depression. Underdiagnosis and misdiagnosis can be reduced by being alert to ethnic and cultural specificity in the presenting complaints of a major depressive episode. For example in some cultures depression may be experienced largely in somatic terms rather than with sadness or guilt. Complaints of "nerves" and headaches (in Latino or Mediterranean cultures), of weakness, tiredness or imbalance (in Chinese or Asian cultures), of problems of the heart (in Middle Eastern cultures) or of being heartbroken (among the Hopi) may all express the depressive experience. Such presentations frequently combine features of Depressive, Anxiety and Somatoform disorders. Cultures may also differ in judgments about the seriousness of particular symptoms (for example irritability may provoke greater concern in some cultures than sadness or withdrawal). Culturally distinctive experiences (e.g., such as fear of being hexed or bewitched, feelings of "heat in the head" or crawling sensations of ants or vivid feelings of being visited by those who have died) must be distinguished from actual delusions and hallucinations that may form part of a Major depressive episode with psychotic features. It is imperative that the clinician should not dismiss a symptom merely because it is viewed as the "norm" for a culture.' (p. 324)

Epidemiology and risk factors

Two major multinational studies of CMDs have been carried out: the World Mental Health Surveys in a large number of developing and developed countries (some of these surveys are still in progress) (WHO World Mental Health Survey Consortium, 2004) and the WHO multinational study of mental disorders in general healthcare settings in 15 centres (Ustun & Sartorius, 1995; and see Box 31.1). These studies used a similar methodology. In the WHO study in general healthcare participants were screened with the General Health Questionnaire and those with a positive screen were interviewed with the Primary Healthcare version of the Composite International Diagnostic Interview (CIDI–PHC) schedule, which yields ICD–10 diagnoses. The overall rate for ICD–10 disorders was 24% and for sub-threshold disorders was 9%, indicating a very high degree of burden due to CMDs in general healthcare. In all centres the most common diagnoses were anxiety, depression and alcoholism. There was, however, a huge variation in rates between centres: the highest rate for CMDs was 52.5%, among primary care attendees in Santiago, Chile; the lowest rates were 7.3%, in Shanghai, China, and 9.4%, in Nagasaki, Japan. There was also considerable variation in the prevalence of individual diagnoses.

Because the investigation was an 'etic' study on a grand scale, the report gives little information on the reasons for these wide variations in prevalence. Apart from methodological problems, there is consistent cross-cultural evidence that regional factors, such as poverty and income inequality, are major risk factors for CMDs, and these may partially explain the dramatic variation. Other international studies of depression have shown that poor education, poverty and female sex are all significant risk factors for depression; the last two of these are discussed further below.

Gender and common mental disorders

Both community-based studies and studies of treatment seekers indicate that women are disproportionately affected by depression (World Health Organization, 2000). The reasons underlying the female vulnerability to depression in Western societies are discussed in Chapter 3 (page 50) and Chapter 30 (page 749); here we are concerned with cultural and social factors that contribute to this increased vulnerability in developing nations.

The WHO study on mental illness in primary care as described above (Ustun & Sartorius, 1995) found an overall sex ratio of 1.89 (based on the 25 000 people who were screened); that is, the overall female rate of depression was almost double the male rate. There was considerable variation between centres, which suggests a cultural basis for some of this variation. The highest ratios were in Santiago, Chile, where the female:male ratio for depression was 4.73:1. This may be partially explained by the high rates of alcoholism among the men in Santiago (the ICD–10 diagnoses of harmful use of alcohol and alcohol dependence were together given to 39.4% of the men but to only 1.6% of the women). In contrast, in Ibadan, Nigeria, an ICD–10 diagnosis of current depression was more common among men (5.3%) than among women (3.8%) (a sex ratio of 0.72). In this centre the rates for alcoholism were low for both men (3%) and women (0%). The reversed sex ratio found in this centre, with men suffering more from depression than women, may be a chance finding, but the huge cross-cultural variability in the sex ratio for depression does call into question any over-simplistic biological or hormonal explanations for the increased vulnerability shown by women for depression.

Sociocultural explanations for the increased vulnerability of women to depression in developing countries may include:

- the pervasive influence of boy preference from birth and the perceived life roles for men and women in South Asia (Patel *et al*, 2002)
- the effects of oppression and reduced opportunities for women for education and healthcare
- the lack of access to better occupations and many other spheres of life as a result of gender inequality.

The reproductive roles of women in developing countries, such as their expected role of bearing children, the severe adverse consequences of infertility and a failure to produce a male child, have been linked to wife battering. Women are far more likely to be victims of violence in their homes and in many developing countries there is also a raised rate of female suicide (Davar, 1999). Box 31.5 looks at the connection between life events and depression among women in one African study. The sex ratio for depression in the Bangalore centre of the WHO study was 3:1; in this centre the rates of alcoholism for both men and women were negligible, and so an excess of alcohol problems among males could not explain the sex rates for depression. Thus, the adverse position of women in Indian society may have explained most of the increased prevalence of depression among women in this centre.

Box 31.5 Life events and depression in women in Harare, Zimbabwe

Broadhead & Abas (1998) looked at the social origins of depression in women in townships of Harare in Zimbabwe. That study provides an important contribution to our understanding of the universal role of life difficulties in the aetiology of depression. The authors screened 172 women with the Present State Examination (PSE) and the Bedford Life Events and Difficulties Scale (LEDS) and found that nearly 31% had a current episode of depression or anxiety. Around 18% were suffering from a depressive disorder, compared with 9% in Camberwell, a deprived inner-London district thought to have a relatively high rate of depression for the UK.

The researchers sought to investigate the reasons for the high rates of depression found in Harare using the LEDS. More women in Harare had suffered from a severe life event (54%) than in Camberwell (31%) in the preceding 12 months. The proportion of women recording both 'severe events' and 'major difficulties', a combination known to predispose to depression, was 55% in Harare but was only 28% in Camberwell. It appeared that the doubling of the rate of depression in Harare could be largely explained by the increased rates for life events and major difficulties found in Zimbabwe. Most of the 'events' were rated severe in Harare, whereas most were rated non-severe in London. In Harare, beliefs in witchcraft and the power of the spirit world were widespread. Thus, certain events such as a lightning strike on one's house would be rated as severe, with high levels of danger. A notable finding in Harare was the high proportion of events involving humiliation and entrapment, related to marital crises such as being deserted with several children, premature death, illness in family members and severe financial difficulties in the absence of an adequate welfare safety net.

The study confirmed that life events and long-term difficulties are universally important causes of depression. The increased rates of depression in the African women could largely be accounted for by the greater number of adverse life experiences of the women in Harare.

Poverty and common mental disorders

A large body of evidence supports the association between poverty and depression in developed countries (see Chapter 30 and the section on Jarman indexes, pages 751–753). Population-based research has demonstrated a higher risk of depression in those who are unemployed (Lewis & Sloggett, 1998), those who have relatively lower income (Weich & Lewis, 1998) and those who have a low standard of living (Lewis *et al*, 1998).

Such links are also evident in developing countries. Five cross-sectional surveys of treatment seekers and community samples from Brazil, Zimbabwe, India and Chile were collated to examine the economic risk factors for depression. In all five studies, there was a consistent, and significant, relationship between low income and risk of CMDs (Patel *et al*, 1999). There was also a relationship between proxy indicators of impoverishment and depression; for example, those who had experienced hunger recently and those who were in debt were more likely to suffer depression. Thus, Todd *et al* (1999) found that respondents in Zimbabwe who reported difficulty in finding money for food were four times more likely to suffer from a CMD in the next 12 months.

Other studies have demonstrated the relationship between CMD and other indicators of poverty, such as poor education and a lack of household amenities (Bahar *et al*, 1992; Mumford *et al*, 1997; Amin *et al*, 1998). Culture also plays a role in determining the vulnerability of the poor to depression in non-financial ways, such as the caste system of South Asia, which relegates a section of the population, such as 'the untouchables', to subservient roles, and the economic disadvantages experienced by ethnic minorities in multicultural societies across the world.

Treatment

The different pathways by which patients sought care in 11 different countries were examined in the 'Pathways to Care' study (Gater *et al*, 1991), which included seven developing countries in Asia, Africa and Latin America. It focused on patients attending psychiatric care, which would be expected to reflect a small, and unrepresentative, fraction of the population suffering from any type of mental disorder. By far the commonest source of referral was the general medical practitioner based in a family practice or in a hospital out-patient clinic.

A study from Harare, Zimbabwe, described the pathways to primary care for patients with conspicuous CMDs attending primary care clinics and traditional medical clinics (Patel, 1998). Other than those patients with an acute illness, most patients consulted more than one care provider; three-quarters of those with a history of prior consultations had consulted both traditional and biomedical care providers. The first care provider sought for the illness was most often a biomedical carer. The finding is consonant with the cultural concepts of illness; thus, illness at onset is considered to be a 'normal' illness and is taken to a biomedical carer. If this treatment fails, or if the patient's expectations are not met, a traditional carer is then consulted. In contrast, depression is rarely considered to be a mental disorder in many developing countries and thus mental health professionals are perceived to have a limited role in its management (Patel, 1996; Patel *et al*, 1998*a*). Thus, attitudes and beliefs about illness causation, which are considerably influenced by culture, will determine the pathways to care.

There is growing evidence of the efficacy and cost-effectiveness of antidepressant and psychological treatments for depression, delivered in community or primary care settings (Patel *et al*, 2004). Despite this evidence, the typical treatment responses by general physicians in developing countries is to prescribe non-efficacious medications (e.g. benzodiazepines) and vitamins. The WHO Multinational Study in General Health Care reported that nearly 10% of primary care attenders in an Indian centre were prescribed psychotropic drugs, a figure similar to that in many European and North American centres (Linden *et al*, 1999). However, the majority of prescriptions were for tranquillisers rather than antidepressants; for example, while 50% of patients with anxiety disorders received tranquillisers, none received antidepressants. A similar, if less marked, imbalance was also recorded for patients with depressive syndromes. As might be expected, prescription of psychotropic drugs was maximum in those patients whose mental disorder was recognised by the physician; recognition in turn was influenced by the severity of symptoms and the presence of overt psychological symptoms. A remarkable finding of the study was that nearly 80% of all prescriptions were for 'drugs of unproven clinical efficacy', such as tonics and tranquillisers. These findings resonate with the earlier discussion on somatisation in primary care (Patel *et al*, 1998*b*); thus, physicians are more likely to diagnose a mental illness when patients present with psychological symptoms, but tend to use inappropriate medications, which suggests a lack of knowledge or confidence in psychopharmacology.

There is some clinical evidence that the effective dose of psychotropic drugs, particularly antidepressants, may vary, with lower doses being reported to be effective in non-European patients (Kilonzo *et al*, 1994). The enzymes involved in the metabolism of psychotropic drugs, the CYPD enzyme system, with more than 50 subtypes of enzyme, show very wide variations between ethnic groups. This may explain some of the variability in drug responsiveness. The subject is discussed for the antidepressants in Chapter 4 and for the antipsychotics in Chapter 11, and also in the review by Lin *et al* (2001). There is also some evidence that neurotransmitter receptor and transporter genes show ethnic variation in their distribution. Thus, the dopamine-2 receptor A1 allele is found in only 9% of Yemenite Jews but 79% of the American native Cheyenne tribe. A region of polymorphism linked to the serotonin transporter gene also shows wide cross-ethnic variation. Thus, the L-allele is found in 17% of East Asians, 45% of Europeans and 70% of those of African ancestry (Lin *et al*, 2001).

These biological differences are of unknown significance and attempts to link these variations to clinical effects in the different ethnic groups have not yielded any positive findings. Of far greater importance is the effect of culture on the expectations of pharmacotherapy, compliance and the ability to understand the need to take drugs over the long term, which is essential for many conditions. Thus, Kinzie *et al* (1987) examined the serum tricyclic levels of a group of Cambodian refugees medicated for their depression and found that 61% had no tricyclics in their blood at all and a further 24% had very low levels.

The influence of culture on severe mental disorders

Symptoms

The classic multinational studies on schizophrenia conducted by the WHO (discussed below) and the considerable clinical experience of psychiatrists in developing countries lend support to the general consensus that the symptoms of schizophrenia, especially thought disorder and perceptual symptoms, are identifiable in all cultures. In the International Pilot Study of Schizophrenia (IPSS), for example, high scores were recorded in all centres for patients with schizophrenia on lack of insight, suspiciousness, delusional mood, delusions or ideas of reference and persecution, flatness of affect, auditory hallucinations and delusions of being controlled by an external agent.

However, the relative importance of certain other symptoms did differ between cultures (see for example Box 31.6). For instance, visual hallucinations or specific types of auditory hallucinations may not signify a psychotic process in those cultures where such phenomena also occur in specific social or religious contexts, as in the Arab nations (Al-Issa, 1995). Catatonia, once common in the developed world, is now very unusual there, but it is still a common symptom of schizophrenia in developing nations. Similarly, the relative value of first-rank symptoms may differ between the developed and developing world.

The content of delusions also varies considerably according to culture; thus, a content pertaining to interference by aliens from other worlds may be encountered more frequently in Western cultures, whereas delusions pertaining to black magic or witchcraft are more common in some African cultures. It is obvious that affected individuals develop delusional explanations in terms of cultural beliefs about forces that operate invisibly over a distance.

Much less is know about the symptoms of manic illnesses across cultures, although it seems quite likely that the behavioural symptoms are similar in different ethnic groups. However, one comparison of symptoms of mania between African–Caribbean and Whites in the UK found that the former were significantly more likely to express delusions than the latter. In particular, delusions of special abilities, grandiose identity and a special mission were more common among African–Caribbeans (Leff *et al*, 1976).

Box 31.6 Culture and hallucinations

Johns *et al* (2002) reported the results of a cross-sectional survey of more than 8000 adults living in the UK. Participants were screened for mental health problems and those who were positive underwent a further diagnostic interview with the Present State Examination. The rates for hallucinations were:

- 4% in the White population
- 9.8% among Caribbean persons
- 2.3% in the South Asians population.

In all ethnic groups, only a minority of those who reported hallucinations were found to suffer from a psychotic illness; however, here too there was a marked ethnic variation, from 11.4% of Whites to 6.7% of South Asians, to just 1.9% of Caribbeans who had such experiences suffering from a probable psychotic illness. Cultural factors, not fully explored in this study, are likely to be a major factor in explaining these marked ethnic variations both in the prevalence of hallucinatory experiences and in their diagnostic significance for psychoses.

Diagnosis and classification

Striking international differences in the classification and diagnosis of severe mental disorders were first studied in the 1960s, when it was noted that first-admission rates for the diagnosis of schizophrenia were much higher in the USA than in the UK. This was attributed to differences in the diagnostic constructs being used in these two basically similar cultures. In the UK, and most of Europe, first-rank symptoms were used as the core diagnostic elements for making a diagnosis of schizophrenia, so that only a narrow segment of psychotic disorders was considered to be schizophrenic, whereas in the USA at that time psychodynamic formulations were the norm, resulting in a much wider net being cast. The US–UK Diagnostic Project (Cooper *et al*, 1972) and the IPSS confirmed this discrepancy and paved the way for the development of internationally accepted criteria for the diagnoses of severe and, in due course, all mental disorders.

Ethnographic studies of the concepts of mental illness have shown that the psychotic disorders are considered mental illnesses in almost all cultures; however, they are often attributed to supernatural causes such as spirit possession (Patel, 1995). The separation of schizophrenia from bipolar disorder, a central tenet of biomedical nosology, does not figure in most indigenous classifications.

Epidemiology and risk factors

Recent systematic reviews have shown that there are wide variations in the prevalence and incidence rates of schizophrenia across cultures and countries (McGrath *et al*, 2004; Saha *et al*, 2005). Longitudinal multinational WHO studies (see below) have also demonstrated international variations in the course and outcome of schizophrenia; perhaps surprisingly, these studies have shown that despite much more limited access to evidence-based care, people with schizophrenia in developing countries appear to have better clinical outcomes.

Since the 1960s, the WHO has been conducting a series of multinational epidemiological studies of schizophrenia. These have been reviewed in the context of cultural influences by Kulhara & Chakrabarti (2001). The first study was the IPSS (World Health Organization, 1979), which investigated 1202 young people with recent-onset functional psychosis in nine countries across the globe (China, Colombia, Czechoslovakia, Denmark, India, Nigeria, the USSR, the UK and the USA). Quite apart from the results, the IPSS was one of the first studies to demonstrate the feasibility of such large multinational studies, provided there was an adequate standardisation of instruments.

The main finding on follow-up of the samples was that those who lived in developing countries seemed to have a better clinical and social outcome. The IPPS also demonstrated that four key symptoms – auditory hallucinations, delusions, social withdrawal and flat affect – are universal. In developing countries higher rates of acute and catatonic schizophrenia were reported, whereas paranoid schizophrenia was more frequent in developed nations.

Because the IPSS involved participants who had been recruited only from psychiatric facilities, the results might have been confounded by the wide variety of different help-seeking patterns in different countries. The Determinants of Outcome of Severe Mental Disorders (DOSMeD) study (Jablensky *et al*, 1992) sought to correct this by recruiting participants who were making their first contact with any helping agency and who had also received a diagnosis of schizophrenia. The DOSMeD study recruited 1379 patients in 12 centres. Age- and sex-specific prevalence rates were similar for the narrow diagnostic category (CATEGO S+), but there was considerable variation in the prevalence of the broader diagnostic categories. At 2-year follow-up, the DOSMeD study confirmed the IPSS findings of a more favourable outcome in developing countries and this could not be explained by clinical confounders such as more cases of acute-onset psychoses in these settings. The improved outcome in developing countries was attributed largely to undefined cultural factors such as greater family support combined with better integration of people with a mental illness into the community.

There are several hypotheses about how social and cultural factors contribute to a less severe course of illness (Desjarlais *et al*, 1995):

1 It has been suggested that models of illness that invoke external causes, such as supernatural explanations, reduce the burden on the self and so diminish guilt and criticism by family members.

2 Another hypothesis is that greater family support improves prognosis. Extended families have often been endowed with almost mythical powers of support and care, although there is in fact rather little evidence to support this. In any event, family structures in most cultures are changing rapidly as industrialisation leads to a reduction in family size and a trend towards nuclear families.

3 A more likely reason is that the types of work available to persons with severe mental disorders in developing countries, such as simple agricultural work, may be less stressful and more available than the more sophisticated occupations found in the industrialised societies, which few patients with schizophrenia are able to cope with. Being able to work, earn money and contribute to the family economy are enormously important in terms of feelings of personal dignity and self-worth.

4 The characteristics of treatment settings may also influence outcome; the greater reliance on formal mental health services in developed countries may lead to states of dependency and inadvertently result in passivity.

The only factor that has been systematically investigated in relation to the better outcomes for schizophrenia in developing countries is the role of the relatives' expressed emotion (EE) (see page 228 for an explanation of EE). A 1-year follow-up of patients with schizophrenia who had made a first contact with psychiatric services in Chandigargh, north India, assessed the influence of EE on outcome (Leff *et al*, 1987). Only the EE construct of 'hostility' showed any link with relapse, while the EE constructs of 'criticism' and 'emotional over-involvement' failed to show any correlation. There was, though, an *overall* correlation between EE and relapse of schizophrenia (as found in the previous Anglo-American studies), with the lower relapse rates in Chandigargh being accounted for by there being fewer high-EE families in north India.

The whole concept of EE may be strongly culturally determined, as it hinges on what is considered to be 'normal' in family life, and this shows wide variation between cultures. In the Indian population the EE construct of 'emotional over-involvement' was almost impossible to assess because Indian families are usually very involved in the lives of their sick relatives and so exactly what constitutes a pathological or inappropriate emotional involvement – something that surpasses the cultural boundaries for family life in north India – is unclear, as family 'intrusiveness' is accepted to a much greater extent in India than in the West (Wig *et al*, 1987).

More recently there has been a failure to replicate these well-known findings of the large WHO studies. There is new evidence contradicting the apparently good prognosis in many developing countries. For example, in the 15- to 25-year outcome studies of participants recruited in the WHO studies across different countries, the proportion of those who died or were lost to follow-up ranged from 23% in Chennai to over 50% in Chandigarh and Agra. An analysis of the cohort from the Chennai study showed a 10% mortality rate and only a 14% rate of full recovery after 10 years (Thara *et al*, 1994).

Ran *et al* (2002) reported the 2-year outcome of a community sample of never-treated persons with schizophrenia in rural China. They identified 510 persons with a lifetime history of schizophrenia, of whom 156 had never been treated. Over the 2 years, only 3.7% of males and 16% of females achieved complete remission. More than 80% of all patients continued to show 'marked symptoms'. These observations question the earlier IPSS and DOSMed findings of an apparently benign outcome for schizophrenia in developing countries.

Treatment

In most developing countries, the overwhelming bulk of clinical work in psychiatric clinics is taken up with the care of persons with severe mental disorders, leading some observers to comment that psychiatry in these countries is virtually synonymous with the 'psychiatry of psychoses' (Asuni, 1991). Most presentations are acute, with families bringing a patient with severe behavioural disturbances to the casualty department or directly to mental health services. Although small differences in presentation or clinical outcomes between societies may excite epidemiologists, a large number of patients in developing countries with schizophrenia remain symptomatic and disabled purely because there are so few psychiatrists and no facilities. The conditions of care in mental hospitals are often grotesquely out of keeping with contemporary standards of medical care, and in this context it is important not to forget that human rights violations and abuse are overwhelmingly more likely to occur in developing countries (National Human Rights Commission, 1999). Large numbers of patients continue to seek care from traditional and religious healers in temples, for example, but these facilities are not without risk: in the Erwadi tragedy in

Box 31.7 An ethnographic study of psychiatric admissions in Uttar Pradesh, India

Nunley (1998) describes the way in which patients and their relatives are treated in two psychiatric units, one at the hospital in Lucknow and the other at Varanasi, in the Indian state of Uttar Pradesh. The total numbers of hospital beds and professionals available in India are far lower than in the West. Nunley estimates 3 beds and 0.13 psychiatric nurses per 100000 population, and 2000 psychiatrists for a population of 1 billion (a rate of 1/500000).

Out-patients were always accompanied by relatives, with the bulk of the interaction taking place between the doctor and the relative rather than between the doctor and the patient. Records were sparse for out-patients and the interview culminated with the doctor usually handing the prescription to the relative rather than the patient, and this also served as the record of the contact (it was not uncommon to see out-patients return for follow-up visits bringing clutches of prescriptions).

For the in-patients there was only one nurse on each ward of 40 patients, so much of the nursing care depended on the first-degree relatives who accompanied the patients during their admission (they usually slept on a mat on the floor beside the patient's bed).

A consultant in Lucknow listed the five tasks of the relative:

1 to make sure the patient did not run away
2 to take physical care of the patient (e.g. washing and dressing, and preparing food, which was usually done on the lawn outside the ward)
3 to take the patient to any treatment, such as electroconvulsive therapy (ECT) or occupational therapy
4 to ensure drug compliance
5 to report any abrupt changes in the patient's condition.

In the process of caring for the patient in the presence of many other relatives, together with some guidance from the clinical staff, the relatives derived support and also learned a great deal about the patient's illness and its management, a function that in Western settings is often assumed by relatives' groups.

Families had to pay for prescriptions but ECT was free, so ECT was much more commonly used. Discharge difficulties, which are common in Western psychiatry, were virtually unheard of because there were very powerful taboos against family rejection.

India in August 2001, 28 patients in a religious healing site who were chronically mentally ill burned to death because they were chained.

In developing countries the vast majority of patients with severe mental disorders will receive only drug treatments or electroconvulsive therapy; few are able to access rehabilitation or psychosocial treatments. The pattern of hospital care for patients with a psychosis is very different from the typical European hospital ward, as the description by Nunley (1998) given in Box 31.7 demonstrates.

The practice of relatives accompanying their patients to hospital as described by Nunley is not unique to India. For example, in Senegal, in Africa, Franklin *et al* (1996) found that only 3.4% of the patients admitted were unaccompanied: 47% had one relative accompanying them and 33% had two companions. This pattern of informal and family care within the hospital set-up contrasts sharply with the Western pattern of separation from family, with contact only during visiting hours, aetiological theories suggesting family causation of illness, wards being run bureaucratically with numerous detailed written policies, nurses spending much of their time writing, repeated inspections, and an over-preoccupation with extensive written records for medico-legal or insurance purposes.

A study in South Africa by Gillis *et al* (1987) on the long-term use of maintenance antipsychotics showed that, 2 years after discharge, the non-compliance rate for White patients was around 25%, for Indian patients 50% and for Black African patients 66%. Such within-country and within-hospital variation could be explained only by widely differing beliefs concerning medication in these three ethnic groups. Such beliefs will obviously affect relapse rates and are therefore topics of great clinical relevance.

Immigration and mental health

The process of immigration can produce huge psychological and social strains on both the immigrant and the host society. Sometimes great literature can convey these difficulties far more eloquently than a whole clutch of scientific papers and there can be few better descriptions of this phenomenon than in Steinbeck's novel *The Grapes of Wrath* (1939). Steinbeck describes the migration of the starving farmers fleeing the dust-bowls of Oklahoma and Tennessee ('the Okies') and their struggles and aspirations in their quest to seek out the supposed paradise of California, as well as the fears and prejudices of the host community:

> 'The moving people were migrants now. And they scampered about looking for work; and the highways were streams of people, and the ditch banks were lines of people. Behind them more were coming. The great highways streamed with moving people. The movement changed them; the highways, the camps along the road, the fear of hunger and the hunger itself changed them. The children without dinner changed them, the endless moving changed them. They were migrants. And the hostility changed them, welded them and united them, hostility that made the little towns group and arm as though to repel an invader.... They said, these goddamned Okies are dirty and ignorant. They're degenerate, sexual maniacs. These goddamned Okies are thieves They'll steal anything. They've got no sense of property rights. And the latter was true, for how can a man without property know the ache of ownership?
>
> In the West there was panic when the migrants multiplied on the highways. Men of property were terrified for their property. Men who had never been hungry saw the eyes of the hungry. Men who had never wanted very much saw the flare of want in the eyes of the migrants. And the men of the towns and the soft suburban country gathered to defend themselves; and they reassured themselves that they were good and the invaders were

bad, as a man must do before he fights. The local people whipped themselves into a mould of cruelty. Then they formed units, squads and armed them with clubs, with gas, with guns. We own this country. We can't let these Okies get out of hand.... And the migrants streamed in on the highways and their hunger was in their eyes and their need was in their eyes. They had no argument, no system, nothing but their numbers and their needs. When there was work for a man, ten men fought for it – fought for a low wage. If that fella'll work for thirty cents, I'll work for twenty-five. And this was good, for wages went down and prices stayed up. And pretty soon we'll have serfs again....

And the companies, the banks worked at their own doom and they did not know it. The fields were fruitful and the starving men moved on the roads. The granaries were full and the children of the poor grew up rachitic and the pustules of pellagra swelled on their sides. The great companies did not know that the line between hunger and anger is a thin line. And money that might have gone to wages went for gas, for guns, for agents and spies, for blacklists, for drilling. On the highways people moved like ants and searched for work, for food. And the anger began to ferment....

Acculturation and mental health

Immigrants, whether refugees or economic migrants, often move to countries that have cultures, languages and customs that are very different to their own. Some will face enormous life transitions, such as moving from a rural agrarian lifestyle to a technologically advanced Western city existence.

The process of acculturation occurs when two cultures are in contact and usually involves a minority immigrant group trying to learn the culture of the host country. For the individual migrant the aim is to achieve cultural competency, which means becoming fluent in the new language as well as achieving occupational, financial and family goals in the new setting. Success will depend on personal attributes such as intelligence and adaptability, and not every immigrant will be able to make the necessary changes; failure will result in stress and perhaps even mental disorder.

Khoa & Van Duesen (1981) describe three common patterns among immigrants who attempt to acculturate:

1 *A rejection of the new culture and a refusal to adapt*. For obvious reasons this pattern is more common among the elderly because they find any change difficult.

2 *Complete assimilation into the new culture with rejection of the culture of origin*. This is more common among children and the young, but can occur in any age or social grouping.

3 *The 'bicultural' pattern*. This is observed among young adults and the middle aged. There is a good adaptation to the new culture, particularly in the realm of work, but for family, social and religious matters the culture of origin is retained.

Adjustment problems may occur in families as well as among individuals, and this may be further complicated among refugee immigrant families, which are less likely to be intact, for example because of the death or incarceration of a male member in the homeland.

Children acculturate far more easily than adults and this may lead to inter-generational conflicts, a well-known example being the reluctance of some young second-generation Indian women to go through with a traditional arranged marriage.

A classic study: emigration and insanity

There has been considerable academic interest in trying to understand the phenomenon of 'immigrant psychoses'. One of the earliest and best-known epidemiological studies of mental disorder following immigration is that of Ødegäard (1932).

At the turn of the 20th century there was great concern in the USA at the large number of immigrants from Europe who seemed to be breaking down. Rumours abounded of a tenfold increase in the rates of insanity among the new migrants and so there was a need to clarify the matter with a sound epidemiological study.

Many Norwegians had settled in Minnesota and Ødegäard (1932) selected a small sector of south-east Minnesota, which had a population of 217000 served by the Rochester State Asylum, the only mental hospital for his study. He compared the admission rates for mental illness for the Norwegian migrants with those of the native-born Americans over four consecutive 10-year periods. His findings were reassuring in that they failed to confirm the rumours of a tenfold increase, but they nevertheless did show that the admission rates for the migrants were 30–50% higher than among the native-born Americans. He was puzzled by this finding and to try to understand this overall increase he compared the admission data in Minnesota with a similar rural catchment area in Norway, the district of Gstaud, which is a little south of Oslo. His results are given in Table 31.3, which shows that the Norwegian immigrants in America were more prone to schizophrenia, syphilis, alcoholism and admissions for senile disorders. The syphilis and the alcoholism are readily explained as part of the more stressful and disorganised life of a migrant. The increased admission rates for the elderly had an obvious social explanation because in Norway the elderly were always cared for by their families and a small portion of the family farm was allocated to them when this was inherited by the eldest son. In America there were many elderly Norwegian immigrants who either had no family or had lost them, so once they could no longer work they soon ended up penniless and homeless. Their admissions were usually the result of social catastrophe rather than psychiatric disorder.

Table 31.3 Comparison between admission rates (per 100000) of Norwegians in America and Norway

	America	Norway
Schizophrenia	27.87	13.80
Depression	6.20	6.75
Mania	1.81	2.66
General paralysis	2.47	1.80
Alcoholic psychoses	2.65	0.90
Senile psychoses	13.11	1.67

Source: Ødegäard (1932).

Table 31.4 Rates of admission by the length of time the patient had been in America

Onset relative to arrival	Rate (%)
Before	8.7
Less than 1 year	4.9
1–2 years	5.8
2–5 years	11.0
5–10 years	18.9
More than 10 years	50.7

Source: Ødegäard (1932).

The real mystery of the study was why the rate of admissions for schizophrenia in Minnesota was double the rate in Norway. To provide some insight into this enigma, Ødegäard conducted a sub-analysis of the rates of admission by the length of time the patient had been in America. This is shown in Table 31.4, in which there are some surprises. The high rate before immigration was probably due to the practice of relatives in the poorer families of 'exporting' sick members by putting them on a boat to get rid of them. However, rates fell in the first 2 years after migration, suggesting a much smaller role for adjustment and acculturation than had been expected. More puzzling was the finding that some 70% of patients experienced their onset of illness more than 5 years after arrival in America; Ødegäard proposed that people with a 'schizoid constitution', which in later life would predispose them to developing schizophrenia, also had a greater tendency to migrate. Such individuals were more likely to be 'frustrated' or 'failing socially' when aged 18–25 years, when decisions regarding immigration were made. This theory has never been proven, but it is of interest, particularly in the light of recent descriptions of the mild personality abnormalities associated with the schizophrenic prodrome.

Other studies on migration and psychosis

An even more puzzling observation among the families of immigrants has been the finding of very high rates of schizophrenia among the second generation of African–Caribbean immigrants to the UK, which was even higher than that found for their parents. This mysterious observation has been explored by Thomas *et al* (1993), who reported psychiatric admissions by ethnic groups in central Manchester over a 4-year period.

Rates of admission, especially for the diagnosis of schizophrenia, were much higher among the African–Caribbean people than among UK-born Europeans. These rates were highest for second-generation (i.e. UK-born) African–Caribbeans, with whom the police were more also more frequently involved than with Europeans or Asians. Asians had similar rates for hospital admission, but had higher rates of diagnoses of psychotic disorders.

Table 31.5 shows a dramatic increase for both first admissions and readmissions for schizophrenia among the second-generation, young adult African–Caribbean immigrants, but not for the second-generation Indian immigrants. The increased rates for psychoses in this group was confined to schizophrenia and did not occur with manic depression. The authors considered nine separate possible explanations for their findings.

This early study by Thomas *et al* (1993) has been followed by a large number of studies focusing on the raised rates of psychosis among African–Caribbeans in the UK and these have recently been reviewed by Sharpley *et al* (2001). The main finding of that review was that, even when strict operational diagnostic criteria are applied, the raised rates remain, particularly in young adults (Table 31.5). The increased rates for schizophrenia found in the UK are not found in Jamaica, where many of the immigrants come from. There was also a suggestion in some studies of higher rates for affective symptoms; the pattern of the illness was more commonly of a relapsing, remitting course, with more social disturbance, but there was less in the way of negative and persistent symptoms.

Studies of the pathways to care have consistently found a raised use of compulsory admission and police involvement for people of African–Caribbean origin. Outcome studies have similarly suggested a differing course, with more imprisonments and compulsory admissions among Africa-Caribbean patients, but these patients had more time in the recovered state and were less likely to develop negative symptoms and continuous unremitting illnesses.

The problem is not unique to African–Caribbean migration to the UK: a similar pattern of raised rates of schizophrenia has been observed among Surinamese immigrants to the Netherlands. Surinam (formerly Dutch Guinea) is a small country in the northern part of South America. It has a population of around 435 000 and of a diverse ethnic mix, consisting of 37% Hindus (whose ancestors migrated from northern India), 31% Creole (mixed White and Black), 15% Javanese, 10% Maroon (descendants of Black African slaves), 2% Amerindian and 2% Chinese. Following independence in 1954 there was a huge migration to the Netherlands, to the extent that almost a third of the Surinamese-born population now live in the Netherlands.

Table 31.5 First-admission and readmission rates for psychoses for persons aged 16–29 years per 100 000 per year

	First admission		Readmission	
	Schizophrenia	Manic depression	Schizophrenia	Manic depression
Caucasian (UK)	35	23	135	62
First-generation Asian	–	33	49	33
Second-generation Asian	35	–	70	140
First-generation African–Caribbean	–	45	301	60
Second-generation African–Caribbean	320	32	1088	96

Source: Thomas *et al* (1993).

Selten *et al* (1997) undertook a large population-based study using the Dutch psychiatric register and found raised rates for schizophrenia among both male (odds ratio 4.5) and female (odds ratio 2.8) Surimanese immigrants. Raised rates schizophrenia were also found for immigrants to the Netherlands from the Netherland Antilles (a group of former Dutch Islands in the West Indies) and for male immigrants from Morocco but not from Turkey.

The authors ruled out selective migration as the cause because almost a third of the population of Surinam had migrated, and they also excluded ethnicity itself as a cause because the ratio of patients with schizophrenia between the Hindus and African–Surinamese population was 3:1, which was the same as the ratio of their respective populations.

Social selection or social causation?

Murphy (1973) postulated that there were three reasons for the differing rates of mental disorder among migrants:

1 The stress of migration and acculturation might itself cause higher (or lower rates) of mental disorder among the immigrants, compared with the host population.
2 The decision to emigrate might be made by those who are more (or less) prone to particular mental disorders.
3 The migrant population might reflect either higher (or lower) morbidity of the country of origin.

Sharpley *et al* (2001) reviewed the evidence for numerous and diverse theories that might explain the raised rates of psychosis found among African–Caribbean immigrants to Europe and further references are given in their extensive review.

- *Isolated psychotic symptoms*. Even in the absence of a mental illness, these may be more common among the immigrant groups. There may be more hallucinations (see above) and delusional thinking, and this may be a background factor.
- *More affective profile*. Several studies have shown that affective symptoms are more common in the 'schizophrenic' illnesses of African–Caribbeans, with increased rates of mania, secondary mania and schizo-mania.
- *Selective migration*. Ødegäard's hypothesis of selective migration proposes that those genetically predisposed to schizophrenia are more likely to migrate. Intermarriage between first-generation migrants might then explain raised rates in the second generation. However, the enormous migration from Suriname to the Netherlands could not have been selective, yet it was associated with a fourfold increase in the rate for schizophrenia.
- *Prenatal viral infections*. African–Caribbean patients had no immunity to rubella and this resulted in high rates of congenital rubella in their offspring. Similar mechanisms have been suggested for schizophrenia but no evidence has been produced.
- *Perinatal complications*. These appear to be twice as frequent among White patients than among African–Caribbeans and so perinatal complications are an unlikely cause.
- *Social deprivation in childhood*. African–Caribbean children are more likely to be exposed to poverty, to have one-parent families, to experience foster care and to have low educational achievement – all of which predispose generally to psychiatric disorder, although evidence linking these deprivations to schizophrenia is lacking.
- *Social deprivation in adult life*. High rates of unemployment, or living alone, and higher rates of imprisonment occur among African–Caribbeans, but these have not been specifically associated with the onset of schizophrenia (although they may occur as a consequence).
- *An urban effect*. There is increasing evidence that urban rates for schizophrenia are considerably increased, although the underlying mechanisms are obscure and probably due to an accumulation of other genetic and environmental risk factors.
- *Racism*. This is a controversial and political issue, but studies among African–Americans have linked racism more to thwarted aspirations and consequent depression than to psychoses.
- *Cannabis use*. Excessive cannabis use is associated with raised rates of psychosis, particularly among those with a family history of psychosis, and cannabis use is relatively common among young African–Caribbeans. However, research from the Netherlands indicated a lower rate of cannabis use among immigrants, even though their rates of schizophrenia were greatly elevated.

Sharpley *et al* (2001) did not attempt to favour one explanation over any other and the reason for the raised rates of schizophrenia in the immigrants remains unknown. They did, however, note that these rates of psychosis probably represent a considerable burden on an already deprived population.

The mental health of refugees

With a growing degree of turmoil in many parts of the world, the study of immigrants and mental illness has been fuelled by an increasing number of refugees from war-torn countries or displaced persons fleeing from economic collapse and conflict in their home countries. There are an estimated 20 million refugees who have fled their own countries, and another 20 million who are internally displaced persons (Ekblad *et al*, 1998). Many of these refugees will have experienced enormous trauma in the form of violence, crime or other humiliations, physical injury, economic dispossession and disruption of family and community structures. In this context, the social cause for the mental disorder is the same as has led to the migration, and so rates of mental disorder among these people would be expected to be at least as high and probably higher than for migrants in general.

Differences in the rates of mental disorder among refugees may relate to the severity of the trauma that the population has been exposed to. The form of any disorder tends to be coloured by the culture of origin, as has been demonstrated in the studies of refugees coming from the war-torn countries of South East Asia. Hinton *et al* (1993) compared the rates of psychiatric disorder, particularly PTSD, among ethnic Vietnamese and ethnic Chinese populations who had fled from Vietnam to the USA. The Vietnamese had mainly fled immediately after the war between the USA and Vietnam, which ended in 1975. The ethnic Chinese, who had been settled in Vietnam for several generations as merchants, fled from Vietnam when hostilities broke out between China and Vietnam in 1978, when the local Vietnamese population turned on them. The ethnic Vietnamese refugees appeared to have had a much harsher time before entry to the USA, reporting more traumatic events (56%) than the Chinese (25%) and the ethnic Vietnamese had more often been boat people (48% versus 18%) before their entry to the USA. Using the Structured Clinical Interview for DSM they found that the prevalence of DSM–III–R diagnoses among the ethnic Vietnamese group was 24%, and 7% of the participants had PTSD, whereas among the ethnic Chinese group the rate for DSM–III-R diagnoses was 14%, with only 1% having PTSD.

The situation in Cambodia during the Khmer Rouge regime was even more terrifying than in Vietnam. Under Pol Pot a quarter of the population died (through executions, starvation or disease). Children aged over 6 years were separated from their parents and placed in work camps; many watched members of their own families being executed. Following the Vietnamese invasion of Cambodia in 1979, the Khmer Rouge regime came to an end and around 150000 Cambodians fled, many of them to the Western parts of the USA. Sack *et al* (1994) interviewed a group of these Cambodian adolescents with the Schedule for Affective Disorders and Schizophrenia and found a point prevalence rate of 37% for PTSD for those in the 22- to 25-year age group. The mothers of these young people had a rate of 53% for the full-blown PTSD syndrome, while the fathers had a rate of 29% for PTSD. These figures should be set against the base rate of PTSD in the USA of around 1–2% using DSM–III criteria. It should be noted that these very high rates were all diagnosed some 10 years after the collapse of the Khmer Rouge regime, when the refugees had been in the USA for more than 8 years, indicating that after very severe trauma PTSD may become a chronic (almost lifelong) condition.

The universal application of one Western type of trauma-related mental disorder, in particular the PTSD concept, has been criticised because it is itself based on culturally influenced notions of how a person is supposed to react to trauma (Guarnaccia *et al*, 1990). Thus, in narrating the experience of Cambodian refugees, Eisenbruch (1991) describes patients who were 'possessed by spirits, troubled by visitations of ghosts from the homeland ... and feels he or she is being punished for having survived'. The cultural construction of the symptoms is also an important determinant of help-seeking behaviour; thus, Buddhist monks would work as 'allies to the clinician in clarifying the diagnosis of cultural bereavement'.

Apart from trauma, Ekblad *et al* (1998) list the types of difficulties encountered by immigrants and refugees that may contribute to mental disorder, describing in a more scientific way the stresses that Steinbeck described in *The Grapes of Wrath*:

- *Marginalisation and minority status*. Others perceive the new immigrants as aliens who are either undesirable or inferior, and as a consequence refugees may develop low self-esteem and depression.
- *Socio-economic disadvantage*. Most refugees will arrive in an impoverished state, although usually the host nation will provide the basic necessities. However, in Africa, for some of the recent waves of migration the receiving country has also been in a state of severe impoverishment and external agencies such as the United Nations have had to deal with the problems of imminent starvation and malnutrition. There may also be profound effects on the developing brain of small children.
- *Poor physical health*. The journey as well as months in transit camps may predispose to physical illness. Poor physical health may be catastrophic to some male migrants who are sending much of their wages home to support families in the homeland.
- *Collapse of social support*. The loss of the extended family, social isolation and states of anomie, particularly among single men, may all contribute to depression.
- *Adaptation to the new culture*. Language difficulties, unemployment, exploitation in the labour market, housing and other social difficulties may all contribute to psychiatric disorder.

For illegal immigrants all of the above may apply, but in addition there is the constant fear of being found out and repatriated, so access to possible sources of help is severely limited.

Some authors have suggested that there is a great danger in the medicalisation of these predominantly social problems and in labelling them as mental disorders, since this leads to sufferers losing the context of their experience and at the same time removing an obligation from the host society to respond appropriately (Kleinman & Kleinman, 1985). From an international perspective, many of the issues discussed above form the basis of a recent critique on the 'etic' assumptions that underlie mental health interventions or trauma programmes in war-affected areas (Summerfield, 1999).

Treatment in multicultural settings

There are two main areas of interest in the treatment literature in cross-cultural psychiatry. The first concerns the management of particular psychiatric disorders among ethnic minorities within Western host countries, and in this area there is considerable knowledge, while the second concerns the problems associated with services and treatment in developing nations. In the latter case the literature is much smaller, but the problems are very much greater and the lack of an informative literature probably reflects no more than the paucity of the services and the poverty of these nations.

Because there are so many combinations of ethnic minority and host nation, it is not possible here to summarise the vast array of publications describing the particular problems that one immigrant community is facing in a particular host country. However, certain

Box 31.8 A culturally competent service

Cross *et al* (reported by Trujillo, 2001, p. 544) tried to see exactly what cultural competence means in the setting of managing disturbed children in a cross-cultural setting, but the principles outlined in their paper (and set out below) apply equally to the situation in adult psychiatry.

- The family is usually the preferred point of intervention. Understanding family structure and dynamics for a particular ethnic group will be helpful in service delivery. This is clearly primary in child psychiatry, but applies in adult psychiatry as well.
- Individuals from minority groups will be struggling with the demands and ideals of at least two cultures and the mental health system should take into account this unique difficulty, which may be more stressful to some people than to others.
- Individuals will make choices, life decisions and treatment decisions, and these will be based on cultural forces that may be very different from those of the host society. Clinicians need to be aware of and respect these cultural forces.
- Inherent in the cross-cultural interaction during psychological treatment are psychodynamic considerations, which should be acknowledged and adjusted for. For example, in dynamic psychotherapy, where transference issues arise, a Vietnamese refugee may have stereotyped (and largely unconscious) fantasies of what an American might be like and these might arise in the transference. Conversely, a Western therapist might have quite different fantasies as to what a Vietnamese, Albanian or African refugee was like and these stereotypes might feed into the countertransference.
- Where there are large ethnic minority populations, appropriate pieces of cultural knowledge should be incorporated into day-to-day clinical practice and policy making.
- Cultural competence will involve working closely with the natural informal network of a particular minority, for example local religious leaders or spirit healers.
- Cultural competence extends the concept of self-determination to the whole minority community, so wherever possible minority groups should be encouraged to participate on hospital boards and serve in the administrative team and be recruited to staff in the mental health teams at all levels.
- Culturally competent services should practise equal and non-discriminatory policies. This point is vital in ensuring that members of minority groups do not feel they are being unfairly treated. In most countries it is therefore enforced by law. Responsive and special outreach services for particular minority groups may also be helpful.

principles are beginning to emerge as to what a good cross-cultural treatment service should be aiming for. Fundamental to this is the concept of being able to deliver a 'culturally competent service' – a term that was drawn up in a position paper for the American Psychological Society by Sue *et al* (1988). In that paper cultural competence was defined as:

> 'the ability to participate in the everyday web of social relationships even if at a limited or reduced level of a particular social group. It means having a sufficient cultural knowledge, reasonable mental blueprints for culturally appropriate behavior so as to be able to act as an insider.'

Achieving complete cultural competence is difficult (Box 31.8), but it is important in the cross-cultural treatment situation, where there is clearly a need for both patient and therapist to be conversant with each other's cultures.

The use of interpreters

When an immigrant is fluent in the language of the host nation, a degree of cultural competence can be assumed. However, when the patient cannot speak or understand the tongue of the host community it is unlikely that much adjustment to the new culture has been made, and the services of an interpreter will be needed. Because psychiatric diagnosis is based exclusively on history and interview, and therefore language, and there are no other confirmatory physical or biological tests, the quality of the translation is crucial. Tribe & Raval (2003) describe the many different roles and functions that an interpreter may have to fulfil and principles to follow while working in a mental health setting. These include:

1 *Impartial and accurate translation.*

2 *Acting as a 'cultural broker' or 'cultural consultant' to both parties.* This entails explaining to the clinician specific aspects of the patient's culture that may impinge on the case, and equally explaining to the patient the doctor's diagnosis and treatment plans, as well as any specific institutional or host country customs or regulations that may be relevant. For example, sexual mores vary widely between cultures and the interpreter will have to be acquainted with what is and is not acceptable in both cultures.

3 *Acting as an advocate for the patient.* Because the only meaningful contact the patient will have with the services will be that in the presence of the interpreter, the only way the patient has of advancing a cause (e.g. pressing for an earlier discharge, or seeking a letter of support for the housing department) will be through the interpreter, who may have to argue the case on behalf of the client.

4 *Acting as an intermediator or conciliator.* Conflicts and strong emotions are an everyday part of work in acute general psychiatry. For example, when a patient is going to be sectioned, or in an acute suicidal episode, the interpreter may have to bear the brunt of the negative emotions – a task interpreters are not trained for and which usually falls to the clinician.

5 *As a link worker helping to coordinate the patient to other agencies and also as a bilingual case worker, especially when treatment is delivered through the multidisciplinary team.* There will usually be no one else who is linguistically competent to carry on some of the basic tasks of the case worker.

Because the more sensitive aspects of psychiatric diagnosis often hinge on the clarification of ambiguities of language (e.g. patients may say their 'marriage is OK' or that they are 'a bit suicidal') the interpreter should have at least a rudimentary knowledge of mental health issues, so that such statements can be properly explored with the guidance of the clinician. Most interpreters find it helpful to have a pre-interview meeting with the clinician, so that they can understand the areas the clinician is seeking to explore; this is followed by the interview itself, which should be conducted quite slowly, to ensure that all parties understand every sentence that has been translated, with the clinician facing the patient and acknowledging that the patient's responses have been understood. After the clinical interview the interpreter should meet again with the clinician to explain any further subtleties of meaning, the significance of any non-verbal expressions and any general impression derived from the interview.

Culturally valid classifications

ICD and DSM

The two main systems of psychiatric classification – at present ICD–10 (World Health Organization, 1992) and DSM–IV (American Psychiatric Association, 1994) (see Chapter 28) – reflect the psychiatric nosologies of Euro-American medicine. Diagnostic criteria of syndromes can and do change over time, as is well demonstrated by the regular revisions of international psychiatric classifications; these revisions are considerably influenced by attitudinal, political and historical factors. Many cross-cultural and psychiatric researchers in low-income countries have argued for greater effectiveness and universal applicability of current classification systems. Indeed, there have been considerable efforts to improve the cultural validity of these international classifications.

ICD–10 was developed with the explicit purpose of being an international classification, in contrast to DSM–IV, whose primary audience was North American. Thus, efforts were made to ensure that the 'experts' who drafted ICD–10 were drawn from as many countries as was feasible. The classification itself was field tested in 39 countries from all continents, by over 700 clinicians, though the largest number of centres were in European or developed countries. In these field trials two or more clinicians rated consecutive new patients presenting to the service and made an ICD–10 diagnosis according to the manual. The inter-rater reliability coefficient (kappa – see Chapter 27, page 698) for each disorder was then calculated. The vast majority of ICD–10 conditions had reasonable reliability (i.e. high kappa values) but a small number of conditions did not, and therefore these definitions may not be very reliable. These included most of the individual personality disorder subtypes, hypochondriasis, mixed anxiety and depressive disorder, recurrent mild depressive disorder, mixed episodes of bipolar disorder, organic depressed state, organic personality disorder, acute schizophrenia-like episode and, somewhat surprisingly, catatonic schizophrenia (Sartorius *et al*, 1993).

Cultural influences on psychiatric classification have been accounted for in DSM–IV in three key areas:

1 In many 'universal' diagnostic categories, such as depression, there are descriptions of the cultural variations in the clinical presentations (see page 791).

2 There is an appendix that lists culture-bound syndromes (these are discussed below).

3 Perhaps the most important of all, there is a recommendation that clinicians make a 'cultural formulation' when assessing a patient whose culture is very different from the host nation (see Box 31.9).

Box 31.9 Cultural formulation in DSM–IV

The DSM cultural formulation requires the clinician to provide a narrative summary on:

- the cultural identify of the individual (e.g. language abilities, cultural preference group, degree of involvement with other cultures in community)
- cultural explanations of the illness (similar to the explanatory models described earlier and including prominent idioms of distress, causal models and treatment preferences)
- cultural factors related to the psychosocial environment and functioning (culturally relevant interpretations of social stressors, available social support and disability)
- cultural elements of the relationship between the individual and the clinician (identifying differences and similarities in cultural and social status that may influence diagnosis and treatment)
- overall cultural assessment (a conclusion formulating how these cultural considerations influence diagnosis and treatment decisions).

Other systems

Although anthropologists have often highlighted the importance of indigenous classifications of illness, in reality there are few enthusiasts for or users of them, even within the developing nations. Indigenous classifications have been mainly based on causal theories, and include spiritual, supernatural or humoral aetiologies (Murdock *et al*, 1980).

The Chinese classificatory system

Although ICD–10 is an international system, it was not (at least initially) intended to supplant local classificatory systems. However, gradually most countries have shed their own national classification schemes and of the few that remain there has been an attempt to make them conform to the ICD as closely as possible. One traditional system of medicine that has managed to avoid being totally pushed into the background is traditional Chinese medicine.

China is, possibly, the only country that has its own, separate classification of mental disorders. The first Chinese Classification of Mental Disorders (CCMD) appeared in 1979 and since then has undergone several revisions. The most recent version, the third (CCMD–3), has been heavily influenced by ICD–10 and DSM–IV, but it still retains certain local features.

The main differences between ICD–10 and CCMD–3 are summarised by Lee (2001). Notable among these are the retention of the term 'neurosis' (which, as discussed above, appears to be the most valid construct to describe depression and anxiety disorders) and the presence of specific categories of mental neurotic disorder such as neurasthenia. This disorder is included in ICD–10 but not in DSM–IV; it is a very common diagnosis among Chinese people. CCMD–3 emphasises insomnia and headache as its core symptoms, whereas in ICD–10 fatigue is regarded as the central symptom of the disorder. The Chinese have also retained the category of unipolar mania.

Personality disorder is less often diagnosed in Chinese populations, possibly because deviant behaviour is dealt with by the penal system. Thus, two categories of personality disorder, borderline and avoidant, are excluded from the Chinese scheme. The Chinese task force who drafted the classification excluded borderline personality disorder from CCMD–3 because they felt that impulsivity and emotional instability were just bad character traits, which should not be medicalised.

Criteria for ICD–10 avoidant personality disorder include 'excessive preoccupation with being criticised or socially rejected in social situations' and 'Unwillingness to become involved with people unless certain of being liked' and 'belief that one is socially inept'. Because self-effacement is such an integral part of the shame-oriented precept of Confucianism, these features may represent a cultural norm in China, making it difficult or almost impossible to discern individuals who might be pathological in this respect. Because of this, the Western concept of avoidant personality disorder cannot be applied to a Chinese population as its criteria represent a pattern of normal and indeed worthy behaviour.

The category of pathological gambling is also excluded from CCMD–3 because gambling is ubiquitous in Chinese society and those who ruin their lives through gambling are regarded as bad rather than ill.

CCMD–3 includes a section on culture-related mental disorders, such as *qigong*-induced mental disorder. *Qigong* is a trance-based form of a traditional Chinese healing system. The disorder is similar to a dissociative state, with identity disturbance, irritability, hallucinations, and aggressive and bizarre behaviours. These are often acute, brief episodes and are linked to too much *qigong* meditation by physically or psychologically ill people.

'Travelling psychosis' (Box 31.10) has been reported only in China and is included in CCMD-3 under the category 'Other psychotic disorders'. It may be an example of a pathoplastic condition occurring at a time of rapid social stress (Lee, 2001).

Although homosexuality on its own is no longer regarded as a psychiatric disorder in the Chinese system, the category of 'Homosexuality with distress' is included. Homosexuality was removed from the Western nosologies only as a result of campaigns from gay pressure groups and these are not so prominent in China. Also, as a result of the Chinese government's one-child policy to limit population growth, the category of sibling rivalry has been omitted from CCMD–3.

Box 31.10 Travelling psychoses – an example of a pathoplastic condition

China is a rapidly changing society subject to huge internal migrations, with millions of people a year migrating from impoverished rural villages to the cities, seeking work. Trains are generally very overcrowded, with people crammed into the toilets, on the luggage racks and even under the seats. Under these conditions people avoid going to the toilet and often stand for long periods. In the mid-1980s reports of a condition called *lutu jingshen Bing*, 'travelling psychosis', began to appear. The term described patients who might suddenly jump off the train in a suicide attempt or even attack a fellow traveller. The condition was manifested by an acute onset of terrifying illusions and hallucinations, panic, motor excitement, and impulsive or suicidal acts.

Research showed that the combination of sleep deprivation, cold weather, hunger and prolonged standing resulted in dehydration, hypoglycaemia and severe fatigue. The termination of travel combined with rest and adequate nutrition led to a spontaneous recovery in almost all cases and most sufferers had either remorse or amnesia for the episode afterwards. Because the condition had occasional forensic implications, regional governments sought to improve conditions on the railways by lessening the overcrowding and so the condition is now less frequently reported.

Culture-specific disorders

The concept of culture-bound syndromes, as currently understood in psychiatry, was first introduced by P. M. Yap, a Western-educated Chinese psychiatrist. In a critique of the previous term 'exotic psychoses' he wrote:

> 'The term exotic psychoses is an unfortunate one. It does not denote all the psychoses found in non-Western countries, but refers only to certain atypical psychogenic psychoses in a number of non-Western populations. Conditions similar to possession states may be seen in Western cultural groups, for example the unnamed condition in which adolescent girls swoon at the voice of a crooner.... The growing importance of cross-cultural studies presages the demise of the term. It should be replaced by "atypical culture-bound psychogenic psychoses". The term is admittedly cumbersome.' (Yap, 1962, p. 163)

Conditions included under this rubric were later to include many neurotic conditions and so 'atypical' and 'psychoses' were dropped, as was 'psychogenic', presumably on the grounds that this was implicit, leaving the rather neater phrase 'culture-bound syndromes', which has remained and is generally accepted.

The number of such syndromes described in the literature exceeds 100, but ICD–10 has reduced this number to a more manageable 12. These are described in an annex to the main text, which is not even in the main volume, but only in the 'Diagnostic criteria for research' section, which is published as an additional book. As noted earlier, DSM–IV also recognises the existence of culture-bound syndromes but likewise relegates them to an appendix. This ambivalent attitude of both classification systems suggests that neither is quite certain about the nosological status of these disorders. The ICD–10 definition of 'culture-specific disorders' states that they should share the following two cardinal characteristics:

1 They are not 'easily' accommodated by the categories in established and internationally used psychiatric classifications.

2 They were first described in, and subsequently closely or exclusively associated with, a particular population or cultural area.

Despite the inclusion of culture-bound syndromes in ICD–10, it is important to note that the use of the term has been criticised by some cross-cultural psychiatrists as an artefact or etic observation, leading to a category fallacy (i.e. creation of a false category based on misrepresentation or misunderstanding of behaviours and emotions in different cultural settings). Furthermore, some of the early descriptions of culture-bound syndromes have been discredited, while the nosological status of those that still remain is uncertain.

Space does not permit a detailed description of all the culture-bound syndromes but in the summary below the more common ones are described in a little more detail, to give the reader a better understanding of this group of conditions.

Amok

Amok is an indiscriminate, unprovoked episode of severely aggressive behaviour, which may culminate in multiple homicide or suicide. The origins of amok are probably to be found in the trance states of the ancient Hindu warriors as they entered battle (Castillo, 1997). In this trance they believed warrior gods possessed them and in effect it was the warrior gods who did the fighting. This aspect of Indian culture was transferred to the Malayan archipelago during the period of Indian colonisation, in the fourth and fifth centuries. Malay warriors adopted the tactic and would attack the enemy en masse, screaming 'Amok! Amok!' and proceeding to kill everyone in sight.

In a typical case of Malaysian amok the person, usually a young man, sits and broods quietly for several hours in a tense and dysphoric state and then suddenly picks up a knife or sword and proceeds to attack anyone within sight. The attack goes on for several hours until the person is killed, subdued or collapses in a state of exhaustion; there is amnesia for the event afterwards. The word *amok* is probably derived from the Sanskrit *amuc*, meaning 'no freedom', although the origin may be in the Portuguese-Indian word *amuco*, which refers to 'heroic warriors ready to die in battle'.

The amok man usually has an intense sense of grievance and the act of amok is seen as seeking revenge for this humiliating position. States similar to amok have been described in Indonesia, southern Africa, Korea, Scandinavia (the *berserker* of the ancient Norse sagas) and among indigenous North Americans. The recent spate of school massacres in America, such as Columbine, or the Hungerford massacre in England, are all related to amok, where the slighted young man with a strong sense of vengeance indulges in an indiscriminate killing spree.

The dhat syndrome

The dhat syndrome (*shen-kui* in China) is a form of anxiety disorder in young men in the 15- to 30-year age group. It has been mostly described in South Asia. The sufferer characteristically presents with a complaint of a whitish discharge in the urine, which is believed to be semen. The word is derived from the Sanskrit *dhatu*, which means essential bodily fluid, of which there are five in ancient Indian medicine; of these, semen is held to be the most important for the maintenance of physical and mental health (Castillo, 1997). Associated symptoms include fatigue, muscle pains, complaints of distortion of the shape of the penis, loss of libido, impotence, anxiety and depressive symptoms. The condition is attributed by men to a loss of semen via any route, but in particular non-procreative routes such as masturbation and nocturnal emissions. It is conceptualised by some authors as a 'sexual neurosis' and has been described in all South Asian societies, though particularly India.

A condition similar to the dhat syndrome has also been described in women in South Asia, who complain of a white vaginal discharge, although this condition has no named diagnostic category at present.

In both genders, the illnesses are considered to be related to the belief that sexual fluids are endowed with considerable potency and vitality, and their loss leads to fatigue and ill health.

A study by Chadda (1995) of 50 male patients complaining of the dhat syndrome found that around two-thirds met the DSM–III–R criteria for major depression (40%), anxiety disorder not otherwise specified (30%) or somatoform disorder not otherwise specified (40%). Psychometric testing with the Illness Behaviour Questionnaire of the whole dhat cohort (compared with a group of psychiatric controls) showed high scores on the factors of general hypochondriasis and affective discomfort but low scores on denial, which suggests that a hypochondriacal temperament combined with cultural beliefs were important aetiological factors.

Koro

Koro is a culture-bound syndrome that presents as an acute panic reaction in men, associated with a strong fear of death as a result of the patient's firm conviction that his penis is retracting and shrinking into his abdomen. The word *koro* is thought to derive from the Malay word *Kura*, which means 'tortoise', with the symbolic meaning that the retraction of the penis is compared to the retraction of the head of the tortoise into its shell. In many Asian countries the penis is sometimes referred to as the 'turtle's head'.

The history of this disorder goes back to ancient times. Koro may have been one of the very first psychiatric disorders ever to have been reported, because there is a description of *suo-yang* (an older Chinese name for koro) in the Yellow Emperor's Classic of Internal Medicine. This was a series of dialogues held between the Yellow Emperor and his court physician,

Ch'i Po, thought to have been written during the period of the warring states (476–221 BC). It is quoted here because of its great antiquity:

> 'When the pulse corresponding to the liver is slightly big there is numbness in the liver. The penis will shrink and there is persistent cough which causes abdominal pain. Illness due to internal pathogenic factors causes impotence; illness due to cold causes retraction of the penis. In the case of the liver, grief moves the innermost self and causes harm to the mind resulting in madness, amnesia, and lack of sperm. Without sperm a person will not be well and the manifestation is one of retraction of the genitals with spasm of the muscles, the bones of the chest are depressed and hair colour is poor. Death usually occurs in the autumn.' (From Ng & Kua, 1996)

Although the condition is much commoner in men it may also present in women, as a fear that the breasts or genitalia will retract. Onset is rapid, intense and unexpected, and is associated with panic, although it would be wrong to designate koro as a simply a type of panic disorder.

Responses may include grasping of the genitals by the victim or a family member, application of splints or devices to prevent retraction, herbal remedies, massage or fellatio. Victims expect the consequences to be fatal. Because they apply splints and tie their penis with string they sometimes cause penile damage, resulting in a urological presentation.

The condition cannot really be categorised in terms of Western terminology but has elements of panic disorder, depersonalisation, castration anxiety and dissociation; it is not usually thought to have a psychotic element.

In areas where belief in koro is widespread, relatives also usually take fright and join in with the sufferer in trying to reverse the retraction of the penis into the abdomen; when whole communities are under stress koro epidemics may occur. The Singapore epidemic of 1967 followed from race riots in the two preceding years, when Singapore left the Malaysian federation. Epidemics in China were prominent in the 'great leap forward' (1957–58), the cultural revolution (1966–69) and more recently in 1984 and 1987 on Hainan Island, especially among the Han people. Epidemics have also followed on from rumours of mass poisoning through pork infected by swine fever, because pork is a staple food in the Chinese diet. In the Haiking County Survey on Hainan Island, the typical koro victim was a Han male (there are also other ethnic groups on the Island) who was young (aged between 15 and 30 years), single, poorly educated and fearful of supernatural forces. Interpersonal conflict and sociocultural demands also contribute and the condition has been reported in most countries in South-East Asia (Cheng, 1996).

Latah

Latah is a highly exaggerated stereotyped response to fright or trauma, followed by echolalia, echopraxia, coprolalia, automatic obedience or trance-like states. Habituation to the stimuli that provoke the startle does not occur. The condition is rare, even in the areas it is reported to exist in, but similar conditions appear to be widely distributed, occurring among the Lapps of Scandinavia, in some communities in Mexico, South America and South-East Asia, and among the Inuit of North America, while in the southern state of Louisiana a group known as the 'Ragin Cajuns' has been described. Among the Ainu of Japan, latah is most commonly precipitated by the sudden recognition of having stepped on a snake (or imagining having done so).

Gilles de la Tourette (1884) took an interest in the condition, which he distinguished from his own syndrome. He proposed calling the condition *tic convulsive*, and suggested that the 'jumping Frenchmen of Maine' and the condition of *myriachit* in Siberia might both be latah equivalents.

The origin of the word latah is unknown but is thought to derive from Malay words meaning ticklish, creeping and love madness.

The aetiology is uncertain but latah is sometimes considered to be most closely related to a dissociative disorder. However, some familial cases have been observed, which suggests a genetic component.

Nervois

Nervois (or nerves, *nevra, nerfiza*) are attacks or episodes of extreme sadness or anxiety comprising emotional distress accompanied by somatic complaints such as head and muscle pain, 'brain aches', sleep disturbances, fatigue, appetite loss and agitation, tingling and 'mareos' (dizziness with occasional vertigo).

The condition is more common in women and is linked to stress and low self-esteem. It is prevalent in South and Central America and some parts of southern Europe. The features are almost identical to mixed states of anxiety and depression, so it represents a general neurotic presentation. Similar syndromes have been described in Africa, Korea, China and Iran.

Susto

'Susto' or 'espanto' literally means fright or soul loss, and is attributed to a frightening event that causes the soul to leave the body. The condition may be chronic and sufferers believe that it can sometimes be fatal. It has diverse symptoms, including agitation, depression, confusion, apathy, anorexia, fever, diarrhoea, troubled sleep with dreams, lack of motivation, low self-esteem and feelings of dirtiness. The syndrome appears to resemble a picture of mixed anxiety, with depressive and somatic symptoms. It is common in Mexico, Central and South America and among the Latino immigrants from these countries to the United States. Ritual healing entails calling the soul back to the body and cleansing the person to restore bodily and spiritual balance.

The condition has been variously attributed to both organic (e.g. hypoglycaemia) and psychosocial (e.g. social conflict) causes, but all cases should be investigated because the long-term mortality of the sufferers may be raised, as it may sometimes be a presentation of a serious physical illness.

Brain fag syndrome

The brain fag syndrome has been extensively described

in West Africa and is attributed to the stress resulting from the pressure on young adults or adolescents to perform well at high school or university in examinations where the emphasis is on rote knowledge from books rather than practical knowledge as learned from elders through oral traditions.

The condition is associated with a variety of medically unexplained physical symptoms, anxiety and depression, blurring of vision and tightness or pain around the head. Students complain that their 'brain is fatigued'. Symptoms are often triggered by the mere effort of reading.

In some developing nations education is seen as one of the few ways of escaping from the grinding poverty and a sociocultural explanation for the phenomenon appears to be most likely.

Frigophobia

Frigophobia (*Wei han zheng*) is a rare type of chronic anxiety state characterised by obsessive fear of the cold (*pa-leng*) and fear of the wind (*pa-feng*). The origins of these beliefs are to be found in ancient Chinese notions of yin and yang, which should always be in a state of harmony if health is to be maintained. According to the Neiching, mental illness is caused by five harmful emanations of yin and yang. These five disturbances are numbness, wildness, insanity, disturbance of speech, and anger. Climatic changes can result in harmful effects on the balance between yin and yang, with wind causing headache, apoplexy and dizziness, while cold causes coughing, heartache and stomach ache, so these climatic extremes should be avoided. Wind is also believed to refer to a pathogenic force that acts quickly and is responsible for many diseases with an acute onset (Ng, 1998).

Frigophobia leads sufferers to dress compulsively in heavy or excess clothing and avoid going outside, and even avoid buildings with air conditioning. The condition, which is rare, takes the form of a specific phobia. It has been mainly described in China, and among Chinese immigrants in Australia, but similar states are described in Central and South America.

Taijin kyofusho

Taijin kyofusho or anthropophobia has received considerable attention in recent years in Japanese and other Eastern cultures because of the crippling nature of its symptoms. The term literally means the disorder (*sho*) of fear (*kyofu*) of interpersonal relations (*taijin*). There is a severe obsession of shame and fear of social contact and extreme self-consciousness regarding appearance. It is characterised by fears of offending others, by blushing, stuttering, emitting offensive odours, staring inappropriately, presenting improper facial expressions, blemishes or physical deformity. Somatic symptoms include aches and pains, fatigue and insomnia. Raised anxiety levels are experienced in places frequented by the sufferers, such as schools, commuter trains and the work place, but not usually at home with family.

The condition tends to affect young people, with a male:female ratio of 3:2. The condition varies in severity from a mild transient disorder sometimes presenting as a social phobic disorder to a delusional disorder or prodrome for schizophrenia. A diagnostic study using the Schedule for Affective Disorders in a cohort of people with taijin kyofusho (Matsunaga *et al*, 2001) found that a variety of axis 1 DSM–IV disorders could present in this way, most commonly social phobia (38%), major depression (27%) and delusional disorder (somatic type) (15%). These people also had high rates of comorbid personality disorders, particularly schizotypal, paranoid and avoidant subtypes. Some of these patients did well with selective serotonin reuptake inhibitors (SSRIs), as might be expected if the underlying conditions are social phobias or depression.

Although taijin kyufusho shows greatest resemblance to the Western condition of social phobia, the symptoms in the Japanese condition usually include a hypersensitivity to certain bodily parts, such as the eyes or a bodily deformity, and this is uncommon in social phobia.

The condition of taijin kyofusho was first described by Morita in the 1930s (Maeda & Nathan, 1999) and he postulated the existence of a hypochondriacal temperament in affected individuals, who would tend to fixate on their weaknesses and focus on their hypochondriachal fears and sensations, particularly in interpersonal situations, and thereby become anxious and depressed. Morita therapy, which was originally devised to treat taijin kyofusho, aims to direct the patient's energy from somatic symptoms to more here-and-now concerns and seems to share a great deal with modern cognitive therapy. A more comprehensive account of Morita therapy is given by Kitanishi & Mori (1995).

Ufufyane

Ufufyane, or saka, is a trance-like state described in southern Africa in which the victim falls under the spell of magic potions administered by rejected lovers or spirit possession. The victim may show emotional lability and conversion symptoms (e.g. convulsions). The condition typically affects young, unmarried women and may last for days or weeks. It appears phenomenologically close to conversion disorders.

Uqamairineq

Uqamairineq is a condition typically described in the Iniut people of the Arctic. It presents with sudden paralysis, accompanied by anxiety, agitation and hallucinations. Most attacks last only minutes and are followed by complete remission. However, attacks often recur, and are alleged to be the result of spirit possession. The phenomenological similarity with ufufyane and a variety of other conversion-like states in other parts of the world is recognised.

Piboloktoq

Piboloktoq or 'Arctic hysteria' is an acute episode of disruptive behaviour that has some resemblances to both latah and amok. Typically there is a prodrome in which the sufferer is observed to be irritable or withdrawn and complains of confusion or depression. Then suddenly without warning the sufferer becomes wildly excited, tears off his clothes, develops severe agitation, echolalia, echopraxia, violence and coprophagia. He then leaves the shelter and runs off frantically into the tundra, plunges into snow drifts, or climbs onto icebergs, placing himself and those trying to pursue him in considerable danger. Fortunately, the sufferer is usually caught and the episode ends with either seizures or collapse, followed by a prolonged sleep, with amnesia for the event afterwards and complete recovery. The condition has been described mainly among the Inuits living in Canada and Greenland, who also apply the term to similar behaviour in their husky dogs (Landy, 1985).

A similar syndrome has been described among a number of indigenous groups in Africa and Asia. It appears to be a dissociative disorder, possibly triggered by interpersonal difficulties, although Landy (1985) suggested that hypervitaminosis of vitamin A owing to the Eskimo diet of eating polar bear liver may be a contributory factor. Although true arctic hysteria is probably very rare and has no Western equivalent, walking off into the snow, in the expectation of dying, has been reported to be a method of attempting suicide in northern Norway (Nissen & Haggag, 1988).

Windigo

Windigo is described among the indigenous peoples of the north-eastern Canadian forests, particularly the Obijwa and Cree, and bears some resemblance to amok. Sufferers behave in a bizarre fashion, eating human flesh and developing homicidal impulses, usually directed at members of the immediate family. It is said to be accompanied by delusions of transformation into the Windigo monster, a mythical man-eating beast that is prominent in the local folklore. Historical research suggests the condition was a form of conversion disorder, but only 70 cases were collected in the world literature up until 1960 (Boag, 1970) and virtually none since, so it is doubtful if the condition still exists, except of course in textbooks of psychiatry, where it continues to flourish, with its description being faithfully reproduced for each new succeeding edition.

Overview

It is easy to scan the above list of conditions and make some stark observations. None of the culture-specific syndromes resembles severe mental disorders; all occur in the context of severe stress and are phenomenologically closest to the neurotic and dissociative disorders. Many bear considerable similarity with one another and with a multitude of other conditions described in very diverse cultures. Jilek (2000) has categorised these syndromes according to their cultural contexts; thus, susto and nervois are folk idioms of distress, Arctic hysteria and windigo are culturally stereotyped reactions to extreme environmental conditions, koro and dhat are related to a cultural concern regarding fertility and procreation, latah and amok are related to a cultural emphasis on learned dissociation, and brain fag is an example of syndromes related to acculturative stress on adolescents (the pressure of academic performance in some cultures).

A culture-bound syndrome should not in itself comprise a complete psychiatric diagnosis. Just as a diagnosis of anxiety disorder can signify anything from a hidden malignancy to a marital problem, all patients must be fully investigated to clarify any underlying pathology.

In ICD–10 it is rightly pointed out that there is much controversy regarding these categories. Some conditions, such as amok, have been described in many more cultures than the condition of multiple personality disorder, which has almost entirely been a White American diagnosis, yet this is listed in the main text, while amok is listed only in an annex. Yet, viewed from the perspective of a psychiatrist in a developing nation, multiple personality disorder has all the features of an exotic culture-bound syndrome, limited in its expression to the White population of North America. It also remains a valid argument that many of the so-called culture-bound syndromes are simply different presentations of 'universal' psychiatric categories, a view that Kraepelin (1904) took of amok and latah as early as the turn of the 19th century, and one that still has a substantial following.

Conclusions

The debate on the role of culture in mental disorders has its historical roots in the observations made by psychiatrists from Western countries, such as Kraepelin, who travelled to other countries and observed similarities and differences in the presentation of psychiatric disorders. A separate route of enquiry was made through the comparative study of mental illness in migrants in developed countries, exemplified by the classic studies by Ødegäard (1932). Since the 1950s, however, cultural psychiatry has become a major force within the mainstream of psychiatric theory and practice. There is now a general consensus that the integration of the universalist (or etic) and culturally relativist (or emic) approaches, and their methodologies, is required to generate a truly international psychiatry.

The prevalence of CMDs varies considerably across countries, and although there is no substantive evidence to explain these variations, it is generally assumed that cultural factors may play a key role. However, it is also evident that culture is only one factor that might explain the differences in the epidemiology of mental disorder between, and within, human societies. Other factors, such as civil strife, war, natural disasters, poverty and endemic physical illnesses, may all interact with culture, and are major risk factors for psychiatric disorder.

For the psychoses, the research evidence has shown that the incidence and prevalence of schizophrenia varies considerably in different cultures, and cultural influences are apparent in the content and diagnostic specificity of symptoms such as hallucinations. The much publicised findings of the large multinational studies that the outcome of schizophrenia is better in developing countries, suggesting some undefined sociocultural influence has not been substantiated in a number of recent studies.

Mental illness has achieved considerable global public health attention as a result of recent reports on the high prevalence and associated disability of mental disorders (World Health Organization, 2001). However, much of the research on mental illness is derived from a small fraction of the world's population in developed countries (Patel & Sumathipala, 2001). This situation is gradually changing and this is reflected in the changing content of cross-cultural studies.

Over the past two decades there has been a paradigm shift, moving away from examining the minutiae of obscure mental disorders in exotic and isolated societies and towards an attempt to grapple with the truly enormous psychiatric morbidity found in developing nations. Thus, the objectives of a truly international psychiatry would be to establish psychiatry as a relevant medical discipline with strong public health roots in all nations of the world.

Acknowledgements

We are grateful to Anne Becker for having provided a copy of her paper while in press and Julian Leff for reviewing an earlier draft of this chapter.

References

Al-Issa, I. (1995) The illusion of reality or the reality of illusion: hallucinations and culture. *British Journal of Psychiatry*, **166**, 368–373.

American Psychiatric Association (1980) *Diagnostic and Statistical Manual of Mental Disorders* (3rd edn) (DSM–III). Washington, DC: APA.

American Psychiatric Association (1987) *Diagnostic and Statistical Manual of Mental Disorders* (3rd edn, revised) (DSM–III–R). Washington, DC: APA.

American Psychiatric Association (1994) *Diagnostic and Statistical Manual of Mental Disorders* (4th edn) (DSM–IV). Washington, DC: APA.

American Psychiatric Association (2000) *Diagnostic and Statistical Manual of Mental Disorders* (4th edn, text revision) (DSM–IV–TR). Washington, DC: APA.

Amin, G., Shah, S. & Vankar, G. K. (1998) The prevalence and recognition of depression in primary care. *Indian Journal of Psychiatry*, **40**, 364–369.

Araya, R., Robert, W., Richard, L., *et al* (1994) Psychiatric morbidity in primary health care in Santiago, Chile. Preliminary findings. *British Journal of Psychiatry*, **165**, 530–532.

Asuni, T. (1991) Development of psychiatry in Africa. In *Mental Health in Africa and the Americas Today* (ed. S. O. Okpaku), pp. 17–32. Nashville, TN: Chrisolith Books.

Bahar, E., Henderson, A. S. & Mackinnon, A. J. (1992) An epidemiological study of mental health and socioeconomic conditions in Sumatera, Indonesia. *Acta Psychiatrica Scandinavica*, **85**, 257–263.

Bebbington, P. (1993) Transcultural aspects of affective disorders. *International Review of Psychiatry*, **5**, 145–156.

Becker, A. E., Burwell, R. A., Gilman, S. E., *et al* (2002) Eating behaviours and attitudes following prolonged exposure to television among ethnic Fijian adolescent girls. *British Journal of Psychiatry*, **180**, 509–514.

Beiser, M., Cargo, M. & Woodbury, M. (1994) A comparison of psychiatric disorder in different cultures: depressive typologies in South-East Asian refugees and resident Canadians. *International Journal of Methods in Psychiatric Research*, **4**, 157–172.

Bhatt, A., Tomenson, B. & Benjamin, S. (1989) Transcultural patterns of somatization in primary care: a preliminary report. *Journal of Psychosomatic Research*, **33**, 671–680.

Boag, T. J. (1970) Mental health of native peoples of the Arctic. *Canadian Psychiatric Association Journal*, **15**, 115–120.

Broadhead, J. & Abas, M. (1998) Life events and difficulties and the onset of depression among women in a low-income urban setting in Zimbabwe. *Psychological Medicine*, **28**, 29–38.

Castillo, R. J. (1997) *Culture and Mental Illness*. Pacific Grove, CA: Brooks Cole.

Chadda, R. K. (1995) Dhat syndrome: is it a distinct clinical entity? *Acta Psychiatrica Scandinavica*, **91**, 136–139.

Channabasavanna, S. M., Raguram, R., Weiss, M., *et al* (1993) Ethnography of psychiatric illness: a pilot study. *NIMHANS Journal*, **11**, 1–10.

Cheng, S. T. (1996) A critical review of Chinese koro. *Culture Medicine and Psychiatry*, **20**, 67–82.

Cooper, J. E., Kendell, R. E., Gurland, B. J., *et al* (1972) *Psychiatric Diagnosis in New York and London*. Oxford: Oxford University Press.

Davar, B. (1999) *The Mental Health of Indian Women: A Feminist Agenda*. New Delhi: Sage (India).

de la Tourrette, G. (1884) Jumping, latah and myriacahit. *Archives de Neurologie*, **8**, 68–74.

Desjarlais, R., Eisenberg, L., Good, B., *et al* (1995) *World Mental Health: Problems and Priorities in Low-Income Countries*. Oxford: Oxford University Press.

Eisenbruch, M. (1991) From post-traumatic stress disorder to cultural bereavement: diagnosis of Southeast Asian refugees. *Social Science and Medicine*, **33**, 673–680.

Ekblad, S., Kohn, R. & Jansson, B. (1998) Psychological and clinical aspects of immigration and mental health. In *Clinical Methods in Transcultural Psychiatry* (ed. S. O. Okpaku), pp. 42–65. Washington, DC: American Psychiatric Association.

Fernando, S. (1991) *Mental Health, Race & Culture*. London: Macmillan & MIND.

Franklin, R. R., Dondon, S., Guege, M., *et al* (1996) Cultural response to mental illness in Senegal. Reflections through patient companions. *Social Science and Medicine*, **42**, 325–338.

Gater, R., De Almeida, E., Sousa, B., *et al* (1991) The pathways to psychiatric care: a cross-cultural study. *Psychological Medicine*, **21**, 761–774.

Gillis, L., Trollip, D., Jakoet, A., *et al* (1987) Non compliance with psychotropic medication. *South African Medical Journal*, **72**, 602–606.

Goldberg, D. & Lecrubier, Y. (1995) Form and frequency of mental disorders across cultures. In *Mental Illness in General Health Care: An International Study* (eds T. B. Ustun & N. Sartorius), pp. 323–334. Chichester: John Wiley & Sons.

Good, B., Good, M. D. & Moradi, R. (1985) The interpretation of Iranian depressive illness and dysphoric affect. In *Culture and Depression* (eds A. Kleinman & B. Good), pp. 369–428. Berkeley, CA: University of California Press.

Greenlees, T. D. (1895) Insanity among the natives of South Africa. *Journal of Mental Science*, **41**, 71–82.

Guarnaccia, P. J., Good, B. & Kleinman, A. (1990)'A critical review of epidemiological studies of Puerto Rican mental health. *American Journal of Psychiatry*, **147**, 1449–1456.

Helman, C. (1991) Limits of biomedical explanation. *Lancet*, **337**, 1080–1082.

Hinton, W. L., Chen, Y. J. & Du, N. (1993) DSM.IIIR disorders in Vietnamese refugees. *Journal of Nervous and Mental Disease*, **186**, 113–122.

Hippius, H., Peters, G. & Ploog D. (eds) (1987) *Emil Kraepelin, Memoirs* (trans. C. Wooding-Deane). New York: Springer-Verlag.

Jablensky, A., Sartorius, N., Ernberg, G., *et al* (1992) Schizophrenia: manifestations, incidence and course in different cultures: a World Health Organization ten-country study. *Psychological Medicine*, monograph suppl. 20, 1–97.

Jilek, W. G. (2000) Culturally related syndromes. In *The New Oxford Textbook of Psychiatry* (eds M. G. Gelder, J. J. Lopez-Ibor & N. Andreasen), vol. I, pp. 1061–1065. Oxford: Oxford University Press.

Johns, L., Nazroo, J. Y., Bebbington, P., *et al* (2002) Occurrence of hallucinatory experiences in a community sample and ethnic variations. *British Journal of Psychiatry*, **180**, 174–178.

Kakar, S. (1982) *Shamans, Mystics and Doctors*. New Delhi: Oxford University Press.

Katon, W. & Walker, E. A. (1998) Medically unexplained symptoms in primary care. *Journal of Clinical Psychiatry*, **59**, suppl. 20, 15–21.

Katon, W., Kleinman, A. & Rosen, G. (1982) Depression and somatisation: I and II. *American Journal of Medicine*, **72**, 127–135, 241–247.

Khoa, L. X. & Van Duesen, J. M. (1981) Social and cultural customs: their cultural customs, their contribution to resettlement. *Journal of Refuge Resettlement*, **1**, 48–51.

Kiev, A. (1964) The study of folk psychiatry. In *Magic, Faith & Healing* (1st edn) (ed. A. Kiev), pp. 3–35. New York: Free Press.

Kilonzo, G., Kaaya, S., Rweikiza, J., *et al* (1994) Determination of appropriate clomipramine dosage among depressed African outpatients in Dar es Salaam, Tanzania. *Central African Journal of Medicine*, **40**, 178–182.

Kinzie, J. D., Leung, P., Bohehnlein, J., *et al* (1987) Tricyclic antidepressant plasma levels in Indo-Chinese refugees. Clinical implications. *Journal of Nervous and Mental Disease*, **175**, 480–485.

Kirmayer, L. J., Dao, T. H. T. & Smith, A. (1998) Somatization and psychologization: understanding cultural idioms of distress. In *Clinical Methods in Transcultural Psychiatry* (ed. S. O. Okpaku), pp. 233–265. Washington, DC: American Psychiatric Press.

Kitanishi, K. & Mori, A. (1995) Morita therapy 1919–95. *Psychiatry Clinics and Neurosciences*, **49**, 245–254.

Kleinman, A. (1987) Anthropology and psychiatry: the role of culture in cross-cultural research on illness. *British Journal of Psychiatry*, **151**, 447–454.

Kleinman, A. & Kleinman, J. (1985) Somatization: the interconnections in Chinese society among culture, depressive experiences, and the meanings of pain. In *Culture and Depression* (eds A. Kleinman & B. Good), pp. 429–490. Berkeley, CA: University of California Press.

Kraepelin, E. (1904) Vergleichende psychiatrica. Trans. Wittkower, E. (1974) Comparative psychiatry. *Transcultural Psychiatric Research Review*, **11**, 108–112.

Kulhara, P. & Chakrabarti, S. (2001) Culture and schizophrenia and other psychotic disorders. *Psychiatric Clinics of North America*, **24**, 449–464.

Landy, D. (1985) Pibloktoq (hysteria) and Inuit nutrition: possible implication of hypervitaminosis A. *Sociology Science and Medicine*, **21**, 173–185.

Le Roux, A. G. (1973) Psychopathology in Bantu culture. *South African Medical Journal*, **47**, 2077–2083.

Lee, S. (2001) From diversity to unity: the classification of mental disorders in 21st century China. *Psychiatric Clinics of North America*, **24**, 421–431.

Leff, J. P., Fischer, M. & Bertelsen, A. (1976) A cross-national epidemiological study of mania. *British Journal of Psychiatry*, **129**, 428–437.

Leff, J., Wig, N., Ghosh, A., *et al* (1987) Expressed emotion and schizophrenia in north India. III. Influence of relatives' expressed emotion on the course of schizophrenia in Chandigarh. *British Journal of Psychiatry*, **151**, 166–173.

Leighton, A. H., Lambo, T. A., Hughes, C. C., *et al* (1963) *Psychiatric Disorder Among the Yoruba*. New York: Cornell University Press.

Lewis, G. & Sloggett, A. (1998) Suicide, deprivation and unemployment: record linkage study. *BMJ*, **317**, 1283–1286.

Lewis, G., Bebbington, P., Brugha, T. S., *et al* (1998) Socioeconomic status, standard of living and neurotic disorder. *Lancet*, **352**, 605–609.

Lin, K. M., Smith, M. W. & Oritz, V. (2001) Culture and psychopharmacology. *Psychiatric Clinics of North America*, **24**, 523–538.

Linden, M., Lecrubier, Y., Bellantuono, C., *et al* (1999) The prescribing of psychotropic drugs by primary care physicians: an international collaborative study. *Journal of Clinical Psychopharmacology*, **19**, 132–140.

Maeda, F. & Nathan, J. H. (1999) Understanding taijin kyofusho through its treatment: Morita therapy. *Journal of Psychosomatic Research*, **46**, 525–530.

Mari, J., Sen, B. & Cheng, T. A. (1989) Case definition and case identification in cross-cultural perspective. In *The Scope of Epidemiological Psychiatry* (1st edn) (eds P. Williams, G. Wilkinson & K. Rawnsley), pp. 489–508. London: Routledge.

Matsunaga, H., Kiriike, N., Matsui, T., *et al* (2001) Taijin kyofusho: a form of social anxiety that responds to serotonin re-uptake inhibitors. *International Journal of Neuropsychopharmacology*, **4**, 231–237.

McGrath, J., Saha, S., Welham, J., *et al* (2004) A systematic review of the incidence of schizophrenia, the distribution of rates and the influence of sex, urbanicity and migration status. *Biomed Central Medicine*, **28**, 2–13.

Mumford, D. B., Saeed, K., Ahmad, I., *et al* (1997) Stress and psychiatric disorder in rural Punjab. A community survey. *British Journal of Psychiatry*, **170**, 473–478.

Murdock, G. P., Wilson, S. F. & Frederick, V. (1980) World distribution of theories of illness. *Transcultural Psychiatric Research Review*, **17**, 37–64.

Murphy, H. D. M. (1973) Migration and mental health. In *An Appraisal of Uprooting and After* (ed. C. Zwingmann & M. Pfister-Ammende). New York: Springer-Verlag.

Murphy, H. D. M. (1977) Transcultural psychiatry should begin at home. *Psychological Medicine*, **7**, 369–371.

Murphy, H. B. M. (1982) *Comparative Psychiatry: The International and Intermittent Distribution of Mental Illness*. New York: Springer.

National Human Rights Commission (1999) *Quality Assurance in Mental Health*. New Delhi: NHRC.

Ng, B. Y. (1998) Wei hang Zheng (frigophobia): a culture-related psychiatric syndrome. *Australia and New Zealand Journal of Psychiatry*, **32**, 582–585.

Ng, B. Y. & Kua, E. H. (1996) Koro in ancient Chinese history. *History of Psychiatry*, **7**, 563–570.

Nissen, T. & Haggag, A. (1988) Parasuicidal snow wandering in the Arctic. Disorders in 21st century clima. *Psychiatric Clinics of North America*, **24**, 421–432.

Nunley, M. (1998) The involvement of families in Indian psychiatry. *Culture, Medicine and Psychiatry*, **22**, 316–353.

Ødegäard, O. (1932) Emigration and insanity: a study of mental disease in Norwegian born population in Minnesota. *Acta Psychiatrica et Neurologica Scandinavica*, vol. suppl. 4, 1–206.

Okpaku, S. O. (ed.) (1998) *Clinical Methods in Transcultural Psychiatry*. Washington, DC: American Psychiatric Press.

Ormel, J., Von Korff, M., Ustun, T. B., *et al* (1994) Common mental disorders and disability across cultures. *JAMA*, **272**, 1741–1748.

Patel, V. (1995) Explanatory models of mental illness in sub-Saharan Africa. *Social Science and Medicine*, **40**, 1291–1298.

Patel, V. (1996) Recognizing common mental disorders in primary care in African countries: should 'mental' be dropped? *Lancet*, **347**, 742–744.

Patel, V. (1998) *Culture and Common Mental Disorders in Sub-Saharan Africa: Studies in Primary Care in Zimbabwe*. Hove: Psychology Press.

Patel, V. (2000) Health systems research: a pragmatic model for meeting mental health needs in low-income countries. In *Unmet Need in Psychiatry* (eds G. Andrews & S. Henderson), pp. 353–377. Cambridge: Cambridge University Press.

Patel, V. & Sumathipala, A. (2001) International representation in psychiatric journals: a survey of 6 leading journals. *British Journal of Psychiatry*, **178**, 406–409.

Patel, V., Gwanzura, F., Simunyu, E., *et al* (1995) The explanatory models and phenomenology of common mental disorder in Harare, Zimbabwe. *Psychological Medicine*, **25**, 1191–1199.

Patel, V., Todd, C. H., Winston, M., *et al* (1998*a*) The outcome of common mental disorders in Harare, Zimbabwe. *British Journal of Psychiatry*, **172**, 53–57.

Patel, V., Pereira, J. & Mann, A. (1998*b*) Somatic and psychological models of common mental disorders in India. *Psychological Medicine*, **28**, 135–143.

Patel, V., Araya, R., Lima, M. S., *et al* (1999) Women, poverty and common mental disorders in four restructuring societies. *Social Science and Medicine*, **49**, 1461–1471.

Patel, V., Rodrigues, M. & De Souza, N. (2002) Gender, poverty and post-natal depression: a cohort study from Goa, India. *American Journal of Psychiatry*, **159**, 43–47.

Patel, V., Araya, R. & Bolton, P. (2004) Treating depression in developing countries. *Tropical Medicine and International Health*, **9**, 539–541.

Prince, R., Okpaku, S. O. & Merkel, R. L. (1998) Transcultural psychiatry: a note on origins and definitions. In *Clinical Methods in Transcultural Psychiatry* (ed. S. O. Okpaku), pp. 3–17. Washington, DC: American Psychiatric Press.

Ran, M., Xiang, M., Huang, M., *et al* (2002) Natural course of schizophrenia: 2-year follow-up study in a rural Chinese community. *British Journal of Psychiatry*, **178**, 154–158.

Sack, W. H., McSharry, S., Clarke, G. N., *et al* (1994) The Khmer adolescent project. I: Epidemiological findings in two generations of Cambodian refugees. *Journal of Nervous and Mental Disease*, **182**, 387–395.

Saha, S., Chant, D., Welham, J., *et al* (2005) A systematic review of the prevalence of schizophrenia *Public Library of Science Medicine*, **2**, e141.

Sartorius, N., Kaelber, C. T., Cooper, J. E., *et al* (1993) Progress towards achieving a common language in psychiatry. Results from the field trial of the clinical guidelines accompanying the WHO classification of mental and behavioral disorders in ICD.10. *Archives of General Psychiatry*, **502**, 115–124.

Sen, B. & Williams, P. (1987) The extent and nature of depressive phenomena in primary health care: a study in Calcutta, India. *British Journal of Psychiatry*, **151**, 486–493.

Selten, J. P., Slaets, J. P. & Khan, R. S. (1997) Schizophrenia in Surinamese and Dutch Antillean immigrants to the Netherlands: evidence of an increased incidence. *Psychological Medicine*, **27**, 807–811.

Sharpley, M., Hutchinson, G., Makenzie, K., *et al* (2001) Understanding the excess of psychosis among the African-Caribbean population in England. A review of current hypothesis. *British Journal of Psychiatry*, **178**, suppl. 40, 560–568.

Skultans, V. (1991) Women and affliction in Maharashtra: a hydraulic model of health and illness. *Culture, Medicine and Psychiatry*, **15**, 321–359.

Somasundaram, D. J., van de Put, W., Eisenbruch, M., *et al* (1999) Starting mental health services in Cambodia. *Social Science and Medicine*, **48**, 1029–1046.

Sue, D. W., Carter, R. D., Manuela Casa, J., *et al* (1988) *Multicultural Counselling Competencies: Individual and Organisational Development*. Thousand Oaks, CA: Sage.

Summerfield, D. A. (1999) A critique of seven assumptions behind psychological trauma programs in war afflicted areas. *Sociology, Science and Medicine*, **48**, 1449–1462.

Thara, R., Henrietta, M., Joseph, A., *et al* (1994) Ten-year course of schizophrenia – the Madras longitudinal study. *Acta Psychiatric Scandinavica*, **90**, 329–336.

Thomas, C. S., Stone, K., Osborn, M., *et al* (1993) Psychiatric morbidity and compulsory admission among UK-born Europeans, Afro-Caribbeans and Asians in central Manchester. *British Journal of Psychiatry*, **163**, 91–99.

Todd, C., Patel, V., Simunyu, E., *et al* (1999) The onset of common mental disorders in primary care attenders in Harare, Zimbabwe. *Psychological Medicine*, **29**, 97–104.

Tribe, R. & Raval, H. (2003) *Working with Interpreters*. Hove: Brunner–Routledge.

Trujillo, M. (2001) Culture and the organisation of psychiatric care. *Psychiatric Clinics of North America*, **24**, 539–555.

Tyrer, P. (2001) The case for cothymia: mixed anxiety and depression as a single diagnosis. *British Journal of Psychiatry*, **179**, 191–193.

Ustun, T. B. & Sartorius, N. (1995) *Mental Illness in General Health Care: An International Study*. Chichester: John Wiley & Sons.

Van Moffaert, M. (1998) Somatization patterns in Mediterranean migrants. In *Clinical Methods in Transcultural Psychiatry* (ed. S. O. Okpaku), pp. 301–319. Washington, DC: American Psychiatric Press.

Weich, S. & Lewis, G. (1998) Poverty, unemployment and the common mental disorders: a population based cohort study. *BMJ*, **317**, 115–119.

Weich, S., Lewis, G., Donmall, R., *et al* (1995) Somatic presentation of psychiatric morbidity in general practice. *British Journal of General Practice*, **45**, 143–147.

WHO World Mental Health Survey Consortium (2004) Prevalence, severity, and unmet need for the treatment of mental disorders in the World Health Organization world mental health surveys. *JAMA*, **291**, 2581–2590.

Wig, N. N., Menon, D. K., Bedi, H., *et al* (1987) Distribution of expressed emotion components among relatives of patients in Aarhus and Chandigarh. *British Journal of Psychiatry*, **151**, 160–165.

World Health Organization (1979) *Schizophrenia: An International Follow-Up Study*. Chichester: John Wiley & Sons.

World Health Organization (1992) *The Tenth Revision of the International Classification of Diseases and Related Health Problems* (ICD–10). Geneva: WHO.

World Health Organization (2000) *Women's Mental Health: An Evidence-Based Review*. Geneva: WHO.

World Health Organization (2001) *The World Health Report 2001: Mental Health: New Understanding, New Hope*. Geneva: WHO.

Yap, P. M. (1962) Words and things in comparative psychiatry with special reference to the exotic psychoses. *Acta Psychiatrica Scandinavica*, **38**, 163–169.

Index

Compiled by Caroline Sheard